YO-CD I-899

Disorders of Bone and Mineral Metabolism

Disorders of Bone and Mineral Metabolism

Edited by

Fredric L. Coe, M.D.

Professor of Medicine and Physiology
Chief, Program in Nephrology
Pritzker School of Medicine
The University of Chicago
Chicago, Illinois

Murray J. Favus, M.D.

Professor of Medicine and
Director of the Bone Program
Pritzker School of Medicine
The University of Chicago
Chicago, Illinois

Raven Press   New York

Raven Press, Ltd., 1185 Avenue of the Americas, New York, New York 10036

Made in the United States of America

Disorders of bone and mineral metabolism/edited by Fredric L. Coe,
  Murray J. Favus.
      p. cm.
    Includes bibliographical references.
    Includes index.
    ISBN 0-88167-749-3
      1. Mineral metabolism—Disorders. 2. Bones—Metabolism—Disorders.
    3. Bones—Diseases. I. Coe, Fredric L. II. Favus, Murray J.
      [DNLM: 1. Bone and Bones—metabolism. 2. Bone Diseases, Metabolic.
    3. Minerals—metabolism.   WE 250 D612]
    RC632.M56D56   1991
    616.7′1—dc20
    DNLM/DLC
    for Library of Congress   91-7862
                                                                        CIP

9 8 7 6 5 4 3 2 1

To our wives,
Eleanor Brodny Coe and Barbara Barnett Favus,
and to our children,
Brian and Laura Coe and Abigail and Elliot Favus

Contents

Contributing Authors xi

Preface xv

I. NORMAL MINERAL METABOLISM

1. Renal Handling of Calcium and Phosphorus 3
Norimoto Yanagawa and David B. N. Lee

2. Regulation of Magnesium Excretion 41
Christian de Rouffignac

3. Intestinal Absorption of Calcium, Magnesium, and Phosphorus 57
Murray J. Favus

4. Regulation of Parathyroid Hormone Synthesis and Secretion 83
Justin Silver

5. Metabolism and Assay of Parathyroid Hormone 107
Claude D. Arnaud and Kin-Kee Pun

6. The Target Tissue Actions of Parathyroid Hormone 123
Lorraine A. Fitzpatrick, Daniel T. Coleman, and John P. Bilezikian

7. Metabolism of Vitamin D 149
Helen L. Henry and Anthony W. Norman

8. Molecular Mechanisms of Cellular Response to the Vitamin D_3
Hormone 163
J. Wesley Pike

9. Clinical Aspects of Measurements of Plasma Vitamin D Sterols and the
Vitamin D Binding Protein 195
John G. Haddad, Jr.

II. BONE STRUCTURE AND BIOLOGY

10. Embryology, Anatomy, and Microstructure of Bone 219
Robert R. Recker

11. The Cellular Biology and Molecular Biochemistry of Bone Formation 241
Pamela Gehron Robey, Paolo Bianco, and John D. Termine

12. The Nature of the Mineral Component of Bone and the Mechanism
of Calcification 265
Melvin J. Glimcher

13. Mechanisms and Regulation of Bone Resorption by Osteoclastic Cells 287
Lawrence G. Raisz

14. The Biology, Chemistry, and Biochemistry of the Mammalian Growth Plate 313
   David S. Howell and David D. Dean

15. Bone Remodeling 355
   David W. Dempster

III. MINERAL METABOLISM DURING THE HUMAN LIFE CYCLE

16. Mineral Metabolism During Pregnancy and Lactation 383
   Russell W. Chesney, Bonny L. Specker, Francis Mimouni, and Charles P. McKay

17. Mineral Metabolism During Childhood 395
   Charles P. McKay, Bonny L. Specker, Reginald C. Tsang, and Russell W. Chesney

18. Integration of Calcium Metabolism in the Adult 417
   David A. Bushinsky and Nancy S. Krieger

IV. INTRODUCTION TO CLINICAL MINERAL DISORDERS

19. Clinical and Laboratory Approach to the Patient with Disorders of Bone and Mineral Metabolism 435
   Fredric L. Coe and Murray J. Favus

20. The Imaging and Quantitation of Bone by Radiographic and Scanning Methodologies 443
   Charles H. Chesnut III

21. Clinical Use of Bone Biopsy 455
   Robert S. Weinstein

22. The Physiologic and Pathogenetic Significance of Bone Histomorphometric Data 475
   A. M. Parfitt

V. DISORDERS OF SERUM MINERAL LEVELS

23. Hypercalcemic States: Their Differential Diagnosis and Acute Management 493
   John P. Bilezikian

24. Asymptomatic Primary Hyperparathyroidism 523
   Neil A. Breslau and Charles Y. C. Pak

25. Disorders of Serum Minerals Caused by Cancer 539
   John J. Orloff and Andrew F. Stewart

26. Hypercalcemia and Abnormal Vitamin D Metabolism 563
   Daniel P. DeSimone and Norman H. Bell

27. The Hypocalcemic States: Their Differential Diagnosis and Management ... 571
   Richard Eastell and Hunter Heath III

28. Disorders of Phosphate and Magnesium Metabolism 587
   Moshe Levi, Robert E. Cronin, and James P. Knochel

VI. DISORDERS OF STONE FORMATION

29. Physical–Chemical Processes in Kidney Stone Formation 613
Charles M. Brown and Daniel L. Purich

30. Mechanisms of Stone Disruption and Dissolution 625
James E. Lingeman

31. Primary Hyperparathyroidism as a Cause of Calcium Nephrolithiasis 671
Aaron Halabe and Roger A. L. Sutton

32. Pathogenesis of Idiopathic Hypercalciuria and Nephrolithiasis 685
Jacob Lemann, Jr.

33. Hyperoxaluric States 707
Lynwood H. Smith

34. Calcium Nephrolithiasis and Renal Tubular Acidosis 729
Vardaman M. Buckalew, Jr.

35. Inhibitors and Promoters of Calcium Oxalate Crystallization: Their Relationship to the Pathogenesis and Treatment of Nephrolithiasis 757
Fredric L. Coe, Joan H. Parks, and Yashushi Nakagawa

36. Noncalcium Nephrolithiasis 801
Malachy J. Gleeson, Kyoichi Kobashi, and Donald P. Griffith

VII. DISORDERS OF BONE

37. Primary Osteoporosis 831
Robert Lindsay and Felicia Cosman

38. Secondary Forms of Osteoporosis 889
Robert Marcus

39. Bone Disease in Chronic Renal Failure and After Renal Transplantation ... 905
Eduardo Slatopolsky and James Delmez

40. Bone Disease Resulting From Inherited Disorders of Renal Tubule Transport and Vitamin D Metabolism 935
Michael J. Econs and Marc K. Drezner

41. Bone Disease Due to Nutritional, Gastrointestinal, and Hepatic Disorders .. 951
Daniel D. Bikle

42. Hereditary Metabolic and Dysplastic Skeletal Disorders 977
Michael P. Whyte

43. Paget's Disease of Bone 1027
Roy D. Altman

44. Primary Cystic and Neoplastic Diseases of Bone 1065
Robert E. Turcotte, Lester E. Wold, and Franklin H. Sim

Subject Index 1089

Contributing Authors

Roy D. Altman, M.D.   *Professor of Medicine, Department of Medicine, University of Miami School of Medicine, P.O. Box 016960, Miami, Florida 33101, and Chief, Arthritis Section, Miami Veterans Administration Medical Center, Miami, Florida 33101*

Claude D. Arnaud, M.D.   *Professor of Medicine and Physiology, Department of Medicine, University of California at San Francisco, and Director, Center for Biomedical Research on Aging, 1710 Scott Street, Box 7921, San Francisco, California 94120*

Norman H. Bell, M.D.   *Professor of Medicine and Pharmacology, Medical University of South Carolina, and Staff Physician, VA Medical Center, 109 Bee Street, Charleston, South Carolina 29403*

Paolo Bianco, M.D.   *Dipartimento di Biolopatologia Umana, Sessione Anatomia Patologica, Universita "La Sapienza," Via Regina Elena 324, I-100161 Rome, Italy*

Daniel D. Bikle, M.D., Ph.D.   *Assistant Professor of Medicine, University of California at San Francisco, and Endocrine Section, VA Medical Center, 4150 Clement Street 111N, San Francisco, California 94121*

John P. Bilezikian, M.D.   *Professor, Departments of Medicine and Pharmacology, Columbia University, College of Physicians and Surgeons, 630 W. 168th Street/P&S 8-405, New York, New York 10032*

Neil A. Breslau, M.D.   *Associate Professor of Medicine, and Director of Clinical Research Center, University of Texas Southwestern Medical Center at Dallas, 5323 Harry Hines Boulevard, Dallas, Texas 75235*

Charles M. Brown, B.S.   *Senior Chemist, Center for the Study of Lithiasis and Pathological Calcification, and Department of Biochemistry and Molecular Biology, University of Florida College of Medicine, Box J-245, J. Hillis Miller Health Center, Gainesville, Florida 32610*

Vardaman M. Buckalew, Jr., M.D.   *Professor of Medicine and Physiology, and Chief of Nephrology, Bowman Gray School of Medicine, Wake Forest University, 300 South Hawthorne Road, Winston–Salem, North Carolina 27103*

David A. Bushinsky, M.D.   *Head, Nephrology Unit, University of Rochester Medical Center, 601 Elmwood Avenue, Box MED, Rochester, New York 14642*

Russell W. Chesney, M.D.   *Professor, Department of Pediatrics, University of Tennessee Health Sciences Center, Memphis, Tennessee 38103*

Charles H. Chesnut III, M.D.   *Professor of Medicine and Radiology, Division of Nuclear Medicine, RC-70, MN 203, University of Washington, School of Medicine, Seattle, Washington 98195*

Fredric L. Coe, M.D.   *Professor, Departments of Medicine and Physiology, and Chief, Nephrology Program, University of Chicago, Pritzker School of Medicine, 5841 S. Maryland Avenue, Box 28, Chicago, Illinois 60637*

Daniel T. Coleman, Ph.D.   *IRTA Fellow, Metabolic Diseases Branch, NIDDK, National Institutes of Health, Bethesda, Maryland 20892*

Felicia Cosman, M.D.   *Assistant Professor of Clinical Medicine, Department of Medicine, Columbia University, College of Physicians and Surgeons, New York, New York 10032*

Robert E. Cronin, M.D. *Associate Professor of Medicine, Departments of Internal Medicine and Nephrology, The University of Texas Southwestern Medical Center at Dallas, and Veterans Affairs Medical Center, 4500 South Lancaster Road (111G1), Dallas, Texas 75216*

David D. Dean, Ph.D. *Professor of Medicine and Biochemistry, Departments of Medicine and Biochemistry—Molecular Biology, University of Miami School of Medicine, P.O. Box 016960, Miami, Florida 33101*

James Delmez, M.D., F.A.C.P. *Associate Professor of Medicine, Washington University School of Medicine, and Attending Physician, Barnes Hospital, and Medical Director, Chromalloy American Kidney Center, St. Louis, Missouri 63110*

David W. Dempster, Ph.D. *Associate Professor of Clinical Pathology, College of Physicians and Surgeons, Columbia University, and Director, Regional Bone Center, Helen Hayes Hospital, Route 9W, West Haverstraw, New York 10993*

Christian de Rouffignac, M.D. *Commissariat a l'Energie Atomique, Departement de Biologie Cellulaire et Moleculaire, Service de Biologie Cellulaire, Centre d'Etudes Nucleaires de Saclay, F-91191 Gif-sur-Yvette, France*

Daniel P. DeSimone, Ph.D. *Medical University of South Carolina, Veterans Administration Medical Center, Charleston, South Carolina 29403*

Marc K. Drezner, M.D. *Professor of Medicine, Departments of Medicine and Cell Biology, Box 3285, Duke University Medical Center, Durham, North Carolina 27710*

Richard Eastell, M.D. *Senior Clinical Fellow, Division of Endocrinology, Metabolism, and Internal Medicine, Mayo Clinic and Mayo Foundation, Rochester, Minnesota 55905*

Michael J. Econs, M.D. *Professor of Medicine, Departments of Medicine and Cell Biology, Box 3285, Duke University Medical Center, Durham, North Carolina 27710*

Murray J. Favus, M.D. *Professor of Medicine, Endocrinology Section and the Nephrology Program, and Director, Bone Program, University of Chicago, Pritzker School of Medicine, 5841 S. Maryland Avenue, Box 28, Chicago, Illinois 60637*

Lorraine A. Fitzpatrick, M.D. *Director, Bone and Histomorphometry Laboratory, Associate Professor of Medicine, Endocrine Research Unit, Mayo Clinic and Foundation, 5-164 West Joseph Building, Rochester, Minnesota 55905*

Malachy J. Gleeson, M.D. *Scott Department of Urology, 6560 Fannin, Suite 1004, Baylor College of Medicine, Houston, Texas 77030*

Melvin J. Glimcher, M.D. *Harriet M. Peabody Professor of Orthopedic Surgery, Harvard Medical School, and Director, Laboratory for the Study of Skeletal Diseases and Rehabilitation, Children's Hospital Medical Center, 300 Longwood Avenue, Boston, Massachusetts 02115*

Donald P. Griffith, M.D. *Professor of Urology, Scott Department of Urology, Baylor College of Medicine, 6560 Fannin, Suite 1004, Houston, Texas 77030*

John G. Haddad, Jr., M.D. *Professor of Medicine, and Chief, Endocrinology Section, University of Pennsylvania School of Medicine, 611 Clinical Research Building, 422 Curie Boulevard, Philadelphia, Pennsylvania 19104-6149*

Aaron Halabe, M.D. *Visiting Scientist for the University of British Columbia, Department of Medicine, Vancouver General Hospital, Vancouver, British Columbia, Canada V5Z 1M9*

Hunter Heath III, M.D. *Consultant in Endocrine Research, and Professor of Medicine, Mayo Clinic and Mayo Medical School, 200 First Street S.W., Rochester, Minnesota 55905*

Helen L. Henry, Ph.D. *Associate Professor, Department of Biochemistry, University of California —Riverside, Riverside, California 92521*

David S. Howell, M.D. *Professor of Medicine, Department of Medicine, D26, University of Miami Medical School, P.O. Box 016960, Miami, Florida 33101*

James P. Knochel, M.D.   *Clinical Professor, Department of Internal Medicine, University of Texas Southwestern Medical Center at Dallas, Dallas, Texas 75216, and Chairman, Department of Internal Medicine, Presbyterian Hospital of Dallas, 8200 Walnut Hill Lane, Dallas, Texas 75231*

Kyoichi Kobashi, Ph.D.   *Department of Biochemistry, Toyama Medical and Pharmaceutical University, Toyama-Shi, Japan*

Nancy S. Krieger, Ph.D.   *Scientist, Departments of Medicine and Pharmacology, University of Rochester, School of Medicine and Dentistry, Rochester, New York 14642*

David B. N. Lee, M.D.   *Professor and Head of Nephrology, Veterans Administration Hospital, 16111 Plummer Street, Sepulveda, California 91343*

Jacob Lemann Jr., M.D.   *Professor of Medicine, Chief, Nephrology Division, Medical College of Wisconsin, Froedfert Memorial Lutheran Hospital, 9200 West Wisconsin Avenue, Milwaukee, Wisconsin 53226*

Moshe Levi, M.D.   *Assistant Professor of Medicine, Departments of Internal Medicine and Nephrology, The University of Texas Southwestern Medical Center at Dallas, and Veterans Affairs Medical Center, 4500 South Lancaster Road (111G1), Dallas, Texas 75216*

Robert Lindsay, M.B.Ch.B., Ph.D., F.R.C.P.   *Professor of Clinical Medicine, Columbia University, College of Physicians and Surgeons, and Director of Research and Chief, Internal Medicine, Helen Hayes Hospital, Route 9W, West Haverstraw, New York 10993*

James E. Lingeman, M.D.   *Director of Research, Methodist Hospital of Indiana, Institute for Kidney Stone Disease, 1801 N. Senate Boulevard, Suite 655, Indianapolis, Indiana 46202*

Robert Marcus, M.D.   *Professor of Medicine, Stanford University School of Medicine, and Director, Aging Study Unit, GRECC 182-B, VA Medical Center, 3801 Miranda, Palo Alto, California 94304*

Charles P. McKay, M.D.   *Department of Pediatrics, University of Tennessee Health Sciences Center, Memphis, Tennessee 38103*

Francis Mimouni, M.D.   *Professor of Pediatrics, University of Tennessee Health Sciences Center, Memphis, Tennessee 38103*

Yashushi Nakagawa, Ph.D.   *Professor of Medicine and Physiology, University of Chicago, Pritzker School of Medicine, 5841 South Maryland Avenue, Box 28, Chicago, Illinois 60637*

Anthony W. Norman, Ph.D.   *Professor, Department of Biochemistry, and Division of Biomedical Sciences, University of California—Riverside, Riverside, California 92521*

John J. Orloff, M.D.   *Staff Physician, West Haven VA Medical Center, and Assistant Professor of Internal Medicine, Yale University School of Medicine, New Haven, Connecticut 06510*

Charles Y. C. Pak, M.D.   *Professor of Medicine, University of Texas Southwestern Medical School, 5323 Harry Hines Boulevard, Dallas, Texas 75235*

A. M. Parfitt, M.D.   *Clinical Professor of Medicine, University of Michigan Medical School, and Fifth Medical Division, Bone and Mineral Research Laboratory, Henry Ford Hospital, 2799 West Grand Boulevard, Detroit, Michigan 48202*

Joan H. Parks, M. B. A.   *Research Associate, Assistant Professor of Medicine and Physiology, University of Chicago, Pritzker School of Medicine, Box 28, 5841 S. Maryland Avenue, Chicago, Illinois 60637*

J. Wesley Pike, Ph.D.   *Associate Professor, Departments of Pediatrics and Cell Biology, Baylor College of Medicine, 8080 N. Stadium Drive, Houston, Texas 77054*

Kin-Kee Pun, M.D., Ph.D., F.R.C.P.(E)   *Assistant Adjunct Professor of Medicine, Program in Osteoporosis and Bone Biology, Department of Medicine, University of California, School of Medicine, San Francisco, California 94115*

Daniel L. Purich, Ph.D. *Professor, Center for the Study of Lithiasis and Pathological Calcification, and Professor and Chairman, Department of Biochemistry and Molecular Biology, University of Florida College of Medicine, Box J-245, J. Hillis Miller Health Center, Gainesville, Florida 32610*

Lawrence G. Raisz, M.D. *Professor of Medicine, Head, Division of Endocrinology and Metabolism, University of Connecticut Health Science Center, Room AM047, 263 Farmington Avenue, Farmington, Connecticut 06032*

Robert R. Recker, M.D. *Professor, Department of Medicine, and Director, Center for Hard Tissue Research, Creighton University School of Medicine, 601 North 30th Street, Suite 5740, Omaha, Nebraska 68131-2197*

Pamela Gehron Robey, Ph.D. *Bone Research Branch, NIDR, NIH, Building 30, Room 106, 900 Rockville Pike, Bethesda, Maryland 20892*

Justin Silver, M.D., Ph.D. *Associate Professor of Medicine, and Director, Mineral Metabolism Unit, Hebrew University, Hadassah University Hospital, Ein Karem, Jerusalem 91120, Israel*

Franklin H. Sim, M.D. *Consultant, Department of Orthopedics, and Professor of Orthopedic Surgery, Mayo Clinic and Mayo Foundation, 200 1st Street, S.W., Rochester, Minnesota 55905*

Eduardo Slatopolsky, M.D., F.A.C.P. *Professor of Medicine, Washington University School of Medicine, and Consultant, Jewish Hospital of St. Louis, and Attending Physician, Renal Division, Barnes Hospital, Box 8129, and Director, Chromalloy American Kidney Center, St. Louis, Missouri 63110*

Lynwood H. Smith, M.D. *Professor of Medicine, Nephrology Section, Mayo Clinic, 200 1st Street S.W., Rochester, Minnesota 55905*

Bonny L. Specker, Ph.D. *Professor, Department of Pediatrics, University of Tennessee Health Sciences Center, Memphis, Tennessee 38103*

Andrew F. Stewart, M.D. *Associate Professor of Internal Medicine, Yale University School of Medicine, and Chief of Endocrinology, West Haven VA Medical Center, West Springs Street, West Haven, Connecticut 06516*

Roger A. L. Sutton, D.M., F.R.C.P., F.R.C.P.(C) *Professor and Head, Division of Nephrology, Department of Medicine, University of British Columbia, 910 West 10th Avenue, Vancouver, British Columbia, Canada V5Z 1M9*

John D. Termine, Ph.D. *Lilly Research Laboratories, Eli Lilly and Company, Lilly Corporate Center, Indianapolis, Indiana 46285*

Reginald C. Tsang, M.D. *Professor, Department of Pediatrics, University of Cincinnati College of Medicine, 231 Bethesda Avenue, Cincinnati, Ohio 45267*

Robert E. Turcotte, M.D. *Special Fellow in Orthopedics, Mayo Graduate School of Medicine, Rochester, Minnesota 55905*

Robert S. Weinstein, M.D. *Professor of Medicine, and Director, Metabolic Bone Disease Laboratory, Medical College of Georgia, HB-5027, Augusta, Georgia 30912*

Michael P. Whyte, M.D. *Associate Professor of Medicine, Jewish Hospital of St. Louis, 216 South Kingshighway, St. Louis, Missouri 63110*

Lester E. Wold, M.D. *Consultant, Section of Surgical Pathology, Mayo Clinic and Mayo Foundation, and Associate Professor, Mayo Medical School, Rochester, Minnesota 55905*

Norimoto Yanagawa, M.D. *Associate Professor of Medicine, Veterans Administration Hospital, 16111 Plummer Street, Sepulveda, California 91343*

Preface

In 1948, perhaps to celebrate the 24th year of the Metabolic Ward, or Ward 4, of the Massachusetts General Hospital, Fuller Albright and Edward C. Reifenstein brought out *The Parathyroid Glands and Metabolic Bone Disease* (Williams and Wilkins Co., Baltimore, Maryland), which they called ". . . an incomplete summary of studies on calcium metabolism . . .", yet was, somehow, complete enough for the generation of our youth, and of our teachers, to stand as the principal reference book of mineral disorders. Our copy, from the University library, is very worn, and we believe the book long ago passed out of print. That it displays an evident age and evidence of heavy use satisfy our expectations and our sense of its place as the prime ancestor of this much larger book we offer here as candidate for its successorship.

What Albright and colleagues studied matches closely to the largest portions of this book: The parathyroid glands, the effects of their hormone, the bone disease of primary and secondary hyperparathyroidism, Vitamin D and its actions, Osteoporosis, Osteomalacia, Paget's disease and Fibrous dysplasia. Stone disease occupied only a small fraction of his work and his book, unlike ours, and the basic science foundation of clinical research, then, was smaller than now, and much less evident in their text than ours. Even so, the correspondence of clinical concerns shows how little 40 years have altered the practice of bone and mineral disorders.

Of course, we know more than Albright. Perhaps most importantly we know the amazing complexity of the vitamin D hormone system, the unique endocrine role of the kidneys in producing $1,25(OH)_2D_3$, the regulation of the parathyroid glands by vitamin D, matters he never suspected. Some things, he simply got wrong. He could not accept that parathyroid hormone affected bone directly, for example, and he created a wrong thinking literature by showing what appeared to be normocalcemic hypercalciuria from parathyroid hormone injection. Because, for him, parathyroid hormone must affect bone only indirectly, by acting upon blood mineral levels, he sometimes seems to capture himself in the web of his own arguments like a distracted spider and, looking back, we almost can imagine how hard he had to work to escape the correct answer.

But even if emphasis and some major points of knowledge set us apart from Albright and his times, the text reads as very modern and instructive. That primary hyperparathyroidism raises serum calcium only modestly, despite marked hypercalciuria, and that finding hypercalciuria and mild hypercalcemia with hypophosphatemia makes a strong diagnosis instructs us today; we frequently observe clinicians passing by very mild hypercalcemia and labelling patients as idiopathic hypercalciuria. His descriptions of osteitis fibrosa in primary hyperparathyroidism and chronic renal failure rival modern publications, and surpass many in showing the histology, gross pathology, and radiography. Little that he described needs changing. Concerning stones, his figure of 5% of stone patients having primary hyperparathyroidism matches our own and modern series, as does the commonness of stone disease with no evidence of bone disease and the often neglected tendency to form calcium phosphate stones. In quality of clinical analysis and differential diagnosis his treatments of all topics rival any ever written.

Perhaps the Albright book stands out most for its intense clinical research. Page after page details studies of patients, that settled for the time, and on occasion for all times the behaviors of important diseases. Basic science lay under much of what Albright did. For example in his struggles to understand bone turnover and, in service of that struggle, to place the supersaturations of blood with respect to bone solid phases he made use of physical chemistry that, then, must have seemed as arcane as certain matters of molecular biology seem now; and he used it fluently, as an expert. But he used it to understand phenomena in patients or normal humans, as he used virtually all he knew, and from the book one gets an impression of a group locked into clinical inquiry, the human condition at the very center of the day's work every day.

We know science progresses differently now, that many of us work far from clinics and patient habitations, far from diseases as a main interest, and certainly we rejoice at the new techniques that make medical scientists powerful in discovery; but—and we use this suspicious looking word carefully —in the clinical intensity of Albright one can find, still, a practical and moral education. Nature made his patients in the ingenious way She has of experimenting, and his charts show how much a disease in even just one person can disclose of new and mysterious happenings utterly unforetold by normal physiology. We all know this, all accept it, and use the knowledge that clinical research may bring discovery as well as we can. Albright simply knew a way to learn from patients better than most other persons ever have in this field of ours, brilliantly and with a great creative impulse; and so his book, however old by now and small compared to ours, deserves a moment of consideration, and a place of unending regard.

Would Albright have appreciated this big book, so full of new data and expert analysis? Certainly, to us at least. He would have thanked us for the present, taken it back to Ward 4, and devoured it, especially the references! And then, no doubt, he would have used every scrap of newness on his ward, every new assay he could commandeer, every imaging method, too. And as for DNA, his patients had it, surely, some abnormal; and do we doubt he would have raced to find abnormal strands as he found abnormal metabolic pathways on his balance ward? See them there, Albright, Reifenstein, Bartter, Forbes, Fraser, Benedict, Klinefelter, Talbott, Thorn, and more, reading our book, combing through every page for some new idea; and recognize that if they lived as our contemporaries now, worked now, that band of scholars, they would have done us in, we two, rolled right over us, made a book we could not equal if we gave our whole lives to the task. And they would have written it alone.

Triteness lies in the direction that finds giants only in the past; they walk about today, and in our field, too. In 40 years or more from now, who they were will be most evident, and what they wrote of merit acknowledged respectfully, as treasurable relic. We offer our book in honor of its writers, who we believe number among their ranks some destined for a future recognition, and also in honor of the Ward 4 band, Albright and his group, who were what all of us must wish to be, quintessential scientists, passionate in quest, tending always to preoccupation with the human situation.

Fredric Lawrence Coe
Murray J. Favus
University of Chicago, June 1991

Disorders of Bone and Mineral Metabolism

PART I

Normal Mineral Metabolism

Disorders of Bone and Mineral Metabolism,
edited by Fredric L. Coe and Murray J. Favus,
© 1992 by Raven Press, Ltd. All rights reserved.

CHAPTER 1

Renal Handling of Calcium and Phosphorus

Norimoto Yanagawa and David B. N. Lee

RENAL HANDLING OF CALCIUM

An average Western diet provides a daily calcium (Ca) intake of about 1000 mg. Under normal conditions, around 35% or 350 mg of this Ca is absorbed. Because the intestine also secretes Ca, estimated at 150 mg/day, the *net* Ca absorbed each day approximates 200 mg (1). In a mature, Ca-replete individual, the kidney would excrete this amount of Ca absorbed, and thereby, maintain the Ca balance.

Renal excretion of Ca begins with the filtration of about 8000 mg Ca at the glomerulus. A normal total plasma calcium (Ca) of 10.0 mg/dL is made up of 4.5 mg/dL of non-filtrable, protein-bound Ca and 5.5 mg/dL of filtrable Ca, which is in turn, made up of 5.0 mg/dL of free Ca ions (Ca^{2+}) and 0.5 mg/dL of Ca complexed with a variety of anions, such as citrate, bicarbonate, and phosphate (2). Assuming a GFR of 100 mL/min, i.e., 144 L/day, the filter load of Ca will amount to about 8000 mg/day (5.5 mg/dL or 55 mg/L × 144 L/day). Of this 8000 mg of filtered Ca, 7800 mg is reabsorbed to yield a net urinary excretion of 200 mg.

Thus, the kidney has to reabsorb a large quantity of the filtered Ca while at the same time to excrete, with relative precision, the small amount of Ca absorbed by the gut. Compared to the intestine which is known for its Ca absorptive potential, the renal tubule reabsorbs 40-fold (8000 mg versus 200 mg) more Ca each day. Bulk Ca reabsorption is accomplished in the proximal nephron and the thick ascending limb, in association with Na reabsorption and with no additional energy requirements. Regulation of the smaller amount of Ca excreted in the urine is mainly accomplished in the distal

N. Yanagawa and D. B. N. Lee: Division of Nephrology, (111R), Medical and Research Services, Sepulveda VA Medical Center, 16111 Plummer Street, Sepulveda, California 91343 and Department of Medicine, University of California at Los Angeles, School of Medicine, Los Angeles, California 90024.

nephron, a locus where the active Ca reabsorptive mechanism and the action of important calcitropic hormones congregate.

We shall first examine some general characteristics of epithelial Ca transport citing examples from both the renal tubular and the intestinal epithelium. We will then focus on the fate of Ca as it traverses through sequential segments of the nephron. Finally, some of the more important factors which influence Ca excretion by the kidney will be discussed.

GENERAL CHARACTERISTICS OF EPITHELIAL CA TRANSPORT

In Ca-absorbing epithelia, such as those lining the renal tubule and the intestine, Ca fluxes across the epithelium can occur both between the cells and through the cells. In the intestine, endocytotic, vesicular Ca translocation represents a third pathway, which allows calcium to remain "extracellular" while traversing through the cell.

Ca Reabsorption Through the Intercellular Pathway

Solvent Drag/Convection

The flow of water across the intercellular pathway can carry with it Ca in solution, a process termed solvent drag or convection (Fig. 1A). Under physiological conditions, net water flow across the renal tubular and intestinal epithelia is directed in the absorptive (lumen-to-interstitium) direction, and thus sets up the condition for Ca absorption by solvent drag. Because Ca parallels water reabsorption, the concentration of Ca in the lumen is not expected to change appreciably. A large fraction of Ca reabsorption in the proximal tubule is mediated through this mechanism. Parenthetically, Ca^{2+} and diffusible complexed Ca also get across the glomeru-

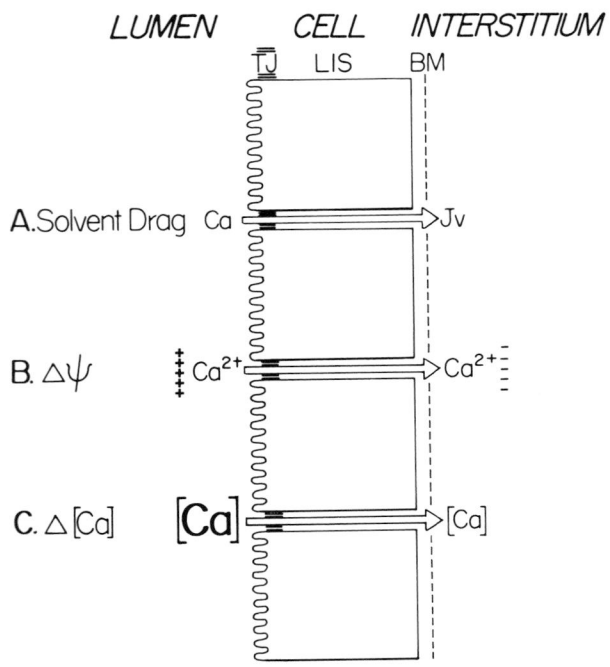

FIG. 1. Schematics of Ca reabsorption through the intercellular pathway. **A:** Reabsorption through solvent drag or convection. Ca is reabsorbed along with net fluid reabsorption (Jv). **B:** Diffusional Ca reabsorption driven by transepithelial voltage (Δψ). Lumen positive potential difference drives positively charged Ca^{2+} across the epithelium into the negatively charged interstitium. **C:** Diffusional Ca reabsorption driven by transepithelial chemical gradient (Δ[Ca]). Higher luminal [Ca] drives Ca in the absorptive direction towards lower [Ca] in the interstitium. TJ, tight junction; LIS, lateral intercellular space; and BM, basement membrane.

lar filtration membrane by solvent drag during glomerular ultrafiltration. Solutes, such as creatinine, which also get across the glomerular filtration membrane unrestricted, are restricted from returning to the interstitium during fluid reabsorption across the tubule.

Diffusion

A second mechanism which moves Ca across the shunt pathway is passive diffusion (3,3a). The force for this mode of transport is the transepithelial electrochemical gradient which can drive ions across the epithelium in the absence of water flow (4). The electrical gradient-driven diffusion plays a major role in Ca reabsorption across the thick ascending limb of the loop of Henle. The net effect of sodium chloride transport and the Na^+ and Cl^- permeabilities across this epithelium is a positive luminal electrical potential (relative to the interstitium) (4a). This would drive the positively charged Ca^{2+} out of the lumen into the interstitium (Fig. 1B). Chemical gradient-driven diffusional reabsorption of Ca (Fig. 1C) probably occurs across most parts of the PCT where the tubular fluid Ca concentration is about 20% higher than that of the plasma or the glomerular filtrate (see below).

In the following discussion the question whether Ca reabsorption in a given nephron segment is passive, active, or both, will often be raised. One approach to deal with such questions is based on the concept of equilibrium concentration. Thus, an electrical gradient-driven passive Ca^{2+} reabsorption would reduce the luminal Ca^{2+} concentration ($[Ca^{2+}]$). The progressive reduction in luminal $[Ca^{2+}]$ would build up a chemical gradient for Ca diffusion in the opposite direction (interstitium-to-lumen). Ultimately a state of equilibrium is reached when the electrical gradient-driven diffusion of Ca out of the lumen equals the chemical gradient-driven diffusion of Ca into the lumen. The luminal $[Ca^{2+}]$ at which this occurs is called the equilibrium Ca concentration. The relationship between the equilibrium Ca concentration and the transmembrane PD is stated by the Nernst equation:

$$PD = -(RT/ZF) \ln (C_2/C_1)$$

where C_2 and C_1 represent the ionic concentrations on the two sides of the membrane at equilibrium. If PD were the only driving force for diffusional Ca reabsorption, then the measured luminal $[Ca^{2+}]$ at equilibrium would be expected to equal, or to remain above the predicted equilibrium $[Ca^{2+}]$. On the other hand, if the measured luminal $[Ca^{2+}]$ is lower than the predicted equilibrium $[Ca^{2+}]$, then additional force(s), such as that generated by an active transport mechanism, must participate in the Ca reabsorptive process.

Direct measurement of the absorptive and secretory fluxes of a solute in the absence of transepithelial electrochemical gradients can also help to distinguish whether it is transported passively or actively. The chemical gradient is eliminated by keeping the solute concentration on both sides of the membrane equal and the electrical gradient can be nullified by using an external voltage clamp. Under such conditions, the two opposing, unidirectional fluxes of a passively transported solute should be equal (since the driving force in each direction is not different), and the flux ratio should be unity. The interrelationship between the fluxes and the electrical driving force across an epithelium of a given permeability is defined by the flux ratio equation of Ussing (5). Changes in transmembrane PD from "zero" would cause predictable changes in the flux ratio from unity. For example, a divalent ion such as Ca would exhibit a 10-fold change in flux ratio in response to a change in transepithelial PD from 0 to 30.7 mV. The transport of a solute which does not demonstrate a flux ratio of 1 at zero transepithelial PD, and whose flux ratio deviates from that predicted by the flux ratio equation at non-zero PD, is not driven by voltage alone, but is most likely mediated by an active process also. However, the interpretation of the flux ratio equation is complex. For example, deviation from the predicted flux ratio can occur if some or all of the Ca is transported as a monovalent ion, $CaCl^+$, rather than the presumed divalent ion, Ca^{2+}. Also, the interaction among the passively driven ions can give rise to phenomena such as the single-file diffusion—the acceleration of the flow of ions in one direction retards the diffusion of ions in the opposite direction (6). Such interactions would cause deviation of the measured flux ratio from the predicted flux ratio without the intervention of any active process.

Ca Absorption Through the Transcellular Pathway

Transcellular transport of Ca across a renal tubular or an intestinal cell would involve at least three steps: entry across the luminal membrane, ferry through the cytoplasm, and exit across the basolateral membrane (Fig. 2).

Luminal Ca Entry

Energetic considerations would predict a non-energy-dependent luminal entry for the cationic Ca, since the cell interior is highly electronegative (-50 to -100 mV), and since the cytosolic $[Ca^{2+}]$ is orders of magnitude lower than the extracellular fluid (ECF) $[Ca^{2+}]$ (nanomolar vs millimolar). Although Ca entry into the cell is favored by both electrical and chemical gradients, its influx across the brush border membrane vesicles demonstrates saturation, rather than simple diffusional, kinetics with a K_m value of around 1 mM (7,8). Saunders and Isaacson using patch electrodes have demonstrated evidence consistent with the presence of apical calcium channel in perfused segments of rabbit proximal straight tubule and cortical collecting duct in vitro (9). Bacskai and Friedman reported that parathyroid hormone activates Ca channels responsible for Ca^{2+} entry into single cultured cells from mouse distal renal tubules (9a). They suggested that the PTH-sensitive, microtubule-dependent exocytosis was responsible for the insertion or activation of Ca^{2+} channels in these cells.

Ca influx can also be modified by changes in brush border membrane lipid composition. Thus, increases in the phosphatidic acid content of brush border membrane is associated with augmentation in Ca influx (10). Brush border membrane vesicles (BBMV) prepared from kidney of PTH-treated dog demonstrated eleva-

tions in both acidic phospholipid content and Ca influx rate (11). Vitamin D also affects phospholipid and fatty acid composition of the renal brush border membrane (12), but correlation between these changes and Ca transport function remains to be established.

Because renal brush border membrane also demonstrates high-affinity binding for Ca (10,11,13), Ca influx measurements using BBMV needs to be carefully distinguished from Ca binding. It also needs to be pointed out that BBMV represent mainly apical membrane fraction of the proximal tubule, a nephron segment in which transcellular Ca transport is not considered to play a major role in Ca reabsorption (see below). Thus, the relevance of such studies to active, transcellular Ca transport in the kidney is uncertain.

Transcytoplasmic Ca Buffering and Ferrying

Following entry at the apical pole, Ca needs to be buffered so that the low intracellular Ca^{2+} environment is protected. It then has to traverse the cytoplasm to the basolateral pole for extrusion. In terms of Ca^{2+} buffering, ATP-dependent Ca uptake by mitochondrial and non-mitochondrial stores has been demonstrated in both rat renal cortical kidney cells (14) and LLC-PK$_1$ cells (15,16). Both inositol 1,4,5-triphosphate (14–16) and angiotensin II (14) have been shown to release Ca from non-mitochondrial store. Moore and associates have demonstrated ATP-dependent Ca^{2+} uptake in microsomal membranes (17) while Parys and associates have reported a Ca^{2+} pump in renal endoplasmic reticulum, distinct from the one in basolateral plasma membrane (18). The question whether these mitochondrial and non-mitochondrial stores also participate in transcytosolic Ca ferrying has not been answered.

Much interest has been focused on the vitamin D-dependent Ca^{2+} binding protein, calbindin-D, as an intracellular system both for buffering and for ferrying Ca^{2+}. Two types of calbindin-D have been described (19). One type with a molecular weight of 28,000 (calbindin-D$_{28}$) and four Ca^{2+} binding sites was first found in avian intestine but was subsequently also found in a variety of mammalian tissue including the kidney, brain, and placenta. The other calbindin-D has a molecular weight of 9000 (calbindin-D$_9$) and two Ca^{2+} binding sites and was found in mammalian intestine. The K_D for calbindin-D$_{28}$ found in rat kidney is estimated at 2.1×10^{-6} M (20) and that for calbindin-D$_9$ found in rat intestine at 0.3 to $0.8 \times 10^{-6} M$ (21,22), values within or close to the range of normal cytosolic $[Ca^{2+}]$. Taylor and associates using immunocytochemical localization technique have also demonstrated the presence of "intestinal" calbindin-D$_9$ in neonatal rat kidney (23). While the higher molecular weight "renal" calbindin-D$_{28}$ is localized in the DCT (see below), the lower molecular weight calbindin-D$_9$ appeared to concentrate in PCT, pars recta and the

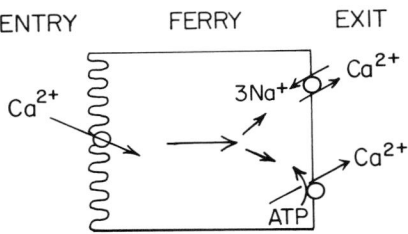

FIG. 2. Schematics of Ca absorption through the transcellular pathway.

thick limb of Henle's loop. Calbindin-D$_9$ in 1-week-old rats is mainly found in the cytoplasm with some located along the brush borders, while in older rats the proportion of localization of this protein at the brush borders increase. The significance of this observation to renal Ca reabsorption remains to be characterized.

Kretsinger and associates proposed that the intestinal calbindin-D facilitates the diffusion of Ca^{2+} within the enterocytes (24), a concept supported by Feher using evidence based on a model system (25). A direct correlation between the amount of intestinal calbindin-D and the rate of active intestinal Ca^{2+} absorption has been documented under a wide variety of physiological conditions (26). Under conditions of maximal active Ca absorption, intestinal calbindin-D content in the enterocytes can attain near millimolar quantities. Less information is available on the relationship between the renal calbindin-D and transcellular Ca transport in the kidney. Based on available data Bronner suggested that this protein may also serve to ferry apical Ca to the basolateral pole of the distal tubular cells for extrusion (27).

In the rat kidney calbindin-D$_{28}$ is demonstrated only in the distal nephron mainly in the DCT (28), where major active Ca reabsorption occurs in the kidney. Three RNA species (1.9, 2.8, and 3.2 kilobase pairs), transcribed from a single gene codes for calbindin-D$_{28}$. 1,25-Dihydroxyvitamin D$_3$ [1,25(OH)$_2$D$_3$] is required for the induction of calbindin-D$_{28}$-mRNA. The effect, first seen two hours following a single injection of 1,25(OH)$_2$D$_3$ peaked after 12 hours. Calbindin-D$_{28}$-mRNA is present in rat kidney before birth and increases markedly in the first week after birth (29–31). In contrast, the intestinal receptor for 1,25(OH)$_2$D$_3$ does not appear till 14–16 days postpartum (32) which is also the period in which the greatest increase in intestinal calbindin-D occurs and when intestinal responsiveness to 1,25(OH)$_2$D$_3$ and intestinal active Ca absorption first ap-

pears (see Ref. 33 for a review). Low dietary phosphorus, a condition which is associated with hypercalciuria (34), has been shown to stimulate calbindin-D$_{28}$-mRNA and calbindin-D$_{28}$ expression (31). Although the effect of a low dietary Ca on stimulating intestinal calbindin-D is well established, its effect on renal calbindin-D expression remains controversial (35).

Basolateral Ca Exit

At the basolateral membrane Ca is actively transported out of the cell against electrochemical gradients. At least two mechanisms may participate in the cellular expulsion of Ca: (i) a Ca-sensitive, Mg-dependent ATPase (Ca ATPase) and (ii) a Ca–Na exchange system (Fig. 2).

Ca is actively pumped out of many cells through the operation of ATP-driven Ca pumps, located in the plasma membrane. These Ca pumps, which have been most extensively studied in erythrocytes, have a high affinity for Ca, with K$_m$, the affinity of the calcium pump for calcium, in the micromolar range, which is within the range of usual cytosolic [Ca^{2+}]. They all have a molecular weight of about 140,000 and are stimulated by calmodulin (36–38).

More recently, the structure of a human plasma membrane Ca^{2+} pump has been deduced from the sequences of cDNA clones (39). A proposed organization and regulatory domains of the Ca^{2+} pump by Gamj and Murer are shown in Fig. 3 (40). The translated sequence of the pump contains 1,220 amino acids, with a calculated molecular weight of 124,683 daltons. Structure–function analysis highlights the presence of a calmodulin-binding domain near the carboxyl terminus and two domains rich in serine and threonine. One of these two domains exhibit sequences which match those found in protein kinase substrates that are cAMP-dependent (41). Close

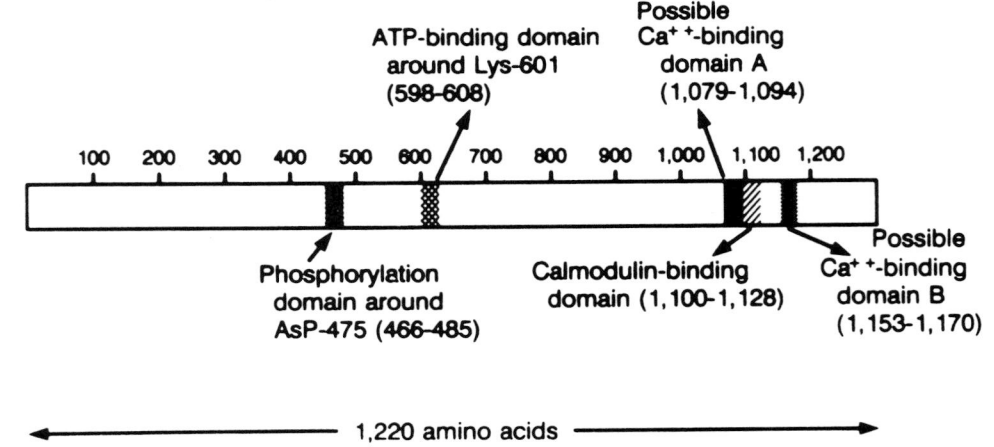

FIG. 3. A proposed organization of the human teratoma plasma membrane Ca^{2+} ATPase-pump. From Gamj and Murer (40).

to the amino terminus are two sequences similar to the E-F hands, i.e., the calcium-binding loci found in molecules such as calmodulin, troponin C, and parvalbumin (42). No structural studies of the renal Ca ATPase have been reported to date.

High affinity Ca ATPase activity has been demonstrated in basolateral plasma membrane preparations (43,44), which, as mentioned earlier, are mostly derived from proximal tubule. Since transcellular Ca transport is not of predominant importance in the proximal tubule (see below), the Ca ATPase may serve a cellular Ca^{2+} homeostasis role rather than a transcellular Ca transporting role. Doucet and Katz found Ca^{2+} ATPase activity along the whole length of the nephron, with maximal activity in the distal tubule, where major active Ca reabsorption occurs in the kidney (45). This observation would suggest that Ca ATPase is not only important in cellular Ca^{2+} homeostasis but also in transcellular transport of Ca. On the other hand, Borke and associates using monoclonal antibodies against erythrocyte Ca^{2+}, Mg^{2+} ATPase recognized an epitope in the basolateral membrane of only the distal convoluted tubule (46), suggesting a more restricted function of the enzyme to active, transcellular Ca reabsorption.

A second process which extrudes Ca from cells is mediated through a Na^+/Ca^{2+} exchanger (46a). This exchanger can move Ca^{2+} in either direction across the cell membrane depending on the electrochemical Na^+ gradient that provides the free energy for the exchange process. Under usual circumstances, Ca is extruded from cells, energized by the inwardly directed electrochemical potential gradient for Na^+, which in turn is established by the activity of the Na^+-K^+ ATPase. Although this process is not driven by direct ATP hydrolysis, its affinity is increased by ATP (47). As one would anticipate, this Na^+-driven Ca^{2+} uptake is inhibited by Na^+ ionophores and ouabain, both of which would reduce the Na gradient directed into the cell. In excitable cells this exchanger is electrogenic, countertransporting three (47) or four (48) Na^+ for one Ca^{2+}, and is thus sensitive to transmembrane voltage changes.

Recently, Nicoll, Longoni, and Philipson have reported the molecular cloning and functional expression of the canine cardiac Na^+/Ca^{2+} exchanger (48a). A sequence of 970 amino acids deduced from a cDNA yielded a relative molecular mass of 108,000 daltons. The difference between this estimate and the purified exchanger protein with relative molecular mass of 160 kD (Kilodaltons), is attributed to glycosylation. The hydropathy plot of the exchanger indicates that it contains 12 membrane-spanning segments and 11 loops connecting these transmembrane segments (Fig. 4). Part of the long cytoplasmic region (*loop f*) resembles a calmodulin-binding domain and may represent a locus where Ca^{2+}-dependent modulation of the exchanger activities reside.

A recent report of Niggli and Lederer provided insights into the molecular operation of the Na^+/Ca^{2+} exchanger in heart myocytes (48b). A rapid increase in intracellular $[Ca^{2+}]$ by photolysis of caged Ca^{2+} produced a transient current that preceded the Na^+/Ca^{2+} exchange current. They proposed that the transient current was a conformational current, I_{conf}, reflecting the binding of Ca^{2+} to the exchanger protein. The observation that I_{conf}

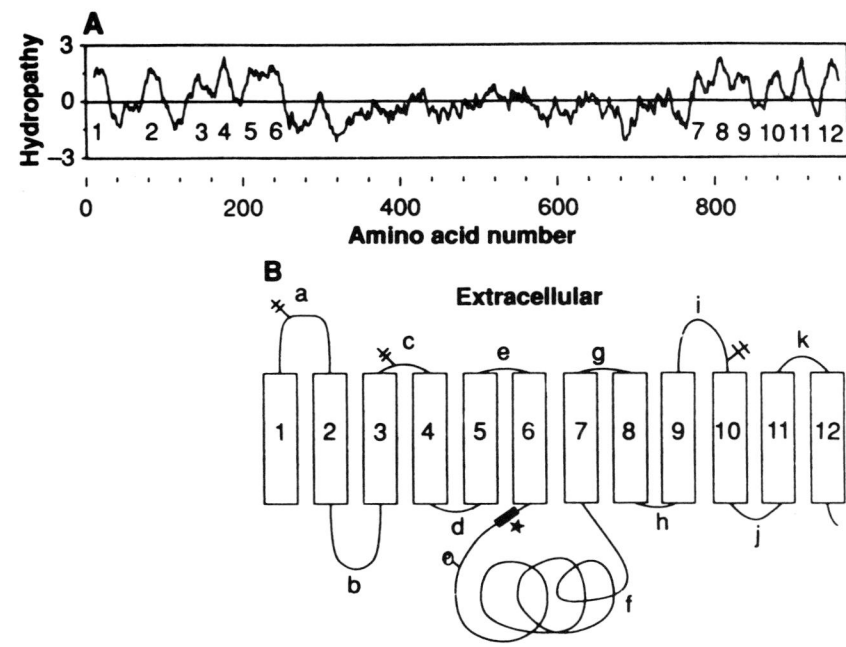

FIG. 4. Hydropathy map (**A**) and model (**B**) for the Na^+-Ca^{2+} exchanger. **A:** Hydrophobicity is indicated by positive numbers and hydrophilicity by negative numbers. Potential membrane-spanning regions are indicated with numbers 1 to 12. **B:** A proposed model for the protein exchanger based on the hydropathy map. One to 12, membrane-spanning segments; a to k, loops connecting transmembrane segments. ‡, possible sites of extracellular asparagine-linked oligosaccharide binding; *, calmodulin binding site; and P, phosphorylation site. From Nicoll et al. (48a).

and the Na^+/Ca^{2+} exchange current were consecutive in time clearly indicates that ion-binding and translocation do not occur in a single step. They calculated that there were at least 250 exchangers per μm^2, turning over up to 2500 times per second. It is important to point out that Na^+/Ca^{2+} exchangers are not necessarily identical in different cell types. For example, unlike the cardiac Na^+/Ca^{2+} exchanger, the Na^+/Ca^{2+} exchanger of the cells of the rod's outer segments of the retina use not only the electrochemical inward Na^+ gradient to extrude Ca^{2+}, but also the outward K^+ gradient. The exchange stoichiometry is $4Na^+:1Ca^{2+},1K^+$, allowing rapid Ca^{2+} extrusion and reduction of intracellular $[Ca^{2+}]$ to very low levels. The relative molecular mass of the rod exchange protein, 220 kD, is also much larger than the cardiac exchange protein (46a).

Na^+/Ca^{2+} exchanger activities have been reported in renal basolateral membranes (49–51). The kinetics of this exchanger have been studied in the rat. Van Heeswijk et al. (49) reported a V_{max} of 3.2 nmol $Ca^{2+} \cdot min^{-1} \cdot mg^{-1}$ protein and a Km of 0.2 μM, while Jayakumar et al. (50) reported a similar V_{max} of 5.4 nmol $Ca^{2+} \cdot min^{-1} \cdot mg^{-1}$ protein, but a higher Km of 8 μM. Scoble et al. (51) in canine renal basolateral membrane also found a V_{max} and Km of 3.2 and 10, respectively. The lower affinity found in the latter two studies have

been attributed to the buffer system used which did not buffer Ca^{2+} below 1 μM, raising the possibility of underestimating or missing a high affinity site (52). Although most studies point to the presence of Na^+/Ca^{2+} activities in both the proximal and distal tubules, recent report from Ramachandran and Brunette localized this exchanger exclusively to the distal tubule in both the rat and the rabbit (53).

Calcium Absorption Through the Endocytotic, Vesicular Pathway

Jande and Brewer first proposed the participation of lysosomes in intestinal calcium transport in 1974 (54). Vesicular Ca transport in the intestine has recently been reviewed by Nemere and Norman (55) and is summarized in Fig. 5, reproduced from the work of the same authors (56). In the left panel, luminal Ca^{2+} enters the cell through brush border Ca channels, activated by conformational changes induced by alteration in membrane fluidity or the presence of membrane-associated Ca-binding complex. The internalized Ca^{2+} is first complexed to Ca-binding protein, which then translocates the Ca^{2+} to Golgi vesicles. Subsequent fusion of these vesicles with the basolateral membrane led to the exocytosis of Ca^{2+} into the antiluminal side of the enterocyte.

$+D_3 [+1,25(OH) D_3]$

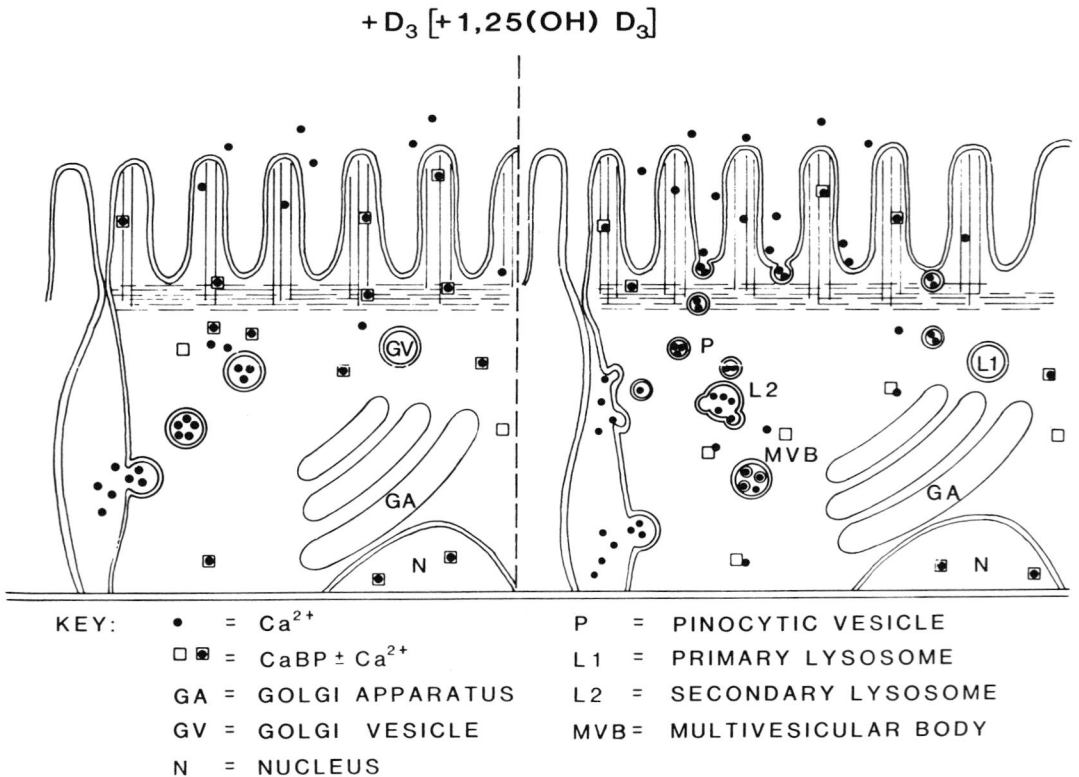

KEY:

•	= Ca^{2+}		P	= PINOCYTIC VESICLE
□ ▣	= CaBP $\pm$ Ca^{2+}		L1	= PRIMARY LYSOSOME
GA	= GOLGI APPARATUS		L2	= SECONDARY LYSOSOME
GV	= GOLGI VESICLE		MVB	= MULTIVESICULAR BODY
N	= NUCLEUS			

FIG. 5. Calcium absorption through the endocytotic, vesicular pathway. See text for details. From Nemere and Norman (56).

In the right panel Ca entry across the brush border membrane is postulated to occur through pinocytotic vesicles. Transport is then completed through direct fusion of these vesicles with the basolateral membrane and exocytosis of Ca^{2+}. An alternate pathway requires the fusion of the pinocytotic vesicles with primary lysosomes, packaged by the Golgi apparatus, to form secondary lysosomes, including multivesicular bodies. The fusion of these Ca-bearing lysosomes with the basolateral membrane completes the transport process.

Vesicular Ca transport has the virtue of moving significant quantities of Ca through the cell while imposing no threat to the fine-tuned homeostasis of the cellular Ca environment. The possible participation of this mechanism in renal Ca transport needs to be explored. Occurrence of endocytosis and the formation of pinocytotic vesicles have been reported in the kidney (57).

CA TRANSPORT IN DIFFERENT SEGMENTS OF THE NEPHRON

Figure 6 depicts the major sites of Ca reabsorption along the nephron. About 70% of the filtered Ca is reabsorbed in the proximal tubule, 20% in the thick ascending limb, up to 10% in the distal tubule, and up to 5% in the collecting duct.

Glomerular Filtration of Ca

Direct measurement of Ca concentrations in glomerular ultrafiltrate (UF_{Ca}) and in plasma (P_{Ca}) gave a UF_{Ca}/P_{Ca} value ranging between 0.63 and 0.70 (58,59), which approximates the filtrable fraction of plasma Ca. The

ultrafilterability of Ca can be modified by factors such as Ca infusion and hypercalcemia (see below).

Proximal Convoluted Tubule

Most available evidence suggest that the bulk of the Ca reabsorbed in the "leaky" proximal convoluted tubule (PCT) is mediated passively through the intercellular pathway (60,61). The ratio of the tubular fluid (TF) calcium concentration to that of ultrafiltrate calcium concentration $(TF/UF)_{Ca}$ is close to 1.0 in the early convolutions of the PCT indicating that the reabsorption of Ca keeps in pace with the reabsorption of Na (and fluid). As mentioned earlier, this is most likely mediated by convection (solvent drag) across the tight junction. Beyond the early convolutions, Ca reabsorption lags slightly behind Na reabsorption, leading to an increase in $(TF/UF)_{Ca}$ to 1.2. This 20% increase in TF Ca concentration relative to that of ultrafiltrate Ca concentration, most likely, reflects molecular sieving of Ca at the apical tight junctions in association with fluid reabsorption. The chemical gradient sets up an additional driving force for Ca reabsorption across the intercellular pathway.

As the tubular fluid traverses from S1 segment into the cortical S2 segment, a third reabsorptive force materializes. The transepithelial voltage, which was lumen negative in the S1 segment, is now lumen positive because of a chloride-bicarbonate bi-ionic electrical potential difference (61a). This lumen positive potential difference would drive the positively charged Ca^{2+} in the absorptive direction. In rabbit PCT (S2 segment), Ng and associates have demonstrated no net Ca flux in the absence of transepithelial water transport and electrochemical gradient

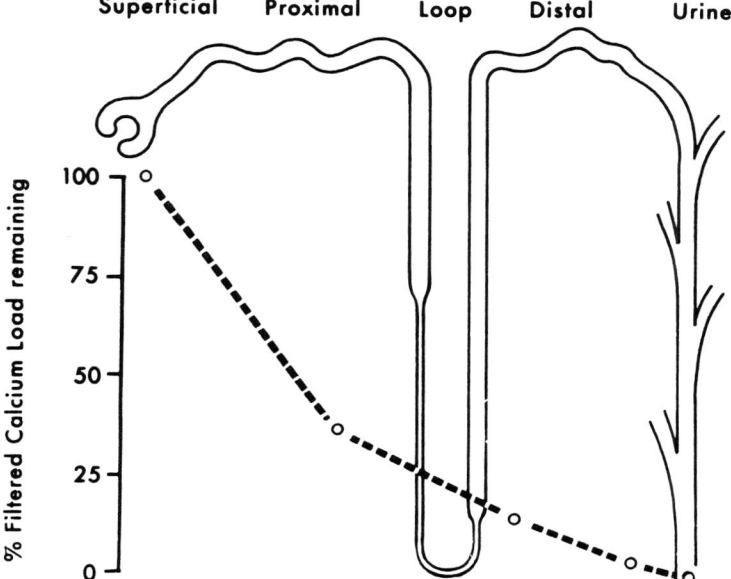

FIG. 6. Calcium reabsorption along the mammalian nephron. Data derived from a number of micropuncture studies in the rat and the dog. From Sutton and Dirks (60).

(62). Induction of lumen-positive PD was associated with net Ca efflux (reabsorption) while induction of lumen-negative was associated with net Ca influx (secretion). The presence of passive, voltage-dependent Ca transport has also been shown using in vivo microperfusion of the rat superficial PCT (63).

Although most studies support the passive nature of Ca reabsorption in the proximal nephron, a number of studies have provided evidence for the existence of active Ca reabsorption in this location (4,64,65). Such mechanisms may be important especially in the earliest convolutions of the PCT where substantial Ca reabsorption occurs in the face of a lumen-negative PD and a (TF/UF)$_{Ca}$ ratio close to unity. As mentioned earlier, while some studies suggest the presence of Ca-ATPase and Na/Ca exchange activities (functions required for active transcellular Ca transport) in the PCT, more recent studies localized the activities of these transporters exclusively to the distal nephron.

Proximal Straight Tubule

The S2 portion of the proximal straight tubule (PST) appears to have electrochemical gradient-dependent, passive Ca reabsorption similar to that observed in the S2 segment of the PCT (66). Analysis of TF collected by micropuncture studies from the end of the superficial proximal tubule and the bend of the loop of Henle indicates that Na and Ca may no longer be reabsorbed in parallel in tubular segments between these two locations, i.e., the PST and the descending limb of the loop of Henle (58,67,68). Rather, the data indicate Ca transport in excess of Na. Substantial active Ca reabsorptive process (7.0–13.0 pEq · min · mm^{-1}) has indeed been demonstrated in the S3 segment of the PST (69,70). In contrast to other cellular Ca transport mechanisms in the nephron, the mechanism in this segment is not affected by the removal of Na from the perfusate (69) or the addition of ouabain to the bathing solution (69,70). Exit at the basolateral membrane must also be different since there is no evidence for Ca-ATPase or Na/Ca exchange activities in this portion of the nephron. It should be noted that the observed dissociation between Na and Ca transport in these studies can also be explained by the heterogeneity in the nephron populations sampled, i.e., the proximal sample was collected from a superficial, cortical nephron while the distal loop sample was collected from a different, deep, juxtaglomerular nephron.

The Descending and the Thin Ascending Loops of Henle

Available information suggests that the descending and the thin ascending limbs of Henle have very low Ca permeability and have negligible effect on net transepithelial Ca transport activities (70,71).

The Thick Ascending Limb of the Loop of Henle (TALH)

The mechanism of Ca transport in this nephron segment has been actively debated (71a). Data from one series of studies (72–74) support the thesis that Ca reabsorption is accomplished through passive, voltage-driven process. The slope of the regression line relating the unidirectional efflux to influx ratios and voltage was greater than that predicted for simple passive diffusion, but was consistent with the single-file diffusion mechanism originally described by Hodgkin and Keynes (6). Other studies however, have found Ca flux ratio greater than that predicted from the transepithelial PD, suggesting the presence of active transport in addition to the gradient-driven passive transport (71). Rouse and Suki proposed that axial heterogeneity may account for some of the differences observed among the studies reported (61). Studies from their laboratory suggest the presence of active Ca transport in the cortical TALH while the medullary TALH exhibited Ca transport characteristics more consistent with a passive mechanism (75). Furosemide in the bathing solution depressed PD without affecting Ca efflux in cortical TALH while in the medullary TALH, Ca efflux was inhibited by similar treatment. Earlier, Imai also demonstrated active, saturable Ca transport in the cortical TALH segments. This mechanism appeared to be independent of anaerobic metabolism, Na transport, and Ca ATPase (76). Other studies have demonstrated that the cortical Ca efflux (reabsorption) is increased, in a PD-independent manner, by the presence of PTH in the bath (77,78), while medullary Ca efflux is stimulated by calcitonin or cyclic AMP (78).

Distal Convoluted Tubule

Available evidence suggests that major regulation of urinary Ca excretion occurs in this portion of the nephron. In free-flow micropuncture studies, (TF/UF)$_{Ca}$ has been shown to drop from 0.6 to 0.3 from the early to the late puncture site (79). Higher Ca transport capacity was demonstrated during in situ perfusion (when luminal Ca availability is not a limiting factor) than under free-flow conditions (when luminal Ca availability is limited by the delivery from the proximal nephron). This suggests that in vivo Ca reabsorption in this segment is limited by the availability of transportable ions. Because only ionic Ca is transported by the tubular cells, the luminal concentration of the complexed Ca may increase. When not limited by the presence of complexed Ca, ionized Ca concentration falls to 0.1 mM and reabsorption in this segment was not saturated with Ca load up to 30 pmole/min (80). This reabsorption, which occurs in the face of a luminal Ca concentration much lower than that of plasma and a PD which is highly lumen-negative, is almost certainly mediated by an active, transcellular process. The mechanism of luminal entry, which is not Na-dependent remains to be characterized (72,79). A recent study using single cultured cortical ascending limb (CAL) and distal convoluted tubule (DCT) cells from the mouse has provided insights into this entry process (9a). It appeared that the PTH-stimulated increase in intracellular Ca^{2+} concentration $[(Ca^{2+})_i]$ began with the insertion or activation of dihydropyridine-sensitive Ca channels in the plasma membrane. This process probably accounted for the delay of 10–12 min before $(Ca^{2+})_i$ began to rise and peaked at 30 min. The increases in $(Ca^{2+})_i$ was shown to result from the influx of extracellular Ca^{2+}. As pointed out by the authors, the response pattern to PTH in these Ca-transporting distal tubular cells is quite different from that exhibited by the proximal tubular cells. In these latter cells, the PTH-induced increase in $(Ca^{2+})_i$ is rapid, transient and has its source from intracellular stores. It is likely that such Ca^{2+} transients reflect signal transduction rather than transcellular Ca transport.

As mentioned earlier renal calbindin-D is preferentially localized in this portion of the nephron and may function as a buffer, a ferry, and an activator of the Ca ATPase. Also discussed earlier, for basolateral exit, Ca ATPase and Na/Ca exchange activities are located maximally, or exclusively in this tubular segment.

Morel and associates have emphasized that the DCT has four morphologically and functionally distinct portions: an ascending limb portion, a "bright" portion, a "granular" portion, and a "light" portion which is morphologically similar to the cortical collecting tubule (81). The "granular" portion has since assumed the new name of the connecting tubule (CNT), and is believed to play an important role in the regulation of urinary Ca excretion. The portion of this connecting tubule which surfaces in the cortex has been identified, for micropuncture purpose, as the late DCT. In isolated segments of rabbit CNT, Imai has measured a net Ca efflux rate of 4.0 pEq · min^{-1} · mm^{-1} (82).

Collecting Duct

Several studies have shown that the Ca in the final urine is less than that measured at the end of the accessible portion of the DCT (58,83,84). One explanation is that the final urine Ca is diluted by the outflow from the deeper, juxtamedullary nephron (not accessible to micropuncture), which may have greater Ca reabsorptive capability and thus produces urine with lower Ca content. An additional possibility is further Ca reabsorption occurs in the collecting duct system. Using isolated, perfused cortical collecting duct segments, several studies have reported very low net efflux, 0.06 to 0.20 pEq · min^{-1} · mm^{-1}, which appeared to be voltage-driven and was not sensitive to PTH or cAMP (85,86).

Others have observed substantial active Ca efflux which was also not sensitive to PTH and cyclic AMP, but was abolished by ADH (82,87). Both calbindin-D (28) and Ca ATPase activity (45) have been reported in this segment.

Little is known about Ca transport in the medullary collecting duct. Using in vivo microcatheterization techniques, Bengele, Alexander, and Lechene have reported the reabsorption of 1.4% of the filtered Ca load in this portion of the nephron (88). The mechanism has not been characterized. Since the PD in this nephron segment is usually lumen-positive, passive Ca absorption is a possibility.

FACTORS INFLUENCING RENAL HANDLING OF CALCIUM

Dietary (Enteral and Parenteral) Factors

Sodium

Walser demonstrated that with acute saline infusion (in the dog), the clearance of Ca increased in parallel with that of Na over a wide range of Na excretion (89). One explanation for this observation is that saline infusion, and the consequent volume expansion, causes reduction in Na (90) and Ca (91) reabsorption in the proximal tubule, where the bulk of these ions are reabsorbed and where the reabsorption of these two ions appears linked. However, further studies have clearly established that urinary excretion of Na and Ca, in general, does not reflect proximal reabsorptive activities, but instead, parallels the transport activities of the distal nephron. Thus, depression of proximal Na reabsorption does not increase urinary Na excretion unless distal reabsorption is also inhibited (92,93). Agus and associates further observed that fractional Ca delivery to the late distal tubule is not different in hydropenic (nonexpanded) and saline-loaded (volume expanded) rats, suggesting that the calciuric effect of saline-loading is the result of inhibition of Ca reabsorption beyond the late distal tubule (94). This effect is not PTH-dependent.

Kleeman and associates reported on the effect of variation in Na intake on Ca excretion in normal humans (95). Maneuvers that increased urinary Na excretion also increase urinary Ca excretion. Parenthetically, it is interesting to note that high dietary Ca intake can also cause marked natriuresis (96). Although, the calciuric effect of chronic increases in dietary Na is now well recognized (97), the transport mechanism and the intrarenal site(s) that are responsible for the altered Ca excretion are still not defined. The rise in urinary Ca following increases in dietary Na intake may also be mediated through extrarenal causes. Increasing Na intake is also associated with increases in circulating levels of immunoreactive PTH (98), which could in turn, stimulate 1,25(OH)$_2$D production and intestinal Ca absorption.

The increments in PTH and 1,25(OH)$_2$D could, in theory, also cause increases in Ca mobilization from the skeleton and thus increasing Ca load for renal excretion. The possible relationship between dietary sodium intake and hypercalciuria and nephrolithiasis is discussed in Chapter 31.

Volume contraction associated with increased proximal tubular reabsorption of Na and Ca is associated with reduced urinary Ca excretion. This has been postulated to participate in the genesis of hypocalciuria associated with thiazide administration (see below) and the nephrotic syndrome (99).

Inorganic Phosphate

It is a long-established observation that oral and parenteral phosphate administration is associated with a fall in urinary Ca (100). The effect is delayed (101) and is manifested even in the face of volume expansion (102). The mechanism for this hypocalciuric effect is still not well understood. Micropuncture studies suggest increases in Ca reabsorption in the distal or terminal portions of the nephron (103). Phosphate administration or excess can also reduce urine Ca through extrarenal mechanisms (104). Thus, phosphate loading is associated with increased Ca sequestration in bone and/or soft tissues, which in turn, could reduce the Ca load for urinary excretion. Phosphate can also stimulate PTH secretion (possibly through reducing plasma ionized Ca concentration) and thereby augments distal Ca reabsorption. Increased phosphate ingestion can also reduce intestinal Ca absorption through complexing and rendering Ca less absorbable.

Phosphorus depletion is associated with hypercalciuria in both humans and animals (104). Proximal tubular fluid reabsorption has been reported both as decreased (84) and normal (105). Phosphate infusion reduced the hypercalciuria without correcting this proximal abnormality, suggesting that this proximal defect is not the causation of the observed hypercalciuria. A re-

duction in Ca reabsorption in the loop of Henle has also been suggested (106,107). This defect may or may not be corrected by PTH infusion, indicating that the hypercalciuria is not necessarily the result of suppression of PTH secretion associated with phosphorus depletion. In microperfusion studies, Imai observed that PTH effect on cortical TALH Ca transport is aborted when bath phosphate concentration is reduced from 3.0 to 1.0 mM (82). Impaired Ca reabsorption has also been reported in distal nephron, beyond the last accessible micropuncture site (108). This defect is completely reversed with phosphate infusion. In addition to a possible direct effect on renal Ca reabsorption, phosphorus depletion is known to increase 1,25(OH)$_2$D$_3$ synthesis, intestinal Ca absorption, and increase mobilization of Ca from the bone, all factors which augment Ca influx into the ECF and thereby increases the Ca load for urinary excretion (104).

Calcium

As discussed earlier, in a normal individual who is in Ca balance, the kidney is obligated to excrete the amount of Ca absorbed by the intestine. When the relationship between urinary Ca excretion and dietary Ca intake is scrutinized in normal individuals, Lemann and associates found that only 6% of an oral Ca load appeared in the urine (109). The relatively modest effect of Ca intake on urine Ca can be predicted from the observations summarized in Fig. 7, which depicts the relationship between net Ca absorbed and dietary Ca intake in humans (110). The slope of the curve at normal Ca intake (around 15 mg/kg/day) is relatively flat when compared to that for lower Ca intake. As discussed elsewhere (111), an oral Ca load may also reduce Ca absorption acutely through a direct mucosal effect. Thus, variation of dietary Ca in a normal population with an adequate dietary Ca intake has relatively little effect on urinary Ca excretion. Factors which modulate intestinal Ca absorption, however, would be expected to have profound influence on urinary Ca excretion (see below).

Other Dietary Factors

Wasserstein and associates have demonstrated that a linear relationship exists between dietary protein intake, estimated by urinary urea nitrogen excretion, and urinary calcium excretion (112). One explanation for this association is that the increases in endogenous acid production, anticipated from an increased protein intake, would increase urinary net acid excretion which is known to augment urinary Ca excretion (109,113). However, Na bicarbonate administration which corrected the urinary pH and ammonium and titratable acid excretion did not completely reverse the hypercalciuria (114). There is evidence to suggest that the calciuric action of protein loading may be related to increases in methio-

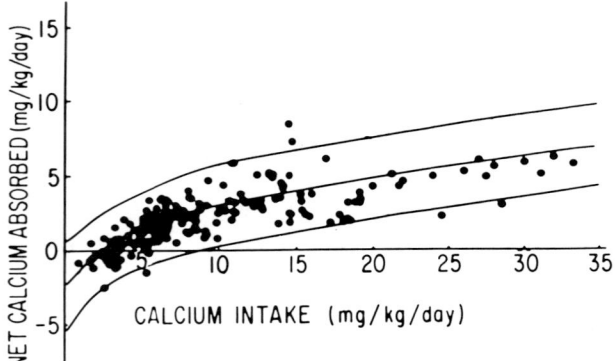

FIG. 7. The relationship between net Ca absorbed and dietary Ca intake in man. From Wilkinson (110).

nine intake and the consequent increases in urinary sulfate excretion (115,116). The calciuric effect of dietary protein appears exaggerated in patients with recurrent nephrolithiasis, i.e., these patients exhibited greater calciuria for a given increment in dietary protein (112). Dietary carbohydrate is also known to augment urinary Ca excretion and this effect may also be magnified in stone formers (117).

Hormonal Factors

Parathyroid Hormone

PTH stimulates renal tubular Ca reabsorption and reduces urinary Ca excretion and is considered a major regulator for renal Ca excretion. PTH reduces GFR, most likely through decreasing the glomerular ultrafiltration coefficient, K_f (118). This would be expected to cause reduction in the filtered load of Ca. Although it is frequently stated that PTH causes parallel reduction in proximal Na and Ca reabsorption (119), both increases (120) or no changes (121,122) in Ca reabsorption in this nephron have been reported with PTH treatment. However, proximal Ca reabsorption, whether decreased, unchanged, or increased, does not appear to influence the hypocalciuric effect of PTH observed in the final urine. A number of studies have demonstrated a stimulatory effect of PTH on Ca reabsorption in the thick ascending limb. The action appears to be localized to the cortical, but not the medullary portion of this segment (72,74,77,78,82), and is dependent on the presence of a lumen-positive PD (77) and normal phosphate concentrations (82). The PTH action can be duplicated by cyclic AMP analogues (77,78,82). PTH also stimulates Ca reabsorption in the DCT segment accessible to micropuncture and beyond (83). This effect appears to be mediated through a PD-independent mechanism and is also not dependent on Na reabsorption (72,82). The effect of PTH on Ca influx into the distal Ca-transporting cells (9a) has been discussed earlier. The highest PTH-sensitive adenylate cyclase activity is located in the PCT and connecting tubules in the rabbit, and in cortical thick ascending limbs and early DCT in the rat (123). Of the many actions of PTH on the PCT is the stimulation of 1,25(OH)$_2$D production, a metabolite of vitamin D whose action on renal Ca handling will now be discussed.

Vitamin D

Clinical and experimental studies have led to divergent observations implicating vitamin D and its metabolites in causing increases (124–129), decreases (130–133), or no changes (134–136) in renal Ca reabsorption. The conflicting results are understandable because the studies were conducted under different experimental conditions and a variety of factors including serum calcium concentrations, vitamin D nutritional status, and parathyroid hormone activities were not independently controlled (137,138). In a study, in which these factors were independently controlled, vitamin D deficiency was clearly shown to reduce tubular Ca reabsorption (139).

Yamamoto and associates further demonstrated that the presence of both PTH and vitamin D are necessary for optimal renal tubular Ca absorption. Figure 8 reproduced from Kurokawa (138) is adapted from the data of Yamamoto (139). An apparent Ca threshold of 9–10 mg/dL is observed under normal conditions (+D+PTH). Increments of serum Ca above this level appears to saturate tubular Ca reabsorptive capacity and urine Ca excretion rose in a linear fashion with further increments in serum Ca. At levels below this threshold, all Ca is reabsorbed and the urine is virtually free of Ca. Absence of either PTH (+D−PTH) or vitamin D (−D+PTH) shifts the "titration" curve to the left, so that the threshold is now around a serum Ca level of 6 mg/dL, reflecting a marked reduction in renal Ca reabsorptive capacity. Absence of both hormones (−D−PTH) leads to further leftward displacement of the curve, reflecting a further drop in threshold and renal Ca reabsorptive capacity.

The precise locus of action of 1,25(OH)$_2$D on renal tubular transport of Ca is still uncertain. Autoradiographic evidence localized nuclear transfer of 1,25(OH)$_2$D-receptor complex to the medullary and cortical thick ascending limbs of Henle's loop and in DCT (140), sites which in general correspond to those where PTH-responsive active Ca transport occurs and also coincide with sites for immunocytochemical localization of calbindin-D, discussed earlier. As discussed elsewhere in the text, vitamin D, through its extrarenal effect, can increase intestinal Ca absorption and bone Ca mobilization, factors known to increase urinary Ca excretion.

Other Hormones

Calcitonin is hypocalciuric in thyro-parathyroidectomized (TPTX) animals (141). Calcitonin-sensitive adenylate cyclase activity has been described in both the cortical and the medullary thick ascending limb of Henle in the rabbit (123). In perfused rabbit tubules, calcitonin has been shown to stimulate both cyclic AMP production and Ca reabsorption in the medullary TALH (78). While PTH stimulates 1-hydroxylase, the enzyme which produces 1,25(OH)$_2$D, in the PCT via a cAMP-dependent mechanism, calcitonin stimulates 1-hydroxylase in the PST via a cAMP-independent mechanism (138). The calcitonin-1-hydroxylase system may play an important role in sustaining 1,25(OH)$_2$D production and renal Ca reabsorption under special physiological conditions of high Ca demand such as during fetal and postna-

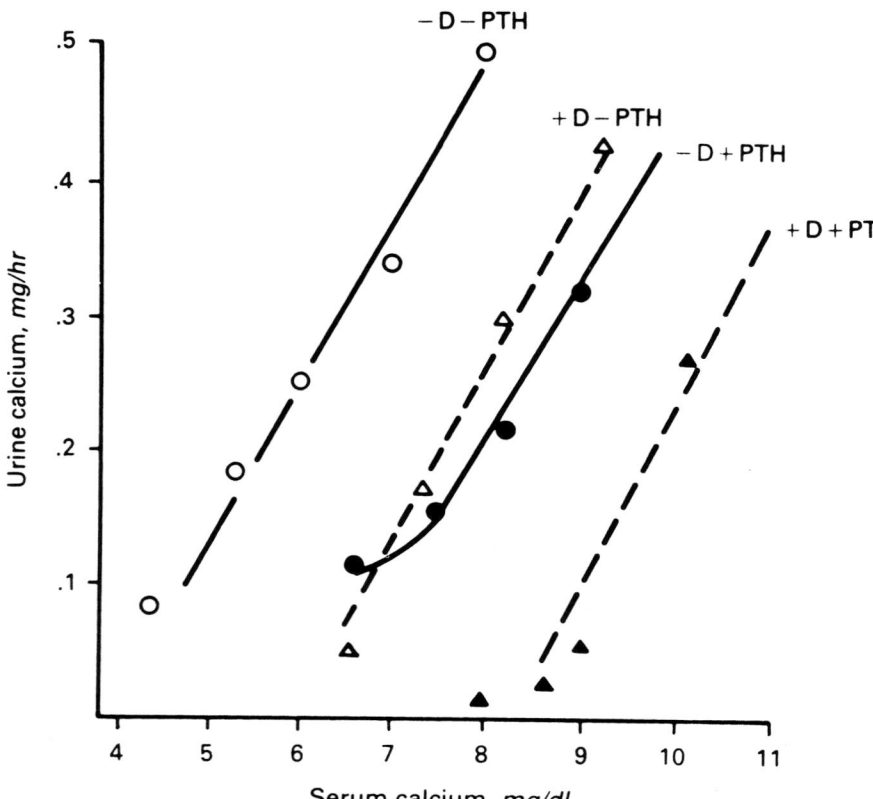

FIG. 8. The effect of PTH and vitamin D on the relationship between serum calcium concentration and urinary calcium excretion in the rat. Both hormones influence the apparent Tm and threshold Ca concentration. From Kurakawa (138).

tal rapid growth and during pregnancy and lactation (138).

Chronic glucocorticoid excess can cause calciuria, probably through a net catabolic effect on the skeleton (142,143). Chronic mineralocorticoid excess can also augment urinary Ca excretion (144,145), possibly mediated through the mechanism of volume expansion. Mineralocorticoids also enhance luminal negativity in the cortical collecting duct, which would be expected to drive Ca^{2+} in the excretory direction.

In clinical and/or laboratory studies, insulin (146), glucagon (146,147), growth hormone (148), thyroid hormone (149), catecholamines (150), and angiotensin (151) have all been reported to increase urine Ca excretion; while antidiuretic hormone causes either an increase (152) or no change (153), and estrogen causes a decrease (154,155) in urine Ca excretion.

Metabolic Pertubations

Acid-Base

Acute and chronic metabolic acidosis is associated with an increase in Ca excretion, which is not attributable to changes in filtered load of Ca or in parathyroid activity (156–158). Metabolic alkalosis results in a decrease in Ca excretion (159,160). Similar changes have been documented in relation to respiratory acidosis and alkalosis (161–163). Micropuncture studies suggest that although acute acidosis reduced proximal Ca (and Na) reabsorption, the hypercalciuria is attributable to an impairment in Ca reabsorption relative to Na reabsorption in the distal nephron (156). Correction of acidosis by bicarbonate infusion, whether in the presence or absence of PTH, reversed both the distal reabsorptive defect and hypercalciuria. Reduction in urinary Ca associated with alkali administration also appeared to be mediated by a distal effect (156). Decreased Ca excretion associated with metabolic alkalosis is more consistently demonstrated with potassium bicarbonate (164) or citrate (165) administration than with the administration of Na salts. This is because Na administration may cause natriuresis with parallel calciuresis, thus masking the alkali-induced hypocalciuria. The effect of acidosis and alkalosis on distal Ca reabsorption raised the possibility of a Ca transport mechanism responsive to distal bicarbonate delivery. Indeed, Peraino and Suki observed an association between urine bicarbonate and renal Ca reabsorption that is independent of systemic acid–base changes (166). Parenthetically, several studies have also suggested that the reduction in proximal Ca reabsorption associated with acute metabolic acidosis may be the result of a lack of bicarbonate in the tubular fluid (166,167). However, in tubule perfusion studies, changes in luminal bicarbonate concentration did not appear to affect Ca transport in the cortical TALH (73).

Hypercalcemia

While hypercalcemia would be expected to increase the Ca filtered load, the net result may be modified by a number of other factors. First, a reduction in the ultrafilterability of both Ca and phosphate has been demonstrated during Ca infusion (168). The mechanism is not well defined. Second, hypercalcemia is known to cause reduction in GFR (169). This has been attributed to a decrease in the glomerular capillary ultrafiltration coefficient, K_f, which occurred only in the presence of PTH (169). PTH can, by itself, cause reductions in K_f and GFR (118), possibly through its effect on mesangial cell contraction and consequent reduction in glomerular capillary surface area (169).

Hypercalcemia affects Ca transport in several segments of the nephron. It reduces the bulk reabsorption in the proximal tubule, leading to parallel increases in the fractional excretion of Ca, Na, and water (94,170). Both in vivo (171) and in vitro (74) microperfusion studies have demonstrated reduction in Ca reabsorption in the TALH with increasing peritubular Ca concentrations, possibly mediated through an inhibition of Ca extrusion at the basolateral membrane. Finally, hypercalcemia also induces a reduction in Ca reabsorption in the distal tubule. Because this last effect is only observed in the presence of parathyroid glands, the effect is most likely mediated through the suppression of PTH secretion (170).

Other Minerals and Ions

Magnesium infusion leads to increased urinary excretion of Ca as well as Mg and Na (172). Quamme and associates have reported that calcium transport in the loop of Henle varied reciprocally with serum magnesium levels (173). Anions including gluconate (174), ferrocyanide (175), and, as mentioned earlier, sulfate can also increase Ca excretion, possibly through complexing ionic Ca and rendering it less reabsorbable.

Hypercalcemia of Malignancy

Renal Ca excretion forms a "safety valve" in the prevention and amelioration of hypercalcemia of malignancy. This function can be compromised by the development of renal failure. In multiple myeloma, the hypercalcemia is more closely related to impaired glomerular filtration than with osteoclast activating factors (OAF) (176). Ralston and associates observed in five patients with malignancy-associated hypercalcemia that renal tubular threshold for Ca reabsorption was elevated (177). In three patients who had successful removal of the primary tumor, the correction of hypercalcemia was associated with the resolution of this abnormality, while bone resorption (as reflected by hydroxyproline excretion) was unchanged. Bone Ca mobilization as an important cause of the observed hypercalcemia was also not supported by histomorphometric analysis of bone biopsy in four patients. Bone resorption was normal in three and slightly increased in one. This line of observations suggest that tumors may produce factors which could increase renal Ca absorption.

Diuretics

Osmotic Diuretics

Osmotic diuresis increases both Na and Ca excretion in the urine (178,179). The mechanism probably involves parallel inhibition of Na and Ca reabsorption in both the proximal tubule and the loop of Henle (180), overwhelming the more distal Ca reabsorptive mechanisms.

Loop Diuretics

Loop-active diuretics, such as furosemide, are potent inhibitors of Na and Cl transport in the TALH (181,182), which in turn, would dissipate the lumen-positive PD (183), the force responsible for the reabsorption of Ca in this nephron segment. The end result is a marked increase in both Na and Ca excretion. The increase in Ca excretion is relatively greater than that of Na. This has been attributed to a greater inhibitory effect of the loop diuretics on the reabsorption of Ca than of Na (184). Alternately, this may be a reflection of greater reabsorption of Na than Ca in the more distal nephron segments. The greater calciuretic effect over the natriuretic effect is further exaggerated when furosemide is given in the presence of metabolic acidosis, a factor which by itself inhibits distal Ca reabsorption (discussed earlier). The calciuretic effect of furosemide is also used clinically for the treatment of hypercalcemia (186). The question whether part or all portions of TALH transport Ca by a passive, voltage-dependent mechanism has been discussed earlier.

Acetazolamide

Although acetazolamide inhibits both Na and Ca reabsorption in the proximal tubule, in the final urine only Na excretion is increased while Ca excretion is either unchanged or reduced (186). This observation clearly suggests a preferential reabsorption of Ca in the distal nephron. Postulated mechanisms include a direct thiazide-like effect on distal Ca reabsorption or a distal inhibitory effect on Na reabsorption with consequent reduction in lumen electronegativity and parallel reduction in PD-driven Ca reabsorption. Since acetazolamide also inhibits proximal bicarbonate reabsorption, the consequent increase in distal delivery of this molecule may increase Ca reabsorption similar to that observed in metabolic alkalosis discussed above.

The Thiazides

Acute administration of thiazide diuretics is associated with a marked natriuresis and a small increase (187) or a decrease (188) in Ca excretion. Based on in vivo microperfusion studies in the rat, Costanzo and Windhager demonstrated that chlorothiazide, in addition to its known inhibitory effect on Na reabsorption, also exhibited an acute stimulatory effect on Ca reabsorption in the DCT (79). This effect on Ca reabsorption is not associated with changes in transepithelial PD (79). This hypocalciuric effect of thiazides appeared to be mediated through a PTH-independent mechanism (189).

Hypocalciuric effect of thiazides is more consistently demonstrated with chronic administration, a property which has led to their use in the management of Ca nephrolithiasis with or without hypercalciuria (190,191). This effect can be prevented or reversed with quantitative replacement of the urinary Na loss, suggesting a possible role of ECF volume contraction (192). In contrast to normal subjects, hypoparathyroid patients failed to develop hypocalciuria, despite exhibiting a similar degree of natriuresis and negative Na balance, suggesting a need for PTH in the expression of thiazide-induced hypocalciuria (192). However, thiazides have been found to reduce Ca excretion in TPTX rats (193). Because the secretion of thiazides into the tubular lumen is a prerequisite for their action, it has been postulated that the tubular secretion of thiazides may be impaired by the absence of PTH, and hence the failure to observe the anticipated hypocalciuric effect (188). While such a defect may be present in the dog (188), it has not been found in humans (189). Moreover, as mentioned earlier, the natriuretic effect of thiazides remained intact in hypoparathyroid patients.

The Potassium-Sparing Diuretics

The potassium-sparing diuretics, amiloride, triamterene, and spironolactone, cause a greater increase in Na than Ca clearance, i.e., reducing the ratio of Ca clearance to Na clearance (193). Amiloride, like the thiazides, has been shown to cause absolute reduction in Ca clearance. The mechanism, however, appeared to be different from that of the thiazides since the effect of the two diuretics is additive (194,195). In perfusion studies the effect of amiloride is mainly observed in the latter half of the DCT, while the effect of thiazides is observed in the first portion of the DCT (194). Also unlike chlorothiazide, amiloride reduced distal tubule and collecting duct negative PD (189,195) and may thus reduce Ca back flux into the lumen, and thereby increase net Ca reabsorption.

Other Factors and Conditions

Familial hypocalciuric hypercalcemia (FHH), a subgroup of Bartter's syndrome, and cisplatin nephropathy are three examples of renal tubular disorders associated with hypocalciuria (196). The inappropriately low urinary Ca excretion in FHH has been attributed to an enhanced reabsorption of Ca in the TALH. In the other two conditions, hypocalciuria may represent part of the primary tubular abnormality or, because these conditions are also associated with magnesium wasting, hypocalciura may occur secondary to hypomagnesemia (173).

Johns and Manitius reported that renal nerve activities can modulate excretion of Ca by a mechanism independent of renal hemodynamics. Whether this represents a direct neural control on Ca transport or an indirect effect, secondary to changes in Na transport, remains to be determined (197).

Immobilization (198) and weightlessness (199) increase urinary Ca excretion, while exercise reduces urinary Ca excretion (200). Cardiac glycosides increase (201) and lithium decreases (202) renal Ca excretion. Ca excretion also exhibits a diurnal variation with peak excretion around midday, at about the same time as peak Na excretion (203).

RENAL HANDLING OF PHOSPHATE

Plasma and intracellular phosphate plays an important role in many metabolic processes involving intermediary metabolisms and energy transfer mechanisms. Of the total body phosphate content (500 to 800 mg) 90% is in the skeleton and 10% is in soft tissue. The adult man is normally in phosphate balance with intake equal to output. Approximately 60% of the dietary intake is absorbed by the intestine over a wide range of phosphate intake (800 to 1500 mg/day). The kidneys account for 65% of the output, the remainder appears in the feces.

PHOSPHATE COMPOSITION IN THE PLASMA

The inorganic orthophosphate comprises approximately one-third of the total plasma phosphorus. Orthophosphates are derived from sequential dissociation of orthophosphoric acid:

$$H_3PO_4 \rightleftarrows H^+ + H_2PO_4^- \rightleftarrows H^+ + HPO_4^{2-} \rightleftarrows H^+ + PO_4^{3-}.$$

Within the physiological range of body fluid pH, the quantities of undissociated orthophosphoric acid and of the completely dissociated trivalent phosphate in the plasma are negligible. Therefore, for practical purposes the term *plasma (inorganic) phosphate* embraces two orthophosphate components, i.e., $H_2PO_4^-$ and HPO_4^{2-}.

The relative proportion of the two ionic species in the circulation may be derived as follows:

$$H_2PO_4 \rightleftharpoons H^+ + HPO_4^{2-}.$$

From the law of mass action and where K_a represents the dissociation constant, it follows that:

$$[H^+] = K_a \times [H_2PO_4^-]/[HPO_4^{2-}].$$

This can be further transformed to

$$-\log [H^+] = -\log K_a - \log [H_2PO_4^-]/[HPO_4^{2-}], \quad \text{or}$$

$$pH = pK_a + \log [HPO_4^{2-}]/[H_2PO_4^-]$$

where pKa represents $-\log Ka$. With pKa value of 6.8, the proportion of the two inorganic phosphate species in the plasma at normal pH 7.4 can be calculated as

$$7.4 = 6.8 + \log [HPO_4^{2-}]/[H_2PO_4^-], \quad \text{or,}$$

$$[HPO_4^{2-}]/[H_2PO_4^-] = 4.$$

Thus, at normal plasma pH, there are 4 of the divalent HPO_4^{2-} phosphates to every monovalent $H_2PO_4^-$. With this mixture of monovalent and divalent ionic species, the plasma phosphate has an intermediate valence of 1.8 ($2 \times 4 + 1$ negative charges per 5 molecules of plasma phosphate). The interconversion of plasma phosphate from millimole (mM) to milliequivalent (mEq) can thus be calculated as m$M \times 1.8 =$ mEq.

Plasma phosphate concentration is measured in terms of the elemental *phosphorus* contained in the *phosphate* molecules. Hence, a normal plasma phosphorus concentration of 3.1 mg/dL is equivalent to 1 mM of phosphorus (atomic weight 30.98), which is the same as 1 mM or 1.8 mEq/L of phosphate. It is to be noted, however, that this simple conversion between *phosphorus* and *phosphate* concentrations may not apply when the unit of mg/dL is used. For example, a plasma *phosphorus* concentration of 3.1 mg/dL is quite different from a plasma *phosphate* concentration of 3.1 mg/dL. The former represents 1 mM of phosphorus while the latter represents 31/96.3 or 0.32 mM of phosphorus or phosphate. The number 96.3 derived from the composite molecular weight of the two phosphate species at pH 7.4. The molecular weight of HPO_4^{2-} and $H_2PO_4^-$ are 96 and 97, respectively, and therefore the composite molecular weight, $2 \times 96/3 + 97/3 = 96.3$. In the following discussion, the abbreviation Pi will be used interchangeably for either phosphorus or phosphate.

CHARACTERISTICS OF RENAL PHOSPHATE EXCRETION

Clearance Characteristics

Under conditions of normal Pi diet and intact parathyroid glands, approximately 20% of the filtered load is excreted. The other 80% of the filtered load is reabsorbed by the renal tubules. The bulk of the current evidence indicates that Pi transport by renal tubules involves essentially a unidirectional reabsorptive process (204). Therefore, the elements of renal function regulating Pi excretion are filtration and reabsorption. Any factor that alters renal Pi excretion is therefore likely to do so by changing either the filtered load (GFR $\times$ plasma Pi), or the tubular reabsorption rate.

The ultrafilterability of Pi can be influenced by several factors such as protein-binding and calcium. Approximately 15 to 20% of the plasma Pi is bound to protein and is not filtered. This, however, is offset by effects related to the unequal distribution of plasma proteins across the glomerular filtration membrane. First, the presence of impermeant, anionic proteins on the blood side results in a Gibbs-Donnan distribution such that on the protein side there is a lesser concentration of diffusible anions such as Pi. The Gibbs-Donnan correction factor for Pi is 0.915 (205) which would raise Pi concentration in the ultrafiltrate by 9.3% (1/0.915). Secondly, the correction of volume occupied by plasma proteins (7%) would also raise the ultrafiltrate Pi concentration by 7.5% (1/0.93). These two effects, when combined (16.8%), can nullify the effect of protein-binding. Indeed, both in vivo and in vitro measurements showed that the ratio of ultrafilterable Pi to total plasma Pi is close to unity (206). Thus, the filtered load of Pi can be appropriately calculated as the product of plasma Pi and the glomerular filtration rate.

In addition to protein-binding, calcium and pH can also affect the ultrafilterability of Pi. Raising the serum calcium has been found to lower the ultrafilterable fraction of Pi, probably due to the formation of a nondiffusible calcium-Pi/protein colloid complex (207). In spite of this effect of calcium on Pi filterability, the filtered load of Pi was found to be increased during calcium infusion (208). Although not clear, this is probably due to the concomitant effect of calcium infusion to release tissue Pi and raise the plasma Pi concentration (208). The pH profile along the glomerular capillary may also affect Pi ultrafilterability through either the differential protein-binding or electrical charge of the monovalent and divalent Pi.

The classic studies by Pitts and associates demonstrated the saturability of Pi reabsorption (209). As plasma Pi concentration was increased, the amount of Pi reabsorbed also increased until the transport capacity was reached. This is demonstrated in Fig. 9. Since inulin is filtered entirely at the glomerulus and is not reabsorbed or secreted by the tubules, its excretion rate ($U_{in}V$) is equal to its filtration rate at the glomerulus. If all the filtered Pi were also excreted without reabsorption, the Pi excretion rate (U_pV) would follow the same line as for inulin. However, in measurements where plasma Pi concentration (PL_p) is progressively increased

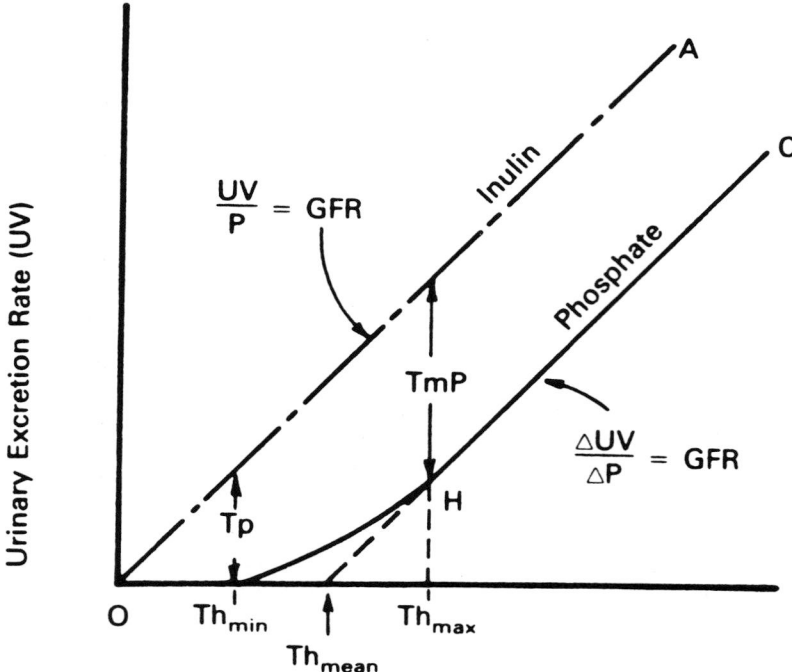

FIG. 9. Schematic relations between urinary Pi excretion rate (UV) and plasma Pi concentrations (PL). Th_{min}, minimal threshold; Th_{mean}, theoretical mean threshold, and Th_{max}, maximal threshold. See text for details. From Lee and Kurakawa (441).

by Pi infusion, U_pV (represented by the curve O-Th_{min}-H-C) is always less than the rate filtered (represented by the line O-A) by an amount indicated by the vertical line depicted as T_p or T_mP. The magnitude of this line reflects the rate of tubular Pi reabsorption. As PL_p increases from O to Th_{min} the tubular Pi reabsorption rate increases in step with the filtration rate so that no Pi is excreted. As PL_p increases further above Th_{min}, T_p continues to increase but no longer at the same rate as the increase in Pi filtration rate so that Pi begins to appear in the urine in increasing quantities. Finally, as PL_p reaches Th_{max} or above, T_p reaches a maximum rate and ceases to increase with further increase in PL_p. This maximum rate is generally known as the maximum tubular reabsorptive rate for Pi or T_mP. When PL_p is raised above Th_{max}, the slope of the U_pV curve (line HC) is identical to that for inulin (line OA), or GFR. The intersect at abscissa by downward extrapolation of line CH is called the mean Pi threshold (Th_{mean}), also known as the theoretical Pi threshold. This represents the PL_p below which most of the filtered Pi is reabsorbed and above which most of the filtered Pi is excreted. It is also evident from Fig. 9 that $Th_{mean} = T_mP/GFR$.

Thus, the renal Pi threshold is equal to the maximum tubular Pi reabsorptive rate per unit volume of GFR, and the measurement of T_mP/GFR provides a useful index for accessing renal tubular Pi reabsorptive activity. A nomogram has been constructed so that T_mP/GFR can be easily derived from the values of both fractional Pi reabsorption (TRP) and plasma Pi concentration (Fig. 10).

Nephron Sites of Phosphate Transport

The major portion of the filtered Pi is reabsorbed in the early proximal convoluted tubule. Micropuncture studies show that 60% to 70% of the filtered Pi load is reabsorbed by the time the filtrate reaches the late proximal convoluted tubule (210,211). In the first 10% to 20% of proximal tubule length, where 15% of the filtered sodium and fluid is reabsorbed, the tubular fluid to ultrafiltrate concentration ratio of Pi (TF/UF_{Pi}) has already fallen significantly from 1.0 to approximately 0.7. This indicates that in the early proximal convoluted tubule, up to 40% of the filtered Pi (or 50% of the Pi reabsorbed by the whole nephron—assuming an overall fractional Pi reabsorption of 80%) is avidly reabsorbed in excess of that for sodium and fluid. The TF/UF_{Pi} remains roughly constant in the remainder of the accessible proximal tubule, indicating that Pi reabsorption continues in the more distal portion of the proximal tubule but at a rate proportional to sodium and fluid reabsorption. The higher Pi transport rate by the early proximal convoluted tubule than by the proximal straight tubule was confirmed by the in vitro isolated perfused rabbit proximal tubules (212).

In addition to this *intranephron* heterogeneity, i.e., the differences in Pi reabsorptive rate along the length of the proximal tubule, the *internephron* heterogeneity in Pi reabsorptive rate between superficial and deep nephrons has also been suggested. Thus, the results from micropuncture studies showed a greater deep nephron Pi reabsorption under the conditions of dietary Pi deprivation

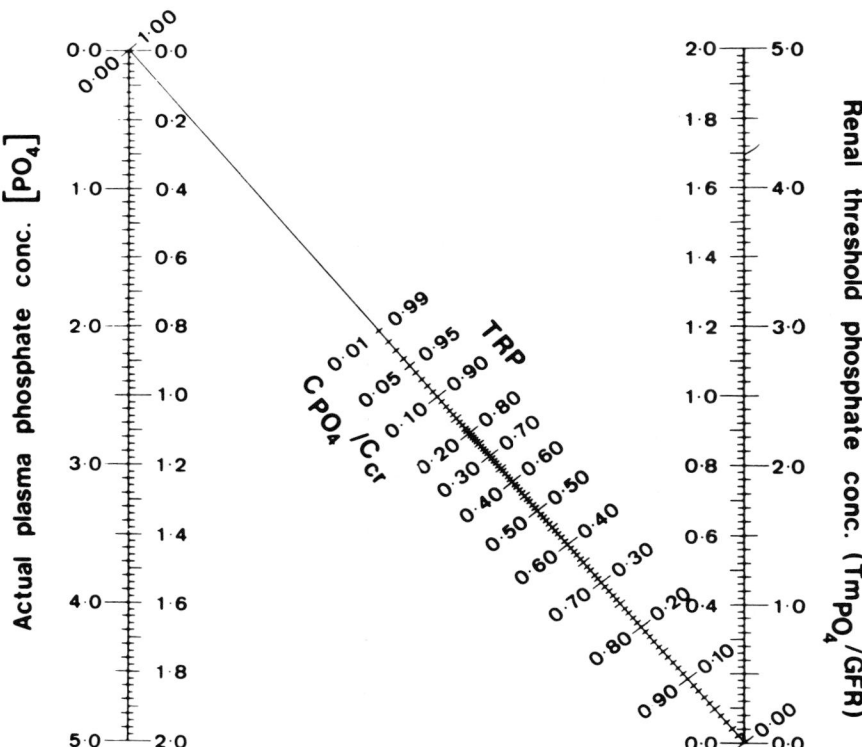

FIG. 10. Nomogram for the derivation of the renal threshold concentration for phosphate. From Bijvoet (454).

or absence of PTH, and a greater rejection of Pi reabsorption under the conditions of dietary Pi loading or PTH infusion (213,214). Results from an in vitro isolated tubule perfusion study, however, revealed no difference in net Pi reabsorption by rabbit proximal convoluted tubules from these two nephron populations (215).

There is little Pi reabsorption between the late accessible proximal tubule and the early distal tubule in animals with intact parathyroid glands (210,211,216,217). However, in the absence of PTH, Pi is reabsorbed between the late proximal tubule and early distal tubule, reflecting Pi reabsorption in the pars recta (216,217). Pi is not reabsorbed in other segments of the loop of Henle. Both in vivo and in vitro microperfusion studies failed to detect reabsorption in the thin descending, thin ascending, and thick ascending limbs of the loop of Henle (218,219).

The existence and significance of distal Pi reabsorption have been debated considerably in recent years. Direct micropuncture evidence suggests that up to 10% of the filtered Pi is reabsorbed by the distal convoluted tubule in the absence of PTH (220). The existence of Pi transport beyond the distal convoluted tubule was suggested by micropuncture studies that showed a higher fraction of the filtered Pi remaining in the late distal tubule than that appearing in the urine (217,220,221). This can be explained either by greater reabsorption in the deep inaccessible nephrons or by reabsorption in the collecting-duct segments. In the isolated perfused rabbit

collecting tubules, a significant Pi absorption rate up to 2–3% of the filtered load has been described by some, but not all, investigators (222,223). Similar controversy also exists concerning Pi transport along the medullary and papillary segments of the collecting duct. A small amount of Pi absorption has been demonstrated by in vivo microcatheterization (224), but not by micropuncture techniques (217). Pi absorption was demonstrated by microcatheterization only in the absence of PTH when the distal delivery of Pi is normally low. In contrast, no discernible Pi reabsorption was observed in control animals with intact parathyroid glands when distal delivery of Pi was relatively higher. Thus, the discrepancy between these studies may be due to differences in species and methodology.

In summary, the proximal convoluted tubule and pars recta are the major sites of Pi reabsorption. In addition, a growing body of evidence also indicates Pi reabsorption along the distal and terminal part of the nephron. However, the relative significance of Pi reabsorption by the distal segments and the role of internephron heterogeneity under various physiological and pathophysiological situations, still remains to be clarified.

Cellular Mechanisms of Phosphate Transport

The cellular events involved in Pi movement from the luminal fluid to the peritubular capillary blood have received more attention in recent years. These studies have focused on the proximal tubules where the principal portion of the filtered Pi is reabsorbed. In the renal proximal tubule, Pi reabsorption occurs principally through a unidirectional process which proceeds transcellularly with minimal intercellular backflux from the plasma to the lumen (Fig. 11). As discussed previously, the Pi concentration in the luminal fluid when it enters the proximal tubule is similar to that in the plasma, i.e., 2.0–2.5 mM, and is normally lowered to 1.0–1.5 mM when it leaves the proximal tubule. In contrast, the cytosolic Pi content in the proximal tubular cells is less well defined. The Pi content in freeze-clamped kidney tissue is approximately 5 mM/kg tissue water (225,226). Measurements of ^{31}P-NMR in isolated perfused kidney revealed that about 27% of the total cellular Pi is free in solution (227). Therefore, the concentration of cytosolic free Pi in the proximal tubular cells can be estimated to be approximately 1 mM. Since there exists a 60–65 mV potential difference (intracellularly negative) across the proximal tubular cell membrane, the free cellular Pi concentration at equilibrium is expected to be 10 times lower than that in the extracellular fluid. The estimated free Pi concentration in the proximal tubular cells thus seems to be higher than the predicted equilibrium value. This would imply that Pi enters the cell from the lumen against its electrochemical gradient by an energy-requiring mechanism, and leaves the cell on the contraluminal membrane down the electrochemical gradient. Thus, Pi absorption by proximal tubular cells is not determined passively by thermodynamic driving forces but rather by the specific transport systems located on the brush border and the basolateral membranes (Fig. 11).

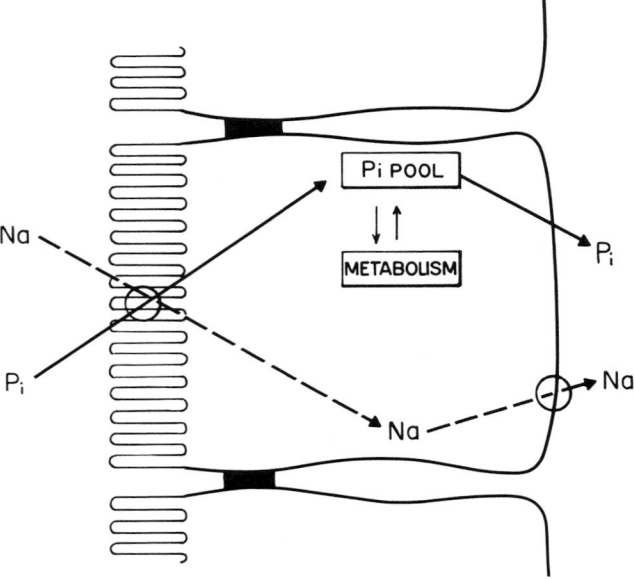

FIG. 11. Schematics of transcellular Pi transport across the proximal tubule cell. See text for details.

Brush Border Membrane

Sodium-Phosphate Cotransporter

The lipid bilayer structure of the brush border membrane consists of a hydrophobic inner core of hydrocarbons. This forms a barrier for hydrophilic molecules such as Pi to traverse the membrane and provides a framework for protein anchoring. Thus, Pi can cross the membrane more rapidly via a specific transport system associated with one or more membrane proteins. Current evidence indicates that most of the proteins involved in transmembrane transport processes are "intrinsic" membrane proteins which span the lipid bilayer in a fixed and asymmetric orientation. The process of movement of Pi is thought to involve subtle conformational changes in the transport protein assembly. Thus, Pi may have access to a polar pocket in a protein that traverses the membrane and releases Pi on the other side. Alternatively, the tertiary structure of the protein may form a channel which spans the membrane and opens upon Pi binding to a site exterior to the bilayer.

Until recently, attempts to identify the brush border membrane Pi transporter have been reported with limited success. Alkaline phosphatase, a known brush border membrane enzyme, was once proposed to be involved in Pi transport across the brush border membrane. This proposal was based essentially on the observations of parallel changes of alkaline phosphatase and Pi transport activity under various experimental conditions (228–231). However, further in vitro studies demonstrated that inhibition of alkaline phosphatase by treatments with levamisole or proteases did not affect the brush border membrane Pi transport and rendered the role of alkaline phosphatase highly unlikely (232–235). Covalent labeling of brush border membrane Pi transport proteins by reagents reacting with different amino acids has also been attempted. For example, brush border membrane Pi transport has been shown to be inhibited by reagents which react with carboxyl (carbodiimides), tyrosine (fluorodinitrobenzene), arginine (phenylglyoxal), and lysine (pyridoxal phosphate) residues, indicating the functional importance of these residues (236–239). A Pi-binding proteolipid, "phosphorin," has also been extracted and purified from the brush border membranes (240,241). While some common properties of Pi binding to this proteolipid and of Pi transport in brush border membrane suggest its involvement in Pi transport, it lacks other important features of the Pi transporter such as sodium-dependency of Pi binding. Recently, by using molecular biology techniques, a single clone mRNA isolated from rabbit renal cortex was found to express Pi transport activity similar to that of brush border membrane when injected into *Xenopus laevis* oocytes (242). It is clear that the success in the isolation of this Pi transporter will provide a useful tool for future studies in this field.

Brush border membrane Pi transport is sodium-dependent. Numerous studies have demonstrated that Pi transport by the brush border membrane is active and secondary to sodium transport. Figure 12 shows a typical experiment demonstrating Na$^+$-Pi cotransport by the isolated brush border membrane vesicles. In the presence of an inward Na$^+$ gradient, Pi is rapidly accumulated in the vesicles to concentrations that transiently exceed the equilibrium values and released back to the medium when the sodium gradient is dissipated. The sodium-dependency has also been found for the transport systems for other solutes such as glucose and amino acids. In proximal tubular cells, the energy required to maintain the favorable electrochemical gradient for sodium is generated by Na,K-ATPase at the basolateral membrane. It thus appears that the sodium gradient across the brush border membrane that favors sodium transport provides a common force for these transport activities. However, the exact mechanism coupling sodium to Pi transport remains unknown. It is possible that the structure of Pi transporter is such that binding of sodium to an adjacent site enhances the binding of Pi to the transporter. At pH 7.4, the Na$^+$-Pi cotransport in brush border membrane is not sensitive to membrane potential. However, at more acid extravesicular pH values, an electrogenic component of Pi transport becomes apparent, which transfers positive charges from luminal to cytoplasmic membrane surface (243). These findings may thus suggest an electroneutral cotransport of two Na$^+$ ions and one divalent Pi ion at physiological pH and an electrogenic cotransport of two Na$^+$ ions and one monovalent Pi ion at acid pH.

It is not known if the electroneutral and the electrogenic components of Na$^+$-Pi cotransport are mediated by one transporter molecule or by two different transporter molecules. The observation of different kinetic characteristics of Pi uptake by brush border membrane vesicles derived from either the same region or different regions of the kidney indicates the existence of heterogeneity in the Na$^+$-Pi cotransport system. The Na$^+$-Pi cotransport in brush border membranes isolated from superficial kidney cortex was found to be resolved into two kinetic components having similar V_{max} but significantly different K_m for Pi (244). In contrast, in vesicles isolated from deep kidney cortex, only one system with high Pi affinity was found. The Pi transport system in vesicles isolated from deep cortex was also found to be more susceptible to the regulation by Pi content in the diet (244).

Regulation of Na$^+$-Pi Cotransporter

Allosteric Regulation by Na$^+$ and H$^+$. In general, the rate of Pi reabsorption in the proximal tubule increases with increasing pH of the tubular fluid (245). With isolated brush border membrane vesicles, the rate of Pi uptake also increases when the extravesicular (or luminal) pH increases (246,247). Since pH changes alter the composition of Pi between the monovalent form, H$_2$PO$_4^-$, and divalent form, HPO$_4^{2-}$, the apparent inhibitory effect of luminal H$^+$ on Pi transport was initially interpreted as to indicate that the divalent form is the preferred species for renal brush border membrane Pi transporter (246–250). However, further studies showed that the effect of pH was sodium dependent; i.e., the effect of pH was greatest at low sodium concentrations. At high sodium concentrations, the pH effect was diminished (251). Kinetic analysis revealed that pH affects the affinity of the brush border membrane Pi transport system for sodium but not for Pi. The K_m for sodium was 70 mM at pH 7.4 and 190 mM at pH 6.4, while the K_m for Pi was the same at both high and low pH. Irrespective of pH value, the affinity of the transporter for Pi was strongly increased by sodium while the affinity for sodium was not affected by Pi. The Hill coefficient for so-

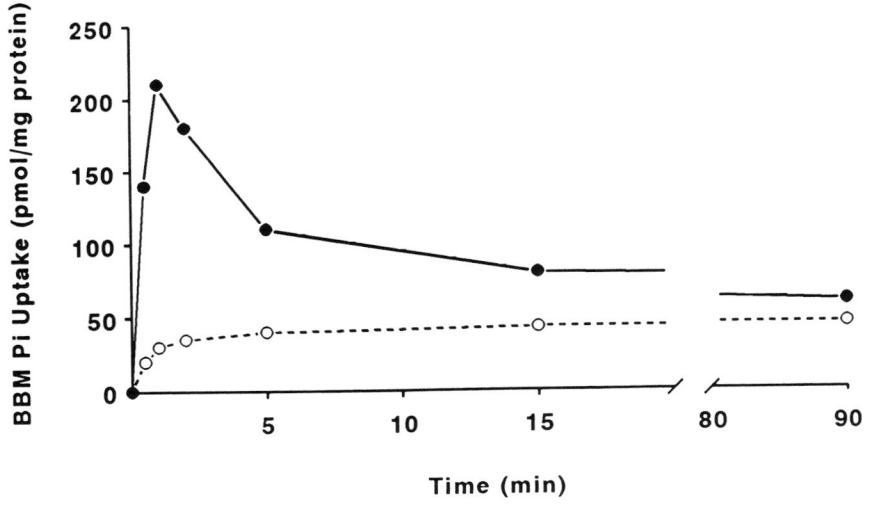

FIG. 12. Uptake of Pi by renal brush border membrane vesicles in the presence of inward-directed Na$^+$ gradient (●——●), or in the absence of Na$^+$ (○--○). See text for details.

dium interaction was 2 and for Pi interaction was 1 under different pHs, suggesting that the two sodium to one Pi stoichiometry of Na$^+$-Pi cotransport was not changed by pH. Collectively, these results indicate that sodium and H$^+$ are powerful allosteric modulators of brush border membrane Pi transport that interact with the transporter at sites different from the Pi-binding site and, by mutual interaction, control the affinity for Pi. Since the estimated K$_m$ for Pi in the proximal tubule in vivo (0.7–1.7 mM) is close to the physiological Pi concentration in the proximal tubule luminal fluid, it is conceivable that changes in luminal fluid pH can effectively modulate the Pi reabsorption rate.

The interactions of sodium and proton with the cytosolic side of the Pi transporter are less well characterized. In isolated brush border membrane vesicles, Pi transport is stimulated when the pH of the intravesicular space (or cytosolic side of the membrane) is lowered (247,251). These results may suggest that H$^+$ has similar effects on the internal and external membrane surface; i.e., a decrease of intravesicular pH would reduce the affinity for Na$^+$ and facilitate the discharge of Na$^+$, followed by the discharge of Pi at the cytosolic side of the membrane, and accelerates the transport cycle (251). Alternatively, these results may provide evidence for a preferential transport of divalent Pi, because at low intravesicular pH, Pi may be trapped inside the vesicles as H$_2$PO$_4^-$ and facilitate the uptake of HPO$_4^{2-}$ (247).

Regardless of the underlying mechanism, these results suggest that H$^+$ acts on both sides of the brush border membrane and influences Pi transport. Fluctuations of cytosolic pH may be expected to have more pronounced effects on Pi transport than changes of luminal pH, because the sensitivity of Pi transporter to pH is higher at the low Na$^+$ concentrations that prevail inside the cell. However, in contrast to the direct effect of luminal pH, the effect of intracellular pH on Pi transport across proximal tubular cell is probably more complex, because in addition to its direct interaction with Pi transporter from the cytosolic side of the brush border membrane, intracellular pH may interact with Pi transport through changes in other parameters such as cellular metabolism and membrane composition. Indeed, as will be discussed later, conflicting evidence has been reported regarding the effect of intracellular pH on Pi transport (252,253).

Covalent Modification by Phosphorylation, ADP-Ribosylation, and Thiol Redox. Studies on the inhibition of proximal tubule Pi transport by PTH and cAMP led to the proposition that cAMP-dependent protein phosphorylation may correlate with a decreased Na$^+$-Pi cotransport in brush border membrane. PTH-sensitive adenylate cyclse is present on basolateral membrane of the proximal tubule (254,255), and cAMP-dependent protein kinase exists in both the cytosol and the brush border membrane (256,257). The Na$^+$-Pi cotransport was decreased in brush border membranes isolated from

kidneys of animals treated with PTH (244,258,259), and the cAMP-dependent phosphorylation of several protein bands was demonstrated in brush border membrane vesicles in vitro (260–264). Based on these observations, experiments were performed to demonstrate a correlation between cAMP-dependent phosphorylation and decreased Na$^+$-Pi cotransport in brush border membrane vesicles in vitro. In some studies, a modest inhibition (up to 15%) of the Na$^+$-dependent Pi uptake was observed when brush border membranes were phosphorylated by cAMP in the presence of ATP (263,265). However, in other studies, when the kinetics of Na$^+$-Pi cotransport were measured, no effect of cAMP on either K$_m$ or V_{max} of the Na$^+$-Pi cotransport system could be demonstrated (260,264). The interpretation of these results is complicated by the methodological difficulties involved in the measurements of the effects of nucleotides on Pi transport in the isolated brush border membrane vesicles where the added nucleotides are rapidly hydrolyzed by alkaline phosphatase, 5′-nucleotidase and nucleotide pyrophosphatase (266–270). The hydrolysis of nucleotides results not only in the rapid depletion of the added nucleotides but also in isotope dilution during the subsequent ^{32}Pi-uptake measurements. The other difficulty involves the need to open the sealed vesicles to let the added nucleotides into the intravesicular space since their effects are relevant only when they locate at the cytosolic side of the membrane. On one hand, this maneuver may adversely affect the regulatory systems of the Na$^+$-Pi cotransport system. On the other hand, it is possible that protein phosphorylation may occur in leaky vesicles while the ^{32}Pi uptake is measured in sealed vesicles. Furthermore, it is not certain if the phosphorylated proteins represent the intrinsic membrane proteins or other nonmembrane cytoskeletal elements which are contained in the vesicles. With these pitfalls and the inconsistent results reported so far, the involvement of protein phosphorylation in the regulation of Na$^+$-Pi cotransport remains to be verified.

Another covalent modification proposed to be involved in the regulation of the Na$^+$-Pi cotransport system is the ADP-ribosylation related to the NAD-hypothesis (228,265,269–274). According to this concept, brush border membrane proteins are ADP-ribosylated by intracellular NAD catalyzed by membrane-bound ADP ribosyltransferase, which results in an inhibition of Na$^+$-Pi cotransport (265,271,273). This hypothesis arose from the observed inverse correlation between gluconeogenesis and Pi transport in renal proximal tubules. Stimulation of renal gluconeogenesis was associated with reduced Pi reabsorption under various conditions, such as administration of PTH or glucocorticoid, starvation, and chronic metabolic acidosis (228,272). Since gluconeogenesis occurs in the direction of utilizing the reducing equivalents of NADH in the cytosol, stimulation of gluconeogenesis is expected to be associated with an increased NAD/NADH ratio, or an increased free NAD in the cytosol of the proximal tubular cells (228,272,275). In an in vitro study, brush border membrane ^{32}Pi uptake was inhibited when NAD was added to the suspension of the brush border membrane vesicles (262). The ^{32}P from ^{32}P-NAD was further demonstrated to be incorporated into brush border membrane proteins, suggesting that ADP-ribosylation occurs in association with a decrease of brush border membrane Pi uptake (265,273). The inhibition of Pi uptake by ADP ribosylation was also suggested to be involved in the effect of cholera toxin (276). However, the methodological pitfalls that complicated the studies of protein phosphorylation also apply to these studies with NAD; i.e., NAD was rapidly hydrolyzed by the brush border membrane vesicles in vitro. The subsequent release of Pi from NAD could result in isotope dilution of ^{32}Pi during the uptake measurements. Indeed, ^{32}Pi uptake was not inhibited by NAD when hydrolysis of the nucleotide had been prevented (268). When NAD was introduced into the intravesicular space and removed from the extravesicular space, no inhibition of Pi uptake was observed (277). Moreover, in isolated perfused kidney (278) and in isolated perfused proximal tubules (279,280) the oxidation and reduction of intracellular NAD with pyruvate and lactate resulted in no appreciable changes in Pi reabsorption. In isolated perfused proximal tubules (279), it was also demonstrated that gluconeogenesis activity can be dissociated from Pi transport, therefore negating a direct cause-effective correlation between gluconeogenesis and Pi transport in proximal tubules.

Results from these studies thus make the proposed scheme that proximal tubule gluconeogenesis activity directly regulates brush border membrane Pi transport through changes in cellular NAD content highly unlikely. The widely observed inverse correlation between brush border membrane Pi transport and cellular gluconeogenesis and NAD content thus remains unexplained. As an alternate mechanism, it is of interest to note that recent studies showed that modification of brush border membrane thiol redox by reducing or oxidizing thiol reagents caused a respective increase or decrease in Na$^+$-dependent Pi uptake (281). Since the cellular NAD content is intimately linked to that of NADP and oxidized glutathione (GSSG), which in turn governs the thiol redox of various cellular proteins, it is possible that changes in cellular NAD content may indirectly alter the brush border membrane thiol redox and affect its Pi uptake. In support of this possibility, it was further found that preincubation of proximal tubules with nicotinamide, an agent which raises cellular NAD content, caused an oxidation of the thiol redox as well as an inhibition of Na$^+$-dependent Pi uptake in the subsequently isolated brush border membrane vesicles (281).

In summary, although cAMP-dependent protein phosphorylation, NAD-dependent ADP ribosylation,

and thiol redox have been demonstrated to modulate brush border membrane Pi uptake, their definitive regulatory roles remain uncertain. The mechanisms underlying the reciprocal correlation between gluconeogenesis and cellular NAD content with Pi reabsorption in renal proximal tubules remain to be elucidated.

Other Regulatory Factors. The lipid microenvironment in which the Na$^+$-Pi cotransporters are immersed may play an important role in the regulation of their transport rate (282). Fluorescence polarization and electron spin resonance experiments indicated a higher order of membrane lipid orientation in the brush border membrane compared with the basolateral membrane. Lipid analyses demonstrated that the cholesterol to phospholipid molar ratios are significantly higher in the brush border membrane than in the basolateral membrane, which may explain the higher order of lipid orientation, or the lower fluidity, of the brush border membrane (283,284). Changes in membrane lipid composition may therefore alter its fluidity state, which in turn may affect the rate of movement of the transport proteins. Indeed, changes in brush border membrane lipid composition and fluidity state have been shown to be associated with changes in its Pi transport rate under the conditions such as dietary Pi deprivation (285) or direct addition of 1,25(OH)$_2$D$_3$ to the brush border membrane (286).

The membrane recycling by endocytosis and exocytosis can be a rapid process effecting membrane protein insertion and removal. In renal proximal tubules, reabsorption of the filtered proteins occurs through endocytosis at the brush border membrane (287,288), and it has been demonstrated that exocytosis accounts for the insertion of proton pumps into the brush border membrane (289). Recent studies in an established renal cell line derived from opossum kidney (OK) cells, which retain proximal tubule transport characteristics, have demonstrated a reciprocal relationship between the changes in endocytosis and that in Na$^+$-dependent Pi uptake and suggested that membrane recycling may play a role in the regulation of Na$^+$-Pi cotransport (190). Evidence has also been provided to suggest the role of membrane-protein transport in the PTH action and the early adaptation to Pi deprivation. Exposure of OK cells to PTH was found to alter apical membrane protein content (291), and inhibition of endocytosis by exposing these cells to hyperosmolar medium was found to attenuate the inhibitory effect of PTH on Na$^+$-dependent Pi uptake (292). On the other hand, exposure of renal epithelial cells to Pi-free medium has been found to induce a rapid increase in Na$^+$-dependent Pi uptake independent of new protein synthesis (293,294). Recent studies showed that this adaptive response was abolished when intracellular protein transport was inhibited by brefeldin, suggesting the participation of membrane protein transport in the early response of Pi uptake to Pi deprivation (295).

Basolateral Membrane

Pi transport across the basolateral membrane is less well characterized. This is mainly because of the technical difficulties involved in the studies on ion transport by the isolated basolateral membrane. In contrast to the brush border membranes, which form a mostly uniform population of tightly sealed, right-side-out-oriented vesicles, the basolateral membrane preparations consist of a mixture of open sheets, inside-out and right-side-out vesicles, and only a small fraction of tightly sealed, transport-competent vesicles (296). In addition, the preparations are usually contaminated with a small but significant amount of brush border membranes. These and other methodological considerations preclude the exact interpretation of the results obtained so far in the isolated basolateral membranes. Nevertheless, the available data suggest the existence in the basolateral membranes of both Na^+-independent (250) and -dependent (297) Pi transport pathways. The Na^+-independent uptake of Pi by basolateral membrane vesicles isolated from rat kidney cortex was found to be inhibited by DIDS, suggesting the involvement of an anion-exchange mechanism (298). However, contradictory reports exist regarding whether Pi and other anions are transported through a common anion transport pathway or through separate transport pathways. In dog kidney basolateral membrane preparation, a Na^+-dependent Pi transport pathway was described (297). As compared to brush border membrane, this transport system was electrogenic and insensitive to pH changes. Kinetic parameters showed that the Na^+-dependent Pi transport system represents a high affinity, low capacity transport system whereas the Na^+-independent Pi transport system is that of low affinity, high capacity. Since the driving forces of Na^+ gradient and cell potential are always directed toward the cell interior, the Na^+-dependent Pi transport system in the basolateral membrane probably functions not for Pi exit from the cell but rather for Pi entry from the contraluminal side when the Pi entry from the lumen becomes restricted (297). On the other hand, the Na^+-independent Pi transport system probably is involved mainly for Pi exit from the cell. The kinetic characteristics found for the Na^+-independent and -dependent Pi transport systems thus seem to be appropriate for their respective functions.

Transcellular Phosphate Transport

Since intracellular Pi plays a major role in governing various aspects of cell metabolism and functions, it is expected that the net Pi transport across the proximal tubular cell will take place without large fluctuations of free Pi concentrations in the cytosol. This implies that Pi entry into the cell across the brush border membrane must be tightly coupled with its exit across the basolateral membrane (Fig. 11). The mechanisms involved in the maintenance of constant free Pi concentrations in the cytosol are not clear. Although it is likely that most of the Pi absorbed across the brush border membrane is rapidly discharged into the blood across the basolateral membrane, the small portion of the Pi which may be esterified into organic Pi compounds probably plays a critical role in the cell function. Informations on the respective importance of Pi entry from the brush border membrane versus that from the basolateral membrane can be derived from studies in isolated perfused kidneys and in isolated perfused proximal tubules (227,299,300). When isolated rat kidneys were perfused with Pi-free medium, the total tissue Pi and the cytosolic free Pi concentration, as determined by ^{31}P-NMR, decreased initially and then remained constant for hours (227). The kidney remained viable under these conditions as indicated by the normal Na^+ reabsorption and O_2 uptake. Thus it appears that the net Pi efflux from the cell was completely inhibited after Pi supply was stopped and a certain amount of Pi had been lost. In the isolated perfused rabbit proximal tubule, omission of Pi from the luminal fluid resulted in an inhibition of net fluid absorption, whereas omission of Pi from the peritubular fluid had no effect on fluid absorption rate (300). The inhibition of fluid absorption and respiration was dependent on the presence of glucose in the luminal fluid and did not occur when glucose transport was inhibited by phloridzin or when glycolysis was inhibited by 2-deoxyglucose. This suggests the occurrence of the so-called Crabtree effect, i.e., hexose-induced inhibition of respiration which occurs when intracellular Pi is incorporated into glycolytic intermediates and becomes a limiting factor for oxidative phosphorylation. Results from these studies also indicate that Pi transport across the brush border membrane is necessary for the maintenance of normal Pi concentration in the cell, and that Pi entry across the basolateral membrane cannot fully compensate for the reduced Pi transport across the brush border membrane.

REGULATION OF RENAL PHOSPHATE EXCRETION

Dietary Effects

The renal tubule has an intrinsic ability to adjust the reabsorption rate of Pi according to the need and the availability of Pi to the body. Pi reabsorption is increased under the conditions of greater Pi need, such as rapid growth, pregnancy, lactation, and dietary restriction. Conversely, in time of surfeit, such as slow growth, chronic renal failure, or dietary excess, the renal phosphate reabsorption is curtailed. Micropuncture and microperfusion studies have shown that these adaptive responses occur in, although not limited to, the proximal tubule (301–305). Once these changes were induced in vivo, they persisted in vitro. Segments of proximal tubules from rabbits fed a low Pi diet showed an enhanced Pi (but not Na$^+$ or glucose) transport rate, whereas proximal tubules from rabbits fed a high Pi diet exhibited a low Pi transport rate (301). The degree of adaptation may be greater in the deep than in the superficial nephrons (306). The adaptation to Pi deprivation is independent of PTH, and the phosphaturic response to PTH and cAMP is severely blunted in Pi-depleted animals (304,307,308). In rats fed a low Pi diet the response to PTH disappears in the early proximal tubule but is retained in the late proximal tubule (305). In fasted hamsters, the response to PTH can be restored by metabolic acidosis and by acetazolamide administration (309,310). The adaptation to the low Pi diet is fast; enhanced Pi transport can be detected after 2–4 hours of Pi deprivation (311,312). The reaction to Pi overload also occurs with similar promptness (313).

The adaptive response to dietary Pi intake can clearly be demonstrated in the brush border membrane. The Na$^+$-dependent Pi uptake across the brush border membrane is markedly increased within hours of dietary Pi restriction or conversely, decreased with short-term elevation of dietary Pi (229,231,249,273,313–315). The triggering mechanism and the intracellular response to dietary Pi restriction are not known. Characteristically, the adaptation is expressed as an increase of V_{max} of Na$^+$-Pi cotransport while K_m is not changed (244,249,312,316), which suggests that the number of Pi transport system in the membrane is increased. A similar adaptive response to Pi restriction has also been demonstrated in renal epithelial cells grown in culture (293,294,317–319). These studies showed that the Na$^+$-dependent Pi uptake by these cells was increased when they were maintained in media low in Pi. These studies also suggested that the adaptive response consisted of an immediate response involving activation of Pi transporters on the apical membrane and a second, long-term response involving new protein synthesis (293,294). It is not clear if the activation of Pi transporters on the apical membrane is due to the uncovering of latent carriers within the membrane, an exocytic insertion of transport assemblies, either from a readily available intracellular reservoir or from de novo synthesis, or a combination of all three processes. Further evidence has also been provided suggesting a role for an increase in brush border membrane fluidity resulting from alterations in its lipid composition (285). Recently, a role for insulin has been proposed in the acute response to dietary Pi restriction (320). Thus, in rats fed a low Pi diet, suppression of endogenous insulin secretion by infusion of somatostatin was found to prevent the adaptive increase in Pi reabsorption despite a lower plasma Pi. The addition of exogenous insulin to these rats restored the antiphosphaturic effect of a low Pi diet (320).

It is of interest that Pi deprivation by fasting does not result in similar Pi handling by the kidney. Pi excretion is higher in fasted rats than in rats fed either a normal or low Pi diet (221,222). Moreover, the fasted rats retain partial responsiveness to PTH, in contrast to the resistance present in rats on a low Pi diet (321). The higher excretion rate of Pi in fasting is likely to be due to effects at the proximal tubule cell, because fasting does not increase the Pi uptake into brush border membrane vesicles (322). Furthermore, when rats adapted to a low Pi diet are subsequently starved, fasting reverses the increased uptake of Pi by the brush border membrane vesicles (322). How the kidneys differentiate between selective and total dietary intake is not known.

Acid-Base Status

It has been well demonstrated that changes in acid–base balance result in changes in urinary Pi excretion. However, the precise relationships are complex and the results obtained by different experimental techniques are divergent or even contradictory. Considering the fact that systemic acid-base balance is likely to affect the pH of different compartments in and around the proximal tubule, such as luminal fluid, cytosol and peritubular fluid, and that these pH changes may have diverse effects on Pi reabsorption, the inconsistent results reported in these studies can probably be attributed to the complex interactions from these different components.

Effect of Luminal pH

In microperfusion experiments in rat proximal tubules, Bank et al. (323) found that the reabsorption of 2 mM Pi was greater at acid than at alkaline pH of the perfusion solution. In another microperfusion study in rat proximal tubule but with much higher Pi concentration (100 mM) in the perfusion solution, Cassalo and Malnick (324) also found that the rate of Pi reabsorption was enhanced at acid than at alkaline perfusion solution. Similar results were also reported in isolated perfused rabbit proximal tubules by Ham et al. (325). In these studies, the reabsorption of 10 mM Pi was found to be higher at acid than at alkaline pH in the lumen.

In contrast to these reports, other studies showed an opposite effect of luminal pH on Pi reabsorption. In microperfusion experiments in rat proximal tubules, Baumann et al. (326) found the reabsorption of 2 mM Pi was twice as high at pH 7.4 as at pH 6.8 in the lumen. In double-microperfusion experiments of rat proximal tubules and peritubular capillaries, Ullrich et al. (253) found that the reabsorption of 4 mM Pi was higher at alkaline than at acid luminal pH. In another microperfusion study in rat proximal tubules, Quamme et al. (327) also showed that Pi reabsorption was twice as high at pH 7.6 than at pH 6.5 in the lumen.

The apparent discrepancies between these results were

in part resolved by the studies reported by Lang et al. (328). These studies showed that Pi reabsorption in rat proximal tubule was stimulated by alkaline luminal pH when Pi concentration in the lumen was low, but it was inhibited by pH increase at high luminal Pi concentration. In the studies reported by Quamme et al. (327), it was also found that systemic infusion of Pi or administration of high-Pi diet diminished the dependency of Pi reabsorption on luminal pH. It thus appears that the luminal pH dependence of Pi reabsorption is under the influence of Pi availability to the proximal tubular cells. Alkaline pH in the lumen enhances Pi reabsorption only when Pi is not in excess to the proximal tubular cells. These observations are in good agreement with the properties of Na^+-Pi cotransporter described in the isolated brush border membrane. In isolated brush border membrane vesicles, alkaline pH at the outer (or luminal) solution stimulates the Na^+-dependent Pi uptake by increasing the affinity of the Na^+-Pi cotransporter for Na^+ and, consequently, for Pi. Thus, at Pi concentration in the lumen above saturation, the luminal pH will no longer have a direct effect on Pi reabsorption.

Effect of Intracellular pH

Changes in intracellular pH may play a key role in regulating proximal tubule Pi reabsorption. Unfortunately, no direct evidence exists to evaluate this possibility or its mechanism. In isolated brush border membrane vesicles, acidic pH in the intravesicular space (or cytosolic side of the membrane) enhances Pi uptake (247,251). As discussed earlier, this is considered to be due to either an increased rate of Pi dissociation from the carrier or the trapping of the monovalent Pi. The effect of intracellular pH, however, may be more complex than its direct effect on brush border membrane because changes in intracellular pH can produce profound metabolic changes, which in turn may exert additional effects on Pi reabsorption.

Ullrich et al. (253) observed that Pi reabsorption was decreased after acetazolamide infusion, and concluded that intracellular alkalosis reduces Pi reabsorption. On the contrary, by using citrate reabsorption and cellular citrate content as an intracellular pH indicator, Knox et al. (252) suggested that intracellular alkalosis enhances, while intracellular acidosis suppresses, proximal tubule Pi reabsorption. On the other hand, results from the systemic acid–base effects have frequently been used to infer the effects of intracellular pH on Pi reabsorption. Such practice, however, could also be misleading because changes in systemic bicarbonate concentration and pH do not necessarily reflect changes in intracellular pH. For example, the systemic metabolic alkalosis in potassium depleted subjects may in fact be associated with an intracellular acidosis. Reciprocally, the systemic meta-

bolic acidosis after acute lithium administration could actually accompany intracellular alkalosis. It is clear that studies which allow simultaneous measurements of intracellular pH and Pi transport are needed to clarify these issues.

Effect of Systemic Acid-Base Balance

Changes in respiratory acid-base balance have direct effects on renal Pi handling. Respiratory acidosis leads to a consistent depression in renal Pi reabsorption (329). This occurs independent of other factors such as PTH, filtered Pi load, bicarbonate reabsorption, or extracellular pH (329). Respiratory alkalosis, on the other hand, results in an increased renal Pi reabsorption (226). This again appears to be dependent on pCO_2 tension rather than extracellular alkalosis, because HCl infusion did not affect the respiratory effect. Furthermore, respiratory alkalosis blunts the phosphaturic effect of PTH and cAMP, suggesting an effect independent of PTH. These observations may suggest a yet unknown but potentially important role of intracellular pCO_2 in controlling Pi reabsorption.

Acute metabolic acidosis induced by acute acid infusion does not alter basal Pi excretion, but does attenuate the phosphaturic effect of PTH (330). In contrast, chronic metabolic acidosis causes a significant decrease in Pi reabsorption (331). Studies in isolated brush border membrane vesicles showed that chronic metabolic acidosis leads to a lower Na^+-dependent Pi uptake with a decrease in V_{max} (332). This is quite different from the direct stimulatory effect of intravesicular H^+ on brush border membrane Pi uptake. The mechanisms leading to this change in the brush border membrane are not known, but an increase in glucocorticoid hormone levels have been implicated to be involved in this down-regulation of Pi transport (333). In addition, the simultaneous increase in Na^+/H^+ exchange activity induced by metabolic acidosis and the resultant changes in luminal as well as intracellular pH could also contribute to the inhibition of Pi reabsorption. Acute metabolic alkalosis by sodium bicarbonate infusion also reduces Pi reabsorption by a mechanism independent of PTH, extracellular fluid volume expansion, or plasma calcium (334,335). This effect, however, is critically dependent on the antecedent dietary Pi intake (336,337), so that bicarbonate infusion in animals on normal dietary Pi intake leads to an enhanced Pi reabsorption, but causes a decrease in Pi reabsorption in animals on high Pi dietary intake. This is similar to the effect of luminal alkalinization as discussed earlier and suggests a possible role of luminal pH in mediating the effect of acute metabolic alkalosis. Chronic alkalosis, on the other hand, increases Pi reabsorption presumably by similar mechanisms as chronic acidosis but working in an opposite direction (338).

Hormones

PTH

It is widely recognized that PTH is the major hormonal regulator of renal Pi reabsorption. Parathyroidectomy decreases renal Pi excretion and, conversely, injection of PTH increases urinary Pi excretion (339). Administration of PTH leads to phosphaturia by reducing the maximal transport rate of Pi reabsorption, TmP/GFR.

Proximal tubules appear to be the main site where PTH exerts its action on Pi reabsorption. Micropuncture studies show that PTH decreases and parathyroidectomy increases Pi reabsorption in the proximal tubule (340–342). In addition to the proximal tubule, Pi transport in the distal tubule may be sensitive to PTH (220). In TPTX animals, the increased fractional excretion of Pi from proximal tubules was not translated into a similar increase in urinary Pi excretion, suggesting that TPTX unmasked a PTH-sensitive Pi reabsorptive mechanism distal to the last accessible proximal tubule. Studies with dissected segments along the nephron showed that PTH-sensitive adenylate cyclase exists in segments such as proximal convoluted and straight tubules, cortical ascending limbs of Henle, distal convoluted and connecting tubules, and the early branched segments of collecting ducts (343). However, the presence of PTH-sensitive adenylate cyclase does not necessarily imply the simultaneous existence of a PTH-sensitive Pi transport system. Whether or not the stimulation of adenylate cyclase in distal tubules correlates with changes in Pi transport or is primarily associated with the known changes in calcium transport is not known. In TPTX animals, the discrepancy between proximal tubule Pi excretion and urinary Pi excretion can also be explained by the heterogeneous PTH effect between nephron populations. Indeed, in TPTX rats, Pi reabsorption is greater in deep than in superficial proximal tubules (344,345). Following an acute infusion of a high dose of PTH, fractional Pi reabsorption decreased to similar levels in both superficial and deep nephrons, suggesting a possibly greater PTH effect in deep nephrons.

In renal proximal tubule, PTH inhibits Pi, bicarbonate, Na^+, and fluid reabsorption (346–349), and stimulates glucose (350–352) and ammonia production (353–355). The sequence of biochemical steps involved with PTH action begins with receptor binding and activation of adenylate cyclase on the basolateral membrane. The PTH-sensitive adenylate cyclase complex in the basolateral membrane consists of a membrane receptor, a nucleotide regulatory component (G protein), and a catalytic subunit (356,357). Guanine nucleotides interact with G protein and promote the coupling between PTH receptor and the catalytic subunit. Activation of adenylate cyclase catalyzes the conversion of adenosine triphosphate to cyclic AMP. Since many of the biological effects of peptide hormones are mediated through cAMP-dependent protein phosphorylation, it has been postulated that PTH-stimulated cAMP may lead to phosphorylation of renal brush border membranes and mediate the hormonal effect on Pi transport (262,263, 265). In support of this thesis, the Pi uptake was found to be decreased in brush border membranes isolated from kidneys of animals treated with PTH (244,258,259), and cAMP-dependent protein kinase was found to be present in the brush border membrane (256,257), which phosphorylates several protein bands in brush border membrane in vitro (260,261,263–265). Furthermore, phosphorylation of brush border membranes by cAMP in the presence of ATP was found to reduce Pi uptake, and the effect of cAMP was reversed when brush border membranes were dephosphorylated by phosphoprotein phosphatase (262,263).

In contrast to these observations, an increasing body of evidence has accumulated to indicate that cAMP-dependent protein phosphorylation alone cannot fully account for the PTH effect on Pi transport. For example, in rabbit kidneys, PTH-sensitive adenylate cyclase has been identified in both proximal convoluted and straight tubules (343). However, the in vitro perfusion of these segments showed that PTH and cAMP, although they inhibit Na^+/H^+ exchange system in both segments, affect Pi transport only in the straight, but not in the convoluted portion of the proximal tubule (352,358). In isolated brush border membrane, despite the phosphorylation of several protein bands by cAMP in the presence of ATP, no effect of cAMP on either the K_m or V_{max} of the Na^+-Pi cotransport system could be demonstrated (260,264). Resistance to phosphaturic effect of PTH and cAMP has been observed in starvation (309,310), in Pi depletion (304,307,308), in respiratory alkalosis (226), after lithium administration (359), and in type II pseudohypoparathyroidism (361). The responsiveness to PTH under these conditions can be restored by various means without affecting the PTH-cAMP axis (359,361–363).

Besides activation of adenylate cyclase, alternate pathways of PTH-stimulated signal generation in the proximal tubule has been reported. In particular, intracellular calcium-dependent mechanisms have received increasing attention. It has been well demonstrated that an increase in intracellular calcium is important in mediating the effect of PTH to stimulate proximal tubule glucose production (350–352). The involvement of intracellular calcium-dependent mechanisms in mediating the effect of PTH on proximal tubule Pi transport has also been suggested recently. Thus, in isolated perfused rabbit proximal convoluted tubule, PTH inhibits bicarbonate reabsorption but fails to stimulate glucose production or inhibit Pi reabsorption (352,358). It was found that the resistance to these PTH responses could be restored by raising the extracellular calcium concentration (358). Furthermore, addition of intracellular calcium antagonists was found to abolish these PTH actions in proximal tubules and in brush border membranes (358,364). The involvement of calcium-dependent mechanisms has been further strengthened by the discovery of a calcium, phospholipid-dependent protein kinase, protein kinase C (365). Thus, in renal proximal tubular cells, PTH activates phospholipase C and stimulates inositol 1,4,5-triphosphate (IP$_3$) and diacylglycerol production (366). The IP$_3$ thus produced releases calcium from intracellular storage and raises cytosolic calcium levels (367,368). The increase in cytosolic calcium and the formation of diacylglycerol concertedly lead to the activation of protein kinase C (365). Similar to cAMP-dependent protein kinase, protein kinase C is present in brush border membrane (369) and may inhibit Pi transport through protein phosphorylation. The possibility that activation of protein kinase C leads to inhibition of Pi transport has been examined in an established renal cell line from opposum kidneys (OK) cells. These cells contain PTH-sensitive adenylate cyclase, and both PTH and cAMP inhibit Pi uptake by these cells (291,292,370–372). However, the concentration of PTH required for adenylate cyclase activation was found to be higher than that required for Pi uptake inhibition by threefold of magnitude (373,374). On the other hand, in OK cells, it was found that PTH activates phospholipase C and increases IP$_3$ and diacylglycerol formation (366), and that activation of protein kinase C by phorbol esters inhibited Pi uptake by these cells (375,376). Recently, it was also found that, although PTH increases cAMP production in all clones of OK cells, there exist certain clonal sublines that show resistance to PTH inhibition of Pi uptake (377). By monitoring changes in intracellular calcium in response to PTH, a close correlation has been observed between the stimulation of transient elevations in cytosolic calcium and the inhibition of Pi uptake by PTH (378). These studies therefore strongly suggest that PTH regulates Pi transport in proximal tubular cells through dual mechanisms, one involves activation of adenylate cyclase and cAMP-dependent protein kinase A, the other involves activation of phospholipase C and protein kinase C.

The inhibition of proximal tubule Pi transport by PTH is associated with a decrease in the apparent maximal rate of Pi transport (V_{max}). Protein phosphorylation, through either protein kinase A or protein kinase C, can conceivably phosphorylate and modify the activity of Pi transport proteins which are already present in the brush border membrane. An alternative possibility, which is also consistent with a V_{max} change, is that PTH may influence membrane recycling. There is good evidence that active membrane recycling, including both endocytosis and exocytosis, occurs in renal proximal tubule (287–

289). The recycling of membrane transport proteins could allow for rapid up- or down-regulation of the capacity of the brush border membrane for solute transport. Indirect support for the involvement of membrane recycling in the proximal tubule response to PTH has been provided by the observations that pretreatment of rats with colchicine, a microtubule disrupting agent, blocked the normal inhibitory action of PTH on renal Pi transport (379). In OK cells, stimulation of endocytosis caused an inhibition of Pi take (290) and abrogated the inhibitory effect of PTH (292).

Vitamin D Metabolites

Considerable controversy exists concerning the effects of vitamin D metabolites on renal Pi excretion (380–382). This is probably related to the complex interaction between their direct actions on renal tubular Pi transport and indirect actions on systemic Pi balance. Short-term administration of vitamin D metabolites has been reported to exert diverse effects on the renal reabsorptive capacity for Pi. Thus, vitamin D is antiphosphaturic in hypophosphatemic states (e.g., vitamin D deficiency or Pi deprivation) or in situations where basal urinary Pi excretion is high (e.g., volume expansion or administrations of PTH or calcitonin). On the contrary, vitamin D is phosphaturic in hyperphosphatemic or Pi-repleted states. Recent studies suggest that vitamin D may increase brush border membrane Pi transport by directly altering membrane lipid composition (286,383). Unlike the controversies surrounding short-term vitamin D effects, the chronic, long-term effects are more universally accepted. Chronic administration of vitamin D enhances intestinal Pi absorption and results in a positive Pi balance (384). The proximal tubules respond appropriately to the abundance of Pi and lowers Pi reabsorption (380,385).

Growth Hormone

Growth hormone has been reported to promote Pi reabsorption by the kidney (386,387). Injection of growth hormone leads to increased renal Pi reabsorption (387,388), whereas hypophysectomy is associated with reduced rates of Pi reabsorption (389,390). Although growth hormone may suppress PTH secretion by its effect to stimulate intestinal calcium absorption (387) and 1,25(OH)$_2$D$_3$ synthesis (391), the antiphosphaturic effect of growth hormone is not mediated through the PTH-axis. Thus, growth hormone was found to enhance renal Pi reabsorption in TPTX animals, and the effect of PTH in lowering renal Pi reabsorption was not modified by growth hormone (387). Since growth hormone raises TmP/GFR, it is likely that growth hormone affects the intrinsic tubular reabsorptive capacity for Pi. Such a notion was further supported by the finding that administration of growth hormone increased Pi uptake by renal brush border membrane (392). The cellular mechanism of growth hormone action is not known, however.

Thyroid Hormone

Altered thyroid function states have diverse effects on urinary Pi excretion (393–395), this is probably related to the extensive extrarenal actions of thyroid hormone on Pi metabolism as well as its complex interactions with other hormone systems. In general, thyroid hormone increases the renal reabsorption of Pi, independent of the actions of PTH (396). Available evidence indicates a direct tubule effect of thyroid hormone. Thus, in primary cultured renal cells, addition of triiodothyronine or thyroxine was found to stimulate Pi uptake (397). On the other hand, pretreatment of thyroid hormone also enhances Pi uptake by the renal brush border membrane (398–400). The increase in cellular and brush border membrane Pi uptake in response to thyroid hormone is sensitive to RNA and protein synthesis inhibitors, suggesting an involvement of protein synthesis in its effect (397).

Glucocorticoid

Glucocorticoids are strongly phosphaturic, even in animals stabilized on a low-Pi diet that normally do not excrete Pi in the urine (274,401). The Pi uptake is reduced in brush border membrane isolated from glucocorticoid-treated animals (274,402). On the other hand, the simultaneous increase in brush border membrane Na^+/H^+ exchange and the resultant luminal acidification could also contribute to the phosphaturic effect of glucocorticoids (402). Glucocorticoids have also been implicated in mediating the phosphaturic effect of metabolic acidosis (333).

Insulin

Insulin decreases plasma Pi concentration because of shifts from the extracellular space into intracellular space (403). Despite this profound extrarenal effect, insulin exerts only a modest antiphosphaturic effect (403). Pretreatment of proximal tubules with insulin leads to an increase in Pi uptake by the subsequently isolated brush border membrane vesicles (404,405), providing evidence of a direct tubular effect. This has been substantiated further by the observation that insulin stimulates Pi transport in OK cells (407). As discussed earlier, insulin may play an important role in mediating the antiphosphaturic effect of Pi deprivation (320).

Calcitonin

Calcitonin is a strongly hypophosphatemic agent (406). When hypophosphatemia is prevented by Pi infusion, administration of calcitonin results in a reduction of renal Pi transport capacity (408). The phosphaturic effect of calcitonin is independent of the concomitant hypocalcemia and PTH secretion (403). Although it is likely that calcitonin causes phosphaturia through its effect on tubule Pi reabsorption, the nephron site and the cellular mechanisms involved remain uncertain. Calcitonin receptor and calcitonin-dependent adenylate cyclase have been localized in medullary and cortical portions of the thick ascending limb of the loop of Henle and the bright portion of the distal convoluted tubule (343). However, it is not clear if the increase in renal cAMP production mediates the effect of calcitonin (403). A recent report that calcitonin treatment causes a reduction in Pi uptake by isolated brush border membrane vesicles would indicate proximal tubule as one of the nephron segments where calcitonin may modulate Pi transport (409).

Atrial Natriuretic Factor (ANF)

In addition to its natriuretic effect, ANF infusion increases urinary excretion of many other solutes including Pi (410,411). The phosphaturic effect of ANF occurs through its inhibition of Pi transport in proximal tubule brush border membranes (412,413). The cellular mechanisms through which ANF causes inhibition of brush border membrane Pi transport are not clear, but recent studies suggest a potential role of ANF in the higher fractional excretion of Pi in rats with reduced renal mass (414).

Catecholamines

Epinephrine decreases plasma Pi, presumably by shifting Pi to the intracellular space (403). The hypophosphatemic response was also observed after isoproterenol (415) and was blocked by propranolol (416), suggesting the involvement of a beta-adrenergic receptor mechanism. Epinephrine, norepinephrine, and isoproterenol are all hypophosphaturic (417). Although the decrease in Pi excretion occurs in the absence of changes in renal hemodynamics, it is difficult to separate these effects from changes in the filtered load of Pi due to the concomitant hypophosphatemia. On the other hand, dopamine increases Pi excretion without changing plasma Pi concentration (418). The role of the renal nerves in Pi handling has also been examined (419). Renal denervation results in a phosphaturia. This effect is believed to be part of a general effect of denervation on proximal transport processes and thus a consequence of decreased sodium reabsorption.

Miscellaneous Factors Influencing Phosphate Excretion

Extracellular Fluid Volume

Expansion of the extracellular fluid volume causes phosphaturia (420–423). Conversely, contraction of the extracellular fluid volume decreases the excretion of Pi. Since acute reduction in GFR does not abort the increase in Pi excretion, it was concluded that volume expansion inhibits tubular Pi reabsorption independent of the filtered load. In whole animal studies, the effect of volume expansion on Pi excretion occurs both in the presence and absence of parathyroid glands, although the magnitude of phosphaturia is greater in intact than in TPTX animals (424–427). This suggests that the full expression of volume expansion-induced phosphaturia requires not only the presence of a natriuresis but also the presence of intact parathyroid glands. Micropuncture studies indicate that volume expansion leads to a decrease in proximal reabsorption of both Na^+ and Pi (340,342,424,426,428–430). However, the magnitude of inhibition is not significantly influenced by the removal of parathyroid glands. Thus, the mitigated phosphaturic effect of volume expansion in TPTX animals relates to enhanced reabsorption of Pi beyond the accessible proximal tubule. Pi reabsorption in the distal convoluted tubule has been shown not to be directly altered by volume expansion (431). Therefore, the increased load of Pi out of the proximal convoluted tubule induced by volume expansion appears to be largely reabsorbed in the proximal straight tubule.

Diuretics

Many diuretics increase urinary Pi excretion. Of all the diuretics, the greatest phosphaturia is produced by the carbonic anhydrase inhibitor, acetazolamide (432–434). Administration of acetazolamide markedly increases the fractional excretion of Pi in relation to that for Na^+. The effect of acetazolamide does not appear to be mediated by PTH, because it also induces phosphaturia in TPTX animals (435). However, because acetazolamide and PTH have similar effects on Pi, bicarbonate, and Na^+ excretion, a number of studies have examined the effect of acetazolamide on the adenylate cyclase system in the kidney. Indeed, both in vivo and in vitro studies demonstrate that acetazolamide increases renal cAMP production (436). The observation that inhibition of adenylate cyclase by lithium blocked the phosphaturic effect of acetazolamide provides indirect evidence for a role of the adenylate cyclase system in the phosphaturic effect of acetazolamide (437). Acetazolamide administration led to natriuresis and bicarbonaturia in both normal and lithium-treated animals. On the other hand, phosphaturia was only observed in the normal, but not in the lithium-treated animals (437). These data suggest that acetazolamide causes natriuresis and bicarbonaturia through inhibition of carbonic anhydrase and causes phosphaturia through activation of adenylate cyclase. On the other hand, the infusion of acetazolamide in patients with hypoparathyroidism or pseudohypoparathyroidism has been shown to result in augmented excretion of Pi without an increase in urinary cAMP (438).

Whether or not inhibition of carbonic anhydrase contributes to the phosphaturic effect of acetazolamide is not clear. However, what appears to be clear is the requirement of the presence of bicarbonate for the phosphaturic effect of acetazolamide. In studies of the isolated perfused kidney, the presence or absence of bicarbonate in the perfusion medium did not alter the basal fractional excretion of Pi. The fractional excretion of Pi remained unaltered when acetazolamide was added in the absence of bicarbonate, but increased following acetazolamide in the presence of bicarbonate (439). Inhibition of carbonic anhydrase by acetazolamide may cause an alkalinization of the luminal fluid, which in turn may also contribute to inhibit proximal tubule Pi reabsorption.

Thiazides also cause significant phosphaturia with fractional excretion of Pi approaching that attained with acetazolamide (435). Although the major site of action of thiazides is in segments beyond the proximal tubule, these diuretics also inhibit carbonic anhydrase and suppress proximal tubule Na^+ and bicarbonate reabsorption. As in the case of acetazolamide, it is uncertain whether the phosphaturic effect of thiazide is a direct result of carbonic anhydrase inhibition or is mediated through separate mechanisms.

Furosemide and ethacrynic acid both have their major action in the ascending limb of loop of Henle. However, these diuretics also exhibit detectable inhibition on carbonic anhydrase activity and reduce proximal tubule bicarbonate reabsorption (434,440). The modest carbonic anhydrase inhibitory activity of furosemide has been proposed as a possible mechanism for its phosphaturic action. In this context, it is interesting to note that the relative potency of these diuretics on carbonic anhydrase inhibition correlates with their potency to inhibit Pi reabsorption (441). Moreover, the phosphaturic effect of furosemide is not additive to that of acetazolamide (442). Furosemide, however, differs from acetazolamide in that it has no effect on urinary cAMP excretion or the adenylate cyclase activity (436). A further difference from acetazolamide is the observation that in acute parathyroidectomized (PTX) dogs, furosemide did not increase Pi excretion except when given during the constant infusion of PTH (442). On the other hand, the dependency of furosemide on PTH in mediating its phosphaturic action has been challenged by the observation that this agent inhibits Pi reabsorption in isolated perfused kidney, obviously in the total absence of PTH (443).

A phosphaturic effect of mannitol was reported that was dependent on the presence of PTH (444). The phosphaturia was believed to be the result of dilutional hypocalcemia stimulating PTH secretion.

Calcium

The circulating calcium concentration may modify renal Pi reabsorption through a number of different mechanisms, including its effect on PTH secretion, plasma Pi concentration, renal hemodynamics, and a possible direct effect on renal tubular Pi reabsorption. Infusion of calcium in normal subjects results in an increase in both renal Pi reabsorption and plasma Pi concentration. Since the absolute urinary Pi excretion was also increased during infusion, the possibility of net Pi mobilization from bone and soft tissue was suggested (445,446). The change in renal Pi reabsorption has been attributed to secondary inhibition of PTH secretion since the antiphosphaturic effect was reversed when exogenous PTH was given simultaneously (445). Moreover, in some hypoparathyroid patients, calcium infusion did not reduce renal Pi excretion (445–447). On the other hand, the existence of a PTH-independent, Pi reabsorptive mechanism that is sensitive to calcium infusion has also been suggested. In micropuncture studies, elevating calcium concentration from the basal hypocalcemic level was found to increase Pi reabsorption by the proximal tubule, loop of Henle, and the distal nephron of PTX rats (448). In isolated perfused rabbit proximal convoluted tubules, elevating the calcium concentration in both the perfusate and the bathing medium from 1.8 mM to 3.6 mM was found to lead to an increase in Pi reabsorption, and lowering ambient calcium to 0.2 mM exerted the opposite effect (449). This calcium-associated action on Pi reabsorption was not observed in the proximal straight tubule.

Induction of hypocalcemia by calcium-chelator infusion leads to an increase in Pi excretion through both PTH-dependent and independent mechanisms (450). Thus, in one study, EDTA infusion failed to cause a phosphaturia when PTH level was held constant by infusion of exogenous hormone in TPTX dogs (451). In other studies, EGTA infusion in TPTX rats caused a clear phosphaturic effect (452). However, in contrast to these studies, recent studies with cultured renal epithelial cells, lowering the extracellular calcium from 2 mM to 0.02 mM was actually found to increase the cellular Pi uptake (453).

ACKNOWLEDGMENTS

The study was supported by grants from NIH, Veterans Administration, National and Southern California Kidney Foundation, and American Heart Association of Greater Los Angeles.

REFERENCES

1. Lustig S, Chan DWS, Lee DBN. Intestinal absorption of calcium. In: Massry SG, Glassock RJ, eds. *Textbook of nephrology,* 2nd ed. Baltimore: Williams & Wilkins, 1989;284–92.
2. Moore EW. Ionized calcium in normal serum, ultrafiltrates and whole blood determined by ion-exchange electrodes. *J Clin Invest* 1970;49:318–34.
3. Agus ZS, Goldfarb S. Renal regulation of calcium balance. In: Seldin DW, Giebisch G, eds. *The kidney: physiology and pathophysiology,* New York: Raven Press, 1985;1323–35.
3a. Wright E, Schulman G. Principles of epithelial transport. In: Maxwell MH, Kleeman CR, Narins RG, eds. *Clinical disorders of fluid and electrolyte metabolism,* 4th ed. New York: McGraw-Hill, 1987;15–31.
4. Bomsztyk K, Wright FS. Contribution of diffusion to transport of calcium by renal proximal tubule. *Clin Res* 1982;30:443A.
4a. Burg MB. Thick ascending limb of Henle's loop. *Kidney Int* 1982;22:454–64.
5. Ussing HH. The distinction by means of tracers between active transport and diffusion. The transfer of iodide across isolated frog skin. *Acta Physiol Scand* 1949;19:43–56.
6. Hodgkin AL, Keynes RD. The potassium permeability of a giant nerve fibre. *J Physiol* 1955;128:61–88.
7. Gmaj P, Murer H, Kinne R. Calcium ion transport across plasma membranes isolated from rat kidney cortex. *Biochem J* 1979;178:549–57.
8. Somermeyer MG, Knauss TC, Weinberg JM, Humes HD. Characterization of Ca^{2+} transport in rat renal brush-border membrane and its modulation by phosphatidic acid. *Biochem J* 1983;214:37–46.
9. Saunders JCJ, Isaacson LC. Non-selective cation and Ca permeable apical channels in rabbit renal tubules. *Int Congr Physiol Sci Helsinki,* 1989.
9a. Bacskai BJ, Friedman PA. Activation of latent Ca^{2+} channels in renal epithelial cells by parathyroid hormone. *Nature* 1990;347:388–91.
10. Somermeyer MG, Knauss TC, Weinberg JM, Humes HD. *Biochem J* 1983;214:37–46.
11. Khalifa S, Mills S, Hruska KA. Stimulation of calcium uptake by parathyroid hormone in renal brush-border membrane vesicles. *J Biol Chem* 1983;258:14400–6.
12. Tsutsumi M, Alvarez U, Avioli LV, Hruska KA. Effect of 1,25-dihydroxyvitamin D_3 in phospholipid composition of rat renal brush border membrane. *Am J Physiol* 1985;249:F117–23.
13. Talor Z, Richison G, Arruda JAL. High-affinity calcium binding sites in luminal and basolateral renal membranes. *Am J Physiol* 1985;246:F472–81.
14. Thevenod F, Streb H, Ullrich KJ, Schulz I. Inositol 1,4,5-triphosphate release Ca^{2+} from non-mitochondrial store in permeabilized rat cortical kidney cells. *Kidney Int* 1986;29:695–702.
15. Parys JB, De Smedt H, Borghgraef R. Calcium transport system in the LLC-PK$_1$ renal epithelial established cell line. *Biochim Biophys Acta* 1986;888:70–81.
16. Cheung JY, Constantine JM, Bonventre JV. Regulation of cytosolic free calcium concentration in cultured renal epithelial cells. *Am J Physiol* 1986;251:F690–701.
17. Moore L, Fitzpatrick DF, Chan TS, Landon EJ. Calcium pump activity of the renal plasma membrane and renal microsomes. *Biochim Biophys Acta* 1974;345:405–18.
18. Parys JB, De Smedt H, Vandenberghe P, Borghgraef R. *Cell Calcium* 1985;6:413–29.
19. Henry HL, Norman AK. Vitamin D: metabolism and biological actions. *Annu Rev Nutr* 1984;4:493–520.
20. Pansini AR, Christakos S. Vitamin D-dependent calcium-binding protein in rat kidney. *J Biol Chem* 1984;259:9735–41.
21. Bruns ME, Fleisher EB, Avioli LV. Control of vitamin D-dependent calcium-binding protein in rat intestine by growth and fasting. *J Biol Chem* 1977;252:4145–50.
22. Ueng TH, Golub EE, Bronner F. The effect of age and 1,25-dihydroxy-vitamin D_3 treatment on the intestinal calcium-binding protein of suckling rats. *Arch Biochem Biophys* 1977;196:624–30.
23. Taylor AN, Gleason WA Jr, Lankford GL. Renal distribution of 10,000 dalton vitamin D-dependent calcium-binding protein in neonatal rats. In: Bronner F, Meinrad Peterlik, eds. *Epithelial calcium and phosphate transport: molecular and cellular aspects.* New York: Alan R. Liss, 1984;199–204.
24. Kretsinger RJ, Mann JE, Simmons JG. Model of the facilitated diffusion of calcium by the intestinal calcium binding protein. In: Norman AW, Schaefer K, Herrath DV, Grigoleit H-G, eds. *Vitamin D: chemical, biochemical and clinical endocrinology of calcium metabolism.* Berlin: Walter deGruyter, 1982;233–46.
25. Feher JJ. Measurement of facilitated calcium diffusion by a

soluble calcium-binding protein. *Biochim Biophys Acta* 1984;773:91–8.

26. Bronner F, Pansu D, Stein WD. An analysis of intestinal calcium transport across rat intestine. *Am J Physiol* 1986;250:G561–9.
27. Bronner F. Renal calcium transport: mechanisms and regulation —an overview. *Am J Physiol* 1989;257:F707–11.
28. Taylor AN, McIntosh JE, Bourdeau JE. Immunocytochemical localization of vitamin D-dependent calcium-binding protein in renal tubules of rabbit, rat and chick. *Kidney Int* 1982;21:765–73.
29. Varghese S, Lee S, Huang YC, Christakos S. Analysis of rat vitamin D-dependent calbindin-D_{28K} gene expression. *J Biol Chem* 1988;263:9776–84.
30. Wood TL, Kobayashi Y, Frantz G, Varghese S, Christakos S, Tobin AJ. Molecular cloning of mammalian 28,000 M_r vitamin D-dependent calcium binding protein (calbindin-D_{28K}) RNAs in rodent brain and kidney. *DNA* 1988;7:585–93.
31. Huang YC, Christakos S. Modulation of rat calbindin-D_{28} gene expression by 1,25-dihydroxyvitamin D_3 and dietary alteration. *Mol Endocrinol* 1988;2:928–35.
32. Halloran BP, HF DeLuca. Appearance of the intestinal cytosolic receptor for 1,25-dihydroxyvitamin D_3 during neonatal development in the rat. *J Biol Chem* 1981;256:7338–42.
33. Lee DBN, Hardwick LL, Hu MS, Jamgotchian N. Vitamin D-independent regulation of calcium and phosphate absorption. *Miner Electrolyte Metab* 1990;16:167–73.
34. Lee DBN, Brautbar N, Kleeman CR. Disorders of phosphorus metabolism. In: Bronner F, Coburn JW, eds. *Disorders of mineral metabolism, vol III*. New York: Academic Press, 1981;283–421.
35. Buckley M, Bronner F. Calcium-binding protein biosynthesis in the rat: regulation by calcium and 1,25-dihydroxyvitamin D_3. *Arch Biochem Biophys* 1980;202:235–41.
36. Niggli V, Penniston J, Carafoli E. Purification of the (Ca^{2+}-Mg^{2+})-ATPase from human erythrocyte membranes using a calmodulin affinity column. *J Biol Chem* 1979;254:9955–8.
37. Hakim G, Itano T, Verma A, et al. Purification of the Ca^{2+} and Mg^{2+} requiring ATPase from rat brain synaptic plasma membrane. *Biochem J* 1982;207:225–31.
38. Caroni P, Carofoli E. The Ca^{2+}-pumping ATPase of heart sarcolemma. Characterization, calmodulin dependence, and partial purification. *J Biol Chem* 1981;256:3263–70.
39. Verma AK, Fileoto AG, Stanford DR, et al. Complete primary structure of a human plasma membrane Ca^{2+}-pump. *J Biol Chem* 1988;263:14152–9.
40. Gamj P, Murer H. Ca^{2+} ATPase; Na^+-Ca^{2+} exchange; brush border membrane; basolateral membrane. *Miner Electrolyte Metab* 1988;14:22–30.
41. Carafoli E, James P, Strehler EE. Structure-function relationships in the calcium pump of plasma membranes. In: Peterlik M, Bronner F, eds. *Molecular and cellular regulation of calcium and phosphate metabolism*. New York: Alan R. Liss, in press.
42. Kretsinger RH. Structure and evolution of calcium-modulated proteins. *Crit Rev Biochem Mol Biol* 1980;8:119–74.
43. Gamj P, Murer H, Kinne R. Calcium ion transport across plasma membranes isolated from rat kidney cortex. *Biochem J* 1979;178:549–77.
44. Tsakamoto Y, Suki WN, Yang TC, et al. Ca^{2+}-dependent ATPases in basolateral membranes of rat kidney cortex. *J Biol Chem* 1986;261:2718–24.
45. Doucet A, Katz AI. High-affinity Ca^{++}-Mg^{++}-ATPase along the rabbit nephron. *Am J Physiol* 1982;242:F346–52.
46. Borke JL, Minami J, Verma AK, et al. Monoclonal antibodies to human erythrocyte Ca^{++}-Mg^{++} adenosine triphosphatase pump recognize an epitope in the basolateral membrane of human kidney distal tubule cells. *J Clin Invest* 1987;80:1225–31.
46a. Reuter H. Sodium-calcium exchange. Ins and outs of Ca^{2+} transport. *Nature* 1991;349:567–8.
47. Blaustein MP. The effects of internal and external cations and of ATP on sodium-calcium and calcium-calcium exchange in squid axons. *Biophys J* 1977;20:79–111.
48. Mullins LJA. A mechanism for Na/Ca transport. *J Gen Physiol* 1977;70:681–95.
48a. Nicoll DA, Longoni S, Philipson KD. Molecular cloning and functional expression of the cardiac sarcolemmal Na^+-Ca^{2+} exchanger. *Science* 1990;250:562–5.
48b. Niggli E, Lederer WJ. Molecular operations of the sodium-calcium exchanger revealed by conformation currents. *Nature* 1991;349:621–4.
49. Van Heeswijk MPE, Geertsen JAM, Van Os CH. Kinetic properties of ATP-dependent Ca^{2+} pump on the Na^+/Ca^{2+} exchange system in basolateral membranes from rat. *J Membr Biol* 1984;79:19–31.
50. Jayakumar A, Cheng L, Liang CT, Sacktor B. Sodium gradient-dependent calcium uptake in renal basolateral membrane vesicles. *J Biol Chem* 1984;259:10827–33.
51. Scoble JE, Mills S, Hruska KA. Calcium transport in canine renal basolateral membrane vesicles. *J Clin Invest* 1985;75:1096–105.
52. Van Os CH. Transcellular calcium transport in intestinal and renal epithelial cells. *Biochim Biophys Acta* 1987;906:195–222.
53. Ramachandran C, Brunette MG. The renal Na^+/Ca^{2+} exchange system is located exclusively in the distal tubule. *Biochem J* 1989;257:259–64.
54. Jande SS, Brewer LM. Effects of vitamin D_3 on duodenal absorptive cells of chicks. *Z Anat Entwgesch* 1974;144:249–65.
55. Nemere I, Norman AW. Transcaltachia, vesicular calcium transport, and microtubule-associated calbindin-D_{28K}: emerging views of 1,25-dihydroxyvitamin D_3-mediated intestinal calcium absorption. *Miner Electrolyte Metab* 1990;16:109–14.
56. Nemere I, Norman AW. Vitamin D and intestinal membranes. *Biochim Biophys Acta* 1982;694:307–27.
57. Christensen EI. Recycling of membrane in renal proximal tubule cells (Abstract). *J Ultrastruct Res* 1981;76:322.
58. Lassiter WE, Gottschalk CW, Mylle M. Micropuncture study of tubular reabsorption of calcium in normal rodents. *Am J Physiol* 1963;204:771–5.
59. Harris CA, Baer PG, Chirito E, Dirks JH. Composition of mammalian glomerular filtrate. *Am J Physiol* 1974;227:972–6.
60. Sutton RAL, Dirks JH. Calcium and magnesium: renal handling and disorders of metabolism. In: Brenner BM, Rector FC Jr, eds. *The kidney*, 3rd ed. Philadelphia: WB Saunders, 1986;551–618.
61. Rouse D, Suki WN. Renal control of extracellular calcium. *Kidney Int* 1990;38:700–8.
61a. Burg MB. Renal handling of sodium, chloride, water, amino acids and glucose. In: Brenner BM, Rector FC Jr, eds. *The kidney*, 2nd ed. 1981;328–70.
62. Ng RCK, Rouse D, Suki WN. Calcium transport in the rabbit superficial proximal convoluted tubule. *J Clin Invest* 1984;74:834–42.
63. Bomsztyk K, George JP, Wright FS. Effect of luminal fluid anions on calcium transport by proximal tubule. *Am J Physiol* 1984;256:F600–8.
64. Ullich KJ, Rumrich G, Kloss S. Active Ca^{2+} reabsorption in the proximal tubule of the rat kidney. *Pflugers Arch* 1976;364:223–8.
65. Bomsztyk K, Wright FS. Effects of transepithelial fluid flux on transepithelial voltage and transport of calcium, sodium chloride and potassium by renal proximal tubule (Abstract). *Kidney Int* 1982;21:269.
66. Bourdeau JE. Calcium transport across the pars recta of cortical segment 2 proximal tubules. *Am J Physiol* 1986;251:F718–24.
67. Jamison RL, Frey NR, Lacy FB. Calcium reabsorption in the thin loop of Henle. *Am J Physiol* 1974;227:745–51.
68. de Rouffignac C, Morel F, Moss N, et al. Micropuncture study of water and electrolyte movements along the loop of Henle in Psammomys with special reference to magnesium, calcium and phosphorus. *Pflugers Arch* 1973;344:309–26.
69. Almedia ALJ, Kudo LH, Rocha AS. Calcium transport in isolated perfused pars recta of proximal tubule (Abstract). *Meeting of the 7th International Congress of Nephrology*. Montreal, 1976;E16.
70. Rouse D, Ng RCK and Suki WN. Calcium transport in the pars recta and thin descending limb of Henle of the rabbit. *J Clin Invest* 1980;65:37–42.
71. Rocha RS, Migaldi JB, Kokko JP. Calcium and phosphate transport in isolated segments of rabbit Henle's loop. *J Clin Invest* 1977;59:975–83.
71a. Bourdeau JE. Renal handling of calcium. In: Brenner BM, Stein JH, eds. *Contemporary issues in nephrology, vol 11: Divalent ion homeostasis*. New York: Churchill Livingstone, 1983;1–31.
72. Shareghi GR, Stoner LC. Calcium transport across segments of

the rabbit distal nephron in vitro. *Am J Physiol* 1978;235:F367–75.

73. Bourdeau JE, Burg MB. Voltage dependence of calcium transport in the thick ascending limb of Henle's loop. *Am J Physiol* 1979;236:F357–64.

74. Shareghi GR, Agus ZS. Magnesium transport in the cortical thick ascending limb of Henle's loop of the rabbit. *J Clin Invest* 1982;69:759–69.

75. Suki WN, Rouse D, Ng RCK, Kokko JP. Calcium transport in the thick ascending limb of Henle. Heterogeneity of function in the medullary and cortical segments. *J Clin Invest* 1980;66:1004–9.

76. Imai M. Calcium transport across the rabbit thick ascending limb of Henle's loop perfused in vitro. *Pflugers Arch* 1978;374:255–63.

77. Bourdeau JE, Burg MB. Effect of PTH on calcium transport across the cortical thick ascending limb of Henle's loop. *Am J Physiol* 1980;239:F121–6.

78. Suki WN, Rouse D. Hormonal regulation of calcium transport in thick ascending renal tubules. *Am J Physiol* 1981;241:F171–4.

79. Costanzo LS, Windhager EE. Calcium and sodium transport by the distal convoluted tubule of the rat. *Am J Physiol* 1978;235:F492–506.

80. Swanson J, Costanzo L, Lee CO, Windhager EE. Calcium ion concentration in rat distal tubular fluid (DTF) in vivo (Abstract). *Fed Proc* 1981;40:462.

81. Morel F, Chabardes D, Imbert M. Functional segmentation of the rabbit distal tubule by microdetermination of hormone dependent adenylate cyclase activity. *Kidney Int* 1976;9:264–277.

82. Imai M. Effects of parathyroid hormone and N^6,O^2-dibutyryl cyclic AMP on Ca transport across the rabbit distal nephron segments perfused in vitro. *Pflugers Arch* 1981;390:145–51.

83. Greger R, Lang F, Oberleither H. Distal site of calcium reabsorption in the rat nephron. *Pflugers Arch* 1978;374:153–7.

84. Goldfarb SW, Westby GR, Goldberg M, Agus ZS. Renal tubular effects of chronic phosphate depletion. *J Clin Invest* 1977;59:770–9.

85. Shareghi GA, Agus ZS. Phosphate transport in the light segment of the rabbit cortical collecting tubule. *Am J Physiol* 1982;242:F379–84.

86. Bourdeau JE, Hellstrom-Stein RJ. Voltage-dependent calcium movement across the cortical collecting duct. *Am J Physiol* 1982;242:F285–92.

87. Holt WF, Lechene C. ADH-PEG$_2$ interactions in cortical collecting tubule. II. Inhibition of Ca and P reabsorption. *Am J Physiol* 1981;241:F461–7.

88. Bengele HH, Alexander EA, Lechene CP. Calcium and magnesium transport along the inner medullary collecting duct of the rat. *Am J Physiol* 1980;239:F24–9.

89. Walser M. Calcium clearance as a function of sodium clearance in the dog. *Am J Physiol* 1961;200:1009–1014.

90. Dirks JH, Cirksena WJ, Berliner RW. The effect of saline infusion on sodium reabsorption by the proximal tubule of the dog. *J Clin Invest* 1965;44:1160–70.

91. Duarte CG, Watson JF. Calcium reabsorption in proximal tubule of the dog. *Am J Physiol* 1967;212:1355–60.

92. Howards SS, Davis BB, Knox FG, Wright FS, Berliner RW. Depression of fractional sodium reabsorption by the proximal tubule of the dog without sodium diuresis. *J Clin Invest* 1968;47:1561–72.

93. Stein JH, Reineck HJ. The role of the collecting duct in the regulation of excretion of sodium and other electrolytes. *Kidney Int* 1974;6:1–9.

94. Agus ZS, Chiu PJS, Goldberg M. Regulation of urinary calcium excretion in the rat. *Am J Physiol* 1977;232:F545–9.

95. Kleeman CR, Bohannan J, Bernstein D, Ling S, Maxwell MH. Effect of variation in sodium intake on calcium excretion in normal humans. *Proc Soc Exp Biol Med* 1964;115:29–32.

96. Stern N, Lee DBN, Silis V, Beck FWJ, Deftos LJ, Manolagas SC, Sowers JR. The effects of high calcium intake on blood pressure and calcium metabolism in the young spontaneously hypertensive rat. *Hypertension* 1984;6(3):639–46.

97. Goldfarb S. Dietary factors in the pathogenesis and prophylaxis of calcium nephrolithiasis. *Kidney Int* 1988;34:544–55.

98. Doris PA, Harvey S, Pang PKT. Parathyroid hormone in sodium-dependent hypertension. *Life Sci* 1987;61:1383–9.

99. Jones JH, Peters DK, Morgan DB, Coles GA, Mallick NP. Observations on calcium metabolism in the nephrotic syndrome. *Q J Med* 1967;36:301–20.

100. Albright F, Bauer W, Cockrill JR. Studies in parathyroid physiology. III. The effect of phosphate ingestion in clinical hyperparathyroidism. *J Clin Invest* 1932;11:411–35.

101. Hulley SB, Goldsmith RS, Ingbar SH. Effect of renal arterial and systemic infusion of phosphate on urinary Ca excretion. *Am J Physiol* 1969;217:1570–7.

102. Coburn JW, Hartenbower DI, Massry SG. Modification of calciuretic effect of extracellular volume expansion by phosphate infusion. *Am J Physiol* 1971;220:371–7.

103. Wong NLM, Quamme GA, Sutton RAL, O'Callaghan T, Dirks JH. Effect of phosphate infusion on renal phosphate and calcium transport. Renal Physiol, Basel, 1985:8:30–37.

104. Lee DBN, Brautbar N, Kleeman CR. Disorders of phosphorus metabolism. In: Bronner F, Coburn JW, eds. *Disorders of mineral metabolism, vol III*, New York: Academic Press, 1981;283–421.

105. Sutton RAL, Quamme GA, O'Callaghan T, Wong NLM, Dirks JH. Renal tubular phosphate reabsorption in the phosphate depleted dog. *Adv Exp Med Biol* 1978;103:405–12.

106. Wong NLM, Quamme GA, Sutton RAL, O'Callaghan TJ, Dirks JH. Renal tubular transport in phosphate depletion. *Can J Physiol Pharmacol* 1980;58:1063–71.

107. Guruprakash GH, Babino H, Duffy WB, Krothapalli R, Senekjian HO, Eknoyan G, Suki WN. Microinjection study of renal calcium absorption in the phosphate-depleted rat. *Miner Electrolyte Metab* 1985;11:262–6.

108. Lau K, Agus ZS, Goldberg M, Goldfarb S. Renal tubular sites of altered calcium transport in phosphate-depleted rats. *J Clin Invest* 1979;64:1681–7.

109. Lemann J Jr, Adams ND, Gray RW. Urinary calcium excretion in human beings. *N Engl J Med* 1979;301:535–41.

110. Wilkinson R. Absorption of calcium, phosphorus and magnesium. In: Nordin BEC, ed. *Calcium, phosphate and magnesium metabolism.* London: Churchill Livingstone, 1976;36–112.

111. Lee DBN, Hardwick LL, Hu MS, Jamgotchian N. Vitamin D-independent regulation of calcium and phosphate absorption. *Miner Electrolyte Metab* 1990;16:167–73.

112. Wasserstein AG, Stolley PD, Soper KA, Goldfarb S, Agus ZS. Case-control study of risk factors for idiopathic calcium nephrolithiasis. *Miner Electrolyte Metab* 1987;13:85–95.

113. Lemann J Jr, Gray RW, Maierhofer WJ, Cheung HS. The importance of renal net acid excretion as a determinant of fasting urinary calcium excretion. *Kidney Int* 1986;29:743–6.

114. Lutz J. Calcium balance and acid-base status of women as affected by increased protein intake and by sodium bicarbonate ingestion. *Am J Clin Nutr* 1984;39:281–8.

115. Whiting SJ, Draper HH. The role of sulfate in the calciuria of high protein diets in adult rats. *J Nutr* 1980;110:212–22.

116. Schuette SA, Zemel MB, Linkswiler HM. Studies on the mechanism of protein-induced hypercalciuria in older men and women. *J Nutr* 1980;10:305–15.

117. Lemann J Jr, Piering WF, Lennon EJ. Possible role of carbohydrate-induced calciuria in calcium oxalate kidney-stone formation. *N Engl J Med* 1969;280:232–7.

118. Ichikawa I, Humes HD, Dousa TP, Brenner BM. Influence of parathyroid hormone on glomerular ultrafiltration in the rat. *Am J Physiol* 1978;234:F393–401.

119. Agus ZS, Gardner LB, Beck LH, Goldberg M. Effects of parathyroid hormone on renal tubular reabsorption of calcium, sodium and phosphate. *Am J Physiol* 1973;224:1143–8.

120. Harris CA, Burnatowska MA, Seely JF, Sutton RAL, Quamme GA, Dirks JH. Effects of parathyroid hormone on electrolyte transport in the hamster nephron. *Am J Physiol* 1979;236:F342–8.

121. Sutton RAL, Wong NLM, Dirks JH. Effects of parathyroid hormone on sodium and calcium transport in the dog nephron. *Clin Sci Mol Med* 1976;51:345–51.

122. Frick A, Rumrich G, Ullrich KF, Lassiter WE. Microperfusion study of calcium transport in the proximal tubule of the rat kidney. *Pflugers Arch* 1965;286:109–17.

123. Morel F, Doucet A. Hormonal control of kidney functions at the cell level. *Physiol Rev* 1986;66:377–468.

124. Gran FC. The retention of parenterally injected calcium in rachitic dogs. *Acta Physiol Scand* 1960;50:132–9.

125. Ney RL, Kelly G, Bartter FC. Actions of vitamin D independent of the parathyroid glands. *Endocrinology* 1968;82:760–6.

126. Puschett JB, Moranz J, Kurnick WS. Evidence for a direct action of cholecalciferol and 25-hydroxycholecalciferol on the renal transport of phosphate, sodium and calcium. *J Clin Invest* 1972;51:373–85.

127. Puschett JB, Fernandez PC, Boyle IT, Gray RW, Omdahl JL, DeLuca HF. The acute renal tubular effects of 1,25-dihydroxycholecalciferol (36781) *Proc Soc Exp Biol Med* 1972;141:379–84.

128. Costanzo LS, Sheehe PR, Weiner IM. Renal actions of vitamin D in D-deficient rats. *Am J Physiol* 1974;226:1490–5.

129. Bonjour J-P, Trechsel U, Fleisch H, Sehenk R, DeLuca HF, Baxter LA. Action of 1,24-(OH)$_2$D$_3$ and a diphosphonate on calcium metabolism in the rat. *Am J Physiol* 1975;229:489–95.

130. Litvak J, Moldawer MP, Forbes AP, Hanneman PH. Hypocalcemic hypercalciuria during vitamin D and dihydroxytachsterol therapy in hypoparathyroidism. *J Clin Endocrinol Metab* 1958;18:246–52.

131. Brickman AS, Coburn JW, Norman AW, Massry SG. Short-term effects of 1,25-dihydroxycholecalciferol on disordered calcium metabolism of renal failure. *Am J Med* 1974;57:28–33.

132. Rizzoli R, Freisch H, Bonjour J-P. Effect of thyroparathyroidectomy on calcium metabolism in rats: role of 1,25(OH)$_2$D$_3$. *Am J Physiol* 1977;233:E160–4.

133. Hugi K, Bonjour J-P, Fleisch H. Renal handling of calcium: influence of parathyroid hormone and 1,25-dihydroxyvitamin D$_3$. *Am J Physiol* 1979;236:F349–56.

134. Bernstein D, Kleeman CR, Maxwell MH. The effect of calcium infusions, parathyroid hormone, and vitamin D on renal clearance of calcium. *Proc Soc Exp Biol Med* 1963;112:353–5.

135. Steel TH, Engle JE, Tanaka Y, Lorenc RS, Dudgeon KL, DeLuca HF. Phosphaturic action of 1,25-dihydroxyvitamin D$_3$. *Am J Physiol* 1975;229:489–95.

136. Burnatowska MA, Harris CA, Sutton RAL, Seely JF. Effects of 1,25(OH)$_2$D$_3$ on Ca, Mg and P$_i$ excretion in the hamster (Abstract). *Kidney Int* 1977;12:454.

137. Kawashima H, Kurokawa K. Metabolism and sites of action of vitamin D in the kidney. *Kidney Int* 1986;29:98–107.

138. Kurakawa K. Calcium-regulating hormones and the kidney. *Kidney Int* 1987;32:760–71.

139. Yamamoto M, Kawanobe Y, Takahashi H, Shimazawa E, Kimura S, Ogata E. Vitamin D deficiency and renal calcium transport in the rat. *J Clin Invest* 1984;74:507–13.

140. Stumpf WE, Sar M, Narbaitz R, Reid FA, DeLuca HF, Tanaka Y. Target cells for 1,25-dihydroxyvitamin D$_3$ in intestinal tract, stomach, kidney, skin, pituitary and parathyroid. *Proc Natl Acad Sci USA* 1980;77:1149–53.

141. Berndt TJ, Knox FG. Effect of parathyroid hormone and calcitonin on electrolyte excretion in the rabbit. *Kidney Int* 1980;17:473–8.

142. Laake H. The action of corticosteroids on the renal reabsorption of calcium. *Acta Endocrinol (Copenh)* 1960;34:60–4.

143. Collins EJ, Garrett ER, Johnston RI. Effect of adrenal steroids on radio-calcium metabolism in dogs. *Metabolism* 1982;11:716–26.

144. Massry SG, Coburn JW, Chapman LW, Kleeman CR. The effect of long-term desoxycorticosterone acetate administration on the renal excretion of calcium and magnesium. *J Lab Clin Med* 1968;7:212–9.

145. Suki WN, Schwettmann RS, Rector FC Jr, Seldin DW. Effect of chronic mineralocorticoid administration on calcium excretion in the rat. *Am J Physiol* 1968;215:71–4.

146. DeFronzo RA, Cooke CR, Andres R, Faloona GR, Davis PJ. The effect of insulin on renal handling of sodium, potassium, calcium and phosphate in man. *J Clin Invest* 1975;55:845–55.

147. Elrick H, Huffman ER, Hlad CJ Jr, Whipple N, Staub A. Effects of glucagon on renal function in man. *J Clin Endocrinol Metab* 1958;18:813–24.

148. Henneman PH, Forbes AP, Moldawer M, Dempsy EF, Carroll EL. Effects of human growth hormone in man. *J Clin Invest* 1960;39:1223–38.

149. Krane SM, Brownell GL, Stanbury JB, Corrigan H. The effect of thyroid disease on calcium metabolism in man. *J Clin Invest* 1956;35:874–87.

150. Morey ER, Kenny AD. Effects of catecholamines on urinary calcium and phosphorus in intact and parathyroidectomized rats. *Endocrinology* 1964;75:78–85.

151. Gantt CL, Carter WJ. Acute effects of angiotensin on calcium, phosphorus, magnesium and potassium excretion. *Can Med Assoc J* 1964;90:287–91.

152. Thorn NA. An effect of antidiuretic hormone on renal excretion of calcium in dogs. *Dan Med Bull* 1960;7:110–2.

153. Vorherr H, Huter J. Die Wirkung von Dolantin auf die Diurese bed Mensch und Ratte. *Klin Wochenschr* 1965;43:1053–7.

154. Ackermann PG, Toro G, Kountz WB, Kheim T. The effect of sex hormone administration of calcium and nitrogen balance in elderly women. *Gastroenterology* 1954;9:450–5.

155. Gallagher JC, Nordin BEC. Oestrogen and calcium metabolism. In: Van Keep PA, Lauritzen C, eds. *Aging and estrogens. Frontiers in hormone research*, vol 2. Basel: S Karger, 1973;98.

156. Sutton RAL, Wong NLM, Dirks JH. Effects of metabolic acidosis and alkalosis on sodium and calcium transport in the dog kidney. *Kidney Int* 1979;15:520–33.

157. Lemann J Jr, Litzow JR, and Lennon EJ. Studies of the mechanism by which chronic metabolic acidosis augments urinary calcium excretion in man. *J Clin Invest* 1967;46:1318–28.

158. Stacy BD, Wilson BW. Acidosis and hypercalciuria: renal mechanism affecting calcium, magnesium, and sodium excretion in the sheep. *J Physiol* 1970;210:549–64.

159. Parfitt AM, Higgins BA, Nassim JR, Collins JA, Hilb A. Metabolic studies in patients with hypercalciuria. *Clin Sci* 1964;27:463–82.

160. Edwards NA, Hodgkinson A. Metabolic studies in patients with idiopathic hypercalciuria. *Clin Sci* 1965;29:143–57.

161. Anderson OS. Acute experimental acid-base disturbances in dogs. *Scand J Clin Lab Invest* 1962;66(Suppl):1–20.

162. Gray SP, Morris JEW, Brooks CJ. Renal handling of calcium, magnesium, inorganic phosphate and hydrogen ions during prolonged exposure to elevated carbon dioxide concentration. *Clin Sci Mol Med* 1973;45:751–64.

163. Wong NML, Sutton RAL, Quamme GA, Dirks JH. The effect of alkalosis on renal tubular calcium reabsorption in the dog (Abstract). *Clin Res* 1978;24:687A.

164. Lemann J, Gray RW, Pluess JA. Potassium bicarbonate, but not sodium bicarbonate, reduces urinary calcium excretion and improves calcium balance in healthy men. *Kidney Int* 1989;35:688–95.

165. Sakhaee K, Nicar M, Hill K, Pak CYC. Contrasting effects of potassium citrate and sodium citrate therapies and crystallization of stone-forming salts. *Kidney Int* 1983;24:348–52.

166. Peraino RA, Suki WN. Urine HCO$_3$ augments renal Ca^{2+} absorption independent of systemic acid-base changes. *Am J Physiol* 1980;238:F394–8.

167. Bomsztyk K, Calalb MB. Bicarbonate absorption stimulates active calcium absorption in the rat proximal tubule. *J Clin Invest* 1988;81:1455–61.

168. Harris CA, Sutton RAL, Dirks JH. Effects of hypercalcemia on calcium and phosphate ultrafilterability and tubular reabsorption in the rat. *Am J Physiol* 1977;233:F201–6.

169. Humes HD, Ichikawa I, Troy JL, Brenner BM. Evidence for a parathyroid hormone-dependent influence of calcium on the glomerular filtration. *J Clin Invest* 1978;61:32–40.

170. Edwards BR, Sutton RAL, Dirks JH. Effect of calcium infusion on renal tubular reabsorption in the dog. *Am J Physiol* 1974;227:13–8.

171. Quamme GA. Effect of hypercalcemia on renal tubular handling of calcium and magnesium. *Can J Physiol Pharmacol* 1982;60:1275–80.

172. Massry SG, Ahumada JJ, Coburn JW, Kleeman CR. Effect of MgCl$_2$ infusion on urinary Ca and Na during reduction in their filtered loads. *Am J Physiol* 1970;219:881–5.

173. Quamme GA, Dirks JA. Intraluminal and contraluminal magnesium on magnesium and calcium transfer in the rat nephron. *Am J Physiol* 1979;238:187–98.

174. Howard PJ, Wilde WS, Malvin RL. Localization of renal calcium transport; effect of calcium loads and of gluconate anion on water, sodium and potassium. *Am J Physiol* 1959;197:337–41.

175. Le Grimellec C, Roinel N, Morel F. Simultaneous Mg, Ca, P, K, Na and Cl analysis in rat tubular fluid. I. During perfusion of either inulin or ferrocyanide. *Pflugers Arch* 1973;340:181–96.

176. Durie BGM, Salmon SE, Mundy GR. Relation of osteoclast activating factor production to the extent of bone disease in multiple myeloma. *Br J Haematol* 1981;47:21–30.

177. Ralston SH, Boyce BF, Cowan RA, et al. Humoral hypercalcemia of malignancy: metabolic and histomorphometric studies during surgical management of the primary tumor. *Q J Med* 1986;58(227):325–35.

178. Wesson LG. Magnesium, calcium and phosphate excretion during osmotic diuresis in the dog. *J Lab Clin Med* 1962;60:422–32.

179. Better OS, Gonick HC, Chapman LC, Varrady PD, Kleeman CR. Effect of urea-saline diuresis on renal clearance of calcium, magnesium, and inorganic phosphate in man (30839) *Proc Soc Exp Biol Med* 1966;121:592–6.

180. Wong NLM, Quamme GA, Sutton RAL, Dirks JH. Effects of mannitol on water and electrolyte transport in the dog kidney. *J Lab Clin Med* 1979;94:683–92.

181. Seldin DW, Eknoyan G, Suki WN, Rector FC Jr. Localization of diuretic action from the pattern of water and electrolyte excretion. *NY Acad Sci* 1966;139:328–43.

182. Edwards BR, Baer PG, Sutton RAL, Dirks JH. Interrelationships of chlorothiazide and parathyroid hormone: a micropuncture study. *J Clin Invest* 1973;52:2418–27.

183. Bourdeau JE, Buss SL, Vurek GG. Inhibition of calcium absorption in the cortical thick ascending limb of Henle's loop by furosemide. *J Pharmacol Exp Ther* 1982;221:815–9.

184. Quamme GA. Effect of intraluminal furosemide (F) on Ca and Mg transport in the loop of Henle and the role of parathyroid hormone (PTH). (Abstract) 11th Annual Meeting of the American Soc Nephrol 1978;p 8A.

185. Suki WN, Yium JJ, Von Minden M, Saller-Herbert C, Eknoyan G and Martinez-Maldonado M. Acute treatment of hypercalcemia with furosemide. *N Engl J Med* 1970;283:836–40.

186. Beck LH and Goldberg M. Effect of acetazolamide and parathyroidectomy on renal transport of sodium, calcium and phosphate. *Am J Physiol* 1973;224:1136–42.

187. Popovtzer MM, Subryan VL, Alfrey AC, Reeve EB, Schrier RW. The acute effect of chlorothiazide on serum-ionized calcium. Evidence for a parathyroid hormone-dependent mechanism. *J Clin Invest* 1975;55:1295–1302.

188. Costanzo LS, Weiner IM. On the hypocalciuric action of chlorothiazide. *J Clin Invest* 1974;54:628–37.

189. Costanzo LS, Weiner IM. Relationship between clearances of Ca and Na: Effect of distal diuretics and PTH. *Am J Physiol* 1976;230:67–73.

190. Coe FL. Treated and untreated recurrent calcium nephrolithiasis in patients with idiopathic hypercalciuria, hyperuricosuria, or no metabolic disorders. *Ann Intern Med* 1977;87:404–10.

191. Yendt ER, Cohanim M. Prevention of calcium stones with thiazides. *Kidney Int* 1978;13:397–409.

192. Brickman AS, Massry SG, Coburn JW. Changes in serum and urinary calcium during treatment with hydrochlorothiazide. Studies on mechanisms. *J Clin Invest* 1972;51:945–54.

193. Jorgensen FS. The effect of bendroflumethiazide (Centyl®) on the renal excretion of calcium and sodium in normal, parathyroidectomized rats. *Acta Pharmacol Toxicol* 1971;30:296–307.

194. Costanzo LS. Comparison of calcium and sodium transport in early and late distal tubules: effect of amiloride. *Am J Physiol* 1984;246:F937–45.

195. Stoner LC, Burg MB, Orloff J. Ion transport in cortical collecting tubule: effect of amiloride. *Am J Physiol* 1974;227:453–9.

196. Sutton RAL. Renal tubular disorders associated with hypocalciuria. *Adv Exp Med Biol* 1986;208:187–91.

197. Johns EJ, Manitius J. An investigation into the neural regulation of calcium excretion by the rat kidney. *J Physiol* 1987;383:745–55.

198. Deitrick JE, Whedon GD, Shorr E. Effects of immobilization upon various metabolic and physiologic functions of normal man. *Am J Med* 1948;4:3–36.

199. Lutwak L, Whedon G, Lachance PA, Reid JM, Lipscomb HS. Mineral, electrolyte and nitrogen balances studies of the Gemini-VII fourteen-day orbital space flight. *J Clin Endocrinol Metab* 1969;29:1140–56.

200. Heaton FW, Hodgkinson A. External factors affecting diurnal variation in electrolyte excretion with particular reference to calcium and magnesium. *Clin Chim Acta* 1963;8:246–54.

201. Kupfer S, Kosovsky JD. Effects of cardiac glycosides on renal tubular transport of calcium, magnesium, inorganic phosphate and glucose in the dog. *J Clin Invest* 1965;44:1132–43.

202. Miller PD, Dubovsky SL, Schrier RW. McDonald KM, Arnaud C. Hypocalciuric effect of lithium in man. *Adv Exp Med Biol* 1976;81:157–72.

203. Briscoe AM, Ragan C. Diurnal variation in calcium and magnesium excretion in man. *Metabolism* 1966;15:1002–10.

204. Schneider EG, Hanson RC, Childers JW, Fitzgerald EM, Gleason SD. Is phosphate secreted by the kidney? In: Massry SG, Fliesch H, eds. *Renal handling of phosphate.* New York: Plenum Press, 1980;59–78.

205. Van Slike DD. Studies of gas and electrolyte equilibria in the blood. V. Factors controlling electrolyte and water distribution in the blood. *J Biol Chem* 1923;56:765.

206. Harris CA. Composition of mammalian glomerular filtrate. *Am J Physiol* 1974;227:972–6.

207. Hopkins T, Howard JE, Eisenberg H. Ultrafiltration studies on calcium and phosphorus in human serum. *Bull Johns Hopkins Med J* 1952;91:1–21.

208. Peraino RA, Suki WN. Influence of calcium on renal handling of phosphate. In: Massry SG, Fleisch H, eds. *Renal handling of phosphate.* New York: Plenum Press, 1980;287–306.

209. Pitts, RF. The excretion of urine in the dog. *Am J Physiol* 1933;106:1–8.

210. Staum BB, Hamburger RJ, Goldberg M. Tracer microinjection study of renal tubular phosphate reabsorption in the rat. *J Clin Invest* 1972;51:2271–6.

211. Strickler JC, Thompson DD, Klose RM, Giebisch G. Micropuncture study of inorganic phosphate excretion in the rat. *J Clin Invest* 1964;43:1596–1607.

212. Dennis VW, Woodhall PB, Robinson RR. Characterization of phosphate transport in isolated proximal tubule. *Am J Physiol* 1976;231:979–85.

213. Knox FG, Osswald H, Marchand GR, et al. Phosphate transport along the nephron. *Am J Physiol* 1977;233:F261–8.

214. Lang F, Greger R, Knox FG, Oberteithner H. Factors modulating renal handling of phosphate. *Renal Physiol* 1981;4:1–16.

215. McKeown JW, Brazy PC, Dennis VW. Intrarenal heterogeneity for fluid, phosphate and glucose absorption in the rabbit. *Am J Physiol* 1979;237:F312–8.

216. Amiel C, Kuntziger HE, Richet G. Micropuncture study of handling of phosphate by proximal and distal nephron in normal and parathyroidectomized rat. Evidence for distal reabsorption. *Pflugers Arch* 1970;317:92–109.

217. Greger R, Lang F, Marchand G, Knox FG. Site of renal phosphate reabsorption: micropuncture and microinfusion study. *Pflugers Arch* 1977;369:111–8.

218. Lang F, Greger R, Marchand GR, Knox FG. Stationary microperfusion study of phosphate reabsorption in proximal and distal nephron segments. *Pflugers Arch* 1977;368:45–8.

219. Rocha AS, Magaldi JB, Kokko JP. Calcium and phosphate transport in isolated segments of rabbit's Henle's loop. *J Clin Invest* 1977;59:975–84.

220. Pastoriza-Munoz E, Colindres RE, Lassiter WE, Lechene C. Effect of parathyroid hormone on phosphate reabsorption in rat distal convolution. *Am J Physiol* 1978;235:321–30.

221. de Rouffignac C, Morel F, Roinel N. Micropuncture study of water and electrolyte movement along the loop of Henle in Psammomas with special reference to magnesium, calcium and phosphorus. *Pflugers Arch* 1973;344:309–26.

222. Dennis VW, Bello-Reuss E, Robinson R. Response of phosphate transport to parathyroid hormone in segments of rabbit nephron. *Am J Physiol* 1977;233:F29–38.

223. Peraino RA, Suki WN. Phosphate transport by isolated rabbit cortical collecting tubule. *Am J Physiol* 1980;238:F358–62.

224. Bengele HH, Lechene CP, Alexander EA. Phosphate transport

along the inner medullary collecting duct of the rat. *Am J Physiol* 1979;237:F48–54.

225. Hems DA, Gaja G. Carbohydrate metabolism in the isolated perfused rat kidney. *Biochem J* 1972;128:412–26.

226. Hoppe A, Metler M, Berndt TJ, Knox FG, Angielski S. Effect of respiratory alkalosis on renal phosphate excretion. *Am J Physiol* 1982;243:F471–5.

227. Freeman D, Bartlett S, Radda G, Ross B. Energetics of sodium transport in the kidney. Saturation transfer ^{31}P-NMR. *Biochim Biophys Acta* 1983;762:325–36.

228. Dousa TP, Kempson SA. Regulation of renal brush border membrane transport of phosphate. *Miner Electrolyte Metab* 1982;7:113–21.

229. Dousa TP, Kempson SA, Shah SV. Adaptive changes in renal cortical brush border membrane. *Adv Exp Med Biol* 1980;128:69–76.

230. Kempson SA, Dousa TP. Phosphate transport across renal cortical brush border membrane vesicles from rats stabilized on a normal, high or low phosphate diet. *Life Sci* 1979;24:881–8.

231. Shah SV, Kempson SA, Northrup TE, Dousa TP. Renal adaptation to low phosphate diet in rats. Blockade by actinomycin D. *J Clin Invest* 1979;64:955–46.

232. Brunette MG, Dennis VW. Effects of L-bromotetramisole on phosphate transport by the proximal renal tubule: failure to demonstrate a direct involvement of alkaline phosphatase. *Can J Physiol Pharmacol* 1982;62:229–34.

233. Storelli C, Murer H. On the correlation between alkaline phosphatase and phosphate transport in rat renal brush border membrane vesicles. *Pflugers Arch* 1980;384:149–53.

234. Tenenhouse HS, Scriver CR, Vizel EJ. Alkaline phosphatase activity does not mediate phosphate transport in the renal-cortical brush border membrane. *Biochem J* 1980;190:473–6.

235. Rohn R, Biber J, Haase W, Murer H. Effect of protease treatment on enzyme content, protein content and transport function of brush border membrane isolated from rat small intestine and kidney cortex. *Mol Physiol* 1983;3:3–18.

236. Craik JD, Reithmeier RAF. Inhibition of phosphate transport in human enthrocytes by water-soluble carbodiimides. *Biochim Biophys Acta* 1984;778:429–34.

237. Strevey J, Brunette MG, Belivenu R. Effect of arginine modification on kidney brush border membrane transport activity. *Biochem J* 1984;223:793–802.

238. Lin JT, Stroh A, Kinne. Structural state of the Na$^+$/D-glucose cotransporter in calf kidney brush-border membranes. *Biochim Biophys Acta* 1985;819:66–74.

239. Wuarin F, Wu K, Murer H, Biber J. The Na$^+$/Pi-cotransporter of OK cells: reaction and tentative identification with N-acetylimidazole. *Biochim Biophys Acta* 1989;981:185–92.

240. Kessler RJ, Vaughn DA. Divalent metal is required for both phosphate transport and phosphate binding to phosphorin, a proteolipid isolated from brush border membrane vesicles. *J Biol Chem* 1984;259:9059–63.

241. Kessler RJ, Vaughn DA, Fanestil DD. Phosphate-binding proteolipid from brush border. *J Biol Chem* 1982;257:14311–7.

242. Werner A, Biber J, Murer H. Cloning of the renal Na$^+$/Pi co-transporter system. *J Am Soc Nephrol* 1990;1:746A.

243. Burckhardt G, Stern H, Murer H. The influence of pH on phosphate transport into rat renal brush border membrane vesicles. *Pflugers Arch* 1981;390:191–7.

244. Brunette MG, Chan M, Maag V, Beliveau R. Phosphate uptake by superficial and deep nephron brush border membranes. Effect of dietary phosphate and parathyroid hormone. *Pflugers Arch* 1984;400:356–62.

245. Murer H, Burckhardt G. Membrane transport of anions across epithelia of mammalian small intestine and kidney proximal tubule. *Rev Physiol Biochem Pharmacol* 1983;96:1–53.

246. Cheng L, Sacktor B. Sodium gradient-dependent phosphate transport in renal brush border membrane vesicles. *J Biol Chem* 1981;256:1556–64.

247. Sacktor B, Cheng L. Sodium gradient-dependent phosphate transport in renal brush border membrane vesicles. Effect of an intravesicular greater than extravesicular proton gradient. *J Biol Chem* 1981;256:8080–4.

248. Brunette MG, Beliveau R, Chan M. Effect of temperature and pH on phosphate transport through brush border membrane vesicles in rats. *Can J Physiol Pharmacol* 1984;62:229–34.

249. Chen L, Liang CT, Sacktor B. Phosphate uptake by renal membrane vesicles of rabbits adapted to high and low phosphorus diets. *Am J Physiol* 1983;F175–80.

250. Hoffmann N, Thees M, Kinne R. Phosphate transport by isolated renal brush border vesicles. *Pflugers Arch* 1976;362:147–56.

251. Amstutz M, Mohrmann M, Gmaj P, Murer H. The effect of pH on phosphate transport in rat renal brush border membrane vesicles. *Am J Physiol* 1985;248:F705–10.

252. Knox FG, Hoppe A, Kempson SA, Shah SV, Dousa TP. Cellular mechanisms of phosphate transport. In: Massry SG, Fleisch H, eds. *Renal handling of phosphate.* New York: Plenum Press, 1980;79–114.

253. Ullrich KJ, Rumrich G, Kloess S. Phosphate transport in the proximal convolution of the rat kidney. III. Effect of extracellular and intracellular pH. *Pflugers Arch* 1978;377:33–42.

254. Chabardes D, Imbert M, Clique A, Montegut M, Morel F. PTH sensitive adenyl cyclase activity in different segments of the rabbit nephron. *Pflugers Arch* 1975;354:229–39.

255. Shlatz LJ, Schwartz IL, Kinne-Safran E, Kinne R. Distribution of PTH stimulated adenylate cyclase in plasma membranes of cells of the kidney cortex. *J Membr Biol* 1975;24:131–44.

256. George ER, Balakir RA, Filburn CR, Sacktor B. Cyclic adenosine monophosphate dependent and independent protein kinase activity of renal brush border membranes. *Arch Biochem Biophys* 1977;180:429–43.

257. Kinne R, Shlatz LJ, Kinne-Safran E, Schwartz IL. Distribution of membrane bound cyclic AMP-dependent protein kinase in the plasma membrane of cells of the kidney cortex. *J Membr Biol* 1975;24:145–59.

258. Evers C, Murer H, Kinne R. Effect of parathyrin on the transport properties of isolated renal brush border vesicles. *Biochem J* 1978;172:49–56.

259. Hruska KA, Hammerman MR. Parathyroid hormone inhibition of phosphate transport in renal brush border vesicles from phosphate-depleted dogs. *Biochim Biophys Acta* 1981;645:351–6.

260. Biber J, Malmstroem K, Scalera V, Murer H. Phosphorylation of rat kidney proximal tubular brush border membranes. Role of cAMP-dependent protein phosphorylation in the regulation of phosphate transport. *Pflugers Arch* 1983;398:221–6.

261. Hammerman MR, Cohn DE, Tamayo J, Martin KJ. Effect of parathyroid hormone on Na$^+$-dependent phosphate transport and cAMP-dependent ^{32}P phosphorylation in brush border vesicles from isolated perfused canine kidneys. *Arch Biochem Biophys* 1983;227:91–7.

262. Hammerman MR, Schwab SJ. Phosphate transport in the kidney. Studies with isolated membrane vesicles. In: Bronner F, Peterlik M, eds. *Epithelial calcium and phosphate transport: molecular and cellular aspects.* New York: Alan R. Liss, 1984;325–30.

263. Hammerman MR, Hruska KA. Cyclic AMP-dependent protein phosphorylation in canine renal brush border membrane vesicles is associated with decreased phosphate transport. *J Biol Chem* 1982;257:992–9.

264. Malmstroem K, Biber J, Gmaj P, Murer H. Possible mechanisms for the regulation of the Pi transport in brush border membrane vesicles. In: Bronner F, Peterlik M, eds. *Epithelial calcium and phosphate transport: molecular and cellular aspects.* New York: Alan R. Liss, 1984;325–30.

265. Hammerman MR, Hansen VA, Morrissey JJ. ADP ribosylation of canine renal brush border membrane vesicle proteins is associated with decreased phosphate transport. *J Biol Chem* 1982;257:12380–6.

266. Angielski S, Zielkiewicz J, Dziezko G. Metabolism of NAD by isolated rat renal brush border membranes. *Pflugers Arch* 1982;395:159–61.

267. Lang RP, Yanagawa N, Nord EP, Sakhrani L, Lee SH, Fine LG. Nucleotide inhibition of phosphate transport in the renal proximal tubule. *Am J Physiol* 1983;245:F263–71.

268. Tenenhouse HS, Chu YL. Hydrolysis of nicotinamide adenine dinucleotide by purified renal brush border membranes. *Biochem J* 1982;204:635–8.

269. Braun-Werness JL, Jackson BA, Werness PG, Dousa TP. Binding of nicotinamide adenine dinucleotide by the renal brush

border membrane fraction from rat kidney cortex. *Biochim Biophys Acta* 1983;732:553–61.

270. Brendt TJ, Knox FG, Kempson SA, Dousa TP. Nicotinamide adenine dinucleotide and renal response to parathyroid hormone. *Endocrinology* 1981;108:2005–7.

271. Hammerman MR, Corpus VM, Morrissey JJ. NAD+-induced inhibition of phosphate transport in canine renal brush border membranes. Mediation through a process other than or in addition to NAD+ hydrolysis. *Biochim Biophys Acta* 1983;732:110–6.

272. Kempson SA, Colon-Otero G, Ou SY, Turner ST, Dousa TP. Possible role of nicotinamide adenine dinucleotide as an intracellular regulator of renal transport of phosphate in the rat. *J Clin Invest* 1981;67:1347–60.

273. Kempson SA, Curthoys NP. NAD+-dependent ADP-ribosyltransferase in renal brush border membranes. *Am J Physiol* 1983;245:C449–56.

274. Turner ST, Kiebzak GM, Dousa TP. Mechanism of glucocorticoid effect on renal transport of phosphate. *Am J Physiol* 1982;243:C227–36.

275. Rasmussen HD, Goodman BP, Friedmann N, Allen JE, Kurokawa K. Ionic control of metabolism. In: Greep RO, Astwood EB, eds. *Handbook of physiology. Endocrinology.* Washington, DC, American Physiology Society, 1976;7:225–64.

276. Al-Mahrouq HA, McAteer JA, Kempson SA. Cholera toxin action on rabbit renal brush border membranes inhibits phosphate transport. *Biochim Biophys Acta* 1988;981:200–6.

277. Gmaj P, Biber J, Angielski S, Stange G, Murer H. Intravesicular NAD has no effect on sodium-dependent phosphate transport in isolated renal brush border membrane vesicles. *Pflugers Arch* 1984;400:60–5.

278. Baines AD, Ross BD. Gluconeogenesis and phosphate reabsorption in isolated lactate or pyruvate-perfused rat kidneys. *Miner Electrolyte Metab* 1984;10:286–91.

279. Yanagawa N, Nagami GT, Jo OK, Iemasu J, Kurokawa K. Dissociation of gluconeogenesis from fluid and phosphate reabsorption in isolated rabbit proximal tubules. *Kidney Int* 1984;25:869–73.

280. Yanagawa N, Nagami GT, Kurokawa K. Cytosolic redox potential and phosphate transport in the proximal tubule of the rabbit. A study in the isolated perfused tubules. *Miner Electrolyte Metab* 1985;11:57–61.

281. Suzuki M, Capparelli AW, Jo OK, Yanagawa N. Thiol redox and phosphate transport in renal brush-border membrane. Effect of nicotinamide. *Biochim Biophys Acta* 1990;1021:85–90.

282. Molitoris BA. Membrane fluidity: Measurement and relationship to solute transport. *Semin Nephrol* 1987;7:61–71.

283. LeGrimellec C, Carriere S, Cardinal J, Giocondi MC. Fluidity of brush border and basolateral membranes from human kidney cortex. *Am J Physiol* 1983;245:F227–31.

284. Molitoris BA, Simon FR. Renal cortical brush border and basolateral membranes: cholesterol and phospholipid composition and relative turnover. *J Membr Biol* 1985;83:207–15.

285. Molitoris BA, Alfrey AC, Harris RA, Simon FR. Renal apical membrane cholesterol and fluidity in regulation of phosphate transport. *Am J Physiol* 1985;249:F12–9.

286. Kurnik BRC, Huskey M, Hruska KA. 1,25-Dihydroxycholexcalciferol stimulates renal phosphate transport by directly altering membrane phosphatidylcholine composition. *Biochim Biophys Acta* 1987;917:81–5.

287. Maack T, Park CH, Camargo MJF. In: Seldin DW, Giebisch G, eds. *The kidney, physiology and pathophysiology.* New York: Raven Press, 1985;1773–803.

288. Coudrier E, Kerjaschki D, Louvard D. Cytoskeleton organization and submembranous interactions in intestinal and renal brush borders. *Kidney Int* 1988;34:309–20.

289. Schwartz GJ, Al-Awqati Q. Carbon dioxide causes exocytosis of vesicles containing H+ pumps in isolated perfused proximal and collecting tubules. *J Clin Invest* 1985;75:1638–44.

290. Kempson SA, Ying AL, McAteer JA, Murer H. Endocytosis and Na+/solute cotransport in renal epithelial cells. *J Biol Chem* 1989;264:18451–6.

291. Reshkin SJ, Wuarin F, Biber J, Murer H. Parathyroid hormone-induced alterations of protein content and phosphorylation in enriched apical membranes of opossum kidney cells. *J Biol Chem* 1990;265:15261–6.

292. Kempson SA, Helmle C, Abraham MI, Murer H. Parathyroid hormone action on phosphate transport is inhibited by high osmolality. *Am J Physiol* 1990;258:F1336–44.

293. Biber J, Murer H. Na-Pi cotransport in LLC-PK1 cells: fast adaptive response to Pi deprivation. *Am J Physiol* 1985;249:C430–4.

294. Caverzasio J, Brown CDA, Biber J, Bonjour JP, Murer H. Adaptation of phosphate transport in phosphate-deprived LLC-PK1 cells. *Am J Physiol* 1985;248:F122–7.

295. Yanagawa N, Roh D, Jo OD. Intracellular protein transport and the adaptation to phosphate deprivation in OK cells. *J Am Soc Nephrol* 1990;1:736A.

296. Gmaj P, Ghijsen W, Murer H, Carafoli E. Calcium transport in isolated and reconstituted basolateral plasma membranes of rat kidney cortex. In: Bronner F, Peterlik M, eds. *Epithelial calcium and phosphate transport: molecular and cellular aspects.* New York: Alan R. Liss, 1984;337–42.

297. Schwab SJ, Klahr S, Hammerman MR. Na+ gradient-dependent Pi uptake in basolateral membrane vesicles from dog kidney. *Am J Physiol* 1984;246:F663–9.

298. Grinstein S, Turner RJ, Silverman M, Rothstein A. Inorganic anion transport in kidney and intestinal brush border and basolateral membranes. *Am J Physiol* 1980;238:F452–60.

299. Brazy PC, Balaban RS, Gullans SR, Mandel LJ, Dennis VW. Inhibition of renal metabolism. Relative effects of arsenate on sodium, phosphate and glucose transport by the rabbit proximal tubule. *J Clin Invest* 1980;66:1211–21.

300. Brazy PC, Gullans SR, Mandel LJ, Dennis VW. Metabolic requirement for inorganic phosphate by the rabbit proximal tubule. *J Clin Invest* 1982;70:53–62.

301. Brazy PC, McKeown JW, Harris RH, Dennis VW. Comparative effects of dietary phosphate, unilateral nephrectomy, and parathyroid hormone on phosphate transport by the rabbit proximal tubule. *Kidney Int* 1980;17:778–800.

302. Knox FG, Haas JA, Haramati A. Nephron sites of adaptation to changes in dietary phosphate. *Adv Exp Med Biol* 1982;151:13–9.

303. Muhlbauer RC, Bonjour JP, Fleisch H. Tubular localization of adaptation to dietary phosphate in rats. *Am J Physiol* 1977;233:F342–8.

304. Pastoriza-Munoz E, Mishler DR, Lechene C. Effect of phosphate deprivation on phosphate reabsorption in rat nephron: role of PTH. *Am J Physiol* 1983;244:F140–9.

305. Ullrich KJ, Rumrich G, Kloess S. Phosphate transport in the proximal convolution of the rat kidney. I. Tubular heterogeneity, effect of parathyroid hormone in acute and chronic parathyroidectomized animals and effect of phosphate diet. *Pflugers Arch* 1977;372:269–74.

306. Haramati A, Haas JA, Knox FG. Adaptation of deep and superficial nephrons to changes in dietary phosphate intake. *Am J Physiol* 1983;244:F265–9.

307. Gloor HJ, Bonjour JP, Caverzasio J, Fleisch H. Resistance to the phosphaturic and calcemic actions of parathyroid hormone during phosphate depletion. Prevention by 1,25-dihydroxy-vitamin D3. *J Clin Invest* 1979;63:371–7.

308. Steel TH. Renal resistance to parathyroid hormone during phosphate deprivation. *J Clin Invest* 1976;58:1461–4.

309. Hoppe A, Destro M, Knox FG. Effect of NH4Cl on phosphaturic response to PTH in the hamster: dissociation from acidemia. *Am J Physiol* 1980;239:E328–32.

310. Knox FG, Preiss J, Kim JK, Dousa TP. Mechanisms of resistance to the phosphaturic effect of the parathyroid hormone in the hamster. *J Clin Invest* 1977;59:675–83.

311. Caverzasio J, Bonjour JP. Mechanism of rapid phosphate transport adaptation to a single low Pi meal in rat renal brush border membrane. *Pflugers Arch* 1987;409:333–6.

312. Levine BS, Ho K, Hodsman A, Kurokawa K, Coburn JW. Early renal brush border membrane adaptation to dietary phosphorus. *Miner Electrolyte Metab* 1984;10:222–7.

313. Cheng L, Dersch C, Kraus E, Spector D, Sacktor B. Renal adaptation to phosphate load in the acutely thyroparathyroidectomized rat: rapid alteration in brush border membrane phosphate transport. *Am J Physiol* 1984;246:F488–94.

314. Stoll R, Kinne R, Murer H. Effect of dietary phosphate intake on phosphate transport by isolated rat renal brush border vesicles. *Biochem J* 1979;180:465–70.

315. Stoll R, Kinne R, Murer H, Fleisch H, Bonjour JP. Phosphate transport by rat renal brush border membrane vesicles: influence of dietary phosphate, thyroparathyroidectomy, and 1,25-dihydroxy D₃. *Pflugers Arch* 1979;380:47–52.

316. Murer H, Stern H, Burckhardt G, Storelli C, Kinne R. Sodium-dependent transport of inorganic phosphate across the renal brush border membrane. *Adv Exp Med Biol* 1980;128:11–23.

317. Biber J, Brown CD, Murer H. Sodium-dependent transport of phosphate in LLC-PK₁ cells. *Biochim Biophys Acta* 1983;735:325–30.

318. Brown CD, Bodmer M, Biber J, Murer H. Sodium-dependent phosphate transport by apical membrane vesicles from a cultured renal epithelial cell line (LLC-PK₁). *Biochim Biophys Acta* 1984;769:471–8.

319. Biber J, Forgo J, Murer H. Modulation of Na⁺-Pi cotransport in opossum kidney cells by extracellular phosphate. *Am J Physiol* 1988;255:C155–61.

320. Allon M, Rodriguez M, Llach F. Insulin in the acute renal adaptation to dietary phosphate restriction in the rat. *Kidney Int* 1990;37:14–20.

321. Beck N, Webster SK, Reineck HJ. Effect of fasting on tubular phosphorus reabsorption. *Am J Physiol* 1979;237:F241–6.

322. Kempson SA, Shah SV, Werness PG, et al. Renal brush border membrane adaptation to phosphorus deprivation: effects of fasting versus low phosphorus diet. *Kidney Int* 1980;18:36–47.

323. Bank N, Aynedjian S, Weinstein SW. A microperfusion study of phosphate reabsorption by the rat proximal renal tubule. *J Clin Invest* 1974;54:1040–8.

324. Cassola AC, Malnic G. Phosphate transfer and tubular pH during renal stopped flow microperfusion experiments in the rat. *Pflugers Arch* 1977;367:249–55.

325. Ham LL, Kokko JP, Jacobson HR. Effect of luminal pH and HCO₃⁻ on phosphate reabsorption in the rabbit proximal convoluted tubule. *Am J Physiol* 1984;247:F25–34.

326. Baumann K, Rumrich G, Papavassiliou F, Kloss S. pH dependence of phosphate reabsorption in the proximal tubule of rat kidney. *Pflugers Arch* 1975;360:183–7.

327. Quamme GA, Wong NLM. Phosphate transport in the proximal convoluted tubule: effect of intraluminal pH. *Am J Physiol* 1984;246:F323–33.

328. Lang F, Greger R, Knox FG, Oberteithner H. Factors modulating renal handling of phosphate. *Renal Physiol* 1981;4:1–16.

329. Webb RK, Woodhall PB, Tischer CC, Glaubiger G, Neelon FA, Robinson RR. Relationship between phosphaturia and acute hypercapnia in the rat. *J Clin Invest* 60:829–37.

330. Beck N. Effect of metabolic acidosis on renal action of parathyroid hormone. *Am J Physiol* 1975;228:1483–8.

331. Beck N. Effect of metabolic acidosis on renal response to parathyroid hormone in phosphorus deprived rats. *Am J Physiol* 1981;241:F23–7.

332. Kempson SA. Effect of metabolic acidosis on renal brush border membrane adaptation to low phosphate diet. *Kidney Int* 1982;22:225–33.

333. Boross M, Kinsella J, Cheng C, Sacktor B. Glucocorticoid and metabolic acidosis-induced renal transport of inorganic phosphate, calcium and NH₄. *Am J Physiol* 1986;250:F827–33.

334. Kuntziger H, Amiel C, Couette S, Coureau C. Localization of parathyroid hormone independent sodium bicarbonate inhibition of tubular phosphate reabsorption. *Kidney Int* 1980;17:749–55.

335. Zilenovski AM, Kuroda S, Bhat S, Bank DE, Bank N. Effect of sodium bicarbonate on phosphate excretion in acute and chronic PTX rats. *Am J Physiol* 1979;236:F184–91.

336. Quamme GA. Effects of metabolic acidosis, alkalosis and dietary hydrogen ion intake on phosphate transport in the convoluted tubule. *Am J Physiol* 1985;249:F769–79.

337. Steele TH. Bicarbonate induced phosphaturia dependence upon the magnitude of phosphate reabsorption. *Pflugers Arch* 1977;370:291–4.

338. Mizgala CL, Quamme GA. Renal handling of phosphate. *Physiol Rev* 1985;65:431–66.

339. Greenwald I, Gross J. The effect of the administration of a potent parathyroid extract upon the excretion of nitrogen, phosphorus, calcium and magnesium with some remarks on the solubility of calcium phosphate in serum and on the pathogenesis of tetany. *J Biol Chem* 1925;66:217–27.

340. Agus ZS, Puschett JB, Senesky D, Goldberg M. Mode of action of parathyroid hormone and cyclic AMP on renal tubular phosphate reabsorption in the dog. *J Clin Invest* 1971;50:617–26.

341. Agus ZS, Gardner LB, Beck LH, Goldberg M. Effects of parathyroid hormone on renal tubular reabsorption of calcium, sodium and phosphate. *Am J Physiol* 1973;224:1143–8.

342. Wen SF. Micropuncture studies of phosphate transport in the proximal tubule of the dog: the relationship to sodium reabsorption. *J Clin Invest* 1974;53:143–53.

343. Morel F. Sites of hormone action in the mammalian nephron. *Am J Physiol* 1981;240:159–64.

344. Haas JR, Berndt T, Knox FG. Nephron heterogeneity of phosphate reabsorption. *Am J Physiol* 1978;234:F287–300.

345. Goldfarb S. Juxtamedullary and superficial nephron phosphate reabsorption in the cat. *Am J Physiol* 1980;239:F336–42.

346. Dennis VW, Brazy PC. Divalent anion transport in isolated renal tubules. *Kidney Int* 1982;22:498–506.

347. Iino Y, Burg MB. Effect of parathyroid hormone on bicarbonate absorption by proximal tubules in vitro. *Am J Physiol* 1979;236:F387–91.

348. Karlinsky ML, Sagner DS, Kurtzman NA, Pillay VKG. Effect of parathormone and cyclic AMP on renal bicarbonate reabsorption. *Am J Physiol* 1974;227:1226–31.

349. McKinney TD, Myers P. PTH inhibition of bicarbonate transport by proximal convoluted tubules. *Am J Physiol* 1980;239:F127–34.

350. Nagata N, Rasmussen H. Parathyroid hormone, cAMP, Ca⁺⁺ and gluconeogenesis. *Proc Natl Acad Sci USA* 1970;64:368–74.

351. Kurokawa K, Ohno T, Rasmussen H. Ionic control of renal gluconeogenesis. II. The effects of Ca⁺⁺ and H⁺ upon the response to parathyroid hormone and cyclic AMP. *Biochim Biophys Acta* 1973;313:32–41.

352. Yanagawa N, Jo OD. Possible role of calcium in parathyroid hormone actions in rabbit renal proximal tubules. *Am J Physiol* 1986;250:F942–8.

353. Pfeifer U, Guder WG. Stimulation of cellular autophagy by parathyroid hormone and cAMP in isolated tubular fragments from the rats kidney cortex. *Virchows Arch* [B] 1975;19:51–67.

354. Chobanian MC, Hammerman MR. Parathyroid hormone stimulates ammoniagenesis in canine renal proximal tubular segments. *Am J Physiol* 1988;255:F847–52.

355. Chen WYC, Chen A, Rodrigues M, et al. Role of parathyroid hormone in renal ammonia metabolism in uremic rat. *Miner Electrolyte Metab* in press.

356. Bellorin-Font E, Martin KJ. Regulation of the PTH receptor cyclase system of canine kidney: effects of calcium, magnesium and guanine nucleotides. *Am J Physiol* 1981;241:F364–73.

357. Bellorin-Font E, Tamayo J, Martin KJ. Regulation of PTH receptor adenylate cyclase system of canine kidney: influence of Mn²⁺ on effects of Ca²⁺, PTH and GTP. *Am J Physiol* 1982;242:F457–62.

358. Dennis VW, Bello-Reuss E, Robinson RR. Response of phosphate transport to parathyroid hormone in segments of rabbit nephron. *Am J Physiol* 1977;233:F29–38.

359. Angielski S, Drewnowska K, Rybczynska A, Szczepanska-Konkel M. Reversible resistance to the phosphaturic effect of cAMP in lithium treated rats. *Acta Physiol* 1982;33:463–74.

360. Drezner M, Nelson FA, Lebovitz HE. Pseudohypoparathyroidism type II: a possible defect in the reception of the cAMP signal. *N Engl J Med* 1972;289:1056–60.

361. Angielski S, Pempkowiak L, Gmaj P, Hoppe A, Nowicka C. The effect of maleate and lithium on renal function and metabolism. In: Schmidt V, Dubach VC, eds. *Renal metabolism in relation to renal function.* 1976;142–51.

362. Stepinski J, Pawlowska A., Angielski S. Effect of lithium on renal gluconeogenesis. *Acta Biochim Pol* 1984;31:229–40.

363. Stepinski J, Rybczynska A, Angielski S. Inhibition of 2-oxoglutarate metabolism by lithium in the isolated rat kidney cortex tubules. *Acta Biochim Pol* 1984;31:241–49.

364. Yanagawa N, Jo OD. Possible role of calcium in parathyroid hormone action on phosphate transport by rabbit renal brush

border membrane. *Biochem Biophys Res Commun* 1985; 128:278–84.

365. Nishizuka Y. Studies and perspectives of protein kinase C. *Science* 1984;225:1365–70.

366. Hruska KA, Moskowitz D, Esbrit P, Civitelli R, Westbrook S, Huskey M. Stimulation of inositol triphosphate and diacylglycerol production in renal tubular cells by parathyroid hormone. *J Clin Invest* 1987;79:230–9.

367. Goligorsky MS, Loftus D, Hruska KA. Cytoplasmic Ca^{2+} in individual proximal tubular cells in culture: effects of parathyroid hormone. *Am J Physiol* 1986;251:F938–44.

368. Hruska KA, Goligorski M, Scoble J, Tsutsumi M, Westbrook S, Moskowitz D. Effects of parathyroid hormone on cytosolic calcium in renal proximal tubular primary cultures. *Am J Physiol* 1986;251:F188–98.

369. Boneh A, Tenenhouse HS. Protein kinase C in mouse kidney: subcellular distribution and endogenous substrates. *Biochem Cell Biol* 1988;66:262–72.

370. Caverzasio J, Rizzoli R, Bonjour JP. Sodium dependent phosphate transport inhibited by parathyroid hormone and cyclic AMP stimulation in an opossum kidney cell line. *J Biol Chem* 1986;261:3233–7.

371. Malmstrom K, Murer H. Parathyroid hormone inhibits phosphate transport in OK cells but not in LLC-PK$_1$ and JTC-12.P3 cells. *Am J Physiol* 1986;251:C23–31.

372. Quamme G, Biber J, Murer H. Sodium phosphate cotransport in OK cells: inhibition by PTH and adaptation to low phosphate. *Am J Physiol* 1989;257:F967–73.

373. Cole JA, Eber SL, Poelling RE, Thorne PK, Forte LR. A dual mechanism for regulation of kidney phosphate transport by parathyroid hormone. *Am J Physiol* 1987;253:E221–7.

374. Cole JA, Forte LR, Eber S, Thorne PK, Poelling RE. Regulation of sodium dependent phosphate transport by parathyroid hormone in opossum kidney cells: adenosine 3'5'-monophosphate dependent and independent mechanisms. *Endocrinology* 1988;122:2981–9.

375. Nakai M, Kinoshita Y, Fukase M, Fujita T. Phorbol esters inhibit phosphate uptake in opossum kidney cells: a model of proximal tubular cells. *Biochem Biophys Res Commun* 1987;145:303–8.

376. Malmstrom K, Stange G, Murer H. Intracellular cascades in the parathyroid hormone dependent regulation of Na$^+$/phosphate cotransport in OK cells. *Biochem J* 1988;251:207–13.

377. Cole JA, Forte LR, Krause WJ, Thorne PK. Clonal sublines that are morphologically and functionally distinct from parental OK cells. *Am J Physiol* 1989;256:F672–9.

378. Miyauchi A, Dobre V, Rickmeyer M, Cole J, Forte L, Hruska KA. Stimulation of transient elevations in cytosolic Ca^{2+} is related to inhibition of Pi transport in OK cells. *Am J Physiol* 1990;259:F485–93.

379. Dousa TP, Duarte CG, Knox FG. Effect of colchicine on urinary phosphate and regulation by parathyroid hormone. *Am J Physiol* 1976;231:61–5.

380. Stoll R, Kinne R, Murer H, Fleisch H, Bonjour JP. Phosphate transport by rat renal brush border membrane vesicles: influence of dietary phosphate, thyroparathyroidectomy and 1,25-dihydroxyvitamin D$_3$. *Pflugers Arch* 1979;380:47–52.

381. Bonjour JP, Preston C, Fleisch H. Effect of 1,25-dihydroxyvitamin D$_3$ on the renal handling of Pi in the thyroparathyroidectomized rats. *J Clin Invest* 1977;60:1419–28.

382. Gloor HJ, Bonjour JP, Caversazio J, Fleisch H. Resistance to the phosphaturic and calcemia actions of parathyroid hormone during phosphate depletion: prevention by 1,25-dihydroxyvitamin D$_3$. *J Clin Invest* 1979;63:371–7.

383. Elganish A, Rifkind J, Sacktor B. In vitro effects of vitamin D3 on the phospholipids of isolated renal brush border membranes. *J Membr Biol* 1983;72:85–91.

384. Lang F. Renal handling of calcium and phosphate. *Klin Wochenschr* 1980;58:985–1003.

385. Bonjour JP, Preston C, Fleisch H. Effect of 1,25-dihydroxyvitamin D3 on the renal handling of Pi: effect of dietary Pi and diphosphates. *J Clin Invest* 1977;60:1419–28.

386. Corvilain J, Abramow M. Some effects of human growth hormone on renal hemodynamics and on tubular phosphate transport in man. *J Clin Invest* 1962;41:1230–5.

387. Corvilain J, Abramow M. Effect of growth hormone on tubular transport of phosphate in normal and parathyroidectomized dogs. *J Clin Invest* 1964;43:1608–12.

388. Caverzasio J, Bonjour JP, Fleisch H. Tubular handling of Pi in young, growing and adult rats. *Am J Physiol* 1982;242:F705–10.

389. Caverzasio J, Faundez R, Fleisch H, Bonjour JP. Tubular adaptation to Pi restriction in hypophysectomized rats. *Pflugers Arch* 1981;392:17–21.

390. Lee DBN, Brautbar N, Walling MW, et al. Role of growth hormone in experimental phosphate deprivation in the rat. *Calcif Tissue Int* 1980;32:105–12.

391. Spanos E. Effect of growth hormone on vitamin D metabolism. *Nature* 1978;273:246–7.

392. Hammerman MR, Karl IE, Hruska KA. Regulation of canine renal vesicle Pi transport by growth hormone and parathyroid hormone. *Biochim Biophys Acta* 1980;603:322–35.

393. Adams PH. Effects of hyperthyroidism on bone and mineral metabolism in man. *Q J Med* 1967;36:1–15.

394. Bijvoet OLM, Majoor CLH. The renal tubular reabsorption of phosphate in thyrotoxicosis. *Clin Chim Acta* 1965;11:181–3.

395. Harden RM. Phosphate excretion and parathyroid function in thyrotoxicosis. *J Endocrinol* 1964;28:281–8.

396. Bommer J, Bonjour JP, Ritz E, Fleisch H. Parathyroid independent change in renal handling of phosphate in hyperthyroid rats. *Kidney Int* 1979;15:325–34.

397. Noronha-Blob L, Lowe V, Sacktor B. Stimulation by thyroid hormone of phosphate transport in primary cultured renal cells. *J Cell Physiol* 1988;137:95–101.

398. Espinosa RE, Keller MJ, Yusufi ANK, Dousa TP. Effect of thyroxine administration on phosphate transport across renal cortical brush border membrane. *Am J Physiol* 1984;246:F133–9.

399. Kinsella J, Sacktor B. Thyroid hormones increase Na$^+$-H$^+$ exchange activity in renal brush border membranes. *Proc Natl Acad Sci USA* 1985;82:3606–10.

400. Yusufi ANK, Murayama N, Keller MJ, Dousa TP. Modulatory effect of thyroid hormones on uptake of phosphate and other solutes across luminal brush border membrane of kidney cortex. *Endocrinology* 1985;116:2438–49.

401. Durasin I, Frick A, Neuweg M. Glucocorticoid induced inhibition of the reabsorption inorganic phosphate in the proximal tubule in the absence of parathyroid hormone. *Renal Physiol* 1984;7:115–23.

402. Freiberg JM, Kinsella J, Sacktor B. Glucocorticoids increase the Na$^+$-H$^+$ exchange and decrease the Na$^+$-gradient dependent phosphate uptake system in renal brush border membrane vesicles. *Proc Natl Acad Sci USA* 1982;79:4932–6.

403. Ritz E, Kreusser W, Bommer J. Effects of hormones other than PTH on renal handling of phosphate. In: Massry SG, Fleisch H, eds. *Renal handling of phosphate.* New York: Plenum, 1980;137–95.

404. Hammerman MR, Rogers S, Hansen VA, Gavin JR. Insulin stimulates Pi transport in brush border vesicles from proximal tubular segments. *Am J Physiol* 1984;247:E616–24.

405. Hammerman MR. Interaction of insulin with renal proximal tubular cell. *Am J Physiol* 1985;249:F1–11.

406. Anderson JB, Talmage RV. The effect on calcium infusion and calcitonin on plasma phosphate in sham operated and thyroparathyrodectomized dogs. *Endocrinology* 1973;93:1222–6.

407. Abraham MI, McAteer JA, Kempson SA. Insulin stimulates phosphate transport in opossum kidney epithelial cells. *Am J Physiol* 1990;258:F1592–8.

408. Zalups RK, Knox FG. Calcitonin decreases the renal tubular capacity for phosphate reabsorption. *Am J Physiol* 1983;245:F345–8.

409. Yusufi ANK, Berndt TJ, Murayama N, Knox FG, Dousa TP. Calcitonin inhibits Na$^+$ gradient dependent phosphate uptake across renal brush border membranes. *Am J Physiol* 1987;252:F598–604.

410. Burnett JC, Granger JP, Opgenorth TJ. Effects of synthetic atrial natriuretic factor on renal function and renin release. *Am J Physiol* 1984;247:F863–6.

411. Hammond TG, Haramati A, Knox FG. Synthetic atrial natriuretic factor decreases renal tubular phosphate reabsorption in rats. *Am J Physiol* 1985;249:F315–8.

412. Hammond TG, Yusufi ANK, Knox FG, Dousa TP. Administration of atrial natriuretic factor inhibits sodium-coupled transport in proximal tubules. *J Clin Invest* 1985;75:1983–9.

413. Yusufi ANK, Hammond TG, Dousa TP, Knox FG. Effect of atrial natriuretic factor on brush border membrane transport of phosphate in phosphate deprived rats. *Biochem Pharmacol* 1988;37:4027–9.

414. Ortola FV, Ballermann BJ, Brenner BM. Endogenous ANP augments fractional excretion of Pi, Ca and Na in rats with reduced renal mass. *Am J Physiol* 1988;255:F1091–7.

415. Kenny AD. Effect of catecholamines on serum calcium and phosphorus levels in intact and parathyroidectomized rats. *Naunyn Schmiedebergs Arch Pharmacol* 1964;248:144–52.

416. Massara F, Camanni F. Propranolol block of adrenalin induced hypophosphatemia in man. *Clin Sci* 1970;38:245–50.

417. Morey ER, Kenny AD. Effects of catecholamines on urinary calcium and phosphorus in intact and parathyroidectomized rats. *Endocrinology* 1964;75:78–85.

418. Cuche JL, Marchand GR, Greger RF, Lang FC, Knox FG. Phosphaturic effect of dopamine in dogs: possible role of intrarenally produced dopamine in phosphate regulation. *J Clin Invest* 1976;58:71–6.

419. Szenasi G, Bencsath P, Lehoczy E, Takacs L. Tubular transport and urinary excretion of phosphate after renal denervation in the anesthetized rat. *Am J Physiol* 1981;240:F481–6.

420. Frick A. Reabsorption of inorganic phosphate in the rat kidney. I. Saturation of transport mechanism. II. Suppression of fractional phosphate reabsorption due to expansion of extracellular fluid volume. *Pflugers Arch* 1968;304:351–64.

421. Frick A. Mechanism of inorganic phosphate diuresis secondary to saline infusion in the rat. *Pflugers Arch* 1969;313:106–22.

422. Massry SG, Coburn JW, Kleeman CR. The influence of extracellular volume expansion on renal phosphate reabsorption in the dog. *J Clin Invest* 1969;48:1237–45.

423. Suki WN, Martinez-Maldonado M, Rouse D, Terry A. Effect of expansion of extracellular fluid volume on renal phosphate handling. *J Clin Invest* 1969;48:1888–94.

424. Beck LH, Goldberg M. Mechanism of the blunted phosphaturia in saline loaded thyroparathyroidectomized dogs. *Kidney Int* 1974;6:18–23.

425. Gradowska L, Caglar S, Rutherford E, Harter H, Slatopolski E. On the mechanism of the phosphaturia of extracellular fluid volume expansion in the dog. *Kidney Int* 1973;3:230–7.

426. Maesaka JK, Levitt MF, Abramson RG. Effect of saline infusion on phosphate transport in intact and thyroparathyroidectomized rats. *Am J Physiol* 1973;225:1421–9.

427. Schneider EG, Goldsmith RS, Arnaud CD, Knox FG. Role of parathyroid hormone in the phosphaturia of extracellular fluid volume expansion. *Kidney Int* 1975;7:317–24.

428. Frick A. Proximal tubular reabsorption of inorganic phosphate during saline infusion in the rat. *Am J Physiol* 1972;223:1034–40.

429. Puschett JB, Agus ZS, Senesky D, Goldberg M. Effects of saline loading and aortic obstruction on proximal phosphate transport. *Am J Physiol* 1972;223:851–7.

430. Poujeol P, Chabardes D, Roinel M, de Rouffignac C. Influence of extracellular fluid volume expansion on magnesium, calcium and phosphate handling along the rat nephron. *Pflugers Arch* 1976;365:203–11.

431. Pastoriza-Munoz E, Colindres RE, Lassiter WE, Lechene C. Effect of state of hydration on segmental phosphate reabsorption in rat nephron. *Min Elect Metab* 1980;4:246–57.

432. Beck LH, Goldberg M. Effects of acetazolamide and parathyroidectomy on renal transport of sodium, calcium and phosphate. *Am J Physiol* 1973;224:1136–42.

433. Fulop M, Brazeau P. The phosphaturic effect of sodium bicarbonate and acetazolamide in dogs. *J Clin Invest* 1968;47:983–91.

434. Puschett JB, Goldberg M. The acute effects of furosemide on acid and electrolyte excretion in man. *J Lab Clin Med* 1968;71:666–77.

435. Eknoyan G, Suki WN, Martinez-Maldonado M. Effect of diuretics on urinary excretion of phosphate, calcium and magnesium in thyroparathyroidectomized dogs. *J Lab Clin Med* 1970;76:257–66.

436. Rodriguez HJ, Walls J, Yates J, Klahr S. Effect of acetazolamide on the urinary excretion of cyclic AMP and on the activity of renal adenylate cyclase. *J Clin Invest* 1974;53:122–30.

437. Arruda JAL, Richardson JM, Wolfson JA, Nascimento L, Rademacher DR, Kurtzman NA. Lithium administration and phosphate excretion. *Am J Physiol* 1976;231:1140–6.

438. Sinha PK, Allen DO, Cleaner SF, Bell NH. Effect of acetazolamide on the renal excretion in hypoparathyroidism and pseudohypoparathyroidism. *J Lab Clin Med* 1977;89:1188–97.

439. Besarb A, Silva P, Ross B, Epstein FH. Bicarbonate and sodium reabsorption by the isolated perfused kidney. *Am J Physiol* 1975;228:1525–30.

440. Fernandez PC, Puschett JB. Proximal tubular action of metolazone and chlorothiazide. *Am J Physiol* 1973;225:954–61.

441. Lee DBN, Kurokawa K. Physiology of phosphorus metabolism. In: Maxwell MH, Kleeman CR, eds. *Clinical Disorders of Fluid and Electrolyte Metabolism.* New York: McGraw-Hill, 1987; 245–95.

442. Haas JA, Larson MV, Marchand GR, Lang FC, Greger FC, Knox FG. Phosphaturic effect of furosemide: role of PTH and carbonic anhydrase. *Am J Physiol* 1977;232:F105–10.

443. Nizet A. Excretion and tubular reabsorption of sodium, glucose and phosphate by isolated dog kidneys. Influence of blood dilution. *Pflugers Arch* 1972;36:267.

444. Maesaka JK, Berger ML, Bornia ME, Abramson RG, Levitt MF. Effect of mannitol on phosphate transport in intact and thyroparathyroidectomized rats. *J Lab Clin Med* 1976;87:680–91.

445. Hiatt HH, Thompson DD. Some effects of intravenously administered calcium on inorganic phosphate metabolism. *J Clin Invest* 1957;36:573–80.

446. Eisenberg E. Effects of serum calcium level and parathyroid extracts on phosphate and calcium excretion in hypoparathyroid patients. *J Clin Invest* 1965;44:942–6.

447. Goldman R, Bassett SH. Effect of intravenous calcium gluconate upon the excretion of calcium and phosphorus in patients with idiopathic hypoparathyroidism. *J Clin Endocrinol Metab* 1954;14:278.

448. Amiel C, Kuntziger H, Couette, S, Coureau C, Bergounioux N. Evidence for a parathyroid hormone independent calcium modulation of phosphate transport along the nephron. *J Clin Invest* 1976;57:256–63.

449. Rouse D, Suki WN. Calcium mediated phosphate transport in proximal convoluted tubule of the rabbit. *Miner Electrolyte Metab* 1983;9:178.

450. Rosenbaum JL. Effect of sudden blood calcium depletion on phosphorus excretion. *Endocrinology* 1964;74:266–72.

451. Cuche JL, Ott CE, Marchand GR, Knox FG. Lack of effect of hypocalcemia on renal phosphate handling. *J Lab Clin Med* 1976;88:271–5.

452. Peraino RA, Suki WN. Influence of calcium on renal handling of phosphate. In: Massry SG, Fleisch H, eds. *Renal handling of phosphate.* New York: Plenum Press, 1980;287–306.

453. Caverzasio J, Bonjour JP. Influence of calcium on phosphate transport in cultured kidney epithelium. *Am J Physiol* 1988;254:F217–22.

454. Bijvoet OLM. Indices for the measurements of the renal handling of phosphate. In: Massry SG, Fleisch H, eds. *Renal handling of phosphate.* New York: Plenum Press, 1980;1–37.

Disorders of Bone and Mineral Metabolism,
edited by Fredric L. Coe and Murray J. Favus,
© 1992 by Raven Press, Ltd. All rights reserved.

CHAPTER 2

Regulation of Magnesium Excretion

Christian de Rouffignac

Magnesium plays an important part in the life of organisms by its participation in many biological events: it acts as a cofactor to enzymatic reactions, enters into bone mineralization, or forms complexes with intra- and extracellular proteins. The factors that are involved in the maintenance of magnesium balance are not fully understood. It is clear, however, that the kidneys play an important role in these homeostatic mechanisms. As with the other constituents of body fluids, the kidneys adapt (through hormonal and nonhormonal controls) the excretion of magnesium to the variations in intake. During magnesium deprivation, the kidneys reabsorb most of the filtered load while the magnesium delivery into urine falls to very low levels; however, during high dietary magnesium intake, the excretion of magnesium is increased to maintain the concentration in body fluids.

For a long time, studies on the renal handling of magnesium were hampered by the lack of microanalytical methods applicable at the tubular level. A decisive impetus was given when it became possible to determine the magnesium content in volumes of biological fluids in the range of nanoliters. This was achieved at the end of the 1960s by the establishment of a new methodology using an electron probe (65,85,86), which made it possible to measure simultaneously the various concentrations of the most important cations of the *milieu interieur,* including magnesium. This was a decisive bit of progress, since the technique was sensitive enough to be applied to the analysis of fluid microsamples collected either in vivo or in vitro by microperfusion of isolated nephron segments.

Several reviews have been devoted to the renal handling of magnesium (57,75,78,80,81,82,105,107). Since the publication of these articles, new information regarding the specific sites and regulation of magnesium transport have become available. In the present chapter, these new observations will be integrated into the general framework of renal magnesium handling, which will first be considered in the normal laboratory animal (either young, adult, or senescent) and also in the "wild" animal. Subsequently, the effects of several nonhormonal factors (such as alteration of Mg, Ca, phosphate, NaCl, acid–base, and water balance) on renal magnesium handling will be considered. In a final section, the influence of hormones, essentially peptide hormones, on Mg transport will be examined.

THE RENAL HANDLING OF MAGNESIUM

Glomerular Filtration

Figure 1 shows the main sites of transport of magnesium along the rat nephron. In the final urine, 5–20% of filtered magnesium remains, indicating that up to 95% of filtered magnesium can be reabsorbed by the nephrons.

Plasma magnesium is filtered by the glomeruli. Part, however, is bound to non-ultrafilterable proteins (59). The fraction of total plasma magnesium that is filtered by the glomerular membranes was experimentally determined by collecting the fluid in Bowman's capsule and comparing its magnesium content to that simultaneously collected in the arterial plasma (13,50). These experiments, done on Munich Wistar rats in which some of the glomeruli were accessible at the kidney surface, indicated that approximately 70% of the plasma magnesium is ultrafilterable. Of this diffusible magnesium, 70% is thought to be in the ionic form, with the remaining magnesium being complexed—particularly to oxalate, phosphate, and citrate ions (107).

C. de Rouffignac: Département de Biologie Cellulaire et Moleculaire, Service de Biologie Cellulaire, Centre d'Études Nucléaires de Saclay, F-91191 Gif-Sur-Yvette, France.

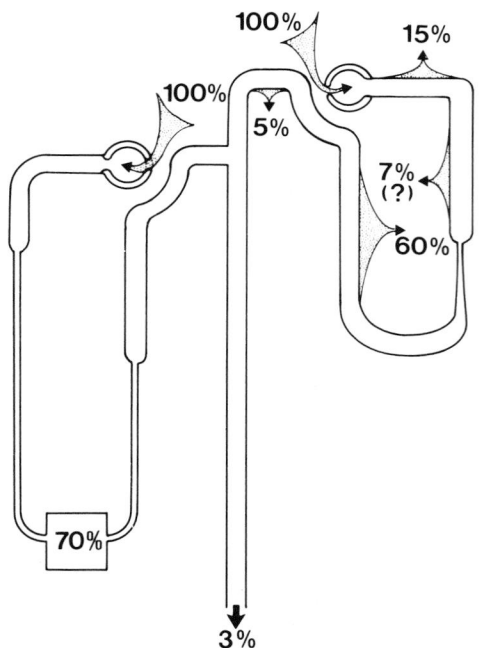

FIG. 1. Tubular handling of magnesium. A superficial nephron and a juxtamedullary nephron are schematically depicted. Arrows represent net reabsorptive fluxes from the lumen to the interstitial space. The net fluxes are expressed as percentages of the amounts of filtered magnesium. At the tip of the loop of the juxtamedullary nephron is indicated the fraction of the filtered magnesium remaining at this site. Data from different studies carried out on the rat in our laboratory (32–37,51–54,89).

Proximal Tubule

The amount of solutes transported through the epithelium—the transepithelial net flux—is the algebraic sum of the fluxes (influx directed from the apical to the baso-

lateral face, and outflux or backflux directed in the reverse direction) that traverse either the cells (transcellular fluxes) or the intercellular spaces (paracellular fluxes).

Only the proximal convoluted tubule (but not the straight tubule) is accessible to micropuncture. Morel et al. (66) were the first to demonstrate in the rat that magnesium reabsorption along this tubule is very limited. This observation has been repeatedly confirmed (4,14,34,51–54,69,97), and it is now generally admitted that only a very small fraction of filtered magnesium (approximately 10–15%) is reabsorbed along the proximal convoluted tubule in the rat. A limited magnesium reabsorption has also been found in other species studied so far, including the rabbit (83), the dog (64,114–116), the golden hamster (17,42), the monkey (117), and in desert rodent species such as the sand rat (94) (*Psammomys obesus*), the pocket mouse (10), and the goundi (*Ctenodactylus valii*) (88).

The magnesium concentration rises along the proximal tubule as a function of water removal (79). This is due to the low permeability to magnesium of the paracellular pathway (12,67,79,90) and is likely due to the low density of magnesium transport systems in the cellular membranes. As indicated in Table 1, the magnesium handling in this nephron segment is very different from that of sodium, of which 60% of the filtered amount is reabsorbed at the end of the proximal convoluted tubule, accompanied by an equivalent amount of water. The magnesium handling is also different from that of calcium. Clearly, calcium is reabsorbed along the proximal tubule in the rat. It is difficult, however, to ascertain the exact fluid-over-plasma ultrafiltrate (F/UF) value reached by calcium at the proximal end tubule site, and more generally at any site along the nephron, partly because of the uncertainty of its concentration in the ultra-

TABLE 1. *Reabsorption of water, Na, Cl, Ca and Mg along the nephron in the rat during antidiuresis*[a]

Tubular sites	F/P, In	F/UF, Na	F/UF, Cl	F/UF, Ca	F/UF, Mg	Fractional deliveries				
						H₂O	Na	Cl	Ca	Mg
End proximal[b]	2.25	0.96	1.15	*1.3*	1.9	44	43	51	*58*	85
Hairpin turn[c]	5.0	1.5	2.0	*2.5*	3.5	20	40	50	*50*	70
Early distal[d]	6.0	0.3	0.4	*0.4*	0.5	17	5.0	6.5	*6.5*	8.5
Late distal[d]	15.0	0.2	0.3	*0.4*	0.6	7.0	1.0	2.0	*2.5*	3.5
Urine[b–d]	200	0.4	0.6	*0.6*	6.0	0.5	0.2	0.3	*0.3*	3.0

[a] This table gives the ratio of fluid (F = either tubular fluid or final urine) to plasma (P) or plasma ultrafiltrate (UF) concentrations, for inulin (In) or the indicated ions. "Fractional deliveries" expresses the amounts of water or electrolytes delivered at the site considered, as a function of filtered amounts. *Hairpin turn:* These values were obtained from juxtamedullary nephrons at the tip of Henle's loop. The other values came from superficial nephrons. The fact that the F/P$_{In}$ was lower at the hairpin turn of these nephrons than at the early distal site of superficial nephrons does not mean that some water is reabsorbed along the ascending limb; more likely, it means that the F/P at the end proximal site (i.e., at the end of the pars recta) is lower in the juxtamedullary nephrons than in the superficial ones (see discussion in Ref. 35). The calcium parameters are given in italics to indicate that the determinations of concentration in plasma ultrafiltrate are generally not as accurate as those of the other ions. These parameters could be overestimated.
[b] Data from Ref. 51.
[c] Data from Ref. 35.
[d] Data from Ref. 33.

filtrate samples. This uncertainty results from the use of micro-ultrafiltration devices, necessitated by the relatively small volume of plasma samples collected in the rat (50), which are not as accurate as those used for ultrafiltrating macrosamples. It seems, however, that Ca concentration at the proximal end tubule site may be subject to variation according to the physiological conditions (78,105).

In the young rat (aged 13–15 days), in contrast to the adult, 50–60% of filtered magnesium is reabsorbed in the proximal tubule, along with sodium and water (55). This fraction progressively declines as a function of age in the case of magnesium, but not in the case of sodium or of water. The most probable explanation for the decrease in proximal tubule permeability to magnesium is that it might be correlated with maturational changes in the paracellular permeability at the tight junction level. In the senescent rat, fractional magnesium reabsorption appears to be unchanged compared to the adult rat (21), fractional magnesium delivery at the end proximal site being analogous in the 10- and 30-month-old rats.

Henle's Loop

General Characteristics of Magnesium Transport in Henle's Loop

Information regarding Henle's loop can be obtained in vivo by micropuncture of either superficial nephrons (at the proximal end and early distal sites) or juxtamedullary nephrons (in the thin descending and ascending limbs accessible at the surface of the papilla in some species such as desert rodents or young rats). In vitro, one can study the functions of individual segments by perfusion of tubules obtained by microdissection.

Micropuncture experiments indicate that a large fraction, approximately 60%, of the filtered magnesium is reabsorbed in the short Henle's loops in all the species thus far studied (4,10,14,17,29,34,42,51–54,69,70,84, 88,89,94,97,117). At the hairpin turn of the long-looped nephrons of the rat, the fraction of filtered magnesium remaining (16,35–37,48,96) is very close to that found at the proximal end tubule of superficial nephrons (51). If we assume that the proximal convoluted tubule of deep nephrons is as poorly permeable to magnesium as that of the superficial nephrons, it is likely that the net movements of magnesium along the descending limb are very limited. By analogy with sodium and water transport values, which in the proximal straight tubule are only half of those measured in the proximal convoluted tubule, it is probable that the fraction of filtered magnesium transported in the proximal straight tubule is smaller than that transported in the proximal convoluted tubule. In vitro microperfusion of isolated segments indicated that in the rabbit proximal straight tubule, magnesium concentration rises with water abstraction, as in the proximal convoluted tubule (83).

To examine the possibility of magnesium entry into the loop, a magnesium-free isotonic saline solution was microperfused at the proximal end tubule in the rat (56). A significant amount of magnesium was present in the fluid collected at the early distal site, with the rate of magnesium influx into the loop being proportional to the perfusion rate. In contrast, Quamme and Dirks (79) failed to detect significant magnesium entry into Henle's loop in rats studied under very similar conditions. We must recognize that in the former experiment, the concentration of magnesium in the collected fluid was as low as 0.12 ± 0.2 mmol·L^{-1}, and it is possible that the sensitivity of analytical technique may explain the discrepancies between the two studies. In some instances, such as after magnesium loading in the rat (15), and in some other rodents, such as the sand rat (94), the data strongly suggest that a significant amount of magnesium can be added to the fluid reaching the hairpin-turn of the long loops, indicating that there is a segment permeable to magnesium along the descending limb. The precise site of magnesium addition, however, remains to be determined.

Integration of segmental functions to account for Mg^{2+} transport in Henle's loop is still impossible because the magnesium transport capacities of the thin descending and ascending limbs are totally unknown. As far as the thick ascending limb is concerned, the picture is now more accurate. The thick ascending limb consists of two portions: the cortical (cTAL) and medullary (mTAL) segments. The mTAL does not reabsorb magnesium in the mouse (3,25,26,113) and rat (M. Imbert-Teboul, B. Mandon, and C. de Rouffignac, unpublished observations). Ca^{2+} reabsorption followed a similar pattern as that of Mg^{2+} in these studies, although one work carried out in the mouse reported a consistent calcium reabsorption in the mTAL (39). The reasons for this discrepancy were discussed elsewhere (3,25,26,113). In the rabbit, however, the mTAL seems to reabsorb some calcium (103).

Mechanisms of Transepithelial Magnesium Transport in the Thick Ascending Limb of Henle's Loop

Magnesium reabsorption across the thick ascending limb epithelium may occur through two pathways: the cellular and transcellular routes. Figure 2 depicts the general characteristics of NaCl and K transport in this epithelium. These are valid for both the cortical and medullary portions (40,43). From these characteristics, it readily emerges that in the cTAL the transcellular route needs the presence of an active step to ensure magnesium transfer from the luminal to the basolateral site. Nothing is known, however, about the transmembrane processes. To date, neither the presence of magnesium channels nor that of a magnesium pump in either membrane has been evidenced.

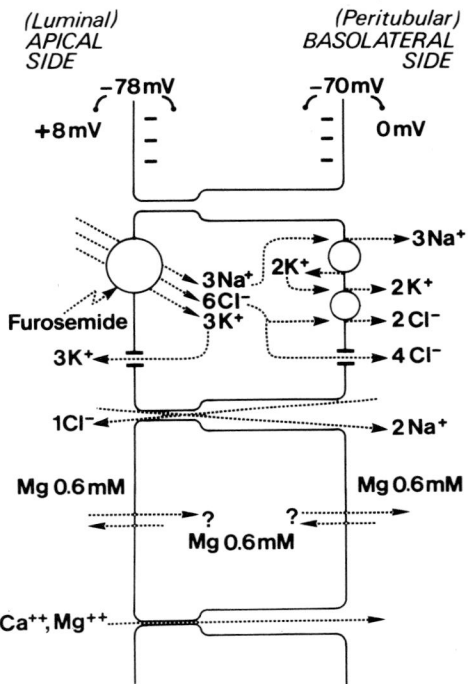

FIG. 2. Cellular mechanisms of Na, Cl, and K transport in the thick ascending limb of Henle's loop. The lumen-positive transepithelial voltage is approximately 8 mV in the rabbit cTAL. The figures indicate the relative values of the fluxes according to Greger (40). "Mg 0.6 mM" indicates the concentration of magnesium ions generally found by micropuncture in the luminal fluid and plasma ultrafiltrate, and the intracellular activity of the magnesium ions as determined by Quamme and Dai (77) on primary cultures of cTAL cells. (Data from Refs. 40 and 77.)

In primary cultures of cTAL cells, however, Quamme and Dai (77) found with a fluorescence method using Mg-Fura 2 that the intracellular magnesium activity was approximately 0.6 mmol·L^{-1}, a value similar to that existing in the culture medium. In cells cultured in low-magnesium media, the intracellular magnesium was around 0.3 mmol·L^{-1}. This was associated with an increase in magnesium transport, in accordance with the process observed in Henle's loop during magnesium deficiency (see section entitled "Factors Decreasing Magnesium Excretion," below). When the cells were placed in high-magnesium media, the intracellular magnesium rose slowly. The refilling of the cell took 6–8 h. According to the authors, this could indicate either (a) a slow entry rate of magnesium, relative to the magnesium pool, or (b) an entry rate matched by a high exit rate. A high exit rate could be maintained for the time necessary for the reversion of the adaptive processes at the time of the cell exposure to low-magnesium media. In any event, these observations indicate that magnesium may penetrate from the extracellular medium into the cytosol. If the refilling process reflects passive cellular entry of magnesium, it is evident that this process is too slow to ac-

count for the magnesium net fluxes measured across cTAL segments (0.5 pmol·min^{-1}·mm^{-1}) (3,25,26,113). If transcellular, such fluxes could refill the cytosol space from zero to 0.6 mmol·L^{-1} within less than 10 s. Of course, such kind of calculation does not take into account the active cellular exit of magnesium that should simultaneously take place, but it emphasizes the magnitude of the difference between the refilling process (6–8 h) and the amplitude of the transepithelial net flux. In fact, the data presently accumulated strongly suggest that magnesium is passively reabsorbed, through the paracellular route.

Shareghi and Agus (101) perfused rabbit cTAL segments in the presence of furosemide to inhibit the activity of the apical Na–2Cl–K cotransport, thereby inhibiting active NaCl transport (see Fig. 2). These authors varied the transepithelial voltage (PD$_{te}$) from +30 mV to −20 mV by using bath-to-lumen or lumen-to-bath Na gradients to generate dilution potentials through the paracellular pathway [permselectivity: PNa$^+$/PCl$^-$ = 1.7 (40)]. With lumen-positive PD$_{te}$, magnesium was reabsorbed from the lumen, whereas with lumen-negative potentials, this ion was secreted into it. The flux-to-voltage relationship indicated that at zero voltage the net transport of magnesium was zero, consistent with passive transport (101).

These studies, however, do not rule out the participation of active processes, because furosemide could also inhibit some active (or secondary active) transport of magnesium as it does for NaCl and K. Nevertheless, if one compares the net magnesium fluxes under control conditions (111) (i.e., in the presence of a PD$_{te}$ generated by active NaCl transport) with those generated by dilution potentials (112) (in the presence of furosemide) of similar magnitude as the control PD$_{te}$, Fig. 3 shows that, for identical PD$_{te}$ values (in absolute terms), the net magnesium fluxes are similar (although of opposite sign), independently of the presence of furosemide. Thus, if any active component of magnesium transport works in parallel to those of the other ions, its participation in the total transepithelial net flux should be very modest, except if some rectification occurs through the paracellular pathway—that is, if the permeability coefficients for magnesium are not identical in both directions.

In the cTAL, the net transport of magnesium and Ca follows very similar patterns in both rabbit (101) and mouse (3,25,26,111,113). Bourdeau and Burg (8) found that in the presence of lumen-negative voltages, calcium was secreted into the lumen of rabbit cTAL segments. In the presence of furosemide, these authors found that the calcium fluxes were strongly dependent on the PD$_{te}$. These data were subsequently confirmed by Shareghi and Agus (101). On the other hand, Suki et al. (104) found in rabbit cTAL that furosemide, although decreasing the PD$_{te}$, did not alter the lumen-to-bath calcium efflux; this finding was not reproduced by Imai (46), who

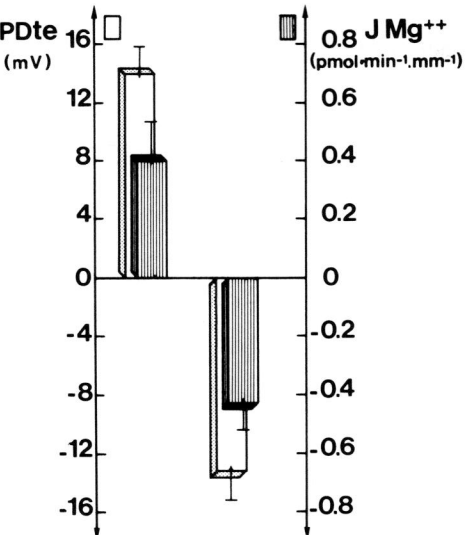

FIG. 3. Voltage dependency of magnesium transport in the mouse cortical thick ascending limb of Henle's loop (cTAL). **Top:** Transepithelial potential difference (PD_{te}) and net reabsorption flux of magnesium (JMg^{++}) measured under control conditions. **Bottom:** PD_{te} and JMg^{++} were measured in the presence of furosemide (10^{-5} M, to inhibit NaCl transport), and PD_{te} was reversed by a dilution potential generated by NaCl gradients (lumen = 150 mmol·L^{-1}, bath = 50 mmol·L^{-1}). (Data from Refs. 111 and 112.)

found that in this species both the lumen-to-bath efflux and the voltage were inhibited by furosemide. Friedman (39) reported that in the mouse cTAL, furosemide, although decreasing the PD_{te} to almost zero, left a substantial net reabsorption of calcium. The literature is thus very confusing. We tend to believe that an active transport process, if it does exist, should participate only moderately in the transepithelial net reabsorption of either calcium or magnesium ions, but further investigations in that domain are clearly warranted. In the rabbit mTAL, the mechanisms of magnesium and calcium transport were never explored. The mouse and rat mTAL do not transport magnesium. The reasons for this remain to be elucidated.

Terminal Nephron Segments

The terminal nephron segments are those located beyond Henle's loop. These segments consist of the distal convoluted tubule (DCT), followed by the connecting tubule and the collecting duct system.

Magnesium transport in the terminal nephron segments has been studied in vivo by micropuncture, essentially in the DCT. Few in vitro data are available.

In vivo, the DCT reabsorbs approximately 5% of the filtered magnesium in the rat (5,32,33,72,79). This amount represents approximately 50–60% of the magne-

sium delivered to the DCT by Henle's loop. It is very likely that a fraction of this reabsorption takes place in the DCT (C. de Rouffignac, unpublished observations). It is undecided whether the connecting tubule reabsorbs a significant amount of magnesium. The reabsorption of magnesium in the DCT is load-dependent (79). Elevation of magnesium delivery to the DCT, either by perfusing artificial solutions (72,79) or by inhibiting magnesium reabsorption in Henle's loop (74), resulted in an increase in magnesium reabsorption. However, the fractional reabsorptions fell significantly for magnesium, whereas it remained unchanged for sodium and calcium (72).

According to Quamme and Dirks (81), distal magnesium reabsorption is close to maximal capacity under normal conditions, whereas that of calcium and sodium is ordinarily unsaturated. The portion of the DCT accessible to micropuncture reabsorbs NaCl, and Ca and secretes K (119). Fractional magnesium reabsorption in the DCT of the rat was found to be similar to NaCl and Ca reabsorption in our laboratory (32,33), whereas it was reported to be two to three times lower than NaCl by Quamme (72). The cellular mechanisms of magnesium reabsorption are totally unknown, because of the heterogeneity of this nephron segment and because of our ignorance about the magnitude of the electrochemical gradient of magnesium across the apical and basolateral membranes. Such is not the case for calcium, which behaves like magnesium along the accessible DCT.

The transport mechanism of calcium in the DCT was recently reviewed by Bronner (11). The salient points are the following: The data of Costanzo and Windhager (22) show that the amount of Ca reabsorbed along the DCT exceeds by two orders of magnitude what could be accounted for by passive diffusion (10 pmol·min^{-1}·mm^{-1} in one case versus 0.13 pmol·min^{-1} in the other) and that calcium is reabsorbed against a transepithelial electrochemical gradient. Thus, some active (transcellular) calcium transport must be present in the DCT cells. Since the cytosol of these cells is electronegative with respect to the apical side, and since intracellular calcium activity is in the nanomolar range whereas it is in the millimolar range in the tubular lumen, calcium entry at the apical side can be purely passive. It does not necessitate a pump, and it is more likely mediated by calcium channels. But the extrusion of calcium at the basolateral site, against an electrochemical gradient of about 100 mV, is necessarily active. The active components at this site could be an Na–Ca exchanger and/or a Ca-ATPase, although their function in the calcium transport by the DCT cells has not been established.

In a recent study, Taniguchi et al. (106) presented several arguments suggesting the presence of an Na–Ca exchanger in the basolateral membrane of cortical collecting tubule (CCT) cells in rat kidney. In the intracellular space, calcium must move from the apical to the basolateral membrane. It is believed that calcium-binding proteins act to ferry calcium across this space (11). All these cellular events remain to be examined not only for calcium but also for magnesium in the DCT and/or the connecting tubule cells.

Transport processes along the collecting duct system can be estimated by comparing the amounts delivered by the connecting tubules to the cortical collecting duct and the amounts recovered in the final urine. However, this is only a very rough method of estimation, since the amounts delivered to the collecting ducts by the deep nephrons, which are inaccessible to micropuncture, are unknown. At any rate, under normal conditions, no important difference was noted between the magnesium remaining at the end distal tubule of superficial nephrons and that in the final urine. This suggests that magnesium transport along the collecting duct system is limited. A microperfusion study of cortical collecting ducts (100) and a micropuncture study along the inner medullary collecting ducts accessible to micropuncture at the surface of the papilla (6,16), indicate that there is no net magnesium transport in these structures, supporting the above conclusion. The fact that the PD_{te} is lumen-negative along the terminal nephron segments [except in the inner stripe portion of the outer medullary collecting tubule, where the Pd_{te} is lumen-positive (see, for example, ref. 91)] could favor passive magnesium secretion towards the tubular lumen. Thus, definitive conclusions about the transport properties of the collecting duct system are not warranted.

FACTORS INFLUENCING MAGNESIUM TRANSPORT ALONG THE NEPHRON

Several factors influence magnesium excretion by the kidney; some of these decrease, whereas others increase, renal magnesium reabsorption. The former factors include hypermagnesemia, hypercalcemia, extracellular fluid volume expansion, diuretics, phosphate depletion, and acute metabolic acidosis, whereas the latter include magnesium depletion and hypocalcemia. The effects of hormones on the magnesium tubular handling will be considered in the next section.

Since the thick ascending limb is a major site of reabsorption for magnesium ions, it is relevant that the main regulatory events take place in Henle's loop. Magnesium transport in the proximal tubule is not significantly affected by the above-mentioned factors. Their influence in the terminal nephron segments is still largely unknown. It is interesting to note, however, that during acute elevation of plasma magnesium, the amounts of magnesium excreted in final urine may exceed those entering the CCT (52,108), suggesting the possibility of some net secretion of magnesium somewhere along the collecting duct system. In one study, the amount of mag-

nesium excreted into urine surpassed that of the amounts filtered at the glomerulus (1). In another study, however, neither secretion nor reabsorption were observed in the terminal segments of rats following elevations of ultrafilterable magnesium (15) which were as high as in the other studies (52,108).

Factors Increasing Magnesium Excretion

Le Grimellec et al. (52) described the influence of magnesium, calcium, and phosphate loadings on the renal and tubular handling of electrolytes, including magnesium, in the rat. Loadings were performed by sustained intravenous infusions during the micropuncture experiments. Following magnesium loading, the fraction of filtered magnesium excreted into the urine increased from 8% to 56%, a considerable increase of magnesium excretion, considering that the magnesium concentration in the plasma ultrafiltrate, and thus in the Bowman's capsule, increased only by a factor of 2. In short, the fraction of filtered magnesium remaining at the proximal end tubule was unchanged by magnesium loading, but that at the early distal tubule site was considerably increased. Thus, the decrease in renal magnesium reabsorption was largely the result of inhibition of magnesium transport in Henle's loop.

During acute calcium loading (53), the micropuncture and clearance data were qualitatively similar to those obtained during acute magnesium loading: There was an associated increase in the fraction of filtered magnesium delivered into the urine (from 10% to 26%), which resulted from an impairment of magnesium reabsorption in the loop. In an in vivo microperfusion study in the rat, Quamme and Dirks (79) observed that when the luminal concentration of magnesium was progressively raised, Henle's loop increased its absolute reabsorption as the luminal magnesium concentration rose (up to 5 mmol · L^{-1}) if the magnesemia were normal, whereas this reabsorption fell considerably when the plasma magnesium concentration was elevated (Fig. 4). According to these authors, hypermagnesemia diminishes magnesium reabsorption in Henle's loop by inhibiting magnesium transport at the peritubular site (79).

From these studies, it is clear that peritubular magnesium alters the reabsorption of this ion in Henle's loop (very probably in the cortical thick ascending limb). To decide whether the alteration is the result of the inhibition of the transcellular or of the paracellular component of this transport, further studies are needed, because no convincing evidence for the existence of a transcellular component is presently available (see section entitled "The Renal Handling of Magnesium," above). In addition, in similar in vivo microperfusion studies (73), as well as in micropuncture studies (53), hypercalcemia was also shown to inhibit magnesium transport (but not

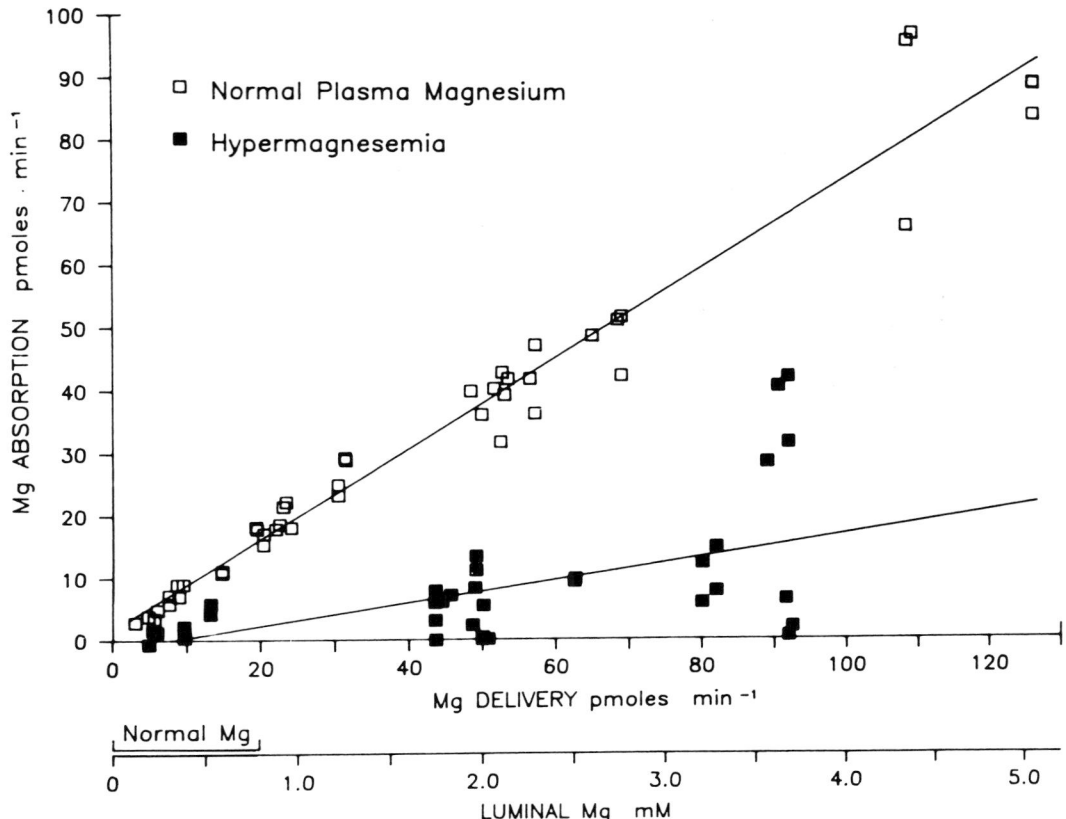

FIG. 4. Effect of luminal magnesium versus peritubular magnesium concentration on net magnesium reabsorption in Henle's loop. Loops were perfused at constant flow rates (25 nL/min) and with solutions containing variable $MgCl_2$ concentrations (0–4 mM) in normal (ultrafilterable Mg 0.55 ± 0.03 mM) or hypermagnesemic (ultrafilterable Mg 3.0 ± 0.2 mM) animals. Absorption was calculated by comparing the delivery rates (perfusion rates × electrolyte concentration) at late proximal tubule with respective deliveries to accessible early distal convoluted tubule. Mg was quantitated by electron microprobe analysis and water absorption with the use of inulin. (Data from Ref 78.)

sodium) transport in Henle's loop. Thus, in vivo, peritubular calcium and magnesium alter magnesium reabsorption in a similar way in the thick ascending limb, by a mechanism acting at the contraluminal side.

At this stage, it is difficult to decide whether or not this inhibition is related to the inhibition of NaCl reabsorption. Shareghi and Agus (101) examined the individual effects of magnesium and calcium in the lumen and in the peritubular medium on the transepithelial net reabsorption fluxes of magnesium and calcium, in isolated perfused cTAL segments of rabbit nephrons. They found that elevation of luminal magnesium increased magnesium transport proportionately, leaving calcium transport unaltered, whereas elevation of peritubular magnesium completely inhibited the magnesium transport, but not the calcium transport. Conversely, elevation of luminal calcium resulted in a proportionate rise of calcium (but not of magnesium) net reabsorption fluxes; elevation of peritubular calcium elicited a marked inhibition of calcium transport, but not magnesium transport. Thus, these in vitro results obtained in the rabbit are at

variance with those obtained in vivo in the rat, which indicated that plasma magnesium or calcium alone can alter *both* magnesium and calcium transports.

During acute phosphate loading, no important changes in magnesium reabsorption along the nephron and no significant changes in magnesium excretion in the final urine were noted (54). Extracellular fluid volume expansion generated by acute hypertonic NaCl loading elicited a significant, although modest, increase in magnesium excretion. This effect was the result of a slight inhibition of magnesium reabsorption along the proximal convoluted tubule and in Henle's loop (69). Administration of furosemide, a loop diuretic known to block the Na–2Cl–K cotransporter present in the luminal membranes of cTAL and mTAL cells, induced a marked diuresis and natriuresis, in a dose-dependent manner, accompanied by an increase in the excretion of magnesium in the urine (27,71,74). This latter effect could result in partial to total inhibition of magnesium transport in the thick ascending limb (according to the concentration of furosemide used; see Fig. 5). In vitro

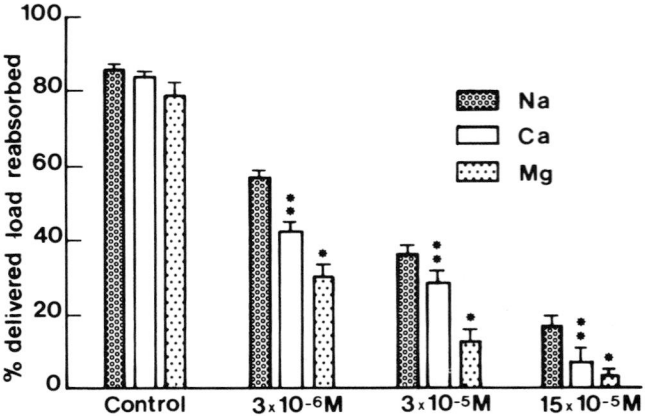

FIG. 5. Dose-dependent effects of intraluminal furosemide on fractional electrolyte reabsorption within rat Henle's loop microperfused in vivo. The loops were perfused from the proximal end site with normal Ringer's solution at 25 nL/min. *Double asterisk: p < 0.05 compared with Na. Single asterisk: p < 0.05 compared with Ca.* (Data from Ref. 74.)

studies were consistent with these findings (112). Dietary phosphate restriction increases magnesium urinary losses, with the defect in magnesium reabsorption occurring in Henle's loop (118). Osmotically active molecules such as mannitol or urea may also inhibit magnesium transport (114,115). Acute acidosis results in increases in magnesium excretion that are reversed by alkali infusion (97).

Finally, it is apparent that every change of Mg transport in Henle's loop is almost entirely reflected in the final urine, as demonstrated by the tight correlation existing between (a) the amount of Mg delivered to the DCT by the loop and (b) the amount of Mg excreted in final urine (31).

Factors Decreasing Magnesium Excretion

The effects of hypomagnesemia and hypocalcemia on magnesium and calcium transport were extensively studied by Quamme and Dirks (81). Briefly, the authors established that during magnesium deficiency of dietary origin the amount of magnesium excreted in the urine decreases to values close to zero (19). In a recent work, Shafik and Quamme (99) reported that the fall in magnesium excretion rate preceded the fall in plasma magnesium concentration. This fall resulted from an enhanced reabsorption of magnesium in Henle's loop. Because the glomerular filtration rate remained constant in these experiments, it appears that the decreases in magnesium excretion during dietary magnesium deficiency result from an increase in magnesium transport. Hypocalcemia also leads to enhanced magnesium reabsorption by the kidney (72). The factor responsible for this stimulation remains to be determined.

HORMONAL CONTROL OF MAGNESIUM TRANSPORT

The nephrons are target sites for many hormones (62), including steroids and hormones stimulating either protein kinase A (cAMP), protein kinase C (Ca, diacylglycerol), or tyrosine kinase (insulin) transduction pathways, among others. Apart from those hormones acting via the cAMP transduction pathway, little is known, at the nephron level, about the effects of the hormones acting through other pathways on magnesium transport.

Proximal Convoluted Tubule

We have seen that the transport of magnesium in this nephron segment is very limited. Neither parathyroid hormone (PTH), glucagon, calcitonin, nor antidiuretic hormone (ADH) modified this situation (5,34,89,95). Kuntziger et al. (49) found in parathyroidectomized rats that magnesium concentration along the PCT rose as a function of water removal, as in normal rats.

Henle's Loop

Henle's loop, and more specifically the thick ascending limb, is a target site for several hormones stimulating the adenylate cyclase system. There are, however, several species differences in this respect.

Table 2 displays the adenylate cyclase activity measured in the presence of various hormones (ADH, glucagon, PTH, calcitonin, and isoproterenol, a β-adrenergic agonist) in the three commonly studied species either (a) in vivo by micropuncture (rat), or (b) in vitro with the microperfusion technique (rabbit, mouse). In the rat and mouse, all five ligands stimulate the cyclase system in the cTAL (3,20,60,62,63). Regarding the mTAL, there are some differences between the two species. This segment is responsive to ADH and glucagon, but not to PTH, in both species, but it is unresponsive to calcitonin in the mouse and to isoproterenol in the rat.

The cyclase responsiveness to hormones (62) in the rabbit is quantitatively different from that recorded in the rat and mouse but shows similarities with regard to sensitivity to ADH and PTH. The rabbit thick ascending limb is unresponsive to isoproterenol (Table 2).

More generally, marked differences may occur among the animal species (64). The V_{max} of the adenylate cyclase response to ADH in the mTAL, relative to that elicited in the medullary collecting tubule (MCT), may largely differ from one species to another. In the hamster and the rat, the maximal response is high and is comparable to that induced in the MCT. It is lower in mouse and jerboa, almost insignificant in the rabbit, and not significantly different from zero in man and dog (98).

Calcitonin stimulates the adenylate cyclase system to

TABLE 2. *Hormonal effects on cyclase responsiveness of isolated segments of rabbit, mouse, and rat cortical and medullary thick ascending limbs of nephron*[a]

Adenylate cyclase activity	Cortical thick ascending limb			Medullary thick ascending limb		
	Rabbit	Mouse	Rat	Rabbit	Mouse	Rat
Basal	0.3	1.1	0.8	0.4	0.7	0.8
ADH	1.0	26.7	7.0	3.7	36.9	27.4
Glucagon	NT	44.3	23.8	NT	37.9	34.6
PTH	4.1	36.0	30.0	NS	NS	NS
Calcitonin	2.8	18.4	24.2	12.6	NS	6.3
Isoproterenol	NS	9.9	6.0	NS	3.9	NS

[a] Adenylate cyclase activities are expressed in $fmol \cdot mm^{-1} \cdot min^{-1}$. They were obtained in the presence of indicated hormones and give the activity due to the hormone (stimulated minus basal activity). NS, not statistically significant; NT, not tested. (Data from Refs. 3, 20, 45, 60, and 62.)

the same extent in the cTAL and mTAL of humans, but to a greater extent in the cTAL than in the mTAL in the rat; in the rabbit, the reverse of the latter situation is true. In the mouse, calcitonin is inactive in the mTAL but active in the cTAL. PTH stimulates the cyclase system in the cTAL but not in the mTAL in all species thus far studied (rat, rabbit, mouse, hamster)—except for humans, in whom this hormone stimulates both nephron segments (64). These differences emphasize the fact that the physiological data obtained in one species may not be entirely valid for another species.

In Vitro Studies

In the mouse, in vitro microperfusion studies with mTAL segments indicated that either arginine vasopressin (AVP) (113), glucagon (25), or isoproterenol (3) [*a fortiori* calcitonin (26), which does not activate the cyclase system] were incapable of inducing a significant increase in magnesium transport in this nephron segment (Fig. 6). In fact, not only magnesium but also calcium transport was unaffected by the hormones, in spite

of marked increases in PD_{te} as well as NaCl transport elicited by either ADH, glucagon, or isoproterenol (3,25,113).

In contrast, all four of the above-mentioned hormones (3,25,111,113), as well as PTH (26), strongly stimulated magnesium (as well as calcium) transport in the cTAL (Fig. 7; in this figure the isoproterenol data are not shown). In the rat, no data are presently available. That PTH stimulates magnesium transport in the rabbit cTAL was demonstrated by Shareghi and Agus (101). Regarding calcium, it is well established that PTH and cAMP analogs stimulate its transport in the rabbit cTAL (9,47,103). Suki and Rouse (103) found that this hormone stimulates calcium transport in the rabbit mTAL but not in the cTAL, whereas the opposite occurs in the mouse (26,110). It seems, therefore, that calcium transport can be stimulated by peptide hormones in cTAL and mTAL segments in the rabbit, whereas transport in the mouse is hormonally stimulated only in the cortical

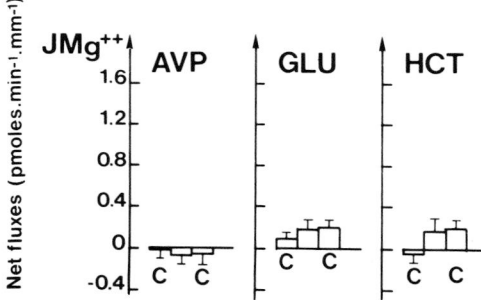

FIG. 6. In vitro microperfusion. Single medullary portions of mouse thick ascending limbs were microperfused in the absence (C) and presence of either ADH (AVP 10^{-10} mol·L^{-1}), glucagon (synthetic porcine glucagon, 1.2×10^{-8} mol), or calcitonin (synthetic human calcitonin, 3×10^{-8} mol·L^{-1}, cibacalcin RC 47175 Ba). The peptides were added to the bath solution. This figure presents the effects of each peptide on magnesium transepithelial net fluxes. C, control. (Data from Refs. 25, 26, and 113.)

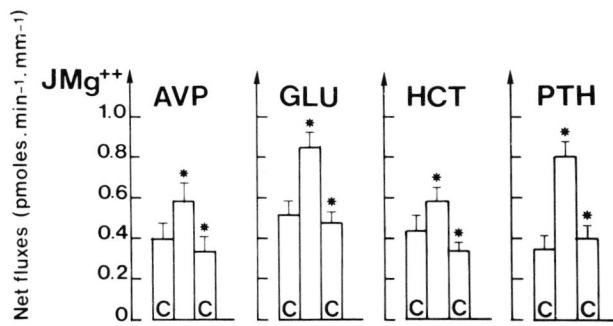

FIG. 7. In vitro microperfusion studies. Single cortical portions of mouse thick ascending limbs were microperfused in the absence (C = control) and presence of either ADH (AVP 10^{-10} mol·L^{-1}); Glu, glucagon (synthetic porcine glucagon, 1.2×10^{-8} mol·L^{-1}); HCT, calcitonin (synthetic human calcitonin, 3×10^{-8} mol·L^{-1}, cibacalcin RC 47175 Ba); or PTH (bovine PTH 1–34 fragments, 10^{-8} mol·L^{-1}, Sigma). The peptides were added to the bath solution. This figure presents the effects of each peptide on magnesium transepithelial net fluxes. *Asterisk:* significantly different from the preceding period. (Data from Refs. 25, 26, 111, and 113.)

part of the TAL. The observation that calcitonin does not stimulate calcium reabsorption in the rabbit cTAL is explained by the absence of an adenylate cyclase system sensitive to calcitonin in this segment (62). Thus, there is good agreement between the effects of PTH and calcitonin on divalent ion transport in the mouse and rabbit.

In the above-mentioned experimental series carried out on mouse cTAL, glucagon, human calcitonin (HCT), PTH, and isoproterenol did not alter the PD_{te} significantly (3,25,26). Does this observation mean that the hormone-mediated increase in magnesium transport in the cTAL is active in nature? We do not think so, for the following reasons.

In the cTAL, time–control experiments showed a spontaneous evolution of the PD_{te} (3,26). When testing a hormone, the voltage measured during the postexperimental (recovery) period was generally lower than that recorded at the beginning of the experiment (3,25,26). The addition of hormone to the bath either slowed or stopped this decline. In only a few cases did the PD_{te} actually rise after the addition of hormone. It would thus seem probable that the spontaneous diminution of the voltage masked, at least in part, the response. The first question was therefore the one raised by the spontaneous decline of PD_{te} with time.

Electrophysiological studies from our laboratory addressed this question (110). It was established that the cTAL displayed high potential and low resistance (R_{te}) values at the beginning of perfusion. Then the PD_{te} decreased and R_{te} increased steadily, reaching stable values after about 60 min. When a hormone (AVP) was added to the bath within the first few minutes of perfusion, during the high-voltage period, the PD_{te} no longer declined. In contrast, when either AVP, PTH, or glucagon (HCT and isoproterenol were not tested) was added after the transitory phase (i.e., after the establishment of steady-state values of PD_{te} and R_{te}), it elicited marked increases in PD_{te} and decreases in R_{te}, indicating that the equivalent short-circuit current, which is proportional to NaCl reabsorption, was indeed stimulated in the cTAL.

These experiments indicate that in studies designed for flux determination in mouse cTAL, it is necessary to include an equilibration period of at least 60 min before experimentation, to allow the tubule to reach a steady state. This was done for the ADH experiments presented in Fig. 7 (111). In these experiments, addition of ADH reversibly increased the PD_{te} from 14.4 ± 1.1 mV during the control period to 17.1 ± 1.4 mV during the experimental period. In previous experiments designed to test the effects of ADH in the mouse cTAL (113), such a delay was not included. Accordingly, the PD_{te} value was high and probably maximal during the pre-experimental periods, relative to that during the postexperimental ones. The variations of PD_{te} on addition of the hormone, therefore, could not be of statistical significance.

From the above observation it seems reasonable to

conclude that not only ADH, PTH, and glucagon, but also HCT and isoproterenol, increase the PD_{te} in the mouse cTAL. In fact, all five hormones increased NaCl transport in these nephron segments (3,25,26,110,111). If magnesium transport is purely passive in the cTAL (through the paracellular pathway), it is likely that the hormone-mediated increase in magnesium (and calcium) transport in the cTAL could be driven by the changes in the electrochemical gradient across the epithelium. However, in the rabbit (9,47,103) and in the mouse (3,25,26,113), hormone-mediated increases in transport were observed in the absence of changes in PD_{te} suggesting either the participation of an active component or an increase in the permeability of the paracellular pathway to divalent cations.

In Vivo Studies

The in vivo effects of four hormones (ADH, PTH, calcitonin, and glucagon) were tested by micropuncture in the rat, using the hormone-deprived model (see legend to Fig. 8). This model was elaborated from the discovery that, in this species, several hormones act on same target cells in several nephron segments (61). In the rat, the distribution (along the thick ascending limb) of the sensitivity of the adenylate cyclase system to these hormones is very similar to that of the mouse; however, in the rat the mTAL is sensitive to calcitonin and insensitive to isoproterenol, whereas the reverse is true in the mouse (Table 2). All four hormones increased potassium, magnesium, and calcium transport in Henle's loop, and only

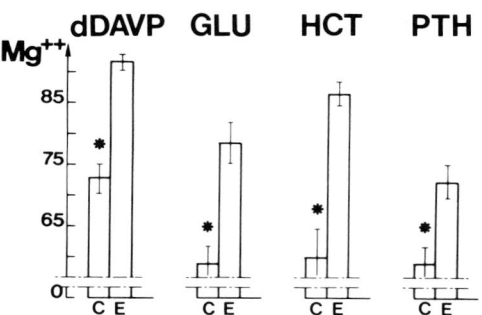

FIG. 8. Effects of 1-desamino-8-D arginine vasopressin (dDAVP), glucagon, calcitonin, and PTH on the fractional reabsorption of magnesium in Henle's loop (reabsorbed amounts are expressed as a percentage of the amounts delivered to the superficial nephrons of Henle's loop. Micropuncture experiments were performed in hormone-deprived (control) rats (Brattleboro D.I. rats which were acutely thyroparathyroidectomized and infused with somatostatin to inhibit glucagon secretion) and in hormone-deprived rats receiving one of the lacking peptides (experimental rats). Administration rates of the peptides were (per 100 g of body weight): dDAVP, 20 pg/min; glucagon, 5 ng/min; human calcitonin, 1 mU/min; PTH, 5 mU/min. C, control; E, experimental. *Asterisk: p* at least <0.05. Each column represents the mean value obtained from five to six different animals. (Data from Refs. 4, 25, 34, and 89.)

PTH failed to increase NaCl transport (4,25,34,89). These findings confirm and extend previous data obtained in the hamster (17,42) showing that PTH and calcitonin stimulate magnesium and calcium transport in Henle's loop. In previous experiments carried out in the rat, however, the stimulatory effect of PTH on magnesium reabsorption in the loop was observed only when magnesium reabsorption was reduced by either hypomagnesemia (76) or furosemide (71). At any rate, it is clear that the effects elicited in vitro by the hormones on the thick ascending limb are fully reflected in vivo in Henle's loop. In the presence of the other hormones the effects still persist, but their detection is not as easy.

In the kidney, the thick ascending limb crosses two regions (the medulla and the cortex), which are anatomically distinct and functionally separated. The fate of electrolytes delivered in these two regions will therefore depend on the local organization of the tubular and vascular structures surrounding the thick ascending limbs. In the rat, at the tip of the long loops (i.e., at the end of their descending thin limbs), magnesium (and calcium) deliveries remained unchanged with either glucagon or PTH (36), as expected in this species if the hormone-mediated increase in calcium and magnesium reabsorption occurs exclusively in the cortex. Calcitonin significantly reduced magnesium and calcium deliveries at the hairpin turn, and dDAVP showed a similar tendency (35,37). It was found that both hormones, in contrast to PTH and glucagon, reduced the fluid delivered at this site by enhancing water removal from the descending thin limb (35,37). We speculate that this water removal resulted in increased calcium and magnesium concentrations in the tubular fluid, allowing these divalent cations to diffuse out of the lumen before reaching the hairpin turn, probably at the same site along the descending limb as that at which NaCl is also escaping—that is, in the inner medulla (for review see Ref. 87).

Distal Convoluted Tubule

The adenylate cyclase system of the rat DCT is also sensitive to many hormones, including ADH, PTH, calcitonin, and glucagon (62). To determine the effects of these four hormones on the DCT, late and early accessible distal convolutions of the same superficial nephrons were punctured in hormone-deprived rats receiving one of the missing hormones. This protocol was used to avoid possible interference between the hormones, although the additivity of these hormones on the cyclase response of the cells was not tested. As shown in Fig. 9, PTH (5), calcitonin (32), and glucagon (5), but not ADH (33), elicited a significant stimulation of magnesium transport in the DCT. The cellular mechanisms of magnesium transport in the DCT are totally unknown. This is complicated because the portion of the DCT accessible

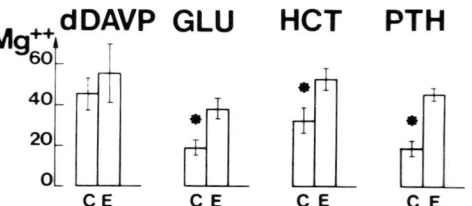

FIG. 9. Effects of 1-desamino-8-D arginine vasopressin (dDAVP), Glucagon, calcitonin, and PTH on the Mg^{2+} fractional reabsorption along the distal convoluted tubule (reabsorbed amounts are expressed as a percentage of the amounts delivered to the distal convoluted tubule of superficial nephrons). Micropuncture experiments were performed in hormone-deprived (control) rats (Brattleboro D.I. rats which were acutely thyroparathyroidectomized and infused with somatostatin to inhibit glucagon secretion) and in hormone-deprived rats receiving one of the lacking peptides (experimental rats). Administration rates of the peptides were (per 100 g of body weight): dDAVP, 20 pg/min; glucagon, 5 ng/min; human calcitonin, 1 mU/min; PTH, 5 mU/min. C, control; E, experimental; *Asterisk: p* at least <0.05. Each column represents the mean value obtained from five to six different animals. (Data from Refs. 5, 32, and 33.)

to micropuncture consists of at least three cell populations showing great differences in morphology, ultrastructural organization, and cyclase responsiveness, and the cell population that is responsible for magnesium transport is unknown.

Hormonal Effects on the Overall Kidney Function

The first data on the hormonal control of magnesium transport in the kidney were obtained in vivo from clearance and micropuncture studies. The first hormone tested was, of course, PTH. This hormone, as well as calcitonin (18,68,70,72,109), was shown to reduce magnesium excretion by enhancing the reabsorption of this ion within the kidney (17,42). Calcitonin was observed to reduce magnesium excretion in magnesium-loaded rats. In these rats, salmon calcitonin (60 mU · min⁻¹ · rat⁻¹) significantly reduced the fractional magnesium excretion from 24.7% during control periods to 15.3% during administration of salmon calcitonin (SCT) (*p* < 0.001) in spite of a slight increase in filtered magnesium during SCT infusions (S. Corraza and C. de Rouffignac, unpublished observations). From the observations reported in Henle's loop and DCT, it is clear that these effects resulted from a direct action of PTH and calcitonin in these structures.

From the data obtained in hormone-deprived rats, it appears that not only PTH (4) and calcitonin (34), but also ADH (89) and glucagon (4), may decrease the urinary excretion of magnesium (Fig. 10). This reduction was dose-dependent within the range of values estimated between 1 and 5 pg/mL (31) (Fig. 11). A dose-dependent response was also noted for HCT (as measured

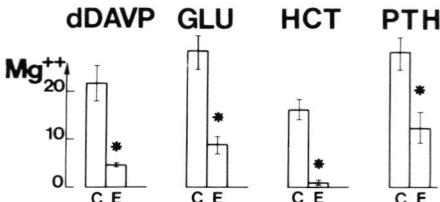

FIG. 10. Effects of 1-desamino-8-D arginine vasopressin (dDAVP), glucagon, calcitonin, and PTH on the fractional Mg^{2+} excretion in final urine (excreted amounts are expressed as a percentage of filtered Mg). Experiments were performed in hormone-deprived (control) rats (Brattleboro D.I. rats which were acutely thyroparathyroidectomized and infused with somatostatin to inhibit glucagon secretion) and in hormone-deprived rats receiving one of the lacking peptides (experimental rats). Administration rates of the peptides were (per 100 g of body weight): dDAVP, 20 pg/min; glucagon, 5 ng/min; human calcitonin, 1 mU/min; PTH, 5 mU/min. C, control; E, experimental. *Asterisk:* p at least <0.05. Each column represents the mean value obtained from five to six different animals. (Data from Refs. 4, 34, and 89.)

by radioimmunoassay) in the range of 0.5 to 5.0 ng/mL (24); both of these concentrations are within the physiological range. During maximal stimulation of endogenous secretion, the concentration of circulating hormones ranges between 20 and 50 pg/mL for ADH (28)

and between 5 and 10 ng/mL for calcitonin (23) as well as for glucagon (38). In addition, in hormone-deprived rats the effects of doses resulting in a maximal reduction of magnesium excretion were additive when dDAVP and glucagon (30) or dDAVP and HCT (but not HCT and glucagon) were used in combination (90). Since the decrease in magnesium excretion in the final urine was shown to be essentially accounted for by hormone-mediated stimulation of magnesium reabsorption in Henle's loop (31), these observations indicate that one hormone can exert its effects on the thick ascending limb, even in the presence of the other hormones.

This was verified by micropuncture studies in either hormone-deprived or intact Brattleboro rats or in Wistar rats), which demonstrated that ionic reabsorption in Henle's loop was increased by one peptide hormone when others were present acting on the same target cells of the thick ascending limb (for review see Refs. 92 and 93). However, as expected, the effects were less marked than in hormone-deprived rats.

At the whole-kidney level, the stimulation effects of either glucagon (2) or dDAVP (7) on calcium and/or magnesium reabsorption were also observed in intact rats—that is, in the presence of other peptide hormones. Thus, all these observations indicate that, in addition to

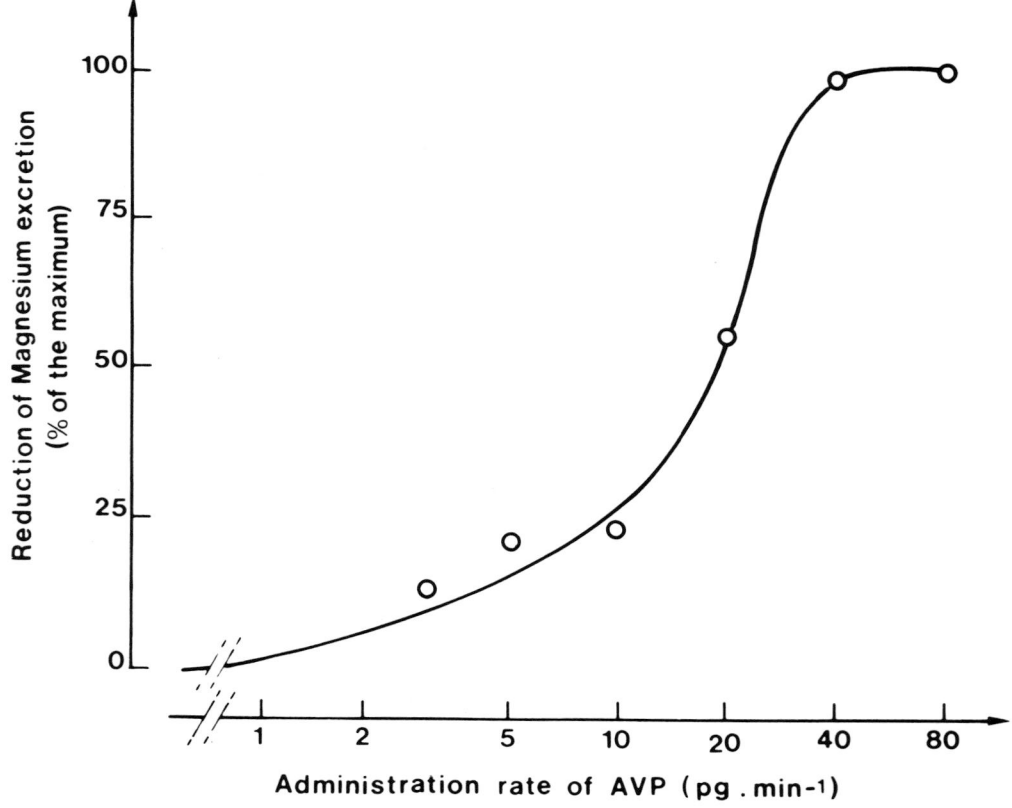

FIG. 11. Dose-dependent effects of AVP on the reduction of Mg excretion rates by the kidney in hormone-deprived rats, expressed as a percentage of maximal reduction. Each point is the mean of the means obtained during clearance experiments in four rats studied at each vasopressin infusion rate. (Data from Ref. 31.)

PTH and calcitonin, glucagon and ADH could potentially participate in magnesium and calcium homeostasis. Before accepting this hypothesis, it will be necessary to discover the physiological or physiopathological circumstances in which these hormones are called into play in homeostatic control of magnesium.

Little is known about steroids and their effects on magnesium excretion. It appears, however, that mineralocorticoids may affect magnesium metabolism. In both normal and adrenalectomized rats, aldosterone increased excretion of magnesium in the urine (44). A similar observation was reported in humans (41). The site of inhibition of magnesium transport by aldosterone is unknown. More generally, chronic administration of either glucocorticoids or mineralocorticoids leads to increased urinary excretion of magnesium (and calcium) in both animals and humans (for reviews see Refs. 58 and 107). Whether these inhibitions result from direct effects of steroids on the tubular epithelium or, more likely, reflect steroid-associated alterations of extrarenal factors, such as extracellular fluid volume expansion, remains to be determined.

ACKNOWLEDGMENT

I gratefully acknowledge the expert secretarial support of Mrs. C. Juillard.

REFERENCES

1. Alfredson KS, Walser M. Is magnesium secreted by the rat renal tubule? *Nephron* 1970;7:241–7.
2. Bailly C, Amiel C. Effect of glucagon on renal magnesium absorption in the rat. *Pflügers Arch* 1982;392:360–5.
3. Bailly C, Imbert-Teboul M, Roinel N, Amiel C. Isoproterenol increases Ca, Mg, and NaCl reabsorption in the mouse thick ascending limb. *Am J Physiol* 1990;258:F1224–31.
4. Bailly C, Roinel N, Amiel C. PTH-like glucagon stimulation of Ca and Mg reabsorption in Henle's loop of the rat. *Am J Physiol* 1984;246:F205–12.
5. Bailly C, Roinel N, Amiel C. Stimulation by glucagon and PTH of Ca and Mg reabsorption in the superficial distal tubule of the rat kidney. *Pflügers Arch* 1985;403:28–34.
6. Bengele HH, Alexander EA, Lechene CP. Calcium and magnesium transport along the inner medullary collecting duct of the rat. *Am J Physiol* 1981;239:24–9.
7. Bouby N, Trinh-Trang-Tan MM, Bankir L. Stimulation of tubular reabsorption of magnesium and calcium by antidiuretic hormone in conscious rats. Study in Brattleboro rats with hereditary hypothalamic diabetes insipidus. *Pflügers Arch* 1984;402:458–64.
8. Bourdeau JE, Burg MB. Voltage dependence of calcium transport in the thick ascending limb of Henle's loop. *Am J Physiol* 1979;236:357–64.
9. Bourdeau JE, Burg MB. Effect of PTH on calcium transport across the cortical thick ascending limb of Henle's loop. *Am J Physiol* 1980;239:F121–6.
10. Braun EJ, Roy DR, Jamison RL. Micropuncture study of the superficial nephron of *Peroganthus penicillatus*. *Am J Physiol* 1982;241:612–7.
11. Bronner F. Renal calcium transport: mechanisms and regulation. An overview. *Am J Physiol* 1989;257:F707–11.
12. Brunette MG, Aras M. A microinjection study of nephron permeability to calcium and magnesium. *Am J Physiol* 221:1442–8.
13. Brunette MG, Crochet MD. Fluoremetric method for the determination of magnesium in renal tubule fluid. *Anal Biochem* 1975;65:79–84.
14. Brunette MG, Vigneault N, Carriere S. Micropuncture study of magnesium transport along the nephron in the young rat. *Am J Physiol* 1974;227:891–6.
15. Brunette MG, Vigneault N, Carriere S. Micropuncture study of renal magnesium transport in magnesium-loaded rats. *Am J Physiol* 1975;229:1695–701.
16. Brunette MG, Vigneault N, Carriere S. Magnesium handing by the papilla of the young rat. *Pflügers Arch* 1978;373:229–35.
17. Burnatowska MA, Harris CA, Sutton RAL, Dirks JH. Effects of PTH and cAMP on renal handling of calcium, magnesium, and phosphate in the hamster. *Am J Physiol* 1977;233:F514–8.
18. Carney S, Thompson L. Acute effect of calcitonin on rat renal electrolyte transport. *Am J Physiol* 1981;240:F12–6.
19. Carney SL, Wong NLM, Quamme GA, Dirks JH. Effect of magnesium deficiency on renal magnesium and calcium transport in the rat. *J Clin Invest* 1981;65:180–8.
20. Chabardes D, Imbert-Teboul M, Gagnan-Brunette M, Morel F. Different hormonal target sites along the mouse and rabbit nephron. In: Guder WG, Schmidt U, eds. *Biochemical nephrology*. Bern: Hubert, 1978;447–54.
21. Corman B, Roinel N. Single nephron filtration rate and proximal reabsorption in aging rats. *Am J Physiol* in press.
22. Costanzo LS, Windhager EE. Calcium and sodium transport by the distal convoluted tubule of the rat. *Am J Physiol* 1978;235:492–506.
23. Cressent M, Bouizar Z, Pidoux E, Moukhtar M, Milhaud G. Effets de l'ovariectomie sur le taux de calcitonine plasmatique chez le rat. *C R Acad Sci (Paris)* 1979;289:501–4.
24. di Stefano A, Elalouf JM, Garel JM, de Rouffignac C. Modulation by calcitonin of magnesium and calcium urinary excretion in the rat. *Kidney Int* 1985;27:394–400.
25. di Stefano A, Wittner M, Nitschke R, Braitsch R, Greger R, Bailly C, Amiel C, Elalouf JM, Roinel N, de Rouffignac C. Effects of glucagon on Na^+, Cl^-, K^+, Mg^{2+}, and Ca^{2+}, transports in cortical and medullary thick ascending limbs of mouse kidney. *Pflügers Arch* 1989;414:640–6.
26. di Stefano A, Wittner M, Nitschke R, Braitsch R, Greger R, Bailly C, Amiel C, Roinel N, de Rouffignac C. Effects of parathyroid hormone and calcitonin on Na^+, Cl^-, K^+, Mg^{2+} and Ca^{2+} transport in cortical and medullary thick ascending limbs of mouse kidney. *Pflügers Arch* 1990;417:161–8.
27. Duarte CG. Effect of ethacrynic acid and furosemide on urinary calcium, phosphate, and magnesium. *Metab Clin Exp* 1968;17:867–76.
28. Dunn FL, Brennan TJ, Nelson AE, Robertson GL. The role of blood osmolality and volume in regulating vasopressin secretion in the rat. *J Clin Invest* 1973;52:3212–9.
29. Edwards BR, Baer PG, Sutton RAL, Dirks JH. Micropuncture study of diuretic effects on sodium and calcium reabsorption in the dog nephron. *J Clin Invest* 1973;52:2418–27.
30. Elalouf JM, Chabane-Sari D, de Rouffignac C. Additive effects of glucagon and vasopressin on renal Mg reabsorption and urine concentration ability in the rat. *Pflügers Arch* 1986;407:566–79.
31. Elalouf JM, di Stefano A, de Rouffignac C. Sensitivities of rat kidney thick ascending limbs and collecting ducts to vasopressin in vivo. *Proc Natl Acad Sci USA* 1986;83:2276–80.
32. Elalouf JM, Roinel N, de Rouffignac C. Stimulation by human calcitonin of electrolyte transport in distal tubules of rat kidney. *Pflügers Arch* 1983;399:111–8.
33. Elalouf JM, Roinel N, de Rouffignac C. Effects of antidiuretic hormone on electrolyte reabsorption and secretion in distal tubules of rat kidney. *Pflügers Arch* 1984;401:167–73.
34. Elalouf JM, Roinel N, de Rouffignac C. ADH-like effects of calcitonin on electrolyte transport by Henle's loop of rat kidney. *Am J Physiol* 1984;246:F213–20.
35. Elalouf JM, Roinel N, de Rouffignac C. Effects of dDAVP in rat juxtamedullary nephrons. Stimulation of medullary K recycling. *Am J Physiol* 1985;249:F291–8.
36. Elalouf JM, Roinel N, de Rouffignac C. Effects of glucagon and

PTH on the loop of Henle of rat juxtamedullary nephrons. *Kidney Int* 1986;29:807–13.

37. Elalouf JM, Roinel N, de Rouffignac C. Effects of human calcitonin on water and electrolyte movements in rat juxtamedullary nephrons: inhibition of medullary K recycling. *Pflügers Arch* 1986;406:502–6.

38. Emmanouel DS, Jaspan JB, Rubinstein AH, Huen AHJ, Fink E, Katz AI. Glucagon metabolism in the rat. Contribution of the kidney to the metabolic clearance of the hormone. *J Clin Invest* 1978;62:6–13.

39. Friedman PA. Basal and hormone activated calcium absorption in mouse renal thick ascending limbs. *Am J Physiol* 1988;254:F62–70.

40. Greger R. Ion transport mechanisms in thick ascending limb of Henle's loop of mammalian nephron. *Physiol Rev* 1985;65:760–97.

41. Hanna S, MacIntyre I. The influence of aldosterone on magnesium metabolism. *Lancet* 1960;706:348–50.

42. Harris CA, Burnatowska MA, Seely JF, Sutton RAL, Quamme GA, Dirks JH. Effects of parathyroid hormone on electrolyte transport in the hamster nephron. *Am J Physiol* 1984;246:F745–56.

43. Hebert SC, Friedman PA, Andreoli TE. Effects of antidiuretic hormone on cellular conductive pathways in mouse medullary thick ascending limbs of Henle. I. ADH increases transcellular conductance pathways. *J Membr Biol* 1984;80:201–19.

44. Horton R, Biglieri EG. Effect of aldosterone on the metabolism of magnesium. *J Clin Endocrinol Metab* 1962;22:1187–92.

45. Imbert M, Chabardes D, Montegut M, Clique A, Morel F. Adenylate cyclase activity along the rabbit nephron as measured in single isolated segments. *Pflügers Arch* 1975;354:213–222.

46. Imai M. Calcium transport across the rabbit thick ascending limb of Henle's loop perfused in vitro. *Pflügers Arch* 1978;374:255–63.

47. Imai M. Effects of parathyroid hormone and dibutyril-cyclic AMP on Ca^{2+} transport across the rabbit distal nephron segments perfused in vitro. *Pflügers Arch* 1980;390:145–51.

48. Jamison RL, Roinel N, de Rouffignac C. Urinary concentrating mechanism in the desert rodent *Psammomys obesus. Am J Physiol* 1979;236(*Renal Fluid Electrolyte Physiol* 5):F448–53.

49. Kuntziger H, Amiel C, Roinel N, Morel F. Effects of parathyroidectomy and cyclic AMP on renal transport of phosphate, calcium and magnesium. *Am J Physiol* 1974;227:905–11.

50. Le Grimellec C, Poujeol P, de Rouffignac C. ³H-inulin and electrolyte concentrations in Bowman's capsule in rat kidney. Comparison with artificial ultrafiltration. *Pflügers Arch* 1975;354:117–31.

51. Le Grimellec C, Roinel N, Morel F. Simultaneous Mg, Ca, P, K, Na and Cl analysis in rat tubular fluid. I. During perfusion of either inulin or ferrocyanide. *Pflügers Arch* 1970;340:181–96.

52. Le Grimellec C, Roinel N, Morel F. Simultaneous Mg, Ca, P, K, Na, and Cl analysis in rat tubular fluid. II. During acute Mg plasma loading. *Pflügers Arch* 1973;340:197–210.

53. Le Grimellec C, Roinel N, Morel F. Simultaneous Mg, Ca, P, K, Na and Cl analysis in rat tubular fluid. III. During acute Ca plasma loading. *Pflügers Arch* 1974;346:171–89.

54. Le Grimellec C, Roinel N, Morel F. Simultaneous Mg, Ca, P, K, and Cl analysis in rat tubular fluid. IV. During acute phosphate plasma loading. *Pflügers Arch* 1974;346:189–204.

55. Lelievre-Pegorier MC, Merlet-Benichou N, Roinel N, de Rouffignac C. Developmental pattern of water and electrolyte transport in rat superficial nephrons. *Am J Physiol* 1983;245:F15–21.

56. Levine DZ, Roinel N, de Rouffignac C. Flow-correlation of K, Ca, P, and Mg influx during continuous microperfusion of the loop of Henle in the rat. *Kidney Int* 1982;22:634–9.

57. Massry SG, Coburn JW. The hormonal and nonhormonal control of renal excretion of calcium and magnesium. *Nephron* 1973;10:66–112.

58. Massry SG, Coburn JW, Chapman LW, Kleeman CR. The acute effect of adrenal steroids on the interrelationship between the renal excretion of sodium, calcium and magnesium. *J Lab Clin Med* 1967;70:563–72.

59. Massry SG, Coburn JW, Kleeman CR. Renal handling of magnesium in the dog. *Am J Physiol* 1969;216:1460–7.

60. Morel F. Sites of hormone action in the mammalian nephron.

Am J Physiol 1981;240(*Renal Fluid Electrolyte Physiol* 9):F159–64.

61. Morel F, Chabardes D, Imbert-Teboul M, Le Bouffant F, Hus-Citharel A, Montegut M. Multiple hormonal control of adenylate cyclase in distal segments of the rat kidney. *Kidney Int* 1982;21:555–62.

62. Morel F, Doucet A. Hormonal control of kidney functions at the cell level. *Physiol Rev* 1986;66:377–468.

63. Morel F, Imbert-Teboul M, Chabardes D. Distribution of hormone-dependent adenylate cyclase in the nephron and its physiological significance. *Annu Rev Physiol* 1981;43:569–81.

64. Morel F, Imbert-Teboul M, Chabardes D. Receptors to vasopressin and other hormones in the mammalian kidney. *Kidney Int* 1987;31:512–20.

65. Morel F, Roinel N. Application de la microsonde électronique à l'analyse élémentaire quantitative d'échantillons biologiques liquides d'un volume inférieur à 10^{-9} l. *J Chim Phys-Chim Biol* 1969;66:1084–91.

66. Morel F, Roinel N, Le Grimellec C. Electron probe analysis of tubular fluid composition. *Nephron* 1969;6:350–64.

67. Murayama Y, Morel F, Le Grimellec C. Phosphate, calcium and magnesium transfers in proximal tubules and loops of Henle, as measured by single nephron microperfusion experiments in the rat. *Pflügers Arch* 1972;333:1–16.

68. Nielsen SP, Buchaman-Lee B, Matthews EW, Moseley JM, Williams CC. Acute effects of synthetic porcine calcitonins on the renal excretion of magnesium, inorganic phosphate, sodium and potassium. *J Endocrinol* 1971;51:455–64.

69. Poujeol P, Chabardes D, Roinel N, de Rouffignac C. Influence of extracellular fluid volume expansion on magnesium, calcium, and phosphate handling along the rat nephron. *Pflügers Arch* 1976;365:203–11.

70. Poujeol P, Touvay C, Roinel N, de Rouffignac C. Stimulation of renal magnesium reabsorption by calcitonin in the rat. *Am J Physiol* 1980;239:F524–32.

71. Quamme GA. Effect of intraluminal furosemide on calcium and magnesium transport in the loop of Henle and the role of PTH. *Kidney Int* 1978;14:642.

72. Quamme GA. Effect of calcitonin on calcium and magnesium transport in rat nephron. *Am J Physiol* 1980;238:E573–8.

73. Quamme GA. Effect of hypercalcemia on renal tubular handling of calcium and magnesium. *Can J Physiol Pharmacol* 1980;60:1275–80.

74. Quamme GA. Effect of furosemide on calcium and magnesium transport in the rat nephron. *Am J Physiol* 1981;241:F340–7.

75. Quamme GA. Control of magnesium transport in the thick ascending limbs. *Am J Physiol* 1989;256:F197–210.

76. Quamme GA, Carney SL, Wong NLM, Dirks JH. Effect of parathyroid hormone on renal calcium and magnesium reabsorption in magnesium deficient rats. *Pflügers Arch* 1980;386:50–65.

77. Quamme GA, Dai LJ. Determination of intracellular Mg^{2+} activity in isolated cortical thick ascending limb cells. *Kidney Int* 1990;37:461.

78. Quamme GA, Dirks JH. Magnesium transport in the nephron. *Am J Physiol* 1980;239:F393–401.

79. Quamme GA, Dirks JH. Effect of intraluminal and contraluminal magnesium on magnesium and calcium transfer in the rat nephron. *Am J Physiol* 1980;238:F187–198.

80. Quamme GA, Dirks JH. Renal magnesium transport. In: Ullrich K, ed. *Review of physiology, biochemistry and pharmacology,* vol 97. Berlin: Springer-Verlag, 1983;69–110.

81. Quamme GA, Dirks JH. Magnesium: cellular and renal exchanges. In: Seldin DW, Giebish G, eds. *The kidney: physiology and pathophysiology.* New York: Raven Press, 1985;1269–80.

82. Quamme GA, Dirks J. The physiology of renal magnesium handling. *Renal Physiol* 1986;9:257–69.

83. Quamme GA, Smith C. Magnesium transport in isolated proximal straight tubule of the rabbit. *Am J Physiol* 1984;246:F544–50.

84. Quamme GA, Wong NLM, Dirks JH, Roinel N, de Rouffignac C, Morel F. Magnesium handling in the dog kidney: a micropuncture study. *Pflügers Arch* 1978;377:95–9.

85. Roinel N. Electron microprobe quantitative analysis of lyophylised 10^{-10} l volume samples. *J Microsc* 1975;22:261–8.

86. Roinel N, de Rouffignac C. X-ray analysis of biological fluids: contribution of microdroplet technique to biology. In: O'Hare AMF, ed. *Scanning electron microscopy.* Chicago: SEM, 1982;1155–71.

87. de Rouffignac C. The urinary concentrating mechanisms. In: Kinne R, ed. *Urinary concentrating mechanisms.* Basel: Karger, 1990;31–102.

88. de Rouffignac C, Bankir L, Roinel N. Renal function and concentrating ability in a desert rodent: the Gundi (*Ctenodactylus vali*). *Pflügers Arch* 1981;390:138–44.

89. de Rouffignac C, Corman B, Roinel N. Stimulation by antidiuretic hormone of electrolyte tubular reabsorption in rat kidney. *Am J Physiol* 1983;244:F156–64.

90. de Rouffignac C, di Stefano A, Wittner M, Chabane-Sari D, Elalouf JM. The renal handling of magnesium. Influences of parathyroid hormone, calcitonin, antidiuretic hormone and glucagon. In: B Lasserre and J. Durlach, eds. *Magnesium, a relevant ion?* John Libbey 1991;145–67.

91. de Rouffignac C, Elalouf JM. Hormonal regulation of chloride transport in the proximal and distal nephron. *Annu Rev Physiol* 1988;50:123–40.

92. de Rouffignac C, Elalouf JM, Roinel N. Physiological control of the urinary concentrating mechanism by peptide hormones. *Kidney Int* 1987;31:611–20.

93. de Rouffignac C, Elalouf JM, Roinel N, Bailly C, Amiel C. Similarity of the effects of antidiuretic hormone, parathyroid hormone, calcitonin and glucagon on rat kidney. In: Robinson RR, ed. *Nephrology.* Springer: Berlin, 1984;340–57.

94. de Rouffignac C, Morel F, Moss N, Roinel N. Micropuncture study of water and electrolyte movements along the loop of Henle in *Psammomys* with special reference to magnesium, calcium, and phosphate. *Pflügers Arch* 1973;344:309–26.

95. de Rouffignac C, Roinel N, Elalouf JM. Comparative effects of peptide hormones on water and electrolyte transport along the proximal and distal tubules of the mammalian nephron. In: Brown JA, Balment RJ, Rankin JC, eds. *New insights into vertebrate kidney function.* New York: Cambridge University Press, 1991; in press.

96. Roy DR. Magnesium absorption in the juxtamedullary loop of Henle: effect of magnesium deprivation. *Can J Physiol Pharmacol* 1987;65:1918–27.

97. Roy DR, Blouch KL, Jamison RL. Effects of acute acid–base disturbances on renal tubule reabsorption of magnesium in the rat. *Am J Physiol* 1982;243:F197–203.

98. Ruggles BT, Murayama N, Werness JL, Gapstur SM, Bentley MD, Dousa TP. The vasopressin-sensitive adenylate cyclase in collecting tubules and in thick ascending limb of Henle's loop of human and canine kidney. *J Clin Endocrinol Metab* 1985;60:914–21.

99. Shafik IM, Quamme GA. Early adaptation of renal magnesium reabsorption in response to magnesium restriction. *Am J Physiol* 1989;257:F974–7.

100. Shareghi GR, Agus ZS. Phosphate transport in the light segment of the rabbit cortical collecting tubule. *Clin Res* 1979;27:430A.

101. Shareghi GR, Agus ZS. Magnesium transport in the cortical thick ascending limb of Henle's loop of the rabbit. *J Clin Invest* 1982;69:759–69.

102. Shirley DJ, Poujeol P, Le Grimellec C. Phosphate, calcium and magnesium fluxes into the lumen of the rat proximal convoluted tubules. *Pflügers Arch* 1976;362:247–54.

103. Suki WN, Rouse D. Hormonal regulation of calcium transport in thick ascending limb renal tubules. *Am J Physiol* 1981;241: F171–4.

104. Suki WN, Rouse D, Ng R, Kokko JP. Calcium transport in the thick ascending limb of Henle. *J Clin Invest* 1980;66:1004–9.

105. Sutton RAL, Quamme GA, Dirks JH. Renal tubular transport of calcium, magnesium and phosphate. In: Giebisch G, Tosteson DC, Ussing HH, eds. *Membrane transport in biology,* vol 4. Berlin: Springer-Verlag, 1979;357–412.

106. Taniguchi S, Marchetti J, Morel F. Na/Ca exchangers in collecting cells of rat kidney. *Pflügers Arch* 1989;415:191–7.

107. Walser M. Divalent cations: physicochemical state in glomerular filtrate and urine and renal extraction. In: Orloff J, Berliner RW, *Handbook of physiology—renal physiology.* Baltimore: Williams and Wilkins, 1973;555–86.

108. Wen SF, Wong NLM, Dirks JH. Evidence for renal magnesium secretion during magnesium infusion in the dog. *Am J Physiol* 1971;220:33–7.

109. Williams CC, Matthews EW, Moseley JM, MacIntyre I. The effects of synthetic human and salmon calcitonins on electrolyte excretion in the rats. *Clin Sci* 1972;42:129–37.

110. Wittner M, di Stefano A. Effects of ADH, PTH and glucagon on transepithelial voltage and resistance of the cortical and medullary thick ascending limb of Henle's loop of the mouse nephron. *Pflügers Arch* 1990;415:707–12.

111. Wittner M, di Stefano A, Mandon B, Roinel N, de Rouffignac C. Effect of ADH on electrolyte transport in the thick ascending limb of the loop of Henle. In: Jard S, Jamison RL, eds. *Proceedings of the 4th International Vasopressin Conference (Montpellier); in press.*

112. Wittner M, di Stefano A, Roinel N, de Rouffignac C. Basal Ca^{++} and Mg^{++} reabsorption in the mouse cTAL is driven by the transepithelial potential difference [Abstract]. *Proc Int Union Physiol Sci* 1989;17:371.

113. Wittner M, di Stefano A, Wangemann P, Nitschke R, Greger R, Bailly C, Amiel C, Roinel N, de Rouffignac C. Differential effects of ADH on sodium, chloride, potassium, calcium, and magnesium transport in cortical and medullary thick ascending limbs of mouse nephron. *Pflügers Arch* 1988;412:516–23.

114. Wong NLM, Quamme GA, Sutton RAL, Dirks JH. Effects of mannitol on water and electrolyte transport in the dog. *J Lab Clin Invest* 1979;94:683–92.

115. Wong NLM, Quamme GA, Dirks JH. Effects of urea on electrolyte transport in the dog kidney. *J Lab Clin Med* 1981;98:741–9.

116. Wong NLM, Quamme GA, Dirks JH. Tubular reabsorptive capacity for magnesium in the dog kidney. *Am J Physiol* 1983;224:62–73.

117. Wong NLM, Reitzik M, Quamme GA. Micropuncture study of the superficial nephron of *Cercopithecus aethiops. Renal Physiol* 1986;9:29–37.

118. Wong NLM, Quamme GA, Sutton RAL, O'Callaghan T, Dirks JH. Renal and tubular transport in phosphate depletion: a micropuncture study. *Can J Physiol Pharmacol* 1980;58:1063–71.

119. Wright FS, Giebisch G. Regulation of potassium excretion. In: Seldin DW, Giebisch G, eds. *The kidney: physiology and pathophysiology.* New York: Raven Press, 1985;1223–50.

Disorders of Bone and Mineral Metabolism,
edited by Fredric L. Coe and Murray J. Favus,
© 1992 by Raven Press, Ltd. All rights reserved.

CHAPTER 3

Intestinal Absorption of Calcium, Magnesium, and Phosphorus

Murray J. Favus

The intestinal absorption of calcium (Ca), magnesium (Mg), and phosphorus (P) are considered together because adequate absorption of all three elements is necessary for normal mineral homeostasis, including control of blood ionized Ca, skeletal growth in childhood, and maintenance of skeletal mass in adulthood. In addition, vitamin D, through its active metabolite 1,25-dihydroxyvitamin D_3 [$1,25(OH)_2D_3$], controls the transport processes of each of these elements.

CALCIUM

Pathways

Evidence that Ca traverses the intestinal epithelium via cellular and paracellular pathways is derived largely from studies in rats and chicks using radioisotopic Ca (^{45}Ca, ^{47}Ca) disappearance from in situ perfused loops of bowel, Ca uptake by in vitro everted gut sacs, or in vitro steady-state Ca bidirectional fluxes across intestinal segments mounted in Ussing chambers. For consistency, this review uses experimental data from mammalian species unless otherwise indicated.

Saturable and Nonsaturable Components

Increasing Ca concentrations ranging from 1 to 200 mM instilled into rat duodenal loops cause a progressive prolongation of the rate of disappearance of Ca from the loops (1–3). Whereas absorption is nearly complete by 20 min with 1–10 mM Ca, 90 min or longer is required for near-complete absorption of 50 mM Ca (Fig. 1).

M. J. Favus: Endocrinology Section and the Nephrology Program, Department of Medicine, University of Chicago, Pritzker School of Medicine, 5841 S. Maryland Avenue, Chicago, Illinois 60637

These observations are consistent with the presence of a saturable transport process, since nonsaturable processes (such as simple or facilitated diffusion) would remove Ca at rates independent of luminal Ca concentration. Michaelis–Menten analysis of this data suggests two components to the rates of disappearance: (i) a saturable component and (ii) augmented rates of disappearance at high Ca concentrations due to a separate, nonsaturable process that is not present at low luminal Ca concentrations (2).

When absorption is measured at a single time point, the amount of Ca absorbed from the loop becomes dependent upon the luminal Ca concentration (Fig. 2). At high Ca concentrations the slope of the line of Ca absorbed versus Ca concentration is linear and is taken to represent the nonsaturable component (4–6). The saturable portion, which is derived by subtracting the linear component from each Ca concentration, becomes evident at low luminal Ca concentrations (Fig. 2). Thus, the Ca absorptive process in duodenum is a result of saturable and nonsaturable components (4–7).

Saturable (Cellular) Transport

While the in situ loop preparation provides evidence for a two-component absorptive process, designation of the observed kinetics of absorption to specific pathways has been determined in other systems. In vitro measurements of bidirectional transmucosal fluxes of Ca across intestinal segments mounted in Ussing chambers (8–10) permit in vivo driving forces (such as Ca concentration, osmotic, and electrical gradients) to be abolished (11,12). Under these conditions the contributions of cellular and paracellular pathways to total transepithelial Ca transport have been determined. Bidirectional transepithelial Ca fluxes measured under these conditions re-

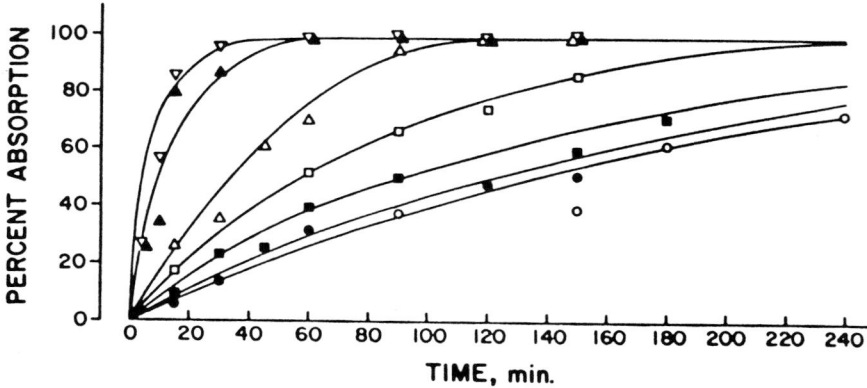

FIG. 1. Time course of Ca absorption by in situ duodenal loops. Male Sprague–Dawley rats (120–150 g) were fed a normal-Ca diet and 2 days before were placed on a low-Ca diet (0.05%). Ca at various concentrations (see figure) was instilled in the intestinal lumen. Absorption, calculated as the amount of ^{45}Ca lost in an indicated time period, is shown as the percent absorbed. Each point represents a mean estimate of two to six loops, with an average SEM of 7%. [From Bronner et al. (3).]

veal an asymmetry, since steady-state mucosal-to-serosal fluxes (J_{ms}) in the absorptive direction increase rapidly at low medium Ca concentrations of 0.1–1.0 mM Ca and then approach a plateau at higher concentration of 2–5 mM (Fig. 3). In contrast, Ca serosal-to-mucosal fluxes (J_{sm}) in the secretory direction increase linearly with medium Ca (0.125–10 mM) without saturation (6,7,9,10,13–17).

Michaelis–Menten kinetic analysis of Ca J_{ms} reveals a saturable component of total Ca J_{ms} across duodenum (10), ileum (13), cecum (14), and colon (18,19). The calculated affinity of the saturable processes ($\frac{1}{2}V_{max}$ or K_d) is in general agreement, ranging from 0.59 to 1.8 mM. The K_d is generally higher when unstirred layers are large, as with in situ perfused loop preparations of rat intestine (3,4) and human perfused segments (20), where calculated K_d may range from 1.9 to 51 mM. The saturable component is present in the absence of concentration, osmotic, and electrical gradients and is abolished by the metabolic inhibitor N-ethylmaleimide (15) or by a nitrogen atmosphere (16,21). Thus, the kinetic characteristics of Ca J_{ms} are consistent with a cellular, carrier-mediated active transport process with a K_d of about 1.0 mM (17).

The Ussing equation (22) predicts a significant passive diffusion component of Ca absorption when luminal Ca (bathing mucosal surface) is greater than 2.0 mM and

blood ionized Ca is 1.25 mM (bathing serosal surface). The Ussing equation also predicts that the contribution of active transport to total transport would be greatest when luminal Ca is below that required for absorption to be driven by diffusional forces. Thus, K_d values below 2.0 mM are consistent with a physiologically significant epithelial transport process when luminal Ca concentrations are low, as during dietary Ca restriction.

Mechanisms of Cellular Transport

Brush-Border Influx. Ca entry across the enterocyte brush-border membrane (Fig. 4) is favored by an electrical gradient of 40–70 mV (cell interior negative) and a chemical gradient of about 10,000 (cytosolic Ca of 100 nM and extracellular or luminal Ca of 1.0 mM). The initial entry process has been investigated using isolated epithelial cells (23), intact epithelium (13,14,24–28), and brush-border membrane vesicles (29–31). Vitamin D and active metabolites increase Ca influx at the mucosal surface (Fig. 4). To distinguish influx across the brush border from movement into the paracellular space, cellular and paracellular pathways for Ca uptake have been identified in rats fed high- or low-Ca diet (13) using voltage clamping and polyethylene glycol as an extracellular marker. Low-Ca diet increases primarily cellular uptake

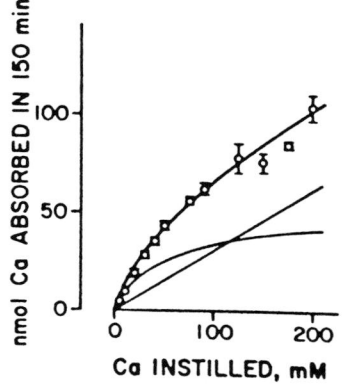

FIG. 2. Calcium absorption in male rats measured by an in situ loop technique 150 min after instillation of Ca at concentrations indicated. Line through mean ± SEM consists of experimental points representing algebraic sum of saturable and nonsaturable components. The straight line has a slope that was obtained by fitting data at the four highest concentrations; the hyperbolic curve was obtained with a best-fit procedure by subtracting the linear component from experimental points. [From Pansu et al. (5).]

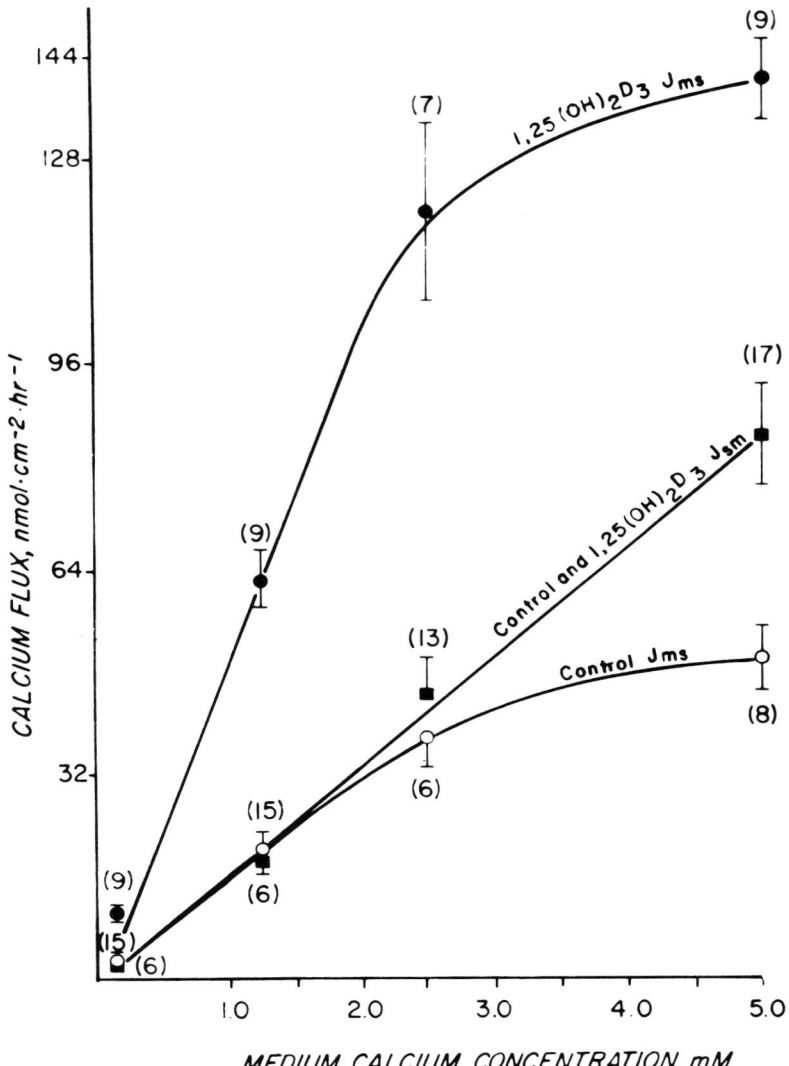

FIG. 3. Steady-state transepithelial Ca fluxes from mucosa to serosa (J_{ms}) and serosa to mucosa (J_{sm}) versus medium calcium concentration across colonic segments from control and $1,25(OH)_2D_3$-treated rats. Numbers in parentheses are numbers of rats per group. Michaelis–Menten kinetic analysis reveals K_d of 1.6 mM and V_{max} of 133 nmol/cm²/h for control animals and 1.8 mM and 236 nmol/cm²/h for $1,25(OH)_2D_3$-treated animals. [From Favus et al. (19).]

via a saturable, carrier-mediated component with (a) a K_d of about 1.0 mM and (b) a transport maximum close to that described for transepithelial Ca J_{ms} (13,14).

Significant cellular uptake also occurs when mediated transport is low, as during high Ca intake (13). While brush-border vesicle Ca influx corresponds to in vivo saturable transport rates (32), brush-border V_{max} is lower than transepithelial fluxes, and response to vitamin D or $1,25(OH)_2D_3$ is only 20–30% of the increase in transepithelial Ca fluxes (29,30). Therefore, brush-border entry appears not to be the rate-limiting step in transcellular Ca transport.

Duodenal cells accumulate more Ca than do jejunal or ileal cells, and duodenal-cell Ca uptake from vitamin-D-deficient rats is lower than that from vitamin-D-replete animals (23). Thus, the higher rate of Ca transport in duodenum as compared to that in jejunum and ileum is probably not due to greater cellularity of duodenum; instead, it is probably due to greater Ca transport by each

duodenal cell. Whether the regional differences in Ca uptake are due to differences in cell capacity at the brush border is unknown.

Ca entry across the brush border consists of binding to the brush-border membrane followed by transport to the cell interior. A small number of high-affinity anionic sites and a large number of low-affinity Ca-binding sites have been identified on the brush-border surface (30,31). Although the specific proteins containing the binding sites have not been identified, the K_d for the high-affinity sites of 10^{-5}–10^{-6} M is similar to affinities for Ca-binding proteins such as brush-border vitamin-D-dependent Ca-binding protein [CaBP or calbindin (32a)], vitamin-D-independent calmodulin (33,34), a calmodulin-binding protein (35,36), and vitamin-D-dependent integral membrane protein [IMCaL (37)]. Ca also binds to the inner aspect of the brush-border membrane, perhaps because of the presence of the vitamin-D-dependent calbindin (38).

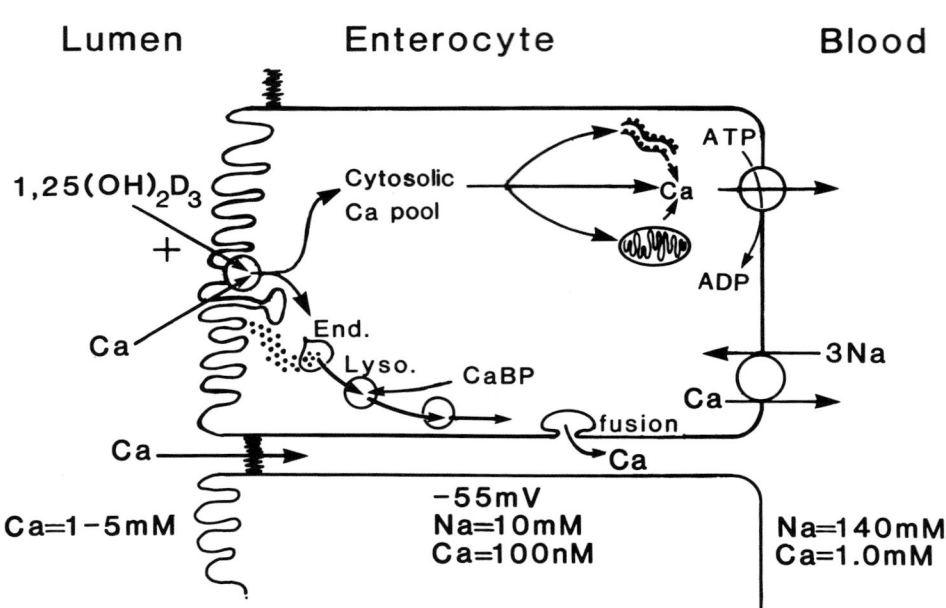

FIG. 4. Schematic of cellular and paracellular pathways for calcium absorption (from lumen to blood) across intestinal epithelium. $1,25(OH)_2D_3$ stimulates brush-border Ca entry. Transcellular pathway may include equilibration with the Ca cytosolic pool, endoplasmic reticulum, or mitochondria. Exit via this pathway would be via ATP-dependent Ca pump or, less likely, Na–Ca exchange. Sequestration of transported Ca may occur with appearance of electron-dense particles below the brush border, with subsequent accumulation in endosomes and lysosomes. The latter structures may contain vitamin-D-dependent calbindin. Exit is via fusion of the lysosomes with the basolateral plasma membrane. Luminal calcium may also traverse the paracellular pathway. Concentration and electrical gradients influence paracellular, but not cellular, pathways.

A brush-border calmodulin has also been described that may participate in the Ca entry process (34,35). Although vitamin D does not increase calmodulin synthesis, it causes a redistribution of calmodulin to the brush-border complex (34,35). The brush-border–calmodulin complex increases Ca uptake by mechanisms other than binding of Ca to the calmodulin.

The molecular basis for Ca entry across brush border is unknown, but initial Ca binding may be an early step in activation of a Ca channel or to increase membrane fluidity. Vitamin D stimulation of brush-border Ca entry does not require new protein synthesis (29,39), and increasing the amount of phosphatidylcholine relative to phosphatidylethanolamine (29,40) may change membrane fluidity. Changes in membrane fluidity by vitamin D and $1,25(OH)_2D_3$ resulting in increased Ca uptake is supported by in vitro incorporation of *cis*-vaccenic acid methyl ester into brush-border membranes which results in increased Ca uptake, whereas the *trans* form of the acid reduced Ca uptake (41). However, direct measurements of membrane fluidity before and after $1,25(OH)_2D_3$ administration have not confirmed changes suggested by the effects of altering membrane lipid composition, with increases (42) or no change (43–45) in fluidity being reported.

Because brush-border alkaline phosphatase activity is increased by vitamin D and $1,25(OH)_2D_3$ (46–48), the role of the enzyme in Ca uptake has been explored. Several lines of evidence indicate that the alkaline phosphatase is probably of secondary importance: Vitamin D activates Ca transport before any detectable increase in alkaline phosphatase activity (46); alkaline phosphatase

and Ca-ATPase activities are due to separate molecular entities (49); the time course of appearance of alkaline phosphatase and Ca-ATPase activities following vitamin D are dissimilar (50); and inhibition of alkaline phosphatase activity by cycloheximide does not inhibit calcium transport activity (29,39).

Basolateral Membrane Exit. The same electrochemical forces that favor Ca entry at the brush border pose potential barriers for Ca extrusion across the plasma basolateral membrane (Fig. 4). These electrochemical barriers to Ca diffusion out of the enterocyte are pertinent if Ca being transported is in equilibrium with the cytosolic Ca pool. However, the electrochemical gradients will not influence Ca transport if Ca is sequestered in vesicles during transcellular transport and is, therefore, not in equilibrium with cytosolic Ca.

Na–Ca exchange has been suggested as a mechanism for Ca efflux across the basolateral membrane. However, recent studies indicate that the ubiquitous Na–Ca exchanger (51–54) can account for only a small fraction of total Ca efflux (55).

A high-affinity Ca- and Mg-activated ATPase (Ca,Mg-ATPase) with specific location in the plasma basolateral membrane has been described (47,49,56,57). The Ca,Mg-ATPase appears to be distinct from Na,Ca-ATPase and alkaline phosphatase, which are located primarily in the brush border (57). ATP-dependent Ca efflux across basolateral membrane has been demonstrated using basolateral membrane vesicles prepared from vitamin-D-deficient (57–61a) and vitamin-D-replete (61,62) rats (Fig. 5). $1,25(OH)_2D_3$, in doses that increase transepithelial Ca J_{ms}, increases ATP-dependent Ca uptake by

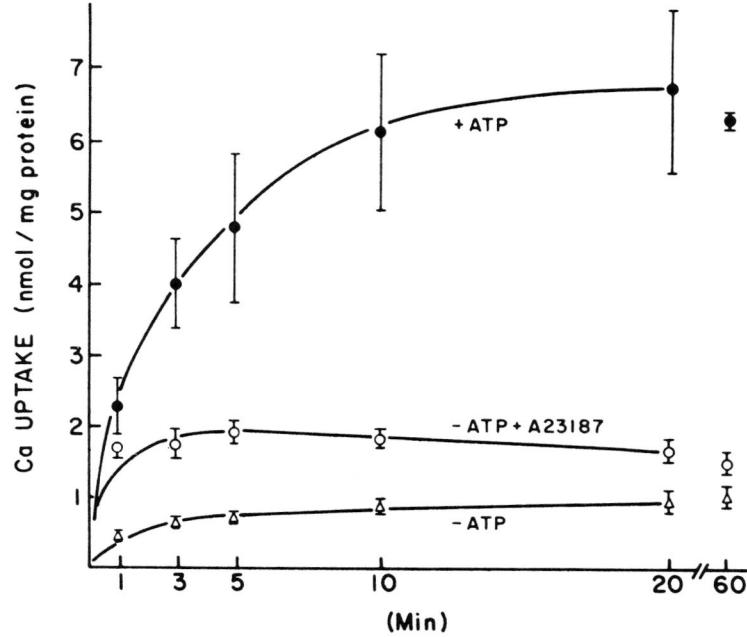

FIG. 5. The effect of ATP and the Ca ionophore A23187 on Ca uptake by rat intestinal epithelial basolateral membrane vesicles. Ca concentration is 0.1 mM; A23187 was added at time 0 at 0.01 mM. Results are mean $\pm$ SEM for three experiments. [From Nellans and Popovitch (61).]

basolateral membrane vesicles from vitamin-D-deficient rats (59–61), but not by vesicles from vitamin-D-replete rats (Fig. 6) (62). Furthermore, increased cellular active transport during chronic dietary Ca restriction is not accompanied by increased ATP-dependent basolateral membrane vesicle Ca uptake (Fig. 6) (62). Thus, 1,25(OH)$_2$D$_3$ activation of the Ca,Mg-ATPase may be

confined to the vitamin-D-deficient state, and the pump may participate in intracellular Ca homeostasis rather than in transcellular Ca transport.

Cellular Events. Under steady-state conditions, net apical Ca influx and net basolateral membrane Ca efflux must be equivalent, and the coordination of apical and basolateral Ca transport is necessary in order to prevent

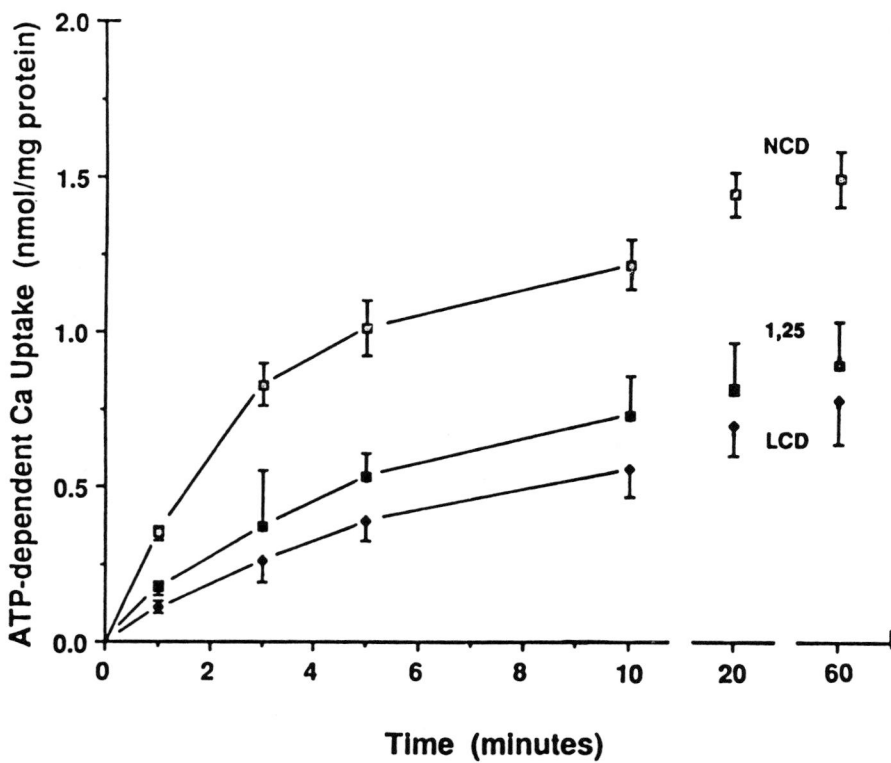

FIG. 6. Initial rates of ATP-dependent Ca uptake by intestinal basolateral membranes prepared from rats fed low-Ca diet (♦), or fed normal-calcium diet and injected with either 1,25(OH)$_2$D$_3$ (■) or vehicle (□) for 4 days. Medium calcium concentration was 0.1 mM; MgATP was 5 mM; and ATP and ^{45}Ca were added at time 0. Values are mean $\pm$ SEM for three experiments. [From Favus et al. (62).]

major fluctuations in the cellular pools of Ca and in cytosolic Ca^{2+} levels. If Ca entering the enterocyte destined for transcellular transport is in equilibrium with the cellular Ca pool, then cytosolic Ca^{2+} concentrations may increase under conditions of high transport rates (Fig. 4). Recent calculations, based upon high rates of epithelial Ca transport across rat cecum (14), indicate that turnover of cytosolic Ca during maximal Ca absorption must approach 25-fold per minute to prevent an increase in cytosolic Ca^{2+}. To maintain a cytosolic Ca concentration that is stable, Ca itself may serve to control brush-border Ca influx or basolateral membrane Ca efflux, or both. It is unlikely that cytosolic Ca^{2+} coordinates Ca transport across the apical and basolateral poles of the enterocyte, since basolateral membrane Ca efflux is not increased during $1,25(OH)_2D_3$-stimulated epithelial Ca transport (62); in addition, Ca ionophores (A23187 and ionomycin) increase brush-border Ca influx and raise cytosolic Ca^{2+} concentrations without increasing transepithelial Ca transport (M. J. Favus and H. N. Nellans, unpublished data). Therefore, the hypothesis that cytosolic Ca^{2+} coordinates Ca transport across apical and basolateral poles of the enterocyte is not supported by available studies.

Transcytotic Ca Transport. An alternative hypothesis for transcellular Ca transport is that Ca translocated across the enterocyte during absorption is not in equilibrium with either cytosolic Ca^{2+} or other noncytosolic Ca pools (63–65). Electron-microscopic examination of duodenal epithelial cells from vitamin-D-deficient rats and chicks show that vitamin D repletion is associated with increased length of brush-border microvilli, number of apical pits at the base of the microvilli, and the number of vesicles in the terminal web region (Fig. 4) (66,67). Following vitamin D or $1,25(OH)_2D_3$ administration, acid-phosphatase-positive vesicular structures in the supranuclear region of chick enterocytes increase in number at the terminal web level and, with time, increase at the basolateral membrane (68–72). Ca has been localized to membrane-bound structures in the enterocyte supranuclear region using microincineration and x-ray microanalysis (68,72), suggesting that these vesicles may participate in transcellular Ca transport. These observations are compatible with, but do not prove, Ca entrance and transcellular transport by receptor-mediated endocytosis.

Although a considerable portion of brush-border Ca binding may be nonspecific, binding of Ca to brush-border membrane may be the initial entry step. Also, unbound Ca movement across brush-border membrane vesicles increases only 30% in response to $1,25(OH)_2D_3$, whereas transcellular Ca J_{ms} increases two- to threefold (28–30). Since the Ca-containing vesicle structures in the submembrane region may arise from the brush border and then detach and move into the cytoplasm, cell Ca entry may occur via an endocytic process rather than influx via membrane pores or Ca channels.

Measurement of cellular Ca movement by fluid-phase pinocytosis using the fluorescent dye Lucifer Yellow indicates that this process can account for only a small portion of total epithelial Ca J_{ms} (M. J. Favus and H. N. Nellans, unpublished observations). The 28-kD CaBP (calbindin) in chick intestine has been found in the cytoplasm near the terminal web and microvillus membrane and may be contained in lysosomes (63). Calbindin (64) and other brush-border-associated Ca-binding proteins such as IMCal (37,73) and calmodulin-associated protein (34–36) could serve to bind Ca within these vesicles during cellular transport. As lysosomal vesicles mature, intravesicular pH decreases to 4.5–4.8, which favors dissociation of calcium from intravesicular binding sites. Quinine and methylamine disrupt lysosomal function by raising intravesicular pH to 5.0 (74,75) and inhibit transcellular Ca J_{ms} (65).

Vitamin D Regulation

Vitamin D, specifically $1,25(OH)_2D_3$, increases intestinal Ca absorption through stimulation of the cell-mediated component of the transport process. The specific mechanism whereby $1,25(OH)_2D_3$ increases Ca transport remains unknown, but there is evidence for a role of genomic and nongenomic events. $1,25(OH)_2D_3$ action is initiated by binding of steroid to the vitamin D receptor. The steroid–receptor complex then interacts with specific genomic sites that initiate expression of specific genes, the products of which are important in initiating or increasing cellular Ca transport. A detailed discussion of the genomic events and regulation of responsive genes is contained in Chapter 8.

Genomic action of $1,25(OH)_2D_3$ also stimulates crypt cell proliferation and accelerates cell migration up the villi (76,76a). Villus tip cell brush-border membrane vesicle Ca uptake is increased by $1,25(OH)_2D_3$, whereas Ca uptake by brush border from villus crypt cells do not respond (77). The vitamin-D-dependent alkaline phosphatase is at its highest concentration in the villus tip cells (77–81), and calbindin concentrations are greatest in villus crypt cells (77). Thus, cellular Ca transport along the villus may occur in villus tip cells, and brush-border vesicle Ca uptake may be dissociated from $1,25(OH)_2D_3$-stimulated alkaline phosphatase and calbindin production (77).

There is also evidence that $1,25(OH)_2D_3$ can stimulate Ca transport rapidly, within minutes of administration, suggesting that nongenomic mechanisms may also be present (82–84). One mechanism whereby $1,25(OH)_2D_3$ may rapidly increase Ca membrane permeability is through alteration of membrane lipid composition. $1,25(OH)_2D_3$ increases phosphatidylcholine and reduces phosphatidylethanolamine (40,85,86). Also, insertion of *cis*-vaccenic acid methyl ester (40) into chick brush-border membranes results in increased Ca uptake. Measurements of membrane fluidity of epithelial brush-border plasma membranes have shown either no effect (43,44) or an increase (42) following vitamin D or 1,25(OH)₂D₃ administration. Because of the high concentrations of $1,25(OH)_2D_3$ used in these studies, further studies are required in order to determine the significance of these early responses.

Nonsaturable (Paracellular) Transport

In situ absorption studies in duodenum show that at high Ca concentrations the nonsaturating component is similar in magnitude throughout the small intestine (2–4,87) and is the dominant pattern of absorption in vitamin-D-deficient rat intestine (7). In contrast, in vitro measurement of Ca J_{ms} shows greater contribution of the nonsaturable component across jejunum and ileum (13,15,16,88) than across duodenum (10), cecum (14), and colon (18,19). The pathways for the saturable and nonsaturable Ca J_{ms} and J_{sm} have been explored in vitro using three techniques: (i) saturation studies discussed above; (ii) simultaneous measurement of fluxes of Ca and neutral molecules confined to the paracellular space, such as mannitol and polyethylene glycol; and (iii) voltage clamping in which Ca fluxes are measured during sustained application of nonzero voltage, resulting in voltage-dependent and voltage-independent fluxes. Application of these techniques provide evidence for a paracellular route for the passive, nonsaturable component of Ca J_{ms}. The nonsaturable components of Ca J_{ms} and J_{sm} are not responsive to vitamin D status or $1,25(OH)_2D_3$ (3,4,6). In ileum, passive ion flux is large,

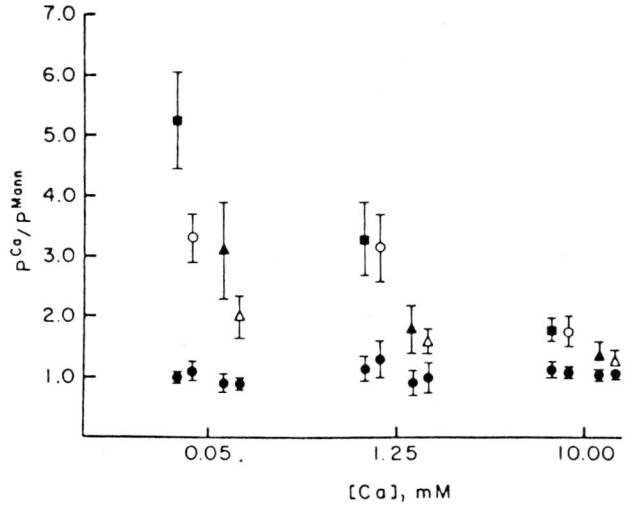

FIG. 8. Ratio of Ca to mannitol permeabilities for mucosal-to-serosal fluxes in the presence (○) and absence (■) of medium D-glucose in ileum from rats fed a low-Ca diet. Data from rats fed a high-Ca diet are shown in the presence (△) and absence (▲) of medium glucose. Corresponding serosal-to-mucosal permeability ratios are denoted by ●. [From Nellans and Kimberg (15).]

with over 93% of total tissue conductance occurring via the paracellular pathway (89). Thus, cellular conductance is only 7% of total conductance, and potential-dependent flux is interpreted as paracellular ion movement. Potential-dependent Ca flux is a major part of total ileal Ca J_{ms}, and there is a linear relationship between the Ca J_{ms} and applied potential (13) (Fig. 7). $1,25(OH)_2D_3$ increases Ca J_{ms} by increasing the potential-independent component and has no effect on the slope of J_{ms} versus applied potential (Fig. 7) (13), as described by the Goldman equation (90).

Membrane permeability (P_{ms} and P_{sm} defined as flux/[Ca or molecule concentration]) of neutral molecules confined to the paracellular space, such as polyethylene glycol and mannitol (15,19,91), are strongly positively correlated with Ca permeability only at high medium Ca conditions (5–10 mM) when Ca carrier-mediated processes are saturated (Fig. 8). In the absence of active transport, such as during a high-Ca diet, the cellular component of Ca J_{ms} is virtually absent. At high Ca concentrations, the permeabilities of Ca P_{ms} and P_{sm} approach equality (Fig. 8) (15,91,92). Passive permeability in ileum is severalfold greater than in cecum (13–16); therefore the voltage-dependent paracellular pathway probably contributes to a larger portion of Ca J_{ms} in ileum than in cecum. In the latter, increased voltage-dependent Ca flux may have a considerable transcellular component as well. In contrast to the largely cellular mucosal-to-serosal Ca fluxes, permeability of the serosal-to-mucosal fluxes of Ca and mannitol are insensitive to temperature and metabolic inhibitors (Fig. 9). Thus, the available data support a paracellular pathway for most, if

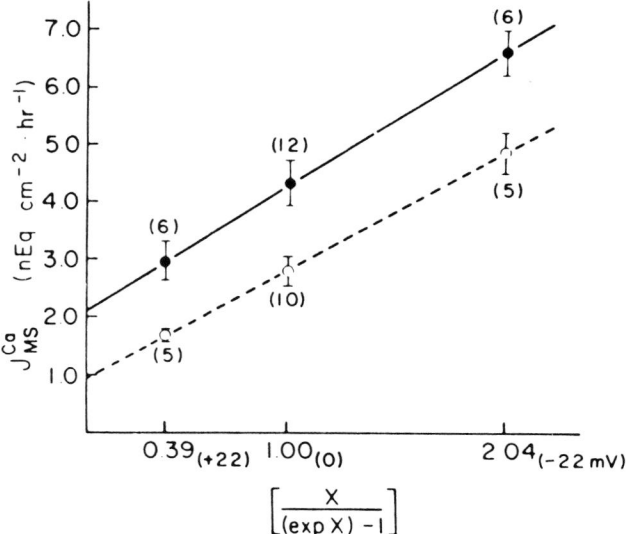

FIG. 7. Relationship between Ca J_{ms} (flux from mucosa to serosa) and potential difference (mV) is indicated by the bracketed expression, where $x = zF(\Delta\psi_{ms})/RT$, where $\Delta\psi_{ms}$ is the potential imposed across the tissue. Lines are mean values of least-squares fit to individual experiments. Number of tissues studied is indicated with SEM at each point for normal-Ca diet (○) and low-Ca diet (●). [From Nellans and Kimberg (13).]

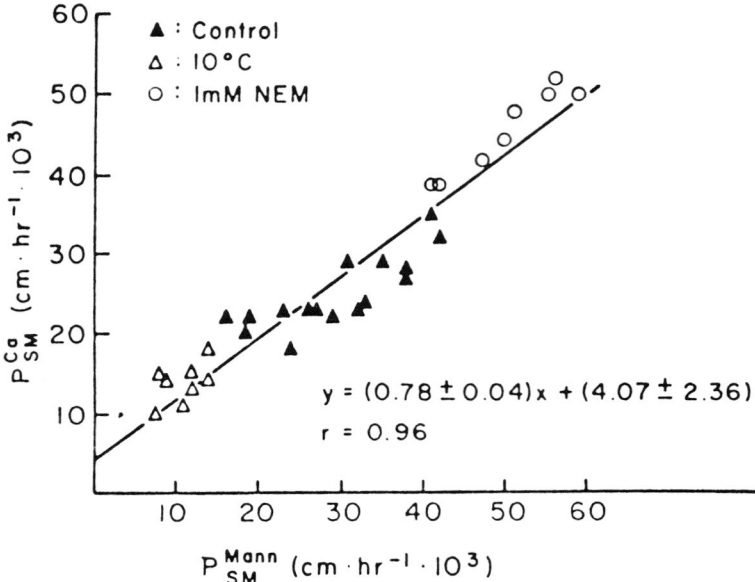

FIG. 9. Permeability for serosal-to-mucosal Ca flux is plotted against simultaneously measured mannitol permeability. Data are from four Ca concentrations (0.05–1.25 m*M*); data from high- and low-Ca diets were pooled, since no significant differences were detected. Values are for control (▲), 10°C (△), and 1 m*M* *N*-ethylmaleimide (○). [From Nellans and Kimberg (15).]

not all, of the diffusive, nonsaturable components of Ca J_{ms} in all regions of the intestine that have been studied.

Ca Secretion

The kinetic characteristics and energetics of Ca secretion (Ca J_{sm}) differ from cellular Ca absorption (Ca J_{ms}), suggesting separate pathways for each. Unlike Ca J_{ms}, which is saturable, Ca J_{sm} increases linearly and fails to reach a plateau over a range of medium Ca from 0.125 to 10.0 m*M* (Fig. 3) (10,13–16,18,19). Also, Ca J_{sm} is not sensitive to metabolic inhibitors or reductions in temperature (Fig. 9) (13), which inhibit J_{ms}. There is variation in Ca secretion along the intestine, with greatest Ca J_{sm} in jejunum and ileum (13,15,16), suggesting that these regions are the major sites of endogenous fecal Ca secretion.

Two lines of evidence support a paracellular pathway for most, if not all, Ca J_{sm}: (i) Ca J_{sm} is positively correlated with mannitol and polyethylene glycol 900 fluxes (Figs. 8 and 9) (15,19,93), which are limited to the intercellular space; and (ii) Ca J_{sm} varies directly with applied current under voltage-clamp conditions (Fig. 7) (15). Since voltage-dependent flow in small intestine is largely paracellular (89), the tight junction (rather than a plasma membrane) may be the resistive barrier to Ca secretion. This assumption has been discussed in the section on the paracellular pathway (see above).

The driving forces for Ca J_{sm} are largely passive diffusional. The transepithelial potential difference of 4–5 mV, lumen negative, favors Ca secretion (Fig. 4); however, the Ca concentration gradient may favor Ca absorption, since luminal Ca may exceed blood ionized Ca.

Therefore, the Ca concentration gradient could overcome or reduce the opposing electrical gradient. Solute and hydrostatic gradients within the epithelium may also drive Ca J_{sm} in the absence of transepithelial gradients. This is suggested by (a) the reduction in Ca J_{sm} when medium sodium is replaced with choline and (b) the increase in Ca J_{sm} in the presence of mucosal glucose (13,15,93). Water recycling from the lateral intercellular space onto the luminal surface may serve to generate the hydrostatic force responsible for solvent drag (15). The greater Ca J_{sm} in small intestine compared to that in colon is due, in part, to the greater resistive barrier to water flow and lower paracellular current across cecum and colon (14,15,89,94).

Regulation of Ca secretion is poorly understood, but luminal factors such as Ca, sodium, and glucose concentrations and blood ionized Ca may influence hydrostatic and concentration-dependent gradients. Chronic dietary Ca restriction (95,96) reduces in vivo plasma-to-lumen Ca flux, but ileal Ca J_{sm} under short-circuit conditions in vitro is not reduced by low-Ca diet or 1,25(OH)$_2$D$_3$ administration (13,15). Somatostatin administration to humans (97,98) and addition to intestinal tissue in vitro stimulate Ca J_{sm} (99). Colon and ileum are most responsive to somatostatin, which is dependent upon the presence of luminal sodium (99). Two other peptide hormones derived from the gut, calcitonin and substance P (100), have no effect on Ca secretion.

Factors Affecting Ca Absorption

Intestinal Ca absorption may be increased or decreased by a variety of hormones or agents, which act either directly on the enterocyte or indirectly through

TABLE 1. *Factors that increase or decrease intestinal Ca absorption*

Increase	Decrease
Vitamin D	Aging
Parathyroid hormone	Glucocorticoids
Low-Ca diet	Thyroid hormone
Growth	Phytate
Lactation	Oxalate
Pregnancy	Thiazide diuretics
Lactose	Gastric surgery
Estrogen	Metabolic acidosis
Alkalosis	

alterations in the circulating levels of $1,25(OH)_2D_3$ (Table 1).

Hormones

Parathyroid Hormone

Parathyroid hormone (PTH) increases intestinal Ca transport through direct stimulation of the renal biosynthesis and secretion of $1,25(OH)_2D_3$ (see Chapter 7). Under conditions of vitamin D deficiency (101,102) or chronic metabolic acidosis (103–107), $1,25(OH)_2D_3$ production is low, and intestinal Ca transport is therefore reduced even though PTH secretion is increased. While PTH may directly stimulate enterocyte Ca transport (108), the weight of evidence argues that PTH increases enterocyte Ca transport indirectly through stimulation of $1,25(OH)_2D_3$ production.

Glucocorticoids

Spontaneous Cushing's syndrome and chronic treatment with pharmacologic doses of glucocorticoids suppress intestinal Ca absorption (109–117) and cause negative Ca balance (112,116; also see Chapter 38). Glucocorticoids suppress Ca active transport (113,115) by decreasing Ca J_{ms} and increasing Ca J_{sm} (115). In chicks (118), basal and $1,25(OH)_2D_3$-stimulated brush-border vesicle Ca uptake are not inhibited by doses of cortisol that inhibit in vivo Ca absorption, suggesting that the site of the inhibition is distal to brush-border Ca entry. In dogs, glucocorticoids increase intestinal vitamin D receptor content (119), whereas the vitamin-D-dependent calcium-binding protein is either increased (113), unchanged (119,120), or decreased (121). Thus, expression of vitamin-D-dependent genes may be altered by glucocorticoids.

The effect of glucocorticoids to inhibit Ca absorption may be part of a general effect on enterocytes, since intestinal sodium and glucose absorption (113) are enhanced by glucocorticoid treatment. Although glucocorticoids may accelerate the metabolic degradation and reduce serum levels of 25-hydroxyvitamin D (117,122), production, degradation, and circulating levels of

$1,25(OH)_2D_3$ are not altered (123,124). Furthermore, pharmacologic doses of $1,25(OH)_2D_3$ can increase Ca J_{ms} (115) and Ca absorption (117) during glucocorticoid therapy and thus overcome the inhibitory actions on Ca transport.

Thyroid Hormone

Intestinal Ca absorption is reduced and Ca balance is negative in patients with hyperthyroidism (125–129) and in experimental animals made hyperthyroid by thyroid hormone ingestion (130–133). The reduction in Ca absorption is probably due to decreased serum $1,25(OH)_2D_3$ as found in hyperthyroid patients (134). The suppressive action of thyroid hormone on enterocyte Ca transport is independent of PTH (127). In rats, hypophysectomy reduces Ca transport (135), which is reduced further by thyroxine administration.

In hypothyroidism, net intestinal calcium absorption may be decreased (136,137) or increased (125,127). The effect of low thyroid hormone levels on $1,25(OH)_2D_3$ production, if any, has not been explored; however, intestinal Ca absorption is restored to normal when hyper- or hypothyroidism is corrected and the euthyroid state is reestablished.

Calcitonin

Variable effects of calcitonin (CT) on Ca absorption have been reported. In experimental animals (138) and in patients with Paget's disease (139), CT acutely inhibits Ca absorption or has no effect (140,141). Acute infusion of salmon CT in healthy humans does not alter Ca movement out of small intestine using the triple-lumen perfusion technique, but it does result in a marked secretion of chloride, sodium, potassium, and water (100,142). Long-term CT infusion (100 h) in sheep reduces Ca absorption only after the infusion is stopped (143). The acute hypocalcemic action of CT is independent of intestinal absorption (144).

Growth Hormone

Administration of growth hormone (GH) to healthy humans and pituitary dwarfs (145–147) and adult rats (133,148) increases net intestinal Ca absorption (145,147). In rats, hypophysectomy reduces Ca active transport (133), and administration of bovine GH or ovine prolactin restores transport activity. The increase in Ca transport occurs within 12 h after GH administration and before changes in body weight or other gross metabolic effects are evident. GH may increase Ca transport by increasing $1,25(OH)_2D_3$ synthesis in intact (149), but not hypophysectomized (150,151), rats. GH also increases Ca transport in vitamin-D-deficient rats in the presence and absence of $1,25(OH)_2D_3$ (152). The dose of $1,25(OH)_2D_3$ required to restore Ca transport in the absence of GH is much greater, suggesting possible synergism between GH and $1,25(OH)_2D_3$ (153). Thus, GH appears to influence the intestinal response to $1,25(OH)_2D_3$ as well as increasing its synthesis.

Estrogens and Androgens

In healthy humans, testosterone administration increases Ca retention, which is further enhanced by estradiol (154). Testosterone increases intestinal Ca absorption in normal subjects and elderly men (155). In postmenopausal women, estrogen increases Ca absorption (156) and converts Ca balance from negative to positive (154).

Ca absorption declines with aging (157) and the menopause (158,159), but it increases towards premenopausal levels following estrogen administration (160). Serum $1,25(OH)_2D_3$ levels decrease (160–162) following estrogen removal and increase within 2 weeks after beginning estrogen (160,163). Also, estrogen has a direct effect on renal proximal tubules to increase $1,25(OH)_2D_3$ synthesis (164).

In experimental animals, the effects of estrogen and testosterone are variable. Injection of estradiol into hypophysectomized or intact male rats for 7 days reduces Ca active transport by everted duodenal gut sacs, whereas testosterone or progesterone have no effect (135).

Drugs

Diuretics

Using balance techniques, thiazide diuretics and chlorthalidone may increase (165,166), decrease (167,168), or have no effect on (169) Ca balance in normal subjects and patients with idiopathic hypercalciuria and kidney stone (see Chapter 32) and may decrease balance in normal children (167). Measurement of unidirectional lumen-to-blood flux of Ca by radioisotopic techniques also shows that thiazide and chlorthalidone reduce Ca absorption in some patients (170–172) but not in others (170–174). In general, Ca absorption is reduced by thiazide and chlorthalidone, and overall Ca balance is improved to the extent that urine Ca is reduced more than intestinal absorption. In rats, chlorthalidone decreases intestinal Ca absorption without altering serum $1,25(OH)_2D_3$ levels (175). Thiazides appear to reduce Ca absorption by mechanisms other than decreasing serum $1,25(OH)_2D_3$ levels or directly interacting with the enterocyte (173).

Furosemide increases urinary Ca excretion, and intestinal Ca absorption increases to match urine Ca losses (176). The increase in Ca transport is not accompanied by changes in serum $1,25(OH)_2D_3$ levels (176). Ethacrynic acid (93) has no direct action on intestinal Ca transport. Trifluoperazine suppresses Ca J_{ms} (93) through a direct interaction with the enterocyte Ca transport process, whereas ouabain has no direct effect on Ca transport (93). The Ca-channel blockers verapamil and nitrendipine inhibit intestinal Ca J_{ms} in vitro only at high concentrations ($10^{-5} M$), suggesting the Ca channels involved in enterocyte cellular Ca transport may not be analogous to the well-characterized Ca channels in the plasma membranes of excitable tissues (92).

Luminal Factors

Ca absorption by double isotope techniques varies depending upon whether it is given with food. The rate of Ca absorption following ingestion of food is lower than the rate obtained when the isotope is administered with $CaCl_2$ alone (177). The dissociation of Ca from the accompanying anion also influences absorption, so that Ca citrate, which is more completely dissociated than Ca carbonate, is more efficiently absorbed (178). A larger portion of Ca is absorbed per 24 h when divided into several doses taken hours apart (179).

Dietary Ca may form soluble or insoluble complexes with a variety of luminal elements and compounds, including phosphorus, phytate, oxalate, fatty acids, and other anionic constituents of the diet. Because Ca is thought to be absorbed in the ionic form, the less-than-complete absorption of dietary Ca is thought to be partly due to complexation of Ca in the intestinal lumen. Because of the large amount of phosphorus in the diet (180) (often 1.0 g or more, compared to less than 1.0 g of Ca), Ca phosphate is a major complex in the intestinal lumen. Because Ca phosphate formation is pH-dependent with a pK_a of about 6.1, increases in luminal pH above pH 6.1 favor complexation and reduction of the amount of ionic Ca available for absorption.

Ca complexation with oxalate and phytate is not as sensitive to pH and is not readily reversible (180). Ingestion of foods rich in oxalate (rhubarb, spinach, other green vegetables, tea) or phytate (unleavened bread unaccompanied by the enzyme phytase) results in reduced Ca absorption. Phytate may be less effective in that it is usually digested in the small intestine (181). Dietary fiber, including cellulose and noncellulose types (182,183), decrease Ca absorption by binding dietary Ca in proportion to the uronic acid content of the fiber (184).

Dietary protein increases urinary Ca excretion, may reduce Ca absorption (185,186), and may cause negative Ca balance. In contrast, certain amino acids, mainly lysine (187), increase Ca absorption. Ingestion of fatty acids such as linoleic acid decreases Ca absorption, but feeding the methyl ester form of linoleate or triglycerides does not (188), presumably because methyl linoleate and triglycerides are absorbed within micelles and do not readily complex with Ca.

Lactose, the major disaccharide in milk and other dairy products, increases net Ca absorption in humans

(189) by a direct action on the intestinal cell (190,191). In experimental animals, the effect of lactose is not dependent upon the presence of vitamin D or active metabolites (192,193). The breakdown of lactose to glucose and galactose may be important, since lactose fails to stimulate Ca absorption in lactose-intolerant people (194). In rat ileum in vitro, lactose increases Ca J_{ms} in the absence of electrochemical or osmotic tissue gradients (91,195,196) and is abolished by replacement of medium sodium by choline (91).

Bacterial flora metabolize lactose to lactic acid, which acidifies the distal small intestine. The decline in luminal pH may favor Ca absorption by increasing ionized Ca available for absorption.

Luminal pH may have a direct effect on Ca transport. Lowering medium pH from 7.4 to 7.1 by reducing medium bicarbonate results in a decline in duodenal and ileal Ca J_{ms} (197), whereas raising pH from 7.4 to 7.7 by increasing medium bicarbonate has no effect on Ca J_{net}. Increasing medium P_{CO_2} to simulate respiratory acidosis has no effect on Ca transport (197).

In rats, chronic metabolic acidosis induced by ingestion of ammonium chloride reduces Ca J_{ms} by decreasing serum $1,25(OH)_2D_3$ (104,105). $1,25(OH)_2D_3$ is reduced because production rates decline with elevation in blood ionized Ca (106). Increased Ca absorption in acidotic rats (198,199) may be due to phosphorus depletion and secondary stimulation of $1,25(OH)_2D_3$. Ca absorption is decreased in human subjects made acidotic with ammonium chloride (200,201), and large Ca intake maintains Ca absorption by vitamin-D-independent pathways (200). Thus, luminal and systemic pH changes may alter Ca transport through direct effects on the enterocyte and indirectly by suppressing $1,25(OH)_2D_3$ production, respectively.

Dietary Ca Intake and Aging

The fraction of dietary Ca absorbed varies with body Ca requirements, daily Ca intake, and age. The average North American diet contains 400–1200 mg Ca, depending upon use of dairy products or Ca supplements. Most adults maintain Ca balance when intake is as low as 2 mg/kg body weight or about 130–150 mg/day (202). Under conditions of low Ca intake, or when Ca requirements are increased, such as during growth, pregnancy, or lactation, the efficiency of Ca absorption increases (10,157,203–210). This physiologic adjustment in Ca absorption, or adaptation, has been demonstrated in humans using metabolic balance (203,204), single and double Ca isotopic measurement of unidirectional Ca movement from lumen to blood (157,208), and in situ intubation and triple-lumen perfusion of segments of proximal and distal small intestine (209). Under these conditions, fractional Ca absorption may range from 20–40% during periods of adequate Ca intake to over

60% when Ca requirements increase or intake is restricted.

Nicolaysen (203,204) recognized the close coordination of Ca absorption to Ca requirements and hypothesized the presence of an unknown signal, or "endogenous factor," formed in response to Ca needs, that stimulates the intestinal response. Subsequent studies in rats showed that vitamin D was required for the adaptation process (203,206). Following the isolation and identification of $1,25(OH)_2D_3$, considerable evidence has accumulated to support $1,25(OH)_2D_3$ as Nicolaysen's endogenous factor (211). In rats, chronic dietary Ca restriction (2–3 weeks) increases (a) renal 25-hydroxyvitamin D-1α-hydroxylase [1OHase] activity (212–215), (b) circulating $1,25(OH)_2D_3$ levels (216–220), (c) target tissue accumulation of the steroid (217), and (d) intestinal epithelial cell vitamin D receptor number (220). Thus, virtually all of the changes in Ca transport during adaptation can be ascribed to the stimulatory actions of $1,25(OH)_2D_3$ on Ca J_{ms}.

The control of $1,25(OH)_2D_3$ production during adaptation remains incompletely understood. PTH is a major regulator of $1,25(OH)_2D_3$ biosynthesis, and low-Ca diet increases PTH secretion (105,221–223). However, the adaptive increase in intestinal Ca J_{ms} may occur in the absence of the parathyroid glands (206,217–219,224,225). The essential role of several other hormones has also been eliminated, since rats retain their ability to respond to low-Ca diet following ablation of the thyroid, adrenal, and pituitary (206). Chronic metabolic acidosis inhibits the expected increase in $1,25(OH)_2D_3$ production during low-Ca diet despite increased PTH (105).

The intestinal Ca transport adaptation to increased Ca requirements is blunted by aging and loss of estrogen in women. Older men require more time (months) to increase Ca absorption and reestablish Ca balance during chronic low Ca intake (226). Triple-lumen perfusion studies show that the rise in jejunal saturable Ca transport V_{max} during low-Ca diet is blunted in older adults (20). Intestinal Ca absorption and serum $1,25(OH)_2D_3$ levels are lower in postmenopausal women despite their lower Ca intake, which would be expected to provoke an increase in $1,25(OH)_2D_3$ production (159). Young rats adapt more rapidly to low-Ca diet than do older rats (227,228), and the rise in ileal Ca J_{ms} in response to low-Ca diet is delayed in older male breeder rats (88). The reduction in Ca transport (205,229) and delay in adaptation with aging is not due to decreased intestinal responsiveness to $1,25(OH)_2D_3$, since the time course and magnitude of the response of Ca transport to $1,25(OH)_2D_3$ is no different in young and old rats (230). Rather, the delay results from decreased $1,25(OH)_2D_3$ production (229,231) caused either by a lag in the time required to increase $1,25(OH)_2D_3$ production or by poorly responsive renal 1OHase.

MAGNESIUM

Driving Forces for Mg Transport

Studies using perfused loops of bowel and everted gut sacs from rats and sheep provide abundant evidence that a large component of transepithelial Mg absorption is due to passive diffusion (232–235). At low luminal Mg concentrations the progressive increase in Mg lumen-to-plasma flux is suggestive of passive diffusion. At higher luminal Mg concentrations (5–10 mM) the lumen-to-plasma flux approaches a plateau (233,235,236). This saturable component observed in vivo is consistent with either facilitated diffusion or cellular active transport, but these two possibilities cannot be distinguished in the presence of spontaneous electrochemical gradients.

Evidence for both passive diffusion and cell-mediated active transport are obtained from measurements of bidirectional fluxes of ^{28}Mg under short-circuited conditions in vitro (232,237–239). Bidirectional Mg fluxes across rat ileum are asymmetrical, with concentration-dependent fluxes from mucosa to serosa (J_{ms}) over low medium Mg becoming saturable at higher Mg concentrations with a K_d of about 1.2 mM (239), whereas Mg secretory fluxes from serosa to mucosa (J_{sm}) are linear over the same range of medium Mg concentration and exceed Mg J_{ms} at 5.0 mM (Fig. 10).

While Mg J_{ms} has a saturable component both in vitro under short-circuited conditions and under open-circuited conditions in situ, the large saturable component of the absorptive flux in vivo almost disappears when the electrical gradients are abolished by short-circuiting in vitro. Although there is evidence for cell-mediated active transport in vitro, the difference between Mg J_{ms} and Mg J_{sm} is small, less than 20% of total Mg J_{ms} (239) (Fig. 10). Thus, an active transport process appears to be present, but it is not a major pathway for Mg J_{ms} under basal conditions; moreover, the saturable component of Mg absorption in situ probably represents facilitated diffusion. In contrast, studies performed in situ and in vitro indicate that passive diffusion appears to play a major role in net Mg transport.

Response to Vitamin D

In animals, vitamin D increases net Mg absorption in isolated loops of bowel and disappears when the Mg fluxes are measured in vitro. In the only study of short-circuited bidirectional Mg fluxes, 1,25(OH)$_2$D$_3$ failed to increase Mg J_{ms} across rat ileum and colon (238,239). However, 1,25(OH)$_2$D$_3$ also did not increase ileal Ca J_{net}, a well-known action of 1,25(OH)$_2$D$_3$. These studies suggest that diffusional forces abolished by short-circuited conditions in vitro may be important driving forces for Mg absorption in vivo.

Pathways for Mg Transport

Mg J_{ms} has voltage-dependent and voltage-independent components, consistent with both cellular and paracellular pathways (239). Mg J_{sm} is completely voltage-dependent, suggesting a paracellular pathway for most, if not all, of the Mg secretory flux (239). Similar kinetic characteristics for Mg absorptive and secretory fluxes have been observed across rat colon (238,240). These findings are also consistent with in vivo studies in which a large saturable Mg flux increased with vitamin D treatment.

Mg Absorption in Humans

In humans, net Mg absorption is 35–40% of dietary intake (241). True Mg absorption, calculated as the sum of Mg absorbed from diet and intestinal juices, varies from 40% to 50% of available Mg. Over the range of normal Mg intake, there is a linear relationship between intake and absorption (242–244). However, at very high Mg intake (10 mM), absorption is lower than predicted (245), suggesting that the Mg absorptive mechanism in humans may be saturable. Because Mg absorption is strongly dependent upon luminal Mg concentration, changes in luminal fluid volume and water absorption would be expected to influence Mg absorption. However, Mg transport is readily demonstrated in the absence of net water movement from triple-lumen intubation experiments (246).

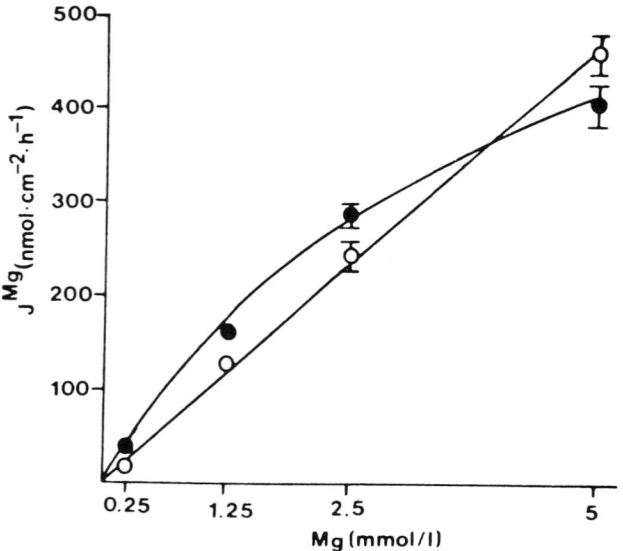

FIG. 10. Concentration-dependence of the mucosal-to-serosal (●) and serosal-to-mucosal (○) Mg fluxes across short-circuited rat ileal epithelium. Medium Ca concentration is 1.25 mM. Values are mean ± SEM for six to eight tissues per group. [From Karbach and Rummel (239).]

Relatively little is known about the sites of intestinal Mg absorption in humans. Based on the appearance of radioactive isotope in blood following oral ingestion, Mg is thought to be absorbed throughout the small intestine, with maximal absorption in the proximal small bowel (245). Mg absorption has been studied in human jejunum and ileum using the triple-lumen perfusion technique (246,247). In jejunum, Mg absorption increases linearly with increasing luminal Mg and approaches a plateau at concentrations approaching 5 mM. Kinetics and rates of Mg absorption are similar in ileum (246). Little information is available on Mg absorption by the large bowel; however, hypermagnesemia following rectal enemas indicates that Mg may also be absorbed by the colon (248).

Role of Vitamin D

PTH increases Mg absorption (249), perhaps indirectly through an increase in renal 1,25(OH)$_2$D$_3$ synthesis. Vitamin D increases Mg balance through an increase in intestinal absorption (250–253). 1,25(OH)$_2$D$_3$ administration increases net Mg absorption in healthy humans (247), in those with a variety of metabolic bone diseases (254), and in those with jejunoileal bypass (253). Patients with low 1,25(OH)$_2$D$_3$, as in chronic renal failure, have lower net Mg absorption, which is restored to normal with 1,25(OH)$_2$D$_3$ (246,247). These estimates of Mg absorption by isotope are not in agreement with studies using metabolic balance, which show that Mg balance is not different between healthy and uremic subjects (255); in addition, 1,25(OH)$_2$D$_3$ and 1α-hydroxyvitamin D$_3$ have no effect on either group, although Ca absorption is increased by both metabolites. The apparent discrepancy may be due to the small changes in net Mg absorption following vitamin D that may be within the error of the balance technique, or it may be a result of the fact that isotope absorption measures unidirectional Mg movement from lumen to blood. Increases in both lumen-to-blood and blood-to-lumen Mg fluxes would not be detected by isotopic techniques, but they would result in no net change by metabolic balance. However, convincing evidence for a stimulatory effect of 1,25(OH)$_2$D$_3$ on Mg net absorption has been obtained using the triple-lumen perfusion technique in healthy humans. Seven days of 1,25(OH)$_2$D$_3$ increases jejunal, but not ileal, net Mg absorption; however, Ca absorption is increased in both segments (Table 2) (256).

Ca and Mg Cotransport

Studies of simultaneous Ca and Mg absorption provide conflicting results. In humans and experimental animals, varying luminal Ca concentration causes reciprocal changes in Mg transport, and the converse has also been observed (234–236,257–263). These studies provide indirect evidence that Ca and Mg are absorbed by a common transport mechanism. In contrast, several lines of evidence suggest that Ca and Mg are transported by separate mechanisms. First, there is a differential effect of vitamin D or 1,25(OH)$_2$D$_3$ on Ca and Mg transport: Vitamin D or 1,25(OH)$_2$D$_3$ increases transport of Ca to a greater extent than that of simultaneously measured Mg in situ (246,254) or in vitro (238–240); in renal failure, absorption of Ca is impaired to a greater degree than that of Mg (255,264); and in vitamin-D-resistant rickets, Ca transport is diminished whereas Mg transport is normal (265). Second, the kinetics of Mg and Ca absorption differ, with Ca reaching a greater V_{max} than does Mg. Third, neither ion appears to be required for the absorption of the other (240), since Ca transport is normal in the absence of Mg, Ca has little or no influence on Mg absorption, and Mg in high concentrations may depress Ca transport only slightly (246).

These divergent results in humans and experimental animals remain unexplained. Anast (265) has suggested that formation of nonabsorbable Mg or Ca complexes with phosphate or oxalate may make more of the noncomplexed cation available for absorption. Reciprocal relations between Ca and Mg absorption may be due to other factors such as complexation and may not be the result of competition for a common transport mechanism.

PHOSPHORUS

Pathways for Inorganic Phosphorus (P) Transport

Isotopic ^{32}P movement across intact intestinal epithelium consists of (a) a small portion that appears in the serosal medium within minutes and (b) a major portion that equilibrates with the serosal medium over a more prolonged period of time. The two kinetic isotopic pools

TABLE 2. *Effect of 1,25(OH)$_2$D$_3$ on net jejunal and ileal Ca and Mg fluxes in healthy subjects*[a]

Segment	Basal	Post Rx	p Value
Calcium			
Jejunum	218 ± 33	377 ± 55	<0.02
Ileum	83 ± 47	296 ± 52	<0.005
Magnesium			
Jejunum	16 ± 25	101 ± 33	<0.05
Ileum	155 ± 63	198 ± 51	NS

Source: After Krejs et al. (256).
[a] Values are mean ± SEM for 10 observations per group. Fluxes are expressed in μmol/30 cm/h. Post Rx is after 1 week of 1,25(OH)$_2$D$_3$ 2 μg/day to healthy males and females. NS, not significant.

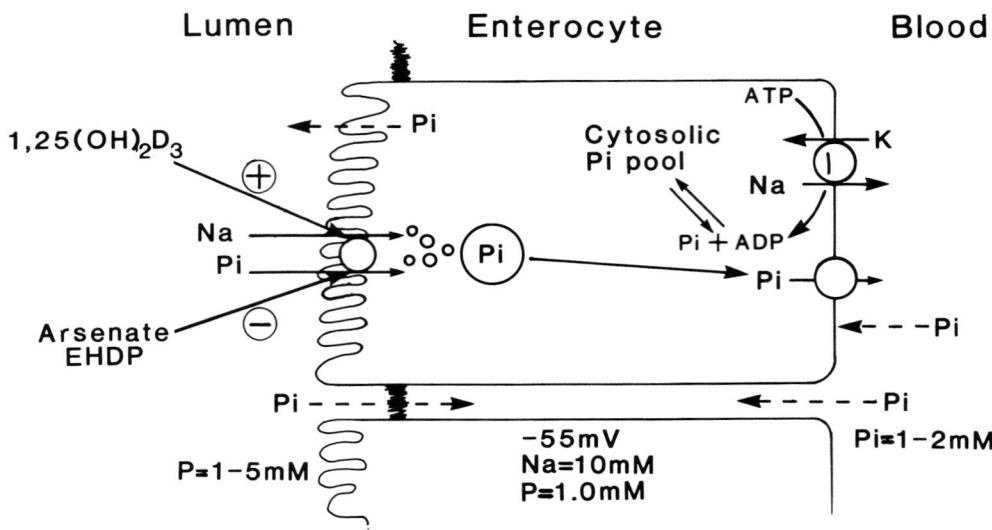

FIG. 11. Schematic of inorganic phosphorus (P_i) absorption (from lumen to blood) and secretion (from blood to lumen) across intestinal epithelium. Broken arrows indicate low-volume pathways. $1,25(OH)_2D_3$ stimulates Na-coupled P_i influx, whereas arsenate and the bisphosphonate EHDP (ethane hydroxy-1-1-diphosphoric acid) inhibit it. Transcellular movement of P_i may be sequestered in structures that are presently unidentified. Exit is down electrical and perhaps concentration gradients.

that develop during transepithelial transport are due to (a) a paracellular pathway represented by the small, rapidly equilibrating pool and (b) a cellular pathway taken by the larger, more slowly equilibrating pool. Thus, most of transepithelial P transport is driven by cellular processes.

Luminal P concentration and estimates of cytosolic P concentration (266) are similar to the P concentration found in the extracellular fluid (1–2 mM), eliminating favorable concentration gradients for P transport. The highly negative charge of the cell interior (−55 mV) retards diffusion of P across brush border (Fig. 11). Therefore, existing electrochemical gradients require either (a) an energy-dependent transport entry process across the brush border or (b) a secondary active process that is driven by the movement of another ion. The same gradients that oppose brush-border P entry permit diffusional exit of P across basolateral membrane; however, the exit process has not been studied.

Cellular Transport Events

Transepithelial P transport across intact epithelium is driven by a cellular active transport process that depends upon sodium (Fig. 11) (266–269). In vivo, P uptake increases linearly with luminal P and Na concentrations (270), supporting the importance of the Na–P cotransport process observed in vitro (Fig. 12). Measurement of transepithelial P fluxes under conditions of electrochemical neutrality in the Ussing apparatus provides the most rigorous evidence for cellular active transport. Under conditions which presumably abolish net diffusional P movement, net P absorption ($J_{ms} > J_{sm}$) has been demon-

strated in proximal and distal rat small intestine (8,271) but not in colon (18,230). In rat jejunum, kinetics of P transport reveal an active saturable process with a K_d for P J_{ms} of 2 mM (272).

Compartmental analysis of P suggest that P ion entering the cell across the brush border is transported

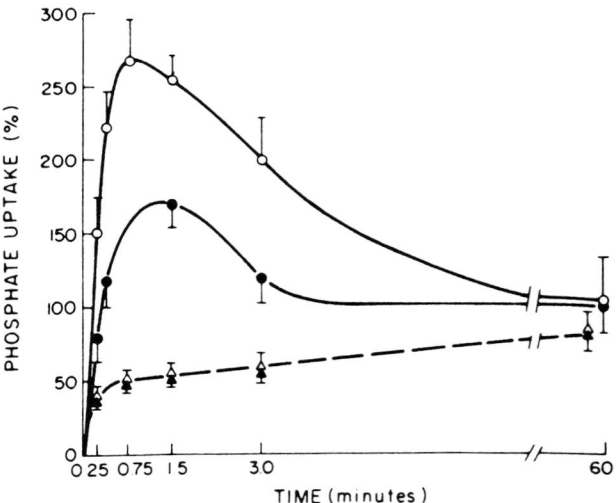

FIG. 12. Time course of phosphate uptake into brush-border membrane vesicles prepared from vitamin-D-deficient chicks treated with $1,25(OH)_2D_3$ (○) or vehicle (●) in the presence of 100 mM NaCl or in the presence of 100 mM choline chloride (▲ treated; △ vehicle). Experiments were performed at pH 7.4, 25°C. Data are percent of 60-min steady-state uptake of vesicles from vehicle-treated chicks in 100 mM NaCl. Values are mean ± SEM for eight experiments. [From Matsumoto et al. (291).]

through the cell sequestered from the intracellular P pool (Fig. 11) (266,273). Cytochalasin inhibits the enterocyte microfilament system and reduces cellular P J_{ms} (274), but it also alters intracellular membrane function; therefore the specificity of cytochalasin action remains to be determined.

Brush-Border P Influx

The sodium-dependence of transepithelial P transport has been demonstrated in studies of P influx across isolated brush border (270). An Na–P cotransport mechanism in intestinal brush-border plasma membrane (52,275–277) is supported by several observations using brush-border membrane vesicles (Figs. 12 and 13): (a) P influx with a transient overshoot is demonstrated in the presence of an inward-directed Na gradient; (b) a decrease in the Na gradient by increasing membrane permeability with Na ionophores decreases P uptake; (c) substitution of choline chloride for sodium chloride reduces P uptake; and (d) a P gradient increases Na influx (275,276). The Na-dependent process can be directly inhibited by mercury, diphosphonate, and arsenate (270) as well as by ouabain, metabolic inhibitors, and anaerobic conditions (273,278,279).

Role of pH

The form of P absorbed is not known, but both luminal pH and ionic strength determine the species of P available for absorption. The pK for the equilibrium between monobasic and dibasic P is 6.8 when ionic strength is that of the extracellular fluid (280). At pH 7.4 the average valence of P is about −1.6; therefore the luminal pH in all but the most proximal duodenum predicts that most P is in the form of HPO_4^{2-}. This is supported by in situ perfusion of rat intestine in which P

absorption (a) increases with increasing medium pH (281) and (b) decreases when luminal pH is reduced (282). The beneficial effects of alkaline pH on P absorption is limited, however, by the formation of insoluble calcium phosphate complexes, which are probably not well-absorbed.

There is evidence for an effect of pH on the Na–P cotransporter. A pH-dependence of brush-border P transport has been observed, where P uptake increases when medium pH is lowered (272,275). At pH 7.4, brush-border membrane vesicle Na-dependent P uptake is almost independent of electrical potential gradients and do not require additional cations; at pH 6.0, however, P transport requires the movement of a net negative charge (275). The pH-dependence of intestinal P transport is not due to the preferential transport of monovalent or divalent P and is not related to an effect of pH on P-binding sites; instead, it is related to changes in the affinity of the transport system for Na and/or direct effects on the transporter (283).

The Na–P Cotransporter

Using a procedure that was employed to characterize the intestinal Na–glucose cotransporter, a 130-kD polypeptide has been identified in rabbit intestinal brush-border membranes that contains both Na and P substrate binding sites and is specifically inhibited by the Na-dependent P transport inhibitors phosphonoxycarboxylic acids and arginine group-specific agents (284). Functional studies of the purified protein, as well as demonstration of a unique primary amino acid sequence of the single band on polyacrylamide gel electrophoresis, are required to confirm that this protein is the Na–P cotransporter.

Effect of Vitamin D

Metabolic balance studies show that both Ca and P absorption increase following vitamin D administration to vitamin-D-deficient animals (285,286). Vitamin D (287,288), 1,25(OH)$_2$D$_3$ (289), and 1α-hydroxyvitamin D$_3$ (289) enhance net intestinal Ca and P absorption in healthy humans and in those with chronic renal failure. Vitamin D increases transepithelial P transport through an increase in the absorptive flux P J_{ms} without a change in secretory flux P J_{sm} (271). Administration of calcitonin inhibits in vivo basal P transport (290), but it is unknown whether vitamin-D-stimulated P absorption is also inhibited by calcitonin.

The site of action of vitamin D to increase cellular P transport appears to be the brush border (Fig. 11). The Na-dependent P uptake process is saturable with a K_d of less than 1 mM (291). Pretreatment with vitamin D or 1,25(OH)$_2$D$_3$ increases Na-dependent P influx into brush-border membrane vesicles (Fig. 11) (270,272,273, 278,291) through an increase in V_{max} without a signifi-

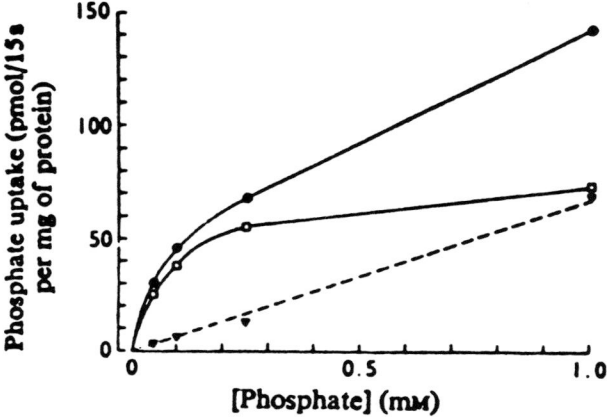

FIG. 13. Phosphate uptake into chick intestinal brush-border membrane vesicles incubated in 100 mM NaCl (●) or 100 mM choline chloride (△). Unfilled squares represent Na-dependent uptake as difference in phosphate uptake in the presence and absence of Na. [From Berner et al. (275).]

cant change in K_d (291). Administration of cyclohexi-mide to vitamin-D-deficient chicks, in doses sufficient to inhibit protein synthesis, blocks an increase in alkaline phosphatase activity but does not block Na-dependent P uptake by brush-border membrane vesicles (291). Thus, the vitamin-D-dependent alkaline phosphatase, which is located in brush border, appears not to be required for Na-dependent P uptake.

Although several vitamin-D-dependent proteins have been implicated in the vitamin-D-mediated Ca transport process, no vitamin-D-dependent proteins have been identified that are specific for P transport.

Phosphate Depletion

Dietary P depletion results in hypercalciuria, reduced urinary P excretion, increased $1,25(OH)_2D_3$ production, circulating levels, and intestinal localization (292–296). In rats fed a low-P diet, Ca balance becomes less positive because of hypercalciuria and a transient increase in Ca absorption which is limited to the proximal small intestine (296). The initial negative P balance is corrected by reduced urinary P and increased duodenal P absorption. Thus, despite low P intake, balance can be maintained by the highly efficient P retention in the kidney and intestine.

Diffusional P Movement

In addition to the evidence for a cellular active P transport process, there is considerable evidence that P can also be absorbed by diffusional forces. Balance studies in rats (297) and humans (298) show a linear relationship between dietary P intake and net P absorption (Fig. 14) (298). In vivo perfusion of rat and chick small intestine also shows a linear increase in P absorption, with no evidence for saturation with increasing luminal P concentrations, although only high concentrations of P were

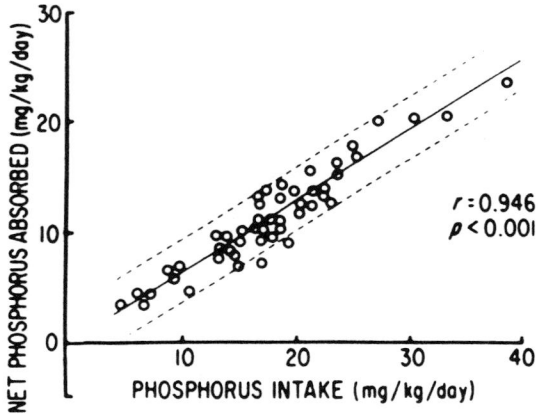

FIG. 14. Relationship between net P absorbed and dietary P intake in normal subjects. [From Wilkinson et al. (298).]

used (281,299). In vivo studies support passive diffu-sional P absorption, whereas the kinetic studies using everted gut sacs yield conflicting results both for (300) and against (301,302) an active transport process. The magnitude of paracellular diffusional P movement has not been measured directly, but the net negative charge of the paracellular space poses a significant barrier to passive P diffusion at low luminal concentrations. Evidence for diffusion at higher concentrations is supported by triple-lumen-tube perfusion of small intestine in healthy humans (303), in which saturation at low luminal P concentrations of 1–3 mM was followed by linear P absorption with no tendency to saturate at higher concentrations. Overall, the evidence favors (a) Na-dependent active cotransport at low luminal P concentrations and (b) passive diffusional forces driving P transport at luminal P concentrations above that which saturates the cotransporter.

Ca and P Cotransport

Because vitamin D and $1,25(OH)_2D_3$ increase intestinal Ca and P absorption, it has been postulated that vitamin D activates a coupled Ca–P transport process. There are data showing a P requirement for Ca active duodenal transport (8) as well as Ca transport that is P-independent (9,304,305). There is also a portion of duodenal and jejunal P transport that requires Ca (268,300).

However, there are several lines of evidence against the presence of a Ca–P cotransporter. Brush-border membrane vesicles from rat, chicken, or rabbit intestine exhibit Na-dependent P transport in the absence and presence of Ca (52,275,291). The polyene antibiotic fili-pin mimics $1,25(OH)_2D_3$ by directly increasing Ca transport, but it has no effect on P transport (29,291).

$1,25(OH)_2D_3$ administration differs in its time course of stimulation for Ca and P active transport (271,291), and intestinal segments respond differentially (271) with maximal Ca J_{ms} in duodenum, maximal P J_{ms} in jejunum, and increased Ca J_{ms} (but not P J_{ms}) in colon (18). However, the P J_{ms}/Ca J_{ms} ratio for each segment in response to $1,25(OH)_2D_3$ remains relatively constant as P J_{ms} and Ca J_{ms} increase twofold. These observations are consistent with coupled Ca–P transport, but they could also reflect a coordinated induction of separate Ca and P transport processes by $1,25(OH)_2D_3$ (271). The differential segmental responses to $1,25(OH)_2D_3$ could reflect the distribution of Ca and P transporting cells, with Ca transporting cells located predominately in duodenum and P transporting cells localized largely in jejunum. If Ca J_{ms} and P J_{ms} were performed by a Ca–P cotransporter, its stoichiometry would have to be quite different for each segment, for example, (P:Ca) 1:3, 3:1, and 1:1 for duodenum, jejunum, and ileum, respectively.

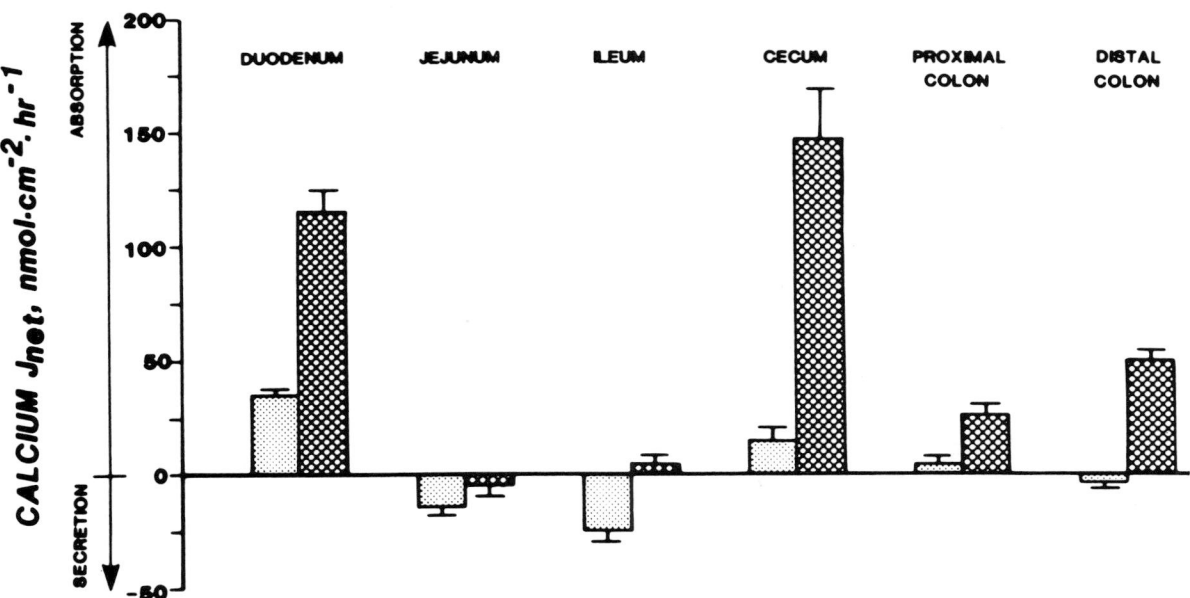

FIG. 15. Net Ca absorption or secretion (above or below horizontal line, respectively) across intestine from vitamin-D-deficient rats treated with $1,25(OH)_2D_3$ (*cross-hatched bars*) or vehicle (*stippled bars*). Net Ca flux ($J_{net} = J_{ms} - J_{sm}$) is calculated from steady-state bidirectional fluxes under short-circuited conditions. [From Favus (17).]

Segmental Ca and P Transport

Proximal Small Intestine

Isotopic Ca appears rapidly in blood after oral administration, indicating absorption by duodenum and proximal jejunum (306,307). Defective proximal intestinal Ca absorption in patients with renal insufficiency suggests that the duodenal absorptive process is $1,25$-$(OH)_2D_3$-dependent (307).

In rats, duodenum normally exhibits net Ca absorption, and J_{ms} decreases during vitamin D deficiency

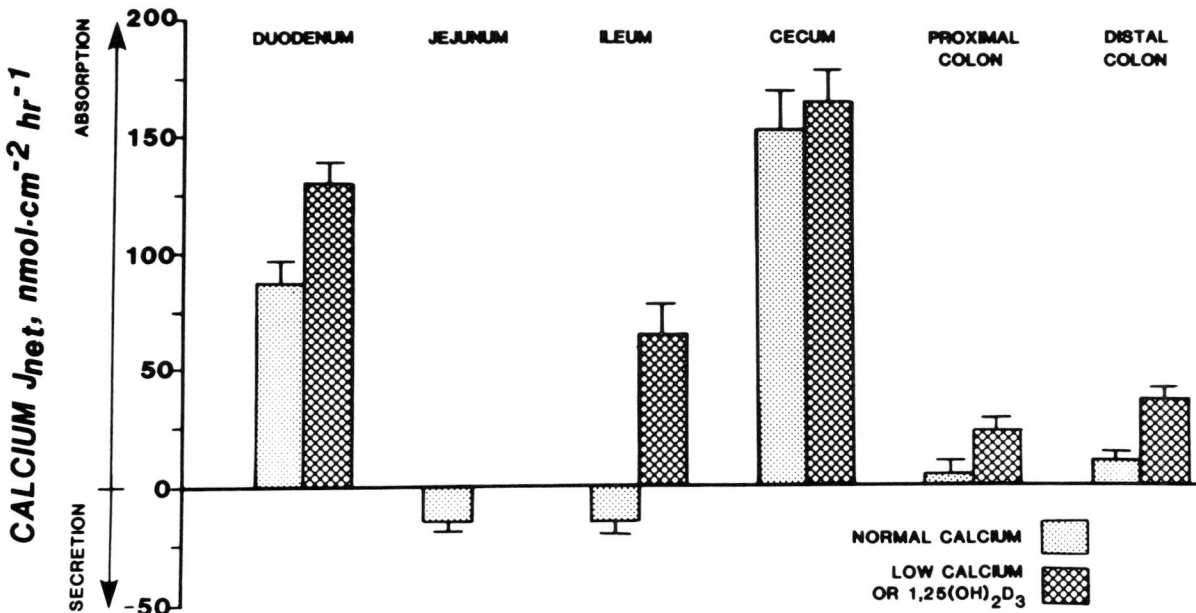

FIG. 16. Net Ca absorption or secretion (above or below horizontal line, respectively) across intestine in rats fed normal chow and injected with vehicle (*stippled bars*) or fed low-Ca diet or injected with $1,25(OH)_2D_3$ to increase endogenous $1,25(OH)_2D_3$ (*cross-hatched bars*). [From Favus (17).]

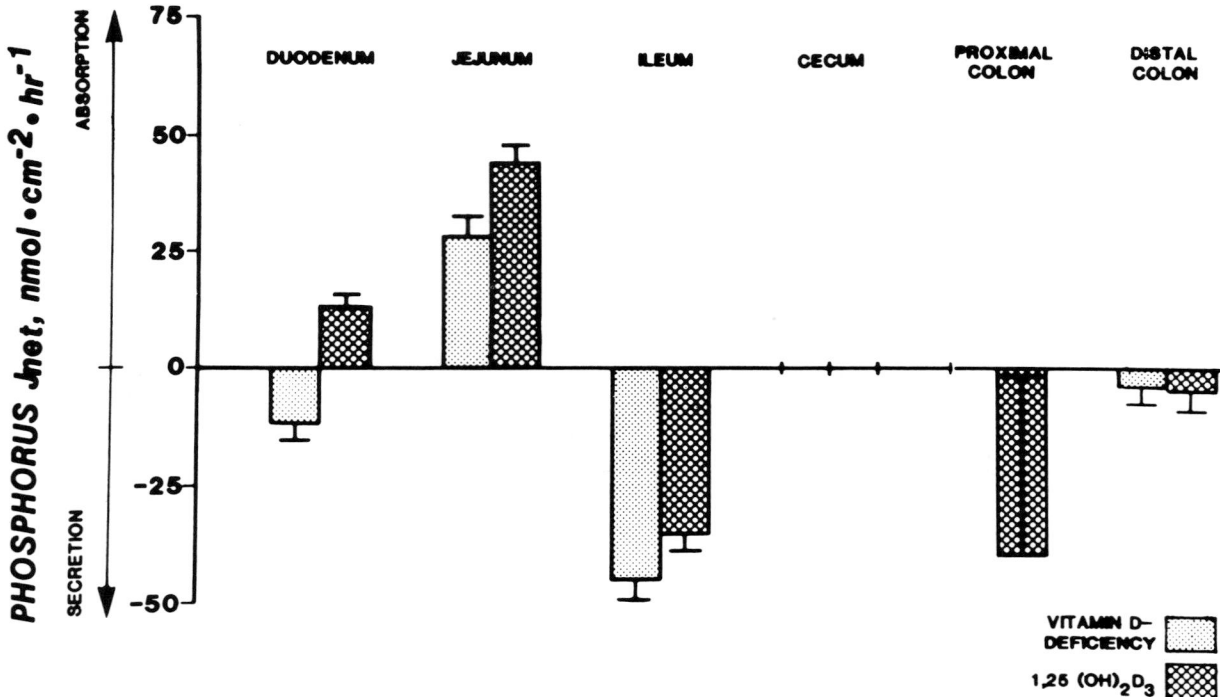

FIG. 17. Net inorganic P absorption or secretion (above or below horizontal line, respectively) from vitamin-D-deficient rats treated with 1,25(OH)$_2$D$_3$ (*cross-hatched bars*) or vehicle (*stippled bars*). [From Favus (17).]

(115,271,308,309) and in older rats (310), resulting in a decrease in J_{net} (Fig. 15). Dietary Ca restriction and 1,25(OH)$_2$D$_3$ administration increase Ca J_{net} through an increase in the absorptive Ca J_{ms} (Fig. 16) (115,271,308,309). Because Ca J_{ms} approaches saturation at about 2.5 mM medium Ca whereas J_{sm} is not saturable, there is net Ca secretion when Ca J_{sm} exceeds Ca J_{ms}, at about 5–10 mM medium Ca (311). In vitamin D deficiency there is net P secretion ($J_{sm} > J_{ms}$). 1,25(OH)$_2$D$_3$ converts net P secretion to net absorption through an increase in J_{ms}. Duodenal P J_{ms} is less than jejunal P J_{ms} (Fig. 17).

Jejunum and Ileum

In humans, triple-lumen-tube perfusion shows net absorption of Ca in response to dietary Ca restriction (20). Administration of 1α-hydroxyvitamin D$_3$ or 1,25-(OH)$_2$D$_3$ increases net Ca absorption of normal subjects and patients with chronic renal failure through an increase in the absorptive flux without a change in secretion (312). In normal adult rats, in vitro Ca J_{sm} exceeds Ca J_{ms}; in addition, 1,25(OH)$_2$D$_3$ increases Ca J_{ms} such that with prolonged stimulation, net secretion may be converted to small net absorption (Fig. 16). The highest basal and 1,25(OH)$_2$D$_3$-stimulated absorptive P fluxes are found in jejunum, with net P absorption present even during vitamin D deficiency (Fig. 17).

Colon

Patients who have undergone small-bowel resection for treatment of inflammatory bowel disease maintain normal radioisotopic Ca absorption when colon is in the fecal stream, whereas ileostomy results in marked reduction in Ca absorption (313). 1,25(OH)$_2$D$_3$ administration can increase Ca net absorption in colon of healthy subjects (314). In rat colon, there is net Ca and P secretion or no net transport ($J_{ms} = J_{sm}$) under basal conditions, and 1,25(OH)$_2$D$_3$ increases Ca J_{ms} and converts net secretion to net absorption (Figs. 15 and 16). In contrast, 1,25(OH)$_2$D$_3$ does not alter P J_{ms} or P J_{sm}. In adult rats, cecum has the highest Ca J_{ms} found in colon or small intestine. Basal Ca J_{ms} is near maximal, since there is no increase with endogenous 1,25(OH)$_2$D$_3$ such as during chronic dietary restriction (Fig. 16), but pharmacologic doses of 1,25(OH)$_2$D$_3$ can increase Ca J_{ms} (315). Vitamin D deficiency reduces cecal Ca J_{ms} to 10% of the vitamin-D-replete state (Fig. 15), and maximal Ca J_{ms} is restored with physiologic doses of 1,25(OH)$_2$D$_3$ that do not cause maximal J_{net} in colon or duodenum (315). Thus, the high Ca J_{ms} in cecum appears to result from increased sensitivity of cecum to 1,25(OH)$_2$D$_3$.

REFERENCES

1. Bellaton CD, Pansu WD, Stein WD, Bronner F. Kinetic analysis of calcium absorption from an in situ duodenal loop [Abstract]. *Fed Proc* 1986;45:180.

2. Zornitzer AE, Bronner F. In situ studies of calcium absorption in rats. *Am J Physiol* 1971;220:1261–6.

3. Bronner F, Pansu D, Stein WD. An analysis of intestinal calcium transport across the rat intestine. *Am J Physiol* 1986;250:G561–9.

4. Pansu D, Bellaton C, Bronner F. The effect of calcium intake on the saturable and non-saturable components of duodenal calcium transport. *Am J Physiol* 1981;240:G32–7.

5. Pansu D, Bellaton C, Bronner F. Developmental changes in the mechanisms of duodenal calcium transport in the rat. *Am J Physiol* 1983;244:G20–6.

6. Pansu D, Bellaton C, Roche C, Bronner F. Duodenal and ileal calcium absorption in the rat and effects of vitamin D. *Am J Physiol* 1983;244:G695–700.

7. Wasserman RH, Taylor AN, Kallfelz FA. Vitamin D and transfer of plasma calcium to intestinal lumen in chicks and rats. *Am J Physiol* 1966;211:419–23.

8. Helbock HJ, Forte JG, Saltman P. The mechanism of calcium transport by rat intestine. *Biochim Biophys Acta* 1966;126:81–93.

9. Walling MW, Rothman SS. Phosphate-independent, carrier-mediated active transport of calcium by rat intestine. *Am J Physiol* 1969;217:1133–48.

10. Walling MW, Rothman SS. Apparent increase in carrier affinity for intestinal calcium transport following dietary calcium restriction. *J Biol Chem* 1970;245:5007–11.

11. Behar J, Kerstein MD. Intestinal calcium absorption: differences in transport between duodenum and ileum. *Am J Physiol* 1976;230:1255–60.

12. Norman DA, Morawski SG, Fordtran JS. Influence of glucose, fructose, and water movement on calcium absorption in the jejunum. *Gastroenterology* 1980;78:22–5.

13. Nellans HN, Kimberg DV. Cellular and paracellular calcium transport in rat ileum: effects of dietary calcium. *Am J Physiol* 1978;235:E726–37.

14. Nellans HN, Goldsmith RS. Transepithelial calcium transport by rat cecum: high-efficiency absorptive site. *Am J Physiol* 1981;240:G424–31.

15. Nellans HN, Kimberg DV. Anomalous calcium secretion in rat ileum: role of paracellular pathway. *Am J Physiol* 1979;236:E473–81.

16. Walling MW, Kimberg DV. Active secretion of calcium by rat ileum and jejunum in vitro. *Am J Physiol* 1973;225:415–22.

17. Favus MJ. Factors that influence absorption and secretion of calcium in the small intestine and colon. *Am J Physiol* 1985;248:G147–57.

18. Lee DBN, Walling MW, Gafter U, Silis V, Coburn JW. Calcium and inorganic phosphate transport in rat colon. Dissociated response to 1,25-dihydroxyvitamin D_3. *J Clin Invest* 1980;65:1326–31.

19. Favus MJ, Kathpalia SC, Coe FL. Kinetic characteristics of calcium absorption and secretion by rat colon. *Am J Physiol* 1981;240:G350–4.

20. Ireland P, Fordtran JS. Effect of dietary calcium and age on jejunal calcium absorption in humans studied by intestinal perfusion. *J Clin Invest* 1973;52:2672–81.

21. Kendrick NC, Kabakoff B, DeLuca HF. Oxygen-dependent 1,25-dihydroxycholecalciferol-induced calcium ion transport in rat intestine. *Biochem J* 1981;1984:178–86.

22. Ussing HH. The distinction by means of traces between active transport and diffusion. *Acta Physiol Scand* 1949;43–56.

23. Bronner F, Pansu D, Bosshard A, Lipton JH. Calcium uptake by isolated rat intestinal cells. *J Cell Physiol* 1983;116:322–8.

24. Walling MW, Rothman SS. Adaptive uptake of calcium at the duodenal brush border. *Am J Physiol* 1973;225:618–23.

25. O'Donnell JM, Smith MW. Influence of cholecalciferol on the initial kinetics of the uptake of calcium by rat small intestinal mucosa. *Biochem J* 1973;134:667–9.

26. Holdsworth ES, Jordan JE, Keenan E. Effects of cholecalciferol on the translocation of calcium by non-everted chick ileum in vitro. *Biochem J* 1975;152:181–90.

27. Patrick G, Sterling C. The dependence of calcium flux into rat intestine on sugars and alkali metals. *Arch Intern Physiol Biochim* 1973;81:453–67.

28. Papworth DG, Patrick G. The kinetics of influx of calcium and strontium in rat intestine in vivo. *J Physiol (Lond)* 1970;210:999–1020.

29. Rasmussen H, Fontaine O, Max EE, Goodman DP. The effect of 1-alpha-hydroxyvitamin D_2 administration on calcium transport in chick intestine brush border membrane vesicles. *J Biol Chem* 1979;254:2993–9.

30. Miller A III, Bronner F. Calcium uptake in isolated brush-border vesicles from rat small intestine. *Biochem J* 1981;196:391–401.

31. Miller A III, Li ST, Bronner F. Characterization of calcium binding to brush border membranes from rat duodenum. *Biochem J* 1982;208:773–82.

32. Schedl HP, Wilson HD. Calcium uptake by intestinal brush border membrane vesicles: comparison with in vivo calcium transport. *J Clin Invest* 1985;76:1871–8.

32a. Miller A III, Ueng T-H, Bronner F. Isolation of a vitamin D-dependent, calcium-binding protein from brush borders of rat duodenal mucosa. *FEBS Lett* 1979;103:319–22.

33. Thomasset M, Molla A, Parkes O, Demaille JG. Intestinal calmodulin and calcium-binding protein differ in their distribution and in the effect of vitamin D steroids on their concentration. *FEBS Lett* 1981;127:13–6.

34. Bikle DD, Munson S, Chafouleas J. Calmodulin may mediate 1,25-dihydroxyvitamin D-stimulated intestinal calcium transport. *FEBS Lett* 1984;174:30–3.

35. Bikle DD, Munson S. 1,25-Dihydroxyvitamin D increases calmodulin binding to specific proteins in the chick duodenal brush border membrane. *J Clin Invest* 1985;76:2312–6.

36. Bikle DD, Munson S. The villus gradient of brush border membrane calmodulin and the calcium-independent calmodulin-binding protein parallels that of calcium-accumulating ability. *Endocrinology* 1986;118:727–32.

37. Kowarski S, Schachter D. Intestinal membrane calcium-binding protein: vitamin D-dependent membrane component of the intestinal calcium transport mechanism. *J Biol Chem* 1980;225:10834–40.

38. Marche P, Leugern C, Cassier P. Immunocytochemical localization of calcium-binding protein in the rat duodenum. *Cell Tissue Res* 1979;197:69–77.

39. Bikle DD, Zolock DT, Morrissey RL, Herman RH. Independence of 1,25-dihydroxyvitamin D_3-mediated calcium transport from de novo RNA and protein synthesis. *J Biol Chem* 1978;253:484–8.

40. Matsumoto T, Fontaine O, Rasmussen H. Effect of 1,25-dihydroxyvitamin D_3 on phospholipid metabolism in chick duodenal mucosal cell. *J Biol Chem* 1981;256:3354–60.

41. Fontaine O, Matsumoto T, Goodman DBP, Rasmussen H. Liponomic control of Ca^{2+} transport: relationship to mechanism of action of 1,25-dihydroxyvitamin D_3. *Proc Natl Acad Sci USA* 1981;78:1751–4.

42. Brasitus TA, Dudeja PK, Eby B, Lau K. Correction by 1,25-dihydroxycholecalciferol of the abnormal fluidity and lipid composition of enterocyte brush border membranes in vitamin D deprived rats. *J Biol Chem* 1986;261:16404–9.

43. Putkey JA, Spielvogel AM, Sauerheber RD, Sunlap CS, Norman AW. Effects of essential fatty acid deficiency and spin label studies of enterocyte membrane lipid fluidity. *Biochim Biophys Acta* 1982;688:177–90.

44. Bikle DD, Whitney J, Munson S. The relationship of membrane fluidity to calcium flux in chick intestinal brush border membranes. *Endocrinology* 1984;114:260–7.

45. Wasserman RH, Chandler JS. Molecular mechanisms of intestinal calcium absorption. In: Peck WA, ed. *Bone and mineral research*, vol 3. Amsterdam: Elsevier, 1985;181–211.

46. Bikle DD, Morrissey RL, Zolock DT. The mechanism of action of vitamin D in the intestine. *Am J Clin Nutr* 1979;32:2322–38.

47. Russell RGG, Monod A, Bonjour J-P, Fleisch H. Relation between alkaline phosphatase and Ca^{2+}-ATPase in calcium transport. *Nature* 1972;240:126–7.

48. Moriuchi S, DeLuca HF. The effect of vitamin D_3 metabolites on membrane proteins of chick duodenal brush borders. *Arch Biochem Biophys* 1976;174:367–72.

49. Ghijsen WEJM, DeJonge MD, Van Os CH. Dissociation between Ca^{2+}-ATPase and alkaline phosphatase activities in plasma mem-

branes of rat duodenum. *Biochim Biophys Acta* 1980;599:538–51.

50. Lane SM, Lawson DEM. Differentiation of the changes in alkaline phosphatase from calcium ion-activated adenosine triphosphatase activities associated with increased calcium absorption in chick intestine. *Biochem J* 1978;174:1067–70.

51. Ghijsen WEJM, DeJong MD, Van Os CH. Kinetic properties of Na/Ca exchange in basolateral plasma membranes in rat small intestine. *Biochim Biophys Acta* 1983;689:85–94.

52. Murer H, Hildmann B. Transcellular transport of calcium and inorganic phosphate in the small intestinal epithelium. *Am J Physiol* 1982;240:G409–16.

53. Hildmann B, Schmidt A, Murer H. Ca^{++}-transport across basal–lateral plasma membranes from rat small intestinal epithelial cells. *J Membr Biol* 1982;65:55–62.

54. Martin DL, DeLuca HF. Influence of sodium on calcium transport by the rat small intestine. *Am J Physiol* 1969;216:1351–9.

55. Nellans HN. Intestinal sodium-dependent calcium transport: role for Na:Ca exchange? In: *Mechanisms of intestinal electrolyte transport and regulation by calcium.* New York: Alan R Liss, 1984;209–20.

56. Ghijsen WEJM, DeJong MD, Van Os CH. Ca-stimulated ATPase in brush border and basolateral membranes of rat duodenum with high affinity sites for Ca ions. *Nature* 1979;279:802–3.

57. DeJonge HR, Ghijsen WEJM, Van Os CH. Phosphorylated intermediates of Ca^{2+}-ATPase and alkaline phosphatase in plasma membranes from rat duodenal epithelium. *Biochim Biophys Acta* 1981;647:140–9.

58. Ghijsen WEJM, DeJong MD, Van Os CH. ATP-dependent calcium transport and its correlation with Ca^{2+}-ATPase activity in basolateral plasma membranes of rat duodenum. *Biochim Biophys Acta* 1982;689:327–36.

59. Ghijsen WEJM, Van Os CH, Heizmann CW, Murer H. Regulation of duodenal Ca^{2+} pump by calmodulin and vitamin D-dependent Ca^{2+}-binding protein. *Am J Physiol* 1986;251:G223–9.

60. Walters JRF, Weiser MM. Calcium transport by rat duodenal villus and crypt basolateral membranes. *Am J Physiol* 1987;252:G170–7.

61. Nellans HN, Popovitch JE. Calmodulin-regulated, ATP-driven calcium transport by basolateral membranes from rat small intestine. *J Biol Chem* 1981;256:9932–6.

61a. Freedman RA, Weiser MM, Isselbacher KJ. Calcium translocation by and lateral–basal membrane vesicles from rat intestine: decrease in vitamin D-deficient rats. *Proc Natl Acad Sci USA* 1977;74:3612–6.

62. Favus MJ, Tembe V, Ambrosic KA, Nellans HN. Effects of $1,25(OH)_2D_3$ on enterocyte basolateral membrane Ca transport in rats. *Am J Physiol* 1989;256:G613–7.

63. Nemere I, Leathers V, Norman AW. 1,25-Dihydroxyvitamin D_3-mediated intestinal calcium transport. Biochemical identification of lysosomes containing calcium and calcium-binding protein (calbindin-28kD). *J Biol Chem* 1986;261:16106–14.

64. Nemere I, Norman AW. 1,25-Dihydroxyvitamin D_3-mediated vesicular calcium transport in intestine: dose–response studies. *Mol Cell Endocrinol* 1989;67:47–53.

65. Favus MJ, Tembe V, Tanklefsky MD, Ambrosic KA, Nellans HN. Effects of quinacrine on calcium active transport by rat intestinal epithelium. *Am J Physiol* 1989;257:G818–22.

66. Jande SS, Brewer LM. Effects of vitamin D_3 on duodenal absorptive cells of chicks. An electron microscopic study. *Z Anat Entwicklungsgesch* 1974;144:249–65.

67. Sampson HW, Krawitt EL. A morphometric investigation of the duodenal mucosa of normal, vitamin D-deficient, and vitamin D-replete rats. *Calcif Tissue Res* 1976;21:213–28.

68. Davis WL, Jones RG, Hagler HK. Calcium containing lysosomes in the normal chick duodenum: a histochemical and analytical electron microscopic study. *Tissue Cell* 1979;11:127–38.

69. Davis WL, Jones RG. Calcium lysosomes in rachitic and vitamin D_3 replete chick duodenal absorptive cells. *Tissue Cell* 1981;13:381–91.

70. Davis WL, Jones RG. Lysosomal proliferation in rachitic avian intestinal absorptive cells following 1,25-dihydroxycholecalciferol. *Tissue Cell* 1982;14:585–95.

71. Warner RR, Coleman JR. Electron probe analysis of calcium transport by small intestine. *J Cell Biol* 1975;64:54–74.

72. Roth J, Bendayan M, Orci L. Ultrastructural localization of intracellular antigens by the use of protein A–gold complex. *J Histochem Cytochem* 1978;26:1074–81.

73. Kowarski S, Cowen LA, Takahashi MT, Schachter D. Tissue distribution and vitamin D dependency of IMCal in the rat. *Am J Physiol* 1987;253:G411–9.

74. Mellman I, Fuchs R, Helenius A. Acidification of the endocytic and exocytic pathways. *Annu Rev Biochem* 1986;55:663–700.

75. Ohkuma S, Poole B. Fluoresence probe measurement of the intralysosomal pH in living cells and the perturbation of pH by various agents. *Proc Natl Acad Sci USA* 1978;75:3327–31.

76. Spielvogel AM, Farley RD, Norman AW. Studies on the mechanism of action of cholecalciferol. V. Turnover time of chick intestinal epithelial cells in relation to the intestinal action of vitamin D. *Exp Cell Res* 1972;74:359–66.

76a. Taylor AN. Intestinal vitamin D-induced calcium binding protein: time-course of immunocytochemical localization following 1,25-dihydroxyvitamin D_3. *J Histochem Cytochem* 1983;31:426–32.

77. Bikle DD, Zolock DT, Munson S. Differential response of duodenal epithelial cells to 1,25-dihydroxyvitamin D_3 according to position on the villus: a comparison of calcium uptake, calcium-binding protein, and alkaline phosphatase activity. *Endocrinology* 1984;115:2077–84.

78. Marche P, Cassier P, Mathieu H. Intestinal calcium-binding protein. A protein indicator of enterocyte maturation associated with the terminal web. *Cell Tissue Res* 1980;212:63–72.

79. Taylor AN, Gleason WA Jr, Lankford GL. Immunocytochemical localization of rat intestinal vitamin D-dependent calcium-binding protein. *J Histochem Cytochem* 1984;32:153–8.

80. Smith MW, Bruns ME, Lawson DEM. Identification of intestinal cells responsive to calcitriol (1,25-dihydroxycholecalciferol). *Biochem J* 1985;225:127–33.

81. Van Corven EJJM, Roche C, Van Os CH. Distribution of Ca^{2+}-ATPase, ATP-dependent Ca^{2+} transport, calmodulin and vitamin D-dependent Ca^{2+}-binding protein along the villus-crypt axis in rat duodenum. *Biochim Biophys Acta* 1985;820:274–82.

82. Nemere I, Szego CM. Early actions of parathyroid hormone and 1,25-dihydroxycholecalciferol on isolated epithelial cells from rat intestine. *Endocrinology* 1981;108:1450–62.

83. Nemere I, Yoshimoto Y, Norman AW. Calcium transport in perfused duodena from normal chicks: enhancement within 14 minutes of exposure to 1,25-dihydroxyvitamin D_3. *Endocrinology* 1984;115:1476–83.

84. Ben Nasr L, Monet JD, Lucas AP, Comte L, Duchambon P, Martin AS. Rapid (10 minute) stimulation of rat duodenal alkaline phosphatase activity by 1,25-dihydroxyvitamin D_3. *Endocrinology* 1988;103:1778–82.

85. Rasmussen H, Fontaine O, Max E, Goodman DBP. The effect of 1-hydroxyvitamin D_3 administration on calcium transport in chick intestine brush border membrane vesicles. *J Biol Chem* 1979;254:2993–9.

86. O'Doherty PJA. 1,25-Dihydroxyvitamin D_3 increases the activity of the intestinal phosphatidylcholine deacylation–reacylation cycle. *Lipids* 1978;14:75–7.

87. Bruns ME, Fleischer EB, Avioli LV. Control of vitamin D-dependent calcium-binding protein in rat intestine by growth and fasting. *J Biol Chem* 1977;252:4145–50.

88. Walling MW, Kimberg DV. Calcium absorption or secretion by rat ileum in vitro: effects of dietary calcium intake. *Am J Physiol* 1974;226:1124–30.

89. Okada Y, Irimajiri A, Inouye A. Electrical properties and active solute transport in rat small intestine. *J Membr Biol* 1977;31:221–32.

90. Goldman DE. Potential impedance, and rectification in membranes. *J Gen Physiol* 1943;27:37–60.

91. Favus MJ, Angeid-Backman E. Effects of lactose on calcium absorption and secretion by rat ileum. *Am J Physiol* 1984;246:G281–5.

92. Favus MJ, Angeid-Backman E. Effects of $1,25(OH)_2D_3$ and calcium channel blockers on cecal calcium transport in the rat. *Am J Physiol* 1985;248:G676–81.

93. Favus MJ, Angeid-Backman E, Breyer MD, Coe FL. Effects of trifluoperazine, ouabain, and ethacrynic acid on intestinal calcium transport. *Am J Physiol* 1983;244:G111–5.

94. Nellans HN. Contributions of cellular and paracellular pathways to transepithelial intestinal calcium transport. *Prog Clin Biol Res* 1988;252:269–76.

95. Petith MM, Schedl HP. Duodenal and ileal adaptation to dietary calcium restriction: in vivo studies in the rat. *Am J Physiol* 1976;231:865–71.

96. Petith MM, Schedl HP. Intestinal adaptation to dietary calcium restriction: in vivo cecal and colonic calcium transport in the rat. *Gastroenterology* 1976;71:1039–42.

97. Scholz D, Schwille PO. Somatostatin and intestinal calcium absorption in man. *Metabolism* 1978;27:1349–52.

98. Evensen D, Hanssen KF, Berstad A. Inhibition of intestinal calcium absorption by somatostatin in man. *Metabolism* 1978;27:1345–7.

99. Favus MJ, Berelowitz M, Coe FL. Effects of somatostatin on intestinal calcium transport in the rats. *Am J Physiol* 1981;241:G215–21.

100. Walling MW, Brasitus TA, Kimberg DV. Effects of calcitonin and substance P on the transport of Ca, Na, and Cl across rat ileum in vitro. *Gastroenterology* 1977;73:89–94.

101. DeLuca HF, Schnoes HK. Metabolism and mechanism of action of vitamin D. *Annu Rev Biochem* 1976;45:631–66.

102. Horiuchi N, Suda T, Takahashi H, Shimazawa E, Ogata E. In vivo evidence for the intermediary role of 3′,5′-cyclic AMP in parathyroid hormone-induced stimulation of 1,25-dihydroxyvitamin D_3 synthesis in rats. *Endocrinology* 1977;101:969–74.

103. Kawashima H, Kraut JA, Kurokawa K. Metabolic acidosis suppresses 25-hydroxyvitamin D_3-1-hydroxylase in the rat kidney. *J Clin Invest* 1982;70:135–40.

104. Langman CB, Bushinsky DA, Favus MJ, Coe FL. Ca and P regulation of 1,25(OH)$_2$D$_3$ synthesis by vitamin D-replete rat tubules during acidosis. *Am J Physiol* 1986;251:F911–8.

105. Bushinsky DA, Favus MJ, Schneider AB, Sen PK, Sherwood LM, Coe FL. Effects of metabolic acidosis on PTH and 1,25(OH)$_2$D$_3$ response to low calcium diet. *Am J Physiol* 1982;243:F570–5.

106. Bushinsky DA, Riera GS, Favus MJ, Coe FL. Response of serum 1,25(OH)$_2$D$_3$ to variation of ionized calcium during chronic metabolic acidosis. *Am J Physiol* 1985;249:F361–5.

107. Gafter U, Kraut JA, Lee DBN, Sillis V, Walling MW, Kurokawa K, Haussler MR, Coburn JW. The effect of metabolic acidosis on intestinal absorption of calcium and phosphorus. *Am J Physiol* 1980;239:G480–4.

108. Birge SJ, Gilbert HR. Identification of an intestinal sodium- and calcium-dependent phosphatase stimulated by parathyroid hormone. *J Clin Invest* 1974;54:710–7.

109. Harrison HE, Harrison HC. Transfer of Ca^{45} across intestinal wall in vitro in relation to action of vitamin D and cortisol. *Am J Physiol* 1960;199:265–71.

110. Williams GA, Bowser EN, Henderson WJ, Uzgiries V. Effects of vitamin D and cortisone on intestinal absorption of calcium in the rat. *Proc Soc Exp Biol Med* 1961;106:664–6.

111. Collins EJ, Garrett ER, Johnston RL. Effect of adrenal steroids on radio-calcium metabolism in dogs. *Metab Clin Exp* 1962;11:716–26.

112. Wajhenberg BL, Periera VG, Kieffer J, Ursic S. Effect of dexamethasone on calcium metabolism and ^{47}Ca kinetics in normal subjects. *Acta Endocrinol* 1969;61:173–92.

113. Kimberg DV, Baerg RD, Gershon E, Grazidusius RT. Effect of cortisone treatment on the active transport of calcium by the small intestine. *J Clin Invest* 1971;50:1309–21.

114. Lukert BP, Stanbury SW, Mawer EB. Vitamin D and intestinal transport of calcium:effects of prednisolone. *Endocrinology* 1973;93:718–22.

115. Favus MJ, Walling MW, Kimberg DV. Effects of 1,25-dihydroxycholecalciferol on intestinal calcium transport in cortisone-treated rats. *J Clin Invest* 1973;52:1680–5.

116. Gallagher JC, Aaron J, Horsman A, Wilkinson R, Nordin BEC. Corticosteroid osteoporosis. *Clin Endocrinol* 1973;2:355–68.

117. Klein RG, Arnaud SB, Gallagher JC, DeLuca HF, Riggs BL. Intestinal calcium absorption in exogenous hypercortisolism. Role of 25-hydroxyvitamin D and corticosteroid dose. *J Clin Invest* 1977;60:253–9.

118. Schultz TD, Bollman S, Kumar R. Decreased intestinal calcium absorption in vivo and normal brush border membrane vesicle calcium uptake in cortisol-treated chickens: evidence for dissocia-

tion of calcium absorption from brush border vesicle uptake. *Proc Natl Acad Sci USA* 1982;79:3542–6.

119. Korkor AB, Kuchibolta J, Arrieh M, Gray RW, Gleason WA. The effects of chronic prednisone administration on intestinal receptors for 1,25-dihydroxyvitamin D_3 in the dog. *Endocrinology* 1985;117:2267–73.

120. Krawitt EL, Stubbert PR. The role of intestinal transport proteins in cortisone-mediated suppression of Ca^{2+} absorption. *Biochim Biophys Acta* 1972;274:179–88.

121. Feher JJ, Wasserman RH. Intestinal calcium-binding protein and calcium absorption in cortisol-treated chicks: effects of vitamin D_3 and 1,25-dihydroxyvitamin D_3. *Endocrinology* 1979;104:547–51.

122. Hahn TJ, Halstead LR, Teitelbaum SL. Altered mineral metabolism in glucocorticoid-induced osteopenia. Effect of 25-hydroxyvitamin D administration. *J Clin Invest* 1979;64:655–65.

123. Favus MJ, Kimberg DV, Millar GN, Gershon E. Effects of cortisone administration on the metabolism and localization of 25-hydroxycholecalciferol in the rat. *J Clin Invest* 1973;52:1328–35.

124. Seeman E, Kumar R, Hunder GG, Scott M, Heath H III, Riggs BL. Production, degradation, and circulating levels of 1,25-dihydroxyvitamin D in health and in chronic glucocorticoid excess. *J Clin Invest* 1980;66:664–9.

125. Bordier P, Miravet L, Matrajt H, Hioco D, Ryckewaert A. Bone changes in adult patients with abnormal thyroid function (with special reference to ^{45}Ca kinetics and quantitative histology). *Proc R Soc Med* 1967;60:1132–4.

126. Shafer RB, Gregory DH. Calcium malabsorption in hyperthyroidism. *Gastroenterology* 1972;63:235–9.

127. Lekkerkerker JFF, Doorenbos H. The influence of thyroid hormone on calcium absorption from the gut in relation to urinary calcium excretion. *Acta Endocrinol* 1973;73:672–80.

128. Singhelakis P, Alevizaki CC, Ikkos DG. Intestinal calcium absorption in hyperthyroidism. *Metabolism* 1974;23:311–21.

129. Haldimann B, Kaptein EM, Singer FR, Nicloff JT, Massry SG. Intestinal calcium absorption in patients with hyperthyroidism. *J Clin Endocrinol Metab* 1980;51:995–7.

130. Friedland JA, Williams GA, Bowser EN, Henderson WJ, Hoffeins E. Effect of hyperthyroidism on intestinal absorption of calcium in the rat. *Proc Soc Exp Biol Med* 1965;120:20–3.

131. Williams GA, Bowser EN, Henderson WJ. Calcium-47 absorption in rats with induced hyperthyroidism. *Isr J Med Sci* 1967;3:639–42.

132. Noble HM, Matty AJ. The effect of thyroxine on the movement of calcium and inorganic phosphate through the small intestine of the rat. *J Endocrinol* 1967;37:111–7.

133. Swaminathan R, Care AD. The effect of thyroxine administration on intestinal calcium absorption and calcium binding protein activity in the chick. *Calcif Tissue Res* 1975;17:257–61.

134. Kaptein EM, Singer FR, Nocoloff JT, Bishop JE, Norman AW. Plasma 1,25-dihydroxycholecalciferol (1,25(OH)$_2$D) is decreased in hyperthyroidism. *Clin Res* 1979;27:369A.

135. Finkelstein JD, Schachter D. Active transport of calcium by intestine: effects of hypophysectomy and growth hormone. *Am J Physiol* 1962;203:873–80.

136. Aub JC, Bauer W, Heath C, Ropes M. Studies of calcium and phosphorus metabolism. III. The effects of the thyroid hormone and thyroid disease. *J Clin Invest* 1929;7:97–137.

137. Krane SM, Brownell GL, Stanbury JB, Corrigan H. The effect of thyroid disease on calcium metabolism in man. *J Clin Invest* 1956;35:874–87.

138. Olson EB, DeLuca HF, Potts JT Jr. Calcitonin inhibition of vitamin D-induced intestinal calcium absorption. *Endocrinology* 1972;90:151–7.

139. Shai F, Baker RK, Wallach S. The clinical and metabolic effects of porcine calcitonin on Paget's disease of bone. *J Clin Invest* 1971;50:1927–40.

140. Cramer CG, Parkes CO, Copp DH. The effect of chicken and hog calcitonin on some parameters of calcium, phosphorus and magnesium metabolism in dogs. *Can J Physiol Pharmacol* 1969;47:181–4.

141. Krawitt EL. Effects of thyrocalcitonin in duodenal calcium transport. *Proc Soc Exp Biol Med* 1967;125:1084–6.

142. Gray TK, Bieberdorf FA, Fordtran JS. Thyrocalcitonin and the

jejunal absorption of calcium, water, and electrolytes in normal subjects. *J Clin Invest* 1973;52:3084–8.

143. Swaminathan R, Ker J, Care AD. Calcitonin and intestinal calcium absorption. *J Endocrinol* 1974;61:83–94.

144. Hirsch PF, Voelkel EF, Munson PL. Thyrocalcitonin–hypocalcemia–hypophosphatemic principle of the thyroid gland. *Science NY* 1964;146:412–3.

145. Beck JC, McGarry EE, Dyrenfurth D, Venning EH. Metabolic effects of human and monkey growth hormone in man. *Science* 1957;125:884–5.

146. Henneman PH, Forbes AP, Moldawer M, Dempsey EF, Carroll EL. Effects of human growth hormone in man. *J Clin Invest* 1960;39:1223–31.

147. Hanna S, Harrison MT, MacIntyre I, Fraser R. Effects of growth hormone on calcium and magnesium metabolism. *Br Med J* 1961;2:12–5.

148. Mainoya JR. Effects of bovine growth hormone, human placental lactogen and ovine prolactin on intestinal fluid and ion transport in the rat. *Endocrinology* 1975;96:1165–70.

149. Braithwaite GD. The effect of growth hormone on calcium metabolism in the sheep. *Br J Nutr* 1975;33:309–14.

150. Spencer EM, Tobiassen O. The mechanism of the action of growth hormone on vitamin D metabolism in the rat. *Endocrinology* 1981;108:1064–70.

151. Spanos E, Barrett D, MacIntyre I, Pike JW, Safilian EF, Haussler MR. Effect of growth hormone on vitamin D metabolism. *Nature (Lond)* 1978;273:246–7.

152. Aloia JF, Yeh JK. Growth hormone and intestinal calcium transport in the rat. *Metab Bone Dis Rel Res* 1980;2:251–5.

153. Yeh JK, Aloia JF. The relationship of growth hormone to 1,25-dihydroxyvitamin D_3 in intestinal calcium transport. *Metab Bone Dis Rel Res* 1981;3:47–9.

154. Albright F, Reifenstein EC. *Parathyroid glands and metabolic bone disease.* Baltimore: Williams & Wilkins, 1948.

155. Lafferty FW, Spencer GE Jr, Pearson OH. Effects of androgens, estrogens and high calcium intakes on bone formation and resorption in osteoporosis. *Am J Med* 1964;36:514–28.

156. Canniggia A, Gennari C, Borrello G, Bencinini M. Intestinal absorption of calcium-47 after treatment with oral oestrogen–gestogens in senile osteoporosis. *Br Med J* 1970;4:30–2.

157. Bullamore JR, Gallagher JC, Wilkinson R, Nordin BEC, Marshall DH. Effect of age on calcium absorption. *Lancet* 1970;2:535–7.

158. Caniggia A, Gennari C, Bianchi V, Guideri R. Intestinal absorption of ^{45}Ca in senile osteoporosis. *Acta Med Scand* 1963;173:613–7.

159. Gallagher JC, Riggs BL, Eisman J, Hamstra A, Arnaud SB, DeLuca HF. Intestinal calcium absorption and serum vitamin D metabolites in normal subjects and osteoporotic patients. *J Clin Invest* 1979;64:729–36.

160. Gallagher JC, Riggs BL, DeLuca HF. Effect of estrogen on calcium absorption and serum vitamin D metabolites in postmenopausal osteoporosis. *J Clin Endocrinol Metab* 1980;51:1359–64.

161. DeLuca HF. Vitamin D metabolism and function. *Arch Intern Med* 1978;138:836–47.

162. Lawoylin S, Zerwekh JE, Glass K, Pak CYC. Ability of 25-hydroxyvitamin D_3 therapy to augment serum 1,25- and 24,25-dihydroxyvitamin D in postmenopausal osteoporosis. *J Clin Endocrinol Metab* 1980;50:593–6.

163. Stock JL, Coderre JA, Mallette LE. Effects of a short course of estrogen on mineral metabolism in postmenopausal women. *J Clin Endocrinol Metab* 1985;61:595–600.

164. Castillo L, Tanaka Y, DeLuca HF, Sunde ML. The stimulation of 25-hydroxyvitamin D_3-1-alpha-hydroxylase by estrogen. *Arch Biochem Biophys* 1977;179:211–7.

165. Yendt ER, Gagne RJA, Cohanim M. The effects of thiazides in idiopathic hypercalciuria. *Am J Med Sci* 1966;261:449–60.

166. Coe FL, Parks JH, Bushinsky DA, Langman CB, Favus MJ. Chlorthalidone promotes mineral retention in patients with idiopathic hypercalciuria. *Kidney Int* 1988;33:1140–6.

167. Donath A, Nordio S, Macagno F, Gatti R. The effect of hydrochlorothiazide on calcium and strontium transport in intestine and kidney. *Helv Pediatr Acta* 1970;25:293–300.

168. Nassim JR, Higgins BA. Control of idiopathic hypercalciuria. *Br Med J* 1965;1:675–81.

169. Harrison AR, Rose GA. The effect of bendrofluazide on urinary and faecal calcium and phosphorus. *Clin Sci* 1968;34:343–50.

170. Barilla DE, Tolentino R, Kaplan RA, Pak CYC. Selective effects of thiazide on intestinal absorption of calcium in absorptive and renal hypercalciuria. *Metabolism* 1978;27:125–31.

171. Ehrig U, Harrison JE, Wilson DR. Effect of long-term thiazide therapy on intestinal calcium absorption in patients with recurrent renal calculi. *Metabolism* 1974;23:139–49.

172. Zerwekh JE, Pak CYC. Selective effects of thiazide therapy on serum 1,25-dihydroxyvitamin D and intestinal calcium absorption in renal and absorptive hypercalciuria. *Metabolism* 1980;29:13–7.

173. Favus MJ, Coe FL, Kathpalia SC, Porat A, Sen PK, Sherwood LM. Effects of chlorthiazide on 1,25-dihydroxyvitamin D_3, parathyroid hormone, and intestinal calcium absorption in the rat. *Am J Physiol* 1982;242:G575–81.

174. Jorgensen FS, Transbol I. The effect of bendroflumethazide on the intestinal absorption of calcium in normocalcemic renal stone formers and in hyperparathyroidism. *Acta Med Scand* 1974;195:33–6.

175. Bushinsky DA, Favus MJ, Coe FL. Mechanism of chronic hypocalciuria with chlorthalidone: reduced calcium absorption. *Am J Physiol* 1984;247:F746–52.

176. Bushinsky DA, Favus MJ, Langman CB, Coe FL. Mechanism of chronic hypercalciuria with furosemide: increased calcium absorption. *Am J Physiol* 1986;251:F17–24.

177. Favus MJ. Transport of calcium by intestinal mucosa. *Semin Nephrol* 1981;1:306–17.

178. Nicar MJ, Pak CYC. Calcium bioavailability from calcium carbonate and calcium citrate. *J Clin Endocrinol Metab* 1985;61:391–3.

179. Phang JM, Kales AN, Hahn TJ. Effects of divided calcium intake on urinary calcium excretion. *Lancet* 1968;2:84–5.

180. Allen LH. Calcium bioavailability and absorption: a review. *Am J Clin Nutr* 1982;35:783–808.

181. Sandberg AS, Hasselblad C, Hasselblad K, Hulten I. The effect of wheat bran on the absorption of minerals in the small intestine. *Br J Nutr* 1982;48:185–91.

182. Ismail-Beigi F, Reinhold JG, Faraji B, Abadi P. Effects of cellulose added to diets of low and high fiber content upon the metabolism of calcium, magnesium, zinc and phosphorus. *J Nutr* 1977;107:510–8.

183. Reinhold JG, Faraji B, Adabi P, Ismail-Beigi F. Decreased absorption of calcium, magnesium, zinc and phosphorus by humans due to increased fiber and phosphorus consumption as wheat bread. *J Nutr* 1976;106:493–503.

184. James WPT, Branch WJ, Southgate DAT. Calcium binding by dietary fibre. *Lancet* 1978;1:638–9.

185. Heaney RP, Recker RR. Effects of nitrogen, phosphorus, and caffeine on calcium balance in women. *J Lab Clin Med* 1982;99:46–55.

186. Anand RC, Linkswiler HM. Effect of protein intake on calcium balance of young men given 500 mg calcium daily. *J Nutr* 104:695–700.

187. Wasserman RW, Taylor AN. Some aspects of the intestinal absorption of calcium with special reference to vitamin D. In: Comar CL, Bronner F, eds. *Mineral metabolism,* vol 3. New York: Academic Press, 1969;320–403.

188. Nordin BEC. Effects of malabsorption syndrome on calcium metabolism. *Proc R Soc Exp Biol Med* 1961;54:497–500.

189. Condon JR, Nassim JR, Millard FJC, Hilbe A, Stainthorpe EM. Calcium and phosphorus metabolism in relation to lactose tolerance. *Lancet* 1970;1:1027–9.

190. Lengemann FW, Comar CL. Distribution of absorbed strontium-85 and calcium-45 as influenced by lactose. *Am J Physiol* 1961;200:1051–4.

191. Leichter J, Tolensky AF. Effect of dietary lactose on the absorption of protein, fat and calcium in the postweaning rat. *Am J Clin Nutr* 1975;28:238–41.

192. Lengemann FW, Wasserman RH, Comar CL. Studies on the enhancement of radiocalcium and radiostrontium. *J Nutr* 1959;68:443–56.

193. Au WY, Raisz RG. Restoration of parathyroid responsiveness in vitamin D-deficient rats by parenteral calcium or dietary lactose. *J Clin Invest* 1967;46:1572–7.

194. Cochet B, Jung A, Griessen M, Bartholdi P, Schaller P, Donath A. Effects of lactose on intestinal calcium absorption in normal and lactose-deficient subjects. *Gastroenterology* 1983;84:935–40.

195. Chang Y-O, Hagsted DM. Lactose and calcium transport in gut sacs. *J Nutr* 1964;82:297–300.

196. Armbrecht HJ, Wasserman RH. Enhancement of Ca uptake by lactose in the rat small intestine. *J Nutr* 1976;106:1265–71.

197. Favus MJ, Bushinsky DA, Coe FL. Effects of medium pH on duodenal and ileal calcium active transport in the rat. *Am J Physiol* 1986;251:G695–700.

198. Goulding A, Campbell DR. Thyroparathyroidectomy exaggerates calciuric action of ammonium chloride in rats. *Am J Physiol* 1984;246:F54–8.

199. Lemann J Jr, Litzow JR, Lennon EJ. The effects of chronic acid loads in normal man: further evidence for the participation of bone mineral in the defense against chronic metabolic acidosis. *J Clin Invest* 1966;45:1608–14.

200. Lemann J Jr, Litzow JR, Lennon EJ. Studies of the mechanism by which chronic metabolic acidosis augments urinary calcium excretion in man. *J Clin Invest* 1967;46:1318–28.

201. Weber HP, Gray RW, Dominguez JH, Lemann J Jr. The lack of effect of chronic metabolic acidosis on 25-OH-vitamin D metabolism and serum parathyroid hormone in humans. *J Clin Endocrinol Metab* 1977;43:1047–55.

202. Coe FL, Favus MJ. Disorders of stone formation. In: Brenner BM, Rector FC, eds. *The kidney.* Philadelphia: WB Saunders, 1981;1950–2007.

203. Nicolaysen R. The absorption of calcium as a function of the body saturation with calcium. *Acta Physiol Scand* 1943;5:201–9.

204. Nicolaysen R, Eeg-Larsen N, Malm OJ. Physiology of calcium metabolism. *Physiol Rev* 1953;33:424–44.

205. Schachter D, Dowdle EB, Schenker H. Active transport of calcium by the small intestine of the rat. *Am J Physiol* 1960;198:263–8.

206. Kimberg DV, Schachter D, Schenker H. Active transport of calcium by intestine: effects of dietary calcium. *Am J Physiol* 1961;200:1256–62.

207. Hansard SL, Comar CL, Plumlee MP. Effect of calcium status, mass of calcium administered and age on Ca^{45} metabolism in the rat. *Proc Soc Exp Biol Med* 1952;78:455–60.

208. Avioli LV, McDonald JE, Lee SW. The influence of age on the intestinal absorption of ^{47}Ca in women and its relation to ^{47}Ca absorption in postmenopausal osteoporosis. *J Clin Invest* 1965;44:1960–7.

209. Ireland P, Fordtran JS. Effect of dietary calcium and age on jejunal calcium absorption in humans studied by intestinal perfusion. *J Clin Invest* 1973;52:2672–81.

210. Malm OJ. Calcium requirement and adaptation in adult men. *Scand J Clin Lab Invest* 1958;10 (Suppl 36).

211. Omdahl JL, DeLuca HF. Regulation of vitamin D metabolism and function. *Physiol Rev* 1973;53:327–72.

212. Omdahl JL, Gray RW, Boyle IT, Knutson J, DeLuca HF. Regulation of metabolism of 25-hydroxycholecalciferol by kidney tissue in vitro by dietary calcium. *Nature* 1972;237:63–4.

213. Henry HL, Midgett RJ, Norman AW. Regulation of 25-hydroxyvitamin D_3 1-hydroxylase in vivo. *J Biol Chem* 1974;249:7584–92.

214. Tanaka Y, DeLuca HF. Rat renal 25-hydroxyvitamin D_3 1- and 24-hydroxylases: their in vivo regulation. *Am J Physiol* 1984;246:E168–73.

215. Favus MJ, Langman CB. Evidence for calcium-dependent control of 1,25-dihydroxyvitamin D_3 production by rat kidney proximal tubules. *J Biol Chem* 1986;261:11224–9.

216. Boyle IT, Gray RW, DeLuca HF. Regulation by calcium of in vivo synthesis of 1,25-dihydroxycholecalciferol and 21,25-dihydroxycholecalciferol. *Proc Natl Acad Sci USA* 1971;68:2131–4.

217. Favus MJ, Walling MW, Kimberg DV. Effects of dietary calcium restriction and chronic thyroparathyroidectomy on the metabolism of [^{3}H]25-hydroxyvitamin D_3 and the active transport of calcium by rat intestine. *J Clin Invest* 1974;53:1139–48.

218. Hughes MR, Brumbaugh PF, Haussler MR, Wergedal JE, Baylink DJ. Regulation of serum 1,25-dihydroxyvitamin D_3 by calcium and phosphate in the rat. *Science* 1975;190:578–80.

219. Rader JI, Baylink DJ, Hughes MR, Safilian EF, Haussler MR.

220. Favus MJ, Mangelsdorf DJ, Tembe V, Coe BJ, Haussler MR. Evidence for in vivo upregulation of the intestinal vitamin D receptor during dietary calcium restriction in the rat. *J Clin Invest* 1988;82:218–24.

221. Garabedian M, Holick MF, DeLuca HF, Boyle IT. Control of 25-hydroxycholecalciferol metabolism by parathyroid glands. *Proc Soc Natl Acad Sci USA* 1972;69:1673–6.

222. Fraser DR, Kodicek E. Regulation of 25-hydroxycholecalciferol-1-hydroxylase activity in kidney by parathyroid hormone. *Nature* 1973;241:163–6.

223. Rasmussen H, Wong M, Bikle D, Goodman DBP. Hormonal control of the renal conversion of 25-hydroxycholecalciferol to 1,25-dihydroxycholecalciferol. *J Clin Invest* 1972;51:2502–4.

224. Pento JT, Waite LC, Tracy PJ, Kenny AD. Adaptation to calcium deprivation in the rat: effects of parathyroidectomy. *Am J Physiol* 1977;232:E336–42.

225. Trechsel U, Eisman JA, Fischer JA, Bonjour J-P, Fleisch H. Calcium-dependent, parathyroid hormone-independent regulation of 1,25-dihydroxyvitamin D. *Am J Physiol* 1980;E119–24.

226. Malm OJ, Nicolaysen R, Skjelkvale L. Calcium metabolism in old age as related to ageing of the skeleton. In: Wolstenholme GEW, Cameron MP, eds. *Ageing—general aspects.* Ciba Foundation Colloquia on Ageing. Boston: Little, Brown, 1955;109–25.

227. Armbrecht HJ, Zenser TV, Bruns ME, Davis BB. Effect of age on intestinal calcium absorption and adaptation to dietary calcium. *Am J Physiol* 1979;236:E769–74.

228. Armbrecht HJ, Zenser TV, Gross CJ. Adaptation to dietary calcium and phosphorus restriction changes with age in the rat. *Am J Physiol* 1980;239:E322–7.

229. Horst RL, DeLuca HF, Jorgensen NA. The effect of age on calcium absorption and accumulation of 1,25-dihydroxyvitamin D_3 in intestinal mucosa of rats. *Metab Bone Dis Rel Res* 1978;1:29–33.

230. Lee DBN, Walling MW, Levine BS, Gafter U, Silis V, Hodsman A, Coburn JW. Intestinal and metabolic effect of 1,25-dihydroxyvitamin D_3 in normal adult rat. *Am J Physiol* 1981;240:G75–8.

231. Armbrecht HJ, Zenser TV, Davis BB. Effect of age on the conversion of 25-hydroxyvitamin D_3 to 1,25-dihydroxyvitamin D_3 by kidney of rat. *J Clin Invest* 1980;66:1118–23.

232. Aldor TAM, Moore EW. Magnesium absorption by everted gut sacs of the rat intestine and colon. *Gastroenterology* 1970;59:745–53.

233. Ross DB. In vitro studies on the transport of magnesium across the intestinal wall of the rat. *J Physiol (Lond)* 1962;160:417–28.

234. Hendrix JZ, Alcock NW, Archbald RM. Competition between calcium, strontium, and magnesium for absorption in isolated rat intestine. *Clin Chem* 1963;9:733–4.

235. Care AD, van't Klooster AT. In vivo transport of magnesium and other cations across the wall of the gastrointestinal tract of sheep. *J Physiol (Lond)* 1965;177:174–91.

236. O'Donnell JM, Smith MW. Uptake of calcium and magnesium by rat duodenal mucosa analyzed by means of competing metals. *J Physiol (Lond)* 1973;229:733–49.

237. Chutkow JG. Sites of magnesium absorption and excretion in the intestinal tract of the rat. *J Lab Clin Med* 1964;63:71–9.

238. Karbach U. Cellular-mediated and diffusive magnesium transport across the descending colon of the rat. *Gastroenterology* 1989;96:1282–9.

239. Karbach U, Rummel W. Cellular and paracellular magnesium transport across the terminal ileum of the rats and its interaction with the calcium transport. *Gastroenterology* 1990;98:985–92.

240. Karbach U, Ewe K. Calcium and magnesium transport and influence of 1,25-dihydroxyvitamin D_3. *Digestion* 1987;37:35–42.

241. King RG, Stanbury SW. Magnesium metabolism in primary hyperparathyroidism. *Clin Sci* 1970;39:281–303.

242. Heaton FW, Pyrah LN. Magnesium metabolism in patients with parathyroid disorders. *Clin Sci* 1963;25:475–85.

243. Seelig MS. Requirements of magnesium by the normal adult. *Am J Clin Nutr* 1964;14:342–90.

244. Jones JE, Manald R, Flink EB. Magnesium requirements in adults. *Am J Clin Nutr* 1967;20:632–5.

245. Graham LA, Caesar JJ, Burgen AASV. Gastrointestinal absorp-

tion and excretion of Mg^{28} in man. *Metab Clin Exp* 1960;9:646–59.

246. Brannan PG, Vergne-Marini P, Pak CYC, Hull AR, Fordtran JS. Magnesium absorption in the human small intestine. *J Clin Invest* 1976;57:1412–8.

247. Schmulen AC, Lerman M, Pak CYC, Zerwekh J, Morawski S, Fordtran JS, Vergne-Marini P. Effect of 1,25(OH)$_2$D$_3$ on jejunal absorption of magnesium in patients with chronic renal disease. *Am J Physiol* 1980;238:G349–52.

248. Fawcett DW, Gens JP. Magnesium poisoning following an enema of epsom salt solution. *JAMA* 1943;123:1028–9.

249. MacIntyre I, Robinson CJ. Magnesium and the gut: experimental and clinical observations. *Ann NY Acad Sci* 1969;162:865–73.

250. Hanna S. Influence of large doses of vitamin D on magnesium metabolism in rats. *Metabolism* 1961;10:737–43.

251. Wasserman RH. Studies on vitamin D$_2$ and the intestinal absorption of calcium and other ions in the rachitic chick. *J Nutr* 1962;77:69–80.

252. Miller ER, Ullery DE, Zutaut DL, Hoefer JA, Luecke RW. Mineral balance studies with the baby pig: effects of dietary vitamin D$_2$ level upon calcium, phosphorus and magnesium balance. *J Nutr* 1965;85:255–9.

253. Charles P, Mosekilde L, Sondergard K, Taagehoj Jensen F. Treatment with high dose oral vitamin D$_2$ in patients with jejunoileal bypass for morbid obesity. *Scand J Gastroenterol* 1984;19:1031–8.

254. Hodgkinson A, Marshall DH, Nordin BEC. Vitamin D and magnesium absorption in man. *Clin Sci* 1979;57:121–3.

255. Coburn JW, Brickman AS, Hartenbower DL, Norman AW. Effect of 1,25(OH)$_2$ and 1-alpha(OH)-vitamin D$_3$ on magnesium metabolism in man. *Program Int Symp Magnesium Summ Commun* 1976;2:36.

256. Krejs GJ, Nicar MJ, Zerwekh JE, Norman DA, Kane MG, Pak CYC. Effect of 1,25-dihydroxyvitamin D$_3$ on calcium and magnesium absorption in the healthy human jejunum and ileum. *Am J Med* 1983;75:973–6.

257. Schachter D, Rosen D. Active transport of Ca^{45} by the small intestine and its dependence on vitamin D. *Am J Physiol* 1959;196:357–62.

258. Cramer CF, Dueck J. In vivo transport of calcium from healed Thiry–Vella fistulas in dogs. *Am J Physiol* 1962;202:161–4.

259. Alcock N, MacIntyre I. Interrelation of calcium and magnesium absorption. *Clin Sci* 1962;22:185–93.

260. Alcock N, MacIntyre I. Some effects of magnesium repletion on calcium metabolism in the rat. *Clin Sci* 1964;26:219–25.

261. MacIntyre I, Hanna S, Booth CC, Read AE. Intracellular magnesium deficiency in man. *Clin Sci* 1961;20:297–305.

262. Toothill J. Effect of certain dietary factors on apparent absorption of magnesium by the rat. *Br J Nutr* 1963;17:125–34.

263. Clarkson EM, Warren RL, McDonald SJ, de Wardener HE. The effect of high intake of calcium on magnesium metabolism in normal subjects and patients with chronic renal failure. *Clin Sci* 1967;32:11–8.

264. Clarkson EM, McDonald SJ, de Wardener HE, Warren R. Magnesium metabolism in chronic renal failure. *Clin Sci* 1965;28:107–15.

265. Anast CS. Magnesium studies in relation to vitamin D-resistant rickets. *Pediatrics* 1967;40:425–35.

266. Kowarski S, Schachter D. Effects of vitamin D on phosphate transport and incorporation into mucosal constituents of rat intestinal mucosa. *J Biol Chem* 1969;244:211–7.

267. Lifshitz F, Harrison HC, Harrison HE. Influence of parathyroid function upon the in vitro transport of calcium and phosphate by the rat intestine. *Endocrinology* 1969;84:912–7.

268. Chen TC, Castillo L, Korychka-Dahl M, DeLuca HF. Role of vitamin D metabolites in phosphate transport of rat intestine. *J Nutr* 1974;104:1056–60.

269. Harrison HE, Harrison HC. Sodium, potassium, and intestinal transport of glucose, *l*-tyrosine, phosphate, and calcium. *Am J Physiol* 1963;205:107–11.

270. Danisi G, Straub RW. Unidirectional influx of phosphate across the mucosal membrane of rabbit small intestine. *Pflugers Arch* 1980;385:117–22.

271. Walling MW. Intestinal Ca and phosphate transport: differential responses to vitamin D$_3$ metabolites. *Am J Physiol* 1977;E488–94.

272. Walling MW. Effects of 1-1,25-dihydroxyvitamin D$_3$ on active intestinal inorganic phosphate absorption. In: Norman AW, Schaefer K, Coburn JW, DeLuca HF, Fraser D, Grigoleit HG, von Herrath D, eds. *Vitamin D. Biochemical, chemical and clinical aspects related to calcium metabolism.* Berlin: de Gruyter, 1977;321–30.

273. Peterlik M, Wasserman RH. Effect of vitamin D on transepithelial phosphate transport in chick intestine. *Am J Physiol* 1978;234:E379–88.

274. Fuchs R, Peterlik M. Vitamin D-induced phosphate transport in intestinal brush border membrane vesicles. *Biochem Biophys Acta* 1980;93:87–92.

275. Berner W, Kinne R, Murer H. Phosphate transport into brush-border membrane vesicles isolated from rat small intestine. *Biochem J* 1976;160:467–74.

276. Hoffmann N, Thees M, Kinne R. Phosphate transport by isolated renal brush border vesicles. *Pflugers Arch* 1976;362:147–56.

277. Murer H, Kinne R. The use of isolated membrane vesicles to study epithelial transport processes. *J Membr Biol* 1980;55:81–95.

278. Birge SJ, Miller R. The role of phosphate in the action of vitamin D on the intestine. *J Clin Invest* 1977;60:980–8.

279. Taylor AN. In vitro phosphate transport in chick ileum: effect of cholecalciferol, calcium, sodium and metabolic inhibitors. *J Nutr* 1974;489–94.

280. Knochel JP, Jacobson HR. Renal handling of phosphorus, clinical hypophosphatemia, and phosphorus deficiency. In: Brenner BM, Rector FC Jr, eds. *The kidney,* 3rd ed. Philadelphia: WB Saunders, 1986;619–62.

281. McHardy GJR, Parsons DS. The absorption of inorganic phosphate from the small intestine of the rat. *Q J Exp Physiol Cogn Med Sci* 1956;41:398–409.

282. Danisi G, Murer H, Straub RW. Effect of pH on phosphate transport into intestinal brush-border membrane vesicles. *Am J Physiol* 1984;246:G180–6.

283. Cramer CF. Effect of Ca/P ratio and pH on calcium and phosphorus absorption from dog gut loops in vivo. *Can J Physiol Pharmacol* 1968;461:171–3.

284. Peerce BE. Identification of the intestinal Na-phosphate cotransporter. *Am J Physiol* 1989;256:G645–52.

285. Nicolaysen R. Studies upon the mode of action of vitamin D. III. The influence of vitamin D on absorption of calcium and phosphorus. *Biochem J* 1937;31:122–9.

286. Carlsson A. The effect of vitamin D on the absorption of inorganic phosphate. *Acta Physiol Scand* 1954;31:301–7.

287. Stanbury SW. Osteomalacia. *Schweiz Med Wochenschr* 1962;92:883–91.

288. Stanbury SW. The phosphate ion in chronic renal failure. In: Hioco DJ, ed. *Phosphate et metabolisme phosphocalcique.* Paris: Sandoz Editions, 1971;187–208.

289. Brickman AS, Hartenbower DL, Norman AW, Coburn JW. Action of 1-hydroxyvitamin D$_3$ and 1,25-dihydroxyvitamin D$_3$ on mineral metabolism in man. *Am J Clin Nutr* 1977;30:1064–9.

290. Juan D, Liptak P, Gray TK. Absorption of inorganic phosphate in the human jejunum and its inhibition by salmon calcitonin. *J Clin Endocrinol Metab* 1976;43:517–22.

291. Matsumoto T, Fontaine O, Rasmussen H. Effect of 1,25-dihydroxyvitamin D$_3$ on phosphate uptake into chick intestinal brush border membrane vesicles. *Biochem Biophys Acta* 1980;599:13–23.

292. Dominguez JH, Gray RW, Lemann J Jr. Dietary phosphate deprivation in women and men: effects of mineral and acid balances, parathyroid hormone and the metabolism of 25-OH-vitamin D. *J Clin Endocrinol Metab* 1976;43:1056–68.

293. Carlsson A. Experiments with radiocalcium on the interrelationships between vitamin D and dietary calcium and phosphorus. *Acta Pharmacol Toxicol* 1953;9:32–40.

294. Haddad JG Jr, Boisseau V, Avioli LV. Phosphorus deprivation: the metabolism of vitamin D and 25-hydroxycholecalciferol in rats. *J Nutr* 1972;102:269–82.

295. Tanaka Y, DeLuca HF. Intestinal calcium transport: stimulation by low phosphorus diets. *Science* 1973;181:564–6.

296. Lee DBN, Brautbar N, Walling MW, Silis V, Coburn JW, Kleeman CR. Effect of phosphorus depletion on intestinal calcium and phosphorus absorption. *Am J Physiol* 1979;236:E451–7.
297. Clark I. Importance of dietary Ca:PO$_4$ ratios on skeletal Ca, Mg, and PO$_4$ metabolism. *Am J Physiol* 1969;217:865–70.
298. Wilkinson R. Absorption of calcium, phosphorus and magnesium. In: Nordin BEC, ed. *Calcium, phosphate and magnesium metabolism*. Edinburgh: Churchill Livingstone, 1976;36–112.
299. Hurwitz S, Bar A. Site of vitamin D action in chick intestine. *Am J Physiol* 1972;222:761–7.
300. Harrison HE, Harrison HC. Intestinal transport of phosphate action of vitamin D, calcium and potassium. *Am J Physiol* 1961;201:1007–12.
301. Asano T. Transport of calcium and inorganic phosphate across the intestinal wall of the rat. *Seitai No Kagaku* 1960;11:55–8.
302. Noble HM, Matty AJ. The effect of thyroxine on the movement of calcium and inorganic phosphate through the small intestine of the rat. *J Endocrinol* 1967;37:111–7.
303. Walton J, Gray TK. Absorption of intestinal phosphate in the human small intestine. *Clin Sci* 1979;56:407–12.
304. Schachter D, Kimberg DV, Schenker H. Active transport of calcium by intestine: action and bio-assay of vitamin D. *Am J Physiol* 1961;200:1263–71.
305. Martin DL, DeLuca HF. Calcium transport and the role of vitamin D. *Arch Biochem Biophys* 1969;134:139–48.
306. Birge SJ, Peck WA, Berman M, Whedon GD. Study of calcium absorption in man. A kinetic analysis and physiologic model. *J Clin Invest* 1969;48:1705–13.
307. Brickman AS, Coburn JW, Rowe PH. Impaired calcium absorption in uremic man: evidence for defective absorption in the proximal small intestine. *J Lab Clin Med* 1974;84:791–801.
308. Walling MW, Favus MJ, Kimberg DV. Effects of 25-hydroxyvitamin D$_3$ on rat duodenum, jejunum, and ileum. Correlation of calcium active transport with tissue levels of vitamin D$_3$ metabolites. *J Biol Chem* 1974;249:1156–61.
309. Walling MW, Kimberg DV. Calcium absorption. Stimulation in vitamin D-deficient nephrectomized rats by *Solanum glaucophyllum. Gastroenterology* 1975;69:200–5.
310. Helbock HJ, Forte JG, Saltman P. The mechanism of calcium transport by rat intestine. *Biochim Biophys Acta* 1966;126:81–93.
311. Walling MW, Kimberg DV. Active secretion of calcium, sodium and chloride by adult rat duodenum in vitro. *Biochim Biophys Acta* 1975;382:213–7.
312. Vergne-Marini P, Parker TF, Pak CYC, Hull AR, DeLuca HF, Fordtran JS. Jejunal and ileal calcium absorption in patients with chronic renal disease. Effect of 1-hydroxycholecalciferol. *J Clin Invest* 1976;57:961–6.
313. Hylander E, Ladefoged K, Jarnum S. The importance of the colon in calcium absorption following small-intestinal resection. *Scand J Gastroenterol* 1980;15:55–60.
314. Grinstead WC, Pak CYC, Krejs GJ. Effect of 1,25-dihydroxyvitamin D$_3$ on calcium absorption in the colon of healthy humans. *Am J Physiol* 1984;247:G189–92.
315. Favus MJ, Langman CB. Effects of 1,25-dihydroxyvitamin D$_3$ on colonic calcium transport in vitamin D-deficient and normal rats. *Am J Physiol* 1984;246:G268–73.

Disorders of Bone and Mineral Metabolism,
edited by Fredric L. Coe and Murray J. Favus,
© 1992 by Raven Press, Ltd. All rights reserved.

CHAPTER 4

Regulation of Parathyroid Hormone Synthesis and Secretion

Justin Silver

The normal concentration of calcium in the extracellular fluid is maintained by the concerted action of the calciotrophic hormones: parathyroid hormone (PTH), calcitonin, and vitamin D's biologically active metabolite, 1,25-dihydroxyvitamin D_3 [$1,25(OH)_2D_3$] (1–4). Central to calcium homeostasis is the rapid secretion of PTH after hypocalcemia (5) which then acts to normalize serum calcium. PTH mobilizes calcium from bone, enhances reabsorption of calcium in the kidney at the distal renal tubule and increases production of $1,25(OH)_2D_3$ in the proximal convoluted tubule (6). $1,25(OH)_2D_3$ acts on the intestine to increase calcium absorption from the diet (7) and together with PTH's action on bone and the kidney the concentration of calcium in the extracellular fluid is increased with a subsequent decrease in PTH secretion thus completing the endocrinological feedback loop. The synthesis and secretion of PTH is therefore a crucial factor in calcium and bone metabolism in both health and disease, and in this chapter current knowledge on the subject will be summarized. This chapter focuses on studies of the PTH gene, regulation of PTH gene transcription, biosynthesis of PTH and its secretion in normal physiology and in secondary hyperparathyroidism.

PTH is an 84 amino acid protein that is the cleavage product of its precursor protein preproPTH (1,8) (Fig. 1). Mature PTH is the only form which is secreted from the parathyroid cell, and it has a molecular weight of approximately 9600 daltons. The amino acid sequence has been determined in several species and there is a high degree of identity among species particularly in the amino-terminal region of the molecule (9). The parathy-

roids synthesize another protein which is also secreted (10–12). This protein, secretory protein I is identical to chromogranin A which was isolated from the adrenal medulla, and is present in other endocrine cells and neoplasms (10). Its function is not known but it is stored and secreted with PTH although with a different transcriptional regulation.

THE PARATHYROID GLAND

In man there are two pairs of parathyroid glands in the anterior cervical region. They are of endodermal origin, derived from the third and fourth pharyngeal pouches. In the rat there is a single pair of glands embedded in the cranial part of the thyroid. The chief cell is the predominant cell in man and the only cell in the rat. The second cell type is the oxyphil cell, which has an acidophilic cytoplasm and many mitochondria. Roth and Raisz (13,14) had suggested that the chief cells had a secretory cycle in which they changed from inactive to active cells. However, it has been suggested that the change in cells from dark to light is artifactual due to problems with fixation. For example, Larsson and co-workers (15) used fixation by vascular perfusion and then there were far fewer light cells, and the cells had a much more uniform ultrastructure. The parathyroid cells have secretory granules which contain PTH, but these are limited in number (16,17). There are relatively few mitoses in the parathyroid cells.

THE PTH GENE

Chromosomal Location

The human PTH gene is localized on the short arm of chromosome 11 and is only present once in the genomes

J. Silver: Department of Medicine, Hebrew University–Hadassah Medical School; Mineral Metabolism Unit, Nephrology Services, Hadassah University Hospital, Ein Karem, Jerusalem, Israel 91120.

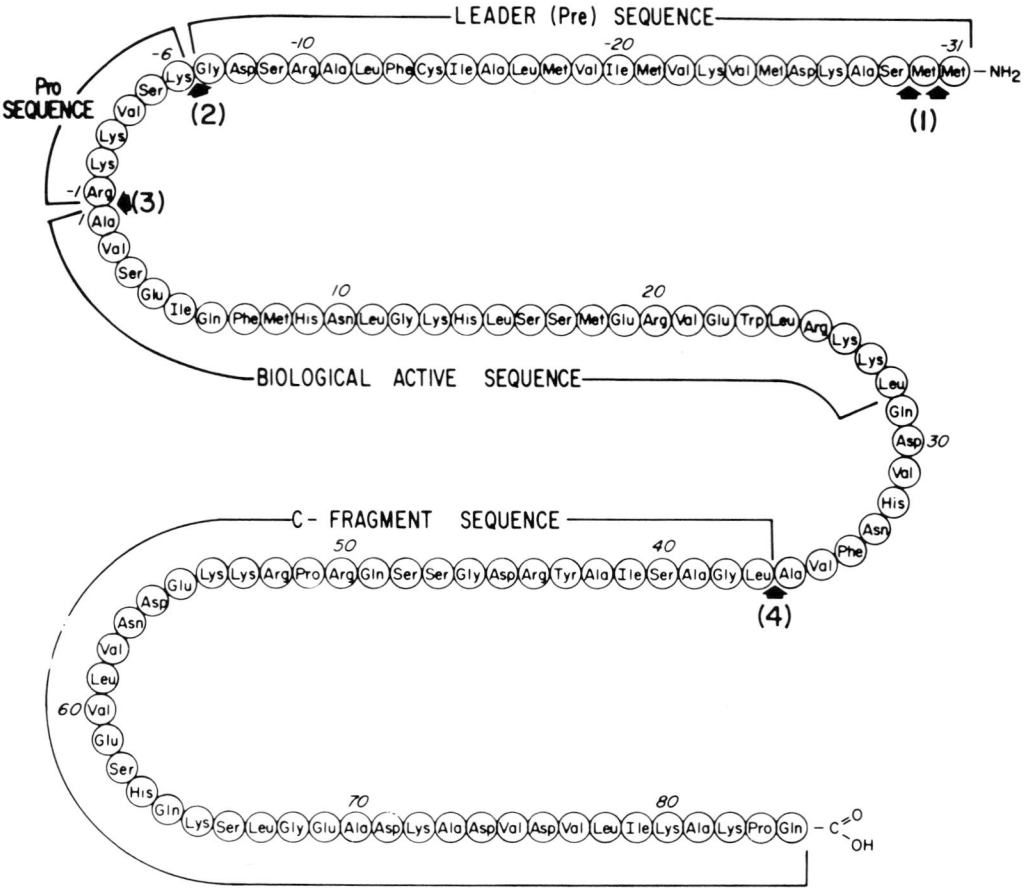

FIG. 1. Primary sequence of preproparathyroid hormone of 115 amino acids. The 84-amino acid sequence of parathyroid hormone (residues 1 through 84) is preceded at NH_2 terminus of 31 amino acids (31 through 1). Arrows indicate peptide bonds cleaved during metabolic processing of precursor and hormone: (1) removal of amino terminal methionines; (2) cleavage of leader (pre-, signal) sequence during growth of nascent polypeptide chain; (3) removal of prosequence during transport of the proparathyroid hormone through Golgi complex of parathyroid cell; and (4) cleavage of hormone into an NH_2-terminal biologically active fragment and an inactive carboxyl (C) fragment, which occurs in the liver. From Habener and Potts (9), with permission.

of humans, rats, and cows (18–20). Interestingly, the gene for calcitonin, the other polypeptide hormone regulating calcium metabolism, is also present on the short arm of chromosome 11, but the two genes are separated by about 8 centimorgans which in terms of base pairs is a relatively long distance. The PTH gene is most closely linked to the β-globulin gene. Zabel and co-workers performed chromosomal in situ hybridization studies that further localized the gene to the region 11p15 (21). Restriction enzyme analysis of the human PTH gene demonstrated polymorphism in their cleavage products in different individuals (18,22). These genetic polymorphisms are useful for genetic analysis, and also for relating parathyroid disease to structural alterations in the PTH gene.

The PTH Gene

The genes for human (23,24), bovine (25–28), rat (29,30), pig (30), and chicken (31,32) PTH have all been cloned. In 1979 Kronenberg and co-workers cloned the bovine PTH cDNA (24), which they then used as a probe to isolate the human and rat PTH cDNAs. The bovine genomic DNA (28) and chicken cDNA (31,32) have also been isolated. The genes all have two introns or intervening sequences, and three exons (33). The primary RNA transcript consists of RNA transcribed from both the introns and exons, and then the RNA sequences derived from the introns are spliced out. The product of this RNA processing, which represents the exons, is the mature PTH mRNA which will then be translated into preproPTH. The laboratories of Kronenberg (33) and Kemper (34) who first cloned the PTH genes also determined their structure. They demonstrated that the first intron separates the 5'-untranslated region of the mRNA from the rest of the gene, and that the second intron separates most of the sequence encoding the precursor specific "prepro" region from that encoding mature PTH (Fig. 2). The three exons that result are thus roughly divided into functional domains. The large first intron in the human gene (3400 base pairs) is much larger than that in the rat and bovine. The second intron is about 100 base pairs in the three species. There is considerable identity among the mammalian PTH genes that is reflected in an 85% identity between the human and bovine proteins, and 75% with the rat protein. There is less identity in the 3'-noncoding region. The human and bovine genes have two functional TATA transcription start sites, and the rat only one. Igarashi and co-workers demonstrated that the two homologous TATA sequences flanking the human PTH gene direct the synthesis of two human PTH gene transcripts both in normal parathyroid glands and in parathyroid adenomas (35). There is a termination codon immediately following the codon for glutamine at position 84 of PTH which indicates that there are no additional precursors of PTH with peptide extensions at the carboxyl position.

Tissue specificity of the expression of a gene is an intriguing question in biology. One of the factors associated with increased gene expression in a particular tissue is decreased methylation of cytosine at particular sites of the gene. Levine and co-workers (36) demonstrated that the DNA from parathyroid glands is hypomethylated at CpG sequences in the neighborhood of the PTH gene but not in the DNA from control tissues. There was no correlation between the degree of hypomethylation of the PTH gene and the level of parathyroid gland secretory activity. Details of the structure of the PTH gene have been reviewed by Kemper (34), who concluded that the PTH gene is a typical eukaryotic gene with consensus sequences for initiation of RNA synthesis, RNA splicing, and polyadenylation, but with a striking characteristic in its stability. It is represented only once in the haploid genome and there are no related genes produced by gene duplication, nor are there pseudogenes (34).

Promoter Sequences

The regions upstream of the transcribed structural gene determine the tissue specificity and contain the regulatory sequences for the gene. For PTH this analysis is by no means complete. Rupp and co-workers (1990) analyzed the human PTH promoter region up to position 805 and identified a number of consensus sequences by computer analysis (37). These included a sequence resembling the canonical cAMP-responsive element 5'-TGACGTCA-3' at position 81 with a single residue deviation. This element was fused to a reporter gene (CAT) and then transfected into different cell lines. Pharmacological agents that increase cAMP lead to an increased expression of the CAT gene, indicating a functional role for the cAMP-responsive element (CRE). These studies need to be repeated in a homologous cell system, namely parathyroid cells, with detailed analysis of protein-DNA interactions at the CRE and other putative regulatory sequences, and with more comprehensive functional analyses. These sequences include, but are not restricted to, the vitamin D response element (VDRE) and elements that recognize the message of hypocalcemia. They are under active investigation in a number of laboratories.

The VDRE has been determined in the promoter of the human and rat (38–40) osteocalcin gene that was facilitated by the availability of an osteoblast-like cell line ROS 17/2.8. The identification of these responsive elements in the PTH gene promoter will allow us to understand with greater clarity the regulation of PTH transcription and synthesis (41,42).

Arnold and co-workers have studied changes in the PTH gene in parathyroid adenomas. They have shown by molecular genetic methods that parathyroid adenomas are monoclonal neoplasms (43). They have also shown in a tumor that there was a DNA rearrangement at the PTH locus that separated the PTH gene's 5'-flanking region from its coding exons (44). The DNA that rearranged involved a recombination at the locus on 11q13 with the PTH locus (on 11p15). Interestingly 11q13 is the known chromosomal location of several oncogenes and the gene for multiple endocrine neoplasia type I (45). In addition Arnold and co-workers have studied the PTH gene of a patient with familial isolated hypo-

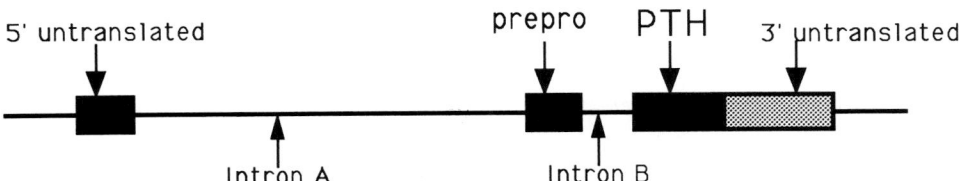

FIG. 2. Schematic diagram of the PTH gene structure. Exons are indicated by the rectangles and the regions of the gene that code for preproPTH are indicated. Modified after Kronenberg (33) and Kemper (34).

parathyroidism (46) and identified a point mutation in the signal peptide encoding region of prepro PTH (47). This T to C point mutation changed the codon for position 18 of the 31 amino acid prepro sequence from cysteine to arginine, and in functional studies they demonstrated that the mutant protein was processed inefficiently.

REGULATION OF TRANSCRIPTION OF THE PTH GENE

The 1980s witnessed an explosion of knowledge in our understanding of gene transcription. Studies on transcriptional regulation of the PTH gene have kept pace. These have been most fruitful in studies on regulation of the PTH gene's expression by calcium and $1,25(OH)_2D_3$.

A low extracellular calcium concentration is the major secretagogue for PTH and calcium was also shown to regulate PTH gene expression both in vitro and in vivo. Russell and co-workers (48) cloned the bovine cDNA for PTH and maintained bovine parathyroid cells in primary culture in the presence of different calcium concentrations. A high calcium concentration (2.5 mM, which in vitro is all ionized and therefore equivalent to 5.0 mM in vivo) led to a decrease in PTH mRNA levels after 16 h with a maximum effect at 72 h. A low calcium concentration had no effect. Brookman and co-workers (49) also studied the effect of calcium on PTH mRNA levels in primary cultures of parathyroid cells. They showed that a low calcium concentration (0.4 mM) increased, and that a high calcium (3 mM) decreased PTH mRNA levels, with a similar time sequence to Russell et al. Farrow and co-workers on the other hand found that most human parathyroid adenomata maintained in culture did not respond to a high calcium concentration by decreasing their PTH secretion despite a modest effect on PTH mRNA levels (50). They suggested that this abnormal regulation was a feature of the adenomatous cells as compared to normal cells. Later Russell and coworkers showed that the effect of calcium was transcriptional in nature (51). These studies were not in agreement with the in vitro studies of Moran et al. (52) that demonstrated that a low calcium concentration increased the synthesis of both PTH and parathyroid secretory protein, and that a high calcium concentration had no effect. In vivo studies of the calcium effect on the PTH gene have been more enlightening (53).

Naveh-Many and co-workers (54) studied rats in vivo. They showed that small decreases in serum calcium from 2.6 to 2.1 mmol/L lead to large increases in PTH mRNA levels reaching 3–5-fold that of controls (Fig. 3). In addition these changes were rapid, occurring within 1 h of the decrease in serum calcium and persisting for 6 h. A high serum calcium had no effect on PTH mRNA

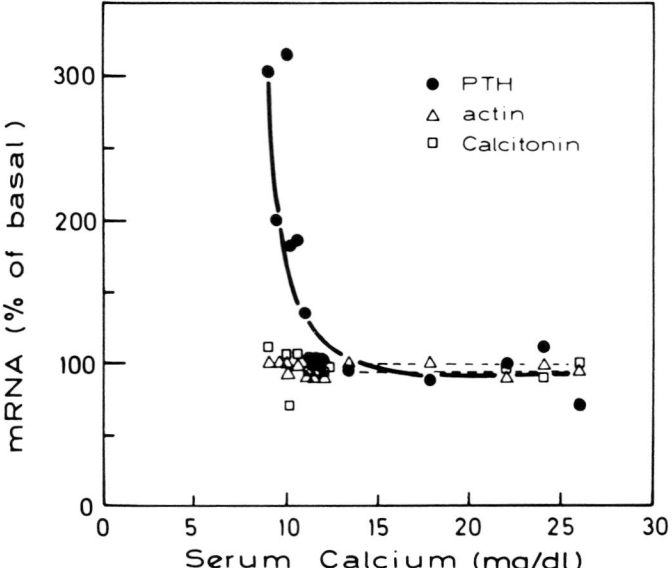

FIG. 3. Effect of changes in serum calcium on mRNA levels for PTH, calcitonin, and actin of rat parathyroid glands at 6 h. The rats were injected with calcium gluconate i.p. to increase the serum calcium, or phosphorus i.p. to decrease the serum calcium. The results at each point are the mean of four rats and expressed as a percentage of basal levels. The cluster of six dots at 11 mg/dL represents the results for groups of control rats. Note that small decreases in serum calcium lead to large increases in PTH mRNA levels, and that a high serum calcium concentration did not affect PTH mRNA. From Naveh-Many et al. (54), with permission of the American Society for Clinical Investigation.

levels even at concentrations as high as 6.0 mmol/L. Interestingly, in these same thyroparathyroid tissue RNA extracts calcium had no effect on the expression of the calcitonin gene. Thus, while a high calcium concentration is a secretagogue for calcitonin it does not regulate calcitonin gene expression. In Fig. 3 the cluster of six dots at 2.5–2.6 mmol/L (11 mg/dL) represents the results for groups of control rats. They are at the bottom of the PTH mRNA vs. calcium relationship. Thus, physiologically PTH biosynthesis is maximally suppressed with respect to calcium, and the gland is geared to respond to falls in serum calcium but not to increases in serum calcium. Yamamoto and co-workers (55) also studied the in vivo effect of calcium on PTH mRNA levels in rats. They confirmed that calcium regulated PTH mRNA levels with hypocalcemia for 48 h due to a calcitonin infusion leading to a sevenfold increase in PTH mRNA levels. Their rats with high serum calcium concentrations (2.9–3.4 mM) had the same PTH mRNA levels as those with normal serum calcium concentrations (2.4–2.6 mM) in agreement with the results of Naveh-Many et al. (54).

The in vivo results on the effect of calcium on the PTH gene's expression are obviously the physiologically relevant observations, and they are supported by studies on the effects of chronic changes in serum calcium which will be presented below. However the differences between the in vivo and in vitro systems need to be addressed. In vitro studies with primary cultures of parathyroid cells are complicated by the loss of calcium responsiveness with time in culture (56–58), and also because a high calcium concentration encourages the growth of fibroblasts at the expense of parathyroid cells (59,60). Therefore studies on the effect of calcium using primary cultures of parathyroid cells are only valid at time periods when the cells are still responsive to changes in serum calcium. This same caveat is less stringent in the in vitro study of the regulation of the PTH gene by sterol hormones.

PTH, calcitonin, and $1,25(OH)_2D_3$ act together to regulate calcium homeostasis. PTH (6) and calcitonin (61) both act on the renal proximal tubules to increase the synthesis of $1,25(OH)_2D_3$ and I shall now present evidence demonstrating that $1,25(OH)_2D_3$ acts on the parathyroid cell and the calcitonin producing C-cell in the thyroid to potently decrease the transcription of these two genes thus completing endocrinological feedback loops.

Parathyroid cells have stereospecific, high affinity receptors for $1,25(OH)_2D_3$ (62–67) similar to the receptors found in the classic target sites for $1,25(OH)_2D_3$, namely intestine and bone (68–70). Moreover, after intravenous administration of radioactively labeled $1,25(OH)_2D_3$ to chicks and rats (71) there was marked accumulation of radioactivity in the parathyroid nuclei. These data suggested that the parathyroid was a target organ for $1,25(OH)_2D_3$. The first studies on this subject were performed in vitro. Silver and co-workers (72,73) added $1,25(OH)_2D_3$ and other vitamin D metabolites to bovine parathyroid cells in primary culture and demonstrated a decrease in PTH mRNA levels to 50% of control at 48–96 h, with no affect on actin mRNA as a control. The effect of $1,25(OH)_2D_3$ was evident at concentrations as low as 1×10^{-11} M with a typical dose response with increasing concentrations of the sterol. The vitamin D metabolites $25(OH)$ D_3 and $24,25(OH)_2D_3$ showed effects only at much higher concentrations, suggesting partial agonist effects. Russell and co-workers later showed that in vitro the effect was transcriptional (74).

Karmali and co-workers confirmed that bovine parathyroid cells in primary culture decreased their levels of both PTH mRNA and secreted PTH after the addition of $1,25(OH)_2D_3$ (75). Interestingly they found that human parathyroid cells derived from human parathyroid adenomas did not respond to $1,25(OH)_2D_3$ by decreasing their PTH mRNA or PTH secretion, despite their normal content of $1,25(OH)_2D_3$ receptors. Cortisol lead to a reduction in the number of $1,25(OH)_2D_3$ receptors in the bovine cells (75), and a decreased responsiveness to $1,25(OH)_2D_3$ (76).

Definitive studies on this subject were performed in vivo by Silver and co-workers (77). They injected normal rats with $1,25(OH)_2D_3$ and measured levels of PTH mRNA. After a single injection of the extremely small dose of 12.5 pmol $1,25(OH)_2D_3$ there was a marked reduction in PTH mRNA levels. The effect of $1,25(OH)_2D_3$ was evident 3 h after 100 pmol $1,25(OH)_2D_3$ and reached less than 1% of basal at 48 h (Fig. 4). The effect of $1,25(OH)_2D_3$ was not on PTH mRNA processing as there were no larger PTH transcripts on Northern blots. There was no affect of $1,25(OH)_2D_3$ on actin mRNA in microdissected rat parathyroids while the decrease in PTH mRNA was maintained, demonstrating the specificity of the effect. In order to determine whether the $1,25(OH)_2D_3$ regulation of PTH mRNA levels was mediated transcriptionally nuclear transcript run-off experiments were performed. In this system RNA synthesis consists of elongation and completion of previously initiated RNA molecules. Thus, the labeling of nascent RNA in vitro accurately reflects the RNA initiation that occurred in vivo. There was a dramatic reduction in PTH transcription in $1,25(OH)_2D_3$ treated rats to 10% of control rats, whereas β-actin transcription in the same $1,25(OH)_2D_3$ treated rats was 100% of control rats. These in vivo results therefore established that $1,25(OH)_2D_3$ regulates PTH mRNA levels through its effect on PTH gene transcription, that $1,25(OH)_2D_3$ is a major factor in the regulation of the PTH gene, and that the parathyroid cell is an important target organ for $1,25(OH)_2D_3$.

Of interest is the interrelationship between the stimuli of low calcium, which increases PTH mRNA levels, and $1,25(OH)_2D_3$ which decreases PTH mRNA levels. When rats were given both these stimuli there was a decrease in PTH mRNA compared to the controls (Fig. 5) (54). This suggests that the effect of $1,25(OH)_2D_3$ is the dominant effect over that of low calcium. The molecular mechanisms involved in such an interaction are of interest and might involve interactions at any of a number of levels, including both a direct genomic effect and a direct effect on transcellular calcium transport. It has been shown that $1,25(OH)_2D_3$ rapidly increases cytosolic calcium in dispersed parathyroid cells due to an increased influx of calcium (78), in which case the dominant role of $1,25(OH)_2D_3$ over a low extracellular calcium might be a result of a direct membrane effect regulating intracellular calcium homeostasis in parathyroid cells. Alternatively, or in addition, the binding of the $1,25(OH)_2D_3$ receptor complex to the 5'-upstream sequence of the PTH gene might activate the low calcium enhancer, or with the ability to immobilize the low calcium enhancer by means of direct contact by looping of the DNA (54).

Okazaki and co-workers studied the effect of $1,25(OH)_2D_3$ on transcription driven by the parathyroid gene promoter (79). They fused 684 base pairs of the 5'-flanking region of the human PTH gene to the bacte-

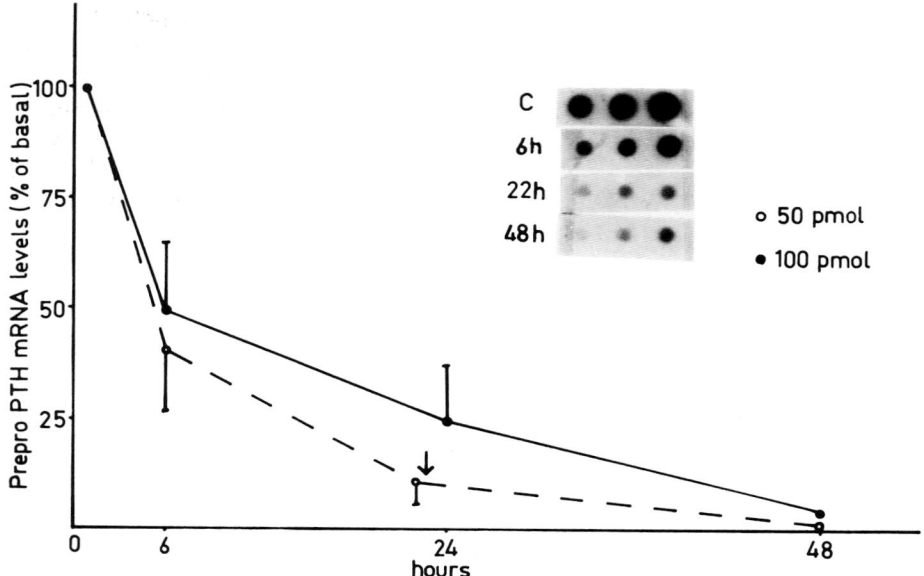

FIG. 4. Time course for the effect of 1,25(OH)$_2$D$_3$ on PTH mRNA levels of rat parathyroid glands. The arrow indicates the second injection of 50 pmol 1,25(OH)$_2$D$_3$. The inset shows representative autoradiographic spots for control (C) and 1,25(OH)$_2$D$_3$ treated rats (100 pmol) at 6, 22, and 48 h. The three dots at each time are from increasing volumes of total RNA extracted from a single rat. Each point gives the mean ± SE for four rats. From Silver et al. (77), with permission of the American Society for Clinical Investigation.

rial neogene, which they transfected into the rat pituitary cell line GH$_4$C$_1$. This cell line has the 1,25(OH)$_2$D$_3$ receptor. After transfection they selected those colonies successfully transfected with the fusion gene by their resistance to the neomycin analog, G418. The level of RNA initiated from the human PTH gene promoter region was suppressed by 1,25(OH)$_2$D$_3$. Synthesis of the same transcript under control of a viral promoter was not regulated by 1,25(OH)$_2$D$_3$. The effect of 1,25(OH)$_2$D$_3$ was detected within 24 h at physiological doses of 1,25(OH)$_2$D$_3$. These studies therefore demon-

strate that 1,25(OH)$_2$D$_3$ decreases PTH transcription by acting on the 5′-flanking region of the PTH gene. As yet the nucleotide sequence in the PTH gene which mediates this action has not been identified in the PTH gene (80,81). The sequence of the vitamin D responsive element has been defined and characterized in the osteocalcin gene (38–40).

Cantley and co-workers correlated the effect of 1,25(OH)$_2$D$_3$ on PTH secretion and PTH mRNA levels in primary cultures of bovine parathyroid cells (82). In short term incubations (30–120 min) 1,25(OH)$_2$D$_3$ had

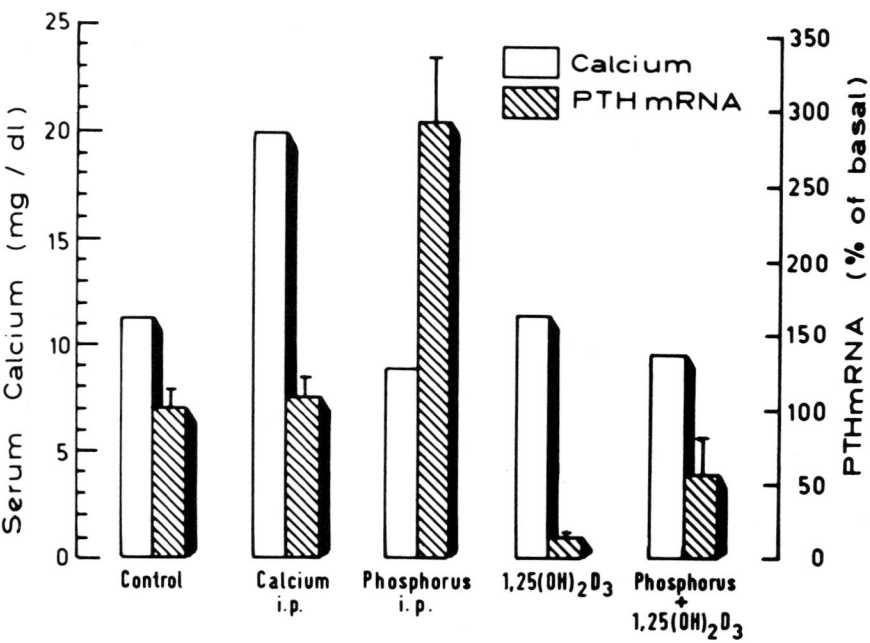

FIG. 5. The effect of calcium, phosphorus, 1,25(OH)$_2$D$_3$, and phosphorus with 1,25(OH)$_2$D$_3$ on serum calcium and PTH mRNA of rat parathyroid glands at 6 h. Rats were injected intraperitoneally with calcium gluconate i.p. or sodium phosphate i.p. or 1,25(OH)$_2$D$_3$ i.p. or phosphorus with 1,25(OH)$_2$D$_3$. The effect of 1,25(OH)$_2$D$_3$ was dominant over the low calcium effect. From Naveh-Many et al. (54), with permission of the American Society for Clinical Investigation.

no effect on PTH secretion, but in long term incubations (24–96 h) there was a dose dependent decrease in PTH mRNA levels and PTH secretion. This study and that of Chan et al. (83) confirms that the 1,25(OH)₂D₃ effect on PTH gene expression is reflected in a decrease in PTH synthesis and subsequent secretion. Earlier studies of the effect of 1,25(OH)₂D₃ on PTH secretion were confounded by the short time sequences used when there would have been no effect of 1,25(OH)₂D₃ on PTH synthesis (84,85), in contrast to studies at longer time intervals that had shown an effect (86). Brown and co-workers studied an analogue of vitamin D, 22-oxacalcitriol, which is reported to have little hypercalcemic effect, on the levels of PTH mRNA in rats (87). Both 1,25(OH)₂D₃ and the analogue led to a decrease in PTH mRNA levels and at the doses used neither caused hypercalcemia, but in detailed studies they showed that oxacalcitriol did not cause hypercalcemia even in larger doses. This and other analogues might have useful effects on PTH synthesis and less effect in increasing the serum calcium.

Naveh-Many and co-workers (88) extended their in vivo study on the PTH gene to an investigation of the effect of 1,25(OH)₂D₃ on calcitonin gene transcription. They were able to do this because the RNA extracts that they had used to determine PTH mRNA were derived from thyroparathyroid tissue, and therefore also contained extracts of the calcitonin producing C-cells. Stripping and rehybridization of their filters for calcitonin mRNA (89,90) and relevant control genes demonstrated for the first time that 1,25(OH)₂D₃ markedly decreased calcitonin mRNA levels with no effect on the control genes actin, thyroglobulin, and somatostatin which is also specific for the C-cells (Fig. 6). This effect was also shown to be transcriptional. These results were confirmed in in vitro studies where in the calcitonin producing C-cell line (TT) Cote and co-workers showed that 1,25(OH)₂D₃ decreased the levels of calcitonin mRNA and the other product of the calcitonin gene, calcitonin gene related peptide (91–93). 1,25(OH)₂D₃ is therefore at the center of endocrinological loops involving PTH, calcitonin, and calcium (Fig. 7).

A further level at which 1,25(OH)₂D₃ might regulate the PTH gene would be at the level of the 1,25(OH)₂D₃ receptor. 1,25(OH)₂D₃ acts on its target tissues by binding to the 1,25(OH)₂D₃ receptor which regulates the transcription of genes with the appropriate recognition sequences, analogous to the action of other small nonpeptide hormones (68,70,94). The concentration of the 1,25(OH)₂D₃ receptor in the 1,25(OH)₂D₃ target sites would allow a modulation of the 1,25(OH)₂D₃ effect (95,96), with an increase in receptor concentration leading to an amplification of its effect and a decrease in receptor concentration dampening the 1,25(OH)₂D₃ effect. Ligand and cation dependent up regulation of the 1,25(OH)₂D₃ receptor has been shown in vivo in rat in-

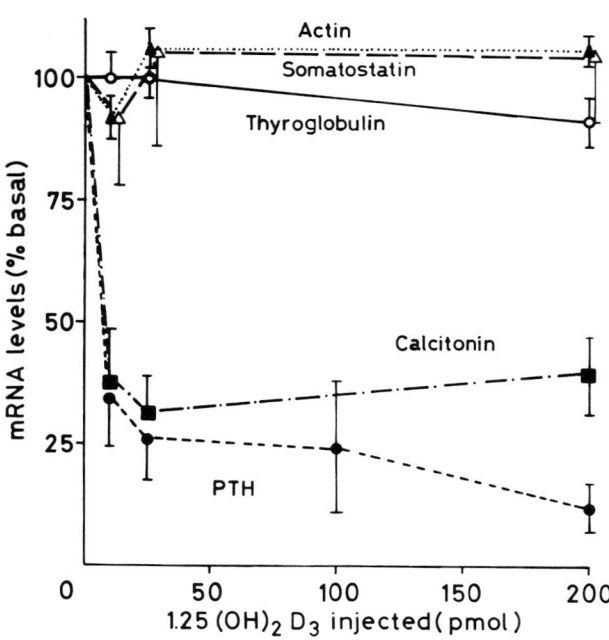

FIG. 6. The effect of 1,25(OH)₂D₃ on mRNA levels for calcitonin, PTH, actin, somatostatin, and thyroglobulin in rat thyroparathyroid glands 24 h after single injections intraperitoneally of 1,25(OH)₂D₃. From Naveh-Many et al. (88), with permission of the American Society for Clinical Investigation.

testine (97–100), and in vitro in a number of systems (100–104).

Naveh-Many and co-workers (105) injected 1,25-(OH)₂D₃ to rats and measured the levels of the 1,25(OH)₂D₃ receptor mRNA (VDR mRNA) and PTH

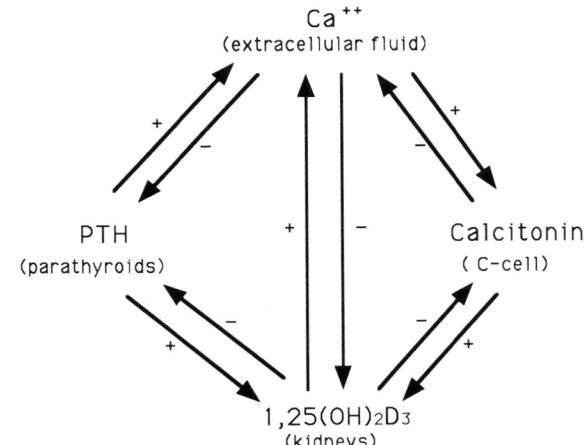

FIG. 7. Interrelationships among extracellular fluid calcium concentration, and the three calcium regulating hormones PTH, calcitonin, and 1,25(OH)₂D₃. Calcium regulates the secretion of PTH and calcitonin, and the synthesis of 1,25(OH)₂D₃. In addition a low calcium concentration increases PTH gene expression. 1,25(OH)₂D₃ decreases the transcription of the PTH and calcitonin genes. Modified from Naveh-Many et al. (88), with permission of the American Society for Clinical Investigation.

mRNA in the parathyro-thyroid tissue. They showed that 1,25(OH)$_2$D$_3$ in physiologically relevant doses led to an increase in VDR mRNA levels in the parathyroid glands in contrast to the decrease in PTH mRNA levels (Fig. 8). This increase in VDR mRNA occurred after a time lag of 6 h, and a dose response showed a peak at 25 pmol.

The VDR mRNA ran as 2 bands at 4.4 kb and 2.2 kb. Duodenum VDR mRNA ran as a single band which also increased after 1,25(OH)$_2$D$_3$ as reported by others. In rats on diets deficient in calcium for 3 weeks after weaning there was no change in VDR mRNA levels, despite large differences in serum calcium and PTH mRNA levels. However, after vitamin D deficiency there were interesting findings in the relative size of the VDR mRNA transcripts as analyzed by agarose gels (Northern blots). In the normal vitamin D rats (ND) there were two VDR mRNA bands and the larger 4.4 kb transcript was the major band, and the 2.2 kb band was less prominent. In contrast in rats on a vitamin D deficient diet for three weeks (−D), the smaller 2.2 kb transcript was the major band. The reason for this difference remains to be explained but in other systems larger transcripts have been shown to be more stable. The larger VDR mRNA band in the normal rats would then be more readily available for translation into the VDR protein, and allow 1,25(OH)$_2$D$_3$ to act. Therapeutically this information might be useful by treating with vitamin D metabolites in order to ensure a stable VDR transcript.

The localization of the VDR mRNA to the parathyroids was demonstrated. A thyroparathyroid cell suspension was sorted by flow cytometry (FACS) into the smaller parathroid cell peak, and the larger thyroid cell peak. VDR mRNA was almost totally in the parathyroid peak. In addition in situ hybridization studies of the thyro-parathyroid and duodenum for the VDR mRNA were performed (Fig. 9). VDR mRNA was localized to the parathyroids in the same concentration as in the duodenum. In in vitro primary cultures of parathyroids there are VDR mRNA bands at 4.4 and 2.2 kb which both increase after 1,25(OH)$_2$D$_3$.

Therefore 1,25(OH)$_2$D$_3$ increases the expression of its receptor's gene in the parathyroid gland, which would result in increased VDR protein synthesis and increased binding of 1,25(OH)$_2$D$_3$. This ligand dependent receptor up regulation would lead to an amplified effect of 1,25(OH)$_2$D$_3$ on the PTH gene, and might help explain the dramatic effect of 1,25(OH)$_2$D$_3$ on the PTH gene.

The regulation of PTH gene transcription is relevant not only in understanding the physiology of the parathyroid gland, but also in the pathophysiology of diseases involving the parathyroid where there is parathyroid hyperplasia (106,107). Secondary parathyroid hyperplasia is a complication of chronic renal disease (108,109) or vitamin D deficiency, and may lead to disabling skeletal complications (110,111). The expression and regulation of the PTH gene has been studied in two models of secondary hyperparathyroidism: (i) with experimental uremia due to 5/6 nephrectomy and (ii) with nutritional secondary hyperparathyroidism due to diets deficient in vitamin D and/or calcium.

5/6 nephrectomy rats had higher serum creatinines, and also appreciably higher levels of parathyroid gland PTH mRNA indicative of their secondary hyperparathyroidism (112). Their PTH mRNA levels decreased after single injections of 1,25(OH)$_2$D$_3$, similar to the response

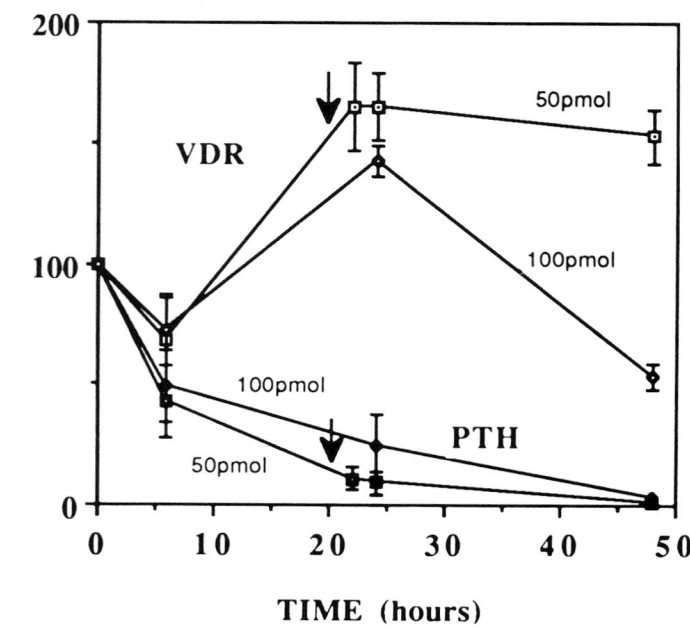

FIG. 8. Time course for the effect of 1,25(OH)$_2$D$_3$ on mRNA levels for PTH and the 1,25(OH)$_2$D$_3$, receptor (VDR) in rat thyroparathyroid glands. Rats were injected with either a single dose of 100 pmol 1,25(OH)$_2$D$_3$, or 50 pmol 1,25(OH)$_2$D$_3$ at 0 and 24 h. The arrow represents the second injection of 1,25(OH)$_2$D$_3$. The data represent the mean ± SE for four rats. From Naveh-Many et al. (105), with permission of the American Society for Clinical Investigation.

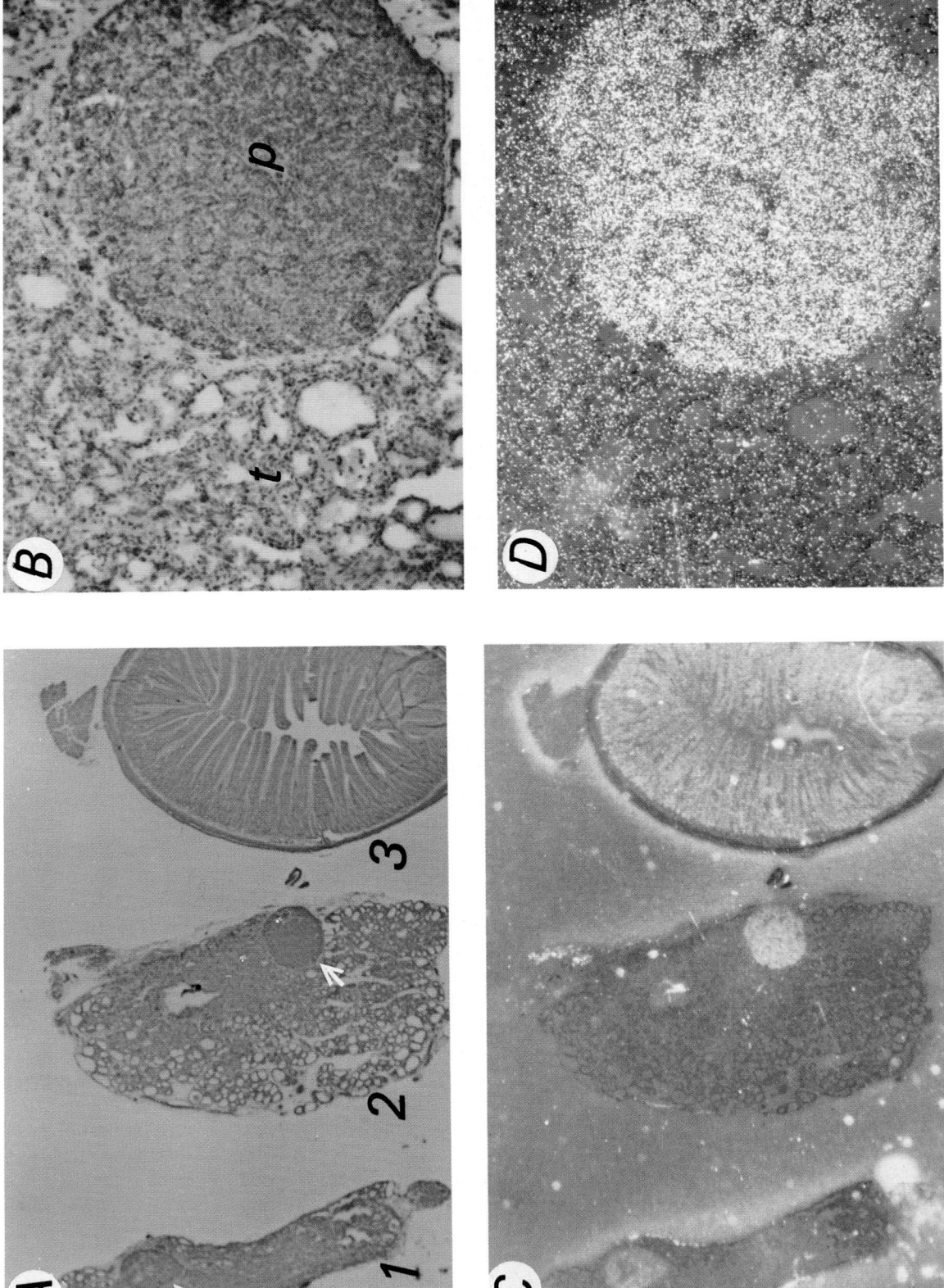

FIG. 9. In situ hybridization of parathyroid-thyroid and duodenum sections with 1,25(OH)$_2$D$_3$, receptor (VDR). (**A**, 1) Parathyroid-thyroid tissue from a control rat. (**A**, 2) Parathyroid-thyroid tissue from a 1,25(OH)$_2$D$_3$ treated rat. The white arrow points at the parathyroid glands. (**A**, 3) Duodenum from the 1,25(OH)$_2$D$_3$ treated rat (100 pmol at 24 h). **A** and **B** were photographed under bright-field illumination, whereas **C** and **D** show dark-field illumination of the same sections. Hybridization was with an antisense VDR probe. After 4 days of autoradiographic exposure, sections were stained with Giemsa stain and photographed. Magnification in **B** is sevenfold the magnification of **A**. From Naveh-Many et al. (105), with permission of the American Society for Clinical Investigation.

of normal rats (Fig. 10). However, their PTH mRNA levels did not increase after the stimulus of acute hypocalcemia, as in normal rats. This might suggest that for the PTH gene to respond to hypocalcemia, normal levels of vitamin D are needed, or alternatively, that the PTH gene expression was already maximally stimulated in the 5/6 nephrectomy rats and therefore could not increase further after acute hypocalcemia. What was of interest in these studies in the 5/6 nephrectomy rats was that the secondary hyperparathyroidism was characterized by an increase in parathyroid gland PTH mRNA but not in VDR mRNA (112). Experimental secondary hyperparathyroidism is characterized by an increase in PTH mRNA per cell and not by an increase in parathyroid cell number (see later), which suggests that in 5/6 nephrectomy rats there was relatively less VDR mRNA per parathyroid cell, or a relative down regulation of the VDR, as has been reported in VDR binding studies (113–115).

The second model of experimental secondary hyperparathyroidism studied was that due to dietary deficiency of vitamin D (−D) and/or calcium (−Ca), as compared to normal vitamin D (ND) and normal calcium (NCa) (116). These dietary regimes were selected to mimic the secondary hyperparathyroidism where the stimuli for the production of hyperparathyroidism are the low serum levels of $1,25(OH)_2D_3$ and ionized calcium. At the center of the pathogenesis of the changes in $1,25(OH)_2D_3$ and ionized calcium levels is the high serum phosphorus which is an early feature of renal failure (Fig. 11). Weanling rats were maintained on these diets for three weeks and then studied. Rats on diets defi-

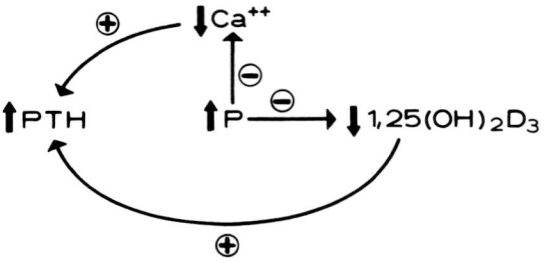

FIG. 11. The pathogenesis of secondary hyperparathyroidism in chronic renal failure. The increase in extracellular phosphorus concentration is an early result of renal failure and this leads to a decrease in the renal production of $1,25(OH)_2D_3$, which together with the direct effect of phosphorus to complex serum calcium, results in a decrease in serum calcium. The low serum calcium and serum $1,25(OH)_2D_3$ lead to secondary hyperparathyroidism.

cient in both vitamin D and calcium (−D−Ca) had a tenfold increase in PTH mRNA as compared to controls (NDNCa) together with much lower serum calciums and also lower serum $1,25(OH)_2D_3$ levels. Calcium deficiency alone (−CaND) led to a fivefold increase in PTH mRNA levels, while a diet deficient in vitamin D alone (−DNCa) led to a twofold increase in PTH mRNA levels (Fig. 12). The effect of injected $1,25(OH)_2D_3$ on PTH mRNA levels in rats with secondary hyperparathyroidism was then studied. Normal rats decreased their PTH mRNA levels after small physiologically relevant doses of $1,25(OH)_2D_3$, such as 12.5–50 pmol. These rats with secondary hyperparathyroidism did not decrease their PTH mRNA levels after single doses of $1,25(OH)_2D_3$ as large as 1000 pmol. However, their PTH mRNA levels did decrease partially after three daily doses of 100 pmol. This might have been a result of up regulation of the $1,25(OH)_2D_3$ receptor (VDR). In addition the effect of acute hypocalcemia on PTH mRNA levels was studied. The rats on a diet of isolated calcium deficiency with a normal vitamin D content (Ca−ND) increased their PTH mRNA after hypocalcemia, but the rats on diets deficient in both vitamin D and calcium (−D−Ca) rats did not. This might have been because their PTH mRNA levels were already maximally stimulated, or that vitamin D is necessary for a normal response to hypocalcemia.

An important clinical question in chronic renal failure patients is whether the secondary hyperparathyroidism is due to an increased number of cells or to an increase in the transcription of PTH per cell. Parathyroid cell number was determined in thyroparathyroid tissue of normal rats and −D−Ca rats. To do this the tissue was enzymatically digested into an isolated cell population that was then passed through a flow cytometer (FACS) and separated by size into two peaks. The first peak of smaller cells contained parathyroid cells as determined by the presence of PTH mRNA, and the second peak contained thyroid follicular cells and calcitonin cells that hybrid-

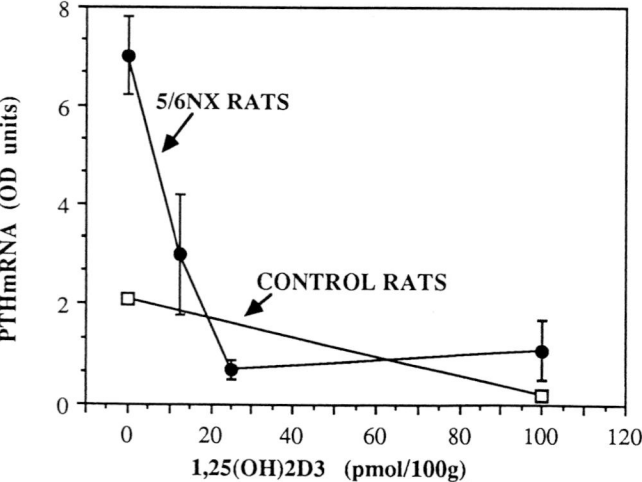

FIG. 10. PTH mRNA levels in the parathyroid glands of control rats and rats with experimental uremia due to 5/6 nephrectomy (5/6 NX). The uremic rats had increased levels of PTH mRNA. After the injection of single doses of $1,25(OH)_2D_3$ there was a decrease in PTH mRNA levels in control and uremic rats. From Shvil et al. (112), with permission of the American Society of Nephrology.

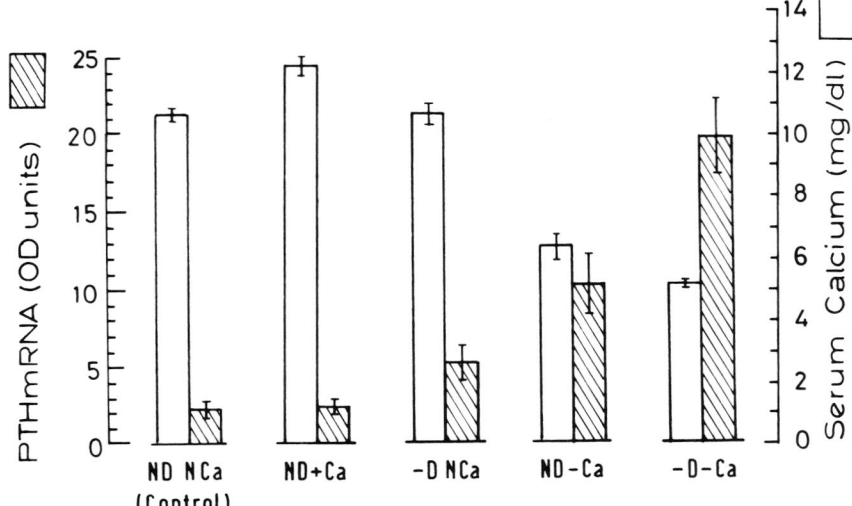

FIG. 12. Effect of dietary calcium and vitamin D given to rats for three weeks from weaning on serum calcium and PTH mRNA levels of rat parathyroid glands. Results are mean ± SEM for four rats on control diet (NDNCa); high calcium (ND+Ca); vitamin D-deficient normal calcium (−DNCa); normal vitamin D, calcium deficient (ND−Ca); vitamin D−, calcium-deficient (−D−Ca). The rats with dietary deficiency of vitamin D (−D) and/or calcium (−Ca) had different degrees of secondary hyperparathyroidism with increased levels of PTH mRNA. Modified from Naveh-Many et al. (116).

ized positively for thyroglobulin mRNA and calcitonin mRNA, but not PTH mRNA. There were 1.6-fold more cells in the −D−Ca rats than in the normal rats, as compared to the tenfold increase in PTH mRNA (Fig. 13). Therefore this model of secondary hyperparathyroidism is characterized by increased transcription per cell, rather than by an increase in cell number.

Wernerson and co-workers have studied parathyroid cell number in dietary secondary hyperparathyroidism (ND−Ca) using stereoscopic electron microscopy and has shown that there is no increase in cell number but that the cells are markedly hypertrophic (117,118). So at least in the secondary hyperparathyroidism of these models, there is parathyroid cell hypertrophy and not hyperplasia. These experimental findings are relevant to the management of patients with secondary hyperparathyroidism. It is possible to regulate the increased transcription of the PTH gene, but it is not possible to decrease the number of parathyroid cells by accelerating cell death or apoptosis (119). For this reason it is appropriate and effective to treat patients with renal failure early with

1,25(OH)₂D₃ and calcium to decrease PTH gene transcription and prevent parathyroid cell proliferation (120,121).

There have been a number of careful and detailed studies in patients with chronic renal failure, on the affect of 1,25(OH)₂D₃ on serum PTH levels as well as on bone histology. Many of these come from the laboratory of Slatopolsky and he discusses them in depth in chapter 39. In brief 1,25(OH)₂D₃ decreases serum PTH levels, and decreases the capacity of PTH to increase after hypocalcemia (122–126). The mechanism of this 1,25(OH)₂D₃ effect is in all probability its effect on PTH gene transcription as discussed above. The end result is to prevent the deleterious effects of PTH on bone.

BIOSYNTHESIS AND INTRACELLULAR PROCESSING OF PTH

The translational product of the PTH mRNA is pre-proPTH, which is the precursor of proPTH. Evidence

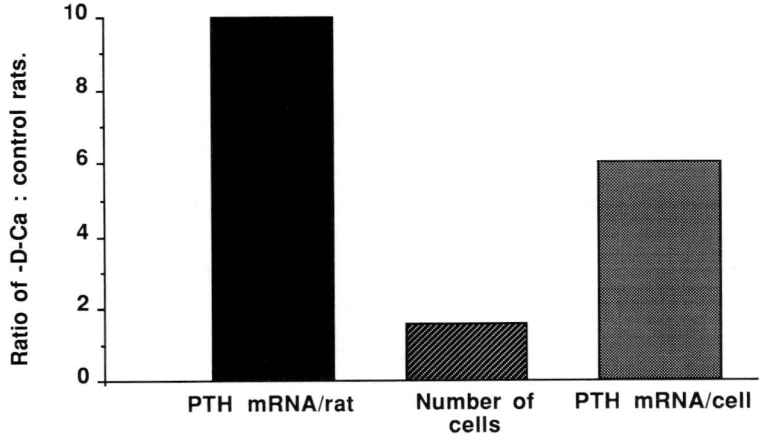

FIG. 13. Comparison of rats with dietary induced secondary hyperparathyroidism due to a vitamin D−, calcium-deficient (−D−Ca) diet to control rats on a normal vitamin D, normal calcium diet. PTH mRNA per rat parathyroid tissue was increased tenfold, with a much smaller increase in parathyroid cells. Therefore increased PTH mRNA per parathyroid cell accounted for most of the increase in PTH mRNA, and this model represents a transcriptional rather than a proliferative model of secondary hyperparathyroidism.

that the translational product of PTH mRNA was larger than proPTH was obtained by translation of a crude preparation of bovine parathyroid RNA in the wheat germ cell-free system (127). The primary translation product migrated slower than proPTH on polyacrylamide gel electrophoresis. A similar precursor had at that time been reported only for immunoglobulin light chains. ProPTH had been identified by the incubation of parathyroid tissue with radioactive amino acids and pulse chase experiments (127–129). The complete primary sequences of both preproPTH (115 amino acids) and proPTH (90 amino acids) were determined by both sensitive protein-sequencing techniques using radioactive amino acids and in cell-free translation of mRNA prepared from parathyroid glands (130–132) (Fig. 1).

PreproPTH, like other proteins that are to be exported from a cell (133), is thought to be synthesized on ribosomes bound to the rough endoplasmic reticulum (127,134,135). This facilitates its specific transport into the cistern of the rough endoplasmic reticulum, and directing it along the secretory pathway of the cell. During protein synthesis the "pre" or signal sequence is cleaved from the precursor protein (135,136). The initiation of preproPTH synthesis occurs on polyribosomes in the cell matrix. During the synthesis of the polypeptide chain the two amino-terminal methionines are removed enzymatically. As the nascent chain continues to grow, the hydrophobic amino-terminal sequence of preproPTH emerges and associates with the endoplasmic reticulum in accord with the signal hypothesis (137). A signal peptidase removes the 23 amino acid single sequence as the protein traverses the membrane of the rough endoplasmic reticulum, leaving the intermediate precursor, proPTH, in the lumen of the endoplasmic reticulum. The signal peptidase acts to enzymatically cleave the glycyl-lysine bond. Almost no intact preproPTH is found in the parathyroid cell indicating a highly efficient conversion to proPTH. PreproPTH is converted to proPTH cotranslationally, and vectorial transport across the endoplasmic reticulum is dependent upon the cleavage of the signal sequence (135,136,138, 139). Within 15 min of its initial formation from preproPTH, the proPTH product moves to the Golgi apparatus where the dibasic residues at the end of the "pro" sequence direct the enzymatic cleavage of the "pro" sequence (Fig. 14). Evidence for the specificity of the intracellular trafficking and processing of preproPTH has come from a number of studies utilizing electron microscopic autoradiography of parathyroid cells labeled with radioactive amino acids (140), amine compounds that disrupt the Golgi complex and inhibitors of microtubule function such as vinblastine and colchicine (141,142). There is little proPTH stored in the parathyroid cell (143) and the small amount present is probably on its way to becoming mature PTH, which might represent its function.

The routing of preproPTH to the endoplasmic reticulum is dependent upon the primary amino acid sequence. Proteins destined for export are synthesized as a larger precursor molecule containing at its amino-terminal end a hydrophobic leader sequence, the so-called signal sequence. This sequence, as it emerges from the ribosome, permits the nascent protein-ribosome-mRNA complex to bind to an 11 S signal recognition particle (SRP). The SRP contains 6 peptides and a 7 S RNA molecule. This complex then binds to an endoplasmic reticulum "docking protein," which then facilitates the nascent protein chain to pass through the membrane and enter the cisternal space (9). The peptide consisting of the leader sequence of preproPTH together with the prohormone specific region was synthesized by Rosenblatt and co-workers (144) and used as a probe to search for receptors in the endoplasmic reticulum. Addition of the synthetic signal peptide to cell-free translation systems containing microsomal vesicles effectively inhibited the conversion of preproPTH to PTH as well as the sequestration of proPTH in the vesicle (145). In addition mutations have been introduced in the amino-terminal domain of the signal peptide of preproPTH and these inhibited translocation without affecting interaction with the signal recognition particle (146). Wiren and co-workers (147–149) have created mutations in the propeptide sequence of preproPTH and have defined their importance in protein translocation, signal sequence cleavage, and membrane binding properties. These results indicate that there are specific saturable receptors or recognition elements that recognize and bind the signal "pre" sequence, and direct it in its passage from the cell. Von Heijne analyzed a number of eukaryotic signal sequences and concluded that signal sequences have a hydrophobic core, which might be responsible for initiating export and for binding to the signal recognition protein, and a second one in the region 5 to 1 conferring processing specificity (137).

After synthesis PTH is packaged in secretory vesicles and may then be secreted, stored, or degraded intracellularly. The parathyroid cell is not rich in secretory granules and Morrisey and co-workers (10,150) demonstrated that as much as 90% of newly generated PTH is neither secreted or stored, but proteolytically degraded within the cell. In cells cultured in the presence of a low extracellular calcium concentration there was less degradation of PTH. As a result of this intracellular degradation of PTH large amounts of carboxy-terminal PTH fragments are present and secreted from parathyroid tissue. A significant proportion of the PTH in the circulation as fragments is derived from the parathyroid gland itself (151). Degradation of PTH in the gland might occur in lysosomes with proteolysis by lysosomal enzymes, such as cathepsin. Calcium by inhibiting secretion would lead to retention of hormone within the gland, where it is more available for proteolysis.

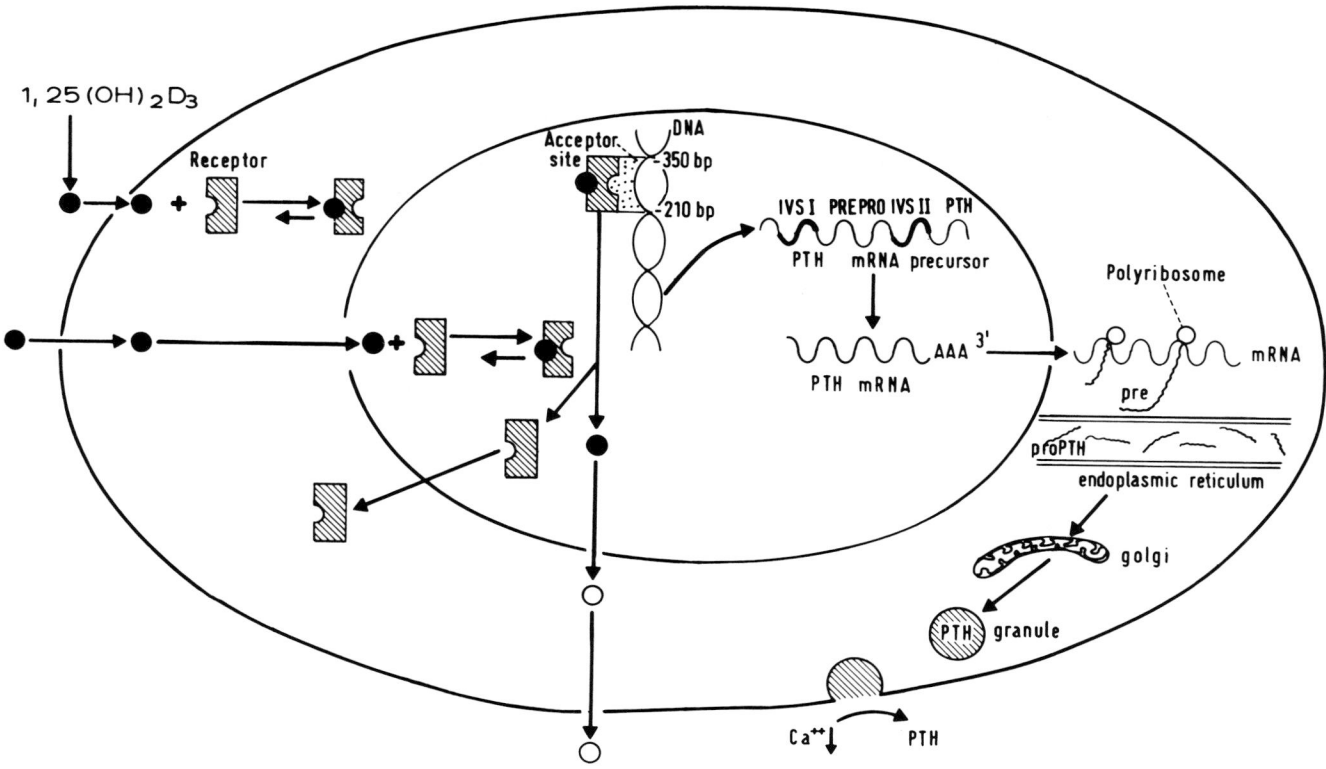

FIG. 14. Model of 1,25(OH)₂D₃ action on the parathyroid cell. 1,25(OH)₂D₃ binds to its receptor (VDR) in the parathyroid cell, which then binds to PTH gene promoter's vitamin D response element (VDRE). In some way this decreases the activity of RNA polymerase II leading to less transcription to the preproPTH mRNA precursor. This precursor is normally processed and spliced to the mature preproPTH mRNA with its polyadenylated tail, which then in the nucleus is attached to polyribosomes where it is translated to preproPTH. The pre sequence of the peptide while still a nascent chain attached to the polysome recognizes and binds to a docking protein, which is a receptor protein located on the cytoplasmic face of the endoplasmic reticulum membrane. The signal peptide is cleaved from the polypeptide chain by signal peptidase before the synthesis of the chain is completed (co-translational cleavage). ProPTH is transported along the Golgi apparatus and the pro sequence is cleaved, leaving the mature PTH in the secretory granule.

PTH SECRETION

In 1942 Patt and Luckardt perfused the isolated thyroparathyroid apparatus of the dog with both low and high concentrations of calcium fluids and measured PTH activity by a bioassay whereby they measured serum calcium in the circulation of the test animal. They showed that secretion was inversely proportional to the calcium content of the perfusate (10). The development of a radioimmunoassay for PTH made it feasible to confirm and extend these studies (152). Sherwood and co-workers (153,154) demonstrated an inverse linear relationship between extracellular calcium or magnesium concentration and PTH secretion. Later Sherwood and co-workers showed that phosphorus itself did not have an independent effect on PTH secretion (5). Mayer and Hurst (155) catheterized the inferior thyroid veins of calves and measured the secretory rate for PTH with

changes in serum calcium. They found that the relationship was sigmoidal and in addition there was a nonsuppressible portion of PTH secretion even at very high levels of serum calcium (156). This sigmoidal relationship has been confirmed in man. Brent and co-workers (157) used a sensitive immunoradiometric assay specific for intact PTH (1–84) to determine the dynamics of the relationship between calcium and serum intact PTH. They confirmed the inverse sigmoidal relationship between PTH and serum total and plasma ionized calcium in men and women, and which was applicable for rapid and slow changes in serum calcium. Johansson and co-workers (158) measured the cytoplasmic calcium concentration of single parathyroid cells and have shown a sigmoidal relationship between sustained changes in cytoplasmic calcium and extracellular calcium concentration in the 0.5–3.0 mM range. The sustained change in calcium concentration is due to the influx of extracellular calcium through calcium channels. The sigmoidal relationship is therefore a property of the parathyroid calcium channel, and perhaps other transduction mechanisms, such as activation of protein kinase A and C. PTH secretion, and perhaps also PTH gene transcription might therefore respond proportionately to the sigmoidal change in cytoplasmic calcium concentration.

Brown has analyzed in detail the sigmoidal relationship between calcium and PTH secretion, defining the so-called set-point which is that calcium concentration producing half of the maximal inhibition of secretion (159). This parameter becomes useful in the analysis of parathyroid tissue from patients with secondary hyperparathyroidism due to renal failure. In tissue from these patients analyzed in vitro they suggested that there was a shift in the set-point to the right indicating a relative insensitivity to calcium (160). Leboff and co-workers have shown that parathyroid cells in culture when rapidly proliferating are also relatively insensitive to a high calcium concentration (56,161,162) demonstrating the importance of rigorously defining in vitro conditions for any study on PTH regulation. Another situation where it has been postulated that there is a shift in the set-point for calcium is in the neonate. Newborn babies (163), as well as newborn calves (164) and pigs (165,166) have higher serum calciums than their mothers together with inappropriately normal or even elevated levels of PTH. Keaton and co-workers (164) showed that a higher serum calcium concentration was needed to reduce serum PTH levels in newborn calves than in older animals, indicating a shift in set-point. Confirmatory evidence was provided in vitro (167–169). In familial hypocalciuric hypercalcemia (FHH) newborn babies may have excessive hypercalcemia related to hyperparathyroidism (170). Marx and co-workers (167) showed that parathyroid cells from such a case when studied in vitro had a marked insensitivity to increases in extracellular fluid calcium.

The secretion of PTH from the parathyroid gland into the extracellular fluid is stimulated by hypocalcemia and is mediated by exocytosis. Habener and co-workers (140) used electron microscopic autoradiography to study the parathyroid cell and concluded that the limiting membrane of granules or vesicles that contain hormone fuse with the plasma membrane, membrane lysis occurs, and the contents of the storage vesicle are released into the circulation. In all other secretory cells apart from the parathyroid and also the juxtaglomerular apparatus's secretion of renin, the stimulus to exocytosis is a high calcium concentration, which serves as a second messenger in the stimulus to secretion. MacGregor and co-workers (171) and Morrissey and Cohn (172) have suggested that more than one secretory pathway may exist in the parathyroid cell. They found that newly synthesized hormone is secreted more rapidly than older hormone, and in addition that certain stimuli

such as cAMP preferentially release newly synthesized hormone.

The mechanism whereby decreases in extracellular calcium stimulate rather than inhibit PTH secretion and PTH gene transcription is an enigma. The parathyroid cell responds to small increases in extracellular calcium with rapid and sustained increases in intracellular calcium concentration, unlike most cells where there is little variation in cytoplasmic ionized calcium concentration (173,174). In the parathyroid cell a high extracellular calcium leads to an increase in intracellular free calcium. This is a receptor mediated process (175).

The earliest evidence for a receptor on the parathyroid cell surface that responds to divalent cation concentration came from electrophysiological studies. Lopez-Barneo and Armstrong (176) showed that a number of divalent and trivalent cations such as lanthanum (La^{3+}), which does not cross the cell membrane, depolarize parathyroid cells by altering plasma membrane conductance to potassium. This alteration in membrane permeability by impermeant cations suggested that there was a polyvalent cation receptor on the external surface of the parathyroid cell membrane. In addition these polyvalent cations also act to inhibit PTH secretion from parathyroid cells in culture with a cation effect of similar rank order to that of their electrophysiological effect (177). However, the issue is not totally clear and Nemeth (175) has concluded that it is still questionable if membrane potential has any significant role in regulating secretion in parathyroid cells.

Other evidence for the presence of a "calcium receptor" has come from the use of monoclonal antibodies to the parathyroid cell and the study of the effect of divalent cations on intracellular calcium concentration. Juhlin and co-workers (178,179) raised monoclonal antibodies to human parathyroid adenoma cells which were reactive against parathyroid tissue and not other human tissue, apart from proximal kidney tubule cells and placental cytotrophoblast cells. Their antibodies were tested in parathyroid cells challenged with a high extracellular calcium and they prevented the anticipated increase in intracellular calcium and inhibition of PTH secretion. Their data suggest that their antibodies either block a calcium receptor or a calcium channel opened by calcium binding to the receptor, rather than interrupt the signal caused by receptor activation (180). Their studies on the calcium receptor using readily available placental material showed that the antiparathyroid antibodies recognized material which also bound lentil lectin, indicating that it is a glycoprotein.

There have been conflicting results of studies on voltage-sensitive calcium channels. Muff and co-workers (174) showed that sustained increases in parathyroid cell intracellular calcium are unaffected by dihydropyridine-type calcium channel agonists or antagonists, suggesting that calcium influx in parathyroid cells is through voltage-insensitive channels that are regulated by activation of the putative "calcium receptor." Different results were obtained by Fitzpatrick and co-workers (181–183) who studied the effect of two types of agonists of voltage-sensitive calcium channels on PTH secretion from dispersed bovine parathyroid cells. Agonists of the L type of calcium channel such as 1,4-dihydropyridine compounds opened the calcium channel and permited entry of extracellular calcium into the cell inhibiting PTH secretion. This effect was inhibited by pertussis toxin which ADP-ribosylates a guanine nucleotide regulatory protein (G-protein), indicating that a G-protein is interposed between the calcium channel and a putative intracellular site controlling PTH secretion (182,184). They also prepared polyclonal, monospecific mouse antibodies against highly purified preparations of α subunits of voltage-sensitive calcium channels from rat muscle transverse tubules (183,185). The antibodies blocked the secretion of PTH from parathyroid cells incubated in a low calcium concentration, and this inhibition was also blocked by pertussis toxin. They concluded that parathyroid cells possess a M_r 150,000 protein analogous to the α_1 subunit of the dihydropyridine sensitive calcium channel. The antibodies open calcium channels by a mechanism that uses a signal-transducing guanine nucleotide regulatory protein (G-protein), resulting in an influx of calcium ions which then inhibits PTH secretion.

Further evidence for a parathyroid cell "calcium receptor" came from studies on the effects of divalent cations on mobilization of intracellular calcium, and on inositol triphosphate (186,187) and diacylglycerol concentrations (188). Nemeth and co-workers (173, 175,189,190) showed in parathyroid cells that a high extracellular calcium lead to a transient spike in intracellular calcium derived from release of intracellular calcium, and a more sustained increase due to influx of calcium through voltage sensitive and insensitive channels. They used impermeant cations such as lanthanum (La^{3+}) which in low concentrations blocked sustained but not transient increases in intracellular calcium caused by an increase in extracellular calcium. In contrast lanthanum at high concentrations led to a rapid and transient increase in intracellular calcium concentration which could not have come from extracellular sources. This is all further support for a calcium receptor on the surface of the parathyroid cell.

Brown and co-workers showed that extracellular calcium and magnesium produced rapid increases in the accumulation of inositol 1,4,5-triphosphate (IP3) and inositol tetrakisphosphate (IP4) (186,191,192) suggesting that they might be the second messengers for the calcium induced spike in intracellular calcium. Moreover, high calcium concentrations lead to an increase in diacylglycerol within 10 sec which persists for 30 min (191). An increase in diacylglycerol concentration usually leads to an increase in protein kinase C activity.

Activators of protein kinase C activity, such as phorbol myristate acetate (PMA) inhibited PTH secretion after 30 min (186,191), and shifted the dose-response curve for extracellular calcium-induced changes in intracellular calcium and PTH secretion to the right without affecting the maximal responses (193). The inhibitor of protein kinase C, staurosporine, reversed the effect of protein kinase C activators. Interestingly when parathyroid cells were treated for 24 h with PMA, they lost >90% of their protein kinase C activity and no longer responded to PMA. However their intracellular calcium concentration and PTH secretion responded normally to changes in extracellular calcium (194). One finding that is difficult to reconcile is that a high calcium decreased rather than increased cytosol protein kinase C activity in parathyroid cells (195).

The parathyroid cell therefore responds like other cells in utilizing the receptor-mediated mobilization of intracellular calcium mediated by inositol phosphates and protein kinase C (196). It is exceptional in that there is an inverse relationship between PTH secretion and extracellular calcium concentration (168,197,198), which must be the function of the elusive "calcium receptor."

Studies with electropermeabilized parathyroid cells have shown that the parathyroid cell loses its unique coupling of hypocalcemia to hormone secretion, and now high calcium concentrations leads to PTH secretion. In these permeabilized cells cAMP and activators of protein kinase C retained their ability to regulate PTH secretion indicating the intactness of the secretory response in these cells and parathyroid cells in general (199,200). In addition in these permeabilized cells, the addition of non-hydrolyzable GTP analogues, such as GppNHp, which activate guanine nucleotide-regulatory proteins, leads to PTH secretion at low but not high calcium concentrations (200). The uniqueness of the parathyroid cell is therefore a function of the cell membrane, or rather a "sensor" or "receptor" located in the plasma membrane.

Enhanced accumulation of cyclic 3',5'-AMP (cAMP) in parathyroid cells due to the addition of agonists that stimulate adenylate cyclase or cholera toxin or inhibitors of cyclic nucleotide phosphodiesterase such as methyl-isobutylxanthine (MIX) lead to rapid increases in PTH secretion (2 min) consistent with a mediatory role for cAMP (192,201). Reduction in extracellular medium content of calcium also is associated with increased cAMP content. The nature of β-adrenergic receptors on parathyroid cells has been studied in detail utilizing the radioactive ligand iodohydroxybenzylpindolol. Parathyroid cells contain about 5,000–10,000 receptors per cell and show saturability and stereospecificity expected of β_2 type adrenergic receptors (202). Other agonists known to act through the adenylate cyclase system such as β-adrenergic catecholamines, dopamine, secretin, and prostaglandin E_2 all cause enhanced cAMP accumulation and increased PTH secretion when tested in bovine parathyroid cells (203–208). Dopaminergic agents such as dopamine cause an up to thirtyfold increase in cAMP accumulation and up to a fourfold increase in PTH secretion from parathyroid cells in vitro. In contrast prostaglandins of the F series inhibit basal as well as agonist-stimulated PTH secretion, associated with a decrease in cAMP content.

Agents which increase intracellular cAMP are potent secretagogues in intact parathyroid cells, even in the virtual absence of extracellular calcium (201). A variety of divalent cations are potent inhibitors of cAMP accumulation (191,209), which is totally reversed by pertussis

toxin's ADP-ribosylation of the inhibitory guanine nucleotide-regulatory-protein, G_i. Pertussis toxin does not reverse the calcium induced increase in cytosolic calcium, suggesting that calcium does not act directly on cAMP accumulation through changes in cytosolic calcium (192). This indicates that divalent cations inhibit adenylate cyclase via G_i through a receptor like mechanism (210). At low extracellular calcium PTH secretion is increased but much less than that due to maximal stimulation by cAMP (169,209,211). A hypothetical model for the regulation of PTH secretion by the cAMP and protein kinase C pathways is shown in Fig. 15.

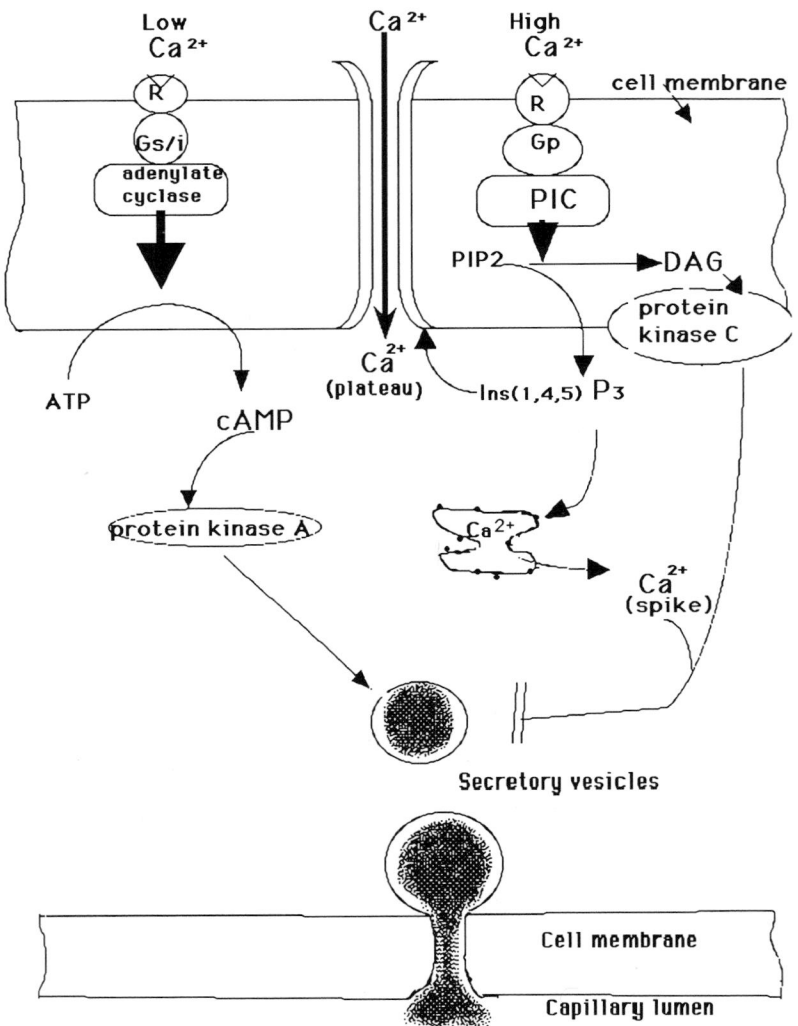

FIG. 15. Diagram depicting cellular events by which changes in extracellular calcium may regulate PTH secretion. Changes in extracellular calcium concentration would be recognized by a plasma membrane "receptor" (R), which would then activate either the adenylate cyclase or inositol phosphate pathways, through different guanine nucleotide-regulatory-protein (G_s, G_i, or G_p). cAMP agonists are potent secretagogues. Phosphoinositidase C (PIC) activation leads to the synthesis of inositol triphosphate [Ins(1,4,5)P_3] and diacylglycerol (DAG) (230). Ins(1,4,5)P_3 raises the intracellular calcium concentration by a transient spike in intracellular calcium derived from release of intracellular calcium from the endoplasmic reticulum, and a more sustained increase due to influx of calcium through voltage sensitive and insensitive channels. An increase in diacylglycerol (DAG) concentration leads to an increase in protein kinase C activity which inhibits PTH secretion.

Rupp and co-workers (37) have shown in a heterologous system (T47D human breast cancer cell line) that after transient transfections of the cAMP response element (CRE) consensus sequence of the human PTH promoter fused to the CAT reporter gene, CAT gene activity was stimulated by forskolin. In addition, DNase 1 protection studies and gel retardation studies, showed protein binding to the PTH-CRE. Therefore the cAMP system is an important transducer not only for PTH secretion but also probably for PTH gene expression.

Although calcium is the principal cation that influences PTH secretion, magnesium can also potentially affect PTH secretion, but only at supraphysiological concentrations, two to three times those found in the extracellular fluid (212,213). The contribution of magnesium compared to calcium is therefore probably small in physiological conditions. Magnesium is however essential for normal PTH secretion. When there is marked hypomagnesemia there is a dramatic inhibition of PTH secretion (214). Patients with hypomagnesemia present with hypocalcemia due to the low PTH levels and after an infusion of magnesium the PTH secretion and serum calcium are corrected.

Other factors which have been reported to increase PTH secretion and synthesis in in vitro studies are cortisol (215,216) and estrogens (217,218). The effect of dexamethasone to increase PTH secretion in cultured bovine parathyroid cells was inhibited by $1,25(OH)_2D_3$ (76). The validity of these observations to physiology remains to be established.

Calcitonin, the other calcium regulating polypeptide hormone is also secreted in response to changes in serum calcium, but in this case to an increase in extracellular calcium concentration. The C-cell intracellular calcium concentration is also regulated by the extracellular calcium concentration but not by the same mechanisms as in the parathyroid cell. Studies with the calcium sensitive fluorescent dyes quin-2 and fura-2 in rat medullary thyroid carcinoma cells (rMTC 6–23) showed that increases in extracellular calcium did not cause increases in inositol 1,4,5-triphosphate (219) nor was there mobilization of intracellular calcium in C-cells, in contrast to the parathyroid cell. The source of the increased intracellular calcium caused by the increase in extracellular calcium was calcium influx through voltage-sensitive calcium channels. This has been confirmed in whole-cell patch clamp experiments (175). The C-cell retains the ability to mobilize intracellular calcium in response to receptor mediated mobilization after the stimulus of vasopressin, bradykinin, or ATP.

With these large differences in the cellular response systems to calcium in the parathyroid and C-cell, it is therefore understandable that their response at the level of gene transcription is also different. Calcium regulates PTH gene transcription (54,116), but does not regulate calcitonin gene transcription (54). In contrast both cells have an intact transduction mechanism for $1,25(OH)_2D_3$ and $1,25(OH)_2D_3$ markedly decreases the transcription of both genes (72,77,88).

REGULATION OF PARATHYROID CELL PROLIFERATION

Parathyroid cells proliferate excessively in parathyroid adenomas, and in both primary and secondary parathyroid hyperplasia. Both parathyroid adenomas (44,45) and the parathyroid hyperplasia of multiple endocrine neoplasia (MEN) are monoclonal neoplasms (220,221). Arnold and co-workers (43) showed that at least six of eight sporadic parathyroid adenomas that they studied contained a large monoclonal component, on the basis of testing of DNA for X-chromosome-inactivation patterns and clonal rearrangement of the parathyroid gene. Primary parathyroid hyperplasia was considered to be of polyclonal origin, but Friedman and co-workers (220) showed that ten tumors from 14 patients with MEN type 1 had losses of alleles from chromosome 11. Most large tumors had allele losses suggesting that a monoclonal adenoma may develop after a phase of polyclonal hyperplasia. The subregion of loss was usually less than the full length of chromosome 11, but always included one copy of the MEN-1 locus (11q13). Genetic abnormalities in patients with MEN-1 had been identified on chromosome 11 with the use of cloned DNA sequences, which had identified restriction-length-polymorphisms (222), and therefore Thakker and co-workers (221) used a similar strategy to study the parathyroid tumors in MEN-1. They found that a single inherited locus on chromosome 11, band q13, caused MEN-1 and that the monoclonal development of parathyroid and pancreatic tumors in patients with MEN-1 involved similar allelic deletions on chromosome 11, specifically on the long arm of chromosome 11, at 11q13. These results are consistent with the hypothesis that a two-stage recessive genetic mutation is responsible for MEN-1, similar to that reported for retinoblastoma. It is hypothesized that the first mutation, which is recessive to the normal dominant allele, does not result in tumor formation but predisposes the cell to tumorigenesis. The growth of a tumor occurs only after a second mutation, which eliminates the normal allele and thereby unmasks the allele altered in the first mutation. Brandi and co-workers (223,224) have found a substance in the plasma of MEN-1 patients which is mitogenic to parathyroid cells and resembles basic fibroblast growth factor. The significance of this factor is not clear.

Secondary hyperparathyroidism in man is usually a consequence of chronic renal failure, but it may also arise in patients with vitamin D deficiency or as a result of the chronically low calcium in patients with X-linked hypophosphatemia treated with phosphorus. In the last condition the phosphorus complexes the calcium and leads to chronic hypocalcemia. In dialysis patients and X-linked hypophosphatemia the glands often become very large and hyperplastic. The hyperparathyroidism not infrequently demands surgical parathyroidectomy, therefore it is important to determine the mechanism of the parathyroid cell proliferation. Hypocalcemia is undoubtedly a causative factor (225).

The factors involved in the proliferation of parathyroid cells in the secondary parathyroid hyperplasia of renal failure probably include a low serum calcium and perhaps also a low serum $1,25(OH)_2D_3$ level. Roth and Raisz (13,16) demonstrated that parathyroid cultures grown in a low extracellular calcium medium had an increased radioactive thymidine uptake indicating enhanced parathyroid cell proliferation. Szabo and co-workers studied rats with experimental uremia due to subtotal nephrectomy, and showed that there was an increase in parathyroid cell mitoses compared to control rats, which was prevented by the prophylactic administration of $1,25(OH)_2D_3$ (226). They also suggested that $1,25(OH)_2D_3$ prevented the cell proliferation of hypocalcemia. However, the detailed transcriptional studies of Naveh-Many et al. (116) and the stereoscopic electron microscopy studies of Wernerson et al. (117,118) demonstrate that the major effect of a low calcium diet given to weanling rats for three to four weeks is to increase PTH transcription per cell with almost no increase in parathyroid cell proliferation. However, this interesting hypothetical property of $1,25(OH)_2D_3$ to inhibit parathyroid cell proliferation needs to be studied in greater detail. There is supportive evidence from the in vitro studies of Nygren et al. (227) for an antiproliferative effect of $1,25(OH)_2D_3$. They studied bovine parathyroid cells in primary culture. After four days of monolayer culture the parathyroid cells increased in both number and size. High concentrations of $1,25(OH)_2D_3$ (10–100 ng/mL) prevented the cell proliferation but not the hypertrophy. Low concentrations of $1,25(OH)_2D_3$ (0.1–100 ng/mL) led to a decrease in PTH release only after four days, probably due to its transcriptional effect. As in other studies at four days PTH secretion was not responsive to a high calcium and there was no increase in intracellular calcium with a high extracellular calcium demonstrating the idiosyncracies of the in vitro system. Kremer and co-workers studied parathyroid cells in primary culture up to eight days after plating when they would not be sensitive to calcium (228). They showed that $1,25(OH)_2D_3$ ($1 \times 10^{-8} M$) delayed but did not prevent the serum induced increase in parathyroid cell proliferation. Interestingly, they showed in these cells that $1,25(OH)_2D_3$ abolished the early rise in c-myc oncogene expression seen in proliferating parathyroid cells, with no effect on c-fos gene expression. This is of interest because $1,25(OH)_2D_3$ added to HL60 leukemia cells decreased c-myc and increased c-fos mRNA levels (229).

Brandi and co-workers have maintained bovine parathyroid cells during many population doublings and shown that in those cells parathyroid cell proliferation was decreased by a high medium calcium (59). Thus $1,25(OH)_2D_3$ and a high calcium might both be inhibitory to parathyroid cell proliferation.

REGULATION OF PTH PRODUCTION

PTH production is regulated at a number of time sequences and at different levels in its production pathway. Regulation is exerted at the stages of secretion, intracellular catabolism, transcription, and proliferation (Fig. 16). The secretion of PTH from its secretory granules is regulated within seconds to minutes. The major regulatory factor is calcium. A further important level of control of preformed PTH is its degradation within the cell to fragments and constituent amino acids by the stimulus of a high calcium. As extensively discussed in this chapter, regulation of PTH gene transcription is a major site of PTH regulation. This occurs within hours and can continue for prolonged periods. The major regulator of transcription is $1,25(OH)_2D_3$ which decreases PTH gene transcription, and in addition hypocalcemia which increases PTH gene transcription. Parathyroid cell proliferation is the final site of regulation and this occurs after the stimulus of prolonged hypocalcemia. $1,25(OH)_2D_3$ very well might have a role in preventing parathyroid cell proliferation but in vivo this property of $1,25(OH)_2D_3$ is not firmly established. The reversal of established parathyroid hyperplasia is a factor of the long half-life of the individual parathyroid cell and is not amenable to pharmacological treatment (119).

There is a large non-suppressible component of both PTH synthesis, as measured by PTH mRNA levels, and PTH secretion. Therefore when there are more parathyroid cells as in secondary parathyroid hyperplasia the non-suppressible contribution from the individual cells

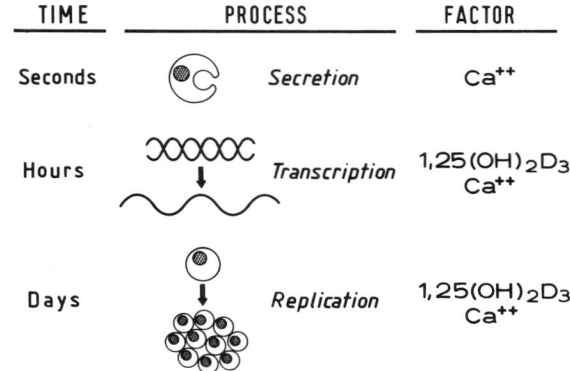

FIG. 16. Regulation of PTH production at different time sequences, and at different levels in its synthesis and secretion. The factors regulating secretion and transcription are more firmly established than those regulating proliferation.

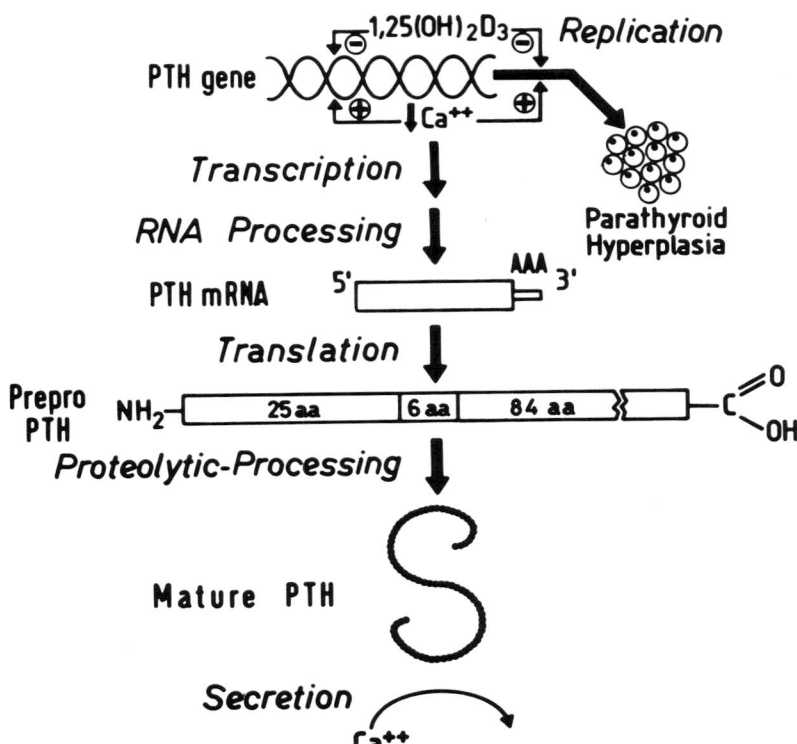

FIG. 17. Diagram depicting cellular events in synthesis and secretion of PTH, and in the replication of parathyroid cells. The regulation of parathyroid cell proliferation by $1,25(OH)_2D_3$ in vivo remains to be firmly established.

results in the production of large amounts of PTH despite the most intensive treatment. However, the use of $1,25(OH)_2D_3$ in such situations has resulted in remarkable reductions in serum PTH levels that must reflect a decrease in PTH gene transcription and PTH production by all the overproducing parathyroid cells (Fig. 17).

Future progress in the regulation of PTH production will continue to come from studies of the molecular biology of the PTH gene and the cell biology of the parathyroid cell, which will rapidly be applied to the pathogenesis of diseases of mineral metabolism and bone. One of the heartening aspects of the basic science studies on the regulation of PTH synthesis and secretion has been their immediate application to patient care with rewarding results.

ACKNOWLEDGMENTS

This work was supported by grants from the National Institutes of Health (grant DK38696), the United States-Israel Binational Science Foundation (BSF), the German-Israel Foundation for Research and Development (GIF), and the Israel Academy of Sciences and Humanities.

REFERENCES

1. Potts JTJ, Kronenberg HM, Habener JF, Rich A. Biosynthesis of parathyroid hormone. *Ann NY Acad Sci* 1980;343:38–55.

2. Habener JF, Rosenblatt M, Potts JT Jr. Parathyroid hormone: biochemical aspects of biosynthesis, secretion, action, and metabolism. *Physiol Rev* 1984;64:985–1053.
3. Norman AW, Roth J, Orci L. The vitamin D endocrine system: steroid metabolism, hormone receptors, and biological response (calcium binding proteins). *Endocr Rev* 1982;3:331–66.
4. DeLuca HF. The metabolism and functions of vitamin D. *Adv Exp Med Biol* 1986;196:361–75.
5. Sherwood LM, Ayer GP, Ramberg CF, Kronfeld DS, Aurbach GD, Potts JT Jr. Regulation of parathyroid hormone secretion: proportional control by calcium, lack of effect of phosphate. *Endocrinology* 1968;83:1043–51.
6. Kawashima H, Torikai S, Kurokawa K. Localization of 25-hydroxyvitamin D_3-1- and -24-hydroxylase along the rat nephron. *Proc Natl Acad Sci USA* 1981;78:1199–203.
7. Fraser DR. Regulation of the metabolism of vitamin D. *Physiol Rev* 1980;60:551–613.
8. Habener JF. Regulation of parathyroid hormone secretion and biosynthesis. *Annu Rev Physiol* 1981;43:211–23.
9. Habener JF, Potts JT Jr. Fundamental considerations in the physiology, biology, and biochemistry of parathyroid hormone. In: Avioli LV, Krane SM, eds. *Metabolic bone disease,* 2nd ed. Philadelphia: WB Saunders Co, 1990:69–130.
10. Cohn DV, Kumarasamy R, Ramp WK. Intracellular processing and secretion of parathyroid gland proteins. *Vitam Horm* 1986;43:283–316.
11. Majzoub JA, Dee PC, Habener JF. Cellular and cell-free processing of parathyroid secretory proteins. *J Biol Chem* 1982;257:3581–8.
12. Cohn DV, Morrissey JJ, Shofstall RE, Chu LL. Cosecretion of secretory protein-I and parathormone by dispersed bovine parathyroid cells. *Endocrinology* 1982;110:625–30.
13. Roth SI, Raisz LG. The course and reversibility of the calcium effect on the ultrastructure of the rat parathyroid gland in organ culture. *Lab Invest* 1966;15:1187–211.
14. Shannon WA, Roth SI. An ultrastructural study of acid phosphatase activity in normal adenomatous and hyperplastic (chief cell type) human parathyroid glands. *Am J Pathol* 1974;77:493–501.
15. Larsson H-O, Lorentzon R, Boquist L. Structure of the parathy-

roid glands as revealed by different methods of fixation. A quantitative light- and electron-microscopic study in untreated Mongolian gerbils. *Cell Tissue Res* 1984;235:51–8.

16. Roth SI, Raisz LG. Effect of calcium concentration on the ultrastructure of rat parathyroid in organ culture. *Lab Invest* 1964;13:331–45.

17. Setoguti T, Inoue Y, Kato K. Electron-microscopic studies on the relationship between the frequency of parathyroid storage granules and serum calcium levels in the rat. *Cell Tissue Res* 1981;219:457–67.

18. Antonarakis SE, Phillips JA, Mallonee RL, et al. Beta-globin locus is linked to the parathyroid hormone (PTH) locus and lies between the insulin and PTH loci in man. *Proc Natl Acad Sci USA* 1983;80:6615–9.

19. Naylor SL, Sakaguchi AY, Szoka P, et al. Human parathyroid hormone gene (PTH) is on short arm of chromosome 11. *Somatic Cell Genet* 1983;9:609–16.

20. Mayer H, Breyel E, Bostock C, Schmidtke J. Assignment of the human parathyroid hormone gene to chromosome 11. *Hum Genet* 1983;64:283–5.

21. Zabel BU, Kronenberg HM, Bell GI, Shows TB. Chromosome mapping of genes on the short arm of human chromosome 11: parathyroid hormone gene is at 11p15 together with the genes for insulin, c-Harvey-ras 1, and beta-hemoglobin. *Cytogenet Cell Genet* 1985;39:200–5.

22. Schmidtke J, Pape B, Krengel U, et al. Restriction fragment length polymorphisms at the human parathyroid hormone gene locus. *Hum Genet* 1984;67:428–31.

23. Hendy GN, Kronenberg HM, Potts JT Jr, Rich A. Nucleotide sequence of cloned cDNAs encoding human preproparathyroid hormone. *Proc Natl Acad Sci USA* 1981;78:7365–9.

24. Vasicek TJ, McDevitt BE, Freeman MW, et al. Nucleotide sequence of the human parathyroid hormone gene. *Proc Natl Acad Sci USA* 1983;80:2127–31.

25. Gordon DF, Kemper B. Synthesis, restriction analysis, and molecular cloning of near full length DNA complementary to bovine parathyroid hormone mRNA. *Nucleic Acids Res* 1980;8:5669–83.

26. Weaver CA, Gordon DF, Kemper B. Introduction by molecular cloning of artifactual inverted sequences at the 5' terminus of the sense strand of bovine parathyroid hormone cDNA. *Proc Natl Acad Sci USA* 1981;78:4073–7.

27. Weaver CA, Gordon DF, Kemper B. Nucleotide sequence of bovine parathyroid hormone messenger RNA. *Mol Cell Endocrinol* 1982;28:411–24.

28. Weaver CA, Gordon DF, Kissil MS, Mead DA, Kemper B. Isolation and complete nucleotide sequence of the gene for bovine parathyroid hormone. *Gene* 1984;28:319–29.

29. Heinrich G, Kronenberg HM, Potts JT Jr, Habener JF. Gene encoding parathyroid hormone. Nucleotide sequence of the rat gene and deduced amino acid sequence of rat preproparathyroid hormone. *J Biol Chem* 1984;259:3320–9.

30. Schmelzer HJ, Gross G, Widera G, Mayer H. Nucleotide sequence of a full-length cDNA clone encoding preproparathyroid hormone from pig and rat. *Nucleic Acids Res* 1987;15:6740–6746.

31. Khosla S, Demay M, Pines M, Hurwitz S, Potts JT Jr, Kronenberg HM. Nucleotide sequence of cloned cDNAs encoding chicken preproparathyroid hormone. *J Bone Miner Res* 1988;3:689–98.

32. Russell J, Sherwood LM. Nucleotide sequence of the DNA complementary to avian (chicken) preproparathyroid hormone mRNA and the deduced sequence of the hormone precursor. *Mol Endocrinol* 1989;3:325–31.

33. Kronenberg HM, Igarashi T, Freeman MW, et al. Structure and expression of the human parathyroid hormone gene. *Recent Prog Horm Res* 1986;42:641–63.

34. Kemper B. Molecular biology of parathyroid hormone. *CRC Crit Rev Biochem* 1986;19:353–79.

35. Igarashi T, Okazaki T, Potter H, Gaz R, Kronenberg HM. Cell-specific expression of the human parathyroid hormone gene in rat pituitary cells. *Mol Cell Biol* 1986;6:1830–3.

36. Levine MA, Morrow PP, Kronenberg HM, Phillips JA. Tissue and gene specific hypomethylation of the human parathyroid

hormone gene: association with parathyroid hormone gene expression in parathyroid glands. *Endocrinology* 1986;119:1618–24.

37. Rupp E, Mayer H, Wingender E. The promoter of the human parathyroid hormone gene contains a functional cyclic AMP-response element. *Nucleic Acid Res* 1990;18:5677–83.

38. Kerner SA, Scott RA, Pike JW. Sequence elements in the human osteocalcin gene confer basal activation and inducible response to hormonal vitamin D3. *Proc Natl Acad Sci USA* 1989;86:4455–9.

39. Demay MB, Gerardi JM, DeLuca HF, Kronenberg HM. DNA sequences in the rat osteocalcin gene that bind the 1,25-dihydroxyvitamin D$_3$ receptor and confer responsiveness to 1,25-dihydroxyvitamin D$_3$. *Proc Natl Acad Sci USA* 1990;87:369–73.

40. Markose ER, Stein JL, Stein GS, Lian JB. Vitamin D-mediated modifications in protein-DNA interactions at two promoter elements of the osteocalcin gene. *Proc Natl Acad Sci USA* 1990;87:1701–5.

41. Liao J, Ozono K, Sone T, McDonnel DP, Pike JW. Vitamin D receptor interaction with specific DNA requires a nuclear protein and 1,25-dihydroxyvitamin D$_3$. *Proc Natl Acad Sci USA* 1990;87:9751–5.

42. Owen TA, Mortell R, Yocum SA, et al. Coordinate occupancy of AP-1 sites in the vitamin D-responsive and CCAAT box elements by fos-jun in the osteocalcin gene: model for phenotype suppression of transcription. *Proc Natl Acad Sci USA* 1990;87:9990–4.

43. Arnold A, Staunton CE, Kim HG, Gaz RD, Kronenberg HM. Monoclonality and abnormal parathyroid hormone genes in parathyroid adenomas. *N Engl J Med* 1988;318:658–62.

44. Arnold A, Kim HG, Gaz RD, et al. Molecular cloning and chromosomal mapping of DNA rearranged with the parathyroid hormone gene in a parathyroid adenoma. *J Clin Invest* 1989;83:2034–40.

45. Friedman E, Bale AE, Marx SJ, et al. Genetic abnormalities in sporadic parathyroid adenomas. *J Clin Endocrinol Metab* 1990;71:293–7.

46. Ahn TG, Antonarakis SE, Kronenberg HM, Igarashi T, Levine MA. Familial isolated hypoparathyroidism: a molecular genetic analysis of 8 families with 23 affected persons. *Medicine (Baltimore)* 1986;65:73–81.

47. Arnold A, Horst SA, Gardella TJ, Baba H, Levine MA, Kronenberg HM. Mutation of the signal peptide-encoding region of the preproparathyroid hormone gene in familial isolated hypoparathyroidism. *J Clin Invest* 1990;86:1084–7.

48. Russell J, Lettieri D, Sherwood LM. Direct regulation by calcium of cytoplasmic messenger ribonucleic acid coding for preproparathyroid hormone in isolated bovine parathyroid cells. *J Clin Invest* 1983;72:1851–5.

49. Brookman JJ, Farrow SM, Nicholson L, O'Riordan JL, Hendy GN. Regulation by calcium of parathyroid hormone mRNA in cultured parathyroid tissue. *J Bone Miner Res* 1986;1:529–37.

50. Farrow SM, Karmali R, Gleed JH, Hendy GN, O'Riordan H. Regulation of preproparathyroid hormone messenger RNA and hormone synthesis in human parathyroid adenomata. *J Endocrinol* 1988;117:133–8.

51. Russell J, Sherwood LM. The effects of 1,25-dihydroxyvitamin D3 and high calcium on transcription of the pre-proparathyroid hormone gene are direct. *Trans Assoc Am Physicians* 1987;100:256–62.

52. Moran R, Born W, Tuchschmid CR, Fischer JA. Calcium-regulated biosynthesis of the parathyroid secretory protein, pro-parathyroid hormone, and parathyroid hormone in dispersed bovine parathyroid cells. *Endocrinology* 1981;108:2264.

53. Silver J, Marks R, Naveh-Many T. Regulation of parathyroid hormone and calcitonin gene expression by 1,25-dihydroxyvitamin D$_3$ and calcium. In: Cohn DV, Glorieux FH, Martin TJ, eds. *Calcium regulation and bone metabolism: basic and clinical aspects.* New York: Excerpta Medica; 1990:140–5.

54. Naveh-Many T, Friedlaender MM, Mayer H, Silver J. Calcium regulates parathyroid hormone messenger ribonucleic acid (mRNA), but not calcitonin mRNA in vivo in the rat. Dominant role of 1,25-dihydroxyvitamin D. *Endocrinology* 1989;125:275–80.

55. Yamamoto M, Igarashi T, Muramatsu M, Fukagawa M, Motokura T, Ogata E. Hypocalcemia increases and hypercalcemia de-

creases the steady-state level of parathyroid hormone messenger RNA in the rat. *J Clin Invest* 1989;83:1053–6.

56. LeBoff MS, Rennke HG, Brown EM. Abnormal regulation of parathyroid cell secretion and proliferation in primary cultures of bovine parathyroid cells. *Endocrinology* 1983;113:277–84.

57. MacGregor RR, Sarras MPJ, Houle A, Cohn DV. Primary monolayer cell culture of bovine parathyroids: effects of calcium, isoproterenol and growth factors. *Mol Cell Endocrinol* 1983;30:313–28.

58. Sakaguchi K, Santora A, Zimering M, Curcio F, Aurbach GD, Brandi ML. Functional epithelial cell line cloned from rat parathyroid glands. *Proc Natl Acad Sci USA* 1987;84:3269–73.

59. Brandi ML, Fitzpatrick LA, Coon HG, Aurbach GD. Bovine parathyroid cells: cultures maintained for more than 140 population doublings. *Proc Natl Acad Sci USA* 1986;83:1709–13.

60. Sakaguchi K, Ikeda K, Curcio F, Aurbach GD, Brandi ML. Subclones of a rat parathyroid cell line (PT-r): regulation of growth and production of parathyroid hormone-related peptide (PTHRP). *J Bone Miner Res* 1990;5:863–9.

61. Kawashima H, Torikai S, Kurokawa K. Calcitonin selectively stimulates 25-hydroxyvitamin D_3-1-hydroxylase in proximal straight tubule of rat kidney. *Nature* 1981;291:327–9.

62. Henry HL, Norman AW. Studies on the mechanism of action of calciferol. VI. Localization of 1,25-dihydroxy-vitamin D_3 in chick parathyroid glands. *Biochem Biophys Res Commun* 1975;62:781–8.

63. Hughes MR, Haussler MR. 1,25-Dihydroxyvitamin D_3 receptors in parathyroid glands: preliminary characterization of cytoplasmic and nuclear binding components. *J Biol Chem* 1978;253:1065–73.

64. Hughes MR, Maussler MR. 1,25-Dihydroxycholecalciferol receptors in parathyroid glands. *J Biol Chem* 1978;253:1065–9.

65. Wecksler WR, Ross FPS, Mason RS, Posen S, Norman AW. Biochemical properties of the 1,25-dihydroxy-vitamin D cytoplasmic receptors from human and chick parathyroid glands. *Arch Biochem Biophys* 1980;201:95–102.

66. Wecksler WR, Henry HL, Norman AW. Studies on the mode of action of calciferol. Subcellular localization of 1,25-dihydroxycholecalciferol in chicken parathyroid glands. *Arch Biochem Biophys* 1977;183:168–73.

67. Brumbaugh PF, Hughes MR, Haussler MR. Cytoplasmic and nuclear binding components for 1,25-dihydroxyvitamin D_3 in chick parathyroid glands. *Proc Natl Acad Sci USA* 1975;72:4871–5.

68. Haussler MR, Mangelsdorf DJ, Komm BS, et al. Molecular biology of the vitamin D hormone. *Recent Prog Horm Res* 1988;44:263–305.

69. Baker AR, McDonnell DP, Hughes M, et al. Cloning and expression of full-length cDNA encoding human vitamin D receptor. *Proc Natl Acad Sci USA* 1988;85:3294–4.

70. Minghetti PP, Norman AW. 1,25(OH)$_2$-Vitamin D_3 receptors: gene regulation and genetic circuitry. *FASEB J.* 1988;2:3043–53.

71. Stumpf WE, Sar M, Reid FA, Tanaka Y, De Luca HF. Target cells for 1,25(OH)$_2$D$_3$ in intestinal tract, stomach, kidney, skin, pituitary and parathyroid. *Science* 1979;206:1188–90.

72. Silver J, Russell J, Sherwood LM. Regulation by vitamin D metabolites of messenger ribonucleic acid for preproparathyroid hormone in isolated bovine parathyroid cells. *Proc Natl Acad Sci USA* 1985;82:4270–3.

73. Russell J, Silver J, Sherwood LM. The effects of calcium and vitamin D metabolites on cytoplasmic mRNA coding for preproparathyroid hormone in isolated parathyroid cells. *Trans Assoc Am Physicians* 1984;97:296–303.

74. Russell J, Lettieri D, Sherwood LM. Suppression by 1,25(OH)$_2$D$_3$ of transcription of the pre-proparathyroid hormone gene. *Endocrinology* 1986;119:2864–6.

75. Karmali R, Farrow S, Hewison M, Barker S, O'Riordan JL. Effects of 1,25-dihydroxyvitamin D3 and cortisol on bovine and human parathyroid cells. *J Endocrinol* 1989;123:137–42.

76. Sugimoto T, Brown AJ, Ritter C, Morrissey J, Slatopolsky E, Martin KJ. Combined effects of dexamethasone and 1,25-dihydroxyvitamin D_3 on parathyroid hormone secretion in cultured bovine parathyroid cells. *Endocrinology* 1989;125:638–41.

77. Silver J, Naveh-Many T, Mayer H, Schmelzer HJ, Popovtzer MM. Regulation by vitamin D metabolites of parathyroid hormone gene transcription in vivo in the rat. *J Clin Invest* 1986;78:1296–301.

78. Sugimoto T, Ritter C, Ried I, Morrissey J, Slatopolsky E. Effect of 1,25-dihydroxyvitamin D_3 on cytosolic calcium in dispersed parathyroid cells. *Kidney Int* 1988;33:850–4.

79. Okazaki T, Igarashi T, Kronenberg HM. 5'-flanking region of the parathyroid hormone gene mediates negative regulation by 1,25-(OH)$_2$ vitamin D_3. *J Biol Chem* 1988;263:2203–8.

80. Minghetti PP, Gibbs PE, Norman AW. Computer analysis of 1,25-dihydroxyvitamin D_3-receptor regulated promoters: identification of a candidate D_3-response element. *Biochem Biophys Res* 1989;162:869–75.

81. Farrow SM, Hawa NS, Karmali R, Hewison M, Walters JC, O'Riordan JL. Binding of the receptor for 1,25-dihydroxyvitamin D_3 to the 5'-flanking region of the bovine parathyroid hormone gene. *J Endocrinol* 1990;126:355–9.

82. Cantley LK, Russell J, Lettieri D, Sherwood LM. 1,25-Dihydroxyvitamin D_3 suppresses parathyroid hormone secretion from bovine parathyroid cells in tissue culture. *Endocrinology* 1985;117:2114–9.

83. Chan YL, McKay C, Dye E, Slatopolsky E. The effect of 1,25 dihydroxycholecalciferol on parathyroid hormone secretion by monolayer cultures of bovine parathyroid cells. *Calcif Tissue Int* 1986;38:27–32.

84. Golden P, Greenwalt A, Martin K, et al. Lack of a direct effect of 1,25-dihydroxycholecalciferol on parathyroid hormone secretion by normal bovine parathyroid glands. *Endocrinology* 1980;107:602–7.

85. Chertow BS, Baker GR, Henry HL, Norman AW. Effects of vitamin D metabolites on bovine parathyroid hormone release in vitro. *Am J Physiol* 1980;238:E384–8.

86. Au WY. Inhibition by 1,25-dihydroxycholecalciferol of hormonal secretion of rat parathyroid gland in organ culture. *Calcif Tissue Int* 1984;36:384–91.

87. Brown AJ, Ritter CR, Finch JL, et al. The noncalcemic analogue of vitamin D, 22-oxacalcitriol, suppresses parathyroid hormone synthesis and secretion. *J Clin Invest* 1989;84:728–32.

88. Naveh-Many T, Silver J. Regulation of calcitonin gene transcription by vitamin D metabolites in vivo in the rat. *J Clin Invest* 1988;81:270–3.

89. Amara SG, David DN, Rosenfeld MG, Roos BA, Evans RM. Characterization of rat calcitonin mRNA. *Proc Natl Acad Sci USA* 1980;77:4444–8.

90. Amara SG, Rosenfeld MG, Birnbaum RS, Roos BA. Identification of the putative cell-free translation product of rat calcitonin mRNA. *J Biol Chem* 1980;255:2645–8.

91. Cote GJ, Rogers DG, Huang ES, Gagel RF. The effect of 1,25-dihydroxyvitamin D_3 treatment on calcitonin and calcitonin gene-related peptide mRNA levels in cultured human thyroid C-cells. *Biochem Biophys Res Commun* 1987;149:239–43.

92. Amara SG, Evans RM, Rosenfeld MG. Calcitonin/calcitonin gene-related peptide transcription unit: tissue-specific expression involves selective use of alternative polyadenylation sites. *Mol Cell Biol* 1984;4:2151–60.

93. Rosenfeld MG, Lin CR, Amara SG, et al. Calcitonin mRNA polymorphism: peptide switching associated with alternative RNA splicing events. *Proc Natl Acad Sci USA* 1982;79:1717–21.

94. McDonnell DP, Mangelsdorf DJ, Pike JW, Haussler MR, O'Malley BW. Molecular cloning of complementary DNA encoding the avian receptor for vitamin D. *Science* 1987;235:1214–7.

95. Marx SJ, Liberman UA, Eil C, Gamblin GT, DeGrange DA, Balsan S. Hereditary resistance to 1,25-dihydroxyvitamin D. *Recent Prog Horm Res* 1984;40:589–620.

96. Silver J, Landau H, Bab I, et al. Vitamin D-dependent rickets types I and II. Diagnosis and response to therapy. *Isr J Med Sci* 1985;21:53–6.

97. Costa EM, Feldman D. Homologous up-regulation of the 1,25(OH)$_2$ vitamin D_3 receptor in rats. *Biochem Biophys Res* 1986;137:742–7.

98. Strom M, Sandgren ME, Brown TA, DeLuca HF. 1,25-dihydroxyvitamin D_3 up-regulates the 1,25-dihydroxyvitamin D_3 receptor in vivo. *Proc Natl Acad Sci USA* 1989;86:9770–3.

99. Favus MJ, Mangelsdorf DJ, Tembe V, Coe BJ, Haussler MR. Evidence for in vivo upregulation of the intestinal vitamin D receptor during dietary calcium restriction in the rat. *J Clin Invest* 1988;82:218–24.

100. Huang Y, Lee S, Stolz R, et al. Effect of hormones and development on the expression of the rat 1,25-dihydroxyvitamin D$_3$ receptor gene. *J Biol Chem* 1989;264:17454–61.

101. Costa EM, Hirst MA, Feldman D. Regulation of 1,25-dihydroxyvitamin D$_3$ receptors by vitamin D analogs in cultured mammalian cells. *Endocrinology* 1985;117:2203–10.

102. Costa EM, Feldman D. Measurement of 1,25-dihydroxyvitamin D$_3$ receptor turnover by dense amino acid labeling: changes during receptor up-regulation by vitamin D metabolites. *Endocrinology* 1987;120:1173–8.

103. Mahonen A, Pirskanen A, Keinanen R, Maenpaa PH. Effect of 1,25(OH)$_2$D$_3$ on its receptor mRNA levels and osteocalcin synthesis in human osteosarcoma cells. *Biochim Biophys Acta* 1990;1048:30–7.

104. Sandgren ME, DeLuca HF. Serum calcium and vitamin D regulate 1,25-dihydroxyvitamin D$_3$ receptor concentration in rat kidney in vivo. *Proc Natl Acad Sci USA* 1990;87:4312–4.

105. Naveh-Many T, Marx R, Keshet E, Pike JW, Silver J. Regulation of 1,25-dihydroxyvitamin D3 receptor gene expression by 1,25-dihydroxyvitamin D$_3$ in the parathyroid in vivo. *J Clin Invest* 1990;86:1968–75.

106. Slatopolsky E, Lopez-Hilker S, Dusso A, Morrissey JJ, Martin KJ. Parathyroid hormone secretion: perturbations in chronic renal failure. *Contrib Nephrol* 1988;64:16–24.

107. Morrissey J, Martin K, Hruska K, Slatopolsky E. Abnormalities in parathyroid hormone secretion in primary and secondary hyperparathyroidism. *Adv Exp Med Biol* 1984;178:389–98.

108. Castleman B, Mallory TB. Parathyroid hyperplasia in chronic renal insufficiency. *Am J Pathol* 1937;13:553–74.

109. Castleman B, Mallory TB. The pathology of the parathyroid gland in hyperparathyroidism. *Am J Pathol* 1932;11:1–72.

110. Slatopolsky E, Lopez-Hilker S, Delmez J, Dusso A, Brown A, Martin KJ. The parathyroid-calcitriol axis in health and chronic renal failure. *Kidney Int Suppl* 1990;29:S41–7.

111. Slatopolsky E, Lopez-Hilker S, Dusso A, Brown A, Delmez J, Martin K. Renal osteodystrophy: past and future. *Contrib Nephrol* 1990;78:38–45.

112. Shvil Y, Naveh-Many T, Barach P, Silver J. Regulation of parathyroid cell gene expression in experimental uremia. *J Am Soc Nephrol* 1990;1:99–104.

113. Brown AJ, Dusso A, Lopez-Hilker S, Lewis-Finch J, Grooms P, Slatopolsky E. 1,25-(OH)$_2$D receptors are decreased in parathyroid glands from chronically uremic dogs. *Kidney Int* 1989;35:19–23.

114. Korkor AB. Reduced binding of [3H]1,25-dihydroxyvitamin D$_3$ in the parathyroid glands of patients with renal failure. *N Engl J Med* 1987;316:1573–7.

115. Merke J, Hugel U, Zlotkowski A, et al. Diminished parathyroid 1,25(OH)$_2$1D$_3$ receptors in experimental uremia. *Kidney Int* 1987;32:350–3.

116. Naveh-Many T, Silver J. Regulation of parathyroid hormone gene expression by hypocalcemia, hypercalcemia, and vitamin D in the rat. *J Clin Invest* 1990;86:1313–9.

117. Wernerson A, Svensson O, Reinholt FP. Parathyroid cell number and size in hypercalcemic rats: a stereologic study employing modern unbiased estimators. *J Bone Miner Res* 1989;4:705–13.

118. Svensson O, Wernerson A, Reinholt FP. Effect of calcium depletion on the rat parathyroids. *Bone Miner* 1988;3:259–69.

119. Parfitt AM. Hypercalcemic hyperparathyroidism following renal transplantation: differential diagnosis, management, and implications for cell population control in the parathyroid gland. *Miner Electrolyte Metab* 1982;8:92–112.

120. Nordal KP, Dahl E. Low dose calcitriol versus placebo in patients with predialysis chronic renal failure. *J Clin Endocrinol Metab* 1988;67:929–36.

121. Pitts TO, Piraino BH, Mitro R, et al. Hyperparathyroidism and 1,25-dihydroxyvitamin D deficiency in mild, moderate, and severe renal failure. *J Clin Endocrinol Metab* 1988;67:876–81.

122. Oldham SB, Smith R, Hartenbower DL, Henry HL, Norman AW, Coburn JW. The acute effects of 1,25-dihydroxycholecalciferol on serum immunoreactive parathyroid hormone in the dog. *Endocrinology* 1979;104:248–54.

123. Slatopolsky E, Weerts C, Thielan J, Horst R, Harter H, Martin KJ. Marked suppression of secondary hyperparathyroidism by intravenous administration of 1,25-dihydroxy-cholecalciferol in uremic patients. *J Clin Invest* 1984;74:2136–43.

124. Delmez JA, Dougan CS, Gearing BK, et al. The effects of intraperitoneal calcitriol on calcium and parathyroid hormone. *Kidney Int* 1987;31:795–9.

125. Andress DL, Norris KC, Coburn JW, Slatopolsky EA, Sherrard DJ. Intravenous calcitriol in the treatment of refractory osteitis fibrosa of chronic renal failure. *N Engl J Med* 1989;321:274–9.

126. Salusky IB, Fine RN, Kangarloo H, et al. "High-dose" calcitriol for control of renal osteodystrophy in children on CAPD. *Kidney Int* 1987;32:89–95.

127. Kemper B, Habener JF, Mulligan RC, Potts JT Jr, Rich A. Preproparathyroid hormone: a direct translation product of parathyroid messenger RNA. *Proc Natl Acad Sci USA* 1974;71:3731–5.

128. Habener JF, Kamper B, Potts JT Jr, Rich A. Preproparathyroid hormone identified by cell-free translation of messenger RNA from hyperplastic human parathyroid tissue. *J Clin Invest* 1975;56:1328–33.

129. Kemper B, Habener JF, Potts JT Jr, Rich A. Pre-proparathyroid hormone: fidelity of the translation of parathyroid messenger RNA by extracts of wheat germ. *Biochemistry* 1976;15:20–5.

130. Niall HD, Keutmann HT, Sauer ML, et al. The amino acid sequence of bovine parathyroid hormone. *Hoppe-Seyler's Z Physiol Chem* 1970;351:1586–8.

131. Sauer RT, Niall HD, Hogan ML, Keutmann HT, O'Riordan JLH, Potts JT Jr. The amino acid sequence of porcine parathyroid hormone. *Biochemistry* 1974;13:1994–9.

132. Keutman HT, Sauer RM, Hendy GN, O'Riordan JLH, Potts JT Jr. Complete amino acid sequence of human parathyroid hormone. *Biochemistry* 1978;17:5723–9.

133. Palade G. Intracellular aspects of the process of protein synthesis. *Science* 1975;189:347–58.

134. Habener JF, Kemper B, Potts JT Jr, Rich A. Proparathyroid hormone: biosynthesis by human parathyroid adenomas. *Science* 1972;178:630–3.

135. Dorner A, Kemper B. Conversion of preproparathyroid hormone to proparathyroid hormone by dog pancreatic microsomes. *Biochemistry* 1978;17:5550–5.

136. Habener JF, Kemper B, Potts JT Jr, Rich A. Parathyroid mRNA directs the synthesis of preproparathyroid hormone and proparathyroid hormone in the Krebs ascites cell-free system. *Biochem Biophys Res Commun* 1975;67:1114–21.

137. Von Heijne G. Patterns of amino acids near signal-sequence cleavage sites. *Eur J Biochem* 1983;133:17–21.

138. Jackson RC, Blobel G. Post-translational cleavage of presecretory proteins with an extract of rough microsomes from dog pancreas containing signal peptidase activity. *Proc Natl Acad Sci USA* 1977;74:5598–602.

139. Perara E, Rothman RE, Lingappa VR. Uncoupling translocation from translation: implications for transport of proteins across membranes. *Science* 1986;232:348–52.

140. Habener JF, Amherdt M, Ravazzola M, Orci L. Parathyroid hormone biosynthesis: correlation of conversion of biosynthetic precursors with intracellular protein migration as determined by electron microscope autoradiography. *J Cell Biol* 1979;80:715–31.

141. Kemper B, Habener JF, Rich A, Potts JT Jr. Microtubules and the intracellular conversion of proparathyroid hormone to parathyroid hormone. *Endocrinology* 1975;96:903–12.

142. Chu H, MacGregor RR, Cohn DV. Energy-dependent intracellular translocation of proparathormone. *J Cell Biol* 1977;72:1–10.

143. Habener JF, Stevens TD, Tregear GW, Potts JT Jr. Radioimmunoassay of human proparathyroid hormone: analysis of hormone content in tissue extracts and in plasma. *J Clin Endocrinol Metab* 1976;42:520–30.

144. Rosenblatt M, Habener JF, Tyler GA, et al. Chemical synthesis of the precursor-specific region of preproparathyroid hormone. *J Biol Chem* 1979;254:1414–21.

145. Majzoub JA, Rosenblatt M, Fennick B, et al. Synthetic preproparathyroid hormone leader sequence inhibits cell-free process-

ing of placental, parathyroid, and pituitary pre-hormones. *J Biol Chem* 1980;255:11478–83.

146. Szczesna-Skorupa E, Mead DA, Kemper B. Mutations in the NH2-terminal domain of the signal peptide of preproparathyroid hormone inhibit translocation without affecting interaction with signal recognition particle. *J Biol Chem* 1987;262:8896–900.

147. Wiren KM, Freeman MW, Potts JT Jr, Kronenberg HM. Preproparathyroid hormone. A model for analyzing the secretory pathway. *Ann NY Acad Sci* 1987;493:43–9.

148. Wiren KM, Ivashkiv L, Ma P, Freeman MW, Potts JT Jr, Kronenberg HM. Mutations in signal sequence cleavage domain of preproparathyroid hormone alter protein translocation, signal sequence cleavage, and membrane-binding properties. *Mol Endocrinol* 1989;3:240–50.

149. Wiren KM, Potts JT Jr, Kronenberg HM. Importance of the propeptide sequence of human preproparathyroid hormone for signal sequence function. *J Biol Chem* 1988;263:19771–7.

150. Morrissey JJ, Hamilton JW, MacGregor RR, Cohn DV. The secretion of parathormone fragments 34–84 and 37–84 by dispersed porcine parathyroid cells. *Endocrinology* 1980;107:164–71.

151. Jung A, Mayer GP, Hurst JG, Neer R, Potts JT Jr. Model for parathyroid hormone secretion and metabolism in calves. *Am J Physiol* 1982;242:R141–50.

152. Silverman R, Yalow RS. Heterogeneity of parathyroid hormone: clinical and physiologic implications. *J Clin Invest* 1973;52:1958–71.

153. Sherwood M, Mayer GP, Ramberg CF Jr, Kronfeld DS, Aurbach GD, Potts JT Jr. Regulation of parathyroid hormone secretion: proportional control by calcium, lack of effect of phosphate. *Endocrinology* 1968;83:1043–51.

154. Sherwood LM, Potts JT Jr, Care AD, Mayer GP, Aurbach GD. Evaluation by radioimmunoassay of factors controlling the secretion of parathyroid hormone. *Nature* 1966;209:52–5.

155. Mayer GP, Hurst JG. Sigmoidal relationship between parathyroid hormone secretion rate and plasma concentration in calves. *Endocrinology* 1978;102:1036–42.

156. Mayer GP, Habener JF, Potts JT Jr. Parathyroid hormone secretion in vivo: demonstration of a calcium-dependent, non-suppressible component of secretion. *J Clin Invest* 1976;57:679–83.

157. Brent GA, LeBoff MS, Seely EW, Conlin R, Brown EM. Relationship between the concentration and rate of change of calcium and serum intact parathyroid hormone levels in normal humans. *J Clin Endocrinol Metab* 1988;67:944–50.

158. Johansson H, Larsson R, Nygren P, et al. Cycloplasmic Ca^{2+} concentration of single normal human and bovine parathyroid cells measured by dual wavelength microfluometry. *Biosci Rep* 1987;7:705.

159. Brown EM. Four-parameter model of the sigmoidal relationship between parathyroid hormone release and extracellular calcium concentration in normal and abnormal parathyroid tissue. *J Clin Endocrinol Metab* 1983;56:572–81.

160. Brown EM, Wilson RE, Eastman RC, Pallotta J, Marynick SP. Abnormal regulation of parathyroid hormone release by calcium in secondary hyperparathyroidism due to chronic renal failure. *J Clin Endocrinol Metab* 1982;54:172–9.

161. Nygren P, Larsson R, Gylfe E, et al. Development of abnormal parathyroid cell function during monolayer culture and its relation to cellular hypertrophy and proliferation. *Acta Pathol Microbiol Immunol Scand [A]* 1987;95:207–14.

162. Nygren P, Larsson R, Johansson H, Gylfe E, Rastad J, Akerstrom G. Inhibition of cell growth retains differentiated function of bovine parathyroid cells in monolayer culture. *Bone Miner* 1988;4:123–132.

163. Allgrove J, Adami S, Manning RM, O'Riordan JLH. Cytochemical bioassay of parathyroid hormone in maternal and cord blood. *Arch Dis Child* 1985;60:110–5.

164. Keaton JA, Barto JA, Moore MP, Gruel JB, Mayer GP. Altered parathyroid response to calcium in hypercalcemic neonatal calves. *Endocrinology* 1978;103:2161–7.

165. Care AD, Ross R. Fetal calcium homeostasis. *J Dev Physiol* 1984;6:59–66.

166. Care AD, Caple IW, Singh R, Peddie M. Studies on calcium ho-

meostasis in the fetal Yucatan miniature pig. *Lab Anim Sci* 1986;36:389–92.

167. Marx SJ, Lasker RD, Brown EM, et al. Secretory dysfunction in parathyroid cells from a neonate with severe primary hyperparathyroidism. *J Clin Endocrinol Metab* 1986;62:445–9.

168. Brown EM, Shoback DM. The relationship between PTH secretion and cytosolic calcium concentration in bovine parathyroid cells. *Prog Clin Biol Res* 1984;168:139–144.

169. Brown EM, Chen CJ, LeBoff MS, Kifor O, Oetting MH, el-Hajj G. Mechanisms underlying the inverse control of parathyroid hormone secretion by calcium. *Soc Gen Physiol Ser* 1989;44:251–68.

170. Marx SJ. Familial hypocalciuric hypercalcemia [editorial]. *N Engl J Med* 1980;303:810–1.

171. MacGregor RR, Hamilton JW, Cohn DV. The bypass of tissue hormone stores during the secretion of newly synthesized parathyroid hormone. *Endocrinology* 1975;917:178–88.

172. Morrissey JJ, Cohn DV. Regulation of secretion of parathormone and secretory protein-I from separate intracellular pools by calcium, dibutyryl cyclic AMP, and (1)-isoproterenol. *J Cell Biol* 1979;82:93–102.

173. Nemeth EF, Scarpa A. Are changes in intracellular free calcium necessary for regulating secretion in parathyroid cells? *Ann NY Acad Sci* 1987;493:542–51.

174. Muff R, Nemeth EF, Haller-Brem S, Fischer JA. Regulation of hormone secretion and cytosolic Ca^{2+} by extracellular Ca^{2+} in parathyroid cells and C-cells: role of voltage-sensitive Ca^{2+} channels. *Arch Biochem Biophys* 1988;265:128–35.

175. Nemeth EF. Regulation of cytosolic calcium by extracellular divalent cations in C-cells and parathyroid cells. *Cell Calcium* 1990;11:323–7.

176. Lopez-Barneo J, Armstrong C. Depolarizing response of rat parathyroid cells to divalent cations. *J Gen Physiol* 1983;82:209–49.

177. Wallace J, Scarpa A. Regulation of parathyroid hormone secretion in vitro by divalent cations and cellular metabolism. *J Biol Chem* 1982;257:10613–6.

178. Juhlin C, Holmdahl R, Johansson H, Rastad J, Akerstrom G, Klareskog L. Monoclonal antibodies with exclusive reactivity against parathyroid cells and tubule cells of the kidney. *Proc Natl Acad Sci USA* 1987;84:2990–4.

179. Juhlin C, Klareskog L, Nygren P, et al. Hyperparathyroidism is associated with reduced expression of a parathyroid calcium receptor mechanism defined by monoclonal antiparathyroid antibodies. *Endocrinology* 1988;122:2999.

180. Nygren P, Gylfe E, Larsson R, et al. Modulation of the Ca^{2+}-sensing function of parathyroid cells in vitro and in hyperparathyroidism. *Biochim Biophys Acta* 1988;968:253–60.

181. Fitzpatrick LA, Brandi ML, Aurbach GD. Prostaglandin F2 alpha and alpha-adrenergic agonists regulate parathyroid cell function via the inhibitory guanine nucleotide regulatory protein. *Endocrinology* 1986;118:2115–9.

182. Fitzpatrick LA, Brandi ML, Aurbach GD. Control of PTH secretion is mediated through calcium channels and is blocked by pertussis toxin treatment of parathyroid cells. *Biochem Biophys Res Commun* 1986;138:960–5.

183. Fitzpatrick LA, Chin H, Nirenberg M, Aurbach GD. Antibodies to an alpha subunit of skeletal muscle calcium channels regulate parathyroid cell secretion. *Proc Natl Acad Sci USA* 1988;85:2115–9.

184. Fitzpatrick LA, Brandi ML, Aurbach GD. Calcium-controlled secretion is effected through a guanine nucleotide regulatory protein in parathyroid cells. *Endocrinology* 1986;119:2700–3.

185. Fitzpatrick LA, Aurbach GD. Control of parathyroid (PTH) secretion is mediated through calcium channels. *Prog Clin Biol Res* 1988;252:47–52.

186. Brown E, Enyedi P, LeBoff M, Rotberg J, Preston J, Chen C. High extracellular Ca^{2+} and Mg^{2+} stimulate accumulation of inositol phosphates in bovine parathyroid cells. *FEBS Lett* 1987;218:113–8.

187. Shoback DM, Membreno LA, McGhee JG. High calcium and other divalent cations increase inositol trisphosphate in bovine parathyroid cells. *Endocrinology* 1988;123:382–9.

188. Kifor O, Brown EM. Relationship between diacylglycerol levels

and extracellular Ca^{++} in dispersed bovine parathyroid cells. *Endocrinology* 1988;123:2723–9.

189. Nemeth EF, Wallace J, Scarpa A. Stimulus-secretion coupling in bovine parathyroid cells. Dissociation between secretion and net changes in cytosolic Ca^{2+}. *J Biol Chem* 1986;261:2668–74.

190. Nemeth EF, Scarpa A. Rapid mobilization of cellular Ca^{2+} in bovine parathyroid cells evoked by extracellular divalent cations. Evidence for a cell surface calcium receptor. *J Biol Chem* 1987;262:5188–96.

191. Brown EM, Fuleihan G, Chen CJ, Kifor O. A comparison of the effects of divalent and trivalent cations on parathyroid hormone release, 3′,5′-cyclic-adenosine monophosphate accumulation, and the levels of inositol phosphates in bovine parathyroid cells. *Endocrinology* 1990;127:1064–71.

192. Brown EM, Chen CJ, Kifor O, et al. Ca^{2+}-sensing, second messengers, and the control of parathyroid hormone secretion. *Cell Calcium* 1990;11:333–7.

193. Morrissey JJ. Effect of phorbol myristate acetate on secretion of parathyroid hormone. *Am J Physiol* 1988;254:E63–70.

194. Racke EK, Nemeth EF. Modulation of cytosolic calcium and hormone secretion by protein kinase C in parathyroid cells [Abstract]. *J Bone Miner Res* 1989;4:105.

195. Kobayashi N, Russell J, Lettieri D, Sherwood LM. Regulation of protein kinase C by extracellular calcium in bovine parathyroid cells. *Proc Natl Acad Sci USA* 1988;85:4857–60.

196. Membreno L, Chen TH, Woodley S, Gagucas R, Shoback D. The effects of protein kinase-C agonists on parathyroid hormone release and intracellular free Ca^{2+} in bovine parathyroid cells. *Endocrinology* 1989;124:789–97.

197. Shoback DM, Thatcher J, Leombruno R, Brown EM. Relationship between parathyroid hormone secretion and cytosolic calcium concentration in dispersed bovine parathyroid cells. *Proc Natl Acad Sci USA* 1984;81:3113–7.

198. Muff R, Fischer JA. Stimulation of parathyroid hormone secretion by phorbol esters is associated with a decrease of cytosolic calcium. *FEBS Lett* 1986;194:215–8.

199. Muff R, Fischer JA. Parathyroid hormone secretion does not respond to changes of free calcium in electropermeabilized bovine parathyroid cells, but is stimulated with phorbol ester and cyclic AMP. *Biochem Biophys Res Commun* 1986;139:1233–8.

200. Oetting M, LeBoff M, Swiston L, Preston J, Brown E. Guanine nucleotides are potent secretagogues in permeabilized parathyroid cells. *FEBS Lett* 1986;208:99–104.

201. Brown EM, Watson EJ, Leombruno R, Underwood RH. Extracellular calcium is not necessary for acute, low calcium- or dopamine-stimulated PTH secretion in dispersed bovine parathyroid cells. *Metabolism* 1983;32:1038–44.

202. Brown EM, Hurwitz S, Woodard CJ, Aurbach GD. Direct identification of beta-adrenergic receptors on isolated bovine parathyroid cells. *Endocrinology* 1977;100:1703–9.

203. Abe M, Sherwood LM. Regulation of parathyroid hormone secretion by adenyl cyclase. *Biochem Biophys Res Commun* 1972;48:396–401.

204. Brown EM, Gardner DG, Windeck RA, Aurbach GD. Cholera toxin stimulates 3′,5′-adenosine monophosphate accumulation and parathyroid hormone release from dispersed bovine parathyroid cells. *Endocrinology* 1979;104:218–25.

205. Brown EM, Hurwitz S, Aurbach GD. Beta-adrenergic stimulation of cyclic AMP content and parathyroid hormone release from isolated bovine parathyroid cells. *Endocrinology* 1977;100:1696–702.

206. Brown EM, Hurwitz SH, Aurbach GD. Alpha-adrenergic inhibition of adenosine 3′,5′-monophosphate accumulation and parathyroid hormone release from dispersed parathyroid cells. *Endocrinology* 1978;103:893–9.

207. Gardner DG, Brown EM, Windeck R, Aurbach GD. Prostaglandin E2 stimulation of 3′,5′-adenosine monophosphate accumulation and parathormone release in dispersed bovine parathyroid cells. *Endocrinology* 1978;103:577–582.

208. Gardner DG, Brown EM, Windeck R, Aurbach GD. Prostaglandin E2 inhibits 3′,5′-adenosine monophosphate accumulation

and parathyroid hormone release from dispersed bovine parathyroid cells. *Endocrinology* 1979;104:1–7.

209. Chen CJ, Anast CS, Brown EM. Effects of fluoride on parathyroid hormone secretion and intracellular second messengers in bovine parathyroid cells. *J Bone Miner Res* 1988;3:279–288.

210. Shoback DM, Brown EM. Forskolin increases cellular cyclic adenosine monophosphate content and parathyroid hormone release in dispersed bovine parathyroid cells. *Metabolism* 1984;33:509–514.

211. Brown EM. PTH secretion in vivo and in vitro. Regulation by calcium and other secretagogues. *Miner Electrol Metab* 1982;8:130–150.

212. Mayer GP, Hurst JG. Comparison of the effects of calcium and magnesium on parathyroid hormone secretion rate in calves. *Endocrinology* 1978;102:1803–1807.

213. Habener JF, Potts JT Jr. Relative effectiveness of magnesium and calcium on the secretion and release of parathyroid hormone. *Endocrinology* 1976;98:197–202.

214. Anast CS, Ohs JM, Kaplan SL, Burns TW. Evidence for parathyroid failure in magnesium deficiency. *Science* 1972;177:606–608.

215. Peraldi MN, Rondeau E, Jousset V, et al. Dexamethasone increases preproparathyroid hormone messenger RNA in human hyperplastic parathyroid cells in vitro. *Eur J Clin Invest* 1990;20:392–7.

216. Au WYW. Cortisol stimulation of parathyroid hormone secretion. *Science* 1976;193:1014–7.

217. Greenberg C, Kukreja SC, Bowser EN, Hargis GK, Henderson WJ, Williams GA. Parathyroid hormone secretion: effect of estradiol and progesterone. *Metabolism* 1987;36:151–4.

218. Greenberg C, Kukreja SC, Bowser EN, Hargis GK, Henderson WJ, Williams GA. Effects of estradiol and progesterone on calcitonin secretion. *Endocrinology* 1986;118:2594–8.

219. Fried RM, Tashjian AH Jr. Actions of rat growth hormone-releasing factor and norepinephrine on cytosolic free calcium and inositol trisphosphate in rat C-cells. *J Bone Miner Res* 1987;2:579–87.

220. Friedman E, Sakaguchi K, Bale AE, et al. Clonality of parathyroid tumors in familial multiple endocrine neoplasia type 1. *N Engl J Med* 1989;321:213–8.

221. Thakker RV, Bouloux P, Wooding C, et al. Association of parathyroid tumors in multiple endocrine neoplasia type I with loss of alleles on chromosome 11. *N Engl J Med* 1989;321:218–24.

222. Larsson C, Skogseid B, Oberg K, Nakamura Y, Nordenskjold MC. Multiple endocrine neoplasia type I gene maps to chromosome 11 and is lost in insulinoma. *Nature* 1988;332:85–7.

223. Brandi ML, Aurbach GD, Fitzpatrick LA, et al. Parathyroid mitogenic activity in plasma from patients with familial multiple endocrine neoplasia type I. *N Engl J Med* 1986;314:1287–93.

224. Brandi ML, Marx SJ, Aurbach GD, Fitzpatrick LA. Familial multiple endocrine neoplasia type I: a new look at pathophysiology. *Endocr Rev* 1988;8:341–405.

225. Lee MJ, Roth SI. Effect of calcium and magnesium on deoxyribonucleic acid synthesis in rat parathyroid glands in vitro. *Lab Invest* 1975;33:72–9.

226. Szabo A, Merke J, Beier E, Mall G, Ritz E. 1,25(OH)$_2$ vitamin D$_3$ inhibits parathyroid cell proliferation in experimental uremia. *Kidney Int* 1989;35:1049–56.

227. Nygren P, Larsson R, Johansson H, Ljunghall S, Rastad J, Akerstrom G. 1,25(OH)2D3 inhibits hormone secretion and proliferation but not functional dedifferentiation of cultured bovine parathyroid cells. *Calcif Tissue Int* 1988;43:213–8.

228. Kremer R, Bolivar I, Goltzman D, Hendy GN. Influence of calcium and 1,25-dihydroxycholecalciferol on proliferation and proto-oncogene expression in primary cultures of bovine parathyroid cells. *Endocrinology* 1989;125:935–41.

229. Brelvi ZS, Christakos S, Studzinski GP. Expression of monocyte-specific oncogenes c-fos and c-fms in HL60 cells treated with vitamin D analogs correlates with inhibition of DNA synthesis and reduced calmodulin concentration. *Lab Invest* 1986;55:269–75.

230. Berridge MJ, Irvine RF. Inositol phosphates and cell signalling. *Nature* 1989;341:197–206.

Disorders of Bone and Mineral Metabolism,
edited by Fredric L. Coe and Murray J. Favus,
© 1992 by Raven Press, Ltd. All rights reserved.

CHAPTER 5

Metabolism and Assay of Parathyroid Hormone

Claude D. Arnaud and Kin-Kee Pun

CIRCULATING FORMS OF PARATHYROID HORMONE

In 1968, Berson and Yalow made the novel observation that parathyroid hormone (PTH) in the circulation of patients with hyperparathyroidism is immunoheterogeneous [1].* Many laboratories have since confirmed and expanded upon their findings [2–7]. Those latter studies showed that the immunoreactive forms of PTH (iPTH) in hyperparathyroid serum consist principally of two forms; intact PTH [PTH (1–84)] and middle (mid) and carboxyl (COOH) fragments of PTH (1–84) [7] with molecular sizes in the 6000–7000 kD range. While no clear evidence is available that amino (NH₂) fragments are present in the general circulation, they have been identified in thyroid and parathyroid venous effluent serum by specific NH₂-terminal radioimmunoassay (RIA) [7]. Whereas intact PTH (1–84) and some NH₂-terminal fragments of PTH are biologically active, COOH-terminal fragments are generally considered to be biologically inert.

The concentration of COOH–PTH fragments in the circulation of normal subjects and of patients with primary hyperparathyroidism is 5–10 times higher than that of PTH (1–84) [8,9], and the concentration of those fragments can be as much as 50–100 times higher than that of PTH (1–84) in patients with secondary hyperparathyroidism associated with chronic renal failure [4]. Whereas those concentration differences are thought to be due to the longer survival time of COOH fragments in the circulation (Fig. 1 and [4,10]; see below), in the case of chronic renal failure they appear to be due principally to the inability of diseased kidneys to excrete them [11–15].

SOURCES OF PARATHYROID HORMONE IMMUNOHETEROGENEITY

Proteolysis of PTH (1–84) occurs normally in the parathyroid gland [16–19] and in peripheral tissues [11–15,20–43] (Fig. 2). The products of PTH degradation are released into the circulation by both sources, but the relative contribution of each to the immunoheterogeneity of PTH in the extracellular fluids is unsettled.

Parathyroid Gland

Before information was available concerning the molecular forms of iPTH in the circulation, two groups of investigators showed independently that PTH fragments were released into the medium by parathyroid adenoma explants cultured in vitro [44–46]. Subsequent studies in vivo by another group of investigators [3] reported that virtually all of the iPTH in venous effluent from parathyroid adenomata in vivo coeluted with [¹²⁵I]PTH (1–84), a finding that tended to impugn those obtained in vitro. Silverman and Yalow [4] found, however, that COOH–PTH fragments had a prolonged half-life as compared with intact PTH and suggested that only a relatively small quantity of COOH fragments, which might not have been adequately resolved from PTH (1–84) by those gel-filtration experiments [3], needed to be released by parathyroid tissue to account for their high concentration in the peripheral circulation. That such was in fact the case was shown by Flueck et al. [7] whose studies of thyroid/parathyroid venous effluents using high resolution fractionation techniques, revealed that COOH fragments comprised as much as 30–50% of the total iPTH output of adenomatous and hyperplastic

---

* For this chapter references are cited in brackets [   ].

C. D. Arnaud and K.-K. Pun: Program in Osteoporosis and Bone Biology, Department of Medicine, University of California, San Francisco, School of Medicine, San Francisco, CA 94115.

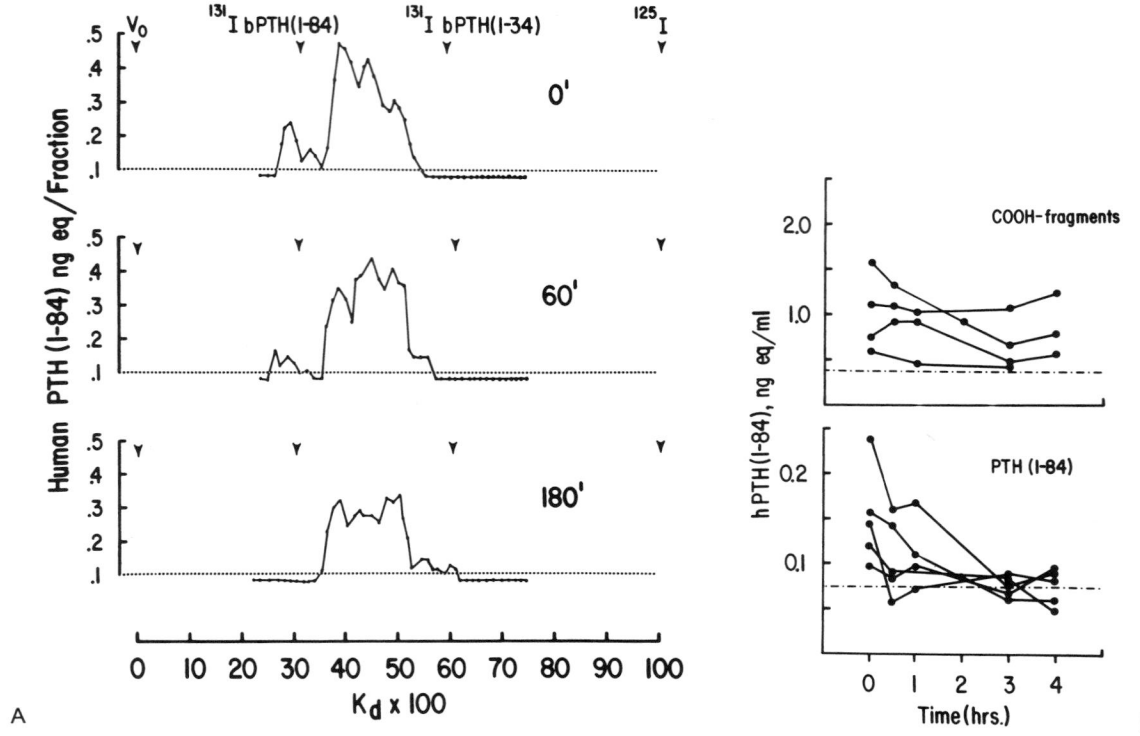

FIG. 1. Survival of various forms of serum immunoreactive parathyroid hormone (iPTH) in the peripheral circulation of 4 patients with primary hyperparathyroidism during 4 h after surgical removal of enlarged parathyroid glands. **A:** Typical elution pattern of mid-region iPTH after peripheral serum was gel filtered on a reverse flow 2.6 × 90 cm Bio Rad P-150 column [7]. Molecular weight markers: *left,* intact [131I]-bovine PTH 1–84 (kD = 9500); *middle,* [131I]bovine PTH 1–34 (kD = 4100); *right,* [125I]. The iPTH component eluting just in advance of [131I]bPTH 1–84 is presumably intact PTH; this component rapidly disappears and is no longer present 3 h after parathyroidectomy (PTX). The iPTH component eluting between [131I]bPTH markers represents at least 3 lower molecular weight mid- and carboxyl-terminal fragments of PTH. Those fragments survive much longer than intact PTH; as much as half of the iPTH present at 0 h remains at 3 h after PTX. **B:** Values for iPTH obtained by integrating areas under curves shown in A plotted as a function of time after PTX (parathyroidectomy). Whereas the iPTH component eluting with [131I]bPTH 1–84 was no longer detectable in 3 patients $\frac{1}{2}$ h after PTX, and in the remaining 2 patients 3 h after PTX, the iPTH components eluting between the markers (COOH fragments) persisted for the full 4 h of the study in 3 of 4 patients.

parathyroid glands (Fig. 3). Those workers calculated that such gland derived fragments could account for between 20% and 100% of the COOH fragments in the peripheral circulation of the patients studied, assuming the fragment half-lives were 5 to 10 times longer than that of PTH (1–84).

Evidence is available supporting roles for two lysosomal enzymes in the intraglandular degradation of PTH; those enzymes have the characteristics of cathepsin B [47,48] and cathepsin D [49]. The cathepsin B-like enzyme cleaves PTH between amino acid residues 36 and 37 yielding a COOH fragment, PTH (37–84), and an NH₂ fragment, presumably PTH (1–36). The cathepsin D-like enzyme cleaves PTH between residues 34 and 35 yielding a COOH fragment (35–84) and an NH₂ fragment, PTH (1–34). Extensive further degradation to smaller peptide fragments and ultimately to free amino acids has been demonstrated [17]. The rate of biosynthe-

sis of PTH increases only slightly, if at all, as the rate of secretion increases [16–18,50]. Instead, the parathyroid gland normally synthesizes more PTH than is needed, degrading an amount of the excess so as to maintain sufficient steady state levels of vesicle-stored hormone for ordinary acute requirements. The only way extraordinary demands for PTH can be met, therefore, is by gland hypertrophy and hyperplasia.

Early studies [51] showing that porcine parathyroid gland extracts contained a calcium-dependent enzyme activity that cleaved PTH prompted the authors of that paper to speculate that the intraglandular degradation of PTH could play an important role in regulating the release of biologically active PTH into the circulation. Indeed, two investigations pursued this possibility within several years of one another; the first [17] showed in vitro that the intracellular degradation of parathyroid hormone stores was dependent upon extracellular calcium

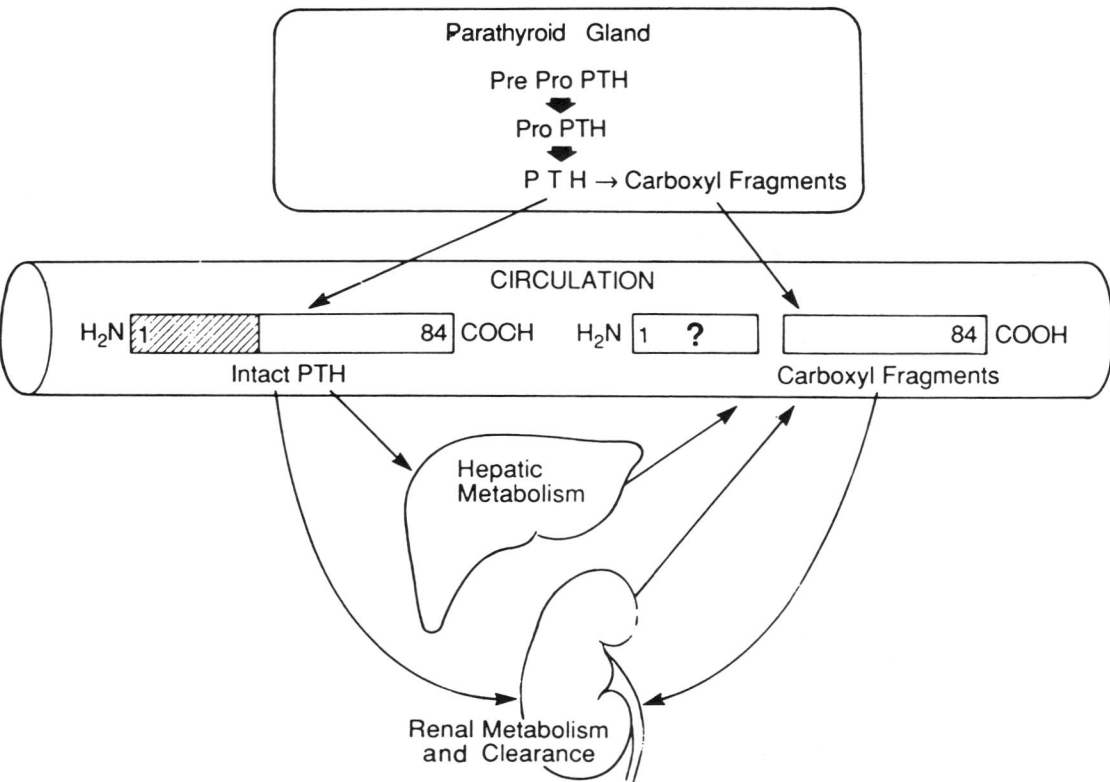

FIG. 2. Secretion, metabolism, clearance, and circulating forms of immunoreactive PTH. PTH is synthesized as a preprohormone, is converted to prohormone, and is secreted as intact hormone, or, it is metabolized into biologically inactive carboxyl fragments prior to secretion. These carboxyl fragments containing both the middle and carboxyl regions are also produced by peripheral metabolism of intact PTH by liver and kidney. The half-life in vivo and the concentration of intact biologically active hormone are small compared with that of inactive carboxyl fragments. Both carboxyl fragments and intact hormone are cleared in the kidney by glomerular filtration. The existence of a significant concentration of amino-terminal fragments is uncertain. From Endres et al. [119].

concentrations, and the second [52] showed that high calcium perfusion of the bovine parathyroid glands caused them to release increased quantities of COOH fragments relative to intact PTH into their venous effluents. Finally, following upon his demonstration that COOH–PTH fragments were released by perifused bovine parathyroid gland in vitro [53], Hanley [54] showed that, using the same system, extracellular calcium regulated the release of COOH fragments from small pieces of hyperplastic parathyroid tissue obtained at surgery from patients with chronic renal failure. When gland pieces were perfused with low calcium medium, the tissue released more intact PTH (55%) than COOH fragments (45%), but under high calcium conditions, proportionally more COOH fragments (63.3%) were released than intact PTH (34.7%).

Several investigators [17,51] have speculated that derangements in the processes connected with PTH degradation in the parathyroid gland might be a reflection of, or even contribute directly to, the pathogenesis of parathyroid gland dysfunction. Two recent studies have addressed this important question. The first [55] compared the calcium suppressibility of dispersed parathyroid cells from 15 individual enlarged parathyroid glands from patients with primary hyperparathyroidism (1° HPT) with the secretion of intact PTH and COOH fragments by those cells. Whereas cells that released predominantly intact PTH were least suppressible, cells that released COOH fragments were most suppressible. Although limited, those data seem to suggest that diminished ability of parathyroid cells to degrade PTH may play a role in the pathogenesis of 1° HPT. The second study [56] tested the hypothesis that decreased degradation of PTH in normal bovine parathyroid cells causes increased PTH secretion. The influence of agents that suppress degradation of intracellular proteins on the release of PTH from those cells was measured. All agents increased the release of PTH under conditions of high calcium inhibition of secretion. These results were interpreted by the authors to indicate that those agents reduced the destruction of PTH secretory vesicles and made more of them available for release. Thus, it follows that a hypothetical naturally

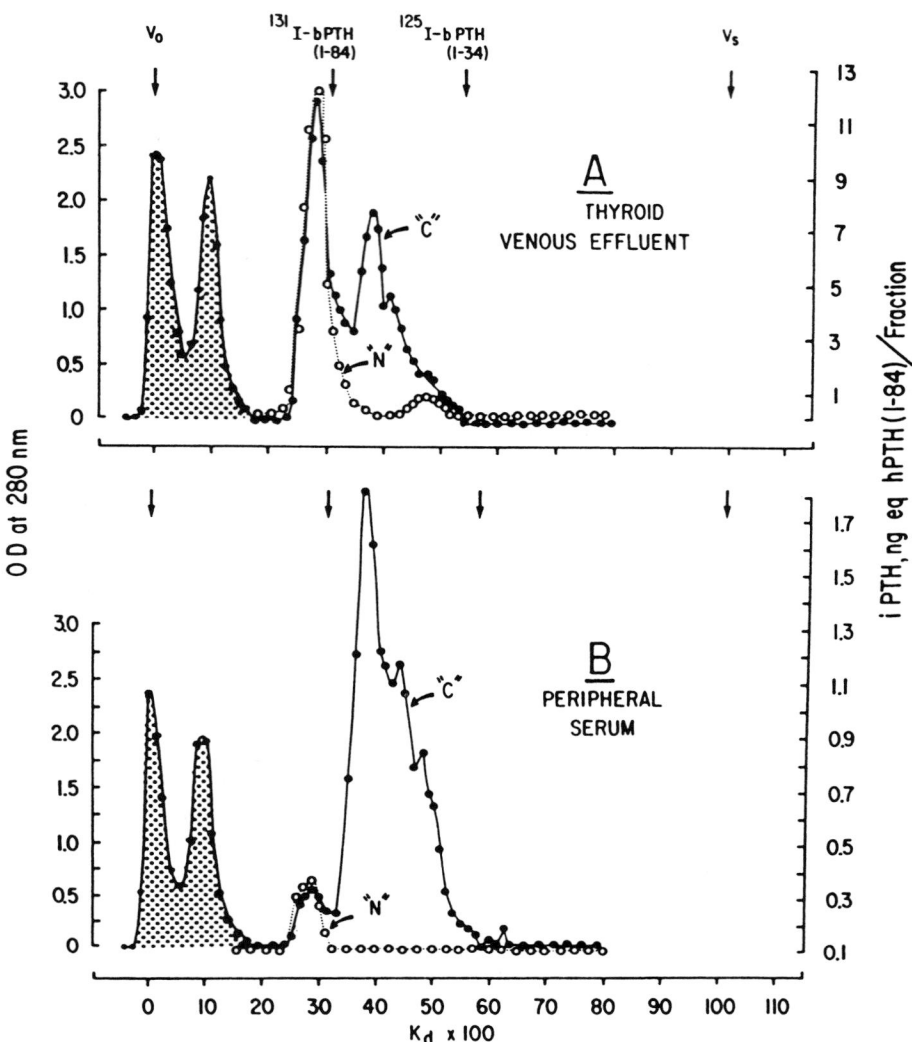

FIG. 3. Elution patterns of iPTH after thyroid venous effluent serum (**A**) and peripheral serum (**B**) was gel filtered on a reverse flow 2.6 × 90 cm Bio Rad P-150 column (7). Molecular weight markers: left, intact [^{131}I]bovine PTH 1–84 ($K_d = 9500$); right, [^{125}I]bovine PTH 1–34 ($K_d = 4100$). The iPTH component eluting just in advance of [^{131}I]bPTH 1–84 is presumably intact PTH; it is recognized by both a NH$_2$-region specific assay ("N") and a mid-region specific assay ("C"). The iPTH component eluting between [^{125}I]-bPTH markers presumably represents at least 3 lower molecular weight mid- and carboxyl-terminal fragments of PTH; it is recognized by the "C" assay but not by the "N" assay. The small component eluting in the position between 40 and 50 K_d in the thyroid venous effluent serum profile (**A**) presumably represents an NH$_2$-terminal PTH fragment. Note the difference in the vertical scale between A and B and the relatively large quantity of mid- and carboxyl-terminal PTH fragments in thyroid venous effluent serum indicating the secretion in vivo of those fragments. The profiles shown are typical of a total of four patients with primary hyperparathyroidism. From Flueck et al. [7].

occurring block of the process of vesicular destruction could induce increased secretion of PTH by individual cells even when they were exposed to levels of extracellular calcium that are ordinarily suppressive.

Peripheral Metabolism of Parathyroid Hormone

Once secreted into the blood, PTH is cleared from the circulation with a $t_{1/2}$ of less than 5 minutes [10,24,57–59]; liver uptake and metabolism of PTH and subsequent renal excretion of liver generated COOH fragments are the principal mechanisms that account for this phenomenon. Binding of PTH to receptors in bone, kidney, and other tissues contributes only minimally.

Technical problems have clouded the interpretation of much of the data derived from studies of the metabolism of administered PTH in whole animals and by isolated organs or tissues in vitro. When unlabeled PTH has been used, unphysiologically high doses have been required so that it and its fragments can be detected by specific immunoassays. When [125I]PTH has been used, most preparations have been biologically inactive (oxidized by the radiolabeling procedure). Most studies have employed PTH of an animal species different from the animal species in which its metabolism is investigated i.e., human PTH in rat kidney or liver perfusions [15]. No studies of the metabolism of administered PTH in humans have been reported.

Those problems notwithstanding, a number of elegant studies reporting upon the peripheral metabolism of PTH have appeared during the past two decades. Segre et al. showed that [125I]bovine PTH (1–84) undergoes rapid metabolism after it is injected into rats [33,37] and dogs [24,28] with the generation of COOH fragments that appear in the plasma. The sites of hormone cleavage were determined in those studies by sequence analysis of isolated 125I-labeled circulating fragments. They were found to occur between residues 33 and 34 and between residues 36 and 37. The resulting COOH fragments therefore had molecular sizes similar to the major endogenously generated circulating fragments [3–7]. One of those fragments (37–84) is identical to that generated by the cathepsin B-like enzyme in porcine parathyroid tissue, but the other (33–84) differs from that generated by the cathepsin D-like enzyme in porcine parathyroid by a single amino acid (34–84). Whether that latter difference is real or an artifact related to the technical difficulties that must have been encountered in the performance of the sequence analyses of circulating [125I]COOH fragments is not clear at the present time. Irrespective of this relatively minor issue, it is clear that all of the described cleavages could result in a NH_2 fragment containing sufficient sequence to be biologically active. Although the early studies of Canterbury and co-workers [25] using isolated liver perfusion suggested that metabolism of PTH by this organ could lead to the generation of a biologically active PTH fragment(s), subsequent studies have not substantiated that finding [42].

There is no question that the COOH fragments of PTH that are generated by peripheral metabolism of PTH find their way into the circulation [24], but it is extremely difficult from available data to assess the quantitative contribution of this process to the overall immunoheterogeneity of PTH in extracellular fluids. One type of experiment that could help provide this important information would be to compare the absolute concentrations of circulating COOH fragments of PTH in normal animals with those produced in surgically parathyroidectomized animals infused constantly with sufficient PTH (1–84) to maintain extracellular calcium concentration in the normal range.

The first studies [60] of the liver as a potential site for the peripheral metabolism of PTH showed little hepatic uptake of oxidized (and probably biologically inactive) [125I]bovine PTH (1–84). However, subsequent work by Neuman et al. [26] showed that hepatic uptake of biologically active preparations of [125I]PTH (1–84) was quite substantial. Furthermore, in earlier studies it had been shown that the clearance of PTH from the circulation of the rat was prolonged by hepatectomy, suggesting a physiological role for the liver in the metabolism of PTH [23].

Canterbury et al. were the first to use isolated perfused rat liver to study the hepatic metabolism of PTH [25]: those workers showed that bovine PTH (1–84) was cleaved during hepatic perfusion into fragments which had elution positions on gel exclusion chromatography that were similar to the immunoreactive forms of PTH in the general circulation of patients with primary hyperparathyroidism. Subsequent studies in the dog in vivo [32] and in perfused rat liver and kidney [15,43] agree that the liver is the organ that clears the circulation of and metabolizes the major portion of secreted intact PTH. Its principal function is therefore to degrade PTH into COOH fragments and release them into the circulation so that they can be quantitatively cleared by glomerular filtration along with relatively smaller amounts of intact PTH. That degradation is probably accomplished by the Kupffer's cells of the liver [39,41].

The question of whether the concentration of extracellular calcium influences the peripheral metabolism of secreted PTH as it appears to do in the parathyroid gland has been addressed in many studies; the results vary widely [15,25,34,58,59,61–64]. Many different experimental models were used in these studies ranging from an assessment of the clearance of bioactive PTH from the circulation of dogs in vivo [58] (no effect of extracellular calcium) to several recent elegant studies of the extraction of synthetic human PTH (1–34) [64] or of synthetic human PTH (1–84) and many of its fragments [15] by isolated perfused rat liver (higher extraction with increased calcium). Although those latter studies used state of the art methodology and are consistent with an intuitively expected result, namely that hypercalcemia stimulates the liver to degrade PTH, the results may not be physiologically relevant because they were obtained in isolated perfused organ systems. However, the definitive nature of data obtained in those studies should prompt future research in whole animal systems using newer technology.

ASSAY OF PARATHYROID HORMONE IN BIOLOGICAL FLUIDS

Immunoassay

The successful development, performance, application, and interpretation of immunoassays of PTH depend upon a thorough understanding of glandular and peripheral metabolism of PTH and how those latter processes relate to the phenomenon of immunoheterogeneity of circulating PTH (see above). Early in the history of PTH radioimmunoassay [5,65–67], at a time when the complexity of the phenomenon was not fully appreciated, the development of a clinically useful assay depended as much on chance as on anything else. Crude extracts of bovine or porcine parathyroid glands were used as immunogens and purified bovine PTH (1–84) was used as labeled ligand in assays for human PTH in serum. As often as not, the failure of an antiserum produced in this way to crossreact sufficiently with human PTH precluded success. Even when crossreaction was adequate, values for immunoreactive PTH (iPTH) in the same serum sample varied widely depending upon the antiserum used in the assay. Distrust in assays in general and in the ability of different laboratories to accurately assay PTH was rife. Physicians were relegated to the difficult position of searching the entire country for an assay that consistently predicted the presence of parathyroid pathology in their patients and once found, to stick with it.

With the recognition that circulating PTH was immunoheterogeneous, some of those serious discrepancies became understandable. First, mid-region and COOH-specific assays measured high levels of PTH because they reacted with both the small amount of intact PTH and the relatively large amount of mid-region and COOH fragments in serum, whereas NH_2-specific assays measured low levels of PTH because they could react only with the small amounts of intact PTH in serum. Second, the concentration of all forms of circulating PTH taken together was considerably lower than those of many other hormones, and the concentration of intact PTH was many times lower than mid-region and COOH fragments. Thus, while very sensitive mid-region and COOH-assays could quantitate serum levels of iPTH in normal subjects, the most sensitive of NH_2-assays could not detect iPTH in normal subjects. As often as not, NH_2-assays gave "noise" readings for normal sera due to nonspecific effects of serum [67], making it difficult to distinguish normal from increased levels of iPTH and impossible to detect decreased levels. That phenomenon even led one of the authors (CDA) to conclude wrongly that COOH-specific assays were vastly superior to NH_2-specific assays in distinguishing normal from hyperparathyroid sera [6].

Currently, several approaches are available for the systematic and purposeful development of mid-region and COOH-specific radioimmunoassays [68–75]. Multivalent antisera raised against crude glandular extracts can be combined with a synthetic mid-region tyrosyl analogue ([43]tyr 44–68) of hPTH for radiolabeling with [125I]. That labeled hPTH fragment is recognized only by antibodies in the multivalent antiserum directed against mid-regional epitopes, thus producing a sequence specific mid-region assay. Another approach is to produce antisera to the synthetic mid-region fragment (44–68) and use the tyrosyl analogue as labeled ligand. This may be less satisfactory than using antisera produced against intact PTH because antisera produced against synthetic fragments may react more vigorously with the fragment used to produce the antiserum than circulating PTH. When this occurs, assays are generally unsatisfactory because dilutions of sera may not produce binding isotherms parallel to curves produced by the synthetic fragment used as immunogen, and values for serum iPTH that are read off such standard curves may be inappropriately high.

Except for a single instance [76], attempts at developing clinically useful radioimmunoassays specific for the NH_2 region of PTH that can assess concentrations of intact iPTH in the peripheral circulation have been discouraging principally because of assay insensitivity. Two site, noncompetitive immunoassays [immunoradiometric (IRMA) and chemiluminometric (ICMA)] [10,77,78] are vastly more sensitive than most competitive assays, and they recently have provided successful alternatives to NH_2-region radioimmunoassays. All of those assays measure intact PTH and use synthetic hPTH (1–84) as a standard.

Originally described by Miles and Hales [79], the principle of IRMA and ICMA is to use two antibodies that recognize two distinct regions of the analyte; one is antibody attached to a solid phase (i.e., plastic) and is used to affinity concentrate the analyte from serum. The other antibody, which is labeled with radioactive, luminescent, fluorescent, or enzymatic compounds, is used to signal the presence of the analyte (Fig. 4). Antibodies used in two-site immunometric assays can be monoclonal or they can be purified from polyclonal antisera by affinity techniques. Usually, the antibody used as the concentration or capture reagent is the one which is in abundant supply because large amounts are generally required to saturate solid phase materials. For most PTH assays, mid- or COOH-region antibodies have been used as capture reagents and NH_2-region antibodies as signal reagents. Antibody labeling has been with either [125I] or a chemiluminescent aryl acridinium ester. The acridinium ester is rendered luminescent after it is exposed to alkaline peroxide. Luminescence is quantitated with an automated luminometer. ICMAs can be as much as 10-fold more sensitive than IRMAs because of the much greater specific activity that can be achieved with luminescence labeling as compared to [125I] labeling of antibodies.

Immunometric assays offer many other advantages over radioimmunoassays. First, standard curves are linear, and virtually all of the analyte in a given sample is used in the assay reaction. Second, shorter "turn around times" can be achieved because maximum assay sensitivity can be realized with vastly shorter incubation times. Third, because serum is not present during the stage of the procedure when labeled antibody is incubated with

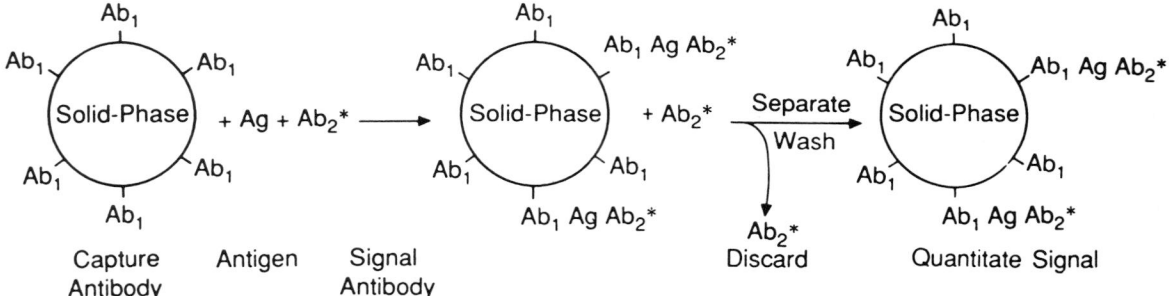

FIG. 4. Two-site, noncompetitive immunoassay. Antigen or hormone is reacted with an immobilized antibody against one antigenic determinant and a labeled signal antibody against a second antigenic determinant. The antigen or hormone forms a bridge between the capture and labeled antibody, producing a "sandwich" complex. Both the capture and signal antibody are added in excess, ensuring that all antigen is measured. Free labeled antibody is conveniently separated from the solid-phase sandwich complexes. The solid-phase-antigen-labeled antibody complex is quantitated with the appropriate detection system. The signal increases with increasing antigen concentration. From Endres et al. [119].

the serum hormone-capture antibody–solid phase complex, many of the nonspecific serum effects that occur in radioimmunoassay are avoided. And finally, immunometric assays are technically easier to perform, more accurate, and more precise.

Bioassay

Bioassays in vivo, such as those that depend upon the prevention by PTH of the development of hypocalcemia in parathyroidectomized rats or the induction by PTH of hypercalcemia in chicks [80,81], are too insensitive to quantitate PTH in serum. Three bioassays in vitro have been developed that depend independently upon the simulation by PTH of: (i) glucose-6-phosphate dehydrogenase activity (cytochemical) in guinea pig renal cortical sections [82], (ii) adenylate cyclase activity in guanyl nucleotide-augmented renal cortical plasma membranes [83], and (iii) cyclic AMP production in cultures of an osteogenic sarcoma cell line [84].

All three assays can measure normal and increased levels of presumably intact PTH in serum. In this sense, they are superior to most NH_2-region radioimmunoassays. The cytochemical assay is even more sensitive than two site assays (see above) routinely using sera diluted to 1:100 and 1:1000. However, its relative lack of precision and accuracy and its large cost have precluded routine clinical use. Although less sensitive, the renal plasma membrane assay is easier to perform and is more accurate, precise, and specific than the cytochemical assay. It is also more convenient than cell culture assay: renal plasma membranes remain stable when frozen at $-70°C$ (at least 6 months) whereas cell cultures require a great deal of labor intensive maintenance.

It is possible that all three bioassays could be made to distinguish between endogenous PTH and parathyroid hormone related polypeptide (PTHrP) (see below) by

immunoextracting serum with appropriate immunoaffinity procedures prior to assay. The feasibility of that approach has been demonstrated; immunoextraction of intact PTH from serum is now performed in the renal plasma membrane assay for PTH [85], and immunoextraction of PTHrP has been described in the performance of radioimmunoassay of this compound in serum [86]. Thus, an approach to distinguishing primary hyperparathyroidism from humoral hypercalcemia of malignancy using bioassay is at hand.

It is not likely that bioassays will ever be used to routinely perform clinical assessments in the future unless they become easier to perform. They will remain, however, powerful research tools that, among other purposes, will be used to validate immunologic procedures claiming to measure biologically active PTH.

Clinical Applications of Parathyroid Hormone Immunoassays

There has been a revolutionary change in the laboratory investigation of persons with hypo- and hypercalcemia in recent years owing to the availability of sensitive and specific immunoassays of serum PTH.

Differential Diagnosis of Hypocalcemia

In the case of hypocalcemia, measurement of serum iPTH segregates patients into two general categories: those with hypoparathyroidism (either parathyroprivic or functional due to magnesium deficiency) and those with other disorders (Fig. 5A). Increased values in a range appropriate to the degree of hypocalcemia essentially excludes the presence of hypoparathyroidism and suggests the possibility of end-organ resistance to PTH [i.e., pseudohypoparathyroidism (Fig. 5B), vitamin D deficiency [87], and vitamin D resistance [88]) or of sec-

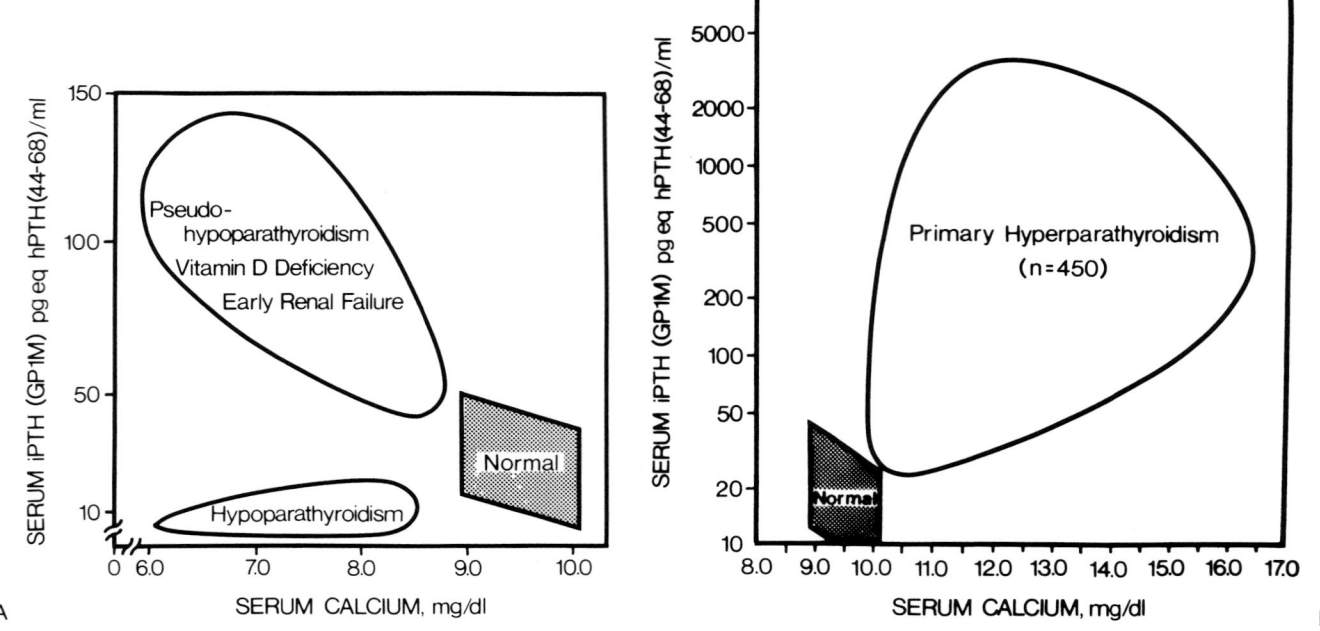

FIG. 5. Serum mid-region immunoreactive PTH in (**A**) hypocalcemic states and in (**B**) primary hyperparathyroidism as a function of the total serum concentration of calcium.

ondary hyperparathyresim resulting from such disorders as renal failure (see below), dietary deficiency of calcium [89], or intestinal malabsorption of calcium [90]. Undetectable serum iPTH confirms the diagnosis of hypoparathyroidism, providing the assay used is sufficiently sensitive to measure serum iPTH in the large majority of normal subjects. Serum iPTH may be barely detectable in some patients with hypoparathyroidism if the assay employed is very sensitive, but such low values may be due to nonspecific effects of serum per se in radioimmunoassays that do not adequately control for this factor [67].

Patients with functional hypoparathyroidism resulting from hypomagnesemia also have low to undetectable levels of serum iPTH [91]. Absolute proof that this condition exists depends upon the demonstration that magnesium salt administration corrects hypomagnesemia, increases serum iPTH, and restores eucalcemia.

Differential Diagnosis of Hypercalcemia

In general, serum iPTH measurements segregate patients with hypercalcemia into two categories. Using a sensitive and specific mid-region assay, serum iPTH is increased in 90% of patients with primary hyperparathyroidism and is inappropriately increased for the level of the serum calcium (upper range of normal) in the remainder (Fig. 5B). In the majority of nonparathyroid disorders causing hypercalcemia, serum iPTH is either undetectable or low unless primary hyperparathyroidism coexists, in which case, it is appropriately increased

for the level of serum calcium. Thus it is possible, using serum iPTH, to diagnose primary hyperparathyroidism, a surgically curable disease, even in the presence of another nonparathyroid disorder which has the potential to produce hypercalcemia on its own.

Nonparathyroid tumors seldom produce sufficient native parathyroid hormone to produce hypercalcemia. Yet many patients with malignancy associated hypercalcemia (MAH) present with a biochemical syndrome indistinguishable in many respects from primary hyperparathyroidism, i.e., they have hypophosphatemia and increased nephrogenous cyclic AMP excretion [92]. This seemingly paradoxical situation was clarified recently when it was shown that a polypeptide could be obtained from the tumors of patients with MAH that was immunologically different from PTH but that stimulated adenylate cyclase in kidney and bone cell preparations [93,94]. Subsequent deduction of the structure of this polypeptide from its cDNA [95–97] revealed it to be a linear 141 amino acid polypeptide homologous with authentic PTH in its amino-terminal first 13 amino acids. Little homology was found in the region of the PTH molecule carboxyl terminal to residue 13. However, the biologic effects of synthetic preparations of the human PTHrP 1–34 fragment are essentially identical in vitro [98–103] and in vivo [99,102,104] to human PTH 1–34, and photoaffinity labeling studies show that PTHrP 1–34 binds to an identical plasma membrane (receptor) component as PTH 1–34 [105–107].

The problem with PTH radioimmunoassays in general is that they cannot always distinguish between primary hyperparathyroidism and malignancy associated hypercalcemia because values for serum iPTH can be normal or even slightly increased in some patients with MAH. This is illustrated in Figs. 6 and 7A. Even though the distributions of values for serum mid-region iPTH as a function of serum total calcium are different in primary hyperparathyroidism and in MAH, there is sufficient overlap (Fig. 6) in those distributions to engender diagnostic bewilderment in a small percentage of cases. The reason this problem exists with radioimmunoassays of PTH but not with immunometric assays of intact PTH (see below and Fig. 7) is not entirely clear. It is thought that radioimmunoassays (particularly mid-region specific) detect the mid- and COOH-region fragments of PTH that are secreted even when the parathyroid glands are maximally suppressed [108] by hypercalcemia, whereas immunometric assays of intact PTH cannot detect those fragments. Another contributing factor could be that certain radioimmunoassays using labeled ligands (i.e., [^{125}I]PTH 1–84) and polyvalent antisera that include and react with the homologous region in PTH and PTHrP (i.e., 1–13) actually detect especially high levels of PTHrP in serum (e.g., the assay used to obtain data shown in Fig. 6). Those assays would be expected to demonstrate immunologic differences between serum containing increased levels of PTH and serum containing increased levels of PTHrP (i.e., different slopes of dilution curves). In fact, such a demonstration [109] was the first clue that there were immunologic differences between the PTH in the sera of patients with primary hyperparathyroidism and patients with MAH. Immunometric assays on the other hand have generally

been developed with mid- or COOH-specific antibodies as capture reagents, making it impossible for them to immunoextract the nonhomologous carboxyl region of PTHrP from serum and include it in the reaction with labeled NH$_2$-terminal antibody.

Utilizing serum immunoextraction procedure and a recently developed radioimmunoassay for PTHrP, Budayr et al. [86] demonstrated increased levels of serum iPTHrP in as many as 60–70% of patients with MAH whereas patients with primary hyperparathyroidism had levels within the normal range. With the development of commercially available assays of serum PTHrP it will be possible to make the laboratory diagnosis of MAH due to excess circulating PTHrP in a direct and specific manner rather than in the way it is done now, namely on negative grounds based on low or undetectable levels of serum iPTH (Fig. 7).

Staging of Renal Osteodystrophy

It is difficult to stage the severity of renal osteodystrophy using any available blood chemistry measurements short of assaying serum mid-region iPTH. For example, serum calcium, phosphorus, magnesium, and alkaline phosphatase are within the reference range early in the course of the development of renal failure (inulin clearance in the range of 20–30 mL/min, stage I, Fig. 8), yet there is histomorphometric evidence of osteitis fibrosa cystica in trephine biopsies of the iliac crest and increased levels of serum iPTH [110]. Thus, because serum iPTH increases as renal function progressively declines below clearances of 40 mL/min [111] it is possible to follow patients with compromised renal function with measurements of serum iPTH to determine when to institute therapeutic measures to prevent or treat secondary hyperparathyroidism (e.g., dietary phosphorus restriction, calcium supplementation, and vitamin D). In this context, it is important to recognize that increases in serum mid-region iPTH may reflect, in part, impaired clearance of mid- and COOH–PTH fragments from the circulation by failing kidneys. This is supported by reports showing that in patients with renal failure, values for serum bioactive PTH [112] and intact iPTH [10] may be within the normal range while serum mid-region iPTH is increased as much as 5- to 10-fold. However, the fact that osteitis fibrosa cystica is present frequently in patients with early renal failure that have increased levels of serum mid-region iPTH [110] strongly suggests that those increases in serum iPTH reflect secondary hyperparathyroidism as well [113]. At this writing, experience with immunometric assays of serum intact PTH are too limited to comment upon their application to the problem of staging renal osteodystrophy, although, as with mid-region assays [110,112,113], it has been possible to demonstrate that serum values of intact iPTH [114,115] correlate highly with quantitative indices of hyperparathyroid bone disease in iliac crest biopsies.

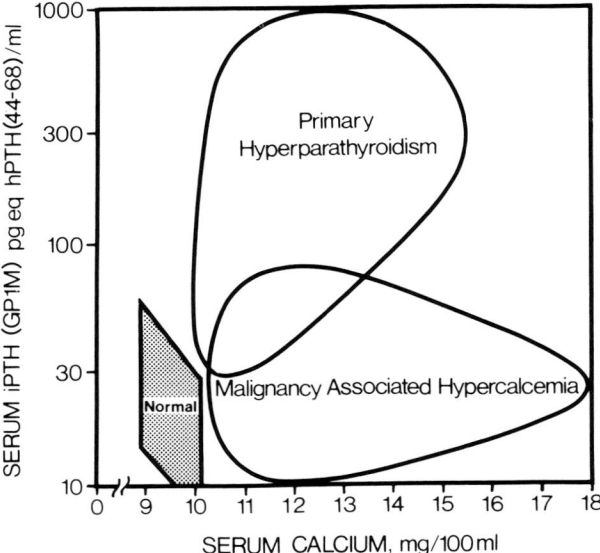

FIG. 6. Comparison of the distributions of serum mid-region immunoreactive PTH values as a function of total serum calcium concentration between patients with primary hyperparathyroidism and malignancy associated hypercalcemia.

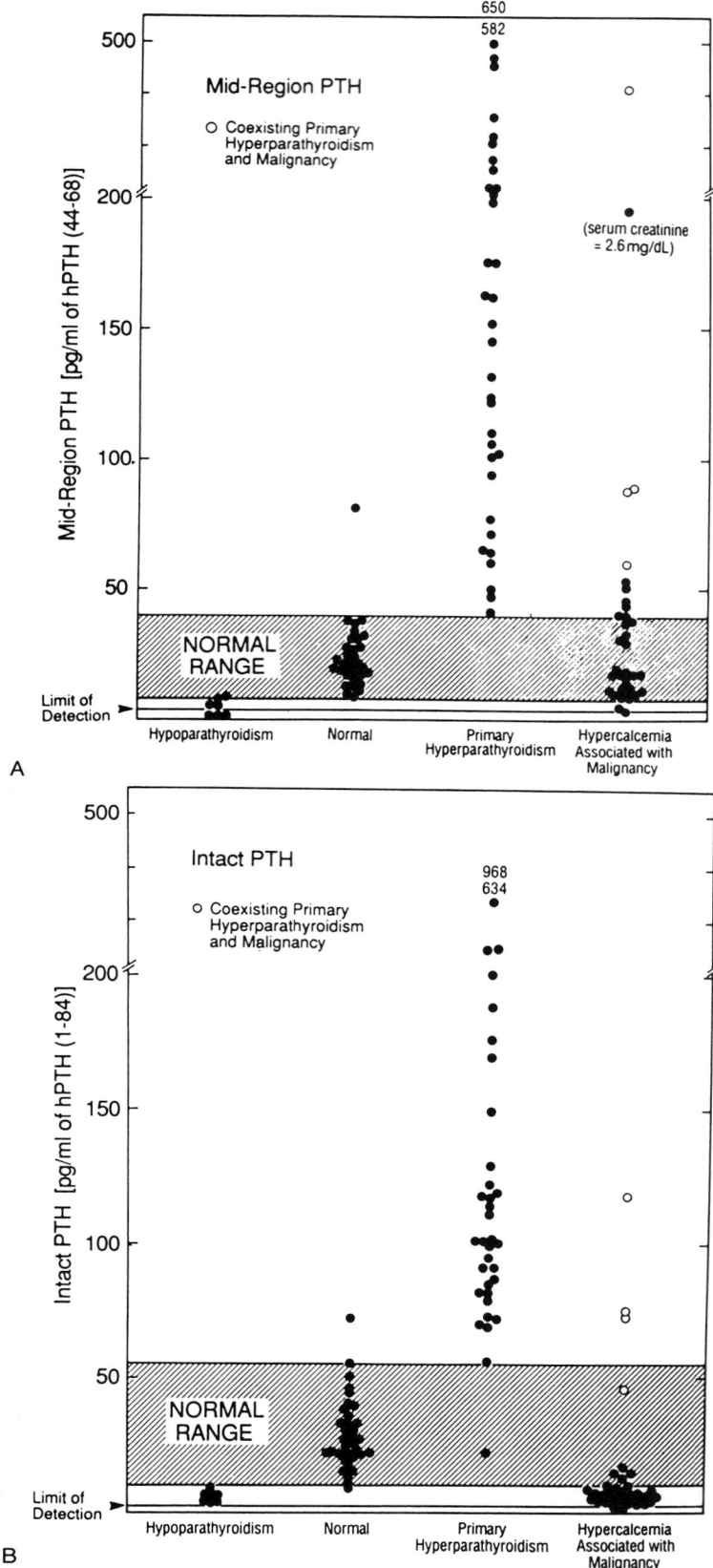

FIG. 7. Clinical utility of parathyroid hormone immunoassays. Serum mid-region (**A**) and intact (**B**) PTH in normal subjects and patients with hypoparathyroidism, primary hyperparathyroidism, and hypercalcemia associated with malignancy. From Endres et al. [119].

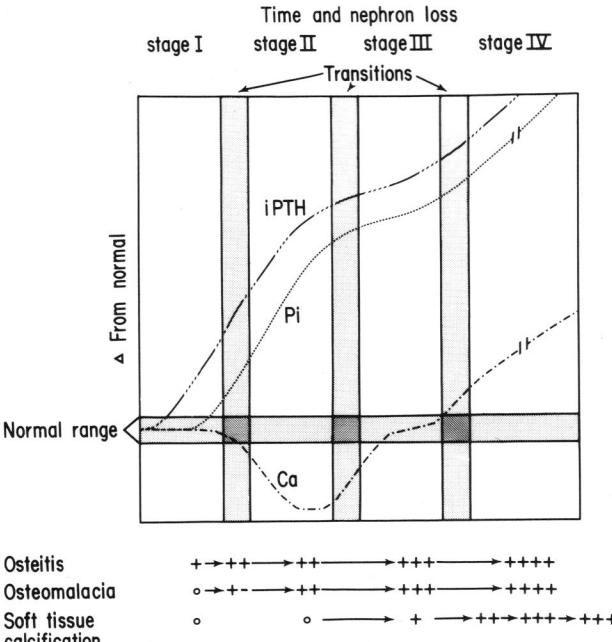

FIG. 8. Stages of biochemical and osseous abnormalities in renal osteodystrophy as a function of time and nephron loss. From Bordier et al. [110].

Patients with stage II disease (Fig. 8) may be easier to spot because they generally have more severe renal functional impairment, hypocalcemia, and hyperphosphatemia. However, hypocalcemia and hyperphosphatemia may be obscured by therapeutic measures, and hyperparathyroidism, detectable only by measurements of serum iPTH, may be of sufficient severity as to warrant more intensive therapy. Untreated stage II hyperparathyroidism is generally identified by serum mid-region iPTH values of 20–30 times the upper limit of the reference range. Those patients are generally amenable to medical therapy.

Patients with stage III disease (Fig. 8) usually have normal levels of total serum calcium but are hyperphosphatemic. They generally have severe osteodystrophy and the beginnings of soft tissue calcification. The severity of those problems are not generally appreciated until serum iPTH measurements are performed and they show values 50–100 times the upper limit of normal. It is important to discover such large increases in serum iPTH because they reflect a degree of hyperparathyroidism which is still reversible with medical therapy but is on the verge of transition to stage IV disease, which generally requires surgical intervention to reduce parathyroid gland mass so that medical therapy will be effective. Stage IV disease (Fig. 8) is characterized by hypercalcemia, hyperphosphatemia, severe osteodystrophy, soft tissue calcification, and serum mid-region iPTH levels 200–1000 times the upper limit of the reference range.

Differential Diagnosis of Hypercalcemia in Association with Renal Failure

It is important to recognize that hypercalcemia in patients with chronic renal failure does not always reflect stage IV secondary hyperparathyroidism. It may reflect primary hyperparathyroidism with associated renal failure. Although that diagnosis is difficult to make, it is usually associated with much lower levels of serum iPTH (mid-region assay, unpublished data) than found in stage IV renal osteodystrophy, i.e., in the range of 5 to 20 times the upper limit of the reference range. Another alternative that must be considered is "aluminum osteodystrophy" [116], which is characterized by severe osteodystrophy, hypercalcemia, and lower levels of serum iPTH, also in the range of 5 to 20 times the upper limit of the reference range (unpublished data). Finally nonparathyroid causes of hypercalcemia, such as sarcoidosis may complicate renal failure. In these instances serum iPTH will also be lower than expected.

Treatment by subtotal parathyroidectomy is the preferred therapy of stage IV secondary hyperparathyroidism and of primary hyperparathyroidism but parathyroidectomy tends to make an "aluminum osteodystrophy" worse [117], and is inappropriate in patients with nonparathyroid hypercalcemia. It is therefore just as important to specifically identify the underlying cause(s) of hypercalcemia in patients with renal failure as it is in patients with normal renal function (see above). The mid-region PTH radioimmunoassay has provided the author with an invaluable diagnostic aid in this regard. Again, there has been too little experience with serum measurements of intact iPTH to know whether they will be similarly helpful.

Comparison of Clinical Utility of Carboxyl (53–84) and Mid (44–68) PTH Radioimmunoassays with an Intact PTH Immunometric Assay

The clinical utilities of a COOH-region-specific (53–84) [73] and a mid-region-specific (43–68) radioimmunoassay [69] have been compared separately [118,119] with the same immunochemiluminometric assay (ICMA) for intact PTH [78] in the differential diagnosis of hypercalcemia. Both sets of investigators in those studies, as well as other investigators who have had experience with both types of assays [10,77,78,118,119; Arnaud and Pun, unpublished], agree that immunometric assays show clear technical advantages over radioimmunoassays. Increased sensitivity and specificity, simplicity of performance, shorter assay time, and stable reagents have been specifically cited.

All three assays (53–84, 44–68, intact) were able to measure iPTH in normal sera and show low or undetectable levels in hypoparathyroid sera. Of 36 sera from patients with proved primary hyperparathyroidism, 35 showed increased levels of intact PTH whereas only 26 of 36 of those same sera showed increased levels of COOH-region (53–84) specific iPTH. By contrast, the intact and the mid-region (44–68) PTH assays were essentially equivalent in this regard (Fig. 7 and [119]). Moreover, the mid-region assay was superior to the intact assay in that PTH levels were more elevated. Whereas 28 of 36 sera showed mid-region values greater than twice normal, intact iPTH was similarly elevated in only 17 of those same 36 sera. Those latter observations strongly suggest the glandular secretion of COOH fragments containing an epitope within the 44–68 amino acid sequence of PTH, and is consistent with the possibility that this epitope is an immunologic marker of abnormal parathyroid tissue.

It is not often that the clinical features of patients with malignancy associated hypercalcemia do not distinguish them from patients with primary hyperparathyroidism. However, serious errors in patient management can occur in the small number of patients in whom that uncertainty is encountered. While the relatively lower values for serum mid-region iPTH in MAH were noted nearly two decades ago (see above, Fig. 6, and [109,120]) to be a powerful means of differentiating those two disease processes, it is very clear that the intact PTH immunometric assay (Fig. 7 and [10,77,78,118,119, Arnaud and Pun, unpublished]) provides a major improvement in this regard.

As commented upon above, serum mid- and COOH-region iPTH may be increased while serum intact iPTH is within the normal range in the presence of renal failure. Although this phenomenon is likely to be due largely to the diminished ability of diseased kidneys to excrete mid- and COOH–PTH fragments, several alternative possibilities should be considered. The first is hypothetical. If the "capture" antibody in an immunometric assay system is mid- or COOH-specific, it is possible that the large quantity of mid- and COOH fragments in the serum of patients with renal failure could saturate that antibody thus leaving few or no sites for the much smaller quantities of intact PTH in serum to be "captured." This would result in spuriously low values for intact PTH. It is important therefore that mid- or COOH–PTH "capture" antibodies be present in vast excess and that the ability of a system to assay intact PTH be tested in the presence of quantities of mid- and COOH–PTH fragments that are expected to be present in sera from patients with renal failure.

The second alternative is that appropriate treatment of even severe secondary hyperparathyroidism (e.g., high dialysate calcium concentrations) may dramatically suppress PTH secretion (so that serum intact iPTH registers in or near the normal range) without altering the size or enormous secretory capacity of greatly enlarged parathyroid glands. In such cases, serum mid- or COOH–iPTH will not be greatly affected by treatment until gland size is decreased, mostly because of the very long half-life of

mid- and COOH fragments in patients with renal failure [4]. Thus, it is likely that serum mid- and COOH–PTH assays may be more consistently reflective of the degree of parathyroid hyperplasia in patients with renal failure than intact PTH assays, especially in those patients undergoing intensive therapy for secondary hyperparathyroidism. Moreover, physicians not recognizing this might be prompted to decrease the intensity of treatment prematurely based on low or normal levels of serum intact iPTH. Not withstanding these considerations, it is fair to say that the interpretation of an elevated serum mid- or COOH–iPTH is problematic in patients with impaired renal function; serum intact iPTH is preferable in their diagnostic evaluation.

Lastly, measurements of iPTH in sera taken from various veins potentially draining enlarged parathyroid glands have been used to localize those glands so that they can be surgically removed [121]. Success in these studies depend upon demonstrating "step up" increases in the concentration of iPTH between peripheral blood and blood draining a parathyroid lesion. Those "step up" differences are less when iPTH measurements are made with mid- or COOH–PTH than with intact PTH assays primarily because of the relatively higher concentrations of mid- or COOH–iPTH as compared with intact iPTH in the peripheral circulation [70,122]. Thus, it is generally recommended that intact or NH_2-terminal PTH assays be used for the measurement of serum iPTH in blood obtained during selective venous catheterization to localize parathyroid pathology.

SUMMARY

Circulating parathyroid hormone (PTH) is immuno-heterogeneous. It consists of small amounts of intact PTH which is biologically active and large amounts of middle (mid)- and carboxyl-terminal (COOH)-PTH fragments which are biologically inert. Those differences in concentrations are due to the longer survival time of mid- and COOH–PTH fragments in the circulation. Both the parathyroid gland and the peripheral degradation of secreted intact PTH constitute the major sources of circulating mid- and COOH–PTH fragments. Biosynthesized intact PTH is degraded by the parathyroid gland by cathepsin-like lysosomal enzymes. The secretory products of the gland include intact PTH and mid- and COOH–PTH fragments in a rough ratio of 7:3. It is possible that very small quantities of amino (NH_2)-terminal fragments are secreted, but most of these fragments are degraded into small peptides and amino acids by the parathyroid gland. There is evidence of a calcium activated PTH degrading enzyme, and studies in vitro and in vivo show that high calcium concentrations increase and low calcium concentrations decrease gland degradation of PTH and secretion of mid- and COOH–PTH fragments. There are interesting new studies that suggest the possibility that a decreased ability of the gland to degrade PTH may increase its secretory capacity, even when exposed to normally suppressive concentrations of extracellular calcium, thus implicating a potential pathological mechanism for the development of secretory autonomy.

The liver and its Kupffer's cell are mainly responsible for PTH degradation, and glomerular filtration by the kidney is responsible for the clearance of intact PTH and its degradative products from the circulation. Recent studies suggest that high calcium concentrations increase hepatic PTH degradation. As in the parathyroid gland, hepatic cathepsin-like enzymes generate mid- and COOH–PTH fragments which are returned to the circulation and added to the pool of PTH fragments secreted by the parathyroid gland. The disposition of companion NH_2 fragments is a mystery. There is little evidence that they circulate under normal conditions. Impaired renal function results in retention of mid- and COOH–PTH fragments and those fragments may confound the interpretation of serum assays of iPTH.

Bioassays, radioimmunoassays, and immunometric assays are available to measure PTH in biological fluids. Bioassays, albeit excellent research tools, are too cumbersome for routine diagnostic use. Radioimmunoassays (RIA) depend upon a immunologic competitive reaction and are limited in sensitivity. The direct measurement of intact PTH by RIA using NH_2-region specific antisera is thus limited by the extremely low concentration of this analyte in serum, even in some patients with moderately severe primary hyperparathyroidism. Radioimmunoassays of mid- and COOH–PTH do not require the same sensitivity because of the relatively higher concentrations of those fragments of PTH in the circulation. Those RIAs measure the mid- and COOH–PTH fragments as well as intact PTH. Immunometric assays have been developed for intact PTH. They use excess PTH antibody to one end of the PTH molecule to capture endogenous PTH from serum and a radioactive or luminescent labeled antibody to the other end of the PTH molecule to signal the presence of the hormone bound to the "capture" antibody. Immunometric assays are exquisitely sensitive and can measure low and normal levels of intact iPTH in serum. They are also more convenient, easy to perform, and have a more rapid turn/around time than RIAs.

Sensitive, specific, and carefully performed mid-region PTH assays still comprise the gold standard in measuring elevated levels of iPTH in primary hyperparathyroidism. This could be because an epitope within the 44–68 amino acid sequence of PTH may represent an immunologic marker of abnormal parathyroid tissue. However immunometric assays of PTH closely rival mid-region PTH assays in segregating normal subjects from those with primary hyperparathyroidism. They also measure lower levels of serum iPTH in malignancy associated hypercalcemia than mid-region assays, thereby providing greater specificity. The extensive experience available in the use of mid-region PTH assay in the staging and clinical follow-up of patients with renal osteodystrophy has not yet accrued with immunometric assays of intact PTH and there may be certain advantages of mid-region assays in revealing the presence of residual parathyroid hyperplasia in patients under intensive treatment of secondary hyperparathyroidism associated with renal failure. Notwithstanding those possible uses of mid-region PTH assays in renal failure, it must be said that their use in diagnostic situations (such as in hypercalcemia) in which renal impairment is present may be limited and that immunometric assays of intact PTH are preferable.

ACKNOWLEDGMENTS

The authors would like to acknowledge the assistance of Sarah Sanchez, M.S., in the preparation of this chapter. The work was supported in part by research grants from the NIH (DK21614 and DK39964).

REFERENCES

1. Berson SA, Yalow RS. Immunochemical heterogeneity of parathyroid hormone in plasma. *J Clin Endocrinol Metab* 1968;28:1037–47.
2. Canterbury JM, Reiss E. Multiple immunoreactive molecular forms of parathyroid hormone in human serum. *Proc Soc Exp Biol Med* 1972;140:1393–1401.
3. Segre GV, Habener JF, Powell D, Tregear GW, Potts Jr JT. Parathyroid hormone in human plasma. Immunochemical characterization and biological implications. *J Clin Invest* 1972;51:3163–72.
4. Silverman R, Yalow RS. Heterogeneity of parathyroid hormone: clinical and physiological implications. *J Clin Invest* 1973;52:1958–71.
5. Fischer JA, Binswanger U, Dietrich FM. Human parathyroid hormone. Immunological characterization of antibodies against a glandular extract and the synthetic amino-terminal fragments 1–12 and 1–34 and their use in the determination of immunoreactive hormone in human sera. *J Clin Invest* 1974;54:794–9.
6. Arnaud CD, Goldsmith RS, Bordier PS, Sizemore GW. Influence of immunoheterogeneity of circulating parathyroid hormone on results of radioimmunoassays of serum in man. *Am J Med* 1974;56:785–93.
7. Flueck JA, DiBella FP, Edis AJ, Kehrwald JM, Arnaud CD. Immunoheterogeneity of parathyroid hormone in venous effluent serum from hyperfunctioning parathyroid glands. *J Clin Invest* 1977;60:1367–75.
8. Dambacher MA, Fischer JA, Hunziker WH, et al. Distribution of circulating immunoreactive components of parathyroid hormone in normal subjects and in patients with primary and secondary hyperparathyroidism: the role of the kidney and of serum calcium concentration. *Clin Sci* 1979;57:435–443.
9. D'Amour P, Labelle F, Lecavalier L, Plourde V, Harvey D. Influence of serum calcium concentration on circulating molecular forms of PTH in three species. *Am J Physiol* 1986;251:E680–7.
10. Blind E, Schmidt-Gayk H, Scharla S, et al. Two-site assay of intact parathyroid hormone in the investigation of primary hyperparathyroidism and other disorders of calcium metabolism compared with a midregion assay. *J Clin Endocrinol Metab* 1988;67:353–60.

11. Hruska KA, Kopelman R, Rutherford WE, Klahr S, Slatopolsky E. Metabolism of immunoreactive parathyroid hormone in the dog: the role of the kidney and the effects of chronic renal disease. *J Clin Invest* 1975;56:39–48.

12. Freitag J, Martin KJ, Hruska K, et al. Impaired parathyroid hormone metabolism in patients with chronic renal failure. *N Engl J Med* 1978;298:29–32.

13. Martin KJ, Hruska KA, Freitag JJ, Klahr S, Slatopolsky E. The peripheral metabolism of parathyroid hormone. *N Engl J Med* 1979;301:1092–8.

14. Hruska KA, Korkor A, Martin K, Slatopolsky E. Peripheral metabolism of intact parathyroid hormone. Role of liver and kidney and the effect of chronic renal failure. *J Clin Invest* 1981;67:885–92.

15. Daugaard K, Egfjord M, Olgaard K. Influence of calcium on the metabolism of intact parathyroid hormone by isolated perfused rat kidney and liver. *Endocrinology* 1990;126:1813–20.

16. Chu LLH, MacGregor RR, Anast CS, Hamilton JW, Cohn DV. Studies on the biosynthesis of rat parathyroid hormone and proparathyroid hormone: adaptation of the parathyroid gland to dietary restriction of calcium. *Endocrinology* 1973;93:915–24.

17. Habener JF, Kemper B, Potts JT Jr. Calcium-dependent intracellular degradation of parathyroid hormone: a possible mechanism for the regulation of hormone stores. *Endocrinology* 1975;97:431–41.

18. Morrissey JJ, Cohn DV. Secretion and degradation of parathormone as a function of intracellular maturation of hormone pools: modulation by calcium and dibutyryl cyclic AMP. *J Cell Biol* 1979;83:521–8.

19. Cohn DV, Elting JJ. Synthesis and secretion of parathormone and secretory protein-I by the parathyroid gland. In: Peck WA, ed. *Bone and mineral research,* annual 2. Amsterdam: Elsevier, 1984;1–64.

20. Segre GV, D'Amour P, Hultman A, Potts JT Jr. Effects of hepatectomy, nephrectomy and nephrectomy/uremia on the metabolism of parathyroid hormone in the rat. *J Clin Invest* 1981;67:439–48.

21. Martin JF, Melick RA, de Luise M. The effect of nephrectomy on the metabolism of labelled parathyroid hormone. *Clin Sci* 1969;37:137–42.

22. Melick RA, Martin TJ. Parathyroid hormone metabolism in man: effect of nephrectomy. *Clin Sci* 1969;37:667–74.

23. Fang VS, Tashjian AH Jr. Studies on the role of the liver in metabolism of parathyroid hormone. I. Effects of partial hepatectomy and incubation of the hormone with tissue homogenates. *Endocrinology* 1972;90:1177–84.

24. Segre GV, Niall HD, Habener JF, Potts JT Jr. Metabolism of parathyroid hormone: physiologic and clinical significance. *Am J Med* 1974;56:774–84.

25. Canterbury JM, Bricker LA, Levey GS, et al. Metabolism of bovine parathyroid hormone. Immunological and biological characteristics of fragments generated by liver perfusion. *J Clin Invest* 1975;55:1245–53.

26. Neuman WF, Neuman MW, Lane K, et al. The metabolism of labeled parathyroid hormone. V. Collected biological studies. *Calcif Tissue Res* 1975;18:271–80.

27. Neuman WF, Neuman MW, Sammon PJ, et al. The metabolism of labeled parathyroid hormone. III. Studies in rats. *Calcif Tissue Res* 1975;18:251–61.

28. Singer FR, Segre GV, Habener JF, et al. Peripheral metabolism of bovine parathyroid hormone in the dog. *Metabolism* 1975;24:139–44.

29. Catherwood BD, Friedler RM, Singer FR. Sites of clearance of endogenous parathyroid hormone in the vitamin D-deficient dog. *Endocrinology* 1976;98:228–36.

30. Goltzman D, Peytremann A, Callahan EN. Metabolism and biological activity of parathyroid hormone in renal cortical membrane. *J Clin Invest* 1976;57:8–19.

31. Habener JF, Mayer GP, Dee PC, Potts JT Jr. Metabolism of amino- and carboxyl-sequence immunoreactive parathyroid hormone in the bovine: evidence for peripheral cleavage of the hormone. *Metabolism* 1976;25:385–95.

32. Martin KJ, Hruska KA, Greenwalt A, et al. Selective uptake of intact parathyroid hormone by the liver: differences between hepatic and renal uptake. *J Clin Invest* 1976;58:781–8.

33. Segre GV, D'Amour P, Potts JR Jr. Metabolism of radioiodinated bovine parathyroid hormone in the rat. *Endocrinology* 1976;99:1645–52.

34. Hruska KA, Martin K, Mennes P, et al. Degradation of parathyroid hormone and fragment production by the isolated perfused dog kidney: the effect of glomerular filtration rate and perfusate Ca^{++} concentrations. *J Clin Invest* 1977;60:501–10.

35. Kau ST, Maack T. Transport and catabolism of parathyroid hormone in isolated rat kidney. *Am J Physiol* 1977;233:F445–54.

36. Martin KJ, Hruska KA, Lewis J, Anderson C, Slatopolsky E. The renal handling of parathyroid hormone. Role of peritubular uptake and glomerular filtration. *J Clin Invest* 1977;60:808–14.

37. D'Amour P, Segre GV, Roth SI, Potts JT Jr. Analysis of parathyroid hormone and its fragments in rat tissues: chemical identification and microscopical localization. *J Clin Invest* 1979;63:89–98.

38. D'Amour P, Huet P, Segre GV, Rosenblatt M. Characteristics of bovine parathyroid hormone extraction by dog liver in vitro. *Am J Physiol* 1981;241:E208–14.

39. Segre GV, Perkins AS, Witters LA, Potts JT Jr. Metabolism of parathyroid hormone by isolated rat Kupffer cells and hepatocytes. *J Clin Invest* 1981;67:449–57.

40. Habener JF, Rosenblatt M, Potts JT Jr. Parathyroid hormone: biochemical aspects of biosynthesis, secretion, action, and metabolism. *Physiol Rev* 1984;64:985–1053.

41. Pillai S, Zull JE. Production of biologically active fragments of parathyroid hormone by isolated Kupffer cells. *J Biol Chem* 1986;261:14919–23.

42. Bringhurst FR, Stern AM, Yotts M, Mizrahi N, Segre GV, Potts JT Jr. Peripheral metabolism of PTH: fate of biologically active amino terminus in vivo. *Am J Physiol* 1988;255:E886–93.

43. Daugaard H, Egfjord M, Olgaard K. Metabolism of intact parathyroid hormone in isolated perfused rat liver and kidney. *Am J Physiol* 1988;254:E740–8.

44. Arnaud CD, Tsao HS, Oldham SF. Native human parathyroid hormone: an immunochemical investigation. *Proc Natl Acad Sci USA* 1970;67:415–22.

45. Sherwood LM, Rodman JS, Lundberg WB. Evidence for a precursor to circulating parathyroid hormone. *Proc Natl Acad Sci USA* 1970;67:1631–8.

46. Arnaud CD, Sizemore GW, Oldham SB, Fischer JA, Tsao HS, Littledike ET. Human parathyroid hormone: glandular and secreted molecular species. *Am J Med* 1971;50:630–8.

47. MacGregor RR, Hamilton JW, Kent GN, Shofstall RE, Cohn DV. The degradation of proparathormone and parathormone by parathyroid and liver cathepsin B. *J Biol Chem* 1979;254:4428–33.

48. MacGregor RR, Hamilton JW, Shofstall RE, Cohn DV. Isolation and characterization of porcine parathyroid cathepsin B. *J Biol Chem* 1979;254:4423–7.

49. Hamilton JW, Jilka RL, MacGregor RR. Cleavage of parathyroid hormone to the 1–34 and 35–84 fragments by cathepsin D-like activity in bovine parathyroid gland extracts. *Endocrinology* 1983;113:285–92.

50. Heinrich G, Kronenberg, Potts JT Jr, Habener JF. Parathyroid hormone messenger ribonucleic acid: effects of calcium on cellular regulation in vitro. *Endocrinology* 1983;112:449–58.

51. Fischer JA, Oldham SB, Sizemore GW, Arnaud CD. Calcium-regulated parathyroid hormone peptidase. *Proc Natl Acad Sci USA* 1972;69:2341–5.

52. Mayer GP, Keaton JA, Hurst JG, Habener JF. Effects of plasma calcium concentration on the relative proportion of hormone and carboxyl fragments in parathyroid venous blood. *Endocrinology* 1979;104:1778–84.

53. Hanley DA, Takatsuki K, Sultan JM, Schneider AB, Sherwood LM. Direct release of parathyroid hormone fragments from functioning bovine parathyroid glands in vitro. *J Clin Invest* 1978;62:1247–54.

54. Hanley DA, Ayer LM. Calcium-dependent release of carboxyl-terminus fragments of parathyroid hormone by hyperplastic human parathyroid tissue in vitro. *J Clin Endocrinol Metab* 1986;63:1075–9.

55. Kubler N, Krause U, Wagner PK, Beyer J, Rothmund M. The secretion of parathyroid hormone and its fragments from dispersed cells of adenomatous parathyroid tissue at different calcium concentrations. *Exp Clin Endocrinol* 1986;88:101–8.

56. MacGregor RR, Bansal DD. Inhibitors of cellular proteolysis cause increased secretion from parathyroid cells. *Biochem Biophys Res Commun* 1989;160:1339–43.

57. Singer FR, Segre GV, Habener JF, Potts JT Jr. Peripheral metabolism of bovine parathyroid hormone in the dog. *Metabolism* 1975;24:139–43.

58. Fox J, Scott M, Nissenson RA, Heath H III. Effect of plasma calcium concentration on the metabolic clearance rate of parathyroid hormone in the dog. *J Lab Clin Med* 1983;102:70–7.

59. Oldham SB, Finck EJ, Singer FR. Parathyroid hormone clearance in man. *Metabolism* 1978;27:993–1001.

60. de Luise M, Martin TJ, Melick RA. Tissue distribution of calcitonin in the rat: comparison with parathyroid hormone. *J Endocrinol* 1970;48:173–9.

61. Neuman MW, Neuman WF, Lane K. The metabolism of labeled parathyroid hormone. VII. Attempts to modify hormone deposition. *Calcif Tissue Res* 1975;19:169–78.

62. D'Amour P, Huet P-M. Serum calcium does not influence the extraction of ^{125}I-bovine parathyroid hormone by the dog liver in vivo. *Clin Invest Med* 1985;8:202–7.

63. Hanano Y, Ota K, Fujita T. Degradation of parathyroid hormone by perfused rat kidney. In: Copp DH, Talmage RV, eds. *Endocrinology of calcium metabolism.* Amsterdam: Excerpta Medica, 1978;359–68.

64. D'Amour P, Huet P-M. Ca^{2+} concentration influences the hepatic extraction of bioactive human PTH-(1–34) in rats. *Am J Physiol* 1989;256:E87–92.

65. Berson SA, Yalow RS, Aurbach GD, Potts JT Jr. Immunoassay of bovine and human parathyroid hormone. *Proc Natl Acad Sci USA* 1963;49:613–7.

66. Reiss E, Canterbury JM. The radioimmunoassay for parathyroid hormone in man. *Proc Soc Exp Biol Med* 1968;128:501–4.

67. Arnaud CD, Tsao HS, Littledike T. Radioimmunoassay of human parathyroid hormone in serum. *J Clin Invest* 1971;50:21–34.

68. Marx SJ, Sharp ME, Krudy A, Rosenblatt M. Radioimmunoassay for the middle region of human parathyroid hormone: studies with a radioiodinated synthetic peptide. *J Clin Endocrinol Metab* 1981;53:76–84.

69. Mallette LE, Tuma SN, Berger RE, Kirkland JL. Radioimmunoassay for the middle region of human parathyroid hormone using an homologous antiserum with a carboxy-terminal fragment of bovine parathyroid hormone as radioligand. *J Clin Endocrinol Metab* 1982;54:1017–24.

70. Hackeng WHL, Lips P, Netenlenbos JC, Lips CJM. Clinical implications of estimation of intact parathyroid hormone (PTH) versus total immunoreactive PTH in normal subjects and hyperparathyroid patients. *J Clin Endocrinol Metab* 1986;63:447–53.

71. Mallette LE, Wilson DP, Kirkland JL. Evaluation of hypocalcemia with a highly sensitive, homologous radioimmunoassay for the midregion of parathyroid hormone. *Pediatrics* 1983;71:64–9.

72. Schmidt-Gayk H, Schmitt-Fiebig M, Hitzler W, Armbruster FP, Mayer E. Two homologous radioimmunoassays for parathyrin compared and applied to disorders of calcium metabolism. *Clin Chem* 1986;32:57–62.

73. Davies CP, Dwyer KP, Riley WJ. C-terminal parathyrin hormone assay: interpretation aided by total urinary cyclic AMP and phosphate excretion indices. *Clin Biochem Revs* 1983;4:81–96.

74. Arnaud C, Zitzner LA. Clinical utility of "mid" and "carboxy" region specific assays of parathyroid hormone. In: Frame B, Potts JT Jr, eds. *Clinical disorders of bone and mineral metabolism.* Amsterdam: Excerpta Medica, 1983;10–3.

75. Zillikens D, Armbruster FP, Stern J, Schmidt-Gayk H, Raue F. Sensitive homologous radioimmunoassay for human parathyroid hormone to diagnose hypoparathyroid conditions. *Ann Clin Biochem* 1987;24:608–13.

76. Segre GV, Potts JT Jr. Differential diagnosis of hypercalcemia. In: DeGroot LJ, ed. *Endocrinology,* vol 2. Philadelphia: WB Saunders, 1989;984–1001.

77. Nussbaum SR, Zahradnik RJ, Lavigne JR, et al. Highly sensitive two-site immunoradiometric assay of parathyrin, and its clinical utility in evaluating patients with hypercalcemia. *Clin Chem* 1987;33:1364–7.

78. Brown RC, Aston JP, Weeks I, Woodhead JS. Circulating intact parathyroid hormone measured by a two-site immunochemiluminometric assay. *J Clin Endocrinol Metab* 1987;65:407–14.

79. Miles LEM, Hales CN. Labelled antibodies and immunological assay systems. *Nature* 1968;219:186–9.

80. Zanelli J, Parson JA. Bioassay of parathyroid hormone. In: Kuhlencordt F, Bartelheimer H, eds. *Handbuch der Inneren Medizin,* vol 6. New York: Springer-Verlag, 1980;599.

81. Zanelli JM, Gaines-Das RE. The first international reference preparation for human parathyroid hormone for immunoassay: characterization and calibration by international collaborative study. *J Clin Endocrinol Metab* 1983;57:462–9.

82. Goltzman D, Henderson B, Loveridge N. Cytochemical bioassay of parathyroid hormone: characteristics of the assay and analysis of circulating hormonal forms. *J Clin Invest* 1980;65:1309–17.

83. Nissenson RA, Abbott SR, Teitelbaum AP, Clark OH, Arnaud CD. Endogenous biologically active human parathyroid hormone: measurement by a guanyl nucleotide-amplified renal adenylate cyclase assay. *J Clin Endocrinol Metab* 1981;52:840–6.

84. Klee GG, Preissner CM, Schloegel IW, Kao PC. Bioassay of parathyrin: analytical characteristics and clinical performance in patients with hypercalcemia. *Clin Chem* 1988;34:482–8.

85. Forero MS, Klein RF, Nissenson RA, et al. Effect of age on circulating immunoreactive and bioactive parathyroid hormone levels in women. *J Bone Min Res* 1987;2:363–6.

86. Budayr AA, Nissenson RA, Klein RF, et al. Increased serum levels of a parathyroid hormone-like protein in malignancy associated hypercalcemia. *Ann Int Med* 1989;111:807–12.

87. Arnaud CD, Glorieux F, Scriver CR. Serum parathyroid hormone levels in acquired vitamin D deficiency of infancy. *Pediatrics* 1972;49:837–40.

88. Arnaud CD, Maijer R, Reade T, Scriver CR, Whelan DT. Vitamin D dependency: an inherited postnatal syndrome with secondary hyperparathyroidism. *Pediatrics* 1970;46:871–80.

89. Calvo MS, Kumar R, Heath H III. Persistently elevated parathyroid hormone secretion and action in young women after four weeks of ingesting high phosphorus, low calcium diets. *J Clin Endocrinol Metab* 1990;70:1334–40.

90. Bordier PJ, Mair P, Arnaud CD, Gueris J, Ferriere C, Norman AW. Early effects of vitamin D_3 and some analogues, 250HD$_3$; 1,25(OH)$_2$D$_3$; 1α(OH)D$_3$ upon resorption, formation and mineralization of bone in nutritional or malabsorption osteomalacia, with reference to serum iPTH, calcium, phosphate and alkaline phosphatase. In: *Vitamin D and problems of uremic bone disease.* New York: Walter de Gruyter, 1975;134–48.

91. Anast CS, Mohs JM, Kaplan SL, et al. Evidence for parathyroid failure in magnesium deficiency. *Science* 1972;177:606–8.

92. Stewart AF, Horst R, Deftos LJ, Lang R, Broadus AE. Biochemical evaluation of patients with cancer-associated hypercalcemia: evidence for humoral and non-humoral groups. *N Engl J Med* 1980;303:1377–83.

93. Strewler GJ, Williams RD, Nissenson RA. Human renal carcinoma cells produce hypercalcemia in the nude mouse and a novel protein recognized by parathyroid hormone receptors. *J Clin Invest* 1983;71:769–74.

94. Rodan SB, Insogna KL, Vignery A, et al. Factors associated with humoral hypercalcemia of malignancy stimulate adenylate cyclase in osteoblastic cells. *J Clin Invest* 1983;72:1511–15.

95. Suva LJ, Winslow GA, Wettehall REH, et al. A parathyroid hormone-related protein implicated in malignant hypercalcemia: cloning and expression. *Science* 1987;237:893–6.

96. Mangin M, Webb AC, Dreyer BE, et al. Identification of a cDNA encoding a parathyroid hormone-like peptide from a human tumor associated with humoral hypercalcemia of malignancy. *Proc Natl Acad Sci USA* 1988;85:597–601.

97. Strewler GJ, Stern PH, Jacobs JW, et al. Parathyroid hormone-like protein from human renal carcinoma cells. Structural and functional homology with parathyroid hormone. *J Clin Invest* 1987;80:1803–7.

98. Kemp BE, Moseley JM, Rodda CP, et al. Parathyroid hormone-related protein of malignancy: active synthetic fragments. *Science* 1987;238:1568–70.

99. Horiuchi N, Caulfield MP, Fisher JE, et al. Similarity of synthetic peptide from human tumor to parathyroid hormone in vivo and in vitro. *Science* 1987;238:1566–8.

100. Rodan SB, Noda M, Wesoloski G, Rosenblatt M, Rodan GA.

Comparison of postreceptor effects of 1–34 human hypercalcemic factor and 1–34 human parathyroid hormone in rat osteosarcoma cells. *J Clin Invest* 1988;81:924–7.

101. Stewart AF, Mangin M, Wu T, et al. Synthetic human parathyroid hormone-like protein stimulates bone resorption and causes hypercalcemia in rats. *J Clin Invest* 1988;81:596–600.

102. Yates AJP, Gutierrez GE, Smoleus P, et al. Effects of synthetic peptide of parathyroid hormone-related protein on calcium homeostasis, renal tubular calcium resorption, and bone metabolism in vivo and in vitro in rodents. *J Clin Invest* 1988;81:932–8.

103. Nakai M, Fukase M, Sakaguchi K, Noda T, Fujii N, Fujita T. Human parathyroid hormone-related protein fragment (1–34) had glucose-6-phosphate dehydrogenase activity on distal convoluted tubules in cytochemical bioassay. *Biochem Biophys Res Commun* 1988;154:146–50.

104. Thompson DD, Seedor JG, Fisher J, Rosenblatt M, Rodan GA. Direct action of the human hypercalcemic factor on bone in thyroparathyroidectomized rats. *Proc Natl Acad Sci USA* 1988; 85:5673–7.

105. Nissenson RA, Karpf D, Bambino T, et al. Covalent labeling of high affinity guanyl nucleotide-sensitive parathyroid hormone receptor in canine renal cortex. *Biochemistry* 1987;26:1874–8.

106. Jueppner H, Abou-Samra AB, Uneno S, Gu WX, Potts JT, Segre GV. The parathyroid hormone-like peptide associated with humoral hypercalcemia of malignancy and parathyroid hormone bind to the same receptor on plasma membrane of ROS 17/2.8 cells. *J Biol Chem* 1988;263:8557–68.

107. Shigeno C, Hiraki Y, Westerberg DP, Potts JT Jr, Segre GV. Photoaffinity labeling of parathyroid hormone receptors in clonal rat osteosarcoma cells. *J Biol Chem* 1988;263:3864–71.

108. Mayer GP, Habener JF, Potts JT Jr. Parathyroid hormone secretion in vivo: demonstration of a calcium-independent, nonsuppressible component of secretion. *J Clin Invest* 1976;57:678–83.

109. Riggs BL, Arnaud CD, Reynolds JC, Smith LH. Immunologic differentiation of primary hyperparathyroidism from hyperparathyroidism due to nonparathyroid cancer. *J Clin Invest* 1971;50:2079–83.

110. Bordier PJ, Marie PJ, Arnaud CD. Evolution of renal osteodystrophy: correlation of bone histomorphometry and serum mineral and immunoreactive parathyroid hormone values before and after treatment with calcium carbonate or 25-hydroxycholecalciferol. *Kidney Int* 1975;7(Suppl 2):S102–12.

111. Arnaud CD, Wilson DM, Smith LH. Primary hyperparathyroidism, renal lithiasis and the measurement of parathyroid hormone in serum by radioimmunoassay. In: Cifuentes-delante L, Rapado A, Hodgkinson A, eds. *Urinary calculi: recent advances in aetiology, stone structure and treatment.* New York: Karger, 1973;346–53.

112. McCarthy JT, Klee GG, Kao PC, Hodgson SF. Serum bioactive parathyroid hormone in hemodialysis patients. *J Clin Endocrinol Metab* 1989;68:340–5.

113. Hruska KA, Teitlebaum SL, Kopelman R, et al. The predictability of the histologic features of uremic bone disease by non-invasive techniques. *Metab Bone Dis Rel Res* 1978;1:39–44.

114. Voigts A, Felsenfeld AJ, Andress D, Llach F. Parathyroid hormone and bone histology: response to hypocalcemia in osteitis fibrosa. *Kidney Int* 1984;25:445–52.

115. Andress DL, Endres DB, Maloney NA, Kopp JB, Coburn JW, Sherrard DJ. Comparison of parathyroid hormone assays with bone histomorphometry in renal osteodystrophy. *J Clin Endocrinol Metab* 1986;63:1163–9.

116. Kopp JB, Andress DL, Maloney N, Sherrard DJ. Bone aluminum accumulation in hemodialysis patients: a longitudinal perspective. *Am J Kidney Dis* 1988;12:214–9.

117. Andress DL, Ott SM, Maloney NA, Sherrard DJ. Effect of parathyroidectomy on aluminum accumulation in chronic renal failure. *N Engl J Med* 1985;312:468–73.

118. St. John A, Davies C, Riley WJ, et al. Comparison of the performance and clinical utility of a carboxyl-terminal assay and an intact assay for parathyroid hormone. *Clin Chim Acta* 1988; 178:215–23.

119. Endres DB, Villanueva R, Sharp CF, Singer FR. Measurement of parathyroid hormone. *Endocrinol Metab Clin North Am* 1989;18:611–29.

120. Benson RC Jr, Riggs BL, Pickard BM, Arnaud CD. Radioimmunoassay of parathyroid hormone in hypercalcemic patients with malignant disease. *Am J Med* 1974;56:821–6.

121. Levin KE, Clark OH. Localization of parathyroid glands. *Annu Rev Med* 1988;39:29–40.

122. Hawker CD, Clark SW, Martin KJ, Slatopolsky E, DiBella FP. Radioimmunoassay of parathyroid hormone: clinical utility and interpretation. Thompson NW, Vinik AI, eds. *Endocrine surgery update.* New York: Grune & Stratton, 1983;321–40.

Disorders of Bone and Mineral Metabolism,
edited by Fredric L. Coe and Murray J. Favus,
Published by Raven Press, Ltd., 1992.

CHAPTER 6

The Target Tissue Actions of Parathyroid Hormone

Lorraine A. Fitzpatrick, Daniel T. Coleman, and John P. Bilezikian

Parathyroid hormone (PTH) helps to maintain calcium homeostasis by regulating the circulating concentration of ionized calcium through key actions at several target organs. The major signal for a change in PTH secretion from the parathyroid glands is the free or ionized calcium concentration. Extremely sensitive to any perturbation of calcium, even within the normal range, the parathyroid cell responds with an increase in PTH secretion if calcium declines, or with a decrease in PTH secretion if calcium increases. The cellular mechanisms in the parathyroid cell responsible for this exquisite and rather unusual sensitivity to calcium have been reviewed in Chapter 4. Knowledge of the circulating species of PTH, their metabolism, and assays developed to measure the circulating concentration of PTH have all been reviewed in Chapter 5. In this chapter we focus upon the biochemical mechanisms utilized by PTH to influence cellular events. A review of the physiological actions of PTH is included to provide perspective on the subject.

PHYSIOLOGICAL ACTIONS OF PTH

Bone

Catabolic Actions

Parathyroid hormone indirectly activates the osteoclast, the bone cell responsible for bone resorption, resulting in short-term and long-term effects. In both situa-

L. A. Fitzpatrick: Endocrine Research Unit, Mayo Clinic and Foundation, Rochester, Minnesota 55905.

D. T. Coleman: Metabolic Diseases Branch, NIDDK, National Institutes of Health, Bethesda, Maryland 20892.

J. P. Bilezikian: Departments of Medicine and Pharmacology, Columbia University, College of Physicians and Surgeons, New York, New York 10032

tions, the result is a net release of calcium into the extracellular space. The complexity of the skeleton as a tissue has made precise evaluation of the cellular effects of PTH on the osteoclast a difficult task. In order to determine how the net actions of PTH can be explained by direct events in bone cells, in vivo and in vitro studies have been utilized. Each study design has advantages and disadvantages. In vitro approaches involving embryonic bone in organ culture preparations allow for quantification of indices of bone resorption, but identification of the cell types involved has been difficult to determine. In in vivo experimental systems, the effects of PTH are not isolated from their familiar physiological milieu, permitting the participation of influential factors and/or mediators such as growth factors, cytokines, and other active agents that are generated locally during the process of bone remodeling. These factors would not necessarily be generated in simple bone cell culture models. Nevertheless, the combination of both kinds of experimental approaches has led to a number of insights into the cellular actions of PTH. This information is briefly reviewed here. More extensive discussion of the topic can be found in Chapters 7, 13, 15, 17, 24 and 31.

Cells lining the endosteal surfaces of bone release radiolabeled calcium in less than 1 h after administration of PTH (1). This initial rapid response to PTH involves structural changes of endosteal surface cells and is an important regulatory mechanism for maintenance of calcium homeostasis. Similarly, PTH rapidly mobilizes calcium in vivo in as early as 3 h after administration, a process that does not require new protein synthesis. This first phase of PTH action is associated with increased metabolic activity of osteoclasts. A second phase of calcium mobilization, which is dependent upon protein synthesis, occurs within 24 h of administration of PTH. This second phase is notable for an increase both in the number and metabolic activity of osteoclasts. It is of interest, however, that a direct effect of PTH on the osteoclast has not been demonstrated (2). On the other hand, PTH is known to have direct effects on the osteoblast, the cell responsible for bone formation (3–12). Key actions of PTH on the osteoblast are inhibition of type I collagen synthesis, stimulation of collagenase synthesis, and reduction of alkaline phosphatase activity (13–15). These actions are dependent upon the concentration of PTH (16).

Increases in osteoclast number and in osteoclast function could occur through intercellular signals generated as a consequence of the direct effects of PTH on the osteoblast (17). In fact, incubation of osteoclasts with osteoblast-like cells induces PTH responsiveness. Abundant evidence obtained by binding and by biochemical studies indicate a direct action of PTH on osteoblast cells. It is also possible that osteoclast activation occurs via an effect of PTH on precursor cells in the lineage of the osteoclast such as skeletal mononuclear cells (18).

These observations have led to the concept of "coupling," a process by which an intercellular signal is generated by PTH's target cell to influence, in turn, a cell (such as the osteoclast) that does not appear to be able to recognize PTH directly. The signal generated by the osteoblast may be definable factors which are released by the activated cell (19–21). One such candidate is interleukin-6, which is produced by osteoblasts in response to PTH (22). Interleukin-6 has been implicated in osteoclastogenesis (23). Several investigators have demonstrated the production of insulin-like growth factor 1 (IGF-1) and insulin-like growth factor 2 (IGF-2) by PTH-stimulated osteoblasts and have proposed a role for these factors in the coupling event (24,25). PTH enhances messenger RNA for IGF-1 in osteoblast-rich cell cultures (26). In addition to the induction of these factors by PTH in osteoblast-like cells, PTH has been shown under other experimental conditions to work synergistically with factors to resorb bone. For example, bone resorption in organ cultures is synergistically enhanced by the simultaneous presence of PTH and interleukin-1. On the other hand, negative interactions between PTH and transforming growth factor beta (TGF-β) have been observed such that PTH prevents binding of TGF-β to osteoblast-like cells (27).

Although it is clear that PTH stimulates osteoclast-mediated bone resorption, biochemical mechanisms of this effect are incompletely understood. Enzymes and other systems released or activated as a result of the metabolic events triggered by PTH include collagenase, lysosomal hydroxylases, acid phosphatases, carbonic anhydrase, H$^+$,K$^+$-ATPases, Na$^+$–Ca^{2+} exchange systems, cathepsin B, and cysteine protease. During bone resorption, an acidic extracellular environment is necessary for protonation of the alkaline salt hydroxyapatite. Ultrastructural studies of the osteoclast indicate that this acidic microenvironment is created by specialized structures in the osteoclast membrane (called "podosomes") that partially seal off the space between the osteoclast and the mineralized surface (see Chapter 10). Several enzymes have been identified in the generation of this acidic microenvironment. H$^+$,K$^+$-ATPase is similar to the proton pump in renal intercalated cells (28). Inhibition of this proton pump by omeprazole blocks PTH-mediated bone resorption (29). This ATPase activity has been localized by immunocytochemistry to the cell-bone attachment site and is present in the ruffled border, the resorptive site of the osteoclast (30). Carbonic anhydrase, another enzyme activated by PTH, may generate hydrogen ion to provide the H$^+$,K$^+$-ATPase proton pump with substrate. It has been documented that patients with osteopetrosis fail to resorb bone properly and are lacking carbonic anhydrase (type II) in skeletal tissue. PTH stimulates the action of carbonic anhydrase II, and PTH-mediated bone resorption is attenuated by the inhibition of this enzyme (31). Several investigators have proposed an important role for Na$^+$–Ca^{2+} exchange in bone resorption by the osteoclast. Amiloride and its analogue, 3'4'-dichlorobenzamil (DCB), inhibited PTH-induced bone resorption in neonatal mouse calvaria (32). DCB can also affect other calcium transport systems such as ATP-dependent calcium pumps, which may also play a role in bone resorption. Other studies indicate that PTH is not required for buffering of protons in neonatal mouse calvaria and that PTH may instead inhibit proton buffering by bone (33).

Anabolic Actions

The catabolic actions of PTH are initiated by effects upon the osteoblasts. PTH has other actions on the osteoblast that lead to its classification as an anabolic agent (34). Under physiological conditions, PTH is important for normal bone remodeling, which could indicate a predominant site of positive action at the level of the osteoblast. In addition, PTH stimulates formation of prostaglandin E$_2$ and 6-keto-prostaglandin F$_{2\alpha}$ in cultured mouse calvarial bone (35,36). Prostaglandin E$_2$ may mediate an increase in osteoblast precursor replication leading to stimulation of bone formation. It is of interest that both catabolic and anabolic actions of PTH appear to be mediated by the osteoblast. The anabolic effects are evident at low doses of PTH and include an increase in osteoblast number, alkaline phosphatase activity, and incorporation of sulfate into cartilage (Chapter 11). These effects are clearly different from the biochemical effects of PTH on the osteoblast when higher doses are employed (see above).

In vivo, anabolic actions can be demonstrated with intermittent, low-dose administration of PTH which, in the experience of some investigators, has led to impressive increases in bone mineral density (37). Under abnormal conditions such as those associated with excess PTH, the signaling mechanisms leading to osteoclast activation predominate, accounting for the resorptive effects of the hormone on bone.

In primary hyperparathyroidism, the physiological actions of PTH on bone formation and bone resorption are exaggerated, leading to clinical and histomorphometric evidence for increased bone turnover (38). It has become apparent that PTH has differential effects on the skeleton depending upon the composition of bone. Most sensitive to the actions of PTH is cortical bone, which constitutes the major structural form in the appendicular skeleton (38,39). In contrast, PTH appears to protect against net bone loss of the axial skeleton, which is comprised predominantly of cancellous bone. This clinical observation has been documented by a number of studies (38–45) and confirmed by detailed analysis of bone biopsy specimens (38,39,44) in primary hyperparathyroidism. The relatively selective actions of PTH on different regions of the skeleton are not understood at the cellular level.

Kidney

The kidney shares the spotlight with bone as a principal target organ of PTH action. PTH is known classically as a phosphaturic agent leading to a decrease in the tubular reabsorption of phosphate. The ability of PTH to induce phosphaturia was the basis for the first clinically useful test to monitor renal PTH responsiveness, the Ellsworth–Howard test (46). Recent studies localized the site of this action of PTH to the proximal convoluted tubule and the pars recta (47). To a lesser extent, phosphate reabsorption is inhibited by PTH in the distal tubule. The action of PTH to induce renal phosphate loss is of interest in light of its actions to mobilize skeletal calcium and phosphate. When PTH secretion is stimulated by a reduction in the ionized calcium, the net effects on the circulating concentrations of calcium and phosphate are to restore the serum calcium level without inducing any change in serum phosphate concentration. The phosphate released from bone is filtered by the kidney; as a result of the renal action of PTH, this phosphate is not reabsorbed. On the other hand, in the pathophysiology of primary hyperparathyroidism, the incompletely regulated secretion of PTH leads to excessive phosphaturia presumably not matched by skeletal phosphate mobilization, resulting in serum phosphate levels in the low to low-normal range.

PTH is a calcium-conserving hormone. This point is best illustrated by its action to increase fractional reabsorption of calcium from the glomerular fluid (Chapter 1). The sites of this effect appear to be in the thick ascending limb of the loop of Henle, in the distal convoluted tubule, and in the early portion of the cortical collecting tubule (48). The physiological importance of this property is obvious because it helps to maintain the serum calcium in response to a reduction in serum calcium concentration. A more complex set of regulatory principles governing both calcium and phosphate handling is illustrated by the example of hypocalcemia induced by a dietary-based increase in serum phosphate levels. Under these conditions, PTH helps to return both the calcium and phosphate concentrations to normal by enhancing and reducing tubular reabsorption of these two ions, respectively.

Under pathophysiological conditions, PTH induces a state of negative calcium balance despite its actions to conserve renal tubular calcium. It is not unusual, in fact, for patients with primary hyperparathyroidism to demonstrate hypercalciuria. The apparent explanation for this observation is the greater filtered load of calcium that accompanies the state of hypercalcemia. The amount of calcium filtered at the glomerulus exceeds even the enhanced capacity for renal tubular calcium conservation. But for any serum calcium level, the presence of PTH will be associated with reduced urinary calcium excretion when compared with urinary calcium excretion seen at the same calcium level in the absence of hormone.

A rapid and consistent increase in urinary cyclic adenosine monophosphate (cAMP) excretion is a characteristic action of PTH. It precedes the phosphaturic actions of PTH. The fundamental observation originally made by Chase and Aurbach (49) gave impetus to the hypothesis that the second messenger responsible for the renal actions of PTH is cAMP. A wealth of data is now available in further support of this hypothesis (see below). The observation has also given rise to a modification of the Ellsworth–Howard test in which urinary cAMP excretion is used instead of phosphate excretion as the renal marker of PTH responsiveness.

Another key renal action of PTH is the stimulation of 1,25-dihydroxyvitamin D_3 [$1,25(OH)_2D_3$] formation. The enzyme responsible for the conversion of 25-hydroxyvitamin D to 1,25-dihydroxyvitamin D, renal 1α-hydroxylase, is located in the proximal tubule (50). PTH appears to be one of the two main stimuli for activation of this enzyme, as shown in studies of PTH administration (51) and in vivo when PTH secretion is stimulated (52) (Fig. 1). The other stimulus to 1,25-dihydroxyvitamin D formation is a reduction in serum phosphate concentration. This renal effect of PTH accounts for the indirect actions of PTH to stimulate gastrointestinal absorption of calcium, an action that is directly mediated by 1,25-dihydroxyvitamin D.

Finally, PTH is known to alter acid–base handling in the kidney. Proximal tubular acidosis is accounted for by the effect of PTH to inhibit bicarbonate transport in the pars recta (34). Although this action is well established, it is rarely of sufficient magnitude to be of pathophysiologi-

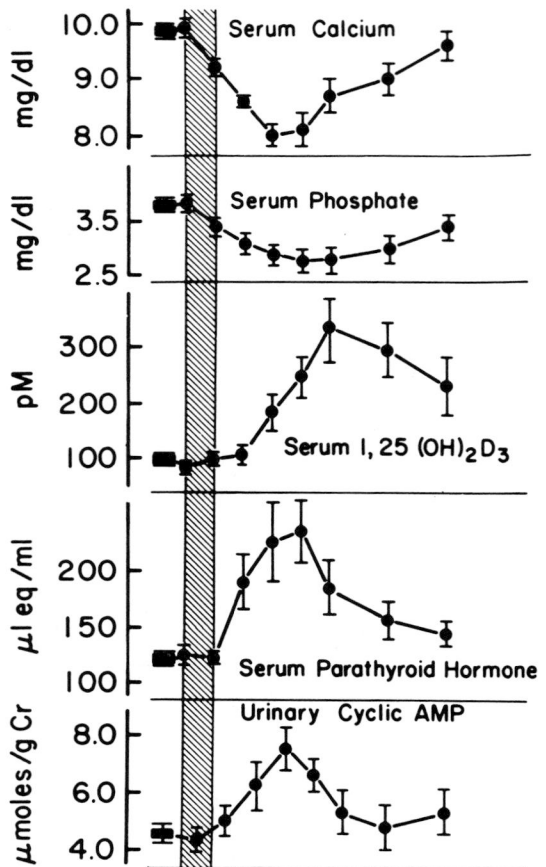

FIG. 1. Response of 1,25(OH)$_2$D$_3$, PTH, and urinary cAMP to hypocalcemia. Eight patients with Paget's disease received plicamycin (25 μg/kg) by intravenous infusion. The rapid decline in serum calcium is followed by increases in PTH and 1,25(OH)$_2$D$_3$. [Modified from Bilezikian et al. (52).]

cal importance in states of PTH excess. Patients with primary hyperparathyroidism tend to show a mild hyperchloremic, compensated metabolic acidosis, but it is of no major clinical significance. The mild acidosis cannot even be used reliably to distinguish between PTH-dependent and PTH-independent hypercalcemic conditions.

Other Tissues

Despite the fact that the overwhelming body of knowledge of PTH action has focused upon the skeleton and the kidney, effects in other tissues have been reported to have potential physiological relevance.

Cartilage

PTH may be responsible for the cellular differentiation of cartilage. The hormone localizes to cartilage growth plates, implicating a role for PTH in growth and differentiation in the zone of transition from cartilage to endochondral bone. In the growth-plate chondrocyte, PTH stimulates proteoglycan synthesis (53). PTH also decreases formation of alkaline-phosphatase-rich matrix vesicles and increases protein synthesis and cell division in chicken epiphyseal growth-plate chondrocytes. The elevation in PTH that occurs with decreasing concentrations of extracellular calcium inhibits mineral deposition and may allow mobilization of calcium from stores in the growth plate (54).

Cardiovascular Effects

PTH causes hypotension in several species of vertebrates, but the effect is selective in the vessels that are affected in each species. This subject has recently been extensively reviewed (55). In humans, an increase in pulse pressure and heart rate occurs within 5–10 min after administration of PTH (56). Purified extract or synthetic analogues of PTH cause hypotension, suggesting that hypotension is a biological property of the PTH molecule and not the results of a contaminant in partially purified preparations. The ability of PTH to cause hypotension is the result of direct vascular relaxation rather than a decrease in cardiac output (57). Within a given species, PTH relaxes only certain blood vessels, with differences in efficacy and potency. It is more effective in relaxing resistance-type vessels than in relaxing conduit-type vessels. In both in vivo and in vitro experiments, PTH is an effective vasorelaxant even when the extracellular calcium concentration is kept constant, suggesting that neither the transient hypocalcemia that occurs after PTH administration nor the subsequent longer-term hypercalcemia is directly responsible for the hypotensive effect. Synthetic bPTH(1–34) and hPTH(1–34) produce hypotension in several species, suggesting that the recognition site of the receptor must be present in the first 34 amino acids. Surprisingly, among a diverse array of peptides tested, PTH is one of the most effective and long-lived peptides to cause hypotension. This area is under intense investigation because the mechanisms of hypotension, as well as their possible physiological implications, remain obscure.

The clinical association between hypertension and primary hyperparathyroidism suggests that PTH may have the opposite effect on the vasculature in the setting of this chronic disorder. In one study, the prevalence rate of hypertension in patients with primary hyperparathyroidism was 48% as compared to 35% in controls (58). Few studies have evaluated the potential causes of hypertension, and some investigators suggest that hypertension does not correlate with increased levels of serum calcium or PTH. One study suggested that plasma levels of cortisol and renin activity were significantly increased in these patients, perhaps accounting for increased blood pressure. Others have suggested a parathyroid origin for a specific hypertension factor. Despite the clinical association between hypertension and primary hyperparathyroidism, one of Koch's postulates has not been fulfilled if there is to be established an etiologic link: Successful surgical removal of the abnormal parathyroid tissue in primary hyperparathyroidism has little effect on the hypertension.

Gastrointestinal Tract

The gastrointestinal tract is regarded as an "indirect" target tissue for PTH. It promotes calcium absorption in the duodenum through its ability to stimulate the production of 1,25-dihydroxyvitamin D. PTH stimulates gastrin release directly (55) and has a relaxant effect on gastrointestinal smooth muscle (59,60). Physiologically, it has been proposed that smooth muscle cells are sensitive to changes in extracellular calcium and that the ability of PTH to relax smooth muscle could counteract an increase in muscle tone or sensitivity as the hormone increases extracellular calcium.

Neuronal Tissue

The effects of uremia on the central nervous system have been attributed, in part, to the increase in PTH that regularly accompanies the uremic state. The available data, however, do not yet present a convincing argument that there is a cause-and-effect relationship between the secondary hyperparathyroidism of renal insufficiency and the dysfunction of the central nervous system. Most of the evidence has focused upon the actions of PTH on cellular calcium metabolism in the central nervous system. Calcium channels are important in the transducing signals generated by neurotransmitters; furthermore, in mouse neuroblastoma cells, bovine PTH(1–34) inhibited (in a concentration-dependent fashion) the L-type calcium current (61). It was suggested that PTH might be an endogenous inhibitor of calcium entry in certain tissues. Perna et al. (62) evaluated the effect of PTH on the metabolism of neurotransmitters in brain synaptosomes of rats with chronic renal failure. Synaptosomes in rats with chronic renal failure have higher calcium content than do synaptosomes in normal rats. Parathyroidectomy reversed these abnormalities. Other investigators have presented evidence that the content of total phospholipids (phosphatidylinositol, phosphatidylserine, and phosphatidylethanolamine) in synaptosomes derived from rats with chronic renal failure is lower than that in normal controls (63).

Fibroblasts

Several investigators have described the presence of PTH receptors in primary cultures of human fibroblasts (64,65). Pun and Ho (65) described two different binding sites for PTH with high ($K_d = 2$ nM) and low ($K_d = 580$ nM) affinities. The IC_{50} for adenylate cyclase activity in fibroblasts is 2 nM, similar to the K_d of the high-affinity binding site. These findings have been confirmed by others (66). The production of cAMP in response to PTH in cultured human dermal fibroblasts has been used to study defects in guanine nucleotide protein activity in pseudohypoparathyroidism (67).

MECHANISMS OF PTH ACTION

Knowledge of the cellular mechanisms responsible for the physiological actions of PTH received great impetus when it was discovered that PTH belongs to the family of polypeptide hormones that stimulate cAMP formation. The second-messenger hypothesis, which states that the external signal generated by hormone is transmitted to a cellular event by cAMP, has dominated hypothetical constructs of PTH action over the past 25 years. The discovery of cAMP and of its role as a second messenger has helped to validate further the receptor theory of hormone action, a hypothesis requiring the existence of a highly specific binding site in the plasma membrane of the cell with which the hormone could interact (68). In contrast to many other adenylate-cyclase-linked hormones for which receptors have been purified, cloned, and expressed, the PTH receptor has proven to be elusive. Nevertheless, it is likely that the general configuration and topography of known receptors that belong to this family will also be shown for the PTH receptor when it is ultimately purified. Understanding of adenylate-cyclase-linked receptors led eventually to a more complete understanding of the hormone receptor unit. We now appreciate that the hormone receptor complex consists of several components besides the hormone receptor and adenylate cyclase. For example, guanine-nucleotide-binding proteins occupy a critical place in transducing the hormonal signal from receptor to effector. In addition, effector systems besides adenylate cyclase are known to be activated as a consequence of hormone-receptor–G-protein interaction. PTH participates as a full member of the family of hormones coupled to adenylate cyclase in that it is dependent upon guanine-nucleotide-binding proteins. Many members of this family of hormones have also been shown to activate other effector systems besides adenylate cyclase. Mounting evidence indicates that PTH activates other second-messenger systems in bone and in kidney. The remainder of this chapter concentrates on this broad area of signal transduction as it relates to PTH.

Stimulation of Adenylate Cyclase Activity by PTH

Although a discussion of adenylate cyclase activation by PTH might logically be considered to belong after a discussion of the PTH receptor and the guanine-nucleotide-binding proteins to which it is linked, it is discussed first because of the primary place the enzyme enjoys in the historical development of our concepts of the PTH receptor unit. The early discovery that administration of PTH leads to an increase in urinary cAMP in human subjects (49) was followed by the demonstration that cAMP can mimic many, if not all, of the renal actions of PTH (69). For example, cAMP is associated with renal phosphate loss, calcium retention, and activation of the 1α-hydroxylase necessary for 1,25-dihydroxyvitamin D synthesis. The effects of PTH in bone cells have also been attributed to cAMP (11,70). In broken-cell preparations of renal cortex and fetal rat calvaria, adenylate cyclase is stimulated directly by PTH (71,72).

As knowledge of the protein structure of PTH became available (Fig. 2), detailed structure–function studies were conducted to determine those aspects of the PTH molecule required for activation of adenylate cyclase. The most fundamental observation in this regard is that the full-length 84-amino-acid polypeptide hormone is not required for complete expression of the adenylate-

cyclase-stimulating properties of the hormone. A much shorter amino-terminal fragment, PTH(1–34), is as potent as the intact molecule (73–77). Fragments consisting of larger carboxy-terminal fragments of PTH, such as PTH(54–84), do not stimulate adenylate cyclase activity. Metabolism of PTH in the liver leads to the generation of several smaller peptides, one of which is PTH(1–34) or an analogue closely related to it. Hepatic metabolism of PTH does not lead to the release of this fragment into the circulation; instead, it leads to further proteolytic digestion. Nevertheless, the demonstration that a fully active but shorter form of PTH is produced in vivo has raised speculation that at target tissues an active fragment might be produced (similar to the metabolism of full-length PTH in the liver) and act locally to affect the cellular consequences of PTH action. It still is not known whether the physiological effects of PTH are due to the 1- to 84-amino-acid polypeptide or whether some, or all, of the actions of PTH can be attributed to the shorter amino-terminal fragment. In view of the fact that

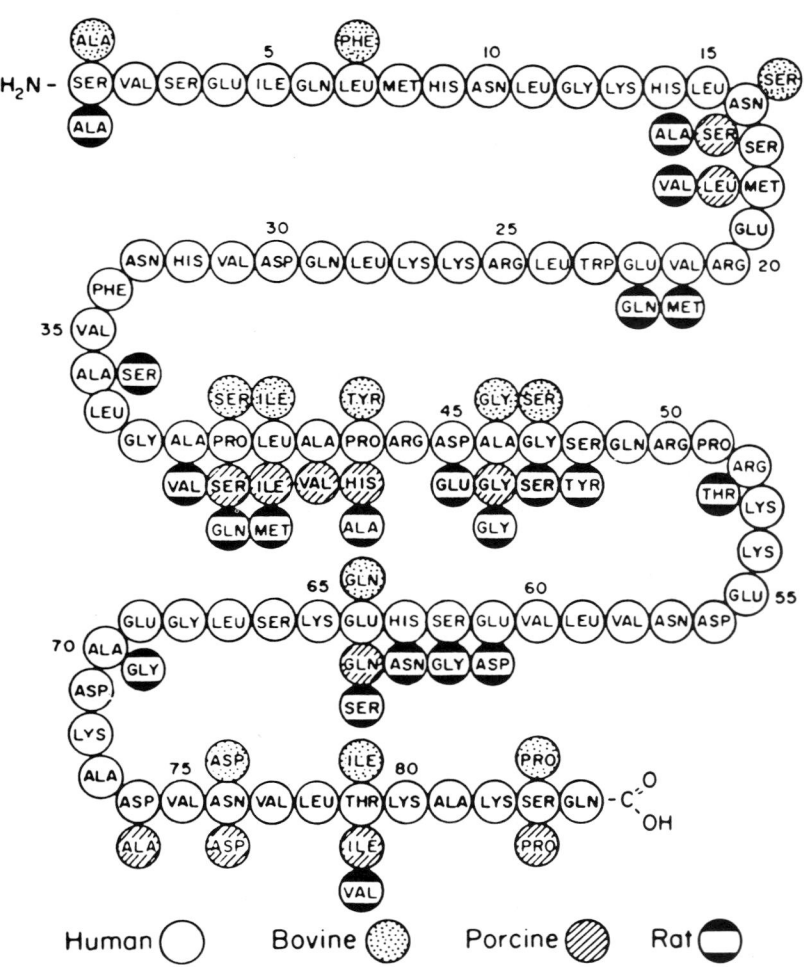

FIG. 2. Primary structure of mammalian PTH. The amino acid sequence of mammalian PTH(1–84) is shown comparing human (backbone sequence) with bovine, porcine, and rat hormones as indicated.

this shorter fragment does not appear to escape from the liver into the circulation, an important physiological role for the amino-terminal fragment is less compelling. In Chapter 5, a more extensive discussion of the peripheral metabolism of PTH is provided.

Stepwise deletion of amino acids from the carboxy-terminal end of the 1–34 fragment of PTH leads to progressive loss in adenylate-cyclase-stimulating properties (74). Amino-terminal fragments of PTH shorter than PTH(1–25) are inactive. It is believed that the region defined by amino acid positions 25–34 facilitates the binding of PTH to its receptor (78–81). In contrast to the gradual loss of adenylate-cyclase-stimulating properties when carboxy-terminal amino acids are sequentially removed from PTH(1–34), stepwise removal of amino-terminal amino acids from position 1 leads to a dramatic loss in adenylate-cyclase-stimulating properties. PTH(2–34), for example, is a markedly weaker agonist than PTH(1–34), highlighting the importance of the amino acid position 1. Presumably, the binding region, 25–34, remains intact in PTH(2–34) despite the loss in bioactivity. These observations have led to the hypothesis that the amino-terminal end of PTH is responsible for activation but is not required for binding to the receptor.

Design of effective PTH antagonists has taken advantage of these points—namely, that foreshortened peptides at the amino-terminal end of the molecule are relatively inactive but probably bind to the PTH receptor. The analogue of PTH lacking the first two amino-terminal amino acids, PTH(3–34), is a very effective competitive antagonist in vitro. This analogue, however, does have weak agonist features in vivo. Further truncation of the amino terminus, along with amidation of the carboxy terminus, leads to even more effective antagonists such as PTH(7–34)amide, a potent antagonist possessing neither in vitro nor in vivo agonist properties. These observations have led to a model of the 1–34 fragment of PTH in which domains of activation, inhibition, and binding have been defined (Fig. 3) (73). The elegant work by Rosenblatt (73) predicted information that was confirmed when it became possible to measure PTH-receptor interactions with specific radioligands (see below).

The gold standard for the structure–function studies that established the importance of various amino acid positions was the adenylate cyclase assay. The relative stimulatory or inhibitory potencies of various fragments of PTH in in vivo bioassays have correlated well in gen-

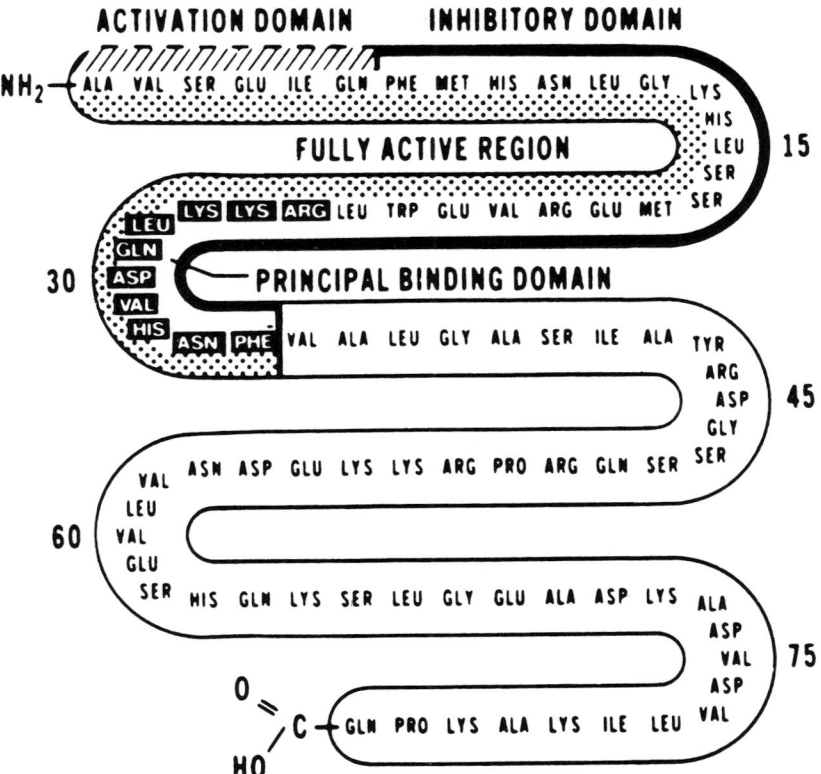

FIG. 3. Model of PTH structure–activity relationships based on binding and adenylate cyclase activation properties. The amino acid sequence of intact bPTH(1–84) is shown. The region containing full biological activity [PTH(1–34)] is indicated by stippling. Within this stippled region are the activation and inhibitory domains as noted. Amino acids indicated by white lettering on a black background are believed to be directly involved in binding to the PTH receptor. [From (73).]

eral with their relative potencies in in vitro assays of adenylate cyclase activity (73,76). However, discrepancies in this relationship are not unexpected, due to major differences in experimental conditions between in vivo and in vitro assay conditions. This point has impeded experimental design of effective PTH antagonists when the in vitro assay for adenylate cyclase is relied upon exclusively. Rosenblatt (73) has demonstrated that the conventional adenylate cyclase assay may not be sensitive enough to detect latent agonist properties of some of these analogues. He has observed that responsiveness of adenylate cyclase to PTH in osteoblast-like ROS 17/2.8 cells is markedly amplified when the cells are previously exposed to dexamethasone and/or pertussis toxin (82). After exposure to dexamethasone and pertussis toxin, the ability of the antagonist peptide [Nleu[8,18]Tyr[34]]b-PTH(3–34)amide to stimulate adenylate cyclase increases from a modest 3-fold to an impressive 10-fold. Even the more specific antagonist [Tyr[34]]bPTH(7–34)amide, which has no agonist properties under conventional assay conditions, becomes a mild agonist when cells are first incubated with dexamethasone and pertussis toxin. This supersensitive in vitro analysis has led to the development of an analogue of PTH that has absolutely no agonist properties in vitro (reference 83). Substitutions at amino acids 10 and 11 led to the development of such a peptide, indicating that the activation domain of PTH previously believed to include amino acids 1–6 should be extended beyond that shown in Fig. 3, to position 12. This kind of analytical approach to in vitro assessment of latent agonist properties of PTH analogues may well lead to the design of peptides that can be shown both in vitro and in vivo to have no agonist properties whatsoever. This approach also has the potential to develop compounds that are superagonists.

Another explanation for discrepancies between agonist properties of PTH in in vitro and in vivo assays for adenylate cyclase is that PTH may utilize second messengers other than cAMP. Several investigators have exploited the fact that PTH(2–34), virtually inactive in the conventional adenylate cyclase assay, can induce substantial hypercalcemia and phosphaturia in various in vivo models (74,84). The well-known antagonist, [Nleu[8,18]Tyr[34]]bPTH(3–34)amide, is a weak agonist in dogs (85) and rats (86) and induces hypercalcemia, phosphaturia, and increased plasma 1,25(OH)₂D₃ concentrations. This peptide can induce the same effects upon urinary phosphate and plasma 1,25(OH)₂D₃ levels as bPTH(1–34) but requires 50- to 100-fold higher concentrations to reach maximal response (85–87). One might account for these observations by the information reviewed above—namely, that the PTH(3–34)amide antagonist can now be shown, under very special conditions, to have in vitro adenylate-cyclase-stimulating properties. However, the special conditions required to demonstrate agonism in the adenylate cyclase assay does

not necessarily indicate that the enzyme is stimulated in vivo or that it is responsible for the physiological effects seen. One might have a situation in which the ability of PTH analogues to stimulate adenylate cyclase activity under these conditions does not reflect the use of the cAMP pathway by these fragments in vivo.

The Phosphatidylinositol Pathway of Hormone Action

Discrepancies in the structure–activity relationships between features required for adenylate cyclase activation and those required for physiological effects are likely to be clues to the structural requirements of putative non-cAMP-mediated responses. Perhaps the most widely recognized response to PTH that cannot be easily ascribed to cAMP mechanisms is that related to changes in intracellular free calcium. At the physiological level, an intriguing transient hypocalcemia noted prior to the hypercalcemic effects of PTH was a prescient observation (Fig. 4) (88,89). The early hypocalcemia can be explained by the action of PTH (which is now well-documented) to induce cellular uptake of calcium (90–96). Evidence that this response does not appear to be mediated by cAMP is supported by five lines of evidence: (i) Cyclic AMP cannot mimic the actions of PTH to raise intracellular free calcium in primary cultures of renal tubular cells (91). (ii) Repeated stimulation of these cells by PTH leads to desensitization of the cAMP response.

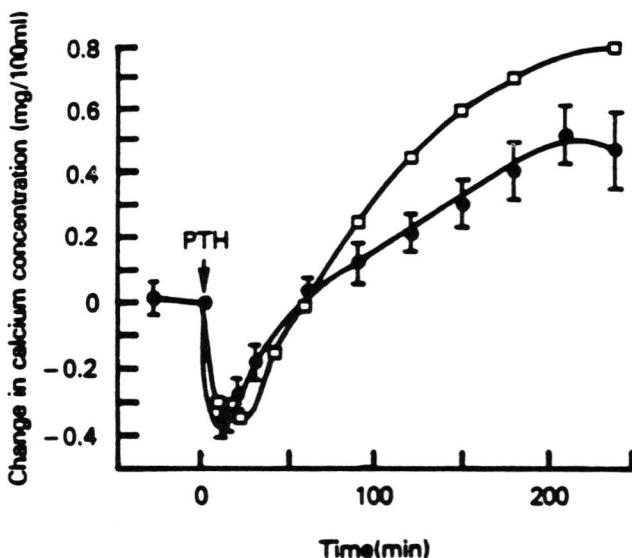

FIG. 4. Initial hypocalcemic actions of PTH. bPTH(1–34) induces a brief, transient hypocalcemia before causing hypercalcemia. Shown are data regarding administration of bPTH(1–34) to dogs in vivo (□) and to mouse calvaria in vitro (●). [From Parsons et al. (88) as modified by Aurbach et al. (245).]

However, the ability of PTH to increase intracellular free calcium is not altered by repeated exposure to PTH (90). (iii) Forskolin stimulates cellular cAMP and can thus mimic actions mediated by cAMP. Yet, the effect of PTH to elevate free calcium in osteoblast-like UMR-106 cells cannot be mimicked by forskolin (97). (iv) Rat brain synaptosomes do not show increases in cAMP after PTH exposure but do show large increases in calcium uptake (92). (v) The PTH analogue [Nleu^{8,18}Tyr^{34}]-PTH(3–34)amide, which inhibits PTH stimulation of adenylate cyclase, can elevate intracellular free calcium (93). In addition to the effects of PTH on intracellular calcium, recent observations of the renal phosphate transport system indicate that here, too, PTH's influence may be, in part, independent of cAMP (98–100).

The data indicating that non-cAMP-mediated actions of PTH are related to changes in intracellular calcium directed attention to a second-messenger system that has as one of its end points changes in cellular calcium. This system is characterized by hydrolysis of phosphoinositides in the plasma membrane of the cell. In the 1980s and now in the 1990s, the phosphatidylinositol pathway of hormone action has received enormous attention, rivaling that of the cAMP pathway in the 1960s and 1970s. It is clear now that hydrolysis of phosphatidylinositides leads to the generation of several messengers that have vitally important functions in transmitting the hormonal signal to the cell (101–104). The list of hormones shown to stimulate this pathway now rivals in length the list of hormones that stimulate cAMP accumulation. An intriguing observation in this regard is that hormones such as glucagon, vasopressin, catecholamines, and many others that stimulate cellular cAMP accumulation also stimulate the hydrolysis of phosphatidylinositides (103,105).

Features of Phosphatidylinositol Hydrolysis

The phosphatidylinositides are present in very small quantities in the plasma membrane of the cell. The three most important compounds are phosphatidylinositol (PI), phosphatidylinositol 4-phosphate (PIP), and phosphatidylinositol 4,5-bisphosphate (PIP$_2$) (Fig. 5). Through the action of PI kinase, PI is phosphorylated to PIP and is then further phosphorylated to PIP$_2$. A phosphatase activity provides for a dynamic steady state, under basal conditions, in which PIP$_2$ can be dephosphorylated to PIP and further dephosphorylated to PI. Also under basal conditions, hydrolysis of these substrates occurs whereby a fraction is converted, by the action of a family of enzymes known as "phospholipase C," to a series of products known as the "inositol phosphates" (IPs) (106–111). PI is hydrolyzed to inositol-1-monophosphate (IP$_1$); PIP is hydrolyzed to inositol 1,4-bisphosphate (IP$_2$); PIP$_2$ is hydrolyzed to inositol 1,4,5-trisphosphate (1,4,5-IP$_3$). In each case, diacylglycerol, another product of the hydrolysis, is formed. Diacylglycerol and its metabolites have their own important actions as a second messenger (112,113). Isomers of these IPs in which the phosphate in position 1 is cyclized to the 2 position are also produced by the action of phospholipase C, leading to the corresponding cyclic IP$_1$, cyclic IP$_2$, or cyclic IP$_3$ compounds (114–117). A pathway exists for further phosphorylation of 1,4,5-IP$_3$ to

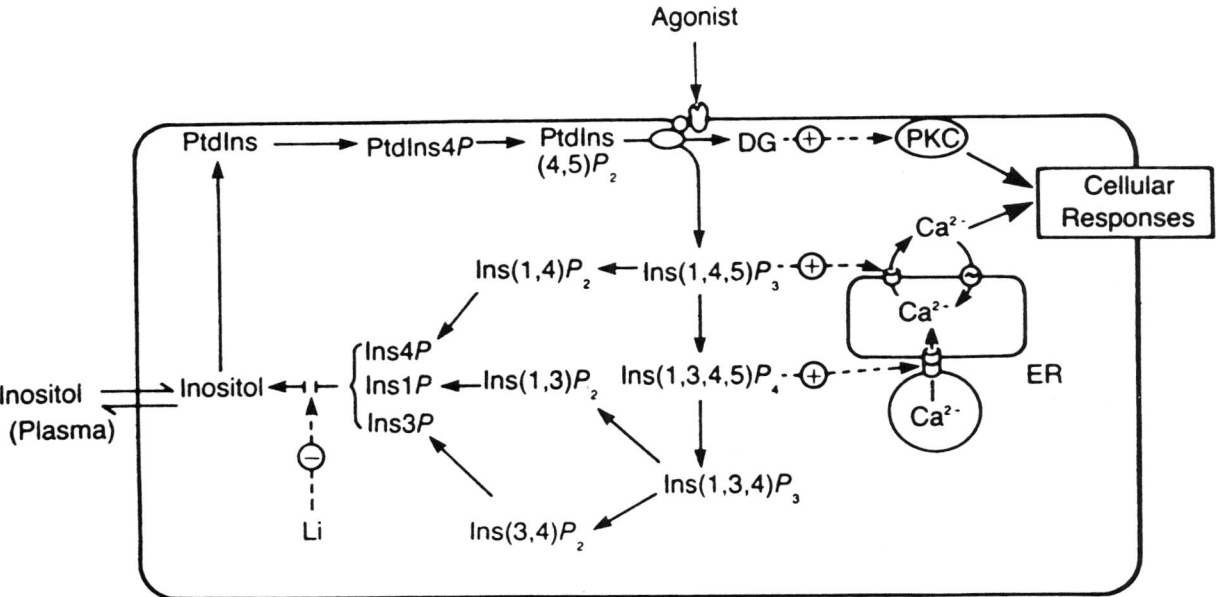

FIG. 5. Summary of major pathways involved in the metabolism of phosphatidylinositol. PtdIns, phosphatidylinositol; DG, diacylglycerol; ER, endoplasmic reticulum; PKC, protein kinase C. [From Berridge (246).]

1,3,4,5-inositol tetrakisphosphate (1,3,4,5-IP$_4$) by inositol 1,4,5-trisphosphate kinase (118–127). It has been shown recently that 1,3,4,5-IP$_4$ can also be formed by direct hydrolysis of a newly discovered substrate for phospholipase C, phosphatidylinositol-3,4,5-trisphosphate (PIP$_3$) (128). Direct hydrolysis of PIP$_3$ to 1,3,4,5-IP$_4$ is believed to be a less important pathway for IP$_4$ formation than phosphorylation of 1,4,5-IP$_3$.

1,3,4,5-IP$_4$ is dephosphorylated to an inactive and isomerically distinct inositol trisphosphate, 1,3,4-inositol trisphosphate (1,3,4-IP$_3$). The kinetics of formation of this product is slower than the formation of the active IP$_3$, namely 1,4,5-IP$_3$. When measures are not taken to distinguish biochemically between these two isomers of IP$_3$, the major product measured is the inactive compound. Although the formation and amount of total 1,3,4-IP$_3$ in a particular experimental setting may indicate the degree of activation of the pathway by agonist, it can be misleading if the kinetics and amount of this product are assumed to represent the time course, presence, or extent of activation of the 1,4,5-IP$_3$ signal (129–134). Direct assay of the active product, 1,4,5-IP$_3$, is a much more reliable indicator of agonist action. 1,3,4-IP$_3$ is subsequently further dephosphorylated to 1,3-IP$_2$ and 3,4-IP$_2$, leading to the monophosphates 1-IP$_1$ and 3-IP$_1$, respectively (127,135).

The active product, 1,4,5-IP$_3$, undergoes a series of dephosphorylation events catalyzed by a family of phosphatases leading to the production of a different set of IPs, namely, 1,4-IP$_2$ and 4-IP$_1$. 1-IP$_1$ [formed by the direct action of phospholipase C upon PI (136)] and 4-IP$_1$ (the product of PIP$_2$ hydrolysis) are subsequently metabolized to inositol. Inositol can then reenter the cycle by serving as a substrate for the formation of PI. Note that the IPs produced by the dephosphorylation of 1,4,5-IP$_3$ are, in general, different from the IPs produced by the direct hydrolysis of PIP and PI.

When this pathway is stimulated by an agonist such as PTH, preferential hydrolysis of the polyphosphoinositide present in the smallest concentration—namely PIP$_2$—occurs, leading to the generation of 1,4,5-IP$_3$. In many cases, another active IP, 1,3,4,5-IP$_4$, is quickly formed by phosphorylation of 1,4,5-IP$_3$. 1,4,5-IP$_3$ has been shown to mediate, in a direct fashion, the intracellular release of calcium from nonmitochondrial stores (113,137–140). The kinetics of 1,4,5-IP$_3$ formation and action are rapid, with peak levels of IP$_3$ and changes in intracellular calcium occurring literally within seconds of hormone exposure.

It is important to note that only a fraction of the phosphoinositides is available to serve as substrates for hormone-stimulated phospholipase C activity (141). Hormone-insensitive pools of PI have been identified in erythrocytes, blowfly salivary glands, WRK-1 mammary tumor cells, pancreatic islets, and GH$_3$ pituitary tumor cells (141–148). The size of the pool of hormone-sensitive PI relative to the total amount of PI appears to differ among tissues. Distinct pools of PIs with different turnover rates and different sites within the cell or even within the membrane itself have been described (141).

As can be appreciated, the activation pathway leading to the production of these IPs is exceedingly complex. It is complex, in part, because activation appears to be an intrinsic aspect of the inactivation pathway. For example, the mono- and diphosphate-containing IPs are believed to be inactive. Similarly, the dephosphorylation of 1,3,4,5-IP$_4$ leads to a series of inactive IPs. The number of IPs that could be produced theoretically as a result of hydroysis, metabolism, and interconversions is an astounding 64 compounds, many of which have already been isolated (118,119,149–153). It is possible that some of these compounds may not be mere metabolic products but may, instead, be active second messengers themselves.

Cellular Consequences of Active Inositol Phosphates

Perturbations in intracellular free calcium trigger many cellular events such as changes in adenylate cyclase, phosphodiesterase, phospholipase A$_2$, and protein kinase activities. These events, in turn, lead to a variety of cellular responses such as smooth muscle contraction, glycogenolysis, hormone secretion, and changes in electrical excitability (138,139,154–157). The means by which the cellular calcium signal is generated include three major mechanisms: (i) second-messenger-mediated release of intracellular calcium stores; (ii) second-messenger-mediated effects upon calcium-channel openings in the plasma membrane; and (iii) direct or guanine-nucleotide-mediated effects on calcium channels. 1,4,5-IP$_3$ is thought to be the second messenger responsible for rapid, transient calcium signals that occur in response to hormones that utilize this pathway. These rapid calcium transients are independent of extracellular calcium (101,112,113,138–140,158). However, calcium release from intracellular stores does become critically dependent upon extracellular calcium for replenishment. After the initial rapid perturbation in cellular calcium, there is a subsequent stimulation of calcium influx across the plasma membrane. The transmembrane flux of extracellular calcium is believed to be triggered by 1,3,4,5-IP$_4$, possibly by 1,4,5-IP$_3$, or by the combined actions of both IP$_4$ and IP$_3$ (159–164). In some tissues there is also evidence for calcium-activated calcium channels which open in response to an elevation in intracellular calcium (165).

The Effects of PTH on Phosphatidylinositol Hydrolysis

Evidence that PTH utilizes the PI pathway has strengthened to the point where it is generally accepted to be a mechanism of PTH action. Several investigators have demonstrated an effect of PTH to stimulate the metabolism of membrane phosphoinositides in a manner that reflects increased turnover of these substrates in renal tissue (166–170). Similar observations have been made in fetal rat limb bones by Rappaport and Stern (171).

In more direct studies, PTH has been shown to increase levels of IPs in intact bone cell preparations as well as in the kidney (172–173). In the opossum kidney (OK) cell line, Hruska et al. (174) have demonstrated a rapid increase in IP_3 release after exposure to PTH. A concomitant decrease in the amount of the substrate PIP_2 was also observed. These investigators have obtained similar data when PTH is exposed to primary cultures of canine proximal tubule cells. In the cultured osteoblast-like cell line ROS 17/2.8, Cosman et al. (175) showed significant stimulation of IP_3 formation by both full-length (1–84) and N-terminal (1–34) PTH.

The observations that PTH may stimulate turnover of the polyphosphoinositides and that net increases in IPs can be measured in response to the hormone suggest that PTH may stimulate the responsible enzyme, namely, phospholipase C. Direct assessment of enzyme activity requires the addition of known amounts of substrate and accurate determination of the amount of product formed. Such studies also require that the product formed is not subject to further metabolism. One might consider in this context the distinction between measuring cellular cAMP and adenylate cyclase activity. Measurement of cAMP does not always reflect the activity of the enzyme; similarly, measurement of IP does not necessarily reflect the activity of phospholipase C. Earlier studies of the IP signaling system were not directed to a measurement of enzyme activity. Studies were usually confined to observations of an increase in radioactivity in chromatographic fractions containing various IPs.

Although the data are still limited for PTH, they do suggest that PTH may be a direct agonist for phospholipase C activity (176,177). In an acute membrane preparation of renal cortical tubules, Coleman showed that PTH(1–34) rapidly increases levels of IP_1, IP_2, and IP_3 within the first 30 s of stimulation (176). The kinetics of the stimulation process indicate, as expected, that the most rapidly increasing IP is IP_3, followed by IP_2 and IP_1. Half-maximal stimulation occurs at approximately 8 nM, which is similar to the concentration required for half-maximal concentration of adenylate cyclase stimulation in the same preparation (Fig. 6). Furthermore, Coleman et al. (178) were able to show that PTH has no effect to alter the metabolism of 1,4,5-IP_3.

Changes in Intracellular Calcium Induced by PTH

The observations leading to the hypothesis that PTH stimulates the hydrolysis of PI were based initially on the ability of PTH to stimulate changes in cellular calcium in the absence of any functional linkage to cAMP. The data implicating PTH in the perturbation of cellular calcium are reviewed in this section.

In the osteosarcoma cell line, UMR-106, PTH induces a three-phase increase in cytosolic calcium: a rapid increase in the first few seconds, followed by a rapid decrease to basal levels within the first minute, followed by a slower increment in cellular calcium (179). The initial rise in intracellular calcium, as measured by fura-2, is inhibited by the calcium-channel blockers lanthanum and verapamil. Increased intracellular levels of cAMP or the addition of a stimulator of protein kinase C, phorbol ester, also blocked channel activity. The slow, incremental rise in intracellular calcium was mediated by intracellular cAMP and was relatively insensitive to calcium-channel antagonists. The authors concluded that UMR-106 cells respond to PTH stimulation by the activation of a cAMP-independent calcium channel. Further classification by this group of investigators led to the description of release of calcium from intracellular pools after activation of protein kinase C by phorbol esters (179). Reid et al. (180) also demonstrated that changes in intracellular calcium after stimulation of UMR-106 cells by PTH were independent of cAMP. The decrement in cytosolic calcium was due to inactivation of calcium channels.

PTH produces transient, concentration-dependent increases in cytosolic calcium in rat osteoblast-like cells (181). Changes in inositol phosphates and diacylglycerol also occur rapidly, consistent with their roles as signals for altering intracellular calcium concentrations. Pertussis toxin exposure reduced the PTH-stimulated elevations in intracellular calcium, suggesting a role for guanine regulatory protein in signal transduction. The fact that analogues of cAMP also reduced intracellular levels of calcium suggests that the adenylate cyclase pathway may serve to dampen the effects of the PI pathway. Using the photoprotein aequorin to determine the changes in intracellular calcium, Donahue et al. (182) showed agonist properties of rat PTH(1–34), bovine PTH(3–34), and bovine PTH(7–34) in ROS 17/2.8 cells. Studies on desensitization of ROS 17/2.8 cells have further underscored the importance of calcium as a physiological effector of PTH-stimulated PI hydrolysis. Exposure of cells to rat PTH(1–34) reduced the cAMP response to PTH but did not attenuate the PTH-induced rise in intracellular calcium (183).

The physiological actions of PTH to regulate the renal tubular handling of calcium, as reviewed in an earlier section, is likely to be directly related to actions of PTH on cellular calcium. In OK* cells, human PTH(1–34) raised intracellular calcium concentration (184). Although hPTH(1–34) also increased cAMP levels in these cells, forskolin and dibutyrl cAMP failed to elicit an increase in cytosolic calcium concentrations. These data suggest that stimulation of intracellular calcium by PTH

---

* OK, opossum kidney.

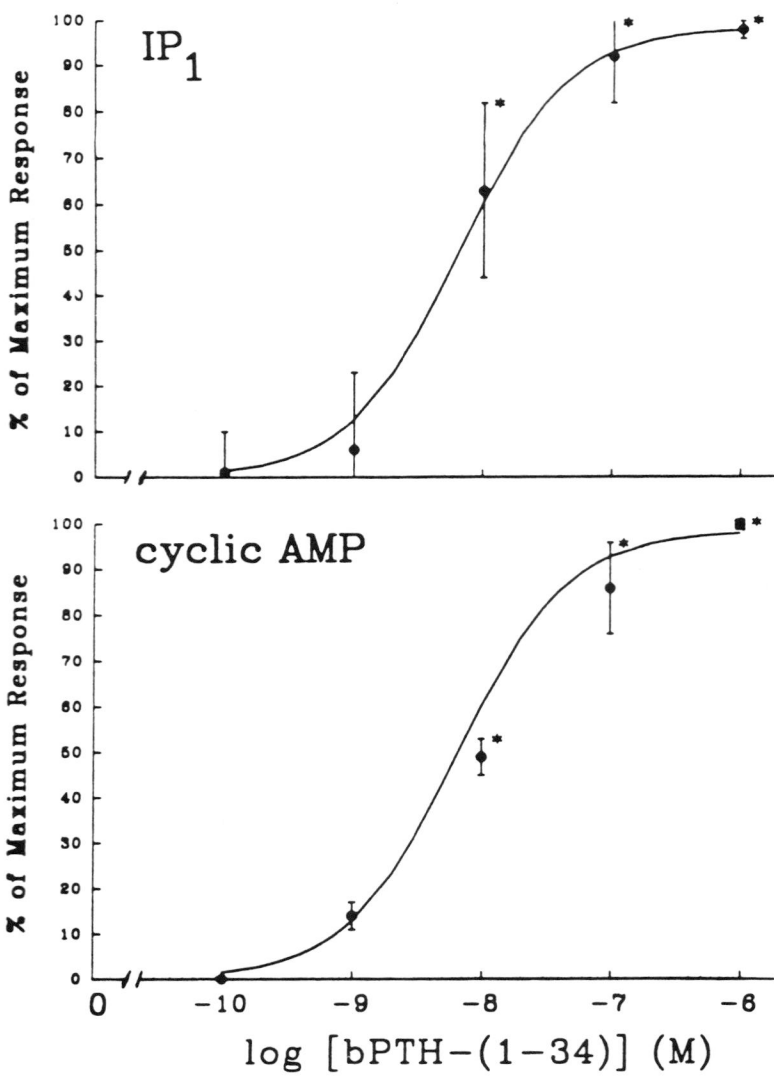

FIG. 6. Relationship of bPTH(1–34) concentration to [³H]IP₁ and cyclic AMP formation. Half-maximal stimulation of [³H]IP₁ is approximately 6 n*M* (**top panel**); half-maximal stimulation of cyclic AMP (**bottom panel**) is approximately 7 n*M*. [From Coleman (247).]

was independent of cAMP activation in these cells. Confirmation of these findings was demonstrated by the fact that rat PTH(1–34) caused a rapid, transient translocation of protein kinase C in concert with the change in intracellular calcium. PTH, however, also led to activation of protein kinase A (185), underscoring the dual nature of the effects of PTH on these two second-messenger systems.

Studies in other systems corroborate these findings. PTH increases cytosolic calcium levels in mouse kidney slices (186) and renal tubular epithelial cells (187) and in primary cultures of canine proximal renal tubule cells (188). Increases in inositol trisphosphate and diacylglycerol production occur in response to PTH in OK cells and in cultured primary proximal tubule cells (174). When these cells are permeabilized, exposure to inositol trisphosphate increases cytosolic calcium concentrations (174).

Specificity of PTH for Effects on Adenylate Cyclase and Phospholipase C

If PTH utilizes two second-messenger systems, one might reasonably ask whether or not the structure–function aspects of PTH, so well worked out for the adenylate cyclase system, is applicable to the PI pathway. A clue that there may be differences in this regard came from Cosman et al. (175) in the ROS 17/2.8 cell line, for which it was shown that when PTH(1–84) is present together with the adenylate cyclase inhibitor, PTH(3–34)amide, there is additive stimulation of IP₃ formation. Thus, the PTH analogue, which is an inhibitor of adenylate cyclase, serves as a co-agonist for phospholipase C activation. In canine renal tubular membranes, structure–function aspects of PTH also differ from the classic observations in the adenylate cyclase assay. In this system, PTH(3–34)amide stimulates the formation of IP. PTH(3–34)amide has also been shown to act directly as an agonist for IP formation in fetal bone (189). In this model, PTH(3–34)amide is more potent than classic PTH fragments.

Demonstration that PTH can stimulate the IP second-messenger system places earlier demonstrations of its ability to perturb cellular calcium in a mechanistic context. It is reasonable to consider the distinct possibility that PTH perturbs cellular calcium by stimulating the intracellular release of IP. In view of the fact that PTH appears to share with a rather large number of polypeptide hormones the ability to activate two major pathways of hormone action, questions of specificity arise. One might expect that PTH might show preferential actions on one or another pathway as a function of the tissue itself. However, both pathways are stimulated by PTH in renal and skeletal tissue so that, at least at a superficial level, one can not make an assignment regarding the ability of PTH to activate one signal transduction pathway in preference to another.

How, then, may specificity be achieved? The model in other hormone systems in which both pathways are stimulated suggests that a critical aspect of specificity might occur at the level of the hormone receptor itself. For example, the alpha-adrenergic receptor can be subclassified into the $alpha_1$ and $alpha_2$ subtypes. The assignment of the PI pathway to the $alpha_1$ receptor, as well as the assignment of adenylate cyclase inhibition to the $alpha_2$ receptor, is generally accepted (190). Even further complexity is possible, however, because it is now known that there are at least two different $alpha_1$ receptors (191). It is not yet clear whether one or both subtypes are linked to PI turnover (192). It is attractive to consider the possibility that the PTH receptor will be shown to consist of subtypes that can account for differential linkage of PTH to adenylate cyclase or phospholipase C activation. The evidence for PTH receptor subtypes is reviewed in the next section of this chapter.

Alternatively, the milieu of the cell could well dictate what pathway will predominate in a given physiological situation. Three observations support this hypothesis. When ROS 17/2.8 cells are grown in the presence of retinoic acid, the distribution of IP products is shifted in favor of the active metabolite IP_3. Lowering the pH of the incubating buffer is associated with a marked increase in phospholipase C activity of ROS 17/2.8 cells (175). It is well known that glucocorticoids enhance adenylate cyclase stimulation by PTH (193). These three observations suggest that experimental conditions that favor the activity of one pathway over the other pathway may be a mechanism of selection. Of course, one does not have to require that only one pathway is stimulated at a given time in the cell. It is likely that each messenger system is regulating a different set of cellular responses. These cellular responses may be mutually important in

some physiological settings and could well be stimulated simultaneously.

The PTH Receptor

The overwhelmingly supportive data pointing to second messengers for PTH that are resident in the plasma membrane of the cell led to the inescapable conclusion that PTH receptors must be present there also. However, the search for appropriate analogues of PTH that could serve as radioligands with which PTH receptors could be detected has been long and hard. Suitable radioligands for PTH were difficult to develop because of several chemical features of the molecule. Standard iodination conditions lead to (a) oxidation of methionine in positions 8 and 18 and (b) inactivation of the hormone (194). Some success has been achieved employing gentler iodination conditions with lactoperoxidase or electrolysis (195). Another useful approach has been to substitute norleucine (which cannot be oxidized) for methionine in positions 8 and 18 and to substitute an iodinatable tyrosine residue for phenylalanine in position 34. To enhance bioactivity, a carboxyamide is provided for the carboxylic acid at the carboxy-terminal end of the molecule. The resulting molecule, [Nleu^{8,18}Tyr^{34}]bPTH(1–34)amide, has been a relatively useful radioligand to detect high-affinity, specific PTH binding sites (196).

One would anticipate that a well-designed ligand for PTH receptors would detect binding sites that fulfill the criteria for a receptor: high affinity, saturability, low capacity, reversibility, and a close relationship to a biochemical or physiological effector. Such criteria for the PTH receptor have been fulfilled in both renal and skeletal tissues. In general, binding affinity is in the range of 1–5 nM. This concentration approximates the concentration required for half-maximal stimulation of adenylate cyclase activity. In renal membranes, binding capacity is approximately 1–5 pmol/mg protein. Radioligand studies have also indicated whether intact PTH can bind to its receptor or whether enzymatic cleavage of PTH to the active 1–34 fragment is necessary prior to binding. When intact PTH is prepared as a radioligand, it binds to cell surface recognition sites in osteoblast-like cells and in renal membranes (195), suggesting that at least up to position 43 (the site of the tracer), intact hormone binds to receptor without the need for further cleavage (9). This observation, along with that indicating that the 1–34 fragment probably does not escape the liver, adds weight to the idea that the full-length peptide is the biologically important one.

Competitive binding studies with PTH analogues confirmed expectations of their relationships to the PTH receptor. The PTH antagonist, [Nleu^{8,18}Tyr^{34}]bPTH(3–34)amide, competes for receptor occupancy in a manner that is indistinguishable from that of fully active PTH. The model predicting that the 25–34 region is the binding domain of the PTH molecule for the PTH receptor has been substantiated further by these binding studies (197–199). Additionally, these studies confirm that positions 1 and 2, although important activation regions for adenylate cyclase, do not influence hormone binding. Of great interest is the observation that the newly discovered PTH-related peptide (PTHrP), implicated as the humoral peptide of malignant hypercalcemia, interacts with binding sites that are indistinguishable from the native PTH receptor (200–202). This subject is reviewed in detail in Chapter 25. PTHrP shows close homology with PTH only in the first 13 amino-terminal amino acids. The region 14–34 and the larger, carboxy-terminal portion of PTHrP are completely divergent from the primary amino acid sequence of PTH. Nevertheless, careful binding studies of peptides in this divergent region of both PTH and PTHrP as well as hybrids between PTH and PTHrP in these areas have recently shown that both peptides bind to the PTH receptor with equal affinity in bovine kidney. What is of particular interest is the fact that despite complete divergence in the so-called binding region of PTH, both peptides appear to be able to bind to the PTH receptor. When these studies are performed in the absence of the amino-terminal region, rat osteosarcoma cells appeared to show a preference for the 19–34 sequence of PTHrP (197). It is evident that binding of the PTH molecule to the PTH receptor requires molecular features beyond what can be gleaned from inspection of the primary sequence of the molecule. It would appear that information providing the "fit" at the binding site will be discovered in the tertiary configuration of both peptides. At this time, there is no evidence for a separate PTHrP receptor.

Although bone and kidney have been the focus of these binding studies, it is noteworthy that PTH-specific binding sites with similar characteristics have been demonstrated in human dermal fibroblasts (203), liver, giant cell tumors, and monocytes. Dermal fibroblasts have been useful in studying the genetic disorder pseudohypoparathyroidism, in which one subtype of the disorder appears to be due to impaired or deficient PTH receptors (see Chapter 27).

Of further interest are data indicating that saturable but relatively low affinity binding with specificity for carboxy-terminal and mid-regions of PTH are seen in renal membranes and in osteosarcoma cells (3,204). Attention to the amino-terminal end of the PTH molecule, vis à vis adenylate cyclase stimulation, might have distracted investigators from exploring the potential for other biological properties of the carboxy-terminal portion of PTH. In this regard, Murray and co-workers (204–206) have shown that the mid-region analogue of PTH is able to stimulate alkaline phosphatase activity in a manner that is distinctive and completely different from the inhibitory actions of the amino-terminal analogue of PTH on alkaline phosphatase.

In contrast to other adenylate-cyclase-linked receptor systems, receptor subtypes for PTH have not yet been conclusively demonstrated. Some binding studies have suggested differential properties of the PTH receptor in comparisons of bovine PTH(1–84) with bovine PTH(1–34)amide binding. Modeling of the receptor sites has suggested either (a) two PTH receptors with similar affinities or (b) a second site for intact PTH on the same receptor (207). Although occasionally a study demonstrates ligand-binding differences between renal and skeletal tissues (208), most studies so far have not been able to distinguish between PTH receptor sites in renal or skeletal tissue. In the few studies that suggest the presence of multiple classes of PTH receptors, it also has not been possible to assign one site to one tissue. Differences in the sensitivities of protein kinase A and protein kinase C to PTH is suggestive of the presence of isoforms of the PTH receptor. Tamura et al. (185) evaluated the effect of PTH on OK cells and noted that translocation of protein kinase C corresponded to changes in intracellular calcium. In contrast, PTH activation of cAMP-dependent protein kinase A occurred at a much lower threshold (0.1 nM PTH) than did protein kinase C activation (10 nM PTH). Bovine PTH(3–34) and bovine PTH(7–34) antagonized rat PTH(1–34)-induced translocation of protein kinase C more effectively than they antagonized PTH activation of protein kinase A. The authors suggested that one or more PTH receptors are linked to adenylate cyclase and phospholipase A.

Autoradiographic studies have localized PTH binding sites to areas of the kidney that are believed to be responsible for the renal actions of PTH. These sites include the basolateral surface of the proximal convoluted tubule, the pars recta, the thick ascending limb of the loop of Henle, and the distal convoluted tubule (10). PTH responsive adenylate cyclase activity also appears to be localized to these renal sites.

Purification of the PTH Receptor

Competitive binding studies have indicated the presence of sites that fulfill the requirements of a bonafide receptor for PTH. Efforts to purify the PTH receptor, however, have proven to be extremely difficult, eluding intense studies by a number of laboratories. In 1990, progress was still limited. Photoaffinity probes have permitted the description of a receptor complex of approximately 70,000 daltons in canine renal membranes, human skeletal cells, and human dermal fibroblasts (209–211). In canine renal membranes, covalent labeling of the PTH receptor with iodinated bovine PTH(1–34) revealed a glycoprotein containing several complex N-linked carbohydrate chains consisting of terminal sialic acid and penultimate galactase in a beta-1,4 linkage to

N-acetyl-D-glucosamine (212). The covalently labeled PTH receptor binds several lectins, including wheat germ agglutinin (WGA), succinylated WGA, and *Ricinus communis* agglutin I. Co-incubation of membranes with WGA produced a dramatic, specific, and concentration-dependent inhibition of PTH(1–34) binding. WGA inhibited PTH-stimulated adenylate cyclase activity, affirming that the terminal sialic acid residues are important in ligand binding.

PTH receptors were affinity-labeled with ^{125}I-bPTH(1–34), derivatized with the heterobifunctional cross-linking agent *N*-hydroxysuccinimidyl 4-azidobenzoate (HSAB), and photolyzed with ultraviolet irradiation to induce covalent bond formation between the receptor and the radioligand. Analysis by sodium dodecyl sulfate–polyacrylamide gel electrophoresis indicated that the major PTH binding component has a molecular weight of approximately 85 kD. Labeling is inhibited by GTP or its analogues, as expected of a G-protein-linked receptor. The 70- and 55-kD species isolated by several laboratories (210,211,213) are probably proteolytic products of the 85-kD receptor. The 70-kD form of the receptor is fully functional with respect to hormone binding and adenylate cyclase activity. The K_d's and K_a's for binding and adenylate-cyclase-associated properties are indistinguishable between the 85- and 70-kD forms. The 50- to 55-kD fragment of the receptor is not functional. Interestingly, this cleavage product is not formed if the receptor remains coupled to the guanine-nucleotide-binding protein, Gs. This observation suggests that the Gs-coupling domain is located within the proteolytic cleavage sites of the 50- and 70-kD moieties.

The hydrodynamic properties of the PTH receptor suggest that it is highly asymmetric. Calculation of the partial specific volume of the receptor–detergent complex suggests a corrected M_r of approximately 166 kD. The covalently labeled 166-kD receptor is oligomeric under denaturing conditions, and the estimated M_r of 85 kD is consistent with the lower molecular form being a homodimer (214).

Disulfide bonds play an important role in many G-protein-linked receptors, and it is not surprising that disulfide bonds also play an important role in the structure and function of the PTH receptor (214). A small, covalently labeled species (<14 kD) is released after exposure of membranes to strong disulfide-reducing agents. This fragment may be in close proximity to the ligand-binding domain of the receptor. The importance of the disulfide bonds is also apparent in the fact that treatment of canine renal membranes with disulfide bond reducing agents such as dithiothreitol abolishes PTH binding (215).

Monoclonal antibodies raised against the PTH receptor bind specifically and with high affinity to renal canine membranes. Western blotting revealed the presence of an 85-kD protein with lectin specificity identical to that of the putative PTH receptor. These antibodies immunoprecipitated covalently labeled PTH receptors in avian bone cells. The antibodies do not inhibit ligand binding nor do they alter PTH-stimulated adenylate cyclase activity; they are therefore unlikely to be directed toward the ligand-binding domain or toward the Gs coupling domain of the receptor. Nevertheless, these monoclonal antibodies may prove useful in identifying PTH receptor cDNAs in expression libraries from kidney and bone (216).

Purification of Other Adenylate-Cyclase-Linked Receptors

It is ironic that PTH was one of the first hormones to be shown to stimulate adenylate cyclase and yet its adenylate-cyclase-linked receptor will be one of the last to be purified. Whereas many hormone receptors belonging to this family have already been purified, cloned, and studied in expression systems, the PTH receptor is an impure preparation. We have with limited insight into its true structure. A number of investigators believe that when the PTH receptor is ultimately purified, it will be shown to share the fundamental properties of all receptors that are linked by guanine-nucleotide-binding proteins to adenylate cyclase. Alternatively, some investigators believe that because of the daunting difficulty in its purification (using techniques that were successful for other hormones of the same family), the purified PTH receptor may prove to be quite different from its cousins in some important ways.

Nevertheless, because it is considered likely that the PTH receptor will share important similarities with the family to which it belongs, a description of these features is provided. A common structural aspect of all bioamine and polypeptide hormone receptors coupled to adenylate cyclase is periodically recurring regions of hydrophobicity. There are a total of seven such regions that are believed to be transmembrane spanning domains. The transmembrane spanning domains are joined by regions of hydrophilicity that form, alternately, intracellular and extracellular loops (Fig. 7) (217,218). The extracellular face of the receptor contains the N-terminus as well as three hydrophilic loops, designated in the figure as E-I, E-II, and E-III. The intracellular face of the receptor contains the C-terminus as well as three additional hydrophilic loops designated C-I, C-II, and C-III. The hydrophobic transmembrane domains are highly conserved among the wide variety of receptors that share this configuration. These regions appear to be important for binding of hormone because site-directed mutagenesis of some of the highly conserved amino acid residues leads to loss or marked reductions in agonist binding properties (219,220). Other shared features include (a) sites of potential N-linked glycosylation near the amino terminus and (b) phosphorylation sites in the cytoplasmic

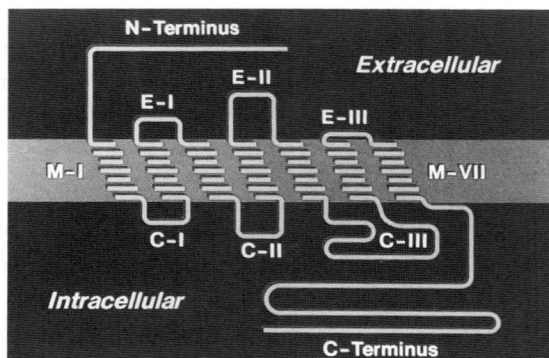

FIG. 7. Model of G-protein-linked receptors. Segments M-I through M-VII are believed to span the lipid bilayer of the plasma membrane. The amino terminus and the connecting loops E-I, E-II, and E-III are adjacent to the extracellular surface, whereas the connecting loops C-I, C-II, and C-III and the carboxyl terminus (C-terminus) are adjacent to the cytoplasmic face of the plasma membrane. [From Lefkowitz and Caron (217).]

domains. The C-I and C-II cytoplasmic loops are conserved, but not to the same extent as the hydrophobic regions. The extracellular domains, the C-III region, and the cytoplasmic carboxy-terminal tail appear to be quite divergent among the different receptors.

Deletion of some hydrophilic regions of the receptor molecule has little or no effect on receptor binding (221). It is believed that the seven transmembrane domains combine in a specific three-dimensional topography to form a ligand-binding pocket. Further work has led to insights which distinguish those receptors that are associated with stimulation or inhibition of adenylate cyclase activity. Receptors that are associated with stimulation of adenylate cyclase have long carboxy-termini and a relatively short intracellular C-III loop. On the other hand, receptors for agonists that are associated with inhibition of adenylate cyclase have short carboxy termini and relatively long C-III loops (Fig. 7). This is also true for agonists that stimulate phospholipase C activity. Mutations or deletions in the C-III region impair the ability of the beta-adrenergic receptor to stimulate adenylate cyclase (221–223). The region which lies between the fifth and the sixth hydrophobic sequences may confer functional specificity to the receptor moiety. This general construct of the adenylate-cyclase-linked receptor contains additional critical features regarding its linkage to the guanine nucleotide proteins (see below).

The structure of the genes encoding several of these adenylate-cyclase-coupled receptors may also have features similar to those of the PTH receptor gene. The beta$_2$-adrenergic and each of the muscarinic receptor genes lack introns in the coding and the 3'-untranslated regions. The lack of introns as well as the intriguing structural primary sequence similarities suggest a common primordial ancestor gene that gave rise to this family of receptors (217,218,224). Corticosteroid-responsive elements are suggested by a steroid-binding hexamer and by marked amplification of the beta-adrenergic signal when rabbit TP3 cells, transfected with the human beta$_2$ gene, are exposed to hydrocortisone (225).

If this information is to be applicable to the PTH receptor, one might use these principles to predict several features. The PTH receptor is likely to share the overall configuration noted above with seven hydrophobic transmembrane spanning domains interrupted by hydrophilic sequences, the latter situating themselves alternatively in the intracellular and extracellular space. One might predict a short C-III region linked on either side by hydrophobic stretches that are unique to the PTH receptor. The speculation of the putative subtype of the PTH receptor which is linked to the activation of phospholipase C is of great interest. According to the model, one might expect there to be a specific PTH receptor subtype linked to phospholipase C activation which differs from the adenylate-cyclase-linked receptor in several critical respects such as the composition and length of the C-III and carboxy-terminal regions. Considering our knowledge of the important effects of glucocorticoids on expression of PTH responsiveness, one would anticipate that steroid response elements should be contained in the regulatory regions of the PTH receptor gene.

Coupling of the Receptor to the Effector: Guanine-Nucleotide-Binding Proteins

This chapter has considered in detail the second-messenger systems for PTH: cAMP and the IP. It has also considered in detail the available information describing PTH receptors. Another very important element in the hormone receptor complex is interposed between this complex and activation of the processes that lead to the generation of cAMP or IP.

This component of the receptor complex, the guanine-nucleotide-binding protein, was discovered by Rodbell and his associates in the early 1970s. The guanine nucleotide guanosine triphosphate (GTP) is an absolute requirement for the stimulation of adenylate cyclase by all hormones that utilize this pathway. Inhibition of adenylate cyclase by hormones that had this effect also required the presence of GTP. GTP was postulated to bind to a guanine-nucleotide-binding protein (G protein) interposed in a functional manner between the hormone receptor and the effector unit. The G protein was believed to transduce the hormonal signal generated by the interaction between the hormone and the receptor.

It is now known that transmembrane signaling utilizes an array of G proteins (226). These G proteins are responsible for modulating the activity of many effectors besides adenylate cyclase, such as cyclic guanosine monophosphate (cGMP) phosphodiesterase, phospholipase C, and ion channels. They convey extracellular signals from receptors for an astonishingly wide array of agonists including neurotransmitters, polypeptides, hormones, drugs, photons, and odorants. They must be regarded as a central element in the hormone receptor unit. In fact, G proteins could be regarded as informational traffic directors with literally a universe of first messengers to guide. G proteins also influence ion channels by direct actions, independent of the hormone-receptor interaction.

Guanine-nucleotide-binding proteins are a large family of structurally and functionally related proteins (227). G proteins involved in transmembrane signaling have a number of common features. They are heterotrimers with subunits designated as alpha, beta, and gamma. The alpha subunit coupled to most hormone receptors range in molecular mass from 39 to 52 kD. Although the alpha subunit is unique to each G protein, providing for structural identification, all alpha subunits are similar in a number of ways. They all bind guanine nucleotides. In the basal, unstimulated state, the G protein is liganded to guanosine diphosphate (GDP), a unit that has a very slow turnover rate and is essentially inactive. The GDP–G-protein complex is believed to reside in the plasma membrane in association with the heterotrimeric holoprotein. It is not physically associated with any receptor or any effector units.

When an agonist such as PTH binds to its receptor, a cascade of dynamically interrelated events is induced (Fig. 8). First, the G-protein unit becomes associated with the high-affinity hormone-receptor complex, forming a so-called ternary complex. The receptor–G-protein interaction leads to the release of GDP and the association of the active guanine nucleotide, GTP, with the G protein. GTP, in turn, facilitates the dissociation of hormone from the receptor by lowering the affinity of these two elements for each other, providing a mechanism to prevent further stimulation by agonist. When the GTP–G-protein complex interacts, the GTPα unit dissociates from the beta–gamma dimer. The GTPα unit is then free to interact directly with an effector, catalytic unit such as adenylate cyclase. It is believed that the GTPα-adenylate-cyclase complex is the complete activation unit.

Regulation of the GTPα unit effector complex is provided for by another intrinsic property of all alpha subunits, namely, GTPase activity. The GTPase activity of the alpha subunit slowly hydrolyzes GTP to the inactive ligand, GDP. The GDPα unit disengages itself from the effector unit and reassociates with the beta–gamma units to re-form the inactive holoprotein.

Another property common to many alpha subunits is their ability to be adenosine diphosphate (ADP)-ribosylated. Transfer of ADP-ribose from nicotinamide-

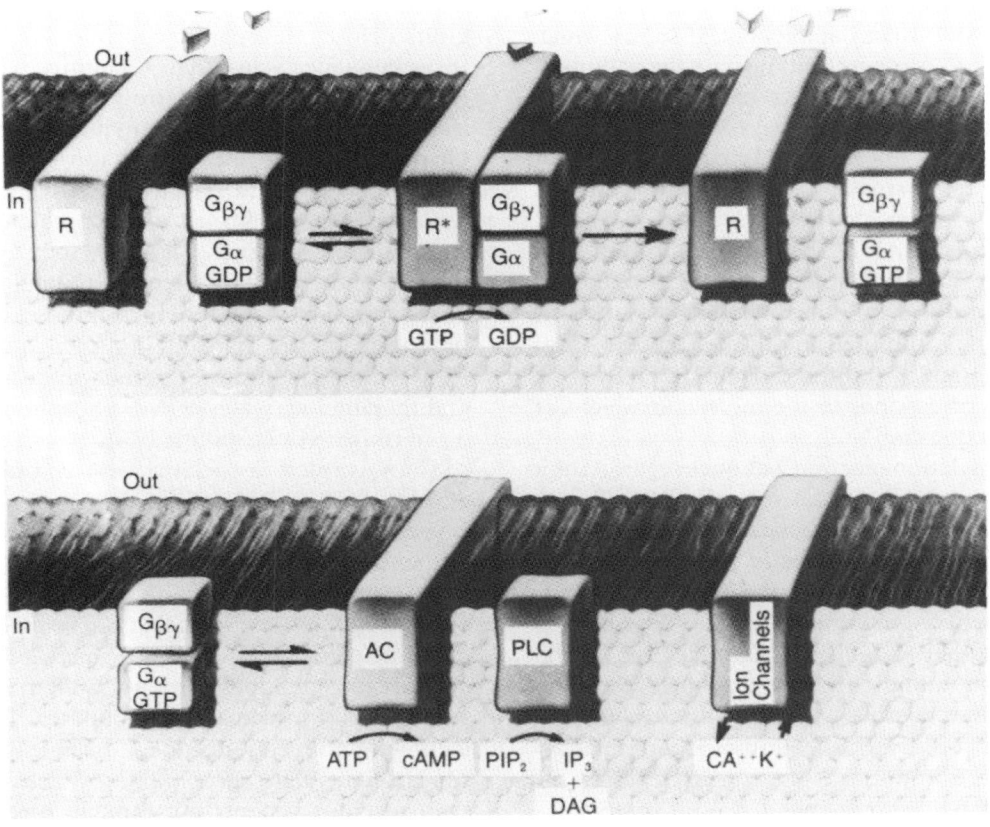

FIG. 8. Schema of G-protein action. [From Graziano and Gilman (248).]

adenine dinucleotide (NAD) is catalyzed by several bacterial toxins. Intracellular ADP-ribosyltransferases have also been described (228). Cholera toxin catalyzes the ADP-ribosylation of G proteins designated Gs (the letter "s" is used to denote the G proteins that serve as a stimulatory link to adenylate cyclase). ADP-ribosylation of Gs is associated with (a) inhibition of the Gs's intrinsic GTPase activity and (b) persistence of the activated GTP–G-protein state. Thus, membrane preparations exposed to cholera toxin demonstrate marked amplification of the adenylate-cyclase-stimulating properties of agonists.

ADP-ribosylation by pertussis toxin, on the other hand, is an inhibitory event in that it disengages the ADP-ribosylated G-protein from the receptor (229). Pertussis toxin was shown first to ADP-ribosylate the family of closely related G proteins known as Gi (the letter "i" is used to denote the G proteins that inhibit adenylate cyclase activity). Pertussis toxin's actions on Gi leads to increased adenylate cyclase activity due to the unopposed action of Gs to stimulate adenylate cyclase. If the pertussis toxin substrate were to mediate a stimulatory event, such as the activation of phospholipase C or a potassium channel, ADP-ribosylation by pertussis toxin would inhibit the response to agonist. In fact, the effect of pertussis toxin to inhibit hormone activation of these other events is now well-described.

Although not extremely useful for functional purposes, G proteins can be classified according to whether or not they are ADP-ribosylatable and, if so, by which toxins (230). Two G proteins that mediate the actions of cGMP phosphodiesterase, the transducins, are substrates for both cholera and pertussis toxins. The G protein known as "Gz" is not believed to be a substrate for cholera or pertussis toxin (231). All Gs, Golf, and Gt proteins, are ADP-ribosylated by cholera toxin. The effect of these toxins to ADP-ribosylate G-protein substrates has been a very useful tool to measure the amount of the alpha subunit in question. ADP-ribosylation of alpha units can be monitored in vitro by the use of (a) ^{32}P-labeled NAD and (b) autoradiographic analysis of the species that corresponds to the molecular weight of the alpha unit in question.

The ADP-ribosylation reaction was once regarded as a quantitative marker of the alpha subunit of the G protein in question. It is now appreciated that it is a better marker of functional competence of the $G\alpha$ unit than the actual amount of G protein in the membrane. Studies utilizing antisera raised against sequence-specific portions of $G\alpha$ have led to accurate quantification of the amount of each subunit in the cell membrane (232). The availability of these relatively specific antisera has permitted a more accurate identification of a particular alpha subunit. This is important when one is dealing with a subset of closely related proteins such as the three func-

tionally and structurally distinct inhibitory G proteins, all designated Gi.

The discrepancy between measured values obtained using immunochemical techniques and the ADP-ribosylation reaction raises a number of mechanistic questions about G proteins that remain unresolved. If the amount of ADP-ribosylatable protein is less that the amount that can be detected by immunochemistry, perhaps there are regions in the membrane that are not available to the ADP-ribosylation reaction. This may indicate that there are regions which are also not available to link with the receptor complex. Alternatively, the immunochemical quantification could be the more accurate index of potential functional ability of the G protein to link to the receptor complex.

The ever-growing family of G proteins has also eluded functional classification. The initial premise that a given G protein would be associated with a specific effector system has given way to the notion that a given G protein mediates multiple functions. For example, Gs is linked to the activation of adenylate cyclase, but it also is associated with stimulation of calcium channels (233). Moreover, at least four Gs proteins are known to be derived from a single gene. Alternate splicing mechanisms related to 15-amino-acid residues encoded by exon 3 of the $Gs\alpha$ gene are responsible for these different translational forms. Except for small changes in kinetic properties of Gs, the four Gs proteins appear to be indistinguishable from each other (234). Golf, a close but separate cousin of Gs, activates olfactory adenylate cyclase. The Gi family, which consists of three genetically distinct proteins, are interchangeable in their ability to inhibit adenylate cyclase. These three Gi proteins also are linked to ion channels for potassium and calcium (235). Go proteins serve as pertussis-sensitive substrates that mediate calcium and potassium currents in diverse tissues. Go proteins are found in great abundance in the brain (236,237). The only G protein, besides Golf, that may be as specific for a given function are the transducins (Gt); one Gt activates cGMP phosphodiesterase activity in retinal rods (Gt,r), and the other activates cGMP phosphodiesterase activity in retinal cones (Gt,c) (230).

The G protein associated with stimulation of phospholipase C activity remains obscure because no specific G protein has yet been identified with this activity. None of the identified G proteins Gs, Gi, or Go appear to be likely candidates. Nevertheless, there is evidence for phospholipase C activities that can be modulated by guanine nucleotides. For example, in receptor systems that enhance phospholipase activity, GTP influences binding affinity and stimulates phospholipase C itself. In experimental microinjection studies, the beta–gamma subunit appears to regulate phospholipase C activity (238). However, receptor systems not thought to be mediated by guanine nucleotides have also been shown to regulate phospholipase C activity.

Structural Features of Gs Units

Among the alpha subunits of G proteins, there is great conservation in primary structure. Gsα is probably the least well conserved, with unique inserts in regions designated by positions 72–86 and 324–336. The other G-protein alpha units characterized so far lack these inserts. In addition, there are 7 residues at the aminoterminal end of Gsα that also account for its larger size. The domains of greatest conservation among all the Gα subunits are those believed to be involved in guanine nucleotide binding: 39–56, 223–226, 243–253, and 288–299. The carboxy-terminal site is involved in binding to a region in the receptor defined by the cytoplasmic loop between the fifth and sixth hydrophobic domains. The amino-terminal site of the alpha subunit is a point of interaction with the beta–gamma dimer. Topographical mapping has suggested that carboxy-terminal and amino-terminal ends of the alpha subunit are in close proximity. This leads to attractive speculation as to how the receptor interaction can lead to holoprotein dissociation.

Knowledge of the primary structure of the G-protein alpha subunit has also led to insights into the sites of ADP-ribosylation by cholera and pertussis toxins. Cholera toxin ADP-ribosylates the Arg[201] in the primary sequence, resulting in inhibition of GTPase activity (239–241). Pertussis toxin ADP-ribosylates a cysteine, four residues from the carboxy terminus (242,243). ADP-ribosylation at this site uncouples G-protein activation catalyzed by the receptor and is, therefore, an inhibitory event. The reason why pertussis toxin is inactive at Gs and Gz is because those alpha units contain tyrosine and isoleucine, respectively, rather than a cysteine residue. It is not clear why cholera toxin does not ADP-ribosylate Gi or Go, because they too have an arginine in position 201 and the contiguous region is moderately well-conserved.

The beta and gamma units of G proteins are tightly associated with each other under physiological conditions. Activation of G leads to dissociation of the holoprotein into free alpha units and a beta–gamma dimer. Until recently, it was believed that the larger, 35-kD beta unit which has a 36-kD counterpart was similar among all G proteins. Similarly, it was believed that there was little, if any, difference among the 8- to 10-kD gamma units. This is probably not the case, however, because subtle but presumably important differences are being appreciated within the family of beta and gamma units. Nevertheless, beta–gamma units appear to be promiscuous in their ability to link to a wide variety of alpha units.

This property has, in fact, led to an alternative hypothesis for Gi action. Upon dissociation of the Gi holoprotein, freed beta–gamma units could scavenge and associate with alpha-s subunits and thereby inactivate them. The inhibitory properties of Gi could thus be realized without a necessary interaction between Giα and the catalytic effector. It is also possible that beta–gamma units have their own functions. Indirect effects of the beta-gamma complex on potassium channels, presumably mediated by direct effects on phospholipase A_2 activity, have been described (238).

G Proteins and PTH Action

PTH shares with all other polypeptide hormones that stimulate adenylate cyclase activity a dependence upon guanine nucleotides. The insights gained in terms of understanding the G proteins and their interactions with hormone receptors appear to be valid for PTH. These features include the ability of guanine nucleotides to alter agonist binding properties. Guanine nucleotides also amplify the agonist properties of PTH upon adenylate cyclase activity. Similar to other systems, the presence of the nonhydrolyzable guanine nucleotide, Gpp(NH)p, leads to a markedly greater stimulation of adenylate cyclase by PTH than can be seen in its absence. The amplification of the signal generated by PTH has been utilized to develop a very sensitive in vitro assay for PTH. This assay differs from assays performed in the absence of Gpp(NH)p by a concentration–response relationship that covers a range of PTH concentrations that is closer to expectations based upon physiological effects (244). The amount of total activity generated by PTH in the presence of Gpp(NH)p is greater, permitting the in vitro assay to show agonist effects more easily. It might be expected that without guanine nucleotides, PTH should not be able to stimulate adenylate cyclase at all. This is likely to be the case for PTH as it is for all adenylate cyclase-linked hormones. However, membrane preparations are impure and contain small amounts of endogenous GTP, accounting (in all likelihood) for the ability of PTH (as well as other hormones) to stimulate adenylate cyclase even when GTP may not be added to the assay mixture.

The cooperative effects of guanine nucleotides upon the other major effector system stimulated by PTH, namely phospholipase C, has been more difficult to establish, a comment that is applicable to a number of other hormones that utilize the PI pathway. In ROS cells, GTP appears to stimulate basal phospholipase C activity, leading to increases in all three inositol phosphates (175). When GTP is present along with PTH, the resultant activity is the sum of the individual stimulation afforded by GTP and PTH. In another osteoblast-like cell line, UMR-106 cells, Babich et al. (177) has shown more conclusively that the stimulation of phospholipase by PTH is dependent upon GTP. They showed an absolute dependence upon GTP, since PTH was unable to stimulate any activity in its absence. Moreover, the GDP analogue, GDPβS (which serves as a stable, inactive guanine nucleotide), was able to inhibit activation afforded by GTP.

Acutely dispersed renal canine tubules have also been examined with respect to the PTH–GTP interrelationships. In this system, GTP stimulates the formation of all three IPs, with a time course which is somewhat slower to develop but which is maintained for a longer period of time. The magnitude of the increases was greater than that observed for PTH alone. The combination of PTH(1–34) and GTP resulted in higher maximal levels for all IPs. The time course of formation appeared to be accelerated. Only for IP$_1$ formation did the magnitude of the increase appear to be greater than additive. Similar to the osteoblast line, GDPβS is able to inhibit the activation afforded by GTP.

One can develop another hypothesis to account for the additive effect of GTP and PTH on IP accumulation without necessarily invoking a G-protein dependence on the phospholipase C enzyme. The increase in IP$_3$ could result from inhibition of the phosphatase responsible for the metabolism of IP$_3$. In recent work, Coleman et al. (178) have shown that under unstimulated conditions, 1,4,5-IP$_3$ is rapidly hydrolyzed, with over 80% metabolized within the first 1 min. In the presence of GTP, the rate of IP$_3$ hydrolysis is slowed by over 70%, and there is a corresponding retardation in the appearance of the breakdown products, IP$_2$ and IP$_1$. In experiments designed to determine whether PTH might also affect the metabolism of 1,4,5-IP$_3$, it was shown that neither PTH(1–34) nor PTH(3–34) had any effects. It is possible, therefore, that the cooperative actions of GTP and PTH on phospholipase C activity reflect independent actions at two different sites. PTH appears to act rather exclusively at the phospholipase C site, whereas GTP appears to act on the site of IP$_3$ hydrolysis and possibly also at phospholipase C. Much more work is needed before a complete understanding of G protein effects on this pathway are appreciated. Even more work will be required to appreciate how this system relates to the actions of PTH to activate PI hydrolysis.

SUMMARY

PTH action is still an area of uncertainty, and many questions remain to be answered. It is clear that PTH activates the adenylate cyclase–cAMP–protein kinase A cascade in classic and nonclassic target tissues. This is the result of (a) PTH binding to its receptor on the cell surface and (b) activation of the adenylate cyclase effector unit by activation of a GTP-binding protein, Gs.

PTH also elicits an increase in intracellular free calcium through multiple mechanisms. The evidence continues to accumulate that PTH stimulates PI hydrolysis, leading to the formation of IPs and diacylglycerol. Several active IPs could well mediate the changes in cellular calcium induced by PTH. In addition, it is possible that PTH is associated with the activation of calcium channels, independent of a biochemical signaling system. Thus, PTH fits into a family of hormones that utilizes several different signaling pathways to influence the cell. The precise cellular mechanisms by which the cell responds in several different ways to a single extracellular signal such as PTH remain to be elucidated by further investigation.

ACKNOWLEDGMENTS

Some of the observations reviewed in this chapter were supported by a grant from the NIH (DK32333).

REFERENCES

1. Talmage RV, et al. The demand for bone calcium in maintenance of plasma calcium concentration. In: Horton JE, Tarplay TM, Davis WF, eds. *Mechanisms of localized bone loss.* Washington, DC: Info Retrieval, 1978;73–92.
2. Chambers TJ, McSheehy PMJ, Thomson BM, Fuller K. The effect of calcium-regulating hormones and prostaglandins on bone resorption by osteoclasts disaggregated from neonatal rat bones. *Endocrinology* 1985;116:234.
3. Demay M, Mitchell J, Goltzman D. Comparison of renal and osseous binding of parathyroid hormone and hormonal fragments. *Am J Physiol* 1985;249:E437.
4. Goltzman D, Peytremann A, Callahan E, et al. Analysis of the requirements for parathyroid hormone action in renal membranes with the use of inhibiting analogues. *J Biol Chem* 1976;250:3199.
5. Horiuchi N, Holick MF, Potts JT Jr, Rosenblatt M. A parathyroid hormone inhibitor in vivo: design and biological evaluation of a hormone analog. *Science* 1983;220:1053.
6. Mahoney CA, Nissenson RA. Canine renal receptors for parathyroid hormone: down-regulation in vivo by exogenous parathyroid hormone. *J Clin Invest* 1983;72:411.
7. Forte LR, Langeluttig SG, Poelling RE, Thomas ML. Renal parathyroid hormone receptors in the chick: downregulation in secondary hyperparathyroid animal models. *Am J Physiol* 1982;242:E154.
8. Tomlinson S, Hendy GN, Pemberton DM, O'Riordan JLH. Reversible resistance to the renal action of parathyroid hormone in man. *Clin Sci Mol Med* 1976;51:59.
9. Rizzoli RE, Somerman M, Murray TM, Aurbach GD. Binding of radioiodinated parathyroid hormone to cloned bone cells. *Endocrinology* 1983;113:1832.
10. Rouleau MF, Warshawsky H, Goltzman D. Parathyroid hormone binding in vivo to renal, hepatic and skeletal tissues of the rat using a radioautographic approach. *Endocrinology* 1986;118:919.
11. Peck WA, Carpenter J, Messinger K, De Bra D. Cyclic 3'5' adenosine monophosphate in isolated bone cells: response to low concentrations of parathyroid hormone. *Endocrinology* 1973;92:692.
12. Majeska RJ, Rodan SB, Rodan GA. Parathyroid hormone-responsive clonal cell lines from rat osteosarcoma. *Endocrinology* 1980;107:1494.
13. Dietrich JW, Canalis E, Maina DM, Raisz LG. Hormonal con-

trol of bone collagen synthesis in vitro: effects of parathyroid hormone and calcitonin. *Endocrinology* 1976;98:943.

14. Heath JK, Atkinson SJ, Mickle MC, Reynolds JJ. Mouse osteoblasts synthesize collagenase in response to bone resorbing agents. *Biochem Biophys Acta* 1984;802(1):151–4.

15. Simon LS, Slovik DM, Neer RM, Krane SM. Changes in serum levels of type I and III procollagen extension peptides during infusion of human parathyroid hormone fragment (1–34). *J Bone Miner Res* 1988;3(2):241–6.

16. Hall AK, Dickson IR. The effects of parathyroid hormone on osteoblast-like cells from embryonic chick calvaria. *Acta Endocrinol* 1985;108(2):217–23.

17. Rodan GA, Martin TJ. Role of osteoblasts in hormonal control of bone resorption—a hypothesis. *Calcif Tissue Int* 1981;33:349.

18. Rouleau MF, Mitchell J, Goltzman D. In vivo distribution of parathyroid hormone receptors in bone. Evidence that a predominant osseous target cell is not the mature osteoblast. *Endocrinology* 1988;123–87.

19. McSheehy PM, Chambers TJ. Osteoblastic cells mediate osteoclastic responsiveness to parathyroid hormone. *Endocrinology* 1986;118(2):824–8.

20. McSheehy PM, Chambers TJ. Osteoblast-like cells in the presence of parathyroid hormone release soluble factor that stimulates osteoclastic bone resorption. *Endocrinology* 1986; 119(4):1654–9.

21. Perry HM III, Skogen W, Chappel J, Kahn AJ, Wilner G, Teitelbaum SL. Partial characterization of a parathyroid hormone-stimulated resorption factor(s) from osteoblast-like cells. *Endocrinology* 1989;125(4):2075–82.

22. Feyen JH, Elford P, Di-Padova FE, Trechsel U. Interleukin-6 is produced by bone and modulated by parathyroid hormone. *J Bone Miner Res* 1989;4(4):633–8.

23. Lowik CWGM, van der Pluijm G, Bloys H, Hoekman K, Bijvoet OLM, Aarden LA, Papapoulos SE. Parathyroid hormone (PTH) and PTH-like protein (PLP) stimulate interleukin-6 production by osteogenic cells: a possible role of interleukin-6 in osteoclastogenesis. *Biochem Biophys Res Commun* 1989;162(3):1546–52.

24. Linkhart T, Mohan S. Parathyroid hormone stimulates release of insulin-like growth factor I (IGF-I) and IGF-II from neonatal mouse calvaria in organ culture. *Endocrinology* 1989; 125(3):1484–91.

25. Canalis E, Centrella M, Burch W, McCarthy TL. Insulin-like growth factor I mediates selective anabolic effects of parathyroid hormone in bone cultures. *J Clin Invest* 1989;83(1):60–5.

26. Bourdeau JE, Lau K. Effects of parathyroid hormone on cytosolic free calcium concentration in individual rabbit connecting tubules. *J Clin Invest* 1989;83(2):373–9.

27. Centrella M, McCarthy TL, Canalis E. Parathyroid hormone modulates transforming growth factor beta activity and binding in osteoblast-enriched cell cultures from fetal rat parietal bone. *Proc Natl Acad Sci USA* 1988;85(16):5889–93.

28. Baron R, Neff L, Roy C, Boisvert A, Caplan M. Evidence for a high and specific concentration of (Na^+K^+)ATPase in the plasma membrane of the osteoclast. *Cell* 1986;46:311–20.

29. Tuukkanen J, Vaananen HK. Omeprazole, a specific inhibitor of H^+-K^+-ATPase, inhibits bone resorption in vitro. *Calcif Tiss Int* 1986;38:123–5.

30. Blair HC, Tietelbaum SL, Ghiselli R, Glick S. Osteoclastic bone resorption by a polarized vacuolar proton pump. *Science* 1989;245:855–7.

31. Hall GE, Kenny AD. Bone resorption induced by parathyroid hormone and dibutyryl cyclic AMP: role of carbonic anhydrase. *J Pharmacol Exp Ther* 1986;238(3):778–82.

32. Krieger NS, Kim SG. Dichlorobenzamil inhibits stimulated bone resorption in vitro. *Endocrinology* 1988;122(2):415–20.

33. Bushinsky DA. Effects of parathyroid hormone on net proton flux from neonatal mouse calvariae. *Am J Physiol* 1987;252(4, part 2):F585–9.

34. Tam CS, Heersche JNM, Murray TM, Parsons JA. Parathyroid hormone stimulates the bone apposition rate independently of its resorptive action: differential effects of intermittent and continual administration. *Endocrinology* 1982;110:506.

35. Ljunggren O, Lerner UH. Parathyroid hormone stimulates prostanoid formation in mouse calvarial bones. *Acta Endocrinol* 1989;120(3):357–61.

36. Raisz LG. Physiology of bone In: Becker KL, ed. *Principles and practice of endocrinology and metabolism.* Philadelphia: JB Lippincott, 1990;468–74.

37. Slovik DM, Rosenthal DI, Doppelt SH, Potts JT Jr, Daly MA, Campbell JA, Neer RM. Restoration of spinal bone in osteoporotic men by treatment with human parathyroid hormone (1–34) and 1,25-dihydroxyvitamin D. *J Bone Miner Res* 1986;1:4.

38. Parisien M, Silverberg SJ, Shane E, et al. The histomorphometry of bone in primary hyperparathyroidism: preservation of cancellous bone structure. *J Clin Endocrinol Metab* 1990;70:930–8.

39. Silverberg SJ, Shane E, De La Cruz L, Dempster DW, Feldman F, Seldin D, Jacobs TP, Siris ES, Cafferty M, Parisien MV, Lindsay R, Clemens TL, Bilezikian JP. Skeletal disease in primary hyperparathyroidism. *J Bone Miner Res* 1989;4:283–91.

40. Kleerekoper M, Villaneuva AR, Mathews CHE, et al. PTH mediated bone loss in primary and secondary hyperparathyroidism. In: Frame B, Potts JT, eds. *Clinical disorders of bone and mineral metabolism.* Amsterdam: Excerpta Medica, 1983;200–3.

41. Parfitt AM. Accelerated cortical bone loss: primary and secondary hyperparathyroidism. In: Uhthoff H, Stahl E, eds. *Current concepts of bone fragility.* Berlin: Springer-Verlag, 1986;279–85.

42. Parfitt AM. Surface specific bone remodeling in health and disease. In: Kleerekoper M, Krane SM, eds. *Clinical disorders of bone and mineral metabolism.* New York: Mary Ann Liebert, 1989;7–14.

43. Parfitt AM, Kleerekoper M, Rao D, et al. Cellular mechanisms of cortical thinning in primary hyperparathyroidism (PHPT). *J Bone Miner Res* 1987;2(Suppl 1):384.

44. Parisien M, Dempster DW, Shane E, et al. Structural parameters of bone biopsies in primary hyperparathyroidism. In: Takahashi HE, ed. *Bone morphometry.* Nagata, Japan: Nishimura, 1990; 228–231.

45. Rao DS, Wilson RJ, Kleerekoper M, Parfitt AM. Lack of biochemical progression or continuation of accelerated bone loss in mild asymptomatic primary hyperparathyroidism: evidence for biphasic disease course. *J Clin Endocrinol Metab* 1988; 67(6):1294–8.

46. Ellsworth R, Howard JE. Studies on physiology of parathyroid glands: some responses of normal human kidneys and blood to intravenous parathyroid extract. *Bull Johns Hopkins Hosp* 1934;55:296.

47. Agus ZS, Wasserstein A, Goldfarb S. PTH, calcitonin, cyclic nucleotides and the kidney. *Annu Rev Physiol* 1981;43:583.

48. Bourdeau JE. Renal handling of calcium. In: Brenner BM, Stein JH, eds. *Contemporary issues in nephrology, vol 2: divalent ion homeostasis.* New York: Churchill Livingstone, 1983.

49. Chase LR, Aurbach GD. Parathyroid function and the renal excretion of 3'5'-adenylic acid. *Proc Natl Acad Sci USA* 1967;58:518.

50. Kawashima H, Jorika S, Kurokawa K. Localization of 25-hydroxyvitamin D_3-1-alpha-hydroxylase and 24-hydroxylase along the rat nephron. *Proc Natl Acad Sci USA* 1981;78:1199.

51. Slovik DM, Daly MA, Potts JT Jr, Neer RM. Renal 1,25 dihydroxyvitamin D, phosphaturic, and cyclic-AMP responses to intravenous synthetic human parathyroid hormone-(1–34) administration in normal subjects. *Clin Endocrinol (Oxf)* 1984;20:369.

52. Bilezikian JP, Canfield RE, Jacobs TP, Polay JS, D'Adamo AP, Eisman JA, DeLuca HF. The response of 1-alpha, 25-dihydroxyvitamin D_3 to hypocalcemia in human subjects. *N Engl J Med* 1978;299:437–41.

53. Iannotti JP, Brighton CT, Iannotti V, Ohishi T. Mechanism of action of parathyroid hormone-induced proteoglycan synthesis in the growth plate chondrocyte. *J Orthop Res* 1990;8(1):136–45.

54. Chin JE, Schalk EM, Kemick ML, Wuthier RE. Effect of synthetic human parathyroid hormone on the levels of alkaline phosphatase activity and formation of alkaline phosphatase-rich matrix vesicles by primary cultures of chicken epiphyseal growth plate chondrocytes. *Bone Miner* 1986;1(5):421–36.

55. Mok LLS, Nickols GA, Thompson JC, Cooper CW. Parathyroid hormone as a smooth muscle relaxant. *Endocr Rev* 1989;10:420–36.

56. Charbon GA, Brummer F, Reneman RS. Diuretic and vascular action of parathyroid extracts in animals and man. *Arch Intern Pharmacodyn Ther* 1968;171:1.

57. Berthelot A, Gairard A. Action of parathormone on arterial pres-

sure and on contraction of isolated aorta in the rat. *Experientia* 1975;31:457.

58. Heath H, Hodgson SF, Kennedy M. Primary hyperparathyroidism: incidence, morbidity and potential economic impact in a community. *N Engl J Med* 1980;302:189–93.

59. Mok LLS, Yang MCM, Pang PKT, Thompson JC, Cooper CW. Parathyroid hormone and gastrointestinal smooth muscle. In: Massry S, Fugita T, eds. *New actions of parathyroid hormone.* New York: Plenum Press, 1989;183–191.

60. Cooper CW, Mok LLS, Seitz PK, Rajaraman S, Thompson JC, ed. *Gastrointestinal endocrinology: receptor and postreceptor mechanisms.* New York: Academic Press, 1990;433–443.

61. Pang PK, Wang R, Shan J, Karpinski E, Benishin CG. Specific inhibition of long-lasting, L-type calcium channels by synthetic parathyroid hormone. *Proc Natl Acad Sci USA* 1990; 87(2):623–7.

62. Perna AF, Smogorzewski M, Massry SG. Effects of verapamil on the abnormalities in fatty acid oxidation of myocardium. *Kidney Int* 1989;36(3):453–7.

63. Islam A, Smogorzewski W, Massry SG. Effect of chronic renal failure and parathyroid hormone on phospholipid content of brain synaptosomes. *Am J Physiol* 1989;256(4, part 2):705–10.

64. Newman W, Beall LD, Levine MA, Cibe JL, Randhawa ZI, Bertolini DR. Biotinylated parathyroid hormone as a probe for the parathyroid hormone receptor. *J Biol Chem* 1989;264:16359–65.

65. Pun KK, Ho PW. Identification and characterization of parathyroid hormone receptors on dog kidney, human kidney, chick bone and human dermal fibroblast. A comparative study of functional and structural properties. *Biochem J* 1989;259(3):785–9.

66. Pun KK, Arnaud CD, Nissenson RA. Parathyroid hormone receptors in human clinical fibroblasts: structural and functional characterization. *J Biomed Mater Res* 1988;3:453–60.

67. Silve C, Santora A, Breslan N, Moses A, Spiegel A. Selective resistance to parathyroid hormone in cultured skin fibroblasts from patients with pseudohypoparathyroidism type Ib. *J Clin Endocrinol Metab* 1986;62:640–4.

68. Robison GA, Butcher RW, Sutherland EW. *Cyclic AMP.* New York: Academic Press, 1971.

69. Goltzman D, Hendy G. Parathyroid hormone. In: *Principles and practice of endocrinology and metabolism.* Becker KL, ed. Philadelphia: JB Lippincott, 1990;402–11.

70. Peck W. Cyclic nucleotides in bone and mineral research. *Adv Cyclic Nucleotide Res* 1979;11:89–130.

71. Chase LR, Aurbach GD. Renal adenyl cyclase: anatomically separate sites for parathyroid hormone and vasopressin. *Science* 1968;159:545.

72. Chase LR, Aurbach GD. The effect of parathyroid hormone on the concentration of adenosine 3′,5′-monophosphate in skeletal tissue in vitro. *J Biol Chem* 1970;245:1520.

73. Rosenblatt M. Peptide hormone antagonists that are effective in vivo. *N Engl J Med* 1986;315:1004.

74. Tregear GW, Van Rietschoten J, Greene E, Keutmann HT, Niall HD, Reit B, Parsons JA, Potts JT Jr. Bovine parathyroid hormone: minimum chain length of synthetic peptide required for biological activity. *Endocrinology* 1973;93:1349.

75. Sabatini S, Yang WC, Kurtzman NA. Effect of parathyroid hormone fragments on calcium transport in toad bladder. *J Pharmacol Exp Ther* 1987;241:448.

76. Calvo MS, Fryer MJ, Laakso KJ, Nissenson RA, Pierce PA, Murray TM, Heath H III. Structural requirements for parathyroid action in mature bone. *J Clin Invest* 1985;76:2348.

77. Pliam NB, Nyiredy KO, Arnaud CD. Parathyroid hormone receptors in avian bone cells. *Proc Natl Acad Sci USA* 1982;79:2061.

78. Kremer R, Bennett HPJ, Mitchell J, Goltzman D. Characterization of the rabbit renal receptor for native parathyroid hormone employing a radioligand purified by reversed-phase liquid chromatography. *J Biol Chem* 1982;257:14048.

79. Nussbaum SR, Rosenblatt M, Potts JT Jr. Parathyroid hormone–renal receptor interactions. *J Biol Chem* 1980;255:10183.

80. Segre GV, Rosenblatt M, Reiner BL, Mahaffey JE, Potts JT Jr. Characterization of the parathyroid hormone receptors in canine renal cortical plasma membranes using a radioiodinated sulfur-free hormone analogue. *J Biol Chem* 1979;254:6980.

81. Rizzoli RE, Somerman M, Murray TM, Aurbach GD. Binding of radioiodinated parathyroid hormone to cloned bone cells. *Endocrinology* 1983;113:1832.

82. McKee RL, Caulfield MP, Rosenblatt M. Treatment of bone derived ROS 17/2.8 cells with dexamechanism and pertussis toxin enables detection of partial agonist activity for parathyroid hormone antagonists. *Endocrinology* 1990;127:76–82.

83. Nutt RF, Caulfield MP, Levy JJ, Gibbons SW, Rosenblatt M, McKee RL. Removal of partial agonism from parathyroid hormone (PTH)-related protein (7–34)NH$_2$ by substitution of PTH amino acids at positions 10 and 11. *Endocrinology* 1990; 127:491–3.

84. Parsons JA, Rafferty B, Grat D, Reit B, Zanelli JM, Keutmann HT, Tregear GW, Callahan EN, Potts JT Jr. Pharmacology of parathyroid hormone and some of its fragments and analogues. In: Talmage RV, Owen M, Parsons JA, eds. *Calcium regulating hormones.* Amsterdam: Excerpta Medica, 1975;33.

85. Segre GV, Rosenblatt M, Tully GL III, Laughan J, Reit B, Potts JT Jr. Evaluation of an in vitro parathyroid hormone antagonist in vivo in dogs. *Endocrinology* 1985;116:1024.

86. Horiuchi N, Rosenblatt M, Keutmann HT, Potts JT Jr, Holick MF. A multi-response parathyroid hormone assay: an inhibitor has agonist properties in vivo. *Am J Physiol* 1983;244:E589.

87. Martin KJ, Bellorin-Font E, Freitag J, Rosenblatt M, Slatopolski E. The arterio-venous difference for immunoreactive parathyroid hormone and the production of adenosine 3′,5′-monophosphate by isolated perfused bone: studies with analogues of parathyroid hormone. *Endocrinology* 1981;109:956–9.

88. Parsons JA, Neer RM, Potts JT Jr. Initial fall of plasma calcium after intravenous injection of parathyroid hormone. *Endocrinology* 1971;89:735.

89. Robertson WG, Peakock M, Atkins D, Webster LA. The effect of parathyroid hormone on the uptake and release of calcium by bone in tissue culture. *Clin Sci* 1972;43:715.

90. Goligorsky MS, Loftus DJ, Hruska KA. Cytoplasmic calcium in individual proximal tubular cells in culture. *Am J Physiol* 1986;251:F938.

91. Hruska KA, Goligorsky M, Scoble J, Tsutsumi M, Westbrook S, Moskowitz D. Effects of parathyroid hormone on cytosolic calcium in renal proximal tubular primary cultures. *Am J Physiol* 1986;251:F188.

92. Reid IR, Civitelli R, Halstead LR, Avioli LV, Hruska KA. Parathyroid hormone acutely elevates intracellular calcium in osteoblastlike cells. *Am J Physiol* 1987;252:E45.

93. Lowik CWGM, van Leeuwen JPTM, van der Meer JM, van Zeeland JK, Scheven BAA, Herrmann-Erlee MPM. A two-receptor model for the action of parathyroid hormone on osteoblasts: a role for intracellular free calcium and cAMP. *Cell Calcium* 1985;6:311.

94. Khalifa S, Mills S, Hruska KA. Stimulation of calcium uptake by parathyroid hormone in renal brush-border membrane vesicles. *J Biol Chem* 1983;258:14400.

95. Scoble JE, Mills S, Hruska KA. Calcium transport in canine renal basolateral membrane vesicles: effects of parathyroid hormone. *J Clin Invest* 1985;75:1096.

96. Boland CJ, Fried RM, Tashjian AH Jr. Measurement of cytosolic free Ca^{++} concentrations in human and rat osteosarcoma cells: actions of bone resorption-stimulating hormones. *Endocrinology* 1986;118:980.

97. Fraser CL, Sarnacki P, Budayr A. Evidence that parathyroid hormone-mediated calcium transport in rat brain synaptosomes is independent of cyclic adenosine monophosphate. *J Clin Invest* 1988;81:982.

98. Cole JA, Forte LR, Eber SL, Thorne PK, Poelling RE. Regulation of sodium-dependent phosphate transport by parathyroid hormone in opossum kidney cells: cAMP dependent and independent mechanisms. *Endocrinology* 1988;122:2981.

99. Cole JA, Eber SL, Poelling RE, Thorne PK, Forte LR. A dual mechanism for regulation of kidney phosphate transport by parathyroid hormone. *Am J Physiol* 1987;253:E221.

100. Murer H, Malmstrom K. Intracellular regulatory cascades: examples from parathyroid hormone regulation of renal phosphate transport. *Klin Wochenschr* 1986;64:824.

101. Berridge MJ. Inositol trisphosphate and diacylglycerol as second messengers. *Biochem J* 1984;220:345.

102. Berridge MJ, Irvine RF. Inositol trisphosphate, a novel second messenger in cellular signal transduction. *Nature* 1984;312:315.

103. Abdel-Latif AA. Calcium-mobilizing receptors, polyphosphoinositides and the generation of second messengers. *Pharmacol Rev* 1986;38:227.

104. Williamson JR, Cooper RH, Joseph SK, Thomas AP. Inositol trisphosphate and diacylglycerol as intracellular second messengers in the liver. *Am J Physiol* 1985;248:C203.

105. Wakelam MJO, Murphy GJ, Hruby VJ, Houslay MD. Activation of two signal-transduction systems in hepatocytes by glucagon. *Nature* 1986;323:68.

106. Rhee SG, Suh PG, Ryu SH, Lee SY. Studies of inositol phospholipid-specific phospholipase C. *Science* 1989;244:546.

107. Suh PG, Ryu SH, Moon KH, Suh HW, Rhee SG. Cloning and sequence of multiple forms of phospholipase C. *Cell* 1988;54:161.

108. Carter HR, Bird IM, Smith AD. Two species of phospholipase C isolated from lymphocytes produce specific ratios of inositol phosphate products. *FEBS Lett* 1986;204:23.

109. Ryu SH, Suh PG, Cho KS, Lee KY, Rhee SG. Bovine brain cytosol contains three immunologically distinct forms of inositol-phospholipid-specific phospholipase C. *Proc Natl Acad Sci USA* 1987;84:6649.

110. Nakanishi H, Nomura H, Kikkawa U, Kishimoto A, Nishizuka Y. Rat brain and liver soluble phospholipase C: resolution of two forms with different requirements for calcium. *Biochem Biophys Res Commun* 1985;132:582.

111. Banno Y, Nakashima S, Nozawa Y. Partial purification of phosphoinositide phospholipase C from human platelet cytosol; characterization of its three forms. *Biochem Biophys Res Commun* 1986;136:713.

112. Berridge MJ. Inositol trisphosphate and diacylglycerol: two interacting second messengers. *Annu Rev Biochem* 1987;56:159.

113. Nishizuka Y. The molecular heterogeneity of protein kinase C and its implications for cellular regulation. *Nature* 1988;334:661.

114. Wilson DB, Connolly TM, Ross TS, Ishii H, Bross TE, Deckmyn H, Brass LF, Majerus PW. Phosphoinositide metabolism in human platelets. *Adv Prostaglandin Thromboxane Leukotriene Res* 1987;17:558.

115. Wilson DB, Connolly TM, Bross TE, Majerus PW, Sherman WR, Tyler AN, Rubin LJ, Brown JE. Isolation and characterization of the inositol cyclic phosphate products of polyphosphoinositide cleavage by phospholipase C. Physiological effects in permeabilized platelets and *Limulus* photoreceptor cells. *J Biol Chem* 1985;260:13496.

116. Connolly TM, Wilson DB, Bross TE, Majerus PW. Isolation and characterization of the inositol cyclic phosphate products of phosphoinositide cleavage by phospholipase C. Metabolism in cell-free extracts. *J Biol Chem* 1986;261:122.

117. Ishii H, Connolly TM, Bross TE, Majerus PW. Inositol cyclic triphosphate [inositol 1,2-(cyclic)-4,5-triphosphate] is formed upon thrombin stimulation of human platelets. *Proc Natl Acad Sci USA* 1986;83:6397.

118. Nahorski SR, Batty I. Inositol tetrakisphosphate: recent developments in phosphoinositide metabolism and receptor function. *Trends Pharmacol Sci* 1986;83:83–85.

119. Hansen CA, Mah S, Williamson JR. Formation and metabolism of inositol 1,3,4,5-tetrakisphosphate in liver. *J Biol Chem* 1986;261:8100.

120. Irvine RF, Letcher AJ, Heslop JP, Berridge MJ. The inositol tris/tetrakisphosphate pathway—demonstration of Ins(1,4,5)P3 3-kinase activity in animal tissues. *Nature* 1986;320:631.

121. Stewart SJ, Prpic V, Powers FS, Bocckino SB, Isaacks RE, Exton JH. Perturbation of the human T-cell antigen receptor–T3 complex leads to the production of inositol tetrakisphosphate: evidence for conversion from inositol trisphosphate. *Proc Natl Acad Sci USA* 1986;83:6098.

122. Balla T, Guillemette G, Baukal AJ, Catt KJ. Metabolism of inositol 1,3,4-trisphosphate to a new tetrakisphosphate isomer in angiotensin stimulated adrenal glomerulosa cells. *J Biol Chem* 1987;262:9952.

123. Biden TJ, Comte M, Cox JA, Wollheim CB. Calcium-calmodu-

124. Rossier MF, Dantand IA, Lew PD, Capponi AM, Vallotton MB. Interconversion of inositol (1,4,5)-trisphosphate to inositol (1,3,4,5)-tetrakisphosphate and (1,3,4)-trisphosphate in permeabilized adrenal glomerulosa cells is calcium sensitive and ATP dependent. *Biochem Biophys Res Commun* 1986;139:259.

125. Tennes KA, McKinney JS, Putney JW Jr. Metabolism of inositol 1,4,5-trisphosphate in guinea-pig hepatocytes. *Biochem J* 1987;242:797.

126. Rossier MF, Capponi AM, Vallotton MB. Metabolism of inositol 1,4,5-trisphosphate in permeabilized rat aortic smooth-muscle cells. Dependence on calcium concentration. *Biochem J* 1987;245:305.

127. Shears SB, Storey DJ, Morris AJ, Cubitt AB, Parry JB, Michell RH, Kirk CJ. Dephosphorylation of *myo*-inositol 1,4,5-trisphosphate and *myo*-inositol 1,3,4-trisphosphate. *Biochem J* 1987;242:393.

128. Traynor-Kaplan AE, Harris AL, Thompson BL, Taylor P, Sklar LA. An inositol tetrakisphosphate-containing phospholipid in activated neutrophils. *Nature* 1988;334:353.

129. Dean NM, Moyer JD. Separation of multiple isomers of inositol phosphates formed in GH3 cells. *Biochem J* 1987;242:361.

130. Tennes KA, McKinney JS, Putney JW Jr. Metabolism of inositol 1,4,5-trisphosphate in guinea-pig hepatocytes. *Biochem J* 1987;242:797.

131. Hansen CA, Mah S, Williamson JR. Formation and metabolism of inositol 1,3,4,5-tetrakisphosphate in liver. *J Biol Chem* 1986;261:8100.

132. Balla T, Guillemette G, Baukal AJ, Catt KJ. Metabolism of inositol 1,3,4-trisphosphate to a new tetrakisphosphate isomer in angiotensin stimulated adrenal glomerulosa cells. *J Biol Chem* 1987;262:9952.

133. Burgess GM, McKinney JS, Irvine RF, Putney JW Jr. Inositol 1,4,5-trisphosphate and inositol 1,3,4-trisphosphate formation in Ca^{2+} mobilizing-hormone-activated cells. *Biochem J* 1985;232:237.

134. Irvine RF, Letcher AJ, Heslop JP, Berridge MJ. The inositol tris/tetrakisphosphate pathway—demonstration of Ins(1,4,5)P3 3-kinase activity in animal tissues. *Nature* 1986;320:631.

135. Berridge MJ, Irvine RF. Inositol phosphates and cell signalling. *Nature* 1989;341:197.

136. Ackermann KE, Gish BG, Honchar MP, Sherman WR. Evidence that inositol 1-phosphate in brain of lithium-treated rats results mainly from phosphatidylinositol metabolism. *Biochem J* 1987;242:517.

137. Streb H, Irvine RF, Berridge MJ, Schulz I. Release of Ca^{2+} from a nonmitochondrial intracellular store in pancreatic acinar cells by inositol-1,4,5-trisphosphate. *Nature* 1983;306:67.

138. Rasmussen H. The calcium messenger system (first of two parts). *N Engl J Med* 1986;314:1094.

139. Rasmussen H. The calcium messenger system (second of two parts). *N Engl J Med* 1986;314:1164.

140. Rasmussen H, Barrett PQ. Calcium messenger system: an integrated view. *Physiol Rev* 1984;64:938.

141. Michell RH, King CE, Guy GR, Hawkins PT, Stephens L. Metabolic pooling of inositol lipids in mature erythrocytes and in hormone-stimulated mammalian cells. *Prog Clin Biol Res* 1987;249:159.

142. Rana RS, Mertz RJ, Kowluru A, Dixon JF, Hokin LE, MacDonald MJ. Evidence for glucose-responsive and -unresponsive pools of phospholipid in pancreatic islets. *J Biol Chem* 1985;260:7861.

143. Monaco ME, Woods D. Characterization of the hormone-sensitive phosphatidylinositol pool in WRK-1 cells. *J Biol Chem* 1983;258:15125.

144. Monaco ME. The phosphatidylinositol cycle in WRK-1 cells evidence for a separate, hormone-sensitive phosphatidylinositol pool. *J Biol Chem* 1982;257:2137.

145. Monaco ME. Inositol metabolism in WRK-1 cells. Relationship of hormone-sensitive to -insensitive pools of phosphoinositides. *J Biol Chem* 1987;262:13001.

146. Koreh K, Monaco ME. The relationship of hormone-sensitive and hormone-insensitive phosphatidylinositol to phosphatidylin-

ositol 4,5-bisphosphate in the WRK-1 cell. *J Biol Chem* 1986;261:88.

147. Rana RS, Kowluru A, MacDonald MJ. Secretagogue-responsive and -unresponsive pools of phosphatidylinositol in pancreatic islets. *Arch Biochem Biophys* 1986;245:411.

148. Imai A, Gershengorn MC. Independent phosphatidylinositol synthesis in pituitary plasma membrane and endoplasmic reticulum. *Nature* 1987;325:726.

149. Dean NM, Moyer JD. Separation of multiple isomers of inositol phosphates formed in GH3 cells. *Biochem J* 1987;242:361.

150. Woodcock EA, Smith IA, Wallace CA, White BL. Evidence for a lack of inositol-(1,4,5)trisphosphate kinase activity in norepinephrine perfused rat hearts. *Biochem Biophys Res Commun* 1987;148:68.

151. Renard D, Poggioli J. Does the inositol tris/tetrakisphosphate pathway exist in the rat heart? *FEBS Lett* 1987;217:117.

152. Majerus PW, Connolly TM, Deckmyn H, Ross TS, Bross TE, Ishii H, Bansal VS, Wilson DB. The metabolism of phosphoinositide-derived messenger molecules. *Science* 1986;234:1519.

153. Heslop JP, Irvine RF, Tashjian AH Jr, Berridge MJ. Inositol tetrakis- and pentakisphosphates in GH4 cells. *J Exp Biol* 1985;119:395.

154. Berridge MJ. Calcium: a universal second messenger. *Triangle* 1985;24:79.

155. Exton JH. Mechanisms involved in calcium-mobilizing agonist responses. *Adv Cyclic Nucleotide Protein Phosphor Res* 1986; 20:211.

156. von Tscharner V, Prod'hom B, Baggiolini M, Reuter H. Ion channels in human neutrophils activated by a rise in free cytosolic calcium concentration. *Nature* 1986;324:369.

157. Steinheardt RA, Epel D. Activation of sea-urchin eggs by a calcium ionophore. *Proc Natl Acad Sci USA* 1974;71:1915.

158. Michell RH. Inositol phospholipids and cell surface receptor function. *Biochim Biophys Acta* 1975;415:81.

159. Kuno M, Gardner P. Ion channels activated by inositol 1,4,5-trisphosphate in plasma membrane of human T-lymphocytes. *Nature* 1987;326:301.

160. Slack BE, Bell JE, Benos DJ. Inositol-1,4,5-trisphosphate injection mimics fertilization potentials in sea urchin eggs. *Am J Physiol* 1986;250:C340.

161. Trimble ER, Bruzzone R, Meehan CJ, Biden TJ. Rapid increases in inositol 1,4,5-trisphosphate, inositol 1,3,4,5-tetrakisphosphate and cytosolic free Ca++ in agonist-stimulated pancreatic acini of the rat. *Biochem J* 1987;242:289.

162. Whitaker M, Irvine RF. Inositol 1,4,5-trisphosphate microinjection activates sea urchin eggs. *Nature* 1984;312:636.

163. Michell B. A second messenger function for inositol tetrakisphosphate. *Nature* 1986;324:613.

164. Irvine RF, Moor RM. Micro-injection of inositol 1,3,4,5-tetrakisphosphate activates sea urchin eggs by a mechanism dependent on external Ca^{2+}. *Biochem J* 1986;240:917.

165. von Tscharner V, Prod'hom B, Baggiolini M, Reuter H. Ion channels in human neutrophils activated by a rise in free cytosolic calcium concentration. *Nature* 1986;324:369.

166. Bidot-Lopez P, Farese RV, Sabir MA. Parathyroid hormone and adenosine-3',5'-monophosphate acutely increase phospholipids of the phosphatidate–polyphosphoinositide pathway in rabbit kidney cortex tubules in vitro by a cycloheximide-sensitive process. *Endocrinology* 1981;108:2078.

167. Wirthensohn G, Lefrank S, Guder WG. Phospholipid metabolism in rat kidney cortical tubules: 1. Effect of renal substrates. *Biochim Biophys Acta* 1984;795:392.

168. Wirthensohn G, Lefrank S, Guder WG. Phospholipid metabolism in rat kidney cortical tubules. 2. Effects of hormones on ^{32}P incorporation. *Biochim Biophys Acta* 1984;795:401.

169. Lo H, Lehotay DC, Katz D, Levey GS. Parathyroid hormone-mediated incorporation of ^{32}P-orthophosphate into phosphatidic acid and phosphatidylinositol in renal cortical slices. *Endocr Res Commun* 1976;3:377.

170. Esbrit P, Navarro F, Manzano F. A possible mechanism whereby parathyroid hormone stimulates phospholipid synthesis in canine renal tubules. *Bone Miner* 1988;4:7.

171. Rappaport MS, Stern PH. Parathyroid hormone and calcitonin

modify inositol phospholipid metabolism in fetal rat limb bones. *J Bone Miner Res* 1986;1:173.

172. Ruth JD, Murray TM. PTH binding and PTH stimulated inositol trisphosphate production in a clonal line of opossum kidney cells [Abstract]. *J Bone Miner Res* 1986;1:S451.

173. Hruska KA, Moskowitz D, Esbrit P, Civitelli R, Westbrook S, Huskey M. Stimulation of inositol trisphosphate and diacylglycerol production in renal tubular cells by parathyroid hormone. *J Clin Invest* 1987;79:230.

174. Hruska KA, Moskowitz D, Esbrit P, Civitelli R, Westbrook S, Huskey M. Stimulation of inositol trisphosphate and diacylglycerol production in renal tubular cells by parathyroid hormone. *J Clin Invest* 1987;79:230.

175. Cosman F, Morrow B, Kopal M, Bilezikian JP. Stimulation of inositol phosphate formation in ROS 17/2.8 cell membranes by guanine nucleotide, calcium and parathyroid hormone. *J Bone Miner Res* 1989;4:413.

176. Coleman DT, Bilezikian JP. Parathyroid hormone stimulates formation of inositol phosphates in a membrane preparation of canine renal cortical tubular cells. *J Bone Miner Res* 1990;5:299.

177. Babich M, King KL, Nissenson RA. G protein-dependent activation of a phosphoinositide-specific phospholipase C in UMR-106 osteosarcoma cell membranes. *J Bone Miner Res* 1989;4:549.

178. Coleman DT, Morrow BS, Bilezikian JP. Effects of guanine nucleotides and parathyroid hormone on inositol 1,4,5-trisphosphate metabolism in canine renal cortical tubular cell membranes. *J Bone Miner Res*, in press.

179. Yamaguchi DT, Hahn TJ, Iida-Klein A, Kleeman CR, Muallem S. Parathyroid hormone-activated calcium channels in an osteoblast-like clonal osteosarcoma cell line. cAMP-dependent and cAMP-independent calcium channels. *J Biol Chem* 1987; 262(16):7711–8.

180. Reid IR, Civitelli R, Halstead LR, Aviok LV, Hruska KA. Parathyroid hormone acutely elevates intracellular calcium in osteoblast-like cells. *Am J Physiol* 1987;253(1, part 1):E45–51.

181. Civitelli R, Reid IR, Westbrook S, Avioli LV, Hruska KA. PTH elevates inositol polyphosphates and diacylglycerol in a rat osteoblast-like cell line. *Am J Physiol* 1988;255(5, part 1):E660–7.

182. Donahue HJ, Fryer MJ, Eriksen EF, Heath H. Differential effects of parathyroid hormone and its analogues on cytosolic calcium ion and cAMP levels in cultured rat osteoblast-like cells. *J Biol Chem* 1988;263(27):13522–7.

183. Bidwell J, Fryer MJ, Firek AF, Donahue HJ, Heath H III. Desensitization of rat osteoblast-like cells (ROS 17/2.8) to parathyroid hormone uncouples the cAMP and cytosolic ionized calcium response links. *Endocrinology* 1991;128:1021.

184. Yamamoto Y, Fukase M, Fujii Y, Fujii T. The effects of human parathyroid hormone-related peptide on cytosolic free calcium and cAMP production in opossum kidney cell. *Bone Miner* 1989;7(3):221–31.

185. Tamura T, Sakamoto H, Filburn CR. Parathyroid hormone 1–34, but not 3–34 or 7–34, transiently translocates protein kinase C in cultured renal (OK) cells. *Biochem Biophys Res Commun* 1989;159(3):1352–8.

186. Fujii Y, Fukase M, Tsutsumi M, Miyauchi A, Tsunenari T, Fujita T. Parathyroid hormone control of free cytosolic Ca^{2+} in the kidney. *J Bone Miner Res* 1988;3(5):525–32.

187. Goligorsky MS, Hruska KA. Hormonal modulation of cytoplasmic calcium concentration in renal tubular epithelium. *Miner Electrolyte Metab* 1988;14(1):58–70.

188. Hruska KA, Goligorsky M, Scoble J, Tsutsumi M, Westbrook S, Moskowitz D. Effects of parathyroid hormone on cytosolic calcium in renal proximal tubular primary cultures. *Am J Physiol* 1986;251(2, part 2):F188–98.

189. Stathopoulos VM, Rosenblatt M, Stern PH. Actions of nleu[8,18]tyr[34]-bPTH-(3-34)amide on resorption and inositol phosphate production in fetal rat limb bones [Abstract]. *J Bone Miner Res* 1988;3:S110.

190. Berthelson S, Pettinger WA. A functional basis for the classification of alpha-adrenergic receptors. *Life Sci* 1977;21:595–606.

191. Minneman KP. Alpha 1-adrenergic receptor subtypes, inositol phosphates and sources of calcium. *Pharmacol Rev* 1988;40:87–119.

192. Han C, Wilson KM, Minnman KP. Alpha 1-adrenergic subtypes and formation of inositol phosphates in dispersed hepatocytes and renal cells. *Mol Pharmacol* 1990;37:903–10.
193. Rodan SB, Rodan GA. Dexamethasone effects on beta-adrenergic receptors and adenylate cyclase regulatory proteins G and G₁ in ROS 17/2.8 cells. *Endocrinology* 1986;118:2510–8.
194. Tashjian AH Jr, Ontjes DA, Munson PL. Alkylation and oxidation of methionine in bovine parathyroid hormone: effects on hormonal activity and antigenicity. *Biochemistry* 1964;3:1175.
195. Goltzman D, Bennett HPJ, Koutsilieris M, et al. Studies of the multiple forms of bioactive parathyroid hormone and parathyroid hormone-like substances. *Recent Prog Horm Res* 1986;42:665.
196. Nussbaum SR, Rosenblatt M, Potts JT Jr. Parathyroid hormone renal receptor interactions: demonstration of two receptor-binding domains. *J Biol Chem* 1980;255:10183.
197. Caulfield MP, McKee RL, Goldman ME, Duong LT, Fisher JE, Gay CT, DeHaven PA, Levy JJ, Roubini E, Nutt RF, Chorev M, Rosenblatt M. The bovine renal parathyroid hormone (PTH) receptor has equal affinity for two different amino acid sequences: the receptor binding domains of PTH and PTH-related protein are located within the 14–34 region. *Endocrinology* 1990;127:83–7.
198. Mahaffey E, Rosenblatt M, Shepard GL, Potts JT Jr. Parathyroid hormone inhibitors determination of minimum sequence requirements. *J Biol Chem* 1979;254:6496.
199. Rosenblatt M, Segre GV, Tyler GA, Shepard GL, Nussbaum SR, Potts JT Jr. Identification of a receptor-binding region in parathyroid hormone. *Endocrinology* 1980;107:545.
200. Nissenson RA, Diep D, Strewler GJ. Synthetic peptides comprising the amino-terminal sequence of a parathyroid hormone-like protein from human malignancies binding to parathyroid hormone receptors and activation of adenylate cyclase in bone cells and kidney. *J Biol Chem* 1988;263:12866.
201. Juppner H, Abou-Samra AB, Uneno S, Gu WX, Potts JT Jr, Segre GV. The parathyroid hormone-like peptide associated with humoral hypercalcemia of malignancy and parathyroid hormone bind to the same receptor on the plasma membrane of ROS 17/2.8 cells. *J Biol Chem* 1988;263:8557.
202. Shigeno C, Yamamoto J, Kitamura N, Noda T, Lee K, Sone T, Shiom K, Ohtaka A, Fujii N, Yajima H, Konishi J. Interaction of human parathyroid hormone-related peptide with parathyroid hormone receptors in clonal rat osteosarcoma cells. *J Biol Chem* 1988;263:18369.
203. Pun KK, Arnaud CD, Nissenson RA. Parathyroid hormone receptors in dermal fibroblasts: structural and functional characterization. *J Bone Miner Res* 1988;3:453.
204. McKee MD, Murray TM. Binding of intact parathyroid hormone to chicken renal plasma membranes: evidence for a second binding site with carboxyl-terminal specificity. *Endocrinology* 1985;117:1930.
205. Murray TM, Rao LG, Muzaffar SA, Ly H. Human parathyroid hormone carboxyterminal peptide (53–84) stimulates alkaline phosphatase activity in dexamethasone-treated rat osteosarcoma cells in vitro. *Endocrinology* 1989;124:1097.
206. Rao LG, Murray TM. Binding of intact parathyroid hormone to rat osteosarcoma cells: major contribution of binding sites for the carboxyl-terminal region of the hormone. *Endocrinology* 1985;117:1632.
207. Garcia JC, McConkey CL, Martin KJ. Separate binding sites for intact PTH 1–84 and synthetic PTH 1–34 in canine kidney. *Calcif Tissue Int* 1989;44(3):214–9.
208. Demay M, Mitchell J, Goltzman D. Comparison of renal and osseous binding of parathyroid hormone and hormonal fragments. *Am J Physiol* 1985;249(5, part 1):E437–46.
209. Coltrera MD, Potts JT Jr, Rosenblatt M. Identification of a renal receptor for parathyroid hormone by photoaffinity radiolabeling using a synthetic analogue. *J Biol Chem* 1981;256:10555–9.
210. Draper MW, Nissenson RA, Winer J, Ramachandran J, Arnaud CD. Photoaffinity labeling of the canine renal receptor for parathyroid hormone. *J Biol Chem* 1982;257:3714–8.
211. Goldring SR, Tyler GA, Krane SM, et al. Photoaffinity labeling of parathyroid hormone receptors: Comparison of receptors across species and target tissues and after desensitization to hormone. *Biochemistry* 1984;23:498–502.
212. Karpf DB, Arnaud CD, King K, Bambino T, Winer J, Nyiredy K, Nissenson RA. The canine renal parathyroid hormone receptor is a glycoprotein: characterization and partial purification. *Biochemistry* 1987;26(24):7825–33.
213. Coltera M, Rosenblatt M, Potts JT Jr. Analogues of parathyroid hormone containing D-amino acids: Evaluation of biological activity and viability. *Biochemistry* 1980;19:4380.
214. Wright BS, Tyler GA, O'Brien R, Caporale LH, Rosenblatt M. Immunoprecipitation of the parathyroid hormone receptor. *Proc Natl Acad Sci USA* 1987;84(1):26–30.
215. Karpf DB, Arnaud CD, Bambino T, Duffy D, King KL, Winer J, Nissenson RA. Structural properties of the renal parathyroid hormone receptor: hydrodynamic analysis and protease sensitivity. *Endocrinology* 1988;123:2611–20.
216. Karpf DB, Bambino T, Arnaud CD, Nissenson RA. Molecular determinants of parathyroid hormone receptor function. In: Cohen DV, Glorieux FH, Martin TJ, eds. *Calcium regulation and bone metabolism: basic and clinical aspects,* vol 10. Excerpta Medica: Amsterdam: 1990;15–23.
217. Lefkowitz RJ, Caron MG. Adrenergic receptors. *J Biol Chem* 1988;263:4993–6.
218. O'Dowd BF, Lefkowitz RJ, Caron MG. Structure of the adrenergic and related receptors. *Annu Rev Neurosci* 1989;12:67–83.
219. Kobilka BK, Frielle T, Dohlman HG, et al. Delineation of the intronless nature of the genes for the human and hamster beta₂-adrenergic receptor and their putative promoter regions. *J Biol Chem* 1987;262:7321–7.
220. Strader CD, Sigal IS, Register RB, et al. Identification of residues required for ligand binding to the beta-adrenergic receptor. *Proc Natl Acad Sci USA* 1987;84:4384–88.
221. Dixon RAF, Sigal IS, Rands E, Register RB, Candelore MR, Blake AD, Strader CD. *Nature* 1987;326:73–7.
222. Strader CD, Candelore MR, Hill WS, et al. Identification of two serine residues involved in agonist activation of the beta-adrenergic receptor. *J Biol Chem* 1989;264:13572–8.
223. Strader CD, Dixon RAF, Cheung AH, et al. Mutations that uncouple the beta-adrenergic receptor from G₅ and increase agonist affinity. *J Biol Chem* 1987;262:16439–443.
224. Kobika BK, MacGregor C, Daniel K, Kobika TS, Caron MG, Lefkowitz RJ. Functional activity and regulation of human beta-adrenergic receptors expressed in *Xenopus* oocytes. *J Biol Chem* 1987;262:15796–802.
225. Einonne LJ, Marullo S, Delavier-Kluteliko C, Kaveri SV, Durieu-Trautmann O, Strosberg AD. Structure of the bone for human beta-adrenergic receptor: expression and promoter characterization. *Proc Natl Acad Sci USA* 1987;34:6995–9.
226. Casey PJ, Gilman AG. G-proteins involvement in receptor–effector coupling. *J Biol Chem* 1988;263:2577–80.
227. Johnson GL, Dhanasekaran N. The G-proteins family and their interaction with receptors. *Endocr Rev* 1989;10:317–31.
228. Moss J, Vaughan M. ADR ribosylation of guanyl nucleotide-binding regulatory proteins by bacterial toxins. *Adv Enzymol* 1987;61:1303–79.
229. Moss J. Signal transduction by receptor-responsive guanyl nucleotide-binding proteins: modulation by bacterial toxin-catalyzed ADP-ribosylation *Clin Res* 1987;35:451–58.
230. Stryer L. Cyclic GMP cascade of vision. *Annu Rev Neurosci* 1986;9:87–119.
231. Fong HKW, Yoshimoto KK, Eversole-Cire P, Simon MI. Identification of a GTP-binding protein a subunit that lacks an apparent ADP-ribosylation site for pertussis toxin. *Proc Natl Acad Sci USA* 1988;85:3066–70.
232. Ransnas LA, Insel PA. Quantitation of the stimulatory guanine nucleotide binding protein G in S49 cell membranes using anti-peptide antibodies to alpha. *J Biol Chem* 1988;263:9482–5.
233. Mattera R, Graziano MP, Yatani A, Zhou Z, Graf R, Codina J, Birnbaumer L, Gilman AG, Brown AM. Splice variants of the alpha subunit of the G protein G₁ activate both adenylyl cyclase and calcium channels. *Science* 1989;243:804–7.
234. Bray P, Carter A, Simons C, et al. Human cDNA clones for four

species of G alpha$_s$ signal transducing protein. *Proc Natl Acad Sci USA,* 1986;83:8893–97.

235. Codina J, Yatani A, Crenet D, Brown AM, Birnbaumer L. The alpha subunit of the GTP-binding protein G$_1$ opens atrial potassium channels. *Science* 1987;236:442–5.

236. Gilman AG. G proteins: transducers of receptor-generated signals. *Annu Rev Biochem* 1987;56:615–49.

237. Jones DT, Reed RR. Molecular cloning of the GTP binding protein cDNA species from rat olfactory neuroepithelium. *J Biol Chem* 1987;262:14241–9.

238. Moriarty TM, Gillo B, Carty D, Premont RT, Landau EM, Iyengar R. Beta subunits of GTP-binding proteins inhibit muscarinic receptor stimulation of phospholipase C. *Proc Natl Acad Sci USA* 1988;85:8865.

239. Gilman AG. G proteins: transducers of receptor-generated signals. *Annu Rev Biochem* 1987;56:615.

240. Casey PJ, Gilman AG. G protein involvement in receptor–effector coupling. *J Biol Chem* 1988;263:2577.

241. Van Dop C, Gsubokawa M, Bourne HR, Ramachandran J. Amino acid sequence of retinal transducin at the site ADP-ribosylated by cholera toxin. *J Biol Chem* 1984;259:696.

242. Hurley JB, Simon MI, Leplow DB, Robishaw JD, Gilman AG. Homologies between signal transducing G proteins and ras gene products. *Science* 1984;226:860.

243. West RE Jr, Moss J, Vaughn M, Lin T, Liu TY. Pertussis toxin-catalyzed ADP-ribosylation of transducin: cysteine 347 is the ADP-ribose acceptor site. *J Biol Chem* 1985;260:14428.

244. Nissenson RA, Abbott SR, Teitelbaum AP, et al. Endogenous biologically active human parathyroid hormone: measurement by a guanyl nucleotide-amplified renal adenylate cyclase assay. *J Clin Endocrinol Metab* 1981;52:840.

245. Aurbach XY, Marx SJ, Spiegel AM. Parathyroid hormone, calcitonin, and the calciferols. In: Wilson JD, Foster DW, eds. *Williams textbook of endocrinology.* Philadelphia: WB Saunders, 1981;1137.

246. Berridge JB. Inositol trisphosphate, calcium, lithium, and cell signaling. *JAMA* 1989;262:1834–41.

247. Coleman DT. Activation of the inositol phosphate second-messenger system in canine renal cortical tubular membranes by parathyroid hormone and guanine nucleotides. PhD. thesis, Columbia University, 1990.

248. Graziano MP, Gilman AG. Guanine nucleotide-binding regulatory proteins: mediators of transmembrane signaling. *Trends in Pharmacol Sci* 1987;8:478–81.

Disorders of Bone and Mineral Metabolism,
edited by Fredric L. Coe and Murray J. Favus,
© 1992 by Raven Press, Ltd. All rights reserved.

CHAPTER **7**

Metabolism of Vitamin D

Helen L. Henry and Anthony W. Norman

Traditionally perceived as an antirachitic vitamin essential for regulation of calcium homeostasis, it is now acknowledged that vitamin D orchestrates a wide array of biological responses via mechanisms analogous to those used by classic steroid hormones. The principal mediator of vitamin D_3 action is a metabolite, $1\alpha,25$-dihydroxyvitamin D_3 [$1,25(OH)_2D_3$], that is derived from its prohormone or precursor form, vitamin D_3. $1,25(OH)_2D_3$ is largely instrumental in mediating the diverse effects of vitamin D in the classical target tissues such as intestine, bone, and kidney. Conceptual advances in the understanding of the biological activity of $1,25(OH)_2D_3$—from the standpoint of its chemistry, biochemistry, regulation, and molecular biology—have unequivocally established its identity as a steroid hormone rather than a vitamin in the classic sense. The interested reader is directed to a number of other reviews which discuss areas of vitamin D endocrinology not emphasized in this chapter (1–4).

Besides its role in mineral homeostasis, $1,25(OH)_2D_3$ has been implicated in the processes of osteogenesis, modulation of immune response, modulation of the process of insulin secretion by the pancreatic B cell, muscle cell function, and the differentiation and growth of epidermal and hemopoietic tissues. From a mechanistic viewpoint, the hormone $1,25(OH)_2D_3$ resembles other classic steroid hormones in that it interacts with specific cytosolic/nuclear receptors—an event that is followed by (a) nuclear localization of the steroid–receptor complex and (b) its subsequent association with selected regions of the regulatory components of genes whose expression can be either up-regulated or down-regulated. The ubiq-

uitous distribution of the vitamin D receptor, coupled with its strong homology with other members of the nuclear transacting receptor family (which includes receptors for thyroid hormone, estrogen, progesterone, glucocorticoid, and retinoic acid), is another additional feature of this hormone that parallels classic steroid hormones. This chapter is aimed at providing a synopsis of the vitamin D endocrine system, and it spans various aspects related to the hormone's biochemistry, metabolism, and regulation.

HISTORY OF DISCOVERY OF VITAMIN D

Any understanding of the history of vitamin D is closely related to the history of rickets (5). The earliest mention of this disease was made by Whistler (in 1645) and later by Glisson (in 1650), who together provided a detailed description of rickets from a clinical perspective. Opinion seems to be divided regarding the etymology of the term "rickets." Some believe that the term "rickets" stems from the term "rucket," implying to breathe with difficulty; ostensibly, breathing was impaired as a result of improper rib development. Others contend that the term originated from the Welsh "wrygaits," meaning "crooked goings" or "twisted legs." The ability of heated, aerated cod liver oil to cure rickets established the existence of a new vitamin which was originally termed "vitamin D" by McCollum.

Nutritional studies by Sir Edward Mellanby later identified rickets as being caused by a dietary deficiency of vitamin D. However, technically, it is erroneous to construe vitamin D as being an essential nutritional substance, since all higher vertebrates have an endogenous mechanism involving the process of sunlight/ultraviolet (UV) irradiation which effects the synthesis of this hormone from its precursor 7-dehydrocholesterol present in the skin (6). UV irradiation of either rachitic children or experimentally induced rachitic rats has also been shown

H. L. Henry: Department of Biochemistry, University of California—Riverside, Riverside, California 92521.
A. W. Norman: Department of Biochemistry and Division of Biomedical Sciences, University of California—Riverside, Riverside, California 92521.

to result in remission of rickets. The knowledge of anti-rachitic properties of irradiated animal foods and animal skins, together with the finding that the activatable factor was present in the sterol fraction, laid the foundation for the eventual isolation and chemical characterization of vitamin D_3 in 1937 in the laboratory of Professor A. Windaus at Göttingen University.

CHEMISTRY OF VITAMIN D AND RELATED COMPOUNDS

Chemically speaking, vitamin D and all its metabolites are seco-steroids. A seco-steroid is one in which the A, B, C, or D rings of the typical cyclopentanoperhydro-phenanthrene ring of cholesterol or 7-dehydrocholesterol backbone (see Fig. 1, top row) is broken; in the case of vitamin D, it is the 9–10 carbon bond of ring B which is broken. If the side chain is equivalent to that of cholesterol, the compound is designated as vitamin D_3; however, if the side chain is that of ergosterol, it is designated as vitamin D_2 (see Fig. 2). The provitamins do not ac-

quire vitamin D activity until the B ring is broken between C-9 and C-10 and a double bond is formed between C-10 and C-19, forming (in the case of vitamin D_3) the 9,10-seco(5Z,7E)-5,7,10(19)-cholestatriene-3β-ol derivative. Because of the 9,10-seco nature of vitamin D compounds, the A ring can become inverted in relation to rings C and D, with rotation occurring around the bond between C-7 and C-8 (see Fig. 1, structure 2). Therefore it is important that the conventional steroid α and β nomenclature for substituent groups on the A ring be indicated with reverse notation, since there is inversion of the A ring.

Vitamin D_2 or ergocalciferol is derived from the provitamin ergosterol upon UV irradiation, similar to the photochemical production of vitamin D_3. It is also a seco-steroid-like vitamin D_3, and the only difference chemically between vitamin D_2 and D_3 is the presence, in vitamin D_2, of a double bond between C-22 and C-23 and an additional methyl group at C-24. It undergoes metabolic conversions similar to those discussed in detail below for vitamin D_3 (see Fig. 2).

A closer analysis of the topology of vitamin D_3 and its

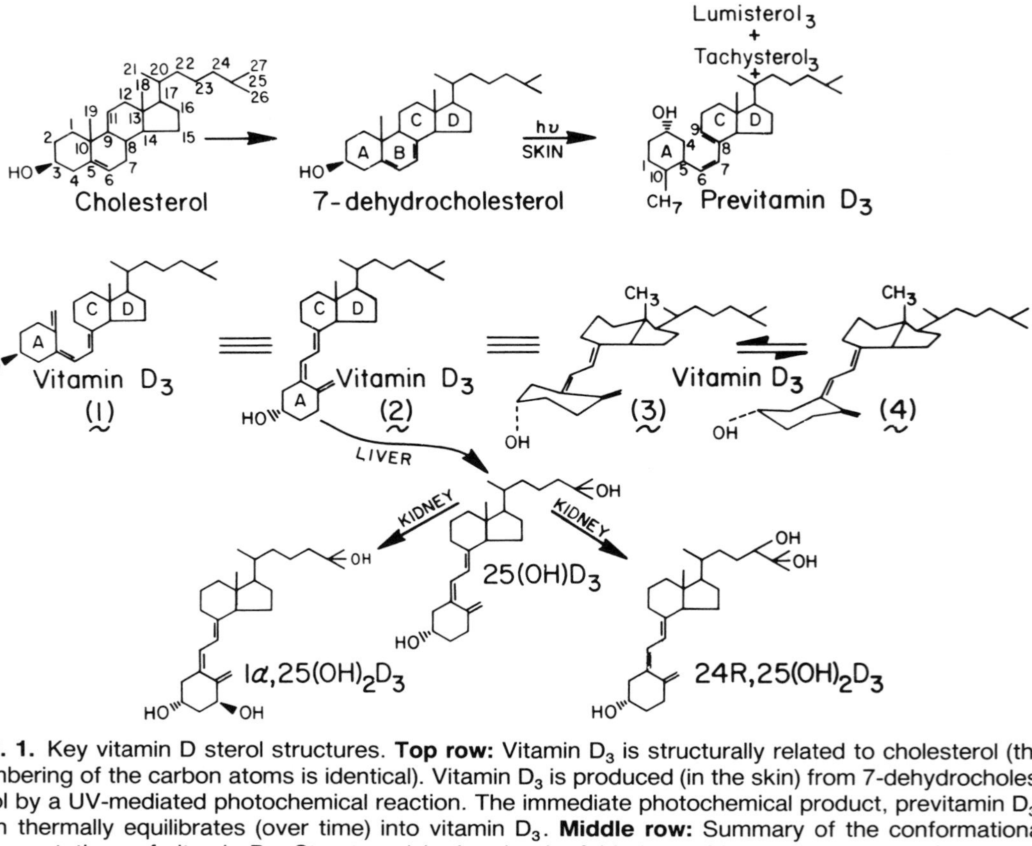

FIG. 1. Key vitamin D sterol structures. **Top row:** Vitamin D_3 is structurally related to cholesterol (the numbering of the carbon atoms is identical). Vitamin D_3 is produced (in the skin) from 7-dehydrocholesterol by a UV-mediated photochemical reaction. The immediate photochemical product, previtamin D_3, then thermally equilibrates (over time) into vitamin D_3. **Middle row:** Summary of the conformational representations of vitamin D_3. Structure 1 is the classic, folded steroid version; structure 2 is an extended version derived from x-ray crystallographic analysis; structures 3 and 4 illustrate the A-ring chair–chair conformer equilibrium present in solution for all vitamin D seco-steroids (including all metabolites) as identified by nuclear magnetic resonance analysis. **Bottom row:** Structures of the three principal metabolites of vitamin D_3.

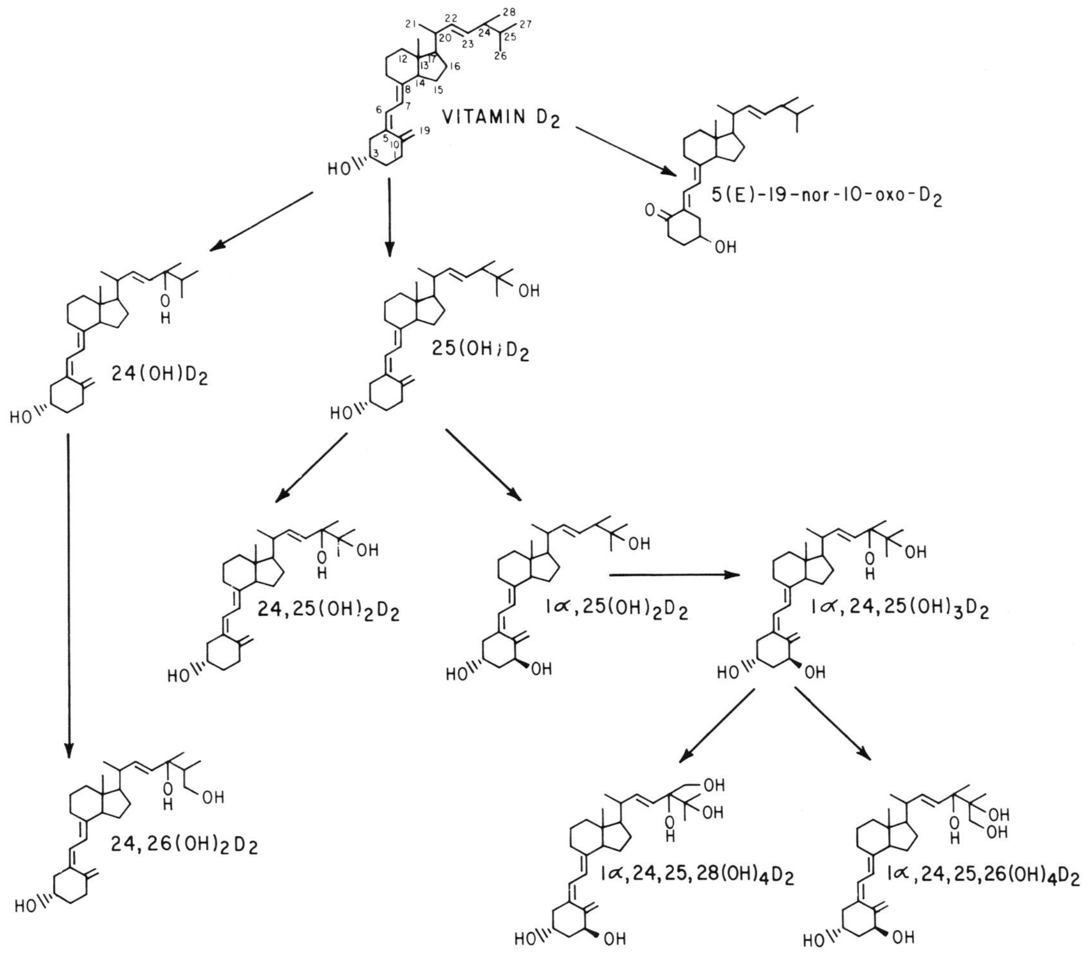

FIG. 2. Summary of the metabolic transformations of vitamin D_3. The structures of all known chemically characterized metabolites are shown.

metabolites in solution by high-resolution proton magnetic resonance spectroscopy, together with lanthanide-induced shift studies (7), indicates that in solution the seco-steroid vitamin D is present in a dynamic equilibration between two chair–chair conformers of the A ring (see Fig. 1, structures 3 and 4); these pair of structures are the most accurate and preferred means of delineating the structure of all vitamin D seco-steroids (8).

Vitamin D and its daughter metabolites share many of the solubility characteristics of classic steroids inasmuch as they are soluble in organic solvents ranging from hexane to methanol and are quite insoluble in aqueous solutions. All the known biologically active D-vitamins possess the *cis*-triene structures which have a UV absorption maximum at 265 nm, with a minimum at 228 nm. Vitamin D is extremely stable when stored in organic solvents in the absence of oxygen and light. Its instability is mostly attributed to oxidative degradation of the *cis*-triene system.

SYNTHESIS OF VITAMIN D

Background

Our understanding of the steroidal mode of action of vitamin D from an endocrine perspective has been facilitated by the elucidation of the complex metabolic pathways and the regulatory mechanisms (9). Metabolic transformation of vitamin D_3 involving hydroxylations at C-1 and C-25 are recognized to be imperative for vitamin D to carry out its biological functions. With the exception of birds and the New World monkey, the biological activities of vitamin D_2 and vitamin D_3 have been shown to be identical in all animals. Although both vitamin D_2 and vitamin D_3 have been utilized as forms of "vitamin D" for supplementation of food (milk, bread, etc.) or vitamin pills, it would appear that utilization of vitamin D_3 is the most appropriate, since this is the naturally occurring form of the D-vitamin in mammals.

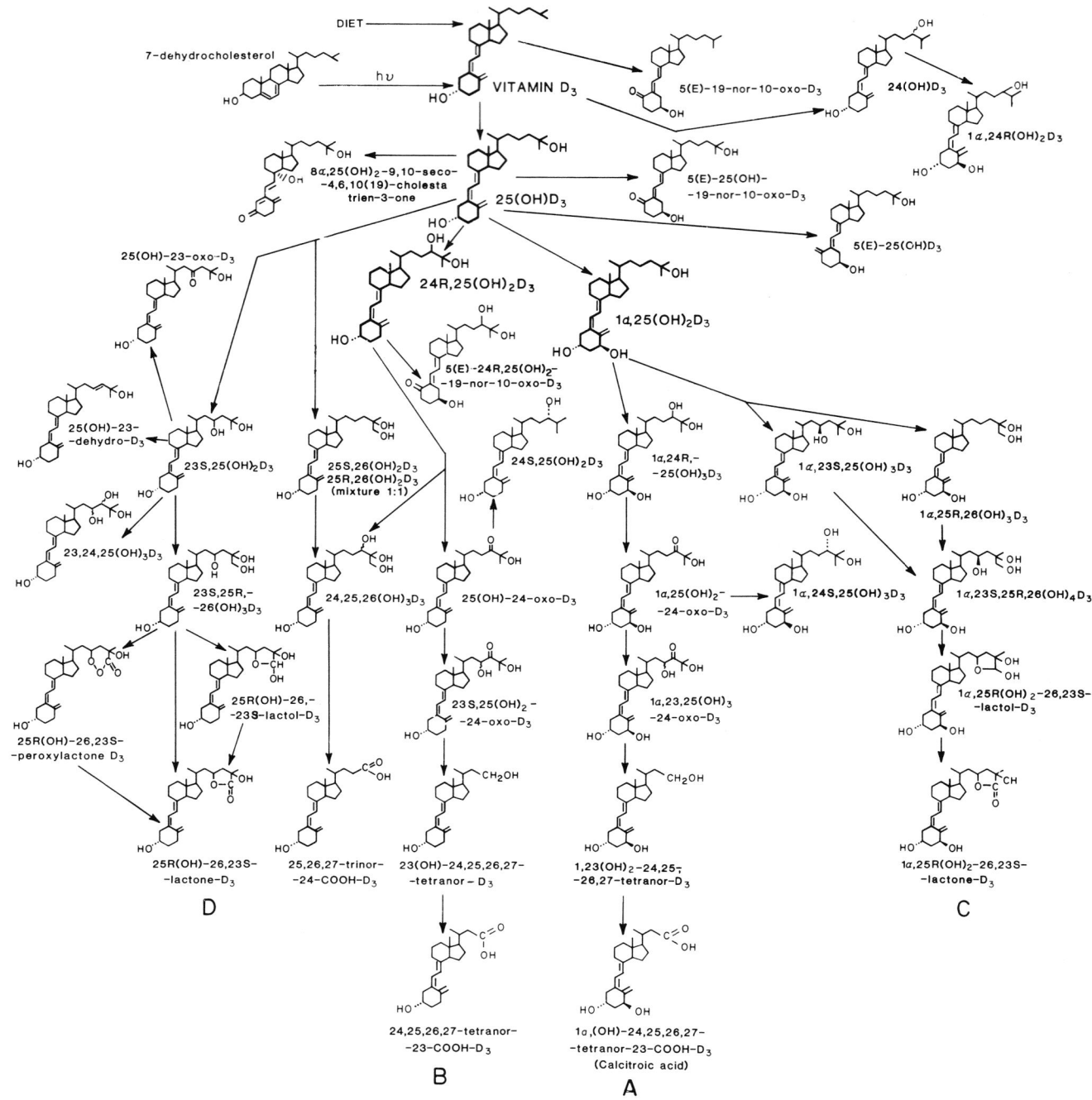

FIG. 3. Summary of the metabolic transformations of vitamin D_3. The structures of all known chemically characterized metabolites are shown.

Figure 3 summarizes our current understanding of the metabolism of vitamin D_3. Altogether, some 37 metabolites of vitamin D_3 have been isolated and chemically characterized. Figure 3 summarizes our current understanding of the metabolism of vitamin D_2; here, nine metabolites have been isolated and characterized. As can be noted by comparison of Figs. 2 and 3, there are many similarities in the metabolism of vitamin D_2, with the

more thorough studies being carried out with vitamin D_3.

Photoproduction of Vitamin D

Though historically vitamin D has been classified as a vitamin that can be obtained from dietary sources, the skin is considered to be the site of photochemical synthesis of vitamin D_3, primarily in the malphigian layer of the epidermis. Upon exposure to sunlight, the epidermal cutaneous reservoir of provitamin D_3 (7-dehydrocholesterol) is photolyzed to previtamin D_3, which undergoes isomerization via a nonphotochemical rearrangement to yield vitamin D_3 at a rate dictated by the temperature of the skin (10). During prolonged exposure to sunlight, the accumulation of previtamin D_3 is delimited by its photoisomerization into two biologically inert sterols, lumisterol and tachysterol. Increased skin concentrations of melanin, as well as changes in geographical locations to more northerly latitudes with lower UV levels, appear to have some ability to reduce the cutaneous production of previtamin D_3 (11).

SYNTHESIS OF 1,25(OH)₂-VITAMIN D₃

Formation of 25(OH)-Vitamin D₃

Background

Vitamin D_3 is transported to the liver and undergoes hydroxylation at C-25 to form $25(OH)D_3$, the major circulating form of vitamin D. This hydroxylation is catalyzed by a mixed function oxygenase(s) enzyme known as "vitamin D_3-25-hydroxylase," localized in liver microsomes and mitochondria.

Characteristics of Vitamin D₃-25-hydroxylase

Tissue and Subcellular Distribution

The liver of the rat was the first reported site of the 25-hydroxylation of vitamin D_3 (12), followed shortly by reports of 25-hydroxylase activity in kidney (13) and intestine (14). Rather broad tissue distribution of the 25-hydroxylation of vitamin D_3 was reported by Ichikawa et al. (15), with activity in lung, ovary, adrenal cortex, and brain, among other tissues; however, the liver was the most abundant source of activity. Although hepatectomized animals have been reported to produce $25(OH)D_3$, it is generally agreed that the liver is the most important site of $25(OH)D_3$ production in vivo under normal physiological circumstances. Hepatoma cell lines retaining parenchymal cell morphology also produce $25(OH)D_3$ (16).

The subcellular distribution of 25-hydroxylation enzyme activity within the liver has been rather more difficult to identify with certainty, but not (as can be seen from Table 1) because of lack of experiments addressing the question. In the majority of those studies in which microsomal and mitochondrial fractions were compared directly, both fractions had substantial activity (15,17). In virtually all tissues and species, there was less than an order of magnitude of difference between apparent 25-hydroxylase activity in the two subcellular fractions.

TABLE 1. *Liver vitamin D_3-25-hydroxylases[a]*

| Species | Reference | 25-Hydroxylase activity | |
		Microsomes	Mitochondria
Rat	8	+	
	15	+	+
	18	−	P
	19	P	−
	20	+	+
Rabbit	24		P
Pig	17	P	
Human	82	−	+

[a] The presence of vitamin D_3-25-hydroxylase activity is indicated by a "+"; a "−" indicates lack of activity. If the subcellular fraction was not assayed, there is no entry. A "P" denotes that a cytochrome P450 capable of supporting 25-hydroxylation was isolated from the fraction indicated.

Furthermore, purified cytochrome P450, which catalyzes the 25-hydroxylation of vitamin D_3 and 1α-OH-D_3, has been obtained from both fractions (17–19).

The uncertainty concerning the physiologically most important subcellular site of $25(OH)D_3$ production in vivo may be the result of one or a combination of the following characteristics of this activity. First, in rats there is a sex difference (20) in both microsomal (male > female by 2.8-fold) and mitochondrial (female > male by 4.6-fold). Whether this sexual dimorphism occurs in other species has not been studied systematically, but if it does it could certainly contribute to variations in experimental observations on the subcellular localization of the 25-hydroxylase. Second, solubilized cytochrome P450s do not always show the same substrate specificity (21–23) as they do when in their intact subcellular organelle. In addition, some P450s show markedly reduced K_m values for their substrates upon solubilization. Thus experimental manipulations and assay conditions can easily influence the observed activity of these enzymes. Finally, a cytochrome P450 preparation purified to homogeneity from rabbit liver (24) also catalyzed the 26-hydroxylation of 5β-cholestane-$3a,7a,12a$-triol; thus substrate specificity is not absolute, and knowing the true physiological substrate of a given cytochrome P450 is not always possible. For these several reasons, a definitive statement on an exclusive subcellular site of 25-hydroxylation cannot be made on the basis of presently available information.

Characteristics of Mixed Function Oxidases in General and of the Vitamin D_3-25-hydroxylase

Regardless of tissue or subcellular origin, the 25-hydroxylation of vitamin D_3 is a cytochrome-P450-dependent process. In these reactions, molecular oxygen is reduced, one molecule to water and one to the hydroxyl group to be incorporated stereospecifically into the steroid—hence, the general term "mixed function oxidase"

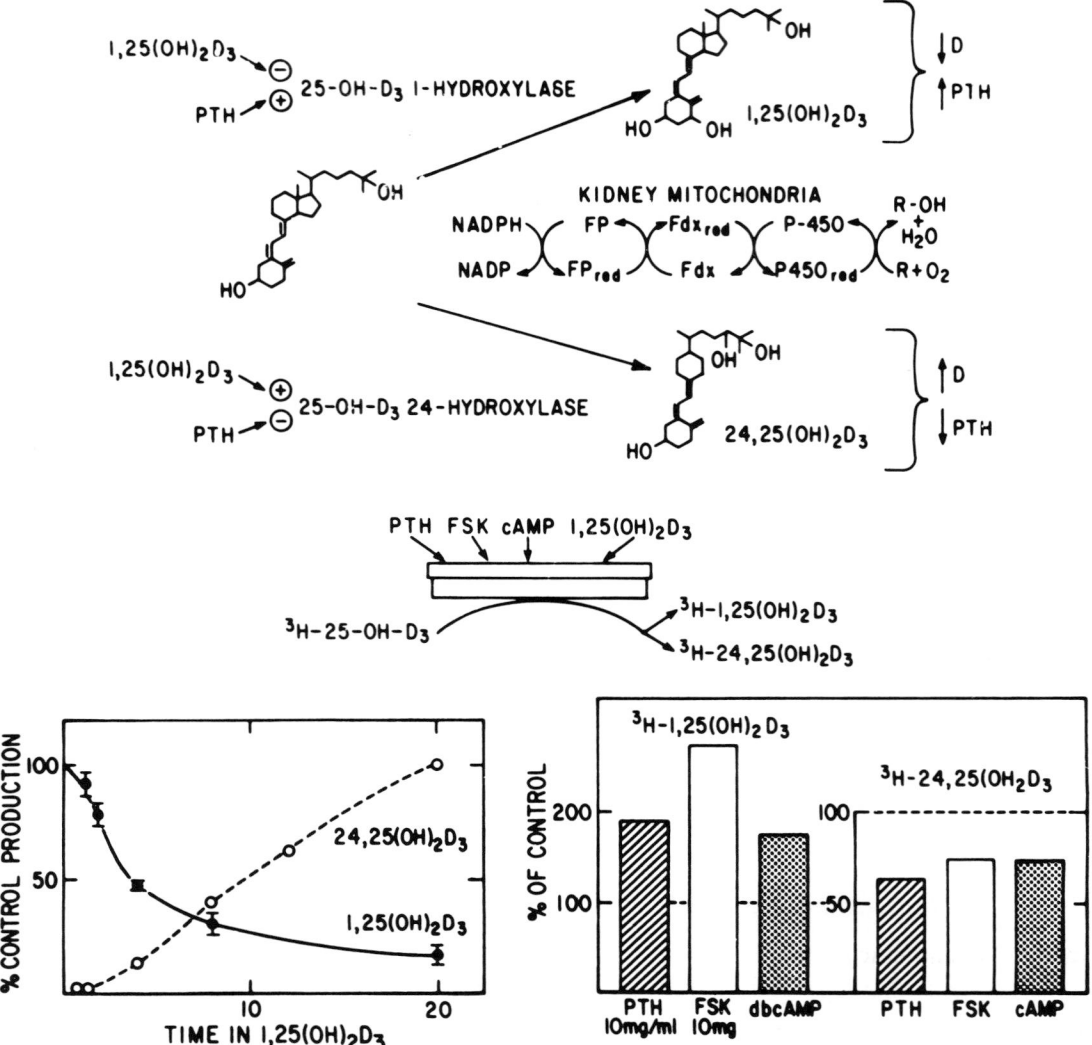

FIG. 4. Regulation of vitamin D metabolism. The components of the mitochondrial 1- and 24-hydroxylases are indicated, along with the nature of the effects of vitamin D or 1,25(OH)₂D₃ and parathyroid hormone (PTH). As indicated in the center and bottom, studies with kidney cell cultures have been particularly useful in elucidating the features of the regulation of 25(OH)D₃ metabolism. FP, flavoprotein; Fdx, ferredoxin; cAMP, cyclic AMP; dbcAMP, dibutyrylcyclic AMP; FSK, forskolin.

(MFO). The electrons for this reductive reaction are, in most instances, ultimately derived from NADPH. In the mitochondria, there are two protein carriers for these electrons. The first, ferredoxin reductase (a protein of about 54 kD), passes electrons, one at a time, to the smaller (12–14 kD) ferredoxin. Ferredoxin is an iron-sulfur protein envisioned to shuttle back and forth between the reductase and cytochrome P450 and is found in the matrix compartment of the mitochondria. In the microsomes, only one electron carrier, the membrane flavoprotein cytochrome P450 reductase, is involved in transferring the electrons between NADPH and cytochrome P450. The relationships between these proteins are illustrated in the upper portion of Fig. 4.

Purified mitochondrial and microsomal P450s catalyzing the 25-hydroxylation of vitamin D have been reported to have molecular weights of 50–52 kD as measured by sodium dodecyl sulfate–polyacrylamide gel electrophoresis. All show the characteristic spectral shift to 450 nm (from which the proteins derive their names) when the reduced hemoprotein is exposed to carbon monoxide.

Regulation of the 25-Hydroxylation of Vitamin D₃

Whether the 25-hydroxylation of vitamin D is subject to feedback regulation was a matter of some controversy in the older literature (25), with evidence existing both for and against a role for $25(OH)D_3$ in this process and no clear resolution of the question. More recent studies (26,27) suggest that $1,25(OH)_2D_3$ can reduce 25-hydroxylase activity in vitro. Using a combination of in vivo and in vitro approaches, however, Haddad et al. (28) showed rather clearly that $1,25(OH)_2D_3$ does not inhibit 25-hydroxylase activity measured in vivo but does alter metabolic handling of $25(OH)D_3$ as well as that of its substrate, vitamin D. These investigators concluded that if $1,25(OH)_2D_3$ does alter 25-hydroxylation, the effect is so modest as to lack physiological meaning. Low calcium levels, on the other hand, clearly elevate the rate at which $25(OH)D_3$ is produced by the liver (28).

The variation in the above observations, along with their interpretation described above, might well lie in the effects of different experimental protocols on serum calcium levels. It should also be pointed out that since the active form of the hormone is $1,25(OH)_2D_3$ (for which $25(OH)D_3$ is the substrate, which usually circulates in more than sufficient amounts to meet the needs of the organism), close regulation at the point of $25(OH)D_3$ production might not be expected to occur.

As alluded to above, there is, in rats at least, sexual dimorphism in the relative activity and subcellular distribution of the 25-hydroxylase (as well as for the handling of other steroids and drugs). This suggests a possible role for the regulation of $25(OH)D_3$ production by the sex steroids, and in fact it has been reported (29) that while 25-hydroxylase activity is independent of hormone status in female rats, it is increased by castration and hypophysectomy in male rats. These investigators concluded that the sexual dimorphism seen in adult rats is the result of differences in the pituitary brought about by exposure to androgens during the neonatal period.

Renal Metabolism of $25(OH)D_3$

Properties of $25(OH)D_3$-1α-hydroxylase and $25(OH)D_3$-24-hydroxylase

It has been known for many years that the chick kidney $25(OH)D_3$-1-hydroxylase is a cytochrome-P450-dependent reaction (30,31) sharing the properties of other mitochondrial MFOs described in section entitled "Formation of 25(OH)-Vitamin D_3," above. That is, it depends on NADPH, a ferredoxin, and a ferredoxin reductase to supply the electrons for the reduction of molecular oxygen. Both enzymes are mitochondrial and undoubtedly share many characteristics with the mitochondrial steroidogenic hydroxylases in the classic steroidogenic tissues such as the adrenal, ovary, and testis. Solubilized cytochrome P450 preparations show complete dependence on NADPH and, depending on the state of partial purification of these proteins, on ferredoxin and ferredoxin reductase as well. These properties have been confirmed for the chick and rat 24-hydroxylase as well (32,33).

Although there is a preliminary report of the purification of porcine kidney 1- and 24-hydroxylases (34), no molecular-weight data were reported. Nevertheless, it appears that the molecular weights will fall within the range of those for other mitochondrial P450s (45–60 kD). A rat kidney cytochrome P450 with 24-hydroxylase activity has been purified (33) and shown to have a molecular weight of about 52 kD.

Regulation of $25(OH)D_3$ Metabolism

$1,25(OH)_2D_3$

It has long been understood that the condition of vitamin D deficiency leads to elevated 1-hydroxylase activity (34,35), and in fact the vitamin-D-deficient chick was the first tissue in which the 1-hydroxylation of $25(OH)D_3$ was demonstrated (35–38). Over the ensuing years of study it has become clear, in fact, that the most effective way of altering the renal metabolism of $25(OH)D_3$ is through manipulation of the vitamin D status—or, more precisely, the $1,25(OH)_2D_3$ status—of the animal. The effect of $1,25(OH)_2D_3$ is to repress renal $1,25(OH)_2D_3$ synthesis and to increase the production of $24,25(OH)_2D_3$. When cell culture systems became available in which to investigate the metabolism of $25(OH)D_3$ (39,40), it was quickly demonstrated that this effect is a direct one on renal cells and not secondary to, for example, effects of $1,25(OH)_2D_3$ on serum calcium, parathyroid hormone (PTH), or serum phosphate. This regulatory process is a dynamic one, being rapidly reversible. When, for example, $1,25(OH)_2D_3$ is removed from the medium, 24-hydroxylase activity returns to basal levels within hours and 1-hydroxylase activity rises to the high levels observed in the hormone-deficient state (see Fig. 4). The actual mechanism of the action of $1,25(OH)_2D_3$ at the subcellular and molecular level to alter the metabolism of $25(OH)D_3$ has not been elucidated, but it likely involves alterations in gene expression. As is clear from the discussion below, many other factors are capable of influencing the renal metabolism of $25(OH)D_3$, but all of these must be considered within the context of the vitamin D status (or in cell culture, the $1,25(OH)_2D_3$ status) of the model being investigated.

Parathyroid Hormone

There is no doubt that elevated parathyroid hormone levels are associated with increased $1,25(OH)_2D_3$ levels and production in vivo (39,41,42,44) and that it stimulates $1,25(OH)_2D_3$ synthesis when added to avian and mammalian cell culture systems (39,40,43,45). In the latter systems, $24,25(OH)_2D_3$ is usually seen to decrease in response to PTH, underscoring the reciprocal nature of the regulation of the production of these two metabolites.

The mechanism of PTH-induced changes in the renal metabolism of $25(OH)D_3$ have not been fully elucidated, and indeed there may be more than one intracellular signaling system mediating these effects. The cyclic AMP (cAMP) pathway, leading to activation of protein kinase A and protein phosphorylation, is certainly involved (46), although evidence for cAMP-independent mechanisms has also been reported (47,48).

Recent observations indicate that 12-O-tetradecanoylphorbol-13-acetate (TPA), presumably by activation of protein kinase C, affects $25(OH)D_3$ in an opposite direction; that is, it causes a decrease in $1,25(OH)_2D_3$ synthesis and an increase in the production of $24,25(OH)_2D_3$.

The factors physiologically responsible for the activation of protein kinase C have not yet been identified, nor have the proteins whose phosphorylation is presumably affected by protein kinase C activation. Although the effects of TPA (the protein kinase C activator) and $1,25(OH)_2D_3$ on $25(OH)D_3$ metabolism are qualitatively similar [both leading to reduced $1,25(OH)_2D_3$ production and increased $24,25(OH)_2D_3$ production], they are additive and therefore likely independent of one another. In addition, the pathways mediated by protein kinases A and C appear to be independent of one another (48).

Other Regulators of 25(OH)D₃ Metabolism

It is likely that $1,25(OH)_2D_3$ and PTH are the most important day-to-day physiological regulators of renal $25(OH)D_3$ metabolism. Although other factors have been implicated from in vivo studies, it is less clear what the direct effect of these on the renal cell might be.

Thus, for example, both decreased serum calcium (in birds and mammals) and phosphate (in mammals) are associated with elevated circulating levels of $1,25(OH)_2D_3$ (reviewed in Ref. 49), but little substantive evidence exists to support physiologically meaningful and direct effects of these ions on renal cell metabolism of $25(OH)D_3$. More complex physiological mechanisms involving other hormones may well be at work in mediating the effects of changes in these blood ions on renal $25(OH)D_3$ metabolism.

Experimentally induced diabetes decreases $1,25$-$(OH)_2D_3$ production (50,51) and is required for the effects of PTH described above (52), but the mechanism of this action of insulin remains to be elucidated. Another observation of potential clinical significance is that ketoconazole and miconazole, the antifungal azoles, decrease renal production of both $1,25(OH)_2D_3$ and $24,25(OH)_2D_3$ (53); these antifungal agents have the same effect on other steroid hormones as well. Thus, high doses of these agents could have implications for calcium metabolism.

Extrarenal 1,25(OH)₂D₃ Synthesis

Originally, synthesis of $1,25(OH)_2D_3$ was postulated to occur exclusively in the kidney (54–56). New data now demonstrate ectopic $1,25(OH)_2D_3$ production in humans under certain circumstances. The best evidence lies in reports of several hypercalcemic patients with either sarcoidosis or tuberculosis who were anephric or who had end-stage renal disease. The hypercalcemia in these patients was associated with elevated serum $1,25(OH)_2D_3$ (57–60). $1,25(OH)_2D_3$ synthesis also takes place during pregnancy when placental and decidual cells synthesize the hormone. This process probably contributes to increased circulating $1,25(OH)_2D_3$ during pregnancy (reviewed in Ref. 61). However, the relevance of placental- and decidual-derived $1,25(OH)_2D_3$ for maternal–fetal calcium exchange is not known. (See Ch. 16.)

The question of whether extrarenal $1,25(OH)_2D_3$ production occurs in nonpregnant anephric individuals without secondary disease has been addressed in several studies. In animal experiments, extrarenal $1,25(OH)_2D_3$ production in vivo by rats could not be demonstrated within 24 h after nephrectomy (62). However, nephrectomized pigs which were maintained on dialysis for several days and which were given large amounts of vitamin D had clearly detectable serum $1,25(OH)_2D$ levels (63). Controversy continues to exist on whether anephric but otherwise normal humans have detectable circulating $1,25(OH)_2D$ levels. More recently, however, low circulating $1,25(OH)_2D$ concentrations (4–16 pg/mL) have been found in the majority of untreated or vitamin-D-treated anephric subjects. The $1,25(OH)_2D$ was measured by radioreceptor assay and bioassay (64) or radioimmunoassay (65). Possibly, improved $1,25(OH)_2D$ assay methodology or examination of larger serum samples will ultimately resolve this issue.

Extrarenal 1-hydroxylase activity has been identified in vitro in a variety of tissues. In sarcoidosis, granulomatous tissue including the macrophage may be the source of the excess $1,25(OH)_2D_3$ that is found in this disorder. A homogenate from a lymph node containing granuloma synthesized a compound indistinguishable from $1,25(OH)_2D_3$ (66), and cultured pulmonary alveolar macrophages (PAMs) from patients with pulmonary sarcoidosis constitutively synthesized $1,25(OH)_2D_3$ from the substrate $25(OH)D_3$ (67,68). Cultured PAMs from normal individuals required activation in vitro by interferon-γ (IFNγ) or bacterial lipopolysaccharide for demonstration of the synthesis of the hormone (69,70). IFNγ-stimulated human bone-marrow-derived macrophages (30) and peritoneal macrophages from peritoneal dialysis patients with a history of peritonitis also produced $1,25(OH)_2D_3$ (71). Likewise, $1,25(OH)_2D_3$ synthesis has been conclusively demonstrated for cultured chicken embryonic calvarial cells (72) and for cultured neonatal human foreskin keratinocytes (73).

Collectively, these results suggest the existence of a vitamin D autocrine–paracrine system involving $1,25(OH)_2D_3$ derived from activated macrophages and hematopoietic target cells in the bone marrow or at the

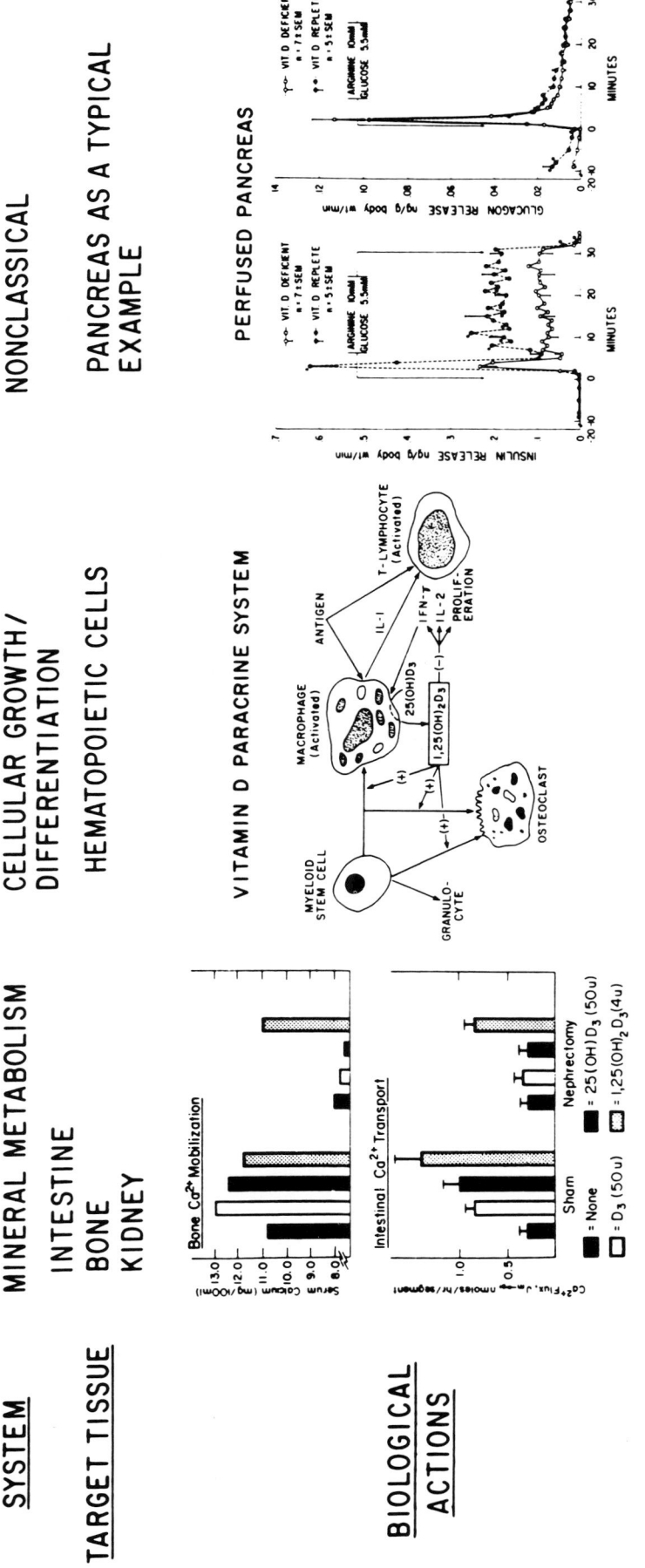

FIG. 5. Summary of the paracrine system for production of 1,25(OH)₂D₃ by activated macrophages.

site of an inflammation (e.g., the alveolites in the sarcoid lung) (see Fig. 5).

CATABOLISM OF VITAMIN D

A number of studies have been carried over the past decade which have contributed to our present understanding of the catabolism of $25(OH)D_3$ and $1,25(OH)_2D_3$. There appear to be two pathways through which the eight-carbon side chain is modified. One, designated by an A at the bottom of Fig. 3, results in the production of $1,25(OH)_2$-24,25,26,27-tetranor-D_3 and its C-23 acid, calcitroic acid. The cleavage of the side chain between C-23 and C-24 follows hydroxylation at the C-24, oxidation of that hydroxyl to the oxo group, and hydroxylation at C-23. The same set of reactions can also occur with $25(OH)D_3$ (pathway B in Fig. 3). Calcitroic acid was initially isolated from the liver (74), but the pathway was elucidated in the kidney (75,76). This catabolic pathway has also been demonstrated in bone cells (76–78), and it probably occurs in other target tissues of $1,25(OH)_2D_3$ as well (76,79,80). Additionally, it should be noted that these pathways are vitamin-D-dependent, since they occur only when the 24-hydroxylase is induced by $1,25(OH)_2D_3$ (76).

The second pathway by which the side chain of $1,25(OH)_2D_3$ and $25(OH)D_3$ can be modified begins with hydroxylation at C-23, and it results in the formation of $1,25(OH)_2$-26,23-lactone D_3 or 25-OH-26,23-lactone D_3 (pathways C and D in Fig. 3). These pathways have been termed "C-23 oxidation pathways" to distinguish them from the pathways beginning with C-24 oxidation, described above.

The $25(OH)D_3$-lactone has been isolated from the plasma of chickens, rats, and pigs given massive doses of vitamin D_3 (83) as well as from incubations of $25(OH)D_3$ with chick kidney homogenates (84). However, the extent to which the pathway occurs in extrarenal tissues has not been clarified. The relative roles of the two pathways (see Fig. 3, A/B versus C/D pathways) in various target tissues and under various physiological conditions remains an area of active investigation.

The biological activity and physiological function(s) of the $25(OH)D_3$-26,23-lactone are still unknown. It seems unlikely that they will be shown to have a unique physiological role, since they appear to be produced only under conditions of vitamin D_3 or $25(OH)D_3$ intoxication. Also, it is not known whether the enzymes which result in the generation of the side-chain lactone ring have a higher affinity for $1,25(OH)_2D_3$ as substrate as compared to $25(OH)D_3$ as substrate.

As shown in Fig. 3 (pathway C), $1,25(OH)_2D_3$ can be converted into $1,25(OH)_2$-26,23-lactone; this steroid was originally isolated from the serum of rats and dogs given large doses of $1,25(OH)_2D_3$ (85,86). Since there are two

asymmetric carbons (C-23 and C-25) in the lactone ring, there then are four diastereoisomers of the lactone which can exist. Wovkulich et al. (87) carried out a total synthesis of 1α-24(R)-$(OH)_2$-vitamin D_3-26,23(S)-lactone and showed that it had physical and biological properties identical to those of the naturally occurring diastereoisomer.

It is intriguing to speculate whether the $1,25(OH)_2$-vitamin D_3-26,23-lactone is an end-product catabolite of $1,25(OH)_2D_3$ or whether it has unique biological properties separate and distinct from its parent $1,25(OH)_2D_3$. Ishizuka et al. (92) reported that the $1,25(OH)_2D_3$-26,23-lactone was a normal metabolite in the plasma of dogs that received only physiological amounts of vitamin D_3 and no additional $25(OH)D_3$ or $1,25(OH)_2D_3$; when the plasma $1,25(OH)_2D_3$ was 36 pg/mL the 1,25-lactone plasma concentration was found to be 100 pg/mL. These results clearly suggest that the $1,25(OH)_2D_3$-26,23-lactone may be a seco-steroid metabolite of vitamin D_3 that can occur under normal physiological circumstances. Ishizuka and Norman (91) have reported the most thorough study of the metabolic pathways (see Fig. 3) contributing to the stereoretention and stereoselectivity of the lactonization of $1,25(OH)_2D_3$. Also, Ishizuka and Norman (84) reported the first biological characterization of the naturally occurring lactone, whereas Wilhelm et al. (89) compared the activities of the four diastereoisomers with respect to the traditional vitamin D biological responses, namely, stimulation of intestinal calcium absorption (ICA) and bone calcium mobilization (BCM) as well as binding to the vitamin-D_3-binding protein (DBP) and intestinal receptors. It was found that the naturally occurring $1,25(S)$-$(OH)_2D_3$-26,23(R)-lactone had a limited ICA and no BCM activity while binding to DBP three times better than $1,25(OH)_2D_3$ but binding to the chick intestinal receptor only 0.8% as well as $1,25(OH)_2D_3$.

More recently, Ishizuka et al. (90–93) have evaluated the biological actions of the four diastereoisomers in the rat osteoblast and bone marrow cells. Interestingly, the naturally occurring isomer, $1,25(S)$-$(OH)_2D_3$-26,23(R)-lactone was found to specifically inhibit the $1,25$-$(OH)_2D_3$-mediated fusion of mouse bone marrow mononuclear cells. These results may point the way to additional studies to evaluate and define the physiological responsibilities of this interesting vitamin D_3 metabolite.

SUMMARY

Metabolism of the parent vitamin D_3 is mandatory so that this molecule is able to generate the spectrum of biological responses [both classic (e.g., intestinal Ca^{2+} absorption) and newly discovered (e.g., cell differentiation, insulin secretion)] that are essential to a normal

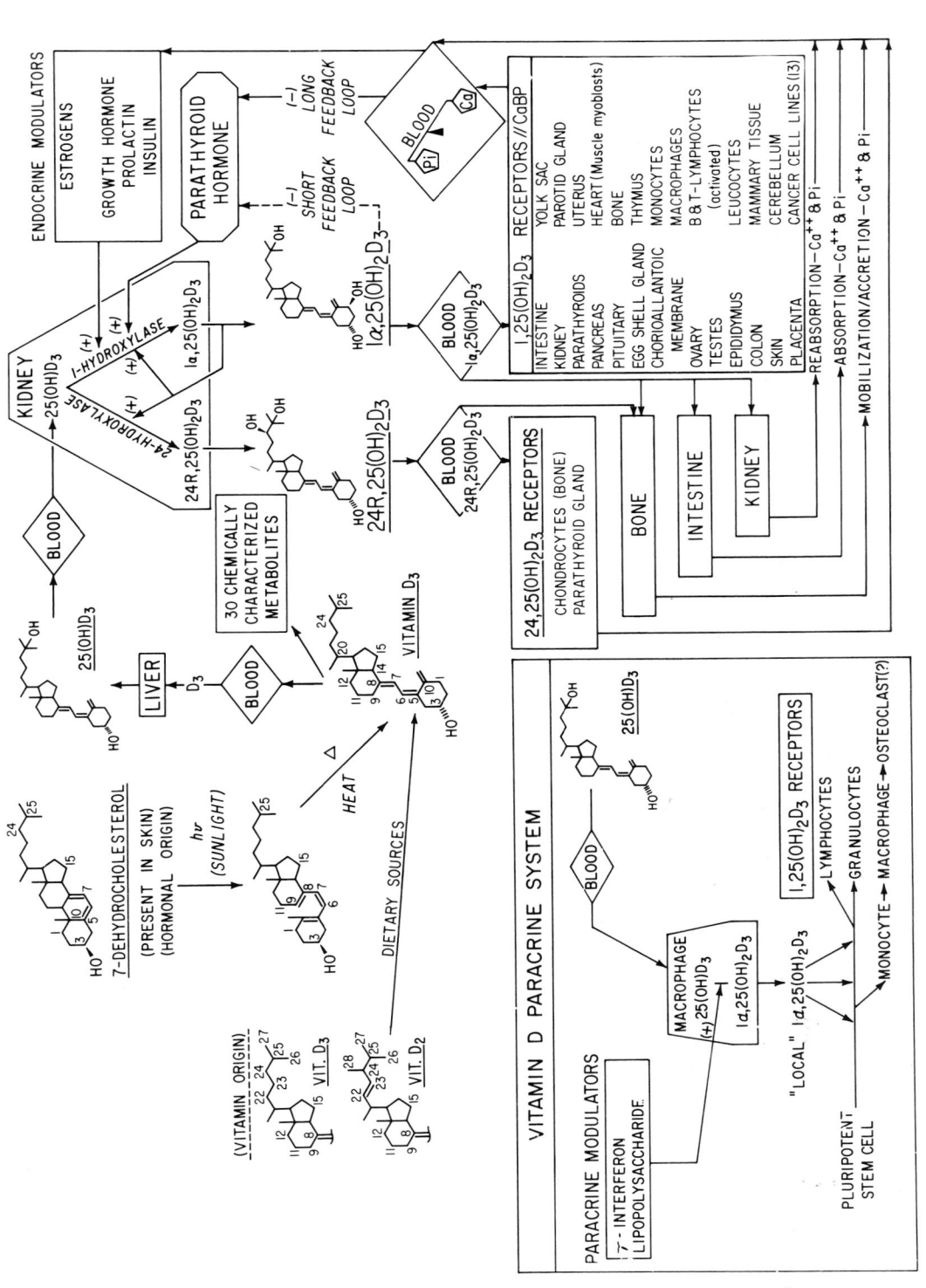

FIG. 6. Summary of the vitamin D₃ endocrine system.

physiologic state. In fact, it seems likely that the parent vitamin D_3 is actually biologically inert; there are no known biological responses that the parent seco-steroid can produce at a concentration lower than that of $1,25(OH)_2D_3$ or $25(OH)D_3$.

Figure 6 summarizes the pivotal role of vitamin D metabolism within the framework of the vitamin D endocrine system. Metabolism by the kidney functioning as an endocrine gland to coproduce $1,25(OH)_2D_3$ and $24,25(OH)_2D_3$ is clearly of major importance. But also the extrarenal production of $1,25(OH)_2D_3$ by activated macrophages and other cells probably contributes to the normal physiological state.

REFERENCES

1. Norman AW, Roth J, Orci L. The vitamin D endocrine system: steroid metabolism, hormone receptors and biological response (calcium binding proteins). *Endocr Rev* 1982;3:331–66.
2. Haussler MR. Vitamin D receptors: nature and function. *Annu Rev Nutr* 1986;6:527–62.
3. Paulson SK, DeLuca HF. Vitamin-D metabolism during pregnancy. *Bone* 1986;331–6.
4. Minghetti PP, Norman AW. $1,25(OH)_2$-Vitamin D_3 receptors: gene regulation and genetic circuitry. *FASEB J* 1988;2:3043–53.
5. Norman AW. *Vitamin D: the calcium homeostatic steroid hormone.* New York: Academic Press, 1979;Chapter 1.
6. Goldblatt H, Soames KN. A study of rats on a normal diet irradiated daily by the mercury vapor quartz lamp or kept in darkness. *Biochem J* 1923;17:294.
7. Wing RM, Okamura WH, Pirio MR, Sine SM, Norman AW. Vitamin D_3 in solution: conformations of vitamin D_3, $1\alpha,25$-dihydroxyvitamin D_3, and dihydrotachysterol$_3$. *Science* 1974; 186:939–41.
8. Okamura WH, Norman AW, Wing RM. Vitamin D: concerning the relationship between molecular topology and biological function. *Proc Natl Acad Sci USA* 1974;71:4194–4197.
9. Henry HL, Norman AW. Vitamin D: metabolism and biological actions. *Annu Rev Nutr* 1984;4:493–520.
10. Holick MF. Skin: site of the synthesis of vitamin D and a target tissue for the active form, 1,25-dihydroxyvitamin D_3. *Ann NY Acad Sci* 1988;548:14–26.
11. Webb AR, Holick MF. The role of sunlight in the cutaneous production of vitamin D_3. *Annu Rev Nutr* 1988;8:375–99.
12. Ponchon G, Kennan AL, DeLuca HF. "Activation" of vitamin D by the liver. *J Clin Invest* 1969;48:2032–7.
13. Tucker G, Gagnon RE, Haussler MR. Vitamin D_3-25-hydroxylase: tissue occurrence and apparent lack of regulation. *Arch Biochem Biophys* 1973;155:47–57.
14. Fukishima M, Suzuki Y, Tohira Y, Matsunaga I, Ochi K, Nagano H, Nishii Y, Suda T. Metabolism of 1α-hydroxyvitamin D_3 to $1\alpha,25$-dihydroxyvitamin D_3 in perfused rat liver. *Biochem Biophys Res Commun* 1975;66:632–8.
15. Ichikawa Y, Hiwatashi A, Nishii Y. Tissue and subcellular distribution of cholecalciferol 25-hydroxylase: cytochrome P-450$_{D25}$-linked monooxygenase system. *Comp Biochem Physiol* 1983; 75B:479–88.
16. Tam S-P, Strugnell S, Deeley RG, Jones G. 25-Hydroxylation of vitamin D_3 in the human hepatoma cell lines Hep G2 and Hep 3B. *J Lipid Res* 1988;29:1637–42.
17. Postlind H, Wikvall K. Purification of a cytochrome P-450 from pig kidney microsomes catalysing the 25-hydroxylation of vitamin D_3. *Biochem J* 1988;253:549–52.
18. Matsumoto O, Ohyama Y, Okuda K. Purification and characterization of vitamin D 25-hydroxylase from rat liver mitochondria. *J Biol Chem* 1988;263:14256–60.
19. Hayashi S, Noshiro M, Okuda K. Isolation of a cytochrome P-450 that catalyzes the 25-hydroxylation of vitamin D_3 from rat liver microsomes. *J Biochem* 1986;99:1753–63.
20. Saarem K, Pedersen JI. Sex differences in the hydroxylation of cholecalciferol and of 5β-cholestane-$3\alpha,7\alpha,12\alpha$-triol in rat liver. *Biochem J* 1987;247:73–8.
21. Suhara K, Takeda K, Katagiri M. P-450$_{11\beta}$-dependent conversion of cortisol to cortisone, and 19-hydroxyandrostenedione to 19-oxoandrostenedione. *Biochem Biophys Res Commun* 1986; 136:369–75.
22. Sato H, Ashida N, Suhara K, Itagaki E, Takemori S, Katagiri M. Properties of an adrenal cytochrome P-450 (P-450$_{11\beta}$) for the hydroxylations of corticosteroids. *Arch Biochem Biophys* 1978; 190:307–14.
23. Wada A, Ohnishi T, Nonaka Y, Okamoto M, Yamano T. Synthesis of aldosterone by a reconstituted system of cytochrome P-450$_{11\beta}$ from bovine adrenocortical mitochondria. *J Biochem* 1985; 98:245–56.
24. Dahlback H, Wikvall K. 25-Hydroxylation of vitamin D_3 by a cytochrome P-450 from rabbit liver mitochondria. *Biochem J* 1988;252:207–13.
25. Fraser DR. Regulation of the metabolism of vitamin D. *Physiol Rev* 1980;60:551–613.
26. Baran DT, Milne ML. 1,25-Dihydroxyvitamin D-induced inhibition of ^{3}H-25-hydroxyvitamin D production by the rachitic rat liver in vitro. *Calcif Tissue Int* 1983;35:461–4.
27. Milne ML, Baran DT. End product inhibition of hepatic 25-hydroxyvitamin D production in the rat: specificity and kinetics. *Arch Biochem Biophys* 1985;242:488–92.
28. Haddad P, Gascon-Barre M, Brault G, Plourde V. Influence of calcium or 1,25-dihydroxyvitamin D_3: supplementation on the hepatic microsomal and in vivo metabolism of vitamin D_3 in vitamin D-depleted rats. *J Clin Invest* 1986;78:1529–37.
29. Saarem K, Pedersen JI. Effect of age, gonadectomy and hypophysectomy on mitochondrial hydroxylation of vitamin D_3 (cholecalciferol) and of 5β-cholestane-$3\alpha,7\alpha,12\alpha$-triol in female and male rat liver. *Biochem J* 1988;251:475–81.
30. Henry HL, Norman AW. Renal 25-hydroxyvitamin D_3-1-hydroxylase: involvement of cytochrome P-450 and other properties. *J Biol Chem* 1974;249:7529–35.
31. Ghazarian JG, Jefcoate CR, Knutson JC, Orme-Johnson WH, DeLuca HF. Mitochondrial cytochrome P-450: a component of chick kidney 25-hydroxycholecalciferol-1-hydroxylase. *J Biol Chem* 1974;249:3026–33.
32. Burgos-Trinidad M, Brown A, DeLuca HF. Solubilization and reconstitution of chick renal mitochondrial 25-hydroxyvitamin D_3-24-hydroxylase. *Biochemistry* 1986;25:2692–6.
33. Pedersen JI, Shobaki HH, Holmberg I, Bergseth S, Bjorkhem I. 25-Hydroxyvitamin D_3-24-hydroxylase in rat kidney mitochondria. *J Biol Chem* 1983;258:742–6.
34. Postlind H. Separation of the cytochromes P-450 in pig kidney mitochondria catalyzing 1α-, 24- and 26-hydroxylations of 25-hydroxyvitamin D_3. *Biochem Biophys Res Commun* 1990;168: 261–6.
35. Fraser DR, Kodicek E. Unique biosynthesis by kidney of a biologically active vitamin D metabolite. *Nature* 1970;228:764–6.
36. Henry HL, Midgett RJ, Norman AW. Studies on calciferol metabolism X. Regulation of 25-hydroxyvitamin D_3-1-hydroxylase, in vivo. *J Biol Chem* 1974;249:7584–92.
37. Norman AW, Myrtle JF, Midgett RJ, Nowicki HG, Williams V, Popjak G. 1,25-Dihydroxycholecalciferol: identification of the proposed active form of vitamin D_3 in the intestine. *Science* 1975;173:51–4.
38. Gray RW, Boyle I, DeLuca HF. Vitamin D metabolism: the role of kidney tissue. *Science* 1971;173:1232–4.
39. Henry H. Regulation of the hydroxylation of 25-hydroxyvitamin D_3 in vivo and in primary cultures of chick kidney cells. *J Biol Chem* 1979;254:2722–9.
40. Trechsel U, Bonjour J-P, Fleisch H. Regulation of the metabolism of 25-hydroxyvitamin D_3 in primary cultures of chick kidney cells. *J Clin Invest* 1979;64:206–17.
41. Garabedian M, Holick MF, DeLuca HF, Boyle IT. Control of 25-

hydroxycholecalciferol metabolism by parathyroid glands. *Proc Natl Acad Sci USA* 1972;69:1673–6.

42. Baksi SN, Kenny AD. Acute effects of parathyroid extract on renal vitamin D hydroxylases in Japanese quail. *Pharmacology* 1979;18:169–74.

43. Fukase M, Birge SJ, Rifas L, Avioli LV, Chase LR. Regulation of 25-hydroxyvitamin D₃ 1-hydroxylase in serum-free monolayer culture of mouse kidney. *Endocrinology* 1982;110:1073–5.

44. Armbrecht HJ, Wongsurawat N, Zenser TV, Davis BB. Differential effects of parathyroid hormone on the renal 1,25-dihydroxyvitamin D₃ and 24,25-dihydroxyvitamin D₃ production of young and adult rats. *Endocrinology* 1982;111:1339–44.

45. Kramer R, Goltzman D. Parathyroid hormone stimulates mammalian 25-hydroxyvitamin d3-1-α-hydroxylase in vitro. *Endocrinology* 1982;110:294–6.

46. Henry HL. Parathyroid hormone modulation of 25-hydroxyvitamin D₃ metabolism by cultured chick kidney cells is mimicked and enhanced by forskolin. *Endocrinology* 1985;116:503–7.

47. Henry HL. Influence of a tumor promoting phorbol ester on the metabolism of 25-hydroxyvitamin D₃. *Biochem Biophys Res Commun* 1986;139:495–500.

48. Henry HL, Luntao EM. Interactions between intracellular signals involved in the regulation of 25-hydroxyvitamin D₃ metabolism. *Endocrinology* 1989;124:2228–34.

49. Henry HL, Norman AW. Vitamin D: metabolism and biological actions. *Annu Rev Nutr* 1984;4:493–520.

50. Ishida H, Cunningham NS, Henry HL, Norman AW. The number of 1,25-dihydroxyvitamin D₃ receptors is decreased in both intestine and kidney of genetically diabetic db/db mice. *Endocrinology* 1988;122:2436–43.

51. Schneider LE, Schedl HP, McCain T, Haussler MR. Experimental diabetes reduces circulating 1,25-dihydroxyvitamin D in the rat. *Science* 1977;196:1452.

52. Henry HL. Insulin permits parathyroid hormone stimulation of 1,25-dihydroxyvitamin D₃ production in cultured kidney cells. *Endocrinology* 1981;108:733–5.

53. Henry HL. Effect of ketoconazole and miconazole on 25-hydroxyvitamin D₃ metabolism by cultured chick kidney cells. *J Steroid Biochem* 1985;23:991–4.

54. Haussler MR, McCain TA. Basic and clinical concepts related to vitamin D metabolism and action. *N Engl J Med* 1977;297:974–83 and 1041–50.

55. Norman AW, Roth J, Orci L. The vitamin D endocrine system: steroid metabolism, hormone receptors, and biological response (calcium binding proteins). *Endocr Rev* 1982;3:331–66.

56. DeLuca HF, Schnoes HK. Vitamin D: recent advances. *Annu Rev Biochem* 1983;52:411–39.

57. Barbour GL, Coburn JW, Slatopolsky E, Norman AW, Horst RL. Hypercalcemia in an anephric patient with sarcoidosis: evidence for extrarenal generation of 1,25-dihydroxyvitamin D. *N Engl J Med* 1981;305:440–3.

58. Maesaka JK, Batuman V, Pablo NC, Shakamuri S. Elevated 1,25-dihydroxyvitamin D levels: occurrence with sarcoidosis with end-stage renal disease. *Arch Intern Med* 1982;142:1206–7.

59. Gkonos PJ, London R, Hendler ED. Hypercalcemia and elevated 1,25-dihydroxyvitamin D levels in a patient with end-stage renal disease and active tuberculosis. *N Engl J Med* 1984;311:1683–5.

60. Felsenfeld AJ, Drezner MK, Llach F. Hypercalcemia and elevated calcitriol in a maintenance dialysis patient with tuberculosis. *Arch Intern Med* 1986;146:1941–5.

61. Gray TK, Lowe W, Lester GE. Vitamin D and pregnancy: the maternal–fetal metabolism of vitamin D. *Endocr Rev* 1981;2:264–74.

62. Shultz TD, Fox J, Heath H III, Kumar R. Do tissues other than the kidney produce 1,25-dihydroxyvitamin D₃ in vivo? A reexamination. *Proc Natl Acad Sci USA* 1983;80:1746–50.

63. Littledike ET, Horst RL. Metabolism of vitamin D₃ in nephrectomized pigs given pharmacological amounts of vitamin D₃. *Endocrinology* 1982;111:2008–13.

64. Lambert PW, Stern PH, Avioli RC, et al. Evidence for extrarenal production of 1α,25-dihydroxyvitamin D in man. *J Clin Invest* 1982;69:722–5.

65. Jongen MJ, van der Vijgh WJ, Lips P, Netelenbos JC. Measure-

66. Mason RS, Frankel T, Chan Y-L, Lissner D, Posen S. Vitamin D conversion by sarcoid lymph node homogenate. *Ann Intern Med* 1984;100:59–61.

67. Adams JS, Singer FR, Gacad MA, et al. Isolation and structural identification of 1,25-dihydroxyvitamin D₃ produced by cultured alveolar macrophages in sarcoidosis. *J Clin Endocrinol Metab* 1985;60:960–6.

68. Reichel H, Koeffler HP, Barbers R, Norman AW. Regulation of 1,25-dihydroxyvitamin D₃ production by cultured alveolar macrophages from normal human donors and from patients with pulmonary sarcoidosis. *J Clin Endocrinol Metab* 1987;65:1201–9.

69. Reichel H, Koeffler HP, Bishop JE, Norman AW. 25-Hydroxyvitamin D₃ metabolism by lipopolysaccharide-stimulated normal human macrophages. *J Clin Endocrinol Metab* 1987;64:1–9.

70. Reichel H, Koeffler HP, Norman AW. Synthesis in vitro of 1,25-dihydroxyvitamin D₃ and 24,25-dihydroxyvitamin D₃ by interferon-γ-stimulated normal human bone marrow and alveolar macrophages. *J Biol Chem* 1987;262:10931–7.

71. Hayes ME, O'Donoghue DJ, Ballardie FW, Mawer EB. Peritonitis induces the synthesis of 1α,25-dihydroxyvitamin D₃ in macrophages from CAPD patients. *FEBS Lett* 1987;220:307–10.

72. Turner RT, Howard GA, Puzas JE, Baylink DJ, Knapp DR. Calvarial cells synthesize 1α,25-dihydroxyvitamin D₃ from 25-hydroxyvitamin D₃. *Biochemistry* 1983;22:1073–6.

73. Bikle DD, Nemanic MK, Whitney JO, Elias PW. Neonatal human foreskin keratinocytes produce 1,25-dihydroxyvitamin D₃. *Biochemistry* 1986;25:1545–8.

74. Esvelt RP, DeLuca HF. Calcitroic acid: biological activity and tissue distribution studies. *Arch Biochem Biophys* 1981;206:403–13.

75. Reddy GS, Tserng K-Y. Calcitroic acid, end product of renal metabolism of 1,25-dihydroxyvitamin D₃ through C-24 oxidation pathway. *Biochemistry* 1989;28:1763–9.

76. Jones G, Vriezen D, Lohnes D, Palda V, Edwards NS. Side-chain hydroxylation of vitamin D₃ and its physiological implications. *Steroids* 1987;49:29–53.

77. Reinhardt TA, Horst RL. Self-induction of 1,25-dihydroxyvitamin D₃ metabolism limits receptor occupancy and target tissue responsiveness. *J Biol Chem* 1989;264:15917–21.

78. Lohnes D, Jones G. Side chain metabolism of vitamin D₃ in osteosarcoma cell line UMR-106. *J Biol Chem* 1987;262:14394–401.

79. Haussler MR. Vitamin D receptors: nature and function. *Annu Rev Nutr* 1986;6:527–62.

80. Pols HA, Schilte HP, Nijweide PJ, Visser TJ, Birkenhager JC. The influence of albumin on vitamin D metabolism in osteoblast-like cells. *Biochem Biophys Res Commun* 1984;125:265–72.

81. Bhattacharyya MH, DeLuca HF. Subcellular localization of rat liver calciferol 25-hydroxylase. *Arch Biochem Biophys* 1974; 160:58–62.

82. Saarem K, Bergseth S, Oftebro H, Pedersen JI. Subcellular localization of vitamin D₃ 25-hydroxylase in human liver. *J Biol Chem* 1984;259:10936–40.

83. Horst RL. 25-OH-D₃-Lactone: a metabolite of vitamin D₃ that is 5 times more potent than 25-OH-D₃ in the rat plasma competitive protein binding assay. *Biochem Biophys Res Commun* 1979; 89:286–93.

84. Ishizuka S, Norman AW. The stereochemical configuration of the natural 23,25,26-trihydroxyvitamin D₃. *FEBS Lett* 1983; 4156:321–4.

85. Ohnuma N, Kiyoki M, Bannai K, Naruchi T, Hashimoto Y, Noguchi T, Norman AW. Studies on vitamin D metabolism: catabolism of 1α,25-dihydroxyvitamin D₃ and 1α-hydroxyvitamin D₃ to a metabolite inactive on bone mineral mobilization. *Steroids* 1980;36:27–39.

86. Ishizuka S, Ishimoto S, Norman AW. Isolation and identification of 1α,25-dihydroxy-24-oxo-vitamin D₃, 1α,25-dihydroxyvitamin D₃-26,23-lactone and 1α,24(S)25-trihydroxyvitamin D₃: in vivo metabolites of 1α,25-dihydroxyvitamin D₃. *Biochemistry* 1984; 23:1473–8.

87. Wovkulich PM, Baggiolini EG, Hennessy BM, Uskokovic MR, Mayer E, Norman AW. Total synthesis of 1α,25(R)-dihydroxyvi-

ment of vitamin D metabolites in anephric subjects. *Nephron* 1984;36:230–4.

tamin D_3 26,23(S)-lactone (calcitriol lactone), a natural metabolite of vitamin D_3. *J Org Chem* 1983;48:4433–6.

88. Ishizuka S, Ishimoto S, Norman AW. Biological activity assessment of 1α,25-dihydroxyvitamin D_3-26,23-lactone in the rat. *J Steroid Biochem* 1984;20:611–5.

89. Wilhelm F, Mayer E, Norman AW. Studies on the mode of action of calciferol. LII. Biological activity assessment of the 26,23-lactones of 1,25-dihydroxyvitamin D_3 and 25-hydroxyvitamin D_3 and their binding properties to chick intestinal receptor and plasma vitamin D binding protein. *Arch Biochem Biophys* 1984;233:322–9.

90. Ishizuka S, Kiyoki M, Kurihara N, Hakeda Y, Ikeda K, Kumegawa M, Norman AW. Effects of diastereoisomers of 1,25-dihydroxyvitamin D_3-26,23-lactone on alkaline phosphatase and colla-gen synthesis in osteoblastic cells. *Mol Cell Endocrinol* 1988;55:77–86.

91. Ishizuka S, Norman AW. Metabolic pathways of 1α,25-dihydroxyvitamin D_3 to 1α,25-dihydroxyvitamin D_3-26,23-lactone: stereo-retained and stereo-selective lactonization. *J Biol Chem* 1987;262:7165–70.

92. Ishizuka S, Ohba T, Norman AW. 1α,25(OH)$_2$D$_3$-26,23-lactone is a major metabolite of 1α,25(OH)$_2$D$_3$ under physiological conditions. In: Norman AW, Schaefer K, Grigoleit HG, Herrath DV, eds. *Vitamin D: molecular, cellular and clinical endocrinology.* Berlin: Walter de Gruyter, 1988;143–4.

93. Ishizuka S, Kurihara N, Hakeda S, Maeda N, Ikeda K, Kumegawa M, Norman AW. 1α,25-Dihydroxyvitamin D_3 [1α,25-(OH)$_2$D$_3$]-26,23-lactone inhibits 1,25(OH)$_2$D$_3$-mediated fusion of mouse bone marrow mononuclear cells. *Endocrinology* 1988;123:781–6.

CHAPTER 8

Molecular Mechanisms of Cellular Response to the Vitamin D₃ Hormone

J. Wesley Pike

Several decades of basic and clinical research support the current concept that 1,25-dihydroxyvitamin D_3 represents the hormonal component of a vast endocrine system that controls numerous biologic functions in a myriad of target tissues and cells. Many of the actions of vitamin D_3 are directed toward control of cellular mechanisms that facilitate calcium and phosphorus homeostasis in birds and mammals. Nonetheless, more recent research efforts have uncovered functional roles for the vitamin D_3 hormone in biologic processes as diverse as regulation of cellular growth and differentiation and control of immune function. The primary purpose of this chapter is to summarize both historical and current studies that have shaped our present understanding of the general mechanisms by which the vitamin molecule exerts its rather pleiotropic effects on target cells. This discussion will be based upon three important tenets. First, 1,25-dihydroxyvitamin D_3 represents the metabolically active form of the vitamin. Second, the activity of the hormone is carried out through mechanisms that involve the regulation of gene expression. And third, the vitamin D_3 receptor mediates the action of 1,25-dihydroxyvitamin D_3 through direct and selective actions on the genome. As will be noted, major strides in the latter area have been made recently through the use of modern molecular biologic techniques. This chapter will conclude with a discussion of the pathophysiology of 1,25-dihydroxyvitamin D_3 as it pertains to aberrations in the effector system for this hormone in the human syndrome of hereditary 1,25-dihydroxyvitamin D_3 resistance.

J. W. Pike: Departments of Pediatrics and Cell Biology, Baylor College of Medicine, Houston, Texas, 77030.

HISTORICAL CONSIDERATIONS SUPPORTING THE GENOMIC MECHANISM OF ACTION OF VITAMIN D₃

Studies Antedating the Discovery of 1,25-Dihydroxyvitamin D₃

The causal relationship between vitamin D_3, serum calcium, and the absorption of calcium and phosphorus by the intestine was known for many years. Nevertheless, the first studies that provided insight into the mechanism by which the vitamin functions came in 1964 by Eisenstein and Passavoy (1), who found that actinomycin D, an inhibitor of transcription, was able to prevent hypercalcemia induced by large doses of vitamin D_3. These studies were followed quickly by a number of experiments that focused upon the antibiotic's effects on calcium transport in the intestine. Blockade of calcium uptake into serum and of intestinal transport of calcium was achieved by actinomycin D in several laboratories (2–4), leading to the possible conclusion that the biologic effect of vitamin D_3 in the intestine was a result of the stimulation of RNA synthesis through transcriptional events. These studies were supported by the observation that an intraperitoneal dose of the vitamin enhanced severalfold the incorporation of [^{3}H]orotic acid into the nuclear RNA of intestinal mucosa (5). Furthermore, vitamin D administration markedly increased the template activity of DNA-dependent RNA synthesis in rat intestinal chromatin (6). Simultaneously, it was noted that an accumulation of tritium from vitamin D_3 injection into chicks was observed in the crude nuclear and chromatin fractions of intestinal mucosa (7). While current knowledge of vitamin D_3 metabolism, transcriptional activation, and the methodologies utilized during those studies would allow less definitive interpretations than the ones advanced at that time, collectively the data supported the concept that the biologic action of vitamin D_3 was a result of its effects within the nucleus of target cells. Indeed, the observation that vitamin D_3 functioned through modification of the genetic machinery prompted the hypothesis (8) that vitamin D_3 operated through mechanisms analogous to those for steroid hormones such as estrogen, progesterone, and the glucocorticoids (9).

Discovery of 1,25-Dihydroxyvitamin D_3

A major problem associated with the studies outlined above was the continued observation that biologic response to vitamin D_3—and indeed even to its proximal precursor 25-hydroxyvitamin D_3—was apparent following administration to animals only after a significant time lag (2–6,10,11). The discovery in the late 1960s and early 1970s that vitamin D_3 required hydroxylation not only in the liver but also in the kidney, and that the active form of vitamin D_3 was in fact 1,25-dihydroxyvitamin D_3, provided the explanation for that retarded response (see Fig. 1). 1,25-Dihydroxyvitamin D_3 was identified initially simply as a more polar, yet unknown, metabolite of vitamin D_3 that appeared to localize in chicken intestinal chromatin (7). Clues to the structure of this active form of vitamin D_3 began to emerge as a result of the studies of Lawson et al. (12); these investigators showed, on the basis of loss of tritium from [1-^{3}H]cholecalciferol substrate, that a modification likely occurred at carbon 1 of the 1,25-dihydroxyvitamin D_3 molecule. This loss was preferential to the intestinal nuclei of vitamin-D_3-deficient chickens. Subsequent studies suggested that the active metabolite was produced by kidney and was considerably more active than 25-hydroxyvitamin D_3 (13). In 1971, material was isolated independently in several laboratories by two methods—one through incubation of 25-hydroxyvitamin D_3 with renal homogenates (14,15), and the other directly from intestinal tissue (16)—and structurally determined to be 1,25-dihydroxyvitamin D_3 shortly thereafter (17).

In the decade that followed, numerous studies were carried out that supported the concept that 1,25-dihydroxyvitamin D_3 was the form of vitamin D_3 that was functional in biologic processes associated with mineral metabolism. Immediate studies showed that 1,25-dihydroxyvitamin D_3 was the most potent of vitamin D_3 metabolites in inducing calcium absorption and in promoting bone calcium resorption activity (18). Perhaps the most compelling was the observation that administration of this metabolite—and only this metabolite—to animals fed a vitamin-D_3-deficient diet led to the prevention of rickets and allowed the maintenance of normal mineral metabolism (19). In addition, only administration of 1,25-dihydroxyvitamin D_3 abrogated the loss

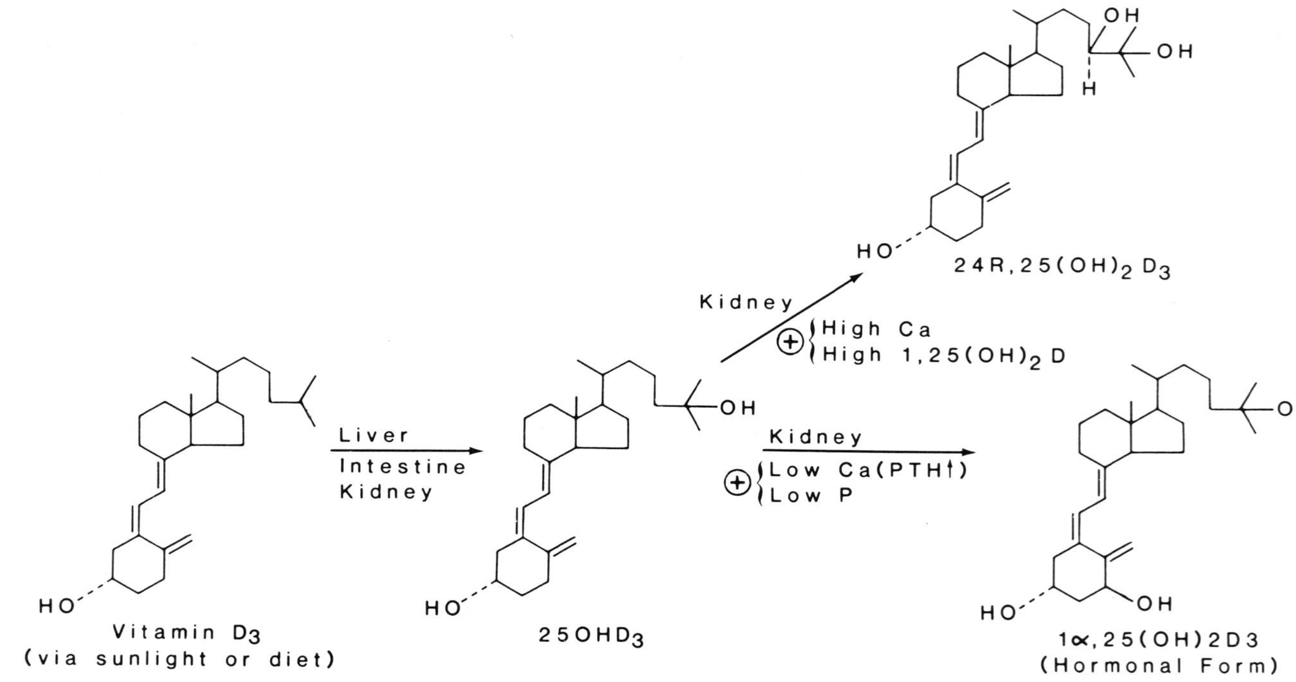

FIG. 1. Metabolism of vitamin D_3 to hormonally active 1,25-dihydroxyvitamin D_3. The physiologic conditions that preferentially enhance the production of 1,25-dihydroxyvitamin D_3 or 24,25-dihydroxyvitamin D_3 are indicated by a circled plus sign. The function of the latter metabolite is controversial.

of intestinal calcium transport and bone calcium mobilization seen upon total nephrectomy in animals (20,21).

1,25-Dihydroxyvitamin D₃ as a Hormonal Signal

The observation that 1,25-dihydroxyvitamin D₃ was produced in the kidney but exhibited profound biologic actions on extrarenal tissues such as the intestine and bone (the classic definition of a hormone) strengthened the early hypothesis that vitamin D₃ might be the essential component of a vast endocrine system. The potent activity of 1,25-dihydroxyvitamin D₃, in turn, suggested that it might indeed be the vitamin D₃ hormone. While numerous experiments were carried out to suggest that 1,25-dihydroxyvitamin D₃ was a hormone, the strongest evidence was derived from studies that identified and clarified the pivotal role of the renal 25-hydroxyvitamin D₃-1-hydroxylase (1-hydroxylase) enzyme, discovered in 1970 by Fraser and Kodicek (13), in the biosynthesis of 1,25-dihydroxyvitamin D₃. This evidence was enhanced through elucidation of many of the exquisite mechanisms by which this enzyme is regulated. As a result of these mechanisms, only small amounts of 1,25-dihydroxyvitamin D₃ are produced and circulate in blood, and this level is precisely controlled and allowed to fluctuate modestly only in response to the mineral needs of the organism (22). Indeed, direct measurement of circulating levels of 1,25-dihydroxyvitamin D₃ by radioreceptor assay confirm that this metabolite increases specifically under conditions of calcium or phosphorus shortage (22,23). In contrast, 25-hydroxyvitamin D₃, the proximal precursor of 1,25-dihydroxyvitamin D₃, as well as many other metabolites of vitamin D₃, circulate

in much higher concentrations; their biosyntheses are, to a large degree, unregulated (24,25).

Both serum calcium and phosphorus levels represent strong signals that enhance the activity of the 1-hydroxylase, leading to increased synthesis of 1,25-dihydroxyvitamin D₃ (Fig. 2) (26–28). Serum calcium is monitored directly by the parathyroid gland, and it responds to lowered calcium levels through an elaboration of parathyroid hormone (PTH). Indeed, 1-hydroxylase activity is not elevated in thyroparathyroidectomized rats maintained on a low-calcium diet (29). Administration of PTH, in turn, has a direct effect on the 1-hydroxylase (29) as well as on the production of 1,25-dihydroxyvitamin D₃ (28). The action of phosphorus is less clear, having potentially both direct and hormone-mediated actions on the renal enzyme independent of PTH. Concomitantly, 1,25-dihydroxyvitamin D₃ exerts negative feedback control on the 1-hydroxylase enzyme, through actions on the kidney enzyme as well as on the parathyroid gland. This effect in the kidney has been demonstrated in numerous ways, but perhaps the most striking is the fact that animals which are fed a vitamin-D-deficient diet and which are thus depleted of circulating vitamin D₃ metabolites exhibit a rather striking increase in renal 1-hydroxylase activity (30). In the parathyroid gland, 1,25-dihydroxyvitamin D₃ action leads to negative regulation of PTH synthesis and secretion (31), thus suppressing the level of this calciotropic signal and, in turn, suppressing the activity of the 1-hydroxylase. Irrespective of mechanism, the positive effects of primary stimuli (such as calcium and phosphate ions) on 1-hydroxylase activity, along with the negative effects of 1,25-dihydroxyvitamin D₃ on its own synthesis, provide strong supportive evidence for the concept that

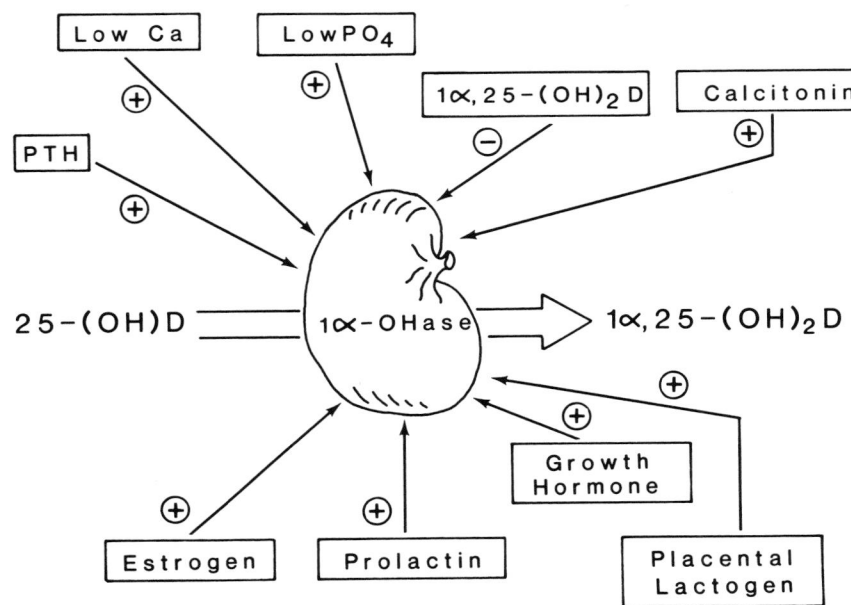

FIG. 2. Regulation of 1,25-dihydroxyvitamin D₃ formation in the kidney by mineral ions, hormones, and 1,25-dihydroxyvitamin D₃ itself. Synthesis of 1,25-dihydroxyvitamin D₃ from 25-hydroxyvitamin D₃ by renal 1-hydroxylase (1α-OHase) is shown. Regulators are boxed, and their positive or negative effects are indicated by a circled plus or minus sign, respectively. The mechanisms by which these modulators affect 1-hydroxylase activity vary.

1,25-dihydroxyvitamin D_3 is not only the active form, but also a hormonal form, of vitamin D_3.

Further investigation of 1,25-dihydroxyvitamin D_3 biosynthesis has revealed additional factors that exert control over the 1-hydroxylase, as outlined in Fig. 2. While the mechanisms by which this regulation takes place are ill-defined and probably diverse, studies have shown that reproductive hormones such as prolactin (32) and estrogen (33–35) are capable of positive modulation of 1,25-dihydroxyvitamin D_3 biosynthesis. Pituitary hormones may also modulate the enzyme's activity and thus influence 1,25-dihydroxyvitamin D_3 levels (36). Interestingly, the dominant effects of these hormones emerge principally during natural periods of mineral stress that occur during physiologic states characterized by enhanced mineral requirements. Specific examples include mammalian growth, pregnancy, and lactation, as well as avian egg-laying (32,37–39). Finally, experimentally induced diabetes in rats leads to a reduction in serum levels of 1,25-dihydroxyvitamin D_3, a reduction restored to normal levels by administration of insulin (40). These experiments reveal an additional interplay between polypeptides such as insulin and normal control of mineral metabolism.

1,25-Dihydroxyvitamin D_3 Action in General Transcription

The discovery that 1,25-dihydroxyvitamin D_3 was capable of inducing biologic response within several hours refocused attention on the mechanism by which the active form of vitamin D_3 functioned to promote calcium transport. Several studies were accomplished using transcriptional inhibitors such as actinomycin D (41,42), although the results were inconsistent and compromised by the uncertainty associated with the use of these potentially toxic inhibitors in vivo. Nevertheless, inhibitory effects by actinomycin D were observed on RNA synthesis in intestine, kidney, and bone, primary targets of vitamin D_3 action. Perhaps the most definitive studies of this nature that addressed the mechanism of 1,25-dihydroxyvitamin D_3 response were carried out in vitro by Corradino (43–46) using the embryonic chick intestinal organ culture system. This experimental model was shown to exhibit a calcium uptake phenomenon consistent with that of the normal mature intestine and, most importantly, was sensitive to external administration of 1,25-dihydroxyvitamin D_3. Corradino revealed that this transport process could be blocked with actinomycin D, alpha-amanitin, or cycloheximide after 24–48 h in culture. No apparent side effects of this treatment were evident, thus allowing the conclusion that both RNA and protein synthesis were also prerequisites to normal functioning of the hormonal form of vitamin D_3. These results were largely confirmed through experiments performed nearly a decade later (47).

The effectiveness of alpha-amanitin, a specific inhibitor of RNA polymerase II, in blocking 1,25-dihydroxyvitamin-D_3-sensitive calcium transport prompted an immediate investigation of the in vivo effect of the hormone on the enzyme. In studies carried out by Zerwekh et al. (48), administration of 1,25-dihydroxyvitamin D_3 to chickens, followed by evaluation of RNA polymerase I and II activity in isolated intestinal mucosal nuclei in vitro, revealed a significant enhancement of the latter enzyme within 2 h of hormone administration. Subsequently, Zerwekh et al. (49) were able to demonstrate that in addition to apparent activation of RNA polymerase II activity, in vivo administration of 1,25-dihydroxyvitamin D_3 to chickens also initiated an increase in intestinal mucosal chromatin template activity. The elevation in template activity by the hormone could also be observed through reconstitution of control chromatin with chicken intestinal cytosols preincubated with 1,25-dihydroxyvitamin D_3 in vitro.

The proposed nuclear mechanism of action of the vitamin D_3 hormone was also supported by the tendency for 1,25-dihydroxyvitamin D_3 to localize in the nucleus of target tissues both in vivo and in vitro. As indicated earlier, the initial observation in this regard was made following administration of vitamin D_3 and prior to the identification of the active metabolite 1,25-dihydroxyvitamin D_3 (7). Several approaches were taken to investigate the localization of hormone in the nuclear fraction of intestinal mucosa. First, utilizing enzymatically synthesized 1,25-dihydroxyvitamin D_3, several groups were able to observe tritiated 1,25-dihydroxyvitamin D_3 in isolated nuclear fractions following administration of hormone to chickens (50,51). These biochemical fractionation experiments were complemented several years later through sterol autoradiography. In experiments carried out simultaneously, Zile et al. (52) and Jones and Haussler (53) observed that specific autoradiographic grains representative of 1,25-dihydroxyvitamin D_3 were evident in high concentration in the nuclei of intestinal crypt and villus cells several hours following administration of tritiated 1,25-dihydroxyvitamin D_3 to rachitic chickens. Tissues insensitive to the hormone exhibited no specific accumulation. The time course of accumulation strongly correlated with the uptake of 1,25-dihydroxyvitamin D_3 into intestinal chromatin, suggesting that both were manifestations of the same phenomenon.

1,25-Dihydroxyvitamin D_3 Action in Specific Protein Induction

The strong dependency of intestinal calcium transport on vitamin D_3 and 1,25-dihydroxyvitamin D_3, particularly in chickens, stimulated an early search for proteins that participated in the uptake process. While several proteins have been characterized over the years and have been proposed to retain a functional involvement in the absorption process, perhaps the most important has been the vitamin-D$_3$-dependent calcium-binding proteins or calbindins. The chicken homologue of this macromolecule was discovered and purified by Wasserman and colleagues (54,55) in 1968 as an approximately 28-kD protein whose synthesis was dependent upon the presence of vitamin D$_3$. Mammalian tissues retain two vitamin-D$_3$-stimulated calbindins, a 28-kD species as well as a 9-kD version, which generally do not share a similar tissue distribution (56). Subsequent experiments revealed that the production of these proteins was strongly influenced by 1,25-dihydroxyvitamin D$_3$ as well as by serum levels of calcium (57,58). Most importantly, the synthesis of calcium-binding protein in response to either vitamin D$_3$ or 1,25-dihydroxyvitamin D$_3$ is blocked in the intestinal organ culture system by actinomycin D (44). These studies were crucial, because they provided the first evidence that 1,25-dihydroxyvitamin D$_3$ not only functions at the level of the nucleus to stimulate calcium absorption, but has direct effects on the synthesis of a specific protein product as well. Unfortunately, despite numerous studies carried out during the course of over two decades since the discovery of calcium-binding protein, the functional role of the calbindins and their relationship to the calcium transport process remain unclarified. Equally uncertain today are the exact mechanisms by which 1,25-dihydroxyvitamin D$_3$ exerts genetic control over the expression of these interesting protein products.

An extensive number of protein products have been found directly responsive to the vitamin D$_3$ hormone. Proteins of unknown identity include those found to exhibit increased or decreased concentration through biochemical analyses in a tissue following 1,25-dihydroxyvitamin D$_3$ administration in vivo. The protein products modulated by 1,25-dihydroxyvitamin D$_3$ have recently been reviewed (59), and some of the more completely described ones are listed in Table 1. They include the following: the calbindins discussed above; alkaline phosphatase; collagen; osteocalcin; matrix gla protein; osteopontin; the PTH precursor; fibronectin; carbonic anhydrase; 25-hydroxyvitamin D$_3$-24-hydroxylase and other vitamin D$_3$ catabolic enzymes; calcitonin; prolactin; and the c-myc and c-fos proto-oncogenes. Despite this long list of proteins that are apparently modulated by vitamin D$_3$, the evidence that has accumulated with regard to mechanism of induction is highly variable, and only a few have been clearly demonstrated to arise directly as a result of increased transcription. Perhaps the best-characterized example of transcriptional control by 1,25-dihydroxyvitamin D$_3$ has emerged through examination of the regulation of the noncollagenous bone protein osteocalcin. This model system for elucidating the transcriptional mechanism of action of vitamin D$_3$ will be considered in depth later in this chapter. However, early studies by Price and Baukol (60) revealed the

TABLE 1. *Partial list of protein products induced by 1,25-dihydroxyvitamin D$_3$*

Category and gene product
Mechanism
1,25-Dihydroxyvitamin D$_3$ receptor
Mineral metabolism
Calbindin D9k
Calbindin D28k
Carbonic anhydrase
Alkaline phosphatase
Osteocalcin
Osteopontin
Matrix gla protein
Collagen
Fibronectin
Vitamin D metabolism
25-Hydroxyvitamin D$_3$-1-hydroxylase
25-Hydroxyvitamin D$_3$-24-hydroxylase

sensitivity of the synthesis and secretion of this protein to the vitamin D$_3$ hormone in culture bone cells. Subsequent studies, following the molecular cloning of the structural gene for osteocalcin (61–64), led to the important observation, as with the calbindins (65,66), that 1,25-dihydroxyvitamin D$_3$ treatment resulted in an increase in the mRNA for these protein species. Thus, as a historical perspective, from the early actions of vitamin D$_3$ on specific gene products progressively down to the actions of its functional, hormonal form on these genes, all evidence has led to the inescapable conclusion that the mechanism of action of the vitamin D$_3$ hormone involves control of gene expression in target cells. Thus, the data continue to be compatible with the earlier hypothesis that 1,25-dihydroxyvitamin D$_3$ acts through mechanisms analogous to those of the steroid hormone family of endocrine signals.

Discovery of a Receptor for the 1,25-Dihydroxyvitamin D$_3$ Hormone

The preferential localization of an active metabolite of vitamin D$_3$, and indeed 1,25-dihydroxyvitamin D$_3$, in target tissues precipitated the search for a macromolecule that could be responsible for selectively binding 1,25-dihydroxyvitamin D$_3$ and that might serve as a receptor for the hormone. Experiments by Haussler and Norman (67) provided the first suggestive evidence that 1,25-dihydroxyvitamin D$_3$ in intestinal mucosal nuclei of chickens is bound to a protein component that might serve this role (see Fig. 3). Additional evidence accumulated from studies in vivo and in vitro revealed that the activity requires high salt concentrations for solubility, is sensitive to proteolytic enzymes, and has a sedimentation coefficient of 3.2 (68,69). The characterization of this receptor protein for 1,25-dihydroxyvitamin D$_3$ was

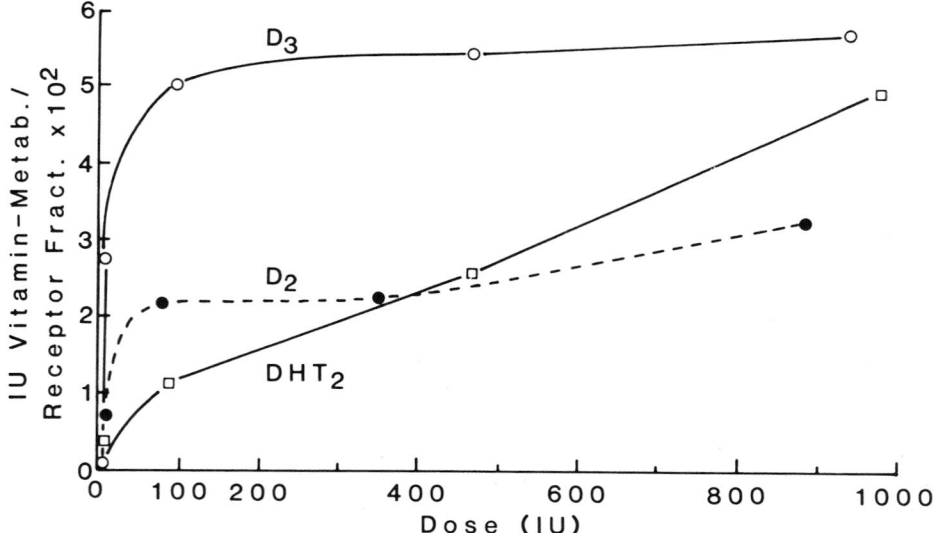

FIG. 3. Saturation of the chromatin-associated receptor fraction as a function of dose of the various D vitamins. The indicated amount of G-^{3}H-vitamin D_3 (D_3), G-^{3}H-vitamin D_2 (D_2), or G-^{3}H-dihydrotachysterol$_2$ (DHT$_2$) was administered to rachitic chicks 15 h prior to sacrifice. Intestinal chromatin (washed once with 1.0% Triton X-100) was then extracted with 0.3 M KCl, and the solubilized receptor fraction was assayed for tritium. Each number is the average of eight determinations on receptor fractions isolated from eight separate chicks. [From Haussler and Norman (67).]

aided significantly by the observation that coincubation of radiolabeled 1,25-dihydroxyvitamin D_3 with chicken intestinal mucosal homogenates resulted in the association of the hormone with nuclear and chromatin fractions in vitro (70). Thus, Brumbaugh and Haussler (70) combined intestinal cytosols with nuclear or chromatin fractions in the presence of 1,25-dihydroxyvitamin D_3 in vitro, and they identified a proteolytically sensitive macromolecule that bound the hormone with high affinity and specificity and that had a sedimentation coefficient, as in in vivo studies, of 3 to 3.5. These studies in the chicken intestine, together with the earlier study that suggested the presence of a vitamin-D_3-binding protein in the same tissue, constitute the discovery of the receptor for 1,25-dihydroxyvitamin D_3. This discovery provided the final experimental tie linking the action of the hormone to nuclear events and, in turn, provided strong support for the proposal that vitamin D_3 acts mechanistically as a steroid hormone.

Early experimenters sought to characterize the affinity and specificity with which the protein in chicken intestine bound 1,25-dihydroxyvitamin D_3, and they also sought to correlate this binding specificity with that of biologic response. Brumbaugh and Haussler (68) reported that the equilibrium dissociation constant of the receptor for hormone was approximately 10^{-9} M when assessed at 4°C. Subsequent studies carried out under more optimal conditions of equilibrium led to more precise estimates of 10^{-10} M (71,72), estimates that continue to be reproduced in studies presently being performed. Moreover, several groups determined the kinetics of receptor association and dissociation with 1,25-dihydroxyvitamin D_3 and calculated their respective kinetic parameters (71,72). Early assessments of the relative binding affinity of the receptor for vitamin D analogues were carried out as competition assays with radiolabeled 1,25-

dihydroxyvitamin D_3 and unlabeled vitamin D_3 metabolites. In all cases, metabolites of the hormone exhibited substantially reduced capacity to compete with the vitamin D_3 hormone for receptor binding, with vitamin D_3 itself and 25-hydroxyvitamin D_3 exhibiting little or no competitive ability (73–75). Within several years, a rather thorough evaluation of the specificity of chicken intestinal receptor binding properties had been accomplished, using not only naturally occurring vitamin D_3 metabolites but synthetic ones as well. All confirmed the unique specificity of the receptor protein for the 1,25-dihydroxyvitamin D_3 ligand and the essentiality of hydroxyl groups at the 1-alpha and carbon-25 positions (76). Importantly, this specificity correlated well with the in vivo response of the intestine to the induction of calcium transport (77).

Simultaneously, the actions of the vitamin D_3 hormone on chicken parathyroid gland, bone, and kidney stimulated evaluation of these tissues for the presence of receptor-like molecules. Accordingly, Brumbaugh et al. (78) identified a protein in the parathyroid gland whose properties were similar to that of the intestinal receptor. Shortly thereafter, receptors for 1,25-dihydroxyvitamin D_3 were identified in bone (79) and kidney (80,81).

Receptor-like molecules were also identified and characterized in mammalian tissues following discovery of the protein in the chicken. Early studies failed to obtain evidence for a receptor-like macromolecule in rat intestine; this was apparently due to the sensitivity of the protein to proteolysis and to the presence of serum-derived vitamin-D-binding protein that also bound 1,25-dihydroxyvitamin D_3 with lower affinity. Nevertheless, Kream et al. (82) overcame these technical problems and provided the first evidence for a mammalian receptor. The characteristics of the protein were very similar to those of the chicken homologue, although sedimentation analysis suggested that the protein exhibited a reduced size (82,83). The rat intestinal receptor became the focus of considerable subsequent research following its discovery. Moreover, this success provided the impetus for investigation of other mammalian tissues that represented targets of vitamin D₃ action. Indeed, biochemical evidence rapidly accumulated for the presence of 1,25-dihydroxyvitamin D₃ receptors in mammalian bone (84,85) and kidney (86,87), sites comparable to those for which receptors had been found in chicken tissues.

Identification of a receptor protein in the chicken intestine precipitated further studies aimed at characterizing the protein's hydrodynamic properties as well as physical structure, both clear prerequisites to its eventual isolation. Initial studies suggested that the concentration of the receptor for 1,25-dihydroxyvitamin D₃ comprised less than 0.002% of the soluble fraction of chicken intestinal mucosal homogenates (68,88). The protein was also extremely sensitive to endogenous proteases. Nevertheless, sucrose gradient analysis and gel filtration chromatography revealed that the receptor had a sedimentation coefficient of 3 to 3.5, a molecular mass of approximately 50,000 to 70,000 (68,70), and a Stokes' radius of 36 Å. The capacity of the receptor to bind 1,25-dihydroxyvitamin D₃ was enhanced and preserved in the presence of reducing agents (82), but it was compromised in the presence of alkylating or sulfhydryl-blocking reagents such as iodoacetamide (83,89). Chromatography of the 1,25-dihydroxyvitamin-D₃-receptor complex revealed it to interact with (a) anion- and cation-exchange columns, (b) hydroxylapatite, and (c) the chromophore dye cibacron blue (88). The receptor also was capable of interacting with immobilized heparin and calf thymus DNA. The latter observation was extremely important because it appeared to substantiate the hypothetical role of the receptor to bind to DNA and to regulate gene transcription. This interaction will be discussed in more detail later in this chapter, although it is worth noting that it remains currently unclear whether the interaction of the receptor with nonspecific calf thymus DNA represents a manifestation of true DNA binding.

The capacity of the chick intestinal receptor to interact with a variety of chromatographic media led rapidly to efforts to purify the protein from intestinal homogenates. Accordingly, McCain et al. (88) reported a minor purification of the intestinal receptor using anion- and cation-exchange columns as well as dye-selective affinity chromatography. Subsequently, Pike and Haussler (90) exploited the affinity of the receptor for DNA to extend that purification to an estimated 40% purity based upon specific activity measurements. Several protein products were present following denaturing gel analysis of total purified protein, although the analysis at the time failed to identify clearly which of the several species present in the preparation represented the 1,25-dihydroxyvitamin

D₃ receptor. Several additional efforts were made to purify the chicken receptor (91,92), all representing minor adaptations of the techniques and procedures indicated above. In 1982, Pike et al. (92,93) prepared sufficient quantities of partially pure intestinal receptor to generate serum antibodies and (subsequently) monoclonal antibodies to the chick receptor for 1,25-dihydroxyvitamin D₃. The use of these antibodies, as well as additional monoclonal antibodies prepared against the purified porcine receptor by Dame et al. (94,95) several years afterward, became instrumental in further characterization of receptor protein from a variety of tissues and in the eventual molecular cloning of both chicken and mammalian forms, an area that will be discussed in depth later. However, despite considerable efforts to characterize the receptor for the vitamin D₃ hormone, our understanding of the structure and function of the protein remained extremely limited during the 1970s and early 1980s.

CONTEMPORARY RESEARCH ON THE GENOMIC MECHANISM OF ACTION OF VITAMIN D₃

The Cellular Distribution of the 1,25-Dihydroxyvitamin D₃ Receptor

The decade of the 1970s closed with the biochemical identification of the 1,25-dihydroxyvitamin D₃ receptor in all avian and mammalian tissues that played a recognized role in mineral metabolism. These tissues included the intestine, bone, parathyroid gland, and kidney. However, experimental evidence was beginning to emerge during that time suggesting a biologic role for the hormone in cellular phenomena apparently unrelated to mineral metabolism, prompting investigators to examine tissues with incidental or nonapparent roles in mineral homeostasis. The bulk of this effort was facilitated by the introduction and commercial availability of tritiated 1,25-dihydroxyvitamin D₃ of very high specific activity. The sensitivity afforded by the use of this reagent was able to overcome the lower concentrations as well as instability of the 1,25-dihydroxyvitamin D₃ receptor inherent to many of the more novel tissues evaluated. As a result, 1,25-dihydroxyvitamin D₃ receptors began to appear through biochemical means in tissues such as the pancreas (81,96,97), placenta (97), pituitary (97,98), ovary (99), testis (100), heart (101), and numerous other tissues as documented in Table 2. These tissues included organs of reproduction, endocrine organs, hematopoietic marrow cells, and immune system cells such as the T and B lymphocyte (102,103). In addition, both skin (104) and muscle (105) appear to be targets for the hormone. Although a clear role for some of these tissues in

TABLE 2. *Tissue distribution of the 1,25-dihydroxyvitamin D₃ receptor through biochemical, autoradiographic, and immunohistochemical analyses*

System	Tissues
Gastrointestinal	Esophagus, stomach, small intestine, large intestine, colon
Hepatic	Liver
Renal	Kidney, urethra
Cardiovascular	Heart muscle
Endocrine	Parathyroid gland, thyroid, adrenal, pituitary
Exocrine	Parotid gland, sebaceous gland
Reproductive	Testis, ovary, placenta, uterus, endometrium, yolk sac, avian chorioallantoic membrane, avian shell gland
Immune	Thymus, bone marrow
Respiratory	Lung
Skeletal	Bone, cartilage,
Epidermis/appendage	Skin, breast, hair follicle
Muscle	Striated muscle
Central nervous system	Brain neurons
Connective	Fibroblasts

mineral transport has been described, it is equally evident that others do not participate in this function.

Of considerable importance during this period, using high specific radioactivity 1,25-dihydroxyvitamin D₃, was the observation that the receptor could be identified in primary and established mammalian cell lines maintained in culture. Initial observations were made in fibroblasts derived from human skin biopsies (106,107) as well as in human breast carcinoma cell lines (108), prompted by the identification of receptor in skin (104) and breast tissue (109), respectively. From these early studies, cell lines of rather diverse origin were investigated for receptor content and shown to contain significant, albeit variable, levels of the 1,25-dihydroxyvitamin D₃ receptor. The origin of receptor positive cell lines, either of cancerous or noncancerous source, included fibroblasts, osteoblasts, myoblasts, monoblasts, hematopoietic cells, lymphocytes, kidney, pituitary, and ovary. The results suggested that few cultured cell lines, and indeed the tissues from which they were derived, were entirely devoid of the 1,25-dihydroxyvitamin D₃ receptor. Nevertheless, because patterns of growth and cell division of cells in culture diverge from that of normal tissues and because the determinants of receptor expression remain unknown, the presence of the receptor in these cell lines has not been taken as a predictive measure of their potential existence in normal cellular counterparts. Irrespectively, cultured cell lines have been extremely useful in studying the relationship between hormone administration, receptor occupancy by 1,25-dihydroxyvitamin D₃, and biologic response (110–112). Interestingly, the initial biologic responses identified in cultured cells relate to the effects of the hormone on cellular growth and differentiation.

Perhaps more important to our knowledge of receptor cellular distribution than identification of the receptor in cultured cells has been the early application of 1,25-dihydroxyvitamin D₃ autoradiography to the identification of target tissues and cell types. While these studies did not identify the receptor directly, they were based upon the strongly supported assumption that entry and retention of 1,25-dihydroxyvitamin D₃ into the cell and to the nucleus is dependent upon the presence of the receptor protein. Studies that allowed visualization of the receptor directly using labeled antibodies to the receptor have confirmed both biochemical and autoradiographic assessments. As outlined earlier, Zile et al. (52) and Jones and Haussler (53) presented the first autoradiographic studies using tissue slices from chicken intestine. In follow-up experiments, it was shown through similar protocols that 1,25-dihydroxyvitamin D₃ localized not only in the duodenum, ileum, and jejunum of rat intestine but also in stomach, kidney, skin, and pituitary (113,114) and shortly thereafter in the pancreas (115). These studies were extended in 1982 to localization of the vitamin D₃ hormone to rat brain and spinal cord (116). While these studies confirmed much of the biochemical evidence that had accumulated, and provided evidence for new and unique sites of action of 1,25-dihydroxyvitamin D₃ in certain tissues, perhaps the most important contribution of autoradiography was visualization of the precise cell types within tissues that were the focus of 1,25-dihydroxyvitamin D₃ uptake. Clearly most interesting was the distribution of hormone in neurons of the brain, including cells of the nucleus centralis of the amygdala, the nucleus interstitialis of the stria terminalis, the rostral thalamus, and medulla oblongata. Hormone was also found in the caudal spinal trigeminal nucleus and in the cervical spinal cord lamina II. These findings indicate the existence of specific neuronal circuits in the brain that are modulated by 1,25-dihydroxyvitamin D₃.

Experiments that allowed visualization of the 1,25-dihydroxyvitamin D₃ receptor were developed more recently using monoclonal antibodies directed against the receptor itself. In studies reported by Clemens et al. (117), receptors were identified and localized in the chicken intestinal villus crypt cells, confirmation of the localization of receptor by both biochemical and autoradiographic means (see Fig. 4). These studies were extended to the visualization of receptor in normal fibroblasts and osteocytes as well as in certain regions of the brain, including cerebellar granule cells, hippocampal granule cells, and pyramidal cells. Staining was also apparent in a cloned osteogenic sarcoma cell line and in cloned mouse fibroblasts. Additional studies also fo-

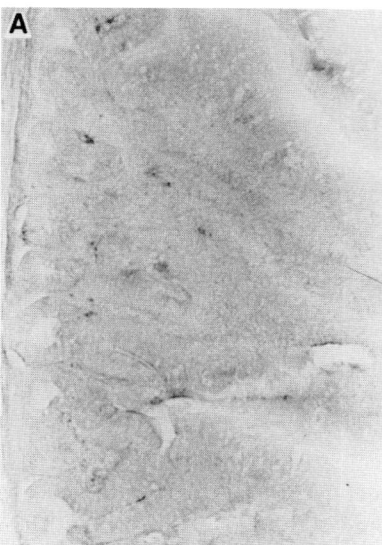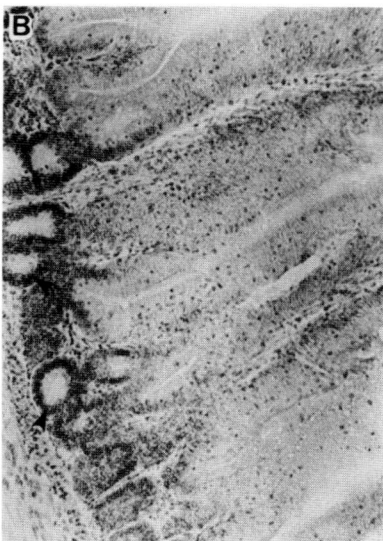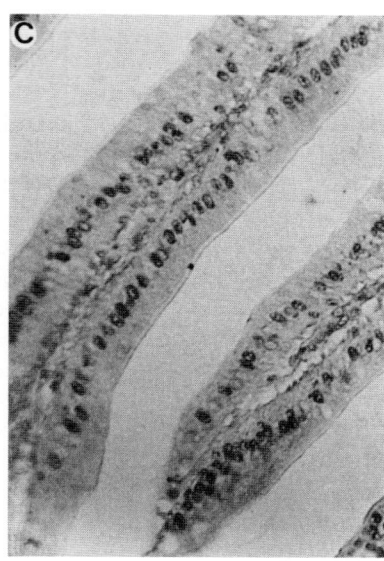

FIG. 4. Immunochemical localization of the 1,25-dihydroxyvitamin D₃ receptor in chick intestine. **A:** Background staining in a tissue section incubated with nonimmune rat IgG. **B:** Staining in a tissue section incubated with the anti-1,25-dihydroxyvitamin-D₃-receptor monoclonal antibody 9A7; initial magnification is ×100. Immunostaining of intestinal epithelial cells is especially apparent in cells in the crypts of Lieberkuhn (*arrows*). **C:** Detail of nuclear staining in epithelial cells of the villus at ×250. The intensity of nuclear staining decreased with increasing dilution of monoclonal antibody and was dependent upon time of fixation. [From Clemens et al. (117).]

cused upon visualization of the receptor in human tissue sections. These experiments resulted in the demonstration of receptor in a wide variety of tissues, all confirming previous biochemical and autoradiographic conclusions (118,119). Receptor was also observed in primary human breast carcinoma biopsies (120). Thus, three independent techniques, largely confirmatory among themselves, have shaped the current concept that the 1,25-dihydroxyvitamin D₃ receptor is almost ubiquitously distributed in tissues, although localized only in selected cell types within those organs and tissues.

Regulation of 1,25-Dihydroxyvitamin D₃ Receptor Expression

Regulation of receptor expression likely represents one mechanism by which cells exert control over both absolute and relative response to 1,25-dihydroxyvitamin D₃ in the face of unchanging or modestly changing serum levels of that hormonal metabolite. Indeed, the cell is conceptually a nontarget for 1,25-dihydroxyvitamin D₃ in the absence of the receptor. For cells that contain the receptor, quantitative changes in the protein's level likely represent determinants of the magnitude of the biologic response. Moreover, absolute expression of the receptor gene as well as quantitative changes in receptor concentration imply the existence of factors that serve to regulate these levels.

Perhaps the most interesting example of specific con-

trol of receptor expression and its effects on biologic response derives from studies of the developing neonatal rat intestine by DeLuca and co-workers (121–124). Rat pups exhibit limited capacity for intestinal transport of calcium during the first several weeks of life. Coincidently, the intestinal mucosa of these pups does not express the 1,25-dihydroxyvitamin D₃ receptor, and not surprisingly the animals are refractory to administration of 1,25-dihydroxyvitamin D₃. The neonatal rat intestine undergoes rapid physiological maturation, however, during the period of transition to a solid diet that precedes weaning at approximately 3 weeks of age. Maturation is characterized by striking changes in intestinal tract morphology, biochemistry, and cellular function (125), and accompanying those changes are (a) the acquisition of capacity to transport mineral, (b) responsivity to 1,25-dihydroxyvitamin D₃, and (c) the synthesis of the 1,25-dihydroxyvitamin D₃ receptor (121). The appearance of receptor was initially determined by the capacity of extracts to bind 1,25-dihydroxyvitamin D₃ (121). More recently, both the protein (126) and its messenger RNA (127,128) have been shown to accumulate during this period in the rat. This physiologic model provides a striking example of how the appearance of the receptor for 1,25-dihydroxyvitamin D₃ leads to acquired sensitivity to the hormone and to the initiation of biologic response. These findings in themselves provide strong evidence for the relationship between receptor, its hormone, and the intestinal absorption of calcium.

An equally interesting model of acquired response to

1,25-dihydroxyvitamin D_3 is the apparent role of the hormone in the biologic responses of certain cells of the immune system. Cells of the monocyte/macrophage lineage express receptors for 1,25-dihydroxyvitamin D_3 that, in response to hormone, promote their differentiation to mature macrophages and also promote their fusion to multinucleated cells that potentially constitute the osteoclast (129,130). In contrast, cells of the lymphoid lineage do not express the receptor and are simultaneously unresponsive to 1,25-dihydroxyvitamin D_3. 1,25-Dihydroxyvitamin D_3 receptors appear, however, following activation by a variety of mitogens (102,131), and this appearance is correlated directly with an acquired sensitivity of the cells to hormonal vitamin D_3. This sensitivity leads to an inhibition of proliferation (perhaps not a direct effect) as well as to reduction in lymphokine production that includes interleukin-2, gamma-interferon, and granulocyte macrophage colony stimulating factor (GM-CSF) (132–134) at the level of RNA and protein. More recent studies suggest that the stimulation of T cells through alternative routes that mimic the physiologic activation pathway, such as with anti-T3 monoclonal antibody, may in fact enhance gamma-interferon synthesis at physiologic levels of 1,25-dihydroxyvitamin D_3 (135). Irrespective of this, the appearance of the receptor is well correlated with an absolute response to 1,25-dihydroxyvitamin D_3.

The appearance of the receptor for 1,25-dihydroxyvitamin D_3 in the above cases is almost certain to be due to induction of receptor gene expression. In the case of receptor appearance in the developing intestine, evidence suggests that glucocorticoids are instrumental in the maturation process that, in turn, leads to receptor expression. Indeed, administration of glucocorticoids to the cultured rat intestine precipitates precocious villus maturation and the concomitant appearance of receptor (123,124). It is unclear, however, whether glucocorticoids directly induce expression of the receptor gene in this system or simply initiate a complex process of cellular reprogramming that, in turn, leads to changes in receptor synthesis (125). Glucocorticoids have been noted to induce receptor in both mature rat (136) and mouse (137) intestine. Direct effects of glucocorticoids were observed in bone cells (138). Little is known, however, of the signals that prompt induction of receptor following T-cell activation. It is presumed that antigen presentation initiates a cascade phenomenon that proceeds via the protein kinase C pathway of gene activation. Perhaps the gene for the 1,25-dihydroxyvitamin D_3 receptor is sensitive to modulation through this effector pathway.

In addition to the above situations, many cellular and physiologic states as well as numerous hormonal factors have been noted to modulate the level of the 1,25-dihydroxyvitamin D_3 receptor. Cell cycle as well as the state of differentiation are determinants of receptor expression (139). In the latter case, osteoclast precursors (mono-cytes and macrophages) are well-endowed with receptors (129,130), whereas terminally differentiated osteoclasts have not been demonstrated to contain the protein. Known agents that alter receptor expression—in addition to the glucocorticoid hormones—include the vitamin A hormone retinoic acid (140,141), 1,25-dihydroxyvitamin D_3 (142,143), dietary calcium (144), and growth factors. The effects of 1,25-dihydroxyvitamin D_3, which will be discussed in a subsequent section, are rather profound and occur at the level of both protein and receptor mRNA. In the case of retinoic acid, a clear up-regulation of the receptor is evident following treatment of osteosarcoma cells in culture with that hormone (140). It has been hypothesized that this accounts for the increase in bone cell responsivity to 1,25-dihydroxyvitamin D_3 with respect to both alkaline phosphatase induction and osteocalcin synthesis (141). While the mechanism of induction by steroid or thyroid hormones and retinoic acid is presumed to be via transcriptional modulation, evidence remains to be gathered to support that hypothesis. Irrespective of the mechanism and modulatory effects, the underlying assumption in these observations is that an increase or decrease in receptor number affects the magnitude of the biologic response to 1,25-dihydroxyvitamin D_3. Several groups have provided evidence that receptor concentration (145) and occupancy (146) are capable of altering bioresponse. More recent studies that will be described later show very clearly that the level of receptor determines the extent of response (147). However, additional factors such as physiologic state of the cell, extent of hormonal metabolism by cells, the abundance of factors that facilitate the transcription of a gene, and the existing level of expression of 1,25-dihydroxyvitamin-D_3-sensitive genes are also likely to contribute significantly to the magnitude of biologic response.

Biochemical and Intracellular Properties of the 1,25-Dihydroxyvitamin D_3 Receptor

Physical Features of the 1,25-Dihydroxyvitamin D_3 Receptor

The 1,25-dihydroxyvitamin D_3 receptor is a protein of trace abundance even in major target tissues such as intestine, kidney, and bone. Estimates based upon hormone-binding studies suggest that the receptor represents less than 0.002% of the soluble fraction of such tissues irrespective of animal source (68,70,90), and at least an order of magnitude less in cultured cells (111). The protein is extremely labile, due to (a) unknown causes, (b) its extreme sensitivity to elevated temperatures, and (c) endogenous and exogenous proteolysis (148–151). The protein also tends to aggregate in the absence of hypertonic salt concentrations (151,152). All of these properties strongly hampered initial efforts to characterize and isolate the protein for precise structural analyses.

Radioactive ligand was essential in tracing the receptor in early biochemical studies, because no direct assays of the protein had been developed. Unfortunately, while the affinity of the receptor for hormone is rather high, as judged by the equilibrium dissociation constant of approximately 10^{-10} M, this interaction is noncovalent in nature and subject to considerable dissociation under both nonequilibrium and denaturing conditions. As a result, only receptors that were capable of binding hormone were detectable, limiting experimental studies to those that favored the integrity of the intact complex. These conditions severely limited receptor characterization and restricted evaluations to the use of nondenaturing techniques such as sedimentation analysis and gel filtration, ion-exchange methods, and group-selective affinity chromatography methods. Despite this, hydrodynamic properties such as sedimentation coefficient, Stokes' radius, and interaction with chromatography media were assessed. With the exception of apparent size, no evidence emerged from these evaluations to suggest that substantial differences exist between receptors from avian and mammalian species. In addition, no evidence accumulated to support a physical or structural difference between receptors from tissue to tissue. Several exchange assays were developed to measure receptors occupied by endogenous ligand, revealing that under normal circumstances, 5–20% of receptors were occupied with hormonal ligand (153,154). The assays, however, were technically difficult and unreliable and were therefore not routinely utilized by investigators.

In 1979, it was discovered that the receptor was capable of interacting with immobilized calf thymus DNA, an observation that suggested that the 1,25-dihydroxyvitamin D₃ receptor is a DNA-binding protein (see Fig. 5) (90). This feature was predictable and entirely consistent with the hypothesis that the receptor mediates the action of the vitamin D₃ hormone through an interaction with the control regions of hormone-sensitive genes. However, despite the fact that intercalating agents such as ethidium bromide blocked receptor interaction with the immobilized DNA ligand (111), the exact nature of the interaction between receptor and this nonspecific DNA remained unclear because of the possibility that the abundance of negatively charged phosphate groups on DNA resulted in nothing more than a polycation-exchange column. Indeed, the receptor was capable of binding tightly to phosphocellulose alone (88). The molecular basis for 1,25-dihydroxyvitamin-D₃-receptor interaction with nonspecific DNA remains to be clarified. In spite of this, the capacity of receptor to bind DNA cellulose emerged as an important technique with which to characterize the receptor. Nevertheless, both it as well as the capacity to bind hormone were taken as representative of two important functions of the receptor and, thus, diagnostic of an intact and functional protein.

The capacity of the receptor to bind to DNA cellulose, along with a wide variety of chromatographic media, afforded the opportunity for several attempts to purify the protein to near-homogeneity. The first successful purification of the receptor from chicken intestine by Pike and Haussler (90) did not lead to the protein's homogeneous isolation nor did it lead to the protein's precise identification following denaturing gel electrophoresis. Nevertheless, this initial study as well as those of Simpson et al. (91) did establish important methodologies under which this extremely rare protein could be collected and iso-

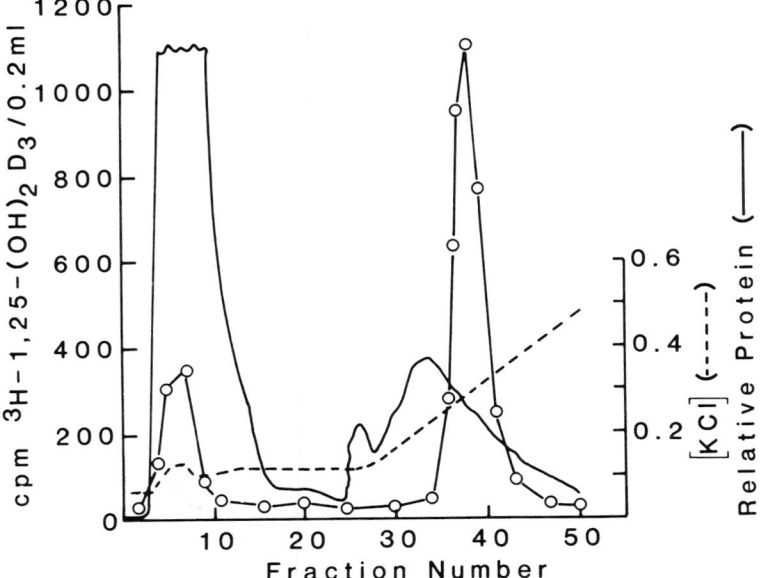

FIG. 5. Chromatography of the chick intestinal 1,25-dihydroxyvitamin D₃ receptor on calf thymus DNA cellulose. Chick intestinal cytosol was incubated with tritiated 1,25-dihydroxyvitamin D₃ and then chromatographed on calf thymus DNA immobilized on cellulose. The receptor–hormone complex was eluted during a linear gradient of potassium chloride at 0.28 M. Solid lines indicate the protein profile, dashed lines indicate the salt gradient, and unfilled circles indicate the tritiated 1,25-dihydroxyvitamin-D₃–receptor complex. [From Pike and Haussler (90).]

lated in relatively significant amounts. One of the most important advances in receptor analysis, which was indeed crucial to the eventual molecular cloning of the protein's structural gene, was the successful generation of anti-receptor monoclonal antibodies. In 1982, Pike et al. (92,93) partially purified the 1,25-dihydroxyvitamin D_3 receptor from large amounts of chicken intestinal mucosa, raised immune responses in rats, and successfully recovered several high-affinity anti-1,25-dihydroxyvitamin D_3 receptor monoclonal antibodies. Subsequent to these experiments, Dame et al. (94,95) partially purified the receptor from porcine intestinal mucosa and generated an extensive series of anti-mammalian receptor monoclonal antibodies from mouse spleen cell fusions. Both sets of antibodies were specific for the 1,25-dihydroxyvitamin D_3 receptor, exhibiting no interaction with receptors for other hormones. In addition, both sets displayed similar immunologic cross-reactivity: Some of the monoclonal antibodies were specific for receptor found in the animal species from which the original antigen was derived, whereas others displayed extensive cross-reactivity with 1,25-dihydroxyvitamin D_3 receptor irrespective of animal origin. None of the antibodies were capable of discriminating receptors from different tissue sources within the same animal species.

Anti-receptor monoclonal antibodies have provided an additional reagent with which to detect and characterize the 1,25-dihydroxyvitamin D_3 receptor. More importantly, they have provided a method whereby receptors could be detected following denaturation irrespective of the presence or absence of hormonal ligand. Denaturing gel electrophoresis followed by Western blot analysis using the monoclonal antibodies as probe revealed that the chicken receptor appeared in two forms: a predominant species of approximately 60 kD and a less abundant species of 58 kD (155). The latter did not appear to arise as a result of proteolysis. In contrast, mammalian forms of the protein were single species ranging in size from 54–55 kD in rat, mouse, and pig to approximately 50–52 kD in the human (94,156,157). Immobilization of the antibodies on insoluble agarose supports, followed by incubation with cellular extracts, permitted direct and efficient immunoadsorption of the receptor from cellular extracts (155,158). These experiments resulted in a facile and rapid purification of the receptor in a single step, although successful elution of the protein from the adsorbent generally resulted in inactive proteins not useful for subsequent functional studies. A modification of this procedure allowed direct precipitation of receptors labeled internally through incubation of cultured cells with radioactive amino acids such as [^{35}S]methionine (157,159,160). Similar experiments carried out with receptor translated in vitro using reticulocyte lysates permitted characterization of receptor mRNA (157). These experiments suggested that while the mammalian receptors were smaller than their avian homologues, the mRNA transcripts were considerably larger. Finally, antibodies were used to detect receptor by both radioligand immunoassay (161) and immunoradiometric assay (162). The former was useful in determining that extracts of cells derived from certain patients with hereditary resistance to 1,25-dihydroxyvitamin D_3 contained defective receptors that were incapable of binding hormone (163; see below). The latter was used to quantitate the effects of 1,25-dihydroxyvitamin D_3 on receptor levels (164). Thus, the use of the antibodies extended the depth of our knowledge of the receptor with respect to both its intracellular biology and its physical characteristics.

Structural Organization of the 1,25-Dihydroxyvitamin D_3 Receptor

Immunologic techniques, together with hormonal ligand assays, provided the first clues as to the structural organization of the 1,25-dihydroxyvitamin D_3 receptor. Initial studies by Pike (165) suggested that the epitope for the anti-receptor monoclonal antibody 9A7 was located within the region of the receptor responsible for binding to DNA, based upon the ability of the antibody to alter the DNA-binding capability of the receptor following formation of a complex. Some of the antibodies raised by Dame et al. (95) were likewise directed toward the DNA-binding domain of the receptor. Allegretto et al. (166) employed limited digestion with trypsin to cleave the protein into two separate domains: (i) a large fragment of 30–40 kD that retained bound 1,25-dihydroxyvitamin D_3 and (ii) a smaller fragment capable of binding DNA cellulose irrespective of the presence of the hormone-binding region. The ability to detect the latter fragment through immunologic reactivity, along with the concomitant loss of immunoreactivity in the hormone-binding fragment, confirmed the relationship between the epitope and the receptor DNA-binding domain. The ability of carboxypeptidase to modestly reduce the receptor's overall mass while simultaneously causing dissociation of the hormone suggested that the steroid-binding region was carboxy-terminal to the DNA-binding domain (167). Taken together, these data led to the simple concept that the receptor was composed of at least two unique functional domains separable by trypsin: (i) an amino-terminal DNA-binding domain and (ii) a carboxy-terminal 1,25-dihydroxyvitamin-D_3-binding domain. As will be discussed later, the molecular cloning of the receptor confirmed this organization.

Intracellular Biology of the 1,25-Dihydroxyvitamin D_3 Receptor

As with other soluble proteins, the synthesis of the receptor occurs in the cytoplasm of the cell following processing and transport of the mRNA from the nucleus. Early studies suggested that the receptor remained in the cytoplasm until hormone complex formation, whereupon it acquired an increased affinity for nuclear components and could subsequently be found localized with the cell nucleus (68,70). Biochemical fractionation techniques initially supported that concept until Kream et al. (82) observed that solubilization of the receptor required the presence of high salt concentrations. Subsequent studies by Walters et al. (168,169) confirmed this requirement through an extensive analysis of the behavior of the receptor under a variety of buffer conditions. These investigators, in turn, advanced the hypothesis that the 1,25-dihydroxyvitamin D_3 receptor was predominantly a nuclear protein regardless of its state of hormone occupancy, very much like the thyroid hormone receptor (170). Given the artifacts associated with biochemical fractionation techniques, the view that the receptor was localized to the nucleus irrespective of hormone occupancy required independent confirmation. In fact, subsequent studies utilizing immunocytochemical techniques supported the contention that the protein was indeed nuclear. Thus, regardless of the state of hormone treatment, both cells in culture and certain tissues exhibited receptor-specific staining predominantly within the nucleus (117). In spite of this, the issue of receptor localization remains to be unequivocally established, principally because, like biochemical studies, immunohistochemical techniques are not without potential artifacts. It is likely that the resolution of this issue will occur upon demonstration, within the receptor, of an amino acid sequence that functions as a signal for nuclear localization.

The suggestion that the receptor localized within the nucleus in the absence of hormone has been supported through additional studies of the behavior of the protein itself. In contrast to several other of the steroid receptors, the receptor for 1,25-dihydroxyvitamin D_3 does not require hormone for low-affinity DNA binding or nuclear binding in vitro (111,171,172). Moreover, no compelling evidence exists for a 1,25-dihydroxyvitamin-D_3-induced activation event analogous to those characteristic of receptors for glucocorticoid, progesterone, androgen, or estrogen hormones. This activation event is believed to occur because the latter proteins appear to be associated with heat shock protein 90 (hsp90) in the absence of ligand (173). Thus, a major role of the cognate hormone in those systems is to cause dissociation of the protein complex, thus liberating a receptor-hormone complex capable of DNA binding and gene activation. Although it is known definitively that the thyroid hormone receptor does not bind to hsp90 (174), no clear evidence exists to date to suggest that the 1,25-dihydroxyvitamin D_3 receptor does or does not form a complex with this macromolecule.

Effect of 1,25-Dihydroxyvitamin D₃ on the Receptor

The binding of 1,25-dihydroxyvitamin D_3 to its receptor in vivo is believed to result in conversion of the pro-tein from an inactive molecule to one fully functional in inducing biologic response. The biochemical events that precede this biomodification are poorly understood, not only for the 1,25-dihydroxyvitamin D_3 receptor but also for the steroid, thyroid hormone, and retinoic acid hormone receptors. It is almost certain, however, that receptor inducibility arises as a result of multiple effects of the cognate ligand. 1,25-Dihydroxyvitamin D_3 exerts a number of phenomenologic effects on its receptor protein, effects that presumably provide clues as to the mechanism by which the hormone functions. Formation of the receptor-hormone complex in vitro appears to stabilize the receptor (88). Thus, the half-life of the complex is considerably extended when compared to that of its unoccupied counterpart. The effect of hormone on receptor half-life in intact cells is unclear. Costa et al. (142) suggested that in cultured kidney cells the presence of hormone reduces this parameter. On the other hand, Pan and Price (175) did not observe a difference in receptor longevity in the presence or absence of hormone. Thus, while it is clear that 1,25-dihydroxyvitamin D_3 exerts an apparently protective effect on the receptor in vitro, its effects on the protein in vivo remain open. Careful studies that utilize assays to examine the receptor protein itself will be required to definitively ascertain the effect of hormone on receptor.

The vitamin D_3 hormone displays a clear ability to affect the receptor's affinity for the cell nucleus, both in vitro and in vivo, as assessed by the ionic strength required to solubilize the protein from the nuclear or chromatin fraction. Extraction of the receptor from the nucleus of cultured cells incubated with 1,25-dihydroxyvitamin D_3 requires a salt concentration significantly higher than that required to extract the receptor from untreated cells (111). Similar studies carried out in chickens treated with 1,25-dihydroxyvitamin D_3 led to an identical conclusion (171,172). Simultaneously, extraction of receptor–hormone complexes formed through in vitro incubation of 1,25-dihydroxyvitamin D_3 with either chromatin or nuclear preparations (both containing the receptor) also require higher ionic strength conditions than do similar preparations without hormone (172). Finally, reconstitution of receptor containing cellular extracts with purified nuclei leads to the nuclear binding of the hormone receptor under salt conditions that prevent identical association of the unoccupied receptor (171). Based upon the assumption that higher salt concentrations required for solubilization are indicative of a higher strength of interaction and, in turn, a higher affinity, all of these experiments suggest that one effect of the hormone on receptor is to modify the protein both in vitro and in vivo to achieve high-affinity binding.

The above phenomenon is similarly reflected in the interaction of the 1,25-dihydroxyvitamin D_3 receptor with immobilized DNA. Early studies suggested that formation of the receptor–1,25-dihydroxyvitamin D_3 complex, whether in vivo or in vitro, resulted in a tighter binding to calf thymus DNA cellulose (111,172). Thus, the occupied 1,25-dihydroxyvitamin D_3 receptor eluted from this affinity ligand at a salt concentration somewhat higher than that of the unoccupied form of the protein. Interestingly, formation of the hormone–receptor complex in vivo resulted in an unanticipated affinity for DNA cellulose which was less than that seen for the complex formed in vitro, although still higher than that for unoccupied receptor (172). Despite these observations, it is unclear whether these findings reflect a physiologic role for the hormone in receptor activation or merely represent an unexplained phenomenon. Thus, as with other steroid receptors, the exact role or roles of the hormone in modulating 1,25-dihydroxyvitamin-D_3-receptor activity remain to be clarified.

Effect of 1,25-Dihydroxyvitamin D_3 on Receptor Regulation

1,25-Dihydroxyvitamin D_3 exerts several additional effects upon the 1,25-dihydroxyvitamin D_3 receptor when administered either in vivo or to cultured organs or cells. In a unique study that allowed estimation of receptor binding activity following induction by a surrogate 1,25-dihydroxyvitamin D_3 (24,25-dihydroxyvitamin D_3), Costa et al. (142) first proposed that treatment of cultured mammalian cells with hormonal vitamin D_3 resulted in an up-regulation of receptor binding activity. These studies suggested the possibility of hormone autoregulation at the level of binding and presumably at the level of the protein. This regulation was multifaceted, exhibiting a rapid response phase during the first hour, followed by a gradual increase over a 20-h period. Actinomycin D was shown to block the extended rise but not the rapid rise in receptor increase. Collectively, these experiments suggested, but did not prove, that the hormone was capable (in cultured cells) of short-term increase in half-life and of simultaneously inducing the receptor gene. A subsequent study in the rat in vivo revealed that the vitamin-D-deficient rat intestine exhibited a significant decrease in receptor number when compared to that of vitamin-D_3-sufficient controls (176). However, additional studies in animals have failed to lead to a consensus regarding (a) the ability of 1,25-dihydroxyvitamin D_3 to induce receptor, (b) the tissue specificity of 1,25-dihydroxyvitamin D_3, or (c) the rapidity with which the induction occurs (128,164). Studies by Pike (156), Mangelsdorf et al. (157), and McDonnell et al. (143), utilizing 1,25-dihydroxyvitamin D_3 directly as an inducer and both 1,25-dihydroxyvitamin D_3 binding and immunoblot assays, provided direct evidence that the protein was up-regulated in response to hormone in cultured mouse fibroblasts (see Fig. 6). This effect was sensitive to cycloheximide and actinomycin

D, suggesting a requirement for continued receptor synthesis. Finally, in studies by both Mangelsdorf et al. (157) and McDonnell et al. (143), examination of the receptor mRNA levels by receptor cDNA hybridization revealed a clear up-regulation at the level of mRNA. This rapid up-regulation by hormone has been confirmed more recently by DeLuca and co-workers in the rat in vivo (164) and in HL-60 cells (177). The lack of induction in chicken intestinal organ culture (160) is consistent with an examination (in this species) of the effect of 1,25-dihydroxyvitamin D_3 on the receptor in vivo, where Hunziker et al. (178) failed to detect significant changes in receptor concentration. Current efforts with regard to receptor regulation focus on determining whether the effects of 1,25-dihydroxyvitamin D_3 are exerted at the level of mRNA stability or on its synthesis.

1,25-Dihydroxyvitamin D_3 treatment in culture cells and in organ culture also leads to enhanced levels of phosphorylation of the receptor. Pike and Sleator (159) demonstrated that the 1,25-dihydroxyvitamin D_3 receptor from cultured mouse fibroblasts treated with 1,25-dihydroxyvitamin D_3 exhibited a retarded migration during sodium dodecyl sulfate–polyacrylamide gel electrophoresis, suggesting a hormone-dependent covalent modification. Coincubation of the cultured cells with 1,25-dihydroxyvitamin D_3 and [^{32}P]orthophosphate, followed by immunoprecipitation, revealed that only the 1,25-dihydroxyvitamin-D_3-dependent retarded band contained radiolabeled [^{32}P], suggesting that the covalent modification was phosphate addition. Time courses suggested that phosphorylation of the receptor coincided with exposure to the hormone itself. Subsequent phosphoamino acid analyses revealed that the phosphorylated amino acid species was limited to a serine residue (179). More recent studies by Brown and DeLuca (160) have shown that 1,25-dihydroxyvitamin D_3 treatment of cultured chicken intestine results in a rapid phosphorylation of receptor in that species as well, again in a fashion coincident with 1,25-dihydroxyvitamin D_3 administration. What is the role of phosphorylation in receptor function? Phosphorylation of the receptor has not been demonstrated to occur in in vitro incubations. Yet the affinity of the receptor for 1,25-dihydroxyvitamin D_3 as well as for calf thymus DNA does not appear to differ if the receptor is occupied in vivo or in vitro (111). Although these studies need detailed confirmation, at present they suggest that the role of hormone-dependent phosphorylation does not involve modification of either of the two binding functions of the protein. Perhaps receptor phosphorylation influences receptor transactivation capabilities, affects turnover, or provides a signal for receptor degradation. A more complete understanding of the role of phosphorylation will only come following (a) identification of the specific serine residue that undergoes phosphorylation and (b) the development of in

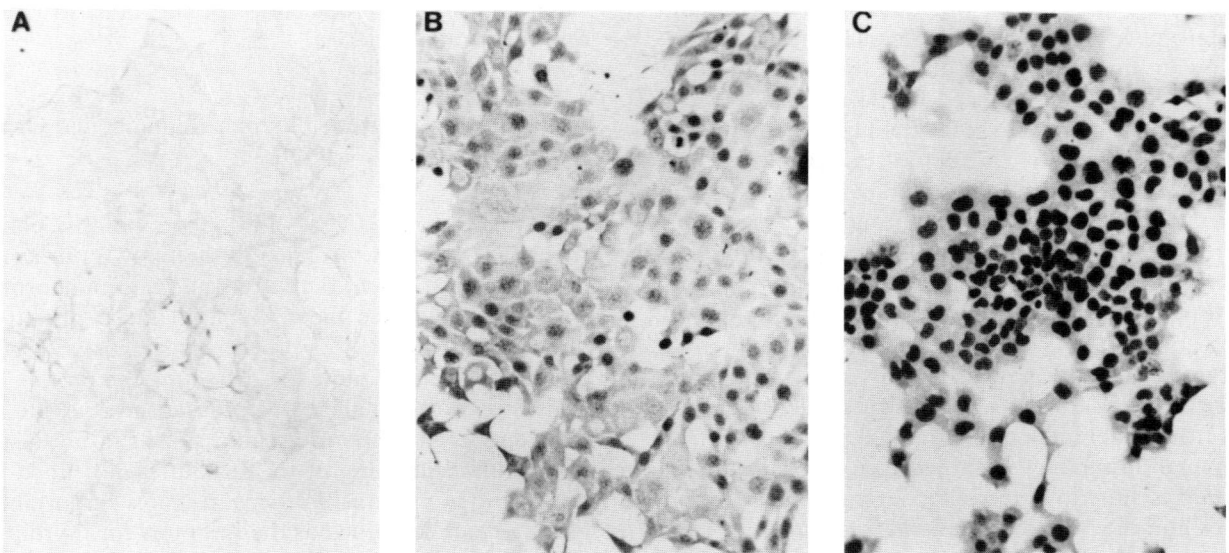

FIG. 6. Visualization of the 1,25-dihydroxyvitamin D_3 receptor in mouse 3T6 fibroblasts, along with up-regulation of this receptor by 1,25-dihydroxyvitamin D_3. **A:** Cells incubated with nonimmune rat IgG. **B:** Cells treated with ethanol and reacted with anti-1,25-dihydroxyvitamin-D_3-receptor monoclonal antibody 9A7. **C:** Cells treated with 1,25-dihydroxyvitamin D_3 for 48 h and then reacted with the 9A7 antibody. Predominantly nuclear staining is evident upon detection with the 9A7 antibody, and it is substantially increased following treatment with 1,25-dihydroxyvitamin D_3. [From Clemens et al. (117).]

vivo and in vitro assays that are capable of assessing the multiple functional capabilities of the receptor itself.

MOLECULAR BIOLOGY OF THE RECEPTOR FOR 1,25-DIHYDROXYVITAMIN D₃

Molecular Cloning of the Receptor for 1,25-Dihydroxyvitamin D₃

The development of antibodies directed toward the 1,25-dihydroxyvitamin D_3 receptor in 1982 and 1985, together with the introduction of a new lambda-phage expression vector in 1983 designated lambda gt11 (180), provided the technical methodology whereby the receptor's rare structural gene could be recovered from a cDNA library. The importance of the molecular cloning of this receptor cannot be underestimated. Because of the receptor's low abundance and labile nature, it was clear to many investigators that insight into the structure and function of the receptor—and, correspondingly, insight into the mechanism of action of 1,25-dihydroxyvitamin D_3—would remain limited until a complementary DNA comprising the receptor structural gene was recovered and its primary sequence deduced. It was on this basis, in fact, that the latter half of the 1980s were witness to the molecular cloning of virtually all the known nuclear receptors, events that have led to an enormous increase in our understanding of the structure and function of these important proteins.

The anti-chicken receptor monoclonal antibody 9A7 was utilized by McDonnell et al. (143) to screen a randomly primed chicken intestinal cDNA expression library prepared in lambda gt11. A single viral clone was identified from a screening of 10^7 recombinants whose protein product was immunologically reactive to 9A7 antibody and, subsequently, to the anti-chicken receptor monoclonal antibody 4A5. A short cDNA was recovered from the lambda clone and utilized to rescreen the library by hybridization, leading to the recovery of a larger cDNA clone. DNA sequence analysis of both cDNAs revealed that they each encoded the domain of a protein that exhibited a high degree of homology to that of the v-erb A gene product as well as to receptors for the glucocorticoid, progesterone, and estrogen hormones. This domain displayed a strong relatedness to the multiple DNA-binding zinc finger domains of the known transcription factor TFIIIA (181), suggesting (a) a role for this domain in DNA binding and (b) a corresponding role for the protein in transcriptional regulation. Both were anticipated observations for the receptor. Hybrid-selected in vitro translation using the cloned cDNA was successfully utilized to confirm that the cDNA recovered by the 9A7 antibody was indeed a portion of the mRNA encoding the chicken 1,25-dihydroxyvitamin D_3 receptor. These experiments constitute the molecular cloning of the receptor for 1,25-dihydroxyvitamin D_3, and they provided the first direct insight into the relationship between it and other bona fide members of the steroid-receptor family of genes that includes the glucocorticoid, progesterone, and estrogen receptors (182).

Following the recovery of cDNA for the chicken receptor, this probe was utilized by Baker et al. (183) to recover the complete cDNA for the human receptor for 1,25-dihydroxyvitamin D_3. Partial cDNA clones were also recovered by Burmester et al. (184) and Pike (185) for the rat receptor—the former through the use of anti-porcine 1,25-dihydroxyvitamin-D_3-receptor monoclonal antibodies prepared by Dame et al. (95), and the latter through hybridization screening utilizing the human receptor cDNA. The complete coding region of the rat receptor cDNA was subsequently recovered by Burmester et al. (127) in 1989. The DNA sequence of these clones from different species revealed extensive regions of very high homology (assumed to represent domains important to function) as well as several smaller regions of lower homology. The functional importance of these domains will be discussed below, but this similarity between the receptors suggests that (as with the other nuclear proteins) the receptor for 1,25-dihydroxyvitamin

D_3 is highly conserved across species, both structurally and functionally.

Cloning of the Steroid, Thyroid, Retinoid, and Orphan Receptor Genes

During the period 1984–1988, representative complementary DNAs for virtually all the known intracellular receptors for the steroid, thyroid, and retinoid hormones were recovered (see Fig. 7). The deduced primary sequences of this class of proteins, together with subsequent experiments aimed at dissecting the protein's domain structure through cDNA mutagenesis, expression, and analysis of receptor function, led to substantial gains in our understanding of the structure and function of these unique proteins. Perhaps the most important initial information gained as the receptors for thyroid hormone, vitamin D_3, and finally the vitamin A hormone retinoic acid were sequentially cloned was the realization that each was structurally and therefore functionally re-

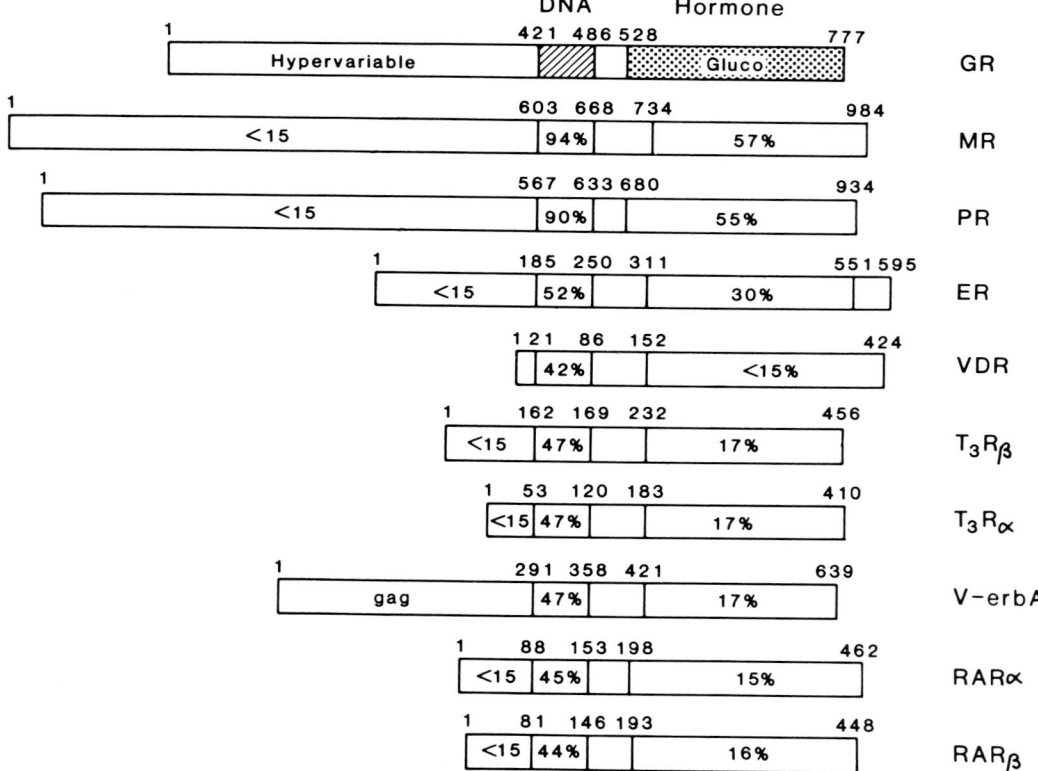

FIG. 7. The steroid-receptor, thyroid-hormone-receptor, and retinoic-acid-receptor superfamily of genes. Schematic comparison of the structural organization of proteins comprising the receptor superfamily. The primary amino acid sequences (numbered above the protein structure) have been aligned on the basis of regions of maximum amino acid sequence identity which are indicated as a percentage relative to the glucocorticoid receptor (GR). DNA- and hormone-binding domains are indicated. GR, glucocorticoid receptor; MR, mineralocorticoid receptor; PR, progesterone receptor; ER, estrogen receptor; VDR, 1,25-dihydroxyvitamin D_3 receptor; T_3R_α and T_3R_β, thyroid-hormone receptors; V-erbA, viral erbA protein receptor; RAR_α and RAR_β, retinoic acid receptors.

lated to each other and to the receptors for estrogen, progesterone, glucocorticoid, and other steroid hormones. As will be discussed below, the relatedness of these gene products suggested that together they comprise a superfamily of proteins, whose functions are to mediate the genomic actions of their respective hormonal ligands (182).

A cDNA encoding the full-length glucocorticoid receptor was the first to be recovered, sequenced, and evaluated by Evans and co-workers (186) and by Yamamoto and co-workers (187). A complete cDNA comprising the human estrogen receptor was reported shortly thereafter (188), followed by recovery of the structural genes for the chicken progesterone receptor (189), human and chicken thyroid hormone receptor (190,191), chicken vitamin D₃ receptor (143), human mineralocorticoid receptor (192), human retinoic acid receptor (193,194), and human and rat androgen receptors (195,196). Molecular cloning of receptors for these hormones from additional species occurred during or following these pioneering efforts. As with the initial cloning of the 1,25-dihydroxyvitamin D₃ receptor, the principal method utilized to recover cDNA clones in the early stages of cDNA recovery relied heavily upon the use of antibodies to recognize receptor produced in recombinant expression libraries. Later studies utilized hybridization screening employing related or partially related cDNAs, oligonucleotides, or fortuitously derived sequences to screen directly for recombinant DNA clones.

The use of partially or fortuitously related cDNAs as probes also led to the identification of a large number of additional members of the steroid-receptor gene family, for which known hormonal ligands remain uncharacterized (197). Indeed, it remains uncertain whether active ligands exist for these interesting proteins, termed *orphan receptors*. Thus, it is possible that these receptors represent constitutively active molecules whose genomic activities are regulated by alternative means, perhaps through transcriptional control of their expression or through post-transcriptional mechanisms. At the present time, there are continuing efforts to identify additional members of the steroid-receptor, thyroid-hormone-receptor, and retinoic-acid-receptor superfamily and to clarify the role that these unique members play in development, differentiation, and cellular homeostasis.

The Structural Organization of the Steroid-Receptor Gene Family

The deduced primary sequences of receptors for the steroid, thyroid, and retinoic acid hormones revealed a similarity in structural organization of the gene family comprised of two major regions of homology (182–197). These regions include both a strong central or amino-terminal core homology domain and a less homologous but more expansive and more complex domain comprised of the carboxy-terminal portion of the proteins. The considerable homology exhibited by this family in these regions suggested that they encoded domains whose functions were similar within the family. As a result, these domains have been the focus of considerable experimental effort.

The DNA-Binding Domain of the Nuclear Receptors

The protein domain that exhibits the greatest degree of amino acid homology from receptor to receptor represents the DNA recognition structure of the steroid-receptor gene family (182,197). This 60- to 70-amino-acid, positionally conserved DNA-binding motif lies at the extreme N-terminus of the 1,25-dihydroxyvitamin D₃ receptor, although it lies more centrally within the receptors for estrogen, progesterone, and glucocorticoids; this is principally due to the latter group's unique N-terminal extension. It is a highly basic region composed of two finger-like projections, each stabilized by a single zinc atom tetrahedrally coordinated by four positionally conserved cysteine residues located at the base of each loop. More recent studies have suggested that the carboxyl sides of each of the two finger structures more likely take the form of two alpha helixes that interface directly with DNA (198). Importantly, the DNA-binding domain of the 1,25-dihydroxyvitamin D₃ receptor has been mapped functionally to this conserved zinc finger region located in the protein's amino terminus, using the protein's affinity for heterologous calf thymus DNA (see Fig. 8) (199). This dual zinc finger motif, as initially exemplified by the *Xenopus* oocyte transcription factor TFIIIA (181), has become the hallmark feature of the steroid-receptor family and has become diagnostic of a DNA-binding transcription factor as well.

Considerable evidence suggests that some of the steroid receptors (in the form of dimers) interact with specific DNA-sequence elements, particularly when the DNA sequences to which they bind exhibit a dyad symmetry. The fact that the DNA-binding domains of the glucocorticoid and progesterone (200) and estrogen (201,202) receptors alone are capable of forming homodimers that interact directly with DNA suggest that important homologous protein–protein contact sites exist within this small domain independent of the regions that interface with DNA. The affinity of these dimers for DNA, however, appears to be considerably less than that of the full-length molecule (201,202), suggesting that other regions of the receptor also participate in the formation of receptor homodimers (see below). Early studies also suggested the possibility that the DNA-binding domain of the glucocorticoid receptor contained inherent transcriptional activating capabilities (203). Regardless, it is clear that while this small, highly conserved region of the steroid receptors may contain several func-

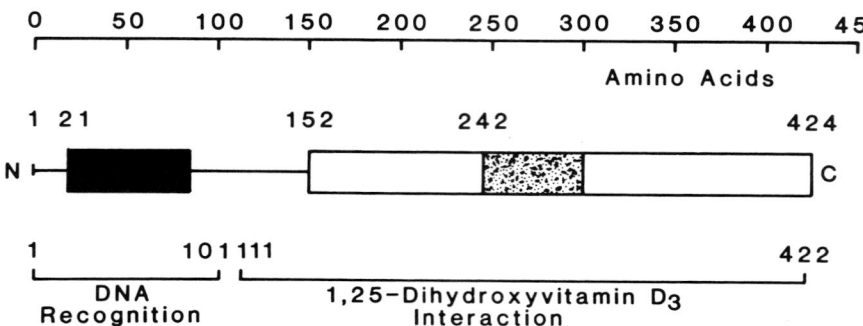

FIG. 8. Binding domains of the 1,25-dihydroxyvitamin D_3 receptor. The 424-amino-acid human protein is illustrated together with the scale indicated. The solid and stippled rectangles within the receptor describe regions of sequence homology with other steroid receptors. The regions between amino acids 1 and 101 and between amino acids 111 and 422 document domains that functionally bind DNA and 1,25-dihydroxyvitamin D_3, respectively.

tional activities, its primary role in all the receptors, including the receptor for 1,25-dihydroxyvitamin D_3, is to direct the protein to appropriate sites located within the promoters for hormone-responsive genes.

The Carboxy-Terminal Steroid-Binding Region of the Receptors

The steroid-binding region of the steroid-receptor gene family is a highly complex domain that extends approximately 200–300 amino acids from the DNA-binding domain to the carboxy terminus of the protein and contains highly hydrophobic regions throughout (see Fig. 8 for the 1,25-dihydroxyvitamin D receptor) (182,197). Its amino-terminal boundary is defined by the presence of a region of homology that exhibits moderate conservation with all members of the steroid-receptor family and that is located 50–150 amino acids downstream of the DNA-binding domain. Mutations introduced into this short homology domain obliterate the capacity of receptors to bind their respective ligands, as do mutations that are introduced into the central portion or extreme carboxy terminus of the protein (204,205). These experiments thus define the general boundaries of the steroid-binding domain. With respect to the 1,25-dihydroxyvitamin D_3 receptor, deletion of regions N-terminal to this secondary homology region also prevent subsequent binding of 1,25-dihydroxyvitamin D_3 (199). This result suggests the possibility that the N-terminal boundary of the hormone-binding domain of this receptor extends further upstream than that of most other members of the receptor gene family. Simultaneously, deletion of approximately 60 amino acids at the carboxy end of the molecule also prevents hormone binding. As a result of these experimental observations in a number of the receptors, it is likely that the domain which forms the hydrophobic hormone-binding pocket of each receptor is a three-dimensional structure created through independent and possibly noncontiguous peptide sequence. A third region of homology within the steroid-receptor family is also present, a region that exhibits the greatest degree of homology among receptor subclasses that appear related [e.g., 1,25-dihydroxyvita-

min D_3 and thyroid hormone receptors (183) or progesterone and glucocorticoid receptors (199)]. While the homology within these regions implies specific functions common to all the members of the receptor gene family, those functions remain to a large extent unclarified. Equally unclear are the amino acid requirements for hormone binding. As stated earlier, numerous deletion, insertion, and point mutations have been introduced into many of the steroid receptors with concomitant loss of ligand binding function. The results of these mutations, however, do not allow distinction between amino acids essential as contact residues and those that precipitate slight changes in structure as the protein is synthesized. Thus, critical features of the steroid-binding region remain to be established.

Despite the uncertainty surrounding the structure of the steroid-binding site within the steroid receptors, it is apparent that this region contains additional functional domains. Functions that have been identified in single members of the receptor family include short peptide regions that represent determinants of nuclear transfer (206,207), regions that participate directly in gene promoter transactivation (205,208,209), and peptide surfaces that are determinants of protein–protein interaction, either with the same receptor (200,202), with other members of the nuclear receptor family (210,211), or with proteins currently uncharacterized (210,212,213). It is likely that a major role of the hormonal ligand upon binding to its receptor is to modify one or more of these functional domains through perturbation of the protein's structure. The complexity of this domain clearly suggests that complete understanding of its complex function will require determination of its three-dimensional structure.

The Human Chromosomal Gene for the 1,25-Dihydroxyvitamin D_3 Receptor

Several of the chromosomal genes for members of the steroid-receptor gene family have been isolated and characterized (214,215). Likewise, genomic clones containing the 1,25-dihydroxyvitamin D_3 receptor were recovered from a human cosmid genomic library, and the structural organization of this gene was recently determined. The gene contains a minimum of 10 exons (ranging in size from approximately 29 to 3595 nucleotides) that, together with intervening intron sequences, span between 60 and 70 kilobases (216). The intronic sequences, in turn, range from 183 base pairs to over 20 kilobases. The first and second exons contain exclusively noncoding sequences located in the mRNA. Exon 3 contains the final 11 base pairs of noncoding sequence, the initiation codon, and sequences encoding the first of the two dissimilar DNA-binding zinc finger structures described above. Exon 4 lies approximately 15 kilobases downstream of exon 3 and encodes the second of the two zinc fingers. The remaining six exons (exons 5–10) comprise the carboxy-terminal two-thirds of the 1,25-dihydroxyvitamin D$_3$ receptor. These include several hinge exons, the second conserved homology region that represents the amino-terminal boundary of the steroid-binding domain (exons 7 and 8), and the largest of the exons (exon 10) that contains over 3200 base pairs of the 3′ noncoding region of the mRNA. Unfortunately, characterization of the promoter region of this gene has not yet been reported. Nevertheless, a comparison of the overall exonic structure of this gene with those for other members of this family suggests that each has evolved from a common primordial gene. Perhaps more importantly, the cloning of this gene from human sources has afforded a detailed analysis of genomic DNA from patients with hereditary resistance to 1,25-dihydroxyvitamin D$_3$ (vitamin-D$_3$-resistant rickets, type II). These studies, which will be described in the final section of this chapter, have established unequivocally that this syndrome can arise as a result of point mutations in essential regions within the gene that compromise the function of the 1,25-dihydroxyvitamin D$_3$ receptor.

CURRENT VIEW OF THE GENOMIC MECHANISM OF ACTION OF 1,25-DIHYDROXYVITAMIN D$_3$

1,25-Dihydroxyvitamin D$_3$ is known to regulate, in a tissue-specific manner, the levels of an extensive number of different proteins. Despite these observations, convincing evidence for regulation at the transcriptional level has emerged for only a few. These include: the peptide hormones calcitonin (217) and parathyroid hormone (218); bone proteins such as osteocalcin (60), osteopontin (219), and collagen (220); the intestinal calbindins (65,66); and several of the proto-oncogenes, such as c-myc (221), c-myb, and c-fos (222). Despite this, with the exception of the osteocalcin gene (which will soon be described in detail) and the osteopontin gene (219), no evidence has emerged to prove unequivocally that the 1,25-dihydroxyvitamin D$_3$ receptor interacts directly with specific DNA sequences within any of these

gene promoters. The clear ability of the receptor to alter levels of unique and well-known transcription factors such as c-fos and c-myc suggests that the modulation of gene expression by 1,25-dihydroxyvitamin D$_3$ may well occur through indirect mechanisms that include both transcriptional and post-transcriptional events. Nevertheless, the fact that the 1,25-dihydroxyvitamin D$_3$ receptor is a member of a family of ligand-controlled transcription factors (182) suggests that 1,25-dihydroxyvitamin D$_3$, through its receptor, is likely to activate at least a subset of genes through direct interactions.

In the past few years, a number of chromosomal genes that encode protein products modulated by the 1,25-dihydroxyvitamin D$_3$ hormone have been recovered and sequenced, and their promoters have been defined. The acquisition of these genes has afforded a direct testing (through molecular biologic methods) of the hypothesis that 1,25-dihydroxyvitamin D$_3$ activates gene expression through DNA sequences to which the receptor directly binds. Perhaps the most advanced studies have involved investigation of the osteocalcin gene promoter. It is clear that transcriptional regulation of this particular gene has emerged as a paradigm for direct 1,25-dihydroxyvitamin D$_3$ modulation. Moreover, research using this model has also enabled studies aimed at determining the molecular basis for both (a) activation of the receptor by 1,25-dihydroxyvitamin D$_3$ and (b) receptor activation of transcription.

Induction of the Osteocalcin Gene Promoter by 1,25-Dihydroxyvitamin D$_3$

Previous studies by Price and co-workers (60,61) revealed that 1,25-dihydroxyvitamin D$_3$ was capable of modulating the bone protein osteocalcin (or bone gla protein) in rat osteosarcoma cells in culture. Following the cloning of the complementary DNA for the rat protein (61), these studies were extended to show that the mRNA was also enhanced by the vitamin D$_3$ hormone. Subsequently, Pan and Price (223) carried out nuclear run-on experiments that demonstrated that the effect of 1,25-dihydroxyvitamin D$_3$ was exerted at the level of transcription. The cloning and characterization of the human osteocalcin gene by Celeste et al. (62) in 1986—and, subsequently, of the rat gene by Yoon et al. (224), Demay et al. (225), and Lian et al. (64)—precipitated investigation of the effect of 1,25-dihydroxyvitamin D$_3$ at the molecular level.

Several groups initially reported that osteocalcin gene promoters themselves were inducible directly by 1,25-dihydroxyvitamin D$_3$. DNA fragments containing the promoter and upstream sequence of either the rat (224,225) or human (147,199,224–228) osteocalcin genes were inserted into plasmids and utilized to direct transcription of the structural gene for chloramphenicol acetyltransferase. These reporter plasmids were introduced by transfection into a variety of mammalian cultured cells, including the rat osteosarcoma cell line (ROS 17/2.8) and the cell lysates examined for enzymatic activity several days later following treatment with 1,25-dihydroxyvitamin D_3. In each of these experiments, the hormone was capable of inducing chloramphenicol acetyltransferase activity by as much as 8- to 10-fold above that observed in cells that did not receive the hormone. Simultaneously, this induction phenomenon was lost when the bulk of the upstream DNA sequence was deleted, leaving only the immediate proximal promoter region to direct transcription. These findings support the hypothesis that a discrete DNA sequence was present in the distal region of the osteocalcin 5' flanking region that was capable of mediating 1,25-dihydroxyvitamin D_3 response in a *cis*-acting fashion.

Kerner et al. (226) localized this *cis*-acting vitamin-D_3-responsive element (VDRE) within the human osteocalcin gene promoter to a region approximately 500 base pairs upstream of the start site of transcription of the gene (see Fig. 9). A DNA fragment containing the promoter and over 1300 base pairs of sequence extending 5' was utilized to create a congenic series of fragments with common 3' ends but progressively decreasing 5' ends. The activity of these DNA fragments was then assessed as described above in response to 1,25-dihydroxyvitamin D_3. Significantly, hormone response was indicated in a fragment whose 5' coordinate was −568, but it was lost when the 5' end was reduced to −418. The sequence between −568 and −413 was further analyzed by introducing a small series of independent internal deletions into the otherwise inducible promoter and examining them for 1,25-dihydroxyvitamin D_3 activation. Loss of hormone inducibility in several, but not all, of the deleted fragments suggested the presence of a short vitamin-D_3-responsive sequence of perhaps 20 base pairs centered around −500 that was fully capable of mediating transcriptional activation by the hormone. Importantly, this DNA sequence was capable of transferring 1,25-dihydroxyvitamin D_3 response when prepared synthetically and introduced into otherwise unresponsive viral promoters such as those for the thymidine kinase gene or the mouse mammary tumor virus. These experiments document the discovery of the first DNA sequence within any gene promoter capable of mediating direct activation by 1,25-dihydroxyvitamin D_3. Subsequent studies by Demay et al. (228) led to the identification of a VDRE located in approximately the same region of the rat osteocalcin gene promoter. As will be discussed shortly, both the rat and human sequences exhibit striking sequence similarity. Perhaps the most important result of these research efforts is that they provide the final evidence and thus confirm the original hypothesis that the mechanism of action of the vitamin D_3 hormone involves direct interactions with genomic sequences located in the promoters of 1,25-dihydroxyvitamin-D_3-inducible genes.

The 1,25-Dihydroxyvitamin D_3 Receptor and Osteocalcin Promoter Induction

The important link between osteocalcin promoter activation by 1,25-dihydroxyvitamin D_3 and the receptor for this ligand was provided by McDonnell et al. (199) and, more recently, by Ozono et al. (147). While the osteocalcin promoter is inducible by 1,25-dihydroxyvitamin D_3 in cells that contain endogenous levels of the receptor, as assessed in studies described above, McDonnell et al. (199) observed that this promoter was unresponsive to 1,25-dihydroxyvitamin D_3 when introduced into a mammalian monkey kidney fibroblast cell line (CV-1) that does not express the 1,25-dihydroxyvitamin D_3 receptor. In contrast, however, when a cDNA expression vector that directed synthesis of the 1,25-dihydroxyvitamin D_3 receptor was introduced together with the osteocalcin promoter plasmid, recovery of 1,25-dihydroxyvitamin D_3 response was immediate. Recovery of response was also evident when the VDRE was inserted

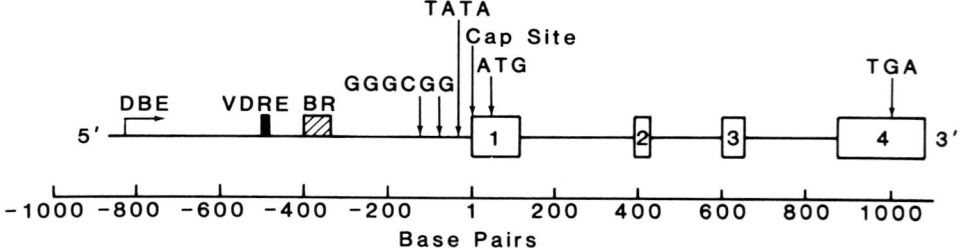

FIG. 9. Structural organization of the human gene for osteocalcin. The four exons that encode the osteocalcin gene product are boxed, and their numbers are indicated. The capsite, initiation (ATG), and termination (TGA) codons are indicated. The promoter and upstream control regions include the TATA box (TATA), two functional SP-1-binding sites (GGGCGG), basal repressor region (BR), vitamin-D-responsive element at nucleotide positions −509 to −485 (VDRE), and a distal basal enhancer region (DBE). The nucleotide base scale is indicated below the gene.

into a heterologous promoter, demonstrating that overall response to 1,25-dihydroxyvitamin D₃ was uniquely dependent upon the VDRE as well as upon the receptor (229). The extent of hormone response was also a direct function of the amounts of receptor expression vector introduced into the cells, suggesting that the magnitude of response was correlated directly with receptor concentration (147). Finally, as will be discussed later, hormonal activation was dependent upon the introduction of a fully functional receptor. Thus, receptors that were dysfunctional as a result of their expression from mutant cDNAs could no longer mediate the action of 1,25-dihydroxyvitamin D₃, despite their presence (229–232). These studies clearly established that the action of 1,25-dihydroxyvitamin D₃ on osteocalcin gene expression and (most likely) on other gene promoters is mediated by its receptor protein. Perhaps as important, these studies also confirmed functionally that the 1,25-dihydroxyvitamin D₃ receptor is indeed a ligand-induced transcription factor, thereby cementing the apparent relationship that existed between this receptor and receptors for the steroid, thyroid, and retinoic acid hormones based upon structure alone. Clearly, the action of 1,25-dihydroxyvitamin D₃ requires the hormone itself, a *cis*-acting VDRE DNA sequence within the promoter of a responsive gene, and the receptor protein acting in *trans*.

Structure and Properties of the 1,25-Dihydroxyvitamin-D₃-Responsive Element

Responsive elements for the steroid, thyroid, and retinoic acid classes of hormone take different sequence conformation, but they are often identified as either short repeated or palindromic sequences (233). As indicated above, the VDRE in the human osteocalcin promoter was localized to a region approximately 500 base pairs upstream of the transcriptional start site of the gene (226). Ozono et al. (147) have recently shown that the VDRE itself is comprised of two directly repeated hexanucleotide sequences separated by three base pairs (see Fig. 10). This organization is highly conserved in the rat osteocalcin VDRE, where 14 of 17 base pairs are identical. A recent report of a VDRE in the osteopontin gene promoter suggests a similar organization of two direct repeats separated by three nucleotide pairs (219). While these repeated sequences do not allow the compilation of a strong consensus sequence, the hexanucleotide AGGT(G/C)A has emerged as a possible candidate for a single half-site. The importance of this consensus sequence is that it is virtually identical to that of estrogen, thyroid hormone, and retinoic acid (233). Interestingly, the osteocalcin promoter is inducible by retinoic acid in osteoblasts through an endogenous retinoic acid receptor but is simultaneously unresponsive to thyroid hormone (229,234). Clearly, the sequence of these elements represents only a single determinant of capacity to respond to specific receptor activation. The spacing and orientation of the repeats, the environment of the promoter, and unique cellular constituents are also significant determinants.

The human VDRE is uniquely juxtaposed to a consensus sequence that represents a binding site for AP-1-binding protein complexes, an example of which are the cellular proto-oncogene members c-Jun and c-Fos (147,234). Recent studies suggest that the presence

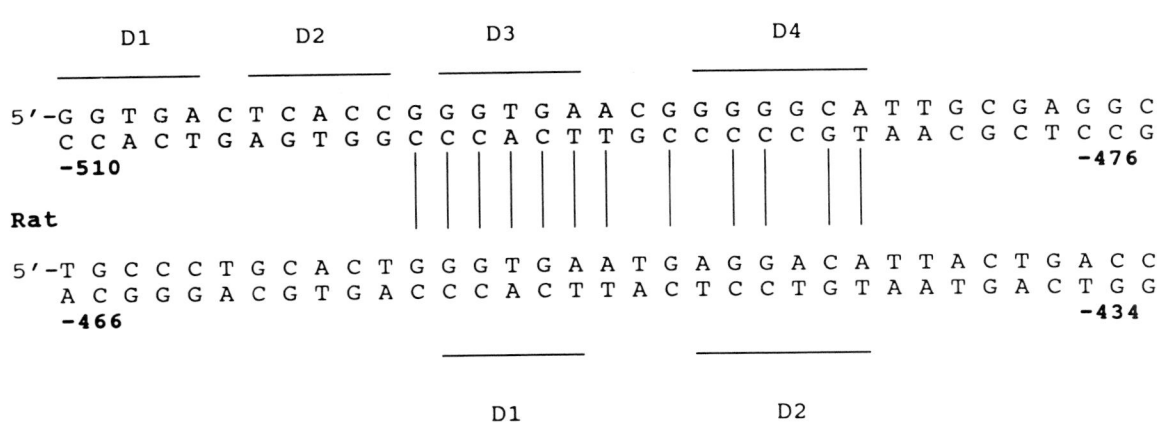

FIG. 10. The nucleotide sequence of the vitamin-D-responsive element located in the 5′ flanking regions of the human and rat osteocalcin genes. The human VDRE sequence is shown as four domains (D1–D4) where D1 and D2 comprise the binding site for AP-1 and where D3 and D4 represent the two tandem repeats that comprise the binding site for the 1,25-dihydroxyvitamin D₃ receptor. The sequence is aligned with the functional tandem repeats of the rat VDRE designated D1 and D2. This alignment reveals nucleotide identity in 12 of 15 base pairs. Nucleotide coordinates within the two osteocalcin promoters are indicated by number.

of this sequence is not essential for vitamin D_3 induction (147). Nevertheless, the presence of this sequence significantly enhances the basal activity of the promoter and synergistically augments the action of 1,25-dihydroxyvitamin D_3. This interesting interaction between two *trans*-activating protein complexes remains to be clarified, although it clearly leads to an increased range of response to the calcemic hormone. While the VDRE region within the rat promoter does not contain this AP-1 element (228), regions significantly upstream of the natural VDRE appear to enhance overall response to 1,25-dihydroxyvitamin D_3 (224,225). Perhaps this upstream region is the functional equivalent of the juxtaposed AP-1 sequence in the human.

The 1,25-Dihydroxyvitamin D_3 Receptor and Osteocalcin Gene Activation

The identification of a gene responsive to 1,25-dihydroxyvitamin D_3 and its receptor at the level of transcription has provided a model system with which to determine the molecular events associated with this activation. More precisely, experiments designed to evaluate the role and mechanism by which 1,25-dihydroxyvitamin D_3 converts the receptor from an inactive to an active molecule are now able to (a) assess the molecular basis for receptor interaction with specific DNA, (b) determine the mechanism by which the receptor alters gene promoter activity, and (c) evaluate the role of additional proteins in the process. Utilizing the transcriptional response assay considered previously, McDonnell et al. (199) evaluated a series of mutant 1,25-dihydroxyvitamin D_3 receptors derived from cDNAs that contained either 3' or 5' deletions of the coding region. The results of this study suggest that transcriptional activation requires the presence of the DNA-binding domain, but that this domain is insufficient to trigger *trans*-activation independently. Consistent with that observation, mutant 1,25-dihydroxyvitamin D_3 receptors containing serine residue substitutions for some of the conserved cysteines responsible for configuring the DNA-binding domain through zinc coordination were also inactive in *trans*-activation (229). Furthermore, mutations that result in alterations in the basic charge of this region also abrogate *trans*-activational capabilities (230–232). Interestingly, a domain that appeared to initiate hormone-independent *trans*-activation was simultaneously localized to a region between the domains for DNA- and hormone-binding (199). However, this *trans*-activation region, together with the DNA-binding domain, exhibited rather weak activity and, as a result, remains to be clarified.

The observation that the DNA-binding domain of the 1,25-dihydroxyvitamin D_3 receptor is essential but insufficient for *trans*-activation prompted a further investigation (in vitro) of the interaction of the receptor with the VDRE. Studies were carried out utilizing the gel retardation or bandshift assay; in this procedure labeled duplex oligonucleotide whose sequence matched the VDRE was incubated with receptor, and then the protein–DNA complexes were resolved from free DNA probe by nondenaturing gel electrophoresis. Demay et al. (228), Ozono et al. (147), Liao et al. (235), and Sone et al. (236) demonstrated that indeed the fully occupied 1,25-dihydroxyvitamin D_3 receptor interacts directly with the VDRE in a manner dependent upon the sequence of the oligonucleotide. Furthermore, in the studies by Liao et al. (235), the formation of the complex was dependent upon 1,25-dihydroxyvitamin D_3, added either in vitro or in vivo. These studies are important because they suggest that the essentiality of hormone in the transcriptional response assay may potentially be exerted at the level of specific DNA binding, an occurrence that would facilitate detailed examination of the role of hormone.

Perhaps even more important is the recent discovery that the ability of the 1,25-dihydroxyvitamin D_3 receptor to interact with the VDRE is cooperatively enhanced in the presence of a nuclear protein found in a number of cultured cells (235,236). While this unknown factor remains to be identified, it is possible that the receptor forms a heterodimer on the VDRE and that this protein complex is capable of activating transcription. This finding is analogous to the DNA-binding enhancement factor recently defined for the thyroid and retinoic acid receptors (212,213), and it may serve as an adapter or bridging factor as recently described by others (237,238). Further studies show definitively that this factor interacts preferentially with the receptor bound to 1,25-dihydroxyvitamin D_3 (T. Sone et al., unpublished data). Thus, the dependence of receptor DNA binding upon hormone and upon the nuclear factor may be related. A hypothesis is therefore emerging that the 1,25-dihydroxyvitamin D_3 receptor acts as a promoter–specifier and that the hormone-binding domain of the protein contains a 1,25-dihydroxyvitamin-D_3-controlled region that initiates contact with an additional protein that facilitates *trans*-activation of the osteocalcin gene and perhaps others. It remains for future studies to prove this new hypothesis regarding the function of accessory proteins and the role of the hormone. It is likely, nevertheless, that complete understanding of the function of the hormone and its influence on DNA binding and transcriptional activation will require determination of the three-dimensional structure of the protein itself.

THE HUMAN SYNDROME OF HEREDITARY 1,25-DIHYDROXYVITAMIN D_3 RESISTANCE

The human syndrome of hereditary 1,25-dihydroxyvitamin D_3 resistance (vitamin-D_3-dependent rickets, type II) is a rare autosomal-recessive disease that occurs early in infancy and is characterized by hypocalcemia, secondary hyperparathyroidism, and osteomalacia or rickets (239–243). These clinical features all persist in parallel with elevated levels of circulating 1,25-dihydroxyvitamin D_3, suggesting that they arise as a result of target organ resistance to the action of this hormonal derivative of vitamin D_3. In addition, subtle but unique biochemical and clinical features of the syndrome from patient to patient suggest the existence of heterogeneity in the nature of the defects that lead to resistance. In view of the complexity of vitamin D_3 action in target tissues, as outlined in detail in this chapter, this observation should not be surprising.

The Vitamin-D₃-Resistant Fibroblast Model

Clinical cases of the syndrome of 1,25-dihydroxyvitamin-D_3-resistant rickets were first documented in the late 1970s. However, it was the discovery that normal skin fibroblasts contain a functional effector system for 1,25-dihydroxyvitamin D_3, as demonstrated by the presence of measurable biologic responses to the hormone in culture, that was key to our eventual understanding of the molecular basis for this disease (106,107). Thus, the subsequent observation that fibroblasts derived from patients resistant to the action of the vitamin D_3 hormone were either qualitatively or quantitatively unresponsive was particularly enlightening (244–250). In light of the foregoing discussion that the 1,25-dihydroxyvitamin D_3 receptor clearly mediates the genomic actions of its ligand, characterization of this protein in defective fibroblasts became the immediate focus of attention. The result of these efforts was the definition of a fibroblastic phenotype in which the binding activity for 1,25-dihydroxyvitamin D_3 normally associated with receptor could not be demonstrated (241,242,244,248). Because immunologic detection methods suggested that receptor expression was normal in these cell types (163), investigators concluded that there was an inability of the receptor to bind 1,25-dihydroxyvitamin D_3. Subsequent experiments defined several additional defects associated with normal receptor activities: (a) defective ability to localize or be retained within the nuclear compartment (243,244,247) and (b) defective ability to bind to heterologous DNA (247,249). Thus, three abnormal receptor phenotypes, as listed in Table 3, have emerged as poten-

TABLE 3. *Phenotypic defects in the 1,25-dihydroxyvitamin D_3 receptor associated with hereditary 1,25-dihydroxyvitamin-D_3-resistant rickets*

Category (References)
1,25-Dihydroxyvitamin D_3 binding   (241, 242, 244, 248)
DNA recognition   (247, 249)
Nuclear retention/translocation   (243, 244, 247)

tially responsible for the disease phenotype of rickets (250).

Genetic Lesions in the 1,25-Dihydroxyvitamin-D₃-Receptor Chromosomal Gene

Messenger RNA transcripts that encode the 1,25-dihydroxyvitamin D_3 receptor are particularly rare species in target cells, and they are therefore difficult to recover and characterize. DNA-dependent techniques, however, have been developed recently that employ pairs of short oligonucleotides to amplify specific nucleotide regions from total genomic DNA (251). Having determined the structural organization and sequence of the human chromosomal gene for the 1,25-dihydroxyvitamin D_3 receptor, as discussed in an earlier section, these techniques were utilized to define precisely the genetic basis for heritable defects associated with 1,25-dihydroxyvitamin D_3 resistance. Hughes et al. (252), Ritchie et al. (231), and Sone et al. (232, and unpublished data) utilized short oligonucleotide sequences complementary to intron sequences to selectively amplify DNA from each of the coding exons of the 1,25-dihydroxyvitamin D receptor gene. The incorporation of restriction sites at the 5′ ends of each synthetic oligonucleotide allowed the subsequent cloning and sequencing of these individually amplified DNAs. In this manner, the presence and nucleotide sequence of each of the exons that encode the human 1,25-dihydroxyvitamin D_3 receptor were determined rapidly for patients with resistance to the hormone.

The search for mutations within the 1,25-dihydroxyvitamin-D_3-receptor gene focused initially upon analysis of patients whose receptors exhibited defects in ability to bind 1,25-dihydroxyvitamin D_3 or to recognize DNA. Three interrelated families that are part of an extended kindred were evaluated for genetic defects related to an inability to bind hormonal 1,25-dihydroxyvitamin D_3 (231). DNA amplification and sequence analysis of exonic regions within the 1,25-dihydroxyvitamin-D_3-receptor chromosomal gene from these patients revealed the presence, in exon 8, of a C-to-A nucleotide substitution that produced a premature termination codon. Parental DNA was heterozygotic for this mutation, and unaffected siblings were either homozygous or heterozygous for the normal gene. The apparent result of this mutation is the synthesis of a protein which is truncated at codon 291 within the hormone-binding domain of the receptor and which is clearly unable to bind the vitamin D_3 hormone. Following the identification of this specific mutation, this genotype has been identified in seven related families (253). Since loss of hormone-binding activity in cells can arise from many different and unrelated defects in the receptor gene, this mutation represents simply one example of many theoretical possibilities. The identification of a mutation such as this within the 1,25-

dihydroxyvitamin D₃ receptor, however, provides important insight into the mechanism by which 1,25-dihydroxyvitamin-D₃-resistant rickets can arise.

Perhaps the most interesting category of receptor defect in patients with resistance to 1,25-dihydroxyvitamin D₃ is that which leads to altered ability to recognize DNA. Importantly, and as outlined above, functional studies have suggested that a region essential, although not sufficient, for DNA-binding activity resides within the N-terminal portion of the 1,25-dihydroxyvitamin D₃ receptor, a region encoded by only two of the 10 exons in the gene. Thus, the search for genetic mutations was initiated by Hughes et al. (252) and Sone et al. (232, and unpublished data) in these two exons with DNA derived from six different families whose receptor proteins appeared normal in ability to bind hormone but exhibited low affinity for immobilized DNA. DNA from the affected patients of these families revealed four independent point mutations within exons 3 and 4 that together encode the DNA-binding region of the 1,25-dihydroxyvitamin D₃ receptor (see Fig. 11). These mutations result in aspartic acid or glutamine substitutions at different sites within or between the dual zinc finger motif that, without exception, result in alterations in the charge of the structure. It is unclear precisely how these changes affect the DNA-binding activity of the 1,25-dihydroxyvitamin D₃ receptor; however, the preponderance of basic amino acids within this region, along with their conservation within the receptor gene family, underlies their importance (182). As discussed earlier, these basic residues are clearly essential for DNA binding and may provide, in part, the basis for general protein–DNA contacts within the major groove of DNA. Regardless of the molecular basis for receptor dysfunction, the identification of natural point mutations located within this region in the receptor, together with a corresponding loss of function in patient cells, suggests that both observations are related to the disease phenotype of rickets.

Transcriptional Activity of Mutant 1,25-Dihydroxyvitamin D₃ Receptors Derived from Patient Genotypes

The identification of mutations within the 1,25-dihydroxyvitamin-D₃-receptor chromosomal gene, the location of these mutations relative to aberrant receptor function in patient cells, and their appropriate genetic distribution among family members each provides strong indirect evidence that the genetic defects defined are responsible for the syndrome of 1,25-dihydroxyvitamin-D₃-resistant rickets. However, to gain additional evidence that the mutations identified within the gene result in aberrant binding functions as well as inability to modify gene transcription, Sone et al. (230,232) and Ritchie et al. (231) recently utilized the technique of site-directed mutagenesis (as described above) to introduce each mutation independently into the normal 1,25-dihydroxyvitamin-D₃-receptor cDNA. Analysis of the

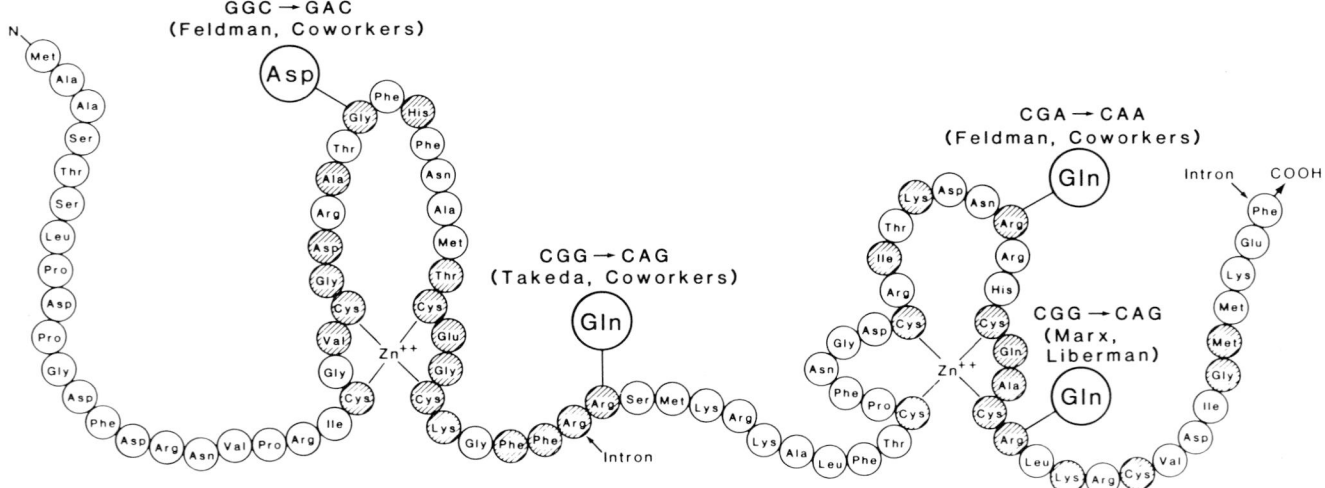

FIG. 11. Genetic mutations identified in the DNA-binding domain of the human 1,25-dihydroxyvitamin-D₃-receptor chromosomal gene of patients with hereditary resistance to 1,25-dihydroxyvitamin D₃. The amino acid sequence of the two coordinated DNA-binding zinc fingers at the amino terminus of the receptor are illustrated. The shaded residues indicate those amino acids that are conserved among the steroid-receptor gene family. Four amino acid substitutions that result from point mutations found in the 1,25-dihydroxyvitamin-D₃ receptor gene in families with hereditary resistance are shown. The mutant nucleotide in the natural codon of each patient DNA that gives rise to the altered residue is summarized over each mutant. [Data are derived from Sone et al. (232, and unpublished data) and Hughes et al. (252).]

mutant receptor products synthesized following transfection into host mammalian fibroblasts revealed that each protein exhibited a functional phenotype identical to that of its corresponding receptor endogenously expressed in patient fibroblasts. Accordingly, introduction of a termination codon resulted in the synthesis (by host cells) of an immunologically detected, 32-kD truncated protein that was unable to bind hormone (231). In addition, the four point mutations introduced individually into the cDNA region encoding the DNA-binding domain of the receptor led to the synthesis of proteins of normal size and ability to bind 1,25-dihydroxyvitamin D₃, but they also led to the synthesis of proteins unable to interact appropriately with nonspecific DNA (230,232) or with the osteocalcin VDRE (T. Sone et al., unpublished data). Thus, the defects associated with these mutated receptors correspond identically to those found in their endogenously synthesized counterparts.

These mutated receptors were also inactive in the response assay (outlined above) to assess the transcriptional activity of the 1,25-dihydroxyvitamin D₃ receptor. Mutant receptor cDNAs were prepared and were then cointroduced, together with the osteocalcin promoter, into cultured cells; the response to 1,25-dihydroxyvitamin D₃ was measured as outlined earlier. The results of these assays suggest that while the normal receptor is fully capable of activating transcription in the presence of 1,25-dihydroxyvitamin D₃, mutant forms of the protein are unable to stimulate the gene promoter, even under conditions of high hormone levels or receptor overexpression (230–232). Thus, receptors synthesized with mutations identified in the chromosomal genes of patients with resistance to hormonal vitamin D₃ display not only abnormal binding functions but aberrant transcriptional functions as well. These data clearly establish the molecular basis for lack of responsiveness to hormone in at least a subset of patients with hereditary 1,25-dihydroxyvitamin-D₃-resistant rickets. They, in turn, strongly support the essential role of this receptor in mediating the biologic functions of hormonal 1,25-dihydroxyvitamin D₃ that have been described in this chapter.

CONCLUSIONS

In this chapter we have described historically the experimental events that have supported the initial hypothesis that the mode of action of 1,25-dihydroxyvitamin D₃ involves modification of specific transcriptional events in the nucleus of target cells. Over the past several decades, the proposal has been proven correct. This mechanism involves a receptor protein located in specific tissues that are responsive to 1,25-dihydroxyvitamin D₃. Extensive investigation suggests that the level of this protein is regulated by a wide variety of hormones and cellular factors. This regulation likely serves to enable the cell to exert a specific degree of control over subsequent biologic response. The 1,25-dihydroxyvitamin D₃ receptor and its chromosomal gene have been cloned. The deduced primary structure of the receptor clearly indicates that it is a member of a large gene family that includes intracellular receptors for other mechanistically similar ligands such as thyroid hormone, retinoic acid, and the sex and adrenal steroids. The 1,25-dihydroxyvitamin D₃ receptor interacts specifically with regulatory DNA elements that control the expression of several genes, and it is likely that these studies will be extended to include additional genes under vitamin D₃ hormone control. The molecular details by which the receptor protein activates transcription remain for future study, as do questions regarding how 1,25-dihydroxyvitamin D₃ controls these activation events in such a precise manner. However, recent experiments related to the role of hormone in facilitating DNA interaction through cooperative binding with accessory proteins may provide clues with regard to the latter events.

The above evidence for the genomic action of 1,25-dihydroxyvitamin D₃ does not preclude the possibility that this hormone, its receptor, or other metabolites of vitamin D may function through additional mechanisms, either directly or indirectly. There is considerable evidence that 1,25-dihydroxyvitamin D₃ is capable of altering the levels of certain proto-oncogene products in target cells, many of which are active transcription factors in themselves. While 1,25-dihydroxyvitamin D₃ and its receptor may modulate these factors directly through gene *trans*-activation, alternative mechanisms are possible. Moreover, a considerable body of evidence not considered in this chapter seems to indicate a possible nongenomic mechanism of action of 1,25-dihydroxyvitamin D₃ that may be exerted at the level of the cellular membrane. The role of the receptor in these events, if any, remains to be demonstrated.

Perhaps the most conclusive evidence for the relevance of 1,25-dihydroxyvitamin D₃, its receptor protein, and the genomic mechanism in the regulation of mineral metabolism derives from studies of the human syndrome of hereditary 1,25-dihydroxyvitamin D₃ resistance. As described in this chapter, considerable derangement of calcium and phosphorus metabolism is evident in the disease phenotype of patients with this disorder. The studies that point to the presence of selective mutations within the gene that encodes the receptor for 1,25-dihydroxyvitamin D₃, as well as the evidence that the protein is incapable of specific genomic actions in vitro, prove unequivocally that the mechanisms developed in this chapter are important to major vitamin D₃ function and that the receptor plays an essential, if not exclusive, role in those functions. Thus, the interplay between both basic and clinical research aimed at understanding the physiology and pathophysiology of vitamin D₃ action has been a success. A discussion of some of the aspects of vitamin D biology not considered in this chapter can be found in additional reviews (59,254).

ACKNOWLEDGMENTS

In this chapter, recent research described by the author was supported by the National Institutes of Health, the March of Dimes Birth Defects Foundation, and the Robert A. Welch Foundation. The author is an Established Investigator of the American Heart Association.

REFERENCES

1. Eisenstein R, Passavoy M. Actinomycin D inhibits parathyroid hormone and vitamin D activity. *Proc Soc Exp Biol Med* 1965;117:77–9.
2. Zull JE, Carnowski-Misztal E, DeLuca HF. Actinomycin D inhibition of vitamin D action. *Science* 1965;149:182–4.
3. Norman AW. Actinomycin D and the response to vitamin D. *Science* 1965;149:184–6.
4. Zull JE, Carnowski-Misztal E, DeLuca HF. On the relationship between vitamin D action and actinomycin-sensitive processes. *Proc Natl Acad Sci USA* 1966;55:177–84.
5. Stohs SJ, Zull JE, DeLuca HF. Vitamin D stimulation of [^{3}H]-orotic acid incorporation into ribonucleic acid of rat intestinal mucosa. *Biochemistry* 1967;6:1304–10.
6. Hallick RB, DeLuca HF. Vitamin D_3-stimulated template activity of chromatin from rat intestine. *Proc Natl Acad Sci USA* 1969;63:528–31.
7. Haussler MR, Myrtle JF, Norman AW. The association of a metabolite of vitamin D_3 with intestinal chromatin in vivo. *J Biol Chem* 1968;243:4055–64.
8. Norman AW. The mode of action of vitamin D. *Biol Rev* 1968;43:97–137.
9. O'Malley BW, Towle HC, Schwartz RJ. Regulation of gene expression in eucaryotes. *Annu Rev Genet* 1977;11:239–77.
10. DeLuca HF. The vitamin D system in the regulation of calcium and phosphorus metabolism. *Nutr Rev* 1979;37:161–93.
11. Morii H, Lund J, Neville PF, DeLuca HF. Biological activity of a vitamin D metabolite. *Arch Biochem Biophys* 1967;120:508–12.
12. Lawson DEM, Wilson PW, Kodicek E. Metabolism of vitamin D: a new cholecalciferol metabolite, involving loss of hydrogen at C-1, in chick intestinal nuclei. *Biochem J* 1969;115:269–77.
13. Fraser DR, Kodicek E. Unique biosynthesis by kidney of a biologically active vitamin D metabolite. *Nature* 1970;228:764–6.
14. Lawson DEM, Fraser DR, Kodicek E, Morrison HR, Williams DH. Identification of 1,25-dihydroxycholecalciferol, a new kidney hormone controlling calcium metabolism. *Nature* 1971;230:228–30.
15. Norman AW, Myrtle JF, Midgett RJ, Nowicki HG, Williams V, Popjak G. 1,25-Dihydroxycholecalciferol: identification of the proposed active form of vitamin D in the intestine. *Science* 1971;173:51–4.
16. Holick MF, Schnoes HK, DeLuca HF. Identification of 1,25-dihydroxycholecalciferol: a form of vitamin D_3 metabolically active in intestine. *Proc Natl Acad Sci USA* 1971;68:803–7.
17. Holick MF, Schnoes HK, DeLuca HF, Suda T, Cousins RJ. Isolation and identification of 1,25-dihydroxycholecalciferol. A metabolite of vitamin D active in intestine. *Biochemistry* 1971;10:2799–804.
18. Haussler MR, Boyce DW, Littledike ET, Rasmussen H. A rapidly acting metabolite of vitamin D_3. *Proc Natl Acad Sci USA* 1971;68:177–81.
19. McNutt KW, Haussler MR. Nutritional effectiveness of 1,25-dihydroxycholecalciferol in preventing rickets in chicks. *J Nutr* 1973;103:681–9.
20. Holick MF, Garabedian M, DeLuca HF. 1,25-Dihydroxychole-calciferol: metabolism of vitamin D_3 active on bone in anephric rats. *Science* 1972;176:1146–7.
21. Wong RG, Norman AW, Reddy CR, Coburn JW. Biologic effects of 1,25-dihydroxycholecalciferol (a highly active vitamin D metabolite) in acutely uremic rats. *J Clin Invest* 1972;51:1287–91.
22. Haussler MR, Brickman AS. Vitamin D: metabolism, actions, and disease states. In: Bronner F, Coburn J, eds. *Disorders of mineral metabolism*, vol 2. New York: Academic Press, 1982;359–431.
23. Brumbaugh PF, Haussler DH, Bressler R, Haussler MR. Radioreceptor assay for 1,25-dihydroxyvitamin D_3. *Science* 1974;183:1089–91.
24. Hughes MR, Baylink DJ, Jones PG, Haussler MR. Radioligand receptor assay for 25-hydroxyvitamin D_2/D_3 and 1,25-dihydroxyvitamin D_2/D_3. Application to hypervitaminosis D. *J Clin Invest* 1976;58:61–70.
25. Hughes MR, Baylink DJ, Gonnerman WA, Toverud SU, Ramp WK, Haussler MR. Influence of dietary vitamin D_3 on the circulating concentration of its active metabolites in the chick and rat. *Endocrinology* 1976;100:799–806.
26. Boyle IT, Gray RW, DeLuca HF. Regulation by calcium of in vivo synthesis of 1,25-dihydroxycholecalciferol and 21,25-dihydroxycholecalciferol. *Proc Natl Acad Sci USA* 1971;68:2131–4.
27. Tanaka H, DeLuca HF. The control of 25-dihydroxyvitamin D metabolism by inorganic phosphorus. *Arch Biochem Biophys* 1973;154:566–74.
28. Hughes MR, Brumbaugh PF, Haussler MR, Wergedal JE, Baylink DJ. Regulation of serum 1,25-dihydroxyvitamin D_3 by calcium and phosphate in the rat. *Science* 1975;190:578–80.
29. Garabedian M, Holick MF, DeLuca HF, Boyle IT. Control of 25-dihydroxycholecalciferol metabolism by parathyroid glands. *Proc Natl Acad Sci USA* 1972;69:1673–6.
30. Tanaka Y, DeLuca HF. Stimulation of 24,25-dihydroxyvitamin D_3 production by 1,25-dihydroxyvitamin D_3. *Science* 1974;183:1198–1200.
31. Russell J, Lettieri D, Sherwood LM. Suppression by 1,25(OH)$_2$D$_3$ of transcription of the preproparathyroid hormone gene. *Endocrinology* 1986;119:2864–6.
32. Spanos E, Pike JW, Haussler MR, Colston KW, Evans IMA, Goldner AM, McCain TA, MacIntyre I. Circulating 1,25-dihydroxyvitamin D in the chicken: enhancement by injection of prolactin and during egglaying. *Life Sci* 1976;19:1751–6.
33. Tanaka Y, Castillo L, DeLuca HF. Control of renal vitamin D hydroxylases in birds by sex hormones. *Proc Natl Acad Sci USA* 1976;73:2701–5.
34. Baksi SN, Kenny AD. Vitamin D_3 metabolism in immature Japanese quail: effects of ovarian hormones. *Endocrinology* 1977;101:1216–20.
35. Pike JW, Spanos E, Colston KW, MacIntyre I, Haussler MR. Influence of estrogen on renal vitamin D hydroxylases and serum 1,25-(OH)$_2$D$_3$ in chicks. *Am J Physiol* 1978;235:E338–43.
36. Spanos E, Barrett D, MacIntyre I, Pike JW, Safilian EF, Haussler MR. Effect of growth hormone on vitamin D metabolism. *Nature* 1978;273:246–7.
37. Pike JW, Toverud S, Boass A, McCain T, Haussler MR. Circulating 1,25-(OH)$_2$D$_3$ during physiological states of calcium stress. In: Norman AW, Schaefer K, Coburn JW, DeLuca HF, Fraser D, Grigoleit HG, von Herrath D, eds. *Vitamin D: biochemical, chemical and clinical aspects related to calcium and metabolism*. Berlin: de Gruyter, 1977:187–9.
38. Boass A, Toverud SU, McCain TA, Pike JW, Haussler MR. Elevated serum levels of 1,25-dihydroxycholecalciferol in lactating rats. *Nature* 1977;267:630–2.
39. Pike JW, Parker JB, Haussler MR, Boass A, Toverud SU. Dynamic changes in circulating 1,25-dihydroxyvitamin D during reproduction in rats. *Science* 1978;204:1427–9.
40. Schneider LE, Schedl HP, McCain TA, Haussler MR. Experimental diabetes reduces circulating 1,25-dihydroxyvitamin D in the rat. *Science* 1977;196:1452–4.
41. Tanaka Y, DeLuca HF, Omdahl J, Holick MF. Mechanism of action of 1,25-dihydroxycholecalciferol on intestinal calcium transport. *Proc Natl Acad Sci USA* 1971;68:1286–8.
42. Tsai HC, Midgett RJ, Norman AW. Studies on calciferol metabo-

lism. VII. The effects of actinomycin D and cycloheximide on the metabolism, subcellular localization, and action of vitamin D₃. *Arch Biochem Biophys* 1973;157:339–47.

43. Corradino RA. Embryonic chick intestine in organ culture. *J Cell Biol* 1973;58:64–78.

44. Corradino RA. 1,25-dihydroxycholecalciferol: inhibition of action in organ-cultured intestine by actinomycin D and alpha-amanitin. *Nature* 1973;243:41–3.

45. Corradino RA. Embryonic chick intestine in organ culture: interaction of adenyl cyclase system and vitamin D₃-mediated calcium absorption mechanism. *Endocrinology* 1974;94:1607–14.

46. Corradino RA. Stimulation of a Cd-binding protein, and inhibition of the vitamin D-dependent calcium binding protein, by zinc or cadmium in organ-cultured embryonic chick duodenum. *Arch Biochem Biophys* 1979;199:43–50.

47. Franceschi RT, DeLuca HF. The effect of inhibitors of protein and RNA synthesis on 1,25-dihydroxyvitamin D₃-dependent calcium uptake in cultured embryonic chick duodenum. *J Biol Chem* 1981;256:3848–52.

48. Zerwekh JE, Haussler MR, Lindell TJ. Rapid enhancement of chick intestinal DNA-dependent RNA polymerase II activity by 1,25-dihydroxyvitamin D₃, in vivo. *Proc Natl Acad Sci USA* 1974;71:2337–41.

49. Zerwekh JE, Lindell TJ, Haussler MR. Increased intestinal chromatin template activity: influence of 1,25-dihydroxyvitamin D₃ and hormone–receptor complexes. *J Biol Chem* 1976;251:2388–94.

50. Tsai HC, Wong RG, Norman AW. Studies on calciferol metabolism. IV. Subcellular localization of 1,25-dihydroxyvitamin D₃ in intestinal mucosa and correlation with increased calcium transport. *J Biol Chem* 1972;247:5511–9.

51. Brumbaugh PR, Haussler MR. 1,25-Dihydroxycholecalciferol receptors in intestine. Association of 1,25-dihydroxycholecalciferol with intestinal mucosa chromatin. *J Biol Chem* 1974;249:1251–7.

52. Zile M, Barsness EC, Yamada S, Schnoes HK, DeLuca HF. Localization of 1,25-dihydroxyvitamin D₃ in intestinal nuclei in vivo. *Arch Biochem Biophys* 1978;186:15–24.

53. Jones PG, Haussler MR. Scintillation autoradiography localization of 1,25-dihydroxyvitamin D₃ in chick intestine. *Endocrinology* 1979;104:313–21.

54. Wasserman RH, Corradino RA, Taylor AN. Vitamin D-dependent calcium-binding protein. Purification and some properties. *J Biol Chem* 1968;243:3978–86.

55. Wasserman RH, Taylor AN. Vitamin D-dependent calcium-binding protein. Response to some physiological and nutritional variables. *J Biol Chem* 1968;243:3987–93.

56. Wasserman RH, Corradino RA, Fullmer CS. Some aspects of vitamin D action; calcium absorption and vitamin D-dependent calcium-binding protein. *Vitam Horm* 1974;32:299–324.

57. Spencer R, Charman M, Wilson P, Lawson DEM. Production and properties of vitamin D-induced mRNA for chick calcium-binding protein. *Eur J Biochem* 1976;71:399–409.

58. Freund T, Bronner F. Regulation of intestinal calcium-binding protein by calcium intake in the rat. *Am J Physiol* 1975; 228:861–9.

59. Minghetti PP, Norman AW. 1,25(OH)₂-Vitamin D₃ receptors: gene regulation and genetic circuitry. *FASEB J* 1988;2:3043–53.

60. Price PA, Baukol SA. 1,25-Dihydroxyvitamin D₃ increases synthesis of the vitamin K-dependent bone protein by osteosarcoma cell. *J Biol Chem* 1980;255:11660–3.

61. Pan L, Price PA. The propeptide of rat bone gamma carboxyglutamic acid protein shares homology with other vitamin K-dependent protein precursors. *Proc Natl Acad Sci USA* 1985;82:6109–13.

62. Celeste AJ, Rosen V, Buecker JL, Kriz R, Wang EA, Wozney JM. Isolation of the human gene for bone gla protein utilizing mouse and rat cDNA clones. *EMBO J* 1986;5:1885–90.

63. Lian JB, Coutts M, Canalis E. Studies of hormonal regulation of osteocalcin synthesis in cultured fetal rat calvariae. *J Biol Chem* 1985;260:8706–10.

64. Lian JB, Stewart C, Puchacz E et al. Structure of the rat osteocalcin gene and regulation of vitamin D-dependent expression. *Proc Natl Acad Sci USA* 1989;86:1143–7.

65. Dupret J-M, Bruns P, Perret C, et al. Transcriptional and post-transcriptional regulation of vitamin D-dependent calcium-binding protein gene expression in the rat duodenum by 1,25-dihydroxycholecalciferol. *J Biol Chem* 1987;262:16553–7.

66. Theophan G, Norman AW. Effects of alpha amanitin and cycloheximide on 1,25-dihydroxyvitamin D₃-dependent calbindin 28K and its mRNA in vitamin D₃-replete chick intestine. *J Biol Chem* 1986;261:7311–5.

67. Haussler MR, Norman AW. Chromosomal receptor for a vitamin D metabolite. *Proc Natl Acad Sci USA* 1969;62:155–62.

68. Brumbaugh PF, Haussler MR. 1,25-Dihydroxycholecalciferol receptors in intestine. Temperature-dependent transfer of the hormone to chromatin via a specific cytosol receptor. *J Biol Chem* 1974;249:1258–62.

69. Lawson DEM, Wilson PW. Intranuclear localization and receptor proteins for 1,25-dihydroxycholecalciferol in chick intestine. *Biochem J* 1974;144:573–83.

70. Brumbaugh PF, Haussler MR. Specific binding of 1,25-dihydroxycholecalciferol to nuclear components of chick intestine. *J Biol Chem* 1975;250:1588–94.

71. Mellon WS, DeLuca HF. An equilibrium and kinetic study of 1,25-dihydroxyvitamin D₃ binding to chicken intestinal cytosol employing high specific activity 1,25-dihydroxy[³H-26,27]-vitamin D₃. *Arch Biochem Biophys* 1979;197:90–5.

72. Wecksler WR, Norman AW. A kinetic and equilibrium binding study of 1,25-dihydroxyvitamin D₃ with its cytosol receptor from chick intestinal mucosa. *J Biol Chem* 1980;255:3571–4.

73. Kream BE, Jose JL, DeLuca HF. The chick intestinal cytosol binding protein for 1,25-dihydroxyvitamin D₃: a study of analog binding. *Arch Biochem Biophys* 1977;179:462–8.

74. Wecksler WR, Okamura WH, Norman AW. Studies on the mode of action of vitamin D-XIV. Quantitative assessment of the structural requirements for the interaction of 1,25-dihydroxyvitamin D₃ with its chick intestinal mucosa receptor system. *J Steroid Biochem* 1978;9:929–37.

75. Wecksler WR, Norman AW. An hydroxylapatite batch assay for the quantitation of 1,25-dihydroxyvitamin D₃-receptor complexes. *Anal Biochem* 1979;92:314–23.

76. Wecksler WR, Norman AW. Biochemical properties of 1,25-dihydroxyvitamin D receptors. *J Steroid Biochem* 1980;13:977–89.

77. Brumbaugh PF, Haussler MR. 1,25-Dihydroxyvitamin D₃ receptors: competitive binding of vitamin D analogs. *Life Sci* 1973;13:1737–46.

78. Brumbaugh PF, Hughes MR, Haussler MR. Cytoplasmic and nuclear binding components for 1,25-dihydroxyvitamin D₃ in chick parathyroid glands. *Proc Natl Acad Sci USA* 1975; 72:4871–5.

79. Mellon WS, DeLuca HF. A specific 1,25-dihydroxyvitamin D₃ binding macromolecule in chicken bone. *J Biol Chem* 1980;255:4081–6.

80. Simpson RU, Franceschi RT, DeLuca HF. Characterization of a specific, high affinity binding macromolecule for 1,25-dihydroxyvitamin D₃ in cultured chick kidney cells. *J Biol Chem* 1980;255:10160–6.

81. Christakos S, Norman AW. Studies on the mode of action of calciferols. XXIX. Biochemical characterization of 1,25-dihydroxyvitamin D₃ receptors in chick pancreas and kidney cytosol. *Endocrinology* 1981;108:140–9.

82. Kream BE, Yamada Y, Schnoes HK, DeLuca HF. Specific cytosol-binding protein for 1,25-dihydroxyvitamin D₃ in rat intestine. *J Biol Chem* 1977;254:9488–91.

83. Wecksler WR, Ross FP, Norman AW. Characterization of the 1,25-dihydroxyvitamin D₃ receptor from rat intestinal cytosol. *J Biol Chem* 1979;254:9488–91.

84. Kream BE, Jose M, Yamada S, DeLuca HF. A specific high-affinity binding macromolecule for 1,25-dihydroxyvitamin D₃ in fetal bone. *Science* 1977;197:1086–8.

85. Chen TL, Hirst MA, Feldman D. A receptor-like binding macromolecule for 1,25-dihydroxycholecalciferol in cultured mouse bone cells. *J Biol Chem* 1979;254:7491–4.

86. Chandler JS, Pike JW, Haussler MR. 1,25-Dihydroxyvitamin D₃ receptors in rat kidney cytosol. *Biochem Biophys Res Commun* 1979;90:1057–63.

87. Colston K, Feldman D. Nuclear translocation of the 1,25-dihy-

droxyvitamin D$_3$ receptor in mouse kidney. *J Biol Chem* 1980;256:7510–3.

88. McCain TA, Haussler MR, Okrent D, Hughes MR. Partial purification of the chick intestinal receptor for 1,25-dihydroxyvitamin D$_3$ by ion exchange and blue dextran–Sepharose chromatography. *FEBS Lett* 1979;86:65–70.

89. Coty W. Reversible dissociation of steroid hormone-receptor complexes by mercurial reagents. *J Biol Chem* 1980;255:8035–7.

90. Pike JW, Haussler MR. Purification of chicken intestinal receptor for 1,25-dihydroxyvitamin D$_3$. *Proc Natl Acad Sci USA* 1979;76:5488–9.

91. Simpson RU, Hamstra A, Kendrick NC, DeLuca HF. Purification of the receptor for 1,25-dihydroxyvitamin D$_3$ from chicken intestine. *Biochemistry* 1983;22:2586–94.

92. Pike JW, Marion SL, Donaldson CA, Haussler MR. Serum and monoclonal antibodies against the chick intestinal receptor for 1,25-dihydroxyvitamin D$_3$. Generation by a preparation enriched in a 64,000 dalton protein. *J Biol Chem* 1983;258:1289–96.

93. Pike JW, Donaldson CA, Marion SJ, Haussler MR. Development of hybridomas secreting monoclonal antibodies to the chicken intestinal 1,25-dihydroxyvitamin D$_3$ receptor. *Proc Natl Acad Sci USA* 1982;79:7719–23.

94. Dame MC, Pierce EA, DeLuca HF. Identification of the porcine intestinal 1,25-dihydroxyvitamin D$_3$ receptor on sodium dodecyl sulfate/polyacrylamide gels by renaturation and immunoblotting. *Proc Natl Acad Sci USA* 1985;82:7825–9.

95. Dame MC, Pierce EA, Prahl JM, Hayes CE, DeLuca HF. Monoclonal antibodies to the porcine intestinal receptor for 1,25-dihydroxyvitamin D$_3$: interaction with distinct receptor domains. *Biochemistry* 1986;25:4523–4534.

96. Pike JW. Receptors for 1,25-dihydroxyvitamin D$_3$ in chick pancreas: a partial physical and functional characterization. *J Steroid Biochem* 1982;16:385–95.

97. Pike JW, Gooze LL, Haussler MR. Biochemical evidence for 1,25-dihydroxyvitamin D receptor macromolecules in parathyroid, pancreas, pituitary, and placental tissues. *Life Sci* 1980;26:407–14.

98. Haussler MR, Manolagas SC, Deftos LJ. Evidence for a 1,25-dihydroxyvitamin D$_3$ receptor-like macromolecule in rat pituitary. *J Biol Chem* 1980;255:5007–10.

99. Dokoh S, Donaldson CA, Marion SL, Pike JW, Haussler MR. The ovary: a target organ for 1,25-dihydroxyvitamin D$_3$. *Endocrinology* 1983;112:200–6.

100. Merke J, Kreusser W, Bier B, Ritz E. Demonstration and characterization of a testicular receptor for 1,25-dihydroxycholecalciferol in the rat. *Eur J Biochem* 1983;130:303–8.

101. Walters MR, Wicker DC, Riggle PC. 1,25-Dihydroxyvitamin D$_3$ receptors identified in the rat heart. *J Mol Cell Cardiol* 1986;18:67–72.

102. Provvedini DM, Tsoukas CD, Deftos LJ, Manolagas SC. 1,25-Dihydroxyvitamin D$_3$ receptors in human leucocytes. *Science* 1983;221:1181–3.

103. Provvedini DM, Tsoukas CD, Deftos LJ, Manolagas SC. 1,25-Dihydroxyvitamin D$_3$-binding macromolecules in human B lymphocytes: effects on immunoglobulin production. *J Immunol* 1986;136:2734–40.

104. Simpson RU, DeLuca HF. Characterization of a receptor-like protein for 1,25-dihydroxyvitamin D$_3$ in rat skin. *Proc Natl Acad Sci USA* 1980;77:5822–6.

105. Costa EM, Blau HM, Feldman D. 1,25-Dihydroxyvitamin D$_3$ receptors and hormonal responses in cloned human skeletal muscle cells. *Endocrinology* 1986;119:2214–20.

106. Feldman D, Chen T, Hirst M, Colston K, Karasek M, Cone C. Demonstration of 1,25-dihydroxyvitamin D$_3$ receptors in human skin biopsies. *J Clin Endocrinol Metab* 1980;51:1463–6.

107. Eil C, Marx SJ. Nuclear uptake of 1,25-dihydroxy[^{3}H]cholecalciferol in dispersed fibroblasts cultured from normal human skin. *Proc Natl Acad Sci USA* 1981;78:2562–6.

108. Eisman JA, Martin TJ, MacIntyre I, Frampton RJ, Moseley JM, Whitehead R. 1,25-Dihydroxyvitamin D$_3$ receptors in a cultured human breast cancer cell line (MCF-7). *Biochem Biophys Res Commun* 1980;93:9–15.

109. Eisman JA, MacIntyre I, Martin TJ, Frampton RJ, King RJB.

110. Sher E, Eisman JA, Moseley JM, Martin TJ. Whole cell uptake and nuclear localisation of 1,25-dihydroxyvitamin D$_3$ by cancer cells (T47D) in culture. *Biochem J* 1981;200:315–20.

111. Pike JW, Haussler MR. Association of 1,25-dihydroxyvitamin D$_3$ with cultured 3T6 mouse fibroblasts. *J Biol Chem* 1983;258:8554–60.

112. Sher E, Frampton RJ, Eisman JA. Regulation of the 1,25-dihydroxyvitamin D$_3$ receptor by 1,25-dihydroxyvitamin D$_3$ in intact human cancer cells. *Endocrinology* 1985;116:971–7.

113. Stumpf WE, Sar M, Reid FA, Tanaka Y, DeLuca HF. Target cells for 1,25-dihydroxyvitamin D$_3$ in intestinal tract, stomach, kidney, skin, pituitary, and parathyroid. *Science* 1979;206:1188–90.

114. Narbaitz R, Stumpf W, Sar M, DeLuca HF, Tanaka Y. Autoradiographic demonstration of target cells for 1,25-dihydroxycholecalciferol in the chick embryo chorioallantoic membrane, duodenum, and parathyroid glands. *Gen Comp Endocrinol* 1980;42:283–9.

115. Clark S, Stumpf WE, Sar M, DeLuca HF, Tanaka Y. Target cells for 1,25-dihydroxyvitamin D$_3$ in the pancreas. *Cell Tissue Res* 1980;209:515–20.

116. Stumpf WE, Sar M, Clark SA, DeLuca HF. Brain target sites for 1,25-dihydroxyvitamin D$_3$. *Science* 1982;215:1403–5.

117. Clemens TL, Garrett KP, Zhou XY, Pike JW, Haussler MR, Dempster DW. Immunocytochemical localization of the 1,25-dihydroxyvitamin D$_3$ receptor in target cells. *Endocrinology* 1988;122:1224–30.

118. Berger U, Wilson P, McClelland RA, Colston K, Haussler MR, Pike JW, Coombes RC. Immunocytochemical detection of 1,25-dihydroxyvitamin D receptors in normal human tissues. *J Clin Endocrinol Metab* 1988;67:607–13.

119. Milde P, Merke J, Ritz E, Haussler MR, Rauterberg EW. Immunohistochemical detection of 1,25-dihydroxyvitamin D$_3$ receptors and estrogen receptors by monoclonal antibodies: a comparison of four immunoperoxidase methods. *J Histochem Cytochem* 1989;37:1609–17.

120. Berger U, Wilson P, McClelland RA, Colston K, Haussler MR, Pike JW, Coombes RC. Immunocytochemical detection of 1,25-dihydroxyvitamin D$_3$ receptors in breast cancer. *Cancer Res* 1987;47:6793–9.

121. Halloran BP, DeLuca HF. Appearance of the intestinal cytosolic receptor for 1,25-dihydroxyvitamin D$_3$ during neonatal development in the rat. *J Biol Chem* 1981;256:7338–42.

122. Massaro ER, Simpson RU, DeLuca HF. Stimulation of specific 1,25-dihydroxyvitamin D$_3$ binding protein in cultured postnatal rat intestine by hydrocortisone. *J Biol Chem* 1982;257:13736–9.

123. DeLuca HF, Franceschi RT, Halloran BP, Massaro ER. Molecular events involved in 1,25-dihydroxyvitamin D$_3$ stimulation of intestinal calcium transport. *Fed Proc* 1982;41:66–71.

124. Massaro ER, Simpson RU, DeLuca HF. Glucocorticoids and appearance of 1,25-dihydroxyvitamin D$_3$ receptor in rat intestine. *Am J Physiol* 1983;244:E230–5.

125. Henning SJ. Functional development of the gastrointestinal tract. In: Johnson LR, ed. *Physiology of the gastrointestinal tract.* New York: Raven Press, 1987;285–300.

126. Pierce EA, DeLuca HF. Regulation of the intestinal 1,25-dihydroxyvitamin D$_3$ receptor during neonatal development in the rat. *Arch Biochem Biophys* 1988;261:241–9.

127. Burmester JK, Wiese RJ, Maeda N, DeLuca HF. Structure and regulation of the rat 1,25-dihydroxyvitamin D$_3$ receptor. *Proc Natl Acad Sci USA* 1988;85:9499–502.

128. Huang Y, Lee S, Stolz R, et al. Effect of hormones and development on the expression of the rat 1,25-dihydroxyvitamin D$_3$ receptor gene. *J Biol Chem* 1989;264:17454–61.

129. Abe E, Miyaura C, Sakagami H, et al. Differentiation of mouse myeloid leukemia cells induced by 1,25-dihydroxyvitamin D$_3$. *Proc Natl Acad Sci USA* 1981;78:4990–4.

130. Shavit ZB, Teitelbaum SL, Reitsma P, Hall A, Pegg LE, Trial J, Kahn AJ. Induction of monocytic differentiation and bone resorption by 1,25-dihydroxyvitamin D$_3$. *Proc Natl Acad Sci USA* 1983;80:5907–11.

131. Bhalla AK, Amento EP, Clemens TL, Holick MF, Krane SM. Specific high affinity receptors for 1,25-dihydroxyvitamin D$_3$ in

human periferal blood mononuclear cells: presence in monocytes and induction in T lymphocytes following activation. *J Clin Endocrinol Metab* 1983;57:1308–10.

132. Matsui TR, Takahashi R, Mihara K, et al. 1,25-Dihydroxyvitamin D3-regulated expression of genes involved in human T lymphocyte proliferation and differentiation. *Cancer Res* 1986;46:5827–31.

133. Reichel H, Koeffler HP, Tobler A, Norman AW. 1α,25-Dihydroxyvitamin D₃ inhibits gamma interferon synthesis by normal human peripheral blood lymphocytes. *Proc Natl Acad Sci USA* 1987;84:3385–9.

134. Lacey PL, Axelrod J, Chappel JC, Kahn AJ, Teitlbaum SL. Vitamin D affects proliferation of a murine T helper cell clone. *J Immunol* 1987;138:1680–6.

135. Manolagas SC. Immunoregulatory properties of 1,25(OH)₂D₃: cellular requirements and mechanisms. In: Norman AW, Schaefer K, Grigoleit HG, von Herrath D, eds. *Vitamin D. Molecular, cellular and clinical endocrinology.* Berlin: de Gruyter, 1988;282–90.

136. Hirst M, Feldman D. Glucocorticoids down-regulate the number of 1,25-dihydroxyvitamin D₃ receptors in mouse intestine. *Biochem Biophys Res Commun* 1982;105:1590–5.

137. Hirst M, Feldman D. Glucocorticoid regulation of 1,25(OH)₂ vitamin D₃ receptors: divergent effects on mouse and rat intestine. *Endocrinology* 1982;111:1400–3.

138. Chen TL, Cone CM, Morey-Holton E, Feldman D. 1,25-Dihydroxyvitamin D₃ receptors in cultured rat osteoblast-like cells. Glucocorticoid treatment increases receptor content. *J Biol Chem* 1983;256:4350–5.

139. Chen TL, Feldman D. Regulation of 1,25-dihydroxyvitamin D₃ receptors in cultured mouse bone cells. Correlation of receptor concentration with the rate of cell division. *J Biol Chem* 1981;256:5561–6.

140. Petkovich PM, Heersche JNM, Tinker DO, Jones G. Retinoic acid stimulates 1,25-dihydroxyvitamin D₃ binding in rat osteosarcoma cells. *J Biol Chem* 1984;259:8274–80.

141. Grigoriadis AE, Petkovich PM, Rosenthal EE, Heersche JNM. Modulation by retinoic acid of 1,25-dihydroxyvitamin D₃ effects on alkaline phosphatase activity and parathyroid hormone responsiveness in an osteoblast-like osteosarcoma cell line. *Endocrinology* 1986;119:932–9.

142. Costa EM, Hirst M, Feldman D. Regulation of 1,25-dihydroxyvitamin D₃ receptors by vitamin D analogs in cultured mammalian cells. *Endocrinology* 1985;117:2203–10.

143. McDonnell DP, Mangelsdorf DJ, Pike JW, Haussler MR, O'Malley BW. Molecular cloning of complementary DNA encoding the avian receptor for vitamin D. *Science* 1987;235:1214–7.

144. Favus MJ, Mangelsdorf DJ, Tembe V, Coe BJ, Haussler MR. Evidence for in vivo upregulation of the intestinal vitamin D receptor during dietary calcium restriction in the rat. *J Clin Invest* 1988;82:218–24.

145. Chen TL, Hauschka PV, Cabrales S, Feldman D. The effects of 1,25-dihydroxyvitamin D₃ and dexamethasone on rat osteoblast-like primary cell cultures: receptor occupancy and functional expression patterns for three different bioresponses. *Endocrinology* 1986;118:250–9.

146. Theophan G, Nguyen AP, Norman AW. Regulation of calbindin-D28K gene expression by 1,25-dihydroxyvitamin D₃ is correlated to receptor occupancy. *J Biol Chem* 1986;261:16943–7.

147. Ozono K, Liao J, Scott RA, Kerner SA, Pike JW. The vitamin D response element in the human osteocalcin gene: association with a nuclear proto-oncogene enhancer. *J Biol Chem* 1990;265:21881–8.

148. Mellon WS, Franceschi RT, DeLuca HF. An in vitro study of the stability of the chicken intestinal cytosol 1,25-dihydroxyvitamin D₃-specific receptor. *Arch Biochem Biophys* 1980;202:83–92.

149. Norman AW, Hunziker W, Walters MR, Bishop JE. Differential effects of protease inhibitors on 1,25-dihydroxyvitamin D₃ receptors. *J Biol Chem* 1983;258:12867–80.

150. Allegretto EA, Pike JW. Trypsin cleavage of chick 1,25-dihydroxyvitamin D₃ receptors. Generation of discrete polypeptides which retain hormone but are unreactive to DNA and monoclonal antibody. *J Biol Chem* 1985;260:10139–45.

151. Franceschi RT, DeLuca HF, Mercado DL. Temperature-dependent inactivation of nucleic acid binding and aggregation of the

152. Franceschi RT, DeLuca HF. Aggregation properties of the 1,25-dihydroxyvitamin D₃ receptor from chick intestinal cytosol. *J Biol Chem* 1979;254:11629–35.

153. Hunziker W, Walters MR, Norman AW. 1,25-Dihydroxyvitamin D₃ receptors: differential quantitation of endogenously occupied and unoccupied sites. *J Biol Chem* 1980;255:9534–7.

154. Massaro ER, Simpson RU, DeLuca HF. Quantitation of endogenously occupied and unoccupied binding sites for 1,25-dihydroxyvitamin D₃ in rat intestine. *Proc Natl Acad Sci USA* 1983;80:2549–53.

155. Pike JW, Sleator NM, Haussler MR. Chicken intestinal receptor for 1,25-dihydroxyvitamin D₃. Immunologic characterization and homogeneous isolation of a 60,000-dalton protein. *J Biol Chem* 1987;262:1305–11.

156. Pike JW. New insights into mediators of vitamin D₃ action. In: Norman AW, Schaefer K, Grigoleit HG, von Herrath D, eds. *Vitamin D. Chemical, biochemical and clinical update.* Berlin: de Gruyter, 1985;97–104.

157. Mangelsdorf DJ, Pike JW, Haussler MR. Avian and mammalian receptors for 1,25-dihydroxyvitamin D₃: in vitro translation to characterize size and hormone-dependent regulation. *Proc Natl Acad Sci USA* 1987;84:354–8.

158. Brown TA, Prahl JM, DeLuca HF. Partial amino acid sequence of porcine 1,25-dihydroxyvitamin D₃ receptor isolated by immunoaffinity chromatography. *Proc Natl Acad Sci USA* 1988;85:2454–8.

159. Pike JW, Sleator NM. Hormone-dependent phosphorylation of the 1,25-dihydroxyvitamin D₃ receptor in mouse fibroblasts. *Biochem Biophys Res Commun* 1985;131:378–85.

160. Brown TA, DeLuca HF. Phosphorylation of the 1,25-dihydroxyvitamin D₃ receptor. A primary event in 1,25-dihydroxyvitamin D₃ action. *J Biol Chem* 1990;265:10025–9.

161. Dokoh S, Haussler MR, Pike JW. Development of a radioligand immunoassay for 1,25-dihydroxycholecalciferol receptors utilizing monoclonal antibody. *Biochem J* 1984;221:129–36.

162. Sandgren M, DeLuca HF. An immunoradiometric assay for 1,25-dihydroxyvitamin D₃ receptor. *Anal Biochem* 1989;183:57–63.

163. Pike JW, Dokoh S, Haussler MR, Liberman UA, Marx SJ, Eil C. Vitamin D₃-resistant fibroblasts have immunoassayable 1,25-dihydroxyvitamin D₃ receptors. *Science* 1984;224:879–81.

164. Strom M, Sandgren ME, Brown TA, DeLuca HF. 1,25-Dihydroxyvitamin D₃ up-regulates the 1,25-dihydroxyvitamin D₃ receptor in vivo. *Proc Natl Acad Sci USA* 1989;86:9770–3.

165. Pike JW. Monoclonal antibodies to chick intestinal receptors for 1,25-dihydroxyvitamin D₃. Interaction and effects of binding on receptor function. *J Biol Chem* 1984;259:1167–73.

166. Allegretto EA, Pike JW, Haussler MR. Immunochemical detection of unique proteolytic fragments of the chick 1,25-dihydroxyvitamin D₃ receptor. Distinct 20-kDa DNA-binding and 45-kDa hormone-binding species. *J Biol Chem* 1987;262:1312–9.

167. Allegretto EA, Pike JW, Haussler MR. C-terminal proteolysis of the avian 1,25-dihydroxyvitamin D₃ receptor. *Biochem Biophys Res Commun* 1987;147:479–85.

168. Walters MR, Hunziker W, Norman AW. Unoccupied 1,25-dihydroxyvitamin D₃ receptors. Nuclear/cytosol ratios depend on ionic strength. *J Biol Chem* 1980;255:6799–805.

169. Walters MR, Hunziker W, Norman AW. Apparent nuclear localization of unoccupied receptors for 1,25-dihydroxyvitamin D₃. *Biochem Biophys Res Commun* 1982;98:990–6.

170. Walters MR, Hunziker W, Norman AW. 1,25-Dihydroxyvitamin D₃ receptors: intermediates between triiodothyronine and steroid hormone receptors. *Trends Biochem Sci* 1981;6:268–71.

171. Pike JW. Interaction between 1,25-dihydroxyvitamin D₃ receptors and intestinal nuclei. Binding to nuclear constituents in vitro. *J Biol Chem* 1982;257:6766–75.

172. Hunziker W, Walters MR, Bishop JE, Norman AW. Unoccupied and in vitro and in vivo occupied 1,25-dihydroxyvitamin D₃ intestinal receptors. Multiple biochemical forms and evidence for transformations. *J Biol Chem* 1983;258:8642–8.

173. Pratt WB. Steroid hormone antagonists at the receptor level: a role for the heat-shock protein MW 90,000 (hsp-90). *J Cell Biochem* 1987;35:51–68.

174. Dalman FC, Koenig RJ, Perdew GH, Massa E, Pratt WB. In contrast to the glucocorticoid receptor, the thyroid hormone receptor is translated in the DNA binding state and is not associated with hsp90. *J Biol Chem* 1990;265:3615–8.

175. Pan LC, Price PA. Ligand-dependent regulation of the 1,25-dihydroxyvitamin D_3 receptor in rat osteosarcoma cells. *J Biol Chem* 1987;262:4670–5.

176. Costa EM, Feldman D. Homologous up-regulation of the 1,25(OH)$_2$ vitamin D_3 receptor in rats. *Biochem Biophys Res Commun* 1986;137:742–7.

177. Lee Y, Inaba M, DeLuca HF, Mellon WS. Immunological identification of 1,25-dihydroxyvitamin D_3 receptors in human promyelocytic leukemic cells (HL-60) during homologous regulation. *J Biol Chem* 1989;264:13701–5.

178. Hunziker W, Walters MR, Bishop JE, Norman AW. Effect of vitamin D status on the equilibrium between occupied and unoccupied 1,25-dihydroxyvitamin D intestinal receptors in the chick. *J Clin Invest* 1982;69:826–34.

179. Haussler MR, Mangelsdorf DJ, Komm BS, et al. Molecular biology of the vitamin D hormone. *Rec Prog Horm Res* 1988;44:263–303.

180. Young RA, Davis RW. Efficient isolation of genes using antibody probes. *Proc Natl Acad Sci USA* 1983;80:1194–8.

181. Miller J, McLachlan AD, Klug A. Repetitive zinc binding domains in the protein transcription factor IIIA from *Xenopus* oocytes. *EMBO J* 1985;4:1609–14.

182. Evans RM. The steroid and thyroid hormone receptor superfamily. *Science* 1988;240:889–95.

183. Baker AR, McDonnell DP, Hughes MR, et al. Cloning and expression of full-length cDNA encoding human vitamin D receptor. *Proc Natl Acad Sci USA* 1988;85:3294–8.

184. Burmester JK, Maeda N, DeLuca HF. Isolation and expression of rat 1,25-dihydroxyvitamin D_3 receptor cDNA. *Proc Natl Acad Sci USA* 1988;85:1005–9.

185. Pike JW. Vitamin D_3 receptors: molecular structure of the protein and its chromosomal gene. In: Norman AW, Schaefer K, Grigoleit HG, von Herrath D, eds. *Vitamin D. Molecular, cellular, and clinical endocrinology.* Berlin: de Gruyter, 1988;215–24.

186. Hollenberg SM, Weinberger C, Ong ES, Cerelli G, et al. Primary structure and expression of a functional human glucocorticoid receptor cDNA. *Nature* 1985;318:635–41.

187. Miesfeld R, Rusconi S, Godowski P, et al. Genetic complementation of a glucocorticoid receptor deficiency by expression of cloned receptor cDNA. *Cell* 1986;46:389–99.

188. Green S, Walter P, Kumar V, et al. Human oestrogen receptor cDNA: sequence, expression and homology to v-erb-A. *Nature* 1986;320:334–9.

189. Conneely OM, Sullivan WP, Toft DO, et al. Molecular cloning of the chicken progesterone receptor. *Science* 1986;233:767–70.

190. Weinberger C, Thompson CC, Ong ES, Lebo R, Gruol DJ, Evans RM. *Nature* 1986;324:641–6.

191. Sap J, Munoz A, Damm K, et al. The c-erb-A protein is a high-affinity receptor for thyroid hormone. *Nature* 1986;324:635–40.

192. Arriza JL, Weinberger C, Cerelli G, et al. Cloning of human mineralocorticoid receptor complementary DNA: structure and functional kinship with the glucocorticoid receptor. *Science* 1987;237:268–75.

193. Giguere V, Ong ES, Segui P, Evans RM. Identification of a receptor for the morphogen retinoic acid. *Nature* 1987;330:624–9.

194. Petkovich M, Brand NJ, Krust A, Chambon P. A human retinoic acid receptor which belongs to the family of nuclear receptors. *Nature* 1987;330:444–50.

195. Chang C, Kokontis J, Liao S. Molecular cloning of human and rat complementary DNA encoding androgen receptors. *Science* 1988;240:324–6.

196. Lubahn DB, Joseph DR, Sullivan PM, et al. Cloning of human androgen receptor complementary DNA and localization to the X chromosome. *Science* 1988;240:327–30.

197. O'Malley BW. The steroid receptor superfamily: more excitement predicted for the future. *Mol Endocrinol* 1990;4:363–9.

198. Hard T, Kellenbach E, Boelens R, et al. Solution structure of the glucocorticoid receptor DNA-binding domain. *Science* 1990;249:157–60.

199. McDonnell DP, Scott RA, Kerner SA, O'Malley BW, Pike JW. Functional domains of the human vitamin D_3 receptor regulate osteocalcin gene expression. *Mol Endocrinol* 1989;3:635–44.

200. Tsai S, Carlstedt-Duke J, Weigel NL, et al. Molecular interactions of steroid hormone receptor with its enhancer element: evidence for receptor dimer formation. *Cell* 1988;55:361–9.

201. Kumar V, Chambon P. The estrogen receptor binds tightly to its responsive element as a ligand-induced homodimer. *Cell* 1988;55:145–56.

202. Fawell SE, Lees JA, White R, Parker MG. Characterization and colocalization of steroid binding and dimerization activities in the mouse estrogen receptor. *Cell* 1990;60:953–62.

203. Godowski PJ, Rusconi S, Miesfeld R, Yamamoto KR. Glucocorticoid receptor mutants that are constitutive activators of transcriptional enhancement. *Nature* 1987;325:365–8.

204. Giguere V, Hollenberg SM, Rosenfeld MG, Evans RM. Functional domains of the human glucocorticoid receptor. *Cell* 1986;46:645–52.

205. Kumar V, Green S, Stack G, Berry M, Jin J-R, Chambon P. Functional domains of the human estrogen receptor. *Cell* 1987;51:941–51.

206. Picard D, Yamamoto KR. Two signals mediate hormone-dependent nuclear localization of the glucocorticoid receptor. *EMBO J* 1987;6:3333–40.

207. Guiochon-Mantel A, Loosfeldt H, Lescop P, et al. Mechanisms of nuclear localization of the progesterone receptor: evidence for interaction between monomers. *Cell* 1989;57:1147–54.

208. Waterman ML, Adler S, Nelson C, Greene GL, Evans RM, Rosenfeld MG. A single domain of the estrogen receptor confers deoxyribonucleic acid binding and transcriptional activation of the rat prolactin gene. *Mol Endocrinol* 1988;2:14–21.

209. Hollenberg SM, Evans RM. Multiple and cooperative trans-activation domains of the human glucocorticoid receptor. *Cell* 1988;55:899–906.

210. Glass CK, Lipkin SM, Devary OV, Rosenfeld MG. Positive and negative regulation of gene transcription by a retinoic acid–thyroid hormone receptor heterodimer. *Cell* 1989;59:697–708.

211. Forman BM, Yang C, Au M, Casanova J, Ghysdael J, Samuels HH. A domain containing leucine-zipper-like motifs mediate novel in vivo interactions between the thyroid hormone and retinoic acid receptors. *Mol Endocrinol* 1989;3:1610–26.

212. Murray MB, Towle HC. Identification of nuclear factors that enhance binding of the thyroid hormone receptor to a thyroid hormone response element. *Mol Endocrinol* 1989;3:1434–42.

213. Burnside J, Darling DS, Chin WW. A nuclear factor that enhances binding of thyroid hormone receptors to thyroid hormone response elements. *J Biol Chem* 1990;265:2500–4.

214. Huckaby CS, Conneely OM, Beattie WG, Dobson AD, Tsai M-J, O'Malley BW. Structure of the chromosomal chicken progesterone receptor gene. *Proc Natl Acad Sci USA* 1987;84:8380–4.

215. Ponglikitmongkol M, Green SM, Chambon P. Genomic organization of the human oestrogen receptor gene. *EMBO J* 1988;7:3385–8.

216. Kesterson RA, Pike JW. The human vitamin D receptor chromosomal gene: structural relationships with the steroid receptor gene family. Submitted for publication, 1991.

217. Nevah-Many T, Silver J. Regulation of the calcitonin gene transcription by vitamin D metabolites in vivo in the rat. *J Clin Invest* 1988;81:270–3.

218. Okazaki T, Igarashi T, Kronenberg HM. 5'-Flanking region of the parathyroid hormone gene mediates negative regulation by 1,25-(OH)$_2$ vitamin D_3. *J Biol Chem* 1988;263:2203–8.

219. Noda M, Vogel RI, Craig AM, Denhardt DT. DNA sequence in murine secreted phosphoprotein I (SPPI, osteopontin, 2AR) gene confers responsiveness to 1,25-dihydroxyvitamin D_3 [Abstract]. *J Bone Miner Res* 1990;5:5.

220. Lichtler A, Stover ML, Angilly J, Kream B, Rowe DW. Isolation and characterization of the rat alpha1(I) collagen promoter. Regulation by 1,25-dihydroxyvitamin D_3. *J Biol Chem* 1989;264:3072–7.

221. Reitsma PH, Rothberg PG, Astrin SM, et al. Regulation of myc gene expression in HL-60 leukemia cells by a vitamin D metabolite. *Nature* 1983;306:492–4.

222. Brelvi CS, Christakos S, Studinski GP. Expression of monocyte-

specific oncogenes c-fos and c-fms in HL-60 cells treated with vitamin D₃ analogs correlates with inhibition of DNA synthesis and reduced calmodulin concentration. *Lab Invest* 1986;55:269–75.

223. Pan LC, Price PA. 1,25-Dihydroxyvitamin D₃ stimulates transcription of bone gla protein [Abstract]. *J Bone Miner Res* 1986;1:A20.

224. Yoon K, Rutledge SJC, Buenaga RF, Rodan GA. Characterization of the rat osteocalcin gene: stimulation of promoter activity by 1,25-dihydroxyvitamin D₃. *Biochemistry* 1988;27:8521–6.

225. Demay MB, Roth DA, Kronenberg HM. Regions of the rat osteocalcin gene which mediate the effect of 1,25-dihydroxyvitamin D₃ on gene transcription. *J Biol Chem* 1989;264:2279–82.

226. Kerner SA, Scott RA, Pike JW. Sequence elements in the human osteocalcin gene confer basal activation and inducible response to hormonal vitamin D₃. *Proc Natl Acad Sci USA* 1989;86:4455–9.

227. Morrison NA, Shine J, Fragonas J-C, Verkest V, McMenemy ML, Eisman JA. 1,25-Dihydroxyvitamin D-responsive element and glucocorticoid repression in the osteocalcin gene. *Science* 1989;246:1158–61.

228. Demay MB, Gerardi JM, DeLuca HF, Kronenberg HM. DNA sequences in the rat osteocalcin gene that bind the 1,25-dihydroxyvitamin D₃ receptor and confer responsiveness to 1,25-dihydroxyvitamin D₃. *Proc Natl Acad Sci USA* 1990;87:369–73.

229. Pike JW. Cis and trans regulation of osteocalcin gene expression by vitamin D and other hormones. In: Cohn DV, Glorieux FH, Martin TJ, eds. *Calcium regulation and bone metabolism.* Amsterdam: Elsevier, 1990;127–36.

230. Sone T, Scott RA, Hughes MR, et al. Mutant vitamin D receptors which confer hereditary resistance to 1,25-dihydroxyvitamin D₃ in humans are transcriptionally inactive in vitro. *J Biol Chem* 1989;264:20230–4.

231. Ritchie HH, Hughes MR, Thompson ET, et al. An ochre mutation in the vitamin D receptor gene causes hereditary 1,25-dihydroxyvitamin D₃-resistant rickets in three families. *Proc Natl Acad Sci USA* 1989;86:9783–7.

232. Sone T, Marx SJ, Liberman UA, Pike JW. A unique point mutation in the human vitamin D receptor chromosomal gene confers hereditary resistance to 1,25-dihydroxyvitamin D₃. *Mol Endocrinol* 1990;4:623–31.

233. Beato M. Gene regulation by steroid hormones. *Cell* 1989;56:335–44.

234. Schule R, Umesono K, Mangelsdorf DJ, Bolado J, Pike JW, Evans RM. Jun-Fos and receptors for vitamins A and D recognize a common response element in the human osteocalcin gene. *Cell* 1990;61:497–504.

235. Liao J, Ozono K, Sone T, McDonnell DP, Pike JW. Vitamin D receptor interaction with specific DNA requires a nuclear protein and 1,25-dihydroxyvitamin D₃. *Proc Natl Acad Sci USA* 1990;87:9751–5.

236. Sone T, McDonnell DP, O'Malley BW, Pike JW. Expression of human vitamin D receptor in *Saccharomyces cerevisiae*: purification, properties and generation of polyclonal antibodies. *J Biol Chem* 1990;265:21997–22003.

237. Pugh BF, Tjian R. Mechanism of transcriptional activation by SP1: evidence for coactivators. *Cell* 1990;61:1187–97.

238. Ptashne M, Gann AAF. Activators and targets. *Nature* 1990;346:329–31.

239. Rosen JF, Fleischman AR, Finberg L, Hamstra A, DeLuca HF. Rickets with alopecia: an inborn error of vitamin D metabolism. *J Pediatr* 1979;94:729–35.

240. Marx SJ, Speigel AM, Brown EM, et al. A familial syndrome of decreased insensitivity to 1,25-dihydroxycholecalciferol. *J Clin Endocrinol Metab* 1978;47:1303–10.

241. Liberman UA, Halabe A, Samuel R, et al. End-organ resistance to 1,25-dihydroxycholecalciferol. *Lancet* 1980;1:504–7.

242. Beer S, Tieder M, Kohelet D, et al. Vitamin D resistant rickets with alopecia: a form of end organ resistance to 1,25-dihydroxyvitamin D. *Clin Endocrinol* 1981;14:395–402.

243. Takeda E, Kuroda Y, Saijo T, et al. 1-Hydroxyvitamin D₃ treatment of three patients with 1,25-dihydroxyvitamin D-receptor-defect rickets and alopecia. *Pediatrics* 1987;80:97–101.

244. Liberman UA, Eil C, Marx SJ. Resistance to 1,25-dihydroxyvitamin D. *J Clin Invest* 1983;71:192–200.

245. Gamblin GT, Liberman UA, Eil C, Downs RW, DeGrange DA, Marx SJ. Vitamin D-dependent rickets type II. *J Clin Invest* 1985;75:954–60.

246. Balsan S, Garabedian M, Liberman UA, et al. Rickets and alopecia with resistance to 1,25-dihydroxyvitamin D: two different clinical courses with two different cellular defects. *J Clin Endocrinol Metab* 1983;57:803–11.

247. Liberman UA, Eil C, Marx SJ. Receptor-positive hereditary resistance to 1,25-dihydroxyvitamin D: chromatography of hormone–receptor complexes on deoxyribonucleic acid-cellulose shows two classes of mutation. *J Clin Endocrinol Metab* 1986;62:122–6.

248. Chen TL, Hirst MA, Cone CM, Hochberg A, Tietze H, Feldman D. 1,25-Dihydroxyvitamin D resistance, rickets, and alopecia: analysis of receptors and bioresponses in cultured fibroblasts from patients and parents. *J Clin Endocrinol Metab* 1984;59:383–8.

249. Hirst MA, Hochman HI, Feldman D. Vitamin D resistance and alopecia: a kindred with normal 1,25-dihydroxyvitamin D binding, but decreased receptor affinity for deoxyribonucleic acid. *J Clin Endocrinol Metab* 1985;60:490–5.

250. Marx SJ, Barsony J. Tissue-selective 1,25-dihydroxyvitamin D₃ resistance: novel applications of calciferols. *J Bone Miner Res* 1988;3:481–7.

251. Saiki RK, Scharf S, Faloona F, et al. Enzymatic amplification of beta-globin genomic sequences and restriction site analysis for diagnosis of sickle cell anemia. *Science* 1985;230:1350–4.

252. Hughes MR, Malloy PF, Kieback DG, et al. Point mutations in the human vitamin D receptor gene associated with hypocalcemic rickets. *Science* 1988;242:1702–5.

253. Malloy PF, Hochberg Z, Tiasno D, et al. The molecular basis of hereditary 1,25-dihydroxyvitamin D₃ resistant rickets in seven related families. *J Clin Invest* 1990;86:2071–9.

254. Haussler MR. Vitamin D receptor: nature and function. *Annu Rev Nutr* 1986;6:527–62.

Disorders of Bone and Mineral Metabolism,
edited by Fredric L. Coe and Murray J. Favus,
© 1992 by Raven Press, Ltd. All rights reserved.

CHAPTER 9

Clinical Aspects of Measurements of Plasma Vitamin D Sterols and the Vitamin D Binding Protein

John G. Haddad, Jr.

VITAMIN D STEROLS IN PLASMA

Although the anti-ricketic principle was recognized long ago (1,2), and this led to important prophylactic and therapeutic strategies, early quantitative techniques for vitamin D depended on laborious chemical assays or difficult and, as it turned out, imprecise and nonspecific bioassays (3–6) of anti-ricketic activity. The studies carried out over the past two decades, however, have identified important vitamin D metabolites, including what is regarded to be the hormonal form (see Chapters 7 and 8). The parent vitamin and the metabolites have unique properties, including their production and clearance rates and plasma concentrations. Techniques have evolved to allow precise quantitation of these sterols and their major transport protein, and their application has led to an improved understanding of the primary and secondary changes in vitamin D metabolism in health and in a variety of clinical disorders.

Vitamin D

Sources

Humans have access to both ergocalciferol (vitamin D_2) and cholecalciferol (vitamin D_3). The ergocalciferol form is found in a variety of foods, dietary supplements, and drugs. Similarly, the cholecalciferol form is utilized in the supplementation of some foods. In different areas of the world, policies differ concerning the supplementa-

tion of foods with vitamin D, as well as the form(s) utilized. Since natural foods, with a few exceptions, contain little vitamin D, the physiological source is believed to derive from cutaneous exposure to effective ultraviolet rays, leading to the production of cholecalciferol (7–10).

Because of its dependence on environmental and/or nutritional factors for vitamin D sufficiency, the vitamin D supply system is unique. This also appears to be the stimulus for the intense economy of these sterols, as reflected by storage forms and the slow release of these sterols from the organism. Thus protracted periods of vitamin D deprivation are required to deplete stores and to cause vitamin D deficiency (9,10).

Regulation of cutaneous sources appears to reflect the degree and duration of ultraviolet exposure and resulting skin pigmentation (11,12). Dark-skinned subjects have less efficient cholecalciferol production for a given amount and intensity of light exposure. Studies indicate that human skin is a remarkably efficient producer (9,13,14), but vitamin D intoxication has not been observed in normal subjects after extensive sunlight exposure.

Both dietary sources of vitamin D and pharmacological amounts are readily absorbed into the intestinal lymphatic system. Diseases of the intestine and biliary tract impair absorption (5,15), as does extensive resection of the small bowel. Patients with such disorders must receive parenteral doses of vitamin D or significant cutaneous production. Intoxication with vitamin D follows the repeated ingestion of large amounts of sterol in a pharmacological form.

Special sources of vitamin D are available to the fetus. In this condition, placental transfer of vitamin D and metabolites is required to provide these sterols. In addi-

J. G. Haddad, Jr.: Department of Medicine, University of Pennsylvania School of Medicine, 422 Curie Boulevard—CRB 611, Philadelphia, Pennsylvania 19104-6149

tion to maternal vitamin D deficiency, premature birth also leads to insufficient transfer of vitamin D to the fetus (16).

Plasma Concentrations

Levels of vitamin D in normal plasma can vary from 0 to 140 ng/mL, depending on recent dietary intake and exposure to effective sunlight (14,17–19). With suitable chromatographic separations, the ergocalciferol (D_2) and cholecalciferol (D_3) content in plasma can be measured (18) (Table 1). Levels are generally higher in summer months and after ingestion or parenteral delivery of vitamin D. Measurements have been directed to studies of the skin responsivity to ultraviolet radiation exposures (11,12,14,19–21). When dietary sources of D_2 are not excessive, D_3 is generally found to be the dominant form.

Kinetics

Depending on the source of vitamin D, its assimilation and disposition will vary considerably. Oral doses are absorbed over 4–10 h, initially associated with chylomicrons in intestinal lymph. In the plasma, some of the vitamin associates with the vitamin D binding protein (DBP), but hepatic entry is favored by its binding to chylomicron remnants (22). Oral ingestion therefore leads to relatively rapid increases in plasma levels and subsequent increases in plasma 25-hydroxyvitamin D [25(OH)D] over several days (23,24). The plasma levels observed after single cutaneous exposures to effective ultraviolet radiation (260–310 nm) increase in hours but do not peak until 48 h after exposure (14,19). Depot injections of D_2 or D_3 in oil are very slowly absorbed into the circulation, providing a long-term source (25).

Clearance of vitamin D from the circulation after intravenous injection occurs with a half-life of 24 hours. The vitamin associates with DBP and lipoproteins after this form of delivery, in contrast to its postabsorptive plasma binding. The precise nature of the escort(s) for D_3 synthesized in skin is not known but is thought to be lipoproteins and DBP (22).

The efficiency of different modes of vitamin D delivery to the body, as judged by 25(OH)D production, appears to be highest for depot injection and cutaneous insolation (7,9,25). For single doses of vitamin D, 25(OH)D production is a power function of vitamin D dosage, with the fractional conversion of the dosage inversely correlated to the level of vitamin D at the time of administration (24). When single doses lead to sustained availability of vitamin D, higher and sustained plasma 25(OH)D levels are seen. Oral doses lead to less-sustained levels of 25(OH)D (25), possibly reflecting non-25-hydroxylation pathways since oral doses lead to formation of other metabolites. Studies in humans reveal 25(OH)D, not vitamin D, to be the major storage form of the vitamin (26).

25-Hydroxyvitamin D

Sources

Although trivial calciferol-25-hydroxylase activities have been demonstrated in other organs in some species, the liver is the important site of the biosynthesis of 25(OH)D (27). No ionic or hormonal control of 25(OH)D production is recognized. Since 25(OH)D is a major storage form of the vitamin, it is conceivable that ingested animal tissues could also provide 25(OH)D, assuming that it was not destroyed during food preparation. In practice, therefore, 25(OH)D availability requires adequate vitamin D (substrate) and adequate hepatic calciferol 25-hydroxylase activity (see Chapter 7). Other, special sources of 25(OH)D are the placental and lactational delivery systems. Of these, the placental mechanism is believed to be most important (28).

Some studies have reported that liver diseases can cause major deficiencies in 25(OH)D production (29,30). However, these interpretations have ignored several factors: (1) Vitamin D sources are threatened in liver disease, since patients are often anorectic and may have limited sunshine exposure; (2) malabsorption of fat-soluble materials occurs in hepatobiliary disorders; and (3) lower total 25(OH)D levels in plasma of patients with liver disease can be proportional to lower plasma levels of DBP (31). Oral challenge doses of vitamin D to such patients may not be absorbed well. In careful studies wherein substrate vitamin D is delivered parenterally,

TABLE 1. *Vitamin D and its metabolites in normal human plasma*

Item	D	25(OH)D	1,25(OH)$_2$
Total concentration	1–300 n*M* (0.4–120 ng/mL)	>10 n*M* (>4 ng/mL)	50–150 p*M* (20–60 pg/mL)
Percent free	—	0.04	0.4
Free concentration	—	5–25 p*M* (2–10 pg/mL)	0.2–0.6 p*M* (80–240 fg/mL)
Body production rate	Up to 250 µg/day	3–12 µg/day	0.5–2.0 µg/day
Plasma half-life	12–24 h	12–20 days	10–15 h

patients with severe liver disease can perform the 25-hydroxylation adequately (32). It appears likely, therefore, that the large constitutive, calciferol 25-hydroxylase capacity is not threatened until end-stage liver insufficiency occurs.

Plasma Concentrations

Plasma levels in normal humans range from 5 to 80 ng/mL, with reasonably good correlation to an individual's sunshine exposure and/or dietary intake of vitamin D (Table 1). Seasonal variations in plasma 25(OH)D concentrations of 50–100% are well recognized (9,23), reflecting the variations in sunlight activation of the provitamin D in skin. In general, lower levels are seen in healthy persons who live in geographical areas characterized by low levels and/or short periods of effective ultraviolet light as well as a policy of not supplementing foods with calciferols (9). Conversely, higher levels are seen in healthy persons who have chronic, high exposure to sunshine (lifeguards) and/or high vitamin D intake values (23,33–35).

With prolonged pharmacological administration of vitamin D, plasma concentrations of 100–600 ng/mL have been observed to correlate with the amount of substrate provided (23,24,34,35). Similarly, the administration of 25(OH)D_3 results in increases of plasma 25(OH)D that are proportional to the amount tendered (36). Most of the circulating 25(OH)D is bound to DBP and albumin.

Kinetics

The plasma half-life of administered 25(OH)D is 10–20 days (36,37). This relatively protracted clearance, together with its positive correlation with substrate availability, results in its plasma concentration being, with few exceptions, an excellent index of body stores of vitamin D and 25(OH)D. 25(OH)D is transformed into other metabolites and catabolic products, but it appears that a significant amount does recirculate from body stores as well (26,38). The apparent clearance of 25(OH)D from plasma is greatly prolonged after prior administration of large amounts of vitamin D (39), and this probably reflects continuing 25(OH)D production from vitamin D stores as well as release of stored 25(OH)D from tissues.

On correction of vitamin D deficiency, the fractional conversion of vitamin D to 25(OH)D is very high, with resulting increases of plasma 25(OH)D over a few days (40,41). With subsequent doses of vitamin D, the fractional conversion is less high, possibly reflecting the higher affinity of calciferol 25-hydroxylase during vitamin D deficiency (9,24).

An important regulation of 25(OH)D clearance from plasma has recently been demonstrated (42,43). Administered 1,25-dihydroxycalciferol [1,25(OH)$_2$D] or in-

creased amounts of endogenously synthesized 1,25-(OH)$_2$D appear to accelerate the hepatic catabolism of 25(OH)D. Thus with 1,25(OH)$_2$ treatment or conditions of increased plasma 1,25(OH)$_2$D, the plasma half-life of 25(OH)D is shortened and plasma 25(OH)D levels can be lowered. The metabolic sluice for the cleared 25(OH)D appears to be aqueous-soluble metabolites that are formed in the liver and cleared into the urine (42).

1,25 Dihydroxyvitamin D

Sources

The major physiological source of plasma 1,25-(OH)$_2$D is the kidney, and this is confirmed by the reduced levels seen in chronic renal disease despite chronic, high substrate levels and the strong stimulus of elevated parathyroid hormone (PTH) to the 25(OH)D-1α-hydroxylase (44,45). The elegant endocrine control of mineral homeostasis depends on the presence of this renal enzyme and various factors that affect its activity.

Extrarenal 25(OH)D-1α-hydroxylase activity has been reported in recent years (46,47). For most of these tissues under normal conditions, it appears unlikely that they contribute substantively to the plasma 1,25(OH)$_2$D content. In some conditions, such as the presence of increased numbers of activated macrophages (46,48–52) and, possibly, certain lymphocyte populations, exaggerated extrarenal production and release of 1,25(OH)$_2$D can occur and provoke excessive bone resorption and/or intestinal absorption of calcium.

Plasma Concentrations

The hormonal form of vitamin D, 1,25(OH)$_2$D, circulates at a concentration of 20–60 pg/mL in normal humans (Table 1). Its plasma level is relatively labile, reflecting the rapid turnover of the sterol and the various influences on its synthesis (53,54). When normal levels are considered together with modestly lowered or raised levels encountered in various disorders, this metabolite correlates positively with indexes of intestinal calcium absorption. Lower plasma 1,25(OH)$_2$D levels are seen in normal subjects with high calcium intakes, and vice versa (44,55).

During the development of vitamin D deficiency, the plasma 1,25(OH)$_2$D levels are maintained at normal levels until profound depletion of substrate occurs, presumably the result of PTH stimulation of the 25(OH)D-1α-hydroxylase. It is noteworthy that provision of vitamin D or 25(OH)D to vitamin D deficient patients will result in striking increases (100–200 pg/mL) of plasma 1,25(OH)$_2$D (40,41). When substrate is increased to patients with primary (56) or secondary (45) hyperparathyroidism, increases in plasma 1,25(OH)$_2$D have been observed. It seems reasonable, therefore, to recognize low and high plasma levels of 25(OH)D when trying to interpret plasma $1,25(OH)_2D$ concentrations. Extremes of substrate availability clearly influence plasma $1,25-(OH)_2D$ levels during high stimulation of the 25(OH)D-1α-hydroxylase.

Kinetics

Estimates of the plasma survivorship of $1,25(OH)_2D$ are in the order of hours, with a turnover of 0.5–1.5 μg/day (53,57). In general, variations of plasma $1,25(OH)_2D$ levels are rapid and attributable to variations in production rates. No diurnal variation has been observed (58). Corroboration of these findings was provided by a model of exaggerated $1,25(OH)_2D$ production in humans wherein effects simulated those found in the disorders mimicked (59).

The practical effect of these considerations appears to be that administered $1,25(OH)_2D$ must be given twice daily to sustain its availability to its tissue receptors. Alternative strategies include utilizing daily doses of $1\alpha(OH)D_3$, since hepatic 25-hydroxylation is required for the relatively sustained production of $1,25(OH)_2D_3$. The widespread distribution and catabolism of $1,25(OH)_2D$ have been studied, but clear examples of disordered clearance of this sterol are not currently known.

Other Sterols

Features

An impressive array of other vitamin D metabolites have been described and measured (60,61). Perhaps best known is $24,25(OH)_2D$ since it was initially recognized to be a renal product that was particularly prominent in experiments with radiolabeled substrate (54). $1,24,25(OH)_2D$ has been identified to have potent activity resembling that of $1,25(OH)_2D$, and can be generated from $24,25(OH)_2D$ or $1,25(OH)_2D$ substrates. $25,26-(OH)_2D$ has also been measured in human samples (41).

None of these sterols, however, have the biological potency, regulated production, and high-affinity receptor system that characterizes $1,25(OH)_2D$ (62). It is possible, however, that specific physiological functions can be identified for some of them, and work in this direction continues in several laboratories. During the correction of vitamin D deficiency, however, none of these metabolites are convincingly altered to suggest their role in repairing disordered mineral homeostasis (40,41). Some investigators have reported selective effects of $24,25(OH)_2D$ on cartilage and bone metabolism, and further work in this area is likely.

Plasma Concentrations

Levels of $24,25(OH)_2D$ and $25,26(OH)_2D$ in humans have been assessed. The former has been reported to range from subnanogram to 4 ng/mL (Table 1). $25,26(OH)_2D$ levels are reportedly lower than $24,25(OH)_2D$ levels. Under unusual circumstances, when plasma 25(OH)D levels are very high, these and other metabolites can become detectable or reach high levels. Positive correlations between plasma 25(OH)D and these metabolites have been observed (63,64). Detectable but lower levels of $24,25(OH)_2D$ are seen in anephric humans (65).

ASSAYS OF VITAMIN D STEROLS IN PLASMA

In recent years considerable attention has been given to improvements in assay specificity, sensitivity, precision, and accuracy. More detailed discussions of these new developments can be found in reviews (60,61).

Extraction Techniques

Since the vitamin D compounds are bound to plasma proteins, most of the effective assays for these sterols require extraction. This usually is accomplished by organic solvent extraction, and a variety of solvents can be used. More recently, solid-phase extraction techniques have become popular (61). Recovery estimates through extraction and chromatography are usually monitored by adding known amounts of the sterol in tracer form to the native plasma.

These sterols are sensitive to light, heat, and oxygen. Procedures are designed to avoid direct ultraviolet light and high temperatures, and utilize vacuum or inert gases such as nitrogen or argon in the drying and storage phases of the assays.

Chromatographic Techniques

Some form of chromatography is required to separate these vitamin D sterols from interfering substances and other vitamin D compounds. With the utilization of stereoselective binding reagents, some assays reported the elimination of chromatographic steps, but several reports have indicated the superiority of assays incorporating chromatography (66,67).

A variety of stationary and mobile phases can be used effectively. More powerful separations are usually effected by high-performance liquid chromatography (HPLC) on silica or octadecylsilanized supports (60,61,65) (Fig. 1). Definitive identifications of isolated materials require mass spectroscopy, and some laboratories are applying such techniques to answer problems in sterol quantitation in certain clinical situations (61). Con-

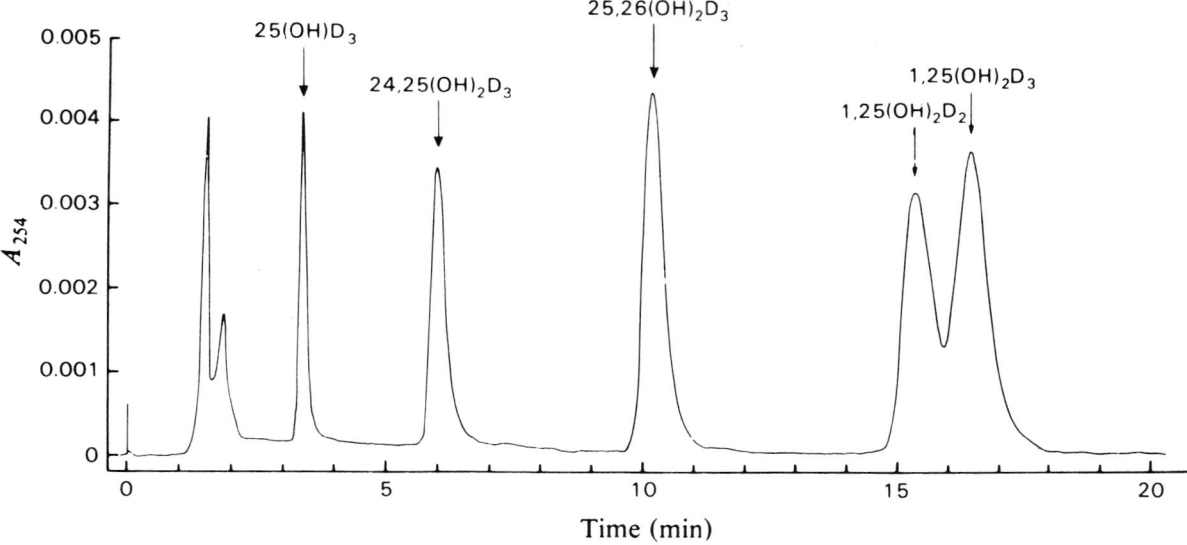

FIG. 1. High-performance liquid chromatography with UV 254 nm detection of the major vitamin D metabolites eluted from a 0.46 × 25 cm column of Zorbax-SIL silicic acid developed in propan-2-ol/hexane (1:9 v/v) at a flow rate of 2 mL/min. (From R. M. Shepard, et al., *Biochem J* 1979;182:55–69.)

venient cartridge forms of straight and reversed-phase supports have become popular (Fig. 2).

Quantitation of Sterols

Physicochemical Assays

Vitamin D

Definitive isolation, identification, and quantitation of vitamin D in foodstuffs and biological fluids usually requires extensive isolation procedures and some form of spectroscopy. Some of these techniques are labor-intensive and have not generally been applied to large numbers of clinical samples. However, some workers have

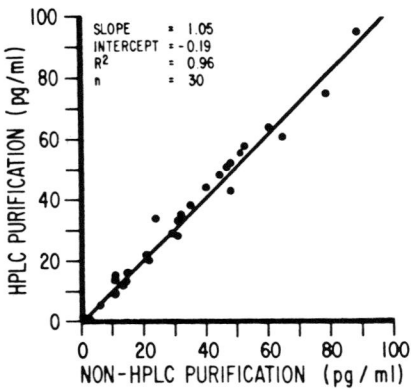

FIG. 2. Comparison of plasma 1,25(OH)$_2$D values obtained using a non-HPLC assay (cartridge chromatography) with an assay that employs both Sephadex LH-20 and HPLC purification before assay by saturation analysis. (From T. A. Reinhardt, et al., *J Clin Endocrinol Metab* 1984;58:91–8.)

utilized multiple steps in assays designed to quantitate D$_2$ and D$_3$ from their HPLC elutions into sensitive detectors (18,60). Other procedures require HPLC separations, derivatizations of the sterols, and gas-liquid chromatography (GLC) and mass spectrometry (MS) (61).

25(OH)D and Other Sterols

HPLC techniques for 25(OH)D and 24,25(OH)$_2$D have been reported (60,64). In general, the abundance and relatively uncluttered chromatographic profile of 25(OH)D have permitted its facile isolation and quantitation. The comparison of 25(OH)D assay results obtained by saturation analyses of chromatographed extracts generally are close to those obtained by HPLC spectroscopy of similar extracts (68). At one time, quantitation of 24,25(OH)$_2$D was popular, and the isolation and quantitation of this sterol was complicated by its coelution with other compounds in plasma. More extensive separations revealed somewhat lower levels of 24,25(OH)$_2$D when contaminating materials were removed (64,65).

Since GLC-MS techniques require expensive instrumentation, their applications have been less extensive than binding assays with comparable or greater sensitivity. However, such definitive technology is obviously helpful in the validation of less specific assay methodology.

Saturation Analyses

Plasma Binding Proteins

Native plasma binding proteins (DBPs) are plentiful, relatively unsaturated with sterols, and provide an inexpensive source of binding reagent in saturation analyses of 25(OH)D, 24,25(OH)$_2$D, and 25,26(OH)$_2$D. The avian plasma protein appears to prefer the cholecalciferol series to the ergocalciferol series, but this degree of specificity has not been developed into a clear-cut, practical advantage for such differential quantitations. The proteins are stable and can provide a high-affinity, specific recognition of the "middle" sterol metabolites in suitably chromatographed extracts of plasma (60,61).

Receptors

Tissue extracts (intestine, thymus, mammary gland) provide the 1,25(OH)$_2$D receptor protein for use in the saturation analyses of this sterol extracted from plasma. The receptor provides a very high affinity, specific binding agent for assay work, although it is relatively labile and requires storage precautions (44,60).

Radioimmunoassays

In recent years several antibodies have been generated to sterol derivative–immunogenic protein complexes. These polyclonal and monoclonal antibodies have been shown to provide excellent binding properties for use in immunoassays of vitamin D and its metabolites (61). In general, however, these reagents have not yet provided the specificity required to permit elmination of chromatographic steps in the preparation of samples for assay. However, these proteins are relatively hardy and their use makes tissue receptor extractions unnecessary.

General

Following extraction and chromatography, the added tracers and native sterols are presented to the binding reagent (binding protein, receptor, antibody) in a buffer containing colloid to minimize sterol adherence to glassware. Incubations are relatively brief, and some form of bound/free separation is effected, usually with an adsorbent. Competition by the unknown sterol is compared with that of pure, reference standard in a displacement curve (Fig. 3). Results are corrected for volume of plasma extracted and the recovery achieved during the extraction and chromatography steps. Some workers have reported excellent results by applying multiple saturation analysis assays to their extensively chromatographed plasma extracts (60,65). A modern bioassay for 1,25(OH)$_2$D depends on its osteolytic properties in bone cultures, after suitable chromatographic isolation (69). In addition, a cytoreceptor assay employs intact cells to reveal the amount of displacement of labeled 1,25(OH)$_2$D by radio-inert 1,25(OH)$_2$D from receptor sites (70).

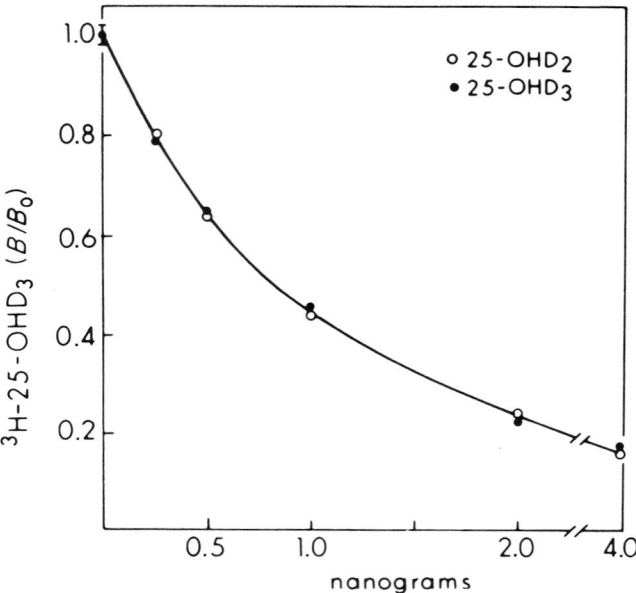

FIG. 3. Competitive binding radioassay of 25(OH)D$_3$ and 25(OH)D$_2$ utilizing a 1:5000 dilution of normal human serum as the source of binding protein. (From J. G. Haddad, *Methods of hormone radioimmunoassay*, 2nd ed., Academic Press, New York, 1979;441.)

PLASMA BINDING PROTEINS

Chylomicrons and Lipoproteins

Oral Route for Vitamin D

After ingestion of vitamin D compounds, they are absorbed into the intestinal chyle, associated with lipid carriers. On entry into the venous circulation, some exchange of vitamin D onto DBP can occur, but the hepatic delivery of ingested vitamin D appears to be aided by its association with chylomicron remnants (22,71). Vitamin D deficiency has not been reported as a result of acquired or genetic disorders of chylomicrons and lipoproteins. This may reflect the existence of non-dietary (cutaneous) sources of the vitamin in such individuals.

Other Transport

Specific information on the nature of egress of cutaneously synthesized vitamin D is not available, although some investigators believe that DBP plays a role since other products and precursors in skin are not as favored ligands as is vitamin D (11,12). However, lipid shuttles from the periphery to the liver can be effected by other carriers, and low-density lipoproteins can facilitate hepatic entry of vitamin D (22,71). Several studies of parenterally injected vitamin D indicate some association of vitamin D with lipoprotein carriers in addition to binding to DBP. In contrast, other vitamin D metabolites appear to be bound by DBP and albumin (31) (Table 2).

Vitamin D–Binding Protein

Physicochemical Features

DBP, a carrier of vitamin D and its metabolites, is a 58-kD α-globulin in human plasma (22). It is identical to group-specific component (Gc-globulin), a plasma protein studied extensively by geneticists (72). DBP has striking homology with α-fetoprotein and serum albumin (73). Codominant alleles are recognized, and although over 100,000 sera have been analyzed, the absence of DBP has never been detected. It is believed that severe mutations or deletions of the DBP gene are lethal events.

DBP is a single-chain polypeptide with a pI value of 4.7, minor carbohydrate components, and a sedimentation coefficient of 3.5S. It is a significant component of plasma α-globulins, with a concentration of approximately 6 μM. The protein is synthesized in the liver and higher plasma concentrations are found during pregnancy and in subjects receiving estrogen treatment (22,73).

Ligand-Binding Characteristics

Sterol-binding preferences of DBP are 25(OH)D = 24,25(OH)$_2$D = 25,26(OH)$_2$D > 1,25(OH)$_2$D > vitamin D. An unusual metabolite, 25(OH)D$_3$-26,23 lactone, has been observed to be more tightly bound than 25(OH)D, but it is a minor constituent of plasma when high substrate levels are present. The D$_2$ and D$_3$ series are equally bound by mammalian DBP (22). Binding affinity for 25(OH)D indicates a K_d of 5 × 10^{-8} M. There is one sterol-binding site per molecule of DBP, and binding to DBP confers aqueous solubility and protection of the sterols. Common DBP alleles appear to have similar, if not identical, binding properties.

Plasma Kinetics and Tissue Distribution

Kinetic studies of the plasma clearance and production of DBP indicate that it turns over more rapidly than the dominant plasma metabolite 25(OH)D (22). The protein constitutes a high-affinity, high-capacity, and high-turnover system for the plasma transport of vitamin D sterols. In humans and animals, DBP undergoes catabolism to small peptides found in urine, and to a lesser extent, in stool. In the rabbit, occupancy of DBP by 25(OH)D$_3$ does not alter its plasma clearance. Similarly, sialidase treatment of DBP does not change its plasma half-life (74). In humans the plasma half-life of DBP is approximately 2.5–3.0 days. The daily production rate in humans is 800 mg/day or 10 mg/kg body weight per day (75).

The precise tissue disposition of plasma DBP is not known, but reports have indicated in some species a more rapid clearance of DBP complexed to actin in the circulation (76–78). Disorders of the metabolism of DBP are not currently known.

Role in Sterol Transport

Compared with its major sterol ligand, 25(OH)D, there is a 40- to 50-fold molar excess of DBP in the plasma of normal humans (22). The normal plasma concentration of DBP is approximately 6 × 10^{-6} M (about 350 μg/mL), whereas vitamin D sterol concentrations usually do not exceed 10^{-7} M (about 40 ng/mL). Variations in sunlight exposure can increase sterol levels severalfold, but even under these conditions only a small fraction of the available binding sites is occupied. Only with pharmacological administration of vitamin D or 25(OH)D will plasma sterol concentrations exceed 10^{-6} M in humans (14,23,34,79). It is important to note that vitamin D intoxication occurs at 25(OH)D concentrations that are well below 6 × 10^{-6} M. It appears, therefore, that full occupancy of plasma DBP does not occur during vitamin D therapy (79,80).

With sterol occupancy of DBP, both the sterol and protein appear to be protected from chemical modifications, and aqueous solubility is conferred to the sterols. There is variable but high affinity for all vitamin D sterols, and many estimates have been made (22,80). There are difficulties in measuring the precise affinity of binding between aqueous and lipid-soluble substances, but estimates under various conditions have provided useful information (22,81). Calculations of the amounts of DBP and sterols and of their binding affinity can provide estimates of the "free" sterol available to tissues (81). When direct analyses of free sterol concentrations were eventually performed (31,82–84), there was a reasonable correlation to the calculated estimates, but the influence of albumin was better assessed with the direct observations (83,84). Although equations for calculating the free concentrations of these sterols in human plasma have been devised, the occupancy of DBP by sterols other than the one under consideration is rarely considered. Further refinement of these estimates can be expected. Occupancy of DBP by favored ligands [e.g., 25(OH)D] would influence the estimate of free 1,25(OH)$_2$D (less avidly bound ligand) derived from calculations independent of 25(OH)D concentrations. A variety of studies appear to support the idea that plasma free 1,25(OH)$_2$D concentration is regulated and reflects the biological effect of this sterol (31,81–88).

Most of the vitamin D metabolites are carried by DBP, with lesser amounts on albumin or lipoprotein carriers (22,71) (Table 2). In a variety of studies in situ (71,87) or in vitro (85,86,88), the presence of DBP appears to slow down or inhibit the tissue or cell entrance of vitamin D sterols. The presence of DBP on the surfaces of various cells has been shown, and suggested that a cell-associated DBP may have a role in the facilitated

TABLE 2. *Features of plasma carriers of vitamin D metabolites*

	DBP	Albumin
Molecular weight	58 kD	67 kD
Plasma concentration	6 μM	600 μM
Sterol binding sites	mol/mol	?
Percent of bound ligand on carrier	88 [25(OH)D] 85 [1,25(OH)$_2$D]	12 [25-OHD] 15 [1,25(OH)$_2$D]
Affinity of ligand for carrier	[25(OH)D$_3$] $5 \times 10^8\ M^{-1}$ [1,25(OH)$_2$D$_3$] $4 \times 10^7\ M^{-1}$	[25(OH)D$_3$] $6 \times 10^5\ M^{-1}$ [1,25(OH)$_2$D$_3$] $5 \times 10^4\ M$
Estrogen effect on carrier concentration	↑	↔

↑, increase. ↔ no change.

delivery of sterols to these cells (89–92). The recent demonstrations of the binding of other steroid-carrying plasma proteins to cells is interesting in this regard (93,94). However, there is no current evidence that cell-associated DBP plays a role in sterol transport into cells.

Actin-Binding Property

For awhile, the vitamin D receptor investigations were hampered by the presence of a large (5–6S) macromolecule in cell extracts that displayed affinities for vitamin D sterols identical to those of DBP. It was later discovered that this molecule represented a mole-per-mole complex of DBP with globular actin (G-actin) (22). Very high affinity binding ($K_d \sim 2 \times 10^{-9}\ M$) has been observed between these proteins. DBP–G-actin has the same affinity and capacity for vitamin D sterols as does DBP alone. The affinity between these proteins is not substantially altered by DBP phenotype, ionic milieu, or physiological changes in pH (95).

Careful analyses of the effects of DBP on actin have revealed that DBP sequesters G-actin and prevents its assembly into filamentous actin (F-actin) (22). Since DBP–actin complexes have been found in the plasma of patients with ongoing tissue destruction (hepatitis, trophoblastic emboli) (73), studies have been directed to understanding a possible role for DBP in preventing intravascular filament formation. Another plasma protein, gelsolin, can sever F-actin, and it is possible that it and DBP constitute a multifunctional actin-scavenger system in plasma. Recently, this system was demonstrated to be saturable, with the formation of intravascular filaments and platelet microthrombi seen after infusion of large amounts of G-actin (96). The action of DBP on G-actin resembles that seen with intracellular proteins, DNase-I, and profilin, but the affinity of G-actin for DBP is 1000-fold higher than for profilin (95).

ASSAYS OF DBP

Saturation Analyses with Ligand

Prior to the isolation of DBP and the development of immunoprobes, information about the titer of DBP in plasma was afforded by estimating the ability of plasma to bind vitamin D sterols. The number of specific and high-affinity binding sites in plasma was determined by techniques alluded to earlier. Aliquots of plasma are incubated with increasing amounts of sterol, usually 25(OH)D$_3$ in radioactive and radio-inert forms, to detect how much sterol is required to saturate the specific binding sites in plasma (Fig. 3). A variety of techniques have been used to separate the bound and free moieties of this sterol (adsorbents, gel filtration, sucrose gradient ultracentrifugation, electrophoresis) (80,97).

Although saturation analyses provide an estimate of binding affinity as well as capacity, there are no known disorders of binding affinity by DBP. Further, the saturation assays appear to underestimate the plasma DBP content by approximately 50% (97), presumably due to the disruptive techniques involved, although occupancy by other ligands has not been excluded completely. Overall, therefore, saturation assays have largely been replaced by immunoassays for plasma DBP.

Immunoassays

The circulating concentration of DBP in healthy persons is approximately 5–8 μM (300–400 μg/mL) by a variety of immunological assay techniques. Earlier precipitation techniques were directed toward the then-known Gc-globulin (98). These have been supplanted by other methods that can be selected for the purposes intended (80,97).

Radial Immunodiffusion

This assay technique is widely used, for it has the sensitivity required for direct serum analyses and is simple and reliable. Suitable antiserum is uniformly dispersed in agar on plates. From wells in the agar, the distance traveled by the DBP prior to its immunoprecipitation is proportional to the amount applied (99–103). Correlations of this technique with radioimmunoassay (102) and nephelometry (103) have been made with good agreement.

Rocket Immunoelectrophoresis

This technique also provides useful information by direct serum applications (104,105). Immunoprecipitation "rocket" heights are proportional to the amount of DBP applied to the gel (Fig. 4). This assay is sensitive to the presence of actin-DBP complexes in plasma, however. The additional negative charge of G-actin results in rocket heights greater than can be explained by DBP concentration alone (105). In the absence of these complexes, as occurs normally, the technique provides reliable information.

Radioimmunoassay

Very sensitive assay methodology has relied on the radioimmunoassay (102,106). For serum analyses, however, considerable dilution of samples is required, and larger experimental errors are encountered (97). The assay relies on the competition between radioactive and radio-inert forms of DBP for binding to anti-DBP antibody. In some studies of fluids in which DBP content is low, the technique would be preferred (107). Other methods, involving enzyme-linked immunosorbancy (ELISA) or immunoradiometric assay (IRMA) could prove useful for extensive screening purposes (108).

FREE STEROL CONCENTRATIONS

In recent years, the importance of estimating (81) and measuring (31,82–84) the free concentrations of vitamin

D metabolites has become apparent. Clinical conditions associated with variations in plasma albumin and DBP imposed the need to consider how much of the measured plasma sterol content was available to the tissues (Table 1).

Estimated Concentration

Calculations of free 25(OH)D or 1,25(OH)$_2$D in plasma depend on estimates of the affinity between these sterols and DBP or albumin (83), as well as the number of binding sites (unknown for albumin) per binding protein, along with the total concentrations of sterols and carriers (Table 2). Initially, only DBP was considered (81), but a model including albumin has been supported by direct experimentation (83). The following affinity constants have been determined for 1,25(OH)$_2$D$_3$:

$$K_A(DBP) = 4.2 \times 10^7 \ M^{-1}$$

$$K_A(albumin) = 5.4 \times 10^4 \ M^{-1}$$

The higher affinity binding was confirmed by direct analyses of the high-affinity binding displayed by human serum, and the lower affinity binding site was observed in analyses of DBP-free serum. The latter analyses correlated with measurements made using human serum albumin alone. Similar analyses for 25(OH)D$_3$ have been made:

$$K_A(DBP) = 7 \times 10^8 \ M^{-1}$$

$$K_A(albumin) = 6 \times 10^5 \ M^{-1}$$

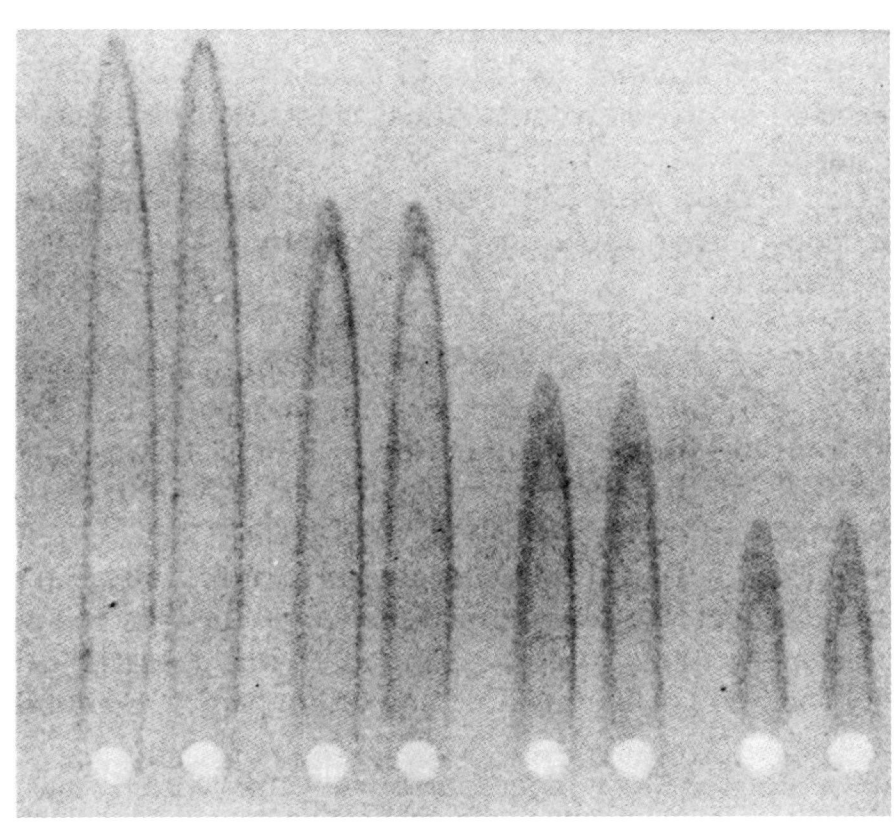

FIG. 4. Rocket immunoelectrophoresis assay of human serum DBP. Duplicate determinations of 0.4, 0.3, 0.2, and 0.1 µg of hDBP are shown. (From P. G. Walsh, et al., *Clin Chem* 1982;28: 1781–3.)

In practice, albumin and DBP are similar in size and charge, and usually their plasma concentrations vary coordinately in diseases characterized by protein losses (nephrotic syndrome) or poor production (liver diseases). However, DBP but not albumin production is enhanced during pregnancy and estrogen therapy (22,81,82). Since most of the total plasma 25(OH)D or 1,25(OH)₂D is bound to DBP, earlier applications of the law of mass action, including DBP alone (81), provided proportional estimates to those that included considerations of the influence of albumin. In brief, the physicochemical equilibrium between sterol and carrier is reflected in these estimates. For estimating the free sterol concentration, an equation reflecting the law of mass action,

$$K_A = \frac{SR}{S_f \cdot R_f}$$

where SR is the concentration of sterol–receptor complexes, R_f is the concentration of unoccupied receptor, and S_f is the concentration of free sterol (109), can be applied. Results have also been expressed as the "free sterol index," or

$$\frac{\text{plasma total sterol concentration (molar)}}{\text{plasma DBP concentration (molar)}}$$

Measured Concentration

The centrifugofiltration technique has been applied to analyses of the free concentrations of 25(OH)D and 1,25(OH)₂D in serum (31,82–84). Purified [³H]sterol and [¹⁴C]glucose (distribution of free water, volume of ultrafiltrate) are dried under N_2 and 0.45 mL of diluted serum are added. After incubation for 45 min at 37°C in a shaking water bath, two 200-μL aliquots are applied to the inner tube of an ultrafiltration vial containing a 12,000-molecular weight dialysis membrane. The samples are centrifuged at 2000g for 90 min, and the contents of the outer vial (ultrafiltrate) and inner tube (serum) are analyzed by dual-label scintillation spectroscopy:

percent free sterol

$$= \frac{[^3H]\text{ultrafiltrate}}{[^{14}C]\text{ultrafiltrate}} \cdot \frac{[^{14}C]\text{serum}}{[^3H]\text{serum}} \times 100$$

The free fraction in this diluted sample is extrapolated to the whole serum by multiplying by the dilution, and carries two assumptions: (1) that the dilution used is on a linear part of the plot of the reciprocal of the free fraction of sterol versus the concentration of the binding components in serum, and (2) that the intercept on the y-axis of this plot is insignificant in relationship to the value of the reciprocal of the free fraction measured in the sample. In general, serum dilutions of 1:10 to 1:100 fit these criteria

for the vitamin D sterol analyses. Additional analyses of the contributions to binding by DBP or albumin have been made (83,84).

Free 25(OH)D levels in normal plasma are approximately 0.03% of total 25(OH)D concentrations and range from 2.5 to 10 pg/mL. About 80% of the bound sterol is bound to DBP, with the remainder mostly on albumin. The percentage of the total sterol that is free or filtrable varies negatively with the DBP and/or albumin concentrations in plasma. Positive correlations are observed between total plasma 25(OH)D and these proteins.

Free 1,25(OH)₂D levels in normal plasma are approximately 0.4% of total 1,25(OH)₂D concentrations and range from 100 to 200 fg/mL (Table 1). About 85% of the bound 1,25(OH)₂D is DBP-bound, with the remainder on albumin. The percentage of the total plasma 1,25(OH)₂D that is free is negatively correlated to DBP concentrations (Fig. 5). The total 1,25(OH)₂D levels correlate positively with DBP concentrations.

At present, direct analyses of free sterol concentrations are research techniques. The influences of plasma carrier concentrations on total sterol levels and their interpretation seems clear, however. Accurate interpretation of total sterol levels necessitates measurement of the plasma protein carriers. In some instances, direct measurement of free sterol levels may be required since other conditions may affect the binding equilibria and these analyses are just beginning to be applied to various clinical conditions. For example, additional studies are needed to evaluate the influence of DBP occupancy by 25(OH)D on the free 1,25(OH)₂D fraction.

Clinical Considerations

At the present time, clinical interest in vitamin D metabolism promotes interest in the quantitation of 25(OH)D and 1,25(OH)₂D assays. Other investigative work can also rely on the quantitation of vitamin D and other metabolites, but the majority of information helpful to the clinician can be derived from the 25(OH)D and 1,25(OH)₂D assays.

For interpretation of assay results, attention certainly must be given to the clinical situation. Information about time outdoors, season, clothing, skin pigmentation, medications, diet, and dietary supplements are useful. Furthermore, the 1,25(OH)₂D assay result can also be helpful since this sterol, in elevated titer, can alter the hepatic metabolism and increase the renal excretion of 25(OH)D (42,43).

Multiple factors appear to influence the production of 1,25(OH)₂D (54). It is helpful, therefore, to make an assessment of blood substrate [25(OH)D] availability, renal function, blood parathyroid hormone, calcium, inorganic phosphorus, as well as diet and hormonal thera-

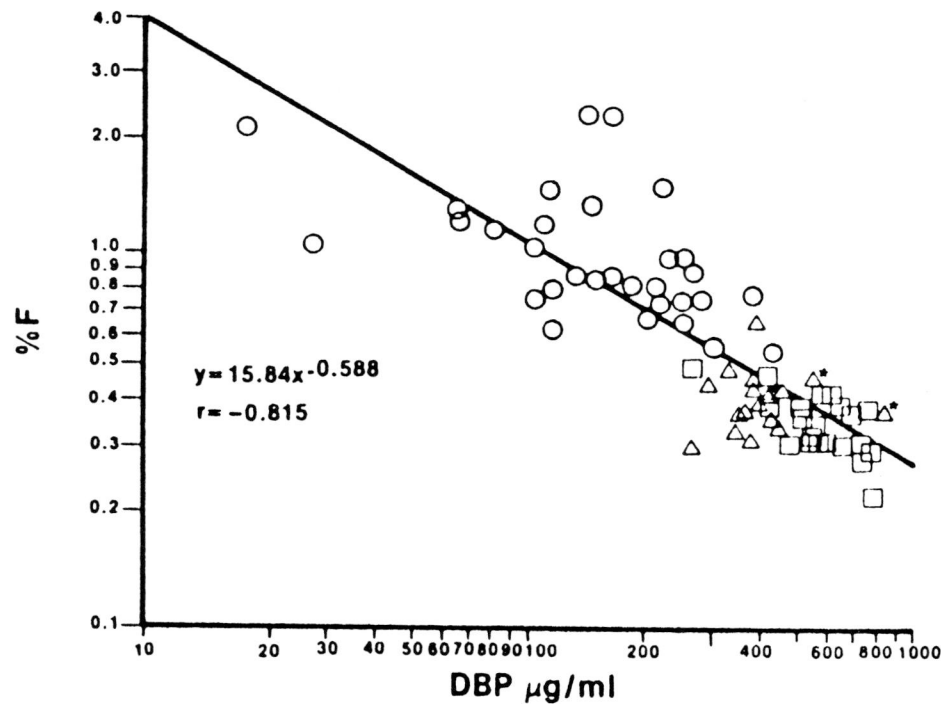

FIG. 5. Log/log plot of the plasma DBP levels and percent free plasma 1,25(OH)$_2$D in 18 normal subjects ($\triangle$), 34 subjects with liver disease (O), 17 pregnant subjects ($\square$), and normal subjects receiving oral contraceptives (*). (From D. D. Bikle et al., *J Clin Invest* 1984; 74:1966–71.)

pies when evaluating blood levels of 1,25(OH)$_2$D. Significant alterations in the blood concentration of DBP and albumin can affect estimates of the "free" vitamin D sterol available to tissues (31,82–84) (Tables 1 and 2).

Age, Sex, and Race

25(OH)D

The plasma 25(OH)D level is a reliable index of vitamin D stores, and values between 5 and 10 ng/mL indicate marginal vitamin D sufficiency. Values below that indicate vitamin D deficiency of some degree. In some areas of the world, a large percentage of the population exhibit marginal sufficiency of vitamin D body stores. Conversely, higher levels are seen in populations exposed to more sunlight and foods fortified with vitamin D (7,40,110).

Advancing age appears to be an indirect factor in lowering plasma 25(OH)D levels. Assuming normal skin synthesis, intestinal absorption, and hepatic metabolism, this sterol's concentration in blood reflects substrate availability. A variety of illnesses, however, can compromise one's appetite, intestinal absorption, and ability and/or desire to spend time outdoors—thereby increasing the likelihood of depleting vitamin D stores by nonreplacement.

On the other hand, prematurity constitutes a threat to vitamin D status in several ways. At premature birth, the placental transfer of sterols from the maternal circulation is lost, and the immature neonatal intestine does not

absorb fats reliably (111). The premature infant cannot reliably take in sufficient breast milk to benefit from that marginal source of vitamin D sterols. Finally, the ability of the immature infant to metabolize vitamin D to 25(OH)D has not been fully characterized.

Although there are no apparent influences of gender on vitamin D sources and 25(OH)D production, the combination of the practice of purdah and a vegetarian diet can increase the probability of vitamin D depletion. Since darker-pigmented skin requires more intense or protracted ultraviolet light exposure for production of cholecalciferol, the relocation of dark-skinned subjects to areas receiving less effective solar irradiation can predispose them to deficient vitamin D production and lower 25(OH)D levels in plasma (11,21).

1,25(OH)$_2$D

In contrast, plasma 1,25(OH)$_2$D concentrations do not reflect vitamin D stores reliably. Rather, they reflect the adequacy of substrate provision to and ionic and hormonal regulation of the 25(OH)D-1α-hydroxylase (54). Feedback regulation by PTH, calcium, and inorganic phosphorus keeps this sterol's plasma concentration fairly constant in the face of wide-ranging amounts of substrate. Some moderate increases have been reported with increased substrate to normal subjects, however.

Although elderly subjects appear to have a reduced 25(OH)D-1α-hydroxylase capacity or responsivity to stimulation (70,112), this appears to be due to the loss of nephrons and/or reduced substrate availability. In older subjects with preserved renal function, perfectly normal

1,25(OH)$_2$D production is seen (113). Premature infants may have a reduced ability to produce 1,25(OH)$_2$D, but this is not certain.

There are no clear-cut differences in 1,25(OH)$_2$D levels attributable to sex or race. Pregnancy can be associated with higher DBP and total 1,25(OH)$_2$D levels in plasma. Free 1,25(OH)$_2$D levels, however, appear to increase in late pregnancy (81,82).

Hormones and Ions

25(OH)D

Extensive investigations have not revealed clear-cut regulation of 25(OH)D production or catabolism by alterations in plasma ions or peptide hormones. Increases of 1,25(OH)$_2$D in plasma, however, can accelerate the conjugation of 25(OH)D into water-soluble esters that are excreted in the urine (42,43). Thus low-calcium diets, hyperparathyroidism (primary and secondary), and 1,25(OH)$_2$D treatment could increase 25(OH)D catabolism and shorten the plasma survivorship of 25(OH)D. Although the precise mechanism is not defined, it appears to be designed to limit 25(OH)D availability during increased 1,25(OH)$_2$D production.

1,25(OH)$_2$D

The major hormonal stimulus to the 25(OH)D-1-α-hydroxylase is parathyroid hormone. In some studies, calcitonin has been shown to stimulate this enzyme in certain parts of the nephron, but the important correlation between a peptide hormone and this enzyme's activity or plasma 1,25(OH)$_2$D concentration is that with parathyroid hormone (114) or the PTH-related peptide (115). Careful studies have shown correlations among bone resorption or calcium absorption efficiency, PTH, and 1,25(OH)$_2$D levels in plasma (55,59,116). The correlations can be influenced by ionic effects (116,117). Increases of plasma calcium can blunt or negate the trophic effect of PTH on 1,25(OH)$_2$D production (114,117). In contrast, lowered calcium levels do not appear to regulate the stimulatory effect of PTH or phosphorus (118).

It is recognized that inorganic phosphorus often has a negative correlation with plasma 1,25(OH)$_2$D levels in plasma (114,116). This can occur in the absence of PTH, reflecting a phosphate-dependent pathway. This also occurs in the absence of sustained decreases in serum phosphate (119). There are sufficient exceptions to convince one that the plasma phosphate level does not always reflect the level of phosphate in the ionic milieu vicinal to the mitochondrial 25(OH)D-1α-hydroxylase (54). Phosphorus deprivation (116,119–121) and the hypophosphatemia of hyperparathyroidism (114,122) are associated with elevated plasma 1,25(OH)$_2$D, but some

genetic disorders of renal phosphate conservation (123,124) and oncogenic osteomalacia (125) are associated with lower levels of this sterol in blood. It therefore seems likely that altered distribution of intracellular phosphate, deranged enzyme regulation, or disturbances in the renal tubular flux of phosphate ions could be responsible for the variety of responses observed.

Vitamin D Deficiency

In the adult, protracted periods of deficient solar exposure and inadequate vitamin D ingestion are required to reach the vitamin D deficient state (Table 3). Assuming reasonably good body stores initially, several months of deficient cutaneous production and dietary vitamin D lack are required to deplete these stores. Additional threats to the economy of vitamin D would be expected when accelerated catabolism of vitamin D occurs, such as when 1,25(OH)$_2$D levels are high (42,43) and when hepatic microsomal P450 enzyme activities are stimulated by drugs such as diphenylhydantoin (126,127).

25(OH)D

With severe depletion, plasma levels of 25(OH)D fall below 2 ng/mL and may become undetectable in routine assays not designed for high sensitivity. Under these circumstances, other metabolites such as 24,25(OH)$_2$D are also undetectably low (41). When 25(OH)D levels fall into this range, the availability of substrate to the 25(OH)D-1α-hydroxylase is insufficient to allow an appropriate amount of 1,25(OH)$_2$D production. It is important to remember that these circumstances are characterized by insufficient intestinal calcium transport and secondary hyperparathyroidism.

1,25(OH)$_2$D

During the initial phase of vitamin D deficiency, plasma levels of 1,25(OH)$_2$D can be normal, and this can be attributed to the stimulation of the 25(OH)D-1α-hydroxylase by parathyroid hormone, overcoming shrinking substrate availability (128,129). Since parathyroid hormone levels are high, however, the calcium and/or 1,25(OH)$_2$D signals to the parathyroid glands are insufficient to reduce the biosynthesis and secretion of PTH (130,131). Provision of substrate rapidly results in a striking increase of plasma 1,25(OH)$_2$D (41,132), clearly indicating that the original 1,25(OH)$_2$D levels were inappropriately low for the needs of the system (Fig. 6). It is also likely that vitamin D deficiency can limit the amount of total plasma 1,25(OH)$_2$D that is available ("free") to enter cells, since a reduction of 25(OH)D would result in an increase in available binding sites for other sterols, including 1,25(OH)$_2$D. With protracted

TABLE 3. *Plasma concentrations[a] of vitamin D metabolites and DBP in various clinical disorders*

Condition	25(OH)D	1,25(OH)$_2$D	DBP
Low calcium intake	↔, ↓	↑	↔
High calcium intake	↔	↓	↔
Low phosphorus intake	↔, ↓	↑	↔
High phosphorus intake	↔	↔, ↓	↔
Vitamin D deficiency			
Early	↓↓	↔	↔
Late	↓↓↓	↓	↔
Treated deficiency (early)	↑	↑↑	↔
Late winter	↓	↔	↔
Late summer	↑	↔	↔
Hypervitaminosis D			
D	↑↑↑	↔, ↓	↔
25(OH)D	↑↑↑	↔, ↓	↔
1,25(OH)$_2$D	↔, ↓	↑↑	↔
Dihydrotachysterol[b]	↔, ↓	"↑"	↔
Pregnancy, estrogen treatment	↔, ↑	↔, ↑	↑
Malabsorption	↔, ↓	↔, ↓	↔, ↓
Cirrhosis of liver[c]	↔, ↓	↔, ↓	↔, ↓
Nephrotic syndromes	↔, ↓	↔, ↓	↔, ↓
Anticonvulsant treatment	↔, ↓	↔, ↓	↔
Hyperparathyroidism	↔, ↓	↔, ↑	↔
Hypercalcemia of malignancy	↔, ↓	↔, ↓	↔, ↓
Hypoparathyroidism	↔	↓	↔
Hyperthyroidism	↔	↓	↔
Chronic renal failure	↔	↓	↔
Hypercalcemia in granulomatous disorders	↔	↑	↔
Tumor-induced osteomalacia	↔	↓	↔
Idiopathic hypercalciuria	↔	↑	↔
X-linked hypophosphatemia	↔	↔, ↓	↔
Vitamin D dependency, I	↔	↓	↔
Vitamin D dependency, II	↔	↑↑↑	↔

[a] ↔, normal; ↑ increased; ↓ decreased. ↑↑, markedly increased; ↓↓ markedly decreased; ↓↓↓ greatly decreased; "↑" increase of 25-hydroxydihydrotachysterol.
[b] A DHT metabolite competes in 1,25(OH)$_2$D CPBA.
[c] Normal free sterol concentrations.

deficiency, however, substrate depletion results in very low 1,25(OH)$_2$D levels in plasma (41,132).

Vitamin D Intoxication

There appears to be a wide margin of safety between vitamin D sufficiency and deleterious excess, as judged by parameters of mineral homeostasis. Physiological routes and sources of vitamin D are not known to cause intoxication. Pharmacological preparations are required, and these are in the order of 1–5 mg (40,000–200,000 IU) daily doses for weeks to months in humans (79,133,134). The bioavailability of such doses varies with the routes and vehicles used (25). Time is required for metabolism to 25(OH)D, but shorter periods to excess are expected if 25(OH)D is the sterol administered. The potent 1,25(OH)$_2$D can produce intoxication very quickly (135).

Studies have shown that vitamin D intoxication can occur in the absence of renal tissue (136,137), and it is generally agreed that a variety of metabolites, in high titer, can stimulate tissues responsible for major

amounts of calcium translocation and hypercalcemia. Under these circumstances, intoxication occurs at high 25(OH)D levels (200–1200 ng/mL) that do not appear sufficient to saturate DBP binding sites (22,80). Plasma 1,25(OH)$_2$D concentrations are normal to low, but little attention has been given to the availability of plasma 1,25(OH)$_2$D when considerably more of the plasma DBP binding sites are taken up by a preferred ligand—25(OH)D. Under these circumstances, a higher percentage of the less-avidly bound ligand, 1,25(OH)$_2$D should be available to the tissues.

Effective therapy of vitamin D intoxication usually reflects interruption of the actions of the sterol at the intestine and bone and is not clearly reflected by alterations in sterol production or catabolism. Adrenocortical steroids are effective (138) by reducing osteolysis and intestinal calcium transfer. Actual reduction of sterol stores requires prolonged abstinence from pharmacological vitamin D preparations (139,140). Shorter periods are required after 1,25(OH)$_2$D toxicity.

The sterols responsible for the intoxication are not always clearly defined since total 1,25(OH)$_2$D levels may be low, normal, or increased (79). However, toxicity in

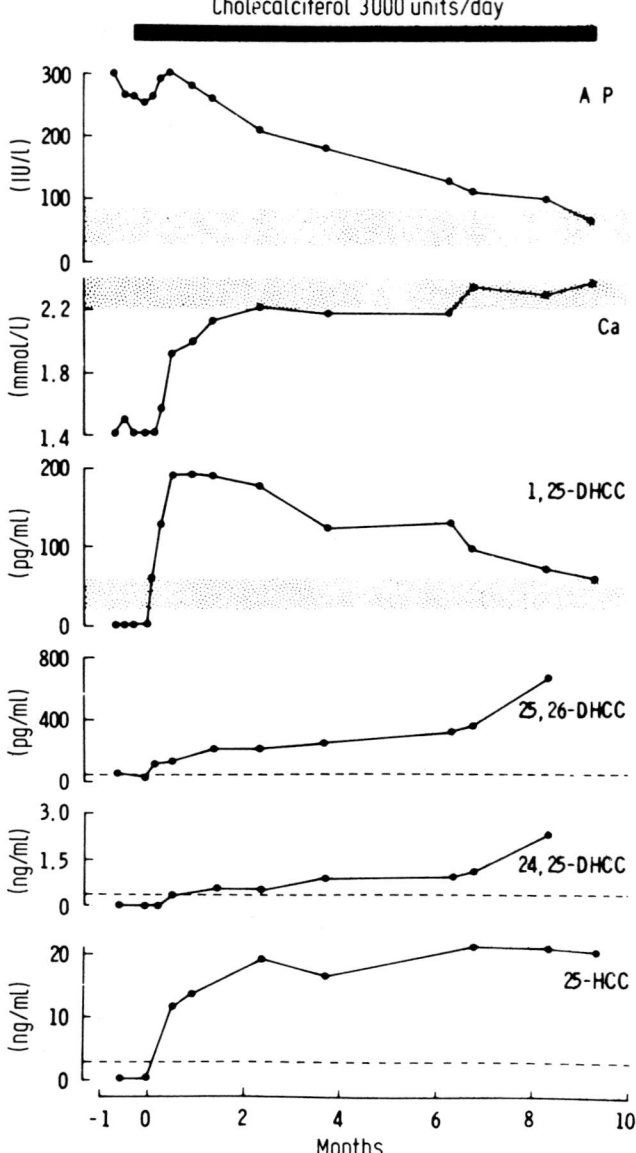

FIG. 6. Sequential observations of serum alkaline phosphatase, calcium, and vitamin D metabolites in a patient with vitamin D deficiency before and after treatment with cholecalciferol. Stippled areas denote the normal ranges. (From S. E. Papapoulos et al., *Lancet* 1980;2:612–15.)

anephric animals and humans (136,137) suggests that sterols without 1α-hydroxyl functions can be causative. Since other sterols can occupy the 1,25(OH)₂D receptor less avidly, logarithmic increases in their titer may explain their ability to overstimulate target tissues through receptor mechanisms.

Other factors can influence sensitivity to vitamin D intoxication. Disorders with extrarenal 25(OH)D-1α-hydroxylase activity (48–52) would sensitize such subjects to increased substrate presentation, as would such enzyme activity in certain lymphomas (141). A common modulator of bone turnover, such as estrogen (142), can be protective against intoxication, but its influence may

also be dependent on its induction of DBP synthesis, thereby requiring larger doses of vitamin D to achieve the metabolite levels associated with intoxication.

Disorders Associated with Vitamin D Therapy

Supplements with vitamin D involve dosages in the range 400–1000 IU/day, but therapeutic applications involve larger doses. Since some delay is required for metabolism in vivo, some physicians have advocated using a loading-dose period prior to estimating the daily dosage required to sustain the desired effect. With the availability of more potent materials, such as $1\alpha(OH)D_3$ and $1,25(OH)_2D_3$, much lower doses are required. Preparations and routes of administration are varied and can be adapted to the needs dictated by a given patient's needs and abilities.

Hypoparathyroidism and Pseudohypoparathyroidism

In these disorders, vitamin D therapy can be considered as a controlled form of intoxication when one realizes that the vitamin forms are being utilized as a PTH surrogate. Of course, vitamin D compounds cannot faithfully substitute for PTH and all of its actions. With regard to providing the $1,25(OH)_2D$ not being synthesized in these disorders because of the lack of sufficient PTH stimulus and high phosphate levels, the treatment with $1,25(OH)_2D$ can be considered a replacement form of treatment. Calcium reclamation at the renal tubule is not restored, however, and many practitioners add a thiazide to the regimen to decrease the hypercalciuria seen during treatment with vitamin D compounds. Often the treatment is to restore serum calcium to the low-normal range to avoid marked hypercalciuria and hypercalcemia.

It is important to remember that some subjects with mild or incomplete hypoparathyroidism may not require vitamin D therapy, and can be managed with large supplements of calcium (143). When therapy with vitamin D is required, there has been an increasing trend toward utilizing $1,25(OH)_2D_3$ since more rapid effects are seen and exaggerated stores of less potent forms can lead to intoxication periods of greater duration. When vitamin D is used, doses of 1–2.5 mg/day are usually sufficient, and higher doses lead to more frequent episodes of hypercalcemia (144). Compliance with dosage recommendations can be checked by assaying the plasma 25(OH)D level, although its correlation to dosage can be considered only a rough correlation (145,146).

Since an important component of such therapy is exaggerated transfer of calcium from the intestinal lumen, the provision of adequate dietary or supplemental calcium is helpful. At higher intakes of calcium, some intestinal transfer occurs by bulk diffusion, and this would complement that absorbed by the active transport mechanism stimulated by vitamin D.

Provision of vitamin D treatment as $1,25(OH)_2D_3$ usually requires 0.5–2.0 μg/dL in divided doses, assuming total elemental calcium daily intake to be 1.5–3.0 g in divided doses. In general, assays of $1,25(OH)_2D$ in plasma are not helpful and can be confusing when estimating the levels obtained during treatment. This is due to the relatively volatile excursions of this plasma sterol across such therapy. Since $1,25(OH)_2D$ treatment can exaggerate 25(OH)D losses (42,43), plasma 25(OH)D could be lowered.

Gastrointestinal and Hepatobiliary Disorders

A variety of disorders of the hepatobiliary and gastrointestinal tracts can impair vitamin D absorption and increase the likelihood of developing vitamin D deficiency (15,147–154) (Table 3). If one assumes the view that cutaneous production of vitamin D_3 is the physiological source (7), only subjects with a heavy dependence on dietary vitamin D are likely to become vitamin D deficient during malabsorption. This is, indeed, the case (151). There have been concerns that an impaired enterohepatic circulation of biologically active vitamin D sterols could imperil sterol stores from any source (155,156). Recent studies appear to indicate that the amount of vitamin D metabolites in bile is small and unlikely to have a substantial impact on vitamin D sufficiency when not absorbed well (157). With protein-losing enteropathies, losses of plasma DBP and 25(OH)D could occur, however. Exaggerated urinary losses of vitamin D metabolites are seen in patients with chronic cholestasis, but normal plasma 25(OH)D responses to ultraviolet light provide adequate sources to prevent osteomalacia (158).

Subjects with prior gastrectomy frequently display low 25(OH)D levels in plasma (159). Since they usually absorb $25(OH)D_3$ well, malabsorption is not thought to play a role in the development of deficiency. Recent work, however, indicates that secondary hyperparathyroidism and increased plasma $1,25(OH)_2D$ can stimulate hepatic catabolism of 25(OH)D (42,43). Calcium malabsorption, therefore, could trigger such a mechanism in such patients. Patients with duodenal exclusion reconstructions (Billroth II) are at greater risk for vitamin D deficiency (160). Lipid malabsorption might therefore occur when bile flow is not constantly effective. Also, plasma DBP levels are lower in patients having undergone total gastrectomy or Billroth II procedures (161). The basis for this is thought to be nutritional and/or hepatic dysfunction.

Treatment to correct deficiency states due to malabsorption can include ultraviolet light (151), parenteral vitamin D, or exaggerated oral doses of vitamin D. Prophylactic strategies include the same programs at lower and less frequent doses. With uncertain absorption,

plasma 25(OH)D levels are normal to low during pharmacological, oral doses of vitamin D. Guaranteed delivery of vitamin D is provided by intramuscular injections of vitamin D in oil preparations, and this can be done with injections of 2.5–12.5 mg (100,000–500,000 IU) every 6 months.

Considerable attention has been given to hepatic disorders since plasma 25(OH)D levels, as well as DBP levels in plasma, are usually lower in such patients (29–31,162,163). Deficiency of vitamin D is not easily attributable to hepatic cirrhosis since 25-hydroxylation is adequate in severe, advanced cases (164,165), and the free 25(OH)D available to tissues is normal (31,163). Since DBP correlates with serum albumin in cirrhosis (162,163), clinicians can interpret 25(OH)D levels in light of the serum content of these carrier proteins. Osteomalacia can occasionally be encountered in liver disease and is probably due to deficient sunlight exposure and poor dietary vitamin D intake or absorption.

Renal Diseases

Advanced renal failure can be associated with clinical features indicating vitamin D deficiency or resistance and secondary hyperparathyroidism (6). Although the osteodystrophy of renal failure is complex, effective vitamin D deficiency is a recognized component, and this is attributable to the inability to provide sufficient $1,25(OH)_2D$. The impairment can be due to loss of nephrons and the negative influence of hyperphosphatemia on the 25(OH)D-1α-hydroxylase activity.

25(OH)D

With heavy protein losses into urine, both 25(OH)D and DBP appear in urine in greater than normal amounts. With marginal sources, such an event can lead to depletion of stores and, on occasion, vitamin D–deficiency osteomalacia (166–168). Not all observers have observed vitamin D deficiency in patients with the nephrotic syndrome, however (167,169), and it seems likely that marked proteinuria and marginal vitamin D sources must coexist to bring about depletion. Plasma half-life of 25(OH)D is reduced by its loss into urine (167), and DBP levels in plasma are reduced (166,167). Strikingly low plasma 25(OH)D levels have been observed in such patients in late summer in a sunny climate, with a negative correlation between the amount of proteinuria and the plasma 25(OH)D concentration (170).

In other renal disorders, the plasma 25(OH)D level is not consistently altered, but increasingly severe renal disease can reduce appetite, impose dietary restrictions, and reduce the desire and ability to go outdoors, thereby threatening vitamin D sources. The turnover rate of plasma 25(OH)D is reduced in anephric patients, however (171). Accordingly, lower 25(OH)D levels in the plasmas of such patients is seen only occasionally

(172,173). During acute renal failure and oliguria, striking decreases in plasma 25(OH)D are seen, with subsequent increases during recovery of renal function (174). Since 25(OH)D is avidly bound to nondialyzable proteins, it is not lost during hemodialysis. Some losses of vitamin D metabolites into peritoneal dialysates have been reported.

1,25(OH)₂D

With advanced loss of nephrons, low plasma 1,25(OH)$_2$D levels are seen despite high plasma PTH levels. There are, however, several factors that appear to modify 1,25(OH)$_2$D production during reduced renal function. The availability of substrate 25(OH)D to the reduced but stimulated 25(OH)D-1α-hydroxylase units is critical, since increases in plasma 25(OH)D have been directly correlated to increases in plasma 1,25(OH)$_2$D under these conditions (45). This may, in part, help us to understand the beneficial effects of providing increased vitamin D to patients with chronic renal disease (6). Studies of the effects of dietary phosphorus also indicate that phosphorus restriction can increase plasma 1,25(OH)$_2$D levels during moderate renal insufficiency (121). Such modulations by diet can be seen in subjects with creatinine clearances of 25–50 mL/min per 1.73 m^2. Lower clearances are usually associated with markedly reduced levels of 1,25(OH)$_2$D in plasma (112,172,175,176).

Selective tubular disorders, both acquired and genetic, have been associated with low (177–179) or high (180) levels of plasma 1,25(OH)$_2$D. In many of these patients, low plasma phosphorus levels are seen, as in the oncogenic osteomalacia syndrome (181). The paradoxically low plasma 1,25(OH)$_2$D in the face of hypophosphatemia may reflect an inordinately high intracellular content of phosphorus in the renal proximal tubule as a result of the greater flux of phosphate during exaggerated losses of this ion into the urine. The opposite circumstances may occur in hyperphosphatemic tumoral calcinosis (180).

Treatment of chronic renal disease with vitamin D currently involves 1,25(OH)$_2$D in divided daily doses of 0.25–1.0 μg, together with calcium supplements, to correct intestinal malabsorption of calcium. In children, daily doses of 15–35 ng/kg have been associated with radiological healing of bone lesions and improved growth when given prior to 12 years of age (182). Following renal transplantation, 1,25(OH)$_2$D levels are restored and, in some instances, increase to very high levels in the first months after transplantation (183).

Endocrine Disorders

Hyperparathyroidism*

On average, patients with primary hyperparathyroidism have elevated levels of 1,25(OH)$_2$D in plasma, but the overlap with normal controls is considerable (114,122,184–189). There appear to be many factors that can modify these levels. Substrate availability can limit or augment the 1,25(OH)$_2$D production (56,114). Dietary influences, such as suppression of 1,25(OH)$_2$ levels with increased calcium intake (190) and increased phosphate (121) and stimulation by decreased phosphate (121), are important. Of course, the nephron population undergoing PTH stimulation must be considered, and the levels of DBP and albumin could be influential.

In addition, however, there are several negative feedback loops that warrant consideration. Hyperparathyroidism leading to moderate to high plasma calcium levels can bring about a suppression of 1,25(OH)$_2$D production, presumably via a direct effect of calcium on the 25(OH)D-1α-hydroxylase (54,114,191,192). Since some suppression of PTH secretion can be seen in hyperparathyroidism (190), the recently described effects of 1,25(OH)$_2$D in reducing PTH biosynthesis and secretion (193,194) can occur. Also, increased 1,25(OH)$_2$D levels can accelerate 25(OH)D catabolism, thereby potentially impairing substrate provision to the 25(OH)D-1α-hydroxylase (42,43).

Secondary hyperparathyroidism, in the absence of renal insufficiency or 25(OH)D deficiency, results in distinctly high 1,25(OH)$_2$D levels in plasma. This is encountered during calcium malabsorption over a protracted period and is associated with higher serum PTH and low to normal serum calcium and inorganic phosphorus levels.

In the hypercalcemia of most malignancies, plasma 1,25(OH)$_2$D levels are normal to low (184,189). This occurs despite PTH-related peptide's ability to stimulate the 25(OH)D-1α-hydroxylase (115) when this peptide is present. Negative influences on 1,25(OH)$_2$D production could be the higher serum calcium levels seen, together with impairment of renal function. With other humoral mediators of hypercalcemia in malignancy, suppression of 1,25(OH)$_2$D would be expected (Table 3).

Thyroid Disease

Hyperthyroidism is associated with low 1,25(OH)$_2$D concentrations in plasma (195) and correspondingly low calcium absorption (196). Increased 1,25(OH)$_2$D levels have been observed in hypothyroid subjects (195). In contrast, 25(OH)D levels in plasma are not altered, nor are the titers of DBP.

Diabetes Mellitus

In the absence of poor control (197), ketoacidosis, and nephropathy (198), vitamin D metabolites are not consistently altered in diabetic patients. With poor control of diabetes in a Bantu population, low serum DBP levels (15% reduction) have been observed along with lowered serum albumin (197). It is possible that the decrease in total serum 1,25(OH)$_2$D seen under these conditions re-

---

* See also Chs. 24 and 31—*Ed.*

flected protein malnutrition and the corresponding decrease in carrier proteins, as has been shown in the rat (199).

Other

Studies of the menstrual cycle (200–202) and male puberty (203) have not demonstrated consistent alterations of vitamin D metabolites during these periods. Estrogen administration increases DBP and $1,25(OH)_2D$ levels in plasma (204,205). When calculated, the free fraction was unchanged by estrogen therapy (204). However, direct measurements have indicated an increase of free $1,25(OH)_2D$ under similar conditions (205). Additional studies are required to resolve this issue. In careful longitudinal studies before and after menopause, no alterations of plasma 25(OH)D, $1,25(OH)_2D$, or DBP were observed in women experiencing bone loss (206). Glucocorticoid excess or treatment appears to reduce plasma $1,25(OH)_2D$ when derived from activated macrophages, but conflicting results have been reported in conditions of renal synthesis of the sterol in children and adults (207,208). The increased $1,25(OH)_2D$ levels of primary hyperparathyroidism do not seem to be affected by glucocorticoid therapy. Plasma 25(OH)D is not affected, in most studies, by such treatment (209,210).

Genetic Disorders

A variety of genetic disorders have been identified to have altered vitamin D metabolite concentrations in plasma (Table 3). A common disorder, idiopathic hypercalciuria, is associated with normal 25(OH)D and increased $1,25(OH)_2D$ levels in plasma (116,185). Exaggerated intestinal calcium absorption can be correlated to the plasma $1,25(OH)_2D$ in such patients. Increased bone resorption can also occur, with negative calcium balance during low-calcium diets. The mechanism of the increased $1,25(OH)_2$ levels is not known but may reflect a primary defect in phosphate homeostasis within the kidney. In pseudohypoparathyroidism, the PTH signal to the renal tubule is not normally received and low plasma $1,25(OH)_2$ and increased serum phosphate are observed (211).

Other genetic disorders affecting the kidney result in lowered plasma $1,25(OH)_2D$. In X-linked hypophosphatemia (XLH), plasma 25(OH)D levels are normal (34) and $1,25(OH)_2D$ levels are inappropriately low, considering the prevailing hypophosphatemia (123,124). In vitamin D dependent rickets type I, the renal enzyme cannot convert normal amounts of substrate to $1,25(OH)_2D$ but can produce slightly increased amounts of $1,25(OH)_2D$ when 25(OH)D levels are increased (212). A role for elevated 25(OH)D in a shift of the binding equilibrium in plasma to favor free $1,25(OH)_2D$ should be considered as well. In vitamin D dependent rickets type II, true resistance to $1,25(OH)_2D$ is seen, with hypocalcemia, second-

ary hyperparathyroidism, and very high levels of $1,25(OH)_2D$ in plasma (213). Since the $1,25(OH)_2D$ levels are the highest seen in any disorder, observers consider that $1,25(OH)_2D$ itself could have a role in determining its plasma level (24).

Recently, a syndrome of hypophosphatemic rickets with hypercalciuria has been identified (214). This autosomal recessive disorder was associated with renal phosphate wasting, high $1,25(OH)_2D$ levels in plasma, and decreased plasma PTH. In contrast to XLH, the hypophosphatemia was accompanied by increased plasma $1,25(OH)_2D$. In other disorders of proximal tubule dysfunction (Fanconi syndrome), $1,25(OH)_2D$ levels in plasma can be normal to low. Acquired disorders of renal tubular phosphate reclamation, such as oncogenic osteomalacia, are associated with low-plasma $1,25(OH)_2D$ (125). An inhibitor of $25(OH)D-1\alpha$-hydroxylase has been suggested, but it is also possible that the effects seen are due to the interference of phosphate handling by the kidney cell.

In familial hypocalciuric hypercalcemia, no clear abnormality of vitamin D metabolism is recognized (215). Although some children with the Williams syndrome have been reported to have exaggerated plasma 25(OH)D responses to vitamin D loading (216) or elevated plasma $1,25(OH)_2D$ (217), these findings have not been confirmed (218). In addition, the plasma DBP levels in the Williams syndrome have been found to be normal (219).

ACKNOWLEDGMENTS

Some of the work cited was supported by PHS Grant AM28292. The author is indebted to Ms. J. Dubbs for preparing the manuscript.

REFERENCES

1. Mellanby E. A further demonstration of the part played by accessory food factors in the aetiology of rickets. *J Physiol* 1918;52:III–IV.
2. Haldschinsky K. Heilung von Rachit's durch Kunsthiche Höhensonne. *Dtsch Med Wochenschr* 1919;45:712–3.
3. Bills CE. Vitamin D group. In: Sehrell W, Harris R, eds. *The vitamins.* New York: Academic Press, 1954;131–266.
4. Warkany J, Guest GM, Grabill EJ. Estimation of vitamin D in blood serum. *J Lab Clin Med* 1941;27:557–65.
5. Haddock L, Vazquez M. Antirachitic activity of the sera of patients with tropical sprue. *J Clin Endocrinol Metab* 1966;26:859–66.
6. Lumb GA, Mawer EB, Stanbury SW. The apparent vitamin D resistance of chronic renal failure. *Am J Med* 1971;50:421–41.
7. Fraser DR. The physiological economy of vitamin D. *Lancet* 1983;1:969–72.
8. Haddad JG, Hahn TJ. Natural and synthetic sources of circulating 25-hydroxyvitamin D in man. *Nature* 1973;244:515–7.
9. Fraser DR. Biochemical and clinical aspects of vitamin D function. *Br Med Bull* 1981;37:37–42.
10. Fraser DR. The physiological economy of vitamin D. In: DeLuca HF, Anast CS, eds. *Pediatric disease related to calcium.* New York: Elsevier, 1980;59–73.

11. Holick MF, MacLaughlin JA, Doppelt SH. Factors that influence the cutaneous production of previtamin D_3. *Science* 1981;211:590–2.

12. Holick MF, MacLaughlin JA, Clark MB, et al. Photosynthesis of previtamin D_3 in human skin and the physiological consequences. *Science* 1980;210:203–6.

13. Stamp TCB, Haddad JG, Twigg CH. Comparison of oral 25-OHD_3, vitamin D and ultraviolet light as determinants of circulating 25-hydroxyvitamin D in man. *Lancet* 1977;1:1341–3.

14. Clemens TL, Adams JS, Nolan JM, Holick MF. Measurement of circulating vitamin D in man. *Clin Chim Acta* 1982;121:301–8.

15. Thompson G, Lewis B, Booth C. Absorption of vitamin D_3-^{3}H in control subjects and patients with intestinal malabsorption. *J Clin Invest* 1966;45:94–102.

16. Hillman LS, Haddad JG. Perinatal vitamin D metabolism. II. Serial blood 25-hydroxyvitamin D concentrations in term and premature infants after birth. *J Pediatr* 1975;86:928–35.

17. Seamark DA, Trafford DJH, Makin HLJ. The estimation of vitamin D and some metabolites in human plasma by mass fragmentography. *Clin Chim Acta* 1980;106:51–62.

18. Jones G. Assay of vitamins D_2 and D_3 and 25-hydroxyvitamin D_2 and D_3 in human plasma by HPLC. *Clin Chem* 1978;24:287–98.

19. Adams JS, Clemens TL, Parrish JA, Holick MF. Vitamin D synthesis and metabolism after ultraviolet irradiation of normal and vitamin D–deficient subjects. *N Engl J Med* 1982;305:722–5.

20. Holmberg I, Larsson A. Seasonal variation of vitamin D_3 and 25-hydroxyvitamin D_3 in human serum. *Clin Chim Acta* 1980;100:173–4.

21. Clemens TL, Adams JS, Henderson SL, Holick MF. Increased skin pigment reduces the capacity of skin to synthesize vitamin D_3. *Lancet* 1982;1:74–6.

22. Haddad JG. Traffic, binding and cellular access of vitamin D sterols. In: Peck WA, ed. *Bone and mineral research,* vol 5. New York: Elsevier, 1987;281–308.

23. Haddad JG, Stamp TCB. Circulating 25-OHD in man. *Am J Med* 1974;57:57–62.

24. Stanbury SW, Mawer EB. Vitamin D metabolism in man: contributions from clinical studies. In: Frame B, Potts, JT, eds. *Clinical disorders of bone and mineral metabolism.* Amsterdam: Excerpta Medica, 1983;72–6.

25. Whyte MP, Haddad JG, Waters DD, Stamp TCB. Vitamin D bioavailability: serum 25-OHD levels in man after oral, subcutaneous, intramuscular and intravenous vitamin D administration. *J Clin Endocrinol Metab* 1979;48:906–11.

26. Mawer EB, Backhouse J, Holman CA. Lumb GA, Stanbury SW. The distribution and storage of vitamin D and its metabolites in human tissues. *Clin Sci Mol Med* 1972;43:413–31.

27. Ponchon G, DeLuca HF. The role of the liver in the metabolism of vitamin D. *J Clin Invest* 1969;48:1273–9.

28. Clements M, Fraser DR. Vitamin D supply to the rat fetus and neonate. *J Clin Invest* 1988;81:1768–73.

29. Wagonfeld JB, Nemchausky BA, Bolt M, VanderHorst J, Boyer JL, Rosenberg IH. Comparison of vitamin D and 25-hydroxyvitamin D in the therapy of primary biliary cirrhosis. *Lancet* 1976;2:391–4.

30. Long RG, Skinner RK, Wills MR, Sherlock S. Serum 25-hydroxyvitamin D in untreated parenchymal and cholestatic liver disease. *Lancet* 1976;2:650–2.

31. Bikle DD, Halloran BP, Gee E, Ryzen E, Haddad JG. Free 25-OHD levels are normal in subjects with liver disease and reduced total 25-OHD levels. *J Clin Invest* 1986;18:748–52.

32. Krawitt EL, Grundman MJ, Mawer EB. Absorption hydroxylation and excretion of vitamin D_3 in primary biliary cirrhosis. *Lancet* 1977;2:1246–9.

33. Haddad JG, Chyu KJ. Competitive protein-binding radioassay for 25-OHD_3. *J Clin Endocrinol Metab* 1971;33:992–5.

34. Haddad JG, Chyu KJ, Hahn TJ, Stamp TCB. Serum concentrations of 25-hydroxyvitamin D in sex-linked hypophosphatemic vitamin D-resistant rickets. *J Lab Clin Med* 1973;81:22–6.

35. Gertner JM, Domenech M. 25-OHD levels in patients treated with high dosage ergo and cholecalciferol. *Clin Pathol* 1977;30:144–50.

36. Haddad JG, Rojanasathit S. Acute administration of 25-hydroxycholecalciferol to man. *J Clin Endocrinol Metab* 1976;42:284–9.

37. Bec P, Bayard F, Louvet JP. 25-Hydroxycholecalciferol dynamics in human plasma. *Rev Eur Etudes Clin Biol* 1972;17:793–6.

38. Omdahl JL, Jelinek G, Eaton RP. Kinetic analysis of 25-OHD_3 metabolism in strontium-induced rickets in the chick. *J Clin Invest* 1977;60:1202–10.

39. Arnaud SB, Meger J. Microassay for 25-OHD: method and interpretation. In: Bikle DD, ed. *Assay of calcium-regulating hormones.* New York: Springer-Verlag, 1983;65–83.

40. Stanbury SW, Taylor CM, Lumb GA, et al. Formation of vitamin D metabolites following correction of human vitamin D deficiency. *Miner Electrolyte Metab* 1981;5:212–27.

41. Papapoulos SE, Clemens TL, Fraher LJ, Gleed J, O'Riordan JLH. Metabolites of vitamin D in human vitamin D deficiency: effect of vitamin D_3 or 1,25-dihydroxycholecalciferol. *Lancet* 1980;2:612–5.

42. Clements MR, Johnson L, Fraser DR. A new mechanism for induced vitamin D deficiency in calcium deprivation. *Nature* 1987;325:62–5.

43. Halloran BP, Bikle DD, Levens MJ, Castro ME, Globus RK, Holton E. Chronic dihydroxyvitamin D_3 administration in the rat reduces serum concentration of 25-hydroxyvitamin D by increasing metabolic clearance rate. *J Clin Invest* 1986;78:622–8.

44. Gray RW. A method for assay of serum or plasma concentrations of 1,25-dihydroxyvitamin D. In: Bikle DD, ed. *Assay of calcium-regulating hormones,* New York: Springer-Verlag, 1983;85–98.

45. Halloran BP, Schaefer P, Lipschitz M, Levens M, Goldsmith R. Plasma vitamin D metabolite concentrations in chronic renal failure: effect of oral administration of 25-hydroxyvitamin D_3. *J Clin Endocrinol Metab* 1984;59:1063–9.

46. Barbour GL, Coburn JW, Slatopolsky E, Norman AW, Horst RL. Hypercalcemia in an anephric patient with sarcoidosis: evidence for extrarenal generation of 1,25-dihydroxyvitamin D. *N Engl J Med* 1981;305:440–3.

47. Howard GA, Turner RT, Sherrard DJ, Baylink DJ. Human bone cells in culture metabolize 25-OHD_3 to 1,25-$(OH)_2D_3$ and 24,25-$(OH)_2D_3$. *J Biol Chem* 1981;256:7738–40.

48. Adams JS, Sharma OP, Gacad MA, Singer FR. Metabolism of 25-OHD_3 by cultured pulmonary alveolar macrophages in sarcoidosis. *J Clin Invest* 1983;72:1856–60.

49. Gkonos PJ, London R, Hendler ED. Hypercalcemia and elevated 1,25-$(OH)_2D$ levels in a patient with end-stage renal disease and active tuberculosis. *N Engl J Med* 1984;311:1683–5.

50. Rolla AR, Granfore A, Balogh K, Khettry U, Davis BL. Case report: granuloma-related hypercalcemia in lipoid pneumonia. *Am J Med Sci* 1986;29:313–6.

51. Kozeny GA, Barbato AL, Bansal VK, Vertuno LL, Hano JE. Hypercalcemia associated with silicone-reduced granulomas. *N Engl J Med* 1984;311:1103–5.

52. Helikson MA, Havey AD, Zerwekh JE, Breslau NA, Gardner DW. Plasma cell granuloma producing calcitriol and hypercalcemia. *Ann Int Med* 1986;105:379–81.

53. Gray RW, Caldos AE, Wilz DR, Lemann J Jr, Smith GA, DeLuca HF. Metabolism and excretion of ^{3}H-1,25$(OH)_2$ vitamin D_3 in healthy adults. *J Clin Endocrinol Metab* 1978;46:756–65.

54. Fraser DR. Regulation of the metabolism of vitamin D. *Physiol Rev* 1980;60:551–613.

55. Adams ND, Gray RW, Lemann J Jr. The effects of oral $CaCO_3$ loading and of dietary calcium deprivation on plasma 1,25-$(OH)_2D$ concentrations in healthy adults. *J Clin Endocrinol Metab* 1979;48:1008–16.

56. LoCascio V, Adami S, Galvanini G, Ferrari M, Cominacini L, Tartarotti D. Substrate product relation of 1-hydroxylase activity in primary hyperparathyroidism. *N Engl J Med* 1985;313:1123–25.

57. Maierhofer WJ, Gray RW, Adams ND, Smith FA, Lemann Jr. Synthesized and metabolic clearance of 1,25-dihydroxyvitamin D as determinants of serum concentration: a comparison of two methods. *J Clin Endocrinol Metab* 1981;53:472–5.

58. Halloran BP, Partale AA, Castro M, Morris RC Jr, Goldsmith RS. Serum concentration of 1,25-$(OH)_2D$ in the human: diurnal variation. *J Clin Endocrinol Metab* 1985;60:1104–10.

59. Maierhofer WJ, Lemann J, Gray RW, Cheung HS. Dietary calcium and serum 1,25-$(OH)_2D$ concentrations as determinants of calcium balance in healthy men. *Kidney Int* 1984;26:752–59.

60. Horst RL. Resolution and quantitation of vitamin D and vitamin D metabolites. In: Bikle DD, ed. *Assay of calcium-regulating hormones.* New York: Springer-Verlag, 1983;21–47.

61. Porteous CE, Caldwell RD, Trafford DJH, Makin HLJ. Recent developments in the measurement of vitamin D and its metabolites in human body fluids. *J Steroid Biochem* 1987;28:785–801.

62. Brommage R, DeLuca HF. Evidence that 1,25-dihydroxyvitamin D_3 is the physiologically active metabolite of vitamin D_3. *Endocr Rev* 1985;6:491–511.

63. Fraher LJ, Clemens TL, Papapoulos SE, Redd J, O'Riordan JLH. Determination of circulating 25,26-dihydroxycholecalciferol in man by radioimmunoassay. *Clin Sci* 1980;59:257–63.

64. Dreyer BE, Goodman DBP. A simple spectrophotometric assay for 24,25-dihydroxyvitamin D_3. *Anal Biochem* 1981;114:37–41.

65. Shepard RM, Horst RL, Hamstra AJ, DeLuca HF. Determination of vitamin D and its metabolites in plasma from normal and anephric man. *Biochem J* 1979;182:55–69.

66. Skinner RK, Wills MR. Serum 25-OHD assay: evaluation of chromatographic and non-chromatographic procedures. *Clin Chim Acta* 1977;80:543–54.

67. Dorantes LM, Arnaud SB, Arnaud CD. Importance of the isolation of 25-OHD before assay. *J Lab Clin Med* 1978;91:791–6.

68. Gilbertson TJ, Stryd RP. HPLC assay for 25-OHD₃ in serum. *Clin Chem* 1977;23:1700–4.

69. Stern PH, Phillips TE, Mavreas T. Bioassay of 1,25-(OH)₂D in human plasma purified by partition, alkaline extraction and HPLC. *Anal Biochem* 1980;102:22–30.

70. Manolagas SC, Culler FL, Howard JE, Brinckman AS, Deftos LJ. The cytoreceptor assay for 1,25-dihydroxyvitamin D_3 and its application to clinical studies. *J Clin Endocrinol Metab* 1983;56:751–60.

71. Haddad J, Jennings A, Aw TC. Vitamin D uptake and metabolism by perfused rat liver: influences of carrier proteins. *Endocrinology* 1988;123:498–505.

72. Cleve H, Constans J. The mutants of the vitamin D binding protein: more than 120 variants of the Gc/DBP system. *Vox Sang* 1988;54:215–25.

73. Cooke NE, Haddad JG. Vitamin D binding protein (Gc globulin). *Endocr Rev* 1989;10:294–305.

74. Haddad J, Fraser DR, Lawson DEM. Vitamin D plasma binding protein: turnover and fate in the rabbit. *J Clin Invest* 1981;67:1550–60.

75. Kawakami M, Blum CB, Ranakrishnan R, Dell RB, Goodman DS. Turnover of the plasma binding protein for vitamin D and its metabolites in normal human subjects. *J Clin Endocrinol Metab* 1981;53:1110–6.

76. Lind SE, Smithe DB, Janmey PA, Stossel TP. Role of plasma gelsolin and vitamin D binding protein in clearing actin from the circulation. *J Clin Invest* 1986;78:736–42.

77. Harper KD, McLeod JF, Kowalski MA, Haddad JG. Vitamin D binding protein sequesters monomeric actin in the circulation of the rat. *J Clin Invest* 1987;79:1365–70.

78. Goldschmidt-Clermont PJ, Van Baelen H, Bouillon R, et al. Role of group specific component (vitamin D-binding protein) in clearance of actin from the circulation in the rabbit. *J Clin Invest* 1988;81:1519–27.

79. Mawer EB, Hann JT, Berry JL, Davies M. Vitamin D metabolism in patients intoxicated with ergocalciferol. *Clin Sci* 1985;68:135–41.

80. Haddad JG. Transport of vitamin D metabolites. *Clin Orthop Rel Res* 1979;142:249–61.

81. Bouillon R, Van Assche FA, Van Baelen H, Heyns W, DeMoor P. Influence of the vitamin D-binding protein on the serum concentration of 1,25-dihydroxyvitamin D. *J Clin Invest* 1981;67:589–96.

82. Bikle DD, Gee E, Halloran B, Haddad JG. Free 1,25-(OH)₂D levels in serum from normal subjects, pregnant subjects and subjects with liver disease. *J Clin Invest* 1984;74:1966–71.

83. Bikle DD, Siiteri BK, Ryzen E, Haddad JG. Serum protein binding of 1,25-(OH)₂D: a re-evaluation by direct measurement of free metabolite levels. *J Clin Endocrinol Metab* 1985;61:969–75.

84. Bikle DD, Gee E, Halloran BP, Kowalski MA, Ryzen E, Haddad JG. Assessment of the free fraction of 25-OHD in serum and its

85. regulation by albumin and the vitamin D binding protein. *J Clin Endocrinol Metab* 1986;63:954–9.

85. Manolagas SC, Deftos LJ. Studies on the internalization of vitamin D_3 metabolites by cultured osteogenic sarcoma cells and their application to a non-chromatographic cytoreceptor assay for 1,25-dihydroxyvitamin D. *Biochem Biophys Res Commun* 1980;95:596–602.

86. Adams J. Specific internalization of 1,25-(OH)₂D by cultured intestinal epithelial cells. *J Steroid Biochem* 1984;20:857–62.

87. Olgaard K, Finco D, Martin K, et al. Extraction of vitamin D metabolites by bones of normal adult dogs. *J Clin Invest* 1980;69:684–90.

88. Vanham G, Van Baelen H, Tan BK, Bouillon R. The effect of vitamin D analogs and of vitamin D binding protein on lymphocytic proliferation. *J Steroid Biochem* 1988;29:381–6.

89. Petrini M, Galbraith RM, Emerson DL, Nel AE, Arnaud P. Structural studies of T-lymphocyte Fc receptors. *J Biol Chem* 1985;260:1804–10.

90. Danan JL, DeLorme AC, Ripoche MA, Bouillon R, Van Baelen H, Marthieu H. Presence of immunoreactive vitamin D–binding protein in rat yolk sac endodermal cells. *Endocrinology* 1985;117:243–7.

91. McLeod JF, Kowalski MA, Haddad JG. Characterization of monoclonal antibody to human serum vitamin D–binding protein (Gc globulin): recognition of an epitope hidden in membranes of circulating monocytes. *Endocrinology* 1986;119:77–83.

92. Nestler JE, McLeod JF, Kowalski MA, Strauss JF III, Haddad JG. Detection of vitamin D–binding protein on the surface of cytotrophoblasts isolated from human placentae. *Endocrinology* 1987;120:1996–2002.

93. Hryb DJ, Khan MS, Romes NA, Rosner W. Specific binding of human CBG to cell membranes. *Proc Natl Acad Sci USA* 1986;83:3253–6.

94. Hsu B, Siiteri PK, Kuhn RW. Interactions between CBG and target tissues. In: Forest MG, Pugeat M, eds. *Binding proteins of steroid hormones,* vol 149. London: Colloque Inserum/John Libbey Eurotext Ltd, 1986;577–91.

95. McLeod JF, Kowalski MA, Haddad JG. Interactions among serum vitamin D binding protein, monomeric actin, profilin and profilactin. *J Biol Chem* 1989;264:1260–7.

96. Haddad JG, Harper KD, Guoth M, Pietra G, Sanger J. Consequences of saturating the circulating actin-scavenger system. *J Cell Biol* 1988;107:31a(abstr 150).

97. Bouillon R, Van Baelen H. Measurement of vitamin D–binding protein by immunological and binding techniques. In: Forest MG, Pugeat M, eds. *Binding proteins of steroid hormones,* vol 149. London: Colloque Inserum/John Libbey Eurotext Ltd, 1986;253–60.

98. Kitchin FD, Bearn AG. Quantitative determination of the group specific protein in normal human serum. *Proc Soc Exp Biol Med* 1965;118:304–7.

99. Cleve H, Dencker H. Quantitative variations of the group-specific component (Gc) and of Barium-α2-glycoprotein of human serum in health and disease. In: Peeters H, ed. *Protides of the biological fluids.* New York: Elsevier, 1966;379–84.

100. Toivanen P, Rossi T, Hirvonen T. The concentration of Gc-globulin and transferrin in human fetal and infant sera. *Scand J Haematol* 1969;6:113–118.

101. Bouillon R, Van Baelen H, DeMoor P. The measurement of the vitamin D-binding protein in human serum. *J Clin Endocrinol Metab* 1977;45:225–31.

102. Imawari M, Goodman DS. Immunological and immunoassay studies of the binding protein for vitamin D and its metabolites in human serum. *J Clin Invest* 1977;59:432–42.

103. Parviainen MT, Harmoinen A, Visakorpi A. Immunophelometric quantification of serum vitamin D–binding globulin. *Scand J Clin Lab Invest* 1982;42:571–5.

104. Walsh PG, Haddad JG. Rocket immunoelectrophoresis assay of vitamin D-binding protein (Gc-globulin) in human serum. *Clin Chem* 1982;28:1781–3.

105. Goldschmidt-Clermont PJ, Galbraith R, Emerson DL, Werner PAM, Nel A, Lee WM. Accurate quantitation of native Gc in serum and Gc: actin complexes by rocket immunoelectrophoresis. *Clin Chim Acta* 1985;148:173–83.

106. Haddad JG, Walgate J. Radioimmunoassay of the binding protein for vitamin D and its metabolites in human serum. *J Clin Invest* 1976;58:1217–22.
107. Dueland S, Bouillon R, Van Baelen H, Pedersen J, Helgerud P, Drevon CA. Binding protein for vitamin D and its metabolites in rat mesenteric lymph. *Am J Physiol* 1985;249:E1–E5.
108. Pierce EA, Dame MC, Bouillon R, Van Baelen H, DeLuca HF. Monoclonal antibodies to human vitamin D–binding protein. *Proc Natl Acad Sci USA* 1985;82:8429–33.
109. Barsano CP, Banmann G. Simple algebraic and graphic methods for the apportionment of hormone (and receptor) into bound and free fractions in binding equilibria; or how to calculate bound and free hormone. *Endocrinology* 1989;124:1101–6.
110. Omdahl JL, Garry PJ, Hunsaker LA, Hunt WC, Goodwin JS. Nutritional status in a healthy elderly population: vitamin D. *Am J Clin Nutr* 1982;36:1225–33.
111. Shaw JCL. Evidence for defective skeletal mineralization in low birth weight infants: the absorption of calcium and fat. *Pediatrics* 1976;57:16–25.
112. Keh-Sung T, Heath H III, Kumar R, Riggs BL. Impaired vitamin D metabolism with aging in women: possible role in pathogenesis of senile osteoporosis. *J Clin Invest* 1984;73:1668–72.
113. Portale AA, Halloran BP, Morris RC Jr. Response of the serum level of 1,25-(OH)$_2$D to restriction of dietary phosphorus: effect of advanced age. *7th Workshop on vitamin D,* Rancho Mirage, CA, 1988;225(abstr).
114. Lalor BC, Mawer EB, Davies M, Lumb GA, Hunt L, Adams PH. Determinants of the serum concentration of 1,25-dihydroxyvitamin D in primary hyperparathyroidism. *Clin Sci* 1989;76:81–6.
115. Horinchi N, Caufield M, Fisher J, et al. Similarity of synthetic peptide from human tumor to PTH in vivo and in vitro. *Science* 1987;238:1566–8.
116. Gray RW, Wilz DR, Caldas AE, Lemann J Jr. The importance of phosphate in regulating plasma 1,25(OH)$_2$-vitamin D levels in humans: studies in healthy subjects, in calcium-stone formers and in patients with primary hyperparathyroidism. *J Clin Endocrinol Metab* 1977;45:299–306.
117. Hulter HN, Halloran BP, Toto RD, Peterson JC. Long term control of plasma calcitrol concentrations in dogs and humans: dominant role of plasma calcium concentrations in experimental hyperparathyroidism. *J Clin Invest* 1985;76:695–702.
118. Bilizekian JP, Caufield RE, Jacobs TP, et al. Response of 1α,25-dihydroxyvitamin D to hypocalcemia in human subjects. *N Engl J Med* 1978;299:437–41.
119. Maierhofer WJ, Gray RW, Lemann J Jr. Phosphate deprivation increases serum 1,25-(OH)$_2$D concentrations in healthy men. *Kidney Int* 1984;25:571–5.
120. Portale AA, Halloran BP, Murphy MM, Morris RC Jr. Oral intake of phosphorus can determine the serum concentration of 1,25-dihydroxyvitamin D by determining its production in humans. *J Clin Invest* 1986;77:7–12.
121. Portale AA, Booth BE, Halloran BP, Morris RC Jr. Effect of dietary phosphorus on circulating concentrations of 1,25-dihydroxyvitamin D and immunoreactive PTH in children with moderate renal insufficiency. *J Clin Invest* 1984;75:1580–9.
122. Thacker RV, Fraher LJ, Adami S, Karmali R, O'Riordan JLH. Circulating concentrations of 1,25-dihydroxyvitamin D in patients with primary hyperparathyroidism. *Bone Miner* 1986;1:137–44.
123. Lyles KW, Clark AG, Drezner MK. Serum 1,25-dihydroxyvitamin D levels in subjects with X-linked hypophosphatemic rickets and osteomalacia. *Calcif Tissue Int* 1981;33:173–5.
124. Delvin EE, Glorieux FH. Serum 1,25-dihydroxyvitamin D concentration in hypophosphatemic vitamin D resistant rickets. *Calcif Tissue Int* 1981;33:173–5.
125. Cotton GE, Van Puffelen P. Hypophosphatemic osteomalacia secondary to neoplasia. *J Bone Joint Surg* 1986;68:129–33.
126. Stamp TCB, Round JM, Rowe DJ, Haddad JG. Plasma levels and therapeutic effect of 25-OHD$_3$ in epileptic patients taking anticonvulsant drugs. *Br Med J* 1972;4:9–12.
127. Hahn TJ. Drug-induced disorders of vitamin D and mineral metabolism. *Clin Endocrinol Metab* 1980;9:107–29.
128. Eastwood JB, deWardener HE, Gray RW, Lemann JL Jr. Nor-mal plasma 1,25-(OH)$_2$ vitamin D concentrations in nutritional osteomalacia. *Lancet* 1979;1:1377–8.
129. Peacock M, Heyburn PJ, Aaron JE, Taylor GA, Brown WB, Speed R. Osteomalacia treated with 1α hydroxy or 1,25-dihydroxyvitamin D. In: Normal AW, Schaefer K, Herrath D, et al., eds. *Vitamin D: basic research and its clinical applications.* Berlin: Walter de Gruyter, 1979;1177–83.
130. Cantley LK, Russell J, Lettieri D, Sherwood L. 1,25-dihydroxyvitamin D suppresses parathyroid hormone secretion from bovine parathyroid cells in tissue culture. *Endocrinology* 1985;117:2114–9.
131. Slatopolsky E, Weerts C, Thielan J, Horst R, Harter H, Martin KJ. Marked suppression of secondary hyperparathyroidism by intravenous administration of 1,25-dihydroxycholecalciferol in uremic patients. *J Clin Invest* 1984;74:2136–43.
132. Stanbury SW, Taylor CM, Lumb GA, et al. Formation of vitamin D metabolites following correction of human vitamin D deficiency. *Miner Electrolyte Metab* 1981;5:212–27.
133. Paterson CR. Vitamin D poisoning: survey of causes in 21 patients with hypercalcemia. *Lancet* 1980;1:1164–5.
134. Schwartzman MS, Franck WA. Vitamin D toxicity complicating the treatment of senile, postmenopausal and glucocorticoid-induced osteoporosis. *Am J Med* 1987;82:224–30.
135. Brickman AS, Coburn JW, Norman AW. Action of 1,25-dihydroxycholecalciferol, a potent, kidney-produced metabolite of vitamin D$_3$, in uremic man. *N Engl J Med* 1972;287:891–5.
136. Pavlovitch H, Garabedian M, Balsan S. Calcium mobilizing effect of large doses of 25-OHD$_3$ in anephric rats. *J Clin Invest* 1973;52:2656–9.
137. Counts SJ, Baylink DJ, Shen FH, Sherrard DJ, Hickman RO. Vitamin D intoxication in an anephric child. *Ann Intern Med* 1975;82:196–200.
138. Vermier J, Engel F, McPherson H. Vitamin D intoxication: a report of 2 cases treated with cortisone. *Ann Intern Med* 1958;48:765–73.
139. Daires M, Mawer EB, Freemont AJ. The osteodystrophy of hypervitaminosis D: a metabolic study. *Q J Med* 1986;61:911–9.
140. Jibani M, Hodges NH. Prolonged hypercalcemia after industrial exposure to vitamin D$_3$. *Br Med J* 1985;290:748–9.
141. Bell NH. Vitamin D-endocrine system. *J Clin Invest* 1985;76:1–6.
142. Verbeelen D, Fuss M. Hypercalcemia induced by oestrogen withdrawal in vitamin D–treated hypoparathyroidism. *Br Med J* 1979;1:522–3.
143. Parfitt AM. Vitamin D treatment in hypoparathyroidism. *Lancet* 1970;2:614–5.
144. Hossain M. Vitamin D-intoxication during treatment of hypoparathyroidism. *Lancet* 1970;1:1149–51.
145. Mason RS, Rosen S. The relevance of 25-hydroxycalciferol measurements in the treatment of hypoparathyroidism. *Clin Endocrinol* 1979;10:265–9.
146. Burns J, Paterson CR. The value of 25-OHD measurements and hypothyroid and pseudohypoparathyroid patients treated with calciferol. *Clin Biochem* 1986;19:49–51.
147. Stamp TCB. Intestinal absorption of 25-hydroxycholecalciferol. *Lancet* 1974;2:121–3.
148. Morgan DB, Hunt G, Paterson CR. The osteomalacia syndrome after stomach operations. *Q J Med* 1970;155:395–410.
149. Kehayoglou AK, Holdsworth CD, Agnew JE, Whelton MJ, Sherlock S. Bone disease and calcium absorption in primary biliary cirrhosis with special reference to vitamin D therapy. *Lancet* 1968;1:715–9.
150. Halverson JD, Teitelbaum SL, Haddad JG, Murphy WA. Skeletal abnormalities after jejunoileal bypass. *Ann Surg* 1979;189:785–90.
151. Jung RT, Davie M, Hunter JO, Chalmers TM. Ultraviolet light: an effective treatment of osteomalacia in malabsorption. *Br Med J* 1978;1:1668–9.
152. Compston JE, Creamer B. Plasma levels and intestinal absorption of 25-hydroxyvitamin D in patients with small bowel resection. *Gut* 1977;18:171–5.
153. Driscoll RH, Meredith SC, Sitrin M, Rosenberg IH. Vitamin D

deficiency and bone disease in patients with Crohn's disease. *Gastroenterology* 1982;83:1252–8.

154. Friedman HZ, Langman CB, Favus MJ. Vitamin D metabolism and osteomalacia in cystic fibrosis. *Gastroenterology* 1985;88:808–13.

155. Kumar R. Hepatic and intestinal osteodystrophy and the hepatobiliary metabolism of vitamin D. *Ann Intern Med* 1983;98:662–3.

156. Compston JE, Marrett AL, Ledger JE, Creamer B. Facial tritium excretion after intravenous administration of ³H-25-hydroxyvitamin D₃ in control subjects and in patients with malabsorption. *Gut* 1982;23:310–5.

157. Clements MR, Chalmers TM, Fraser DR. Enterohepatic circulation of vitamin D: a reappraisal of the hypothesis. *Lancet* 1984;1:1376–9.

158. Jung RT, Davie M, Siklos P, Chalmers TM, Hunter JO, Lawson DEM. Vitamin D metabolism in acute and chronic cholestasis. *Gut* 1979;20:840–7.

159. Gertner JM, Lilburn M, Domenech M. 25-Hydroxycholecalciferol absorption in steatorrhea and post-gastrectomy osteomalacia. *Br Med J* 1977;1:1310–2.

160. Kozawa K, Imawari M, Shimazu H, Kobori O, Osuga T, Morioka Y. Vitamin D status after total gastrectomy. *Dig Dis Sci* 1984;29:411–6.

161. Imawari M, Kozawa K, Akanuma Y, Koizumi S, Itakura H, Kosaka K. Serum 25-OHD and vitamin D-binding protein levels and mineral metabolism after partial and total gastrectomy. *Gastroenterology* 1980;79:255–8.

162. Imawari M, Akanuma Y, Itakura H, Muto Y, Kosaka K, Goodman DS. The effects of diseases of the liver on serum 25-OHD and on the serum binding protein for vitamin D and its metabolites. *J Lab Clin Med* 1979;93:171–80.

163. Bouillon R, Auwerx J, DeKeyser L, Fevery J, Lissens W, DeMoor P. Serum vitamin D metabolites and their binding protein in patients with liver cirrhosis. *J Clin Endocrinol Metab* 1984;59:86–9.

164. Posner DB, Russell RM, Absood S, et al. Effective 25-hydroxylation of vitamin D₂ in alcoholic cirrhosis. *Gastroenterology* 1978;74:866–70.

165. Mobarhan SA, Russell RM, Recker RR, Posner DB, Iber FL, Miller P. Metabolic bone disease in alcoholic cirrhosis: a comparison of the effect of vitamin D₂ 25-OHD, or supportive treatment. *Hepatology* 1984;4:266–73.

166. Auwerx J, DeKeyser L, Bouillon R, DeMoor P. Decreased free 1,25-dihydroxycholecalciferol index in patients with the nephrotic syndrome. *Nephron* 1986;42:231–5.

167. Barragry JM, France MW, Carter ND, et al. Vitamin D metabolism in nephrotic syndrome. *Lancet* 1977;2:629–32.

168. Malluche HH, Goldstein DA, Massry SG. Osteomalacia and hyperparathyroid bone disease in patients with nephrotic syndrome. *J Clin Invest* 1979;63:494–500.

169. Korkor A, Schwartz, Bergfeld M, et al. Absence of metabolic bone disease in adult patients with the nephrotic syndrome and normal renal function. *J Clin Endocrinol Metab* 56:496–500.

170. Goldstein DA, Oda Y, Kurokawa K, Massry SG. Blood levels of 25-OHD in nephrotic syndrome. *Ann Intern Med* 1977;87:664–7.

171. Gray RW, Weber HP, Dominguez JH, Lemann J Jr. The metabolism of vitamin D₃ and 25-OHD₃ in normal and anephric humans. *J Clin Endocrinol Metab* 1974;39:1045–56.

172. Mason RS, Lissner D, Wilkinson M, Posen S. Vitamin D metabolites and their relationship to azotemic osteodystrophy. *Clin Endocrinol* 1980;13:375–85.

173. Bayard F, Bec PH, That HT, Louvet JP. Plasma 25-OHD₃ in chronic renal failure. *Eur J Clin Invest* 1973;3:447–50.

174. Pietrek J, Kokot F, Kuska J. Serum 25-OHD and PTH in patients with acute renal failure. *Kidney Int* 1978;13:178–85.

175. Mawer EB, Backhouse J, Taylor CM, Lumb GA, Stanbury SE. Failure of formation of 1,25-dihydroxycholecalciferol in chronic renal insufficiency. *Lancet* 1973;1:626–8.

176. Chesney RW, Hamstra AJ, Mazess RB, Rose P, DeLuce HF. Circulating vitamin D metabolite concentrations in childhood renal diseases. *Kidney Int* 1982;21:65–9.

177. Baran DT, Marcy TW. Evidence for a defect in vitamin D metab-

olism in a patient with incomplete Fanconi syndrome. *J Clin Endocrinol Metab* 1984;59:998–1001.

178. Drezner MK, Lyles KW, Haussler MR, Harrelson JM. Evaluation of a role for 1,25-(OH)₂D in the pathogenesis and treatment of x-linked hypophosphatemic rickets and osteomalacia. *J Clin Invest* 1980;66:1020.

179. Offerman G, Delling G, Haussler M. 1,25-Dihydroxycholecalciferol in hypophosphatemic osteomalacia presenting in adults. *Acta Endocrinol* 1978;88:408–16.

180. Prince M, Schaefer P, Golsmith R, Chausmer A. Hyperphosphatemic tumoral calcinosis: association with elevation of serum 1,25-dihydroxycholecalciferol concentrations. *Ann Intern Med* 1982;96:586–91.

181. Miyanchi A, Fukase M, Tsutsumi M, Fujita T. Hemangiopericytoma-induced osteomalacia: tumor transplantation in nude mice causes hypophosphatemia and tumor extracts inhibit renal 25-hydroxyvitamin D-1-hydroxylase activity. *J Clin Endocrinol Metab* 1988;67:46–53.

182. Chan JCM, Kodroff MB, Landwehr DM. Effects of 1,25-(OH)₂D₃ on renal function, mineral balance, and growth in children with severe chronic renal failure. *Pediatrics* 1981;68:559–71.

183. Garabedian M, Silve C, Levy-Bentolila D, et al. Changes in plasma 1,25 and 24,25-dihydroxyvitamin D after renal transplantation in children. *Kidney Int* 1981;20:403–10.

184. Haussler MR, Baylink DJ, Hughes MR, et al. The assay of 1α-25-dihydroxyvitamin D₃: physiologic and pathologic modulation of circulating hormone levels. *Clin Endocrinol* 1976;5:151S–65S.

185. Broadus AE, Horst RL, Lang R, Littledike ET, Rasmussen H. The importance of circulating 1,25-dihydroxyvitamin D in the pathogenesis of hypercalcemia and renal stone formation in primary hyperparathyroidism. *N Engl J Med* 1980;302:421–6.

186. Lund B, Sorensen OH, Lund B, Bishop J, Norman AW. Stimulation of 1,25-(OH)₂D production by parathyroid hormone and hypocalcemia in man. *J Clin Endocrinol Metab* 1980;50:480–4.

187. Kaplan RH, Haussler MR, Deftos LJ, Bone H, Pak CYC. The role of 1,25-(OH)₂D in the mediation of intestinal hyperabsorption of calcium in primary hyperparathyroidism and absorptive hypercalciuria. *J Clin Invest* 1977;59:756–60.

188. Duncan WE, Aw TC, Walsh PG, Haddad JG. Normal rabbit intestinal cytosol as a source of binding protein for the 1,25-dihydroxyvitamin D₃ assay. *Anal Biochem* 1983;132:209–14.

189. Stewart A, Horst R, Deftos L, Cadman E, Lang R, Broadus A. Biochemical evaluation of patients with cancer-associated hypercalcemia. *New Engl J Med* 1980;303:1377–83.

190. Insogna KL, Mitnick ME, Stewart AF, Burtis WJ, Mallette LE, Broadus AE. Sensitivity of the parathyroid hormone–1,25-(OH)₂D axis to variations in calcium intake in patients with primary hyperparathyroidism. *N Engl J Med* 1985;313:1126–30.

191. Hove K, Horst RL, Littledike ET, Beitz DC. Infusions of parathyroid hormone in ruminants: hypercalcemia and reduced plasma 1,25-(OH)₂D concentrations. *Endocrinology* 1984;114:897–903.

192. Wortsman J, Haddad JG, Posillico JT, Brown EM. Primary hyperparathyroidism with low serum 1,25-(OH)₂D levels. *J Clin Endocrinol Metab* 1986;62:1305–8.

193. Dietel M, Dorn G, Montz R, Altenahr E. Influence of vitamin D₃, 1,25-dihydroxyvitamin D₃ and 24,25-dihydroxyvitamin D₃ on parathyroid hormone secretion, adenosine 3′, 5′-monophosphate release, and ultrastructure of parathyroid glands in organ culture. *Endocrinology* 1979;105:237–45.

194. Russell J, Lettieri D, Sherwood LM. Suppression by 1,25-(OH)₂D₃ of transcription of the pre-preparathyroid hormone gene. *Endocrinology* 1986;119:2864–6.

195. Bouillon R, Muls E, DeMoor P. Influences of thyroid function on the serum concentration of 1,25-dihydroxyvitamin D₃. *J Clin Endocrinol Metab* 1980;51:793–7.

196. Peerenboom H, Keck E, Kruskemper HL, Strohmeyer G. The defect of intestinal calcium transport in hyperthyroidism and its response to therapy. *J Clin Endocrinol Metab* 1984;59:936–40.

197. Nyomba BL, Bouillon R, Bidingya M, Kandjingu K, DeMoor P. Vitamin D metabolites and their binding protein in adult diabetic patients. *Diabetes* 1986;35:911–5.

198. Storm TL, Sorensen OH, Lund BJ, et al. Vitamin D metabolism

in insulin-dependent diabetes mellitus. *Metab Bone Dis Relat Res* 1983;5:107–10.

199. Nyomba BL, Bouillon R, Lissens W, Van Baelen H, DeMoor P. 1,25-Dihydroxyvitamin D and vitamin D–binding protein and both decreased in streptozotocin-diabetic rats. *Endocrinology* 1985;116:2483–8.

200. Gray TK, McAdoo T, Hatley L, Lester GE, Thierry M. Fluctuation of serum concentrations of 1,25-(OH)₂D₃ during the menstrual cycle. *Am J Obstet Gynecol* 1982;144:880–4.

201. Baran DT, Whyte MP, Haussler MR, Deftos LJ, Slatopolsky E, Avioli LV. Effect of the menstrual cycle on calcium-regulating hormones in normal young women. *J Clin Endocrinol Metab* 1980;50:377–9.

202. Muse KN, Manologas SC, Deftos LJ, Alexander N, Yen SSC. Calcium-regulating hormones across the menstrual cycle. *J Clin Endocrinol Metab* 1986;62:1313–16.

203. Krabbe S, Hummer L, Christiansen C. Serum levels of vitamin D metabolites and testosterone in male puberty. *J Clin Endocrinol Metab* 1986;62:503–7.

204. Aarskog D, Aksnes L, Markestad T, Rodland O. Effect of estrogen on vitamin D metabolism in tall girls. *J Clin Endocrinol Metab* 1983;57:1155–8.

205. Cheema C, Grant BF, Marcus R. Effects of estrogen on circulating free and total 1,25-dihydroxyvitamin D and on the parathyroid–vitamin D axis in postmenopausal women. *J Clin Invest* 1989;83:537–42.

206. Falch JA, Oftebro H, Haug E. Early postmenopausal bone loss is not associated with a decrease in circulating levels of 25-OHD, 1,25-(OH)₂D, or vitamin D-binding protein. *J Clin Endocrinol Metab* 1987;64:836–41.

207. Chesney RW, Mazess RB, Hamstra AJ, DeLuca HF. Reduction of serum 1,25-dihydroxyvitamin D in children receiving glucocorticoids. *Lancet* 1978;2:1123–5.

208. Braum JJ, Juttmann JR, Visser TJ, Birkenhager JC. Short-term effect of prednisone on serum 1,25-(OH)₂D in normal individuals and in hyper- and hypoparathyroidism. *Clin Endocrinol* 1982;17:21–8.

209. Hahn TJ, Halstead LR, Haddad JG. Serum 25-OHD concentrations in patients receiving chronic corticosteroid therapy. *J Lab Clin Med* 1977;90:399–404.

210. Streck WF, Waterhouse C, Haddad JC. Glucocorticoid effects in vitamin D intoxication. *Arch Intern Med* 1979;139:974–7.

211. Lambert P, Hollis B, Bell N, Epstein S. Demonstrations of a lack of change in serum 1,25-dihydroxyvitamin D₃ in response to parathyroid extract in pseudohypoparathyroidism. *J Clin Invest* 1980;66:782–91.

212. Delvin EE, Glorieux FH, Marie PJ, Pettifor JM. Vitamin D-dependency: replacement therapy with calcitriol. *J Pediatr* 1981;99:26–34.

213. Marx SJ, Liberman UA, Eil C, Gamblin GT, DeGrange DA, Balsan S. Hereditary resistance to 1,25-dihydroxyvitamin D. *Recent Prog Horm Res* 1984;40:589–620.

214. Tieder M, Modai D, Samuel R, et al. Hereditary hypophosphatemic rickets with hypercalciuria. *N Engl J Med* 1985;312:611–7.

215. Davies M, Adams PH, Berry JL, et al. Familial hypocalciuric hypercalcemia: observations on vitamin D metabolism and parathyroid function. *Acta Endocrinol* 1983;104:210–5.

216. Taylor AB, Stern PH, Bell NH. Abnormal regulation of circulating 25-OHD in the Williams syndrome. *N Engl J Med* 1982;306:972–5.

217. Garabedian M, Jacoz E, Guillozo H, et al. Elevated plasma 1,25-dihydroxyvitamin D concentrations in infants with hypercalcemia and an elfin facies. *N Engl J Med* 1985;312:948–52.

218. Martin N, Snodgrass G, Cohen R, et al. Vitamin D metabolites in idiopathic hypercalcemia. *Arch Dis Child* 1985;60:1140–3.

219. Daiger S, Miller M, Romeo G, Parsons M, Cavalli-Sforza L. Vitamin D–binding protein in the Williams syndrome and idiopathic hypercalcemia. *N Engl J Med* 1978;298:687–8.

PART II

Bone Structure and Biology

Disorders of Bone and Mineral Metabolism,
edited by Fredric L. Coe and Murray J. Favus,
© 1992 by Raven Press, Ltd. All rights reserved.

CHAPTER 10

Embryology, Anatomy, and Microstructure of Bone

Robert R. Recker

Functionally, the skeleton in humans and higher vertebrates is really two organs. One serves as a reservoir of inorganic elements (such as calcium and magnesium) responding to the needs of internal homeostasis, and the other serves as a structural support permitting movement and locomotion in the gravitational environment of the earth's surface. Ordinarily these two functions do not come in conflict because the mineral reservoir supporting internal homeostasis is bountiful and readily replenished while the strength of the structural component includes a generous margin of safety. However, the reservoir function is dominant and, when subjected to stressful perturbation, has the power to overcome the structural function in attempts to adapt. For example, in conditions of severe external calcium deprivation, the mass of the skeleton will be sacrificed and the mechanical strength will be reduced to dangerous levels to support internal (plasma) homeostasis. On the other hand, demand that might arise in the process of confronting excessive structural needs (increase in skeletal mass in response to heavy mechanical loads) will not ordinarily result in sacrifice of internal (plasma) homeostasis. Thus while the two functions coexist in harmony most of the time, the needs of plasma calcium homeostasis reign supreme.

The cells of the skeleton which work to achieve and maintain the structure of the skeleton and which accomplish the adaptation to mechanical usage are the same ones responsible for the maintenance of plasma calcium homeostasis. This dual role suggests that powerful systems exist to organize and control the numbers, location, and work efficiency of these cells in order to accomplish these widely disparate tasks. Frost (1,2) refers to the system of regulation of bone cell function serving the structural needs of the skeleton as the *intermediary organization* (IO) of the skeleton (described below). This chapter discusses the embryology, anatomy, and structural function of the skeleton at the micro and macro levels in the context of this IO. The discussion will be about the human skeleton except in those areas where information on humans is incomplete or where information regarding an animal or in vitro model helps in understanding the human condition.

DEVELOPMENTAL BIOLOGY

Why is a section on developmental biology of the skeleton included in a textbook such as this? One reason is that it is useful to understand something about prenatal origins of the skeleton when trying to understand mechanisms behind developmental abnormalities encountered in the clinic. Another is that the embryology of the skeleton is fascinating in its own right. Many who study the adult skeleton have a great deal of curiosity about its origins and the interaction of the development of its various parts with the development of the rest of the body. Finally, the cell and molecular biology associated with early development may contain something ultimately useful to the clinical scientist. For example, certain embryonic developmental behavior remains in postembryonic, childhood skeletal development in the form of elongation and sculpting of the skeleton. The adult human even possesses a vestige of this tissue behavior in the form of periosteal modeling in response to mechanical force (1,2). Unfortunately, not much is known about the cell and molecular biology of embryonic development, and thus we cannot readily access the latent potential that might exist in the adult skeleton to increase (or decrease) its mass or rearrange its structure.

R. R. Recker: Center for Hard Tissue Research, Creighton University, Omaha, Nebraska 68131.

The first part of this section focuses on the description of skeletal development, skeletal cells, and the arrangement of tissue in space. It will set the stage for a discussion of the structure and function of skeletal tissue in the ensuing pages.

Origins of Skeletal Tissue

The first stage of embryologic development requires that the simple organism of a few cells differentiate into three layers (3). All of the components of the mature creature can be traced to one of these three basic pluripotential cell layers. Figure 1 is a schematic diagram of a very early human embryo of about 17 days. At this stage, the original solid "ball" of cells that developed in the first week after fertilization has formed two cavities, both lined with cells from the embryo and separated by a septum which contains all the information and cell material that will become the fully developed human. The dorsal–ventral orientation has already been decided, and the three primordial layers can be identified. The cavity above is the amniotic cavity, and the one below is the yolk sac.

Development of the Axial Skeleton

The axial skeleton is made up of the spine, skull, ribs, and sternum. Its formation is presented in schematic transverse sections in Fig. 2 and photographs in Fig. 3. The embryo is still a rather thin plate in Fig. 2A, but the layers can be identified. The dorsum is identified in the ectoderm by the presence of the neural plate and neural groove. The endoderm is below, and sandwiched in between is the mesoderm (which will give rise to the skeleton). The mesoderm is made up of embryonic connective tissue (mesenchyme) which can differentiate in

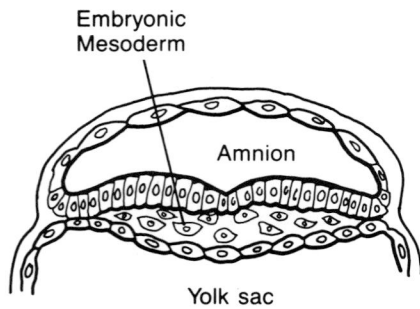

FIG. 1. Schematic diagram of a cross section of a 17-day-old human embryo. The three layers from which the entire fetus will develop are present between the amnion and the yolk sac. The dorsal–ventral orientation has been decided: The amnion is on the dorsal side, and the yolk sac on the ventral side. The embryonic mesoderm, sandwiched between the ectoderm dorsally and the endoderm ventrally, contains the forerunners of the skeletal system.

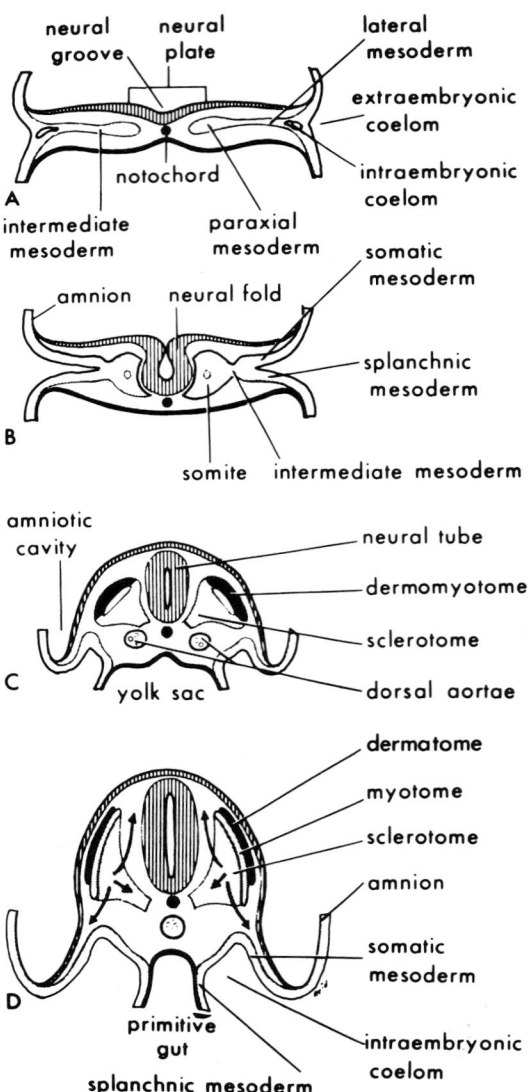

FIG. 2. Transverse sections through embryos of various ages, illustrating the formation and differentiation of somites. A: A presomite embryo (about 18 days); the somites are derived from the paraxial mesoderm. B: A 22-day embryo; C: A 26-day embryo; the dermomyotome later becomes a myotome (future muscle) and a dermatome (future dermis). The sclerotome becomes skeleton. D: A 28-day embryo; the arrows indicate migration of cells from the sclerotome regions of the somites. [From Moore (3), with permission.]

many different ways. For example, mesenchymal cells can develop into fibroblasts, osteoblasts, chondroblasts, and other connective tissue precursors. Some of the mesenchyme in the head region develops from the neural crest, which becomes part of the brachial arches.

The mesoderm is divided into three contiguous areas: paraxial, intermediate, and lateral mesoderm. The somites arise from the paraxial mesoderm, and their development begins by about 22 days as shown in Fig. 2B. The

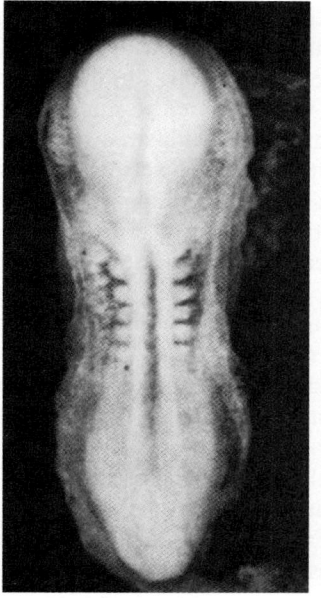 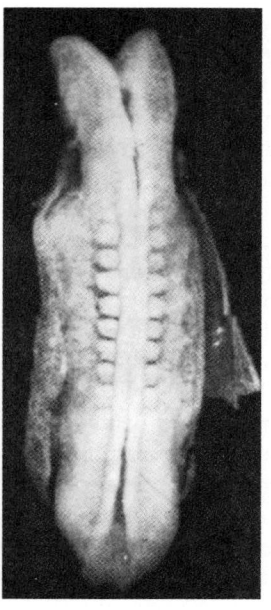

FIG. 3. Photographs of embryos early in the fourth week. These show the somites as the palisades beside the neural tube. **A:** The neural tube is a deep groove in the curved embryo, and it is open throughout its entire extent. **B:** The neural tube is formed opposite the somites, and it is widely open on both ends. [From Moore (3), with permission and courtesy of Professor Hideo Nishimura, Kyoto University, Kyoto, Japan.]

medial area of the somite becomes the sclerotome from which the vertebrae develop.

Development of the Appendicular Skeleton

Limb buds appear at about 28 days of fetal life. These are outpockets of the mesodermal layer containing mesenchyme and possessing a specialized tip of ectoderm, called the *apical ectodermal ridge.* Progression of limb development is shown schematically in Fig. 4. By the sixth week, the entire cartilaginous model of the limb bones are in place. The inductive influence of the apical ridge has been demonstrated in work by Krabbenhoft and Fallon (4) in chicks. Grafts of the lower limb bud onto the upper one result in formation of lower limb elements in the upper limb if the graft is placed within 162 μm of the apical ridge. However, if placed further away, the grafted cells become incorporated into a normal-appearing upper limb.

Histogenesis of Bone

Bone is a biphasic material made up of an organic matrix of collagen fibrils embedded in an amorphous substance, with mineral crystals precipitated within the

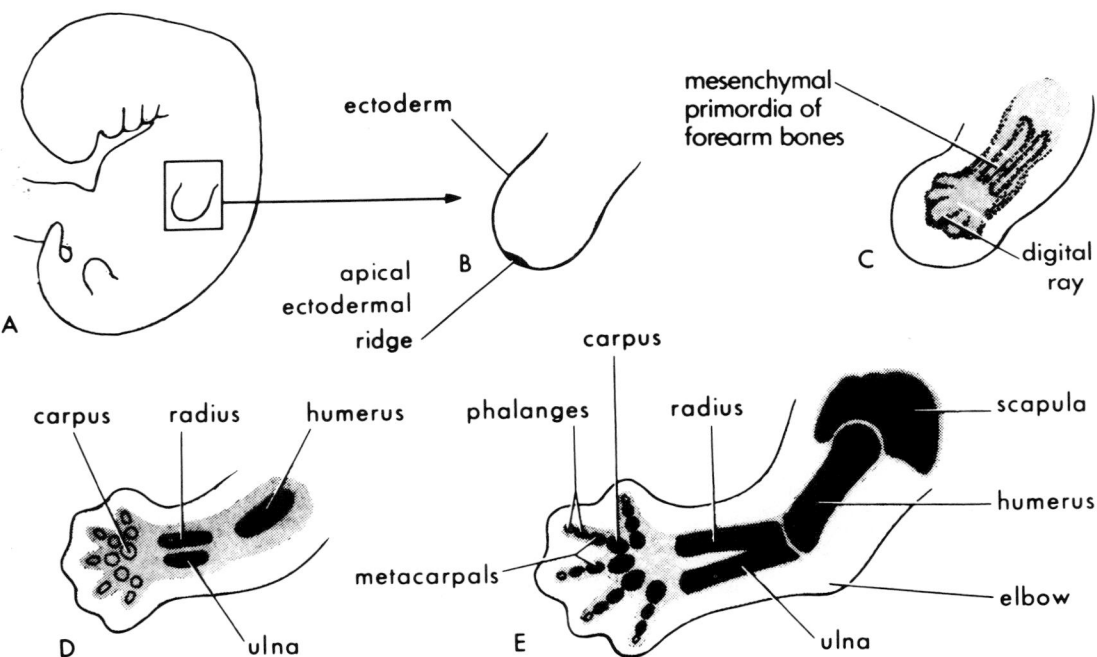

FIG. 4. A: Schematic diagram of an embryo at about 28 days, at the beginning of the formation of limb buds. **B:** Schematic diagram of a longitudinal section through the upper limb bud. The apical ectodermal ridge induces growth of the loose mesenchyme in the limb bud and promotes the ability to form specific cartilaginous elements. **C:** Schematic diagram of an upper limb bud at about 33 days, showing the mesenchymal primordia of the limb bones. The digital rays are mesenchymal condensations that will undergo chondrification and ossification to form the bones of the hand. **D:** At 6 weeks the hyaline cartilage models of the various bones are visible. **E:** Later in the sixth week, the completed cartilaginous models of the bones of the upper limb are visible. [From Moore (3), with permission.]

matrix. The first bone to appear in the embryo comes from one of two precursor tissues, mesenchyme and cartilage.

Intramembranous Ossification

"Membranous bone" is the term used to describe bone that arises directly in mesenchyme which is in the form of a sheet or membrane. This mesenchyme is rather loosely organized, and the cells are relatively far apart (Fig. 5). At the time bone begins to form, some of the cells condense more tightly, leaving thin extensions of their cytoplasm to communicate with one another. Nests of these cells begin to take on the appearance of osteoblasts and begin to secrete the protein matrix of bone, the osteoid. The osteoblasts, along with their thin extensions, bury themselves in the matrix, which then begins to calcify. The collagen fibrils of this matrix are arranged in a haphazard, random manner, and the bone tissue resulting from this process is called *woven bone* or *primitive bone.* Gradually the woven bone engulfs blood vessels as it enlarges, eventually organizing itself into broad, flattened plates that contain an outer and inner shell of compact bone enclosing an inner space containing trabecular bone and marrow. During this process, the woven bone with its randomly arranged collagen fibrils is replaced by highly organized lamellar bone in which the matrix is arranged in tightly packed sheets. The organization of trabecular and compact bone is discussed in greater detail below.

Endochondral Ossification

Endochondral ossification is the term used to describe bone that arises from a cartilaginous mold or template. These templates are laid down by chondrocytes arising from the mesenchyme of the somites (the sclerotomes) or the limb buds as presented schematically in Fig. 6. The primary ossification center of a long bone develops in the middle part of what will become the shaft or diaphysis of the bone. The cartilage in this area begins to calcify, and the chondrocytes begin to die. At the same time, the cells in the collar around the diaphysis differentiate into osteoblasts and begin to form bone, the first appearance of the periosteum. Blood vessels penetrate the periosteum and gain access to the calcified cartilage of the diaphysis, bringing elements that will form marrow along with a new crop of cells called *osteoclasts,* which can remove calcified cartilage. When osteoclasts invade and begin work, osteoblasts follow and begin to replace the calcified cartilage with lamellar bone. This process continues toward the ends of the bone.

At about the time of birth, a secondary ossification center begins in the end of the long bone, the epiphysis. Essentially the same process occurs here as occurred in the primary center of ossification; however, the juncture between the diaphysis and the epiphysis assumes the specialized function of elongation or growth. The epiphyseal plate continues to deposit cartilage which undergoes transformation to bone similar to that described above, and during this process the bone elongates. Ultimately, the epiphyses all become engulfed in the process of forming bone and can no longer produce cartilage and elongation. This "closure" of epiphyses occurs at the end of the growth period in early adult life.

BONE AS A STRUCTURAL ORGAN: MACROSCOPIC ORGANIZATION

The skeleton is an organ of structural support, and the most prominent material property of its tissue is striking rigidity and hardness. This is fortunate and appropriate

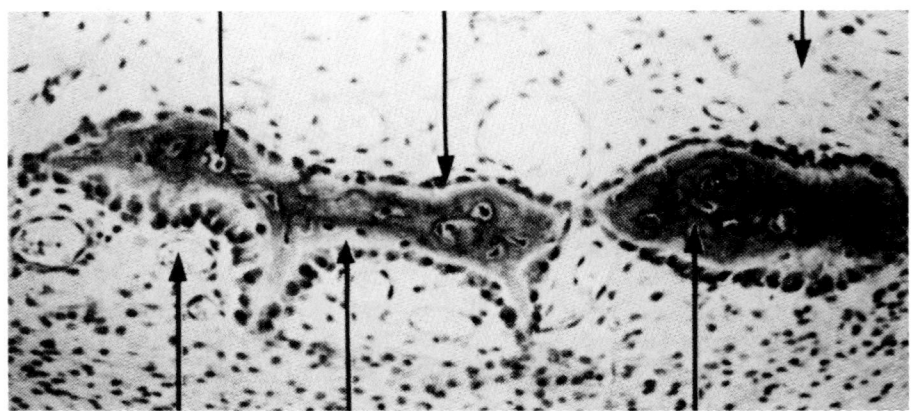

FIG. 5. Photomicrograph showing intramembranous ossification (×100). The section comes from developing bone in the mandible. [From Moore (3), with permission and courtesy of Professor Jean Hay, Department of Anatomy, University of Manitoba, Winnipeg, Canada.]

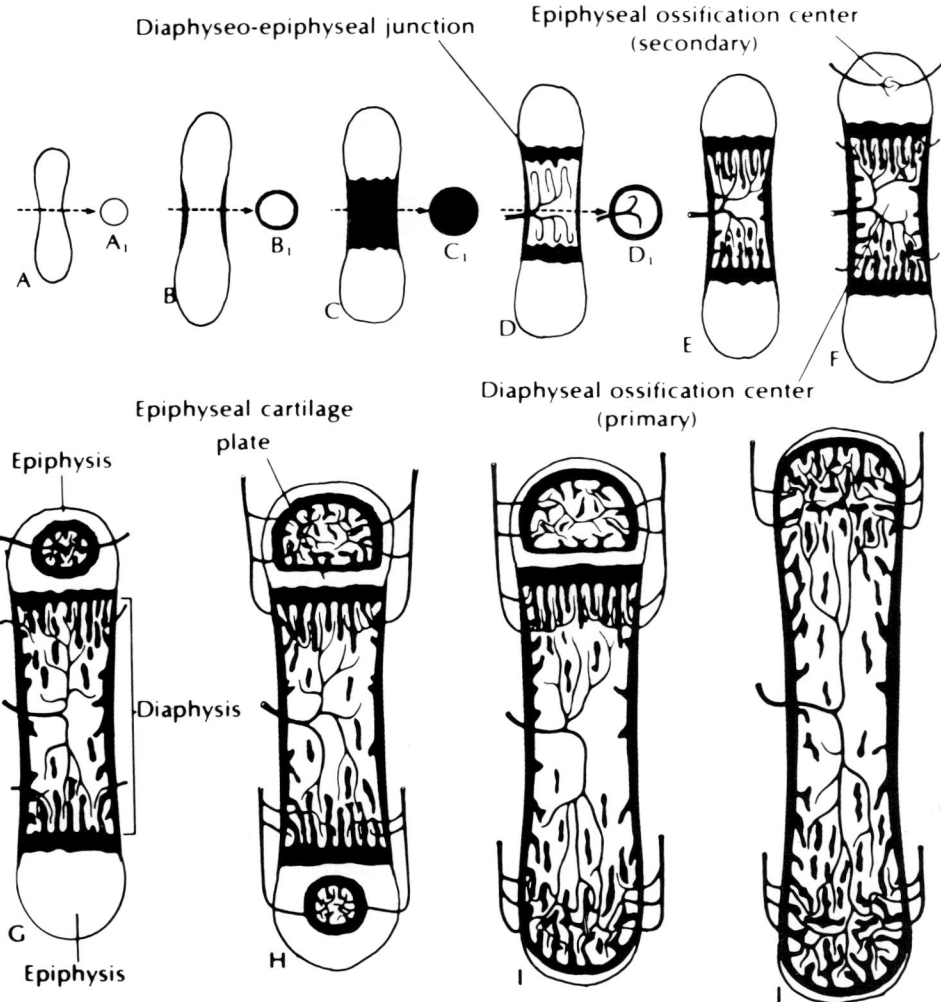

FIG. 6. Schematic diagrams of endochondral ossification and development of a long bone. **A** to **J** are longitudinal sections, and **A₁** to **D₁** are cross sections at the levels indicated. **A:** Cartilage model. **B:** Appearance of subperiosteal ring of bone. **C:** Cartilage begins to calcify. **D:** Vascular mesenchyme enters. **E:** Zone of ossification appears at diaphyseo-epiphyseal junctions. **F:** Blood vessels and mesenchyme enter at superior epiphyseal cartilage. **G:** Growth of epiphyseal ossification center. **H:** Growth of inferior epiphyseal ossification center. **I:** Ossification of inferior epiphyseal cartilage plate. **J:** Ossification of superior epiphyseal cartilage plate, and formation of a continuous bone marrow cavity. Bone elongation stops when the epiphyseal plates ossify. [Modified from Moore (3), with permission.]

because it must support the weight of the body, remaining competent while exposed to repeated small mechanical forces as well as sudden extreme ones without failing. It must provide strong attachment for muscles and must provide various levers and pivots for muscle functions, some of which are capable of generating very considerable amounts of mechanical force. It must protect various cavities such as the cranial vault and chest cavity, which contain delicate and vulnerable organs. A further requirement in the case of the chest is that the rigid cavity remains sufficiently flexible to accommodate ventilation. It does this by an arrangement of "staves" (ribs) and flexible attachments (ligaments and intercostal muscles).

Finally, it provides housing for the bone marrow, with which it maintains a very close association.

All of the bone tissue making up the skeleton exists in either of two general structural categories, compact bone and trabecular bone. Compact bone is the dense outer shell of the skeleton, and trabecular bone is the system of plates, rods, arches, and struts which is encased within the shell. About 80% of the mass of the skeleton is compact bone, and the rest is trabecular bone. Other names for compact bone are haversian bone or cortical bone, and other names for trabecular bone are cancellous bone or spongious bone. Marrow occupies the spaces between and around the plates and struts of trabecular bone, and it is held in place by a network of fine fibrous tissue called a *reticulum,* which is attached to the inner walls of the cortex and to the trabeculae. Figure 7 shows the arrangement of trabecular bone encased within the shell of compact bone and gives a hint of the functional adaptation to mechanical forces that occurs in the skeleton. This photograph of the head of the femur and the accompanying radiograph show that the trabeculae are anisotropic, which means that they are not randomly arranged in space. Instead, they are arranged around the lines of stress that one can imagine must be present during weight-bearing when a person is in the upright posture.

Adult Long Bones or Appendicular Skeleton

The appendicular skeleton is defined as the bones of the extremities, including all of the bones of the limb girdles. The more distal of the bones of the appendicular skeleton are called the *long bones* and are shaped in the form of cylinders or tubes, with the outer walls of the tubes made up of compact bone and the inner cavities filled with trabeculae and marrow. The tubes are not perfect cylinders but show some irregularity in cross-sectional shape due to the combined effects of (a) mechanical forces experienced during development and (b) the genetic blueprint. For example, the cross section of the tibia in the human and most animals is triangular in shape, whereas the metacarpal is more nearly cylindrical.

The cavity of a long bone is called the *medullary canal* or *medullary cavity,* and its boundary is defined as the diameter delimited by the junction of the cortex and marrow. Figure 8 shows the anatomic regions of a long bone. The majority of the long cylindrical part of the bone is called the "diaphysis," and each of the ends is called an *epiphysis.* The region immediately adjacent to the epiphysis, called the *metaphysis,* is a cone-shaped region which tapers to blend into the diaphysis. The epiphysis and metaphysis are delineated by an epiphyseal line, the remnant of the broad cartilaginous growth plate which disappears when growth or elongation is complete in the fully mature animal.

Adult Axial Skeleton and Flat Bones

The spine, ribs, sternum, and skull make up the axial skeleton, which contains bones that are irregularly shaped or flat. (The proximal appendicular skeleton contains parts that are also flat and/or irregular in shape.) Regardless of the shape of these bones or whether they are axial or appendicular, they consist of an outer shell of compact bone surrounding an inner cavity containing trabecular bone and marrow.

The gross anatomy of vertebrae deserves special attention because of the frequency of disease occurring there. The anterior part of each vertebra consists of (a) a cylindrical body containing an outer shell of compact bone and (b) an inner cavity containing trabecular bone and marrow. The posterior part consists of a complex struc-

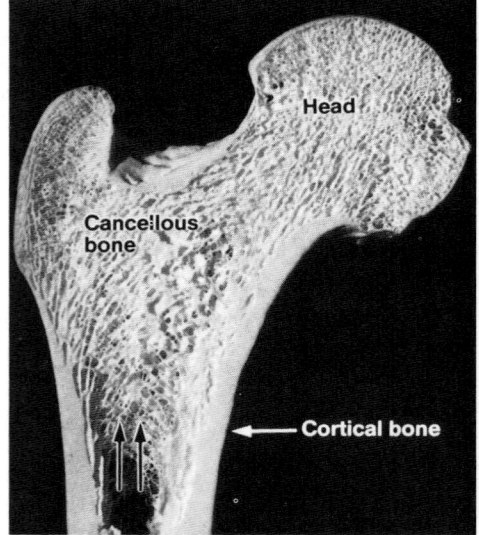
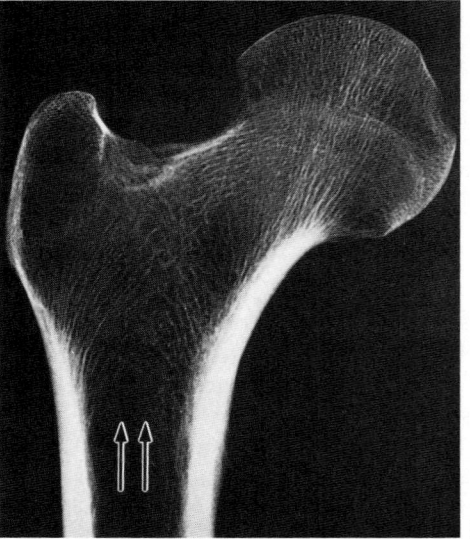

FIG. 7. Bone section and radiograph of dried proximal end of normal human femur. **A:** Photograph of 8-mm-thick proximal femur cut in a frontal plane. The head and greater trochanter are encased in a thin shell of cortical (compact) bone, while the shaft is encased in a thick cylinder of cortical (compact) bone. The arching pattern of trabeculae are arranged around the lines of stress to which the bone was exposed during life. **B:** Radiograph of same bone section. [From Weiss (5), with permission and courtesy of Professor W. S. S. Jee.]

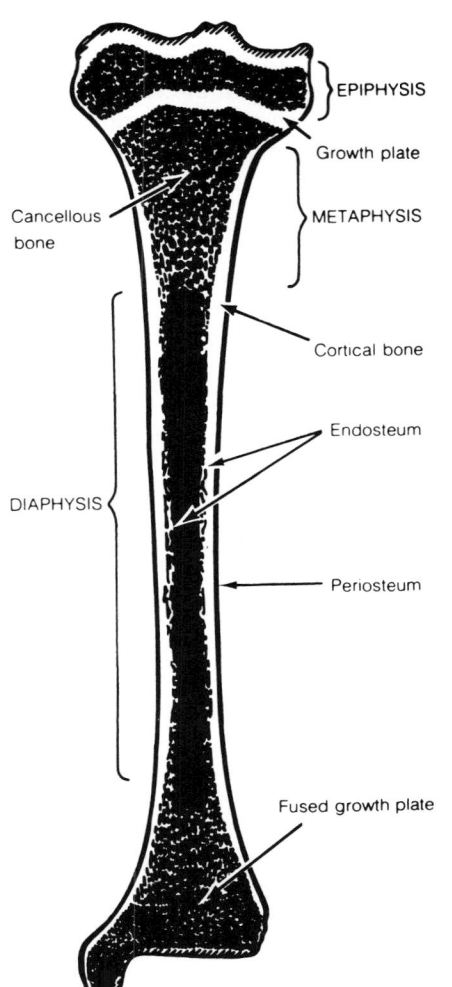

FIG. 8. Schematic diagram of frontal section of a growing human tibia. The proximal epiphyseal plate remains open while at the distal end the epiphysis is fused to the metaphysis. [From Weiss (5), with permission and courtesy of Professor W. S. S. Jee.]

ture which houses the spinal cord within an arch. Protruding from the arch are lateral and posterior spinous processes along with articular facets which connect each vertebra. The vertebral bodies support most of the weight of the person, and they are cushioned by intervertebral disks of gelatinous material located within the confines of the annular ligament. The annular ligament is strongly attached at the margins of each vertebral body above and below.

Whole vertebrae have been thought to consist of 50–75% trabecular bone. This is of particular interest because: (a) there is a high rate of metabolism in trabecular bone compared to that in compact bone; (b) the spine is a major target of disease in osteoporosis; and (c) measurements of bone mineral are commonly made in the spine. Thus spine metabolism, spine disease, and spine mass have been assumed to be largely trabecular metabolism,

trabecular disease, and trabecular mass. However, recent work (6) has shown that the mass of whole vertebrae is no more than about 25% trabecular bone and that the mass of the vertebral body is no more than about 40% trabecular bone. Thus significant changes in mass, as measured in the spine by methods which include entire vertebrae (dual photon absorptiometry), probably include significant changes in the compact, as well as the trabecular, bone of the spine.

BONE AS A TISSUE

The Matrix–Mineral Composite

The structural material of the skeleton is a composite made up of two phases, an organic and an inorganic one. Detailed description of this composite is presented in Chapter 12; however, for the reader's convenience in understanding the following discussion, a brief description is given here. Water makes up about 20% of the wet weight of bone tissue, and of the dry weight about 77% is inorganic and 23% is organic (7). The organic phase is made up of about 89% collagen. The remainder is a complex mixture of noncollagenous proteins such as osteocalcin, osteonectin, sialoproteins, proteoglycans, and others which are discussed in other chapters of the volume, along with small amounts of lipids and carbohydrates. The collagen–mineral composite is the source of the mechanical strength of the skeleton and is the focus of attention here.

The collagen is type I, and each molecule consists of two α_1 chains and one α_2 chain (8). The collagen molecules exist in a helical structure containing considerable cross-linking together with some post-translational attachment of galactose. They are packed end-to-end into fibrils which contain holes or pores in the gaps between the end of one and the beginning of another. The packing of collagen fibrils is illustrated in Fig. 9. The holes measure about 400 Å and are the site of precipitation of about half of the mineral deposited in bone. The remainder of the mineral is deposited along the length of the fibers and between them. The noncollagenous proteins occupy this space as well. The collagen fibrils can be seen by light microscopy in decalcified and undecalcified thin sections as alternating lines of refracted light which parallel the surfaces of the trabeculae or which are distributed concentrically around the haversian canals in compact bone.

The mineral is in the form of hydroxyapatite, a crystalline lattice in which the principal components are calcium and phosphate ions. (Apatite is the form in which most of the earth's calcium phosphate salt is precipitated, whether in biological or nonbiological systems.) The empirical formula for the hydroxyapatite in bone is $Ca_{10}(PO_4)_6(OH)_2$; a number of substitutions are possible

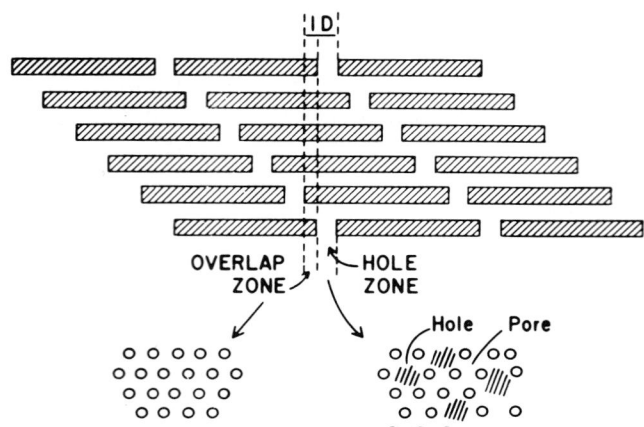

FIG. 9. Schematic view of packing of collagen molecules within a fibril. The overlap zone, hole zone, holes, and pores are demonstrated in longitudinal section above and in cross section below. Holes are spaces present at the ends of collagen molecules, and pores are spaces between collagen molecules. The mineral crystals deposit in the spaces around the collagen molecules and in the holes. The exact composite molecular arrangement of collagen and mineral crystals is not yet known. [Modified from Veis and Sabsay (8), with permission.]

(e.g., fluoride) which can change the material properties. The substitutions may also act to entrap small amounts of various elements and components such as magnesium or carbonate.

Material Properties of Bone Tissue

As materials engineers have known for many years, the composite arrangement of bone tissue yields a material that is very strong for its weight and much stronger than either component would be alone. Because the collagen matrix component is a fiber, the direction of the fiber elements affects the material properties much like the direction of the grain in lumber determines the orientation or direction that it is strongest. The effect of this orientation is illustrated in Table 1, which shows results of experiments on the strength of bone tissue—in this case a human femur (9). As shown here, bone can withstand more force in the longitudinal direction than in the transverse direction in both tension and compression.

Furthermore, bone tends to resist force better in compression than in tension. This corresponds to the function of the femur, where in iife the predominant direction of force is longitudinal compression during weight-bearing and locomotion. The osteoblasts which lay down bone matrix must be fed information on the directions and amounts of force being applied to the tissue they are building during their work, and they must have the machinery to respond in order to produce optimal orientation of the fibers.

Table 2 presents information on the mechanical strength of bone relative to several common structural materials (10). It compares favorably with cast iron and is about half as strong as one form of steel. It compares very favorably with aluminum and an aluminum alloy and is about twice as strong as Lucite or Teflon. The weight of bone is much less than any of the materials in the table, ranging from about 10% the weight of cast iron to about 30–40% the weight of Lucite. Thus the strength/weight ratio of bone is very high compared to that of other common structural materials.

Table 3 illustrates peak functional strains in a number of animals of widely varying size during activities that elicited the highest recorded strains in these animals (11). It is most interesting that these different load-bearing bones from different areas and different species showed maximum peak strains that were remarkably similar. Nature seems to have developed a means of scaling the skeletal dimensions over a very wide range of animal size without changing the intrinsic material properties of bone tissue and without creating a skeleton so massive in large animals that locomotion is restricted. Furthermore, the safety factors for yield failure and for ultimate failure are about 3 and approaching 10, respectively (12). Thus bones from a variety of animals can withstand about three times their usual peak force before damage begins to occur and about 10 times usual peak force before complete failure (fracture) occurs.

Functional Adaptation of the Fiber–Mineral Composite

The phrase "functional adaptation," when used in the field of skeletal science, can have many meanings. Here it refers to the phenomenon of arrangement or rearrangement of the geometry of bone tissue in the living ani-

TABLE 1. *Ultimate properties of human femur*

	Ultimate stress[a]		Yield stress,[b] longitudinal	Strain at fracture[c]	
	Longitudinal	Transverse		Longitudinal	Transverse
Tension	133	51	114	31,000	7,000
Compression	193	133		19,000	28,000

[a] Ultimate stress (megapascals, mPa) = force at which complete failure (fracture) occurs.
[b] Yield stress (megapascals, mPa) = force at which damage begins; bending occurs, but not fracture; fails to return to prebending shape.
[c] Microstrain (μE) = fractional change in dimension of 10^{-6} (9).

TABLE 2. *Typical mechanical properties at room temperature*

	Tensile strength (mPa)	Yield strength (mPa)
Human femur	133	114
Cast iron	124–413	55–276
Steel (SAE 1300 annealed)	483	276
Aluminum (pure, rolled)	90–166	20–145
Aluminum (copper alloy)	131–159	83–110
Lucite (methylmethacrylate)		48
Teflon		14–31

Source: Adapted from Reilly and Burstein (9) and Baumeister (10).

mal to obtain the greatest mechanical strength while retaining the greatest economy of mass. This phenomenon operates at all levels from the submicroscopic to the microscopic and macro levels. The fiber–mineral composite is at the junction between submicroscopic and microscopic; it, too, shows evidence of adaptation to the forces placed on it. For example, Barbos et al. (13) showed that the longitudinal and transverse lamellae of the adult human femur had a rotational distribution consistent with the distribution of the bending forces normally operative in the bone. The lamellae tend to be (a) transverse where the forces tend to be compressive and (b) longitudinal where the forces tend to be tensile (14).

Furthermore, Riggs et al. (15) demonstrated that longitudinal arrays of lamellae in the adult equine radius existed where the strains were predominantly tensile, whereas transverse arrays existed where the strains were predominantly compressive. However, the primary bone, deposited in the absence of mechanical forces prior to birth in the equine radius, contained predominantly longitudinal lamellae. Their conclusion from these findings was that secondary haversian bone (deposited after birth) in the horse is laid down in a strain-sensitive manner corresponding to the fact that it is formed postnatally—that is, when the animal is ambu-

lating and the skeleton is subjected to strain. On the other hand, prenatal primary bone is not subjected to mechanical force during formation and thus is not laid down in a strain-sensitive manner.

The microstructural features of bone tissue and the material properties described in previous sections indicate that bone-forming cells must possess mechanisms for detecting the mechanical environment and responding appropriately to it. At present, we know very little about these mechanisms. Furthermore, as will be seen in later sections of this chapter, the mechanical environment of working bone cells influences the architecture of bone tissue on a scale much larger than the microstructure of the collagen fibers as described above. Mechanisms must exist that regulate and coordinate large groups of bone cells spread over large areas. The challenge for biologists is to discover these mechanisms so that they might be manipulated to inhibit or reverse skeletal fragility in the treatment of patients with bone diseases (1,2,16,17).

BONE ENVELOPES

There are five envelopes that have been described within and surrounding the skeleton. These are called "envelopes" in the sense that each describes a broad surface area of the skeleton containing similar groups of cells coordinated to perform a similar function within a similar relative location. They are important to distinguish because the metabolic activities that occur on each of them are somewhat different and the systems that organize bone cell function on each are also different. Thus functionally they are distinct.

Periosteal Envelope or Periosteum

The periosteal envelope is defined as the envelope which covers or encases the entire skeleton on its outer margin. It is largely covered by a layer of undifferen-

TABLE 3. *Peak functional strains measured from strain gauges[a]*

Bone	Activity	Microstrain	Safety factor	
			Yield	Ultimate
Horse radius	Trotting	−2800	2.4	5.6
Horse tibia	Galloping	−3200	2.1	4.9
Horse metacarpal	Accelerating	−3000	2.3	5.2
Dog radius	Trotting	−2600	2.6	6.1
Dog tibia	Galloping	−2100	3.2	7.4
Turkey tibia	Running	−2350	2.9	6.7

[a] Peak functional strains (μE, in microstrain) were measured from bonded strain gauges in a range of animals of different sizes during their customary activity which elicited the highest recorded strains (11). These different load-bearing bones from different areas and different species showed maximum peak strains that were remarkably similar. Safety factors for yield failure and for ultimate failure were based on values of 6800 and 15,700 microstrain, published by Carter et al. (12).

tiated cells (called a *cambrian layer*) which, in turn, is covered by a sheath of fibrous connective tissue. These layers are not present in areas where tendons and ligaments attach or in areas covered by articular cartilage. The neck of the femur, the subscapular area, and sesamoid bones also do not possess these layers. The periosteal envelope increases in area in most parts of the skeleton throughout life in humans as the outer volume of the skeleton expands. The increase is steady during childhood, accelerates during adolescence, and then continues at a very slow pace until death. It is fundamentally a forming envelope playing a significant role in fracture healing and in the response to intense mechanical usage (18–20).

Haversian Envelope

The haversian envelope encompasses the compact or cortical bone. It is an envelope in the sense that the center of each haversian system contains vessels and a nerve which lie within a fibroblast network surrounded by a membrane which is in apposition to a bone surface. Furthermore, the interface between the osteocyte (or its cytoplasmic extensions) and the adjacent mineralized tissue can be thought of as part of this envelope, and the walls of Volkmann's canals can also be thought of as part of this envelope.

Figure 10 is a schematic diagram showing the arrangement of circumferential lamellae and primary and secondary osteons in the haversian or cortical envelope. Primary osteons are the first haversian systems that were formed. Secondary osteons are haversian systems that were formed later, and they tend to leave parts of primary osteons between them. After a time, successive waves of new osteons convert the entire cortex to secondary osteons.

The haversian envelope is not ordinarily a bone-losing one. Even in patients with osteoporosis and reduced bone mass, the haversian envelope does not tend to develop spaces or voids. Of course, the size of the haversian envelope shrinks with age and with osteoporosis, but

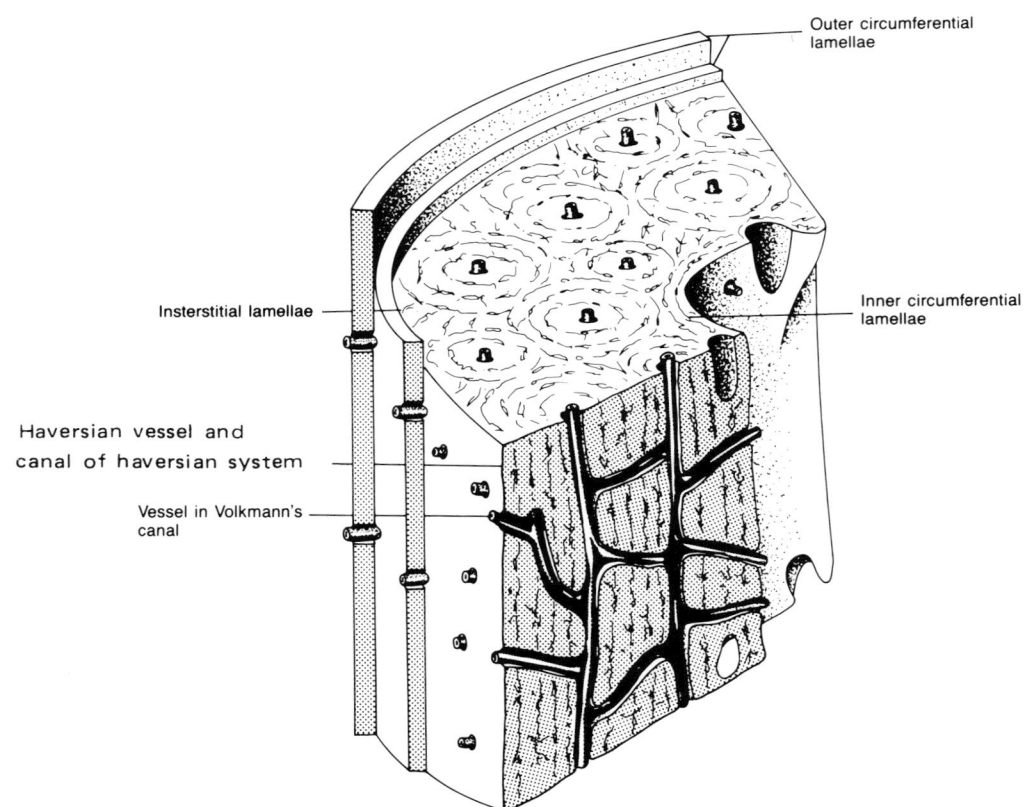

FIG. 10. Schematic diagram of a cutout of compact bone from the diaphysis of an adult long bone showing the haversian envelope. The histological organization is seen showing an outer circumferential layer of lamellae, an inner circumferential layer of lamellae, and the haversian systems in between. The interstitial lamellae are remnants of earlier (primary) haversian systems that were partially removed during remodeling. The newer (secondary) haversian systems are identified by their uninterrupted circumferences. Nutrition is brought to the haversian vessels from the transverse Volkmann's canals, which penetrate the outer circumferential lamellae and the periosteum. The number of osteons has been reduced for simplicity. [Modified from Cormack (48), with permission.]

that is due to either (a) movement of the cortico-endosteal envelope toward the periosteum or (b) expansion of the medullary canal at the expense of the cortex or haversian envelope (21).

Cortico-endosteal Envelope

The cortico-endosteal envelope is defined as the envelope which delimits the outermost boundary of the medullary canal. It is interrupted by connections of trabeculae to the cortex. (It should be noted that all trabeculae are connected to the inner wall of the cortex at the cortico-endosteal envelope.) It is generally a bone-losing envelope, and except for a relatively short period of time in adolescence in young women when it moves centrally toward the marrow cavity (22), it expands throughout life. In the process it outpaces the expansion of the periosteal envelope and thus the cortex tends to thin throughout most of life.

Endosteal Envelope

The endosteal envelope is also referred to as the *trabecular envelope* and can be thought of as the interface between the marrow and trabecular bone. The ratio of endosteal surface to trabecular volume is high compared to the surface-to-volume ratio of the other envelopes. Because most of the metabolic activities in bone occur on surfaces, it is not surprising that the metabolic activity on this envelope, as compared to that on other envelopes, is greater in relation to the volume of bone. This is predominantly a bone-losing envelope, although throughout much of life it shows neither gain or loss.

Transitional Envelope

The transitional envelope is an ill-defined area immediately adjacent to the cortico-endosteal envelope, occupying about one-third of the space of the medullary cavity between the cortico-endosteal surfaces. It was called the *transitional zone* in transileal biopsy specimens by Keshawarz and Recker (21). It does not possess an easily defined boundary, and thus most workers have included it within the endosteal envelope. Reasons to consider it as a separate envelope are as follows: (a) It is an area of trabecular bone where metabolic activity (remodeling) is highest, and (b) it is an area of trabecular bone which is taken from the inner portion of the cortex as the medullary canal enlarges at the expense of the cortex.

BONE SURFACES

There are basically three types of bone surfaces described by bone histologists and histomorphometrists:

resting, forming, and resorbing surfaces. They usually refer to surfaces confined to the endosteal envelope, although the other envelopes also exhibit resting, forming, and resorbing surfaces at various times and under various circumstances as will be seen below.

Resting Surface (Fig. 11)

The resting surface is quiescent because neither forming nor resorbing activities or cells are present. It is smooth and covered by a very thin layer of lining cells (see below). It is in communication with the osteocytes that are distributed throughout the bone tissue. This important surface is the interface between bone tissue on the one hand and bone cell modeling and remodeling activities on the other. Somehow, messages must reach this surface of bone cell activity, and these messages must contain information to select the location for remodeling activity, to trigger the differentiation of bone cells from their precursors at that location, and to regulate the amount of work they do at that location. The resting surface is very important in the intermediary organization of the skeleton, but unfortunately it is not well understood.

Forming Surface

The forming surface (see Fig. 11) is characterized by unmineralized osteoid, with or without overlying osteoblasts. Histomorphometrists also refer to it as the *osteoid surface*. The name infers that bone formation is taking place at the time of the sampling, but that can only be an inference when viewing sections such as those seen in Fig. 11. The forming surface as defined here is a static feature, and measurements of it are referred to as *static measurements* by histomorphometrists. No quantitative or dynamic rate information can be obtained from viewing or measuring these static surfaces. Dynamic measurements of bone appositional rates and their derivative calculations (bone formation rates, bone formation periods, etc.) can be obtained by using fluorochrome tissue–time markers such as tetracycline. These markers are given to subjects (or animals) in two time periods prior to obtaining bone samples. They are deposited at bone-forming sites in vivo and are activated by fluorescent light microscopy of unstained specimens. Knowing the time interval between administration of labels, the measured distance between labels, and the extent of surface covered by labels, one can obtain dynamic information about bone formation at an individual remodeling site and can estimate average bone formation over all surfaces (23). Nevertheless, the presence of unmineralized osteoid is sufficient to refer to a surface as a forming surface even in the absence of markers. The identification of a bone-forming site as defined here requires the

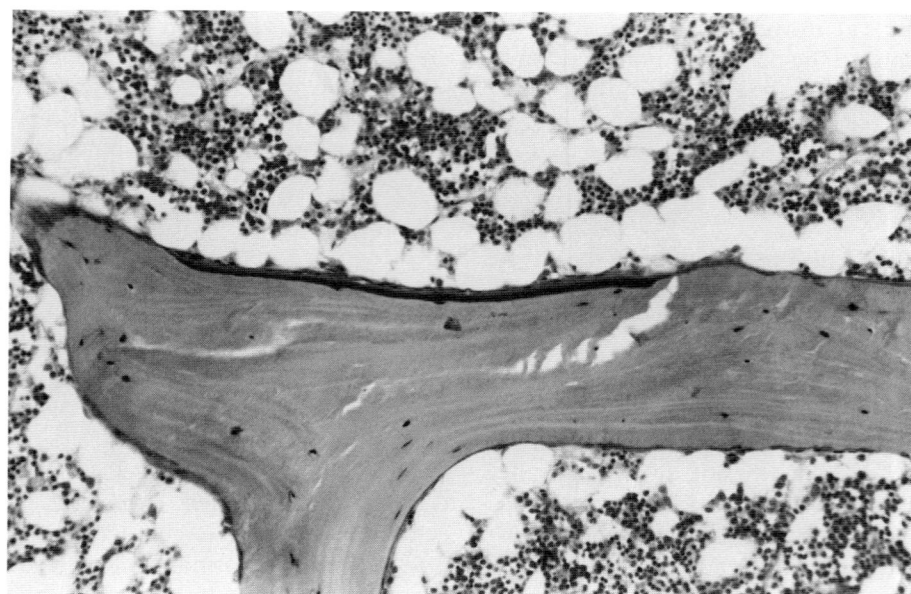

FIG. 11. Photomicrograph (Goldner's stain, ×115) of a thin section from an undemineralized human transileal biopsy specimen. There is a resting trabecular surface in the lower right portion of the figure. It is smooth and there are no osteoblasts or osteoclasts. It is devoid of formation or resorption. The lining cells are few in number and are thin. There is also a forming trabecular surface in the center of the figure. The osteoid is darker than the mineralized bone. Relatively flat osteoblasts are present at the surface of the osteoid.

use of undemineralized sections stained so that mineralized and unmineralized osteoid can be distinguished from one another.

Active bone formation at a forming surface may pause and then resume at a later time (24,25). This pause is called *off-time* by Frost (26), and a method of calculating it has been demonstrated by Kimmel et al. (27). During the off-time, osteoid at the forming site is covered by lining cells and the absence of forming activity is confirmed by the absence of tetracycline label. The importance of the phenomenon of "off-time" is not yet fully understood.

Resorbing Surface

The hallmark of the resorbing surface is the appearance of a scalloped erosion (Fig. 12), also called an *eroded surface* or *Howship's lacuna*. This scalloped surface may or may not have a bone-resorbing cell in contact with it. When there are no bone-resorbing cells, a resorption surface is said to be inactive or in a resting or reversal stage (28); histomorphometrists divide the resorption surface into an active and an inactive component based on the presence or absence of resorbing cells. By using an acid phosphatase stain (29), one can get a more accurate measure of the surface occupied by osteoclasts, since this stain allows identification of mononuclear osteoclasts or even osteoclast cytoplasm devoid of nuclei.

It is important to understand that resorptive activity may or may not be taking place at a resorptive site at the time of sampling regardless of whether an osteoclast is present. Tetracycline markers allow measurements of tissue and cell-level bone formation rates, but there is no counterpart for measurement of tissue- and cell-level bone resorption rates. The histomorphometric measures of resorbing surfaces are static measures and do not give information about resorbing rates (23).

BONE CELLS

Osteoblasts

Any cell that forms bone (Fig. 13)—whether during growth and modeling, during adult remodeling, or during fracture healing—is, by definition, an osteoblast. In all cases these cells appear to be very similar in morphology. Furthermore, the changes in morphology that occur during their lifespan of active bone formation are similar irrespective of their site of activity. They first appear as very plump cuboidal cells lined up in a palisade along the forming site. In most microscopic sections, osteoid had already begun to appear when the sample was obtained, and thus the cells line up on the surface of unmineralized osteoid. It is very rare to see plump osteoblasts in place at a formation site devoid of unmineralized osteoid, since the period of time between differentiation of osteoblasts and the formation of the first matrix is very short. Early

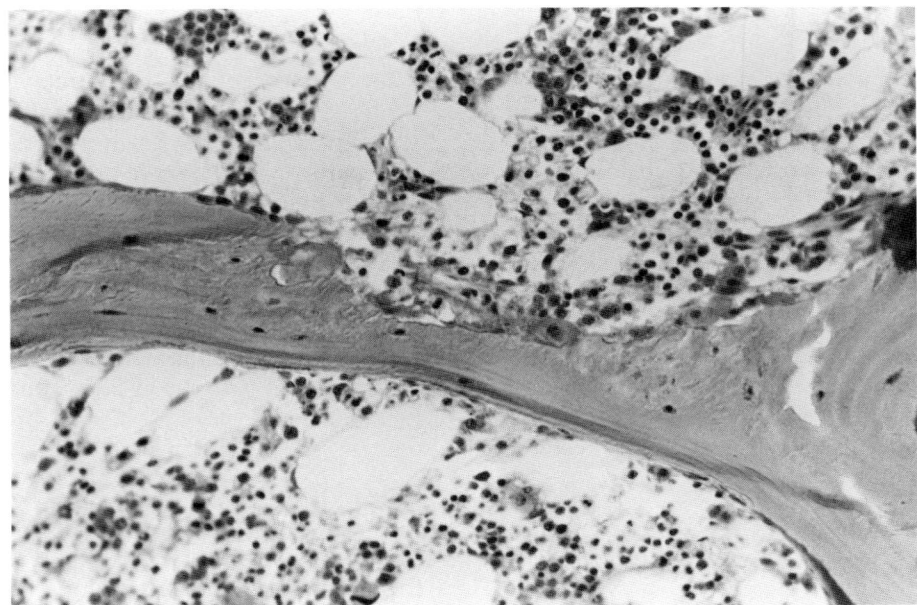

FIG. 12. Photomicrograph (Goldner's stain, ×115) of trabecular resorbing surface in a thin section from an undemineralized human transileal biopsy specimen. The heavily scalloped surface in the right center denotes a large Howship's lacuna. Part of the erosion surface is in contact with osteoclasts. Osteoclasts and their erosion surfaces occupy a much smaller portion of the trabecular surface than do either (i) lining cells and their resting surfaces or (ii) osteoblasts and their forming surfaces. A resting surface is present in the lower left.

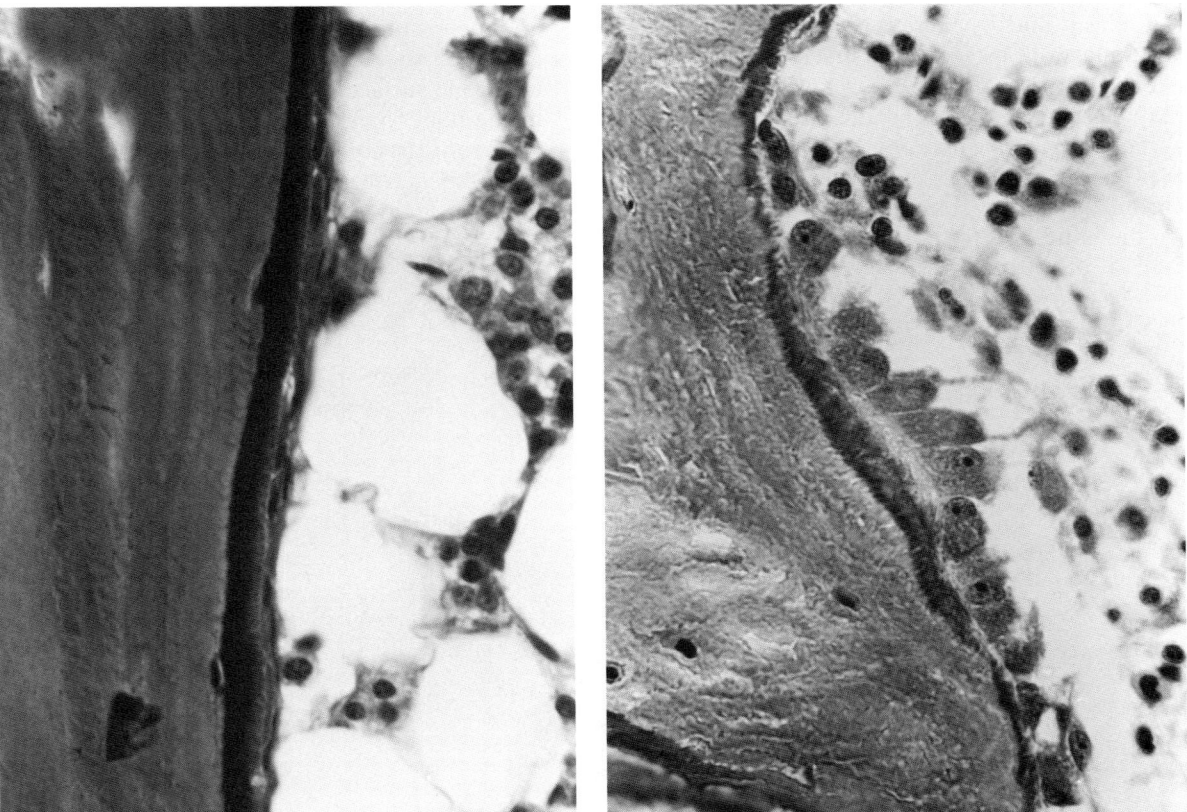

A   B

FIG. 13. Photomicrograph (Goldner's stain, ×325) of trabecular forming surface; thin section from an undemineralized human transileal biopsy specimen. **A:** High-power view of osteoblasts lined up on a surface of unmineralized osteoid. These are newly created osteoblasts as judged by their plump appearance. The eccentric nuclei and prominent Golgi apparatus are visible. **B:** More mature forming site as judged by the more flattened osteoblasts, which are fewer in number and contain a flattened, oblong nucleus. The Golgi apparatus is less visible.

in the process, the nuclei are eccentric and there are prominent Golgi zones. Osteoblasts also have cell processes, gap junctions, endoplasmic reticulum, and collagen-containing secretory vesicles. As formation progresses, the osteoblasts decrease in number at the formation site and they become more flattened. Bone-forming activity slows, and some of the osteoblasts become incorporated into the formed bone as osteocytes. Others remain on the surface as lining cells. The lifespan of the individual osteoblast depends on whether or not it becomes an osteocyte. The functional lifespan of the team of osteoblasts at a given bone remodeling site may range from 3–4 months to 1.5 years. The average is about 5–6 months (30).

Lining Cells

Lining cells (see Fig. 14) are remnants of the team of osteoblasts that previously laid down bone matrix. The cytoplasm is usually not visible on light microscopy, and the nucleus is barely visible, elongated or flattened, and darkly stained by most methods of staining. Lining cells communicate with the syncytium of osteocytes through the osteocytic canaliculi. On exposure to parathyroid hormone, they respond by contracting the boundaries of their cytoplasm and by secreting enzymes which clear away a thin layer of osteoid. The first step seems to permit osteoclasts to begin bone resorption (31). Lining cells may be very important in the selection of specific sites on bone surfaces where modeling or remodeling is to take place.

There has been some confusion regarding the name given to the bone cells found on resting surfaces. Histo-morphometrists have traditionally referred to them as *lining cells*, whereas cell biologists have often called them *osteoblasts*. Although it is true that they are cells left over from the team of osteoblasts that formed bone, they have departed far enough from the osteoblast phenotype in both function and morphology that they should carry a distinct name. The term *lining cells* should be used to distinguish them in thin sections from the plump, metabolically active osteoblasts found in palisades at bone-forming sites, and it should also be used in discussions of both the histology and physiology of bone metabolism.

Osteocytes

Osteocytes are survivors of the group of osteoblasts from each forming site which became entrapped in the bone matrix as it was being laid down (Fig. 15). Describing them as survivors implies that some of the bone-forming cells disappeared or were lost during formation. Indeed, Parfitt (32) has shown that fewer cells survive as osteocytes than were present as osteoblasts during bone formation. The fate of the missing osteoblasts is unknown.

Osteocyte cell bodies are found in lacunae (Fig. 16), and their multiple cytoplasmic processes extend through canaliculi to communicate with neighboring osteocytes and bone surface cells. The canaliculi are small tunnels in the bone, measuring about 1–2 μm in diameter. Osteocyte nutrition probably takes place across the gap junctions between the cytoplasmic extensions of neighboring osteocytes. Ion and nutrient exchange may also occur by flow along the fluid space between the cell walls

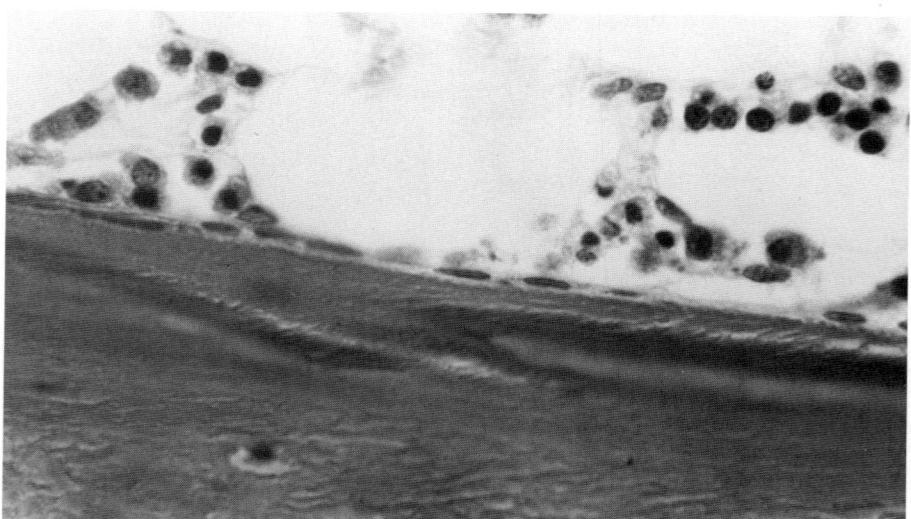

FIG. 14. Photomicrograph (Goldner's stain, ×625) of trabecular lining cells; thin section from an unde-mineralized human transileal biopsy specimen. The nuclei are barely visible and are very thin, flattened, and dark-staining. The cytoplasm of the lining cells is usually not visible at all at this power. A thin line of osteoid is often visible beneath lining cells and is called the "lamina limitans." This may be a small remnant of permanently unmineralized osteoid present in vivo, or it may be due to leaching of a small amount of mineral from the trabecular surface during fixing of the specimen.

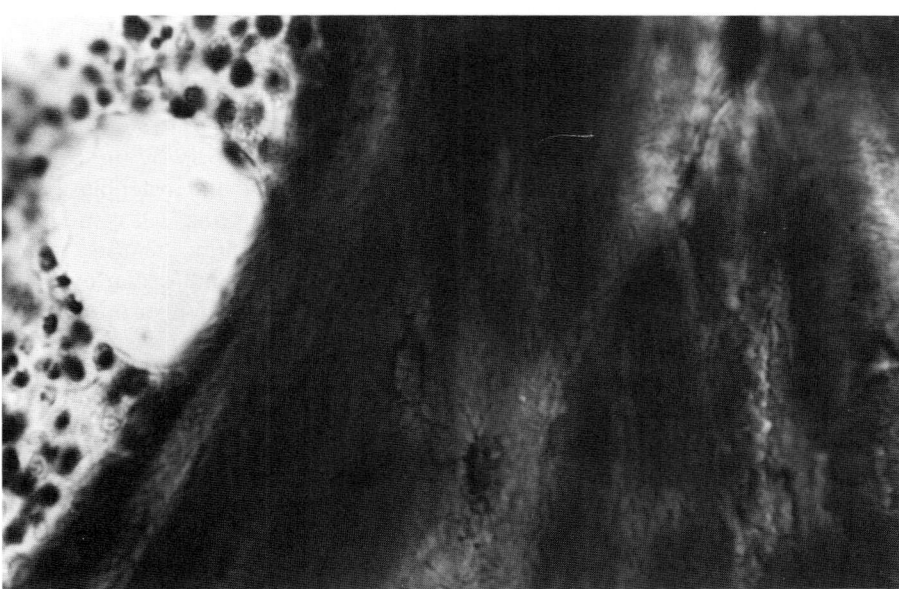

FIG. 15. Photomicrograph (toluidine blue stain, ×710) of osteocytes; thin section from an undemineralized human transileal biopsy specimen. The canaliculi are very small but numerous, and they contain the cytoplasmic extensions of osteocytes. This section shows an osteocyte lacuna, with numerous ones extending as thin, dark, spidery lines, some toward a neighboring osteocyte lacuna. The mineralized bone is stained more darkly here compared to the other sections that are stained with modified Goldner's stain.

of the osteocytic processes and the solid mineralized walls of the canaliculi. The network of canaliculi is very dense; none of the bone tissue is more than a few micrometers away from an osteocytic extension. Osteocytes never divide, and only one normally ever occupies a la-

cuna. Their lifespan varies with the lifespan of the bone tissue in which they are embedded. They are destroyed when bone is resorbed.

The function of osteocytes is not clear. Osteocytic death is associated with a small increase in the mineral-

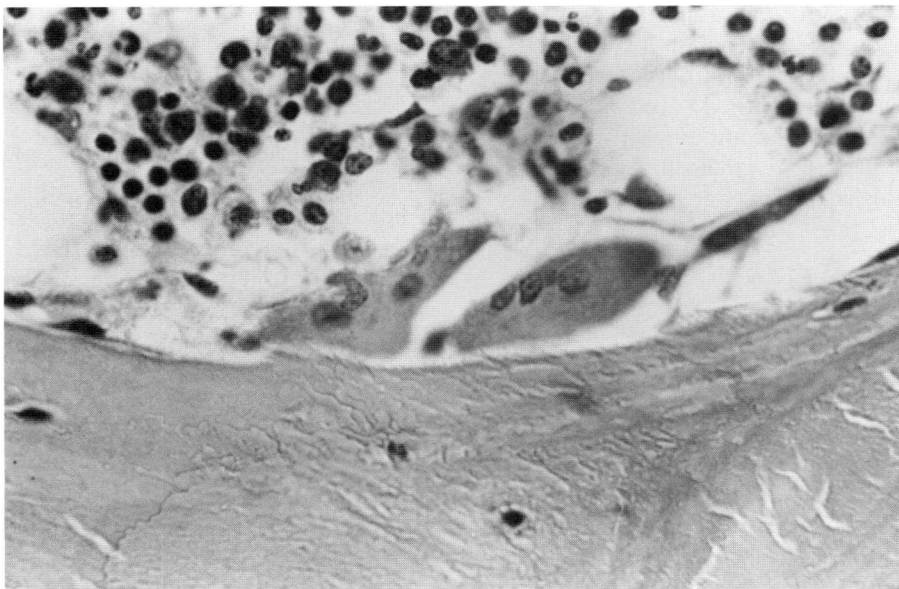

FIG. 16. Photomicrograph (Goldner's stain, ×740) of osteoclasts; thin section from an undemineralized human transileal biopsy specimen. This pair of osteoclasts is in a very shallow Howship's lacuna. Osteoclasts contain multiple nuclei, each with several nucleoli. The cytoplasm stains dark pink with Goldner's stain. They may contain up to 50 nuclei and measure up to 100 μm in diameter. The zone of attachment to the bone surface, where bone resorption is active, is faintly visible in both these osteoclasts. An electron-microscopic examination of this resorption would probably reveal a brush border with a surrounding clear zone.

ization of the neighboring osteoid, the significance of which is not understood. The location of osteocytes, along with their network of cytoplasmic communication, suggests that they may play a role in sensing strain resulting from mechanical force applied to the skeleton during mechanical usage, or they could act as part of a transducer mechanism that converts changes in the strain environment into organized bone cell work.

Osteoclasts

Osteoclasts are multinucleated giant cells which resorb bone (Fig. 16). They range from 20 μm to over 100 μm in cross section and contain 2–50 nuclei. They occupy shallow pits called "Howship's lacunae" on flat bone surfaces, and they are present in the leading edge of cutting cones in haversian bone. Features seen on light microscopy include a foamy acidophilic cytoplasm, a striated appearance at the site of attachment to the bone, and positive staining for tartrate-resistant acid phosphatase. On electron microscopy, the striated zone adjacent to the bone is an area of extensive membrane infoldings called the *ruffled border.* This area is very motile, and bone can be seen dissolving under it in cinematographic studies of living tissue. Surrounding the ruffled border is a clear zone devoid of organelles (called the *podosome* or *filamentous zone*), where the ruffled border is sealed to the bone surface. This seal apparently localizes the highly acidic microenvironment, which is conducive to resorption of bone. The cytoplasm contains numerous mitochondria, rough endoplasmic reticulum, multiple Golgi complexes, pairs of centrioles in a centrosome, vacuoles, and numerous granules. Osteoclasts are very metabolically active and respond to parathyroid hormone, calcitonin, 1,25-dihydroxyvitamin D, and other agonists. Their lifespan is uncertain, although it may be as long as 7 weeks. The average normal duration of a resorption site in humans is about 4 weeks.

INTERMEDIARY ORGANIZATION OF THE SKELETON

Frost (1,2) coined the term *intermediary organization* (IO) of the skeleton to describe the control and regulation of coordinated cellular events that occur in the living human or animal skeleton. These events may be coordinated over wide areas of bone surface, and the coordination may last over surprisingly long expanses of time. Frost recognized that bone cells do not work alone or individually and that the end product of their group activities was very difficult to disrupt by interventions designed to affect the work or lifespan of a single class of bone cells such as osteoclasts. He pointed out that these activities were regulated by an order of control higher than a single cell (osteoclast or osteoblast) or a single

function (resorption or formation). Thus successful pharmacologic inhibition of osteoclastic bone resorption in the human adult would not result in significant increase in bone mass, because the inhibition would eventually affect bone formation by the osteoblasts. This link between osteoclast and osteoblast function has been referred to as "coupling" (33), and investigators have been looking for coupling "factors" to explain the link between resorption and formation. Frost's paradigm holds that the link between resorption and formation is part of a higher-level control system, namely, the IO of the skeleton.

Although many subdivisions of the IO have been described by Frost, at least four discrete functional subdivisions of the general paradigm of an IO can be recognized: growth, modeling, remodeling, and fracture healing. Each of these processes has its own IO, but each utilizes the same bone cells to accomplish its work. In each case, the cells are organized to perform a different task for the organism. Abnormalities can develop in each IO independently of the others, and "coupling" of resorption and formation is very different for each of them. Thus, fracture healing can fail as a result of defects in its IO, yet remodeling can continue unaffected. Most human bone diseases are rooted in abnormalities of the IO, and our ability to cure, prevent, or reverse them depends on developing an understanding of the IO. We know little about how the work of cells on one surface and of those on another surface perhaps several centimeters away can be coordinated, and we know very little about the various subdivisions of the IO beyond descriptions of their operations.

Growth

The function of this IO is elongation of the skeleton and the creation of trabeculae. Both the control and effector mechanisms are located in the growth plate, also known as the epiphysis. A detailed description of the growth plate and its function is contained in Chapter 14 and will not be repeated here. The basic program providing instructions for this IO is genetic, with a lesser dependence on the mechanical environment in the area of the epiphysis. The evidence for this independence comes from the clinical experience that elongation continues, although at a slowed pace, in the paralyzed limb of a child who has suffered paralysis of one lower extremity. The growth IO is modulated or controlled by hormones such as growth, thyroid, and sex hormones and by factors such as insulin-like growth factor 1 (IGF-1). It is coordinated over a long period of time: extremely rapid during fetal and early postnatal life, slower during childhood, rapid again during the adolescent growth spurt, and extinguished at the end of adolescence. This coordination is orchestrated over a period of 20 or more years.

During this extended period of time, numerous factors can affect the growth pattern, but it is really quite robust to most of them. Thus, despite the fact that life during childhood is characterized by nutritional variation, repeated acute illness, environmental toxic exposures, variation in physical activity, changes in climate, and even chronic disease, the IO of growth will still emerge pretty much intact. In spite of these vicissitudes, most persons achieve reasonable adult stature. Furthermore, epiphyseal function is reasonably well coordinated over the entire body. For example, both legs elongate at an even pace even though the epiphyses involved are situated some distance apart. This is fortunate; otherwise the awkwardness of adolescence might be much worse than it is.

Modeling

Modeling is the IO responsible for shaping or sculpting the skeleton during growth. It is a highly integrated, finely tuned system, which is responsive to the mechanical forces that are placed on the skeleton while elongation is taking place at the growth plate during normal development. Figure 17 illustrates how modeling behaves in the growing tibia.

The modeling IO responds to mechanical forces by changing the shape of a bone as it elongates, converting it from the solid, large-diameter cylinder found beneath the epiphysis to the tapered hollow funnel of the metaphysis and the irregularly shaped hollow shaft of the diaphysis. The figures illustrate how in the process of modeling, formation occurs on broad surfaces while resorption occurs on parallel surfaces nearby, resulting in movement of an entire wall of bone in space. The process almost always results in a net *increase* in the amount of bone tissue present, but with its architecture arranged to obtain optimal mechanical strength from the *least* amount of tissue. Table 4 compares some of the important features of modeling with those of remodeling. It is noteworthy that the IO of modeling coordinates and controls bone cell work over large surfaces and over large distances. Furthermore, osteoclast work may occur over a large surface area in the absence of osteoblast work; conversely, osteoblast work may occur over a large surface area in the absence of osteoclast work. Activation of osteoblast precursors can occur on a bone surface to form osteoblasts without prior activation of osteoclasts. Similarly, activation of osteoclast precursors can occur to form osteoclasts without subsequent activation of osteoblasts at that site to form new bone. The concept of "coupling" of resorption and formation has a much different physiologic meaning when it occurs within the IO of modeling than it does when it occurs within the IO of remodeling. In modeling, coupling occurs in the broad sense that the osteoclasts and osteoblasts do the work in

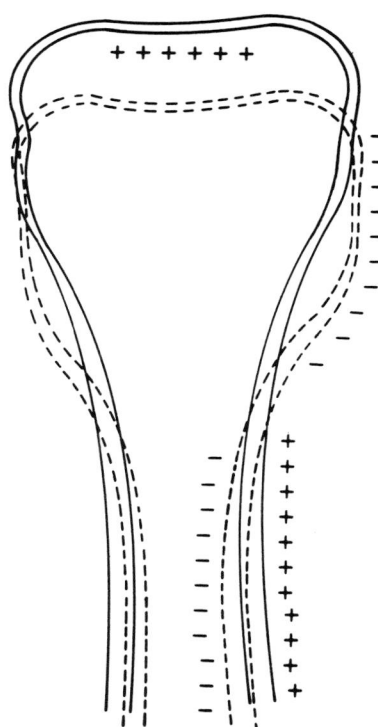

FIG. 17. Diagram of modeling occurring during growth. The dashed image (---) represents a frontal cross section of the proximal end of the tibia. The uninterrupted image represents the same tibia after about 21 days of growth. Bone is (i) added in the long axis at the proximal end, (ii) removed on the outer surface of the diaphysis and added on the inner surface of the diaphysis to shape the funnel of the metaphysis, and (iii) removed on the inner and added to the outer surface of the metaphysis to blend the cylinder of the diaphysis to the funnel of the metaphysis. The wall of the diaphysis is thickened in the process. +, bone added; −, bone removed.

coordination to accomplish the bone sculpting; however, there is usually a bit more work done by the osteoblasts than by the osteoclasts, since the process usually results in a net increase in the amount of bone tissue. In the remodeling IO described below, resorption and formation follow one another and are coupled tightly in a single remodeling site, with a scheduled length of time and a precise volume of bone (A → R → F; see discussion of remodeling, below).

TABLE 4. *Comparison of modeling and remodeling*

	Remodeling	Modeling
Location	Spatially related	Different surfaces
Coupling	A → R → F	A → F; A → R
Timing	Cyclical	Continuous
Extent	Small (<20%)[a]	Large (>90%)
Apposition rate	Slow (0.3–1.0 μm/day)	Fast (2–10 μm/day)
Balance	No change or net loss	Net gain

Source: From Jee (5).
[a] Of available surface.

The modeling IO is characterized by two more features of considerable importance: It is age-dependent, and its bone gain is mostly subperiosteal. The potential for modeling is greatly reduced in humans after adolescence; by the middle twenties, it becomes almost nonexistent. This fact is illustrated by the orthopedic experience in fracture healing in children, where alignment and apposition of fragments in, say, a tibial fracture need not be very strict. The modeling IO will correct a relatively large amount of displacement and angulation during the months and years of modeling following the injury. Conversely, defects in alignment and apposition of a tibial fracture in older adolescents and adults are largely permanent.

The second feature, subperiosteal location of activity, is harder to document, but it seems accurate. In the animal experiments of in vivo strain exposure by Rubin and Lanyon (20), as well as in the rat work now underway in the present author's laboratory (18), increased strain exposure results in periosteal new bone and little endosteal gain. Furthermore, in the present author's clinical experience, increased mechanical usage of the tibiae occurring in runners training for marathons may result in periosteal new bone without endosteal gain. However, the medullary canal is never exposed to a very intense strain environment even when excess strain is applied in bending experiments or in situations of increased physical activity. This is because most of the stress of mechanical force on bone is taken by the outer cortex (34).

Remodeling

Remodeling is the IO which functions to remove bone (described in detail in Chapter 15). The entire volume of bone removed is replaced under usual circumstances, provided that the bone is being subjected to the normal ongoing strains of mechanical usage. The pattern of remodeling in compact bone involves the creation of a resorption tunnel, which is filled in as it moves parallel to the long axis of the bone. In trabecular bone, shallow excavations are formed by osteoclasts and then filled in by a team of osteoblasts. The pattern of cell appearance at a remodeling site is *A*ctivation of osteoclasts followed by *R*esorption of existing bone followed by *F*ormation of new bone (A → R → F), all occurring at the same anatomic surface (35). The time sequence in trabecular bone in normal women is about 1 month for resorption and 5 months for formation, for a total of 6 months to complete a remodeling cycle (30). The time sequence for compact bone is a little longer. The group of cells which carry out the work of a remodeling site has been called the basic multicellular unit (BMU) (36), and the quantum of bone that is formed by a BMU has been called the basic structural unit (BSU) (23).

The remodeling IO involves the concept of "coupling," usually referred to by authors in the field. This linkage of resorption and formation is very tight; formation follows resorption at the resorption site, not at some other location, and the amount of bone formed is almost always very nearly equal to the amount removed. Coupling is also manifest at a higher level of organization; global rate changes in resorption are invariably followed by similar global rate changes in formation. Most agents or situations that inhibit resorption do so by inhibiting activation of osteoclasts. The first thing noticed thereafter is a small increase in bone mass, because the formation ongoing at the beginning of inhibition is left unaffected. Thus, a net gain of bone occurs until leftover formation has been completed. At the end of that period, bone mass will stabilize at a slightly higher level (an increase of about 1–3%), since the remodeling space is reduced. However, no further gain in bone will occur, and bone formation will stabilize at rates equal to the new resorption rates. Measures of remodeling, such as serum osteocalcin, alkaline phosphatase, and urine hydroxyproline, are lower than previous levels.

The period of time between activation of a BMU and its completion is referred to as *Sigma* by Frost (37), and its definition contains a very important inference. Whenever an animal that remodels bone sustains a perturbation changing the activation frequency of new BMUs, a transient state develops which lasts for a period of time equal to one complete Sigma. This transient state cannot "cure" a skeletal disease. In order to judge the long-term effects of a skeletal perturbation, one must wait until at least one complete Sigma has passed before beginning observation, and then one must observe the new steady state for two or more Sigmas. In humans this can take as long as several years, thus resulting in very long periods of observation in order to determine whether a trial of treatment is successful.

The remodeling process replaces aged bone tissue with new bone tissue. With the passage of time, repeated strain (bending) of skeletal tissue that occurs during ordinary mechanical usage (locomotion or any physical activity) results in the development of microdamage and the need to replace or renew bone tissue. Unless microdamage is repaired, it will accumulate and lead to catastrophic structural failure, namely, fracture. A dramatic example of accumulation of microdamage and structural failure of the skeleton occurs in the military recruits who suffer "march fractures" during early training. In these cases, mechanical usage is increased so much that normal remodeling cannot keep pace in repairing the microdamage. It is likely that many clinical syndromes of excess skeletal fragility (osteoporoses) involve defective microdamage repair, since the fragility is out of proportion to the decrease in bone mass (27); in addition, dynamic histomorphometry has demonstrated sluggish or inefficient remodeling. Much more research is needed in order to measure the location and burden of microdamage in the skeletons of humans with excessive skeletal fragility and to discover the mechanism which links activation of BMUs to sites of microdamage.

Fracture Healing

This IO is mentioned here in order to separate it from the others. A detailed description can be found in texts of histology, pathology, and orthopedics and will not be repeated here. However, a few interesting features about this IO should be pointed out. The sequence of events occurring at a fracture involves clot formation, mesenchymal (fibroblast) cell proliferation, appearance of osteoblasts, and the very rapid formation of a large amount of cartilage and woven bone around the fracture site. This is a highly organized group of activities which has the result of restoring mechanical strength to the fracture site in the shortest time possible. After the deposition of a large fracture callus of woven bone, the callus is gradually removed and replaced by normal lamellar bone; the end result is restoration of the fracture site to its previous state. The entire process may take years, but in the meantime the mechanical strength of the site is maintained.

In the immediate postfracture period (and after soft-tissue injury or surgery in the absence of fracture), there is a phenomenon of widespread acceleration of the normal bone remodeling and soft-tissue metabolism, called by Frost (38) the regional acceleratory phenomenon (RAP). This feature of the fracture IO seems to facilitate and speed the fracture and soft-tissue repair process. It has not been taken into account in many clinical and experimental studies and thus has confounded the interpretation of clinical and experimental results of many studies involving bone and/or soft-tissue surgery or injury.

Because it is a discrete IO, fracture healing may be the target of discrete abnormalities. For example, it may fail to appear at all. This results in a nonunion and is recognized by the fact that no fracture callus appears on radiographs. The integrity of the fracture site can be restored by the remodeling IO as it gradually bridges the defect. This takes long-term strict immobilization of the fracture site, and it is a very difficult clinical problem. In other cases, the fracture IO is delayed in appearance as manifest by late appearance of the callus on radiographs, or it may be weak in intensity and be reduced in size on radiographs. Of course this delays the return of mechanical integrity to the fracture site.

STRUCTURAL ADAPTATION TO MECHANICAL USAGE

Introductions to this topic (16,17) must begin by referring to the early ideas of J. Wolff (39). The text of "Wolff's law" has been translated into English (40); because of its importance it is repeated here:

> Every change in the form and function of bones, or of their function alone, is followed by certain definite changes in their internal architecture and equally definite secondary alteration in their external conformation, in accordance with mathematical laws.

A modern adaptation of this expression of Wolff's law might be stated as follows:

> Given that the material properties (strength and stiffness) of normal bone tissue remain constant among vertebrates, the quantity and geometric structure of bone are both regulated so that the needs of mechanical usage are met with the smallest mass of bone tissue.

Thus very large animals are not so burdened by the weight of their skeletons that locomotion is seriously hindered, and very small animals are not endangered by a skeleton so weak that their survival is threatened by an excessively fragile skeleton. Wolff (39) stated that the adaptation of the skeleton followed mathematical laws, but he did not formulate them. Recent workers have proposed mathematical laws to describe the adaptation of the skeleton to mechanical usage (16,17,34,41,42). These will not be covered here in detail, but some generalities concerning them will be put forth in this section.

Stress and Strain

When a mechanical force is applied to a structural material such as bone tissue, a certain amount of deformation will occur depending on its innate stiffness, and the material will resist this bending with internal counterforce. The deformation is called *strain,* and the counterforce that resists deformation is called *stress.* The units used to express force, strain, and stress in the ranges encountered in bone tissue are as follows:

$$\text{Force} = \text{Newtons (N)}$$
$$\text{Newton} = 0.23 \text{ lb}$$
$$\text{Strain} = \text{Change in length/original length}$$
$$\text{One strain} = 100\% \text{ Stretch deformation}$$
$$\text{One microstrain } (\mu E) = 10^{-6} \text{ Strain}$$
$$\text{Stress} = \text{Force/area}$$
$$\text{Stress} = \text{Megapascals (MPa)}$$
$$\text{Megapascal} = \text{N/mm}^2$$

It is not possible to measure directly the stress generated in a material when a force is applied to it, but in most materials such as bone, direct measurements of strain are possible on the surface. The dimensionless numbers for strain represent fractional changes in length, width, or any other dimension. One can think of strain as a unit of deformation which is mathematically related to stress in a material through its stiffness. There is now a growing body of data on the strains generated in vivo on the surfaces of bones during the normal and peak activity of various species (11), and some of them are listed above. These measurements are made by cementing tiny strain gauges (by a surgical procedure) to the surfaces of bone and transmitting their signals by sophisticated telemetry.

The Safety Margin

Peak strains generated in vivo are remarkably consistent among vertebrate species at about 2000–3000 μE, as noted in Table 3. Furthermore, the increase in strain required to cause permanent damage without fracture is about three times peak strain, and that required to cause complete failure or fracture is about 10 times peak strain. Thus, the safety margins for strain are about 3 and 10. (There is some disagreement about the magnitude of peak strains and the safety factors, but everyone's estimates are within the same order of magnitude.) Frost (1,2,16,17) has stated that the magnitude of these safety factors is governed by the fatigue life of bone tissue rather than by the necessity of preventing failure from single overloads. For example, Carter and Caler (43) have shown that with cyclic strains of about 4000 μE, well below failure levels, bone can fail in fatigue with only a few thousand strain cycles, a number of cycles less than 1 month of normal usage. The fatigue life of normal bone is several hundred thousand cycles or more under normal usage. Thus a relatively small reduction in bone mass in an animal or human might lead to an increase in strain which remains well below the safety margin for fracture. However, it may cause a large increase in the rate of accumulation of microdamage, a marked reduction in the fatigue life of the skeletal tissue, and a marked increase in the fragility of the skeleton. This may be the case in osteoporosis, where skeletal fragility is out of proportion to the reduction in bone mass. If these patients have a defect in the ability of their skeletons to respond to strain by increasing or sustaining their mass, then a relatively small reduction in bone mass could result in fragility to a degree which is out of proportion to the reduction in bone mass because of the accumulation of microdamage faster than remodeling can repair it. Studies in this area have been hampered by the lack of a convenient method of locating and quantifying microdamage.

There must be a mechanism for maintaining bone mass and architecture such that the peak strains of ordinary mechanical usage remain at about one-third the damage level; such a mechanism would prevent microdamage from accumulating at a rate beyond the capacity for repair by the remodeling system.

The Mechanostat

Mechanostat is the term coined by Frost (1,2) to describe the mechanism for determining the mass and geo-metric arrangement of skeletal tissue in the living animal. This mechanism has not been demonstrated empirically, yet there is compelling evidence for its existence. It is a mechanism for sensing the peak strains generated in bone by an animal's normal physical activity. When peak strains exceed a certain magnitude, the mechanostat generates signals which initiate cellular events to increase the amount of bone tissue under load and/or rearrange the architecture of the bone tissue so that peak strains return to the normal range. Conversely, when peak strains fall below a certain magnitude, the mechanostat generates signals which initiate cellular events to decrease the amount of bone tissue present. Frost (1,2) has described "windows" of mechanical usage which characterize the behavior of the mechanostat. The underuse window corresponds to peak strains below about 50 μE. Bone is removed when subjected to this degree of disuse. The normal-use window corresponds to strains of about 50–2000 μE, when bone is maintained in a steady state of approximately constant mass and architecture. The overuse window corresponds to strains of about 2000–4000 μE (the upper margin of this window is much less certain than the others); at this point the amount of bone tissue increases until peak strain magnitude returns to the normal-use window, provided that accumulated microdamage does not cause mechanical failure before the new steady state can be reached. The pathological overuse window corresponds to strain magnitudes from above the overuse window to about 15,000–30,000 μE, the strain at failure. At any magnitude of peak strain in the pathological overuse window, there is an exuberant cellular response which results in production of copious amounts of woven bone or even cartilage (18). Skeletal tissue cannot endure this amount of mechanical usage without rapidly progressing to failure, and a vigorous response that resembles fracture healing takes place.

Change in the Mechanostat Setpoint

Changes in the setpoint(s) of the mechanostat would cause predictable changes in the mass (and geometry) of the skeleton (44). For example, a rise in the setpoint would be expected to result in a decrease in bone mass because the system would interpret the situation as mechanical underuse and would respond by removing bone. On the other hand, a lowering of the setpoint would be expected to result in an increase in bone mass because the system would interpret the situation as mechanical overuse and would respond by adding bone. There are situations occurring in nature or experimentally which demonstrate what might happen when the setpoint is changed in an animal which undergoes bone remodeling.

In order to understand the background for this, it is pertinent to recall the morphological changes which occur with underuse or disuse in an adult bone remodeling animal. This information was produced in a series of dog experiments by Uthoff and Jaworski (45), who demonstrated that casting of the forelimb results in bone loss from bone surfaces in contact with marrow. Thus, trabecular and cortical bone both decrease: The trabecular bone decreases by a combination of trabecular thinning and loss of trabecular elements, and cortical bone decreases by loss from the cortico-endosteal surface. The skeleton "erodes" from the inside, but the outer volume of the skeleton does not shrink. Similar findings were reported with immobilization of adult monkeys (46). The pattern of bone loss is similar in adult humans who become paralyzed from trauma or neurologic disease. The pattern of bone loss that occurs in adult humans with removal of estrogens at menopause is similar (21,22,27,47) to that found in disuse. Bone is lost on trabecular and cortico-endosteal surfaces in contact with marrow. The outer volume of the skeleton remains unchanged. Similar morphological changes occur in the bones of adult humans and remodeling animals when exposed to calcium nutritional deficiency.

In both estrogen deprivation and calcium deficiency the skeleton behaves as though it is exposed to underuse. However, in both cases these findings occur in the setting of normal mechanical use. A unified mechanism which explains these findings is that in both cases, the setpoint for detecting mechanical usage has been raised upward and thus the remodeling system responds by ridding the body of what it perceives as an unwanted excess of bone tissue. As mentioned above, we do not yet have direct experimental proof of the existence of such a mechanostat, yet the available data and observations suggest the existence of such a mechanism for maintaining bone mass and architecture. It is important to note that if a mechanostat that responds to strain does exist, then the osteoblasts and osteoclasts are the effectors of the system. It follows that perturbations in the function of these effectors will not cause permanent change in bone mass or architecture, because any such change will be countered by the function of the mechanostat and its setpoint.

Future Directions

The implications of Frost's mechanostat theory are very important. We need details of its workings, and we also need convincing documentation of its existence in living animals and humans. Experiments performed in vitro will not contain the elements of such a system. One can think of a kidney analogy here if we started with the assumption that there was no knowledge of the countercurrent system. Discovery of how urine is formed by the kidney by using only tissue or cell culture methodology would be very difficult or even impossible. (Early micropuncture studies of isolated, perfused kidneys helped because the system was studied with an intact whole organ, thus simulating the in vivo state closely enough.) A similar situation may be present in skeletal research if the analogue of the countercurrent system is the mechanostat, present in vivo but not in vitro. Bone cell culture or bone tissue culture methodology will not provide the means to investigate a system of control which exists only in the intact animal.

Another important implication associated with the idea of a mechanostat or setpoint detecting strain is relevant in designing pharmacologic or therapeutic interventions. Attempts at treating bone loss, for example, by stimulating osteoblast work or inhibiting osteoclast work can be predicted to fail because the mechanostat system will override the attempts. Thus truly successful treatment of pathological bone loss and excessive skeletal fragility in humans would demand that we find a pharmacologic means of changing (lowering) the skeleton's setpoint for detecting and responding to mechanical strain. This exciting possibility will remain elusive until proper research on the paradigm is conducted in vivo.

SUMMARY

This chapter reviewed the developmental biology of the skeleton along with the structural organization at both the macroscopic and microscopic levels. The material properties of skeletal tissue were described along with the functional adaptation of the fiber–mineral composite. The various functional envelopes of the skeleton were described, and the anatomic surfaces were explained in some detail. The microscopic anatomy of the various bone cells seen on surfaces was presented in order to help the reader understand the literature of bone histomorphometry. Finally, the intermediary organization of the skeleton was presented along with some new ideas on the physiology of adaptation to mechanical usage. Future directions of research were pointed particularly at the area of functional adaptation and the concept of a mechanostat. The reader is encouraged to be on the lookout for (a) future developments coming from research directed at understanding the mechanism of skeletal response to strain and (b) attempts at manipulation of the setpoint or mechanostat.

REFERENCES

1. Frost HM. *Intermediary Organization of the Skeleton,* vol I. Boca Raton, FL: CRC Press, 1986.
2. Frost HM. *Intermediary Organization of the Skeleton,* vol II. Boca Raton, FL: CRC Press, 1986.
3. Moore KI. *The developing human.* Philadelphia: WB Saunders, 1988.
4. Krabbenhoft KM, Fallon JF. The formation of leg or wing specific structures by leg bud cells grafted to the wing bud is influenced by proximity to the apical ridge. *Dev Biol* 1989;131:373–82.
5. Jee WSS. The skeletal tissues. In: Weiss L, ed. *Cell and tissue biology.* Baltimore: Urban & Schwarzenberg, 1988;213–53.
6. Nottesdad SY, Baumel JJ, Kimmel DB, Recker RR, Heaney RP. The proportion of trabecular bone in human vertebrae. *J Bone Miner Res* 1987;2:221–9.
7. Carter DR, Spengler DM. Mechanical properties and composition of cortical bone. *Clin Orthop* 1978;135:192–217.
8. Veis A, Sabsay B. The collagen of mineralized matrices. In: Peck

WA, ed. *Bone and mineral research,* vol 5. Amsterdam: Elsevier, 1987;1–64.

9. Reilly DT, Burstein AH. The elastic and ultimate properties of compact bone tissue. *J Biomech* 1975;8:393–405.

10. Baumeister T III, et al. In: Baumeister T, Avallone EA, Baumeister T III, eds. *Mark's standard handbook for mechanical engineers.* New York: McGraw–Hill, 1978.

11. Rubin CT, Lanyon LE. Dynamic strain similarities in vertebrates; an alternative to allometric limb bone scaling. *J Theor Biol* 1984;107:321–7.

12. Carter DR, Caler WE, Spengler DM, Frankel VH. Fatigue behavior of adult cortical bone: the influence of mean strain and strain range. *Acta Orthop Scand* 1981;52:481–90.

13. Barbos MP, Bianco P, Ascenzi A, Boyde A. Collagen orientation in compact bone. II. Distribution of lamellae in the whole of the human femoral shaft with reference to its mechanical properties. *Metab Bone Dis Rel Res* 1984;5:309–15.

14. Ascenzi A, Boyde A, Bianco P, Barbos MP. Relationship between mechanical properties and structure in secondary bone. *Connect Tissue Res* 1986;15:73–6.

15. Riggs CM, Lanyon LE, Boyde A. Preferred orientation of the ultrastructural elements of bone: relationship with strain. Paper presented at Proceedings, 36th annual meeting of the ORS, New Orleans, 1990.

16. Frost HM. Skeletal structural adaptations to mechanical usage (SATMU). 1. Redefining Wolff's law: the bone modeling problem, *Anat Rec* 1990;226:403–13.

17. Frost HM. Skeletal structural adaptations to mechanical usage (SATMU). 2. Redefining Wolff's law: the bone remodeling problem. *Anat Rec* 1990;226:414–22.

18. Turner CT, Kimmel DB, Recker RR. A non-invasive, in vivo model for studying strain adaptive bone modeling. *Bone* 1991;in press.

19. Burr DB, Schaffler MB, Yang KH, Lukoschek M, Sivaneri N, Blaha JD, Radin EI. Skeletal changes in response to altered strain environments: Is woven bone a response to elevated strain? *Bone* 1989;10:223–33.

20. Rubin CT, Lanyon LE. Regulation of bone mass by mechanical strain magnitude. *Calcif Tissue Int* 1985;37:411–7.

21. Keshawarz NM, Recker RR. Expansion of the medullary cavity at the expense of cortex in postmenopausal osteoporosis. *Metab Bone Dis Rel Res* 1984;5:223–8.

22. Garn SM. *The earlier gain and the later loss of cortical bone in nutritional perspective.* Springfield, IL: Charles C Thomas, 1970.

23. Frost HM. Bone histomorphometry: analysis of trabecular bone dynamics. In: Recker RR, ed. *Bone histomorphometry: techniques and interpretation.* Boca Raton, FL: CRC Press, 1983;109–42.

24. Hori M, Takahashi H, Konno T, Inoue J, Haba T. A classification of in vivo bone labels after double labeling in canine bones. *Bone* 1985;6:147–54.

25. Keshawarz NM, Recker RR. The label escape error: Comparison of measured and theoretical fraction of total bone-trabecular surface covered by single label in normals and patients with osteoporosis. *Bone* 1986;7:83–7.

26. Frost HM. Resting seams: "on" and "off" in lamellar bone formation centers. In: Jee WSS, Parfitt AM, eds. *Bone histomorphometry.* Third International Workshop. *Metab Bone Dis Rel Res (Suppl)* 1980;167–70.

27. Kimmel DB, Recker RR, Gallagher JC, Vaswani AS, Aloia JF. A comparison of iliac bone histomorphometric data in post-meno-

pausal osteoporotic and normal subjects. *Bone Miner* 1990;11:217–35.

28. Baron R, Magee S, Silvergate A, Broadus A, Lang R. Estimation of trabecular bone resorption by histomorphometry: evidence for a prolonged reversal phase with normal resorption in post-menopausal osteoporosis, and coupled increased resorption in primary hyperparathyroidism. In: Frame B, Potts JT, eds. *Clinical disorders of bone and mineral metabolism.* Amsterdam: Excerpta Medica, 1983;191–5.

29. Lau KHW, Onishe T, Wergedal JE, Singer FR, Baylink DJ. Characterization and assay of tartrate-resistant acid phosphatase activity in serum: potential use to assess bone resorption. *Clin Chem* 1987;33:458–62.

30. Recker RR, Kimmel DB, Parfitt AM, Davies KM, Keshawarz NM, Hinders SM. Static and tetracycline-based bone histomorphometric data from 34 normal postmenopausal females. *J Bone Miner Res* 1988;3:133–44.

31. McSheehy PMJ, Chambers TJ. Osteoblast-like cells in the presence of parathyroid hormone release soluble factor that stimulates osteoclastic bone resorption. *Endocrinology* 1986;119:1654–9.

32. Parfitt AM. The physiologic and clinical significance of bone histomorphometric data. In: Recker RR, ed. *Bone histomorphometry: techniques and interpretation.* Boca Raton, FL: CRC Press, 1983;144–217.

33. Ivey JL, Baylink DJ. Postmenopausal osteoporosis: proposed roles of defective coupling and estrogen deficiency. *Metab Bone Dis Rel Res* 1981;3:3–7.

34. Cowin SC. Bone remodeling of diaphyseal surfaces by torsional loads: theoretical predictions. *J Biomech* 1987;20:1111–20.

35. Frost HM. Dynamics of bone remodeling. In: Frost HM, ed. *Bone biodynamics.* Boston: Little, Brown, 1964;315–33.

36. Frost HM. Some ABC's of skeletal pathophysiology. III: bone balance and the Delta B. BMU. *Calcif Tissue Int* 1989;45:131–3.

37. Frost HM. Tetracycline-based histological analysis of bone remodeling. *Calcif Tissue Res* 1969;3:211–39.

38. Frost HM. The regional acceleratory phenomenon. *Henry Ford Hosp Med J* 1983;31:3–9.

39. Wolff J. *Das Gesetz der Transformation der knochen.* Berlin: A Hirschwald, 1892;1–126 (English translation, Springer-Verlag, 1986).

40. Rasch PJ, Burke RK. *Kinesiology and applied anatomy,* 2nd ed. Philadelphia: Lee & Febiger, 1963;1–503.

41. Carter DR. Mechanical loading history and skeletal biology. *J Biomech* 1987;20:1095–1109.

42. Lanyon LE. Functional strain in bone tissue as an objective, and controlling stimulus for adaptive bone remodelling. *J Biomech* 1987;20:1083–93.

43. Carter DR, Caler WE. Uniaxial fatigue of human cortical bone. The influence of tissue physical characteristics. *J Biomech* 1981;14:461–70.

44. Turner CH. Homeostatic control of bone structure. *J Bone Miner Res* 1990;5:698.

45. Uthoff KH, Jaworski ZGF. Bone loss in response to long-term immobilization. *J Bone Joint Surg* 1978;60B:420–9.

46. Young DR, Niklowitz WJ, Brown RJ, Jee WSS. Immobilization-associated osteoporosis in primates (*M. nemestrina*). *Bone* 1986;7:109–17.

47. Meema HE. The occurrence of cortical bone atrophy in old age and in osteoporosis. *J Can Assoc Radiol* 1962;13:27–32.

48. Cormack DM. Bone. In: Cormack DM, ed. *Ham's histology,* 9th ed. Philadelphia: Lippincott, 1987;309.

Disorders of Bone and Mineral Metabolism,
edited by Fredric L. Coe and Murray J. Favus,
Published by Raven Press, Ltd., 1992.

CHAPTER 11

The Cellular Biology and Molecular Biochemistry of Bone Formation

Pamela Gehron Robey, Paolo Bianco, and John D. Termine

Bone, or more correctly, the bone–bone marrow organ, is a unique combination of many cell types, all of which synthesize a characteristic subset of connective tissue components. While it is primarily the duty of osteoblastic cells to produce the structural elements of extracellular bone matrix (Fig. 1), proteins synthesized locally (frequently growth factors) by other cells such as those found in the marrow (stromal fibroblasts, hematopoietic stem cells, endothelial cells, etc.), or brought in via the circulatory system, are deposited within the mineralized compartment. The result is a remarkable concoction that confers not only skeletal strength, but also the unique ability of bone to undergo continuous remodeling throughout life.

The advent of procedures for chemical dissection of mineralized matrix components (1,2) and subsequent analysis by microanalytical techniques, combined with in vitro studies of cells within the osteoblastic lineage, has generated an ever-increasing list of endogenously and exogenously produced bone matrix components. Collagen contributes 90% of the total organic matrix. The remaining 10% is composed of various types of molecules. However, the percentage of each component varies with animal species, development; and perhaps the site within the skeleton. (Tables 1 and 2, reviewed in ref. 3). However, the questions still remain—what is the composition of the supermolecular complex (the "bone matrix unit") that will initiate deposition of mineral, and how is this process regulated by osteoblast(s)? Since the major structural element in the organic phase, type I collagen, is found in other connective tissues, the non-collagenous components have been the focus of consider-

able attention in order to determine their role in bone physiology. While it was hoped that these components would be unique to bone, careful examination has indicated that few (only one to date), in fact, seem to be bone specific. Yet the importance of the more widely distributed bone matrix components should not be overlooked, since it is probable that osteoblasts have the ability to make tissue specific modifications, and to regulate the stoichiometry of the bone matrix unit.

Examination of bone formation, either in fetal and postnatal development, or during bone turnover, indicates that it is not a one step process. As exemplified by developing subperiosteal bone, which can be likened to the growth plate of cartilage, the cells pass through a maturation pathway (4; Bianco, Fisher, and Gehron Robey, unpublished results). Thus, cells and the matrix are primed for the ultimate event—mineralization. However, it should be noted that bone remodeling during endochondral bone turnover and bone formation may actually be a condensation of the events seen in subperiosteal bone development, occurring in a discrete location on previously formed mineralized matrix (Fig. 2). Consequently, the factors that regulate these different processes, as well as the ultimate output of the bone-forming cells may differ. The following is a brief description of the potential players and managers of the bone extracellular matrix, listed roughly in order of their appearance in developing bone, and salient features that may be of import.

ENDOGENOUS PROTEINS

Collagen

Collagen is defined as a molecule composed of three polypeptide chains, termed α chains, which associate

P. Gehron Robey, P. Bianco, and J. D. Termine: Bone Research Branch, National Institute of Dental Research, National Institutes of Health, Bethesda, MD 20892.

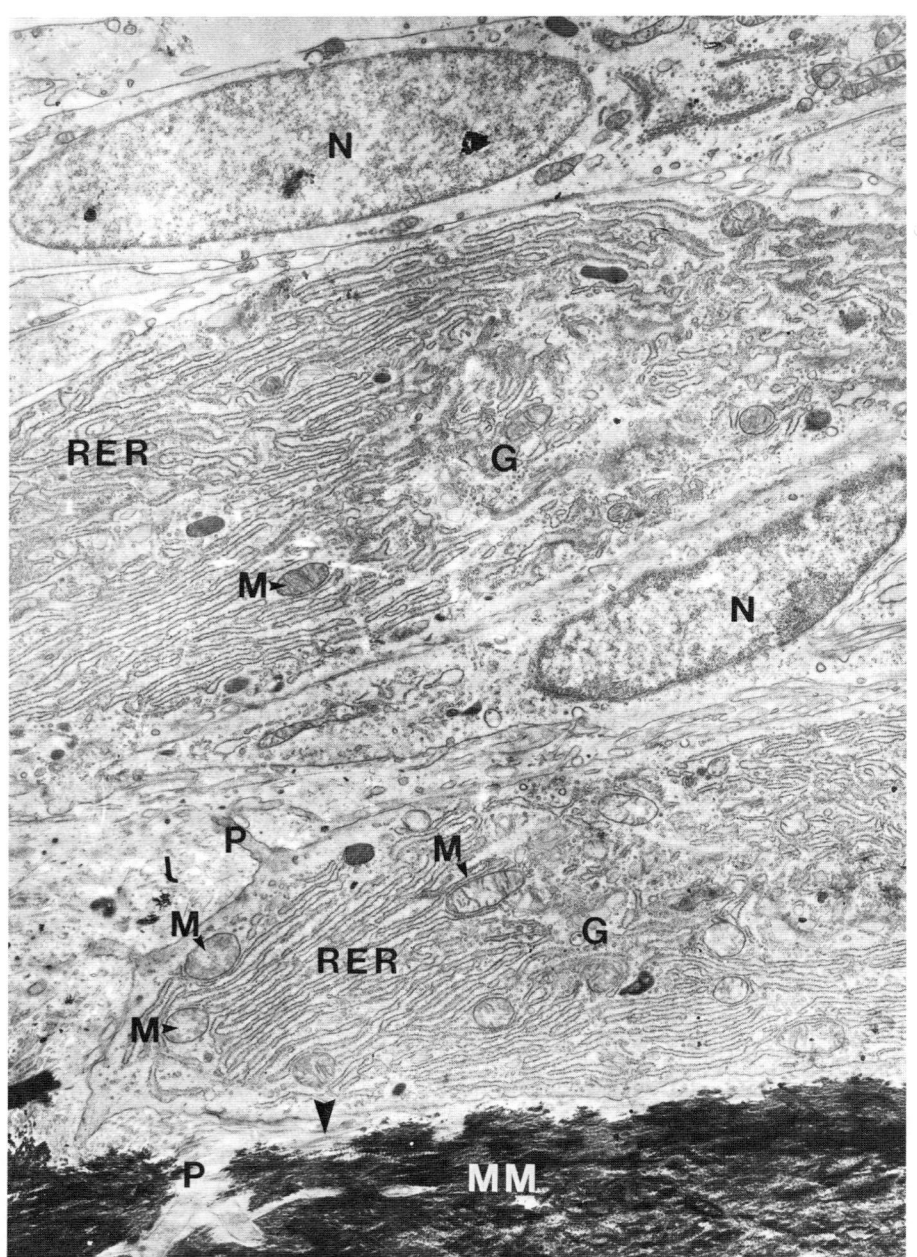

FIG. 1. Ultrastructure of an osteoblast (OB), the primary bone-forming cell. The term osteoblast is basically a histological definition that describes a particular cell in relationship to mineralized matrix and soft tissue. A thin layer of unmineralized osteoid (arrowhead) separates this cell from the mineralized matrix (MM). Ultrastructural features indicate that osteoblasts are highly active metabolically, with numerous mitochondria (M), and secretory in nature; as indicated by extensive Golgi apparati (G) and rough endoplasmic reticulum (RER), which are polarized towards the site of osteoid deposition. (N, nucleus.)

TABLE 1. *Organic composition of mineralized matrix synthesized by bone-forming cells*

Collagen: predominantly type I collagen (possibly trace amounts of types III, V, XI, and XIII)
Proteoglycans: a large condroitin sulfate PG (replaced during switch from mesenchyme to bone), Biglycan, decorin, (perhaps trace amounts of a heparan sulfate PG), Hyaluronan
Glycoproteins (many are sulfated, phosphorylated, and contain RGD): Fibronectin, thrombospondin, osteonectin, alkaline phosphatase, osteopontin, bone sialoprotein, BAG-75
γ-carboxy glutamic acid-containing proteins: matrix gla protein, osteocalcin

TABLE 2. *Non-structural components of mineralized matrix synthesized locally by cells in the osteoblastic lineage and adsorbed from the circulation*

PRODUCED ENDOGENOUSLY

Enzymes and their inhibitors
    Alkaline phosphatase, collagenase and TIMP, plasminogen activator and inhibitor, etc.
Paracrine and autocrine growth factors
    FGFs, IGFs, TGF-βs, etc.
Proteolipids
Bone morphogenetic proteins(?)

ADSORBED FROM EXOGENOUS SOURCES

Growth factors
    FGFs, IGFs, TGF-βs, PDGF, etc.
Serum proteins
    Albumin, α₂-HS glycoprotein (fetuin?), immunoglobulins, transferrin, hemoglobin, etc.

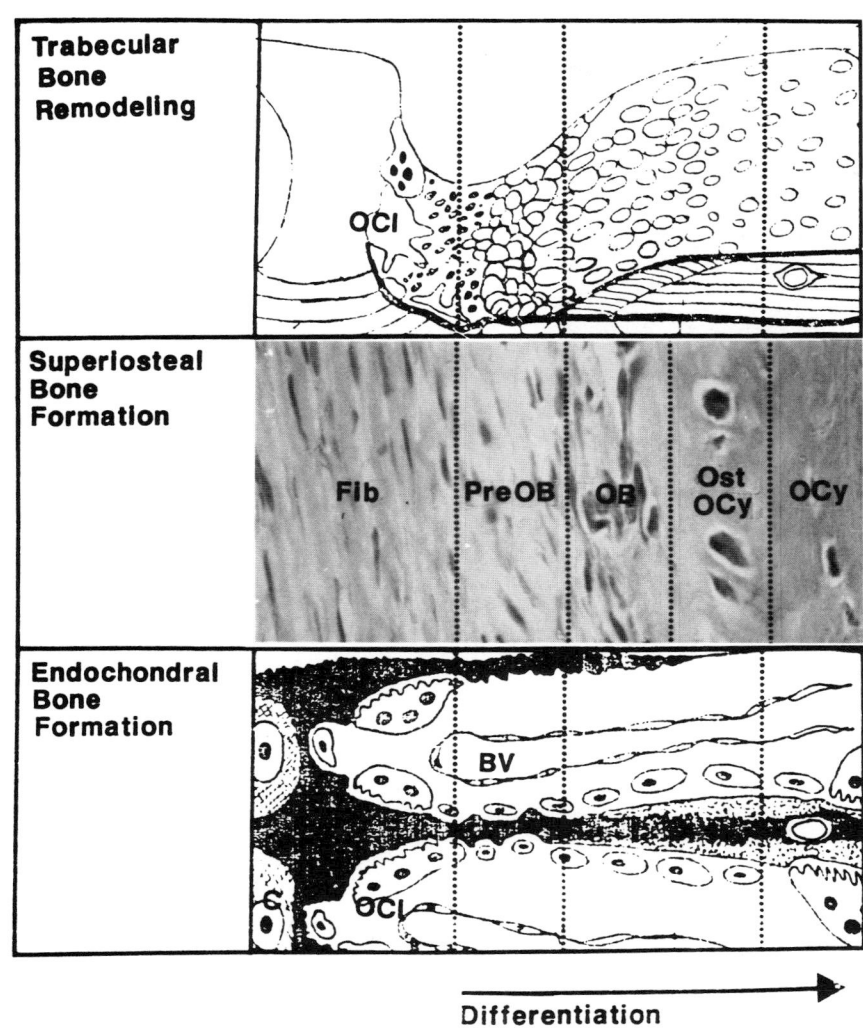

Differentiation

FIG. 2. Patterns of bone formation. Cells in the osteoblastic lineage pass through a series of maturational stages, which can best be identified in subperiosteal bone, but may also be present during trabecular bone remodeling or in endochondral bone formation. Fib, fibroblast or undifferentiated mesenchymal cell; PreOB, preosteoblast; OB, osteoblast; Ost Ocy; osteoid osteocyte; OCy, osteocyte; OCl, osteoclast; and BV, blood vessel.

into a triple helical molecule. These α chains are characteristic in that they are formed of long stretches with the triplet sequence Gly-X-Y, where X is often proline and Y hydroxyproline. Both hydroxyproline and hydroxylysine are formed by posttranslational modification and are somewhat unique to collagen. Interstitial collagen is composed of these rod shaped molecules that associate both end to end and laterally in a quarter-staggered fashion to form fibrils (reviewed in 5). The most abundant collagen, type I, is a hetero trimer containing two $\alpha_1(I)$ chains and one $\alpha_2(I)$ chain. Like many other molecules, collagen is synthesized in a precursor form with extensions at both the amino and carboxy termini. These extensions are, for the most part, cleaved during secretion and fibril formation. In bone, the ratio of type I to other collagens is much higher than in soft connective tissues, so much so that it has been frequently stated that mineralized matrix contains solely type I. Yet trace amounts of types III, V, and XI have been isolated (6), although it is not clear if they are within the mineralized compartment, or from the vasculature which extensively infil-

trates the matrix. In soft tissues, types III and V have been suggested to regulate collagen fibril diameter (7), and recent studies have identified FACITs (fibril associated collagen with interrupted triple helices) such as types IX, XI, and XII (8–10) which are located on the fibril surfaces and may interface with the surrounding environment. Immunohistochemical and in situ hybridization studies have localized small amounts of a FACIT collagen (type XII) (11), and possibly type XIII (12) to developing bone. Although type I collagen fibrils in bone are somewhat larger than in most other tissues, there may be a role for these minor collagen types.

Although there is only one gene encoding for $\alpha_1(I)$ and $\alpha_2(I)$, bone type I collagen has several distinguishing features (Figure 3). The pattern of posttranslational modifications of bone type I collagen differs from that of soft tissues in that it contains predominantly galactosyl hydroxylysyl residues (as opposed to glucosyl-galactosyl-hydroxylysyl residues in skin). There are fewer interchain crosslinks, and these originate via the hydroxyallysine pathway (13). This latter characteristic may be due

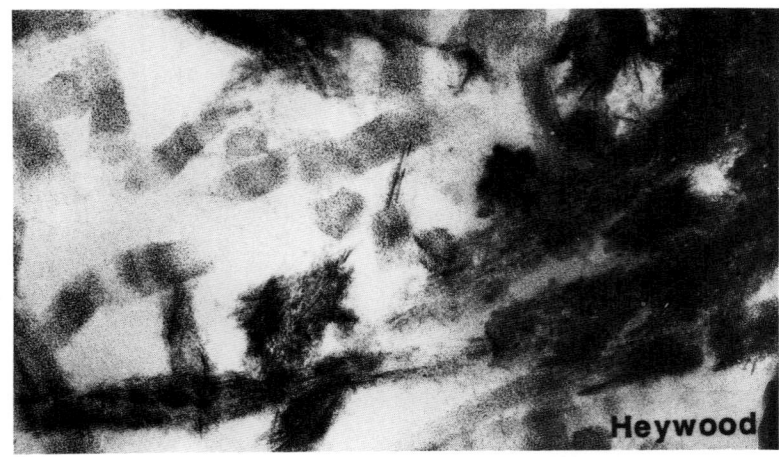

	Bone	Soft Connective Tissues
Glycosylation	Gal-Hyl	Glu-Gal-Hyl
Phosphorylation	24K PP = pN extension	?
X-link Pathway	Hydroxyallysine	Allysine
Mature Crosslink	Lysyl-pyridinoline	Hydroxylysyl-pyridinoline
Fibrils	Type I (III,V,XI,XIII?)	Type I with III, V and FACITS

FIG. 3. Comparison of bone collagen and soft tissue collagen. Electron micrograph of hydroxyapatite deposition on collagen produced by fetal bovine bone cell cultures. Electron micrograph courtesy of Brigid R. Heywood.

to the presence of mineral within the collagen fibril. Collagen in bone may also be phosphorylated. In early studies, a $M_r = 24,000$ phosphoprotein was isolated from bone (2), and has now been identified as the N-terminal precursor extension of collagen (14), however this modification has not been well defined in bone or in soft tissues.

Non-Collagenous Proteins

In toto, 10% of the organic phase in prenatal and neonatal bone is made of a wide variety of non-collagenous proteins including proteoglycans, glycoproteins that can be sulfated, phosphorylated, or both, γ-carboxy glutamic acid containing proteins and proteolipids. The proportion of each protein is dependent on the animal species. In addition, the levels are also age-dependent (15), and as bone matures, all undergo degradation (16). Consequently, in aged bone, which has fewer sites of recent remodeling, they are almost undetectable. While in vitro studies have pointed to possible functions for several of these proteins, their precise functions in vivo are not yet known.

Proteoglycans (Versican, Biglycan, Decorin) and Hyaluronan

A number of proteoglycans, composed of a protein core to which glycosaminoglycans are attached, are found in bone matrix (Fig. 4, Table 3, reviewed in ref. 17). During early bone development, a large chondroitin sulfate proteoglycan (now named versican) is found primarily in the loose interstitial mesenchyme, and its function may be to capture space destined to become bone (18). As development proceeds, it is replaced by two smaller species, biglycan (so-named by virtue of its two chondroitin sulfate side chains, previously called PG-I) and decorin (thought to "decorate" collagen fibrils and regulate fibril growth, previously named PG-II). Based on studies following radioactive sulfate incorporation, it is widely thought that proteoglycans must be removed prior to matrix mineralization. However, it should be pointed out that the large chondroitin sulfate proteoglycan contains a large number of sulfated side chains compared to biglycan and decorin, which contain two and one glycosaminoglycans respectively. Consequently, replacement of the large CSPG by biglycan and decorin would result in a net decrease in sulfate incorporation, but does not rule out involvement of these small PGs in mineralization. In fact, autoradiographic studies indicate an intimate association of sulfate at the initial sites of mineral precipitation (19), and in vivo studies have shown that a population of proteoglycans migrate rapidly to the mineralization front (20). While biglycan and decorin are highly related evolutionarily, they are remarkably divergent in their tissue distribution, which may reflect differences in function. Recent immunohis-

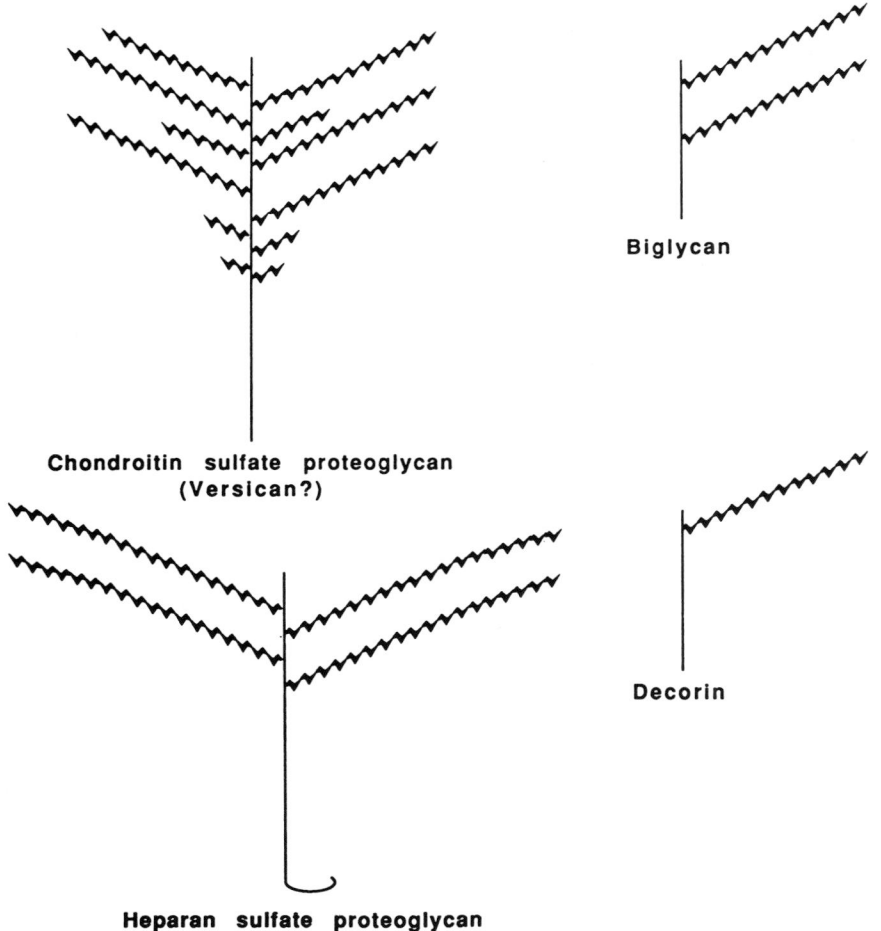

Chondroitin sulfate proteoglycan (Versican?)

Biglycan

Heparan sulfate proteoglycan

Decorin

Hyaluronan

FIG. 4. Schematic representation of proteoglycans produced by bone cells in vitro. Courtesy of Neal S. Fedarko.

tochemical studies have shown that while decorin is fairly uniformly distributed throughout developing bone matrix, biglycan is located in pericellular areas in sites active in morphogenesis, and in osteocytic lacunae (21) (Fig. 5). Analysis of the amino acid sequence of both proteins discloses domains that share homology with a number of morphogenetic proteins such as Drosophila chaoptin and toll, and also (22) fibromodulin (23), and the TGF-β binding protein, OIF (24), originally isolated from bone. In vitro analysis indicates that biglycan is initially cell-associated, and rapidly turned over, while decorin exhibits a pattern similar to that of collagen (25). Although a heparan sulfate proteoglycan is synthesized by bone cells, it generally remains cell surface associated, and may bind growth factors synthesized locally or absorbed from the circulation. The role of the unsulfated glycosaminoglycan, hyaluronan, in bone is virtually unknown, but by analogy to other tissues, may be involved in cellular proliferation and differentiation.

Glycoproteins (Table 4)

Osteonectin(s). This acidic glycoprotein is highly enriched in bone matrix (10,000 times more than in soft connective tissues) (26). While it appears to be induced by in vitro culture conditions in many cell types (27), in vivo, osteonectin is produced *constitutively* in bone (Fig. 6), and in a limited number of non-mineralized tissues such as the periodontal ligament which is tightly adherent to bone (28), and salivary and renal tubule epithelium, which are cells involved in ion transport (29). In addition, it is *transiently* expressed by other cell types undergoing rapid morphological and/or differentiation events [e.g., in decidual cells (30), and in certain basement membrane producing cells such as parietal endoderm (SPARC protein) (31)]. Osteonectin is also found in the α granules of platelets (32), although it has not yet been determined if it is a biosynthetic product of megakaryocytes. There is now evidence that there may be tis-

TABLE 3. *Biochemical features of proteoglycans and hyaluronan found in developing bone and synthesized by bone-forming cells in vitro*

Name	Intact M_r	Protein core	GAG chains
(large CSPG)	$\sim 1 \times 10^{6}$ [a]	$\sim 390,000$ [b]	40,000[a] CS
Biglycan (PG-I)	$\sim 270,000$ [b]	$\sim 38,000$ [b]	45,000[a] CS *in vivo* DS *in vitro*
Decorin (PG-II)	$\sim 135,000$ [b]	$\sim 38,000$ [b]	45,000[a] CS *in vivo* DS *in vitro*
Produced by osteoblastic cells in vitro			
Syndecan (HSPG)	$\sim 400,000$ [b]	$\sim 83,000$ [b]	60,000[a] HS $\sim 1.4 \times 10^{6}$ [a] HA (hyaluronan)

[a] Determined by molecular sieve column chromatography.
[b] Determined by SDS-PAGE.
GAG, glycosaminoglycan; CS, chondroitin sulfate; and DS, dermatan sulfate.

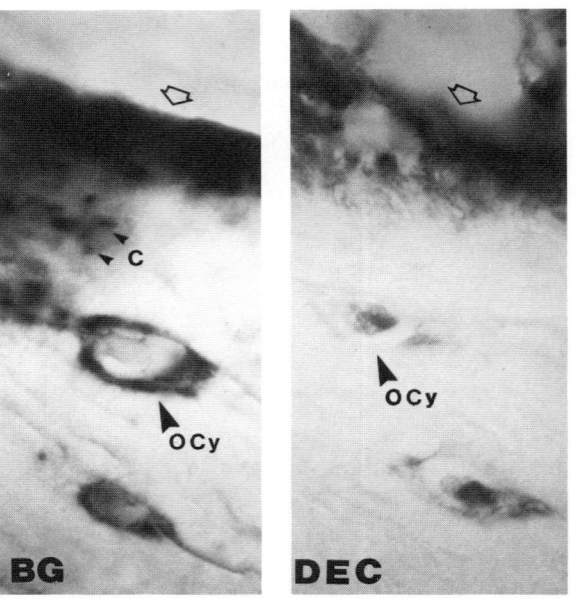

FIG. 5. Immunohistochemical localization of (**A**) biglycan (BG) and (**B**) decorin (DEC) in human developing subperiosteal bone. Biglycan is localized in osteoid (*open arrows*) and in osteocytic lacunae (OCy) and canaliculi (*small arrows,* c). Decorin, also in osteoid, is absent from the lacunae.

sue specific forms (33,34), although it is not yet clear whether they are the result of differing posttranslational modifications, or differences in protein sequence. The molecule binds to collagen, and contains multiple Ca^{2+} binding sites and binds with high affinity (K_d 10^{-8} M) (35,36), properties that point to a role as a moderator of mineralization. The molecule also contains at least one, and possibly two, E-F hand calcium binding sites (37), an unusual finding in a secreted protein (Fig. 7).

RGD (Arg-Gly-Asp)-Containing Proteins (Fibronectin, Thrombospondin, Osteopontin, and Bone Sialoprotein). In addition to type I collagen, bone matrix contains at least four additional proteins that contain the amino acid sequence RGD (Fig. 8), which binds to cell surface receptors (integrins) (reviewed in ref. 32) thereby mediating cell attachment (39). Fibronectin is produced by osteoblastic cells, but may also be brought in via the vasculature, and appears fairly early during osteogenesis (40) and mediates cell attachment and spreading of bone

TABLE 4. *Biochemical features of glycoproteins, RGD-containing proteins, and γ-carboxylated proteins of mineralized bone matrix*

Protein	M_r	Distinguishing features
Glycoproteins		
Osteonectin (SPARC, BM-40)	43–46,000[a] 32,000[b]	Glycosylated, phosphorylated, multiple low affinity Ca^{2+}, two E-F hands, ovomucoid homology
Alkaline phosphatase	S—S dimer, 50–80,000[b]	Ca^{2+} binding
BAG-75	75,000	~50% carbohydrate (7% sialic acid), 8% phosphate
RGD-containing proteins		
Fibronectin	S—S dimer, 250,000	Fibrin, heparin, bacterial, gelatin, collagen, DNA, cell surface binding sites, initial cell attachment
Thrombospondin	S—S trimer, 150,000	Ca^{2+} and hydroxyapatite binding, similar binding sites as FN, binds to osteonectin, cell adhesion without spreading
Osteopontin (BSP-I, 2ar, SPP-I, pp69)	45–75,000[a] 41,500[b]	N- and O-linked oligosaccharides, phospho-serine and tyrosine, cell attachment
Bone sialo-protein	$\sim 75,000$ [a] 33,500[b]	50% carbohydrate (12% sialic acid), tyrosine sulfation in some species, cell attachment
γ-carboxy glutamic acid containing proteins		
Matrix gla protein	15,000	One intramolecular S—S, 5 residues of gla
Osteocalcin	12–14,000[a] 5,800[b]	One intramolecular S—S, 3–5 residues of gla, hydroxyapatite binding dependent on gla

[a] Determined by SDS-PAGE.
[b] From protein sequence.
S—S, disulfide bond.

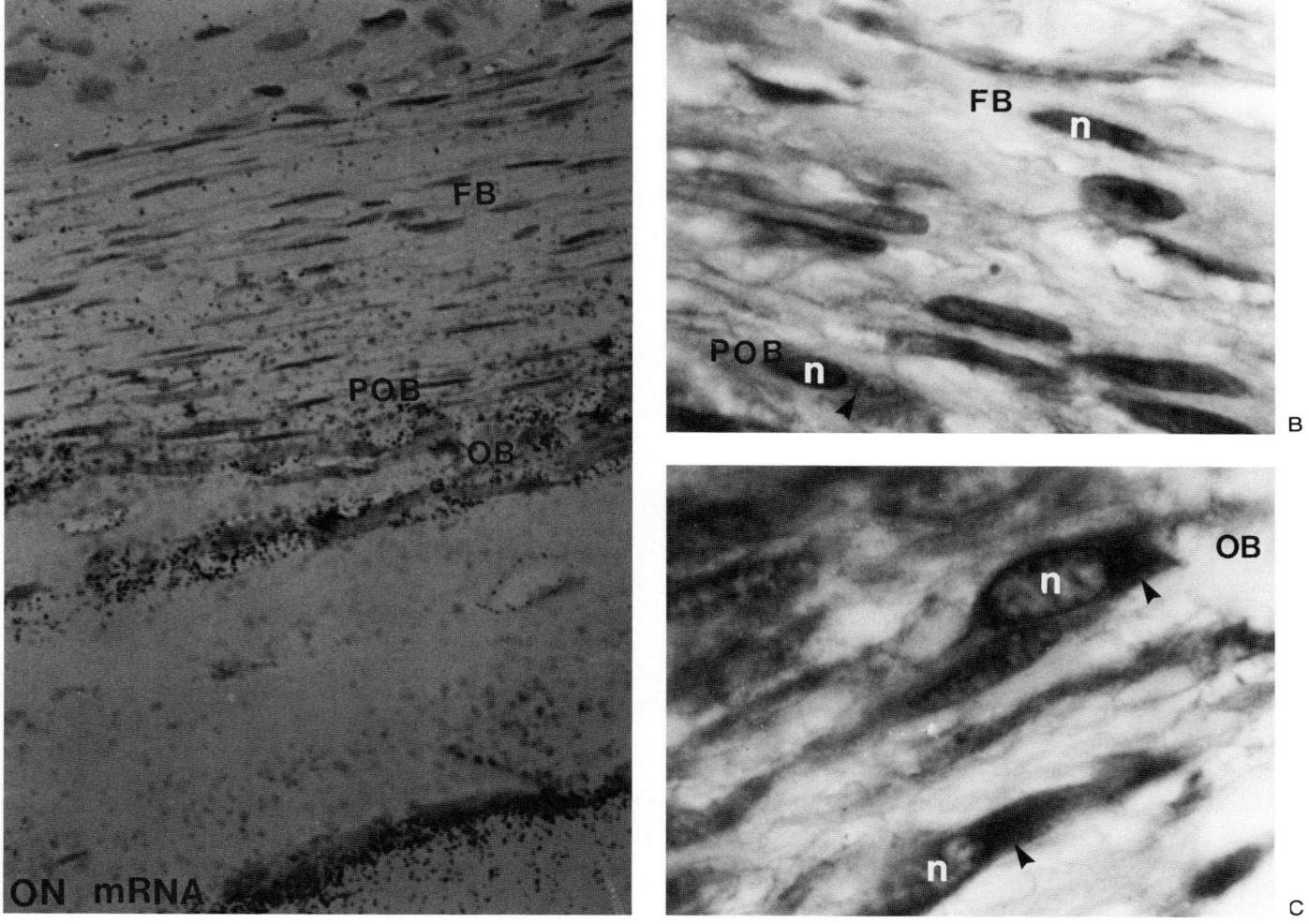

FIG. 6. In situ hybridization (**A**) and immunohistochemical localization (**B** and **C**) of osteonectin (ON) mRNA and protein in human developing subperiosteal bone. Osteonectin mRNA (demonstrated by hybridization with a ^{35}S-labeled ON cDNA probe and autoradiography) is found predominantly in the osteoblastic layer (OB), in relatively lower concentration in preosteoblasts (POB), and virtually absent in fibroblasts (FB). By histochemistry, the nuclei (n) of all cells are intensely stained by hemotoxylin, but immunodetectable ON is absent from the cytoplasm of FB, present at low levels in POBs (*arrow*, **B**), while OB cytoplasm is intensely stained (*arrowheads*, **C**).

cells in vitro. Thrombospondin, an endogenous product, mediates only adhesion of cells, but not spreading (41). It is noteworthy that the RGD sequence is buried in a globular domain that contains multiple Ca^{2+} binding sites, and the availability may be regulated by the prevailing calcium environment (reviewed in ref. 42). The remaining two RGD proteins are the bone matrix sialoproteins, osteopontin (reviewed in ref. 43) [also identified as 2ar (44) and pp69 (45) in other tissues] and bone sialoprotein (46,47), both of which are produced somewhat later in bone development. While immunohistochemistry and in situ hybridization show that osteopontin is constitutively produced by a number of cell types (chondrocytes, certain bone cells and mononuclear cells in the marrow, renal tubule cells) in vivo (48), its level of expression is dramatically increased by tumor promoters

(44) and transformation (49). This protein appears to exist in multiple forms that result from varying levels of phosphorylation (50), and alternate splicing of mRNA (compare sequences in refs. 51 and 52). Osteopontin contains the sequence GRGDS, identical to the attachment sequence found in fibronectin and vitronectin, and mediates cell attachment of a number of cell types (including bone cells) in vitro. Bone sialoprotein, to date, has been found only in osteoblasts, osteocytes (Fig. 9), trophoblasts of the pregnant uterus, and at low levels in fetal hypertrophic chondrocytes (53). Osteoclasts also contain BSP mRNA and protein (53). Unlike osteopontin, the cell attachment sequence is RGDN in humans and the molecule has been shown to bind to a vitronectin-type integrin ($\alpha_v\beta_3$) receptor in rat osteosarcoma cells (54). While in fibroblastic cells, bone sialoprotein is not

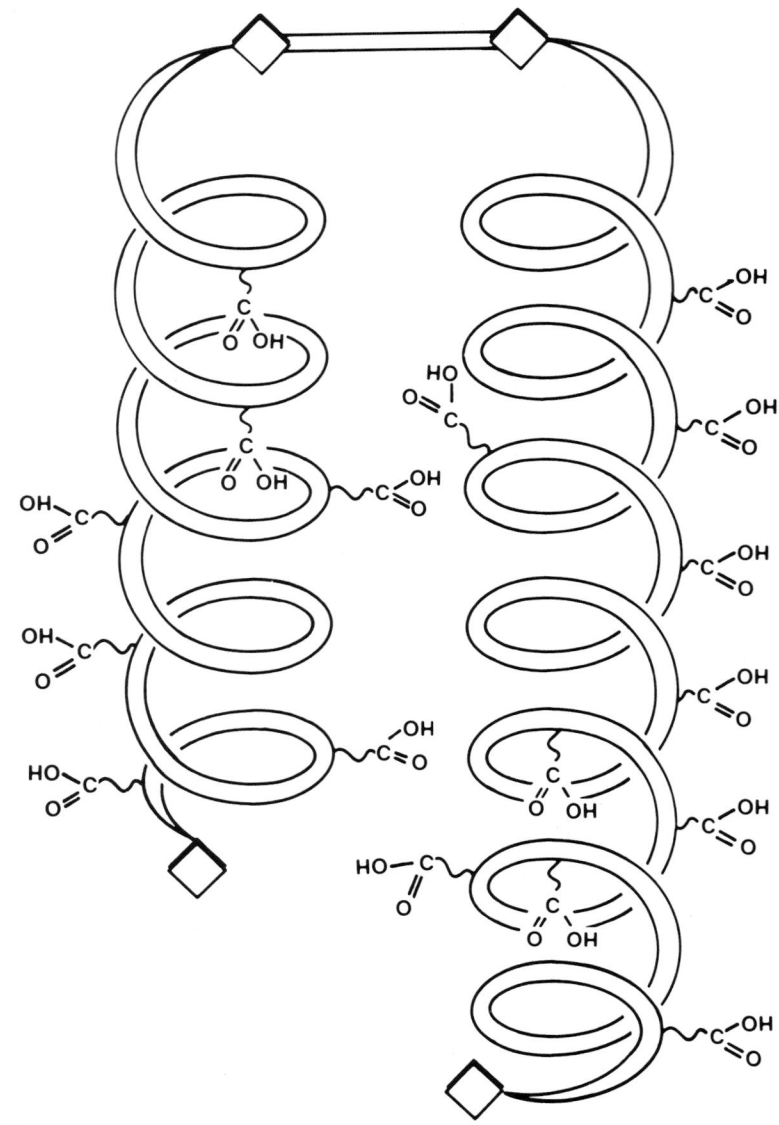

FIG. 7. Schematic representations of the osteonectin molecule. The sequence of the amino terminal region predicts a helical structure with a bend caused by two prolyl residues (**A** and "1" in **B**). This potential structure may expose multiple acidic groups capable of low affinity Ca²⁺ binding. In addition, (**B**) the molecule contains a region homologous to ovomucoid (2), and one E-F hand Ca²⁺ binding structure, (3) and possibly a second (4).

as active in mediating cell attachment as osteopontin (55), it appears to be equally as active in bone cell attachment (Mintz, Grzesik, Gehron Robey, and Fisher, unpublished results). Interestingly, the protein contains multiple tyrosine sulfation consensus sequences (56,57). However, factors regulating the level of sulfation are not clear since bone sialoprotein isolated from human bone is poorly sulfated (L. W. Fisher, National Institutes of Health, personal communication) while that isolated from mouse bone cells (58) and UMR-106-NIH is highly sulfated (59). The degree of sulfation does not appear to influence cell attachment activity in vitro. A third sialo-

protein in bone, BAG (bone acidic glycoprotein)-75, shares common features with osteopontin and bone sialoprotein (60,61), but it is not yet known whether it has cell attachment activity.

While it is understandable that these attachment proteins would be located in pericellular locations, it is not clear how they become distributed throughout bone matrix. It has long been felt that extracellular matrix is a mediator of cellular metabolism. Therefore, it is conceivable that the presence of these proteins at various stages of bone development may influence cellular metabolism, and that they are left behind by cell surface shed-

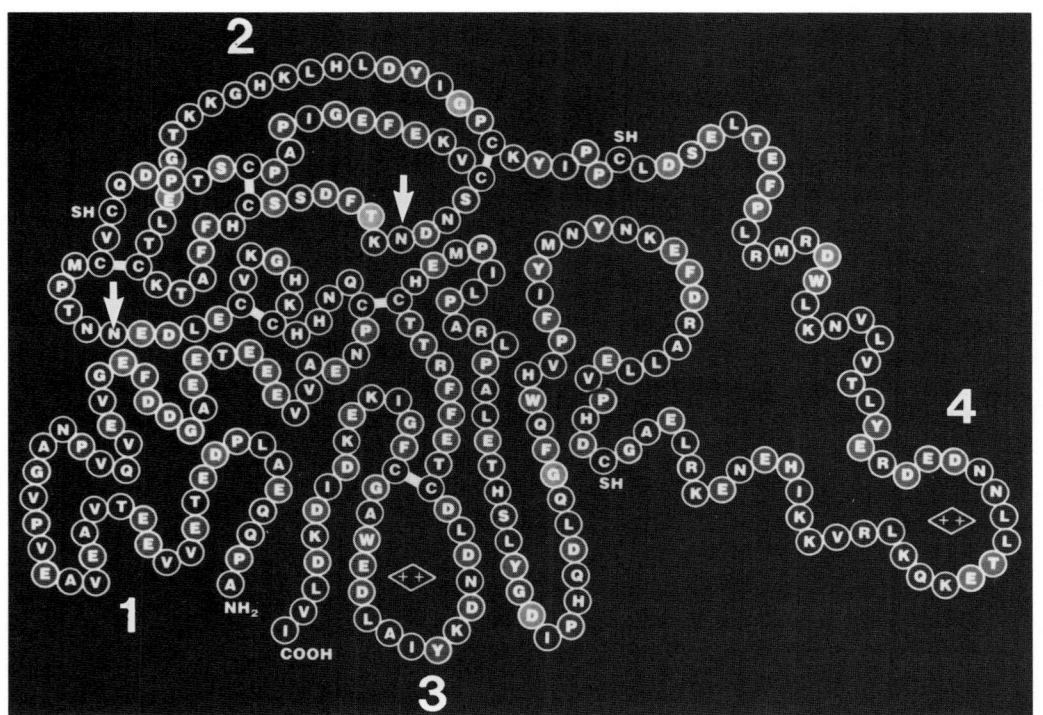

FIG. 7. *Continued.*

ding as bone apposition proceeds. It is also possible that osteoblasts and/or osteoclasts may pick and choose an appropriate attachment protein via expression of a particular cell surface integrin receptor.

γ-Carboxy Glutamic Acid (Gla)-Containing Proteins (Matrix Gla Protein and Osteocalcin). Bone matrix contains two proteins bearing the modified amino acid, γ-carboxy glutamic acid (gla), generated by vitamin K-dependent enzymes (Table 5). Matrix gla protein (MGP) appears at an early stage of cartilage and bone development, and in other tissues as well (62). Little is known about its deposition in bone matrix, or its possible function. Osteocalcin, one of the first described bone matrix proteins, appears late in bone development, and is perhaps the only protein unique to bone (reviewed in ref. 63). Osteocalcin expression is exquisitely regulated by

1,25-dihydroxyvitamin D_3 (64) and its gene promoter has been used to identify vitamin D regulatory elements (65). While the presence of gla confers Ca^{2+} binding properties with a moderate affinity ($K_d = 0.83$ mM), the relatively late appearance (and perhaps even postmineralization deposition) (66) of osteocalcin in developing bone (Fig. 10) points away from a role as a nucleator of mineralization. In fact, correlation of circulating osteocalcin levels with histomorphometric markers of bone turnover indicate that osteocalcin may correlate better with markers of the end phase of bone formation and present a signal to initiate bone turnover at a given bone matrix site. Current studies point to this role since bone deficient in osteocalcin (by means of warfarin inhibition of γ-carboxylation) does not undergo resorption in in vivo model systems (67). It has also been suggested that osteo-

TABLE 5. *Comparison of the two vitamin K-dependent γ-carboxylate proteins of mineralized bone matrix*

	Matrix gla protein	Osteocalcin
Distribution	Broad (cartilage, bone, lung, heart, kidney)	Hard tissue specific
Developmental appearance	Appears early, remains relatively constant	Appears late
Ca^{2+} binding	Presumably yes due to presence of gla	$K_d = \sim 0.83$ mM
Functional aspects	?	Chemotactic for a number of cell types, possible role in formation and function of osteoclasts

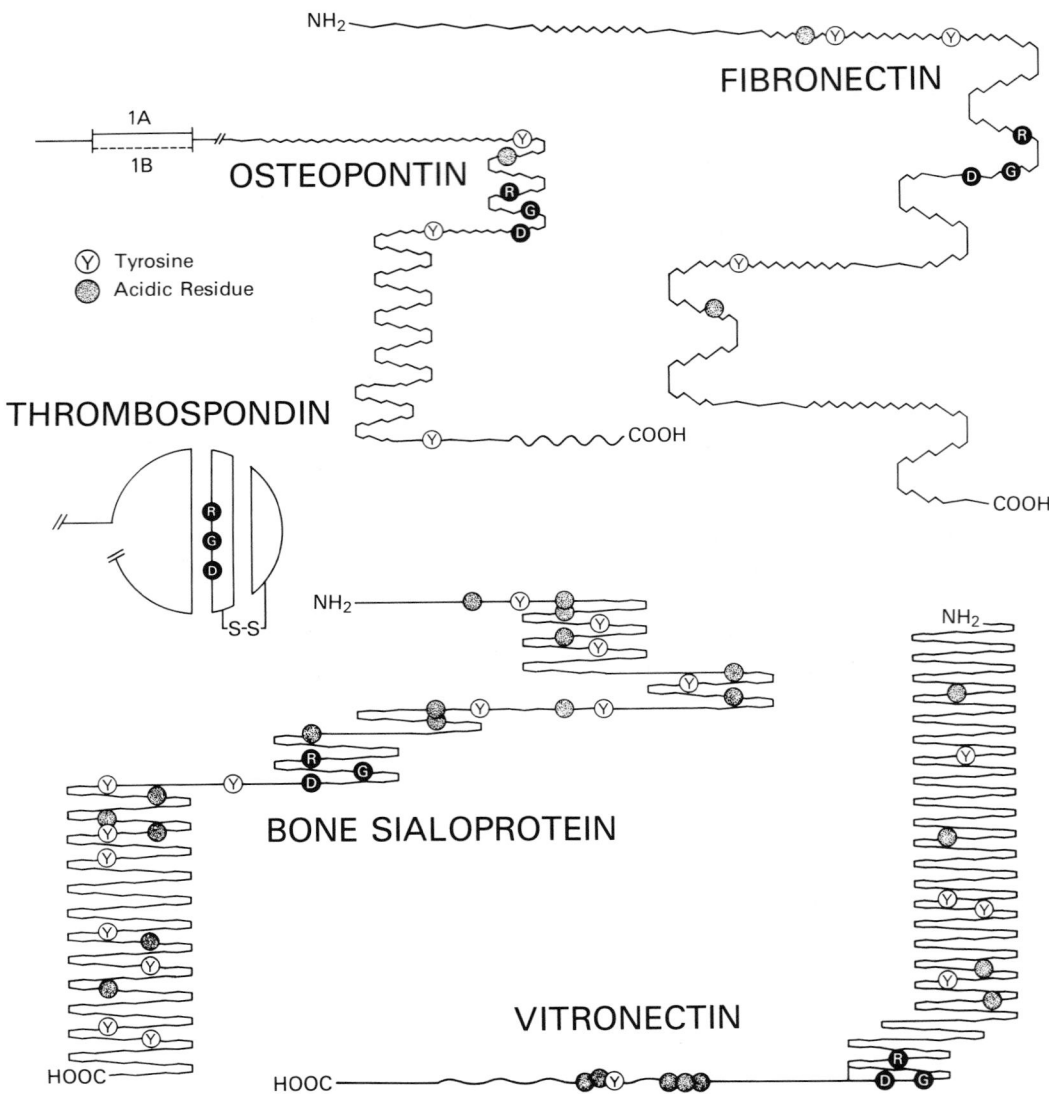

FIG. 8. Predicted conformations of the RGD regions of the RGD-containing proteins of bone. GOR (Garnier, Osguthorpe, and Robson) plots of the sequence surrounding the RGD region predict a similar conformation for fibronectin and osteopontin, whereas bone sialoprotein is more like vitronectin, another RGD-containing protein that may be localized in bone matrix, and in fact, BSP has been found to bind to a vitronectin receptor. Interestingly, there are a number of potential tyrosine sulfates (Y) based on the proximity of acidic residues and beta turns in the molecule. In thrombospondin, the RGD resides in a globular domain, the conformation of which is Ca^{2+} dependent. GOR plots courtesy of Larry W. Fisher.

calcin may be a chemoattractant for osteoclastic precursors (68), and may influence the activity of osteoclasts following fusion of precursor cells.

Other Protein Constituents of the Organic Matrix
(Table 2)

Growth Factors. Mineralized bone matrix is a virtual gold mine of factors that influence cell proliferation and/ or differentiation. Due to the increasing sensitivity of extraction procedures, and microanalytical and microse-

quencing techniques, the identification list of these proteins is ever-increasing. To date, acidic and basic fibroblast growth factors, insulin-like growth factors, a family of transforming growth factor-β molecules, platelet-derived growth factor and bone morphogenetic proteins (osteoinductive factors) have been identified (reviewed in refs. 69,70,71). Many of these are synthesized by cells in the osteoblastic lineage (FGFs, IGFs, TGF-βs, and perhaps PDGF) or by intimately associated cells such as chondrocytic cells, endothelial cells, and fibroblasts (PDGF, FGFs, IGFs). The origin of the family of bone

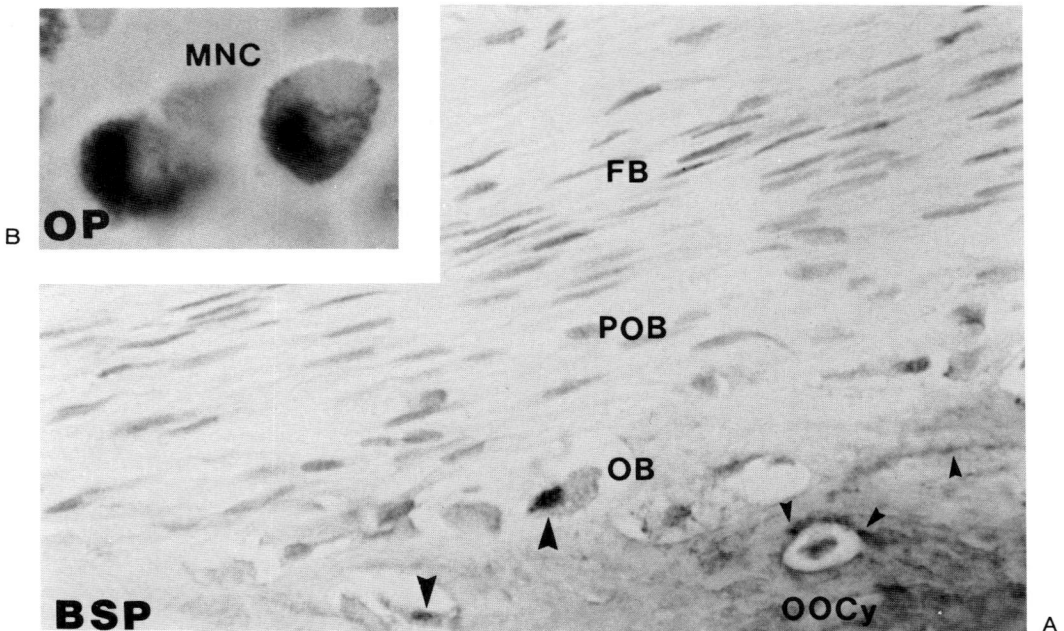

FIG. 9. Immunolocalization of bone sialoprotein (**A**) and osteopontin (**B**) in developing human subperiosteal bone. BSP is found in bone matrix, but is focal in nature (*small arrowheads*) as opposed to the more uniform distribution of other bone matrix proteins. Of the bone forming cells, only osteoblasts (OB) and occasional osteoid osteocytes (OOCy) contain BSP, as shown by the intense staining of the secretory apparati (*large arrowheads*). Osteopontin (OP) exhibits a similar pattern, but is also found in small mononuclear cells (MNC) in newly formed marrow (**B**).

morphogenetic proteins is not definitively known at this time. It is apparent that the same factors that are produced locally are also adsorbed to hydroxyapatite from the circulation (PDGF, FGFs, IGFs, and TGF-βs), as is β_2 microglobulin which was initially described as bone-derived growth factor. It is not known whether the origin (systemic versus local) alters the effectiveness of a given factor on regulation of cellular metabolism.

Enzymes and Their Inhibitors. Although not typically regarded as a matrix component, alkaline phosphatase (a hallmark of cells in the osteoblastic lineage) or a closely related molecule, has been isolated from the mineralized bone matrix (72). This protein is normally bound to cell membranes via a phosphoinositol linkage that is sensitive to phospholipase C, and may be shed from the cell surface either directly or on the surface of matrix vesicles.

Proteins present in mineralized matrix are slowly degraded with time or advancing age (16). The enzymes that are responsible for the removal of the organic matrix are not well defined to date, but may in part be adsorbed from the circulation. Like other connective tissue cells, osteoblasts apparently synthesize matrix degrading enzymes as well as their inhibitors, and many of these are found in the mineralized matrix. Collagenase and its inhibitor, TIMP, plasminogen activator and plasminogen activator inhibitor, have all been isolated from bone. In

addition, enzymes that degrade osteonectin, osteopontin, and bone sialoprotein have been alluded to in a number of studies. It is also possible that lysosomal enzymes (endoglycosidases and cysteine-proteases) secreted by osteoclasts into the "extracellular lysosomal compartment" may also reside in bone matrix, and may exhibit some activity even at neutral pH (reviewed in ref. 3).

PROTEINS ADSORBED FROM THE CIRCULATION

In addition to growth factors, there are a considerable number of other proteins that adsorb to mineralized bone matrix from serum (73). These include transferrin, immunoglobulins, α_1 acid glycoprotein, α_1-antitrypsin, apoA-I lipoprotein, and hemoglobin. However, two proteins, albumin and α_2-HS glycoprotein, are relatively abundant (3% and up to 20% of the total non-collagenous proteins, respectively), and α_2-HS is actually concentrated up to 100-fold above the serum level. It is not known whether these proteins make structural contributions to the bone matrix unit, but α_2-HS has several properties that suggest a function in the recruitment of osteoclastic precursors (74). It is now apparent that fetuin, a protein often used in tissue culture medium for its growth promoting ability, is the fetal bovine analog of

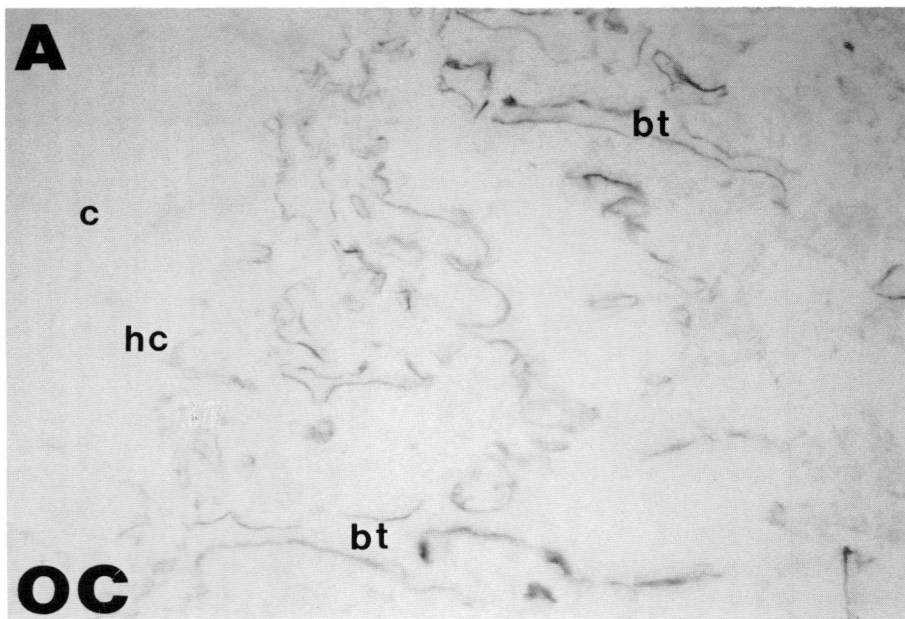

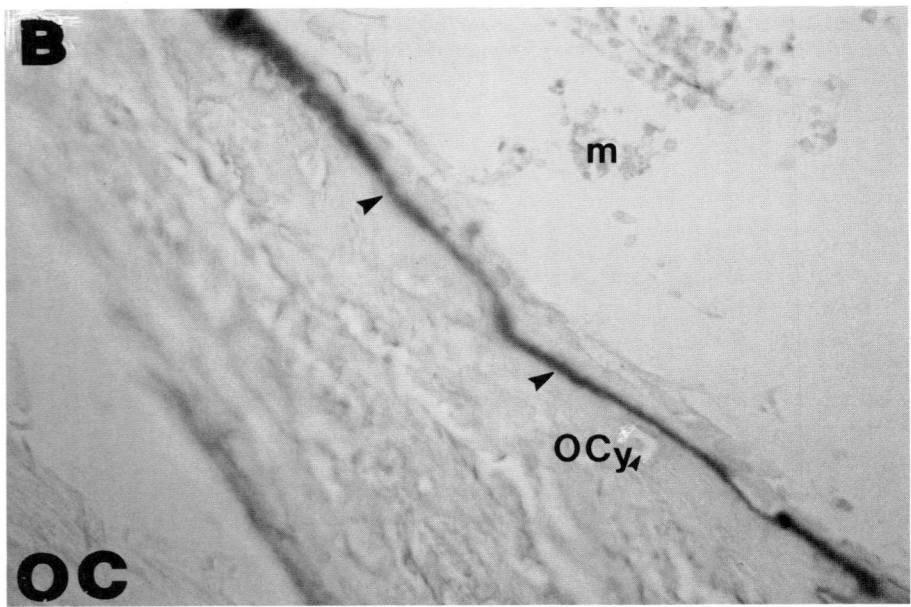

FIG. 10. Immunolocalization of osteocalcin (OC) in developing human endochondral bone. Using an antibody raised against the mature secreted form of osteocalcin, there is a very clear delineation of growth plate cartilage (c) which is negative from the newly formed boney trabeculae (bt) which are sharply positive (A). At higher magnification (B), the mineralization front (*arrows*) overlying osteocytes (OCy) is strongly positive for osteocalcin, indicative of its late appearance in bone formation.

human α_2-HS (75), information that warrants attention in bone physiology.

MATRIX MINERALIZATION

Physiological mineralization, under control of osteoblasts, is temporally and spatially delayed such that an unmineralized matrix (osteoid) is maintained between the cell and the mineralization front. It is postulated that ubiquitous distribution of mineral is prevented by the presence of crystallization inhibitors such as Ca^{2+}-binding serum proteins, matrix proteins, and crystal poisons (e.g., pyrophosphate) that must be removed, either by proteases or by phosphatases. Then, precipitation may proceed with the formation of a precursor amorphous calcium phosphate (which may then be rapidly converted to octacalcium phosphate), mediated by matrix vesicle (homogeneous hydroxyapatite nucleation within the matrix vesicle lumen) and/or collagen-based (heterogeneous nucleation) pathways (reviewed in refs. 76,77). Matrix vesicles appear to be operative in the *initial* stages of hypertrophic cartilage and woven bone mineralization, after which the predominant pathway is collagen mediated. Although newly formed hydroxyapatite crystals are found within the hole regions of collagen fibrils, the role of collagen in this event is still an enigma. Heterogeneous nucleation requires that the nucleator have a high affinity for the precipitating ions and that the molecular topography be complimentary to the surface of the precipitating mineral (suggested to be a β pleated sheet, 78). However, type I collagen does not fulfill either of these two requirements, and may act as a scaffold upon which bona fide nucleators are bound. In fact, the surface of collagen fibrils are most likely not available to the external environment, and is probably "decorated" with molecules such as decorin, osteonectin, and others yet to be identified (perhaps a bone FACIT collagen). However, several non-collagenous bone proteins (proteoglycans, osteonectin, osteocalcin) have been described as inhibitors of mineralization (77) because they inhibit hydroxyapatite precipitation when added to supersaturated calcium phosphate solutions. This interpretation is somewhat misleading since binding of the protein to the surface of seed crystals would prevent further *crystal growth*, and does not really comment on the protein's ability to *initiate* mineral precipitation onto solid phase substrata (79,80). While the function of a particular protein may be to inhibit crystal growth once it has reached a certain size, the ability of a protein (or a set of proteins) to nucleate and regulate the direction of crystal growth may require immobilization in a proper orientation.

MOLECULAR BIOLOGY OF BONE MATRIX PROTEINS

Assembly of an appropriate matrix is regulated by the (i) coordinated transcription of a set of genes to form mRNA; (ii) maintenance of the required steady state levels of mRNA; and (iii) translation into protein, followed by secretion and deposition. The application of molecular biological techniques has provided many of the tools needed to unravel this sequence. To date, virtually all of the abundant, structural bone matrix proteins have been cloned, and the resulting cDNAs have been used to locate and measure mRNA in vivo and in vitro. In addition, genes as well as their promoters have been isolated for α_1 and α_2 of type I collagen (81–84), fibronectin (85), thrombospondin (86), biglycan (87), alkaline phosphatase (88,89), matrix gla protein (90), osteonectin (91–93), and osteocalcin (65,94–96) (Table 6).

Gene activity is regulated by the combined action of cis-acting and trans-acting factors. Cis-acting factors are sequences located either in the promoter region, or elsewhere in the gene (in introns, sequences interspersed within the coding portion of the gene that are removed prior to protein translation) and are structurally required for gene activity. Trans-acting factors are encoded outside of the gene in question and bind to particular sequences, and may be cell or tissue specific. In addition, the genes contain responsive elements, i.e., consensus sequences that have been associated with either gene activation or inhibition by hormonal or environmental manipulation (Fig. 11). A simplistic hypothesis would espy that genes encoding proteins that are required at a particular stage of matrix development contain similar sets of responsive elements, and would respond positively to a particular factor, whereas other genes that are not required may contain the same elements, but respond negatively. This would result in the generation of a particular subset of proteins by cells at various stages of maturity as might be exemplified in Fig. 12.

Responsive elements for several factors known to influence bone such as 1,25-dihydroxyvitamin D_3 and other steroids, retinoic acid, and cAMP have been identified in several bone-related genes. The trans-acting fac-

TABLE 6. *Structural features of bone genes and their transcribed products*

Protein	Chromosome, gene, and mRNA	Promoter
Collagen		
$\alpha1$ (I)	7, 51 exons, 7.2 and 5.9 kb mRNA	TATA box, CCAAT, 1,25(OH)$_2$ D$_3$ element, pos. and
$\alpha2$ (I)	17, 51 exons, 6.25 and 5.5 kb mRNA	neg. elements in 1st intron CCAAT, NF1 binding site
Fibronectin[a]	7, 48 exons, 7.5 kb mRNA	AT, then GC rich, ATATAA, CAAT, cAMP responsive element
Thrombospondin	15 exons, 6.1 kb mRNA	TTTAAA, inverted CCAAT, AP1, AP2 and SP1 sites
Biglycan	X, 8 exons, 2.1 and 2.6 kb mRNA	GC-rich, SP1 and AP2 binding sites
Decorin	12 exons, 1.6 and 1.9 kb mRNA	
Alkaline phosphatase	1 exon, 2.6 kb mRNA	TATA, GC boxes, SP1 binding sites
Osteonectin	5, 10 exons, 2.5 and 3.0 kb mRNA	CCAAT, GAGA; NF1 and SP1 binding sites, growth hormone heta shock, cAMP, metal response elements
Osteopontin[a]	4 exons, 1.6 kb mRNA	
BSP	4 exons, 2.0 and 3.0 kb	
MGP	12, 4 exons, 0.7 kb mRNA	TATA, CAT, retinoic acid and 1,25(OH)$_2$D$_3$ elements
Osteocalcin	1, 4 exons, 0.6 kb mRNA	TATA box, CCAAT; NF1, AP1 and AP2 binding sites, retinoic acid and 1,25(OH)$_2$D$_3$ elements (may be the same), cAMP responsive element

[a] Alternate splicing has been identified.

THE GENERIC GENE

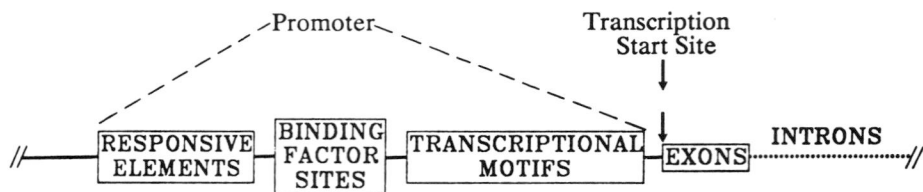

FIG. 11. Structural organization of genes. A gene is composed of three basic regions. The promoter is generally defined as the region preceding the mRNA transcription start site that contains sequences that are structurally required by RNA polymerases (transcriptional motifs), responsive elements (sequences that are associated with factor activity such that if it is deleted, there is no longer an effect), and sequences that bind to nuclear factors that modulate polymerase activity. The sequence following the transcription start site is composed of exons (sequences that encode protein) and introns (sequences that are spliced during transport to the cytoplasm). Characteristics of bone matrix genes are listed in Table 6.

tors in bone cells that mediate activity of the responsive elements are not well known, but in some cases are the hormone receptors themselves, and it has recently been shown that the products of the proto-oncogenes, jun and fos, may also be involved (97). Genes may also have multiple transcription start sites, and it is probable that DNA binding factors regulate which start site is used under certain conditions. Once the precursor mRNA is transcribed, the introns are spliced out to form the mature molecule and it is now apparent in many proteins (including fibronectin and osteopontin), alternate splic-

ing (preferential use of one exon over another, exon skipping, intra-exon splicing) takes place. Again, the factors that regulate alternate splicing are not yet defined, but presumably depend on the availability of the splice sequences at the intron–exon junctions, and may be affected by binding of factors at particular sites along the precursor molecule. Translational controls of the bone-related mRNAs have not been well defined to date. Alteration of the steady state levels of mRNA and translative capacity may be coupled to the proliferative state of the cell (98), and associated with base methylation, tertiary

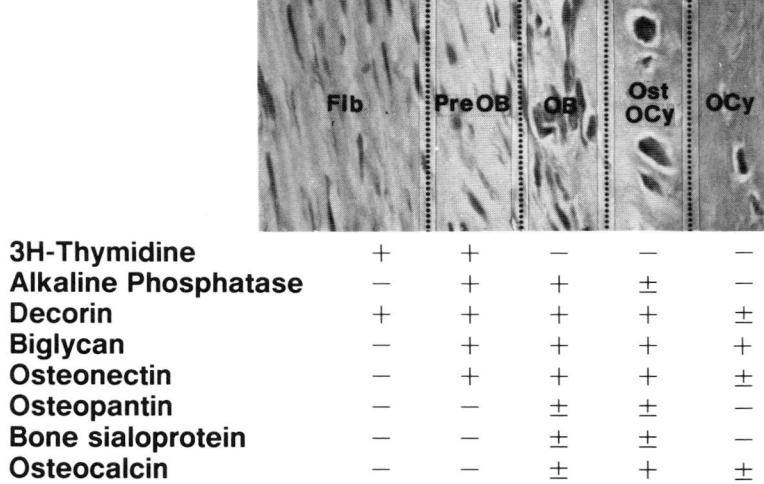

	Fib	PreOB	OB	Ost OCy	OCy
3H-Thymidine	+	+	−	−	−
Alkaline Phosphatase	−	+	+	±	−
Decorin	+	+	+	+	±
Biglycan	−	+	+	+	+
Osteonectin	−	+	+	+	±
Osteopantin	−	−	±	±	−
Bone sialoprotein	−	−	±	±	−
Osteocalcin	−	−	±	+	±

FIG. 12. Pattern of bone matrix gene expression in developing human subperiosteal bone. Through the concerted action of various factors that regulate gene expression, cells at different stages of maturation express different subsets of proteins. Fibroblasts (Fib) (or undifferentiated mesenchyme) are mitotic (indicated by 3H-thymidine uptake) but do not express most of the non-collagenous bone matrix proteins. Preosteoblasts (PreOB), are still proliferative, and expression proteins indicative of early bone formation (alkaline phosphatase, decorin, biglycan, and osteonectin). More mature osteoblasts (OB), for the most part non-mitotic, are beginning to express late markers (osteopontin and bone sialoprotein). Osteoid osteocytes (Ost Ocy) mark a transition state between osteoblasts and osteocytes (OCy), and may be the first cells to express osteocalcin. Both of these maturational stages are for the most part alkaline phosphatase negative.

structure of the 5′ untranslated region, and polyadenylation. Translation of mRNA can also be affected by the encoded protein itself, or parts thereof. For example, both the amino and carboxy terminal precursor peptides of type I collagen inhibit translation of its component chains in vitro (99–101).

REGULATION OF BONE MATRIX FORMATION

The synthesis, deposition, and turnover of extracellular matrix proteins by cells within the osteoblastic lineage is in part regulated by a wide number of growth factors and hormones. There is an enormous amount of information on the in vitro effects of these factors on various bone cell cultures. However, in reviewing the literature, one quickly realizes that there is a great deal of variability in these results. This variability is due to factors including animal species, developmental age, transformation, method of inducing cell culture preparation, and culture conditions (density, length of time in culture, medium supplements, etc.). Consequently, the exact direct or indirect effects of regulatory factors on cells in the osteoblastic lineage are not yet clearly defined, and cannot be discussed fully here. While organ cultures of developing bone take us one step closer to unraveling these complex pathways, it must be noted that such studies are usually performed in serum-free conditions, with only one or a limited number of factors present, and obviously in the absence of intact circulation. The major problems in the design of in vitro experiments results from a lack of information as to when exactly during bone formation the factor is present, where it exerts its effect (i.e., what cell type within the lineage possess the appropriate receptors) and how much is available. Therefore, it may be difficult to discern whether a given regulatory factor plays a role in normal bone formation or bone turnover (as a consequence of liberation of factors from the mineralized matrix by osteoclastic activity). However, many important generalizations have been derived from in vivo and organ culture studies (reviewed in refs. 102–107).

Growth factors found in the bone matrix by bone cells clearly influence bone matrix synthesis and turnover. In addition, growth factors synthesized by other bone-associated cell types, as well as those synthesized by exogenous sources and brought in by the circulation, also play a role in this process. These factors bind to specific receptors either on or in the target cells; in this case, cells that pass through the bone-formation pathway. These binding events trigger either one or several intracellular events including the generation of cAMP (108), inositol trisphosphate, and diacylglycerol (109), and ion fluxes from intracellular stores or through cell membrane ion channels (110). These signals, either singly or in concert, exert an effect on the transacting factors that regulate gene expression, and in some cases the receptor-ligand complex may bind directly to the promoter region of a gene. Through these pathways, growth factors and hormones act to stimulate proliferation of a particular cell type, or to promote differentiation (as determined by characteristics such as alkaline phosphatase activity, cAMP responsiveness, and bone matrix formation) in the absence of proliferation, or both.

Local Factors

Bone-forming cells produce a number of agents that influence proliferation and differentiation either in the same cell type (autocrine) or in other cell types (paracrine) (111). However, there is very little information on the influence of the maturational stage of the cell on the level of factor production, receptor concentration, or on the pattern of matrix protein secretion within the lineage.

Both acidic and basic fibroblast growth factors (aFGF and bFGF) are synthesized by osteoblastic cells, but may also arise from endothelial cells and the circulation (69). Generally, FGFs are not considered to be secreted proteins, and are usually sequestered either within or around cells (112), and the mechanism by which they become localized to the bone matrix is not known. The activities of the FGFs are quite similar, although aFGF activity is increased by the presence of heparin which enhances receptor binding (113). Both forms increase proliferation within bone (114), most likely of an osteoblastic precursor population(s), but bFGF is active at lower concentrations than aFGF. In addition, collagen synthesis is also increased, not only due to the increased number of bone-forming cells, but as a percentage of total protein synthesis. However, the FGFs do not appear to modulate further differentiation (115).

Insulin-like growth factors (previously termed somatomedins) are made locally and are adsorbed from the circulation (116–118). Both IGF-I and IGF-II increase bone cell proliferation and total protein synthesis. IGF-I is more active than IGF-II in most systems, and its major effect appears to be on preosteoblastic proliferation, without affecting subsequent maturation. The overall effect of IGFs is to increase protein content, not only by increasing synthesis but also by decreasing collagen degradation (reviewed in ref. 118). The IGF receptor has recently been identified to be the same as the mannose-6-phosphate directed receptor that binds to most lysosomal enzymes (119), but its location in bone is not yet known. In addition to this receptor, there are a number of binding proteins that may regulate IGF presentation to cells.

There are a number of transforming growth factor-β molecules present in bone including β_1 (120), β_2 (121), and the related bone morphogenetic proteins synthesized locally and/or adsorbed from serum or neighboring cells. The TGF-βs stimulate proliferation of osteoprogenitor cells, and increase the percentage of collagen in this population (122). In addition, TGF-βs also have been reported to influence the maturation of cells by increasing levels of alkaline phosphatase. However, alkaline phosphatase is particularly prominent in preosteoblastic rather than osteoblastic cells. Studies of demineralized bone particle induced bone formation indicates that TGF-β expression occurs subsequent to the endochondral phase and concomitantly with type I collagen expression (123,124). That, along with data showing that subperiosteal injection ultimately leads to an increase in bone mass (125), indicates that TGF-β increases the population of a committed precursor. TGF-β binds to a number of cell-surface proteins, some of which may be partially processed forms of the receptor, reported to be a proteoglycan (betaglycan) (126). The intracellular mechanisms of action have yet to be determined.

Platelet-derived growth factor (PDGF) found in bone matrix is most likely adsorbed from serum, although it has been reported to be synthesized by endothelial cells and osteosarcoma cells. This factor increases proliferation of osteoprogenitors in the periosteum of developing bone, and also increases total protein synthesis (127). Osteoblasts produce, and respond to prostaglandins (128). While most often associated with bone resorption, PGE_2 promotes proliferation of presumptive progenitors in the periosteum and also stimulates collagen synthesis (129). PGE may also mediate the response of bone cells to other growth factors.

Cartilage produces many of the same types of growth factors listed above, and most likely others unique to cartilage that may also influence bone formation. Bone marrow is another rich source of growth factors, and cytokines, the products of hematologic cells, influence bone formation. Interleukin-1 (IL-1), which may be an osteoblast-derived product as well, causes increased bone resorption in organ culture (130), but also increases proliferation. At low doses, it stimulates collagen synthesis, but is inhibitory with increasing concentration (131). The tumor necrosis factors (TNF-α = cachectin, TNF-β = lymphotoxin) stimulate proliferation and collagen synthesis in preosteoblasts, but decrease collagen synthesis in more mature cells (132,133). Colony stimulating factors (CSFs) may also influence matrix formation, in particular GM-CSF (again, also produced by bone-forming cells) (134), which has been implicated in osteoclastic precursor proliferation, and may be involved in the signaling that must take place between blasts and clasts. Interferon-γ (INF-γ) has also been found to decrease proliferation and collagen synthesis, but there is no information on maturational effects (135).

Systemic Factors

The list of systemic factors that have receptors located in or on osteoblasts is increasing almost daily. These factors can directly influence bone matrix protein metabolism, or can influence the production of endogenous factors and/or their receptor binding capacities.

Parathyroid hormone (PTH) can exert variable effects on bone formation that depend on dose and length of time of exposure. PTH is bound to a cell surface receptor apparently located in cells immediately adjacent to but distinct from fully differentiated osteoblasts (136). Once bound, it induces both cAMP production, and a Ca^{2+} flux, which thereby transduces the signal (by pathways that are currently under investigation). These signals can cause an induction in the production of locally produced IGF-I (137) and/or GM-CSF (134), block the effects of locally produced IGF-I (138) or alter growth factor binding to its receptor as exemplified by TGF-β (139). Consequently, PTH-induced regulation of the amount factor presented to receptor-bearing cells can result in a spectrum of effects, which may explain its variability with respect to bone formation versus bone resorption.

1,25-Dihydroxyvitamin D_3, another important regulator of bone turnover, for the most part appears to have a negative effect on the proliferative phase of bone formation, and has been called a maturational factor necessary for normal growth and matrix mineralization (107). In fact, in vitro, it is required for the production of osteocalcin, which is a late appearing product of mature osteoblast and/or early osteocytic cells (64). While there appear to be direct and immediate effects of 1,25-dihydroxyvitamin D_3 on cells (140), the action of 1,25-dihydroxyvitamin D_3 in gene activation may require the binding of the receptor-ligand complex as well as other gene products to the promoter. Conversely, 1,25-dihydroxyvitamin D_3 decreases type I collagen production, again, indicative of shifting cells from one stage to another (141,142). The receptor for this steroid is widely distributed, but within the maturational scheme, has not been well characterized in bone.

As indicated by the loss of bone density in a large percentage of women following menopause, it has long been apparent that there is a role for estrogen in bone metabolism. Although estrogen receptors have not been directly identified on bone-forming cells in situ, in vitro evidence indicates that they are present, albeit in low numbers (143,144). Estrogen has been reported to decrease subperiosteal bone matrix protein production (145) but to increase trabecular bone formation (146). Its beneficial effects in maintaining bone mass may also be related to a decrease in bone turnover, or a slowing of bone resorption.

Other systemic factors may influence bone formation by the modulation of local growth factor synthesis and/or directly. Insulin may stimulate collagen synthesis via the production of IGF-I by the liver (107), or directly increase the production of collagen in central bone (147) independently of an increase in proliferation of progenitor cells. Growth hormone also appears to stimulate IGF-I, but by osteoblastic cells (107). β_2 Microglobulin (originally described in bone as bone-derived growth factor (148), is found on the surface of bone-forming cells and may mediate IGF-I binding (107). The effects of glucocorticoids are dependent on a number of factors. There is an increase in collagen synthesis following brief exposures which may be mediated by increased IGF receptor binding, whereas long-term treatment causes reduced proliferation of preosteoblasts and a subsequent decrease in matrix formation (149). The retinoids most certainly are required for normal bone development and maintenance, however, the direct effects on cells within the lineage are not well established at this time (150).

Because of their ability to alter bone resorption independent of a direct effect on osteoclasts, other systemic factors including thyroid hormones, vasoactive intestinal peptide, and epidermal growth factor have been implicated in altering bone-forming cell metabolism (151). The EGF receptor has been localized in undifferentiated cells in close proximity to osteoclasts and in cells found in mixed spicules of calcified cartilage and bone in the growth plate (152). However, an understanding of the effects of all these factors on bone formation awaits further systematic characterization.

INFLUENCE OF CELL CYCLE ON CELLULAR ACTIVITY

It is now apparent in many cell systems that the position of a cell within the various phases of the cell cycle, (G_1, S, G_2, and M) plays a major role in their metabolic activities (153). In general, protein synthesis can occur throughout G_1 and S, but individual proteins may peak at various points throughout these two phases. DNA synthesis is the hallmark of S phase, which is followed by two relatively short phases, G_2 (preparation for mitosis) and cytokinesis during M phase. In some cases, cells drop out of the cycle, and become arrested or quiescent in a somewhat nebulous state, G_0. As cells mature (or senescence), the doubling time (marked by the length of time between division), and the length of G_1 may increase. In developing bone, osteoprogenitor cells proliferate, but the rate of their proliferation decreases, so much so that an osteoblast is considered to be a non-mitotic cell (although occasional osteoblasts have been detected using ^{3}H-thymidine which is incorporated specifically into newly synthesized DNA). This progression has recently been demonstrated in vitro (reviewed in ref. 154). It has recently been determined that alkaline phosphatase activity is dependent on the cell cycle, with cell surface AP levels increasing during G_1, peaking during S phase, rapidly shed from the surface during G_2, and virtually absent during M phase (155). Preliminary results indicate that synthesis of other bone matrix-related proteins exhibit different patterns throughout the cycle (Fedarko and Gehron Robey, unpublished results). In addition, it is also possible that functional receptors are also cell cycle dependent, however, virtually no information

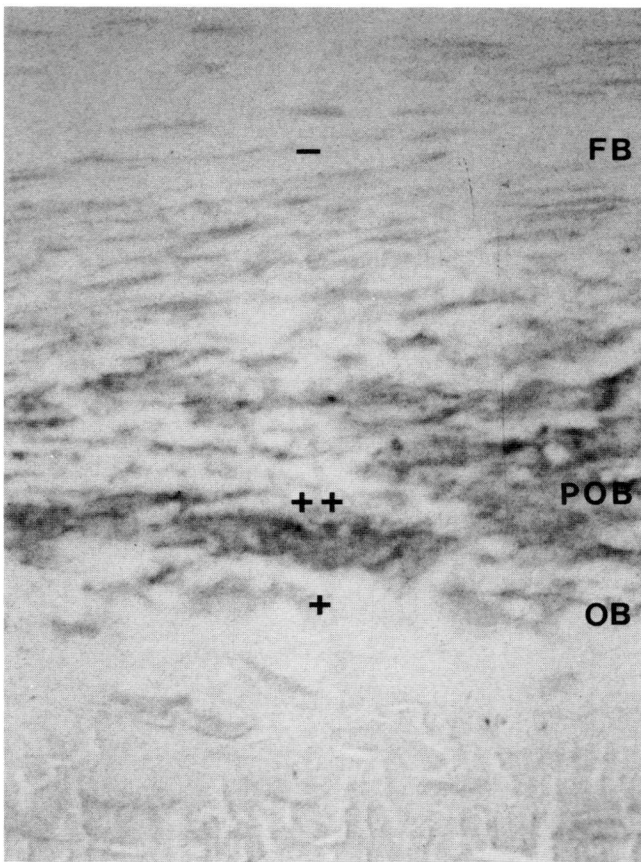

FIG. 13. Alkaline phosphatase activity (AP) in developing human subperiosteal bone. While the osteoblastic (OB) layer is seen to AP positive (+), preosteoblasts (POB) exhibit higher levels of activity (++), and fibroblasts (FB) are negative (−).

is available with respect to bone-forming cells at this time.

Based on this information, it may now be possible to correlate changes in biosynthetic pattern as a function of position in the cycle to different maturational stages of bone-forming cells. For example, in developing subperiosteal bone, preosteoblasts contain higher levels of membrane associated alkaline phosphatase than mature osteoblasts (Fig. 13). It is tempting to speculate that at a certain point a preosteoblast undergoes a division thereby shedding its alkaline phosphatase, and enters G_1 phase and begins to replace cell surface enzyme. But, due to its surrounding environment of extracellular matrix and local factors, and/or availability of functional receptors, this cell does not receive the appropriate signal(s) to progress, or receives signals that cause it to become somewhat arrested in G_1 to form an osteoblast. At this point, some, but not all osteoblasts are surrounded first by unmineralized osteoid and subsequently by mineralized matrix, and are further arrested in a G_0-like or quiescent state to form osteocytes (Fig. 14). In other instances, the osteoblasts do not become entombed, but form quiescent lining cells, although not necessarily with the same

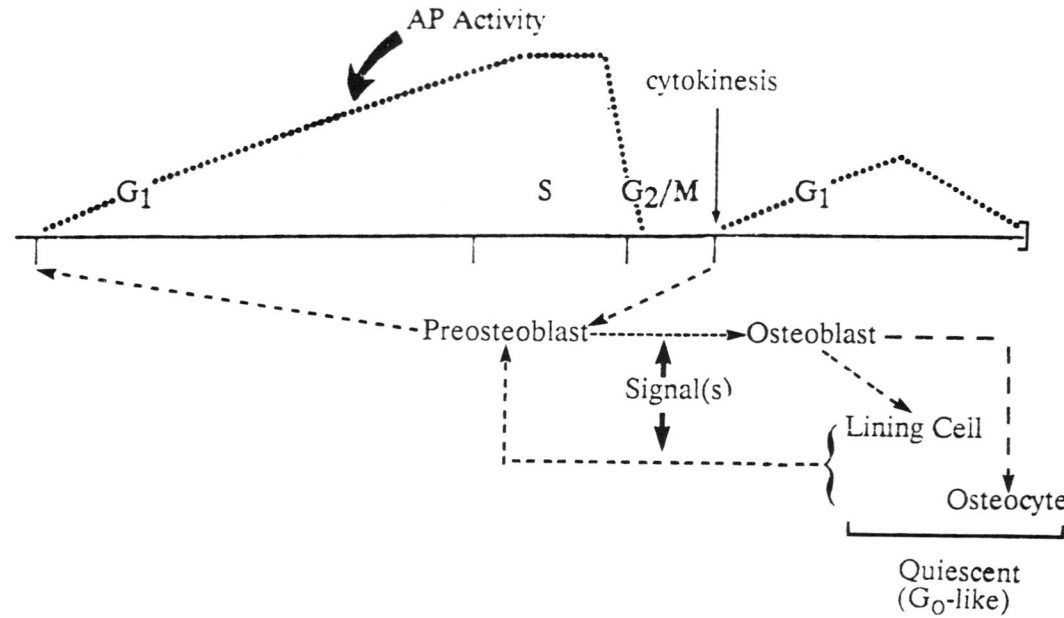

FIG. 14. Potential influence of the cell cycle in osteoblastic maturation.

set of metabolic characteristics as osteocytes. An understanding of metabolic changes dependent on the cell cycle may aide greatly in our understanding and manipulation of the osteoblastic maturation sequence.

BONE MATRIX PROTEINS AS BIOCHEMICAL MARKERS

It has long been the wish of clinicians anxious to assess skeletal status to have biochemical assays available for use on body fluids that specifically mark bone formation versus bone resorption. While many assays have been developed for bone matrix-related proteins, there are a plethora of problems that makes interpretation of the results difficult. First, patient status such as renal function, fasting versus non-fasting, circadian rhythms, etc. can influence the assays independent of skeletal status. Second, most of the bone matrix proteins are also synthesized by non-related soft tissues and contribute a "background" that cannot easily be subtracted. Finally, bone matrix proteins can be present in body fluids either intact (potentially indicative of formation, although it is not precisely known how newly synthesized proteins escape into the circulation) or fragmented (sometimes indicative of formation when precursor portions of molecules are cleaved, or of resorption due to osteoclastic action). In general, assays using antibodies directed against a particular protein do not readily distinguish between these two scenarios.

The complexities of biochemical analysis in a clinical setting have been extensively reviewed elsewhere (156,157). Consequently, what follows here is a brief de-

scription of potential new assays based on recent findings. It is now apparent that there are differences between bone-derived versus soft tissue-derived proteins based on possible differential mRNA splicing (leading to variations in protein sequence) and posttranslational modifications. These discoveries offer the opportunity to generate more specific antibodies, directed against regions of the molecule that are unique to bone, that will be clinically more valuable.

Since collagen is the most abundant of the bone matrix proteins (90% of the organic matrix), much attention has been directed to its assessment. Since it is synthesized in a precursor form, the levels of the pN and pC fragments mark formation, but in soft connective tissue as well as in bone. However, the discovery that the pN fragment in bone collagen is phosphorylated may provide a distinguishing characteristic, but it has yet to be determined if other connective tissues carry out this posttranslational modification. Determination of fragments bearing hydroxyproline and hydroxylysine (somewhat collagen specific amino acids) in serum and urine can be indicative of resorption, but again soft tissue degradation also contributes to these levels. However, a promising assay has recently been developed based on the fact that the crosslinks formed in bone are different from those in soft tissue, such that upon hydrolysis of urine, lysyl-pyridinoline (primarily from bone collagen) and hydroxylysyl-pyridinoline from bone and soft tissue) are generated (158). Correlations of these two moieties with known states of increased bone formation and/or resorption will determine the validity of this assay.

Of the non-collagenous bone matrix proteins, osteocalcin assays has received the most attention to date due to its bone specificity. Consequently, analysis of results from osteocalcin immunoassays under a variety of conditions have provided a valuable learning experience of the potential pitfalls. Since osteocalcin is produced late in the bone formation scheme, it may in fact be a signal for the recruitment of osteoclastic precursors and initiation of bone resorption. It is now apparent that osteocalcin is present in an intact form as well as in fragments, and therefore total immunoreactive osteocalcin may reflect a variable mixture of formation and resorption products. Most available assays utilize antibodies raised against the bovine homolog which cross react with human osteocalcin. However, there appears to be variability between antibodies with respect to reactivity against fragments, although it has been suggested that most antibodies do not recognize the fragments efficiently. But as such, these assays do correlate with *changes* in bone formation rate when uncoupled from resorption in disorders such as Paget's disease and osteoporosis.

A hallmark of early bone formation is alkaline phosphatase, but genetically related isozymes are also produced in liver and kidney. The isozymes differ from one another in sensitivities to inhibitors and heat stability, however these assays are somewhat tedious. Monoclonal antibodies have been generated that recognize bone-specific epitopes, and may be of use. It should be noted that fragments of alkaline phosphatase generated by proteolysis still maintain activity, and a protein with alkaline phosphatase activity has also been found in bone matrix. Consequently, osteoclastic activity may release an active fragment into the circulation as well.

A similar situation exists in the assay of osteonectin as for alkaline phosphatase. Osteonectin is constitutively produced in vivo in bone and associated tissues, salivary and renal epithelia, and apparently megakaryocytes since it is found in the α granules of platelets. Since platelets contain osteonectin, its assessment necessitates the use of carefully prepared plasma (to avoid platelet release reactions). However, platelet and bone osteonectin can be distinguished by monoclonal antibodies, but it is not yet known if there are differences between bone osteonectin and osteonectin derived from the other sources.

Of the bone matrix sialoproteins, bone sialoprotein is the most tissue specific, and in the absence of pregnancy, may be indicative of late stages of bone matrix formation. However, BSP, like osteonectin, may also be in platelets (159). Consequently, further assessment is needed to determine the relevance of circulating bone sialoprotein to bone formation. Osteopontin may also represent a useful marker. Although it is widely distributed, there may be a bone-specific deletion of a stretch of amino acids near the amino terminus, and it appears to be differentially phosphorylated under certain circumstances.

TABLE 7. *Potential functions of components of the bone matrix unit (structural and non-structural)*

Proliferation and maturation of precursor cells
　Growth and morphogenetic factors
　Cell attachment proteins (?) (thrombospondin, fibronectin, osteopontin, bone sialoprotein, vitronectin)
Formation and orientation of matrix scaffolding
　Collagen(s)
　Proteoglycans and hyaluronan
Deposition of hydroxyapatite
　Alkaline phosphatase (?)
　Osteonectin (?)
　Other proteins
Modeling and remodeling of mineralized matrix
　Osteocalcin (?)
　α_2HS-glycoprotein (?)

As can be seen from the above description, virtually all of the currently available assays and those under development absolutely require specific and well characterized antibodies. Reactivity against intact versus fragmented forms of the molecule must be well documented, and antibodies that react with bone specific characteristics of the molecule must be developed. Subsequently, careful correlations between assay levels in plasma, serum, and/or urine with histomorphometric and bone density parameters will be needed to fully establish the value of a given marker.

SUMMARY

Clearly, major advances in the identification of bone matrix components, isolation of the genes for these proteins, and determination of regulatory pathways within cells have been made within a short amount of time. From this body of work, the functions of these proteins are beginning to be identified (Table 7). With continued effort in defining the steps in the assembly of the bone matrix unit and how these steps are regulated by the cells within the osteoblastic lineage, we may begin to intelligently alter these processes to our advantage in the control of both genetic and acquired bone disease.

REFERENCES

1. Termine JD, Belcourt AB, Christner PJ, Conn KM, Nylen MU. Properties of dissociatively extracted fetal tooth matrix proteins. *J Biol Chem* 1980;255:9760–72.
2. Termine JD, Belcourt AB, Conn KM, Kleinman HK. Mineral and collagen-binding proteins of fetal calf bone. *J Biol Chem* 1981;256:10403–8.
3. Gehron Robey P. The biochemistry of bone. *Endocrinol Metab Clin North Am* 1989;18:859–902.
4. Strauss PG, Closs EI, Schmidt J, Erfle V. Gene expression during osteogenic differentiation in mandibular condyles in vitro. *J Cell Biol* 1990;110:1369.
5. Martin GR, Timpl R, Muller PK, Kuhn K. The genetically distinct collagens. *Trends Biochem Res* 1985;251:285–7.

6. Niyibizi C, Eyre DR. Identification of cartilage α_1(XI) chain in type V collagen from bovine bone. *FEBS Lett* 1989;242:314–8.

7. Adachi E, Hayashi T. In vitro formation of hybrid fibrils of type V collagen and type I collagen. *Connect Tissue Res* 1986;14:257.

8. van der Rest M, Mayne R. Type IX collagen proteoglycan from cartilage is covalently cross-linked to type II collagen. *J Biol Chem* 1988;263:1615.

9. Burgeson RE, Hebda PA, Morris NP, Hollister DW. Human cartilage collagens: comparison of cartilage collagens with human type V collagen. *J Biol Chem* 1982;257:7852.

10. Gordon MK, Gerecke DR, Dublet B, van der Rest M, Sugrue SP, Olsen BR. Type XII collagen: a large multidomain molecule with partial homology to type IX collagen. *J Biol Chem* 1989; 264:19772–8.

11. Sugrue SP, Gordon MK, Seyer J, Dublet B, van der Rest M, Olsen BR. Immunoidentification of type XII collagen in embryonic tissues. *J Cell Biol* 1989;109:939–45.

12. Pihlajaniemi T, Tamminen M, Sandberg M, Hirvonen H, Vuorio E. The α_1 chain of type XIII collagen. *Ann NY Acad Sci* 1990;580:440.

13. Eyre DR. Collagen: molecular diversity in the body's protein scaffold. *Science* 1980;207:1315–22.

14. Fisher LW, Gehron Robey P, Tuross N, et al. The M_r 24,000 phosphoprotein from developing bone is the NH$_2$-terminal propeptide of the α_1 chain of type I collagen. *J Biol Chem* 1987;262:13457–62.

15. Conn KM, Termine JD. Matrix protein profiles in calf bone development. *Bone* 1985;6:33–6.

16. Fisher LW, Termine JD. Purification of the non-collagenous proteins from bone: technical pitfalls and how to avoid them. In: Ornoy A, Harell A, Sela J, eds. *Current advances in skeletogenesis.* Amsterdam: Elsevier, 1985;467–72.

17. Ruoslahti E. Proteoglycans in cell regulation. *J Biol Chem* 1989;264:13369–72.

18. Fisher LW. The nature of proteoglycans of bone. In: Butler WT, ed. *The chemistry and biology of mineralized tissues.* Birmingham: EBSCO Media, 1985;188–96.

19. Leblond CP, Wienstock MA. Comparative study of dentin and bone formation. In: *The biochemistry and physiology of bone.* New York: Academic Press, 1976;517.

20. Prince CW, Rahemtulla F, Butler WT. Incorporation of [^{35}S]-sulphate into glycosaminoglycans by mineralized tissues *in vivo*. *Biochem J* 1984;224:941–5.

21. Bianco P, Fisher LW, Young MF, Termine JD, Gehron Robey P. Expression and localization of the two small proteoglycans, biglycan and decorin, in human developing skeletal and non-skeletal tissues. *J Histochem Histocytol,* 1990;38:1549–63.

22. Fisher LW, Termine JD, Young MF. Deduced protein sequence of bone small proteoglycan I (biglycan) shows homology with proteoglycan II (decorin) and several nonconnective tissue proteins in a variety of species. *J Biol Chem* 1989;264:4571–6.

23. Oldberg A, Antonsson P, Lindblom K, Keinegard D. A collagen-binding 50kDa protein (fibromodulin) is structurally related to the small interstitial proteoglycans PG-S1 and PG-S2. *EMBO J* 1989;8:2601–4.

24. Bentz H, Chang R-J, Thompson AY, Glaser CB, Riosen DM. Amino acid sequence of bovine osteoinductive factor. *J Biol Chem* 1990;265:5024–9.

25. Fedarko NS, Young MF, Termine JD, Gehron Robey P. Temporal regulation of hyaluronan and proteoglycan metabolism in human bone cells in vitro. *J Biol Chem* 1990;265:12200–9.

26. Gehron Robey P, Fisher LW, Stubbs JT, Termine JD. Biosynthesis of osteonectin and a small proteoglycan (PG-II) by connective tissue cells in vitro. In: Sen A, Thornhill T, eds. *Development and diseases of cartilage and bone matrix.* New York: Alan R. Liss, 1986;115–25.

27. Sage H, Tupper J, Bramson R. Endothelial cell injury in vitro is associated with increased secretion of an M_r 43,000 glycoprotein ligand. *J Cell Physiol* 1986;127:373–87.

28. Wasi S, Otsuka K, Yao L-L, Tung PS, Aubin JE, Sodek J, Termine JD. An osteonectin-like protein in porcine periodontal ligament and its synthesis by periodontal ligament fibroblasts. *Can J Biochem Cell Biol* 1984;62:470–8.

29. Bianco P, Kopp JB, Fisher LW, Termine JD, Gehron Robey P.

New data on the distribution of osteonectin/SPARC in human and mouse tissues and their potential implications. *J Bone Miner Res* 1989;4(Suppl):S245.

30. Wewer UM, Albrechtsen R, Fisher LW, Young MF, Termine JD. Osteonectin/SPARC/BM-40 in human decidua and carcinoma, tissues characterized by de novo formation of basement membrane. *Am J Pathol* 1988;132:345–55.

31. Holland PWH, Harper SJ, McVey JH, Hogan BR. In vivo expression of mRNA for the calcium-binding protein (SPARC) osteonectin revealed by in situ hybridization. *J Cell Biol* 1987; 105:473–82.

32. Stenner DD, Tracy RP, Riggs BL, Mann KG. Human platelets contain and secrete osteonectin, a major protein of mineralized bone. *Proc Natl Acad Sci USA* 1986;83:6892–6.

33. Malaval LP, Darbouret B, Preaudet C, Delmas PD. Monoclonal antibody recognizing osteonectin from bone but not from platelet. *J Bone Miner Res* 1988;3(Suppl):552.

34. Villareal XC, Malaval L, Mann KG, Delmas P, Long GL. Epitope mapping of two monoclonals antibodies to the central portion of human osteonectin. *Calcif Tissue Int* 1991;48:138–41.

35. Termine JD, Kleinman HK, Whitson SW, Conn KM, McGarvey ML, Martin GR. Osteonectin, a bone-specific protein linking mineral to collagen. *Cell* 1981;26:99–105.

36. Engel J, Taylor W, Paulsson M. Calcium binding domains and calcium-induced conformational transition of SPARC/BM-40/Osteonectin, and extracellular glycoprotein expressed in mineralized and nonmineralized tissues. *Biochemistry* 1987;26:6958–65.

37. Bolander ME, Young MF, Fisher LW, Yamada Y, Termine JD. Osteonectin cDNA sequence reveals potential binding regions for calcium and hydroxyapatite and shows homologies with both a basement membrane protein (SPARC) and a serine proteinase inhibitor (ovomucoid). *Proc Natl Acad Sci USA* 1988;85:2919–23.

38. Hynes RO. Integrins: a family of cell surface receptors. *Cell* 1987;48:549–54.

39. Peirschbacher MD, Ruoslahti E. Cell attachment activity of fibronectin can be duplicated by small synthetic fragments of the molecule. *Nature* 1984;309:30–3.

40. Weiss RE, Reddi AH. Synthesis and localization of fibronectin during collagenous matrix-mesenchymal cell interaction and differentiation of cartilage and bone in vivo. *Proc Natl Acad Sci USA* 1980;77:2074–8.

41. Gehron Robey P, Young MF, Fisher LW, McClain TD. Thrombospondin is an osteoblast-derived component of mineralized extracellular matrix. *J Cell Biol* 1989;108:719–27.

42. Frazier WA. Thrombospondin. *J Cell Biol* 1987;105:625–32.

43. Butler WT. The nature and significance of osteopontin. *Coll Relat Res* 1989;23:123–36.

44. Smith JH, Denhardt DT. Molecular cloning of a tumor promoter-inducible mRNA found in JB6 mouse epidermal cells. *J Cell Biochem* 1987;34:13–22.

45. Laverdure GR, Banerjee D, Chackalaparampil I, Mukerjee BB. *FEBS Lett* 1987;222:261–5.

46. Herring GM. The organic matrix in bone. In: Bourne GH, ed. *The biochemistry and physiology of bone,* New York: Academic Press, 1972;127–89.

47. Fisher LW, Whitson SW, Avioli LV, Termine JD. Matrix sialoprotein of developing bone. *J Biol Chem* 1983;258:12723–7.

48. Nomura S, Wills AJ, Edwards DR, Heath JK, Hogan BLM. Developmental Expression of 2ar (osteopontin) and (SPARC) Osteonectin RNA as revealed by in situ hybridization. *J Cell Biol* 1988;106:441–50.

49. Craig AM, Nemir M, Mukherjee BB, Chambers AF, Denhardt DT. Identification of the major phosphoprotein secreted by many rodent cell lines as 2ar/osteopontin. *Biochem Biophys Res Commun* 1988;157:166–73.

50. Nemir M, DeVouge MW, Mukherjee BB. Normal rat kidney cells secrete both phosphorylated and nonphosphorylated forms of osteopontin showing different physiological properties. *J Biol Chem* 1989;264:18202–8.

51. Kiefer MC, Aauer DM, Barr PJ. The cDNA and derived amino acid sequence for human osteopontin. *Nucleic Acids Res* 1989;17:3306.

52. Young MF, Fisher LW, McBride WO, Termine JD. cDNA clon-

ing, chromosomal location and RFLP Analysis of human osteopontin. *Genomics* 1990;7:491–502.

53. Bianco P, Fisher LW, Young MF, Termine JD, Gehron Robey P. Expression of bone sialoprotein (BSP) in human developing skeletal and nonskeletal tissues as revealed by immunostaining and in situ hybridization. *Calcif Tissue Int.* in press.

54. Oldberg A, Franzen A, Heinegard D, Pierschbacher M, Rouslahti E. Identification of a bone sialoprotein receptor in osteosarcoma cells. *J Biol Chem* 1988;263:19433–6.

55. Somerman M, Fisher LW, Foster RA, Sauk JJ. Human bone sialoprotein I and II enhance fibroblast attachment in vitro. *Calcif Tissue Int* 1988;43:50–3.

56. Oldberg A, Franzen A, Heinegard D. The primary structure of a cell-binding bone sialoprotein. *J Biol Chem* 1988;263:19430–2.

57. Fisher LW, McBride OW, Termine JD, Young MF. Human bone sialoprotein: deduced protein sequence and chromosomal localization. *J Biol Chem* 1990;265:2347–51.

58. Ecarot-Charrier B, Bouchard F, Delloye C. Bone sialoprotein II synthesized by cultured osteoblasts contains tyrosine sulfate. *J Biol Chem* 1989;264:20049–53.

59. Midura RJ, McQuillan DJ, Benham KJ, Fisher LW, Hascall VC. A rat osteogenic cell line (UMR 106-01) synthesizes a highly sulfated form of bone sialoprotein. *J Biol Chem* 1990;265:5285–91.

60. Gorski JF, Shimizu K. Isolation of a new phosphorylated glycoprotein from mineralized phase of bone that exhibits limited homology to adhesive protein osteopontin. *J Biol Chem* 1988;263:15938–45.

61. Gorski JP, Griffin D, Dudley G, et al. Bone acidic glycoprotein-75 is a major synthetic product of osteoblastic cells and localized as 75-and/or 50-kDa forms in mineralized phases of bone and growth plate and in serum. *J Biol Chem* 1990;265:14956–63.

62. Otawara Y, Price PA. Developmental appearance of matrix Gla protein during calcification in the rat. *J Biol Chem* 1986;261:10828–32.

63. Price PA. Osteocalcin. In: Peck WA, ed. *Bone and mineral research.* Princeton: Excerpta Medica, 1983;157–90.

64. Price PA, Baukol SA. 1,25-dihydroxyvitamin D$_3$ increases synthesis of the vitamin K-dependent bone protein by osteocarcoma cells. *J Biol Chem* 1980;255:11660–3.

65. Demay MD, Roth DA, Kronenberg HM. Regions of the rat osteocalcin gene which mediate the effect of 1,25-dihydroxyvitamin D$_3$ on gene transcription. *J Biol Chem* 1989;264:2279–82.

66. Kasai R, Avioli LV, Noguchi A, Bianco P, Gehron Robey P, Kahn AJ. Distribution and regulation of an anti-proBGP cross-reacting protein in human serum, osteosarcoma and normal cells and fetal bone. *J Bone Miner Res* 1989;4(Suppl):S247.

67. Lian JB, Tassinari M, Glowacki J. Resorption of implanted bone prepared from normal and warfarin-treated rats. *J Clin Invest* 1984;73:1223.

68. Malone JD, Teitelbaum SL, Griffin GL, Senior RM, Kahn AJ. Recruitment of osteoblast precursors by purified bone matrix constituents. *J Cell Biol* 1982;92:227–30.

69. Hauschka PV, Mavrakos AE, Iafrati MD, Doleman SE, Klagsbrun M. Growth factors in bone matrix. *J Biol Chem* 1986;261:12665–74.

70. Canalis E, McCarthy T, Centrella M. Isolation of growth factors from adult bovine bone. *Calcif Tissue Int* 1988;43:346–51.

71. Celeste AJ, Iannazzi JA, Taylor RC, et al. Identification of transforming growth factor-β family members present in bone-inductive protein purified from bovine bone. *Proc Natl Acad Sci USA* 1990;87:9843–7.

72. deBernard B, Bianco P, Bonnuci E, et al. Biochemical and immunohistochemical evidence that in cartilage an alkaline phosphatase is a calcium-binding glycoprotein. *J Cell Biol* 1986;103:1615–23.

73. Delmas PD, Tracy RP, Riggs BL, Mann KG. Identification of the noncollagenous proteins of bovine bone by two-dimensional gel electrophoresis. *Calcif Tissue Int* 1984;36:308–16.

74. Malone JD, Richards M. α$_2$-HS glycoprotein is chemotactic for mononuclear phagocytes. *J Cell Physiol* 1987;132:118.

75. Dziegielewska KM, Brown WM, Casey S-J, et al. The complete cDNA and amino acid sequence of bovine fetuin: its homology with α$_2$-HS glycoprotein and relation to other members of the cystatin superfamily. *J Biol Chem* 1990;265:4354.

76. Mann S. Mineralization in biological systems. *Structure Bond* 1983;54:126–74.

77. Anderson HC. Biology of disease: mechanism of mineral formation in bone. *Lab Invest* 1989;60:320–30.

78. Traub W, Jodaikin A, Weiner S. Diffraction studies of enamel protein-mineral structural relations. In: Butler WT, ed. *The chemistry and biology of mineralized tissues.* Birmingham, AL: EBSCO Media, 1985;221.

79. Addadi L, Weiner S. Interactions between acidic proteins and crystals: stereochemical requirements in biomineralization. *Proc Natl Acad Sci USA* 1985;82:4110.

80. Fisher LW, Termine JD. Noncollagenous proteins influencing the local mechanisms of calcification. *Clin Orthop* 1985;200:362.

81. Chu ML, deWet W, Bernard M, Ramirez F. Fine structural analysis of the human proα$_1$(I) collagen gene. *J Biol Chem* 1985;260:2315–20.

82. Lichtler A, Stover ML, Angilly J. Isolation and characterization of the rat α$_1$(I) collagen promoter: regulation by 1,25-dihydroxy-vitamin D$_3$. *J Biol Chem* 1989;264:3072–7.

83. Schmidt A, Rossi P, de Crombrugghe B. Transcriptional control of the mouse α$_2$(I) collagen gene. *Mol Cell Biol* 1986;6:347–54.

84. Vogeli G, Ohkubo H, Sobel ME, Yamada Y, Pastan I, deCrombrugghe B. Structure of the promoter for chicken α$_2$ type I collagen gene. *Proc Natl Acad Sci USA* 1981;78:5534–5540.

85. Dean DC, Bolus CL, Bourgeois S. Cloning and analysis of the promoter region of the human fibronectin gene. *Proc Natl Acad Sci USA* 1987;84:1876–80.

86. Donoviel DB, Framson P, Eldridge CF, Cooke M, Kobayashi S, Bornstein P. Structural analysis and expression of the human thrombospondin gene promoter. *J Biol Chem* 1988;263:18590–3.

87. Fisher LW, Heegaard A-M, Vetter U, et al. Human biglycan gene: putative promoter, intron-exon junctions, and chromosomal localization. *J. Biol. Chem.,* in press.

88. Weiss MP, Kunal R, Henthorn PS, Lamb B, Kadesch T, Harris H. Structure of the human liver/bone/kidney alkaline phosphatase gene. *J Biol Chem* 1988;263:12002.

89. Zernik J, Thiede MA, Twarog K, et al. Cloning and analysis of the 5′ region of the rat bone/liver/kidney/placenta alkaline phosphatase gene. A dual function promoter. *Matrix* 1990;10:38–47.

90. Cancela L, Hsieh C-L, Francke U, Price PA. Molecular structure, chromosome assignment, and promoter organization of the human matrix gla protein gene. *J Biol Chem* 1990;265:15040–8.

91. McVey JH, Nomura S, Kelly P, Mason IJ, Hogan BLM. Characterization of the mouse SPARC/osteonectin gene. *J Biol Chem* 1988;263:11111–6.

92. Young MF, Findlay DM, Dominguez P, et al. Osteonectin promoter: DNA sequence analysis and S1 endonuclease site, potentially associated with transcriptional control in bone cells. *J Biol Chem* 1989;264:450–6.

93. Nomura S, Hashmi S, McVey JH, Ham J, Parker M, Hogan BLM. Evidence for positive and negative regulatory elements in the 5′-flanking sequence of the mouse (SPARC) osteonectin gene. *J Biol Chem* 1989;264:12201.

94. Celeste AJ, Rosen V, Buecker JL. Isolation of the human gene for bone gla protein. *EMBO J* 1986;5:1885–9.

95. Puchacz E, Lian JB, Stein GS, Wozney J, Huebner K, Croce C. Chromosomal localization of the human osteocalcin gene. *Endocrinology* 1989;124:2648–52.

96. Yoon K, Rutledge SJC, Buenaga RF, Rodan GA. Characterization of the rat osteocalcin gene: stimulation of promoter activity by 1,25-dihydroxyvitamin D$_3$. *Biochemistry* 1988;27:8521–6.

97. Schule R, Umesono K, Mangelsdorf DJ, Bolado J, Pike JW, Evans RM. Jun-fos and receptors for vitamin A and D recognize a common response element in the human osteocalcin gene. *Cell* 1990;61:497–504.

98. Holthius J, Owen TA, van Wijnen A, et al. Tumor cells exhibit deregulation of the cell cycle histone gene promoter factor HiNF-D. *Science* 1990;247:1454–7.

99. Paglia L, Wilczek J, Diaz de Leon L, Martin GR, Horlein D, Muller PK. Inhibition of procollagen cell-free synthesis by amino-terminal extension peptides. *Biochemistry* 1979;18:5030–4.

100. Weistner M, Krieg T, Horlein D, Glanville RW, Fietzek PP, Muller PK. Inhibiting effect of procollagen peptides on collagen biosynthesis in fibroblast cultures. *J Biol Chem* 1979;254:7016–23.

101. Wu CH, Donovan CB, Wu GY. Evidence for pretranslational regulation of regulation of collagen synthesis by procollagen propeptides. *J Biol Chem* 1986;261:10482–4.

102. Canalis E, McCarthy TL, Centrella M. Growth factors and the regulation of bone remodeling. *J Clin Invest* 1988;81:277.

103. Canalis E, Lian JB. Effects of bone associated growth factors on DNA, collagen and osteocalcin synthesis in cultured fetal rat calvarie. *Bone* 1988;9:243–6.

104. Canalis E, McCarthy TL, Centrella M. Growth factors and the skeletal system. *J Endocrinol Invest* 1989;12:577–84.

105. Canalis E, McCarthy TL, Centrella M. The role of growth factors in skeletal remodeling. *Endocrinol Metab Clin North Am* 1989;18:903–18.

106. Pfeilschifter J, Oechsner M, Naumann A, Gronwald RG, Minne HW, Ziegler R. Stimulation of bone matrix apposition in vitro by local growth factors: a comparison between insulin-like growth factor I, platelet-derived growth factor, and transforming growth factor-β. *Endocrinology* 1990;127:69–75.

107. Canalis E. Regulation of bone remodeling. In: Favus MJ, ed. *Primer on the metabolic bone diseases and disorders of mineral metabolism* Richmond, VA: William Byrd Ress, 1990;23–8.

108. Chase LR, Aurbach GD. Parathyroid functions and the renal excretion of 5'-adenylic acid. *Proc Natl Acad Sci USA* 1967;58:418–525.

109. Berridge MJ. Intracellular signalling through inositol trisphosphate and diacylglycerol. *Biol Chem Hoppe-Seyler* 1986;367:447–56.

110. Berridge MJ. Calcium oscillations. *J Biol Chem* 1990;265:9583–6.

111. James R, Bradshaw RA. Polypeptide growth factors. *Ann Rev Biochem* 1984;53:259.

112. Abraham JA, Whang JL, Tumolo A, et al. Human basic fibroblast growth factor: nucleotide sequence and genomic organization. *EMBO J* 1986;5:2523–8.

113. Schreiber AB, Kenney J, Kowalski WJ, Friesel R, Mehlman T, Maciag T. Interaction of endothelial cell growth factor with heparin: characterization by receptor and antibody recognition. *Proc Natl Acad Sci USA* 1985;82:6138.

114. Canalis E, Lorenzo J, Burgess WH, Maciag T. Effects of endothelial cell growth factor on bone remodelling in vitro. *J Clin Invest* 1987;79:52–8.

115. Canalis E, McCarthy T, Centrella M. Effects of basic fibroblast growth factor on bone formation in vitro. *J Clin Invest* 1988;81:1572–7.

116. Frolik CA, Ellis LF, Williams DC. Isolation and characterization of insulin-like growth factor II from human bone. *Biochem Biophys Res Commun* 1988;151:1011–8.

117. Mohan JC, Jennings TA, Linkhart T, Baylink DJ. Primary structure of human skeletal growth factor: homology with human insulin-like growth factor II. *Biochem Biophys Acta* 1988;966:44–5.

118. Canalis E, Centrella M, McCarthy TL. Role of insulin-like growth factor I and II on skeletal remodeling. In: Raizada MK, ed. *Molecular and cellular aspects of insulin and IGFI/II: implications for the central nervous system* New York: Plenum, 1989.

119. MacDonald RG, Pfeffer SR, Coussens L. A single receptor binds both insulin-like growth factor II and mannose-6-phosphate. *Science* 1988;239:1134.

120. Seyedin SM, Thompson AY, Bentz H, et al. CIF-A: apparent identity to TGF-β. *J Biol Chem* 1986;261:5693–5.

121. Seyedin SM, Segarini PR, Rosen DM, Thompson AY, Bentz H, Graycar J. Cartilage-inducing factor-β is a unique protein structurally and functionally related to transforming growth factor-β. *J Biol Chem* 1987;262:1946–9.

122. Centrella M, Massague J, Canalis E. Human platelet-derived transforming growth factor-β stimulates parameters of bone growth in fetal rat calvarie. *Endocrinology* 1986;119:2306–12.

123. Carrington JL, Roberts AB, Flanders KC, Roche NS, Reddi AH. Accumulation, localization, and compartmentation of transforming growth factor-β during endochondral bone development. *J Cell Biol* 1988;107:1969–75.

124. Bortell R, Barone LM, Tassinari MS, Lian JB, Stein GS. Gene expression during endochondral bone development: evidence for coordinate expression of transforming growth factor-β_1 and collagen type I. *J Cell Biochem* 1990;44:81–91.

125. Noda M, Camilliere HJ. In vivo stimulation of bone formation by transforming growth factor-β. *Endocrinology* 1989;124:2991–4.

126. Andres JL, Stanley K, Cheifetz S, Massague J. Membrane-anchored and soluble forms of betaglycan, a polymorphic proteoglycan that binds transforming growth factor-β. *J Cell Biol* 1989;109:3137–45.

127. Canalis E. Effect of platelet-derived growth factor on DNA and protein synthesis in cultured rat calvaria. *Metabolism* 1981;30:970–77.

128. Raisz LG, Martin TJ. Prostaglandins in bone and mineral metabolism. In: Peck WA, ed. *Bone and mineral research annual,* vol 2. Amsterdam: Excerpta Medica, 1984;286.

129. Chyun YS, Raisz LG. Stimulation of bone formation by prostaglandin E₂. *Prostaglandins* 1984;27:97–103.

130. Dewhirst FE, Stashenko PP, Mole JE. Purification and partial sequence of human osteoclast activating factor, identity with interleukin-1. *J Immunol* 1985;135:2562.

131. Canalis E. Interleukin-1 has independent effects on DNA and collagen synthesis in cultures of rat calvariae. *Endocrinology* 1986;118:74–81.

132. Bertolini DR, Nedwin GE, Bringman TS. Simulation of bone resorption and inhibition of bone formation in vitro human tumor necrosis factors. *Nature* 1986;319:516–8.

133. Canalis E. Effects of tumor necrosis factor on bone formation in vitro. *Endocrinology* 1987;121:1596–604.

134. Horowitz MC, Coleman DL, Flood PM. Parathyroid hormone and lipopolysaccharide induce murine osteoblast-like cells to secrete a cytokine indistinguishable from granulocyte-macrophage colony-stimulating factor. *J Clin Invest* 1988;83:149–57.

135. Smith D, Gowen M, Mundy, GR. Inhibitory effects of gamma interferon in the presence of other cytokines on collagen and non-collagen protein synthesis in fetal rat calvaria. *Endocrinology* 1986;120:2494–9.

136. Rouleau F, Mitchell J, Goltzman D. In vivo distribution of parathyroid hormone receptors in bone: evidence that a predominant osseous target cell is not the mature osteoblast. *Endocrinology* 1988;123:187–91.

137. McCarthy TL, Centrella M, Canalis E. Parathyroid hormone enhances the transcript and polypeptide levels of insulin-like growth factor I in osteoblast-enriched cultures from fetal rat bone. *Endocrinology* 1989;124:1247–53.

138. Kream BE, Petersen DN, Raisz LG. Parathyroid hormone blocks the stimulatory effect of insulin-like growth factor-I on collagen synthesis in cultured 21-day fetal rat calvariae. *Bone* 1990;11:411–5.

139. Pfeilschifter J, Mundy GR. Modulation of type β transforming growth factor activity in bone cultures of osteotropic hormones. *Proc Natl Acad Sci USA* 1987;84:2024–7.

140. Civitelli R, Kim YS, Gunsten SL, et al. Nongenomic activation of the calcium message system by vitamin D metabolites in osteoblast-like cells. *Endocrinology* 1990;127:2253–62.

141. Raisz LG, Kream BE, Smith MD, Simmons HA. Comparison of the effects of vitamin D metabolites on collagen synthesis and resorption of fetal rat bone in organ culture. *Calcif Tissue Int* 1980;32:135–8.

142. Bringhurst FR, Potts JT Jr. Effects of vitamin D metabolites and analogs of bone collagen synthesis in vitro. *Calcif Tissue Int* 1982;34:103–10.

143. Eriksen EF, Colvard DS, Berg NJ, et al. Evidence of estrogen receptors in normal human osteoblast-like cells. *Science* 1988;241:84–6.

144. Komm RS, Terpening CM, Benz DJ, et al. Estrogen binding, receptor mRNA, and biologic response in osteoblast-like osteosarcoma cells. *Science* 1988;241:81–4.

145. Turner RT, Colvard DS, Spelsberg TC. Estrogen inhibition of periosteal bone formation in rat long bones: down-regulation of gene expression for bone matrix proteins. *Endocrinology* 1990;127:1346–51.

146. Takano-Yamamoto T, Rodan GA. Direct effects of 17β-estradiol

on trabecular bone in ovariectomized rats. *Proc Natl Acad Sci USA* 1990;87:2172–6.

147. Craig RG, Rowe DW, Petersen DN, Kream BE. Insulin increases the steady state level of $\alpha_1(I)$ procollagen mRNA in the osteoblast-rich segment of fetal rat calvaria. *Endocrinology* 1989; 125:1430–7.

148. Canalis E, McCarthy TL, Centrella M. A bone-derived growth factor isolated from rat calvariae is beta$_2$ microglobulin. *Endocrinology* 1987;121:1198–200.

149. Canalis E. Effects of glucocorticoids on type I collagen synthesis, alkaline phosphatase activity, and deoxyribonucleic acid content in cultured rat calvarie. *Endocrinology* 1983;112:931–9.

150. Mellanby E. Vitamin A and bone growth: reversibility of vitamin A deficiency changes. *J Physiol (Lond)* 1947;105:382.

151. Martin TJ, Ng KW, Suda T. Bone cell physiology. *Endocrinol Metab Clin North Am* 1989;18:833–58.

152. Martineau-Doize B, Lai WH, Warshawsky H, Bergeron JJM. In vivo demonstration of cell types in bone that harbor epidermal growth factor receptors. *Endocrinology* 1988;123:841–58.

153. Mitchison JM. In: *The biology of the cell cycle,* New York: Cambridge University Press, 1971.

154. Stein GS, Lian JB, Owen TA. Relationship of cell growth to the regulation of tissue-specific gene expression during osteoblast differentiation. *FASEB J* 1990;4:3111–23.

155. Fedarko NS, Bianco P, Vetter U, Gehron Robey P. Human bone cell enzyme expression and cellular heterogeneity: correlation of alkaline phosphatase enzyme activity with cell cycle. *J Cell Physiol* 1990;144:115–21.

156. Delmas PD. Biochemical markers of bone turnover for the clinical assessment of metabolic bone disease. *Endocrinol Metab Clin North Am* 1990;19:1–18.

157. Gehron Robey P, Termine JD. Biochemical markers of metabolic bone disease. In: Avioli LV, Krane SM, eds. *Metabolic bone disease.* New York: WB Saunders, 1990.

158. Beardsworth JJ, Eyre DR, Dickson IR. Changes with age in the urinary excretion of lysyl- and hydroxylysyl pyridinoline, two new markers of bone collagen turnover. *J Bone Miner Res* 1990;5:671–7.

Disorders of Bone and Mineral Metabolism,
edited by Fredric L. Coe and Murray J. Favus,
1992 by Raven Press, Ltd.

CHAPTER 12

The Nature of the Mineral Component of Bone and the Mechanism of Calcification

Melvin J. Glimcher

The questions pursued in this chapter are: (1) What is the nature of the mineral phase in bone (i.e., the chemical composition and crystal structure of the solid calcium phosphate (CaP) mineral phase in bone), and what changes occur in the mineral phase per se with time and maturation? (2) Where is the mineral phase located ultrastructurally? (3) What, if any, are the structural and chemical relationships between the CaP mineral phase and the individual components of the matrix? (4) Why and how is a solid mineral phase deposited (i.e., the mechanism of calcification and its regulation)?

BIOLOGICAL FUNCTIONS OF THE MINERAL PHASE

The CaP mineral phase in bone performs two major functions, both of which depend to a significant extent on the exact size, shape, chemical composition, and crystal structure of the mineral crystallites. The mineral phase acts on the one hand as an *ion reservoir* and on the other hand as an excellently designed *structural material* that determines in large part the mechanical properties of bone substance, bone tissue, and bone as an organ. The importance of the role of bone mineral as an ion reservoir can be appreciated from the fact that about 99% of the body calcium, about 85% of the body phosphorus, and from 40 to 60% of the total body Na and Mg are associated with the bone crystals, which consequently serve as the major source for the transport of

these ions to and from the extracellular fluids. As a result, the bone crystals play a critical role in maintaining the extracellular fluid concentrations of these ions, which are critical for a variety of physiological functions (e.g., nerve conduction and muscle contraction) and a number of important biochemical reactions, for some of which (e.g., Ca^{2+}) serum concentrations are maintained within a physiologically necessary narrow range.

From a structural standpoint, the impregnation of the otherwise soft, pliable organic matrix of bone tissues by the rocklike CaP crystals of apatite converts the soft organic matrix to a relatively hard, rigid material which now posesses the necessary mechanical properties that permit it to withstand the forces, stresses, and strains imposed on it by the mechanical forces generated by gait, prehension, respiration, and so on. Moreover, this relatively inflexible and rigid material is now able to preserve the shape of the organism as a whole and to protect vital organs such as the brain, spinal cord, lungs, and heart. The mechanical properties of bone as a structural material is clearly highly dependent on both the physical and chemical properties of the mineral phase, its three-dimensional disposition within the bone substance and bone tissue, and on its ultrastructural and molecular relationships to specific structural components of the organic matrix.

Although not a direct function of bone mineral or of bone *tissue,* bone as an *organ* does provide for another important general physiological function: It acts as host to the precursors of the blood cells (marrow). It is precisely because both of the two major biological functions of the bone mineral ultimately depend to a great extent on the precise chemical composition, physical chemical properties, and crystal structure of the mineral phase that so much attention has been directed at elucidating these characteristics. It is important to keep in mind that significant changes in both the chemical composition and structure occur in the mineral phase with time (i.e., the mineral phase changes with time after its initial depo-

M. J. Glimcher: The Laboratory for the Study of Skeletal Disorders and Rehabilitation, The Children's Hospital, Harvard Medical School, 300 Longwood Avenue, Boston, Massachusetts 02115
This chapter appeared previously in L. Alvioli, ed., *Metabolic Bone Disease and Clinically Related Disorders,* New York, Grune & Stratton, 1990. It is reprinted here by permission by Grune & Stratton and Dr. Alvioli.

sition in the tissue). Not only must this fact be kept in mind when attempting to understand the changes in mineral metabolism as a function of the age of the organism, but equally important, one must take this into account when trying to explain the serum and other changes (e.g., 47 Ca uptake and disappearance) observed in normal subjects and patients with metabolic bone diseases. This is especially true in instances in which the rates of bone formation and resorption have been significantly altered, and consequently, the amount and proportion of new bone and old bone (and therefore of young bone and old bone crystals) have also changed markedly. In turn, this significantly alters the population distribution of bone mineral as a function of *bone mineral age* (as opposed to animal age). Unfortunately, such considerations are rarely taken into account in clinical studies and may in part account for some of the discrepancies noted in metabolic studies between predicted serum values and bone turnover values and those actually observed.

THE NATURE OF THE MINERAL PHASE IN BONE AND THE CHANGES THAT OCCUR WITH TIME

The bone mineral has been known by chemical analyses to contain calcium and phosphorus as its principal constitutents for over 150 years and since 1894 to be a calcium phosphate carbonate (1). The first reports of its crystal structure were published by DeJong (2) and Roseberry et al. (3). Both groups of investigators identified the bone mineral as a hydroxyapatite (HA) based on the reflections generated by x-ray diffraction. Unfortunately, progress in identifying in detail the exact chemical composition and specific spatial arrangement of its constituents at any stage of its development (i.e., from its initial deposition to the final mature mineral) has been very slow. Indeed, these parameters are still not known in detail 60 years after the bone mineral was first identified as HA by DeJong (2). The obstacles that have prevented a definite resolution of the problem are many—biological, crystallographic, and technical. (For reviews, see Refs. 4–11.) In the first place, the apatite phase in bone is very poorly crystalline, generating only a few broad peaks which by themselves do not permit one to assign to it a unique crystal structure or composition (i.e., one cannot differentiate by x-ray diffraction and chemical composition between a number of similar apatitic or apatite-like structures). Indeed, a number of what appear to be closely related but distinct chemical and structural CaP compounds give the same apatitic x-ray diffraction pattern. The poor x-ray diffraction pattern generated by the bone mineral has also precluded the detection of small amounts of CaP compounds other than HA that might also be present (i.e., the x-ray diffraction data fail

to distinguish whether such nonapatitic mineral phases are present). Bone mineral is also known by chemical and physical analyses to contain small but significant amounts of extraneous ions such as HPO_4^{2-}, Na, Mg, citrate, carbonate, K, and others, whose positions and configurations are not completely known. The ideal stoichiometry (Ca/P molar ratio of 1.67) is also rarely found in bone, especially in young bone mineral, which usually has a Ca/P ratio of less than 1.67. The bone mineral has also been shown to contain strongly bound or possibly even crystalline water. The latter cannot be a true constituent of HA since it has the structural formula $Ca_{10}(PO_4(OH)_2$. Both the composition of bone mineral and its x-ray diffraction characteristics change with maturation: The mineral phase becomes more crystalline with age and maturation (12) but never approaches the highly crystalline state of naturally occurring, geological HA or synthetic HA made by precipitation and refluxing of CaP in vitro.

Electron micrographs of bone, which have revealed the very small size of the bone crystals [about (15–35 Å) $\times$ (50–100 Å) $\times$ (400–500 Å)] (13,14), help to explain the poor x-ray diffraction pattern generated by the bone mineral. However, other characteristics of bone mineral, such as crystal strain, vacancies, additions to (e.g., carbonate), and adsorption into the lattice of other ions (Na, Mg, etc.), also represent significant differences between bone mineral and crystalline HA and may also contribute to its specific x-ray diffraction characteristics. Most importantly, progressive changes occur in the x-ray diffraction patterns of bone mineral as a function of the age of the tissue, of the animal, and principally of the age of the mineral itself. These x-ray diffraction changes are also accompanied by significant changes in the chemical composition of the mineral phase, namely, an increase in the Ca/P ratio an increase in the content of carbonate, and a decrease in the concentration of HPO_4^{2-} and H_2O (15,16). Recognition that the mineral phase undergoes extensive structural and chemical changes after its initial formation has led investigators to explore the nature of the first solid phase of CaP deposited and the detailed changes that it undergoes during aging and maturation and to search for the reasons why these x-ray and compositional changes occur. It is important to note that there is also no general agreement as to the exact structure and location of all of the carbonate ions even in synthetically prepared carbonate apatites, an indication of the technical and conceptual difficulties of determining the exact crystal structure of this class of CaP compounds.

Biologically, one of the major difficulties that has to be overcome in obtaining bone samples for structural and compositional studies, especially in studying the initial CaP solid phase deposited and the changes that occur in the mineral with time, is the preparation of macroscopic samples that are homogeneous with respect to the age of the bone mineral. This is due to the fact that at any age there is continuous bone formation and resorption. Depending on both the absolute and relative rates of these two processes, a sample of bone will contain different proportions of bone mineral of different ages. Since the chemistry and structure of the bone mineral changes with the age of the bone mineral, sampling techniques need to overcome this difficulty if the nature of the initial mineral phase formed is to be studied as well as the changes that occur in the mineral with time and maturation. Failure to accomplish this and the use of whole bone samples in general result in the data reflecting only the average properties of a *heterogeneous* sample of bone mineral ranging in age from the very youngest to the very oldest crystals.

RECENT THEORIES OF THE NATURE OF THE BONE MINERAL

Amorphous Calcium Phosphate Theory

The first recent, major new concept concerning the nature of the mineral phase in bone was provided in 1966 and in subsequent years by a group of scientists led by Aaron Posner of Cornell Medical School (17–20). In essence, they reasoned that it should be possible to follow both the chemical composition and the x-ray diffraction characteristics of synthetic CaP solid phases as a function of time after their precipitation in vitro. When this was done, they found that the initial solid phase of CaP formed after in vitro precipitation of Ca and P at alkaline pH was not crystalline but rather an *amorphous* calcium phosphate (ACP) (i.e., the solid phase of CaP did not generate a coherent x-ray diffraction pattern), indicating that there was no long-range order of the CaP and other ions in the CaP solid phase.

To explore the possibility that the same sort of kinetic processes and phase changes were occurring in the bone mineral, calculations were carried out comparing the predicted x-ray diffraction intensities of bone mineral based on the CaP contents of the bone specimen used for x-ray diffraction, and the intensities of the x-ray diffraction reflections found experimentally. According to these calculations, it was found that a very significant amount of the CaP solid phase of bone was not contributing to the x-ray diffraction reflections. This was consistent with the conclusion that a significant fraction of the CaP solid phase in bone was in a noncrystalline, nondiffracting, amorphous state (ACP). Further work using bone of various ages and using other techniques, such as infrared spectroscopy (later found to be of doubtful or no value), supported their hypothesis that like the precipitation of CaP in vitro, the initial CaP solid phase deposited in bone is an ACP that gradually transforms with time to poorly crystalline hydroxyapatite (PCHA). Thus they concluded from their experiments that the initial CaP

mineral phase in young, developing bone was ACP, and that with age the amount of ACP decreased and the amount of PCHA increased. The rate of ACP formation was postulated to be greater than the rate at which ACP was converted to PCHA, so that in young bone containing a large proportion of newly formed bone and therefore of newly deposited bone mineral, the *major* CaP solid phase was ACP.

The ACP theory was a very attractive hypothesis: It accounted for the progressive change in chemical composition with age and maturation as the proportions of ACP and PCHA changed. It explained the increasing intensity of the x-ray diffraction intensities with time as more and more of the ACP (which does not generate or contribute to the intensities of the x-ray diffraction reflections at all) was converted to PCHA. The ACP formed in vitro also had a low Ca/P ratio, contained tightly bound or crystalline H_2O, and had other characteristics of newly deposited bone mineral. It is not surprising, therefore, that the ACP theory of the nature of the initial deposits of CaP in bone and the changes that occur in the mineral during maturation received very wide international acceptance for almost 20 years. However, as more and more experimental data were compiled, and other structural and compositional factors taken into account, which like the presence of an ACP phase, would also be expected and were found experimentally to reduce the x-ray diffraction intensity of a poorly crystalline substance such as bone mineral, the calculated proportion of the bone mineral in the form of ACP decreased. Indeed, the ACP content of some samples of very young bone previously calculated to contain 60–70% or more of ACP were now recalculated to be one-half or less of this value. Similarly, the ACP of adult mature bone, earlier calculated to account for at least 35% of the bone mineral, was no longer even detectable within the limits of the methods used. Note that the critical point of the ACP theory is that the initial solid phase of CaP formed in bone is ACP. Consequently, one expects and it was found experimentally by these methods and calculations that the major CaP solid phase in young bone was ACP; indeed, in the very earliest bone mineral deposited in very rapidly turning over young bone, one would predict that the bone mineral would consist entirely or almost entirely of ACP. The finding that *no* ACP was detected in mature bone is not as signficant as it might seem since it is consistent with the ACP theory, that is, by the time this stage of maturity of the bone mineral is reached, the ACP theory might predict that all of the ACP could have reasonably been expected to convert to PCHA.

Problems with the ACP Theory: Alternative Theories

The increasing reservations of the ACP theory expressed by a number of research workers prompted a complete conceptual and experimental reevaluation of the ACP theory. Since the critical point in the ACP theory is the prediction that ACP is by far the major and in the beginning the only CaP solid phase in very young bone mineral, it was necessary to prepare homogeneous bone samples containing only the very youngest and most homogeneous (with respect to age) bone crystals, as well as a series of bone samples containing homogeneous (age) mineral phase of increasing age and maturation.

Another point to emphasize here is that the age of the mineral and the age of the animal are not synonymous, since in bone of any age both new bone formation and bone resorption are occurring simultaneously. Whole bone samples will therefore contain bone mineral of very widely different age, and data from such samples will represent values based on the average age of the bone mineral in the particular samples. In many instances, bone from widely different aged animals will provide widely varying proportions of the very youngest and very oldest bone crystals, in which case the *average* age of the mineral phase varies considerably. Data from such widely different aged animals before and after long bone growth has ceased and bone turnover has decreased will provide qualitative differences in the age of the bone mineral per se. However, except for the very youngest embryonic bone, such samples cannot provide samples of bone mineral that are relatively homogeneous with respect to the age of the bone mineral, and clearly cannot provide the narrow homogeneous (with respect to age) samples of the very early and youngest CaP solid phase deposited.

Bone containing relatively homogeneous samples of very young bone mineral were obtained first by using very young embryonic chick bone which was turning over very rapidly so that the age of the bone tissue and consequently of the bone mineral spanned at most 48 h, and second, by fractionating bone powder from such young embryonic bones by density centrifugation. Density centrifugation produced samples of bone of different densities and therefore of different mineral content and consequently of different bone mineral age (Fig. 1) (21). Not only were the ages of the bone mineral in such samples produced by these techniques even more homogeneous with respect to age of the bone mineral than whole bone samples, but since the samples were derived from very young chick embryos (16–17 days) (22) and more recently, 11-day-old embryonic chicks, and because of the very young age and rapid turnover of the embryos and consequently of the *whole* bone mineral in the bone tissue, the low-density samples from such preparations represent the youngest, macroscopic bone mineral samples ever obtained and studied by gross physical chemical means.

As alluded to earlier, the amounts of ACP in various in vitro CaP preparations and in bone mineral were originally determined by the Cornell group using an *indirect* (17–20) method. The exact amount and proportion of ACP was later found to depend on how one assigned precise values to various chemical and structural functions. To avoid this potential pitfall, in the more recent work on embryonic chick bone, the samples were analyzed for the presence of ACP by a *direct* method using a procedure referred to as x-ray radial distribution function analysis (RDF) (22,23). The important and critical findings were that *no* ACP was found in even the very earliest bone mineral, at an age where one would predict on the basis of the previous studies of ACP calculated by the indirect method, that essentially *all* of the solid CaP mineral phase should be in the form of ACP. Indeed, just such studies were carried out on the youngest samples of chick bone and analyzed by the methods described (18,20). As predicted, essentially all of the mineral phase was calculated to exist as an amorphous CaP solid by this indirect method, while direct analysis by RDF revealed

A   B   C

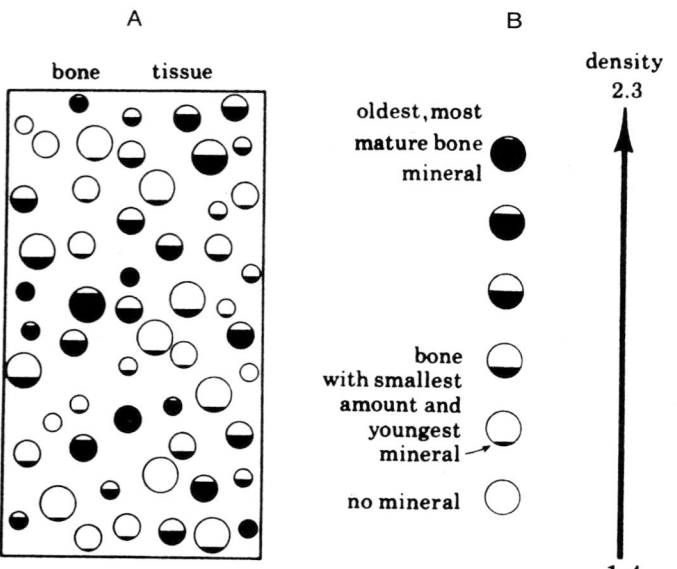

bone tissue

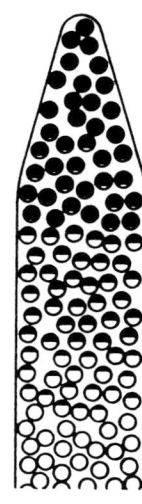

density
2.3

oldest, most
mature bone
mineral

bone
with smallest
amount and
youngest
mineral

no mineral

1.4

FIG. 1. Schema for separating bone powder on the basis of mineral content. The younger mineral phase is in the low-density particles and the oldest mineral phase is in the highest density particles. **A:** Bone tissue is never homogeneous with respect to the age of its mineral particles. **B:** Bone tissue; the amount of bone mineral increases with increasing age and maturation. **C:** To obtain specimens of bone containing mineral particles of different ages, bone is first ground to fine powder and then separated according to its density by centrifugation. (Reproduced with permission from Glimcher MJ: Recent studies of the mineral phase in bone and its possible linkage to the organic matrix by protein-bound phosphate bonds. *Philos Trans R Soc Lond [Biol Sci]* 1984; 304:479–508.)

that essentially all of the CaP mineral phase was poorly *crystalline* with no detectible ACP. Since *no* ACP was found in bone mineral of any age, the two major postulates of the ACP theory could not be substantiated experimentally: (1) that the initial CaP solid phase deposited and remaining in bone as the major, solid CaP mineral phase was an ACP, and (2) that this ACP phase gradually transformed to PCHA with time.

Although the failure to detect ACP in the very youngest bone mineral effectively rules out the premises of the original ACP theory, it does not mean that ACP does not occur as the (or one of the) initial solid CaP phase(s) formed. It is conceivable that the rate of the ACP to PCHA transformation is so rapid with respect to the formation of ACP that very little or no ACP ever appears in the tissue. Under these circumstances, ACP would not be a detectable solid-phase constituent of the CaP mineral phase of bone. Such a concept, however, is completely different from the original ACP theory and from the calculations made from the experimental findings using this concept: namely, that ACP is the *major* solid phase constituent of the bone mineral in young developing bone. Indeed, if the ACP theory is projected to the bone mineral in very young chick embryos, it predicts that ACP constitutes about 100% of the bone mineral when indeed *none* can be demonstrated.

Recent studies using ^{31}P NMR have also failed to detect the presence of ACP (24,25). In addition, the ^{31}P NMR studies of both synthetic CaP solid phases and of bone mineral have revealed the presence of noncrystalline HPO_4^{2-} groups in a brushite ($CaHPO_4 \cdot 2H_2O$)-like configuration in addition to apatite. The amount of the noncrystalline brushite decreases with the age of the bone mineral. The ^{31}P NMR spectrum of bone could be almost completely duplicated by computer modification of synthetic samples of apatite containing about 5% CO_3^- and about 5–10% of noncrystalline HPO_4^{2-} in a brushite-like configuration.

Complementary findings were obtained from several other studies. In one comparative study, the crystallinity or crystal index of the bone mineral was studied as a function of age and maturation (12). These data showed that from the beginning, the CaP solid phase is a PCHA, whose crystallinity increases with time. However, even in the oldest bone samples studied, the PCHA, although more crystalline than younger bone mineral, remains poorly crystalline.

^{1}H NMR and Fourier transform infrared spectroscopy studies have not been able to detect any hydroxyl groups in the bone mineral of very young to very old animals. What substitutes for the hydroxyl groups in these vacancies has not been determined (26).

In summary, at present, the bone mineral can be briefly described as follows: The bone mineral appears to be deposited from the beginning as a (very) poorly crystalline type B (carbonate) apatite (not *hydroxy*apatite), containing about 5% CO_3^- and about 5–10% HPO_4^{2-},

the latter in a noncrystalline brushite configuration. With time, the Ca/P increases to values approximating pure apatite (Ca/P = 1.67), and the context of CO_3^- increases while that of HPO_4^{2-} decreases slightly. The crystallinity of the apatite crystals increases but never beyond a poorly crystalline state.

LOCATION OF THE MINERAL PHASE IN BONE

The ultrastructural location of the mineral phase in bone is a very important parameter in determining its

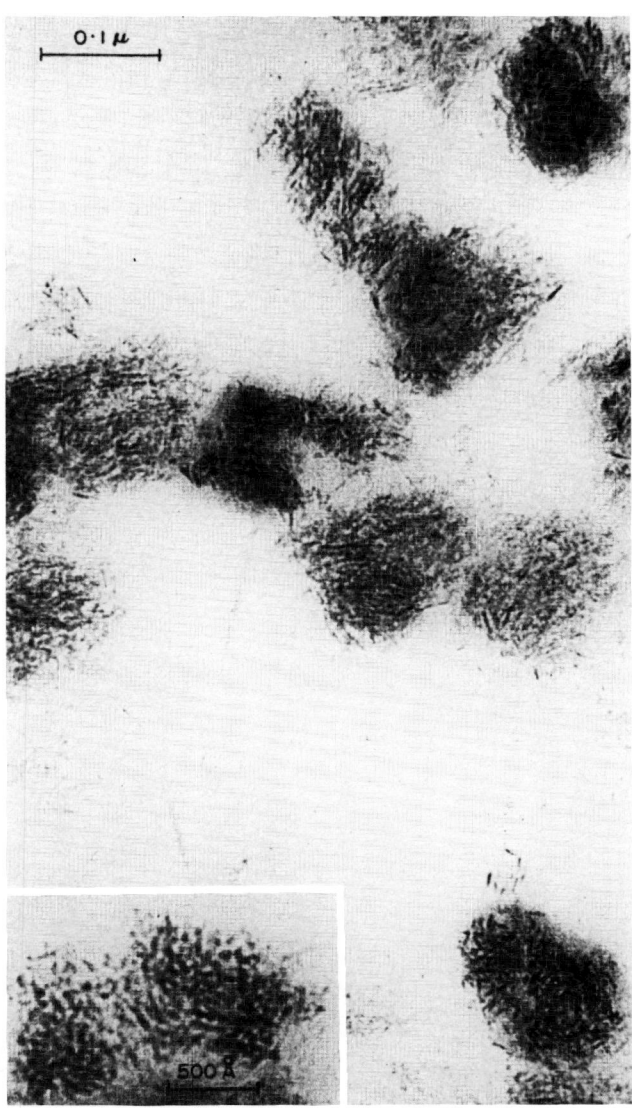

FIG. 2. Unstained fish bone, which was not decalcified. The dense particles, identified by electron diffraction as Ca-P apatite crystals, are located within the collagen fibrils, which are seen primarily in cross-sectional profile. *Insert* shows two adjacent collagen fibrils at higher magnification. Mineral particles are located within the collagen fibrils. (Reproduced with permission from Glimcher MJ: Molecular biology of mineralized tissues with particular reference to bone. *Rev Mod Physics* 1959;31:359–393.)

biological functions: how it functions as an ion reservoir, its effectiveness in changing the mechanical properties of the tissue, and as it turns out, the mechanism of calcification (i.e., how and why the CaP crystals form at all).

Electron micrographs of osteoid and of calcified bone tissue which has been decalcified show that the volume of space between collagen fibrils accounts for at best about 10–15% (or less) of the volume of the extracellular space in most bone, up to 15–20% in certain bone, the remaining volume of the extracellular space being occupied by the collagen fibrils. It is clear from such information alone that the vast majority of the bone mineral must reside within the collagen fibrils; that is, there is nowhere near enough room to house the amount of bone mineral present in the tissue except within the collagen fibrils. This has been confirmed by electron microscopy of undecalcified tissue sections which on cross section show collagen fibrils impregnated with the mineral crystallites (Fig. 2 to 5). In these electron micrographs of the early and late stages of mineralization of fish bone in which tissue the collagen fibrils are widely separated, thus permitting one to clearly observe the collagen fibrils and the extracellular space between them, the mineral phase is observed to be located almost entirely within the collagen fibrils, with the extracellular spaces between the collagen fibrils free of the mineral crystals. In some instances, at the very last stages of calcification, some mineral may be observed outside the collagen fibrils. A similar situation exists in chick bone and other species.

The CaP crystals are not randomly distributed within the collagen fibrils. Electron micrographs, especially of the early stages of mineralization, have shown that the CaP crystals are first deposited within the hole zone region of the fibrils, essentially "staining" the fibrils and imparting about a 700 Å axial period to the fibrils (Figs. 6 and 7). Later, as more and more mineral is deposited within the collagen fibril, the 700-Å axial periodicity of the mineral phase is gradually lost, presumably due to the fact that with increasing calcification, the crystals are also being deposited in the pores of the fibril.

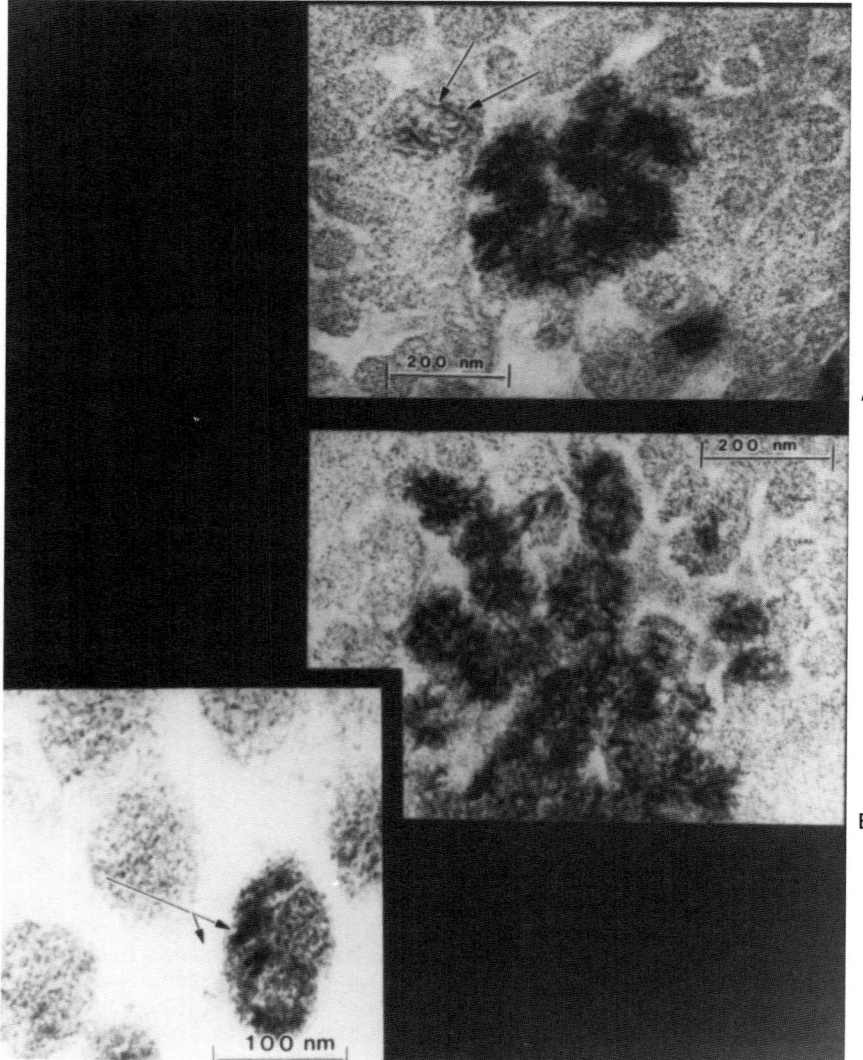

FIG. 3. Successive stages of mineral deposition in herring bone tissue. Thick (1 μm) cross sections of collagen fibrils were prepared using anhydrous technique of specimen preparation. **A:** The first electron-dense deposits (*arrows*) occur within the boundary of the collagen fibril. **B** and **C:** As mineralization progresses further, no mineral particles have been deposited in the extrafibrillar spaces between the fibrils. The deposition of mineral particles in the adjacent collagen fibrils demonstrates that the nucleation of Ca-P crystals in each of the fibrils is an independent physical chemical event. (Reproduced with permission from DD Lee, unpublished).

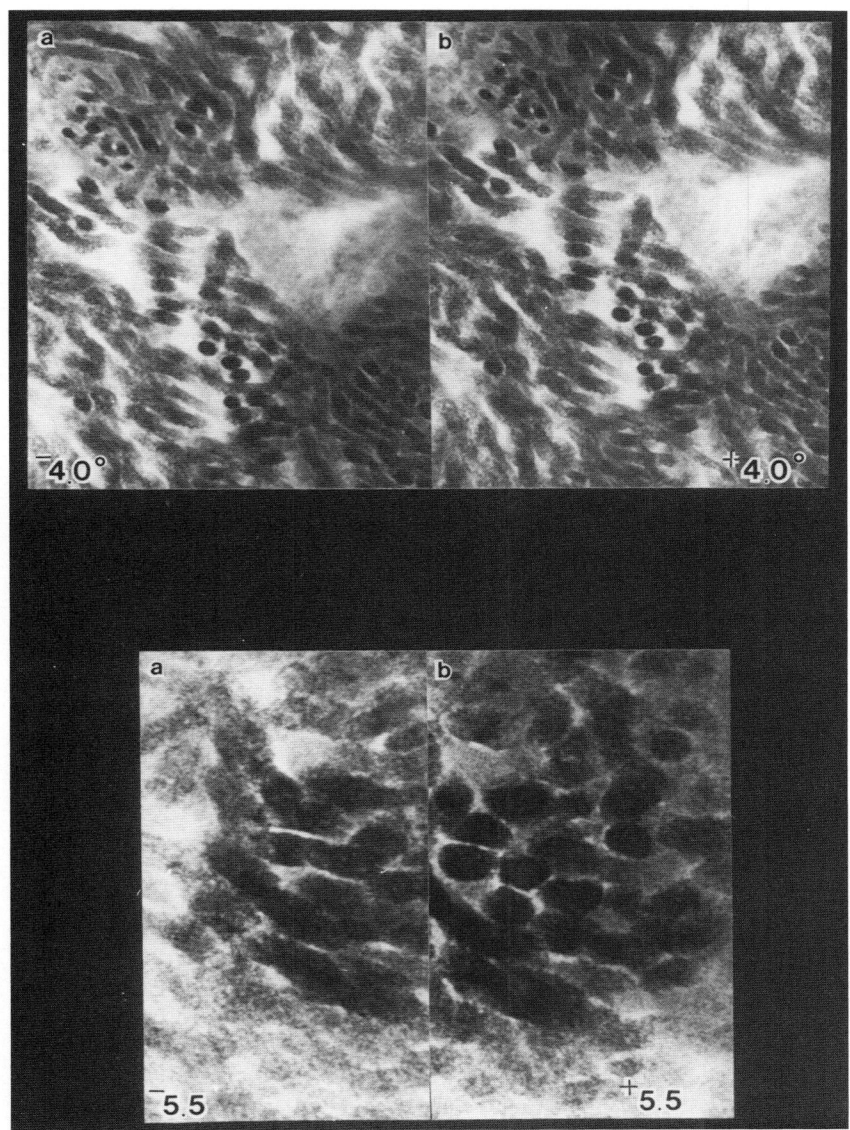

FIG. 4. A pickerel fish bone prepared anhydrously seen in cross-sectional profile (*top*). A higher magnification of the same region (*bottom*) illustrating the electron-dense Ca-P particles located within collagen fibrils. Three-dimensional localization of these mineral crystallites can be fully appreciated by stereoscopic examination, eliminating the possibility that these minerals are located on the surface of the section. (Reproduced with permission from DD Lee, unpublished).

Electron microscopy and electron diffraction of the mineral phase from the beginning of collagen calcification show that the long axis (crystalline *c*-axis) of the crystals within a single fibril are relatively parallel to one another and to the long axis of the fibril in which they are located. The localization of the earliest deposited crystals to the hole zone regions of the collagen fibrils by electron microscopy (Fig. 6 and 7) (27,28) has been confirmed by the elegant low-angle neutron and x-ray diffraction study of intact calcified turkey tendon tissue (29,30) and by reconstruction of the location of the mineral phase in collagen fibrils by optical transforms of low-angle x-ray diffraction data (31).

Another electron microscopic observation of the early stages of calcification which is very important in eventu-

ally formulating a hypothesis of the mechanism of calcification is that the CaP crystals are initiated at sites distinct from one another with unmineralized regions separating the mineralization sites, not only in adjacent fibrils but even within a single collagen fibril. This makes it clear that the eventual deposition of the crystals within the entire length of a single collagen fibril or of groups of fibrils does not occur by a propagation from one site, but rather that there are *independent nucleation sites* along the length of individual fibrils where mineralization is initiated (i.e., in the hole zone regions of the fibrils). This is not to say that secondary crystal formation does not occur locally and extend locally in the hole spaces and to the pores from the initial sites where the CaP crystals are first initiated, only that each of the spaces corresponding

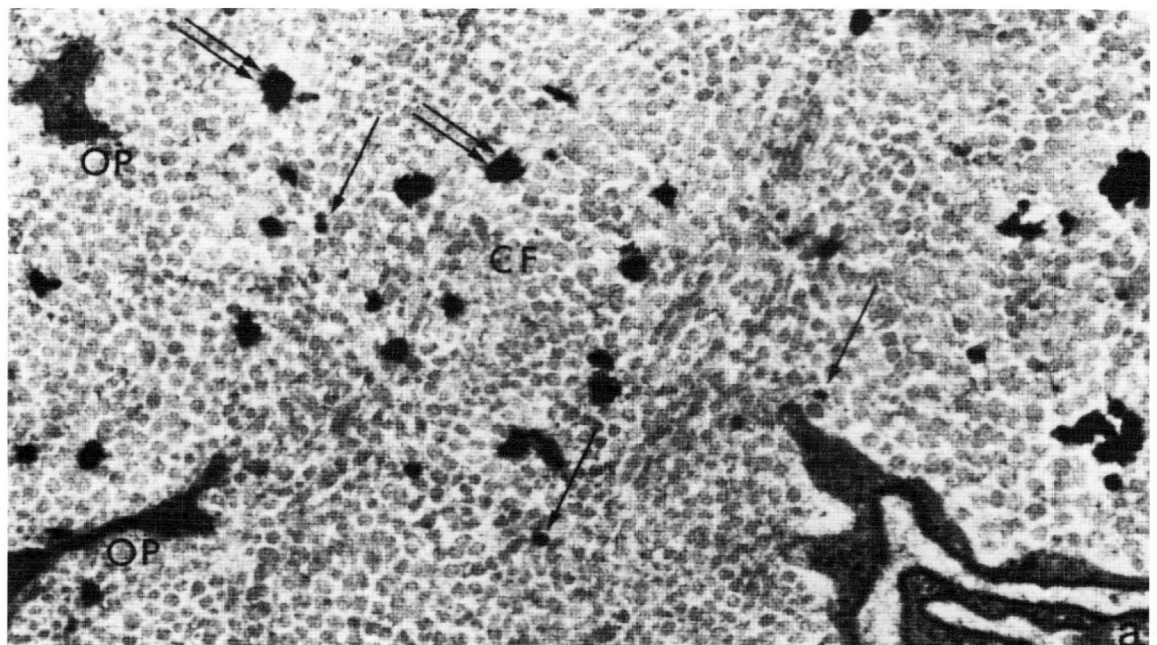

FIG. 5. Early stages of calcification of embryonic chick bone. Collagen fibrils are seen in cross section. Note mineral-free collagen fibrils (C.F.) and fibrils in varying stages of mineralization impregnated with a solid phase of calcium phosphate. The spaces between the fibrils are free of mineral particles. The calcification of each of the fibrils and of the separate sites along the axial length of a single fibril is a physical chemical independent event. Two osteoblast processes (O.P.) are indicated. (Reproduced with permission from Landis WJ, Paine MC, Glimcher MJ: Electron microscopic observations of bone tissue prepared anhydrously in organic solvents. *J Ultrastruct Res* 1977;59:1–30.)

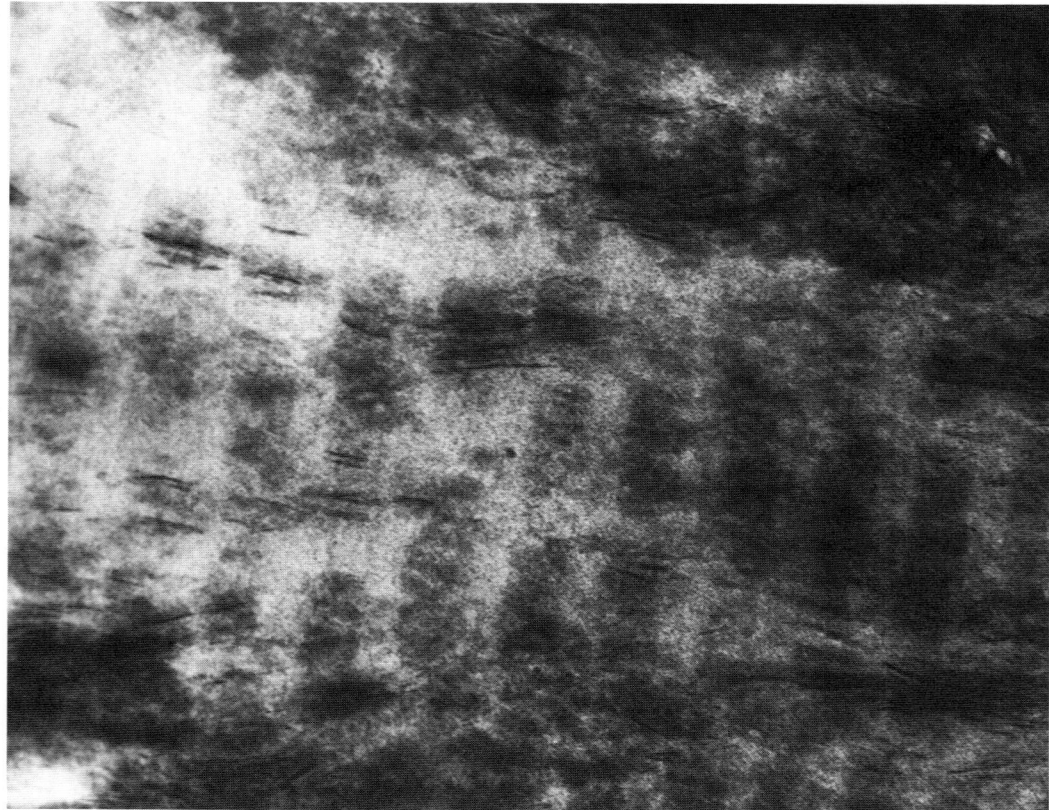

FIG. 6. Electron micrograph of an unstained, longitudinal section of undecalcified embryonic chick bone. The dense mineral phase appears to "stain" the collagen fibril at regular intervals along its axial length. In some areas, the inorganic crystals can be seen on edge as dark lines. Most of the mineral phase is not resolvable into individual crystals.

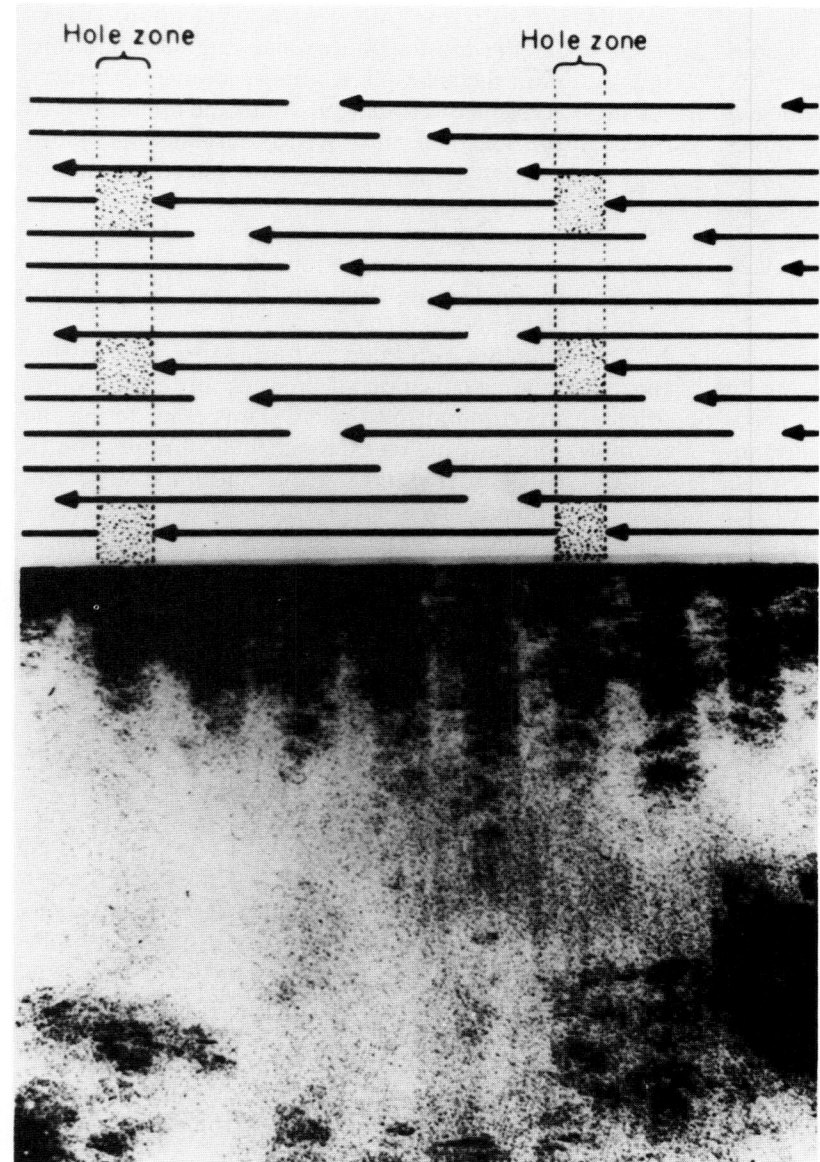

FIG. 7. The identification of the location of the mineral phase in bone collagen between the a^3 and c^3 bands places the crystals in the hole zone. (Reproduced with permission from Glimcher MJ, Krane SM: The organization and structure of bone, and the mechanism of calcification, in Ramachandran GN, Gould BS (eds): *Treatise on Collagen.* New York, Academic Press, Inc. 1968, vol 7B, pp 68–251.)

to the hole zone regions has the potential of being an independent site where the heterogeneous nucleation of crystals can begin.

CURRENT THOUGHTS ABOUT THE MECHANISM OF CALCIFICATION

Regardless of the tissue involved (bone, dentin, enamel, cartilage, etc.) and indeed of the organism involved and the nature of the mineral phase (CaP, $CaCO_3$, $SrSO_4$, etc.), physical chemical principles dictate that the formation of a solid phase from a solution phase represents a *phase transformation* (in this case solution → solid) and is not, as it was once thought to be, a chemical reaction. Biological mineralization, the forma-

tion of an inorganic solid phase in biological tissues, regardless of the nature of the mineral phase, must therefore be governed by the laws of thermodynamics concerned with the stability of phases and with the kinetics of such phase changes. The simplest example illustrating what a phase change is and how it is distinguished from a chemical reaction is the freezing of H_2O: $H_2O_{(l)} \rightarrow H_2O_{(s)}$ (5,10,13).

No chemical reaction is occurring; there are no chemical reaction products, and so on. The H_2O molecules simply change their *state of aggregation* from water in a liquid state $[H_2O_{(l)}]$ to H_2O molecules in a solid (ice) state $[H_2O_{(s)}]$. To accomplish this phase transformation, the water molecules must interact to form aggregates ("embryos") until they reach a critical size after which an increase in size is accompanied by a decrease in free energy and continued growth of the aggregates until a solid state is reached (13,32). If this is accomplished by gradually lowering the temperature in the absence of any external particles, there occurs the formation of a sufficient number of critically sized aggregates of H$_2$O liquid molecules called *embryos,* which grow by the addition of more H$_2$O$_{(l)}$ molecules to form critically sized embryos called nuclei, which then grow with a decrease in free energy to form the first particles of the new phase (ice). This process is called *homogeneous nucleation.* If one carries out the experiment with AgI (or CuI) added to the water before cooling, the process differs from homogeneous nucleation in several very important respects. In the first place the extent to which the temperature needs to be dropped before the crystals are formed is substantially less when AgI (or CuI) is present: to about −39°C without AgI and to only about −4–5°C with AgI or CuI present from the start. Second, without AgI the ice crystals form in one mass throughout the entire vessel. With AgI present, the ice crystals begin to form on the surface of the AgI (or CuI) crystals. The lattice parameters, especially of the basal planes of AgI (and CuI), closely match those of ice. This complementarity of crystal lattice structure between ice and AgI allows the AgI to initiate the phase change from water to ice at a higher temperature (more easily) than occurs in the absence of particles. This process of initiating a phase change by and on an outside agent or substance is called *heterogeneous nucleation* and the substance (AgI) that initiates the heterogeneous nucleation is termed a (heterogeneous) nucleator, nucleation agent, nucleation substrate, and so on. For a nucleator to initiate heterogeneous nucleation, for example, of a solid phase from a solution phase, the solution phase must be in *metastable equilibrium* with respect to the components in solution which will ultimately make up the solid phase. (See also Ch. 29 for a discussion of phase changes and their thermodynamics.)

In conceptual thermodynamic terms, a fluid or any other phase may be stable with regard to adjacent states that differ infinitesimally in their intensive properties from the given state but unstable in regard to states that differ finitesimally from the given state in their intensive properties. Such a fluid is stable with respect to *continuous* changes in state but *unstable* with respect to *discontinuous* changes in state. This is called a *metastable state* (as opposed to a stable state or an unstable state), and a fluid in such a state would be in *metastable equilibrium.* A *metastable solution* therefore refers to a state in which the solution phase is stable for an infinitely long time but still has the potential to form a solid phase under the right conditions, for example, by the intervention of a nucleation agent. In vitro nucleation experiments with a variety of solid salts and inorganic crystals have demonstrated that even under the most careful conditions and despite every effort to remove all solid particles that might act as heterogeneous nucleators, it is virtually impossible to obtain true homogeneous nucleation. That is, even under the most stringent and careful conditions, nucleation of the solid phase almost always takes place by the heterogeneous route and not by the homogeneous mechanism. The nucleation agents (dust and other particles, surface defects in the vessels, etc.) need not be and in almost all cases are not highly specific or effective catalysts—nevertheless, they are sufficiently effective to induce heterogeneous nucleation before it occurs by homogeneous nucleation. (See also Chapter 35 for discussion of nucleation.)

These data are important in formulating any mechanism for the calcification of bone or any of the other biologically mineralized tissues. Thus considering the complexity of any biological tissue that contains a multitude of highly ordered intra- and extracellular structures and components any or all of which can act as heterogeneous nucleators, it would hardly be possible for homogeneous nucleation of a mineral phase to occur in a biological tissue. Instead, any one or a combination of structures or macromolecular components could and would undoubtedly serve as heterogeneous nucleators long before homogeneous nucleation could occur. Indeed, if the phenomenon of calcification follows all other important biological processes, one would expect in most instances that the heterogeneous nucleation agent or substrate would be quite specific, chemically, structurally, and spatially.

Based on the observations that in some tissues and in some organisms, the inorganic crystals are not highly organized but appear to be randomly dispersed with regard to their spatial disposition, and further that in some instances the crystal size and habit are very closely like those observed in in vitro precipitation, a general hypothesis of biological mineralization has been recently proposed (33). Biological mineralization is divided into two general categories: (1) *matrix-mediated mineralization,* by which is meant that certain organic matrix components (principally extracellular) induce and control the deposition of the mineral crystals, their orientation and organization, and their growth and habit; and (2) *biologically induced mineralization,* where the hypothesis appears to imply that unlike matrix-mediated mineralization, the intracellular or extracellular organic (matrix) constituents do not play this role. At first glance, this subdivision of biological mineralization on the descriptive level does have certain attractive features. However, on close inspection, both the semantics and, most important, the biological and physical chemical concepts underlying the thesis and used as an explanation for the differences observed morphologically can be seriously questioned. In the first instance, the separation of the two putative classes of biological mineralization into matrix-mediated and biologically induced on the basis of crystal orientation or the lack of it and the shape and size of the crystals is misleading. This subdivision of biological mineralization on the descriptive level does have certain attractive features. Clearly, if one examines many different mineralized biological tissues, one is struck with the marked difference in how the crystals are organized: highly organized tissue in which the crystals are almost completely parallel with one another in an almost perfect two-dimensional array, while in others the crystals appear to be essentially randomly oriented over macroscopic areas. However, on close inspection, both the semantics and, most important, the physical chemical concepts underlying the thesis used as an explanation for the differences observed morphologically and the biological implications can be questioned seriously.

We believe that *all* biological mineralization is *biologically induced* (i.e., crystal nucleation by organic constituents in the tissue). Only the organic constituents that act as mediators or heterogeneous nucleators vary from tissue to tissue both intra- and extracellularly. As noted earlier, it would hardly be possible for homogeneous nucleation of a mineral phase to occur in a biological tissue. Thus the critical and basic underlying physical chemical mechanism of mineralization in both the classes (biologically induced and matrix-mediated) is the same. There is no physical chemical basis for separating the mineralized tissues on the basis of whether the crystals are oriented or not, with the implication that this reflects some underlying difference in how and why the crystals are nucleated. The same is true for size and shape (habit) of the crystals.

I think that the separation of the biologically mineralized tissues and the cellular and extracellular components of these tissues into two broad classes based on the organization, orientation, and habit of the crystals is potentially an important one, and that investigations as to the underlying bases for such phenomena are likely to shed light on the mechanism of crystal deposition and their growth and development. However, I do not believe that there is any physical, chemical, biological, or biochemical basis that allows one to use these morphological observations to formulate the basis for the initiation of mineralization. Indeed, failure to distinguish between the phenomena of crystal growth and crystal habit and both from crystal nucleation may seriously confuse a number of issues related to the initial and basic underlying mechanism of how and why crystals form at all. The important and critical fact to stress is that in the case of both biologically induced and matrix-mediated calcification, the underlying mechanism of crystallization (i.e., how and why the crystals form at all) is the same: heterogeneous nucleation by a biological substrate or nucleator. To label one group "biologically induced" and the other "matrix-mediated" based on crystal orientation or habit (size and shape) is to obscure this most important point and to confuse factors that may control the subsequent growth and orientation of the crystals, which are themselves completely independent from each other, and why the crystals are formed at all.

In the first place, although it is true that the crystals of many mineralized tissues are not oriented or organized parallel to one another over any significant distance, it does not follow that this lack of crystal alignment precludes their having been initiated by heterogeneous nucleation. In general, formation of crystals by a nucleation agent or substrate in no way implies or demands theoretically or experimentally that the forming crystals, and eventually the formed crystals, be oriented or aligned with respect to each other or to the nucleation substrate. Although the two phenomenon (nucleation and oriented overgrowth or epitaxy) overlap in some instances, they are independent processes and heterogeneous nucleation can occur with or without oriented overgrowth (epitaxy) of the crystals. Indeed, in some cases, relatively poor nucleation substrates readily produce epitaxial growth (orientation) of the nucleated crystals; that is, the nucleated crystals grow with an absolutely perfect alignment along selected planes of the heterogeneous substrate with perfect coorientation of certain planes of the forming crystals and the nucleation substrate (epitaxy). Moreover in the tissues in question, since the exact three-dimensional architecture of the intra- or extracellular matrix and each of its components and therefore of the potential nucleation sites of the components are not known, it is possible that the nucleation sites are themselves relatively randomly organized with respect to the three-dimensional morphology of the tissue or tissue component. In such cases, even if oriented overgrowth (epitaxy) did occur after heterogeneous nucleation, one would still observe a relatively random organization of the inorganic crystals.

Knowledge of the orientation of the exact molecular or macromolecular component of the organic matrix involved and of the presumptive nucleation sites is critical in trying to assess the role of organic matrices on the basis of crystal disposition and orientation. At a somewhat higher morphological level, for example, the collagen fibrils of newly deposited, very young bone in young embryonic animals, which is being rapidly deposited and resorbed, are almost randomly oriented, the extent depending in part on the age and rate of bone synthesis. X-ray diffraction and large field electron diffraction studies show no preferred orientation of the crystals, and routine electron microscopy reveals no distinctive ordering of the crystals over long distances (in relatively large regions) of the tissue. However, careful high-resolution electron microscopy reveals that in local regions where one can visualize only a few collagen fibrils in good longitudinal profile, the crystals are indeed aligned with their long axes (*c* axis) roughly parallel to the individual fibrils within which they are located (13). In summary, orientation of the inorganic crystals appears to be more a matter of the state of aggregation and the orientation and organization of the organic matrix constituents than a reflection of a basic difference in the mechanism by which the crystals are initially formed. Similarly, differences in the size and shape of the inorganic crystals in the various tissues compared with those observed in synthetic crystals made in vitro (which vary tremendously depending on the external conditions under which they are prepared) also appears to be independent of the underlying mechanism that initiates the formation of the inorganic crystals.

Another of the many other possibilities to explain lack of long-range order of the crystals is that there may only be a few nucleation sites within the matrix or intracellular component where crystal formation is initiated by heterogeneous nucleation, the rest and vast majority of the crystals being formed by secondary nucleation from the initial inorganic crystals formed by heterogeneous nucleation. Unless there were physical constraints within the organic matrix or its components which tended to physically direct crystal growth in a specific direction, the majority of the crystals formed by secondary nucleation would be randomly oriented.

Although there are undoubtedly many factors which together control the orientation of the crystals in tissues, one of the most important appears to be the organization of the organic substrate in which the crystals are nucleated and grow. In the case of collagen or the enamel matrix and in certain invertebrate shells, the structural organic matrix molecules are themselves assembled into highly ordered macromolecular aggregates (fibrils, enamel tubules, compartments) which structurally, architecturally, and possibly stereochemically direct the *alignment* and *orientation* of the crystals during their growth (27,34). If such tertiary or quaternary structure is absent, it is clearly possible, in fact probable, that once nucleated by such organic molecules or structures, the crystals would be randomly oriented. Thus the orientation of the crystals in a tissue appears to be more a function of the secondary, tertiary, and possibly quaternary structure of the organic molecules composing the nucleation substrate than any basic difference in the underlying physical chemistry or biology of the basic process of mineralization.

The hypothesis also suggests that the size and shape of the crystals is an indication of whether mineralization is biologically induced or matrix-induced. For example, it is pointed out that in instances of biologically induced calcification, the size and shape of the crystals closely resemble those prepared in vitro, while in matrix-mediated calcification, the size and shape of the crystals is quite different from crystals prepared in vitro. Although this may be true in some instances, it is not true of the major vertebrate calcified tissues. For example, the apatite crystals in bone, dentin, and cementum, which are considered to be initiated by components in their organic matrices (matrix-mediated), are for the most part indistinguishable from those precipitated in the test tube, while those in enamel, which also falls in the class

of matrix-mediated mineralization, contain highly oriented crystals several orders of magnitude greater than those precipitated at 37°C in vitro. In short, there is no general rule that the habit of inorganic crystals formed by clear-cut heterogeneous nucleation via an organic matrix in vivo must differ from the habit of crystals formed by homogeneous nucleation in vitro or in vivo. Moreover, even in vitro, minor changes in the solution phase can markedly alter the habit of crystals formed by either homogeneous or heterogeneous nucleation.

Postulated Role of Collagen in Bone Calcification

Based on the physical chemical principle that calcification of bone is a phase transformation (i.e., that calcium, carbonate and inorganic phosphate, and so on, in solution in the extracellular fluid (ECF) aggregate form a *solid mineral phase* of Ca, inorganic phosphorus (P_2), and carbonate and other ions, and that it is almost certainly initiated by heterogeneous nucleation), and the ultrastructural data, which have revealed a most striking and intimate relationship between the mineral crystals and the highly ordered essentially two-dimensional liquid crystals of collagen fibrils, it is easy to take the next step and hypothesize that the heterogeneous nucleation sites reside in some unique location of the collagen fibril having specific physical, chemical, electrical, steric, and spatial properties (13,28).

Experiments to test this hypothesis have been done both in vitro and in vivo. In vitro, solutions of CaP experimentally demonstrated to be in metastable equilibrium [i.e., stable for at least one month (no crystals formed spontaneously)] were exposed to purified reconstituted soft-tissue collagens and to decalcified bone collagen. Both preparations nucleated apatite crystals within 24–48 h (13,32,34). A variety of other proteins failed to nucleate CaP crystals from the identical solutions. Electron microscopy showed that the initial crystals were formed within the collagen fibrils in a very orderly pattern with an axial period of about 700 Å (i.e., once per collagen period). Later analyses revealed that this location within the collagen fibrils corresponded with the hole zone region similar to what is found in native in vivo calcified bone (27,28). When the collagen molecules were polymerized into fibrils in which the molecules were aggregated differently than they are in the native fibrils of bone, skin, tendon, and so on, these fibrils were not capable of nucleating CaP crystals from the metastable solutions of CaP in vitro. This demonstrated that the ability of collagen fibrils to nucleate CaP crystals in vitro was ultimately dependent on the tertiary structure of collagen; there was something about the specific three-dimensional packing of the collagen molecules in native-type fibrils (about a 700 Å axial period) which resulted in the formation of highly specific chemical, steric, electrochemical, and spatial properties within a particular portion of the fibril (the hole zone region), which together constituted a *heterogeneous nucleation site* for apatite crystals. Further experimental evidence that particular regions within the collagen fibrils act as specific heterogeneous nucleation sites for apatite crystals comes from in vivo experiments in which reconstituted soft-tissue collagen fibrils prepared from the skin of animals, placed back in the peritoneal cavity and subcutaneous regions of the same animals or littermates, were found to calcify in vivo, and in the same manner that they do in vitro and in native bone: the crystals are first deposited within the hole zone regions of the collagen fibrils (35; M. J. Glimcher, J. Barr, and P. Goldhaber, unpublished data).

Several points need to be made, however. The first is that the initiation of calcification of reconstituted soft-tissue collagens both in vitro and especially in vivo is much slower than the recalcification of decalcified bone collagen fibrils in vitro. But even in vitro, the length of time between the exposure of decalcified bone collagen fibrils to a metastable solution of CaP and the nucleation of a CaP solid phase of apatite is longer than one would expect for a very potent nucleation substrate. This raises the possibility that while the collagen fibrils of bone and other mineralized tissues are heterogeneous nucleation substrates and are necessary for the initiation of apatite formation, they may not be biologically sufficient (10).

It will prove useful at this point to distinguish between the chemical nature of the components and other factors (structural, electrochemical, steric, etc.) that define a *nucleation site*, which is the basic mechanism of heterogeneous nucleation and the underlying basis for the initiation of calcification, and those ancillary factors that can control or regulate the nucleation process, subsequent crystal growth, and so on. These would include factors that might facilitate or inhibit nucleation but not be part of the structural nucleation site per se (decreasing or increasing the lag time, for example), either directly by affecting the nucleation site or indirectly by altering the metastability of the extracellular fluids in the immediate vicinity of the nucleation substrate. Failure to make the distinction between the two categories—that is, components which are part of the nucleation site per se which are directly related to the mechanism of nucleation, and those components that regulate and control the rate of nucleation, for example—has caused a certain amount of confusion in the literature. This has been especially true in the assessment of the possible roles of certain tissue components in the nucleation of apatite crystals in certain tissue compartments and in the tissue as a whole, as opposed to their potential function as regulators.

In discussing and exploring some of the factors that may influence the local nucleation of apatite crystals within selected areas of the collagen fibrils, we distinguish between calcification of the *tissue* and calcification of specific intracellular or extracellular compartments and components within the tissue. Tissue calcification includes all of the compartments and components that are calcified (Fig. 8). In addition to collagen fibrils, in which the vast majority of the crystals in bone are located, CaP particles have been observed intracellularly in the mitochondria of osteoblasts (and in the chondroblasts of cartilage), and extracellularly in so-called matrix vesicles, compartments formed by the budding off of portions of the plasma membrane of osteoblasts and chondroblasts.

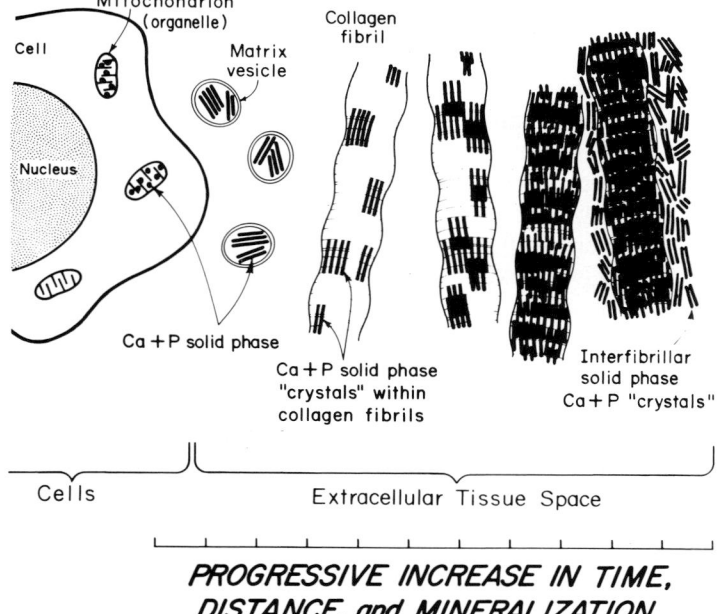

FIG. 8. Diagrammatic representation of bone tissue calcification and of the putative calcification of several of its intra and extracellular compartments and components. The exact and specific physical chemical roles of mitochondria and matrix vesicles in bone tissue calcification have not yet been defined. (Reproduced with permission from Glimcher MJ: Recent studies of the mineral phase in bone and its possible linkage to the organic matrix by protein-bound phosphate bonds. *Philos Trans R Soc Lond* [*Biol Sci*] 1984;304:479–508.)

Lehninger (36), Shapiro et al. (37–40), and Brighton and Hunt (41) have demonstrated that the mitochondria of differentiating cartilage cells in the epiphyseal plate (chondroblasts) as well as the osteoblasts of developing bone (14) contain a significant number of dense granules composed principally of Ca and P_i. Using specific staining for calcium in the mitochondral granules of epiphyseal cartilage cells, it was shown that the number of such granules decreased with increasing maturation of the cartilage cells and with the onset and progression of extracellular calcification. Because the concentration and eventual virtual disappearance of these CaP granules in the mitochondria coincides with the appearance and progressive increase of extracellular calcification in the tissue, investigators (36,41) have suggested that the mitochondrial granules in some way help to initiate calcification of the extracellular matrix. For example, Lehninger (36) has suggested that the solid-phase particles of CaP in the mitochondria of bone and cartilage cells are extruded into and traverse the extracellular space, eventually becoming lodged in the hole zone regions of the collagen fibrils (36). In a similar vein, Anderson (42–44) and Bonucci (45) have described plasma membrane–derived vesicles in the extracellular matrices of both bone and cartilage, many of which appear to contain crystals of HA when observed electromicroscopically (matrix vesicles).

Because calcification of these vesicles appears to occur prior to the calcification of the collagen fibrils, several hypotheses have been presented which postulate that the solid-phase particles or crystals of CaP themselves, which are deposited in the matrix vesicles, *directly* cause the mineralization of the collagen fibrils (42–48). Several different theories have been advanced as to how crystals in one compartment (matrix vesicles) can induce nucleation of new, de novo crystals *in specific locations* of another compartment (collagen fibrils) spatially separated from the first compartment. In one proposal (43,48,49) it is suggested that CaP particles in the matrix vesicles are assumed to pierce the membrane of the matrix vesicles and are extruded in the extracellular space. The extruded crystals then act as nucleation catalysts for the formation of additional crystals of CaP by secondary nucleation and multiplication. The continuous formation of new crystals progressively fills the extracellular tissue spaces between the collagen fibrils with inorganic crystals. When the newly forming crystals reach the collagen fibrils, the crystals enter (and/or form) only within the hole zone regions of the collagen fibrils. Later, continued secondary nucleation and multiplication within the collagen fibrils cause new additional crystals to form within the pore spaces of the collagen as well. In this schema, collagen fibrils are simply a passive repository for the deposition of CaP crystals and subsequent secondary multiplication of CaP crystals, which eventually re-

sults in the almost complete impregnation of the fibrils with a solid mineral phase of CaP. Neither the collagen fibrils nor any of the noncollagenous macromolecules associated with them are considered to play any role in the formation of the crystals of CaP within the fibrils.

Such an explanation seems completely improbable from the standpoints of both physical chemistry and electron microscopic observations. As pointed out, calcification of the collagen fibrils consist of a large number of *independent* nucleation events, at independent nucleation sites, which are independent from each other even within the same fibril, and which therefore must clearly be completely independent of the *direct* influence of crystals deposited in compartments spatially separated from the collagen nucleation sites such as matrix vesicles (50) or mitochondria (38–41).

In the matrix vesicle theory, one would expect to find masses of crystals occupying the space in ECF between the fibrils *before* calcification of the collagen fibrils started. The theory suffers from the fact that the suggested sequence of events does not in any way correspond to what is actually observed during the calcification of bone (or dentin or cementum) by electron microscopy. Indeed, just the opposite is seen. In our extensive studies of embryonic chick bone by nonaqueous as well as aqueous techniques for the preparation of the tissue samples (14,27,51,52) and in countless published and unpublished electron micrographs of others, as well as recent studies of fish bone by high-voltage stereoscopic electron microscopy, we have never observed a stage of calcification in which the extracellular spaces were filled with bone mineral at a time when the collagen fibrils were unmineralized. Indeed, even in the earliest stages of embryonic bone or dentin calcification, at a time when the collagen fibrils are just beginning to mineralize, the most common picture observed is of partially and completely mineralized collagen fibrils separated from one another by *unmineralized* space (see Figs. 2 to 5). At a stage when there are numerous collagen fibrils well mineralized, there is still little or no mineral phase present between the fibrils.

Moreover, the proposal that crystals of CaP, formed randomly by secondary nucleation and multiplication in the extracellular spaces, are somehow able to find their way in the extracellular spaces selectively *only* to the hole zone regions of the collagen fibrils is thoroughly improbable from both the physicochemical and biological standpoints. Instead, if the sequence of events did occur as envisaged by the matrix vesicle theory, it would follow that at the early stages the collagen fibrils would become encrusted in a random fashion by the self-propagating and multiplying mineral-phase particles, which would fill the extracellular tissue spaces. Collagen fibril calcification would then proceed *without* the localization of the crystals to the hole zone regions of the fibrils. This does not correspond to what is actually observed by electron microscopy (27,53) and x-ray and neutron diffraction (29–31).

Electron microscopic studies have shown that matrix vesicles are observed in only the very early stages of embryonic chick bone development. In later stages of embryonic development, matrix vesicles either are not observed at all or are only few in number. These data are consistent with our own observations. Thus the collagen fibrils of all the new bone laid down after this early embryonic bone has been resorbed (50) are calcified in the absence of matrix vesicles (49; W. J. Landis and M. J. Glimcher, unpublished data). Matrix vesicles are therefore *not obligatory* for the calcification of bone tissue. Indeed, if they do play any role in the calcification of bone, their action must be limited to a brief period during the early stages of embryonic development, since bone that is synthesized after this very early stage calcifies in the absence of matrix vesicles.

There are, of course, indirect ways in which calcification in one compartment, such as the mitochondria and matrix vesicle, can influence the formation of solid-phase mineral particles in another spatially distinct compartment: that is, dissolution of the crystals in one compartment (e.g., matrix vesicles or mitochondria), and the pumping out and *specifically* directed transport of the Ca and P ions to and within the second compartment. If sufficient amounts of Ca, P_i are transported, the metastability of the fluid within the second compartment may be increased to the point that a nucleation substrate within the second compartment is capable of initiating the formation of apatite crystals by heterogeneous nucleation more easily. Although this scenario is theoretically possible, it may not be very probable, since there does not appear to be a sufficient amount of mineral in either the mitochondria or matrix vesicles so that when dissolved, the tissue ECF concentration of Ca and P_i will have been raised significantly. Further work and measurements are needed. Another suggestion, offered by Thyberg and Friberg (54), is that the matrix vesicles may function by releasing enzymes that degrade the proteoglycans surrounding the collagen fibrils. The degradation and removal of the proteoglycans, thought by many to be inhibitors of calcification, would then permit the collagen fibrils to initiate calcification (55).

The normal calcification of turkey tendon provides further confirmation that calcification occurs in distinct nucleation sites within the collagen fibrils, each as an *independent* event; that is, the calcification of collagen fibrils does not "spread like a wave" throughout a single fibril from a single nucleation site, but rather by nucleation of crystals at multiple independent spatially separated and distinct sites (hole zone region) within a single fibril and then by secondary nucleation within the pores.

In bone (as with tendon), the initial deposition of the crystals within the holes of the collagen leads to an axial periodicity of the crystals along the long axes of the fibrils identical to that of the collagen itself (13,56). With time and with increasing mineralization, more and more crystals are deposited within the pore space, eventually obliterating the initial axial periodicity of the mineral phase.

The calcifying tendon system also provided additional information. Matrix-bound mineral, presumably in matrix vesicles, was clearly observed. The mineral phase was clearly spatially separated from the sites in the collagen where mineral was initiated. It is clear that in this tissue, the mineral crystals in the putative matrix vesicles do not play a direct role in the initiation of calcification of the collagen fibrils, the crystals in the collagen being formed at a distance from the crystals in the matrix vesicles as events totally independent from the matrix vesicle crystals.

Indeed, there is no evidence that there is even an indirect effect of the mineral crystals of the matrix vesicles on collagen calcification—that there is dissolution of the matrix vesicle crystals with Ca^{2+} and P_i ions pumped out to increase the metastability of the extracellular fluid in the close vicinity of the collagen fibrils. The crystals in the putative vesicles remain in the vesicles during the initiation of collagen calcification. Like the observations in bone, calcification of collagen fibrils in loci separated from one another implies that the initiation of calcification in each of the hole zone regions represents an independent event.

The fact that there is neither a physical chemical basis nor experimental evidence by EM or other techniques that solid-phase particles of CaP in either mitochondria or matrix vesicles *directly* induce calcification of collagen fibrils in no way diminishes the importance of their discovery. The identification of these CaP particles and of the membrane-bound matrix vesicles has opened up an entirely new field of investigation in the mineralized tissues which promises to shed significant information on important biological phenomena in mineralized tissues.

OTHER FACTORS AND COMPONENTS THAT MAY REGULATE CALCIFICATION OF COLLAGEN FIBRILS

As already mentioned, although the specific stereochemistry and spatial organization of the collagen fibrils of bone, dentin, cementum, and so on, result in the formation of nucleation sites within the hole zone regions, these factors, although necessary, may not be sufficient in vivo (10). Even if the conditions in the extracellular fluids are adequate (extent of metastability) for nucleation by the collagen fibrils, there may be other structural and chemical factors intimately related to the collagen fibrils, which, together with the collagen fibrils, constitute the necessary and biologically sufficient conditions for heterogeneous nucleation of CaP crystals. For example, although purified collagen fibrils in dialysis bags (35) or Millipore chambers (M. J. Glimcher, unpublished data) do calcify in vivo when placed in the peritoneum or subcutaneously, calcification does not occur for several weeks compared with the rapid calcification (hours) of collagen fibrils in the osteoid of bone.

There are a number of organic components that have been conceptually postulated to be an integral part of the nucleation site and therefore to be involved directly in the mechanism of nucleation or to regulate collagen calcification and in support of which experimental data have been obtained.

Phosphoproteins

Reasons why organically bound phosphorus (rather than Ca^{2+}) better meets the requirements as the critical ion, which is either an integral part of the nucleation or interacts with the nucleation site in the organic matrix, have been presented in some detail (5,27,34). In brief:

1. Unlike ionic Ca^{2+} bound electrostatically to the organic matrix, the organic phosphate residues would not be randomly oriented but rather, rigidly disposed and sterically organized according to the stereochemistry of the protein(s) with which it was associated. Such organic phosphate groups might therefore be in sterically oriented positions according to the stereochemistry of the protein, and therefore in a three-dimensional array resembling certain planes of the apatite lattice. They would therefore be an integral part of the heterogeneous nucleation site.
2. Although covalently bound to the protein, the organic phosphate groups would still be able to react strongly with free Ca^{2+} in a way that would also permit the bound Ca^{2+} to react further with additional inorganic phosphate ions, thus building up a cluster of Ca and phosphate ions that could function as nuclei of apatite crystals.
3. The phosphorylation of certain amino acid residues in particular locations in the protein would also be possible enzymatically by protein kinases and adenosine triphosphate (ATP), thus assuring exquisite biological control and localization of the process. This precise cellular control and molecular localization of the calcification process makes the potential role of organically bound phosphorus very attractive from both the physical chemical and biological standpoints.

Experimentally, the first step was to determine if phosphoproteins were present in bone and other mineralized tissues. To date, all calcified tissues, both normal and pathological, have been shown to contain phosphoproteins (57–63). All of the phosphoproteins contain O-phosphoserine [Ser(P)]. Bone, cartilage, and cementum contain, in addition, significant amounts of O-phosphothreonine [Thr(P)] (61,64–67). Protein kinases have been isolated from several connective tissues that specifically phosphorylate the Ser(P) residues in vitro using ATP as a source for the phosphoryl groups (27).

Functionally, the phosphoproteins have met a number of the criteria necessary if they are to function to facilitate the nucleation of apatite crystals within the collagen fibrils. For example, the phosphoproteins of dentin strongly bind large amounts of Ca^{2+} (68), and ^{31}P-NMR studies have in addition shown that the Ser(P) residues are able to form ternary complexes with Ca^{2+} and inorganic phosphate ions (69), that is,

$$\text{protein} - \text{O} - \overset{\displaystyle \overset{O}{\diagup}}{\underset{\displaystyle \underset{O}{\diagdown}}{P}} - Ca^{2+} - P_i$$

ternary complex

Similarly, careful calcium-ion-binding studies of dentinal collagen by Katz and Li (70) have clearly shown a significant increase in the number of bound Ca^{2+} ions as a function of the number of phosphoprotein molecules complexed with collagen, and consequently the concentration of Ser(P) in the collagen–phosphoprotein complexes.

Although the physical chemical data demonstrate that the physical chemical properties of the phosphoproteins will permit them to participate in the mineralization of the collagen fibrils, there were at least three important and critical biological questions that had to be answered before any hypothesis could be formulated:

1. Are the phosphoproteins of bone synthesized by bone cells; that is, are they truly bone proteins, or like albumin and others, are they synthesized elsewhere and bound and concentrated in bone?
2. If synthesized by bone cells, by which cells?
3. Where were they located in the tissue? Were they in the region where initiation of mineralization in vivo occurred?

Appropriate answers to all three questions were necessary as minimum requirements if they were even to have the potential for participating in calcification.

Tissue and then cell culture experiments established that the phosphoproteins were synthesized by bone, and in particular by the osteoblasts (71,72). Further, when animals were given ^{33}P (73,74), light and electron microscopy autoradiography showed that the ^{33}P [identified chemically as Ser(P) and Thr(P)] was first located within the osteoblast (and odontoblast in dentin) and then excreted and concentrated at the sites where mineralization was initiated. These findings demonstrating that the phosphoproteins were synthesized in bone and by the appropriate cells and were located in the appropriate place in the tissue (i.e., where mineralization was first occurring) at least met the minimum number of biological requirements necessary for them to even be considered to function as facilitators of the heterogeneous nucleation of apatite crystals by collagen fibrils or to be an integral part of the nucleation site itself.

Analyses of uncalcified and calcifying turkey tendon (before ossification occurs) have shown that there are no detectable phosphoproteins in regions of turkey tendon or in specific turkey tendon "never-to-be-calcified" and put in potentially calcifiable in turkey tendons prior to calcification. However, once mineralization begins, phosphoproteins are detected and increase in concentration as increasing amounts of mineral are deposited (65).

Recent experiments in which the lag time (i.e., time to induce nucleation of a CaP solid phase) was measured during in vitro calcification of bone collagen were consistent with a positive role for the phosphoproteins in facilitating nucleation of apatite crystals by bone collagen fibrils (75). In these experiments, decalcified bone collagen fibrils are placed in metastable CaP solutions and the time it takes to initiate CaP deposition is measured. Collagen preparations complexed with varying amounts of phosphoprotein containing Ser(P) were used. The results clearly demonstrated that there was a very striking correlation of the lag time (time to initiate nucleation) and the amount of phosphoprotein complexed to the collagen as measured by the Ser(P) concentration (Fig. 9).

In summary, while the potential role of the phosphoproteins in facilitating calcification remains a hypothesis and not a proven fact, their theoretical and experimental physical chemical properties and biological characteristics (i.e., the fact that they are synthesized by the osteoblasts in cell culture and in vivo and excreted in vivo at sites in the native tissue where calcification is initiated) and their marked influence in facilitating nucleation by collagen fibrils in vitro are all strong supporting data for their projected role in the initiation of calcification.

Several other components and factors have also been implicated in the initiation or facilitation of mineralization or in its inhibition. Proteolipids and complexed acidic phospholipids (76) have been prepared from a vari-

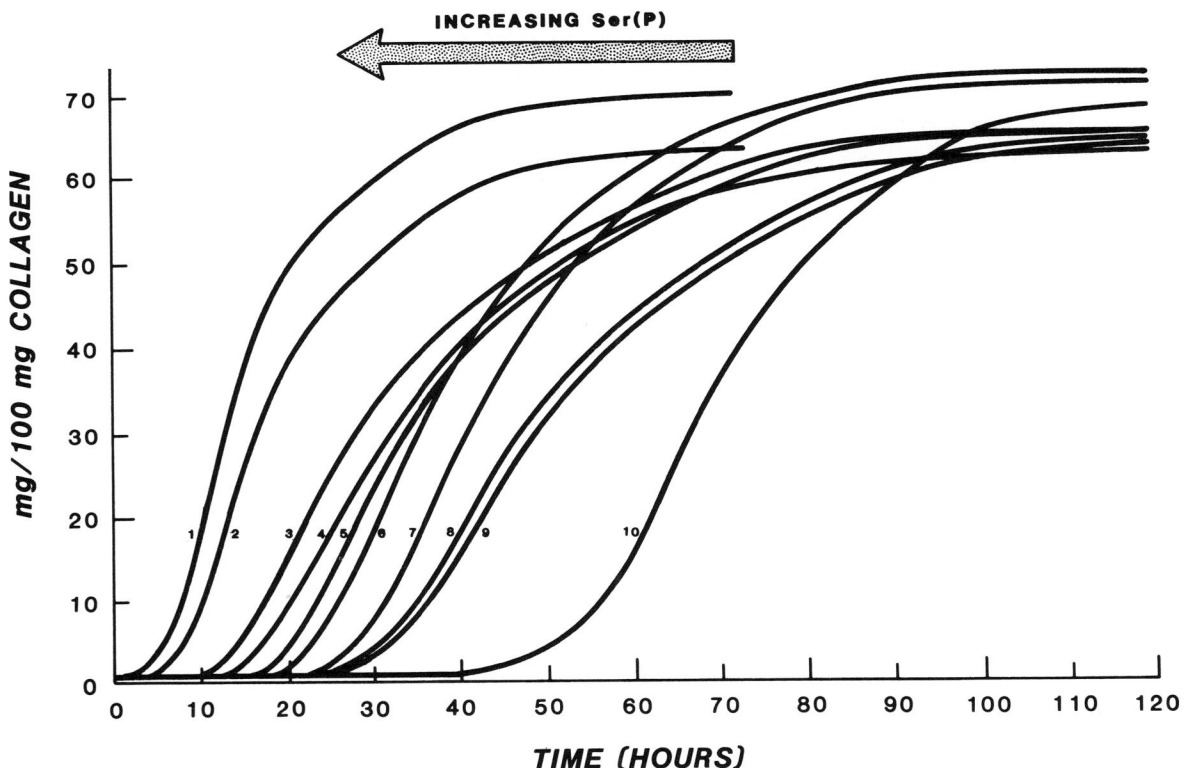

FIG. 9. Lag time in hours of in vitro nucleation of a CaP solid phase from a metastable solution of CaP as a function of the amount of phosphoprotein complexed to collagen as measured by Ser(P) concentrations. Lag time, viz., time for a collagen phosphoprotein complex to initiate mineralization in vitro, decreases with increasing amounts of phosphoprotein complexed to the collagen. (Reproduced with permission from A Endo and MJ Glimcher, unpublished.)

ety of sources and their ability to initiate calcification from metastable solutions of CaP in vitro examined. These lipid components have been found to be very effective heterogeneous nucleators of apatite in vitro (77–79). Although there has been no ultrastructural localization of these lipid components, the most likely source of these components would appear to be cell (plasma) membranes. Therefore, one might expect that they are present in the membranes of the matrix vesicles, which themselves are derived from the plasma membrane. Thus it is possible that they are involved in the calcification of matrix vesicles. Their ability to nucleate apatite crystals in vitro without any additional components suggests that they may be nucleation substrates per se rather than facilitators.

It seems clear that there must also be a number of factors that control calcification of the individual components, and of the tissue as a whole, in a negative sense; that is, they delay or tend to inhibit the deposition of CaP by influencing the rate of nucleation (lag time), number of nucleation sites, or both, diminishing or abolishing secondary nucleation and multiplication, decreasing the metastability of the extracellular fluids bathing the collagen fibrils of bone or, in the case of other tissues, other structural nucleators (50), or all or some combination of these factors. The components that have received most attention conceptually, and which have been most intensely studied experimentally, are the proteoglycans.

The proteoglycans, constituents of all vertebrate mineralized tissues, especially cartilage, are a good example of how important it is, when attempting to postulate whether an organic constituent acts as a nucleation agent, not to rely solely on the point of whether or not the component in question binds Ca^{2+} (5,13,27,34). Among the factors that are equally as important as the Ca^{2+}-binding ability per se are its configuration, whether the component exists in solution or in the solid state, the stereochemistry of the reactive groups, and most important, whether the Ca^{2+} in the reactive groups that form complexes with Ca^{2+} can still react with inorganic phosphate ions. If not, the bound Ca^{2+} will essentially be chelated or clathyrated and, being unable to react with inorganic phosphate ions, be unable to take part in the formation of embryos or nuclei of Ca^{2+} and P_i and thus in nucleation or calcification. Indeed, such components would prevent or inhibit nucleation and other steps in calcification rather than facilitate it. The state of aggregation is particularly important. Aggregates of a macromolecule packed in a very particular way in the solid state might easily form a highly specific three-dimensional steric and electrical array of side-chain groups derived from adjacent macromolecules which would constitute a nucleation site (5,13). The bound Ca^{2+} ions might even be reactive enough to bind P_i ions. However, no further reaction to build up embryos and eventually nuclei occurs because of the lack of the necessary specific three-dimensional steric array of side chains from a significant

number of adjacent closely and specifically packed macromolecules. Thus it is perfectly possible that some components may act to block nucleation when they are in solution, yet facilitate nucleation when in the solid state, and vice versa. Failure to take such factors into account has led to a great deal of confusion in the literature.

The phosphoproteins are examples of such components: When dissolved in a metastable solution of CaP, it essentially delays the onset of spontaneous precipitation (80), whereas bound to collagen fibrils in the solid state, the phosphoprotein (in the solid state) facilitates the nucleation of CaP from solutions of CaP in metastable equilibrium (75).

In the early literature of calcification, the ability of the proteoglycans to bind Ca^{2+} via their carbonyl and sulfate side-chain groups led most investigators to postulate that these components somehow directly initiated formation of the crystals or at least facilitated calcification (see, e.g., Ref. 81–83). Later it was pointed out that this same physical chemical characteristic (Ca^{2+} binding) could serve just as well in making the proteoglycans an inhibitor, that is, by preventing the Ca^{2+} concentration in the extracellular fluid from reaching a level sufficient for heterogeneous nucleation to occur by the collagen fibrils (13,34). The phenomenon was likened to that of tanning skin collagen (34), in which case the process was markedly facilitated when the proteoglycans and other noncollagenous substances were first removed from the skin before tanning was begun (84). The physical chemical similarities between the tanning and calcification of collagen (availability of collagen side chains for chemical and physical interactions with other chemical components) was demonstrated when it was shown that the collagen in native skin failed to calcify in vitro when exposed to metastable solutions of CaP, whereas skin first treated with hyaluronidase and other enzymes and/or extracted with salt solutions of high ionic strength did mineralize (13,34).

The proteoglycans have a number of other physical chemical characteristics which theoretically would also tend to inhibit calcification. In addition to binding Ca^{2+} ions, proteoglycan gels inhibit the diffusion of Ca^{2+} and exclude inorganic phosphate ions (5,27).

Biological evidence also exists that supports an inhibitory role for the proteoglycans in calcification. During the calcification of cartilage in endochondral ossification, the amount of proteoglycans in the tissue decreases progressively starting from the completely uncalcified regions to the regions undergoing calcification (85). Moreover, during this time, the proteoglycan macromolecules are degraded and reduced in size (86). Not only the decrease in size but the decrease in molecular weight and chain length (34) will decrease the number of Ca^{2+} ions that can be bound by the proteoglycans, thus "exposing" the collagen fibrils and permitting them to function as heterogeneous nucleators for the formation of apatite crystals. On the basis of analyses from direct puncture of the epiphyseal cartilage fluid, similar conclusions have been reached by Pita and Howell et al. (87–93) and by Posner, Blumenthal, Boskey, and colleagues (94–96), who have conducted extensive experiments on the function of proteoglycans in in vitro calcification. Similarly, electron probe microanalysis of bone has shown more sulfate in the relatively sparsely mineralized osteoid of bone than in the more mineralized mature regions (97,98). The "protective" function of the proteoglycans in inhibiting the reaction between extracellular fluid components and collagen fibrils by binding and decreasing diffusion is also illustrated in the case of cartilage by marked enhancement of the intensity of reactions between antibodies to type II collagen after reaction of the tissue with hyaluronidase.

On the other hand, there persists some strong feeling that the proteoglycans are directly involved in the nucleation and initiation of calcification based principally on extensive electron micrographic studies (45,99,100). These include studies which showed that a particular protein component, the alpha (II) C-terminal propeptide ("chondrocalcin"; A. R. Poole, personal communication) was intimately associated with the mineral crystals in growth plate cartilage and in the initial deposits of the mineral phase with proteoglycan as well.

As for other structural factors, Katz and Li (70,101) have demonstrated that the collagen molecules in rat tail tendon are so closely packed that the diffusion of ions such as phosphate must be seriously limited. In contrast, the pathways in bone collagen are much larger, allowing diffusion of the hydrated phosphate ions to and within the collagen fibrils of bone without restriction. These

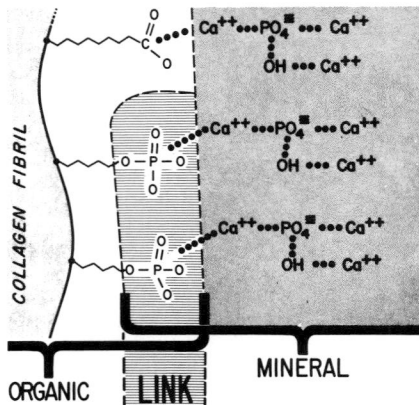

FIG. 10. Schematic diagram illustrating how protein-bound phosphomonoester groups may be constituents of both the organic and the mineral phases and thus serve as a bridge, chemically and physically linking the organic structural molecules of the organic matrix to the inorganic mineral crystals. (Reproduced with permission from Glimcher MJ: Recent studies of the mineral phase in bone and its possible linkage to the organic matrix by protein-bound phosphate bonds. *Philos Trans R Soc Lond* [*Biol Sci*] 1984;304:479–508.)

structural factors would therefore have a tendency to inhibit calcification in some normally uncalcified tissues, such as tendon, while facilitating it in bone.

There are a large number of other substances which allegedly are able to decrease or inhibit mineralization in vitro and in vivo. These include pyrophosphate, fluoride, polypeptides containing phosphorus, magnesium, and others (5,27). Presumably, many of these substances decrease or inhibit calcification by interacting with and effectively decreasing the number or "inactivating" the CaP nuclei of the metastable solution phase (5) rather than by binding Ca^{2+} alone (Fig. 10) (27).

CALCIFICATION IN SUMMARY

From the physical chemical standpoint, the formation of a solid phase of CaP in bone represents a *phase transformation,* a process exemplified by the formation of ice from liquid water. Considering the structural complexity and abundance of highly organized macromolecules in the cells and extracellular tissue spaces of mineralized tissues generally and in bone particularly, it is inconceivable that this phase transformation occurs by homogeneous nucleation (i.e., without the active participation, initiation, and induction by an organic component acting as a nucleation agent). This is almost surely true in biological mineralization in general. Electron micrographs and low-angle neutron and x-ray diffraction studies clearly show that calcification of collagen fibrils occurs in an extremely intimate and highly organized fashion: initiation of crystal formation within the collagen fibrils in the hole zone region, with the long axis (c-axis) of the crystals aligned roughly parallel to the long axis of the fibril within which they are located. Crystals are initially formed in hole zone regions within individual fibrils at distances from one another with unmineralized regions separating them (i.e., spatially distinct nucleation sites where calcification is initiated). This indicates that such regions within a single, indirectional fibril represent independent sites for heterogeneous nucleation.

Clearly, sites where mineralization is initiated in adjacent collagen fibrils are even further spatially separated, emphasizing more clearly that the process of progressive calcification of the collagen fibrils and therefore of the tissue is characterized principally by the presence of increasing numbers of independent nucleation sites within additional hole zone regions of the collagen fibrils. The additional increase in the mass of CaP apatite accrues principally by multiplication of more crystals, mostly by secondary nucleation from the crystals initially deposited in the hole zone region. Very little additional growth of the crystals occurs with time, the additional increase in mineral mass being principally the result of multiplication—increase in the number of crystals not in the size of the crystals (crystal growth). The progressive increase in the number of crystals within the collagen fibrils and possibly the slow growth of the crystals extends to include the overlap zone of the collagen fibrils ("pores") so that all of the available space within the fibrils (possibly expanded in volume from its uncalcified level) is eventually occupied by the mineral crystals.

It is absolutely critical to recognize that the calcification of each of the tissue components and compartments that are spatially separated (collagen, mitochondria, matrix vesicles) must be an independent physical chemical event. That is, there is no way that the solid phase CaP crystals of one component can directly cause or influence the initiation of calcification (nucleation) in another component from which it is physically separated.

Recent Data on Phosphoproteins and Calcification

Several light and high-resolution electron microscopic immunocytochemical technical studies of bone have clearly demonstrated that the phosphoproteins are either limited to or concentrated principally at the site of initial mineralization, in close relationship to the collagen fibrils (102–105). These data which show the location of the phosphoproteins at the site where calcification begins are consistent with earlier autoradiographic studies with ^{33}P at light and electron micrographic levels (74) and provide further strong evidence to support the role of phosphoproteins in calcification.

Gerstenfeld et al. (106) in our laboratories have developed a cell culture system utilizing chick bone osteoblasts which produces a typical bone collagen matrix chemically and which is organized morphologically in lamellae like it is in bone. Electron microscopic examination reveals that calcification occurs in the cell culture system within the collagen fibrils as it does in vivo. Most important, a time study has shown that collagen is synthesized and extruded into the extracellular matrix before any of the noncollagenous matrix constituents. A critical observation was that the phosphoproteins are synthesized at or just prior to the first evidence of Ca and P deposition initial mineralization (107,108). High-resolution electron microscopic and immunocytochemical studies have localized the phosphoproteins to the sites where the crystals are first nucleated, similar to the observations obtained in vivo (104,105,107).

To understand the mechanisms by which these phosphoproteins are phosphorylated, we have studied protein kinases in the strips of periosteal bone isolated from 12-day embryonic chick tibiotarsus in which bone phosphoproteins have already been characterized (109,110). We have detected a protein kinase (110) in the detergent extract of the membranous fractions which phosphorylates the bone phosphoproteins of 12-day-old embryonic chick tibia periosteal bone strips (109). This enzyme, tentatively named *bone phosphoprotein kinase* (BPP kinase), has a catalytic subunit of $M_r \sim 39,000$, utilizes GTP as well as ATP as a phosphoryl donor, and is inhib-

ited by 2,3-diphosphoglycerate and heparin and therefore is similar to casein kinase II. The enzyme can phosphorylate dephosphorylated proteins such as casein, phosvitin, and chicken bone phosphoproteins but prefers the chicken bone phosphoproteins. The in vitro phosphorylation assay products of this enzyme in the extract were indistinguishable on a sodium dodecyl sulfate (SDS) polyacrylamide gel from the major [^{32}P]-phosphoproteins metabolically labeled in the embryonic chick bone tissue. The regulatory mechanisms of the phosphorylation process of bone phosphoproteins by BPP kinase as well as the potential role of this enzyme in mineralization are under investigation.

ACKNOWLEDGMENTS

This work was supported in part by the New England Peabody Home for Crippled Children, Inc., National Institutes of Health Grants AM 34078 and AM 34081, National Science Foundation Grant PCM-8216959, Mineral Grant AR34081, Program Project Grant 5P01AR34078-08, and from an Institutional Grant from the Orthopaedic Research and Education Foundation, funded by the Bristol-Myers/Zimmer Corporation.

REFERENCES

1. Levy M. Chemische untersuchungen über osteomalacische knochen. *Hoppe-Seyler's Z Physiol Chem* 1894;19:239–70.
2. DeJong WF. La substance minérale dans les os. *Recl Trav Chim Pays-Bas Belg* 1926;45:445–8.
3. Roseberry HH, Hastings AB, Morse JK. X-ray analysis of bone and teeth. *J Biol Chem* 1931;90:395–407.
4. Glimcher MJ, Bonar LC, Grynpas MD, Landis WJ, Roufosse AH. Recent studies of bone mineral: is the ACP theory valid? *J Crystal Growth* 1981;53:100–19.
5. Glimcher MJ. Composition, structure, and organization of bone and other mineralized tissues and the mechanism of calcification. In: Greep RO, Astwood EB, eds. *Handbook of physiology*, vol 7, *Endocrinology*. Washington, DC: American Physiological Society, 1976;25–116.
6. Brown WE, Chow LC. Chemical properties of bone mineral. *Annu Rev Mater Sci* 1976;6:213–36.
7. Wadkins CL, Luben R, Thomas M, Humphreys R. Physical biochemistry of calcification. *Clin Orthop* 1974;99:246–66.
8. Termine JD. Mineral chemistry and skeletal biology. *Clin Orthop* 1972;85:207–41.
9. Posner AS. Crystallite chemistry of bone mineral. *Physiol Rev* 1969;49:760.
10. Glimcher MJ. Recent studies of the mineral phase in bone and its possible linkage to the organic matrix by protein-bound phosphate bonds. *Philos Trans R Soc Lond (Biol)* 1984;304:479–508.
11. Elliot JC. The problems of the composition and structure of the mineral components of the hard tissues. *Clin Orthop* 1973;93:313–45.
12. Bonar LC, Roufosse AH, Sabine WK, Grynpas MD, Glimcher MJ. X-ray diffraction studies of the crystallinity of bone mineral in newly synthesized and density fractionated bone. *Calcif Tissue Int* 1983;35:202–9.
13. Glimcher MJ. Molecular biology of mineralized tissues with particular reference to bone. *Rev Mod Phys* 1959;31:359–93.
14. Landis WJ, Glimcher MJ. Electron diffraction and electron probe microanalysis of the mineral phase of bone tissue prepared by anhydrous techniques. *J Ultrastruct Res* 1978;63:188–223.
15. Woodward HQ. The composition of human cortical bone. *Clin Orthop* 1964;37:187–93.

16. Pellegrino ED, Biltz RM. Mineralization in the chick embryo. I. Monohydrogen phosphate and carbonate relationships during maturation of the bone crystal complex. *Calcif Tissue Res* 1972;10:128–35.
17. Eanes ED, Harper RA, Gillessen IH, Posner AS. An amorphous component in bone mineral. In: Gaillard PJ, van der Hoff A, Steendyk R, eds. *4th European symposium on calcified tissues.* Amsterdam: Excerpta Medica, 1966;24–6.
18. Termine JD. Amorphous calcium phosphate: the second mineral of bone [PhD thesis]. Ithaca, NY: Cornell University; 1966.
19. Termine JD, Posner AS. Infrared analysis of rat bone: age dependency of amorphous and crystalline mineral fractions. *Science* 1966;153:1523–5.
20. Termine JD, Posner AS. Amorphous/crystalline inter-relationships in bone mineral. *Calcif Tissue Res* 1967;1:8–23.
21. Roufosse AH, Landis WJ, Sabine WK, Glimcher MJ. Identification of brushite in newly deposited bone mineral from embryonic chicks. *J Ultrastruct Res* 1979;68:235–55.
22. Grynpas MD, Bonar LC, Glimcher MJ. Failure to detect an amorphous calcium phosphate solid phase in bone mineral. *Calcif Tissue Int* 1984;36:291–301.
23. Fawcett RW. A radial distribution function analysis of an amorphous calcium phosphate with calcium to phosphate molar ratio of 1.42. *Calcif Tissue Res* 1973;13:319–25.
24. Aue WP, Roufosse AH, Roberts JE, Glimcher MJ, Griffin RG. Solid state ^{31}P NMR studies of synthetic solid phases of calcium phosphate: potential models of bone mineral. *Biochemistry* 1984;23:6110–4.
25. Roufosse AH, Aue WP, Glimcher MJ, Griffin RG. An investigation of the mineral phases of bone by solid state ^{31}P magic angle sample spinning NMR. *Biochemistry* 1984;23:6115–20.
26. Roberts JE, Bonar LC, Grynpas MD, Glimcher MJ, Griffin RG. Characterization of the youngest mineral phases of bone by solid state phosphorus-31 magic angle sample spinning nuclear magnetic resonance and x-ray diffraction. [In preparation].
27. Glimcher MJ, Krane SM. The organization and structure of bone, and the mechanism of calcification. In: Ramachandran GN, Gould BS, eds. *Treatise on collagen,* vol 7B. New York: Academic Press, 1968;68–251.
28. Glimcher MJ. A basic architectural principle in the organization of mineralized tissues. In: Milhaud G, Owen M, Blackwood HJJ, eds. *Proceedings of the 5th European symposium on calcified tissues, 1967.* Paris: Société d'Edition d'Enseignement Supérieur, 1968;3–26.
29. White SW, Hulmes DJS, Miller A, Timmins PA. Collagen–mineral axial relationship in calcified turkey leg tendon by x-ray and neutron diffraction. *Nature (Lond)* 1977;266:421–5.
30. Berthet-Colominas C, Miller A, White SW. Structural study of the calcifying collagen in turkey leg tendons. *J Mol Biol* 1979;134:431–45.
31. Engstrom A. Apatite–collagen organization in calcified tendon. *Exp Cell Res* 1966;43:241–5.
32. Glimcher MJ, Hodge AJ, Schmitt FO. Macromolecular aggregation states in relation to mineralization: the collagen–hydroxyapatite system as studied in vitro. *Proc Natl Acad Sci USA* 1957;43:860–7.
33. Lowenstam HA. Minerals formed by organisms. *Science (NY)* 1981;211:1126–31.
34. Glimcher MJ. Specificity of the molecular structure of organic matrices in mineralization. In: Sognnaes RF, ed. *Calcification in biological systems.* Washington, DC: American Association for the Advancement of Science, 1960;421–87.
35. Mergenhagen SE, Martin GR, Rizzo AA, Wright DN, Scott DB. Calcification in vivo of implanted collagen. *Biochim Biophys Acta* 1960;43:563–5.
36. Lehninger AL. Mitochondria and calcium ion transport. *Biochem J* 1970;119:129–38.
37. Shapiro IM, Greenspan JS. Are mitochondria directly involved in biological mineralization? *Calcif Tissue Res* 1969;3:100–2.
38. Shapiro IM, Lee NH. Calcium accumulation by chondrocyte mitochondria. *Clin Orthopaed* 1975;106:323–9.
39. Shapiro IM, Wuthier RE. A study of the phospholipids of bovine dental tissue. II. *Arch Oral Biol* 1966;11:513–9.
40. Shapiro IM, Wuthier RE, Irving JT. A study of the phospholipids of bovine dental tissues. I. *Arch Oral Biol* 1966;11:501–12.
41. Brighton CT, Hunt RM. Mitochondrial calcium and its role in calcification. *Clin Orthop* 1974;100:406–16.
42. Anderson HC. Vesicles associated with calcification in the matrix of epiphyseal cartilage. *J Cell Biol* 1969;41:59–72.
43. Anderson HC. Calcium-accumulating vesicles in the intercellular matrix of bone. In: Elliott K, Fitzsimons DW, eds. *Ciba Foundation symposium on hard tissue growth, repair and remineralization.* Amsterdam: Elsevier, 1973;213–46.
44. Morris DC, Vaananen HK, Anderson HC. Matrix vesicle calcification in rat epiphyseal growth plate cartilage prepared anhydrously for electron microscopy. *Metab Bone Dis Relat Res* 1984;5:131–7.
45. Bonucci F. The locus of initial calcification in cartilage and bone. *Clin Orthop* 1971;78:108–39.
46. Ali SY. Analysis of matrix vesicles and their role in the calcification of epiphyseal cartilage. *Fed Proc Fed Am Soc Exp Biol* 1976;35:135–42.
47. Ali SY, Craig-Gray J, Wisby A, Phillips M. Preparation of thin cryosections for electron probe analysis of calcifying cartilage. *J Microsc* 1977;111:65–76.
48. Wuthier RE. A review of the primary mechanism of endochondral calcification with special emphasis on the role of cells, mitochondria and matrix vesicles. *Clin Orthop* 1982;169:219–42.
49. Anderson HC. Evolution of cartilage. In: Slavkin HC, ed. *The comparative molecular biology of extracellular matrices.* New York: Academic Press, 1972;200–5.
50. Glimcher MJ. On the form and function of bone: from molecules to organs. Wolff's law revisited, 1981. In: Veis A, ed. *The chemistry and biology of mineralized connective tissues.* Amsterdam: Elsevier/North-Holland, 1981;618–73.
51. Landis WJ, Hauschka BT, Rogerson CA, Glimcher MJ. Electron microscopic observations of bone tissue prepared by ultracryomicrotomy. *J Ultrastruct Res* 1977;59:185–206.
52. Landis WJ, Paine MC, Glimcher MJ. Electron microscopic observations of bone tissue prepared anhydrously in organic solvents. *J Ultrastruct Res* 1977;59:1–30.
53. Glimcher MJ, Katz EP, Travis DF. The organization of collagen in bone: the role of noncovalent forces in the physical properties and solubility characteristics of bone collagen. In Comte P, ed. *Symp int biochim physiol tissu conjonctif, 1966.* Lyon, France: Société Ormeco et Imprimerie du Sud-Est, 1966;491–503.
54. Thyberg J, Friberg U. Ultrastructure and acid phosphatase of matrix vesicles and cytoplasmic dense bodies in the epiphyseal plate. *J Ultrastruct Res* 1970;33:554–73.
55. Landis WJ. Temporal sequence of mineralization in calcifying turkey leg tendon. In: WT Butler, ed. *The chemistry and biology of mineralized tissues.* Birmingham, AL: Ebsco Media, 1985;360–3.
56. Robinson RA, Watson ML. Collagen–crystal relationships in bone as seen in the electron microscope. *Anat Rec* 1952;114:383–409.
57. Glimcher MJ. Phosphopeptides of enamel matrix. *J Dent Res* 1979;58B:790–806.
58. Veis A, Spector AR, Zamoscianyk H. The isolation of an EDTA-soluble phosphoprotein from mineralizing bovine dentin. *Biochim Biophys Acta* 1972;257:404–13.
59. Linde A, Bhown M, Butler WT. Non-collagenous proteins of rat dentin: evidence that phosphoprotein is not covalently bound to collagen. *Biochim Biophys Acta* 1981;667:341–50.
60. Seyer JM, Glimcher MJ. Isolation, characterization and partial amino acid sequence of a phosphorylated polypeptide (E$_4$) from bovine embryonic dental enamel. *Biochim Biophys Acta* 1977;493:441–51.
61. Glimcher MJ, Kossiva D, Roufosse A. Identification of phosphopeptides and gamma-carboxyglutamic acid-containing peptides in epiphyseal growth plate cartilage: proteins of bone cementum; comparison with dentin, enamel and bone. *Calcif Tissue Int* 1979;27:187–91.
62. Anderson RS, Schwartz ER. Phosphorylation of proteoglycans from human articular cartilage by a cAMP-dependent protein kinase. *Arthritis Rheum* 1984;27:1023–7.
63. Oegema TR Jr, Brown N, Dziewiakowski D. The link protein in proteoglycan aggregates from the Swarm rat chondrosarcoma. *J Biol Chem* 1977;252:6470–7.
64. Cohen-Solal L, Lian JB, Kossiva D, et al. The identification of

O-phosphothreonine in the soluble noncollagenous phosphoproteins of bone matrix. *FEBS Lett* 1978;89:107–10.

65. Glimcher MJ, Brickley-Parsons D, Kossiva D. Phosphopeptides and γ-carboxyglutamic acid-containing peptides in calcified turkey tendons: their absence in uncalcified tendon. *Calcif Tissue Int* 1979;27:281–4.

66. Glimcher MJ, Lefteriou B, Kossiva D. Identification of O-phosphoserine, O-phosphothreonine and γ-carboxyglutamic acid in the noncollagenous proteins of bovine cementum; comparison with dentin, enamel and bone. *Calcif Tissue Int* 1979;28:83–6.

67. Linde A, Bhown M, Butler WT. Non-collagenous proteins of dentin: a re-examination of proteins from rat incisor dentin utilizing techniques to avoid artifacts. *J Biol Chem* 1980;255:5931–42.

68. Lee SL, Veis A. Studies on the structure and chemistry of dentin collagen–phosphoryn covalent complexes. *Calcif Tissue Int* 1980;31:123–34.

69. Lee SL, Glonek T, Glimcher MJ. ^{31}P nuclear magnetic resonance spectroscopic evidence for ternary complex formation of fetal phosphoprotein with calcium and inorganic orthophosphate ions. *Calcif Tissue Int* 1983;35:815–8.

70. Li SH, Katz E. On the state of anionic groups of demineralized matrices of bone and dentin. *Calcif Tiss Res* 1977;22:275–84.

71. Glimcher MJ, Kossiva D, Brickley-Parsons D. Phosphoproteins of chicken bone matrix: proof of synthesis in bone tissue. *J Biol Chem* 1984;259:290–3.

72. Gotoh Y, Sakamoto M, Sakamoto S, et al. Biosynthesis of O-phosphoserine-containing phosphoproteins by isolated bone cells of mouse calvaria. *FEBS Lett* 1983;154:116–20.

73. Weinstock M, Leblond CP. Radioautographic visualization of the deposition of a phosphoprotein at the mineralization front in the dentin of the rat incisor. *J Cell Biol* 1973;56:838–45.

74. Landis WJ, Sanzone CF, Brickley-Parsons D, Glimcher MJ. Radioautographic visualization and biochemical identification of O-phosphoserine- and O-phosphothreonine-containing phosphoproteins in mineralizing embryonic chick bone. *J Cell Biol* 1984;98:986–90.

75. Endo A, Glimcher MJ. The potential role of phosphoproteins in the in vitro calcification of bone collagen. In: VM Goldberg, ed. *Transactions of the 32nd meeting of the Orthopedic Research Society.* Chicago: Adept Printing, 1986;221.

76. Raggio CL, Boyan BD, Boskey AL. In vivo induction of hydroxyapatite formation by lipid macromolecules. *J Bone Joint Surg.* [In press].

77. Odutuga AA, Prout RES, Hoare J. Hydroxyapatite precipitator in vitro by lipids extracted from mammalian hard and soft tissues. *Arch Oral Biol* 1975;20:311–6.

78. Boskey AL, Posner AS. The role of synthetic and bone-extracted Ca–phospholipid–PO$_4$ complexes in hydroxyapatite formation. *Calcif Tissue Res* 1977;23:251.

79. Boyan BD. Proteolipid-dependent calcification, In: Butler WT, ed. *The chemistry and biology of mineralized tissues.* Birmingham, AL: Ebsco Media, 1985;125–31.

80. Nawrot CF, Campbell DJ, Shroaeder JK, van Valkenburg M. Dental phosphoproteins: induced formation of hydroxyapatite during in vitro synthesis of amorphous calcium phosphate. *Biochemistry* 1976;15:3445–9.

81. Sobel AE. Local factors in the mechanism of calcification. *Ann NY Acad Sci* 1955;60:713–32.

82. Sobel AE, Burger M. Calcification. XIV. Investigation of the role of chondroitin sulfate in the calcifying mechanism. *Proc Soc Exp Biol Med* 1954;87:7–13.

83. Sylven B. Cartilage and chondroitin sulfate. II. Chondroitin sulfate and the physiological ossification of cartilage. *J Bone Joint Surg* 1947;29:973–6.

84. Burton D, Reed R. Mucoid material in hides and skins and its significance in tanning and dyeing. *Discuss Faraday Soc* 1954;16:195–201.

85. Lohmander S, Hjerpe A. Proteoglycans of mineralizing rib and epiphyseal cartilage. *Biochim Biophys Acta* 1975;404:93–109.

86. Buckwalter JA. Proteoglycan structure and calcifying cartilage. *Clin Orthop* 1983;172:207–32.

87. Howell DS. Bone formation: biochemistry of calcification. *Israel J Med Sci* 1976;12:91–7.

88. Howell DS, Carlson L. The effect of papain on mineral deposition in the healing of rachitic epiphyses. *Exp Cell Res* 1965;37:582–96.

89. Howell DS, Carlson L. Alterations in the composition of growth cartilage septa during calcification studied by microscopic x-ray elemental analysis. *Exp Cell Res* 1968;51:185–95.

90. Howell DS, Marquez JF, Pita JC. The nature of phospholipids in normal and rachitic costochondral plates. *Arthritis Rheum* 1965;8:1039–46.

91. Howell DS, Pita J, Marquez J. Phosphate concentration and sodium activity of fluids obtained by micropuncture in epiphyseal cartilage. *Fed Proc* 1965;24:566.

92. Pita JC, Cuervo LA, Madruga JE, Muller FJ, Howell DS. Evidence for a role of proteinpolysaccharides in regulation of mineral phase separation in calcifying cartilage. *J Clin Invest* 1970;49:2188–97.

93. Pita JC, Muller F, Howell DS. Disaggregation of proteoglycan aggregates during endochondrial calcification: physiological role of cartilage lysozyme. In: Burleigh M, Poole R, eds. *Dynamics of connective tissue macromolecules.* Amsterdam: North-Holland, 1975;247–58.

94. Posner AS, Blumenthal NC, Boskey AL, et al. Formation and transformation of amorphous calcium phosphate to hydroxyapatite, a bone analogue, in calcified tissue. In: Czitober M, Eschberger J eds., *Calcified Tissue.* Vienna, Facta Publications, 1973;1–4.

95. Chen CC, Boskey AL. The effect of proteoglycans on in vitro hydroxyapatite growth. *Calcif Tissue Int* 1984;36:285–90.

96. Chen CC, Boskey AL. Mechanisms of proteoglycan inhibition of hydroxyapatite growth. *Calcif Tissue Int* 1985;37:395–400.

97. Baylink D, Wergedal J, Stauffer M, Rich C. Effects of fluoride on bone formation, mineralization, and resorption in the rat. In: Vischer TL, ed. *Fluoride in medicine.* Bern: Hans Huber, 1970;37–69.

98. Baylink D, Wergedal J, Thompson E. Loss of proteinpolysaccharides at sites where bone mineralization is initiated. *J Histochem Cytochem* 1972;20:279–92.

99. Bonucci E, Dearden LC, Mosier HD Jr. Effects of glucocorticoid treatment on the ultrastructure of cartilage and bone. *Adv Exp Med Biol* 1984;171:269–78.

100. Poole AR, Pidoux I, Reiner A, Rosenberg L. An immunoelectron microscopic study of the organization of proteoglycan monomer, link protein, and collagen in the matrix of articular cartilage. *J Cell Biol* 1982;93:921–37.

101. Katz EP, Li S-T. Structure and function of bone collagen fibrils. *J Mol Biol* 1973;80:1–15.

102. Prince CW, Oosawa T, Butler WT, et al. Isolation, characterization and biosynthesis of a phosphorylated glycoprotein from rat bone. *J Biol Chem* 1987;262:2900–7.

103. Heinegard D, Hultenby K, Oldberg A, Reinholt F, Wendel M. Macromolecules in bone matrix. *Connect Tissue Res* 1989;21:3–14.

104. Bruder SP, Caplan AI, Gotoh Y, Gerstenfeld LC, Glimcher MJ. Immunohistochemical localization of a ~66kD glycosylated phosphoprotein during development of the embryonic chick tibia. *Calcif Tissue Int.* [In press].

105. McKee MD, Nanci A, Landis WJ, Gotoh Y, Gerstenfeld LC, Glimcher MJ. Developmental appearance and ultrastructural immunolocalization of a major 66kD phosphoprotein in embryonic and post-natal chicken bone. *Anat. Rec.* 1990;228:77–92.

106. Gerstenfeld LC, Chipman SD, Glowacki J, Lian JB. Expression of differentiated function by mineralization cultures of chicken osteoblasts. *Dev Biol* 1987;122:49–60.

107. Gerstenfeld LC, Gotoh Y, McKee MD, Nanci A, Landis WJ, Glimcher MJ. Expression and ultrastructural immunolocalization of the major phosphoprotein synthesized by chicken osteoblasts during mineralization in vitro. *Anat. Rec.* 1990;228:93–103.

108. Gotoh Y, Gerstenfeld LC, Glimcher MJ. Identification and characterization of the major chicken bone phosphoprotein: analysis of its synthesis by cultured embryonic chick osteoblasts. *Eur J Biochem.* 1990;187:49–58.

109. Mikuni-Takagaki Y, Glimcher MJ. Post-translational processing of chicken bone phosphoproteins. I. Identification of the bone phosphoproteins of embryonic tibia. *Biochem J.* 1990;585–591.

110. Mikuni-Takagaki Y, Glimcher MJ. Post-translational processing of chicken bone phosphoproteins. II. Identification of bone [phospho]protein kinase. *Biochem J.* 1990;268:593–597.

Disorders of Bone and Mineral Metabolism,
edited by Fredric L. Coe and Murray J. Favus,
© 1992 by Raven Press, Ltd. All rights reserved.

CHAPTER 13

Mechanisms and Regulation of Bone Resorption by Osteoclastic Cells

Lawrence G. Raisz

During the past 20 years our understanding of the osteoclast has been advanced substantially: first by detailed morphological descriptions and subsequently by functional analysis. Methods for isolating osteoclasts and studying their behavior on mineralized surfaces have been developed. Functional elements of these cells have been identified by histochemical and immunocytochemical methods. The hematopoietic origin of osteoclasts has been confirmed, but the precise relation of the osteoclast to other hematopoietic cells is still not clear. There are other gaps in our knowledge. We believe that cells of the osteoblastic lineage are important with regard to the activation of bone resorption, but we have not yet identified the specific cells and mediators involved. We do not know what stops osteoclastic bone resorption. Multiple local and systemic factors have been identified which can regulate bone resorption in cell and organ culture and in vivo. Such a complex regulation would be expected because osteoclasts must serve both (a) the metabolic function of maintaining movement of calcium from bone to blood and (b) the structural role of remodeling bone at specific sites. This chapter will approach the function and regulation of bone resorption by osteoclasts by asking a series of questions. Some questions will be answered in considerable detail, whereas others will only be speculated upon. This topic has been the subject of a number of recent reviews which provide additional background and references (1–7). The references in the chapter will largely represent recent studies on each question, but earlier key references will also be provided.

L. G. Raisz: Division of Endocrinology and Metabolism, University of Connecticut Health Science Center, Farmington, Connecticut 06032.

WHY ARE OSTEOCLASTS IMPORTANT?

It seems most likely that the osteoclast is the major cell responsible for the skeletal contribution to the regulation of serum calcium concentration. There have been suggestions that osteoblasts or osteocytes might be directly responsible for the movement of calcium from bone to blood, but this has not been supported by convincing experimental data (8). In contrast, all of the agents which have been shown to increase serum calcium concentration in vivo have been shown to increase osteoclastic activity, and the hormones and drugs which lower serum calcium concentration have been shown to inhibit osteoclastic activity. This is true not only for the established calcium-regulating hormones, parathyroid hormone (PTH), 1,25-dihydroxyvitamin D_3 [1,25(OH)$_2$D$_3$], and calcitonin, but also for certain systemic hormones which can alter serum calcium concentration, particularly under pathologic conditions, such as thyroid hormones, glucocorticoids, and the PTH-related peptide of malignancy (PTHrP). Some local regulators can affect serum calcium concentrations. For example, it has been shown that prostaglandin E_2 (PGE$_2$) and interleukin-1 (IL-1) can produce systemic hypercalcemia (9,10). Interestingly, transient hypocalcemia has been reported after bolus injections of IL-1 (11). This effect was blocked by indomethacin, an inhibitor of prostaglandin synthesis, and hence might be due to local release of prostaglandins which can produce a transient initial inhibition of osteoclastic activity (12).

Osteoclasts are critical in the physiologic modeling, as well as remodeling, of bone. For example, osteoclasts are rarely seen on the periosteal surfaces of the tubular portion of long bones in adults, but they do mediate the removal of the metaphyseal flair during the elongation of long bones in children. Bone remodeling involves activation of osteoclasts at specific sites, often determined by changes in mechanical forces (13–15).

Osteoclastic resorption is particularly important in the pathogenesis of metabolic bone disease. In osteoporosis, excessive osteoclastic resorption not only is responsible for loss of bone mass, but probably also results in decreased bone strength because it produces perforations and discontinuities of trabecular plates as well as increased porosity of the cortex. Osteoclasts are responsible for lytic lesions in malignancy, bone loss around sites of inflammation, and the initial bone loss that occurs with immobilization (15). Excessive proliferation and disordered function of osteoclasts is the pathologic lesion in Paget's disease. Failure of osteoclast function can result in osteopetrosis (16,17). Genetic defects in the osteoclasts which occur in various forms of osteopetrosis may help us to understand the regulation of these cells. Thus we must learn more about how osteoclasts work if we are to understand calcium regulation, bone modeling and remodeling, and the pathology of skeletal disease.

WHAT PART DO OTHER CELLS PLAY IN BONE RESORPTION?

Role of Osteoblasts, Osteocytes, and Lining Cells in Bone Resorption

One of the most active areas of current research is the study of the role of cells of the osteoblastic lineage in activating bone resorption. The possible mechanisms are illustrated in Fig. 1. The target cell for activation of resorption is not yet fully defined. The inactive surfaces of bone are covered, somewhat loosely, by a population of lining cells which are thought to be resting or inactive osteoblasts, no longer forming bone matrix (18). In addition to these cells, there may be target cells for bone-resorbing hormones more distant from the bone surface (19). These could represent osteoblast precursors or marrow stem cells.

The importance of cells of the osteoblastic lineage in initiating resorption has been emphasized by recent studies of isolated osteoclasts, which show that cells with osteoblastic phenotype can activate osteoclasts; these studies suggest that there are factors produced by the osteoblasts which are responsible for this activation (20–26). When isolated osteoclasts are treated with PTH, PTHrP, 1,25-dihydroxyvitamin D [1,25(OH)$_2$D], or other stimulators of bone resorption, there is no increase in their ability to produce resorption pits on mineralized bone slices. When osteoblasts or osteosarcoma cells which have osteoblast-like features are added to the system, there is an increase in osteoclastic activity, and this

is further stimulated by these bone-resorbing hormones. Since conditioned medium from osteoblast cultures can increase osteoclastic activity, it has been postulated that there is a specific mediator for this cell interaction. This mediator has not yet been fully identified. On the basis of preliminary studies, which suggest a number of different molecular sizes, there may be more than one chemical entity involved. On the other hand, when co-cultures of marrow stromal cell lines with spleen cells have been shown to produce osteoclasts, the data suggest that osteoclast formation requires cell–cell contact (27,28). Thus a membrane-bound factor or even cytoplasmic exchange through gap junctions may be required for activation. In addition to producing a putative mediator, cells of the osteoblast lineage may prepare the bone surface for resorption. Removal of protein (particularly collagen) from the bone surface, which exposes a fully mineralized matrix, appears to enhance both the attachment and the activity of osteoclasts (29–31). The removal of proteins and proteoglycans on the bone surface is thought to be accomplished by the release of procollagenase and plasminogen activator from osteoblastic cells (32–35). One hypothesis is that there is a cascade in which the plasminogen-activator–plasminogen–plasmin system activates collagenase and other metalloproteinases which degrade matrix components (36). Plasminogen activator has also recently been identified in osteoclasts (37), and this could play a role in enzyme activation.

A final component of the hypothesis concerning the role of lining cells in activating resorption, as presented by Rodan and Martin (38), was that these lining cells, which would normally prevent access of osteoclasts in the bone surface, must also undergo a shape change in order to permit resorption. There is evidence that hormones which stimulate bone resorption can produce shape changes in osteoblastic cells, which is consistent with this hypothesis (39,40).

The possibility that osteoblastic cells, particularly the osteocytes, contribute to osteoclastic resorption by fusing with osteoclasts as active components of that cell has been suggested, but it seems more likely that osteocytes are phagocytized and digested by osteoclasts (41,42). However, there is recent evidence that living osteocytes might enhance osteoclastic bone resorption by contributing proteolytic enzymes (43). Isolated osteoclasts were found to resorb substantially more when applied to bones in which the surfaces were stripped of osteoblasts, but the interior bone cells were allowed to remain alive, compared to bones devitalized by freezing and thawing. This enhanced effect on live bone was blocked by the tissue inhibitor of metalloproteinase (TIMP), which can block collagenase, stromelysin, and gelatinase. In contrast, TIMP had no effect on the resorption of devitalized bone by isolated osteoclasts.

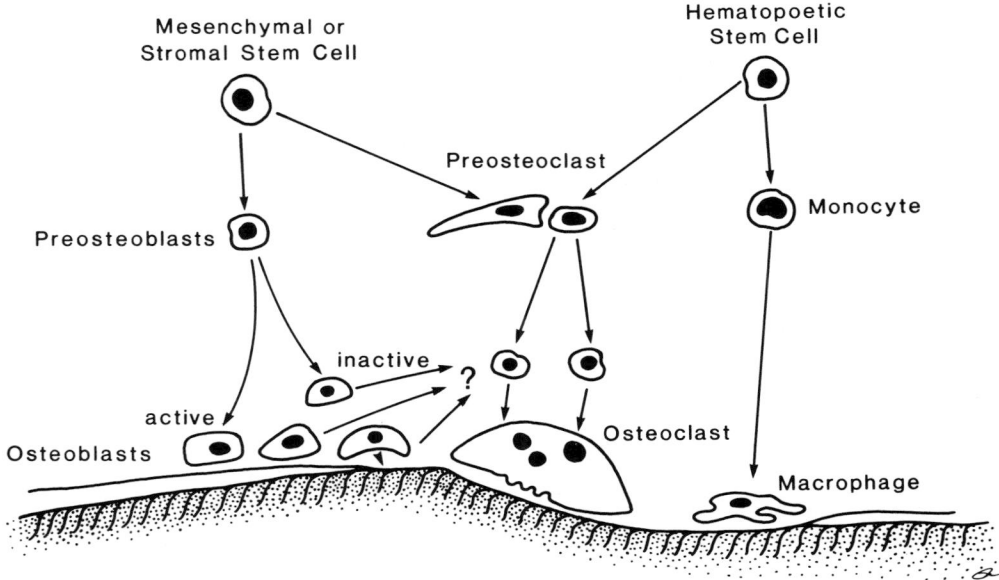

FIG. 1. Cell interactions in bone resorption. This diagram depicts the multiple potential pathways for the activation of osteoclastic bone resorption. Undifferentiated mesenchyme cells or stromal cells from the bone marrow may activate osteoclasts by direct cell contact. They may also differentiate into osteoblasts which could either directly stimulate osteoclast replication, differentiation, and fusion by cell contact or produce a soluble mediator. The inactive osteoblasts or lining cells probably also undergo shape changes and may produce enzymes which degrade proteins on the bone surface to expose the mineralized matrix and facilitate osteoclastic resorption. Macrophages may complete the resorptive process by producing proteolytic enzymes to reverse collagen remnants.

Role of Monocyte–Macrophages in Bone Resorption

There are several possible roles for cells of the monocyte–macrophage lineage in regulating bone resorption. The possibility that the osteoclast is a direct descendent of the monocyte–macrophage line seems unlikely (see below). On the other hand, it does seem likely that macrophage-like mononuclear cells play a role in the completion of the resorptive process during bone remodeling. These cells are found at the base of Howship's lacunae during the reversal phase between resorption and formation. Macrophage-like cells can resorb mineralized matrix particles (44,45), possibly by the release of collagenase, gelatinase, and other enzymes which degrade the matrix. Residual collagen fibers, which are seen at the base of resorption pits made by osteoclasts in vitro, could be removed by these degradative enzymes. Macrophage-like cells might also be important in stopping the resorptive process, either by releasing factors which block further osteoclastic resorption, such as transforming growth factor β (TGF-β), or by blocking access to the mineralized bone. The latter could be accomplished by the production of the special layer of matrix called the "cement line," which differs from the usual bone matrix in having less collagen and more proteoglycan. This layer may also be important in the attachment of new osteoblasts and in

providing an effective seal between old and new bone. Since macrophages are also a source of growth factors, they could play an additional role in the initiation of bone formation at remodeling sites by stimulating replication, differentiation, and migration of new osteoblasts.

ARE OSTEOCLASTS DERIVED FROM HEMATOPOIETIC STEM CELLS?

A number of studies over the past 20 years have established the concept that the osteoclast is derived from a hematopoietic stem cell and not from a mesenchymal stem cell (46). The studies of Walker (47) using spleen cells from osteopetrotic and normal mice were seminal in the development of this concept. Subsequently, marrow cells from a compatible donor were shown to restore osteoclastic resorption in human osteopetrosis (48).

Recently, there have been attempts to characterize the osteoclast lineage more precisely, to define its relationship to other cells of hematopoietic origin, and to identify the factors which stimulate the proliferation, differentiation, and fusion of precursors into multinucleated osteoclasts. Several different models have been used, and there has been some controversy concerning the interpretation of data from these models. Complete characterization by multiple criteria must be used to establish that a specific multinucleated cell is an osteoclast. This should include not only the presence of calcitonin receptors and tartrate-resistant acid phosphatase, but also evidence that the multinucleated cell produces lacunae or resorption pits in mineralized bone through the formation of a typical ruffled border surrounded by a clear or sealing zone, the characteristic resorbing apparatus of this highly specialized cell. Limiting characterization to multinuclearity and the development of tartrate-resistant acid phosphatase may be unreliable (46,49). The presence of calcitonin receptors may be a somewhat more reliable marker (50,51).

Most studies have been carried out in long-term cultures of bone marrow or spleen cells (52–57), although osteoclast-like cells can also be produced from human and blood monocytes (58). Another model which has been useful in identifying osteoclast precursors is a coculture of fetal mouse bone rudiments from which the periosteum has been stripped; hence, osteoclast precursors have been removed, together with putative precursor cells from spleen, liver, or marrow (59–64). Cells with a substantial number of osteoclastic features can also be formed ectopically in vivo in response to implants of mineralized bone (65–69). This model can be used to analyze the components of mineralized matrix which are most important for stimulating osteoclast formation. In fact, it is possible that the osteoclast has (a) specific receptors for hydroxyapatite (or for a combination of minerals) and (b) a specific matrix component such as the bone gamma-carboxyglutamic-acid-containing protein (BGP or osteocalcin) (67,69). In osteopetrotic rats the defect in bone resorption is associated with decreased BGP in bone and increased BGP in the serum (70). In contrast, giant cells which form around unmineralized bone matrix and around other foreign materials do not show a preference for mineralized surfaces and do not develop the typical resorbing apparatus of the osteoclasts (65). These giant cells are presumably derived from the separate monocyte–macrophage lineage and may also be formed in marrow and spleen cultures, so that many of the multinucleated cells produced are not true osteoclasts.

These models have been used to answer a number of specific questions about osteoclasts. Studies of surface antigens have shown that osteoclasts contain a number of the markers for macrophages, megakaryocytes, and other cells of hematopoietic or even mesenchymal origin, but that they also express specific, separate antigens (71–83). Many of the antigens appear to be members of the adhesion receptor family (84). Some osteoclast-specific antigens appear to be common to a number of different species and could be important in elucidating the functions of this cell type (74). Moreover, the antigens which are most characteristic of differentiated macrophages are usually not expressed by osteoclasts, and

vice versa (76,85). These findings are consistent with an early separation of the lineages of osteoclast and macrophage precursors.

A number of factors have now been identified which can facilitate the formation of osteoclasts from hematopoietic precursor cell populations. The studies using bone implants suggest that some component of the matrix and/or the mineral itself is an important stimulus (69), and this has been confirmed in marrow culture (86). Colony-stimulating factors (CSFs) may also be important in enhancing osteoclast formation, possibly by stimulating replication of early precursors (87). Bone-marrow-derived stromal cell lines which produce CSFs have been shown to support osteoclast differentiation (28). The osteopetrotic (op/op) mouse is deficient in macrophage CSF, and this may be important in the pathogenesis of the osteoclast defect in this model (88). However, in marrow cultures CSFs can inhibit (89,90), as well as stimulate (91), osteoclast formation.

Following the initial observation that $1,25(OH)_2D_3$ could promote fusion of macrophages and giant cell formation, a number of studies have examined the role of this hormone in the generation of osteoclasts from hematopoietic cells (92–97). Since the formation of both osteoclastic and nonosteoclastic giant cells can be stimulated by $1,25(OH)_2D_3$ (92), its specific role in osteoclastogenesis is difficult to define. However, there is evidence that some of the $1,25(OH)_2D_3$-stimulated polykaryons are true osteoclasts. Other factors may modulate this response. Retinoic acid can increase osteoclast formation, but its action seems to differ from that of $1,25(OH)_2D_3$ (98). PGE_2 has been shown to increase osteoclast formation, although its initial effect on osteoclast function is inhibitory (99,100).

HOW DO OSTEOCLASTS WORK?

Perhaps the most important advance in our understanding of the osteoclast has been the development of a clearer picture of the mechanisms by which this cell attaches to bone and resorbs mineral and matrix, which has evolved from a combination of morphologic studies, biochemical analyses, and immunocytochemistry (101). The osteoclast has a number of unique structural features which enable it to resorb bone (Figs. 2 and 3). It is a large, multinucleated, polarized cell whose surfaces are divided into three different functional areas. The basolateral membrane, away from the bone surface, is specialized for active transport of the products of bone resorption to the extracellular fluid. The "clear zone" or "sealing zone" is specialized to attach tightly to the mineralized bone surface that is to be resorbed. The former term refers to the absence of mitochondria and other subcellular particles in the cytoplasm of this zone, although it is rich in actin filaments. The ruffled border

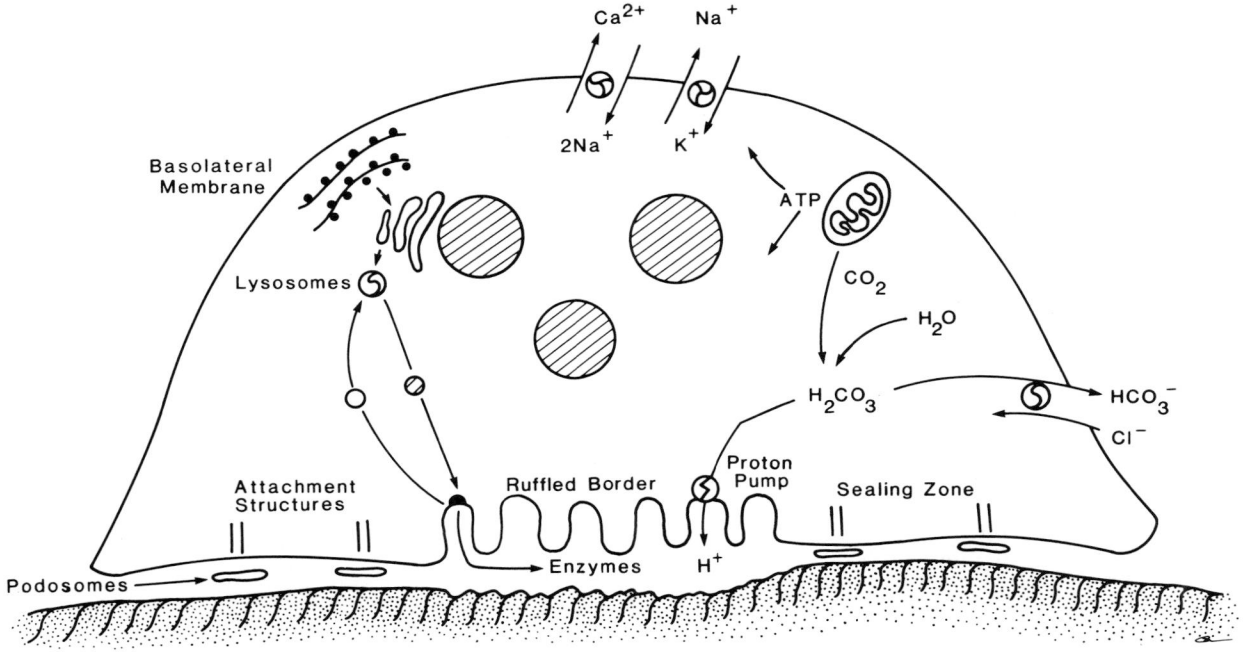

FIG. 2. Functional morphology of the osteoclast. This simplified diagram indicates some of the functional elements of the osteoclast. The basolateral membrane has ATP-dependent ion transport systems to extrude calcium and maintain intracellular potassium, similar to other cells. The osteoclast is enriched in mitochondria to provide the large amount of ATP necessary for these pumps as well as for an electrogenic proton pump which raises the hydrogen ion concentration at the ruffled border area. Lysosomal enzymes are synthesized and taken up in Golgi vesicles which contain mannose-6-phosphate receptors. These vesicles presumably circulate through the cell, discharging their enzyme contents into the ruffled border area. The sealing zone, with its actin filaments and specialized attachment structures (podosomes), surrounds the ruffled border area and separates it from the extracellular fluid. Carbonic acid is generated from the CO_2 produced by mitochondrial metabolism and provides the source for hydrogen ions. The excess HCO_3^- is removed by exchange with chloride.

area carries out the resorption process itself. Although mononuclear osteoclasts have been described, the majority of active cells are polykaryons, having 2–10 nuclei. Larger osteoclasts are seen in certain pathologic states, such as Paget's disease, and under conditions when osteoclast formation is stimulated but function is blocked, such as after treatment with bisphosphonates. The osteoclast is richly endowed with mitochondria to provide the large amount of ATP necessary for its transport functions and has a substantial amount of rough endoplasmic reticulum for the synthesis of transport proteins and lysosomal enzymes. Multiple Golgi complexes are present around each of the nuclei of the cell, and many coated transport vesicles are found between the Golgi and the ruffled border. Just subjacent to the ruffled border, there are large areas which appear to be vacuoles, but these may also represent expanded extracellular recesses of the ruffled border area where the digestive products of resorption have accumulated.

Resorption depends on the ability of this cell to attach itself to bone in such a way as to seal off an area of specialized membrane activity called the "ruffled border." The sealing zone contains a complex adhesion system (102–110). Although the details have not been completely established, this system must involve (a) ligands on the bone surface and (b) receptors on the osteoclast. There are bone proteins which could bind both to mineralized collagen and to adhesion receptors on the osteoclast. Several candidates for such ligand proteins have been identified, including osteonectin, osteopontin, and other glycosylated phosphoproteins in bone which contain the Arg–Gly–Asp (RGD) sequence which can bind to vitronectin receptors (111).

The osteoclast surface has a vitronectin receptor probably in the form of a β_3 integrin which is localized, together with vinculin and talin, in specialized ring-like structures called "podosomes." These, in turn, are attached to the cytoskeletal elements within the cell which contain actin and which presumably provide the force for adherence (107). This attachment apparatus is under hormonal control. Its differentiation appears to be increased by retinol (103), and the structures are disrupted by calcitonin (102). A region similar to the clear or sealing zone is frequently seen when other cells with degradative function are bound to their substrate, such as macrophages and foreign-body giant cells (69). However,

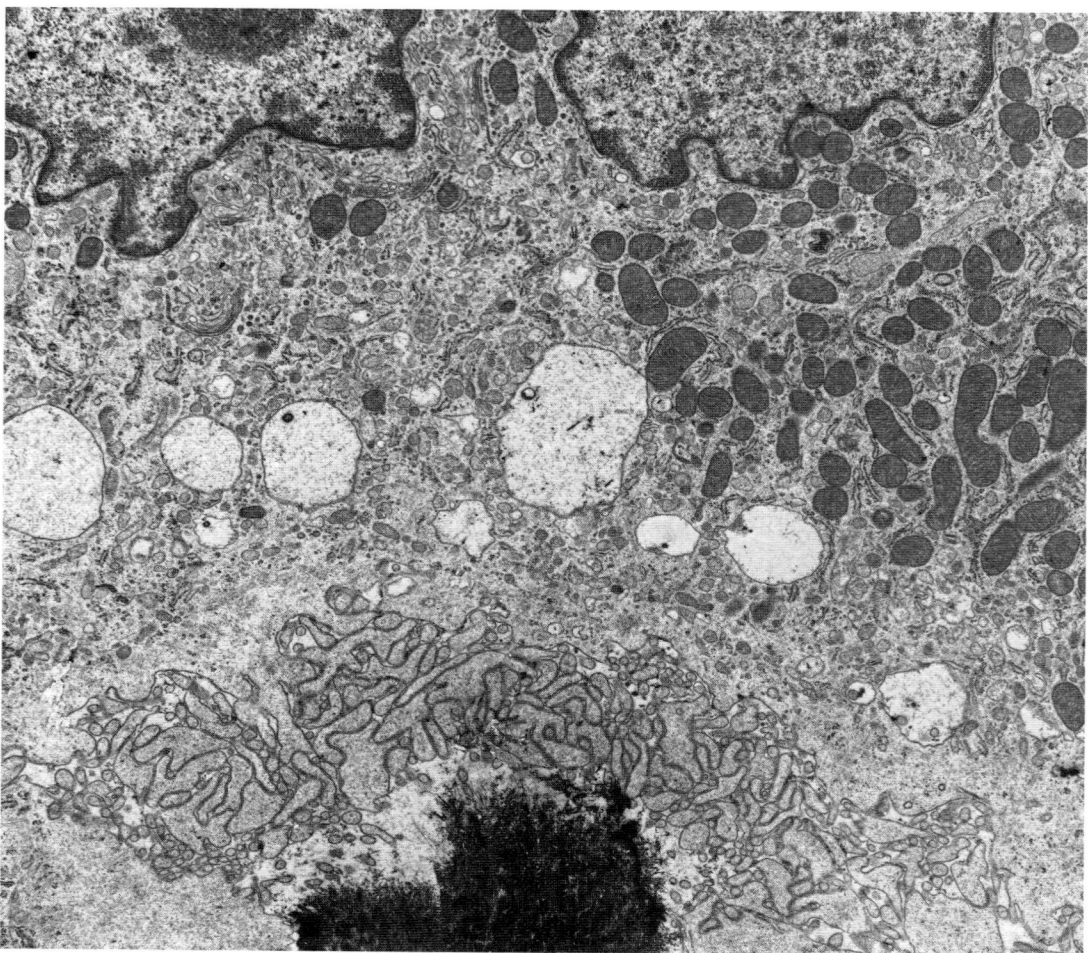

FIG. 3. Electron micrograph of a rat osteoclast. Note the extensive ruffled border area with the disrupted bone surface below it. Clear or sealing zones are seen apposed to the bone at the margins of the ruffled border area. There are many large vacuoles as well as lysosomes subjacent to the ruffled border area. Abundant mitochondria and prominent golgi are seen close to the multiple nuclei. (Figure kindly provided by Dr. Scott C. Miller, Division of Radiobiology, University of Utah).

there must be some difference in the specific attachment process between these cells and osteoclasts to account for the preferential binding of the latter to mineralized surfaces.

The basolateral surfaces of the osteoclast are also specialized. This surface appears to have binding sites for a variety of agglutinins and also appears to contain coated pits (112–114) as well as the transport systems necessary for maintaining osteoclast function, including a calcium extrusion pump, sodium–potassium pumps (Na$^+$,K$^+$-ATPase), and a Cl$^-$–HCO$_3^-$ exchanger (see below).

Perhaps the most remarkable specialization of the osteoclast is the ruffled border. This area contains the elements to resorb both the organic and inorganic components of bone (115). Both activities depend on extracellular acidification of the area under the ruffled border (116–119). This acidification is accomplished by

a proton pump which has been compared to the H$^+$,K$^+$-ATPase at the luminal border of the kidney and in the acid-secreting cells of the stomach. The details of the osteoclast proton pump have not been fully elucidated; however, this pump does appear to be sensitive to *N*-ethylmaleimide, similar to the proton pump of the kidney (120). Recent isolation of the renal proton pump should lead to more information on the similarities and differences between these two hydrogen transport systems (121). Although similarity to the gastric proton pump was initially postulated because of the inhibitory effect of omeprazole, this occurs only at high drug concentrations (122,123). Moreover, the osteoclast pump differs from the gastric H$^+$,K$^+$-ATPase in being resistant to inhibition by vanadate (120). This electrogenic proton pump requires ATP, which is presumably maintained by the abundant mitochondria in osteoclasts. ATP is presumably also important for the sodium–potassium pump and the calcium extrusion pump in the basolateral membrane of the cell (101,124–126).

The main source of hydrogen ion for the proton pump is carbonic acid. Osteoclasts contain large amounts of carbonic anhydrase to facilitate the conversion of CO_2 and H_2O to H_2CO_3 (127–129). The location and amount of this enzyme varies with hormonal changes in osteoclastic activity. Thus carbonic anhydrase is concentrated in the ruffled border area when osteoclasts are stimulated, and it becomes diffusely spread through the cytoplasm when activity is inhibited. The generation of protons from carbonic acid results in an excess of bicarbonate in the cell which, in turn, must be removed at the basolateral border, probably by chloride–bicarbonate exchange (130–132). An Na^+–H^+ antiporter may also be important in proton transport, and this could bypass the anion exchanger (133). Hydrogen ions not only are important for ruffled border function (134), but may also regulate intracellular calcium movement in osteoclasts (135,136).

The degradation of bone matrix is presumably the result of the activity of a number of lysosomal enzymes which can degrade collagen as well as the noncollagenous components of bone at low pH (6,7). Although it may not be the most important of the degradative enzymes, tartrate-resistant acid phosphatase (TRAP)—also known as "purple acid phosphatase"—has been studied extensively because it is abundant in osteoclasts and relatively less prominent in other cells (137–142). This type of acid phosphatase has been isolated and purified from bone and is found not only in osteoclast itself, but in presumptive mononuclear precursors. Tartrate resistance is not specific for osteoclastic acid phosphatase, and similar enzyme activity can be found in other tissues—particularly macrophages (143). Nevertheless, there is a correlation between activation of bone resorption and acid phosphatase movement and release (144,145). This correlation is equally good for other lysosomal enzymes (146). A variety of cathepsins and other lytic enzymes which are produced by the osteoclast are able to degrade collagen at low pH (115). Whether there is a specific collagenase among this family of enzymes has not yet been established, but the classic mammalian collagenase found in fibroblasts and macrophages has not been identified in the osteoclast (6).

The polarized secretion of lysosomal enzymes by osteoclasts has now been described in some detail (101,124,147). The initial step is the targeting of these enzymes from their sites of synthesis in the endoplasmic reticulum to transport vesicles via the Golgi apparatus. The Golgi apparatus and vesicles are enriched in mannose-6-phosphate receptors (101,148), and the lysosomal enzymes themselves have specific recognition markers for this receptor. The exocytic pathway ultimately ends at the ruffled border membrane with which the transport vesicles presumably fuse to release their enzymes into the acid extracellular environment. Thus the usual formation of an intracellular acidic phagolysosome seen in macrophages and neutrophils is essentially exteriorized to the surface of the bone by this process. It seems likely that much of the degradation of the matrix occurs extracellularly in the ruffled border area, but some pinocytotic vesicles may be formed which engulf the extracellular contents of the ruffled border area and continue the degradative process.

There is evidence that oxygen-derived free radicals are produced by osteoclasts and may be localized in the ruffled border area (149,150). Superoxide dismutase, which depletes tissue of superoxide anions, can block bone resorption (149), and this enzyme has been identified in osteoclasts (151). A specific role for superoxide in the resorptive process is not proven, but a defect in its generation by leukocytes has been found in one form of osteopetrosis (152).

Complex transport processes are required to maintain these osteoclast functions. Membrane polarization, selective sodium–potassium transport, active ATPase-dependent calcium extrusion, and multiple K^+ conductances have been identified in this cell (126,153–155). Extracellular calcium may regulate intracellular calcium and stimulate transport in osteoclasts (156,157). The complete series of steps required for calcium transport are still not fully understood. At present, the simplest hypothesis is that the initial dissolution of bone mineral is due to the secretion of protons which convert surface phosphates on hydroxyapatite to more soluble hydrogen phosphate (158). This would release calcium ions but could conceivably also result in the release of undissolved hydroxyapatite crystals. Ion transport through the cell with a calcium extrusion pump on the basolateral membrane would be one mechanism for recovering the ion. Voltage-dependent calcium channels have been identified in isolated osteoclasts, but they have not yet been localized to a functional site (159). Uptake of crystals with dissolution in acidic vacuoles and subsequent extrusion could be another mechanism for calcium removal. Finally, it is possible that some of the calcium escapes through the sealing zone, perhaps facilitated by a carrier molecule. One candidate for such a molecule is hyaluronic acid. It is known that hyaluronic acid production is increased during bone resorption, but its role in the resorptive process has not been identified (160,161).

HOW IS OSTEOCLASTIC BONE RESORPTION REGULATED?

A large number of local and systemic factors which regulate osteoclastic bone resorption have been identified, and these probably act at different sites and by different mechanisms. Before discussing the specific actions of individual agents, we will review some of the general features of regulation. As discussed above, many of the regulatory factors appear to have their primary action on cells of the osteoblast lineage (38). The molecular and biochemical mechanisms of action of PTH, 1,25(OH)$_2$D$_3$, IL-1, PGE$_2$, and other activators of bone resorption on these cells are discussed in greater detail elsewhere in this volume. Multiple cellular mechanisms clearly exist, and the current concept is that the osteoblast responds to these factors through both cyclic-AMP-dependent and cyclic-AMP-independent mechanisms (162–169). Activation of the phosphatidylinositol (PI) pathway and direct effects on calcium channels have been identified in osteoblastic cells, and these presumably could be important in the initial activation process. Although effects of hormones and local factors on cyclic AMP, PI, and calcium entry in osteoblastic cells have been described in some detail, there is only indirect evidence implicating these different pathways in osteoclast activation. Under some circumstances a nonosteoblastic cell pathway may be involved in initiating resorption, since the removal of mineralized cartilage by chondroclasts appears to involve the same final common pathway; that is, the chondroclast and osteoclast are functionally similar, but the typical osteoblastic lining cells are not present. In this situation the activating cell could still be a stromal marrow cell of the osteoblastic lineage. Vascular invasion could be important in resorption of calcified cartilage and also in Haversian remodeling. It is not clear how local or systemic factors regulate this process, nor whether a nonosteoblastic cell such as an endothelial cell could mediate hormonal activation.

Whatever the mechanism of activation, recruitment of new osteoclasts is clearly the vital next step. Under most physiological and pathological circumstances, an increase in bone resorption is accomplished largely by increasing the number of osteoclasts on the bone surface rather than simply activating existing fully differentiated osteoclasts. However, an increase in osteoblast number does not necessarily require cell replication if enough precursor cells are already present. For example, the resorptive response to PTH in fetal rat long-bone organ cultures is not blocked by hydroxyurea or aphidicolin, agents which can inhibit DNA synthesis (170). On the other hand, these inhibitors of cell replication can block the resorptive response to some stimulators, particularly epidermal growth factor (EGF) or transforming growth factor α (TGF-α) and PGE$_2$ (171–174). There is as yet no explanation for this difference among stimulators of bone resorption. It does not appear to depend on whether the agent is local or systemic, since the effect of IL-1, which acts locally, is not markedly inhibited by blocking cell replication. The resorptive response to phorbol esters and the basal level of resorption that occurs in unstimulated control cultures of fetal rat long bones are also decreased by inhibitors of cell replication. This suggests that basal bone resorption is maintained, at least in part, by continued replication of osteoblast pre-

cursors and that perhaps protein kinase C is involved in this response (174). Interestingly, pertussis toxin has effects similar to those of inhibitors of cell replication in this model (175,176), but a pertussis-toxin-sensitive regulatory protein which is involved in cell replication or which activates protein kinase C has not yet been identified in bone.

The differentiation and migration of precursor cells to the bone surface has been examined in in vitro and in vivo model systems, as well as during fetal development (60,137,177). These studies clearly indicate that when bone resorption is stimulated, there is an increase in the number of TRAP-positive mononuclear cells in the periosteum. These may attach to bone as mononuclear cells, but it is not clear that they can actually resorb bone without fusion. It seems more likely that small polykaryons must be formed for the osteoclast to be large enough to produce a sealing zone and ruffled border (178).

The modulation of the activity of fully formed and differentiated osteoclasts appears to be more limited. Inhibition clearly can be demonstrated with calcitonin and high concentrations of prostaglandins. These effects are presumably related to increased cyclic AMP production and can be mimicked by agents which increase cyclic AMP in the osteoclast (179–191). Studies on the role of cyclic AMP in osteoclastic bone resorption have been complicated by the fact that resorption is measured in organ cultures, and that the cyclic AMP effect in osteoblasts may be opposite to that in osteoclasts—that is, the osteoblast response results in increased resorption, although this may be only part of the second-messenger system. Thus agents which increase adenylyl cyclase activity, such as forskolin and cholera toxin, or which increase cyclic AMP levels by inhibiting cyclic nucleotide phosphodiesterase, such as isobutyl methyl xanthine, have often produced biphasic responses in organ culture. Similarly, PGE$_2$ can cause transient inhibition followed by prolonged stimulation of bone resorption (192,193).

Although the inhibitory effects of calcitonin are readily demonstrated in isolated mammalian osteoclasts, it has been difficult to demonstrate these effects in avian osteoclasts (194,195). This may be because they are down-regulated by high endogenous calcitonin levels, since osteoclasts from chicks on a low-calcium diet have been found to respond to calcitonin (196). On the other hand, a recent histochemical study showed that adenylate cyclase was abundant in chick osteoblasts but that it could not be identified in osteoclasts (197).

The first effect of calcitonin on osteoclasts in vivo appears to be a decrease in the ruffled borders (198). The contraction of isolated osteoclasts cultured on glass may reflect this membrane effect (199). Lysosomal enzyme release as well as the high proton concentration in the area within the sealing zone quickly disappear with calcitonin treatment. In organ cultures, ^{45}Ca release decreases to the values seen with dead bones; that is, cell-mediated resorption is completely blocked. In the short term, the attachment apparatus of the sealing zone may still be present; however, in many in vivo studies the osteoclasts are found away from the bone surface after calcitonin treatment, and their number (even in the marrow space) progressively diminishes. These effects may have been most strikingly observed with pathologic osteoclasts in Paget's disease and may not be as significant for normal osteoclasts, which can remain attached, escape from inhibition, and begin to resorb again in organ culture.

Although it has been difficult to increase the activity of isolated osteoclasts with hormones or local factors, this may be an artifact of the culture system used; that is, isolated osteoclasts may already be fully activated or have lost the capacity to respond to stimulators. In organ culture, administration of PTH can produce a rapid increase in ruffled border area which appears to precede the increase in osteoclast number (200). There is evidence that such activation can also occur in mixed cultures of osteoblasts and osteoclasts, but this could be due to recruitment; moreover, the direct activation of a specific individual osteoclast has been difficult to demonstrate. Morphologic studies on the reactivation of osteoclasts which escape from inhibition by calcitonin has supported the concept that individual osteoclasts can increase as well as decrease their activity (182,189).

WHAT ARE THE ACTIONS AND INTERACTIONS OF SYSTEMIC AND LOCAL STIMULATORS OF BONE RESORPTION?

Some of the many agents which can stimulate bone resorption under physiologic or pathologic conditions are listed in Table 1. The most important systemic stimulators are probably PTH and $1,25(OH)_2D_3$, whereas the most important local stimulators are probably PGE_2 and IL-1. Among the other systemic stimulators, thyroid hormones, vitamin A, and PTHrP have clearly been shown to increase osteoclastic activity. There is a much larger list of potential local regulators, including other cytokines and eicosanoids as well as numerous growth factors. Many factors have dual actions in the sense that they stimulate bone resorption both directly and by increasing endogenous prostaglandin production.

A number of synergistic interactions among bone resorbers have also been identified. One of the first to be described was the interaction between bacterial lipopolysaccharide and the major resorbers, PTH, PGE_2, and IL-1 (201). This interaction may be important in the pathogenesis of bone loss in periodontal disease. Subsequent studies showed synergism between IL-1 and PTH or PTHrP, and even between the cytokines which have been identified as osteoclast-activating factors; that is, tumor necrosis factors α and β [TNF-α and TNF-β (lymphotoxins)] were shown to interact synergistically with

TABLE 1. *Physiologic and pathologic regulators of bone resorption*

Stimulators
Parathyroid hormone
Parathyroid-hormone-related peptide
1,25-Dihydroxyvitamin D
Interleukin-1 and tumor necrosis factor
Thyroid hormones
Vitamin A
Transforming growth factor/epidermal growth factor
Fibroblast growth factor
Heparin
Bacterial endotoxin
Thrombin
Bradykinin

Biphasic regulators
Prostaglandin E_2 and other prostanoids
Transforming growth factor β
Lymphocyte inhibitory factor/differentiation inducing factor

Inhibitors
Calcitonin and related peptides
Interferon-gamma
Glucocorticoids
Estrogens and androgens

Possible agonists—effects not established
Interleukin-6
Colony-stimulating factors—GMCSF and MCSF

IL-1 (202–204). Some of these interactions may be dependent on endogenous prostaglandin synthesis. In cultures of osteoblastic cells a synergistic enhancement of PGE_2 production has been demonstrated with several different combinations, including PTH and IL-1, IL-1 and TGF-α/EGF, and IL-1 and TGF-β (205–208). These synergistic interactions occur at low concentrations and may be important in physiologic and pathologic responses. Maximal rates of resorption that can be achieved in organ culture systems are probably limited by the tissue and not by the amount of agonist; thus when maximally effective concentrations are employed, it is usually not possible to demonstrate further stimulation of bone resorption. However, the addition of a high concentration of prostacyclin (PGI_2) was found to enhance the resorptive response to a maximally effective dose of PTH (192).

Parathyroid Hormone

Although PTH is the most extensively studied of the bone resorbers, there are still many questions about its action. In organ culture systems the resorptive response generally requires higher concentrations than are encountered in vivo. This may be due, in part, to rapid degradation or nonspecific binding of PTH in these culture systems. Increased sensitivity to PTH can be achieved in vitro by adding substances which can protect against binding or degradation (209,210). PTH does stimulate endogenous prostaglandin production in bone (211–215), but this is not essential for the resorptive response. PTH can also increase the production of IL-6 by bone cells (216). This cytokine has not been shown to mediate stimulation of bone resorption directly, but it may enhance the response to IL-1 (217).

The bone-resorbing activity of PTH is closely mimicked by PTHrP. Some differences in potency between synthetic PTHrP 1–34 and various forms of PTH have been reported, but in all cases the effects are qualitatively similar (218–225). Moreover, PTHrP and PTH can both increase the production of multinucleated cells in mouse bone marrow cultures (226). Since most of these studies have been carried out with the N-terminal peptides of PTHrP, which have the greatest similarity to PTH, there may be qualitative differences in the effects on resorption with larger forms of the PTHrP molecule, but PTHrP 1–84, 1–108, and 1–141 also stimulate resorption (227). Both PTH and PTHrP have been shown to act on osteoblasts, and there is evidence that they stimulate the secretion of specific mediators of osteoclast activation. However, as noted above, these mediators have not yet been fully characterized, and additional effects on the osteoclast lineage itself have not been ruled out.

Vitamin D

Although $1,25(OH)_2D_3$ is a more potent stimulator of bone resorption on a molar basis in organ culture than is PTH, it is probably not as important in stimulating bone resorption in vivo (228,229). In renal osteodystrophy and vitamin D deficiency, with low levels of $1,25(OH)_2D_3$ and high levels of PTH, bone resorption can be markedly increased. Moreover, in renal failure, resorption is decreased by oral administration of $1,25(OH)_2D_3$, presumably by reducing secondary hyperparathyroidism. The concentrations of $1,25(OH)_2D_3$ which stimulate bone resorption are such that one can assay this hormone in blood using the resorptive response, but this requires that the hormone be extracted to separate it from its plasma-binding proteins (230). Increased levels of $1,25(OH)_2D_3$ are probably sufficient to increase bone resorption in severe calcium deficiency when total concentrations are as high as 10^{-9} M and when free hormone levels are as high as 10^{-11} M.

As noted above, $1,25(OH)_2D_3$ does appear to play an important role in the formation and differentiation of osteoclasts. In vitro studies using a variety of marrow culture systems have shown increased formation of multinucleated cells, some of which clearly have osteoclastic phenotype. The importance of this effect in vivo is not fully established; however, it is of interest that in severe vitamin D deficiency, replacement of calcium and phosphate by infusion restored bone formation to normal,

but remodeling of the metaphysis by osteoclasts appeared to be diminished (231). Structure activity relations for vitamin D metabolites have generally shown that their bone-resorbing activity parallels other activities mediated by the vitamin D receptor. Recently, however, analogs of $1,25(OH)_2D_3$ have been produced in which the bone-resorptive and cell-differentiation activities are dissociated (232,233).

Prostaglandins

There is ample evidence that PGE_2 can play a central role in the local regulation of bone resorption (234,235). In vivo studies have suggested that the resorptive response to immobilization and to orthodontic tooth movement can be blunted by inhibitors of prostaglandin synthesis and increased by local administration of PGE_2 (14,236). On the other hand, as noted above, the initial hypocalcemic response to IL-1 may be due to PGE_2-mediated inhibition of osteoclasts (11). Mechanical forces have complex biphasic effects on prostaglandin production by bone cells which could mediate local resorptive responses to stress (237).

The mechanisms by which mechanical forces modulate bone resorption are poorly understood; however, compressive forces can decrease osteoclastic activity, and immobilization can produce an increase (15,238,239). The latter response is blocked by indomethacin. It is tempting to assign a role for prostaglandins in the inhibitory response to compression, but there is as yet no evidence for this.

PGE_2 is the most abundant eicosanoid produced by bone, but not the only one (240,241). Other prostaglandins of the E series are also potent bone resorbers (242,243). Prostacyclin is the next most abundant product of arachidonic acid in bone after PGE_2, but it does not appear to be an important mediator of the resorptive response in mouse calvarial organ culture (244). Small amounts of $PGF_{2\alpha}$ can also be produced by bone, and exogenous $PGF_{2\alpha}$ can stimulate bone resorption. However, its effect appears to be due, at least in part, to an increase in endogenous PGE_2 production (245). Other products of oxygenated fatty acids, such as the leukotrienes, may have effects on bone metabolism, but here again stimulation of endogenous PGE_2 production may mediate the response (246).

Although nonsteroidal anti-inflammatory drugs (NSAIDs) have been used extensively to analyze the role of prostaglandins in physiologic and pathologic responses in the skeleton (247–250), interpretation is complicated by the fact that the effects of NSAIDs on prostaglandin production in bone may be biphasic, with inhibition of PGE_2 production at high concentrations (10^{-5} to 10^{-7} M) and stimulation of PGE_2 production at low concentrations (10^{-9} to 10^{-11} M) (251). Nevertheless, using high concentrations of indomethacin to inhibit prostaglandin synthesis, a variety of resorptive responses in bone organ culture have been shown to be mediated by increases in endogenous prostaglandin production (252–255).

Interleukin-1 and Other Cytokines

The concept that a cytokine derived from hematopoietic cells could stimulate bone resorption was derived from the finding, almost 20 years ago, that conditioned medium from cultures of antigen- or agglutinin-stimulated human mononuclear cells could increase ^{45}Ca release in organ culture (256,257). This activity was named "osteoclast activating factor" and was subsequently shown to be IL-1, both by direct purification and by studies using specific antisera (258,259). However, it was found that other cytokines derived from leukocytes could stimulate bone resorption, particularly TNF-α and TNF-β (lymphotoxins) (260,261). IL-1α and IL-1β are probably somewhat more potent stimulators of resorption than are the TNFs. All four cytokines have both prostaglandin-independent and prostaglandin-dependent effects on bone resorption which appear to vary with the model used and even in different studies using the same model (252,262,263). This variation may depend, in part, on an early effect of PGE$_2$ to increase the replication of osteoclast precursors. Thus pretreatment with indomethacin can blunt the response to IL-1, whereas simultaneous addition is much less effective (264). Recent studies have shown that human osteoblast-like cells can produce TNF and that this can be stimulated by other cytokines (265). Bone organ cultures can also produce both IL-1α and IL-1β, although the specific cell source has not been identified (266).

The role of other cytokines in mediating bone resorption is less well established. As mentioned above, IL-6 may enhance IL-1-stimulated resorption. A differentiation-inducing factor, which is also a lymphocyte inhibitory factor (LIF), has been found to stimulate bone resorption by a prostaglandin-dependent mechanism, but to inhibit resorption in cultured fetal-rat long bones (267–269). CSF, particularly granulocyte–macrophage CSF (GMCSF) and macrophage CSF (MCSF), have been identified in bone cell cultures (270–272), and their release is stimulated by other cytokines (273,274). The CSFs appear to stimulate cell replication along alternate pathways, which can decrease the formation of multinucleated osteoclasts and inhibit osteoclast activity (275–277). However, the effect on bone resorption in vivo requires further study because, as noted above, a defect in MCSF production has been identified in osteopetrotic animals which also have defective osteoclastic bone resorption (88).

Thyroid Hormones

An increase in bone resorption in hyperthyroidism is apparent from clinical studies, but evidence for direct stimulation of bone resorption is limited. Both thyroxine and triiodothyronine can increase calcium release from fetal rat long bones and neonatal mouse calvaria (278–280). The response in mouse calvaria appears to be partially, but not completely, dependent on endogenous prostaglandin production.

Vitamin A

Vitamin A (retinol) was actually the first agent shown [by Fell and Mellanby (281) in 1952] to stimulate bone resorption in vitro. Retinoids have been used to stimulate bone resorption and produce hypercalcemia in vivo (282). Retinoic acid is also an important differentiating factor for bone cells and can enhance the effect of 1,25(OH)$_2$D$_3$ to produce activation and fusion of mouse alveolar macrophages (283). Retinoic acid is not as effective or as potent as 1,25(OH)$_2$D$_3$ in stimulating osteoclast function and does not show the positive interaction with fetal calf serum that occurs with 1,25(OH)$_2$D$_3$ (284). Retinol has also been shown to have a direct effect on podosome distribution in isolated osteoclasts (103), and both retinol and retinoic acid may stimulate osteoclast activity directly (285).

Growth Factors

As noted above, growth factors have been shown to stimulate bone resorption by increasing endogenous PGE$_2$ production (253,254). In fetal rat long-bone cultures, EGF/TGF-α can stimulate resorption independent of prostaglandin synthesis (286–288); however, under certain conditions, specifically with the addition of IL-1 or hydroxyurea, the response is converted to a prostaglandin-dependent one (171,172). Similar findings have been obtained recently with fibroblast growth factors (FGFs). In mouse calvaria, both acidic and basic FGFs were found to stimulate resorption by a prostaglandin-dependent mechanism (289); in fetal rat long bones, however, FGFs could stimulate bone resorption by both prostaglandin-dependent and prostaglandin-independent mechanisms (290,291). The prostaglandin-independent response to acidic FGF was only obtained in the presence of heparin, and the response to basic FGF was enhanced by heparin. In this connection, it is of interest that heparin has been shown to enhance bone resorption in organ cultures in the presence of serum (292) as well as in vivo, but not in chemically defined medium (291). Thus it is possible that the bone resorption produced by heparin could be due to activation of heparin-binding growth factors, such as FGFs, which are found in skeletal tissue and produced by bone cells (293,294).

Although TGF-β can stimulate bone resorption by increasing prostaglandin production, its major effect appears to be inhibitory (see below). This may also be the case for LIF. There are relatively few studies of the effect of growth factors on bone resorption in vivo. EGF has been shown to produce hypercalcemia and to increase osteoclast number (295,296).

WHAT STOPS OSTEOCLASTIC BONE RESORPTION?

The existence of such a large number of stimuli which can increase the number and activity of osteoclasts makes it all the more remarkable that the number of resorption sites and their size is normally so well-limited. On the other hand, pathologic conditions in which bone resorption is excessive are common; for example, excessive resorption is the major pathogenetic mechanism in hypercalcemia, Paget's disease, localized bone loss associated with inflammation, and most forms of osteoporosis. There are only a few known physiologic inhibitors of osteoclastic bone resorption (Table 1).

Calcitonin

The best-studied and probably the most potent inhibitor of bone resorption is calcitonin, which causes a rapid contraction and loss of motility of osteoclasts and a marked but transient decrease in resorptive activity. The changes in motility and in resorption are not necessarily connected, since a return of motility can occur when resorption is still inhibited (199,297,298). The transient nature of calcitonin inhibition, which has been termed the "escape phenomenon" (299), is still not fully understood. There is evidence that inhibition of cell replication can delay escape (300), suggesting that the phenomenon depends on the formation of new calcitonin-resistant osteoclasts, but isolated osteoclasts have been shown to resume resorptive activity in the presence of high concentrations of the hormone (182,298). Down-regulation of calcitonin receptors has been amply demonstrated in other cell populations (301) and probably occurs in osteoclasts as well. This could explain the observation that osteoclasts from calcium-replete chickens are unresponsive to calcitonin, presumably because they have high endogenous calcitonin secretion, whereas osteoclasts from calcium-deficient chickens show calcitonin receptors and a response to the hormone (302). Escape appears to depend on continuous presence of high concentrations of calcitonin, and sustained effects on resorption can be seen in vivo when the hormone is given intermittently.

Peptides related to calcitonin can inhibit bone resorption. These include not only the calcitonin-gene-related peptides (CGRPs) (303,304), but also amylinamide, a protein that is co-secreted from the beta cells of the pancreas with insulin (305,306). Although high concentrations of these peptides are required to inhibit bone resorption, they could play a role as local regulators. Moreover, CGRPs have effects on cyclic AMP in bone cell populations which do not respond to calcitonin (307).

Glucocorticoids

A direct inhibitory effect on bone resorption has been observed with glucocorticoids both in vivo and in vitro (308–310), although some studies have shown stimulation (311,312). It is possible that glucocorticoids can transiently enhance the formation or function of osteoclasts, but when the hormone is present for longer periods, bone resorptive activity is reduced as a result of decreased replication of precursors. In vivo, increased bone resorption is often seen with glucocorticoids because of impaired calcium absorption and secondary hyperparathyroidism (313). Glucocorticoids can inhibit prostaglandin production, and hence they are particularly effective in blocking resorptive responses which are prostaglandin-dependent. There may also be selective inhibitory effects for specific resorbers. For example, PTH and $1,25(OH)_2D_3$ are relatively resistant, whereas the response to IL-1 can be diminished by relatively low concentrations of glucocorticoids (200); this may be responsible for the effectiveness of glucorticoid therapy in myeloma (314).

Estrogens and Androgens

Sex hormones are clearly important physiologic regulators of bone resorption. Their inhibitory effect has repeatedly been demonstrated in vivo; however, in vitro studies failed to show inhibition at physiologic concentrations (315). Because of this, it was thought that the sex hormone effect was indirect, but recent evidence indicates that sex hormones have direct effects on bones which may involve both inhibition of resorption and stimulation of formation (316). Estrogens and androgens can inhibit PTH-stimulated cyclic-AMP production in bone cells (317,318). The release of calcium from cultured neonatal mouse calvaria can be decreased by 17β-estradiol at concentrations of 10^{-10} to 10^{-12} M, which are similar to the free concentrations present in vivo (319). Estrogens can also decrease prostaglandin release from bone in vitro, but it is possible that the effects on resorption and on prostaglandin production are separate. Prostaglandin production is increased in cultured calvaria from oophorectomized rats, and it is decreased by administration of estradiol in vivo (320). Production of other local factors such as IGF-1 and TGF-β can be affected by sex hormones (321,322), and the latter could mediate inhibition of bone resorption. Estrogen administration has also been found to decrease IL-1, TNF-α, and GM-CSF production by circulating macrophages (323,324). If cells of the monocyte–macrophage series in bone were to release smaller amounts of cytokines in the presence of sex hormones, this could also affect resorption.

Local Inhibitors

One of the most perplexing questions concerning osteoclast regulation is the mechanism by which bone resorption is stopped locally. One possibility is that the depths of Howship's lacunae and the lengths of Haversian canals produced by active osteoclasts are limited by the lifespan of those osteoclasts (325,326). Thus with each activation cycle a generation of osteoclasts appear which can carry out only a limited amount of resorption. In this regard, it has been suggested that pathologic "killer" osteoclasts are responsible for the marked loss of trabecular bone that occurs in rapidly progressive osteoporosis (327). However, it seems likely that there are local humoral regulators which can limit the rate or extent of resorption. One candidate for such a local factor is interferon-gamma (IFN-γ). This cytokine might be produced by the macrophages present on the bone surface during the reversal phase. IFN-γ has been shown to inhibit the formation of osteoclast-like cells in marrow cultures (328) and to block the stimulation of resorption by PTH and PGE$_2$, although its greatest effectiveness appears to be against IL-1 (262,329,330). Inhibition of resorption by IFN-γ appears to be associated with decreased proliferation of osteoclast precursors and does not show the escape phenomenon associated with calcitonin (331). Surprisingly, IFN-γ was found to stimulate production of osteoclast-like cells on implanted bone particles (332).

As noted above, CSF may steer cell replication and differentiation away from osteoclast formation, and these factors are also produced by bone cells and could act to stop further recruitment of osteoclasts at resorbing sites. LIF may also be a local inhibitor, although its effects are biphasic.

A prime candidate for the factor which stops the resorptive process is TGF-β (333). Although TGF-β can stimulate resorption in some organ culture systems by a prostaglandin-dependent mechanism, its direct effect appears to be inhibitory (334,335). Moreover, PTH and other stimulators of bone resorption can increase TGF-β activity in bone organ and cell cultures (336,337). Bone-derived TGF-β is probably released as a latent complex and activated during the resorptive process (338,339).

Both TGF-β and another bone-derived growth factor, osteoinductive factor (OIF), have been shown to inhibit osteoclast function in vitro (340); however, the effects of TGF-β on osteoclast formation are biphasic, with enhancement of 1,25(OH)$_2$ stimulation at low concentrations and inhibition at high concentrations (341). The stimulatory effect appears to depend on PG production.

The ability of PGE$_2$ and other prostaglandins to inhibit the activity of osteoclasts could also play a role in stopping resorption (12). The structure–activity relations for this effect may differ somewhat from those for the slow stimulation of resorption, and it is possible that compounds other than PGE$_2$, particularly PGI$_2$, could play a role. Since prostaglandin production is local, the pattern of responses could vary with the specific eicosanoid produced, the type of responding cell present, and the duration and intensity of the stimulus (342).

Other local inhibitors may exist. Culture medium from bones which have been subjected to intermittent compressive forces can inhibit osteoclastic resorption (238). Specific inhibitors which act selectively against a particular stimulator could be important. For example, macrophages can secrete an IL-1 receptor antagonist which selectively blocks the response to IL-1 (343,344).

HOW DO PHARMACOLOGIC AND PATHOLOGIC AGENTS AFFECT BONE RESORPTION?

A variety of pharmacologic agents have been shown to affect bone resorption. Some of these are agents which affect hormone production or which act on hormone receptors or second messengers. The latter include not only agents which increase cyclic AMP, but also agents which increase cell calcium and activate protein kinase C (345,346). However, these approaches have not yet led to the development of agents that are of potential clinical use as pharmacologic regulators of bone resorption.

Hormone Analogs

Although no practical therapeutic agent has yet emerged, PTH analogs, particularly those which are shortened at the amino terminus and further altered to prevent degradation, can act as potent inhibitors of PTH action in vitro and may be effective in vivo (347–349). Since PTH and PTHrP produce hypercalcemia by acting on the same receptor, such a molecule might also be effective in humoral hypercalcemia of malignancy.

A large number of calcitonin analogs have been synthesized. Some have been used to facilitate identification of the calcitonin receptor (350), whereas others are clinically useful because they are more potent or have a longer half-life. Although many different molecules with remarkably different sequences and structures have been tested (351), none has yet been shown to be free of side effects or to overcome the problem of the escape phenomenon. Calcitonin-gene-related peptide (CGRP), which is an alternative transcript of calcitonin mRNA, does have calcitonin-like activity in bone, but is much less potent. Bones treated with CGRP and PTH still show escape and appear to be cross-desensitized to calcitonin (352).

It may be possible to synthesize analogs of vitamin D which have selective activity on resorption (232,233). It is possible that the lactone form of $1,25(OH)_2D_3$ can act as a biological antagonist to the hormone and block bone resorption (353).

Phosphate Compounds

Although high concentrations of phosphate can inhibit bone resorption, this may be largely a physiochemical effect rather than an effect on cell function (354). Increasing phosphate concentration can decrease the rate of ^{45}Ca release from bone in organ culture, but it does not block the release of lysosomal enzymes or alter the structure of the osteoclast. Presumably, the high extracellular phosphate concentration is reflected in an increased phosphate concentration in the ruffled border area, where it could buffer hydrogen ions and prevent their action on hydroxyapatite crystals.

Another possibility is that a high concentration of inorganic phosphate increases the local concentration of pyrophosphate by slowing its hydrolysis. Pyrophosphate is a more potent inhibitor of hydroxyapatite crystal dissolution than is phosphate, and hence pyrophosphate should be a more potent inhibitor of resorption; however, in organ cultures or in vivo, pyrophosphate is hydrolyzed so rapidly that it is no more effective than phosphate. The effect of pyrophosphate on hydroxyapatite was part of the impetus for the development of the nonhydrolyzable pyrophosphate analogs in which the phosphates are connected by carbon rather than by oxygen. These bisphosphonates (formally called "diphosphonates") bind to hydroxyapatite and inhibit crystal growth and dissolution. However, as more and more of these compounds are synthesized and studied, it is clear that they can have a specific and selective inhibitory effect on osteoclastic bone resorption (355-362). The simplest explanation for the selective effect of bisphosphonates on osteoclasts is that they are first bound to the hydroxyapatite crystals in bone and then taken up by the osteoclasts during resorption. The various bisphosphonates would then be selectively toxic to the cells which have ingested them. However, there is also evidence that bisphosphonates can affect macrophages and osteoclast precursors. Whatever their mechanism, the bisphosphonates are the most potent pharmacologic inhibitors of bone resorption available for clinical use. The new,

highly potent compounds may ultimately supplant etidronate, the first bisphosphonate used extensively for the treatment of Paget's disease, hypercalcemia of malignancy, and osteoporosis.

Potassium peroxydiphosphate (KPDP) is a somewhat different pyrophosphate analog which is partially resistant to pyrophosphatase and which may release hydrogen peroxide or free oxygen radicals during hydrolysis. It can inhibit bone resorption and may also directly inactivate some bone-resorbing agents, presumably by oxidation (363).

Enzyme Inhibitors

Since collagenase, plasminogen activator, and lysosomal enzymes are all implicated in the resorptive process, it is not surprising that inhibitors of these enzymes have been tested as antiresorptive agents. This mechanism probably is the basis for inhibition of resorption by a number of synthetic peptides, antiarthritic agents, and bioflavonoids (364-372). Many of the lysosomal enzyme inhibitors are secondary amines, which might act not only by blocking enzyme activity but also by neutralizing the acidic environment, either in the lysosomal compartment itself or in the ruffled border area (373,374). This mechanism could also explain the antiresorptive effect of NH_4Cl (375).

Inhibitors of Ion Transport

Agents which inhibit hydrogen ion secretion, calcium transport, or chloride–bicarbonate exchange could inhibit bone resorption by blocking one of the essential transport steps required for the function of osteoclasts. Among the calcium antagonists, diphenylhydantoin, diltiazem, amrinone, and diclorbenzamin are inhibitors of bone resorption which may act by blocking calcium transport or sodium–calcium exchange (373,376-378). Omeprazole, an inhibitor of proton secretion, can also inhibit bone resorption, although the H^+,K^+-ATPase upon which it acts does not appear to be the primary proton pump in osteoclasts (122,123). Carbonic anhydrase inhibitors were among the earliest drugs shown to inhibit bone resorption, and there is a good correlation between potency as an enzyme inhibitor and as a resorption antagonist (379,380). Hydrochlorothiazide may act by a similar mechanism (381). The use of carbonic anhydrase inhibitors is limited, however, by the fact that they produce systemic acidosis.

Since chloride–bicarbonate exchange across the basolateral membrane is important in enabling the osteoclast to selectively secrete protons into the ruffled border area, inhibitors of this process might be expected to block resorption, and two stilbenes which can block anion transport were found to inhibit resorption in vitro (382). However, they also inhibit DNA and protein synthesis and are unlikely to be useful pharmacologic agents.

Other Pharmacologic Agents

A number of other agents have been used to inhibit bone resorption in vitro, and a few of these have now been tested clinically. In the past, plicamycin (mithramycin), an inhibitor of DNA-dependent RNA synthesis, was widely used in hypercalcemia of malignancy. Recently, a compound previously tested for use in malignancy, gallium nitrate, was also shown to inhibit osteoclast function and appears to be substantially less toxic than plicamycin (383,384). A radioprotective agent, WY-2721, has an interesting combination of effects which are useful for the treatment of hypercalcemia. It not only inhibits bone resorption, but also inhibits the secretion of PTH and increases the urinary excretion of calcium (385,386). This would make it particularly useful in hypercalcemic states in which excessive renal tubular reabsorption of calcium plays a major role. Immunosuppressive agents of the cyclosporine family have been shown to inhibit bone resorption in vitro (387,388) and in vivo (389), but they were reported to increase bone resorption when administered to oophorectomized rats (390). Thiophene-2-carboxylic acid was found to inhibit bone resorption by presently undefined mechanisms (391). Recently a derivative, thionapthene-2-carboxylic acid, was shown to be substantially more potent both in vivo and in vitro (392,393).

Bacterial lipopolysaccharide (LPS) and other bacterial products can stimulate osteoclastic bone resorption in organ culture and in vivo (394–398). Bacterial products probably act both directly and indirectly on bone cells, since there is evidence for stimulation of IL-1 and prostaglandin synthesis (399). LPS has been found to increase collagenase production in osteoblasts (400). Whatever the mechanism, bacterial products are clearly implicated in the pathogenesis of bone loss in both periodontal disease (401) and osteomyelitis. A role for prostaglandins as the final common pathway has been suggested by the observation that cyclo-oxygenase inhibition can slow bone loss in periodontal disease (250).

A number of ions can affect bone resorption, but it is not known whether they act directly on osteoclasts. Fluoride has been shown to inhibit bone resorption at high concentrations (402,403), but its major effect in humans appears to be to stimulate bone formation (404). Aluminum can increase calcium efflux from bone in culture (405). In vivo aluminum may produce hypercalcemia (406). Cadmium also increases bone resorption (407), possibly by stimulating prostaglandin production (255). While this could play a role in the bone disease produced by cadmium exposure, an effect on vitamin D activation by the kidney is likely to be the major pathogenetic mechanism (408). Lithium was recently found to block the action of calcitonin on osteoclasts (409). On the other hand, lithium can also inhibit the resorptive response to PTH (410). In vivo lithium often produces hypercalcemia, but this may be due to effects on the parathyroid glands and the intestine, rather than bone (411,412).

HOW CAN WE IMPROVE OUR UNDERSTANDING OF BONE RESORPTION?

This overview of osteoclastic bone resorption was presented in the form of a series of questions partly to point out the many gaps in our knowledge. Probably the most important of these is the fact that we have not identified the putative factor (or cell–cell interaction) which initiates osteoclast activity in remodeling. We also have not identified the factors which limit the activity of osteoclasts physiologically.

There are major technical obstacles which limit our understanding of the osteoclast. Local factors which presumably regulate osteoclast function may not be measurable in the blood and are likely to be present in bone only in small amounts and for short periods. We do not yet have in vitro models using fully defined cell populations in which we can examine all the steps in the resorptive process—namely, activation, osteoclast formation, and removal of bone mineral and matrix. However, the cell culture systems currently being used are rapidly approaching this goal.

It should be possible to use newer techniques of molecular biology—such as in situ hybridization, the polymerase chain reaction, and immunocytochemistry—to identify and quantitate local regulatory factors. Through such an analysis, selective inhibitors for specific pathogenetic factors which block abnormal, but not normal, bone remodeling may ultimately be developed and provide a better approach to the therapy of metabolic bone disease.

Finally, in developing strategies for defining the role of the osteoclast in the pathogenesis of the disease and for producing specific therapeutic agents that would control its role, we must not forget that osteoclastic resorption is essential for normal bone remodeling and, hence, for the maintenance of the structural integrity of the skeleton. Osteoclastic bone resorption is probably also necessary to maintain serum calcium concentration, although if intestinal supplies are adequate and bone formation is not rapid, this may require only a small proportion of the osteoclasts normally present.

REFERENCES

1. Boyde A, Jones SJ. Early scanning electron microscopic studies of hard tissue resorption: their relation to current concepts reviewed. *Scan Microsc* 1987;1:369–82.

2. Huffer WE. Morphology and biochemistry of bone remodeling: possible control by vitamin D, parathyroid hormone, and other substances. *Lab Invest* 1988;59:418–42.

3. Marks SC Jr, Popoff SN. Bone cell biology: the regulation of development, structure, and function in the skeleton. *Am J Anat* 1988;183:1–44.

4. Peck WA, Woods WL. The cells of bone. In: Riggs BL, Melton LI, eds. *Osteoporosis: etiology, diagnosis, and management.* New York: Raven Press, 1988;1–44.

5. Raisz LG. Local and systemic factors in the pathogenesis of osteoporosis. *N Engl J Med* 1988;318:818–27.

6. Sakamoto S, Sakamoto S. Degradative processes of connective tissue proteins with special emphasis on collagenolysis and bone resorption. *Mol Aspects Med* 1988;10:

7. Vaes G. Cellular biology and biochemical mechanism of bone resorption. *Clin Orthop* 1988;231:239–71.

8. Sissons HA, Kelman GJ, Marotti G. Bone resorption in calcium-deficient rats. *Bone* 1985;6:345–48.

9. Tashjian AH, Voelkel EF, Robinson DR, Levine L. Dietary menhaden oil lowers plasma prostaglandins and calcium in mice bearing the prostaglandin-producing $HSDM_1$ fibrosarcoma. *J Clin Invest* 1987;74:2042–8.

10. Boyce BF, Aufdemorte TB, Garrett IR, Yates AJP, Mundy GR. Effects of interleukin-1 on bone turnover in normal mice. *Endocrinology* 1989;125:1142–50.

11. Boyce BF, Yates AJP, Mundy GR. Bolus injections of recombinant human interleukin-1 cause transient hypocalcemia in normal mice. *Endocrinology* 1989;125:2780–3.

12. Fuller K, Chambers TJ. Effect of arachidonic acid metabolites on bone resorption by isolated rat osteoclasts. *J Bone Miner Res* 1989;4:209–15.

13. Burr DB, Martin RB, Schaffler MB, Radin EL. Bone remodeling in response to in vivo fatigue microdamage. *J Biomech* 1985;18:189–200.

14. Thompson DD, Rodan GA. Indomethacin inhibition of tenotomy-induced bone resorption in rats. *J Bone Miner Res* 1988;3:409–14.

15. Weinreb M, Rodan GA, Thompson DD. Osteopenia in the immobilized rat hind limb is associated with increased bone resorption and decreased bone formation. *Bone* 1989;10:187–94.

16. Marks SC Jr. Osteoclast biology: lessons from mammalian mutations. *Am J Med Genet* 1989;34:43–54.

17. Marks SC Jr, Popoff SN. Osteoclast biology in the osteopetrotic (op) rat. *Am J Anat* 1989;186:325–34.

18. Miller SC, Saintgeorges L, Bowman BM, Jee WSS. Bone lining cells—structure and function—review. *Scan Microsc* 1990;3:953–62.

19. Rouleau MF, Mitchell J, Goltzman D. In vivo distribution of parathyroid hormone receptors in bone: evidence that a predominant osseous target cell is not the mature osteoblast. *Endocrinology* 1988;123:187–91.

20. McSheehy PMJ, Chambers TJ. Osteoblastic cells mediate osteoclastic responsiveness to parathyroid hormone. *Endocrinology* 1986;118:824–8.

21. McSheehy PMJ, Chambers TJ. Osteoblast-like cells in the presence of parathyroid hormone release soluble factor that stimulates osteoclastic bone resorption. *Endocrinology* 1986;119:1654–9.

22. McSheehy PMJ, Chambers TJ. 1,25-Dihydroxyvitamin-D_3 stimulates rat osteoblastic cells to release a soluble factor that increases osteoblastic bone resorption. *J Clin Invest* 1987;80:425–9.

23. Perry HM, Skogen W, Chappel JC, Wilner GD, Kahn AJ, Teitelbaum SL. Conditioned medium from osteoblast-like cells mediate parathyroid hormone induced bone resorption. *Calcif Tissue Int* 1987;40:298–300.

24. Perry HM, Skogen W, Chappel J, Kahn AJ, Wilner G, Teitelbaum SR. Partial characterization of a parathyroid hormone-stimulated resorption factors from osteoblast-like cells. *Endocrinology* 1989;125:2075–83.

25. Dickson IR, Scheven BAA. Regulation of new osteoclast formation by a bone cell-derived macromolecular factor. *Biochem Biophys Res Commun* 1989;159:1383–90.

26. Morris CA, Mitnick ME, Weir EC, Horowitz M, Kreider BL, Insogna KL. The parathyroid hormone-related protein stimulates human osteoblast-like cells to secrete a 9,000 dalton bone-resorbing protein. *Endocrinology* 1990;126:1783–5.

27. Takahashi N, Akatsu T, Udagawa N, Sasaki T, Yamaguchi A, Moseley JM, Martin TJ, Suda T. Osteoblastic cells are involved in osteoclast formation. *Endocrinology* 1988;123:2600–2.

28. Udagawa N, Takahashi N, Akatsu T, Sasaki T, Yamaguchi A, Kodama H, Martin TJ, Suda T. The bone marrow-derived stromal cell lines MC3T3-G2/PA6 and ST2 support osteoclast-like cell differentiation in cocultures with mouse spleen cells. *Endocrinology* 1989;125:1805–14.

29. Chambers TJ, Darby JA, Fuller K. Mammalian collagenase predisposes bone surfaces to osteoclastic resorption. *Cell Tissue Res* 1985;243:671–5.

30. Shimizu H, Sakamoto S, et al. The effect of substrate composition and condition on resorption by isolated osteoclasts. *Bone Miner* 1989;6:261–76.

31. Shimizu H, Sakamoto S, Sakamoto M. Matrix collagen of devitalized bone is resistant to osteoclastic bone resorption. *Connect Tissue Res* 1989;20:169–75.

32. Delaisse J-M, Eeckhout Y, Vaes G. Bone-resorbing agents affect the production and distribution of procollagenase as well as the activity of collagenase in bone tissue. *Endocrinology* 1988;123:264–76.

33. Hamilton JA, Lingelbach S, Partridge NC, Martin TJ. Regulation of plasminogen activator production by bone-resorbing hormones in normal and malignant osteoblasts. *Endocrinology* 1985;116:2186–91.

34. Allan EH, Hamilton JA, Medcalf RL, Kubota M, Martin TJ. Cyclic AMP-dependent and -independent effects on tissue-type plasminogen activator activity in osteogenic sarcoma cells; evidence from phosphodiesterase inhibition and parathyroid hormone antagonists. *Biochim Biophys Acta* 1986;888:199–207.

35. Jilka PL. Procollagenase associated with the noncalcified matrix of bone and its regulation by parathyroid hormone. *Bone* 1990;10:353–8.

36. Thomson BM, Atkinson SJ, McGarrity AM, Hembry RM, Reynolds JJ, Meikle MC. Type I collagen degradation by mouse calvarial osteoclasts stimulated with 1,25-dihydroxyvitamin D_3: evidence for a plasminogenplasmin–metalloproteinase activation cascade. *Biochim Biophys Acta* 1990;1014:125–32.

37. Grills BL, Gallagher JA, Allan EH, Yumita S, Martin TJ. Identification of plasminogen activator in osteoclasts. *J Bone Miner Res* 1990;5:499–505.

38. Rodan GA, Martin TJ. Role of osteoblasts in hormonal control of bone resorption—a hypothesis. *Calcif Tissue Int* 1981;33:349–51.

39. Shen V, Rifas L, Kohler G, Peck WA. Prostaglandins change cell shape and increase intercellular gap junctions in osteoblasts cultured from rat fetal calvaria. *J Bone Miner Res* 1986;1(3):243–9.

40. Ali NN, Melhuish PB, Boyde A, Bennett A, Jones SJ. Parathyroid hormone, but not prostaglandin E_2, changes the shape of osteoblasts maintained on bone in vitro. *J Bone Miner Res* 1990;5:115–21.

41. Bargsten G, Stanka P. Light and electron microscopic study on the osteoclastic phagocytosis of cells in the rat. *Anat Anz* 1985;159:13–20.

42. Elmardi AS, Katchburian MV, Katchburian E. Electron microscopy of developing calvaria reveals images that suggest that osteoclasts engulf and destroy osteocytes during bone resorption. *Calcif Tissue Int* 1990;46:239–45.

43. Shimizu H, Sakamoto M, Sakamoto S. Bone resorption by isolated osteoclasts in living versus devitalized bone: differences in mode and extent and the effects of human recombinant tissue inhibitor of metalloproteinases. *J Bone Miner Res* 1990;5:411–8.

44. Gray TK, D'Amico C, Kaplan R, Dodd RC, Mesler D, Cohen MS. Mononuclear phagocytes secrete a protein that directly resorbs devitalized bone particles. *Bone Miner* 1986;1:235–45.

45. Leung DYM, Key L, Steinberg JJ, Young MC, Von Deck M, Wilkinson R, Geha RS. Increased in vitro bone resorption by monocytes in the hyper-immunoglobulin D syndrome. *J Immunol* 1988;149:84–8.

46. Chambers TJ. The origin of the osteoclast. In: Peck W, ed. *Bone and mineral research*, vol 6. New York: Elsevier, 1989;1–25.

47. Walker DG. Spleen cells transmit osteopetrosis in mice. *Science* 1975;190:785–6.
48. Coccia PF, Krivit W, Kersey JH, Kim TH, Nesbit ME, Ramsay KC, Warkentin PI, Teitelbaum SL, Kahn AJ, Brown DM. Successful bone marrow transplantation for infantile malignant osteopetrosis. *N Engl J Med* 1980;302:701.
49. Hattersley G, Chambers TJ. Generation of osteoclastic function in mouse bone marrow cultures: multinuclearity and tartrate-resistant acid phosphate are unreliable markers for osteoclastic differentiation. *Endocrinology* 1989;124:1689–96.
50. Hattersley G, Chambers TJ. Calcitonin receptors as markers for osteoclastic differentiation: correlation between generation of bone-resorptive cells and cells that express calcitonin receptors in mouse bone marrow cultures. *Endocrinology* 1989;125:1606–12.
51. Taylor LM, Tertinegg I, Okuda A, Heersche JNM. Expression of calcitonin receptors during osteoclast differentiation in mouse metatarsals. *J Bone Miner Res* 1989;4:751–8.
52. MacDonald BR, Mundy GR, Clark S, Wang EA, Kuehl TJ, Stanley ER, Roodman GD. Effects of human recombinant CSF-GM and highly purified CSF-1 on the formation of multinucleated cells with osteoclast characteristics in long-term bone marrow cultures. *J Bone Miner Res* 1986;1:227–233.
53. Takahashi N, Akatsu T, Sasaki T, Nicholson GC, Moseley JM, Martin TJ, Suda T. Induction of calcitonin receptors by $1\alpha,25$-dihydroxyvitamin D_3 in osteoclast-like multinucleated cells formed from mouse bone marrow cells. *Endocrinology* 1988;123:1504–10.
54. Takahashi N, Kukita T, Macdonald BR, et al. Osteoclast-like cells form in long-term human bone marrow but not in peripheral blood cultures. *J Clin Invest* 1989;83:543–550.
55. Oursler MJ, Osdoby P. Osteoclast development in marrow cultured in calvaria-conditioned media. *Dev Biol* 1988;127:170–8.
56. Fuller K, Chambers TJ. Generation of osteoclasts in cultures of rabbit bone marrow and spleen cells. *J Cell Physiol* 1987;132:441–52.
57. Kurihara N, Chenu C, Miller M, Civin C, Roodman GD. Identification of committed mononuclear precursors for osteoclast-like cells formed in long term human marrow cultures. *Endocrinology* 1990;126:2733.
58. Orcel P, Bielakoff J, de Vernejoul MC. Formation of multinucleated cells with osteoclast precursor features in human cord monocyte cultures. *Anat Rec* 1990;226:1–9.
59. Scheven BAA, Burger EH, Kawilarang-de Haas EWM, Wassenaar AM, Nijweide PJ. Effects of ionizing irradiation on formation and resorbing activity of osteoclasts in vitro. *Lab Invest* 1985;53:72–9.
60. Burger EH, Boonekamp PM, Nijweide PJ. Osteoblast and osteoclast precursors in primary cultures of calvarial bone cells. *Anat Rec* 1986;214:32–40.
61. Scheven BAA, Visser JWM, Nijweide PJ. In vitro osteoclast generation from different bone marrow fractions, including a highly enriched hematopoietic stem cell population. *Nature* 1986;321:79–80.
62. Helfrich MH, Thesingh CW, Mieremet RHP, van-Iperen Gent AS. Osteoclast generation from human fetal bone marrow in cocultures with murine fetal long bones. A model for in vitro study of human osteoclast formation and function. *Cell Tissue Res* 1987;249:125–36.
63. Helfrich MH, Mieremet RHP, Thesingh CW. Osteoclast formation in vitro from progenitor cells present in the adult mouse circulation. *J Bone Miner Res* 1989;4:325–34.
64. Hagenaars CE, van der Kraan AAM, Kawilarang-de Haas EWM, et al. Osteoclast formation from clonation of pluripotent hemopoietic stem cells. *Bone Miner* 1989;6:179–89.
65. Glowacki J, Jasty M, Goldring S. Comparison of multinucleated cells elicited in rats by particulate bone, polyethylene, or polymethylmethacrylate. *J Bone Miner Res* 1986;1:327–31.
66. Glowacki J, Cox KA. Osteoclastic features of cells that resorb bone implants in rats. *Calcif Tissue Int* 1986;39:97–103.
67. Glowacki J, Lian JB. Impaired recruitment and differentiation of osteoclast progenitors by osteocalcin-deplete bone implants. *Cell Differ* 1987;21:247–54.
68. Goldring SR, Roelke M, Glowacki J. Multinucleated cells elicited in response to implants of devitalized bone particles possess receptors for calcitonin. *J Bone Miner Res* 1988;3:117–20.
69. Glowacki J, Rey C, Cox K, Lian J. Effects of bone matrix components on osteoclast differentiation. *Connect Tissue Res* 1989;20:121–9.
70. Lian JB, Marks SC Jr. Osteopetrosis in the rat: coexistence of reductions in osteocalcin and bone resorption. *Endocrinology* 1990;126:955–62.
71. Oursler MJ, Bell LV, Clevinger B, Osdoby P. Identification of osteoclast-specific monoclonal antibodies. *J Cell Biol* 1985;100:1592–1600.
72. Athanasou NA, Heryet A, Quinn J, Gatter KC, Mason DY, McGee JO'D. Osteoclasts contain macrophage and megakaryocyte antigens. *J Pathol* 1986;150:239–46.
73. Athanasou NA, Quinn J, McGee JO'D. Leukocyte common antigen is present on osteoclasts. *J Pathol* 1987;153:121–6.
74. Horton MA, Chambers TJ. Human osteoclast-specific antigens are expressed by osteoclasts in a wide range of non-human species. *Br J Exp Pathol* 1986;67:95–104.
75. Horton MA, Lewis D, McNulty K, Pringle JAS, Chambers TJ. Human fetal osteoclasts fail to express macrophage antigens. *Br J Exp Pathol* 1985;66:103–8.
76. Sminia T, Dijkstra CD. The origin of osteoclasts: an immunohistochemical study on macrophages and osteoclasts in embryonic rat bone. *Calcif Tissue Int* 1986;39:263–6.
77. Horton MA, Lewis D, McNulty K, Pringle JAS, Chambers TJ. Monoclonal antibodies to osteoclastomas (giant cell bone tumors): definition of osteoclast-specific cellular antigens. *Cancer Res* 1985;45:5663–9.
78. Horton MA, Rimmer EF, Chambers TJ. Giant cell formation in rabbit long-term marrow cultures: immunological and function studies. *J Bone Miner Res* 1986;1:5–14.
79. Kukita T, Mcmanus LM, Miller M, et al. Osteoclast-like cells formed in long-term human bone marrow cultures express a similar surface phenotype as authentic osteoclasts. *Lab Invest* 1989;60:532–8.
80. Kukita T, Roodman GD. Development of a monoclonal antibody to osteoclasts formed in vitro which recognizes mononuclear osteoclast precursors in the marrow. *Endocrinology* 1989;125:630–7.
81. Chilosi M, Gilioli E, Lestani M, Menestrina FS, Fiore-Donati L. Immunohistochemical characterization of osteoclasts and osteoclast-like cells with monoclonal antibody MB1 on paraffin-embedded tissues. *J Pathol* 1988;156:251–4.
82. Athanasou NA, Quinn J, Horton MA, McGee JO'D. New sites of cellular vitronectin receptor immunoreactivity detected with osteoclast-reacting monoclonal antibodies 13C2 and 23C6. *Bone Miner* 1990;8:7–22.
83. Davies J, Warwick J, Totty N, Philp R, Helfrich M, Horton M. The osteoclast functional antigen, implicated in the regulation of bone resorption, is biochemically related to the vitronectin receptor. *J Cell Biol* 1989;109:1817–26.
84. Horton MA, Davies J. Perspectives: adhesion receptors in bone. *J Bone Miner Res* 1990;4:803–8.
85. Zambonin-Zallone A, Teti A, Gaboli M, Marchisio PC. Beta 3 subunit of vitronectin receptor is present in osteoclast adhesion structures and not in other monocyte–macrophage derived cells. *Connect Tissue Res* 1989;20:143–9.
86. Fuller K, Chambers TJ. Bone matrix stimulates osteoclastic differentiation in cultures of rabbit bone marrow cells. *J Bone Miner Res* 1989;4:179–83.
87. Schneider GB, Relfson M. Pluripotent hemopoietic stem cells give rise to osteoclasts in vitro: effects of rGM-CSF. *Bone Miner* 1989;5:129–38.
88. Felix R, Cecchini MG, Hofstetter W, Elford PR, Stutzer A, Fleisch H. Impairment of macrophage colony-stimulating factor (M-CSF) production and lack of resident bone marrow macrophages in the osteopetrotic OP/OP mouse. *J Bone Miner Res* 1990;5:700–10.
89. Shinar DM, Sato M, Rodan GA. The effect of hemopoietic growth factors on the generation of osteoclast-like cells in mouse bone marrow cultures. *Endocrinology* 1990;126:1728–35.
90. Hattersley G, Chambers TJ. Effects of interleukin 3 and of granulocyte–macrophage and macrophage colony stimulating

factors on osteoclast differentiation from mouse hemopoietic tissue. *J Cell Physiol* 1990;142:201–9.

91. Barton BE, Mayer R. IL-3 induces differentiation of bone marrow precursor cells to osteoclast-like cells. *J Immunol* 1989;143:3211–6.

92. Abe E, Miyaura C, Tanaka H, Shina Y, Kuribayashi T, Suda S, Nishii Y, DeLuca HF, Suda T. 1α,25-Dihydroxyvitamin D_3 promotes fusion of mouse alveolar macrophages both by a direct mechanism and by a spleen cell-mediated indirect mechanism. *Proc Natl Acad Sci USA* 1983;80:5583–7.

93. Roodman GD, Ibbotson KJ, MacDonald BR, Kuehl TJ, Mundy GR. 1,25-Dihydroxyvitamin D_3 causes formation of multinucleated cells with several osteoclast characteristics in cultures of primate marrow. *Proc Natl Acad Sci USA* 1985;82:8213–8217.

94. Macdonald BR, Takahashi N, McManus LM, Holahan J, Mundy GR, Roodman GD. Formation of multinucleated cells that respond to osteotropic hormones in long term human bone marrow cultures. *Endocrinology* 1987;120:2326–33.

95. Pharoah MJ, Heersche JNM. 1,25-Dihydroxyvitamin D_3 causes an increase in the number of osteoclast-like cells in cat bone marrow cultures. *Calcif Tissue Int* 1986;37:276–81.

96. Takahashi N, Mundy GR, Kuehl TJ, Roodman GD. Osteoclast-like cell formation in fetal and newborn long-term baboon marrow cultures is more sensitive to 1,25-dihydroxyvitamin D_3 than adult long-term marrow cultures. *J Bone Miner Res* 1987;2:311–7.

97. Sasaki T, Takahasi N, et al. Multinucleated cells formed on calcified dentine from mouse bone marrow cells treated with 1α,25-dihydroxyvitamin D_3 have ruffled borders and resorb dentine. *Anat Rec* 1989;224:379–91.

98. Scheven BAA, Hamilton NJ. Retinoic acid and 1,25-dihydroxyvitamin D_3 stimulate osteoclast formation by different mechanisms. *Bone* 1990;11:53–9.

99. Akatsu T, Takahashi N, Debari K, et al. Prostaglandins promote osteoclast-like cell formation by a mechanism involving cyclic adenosine 3',5'-monophosphate in mouse bone marrow cell cultures. *J Bone Miner Res* 1989;4:29–35.

100. Okuda A, Taylor LM, Heersche JNM. Prostaglandin E_2 initially inhibits and then stimulates bone resorption in isolated rabbit osteoclast cultures. *Bone Miner* 1990;7:255–66.

101. Baron R. Molecular mechanism of bone resorption by the osteoclast. *Anat Rec* 1989;224:317–24.

102. Hunter SJ, Schraer H, Gay CV. Characterization of the cytoskeleton of isolated chick osteoclasts: effect of calcitonin. *J Histochem Cytochem* 1989;37:1529–38.

103. Zambonin-Zallone A, Teti A, Carano A, Marchisio PC. The distribution of podosomes in osteoclasts cultured on bone laminae: effect of retinol. *J Bone Miner Res* 1988;3:517–23.

104. Simpson A, Horton MA. Expression of the vitronectin receptor during embryonic development: an immunohistological study of the ontogeny of the osteoclast of the osteoclast in the rabbit. *Br J Exp Pathol* 1989;70:257–66.

105. Turksen K, Kanehisa J, Opas M, Heersche JNM, Aubin JE. Adhesion patterns and cytoskeleton of rabbit osteoclasts on bone slices and glass. *J Bone Miner Res* 1988;3:389–400.

106. Zambonin-Zallone A, Teti A, Grano M, et al. Immunocytochemical distribution of extracellular matrix receptors in human osteoclasts: a β_3 integrin is colocalized with vinculin and talin in the podosomes of osteoclastoma giant cells. *Exp Cell Res* 1989;182:645–52.

107. Lakkakorpi P, Tuukkanen J, Hentunen T, Jarvelin K, Vaananen K. Organization of osteoclast microfilaments during the attachment to bone surface in vitro. *J Bone Miner Res* 1990;4:817–26.

108. Davies J, Warwick D, Totty N, Philp R, Helfrich M, Horton M. The osteoclast functional antigen, implicated in the regulation of bone resorption, is biochemically related to the vitronectin receptor. *J Cell Biol* 1989;109:1817–26.

109. Taylor ML, Boyde A, Jones SJ. The effect of fluoride on the patterns of adherence of osteoclasts cultured on and resorbing dentine: a 3-D assessment of vinculin-labeled cells using confocal optical microscopy. *Anat Embryol* 1989;180:427–35.

110. Akisaka T, Subita GP, Shigenaga Y. Surface modifications at the perosseous region of chick osteoclast as revealed by freeze-substitution. *Anat Rec* 1988;222:323–32.

111. Gotoh Y, Gerstenfeld LC, Glimcher MJ. Identification and characterization of the major chicken bone phosphoprotein—analysis of its synthesis by cultured embryonic chick osteoblasts. *Eur J Biochem* 1990;187:49–58.

112. Pierce A, Lindskog S. Coated pits and vesicles in the osteoclast. *J Submicrosc Cytol Pathol* 1988;20:161–8.

113. Vaananen KK, Malmi R, Tuukkanen J, Sunquist K, Harkonen P. Identification of osteoclasts by rhodamine-conjugated peanut agglutinin. *Calcif Tissue Int* 1986;39:161–5.

114. Popoff SN, Schneider GB. Processing of concanavalin A-receptor complexes by rat osteoclasts in vitro. *Am J Anat* 1986;176:53–64.

115. Blair HC, Kahn AJ, Crouch EC, Jeffrey JJ, Teitelbaum SL. Isolated osteoclast resorb the organic and inorganic components of bone. *J Cell Biol* 1986;102:1164–72.

116. Baron R, Neff L, Louvard D, Courtoy PJ. Cell-mediated extracellular acidification and bone resorption: evidence for a low pH in resorbing lacunae and localization of a 100-kd lysosomal membrane protein at the osteoclast ruffled border. *J Cell Biol* 1985;101:2210–22.

117. Arnett TR, Dempster DW. Effect of pH on bone resorption by rat osteoclasts in vitro. *Endocrinology* 1986;119:119–24.

118. Blair HC, Teitelbaum SL, Ghiselli R, Gluck S. Osteoclastic bone resorption by a polarized vacuolar proton pump. *Science* 1989;245:855.

119. Arnett TR, Dempster DW. Protons and osteoclasts. *J Bone Miner Res* 1990;5:1099–103.

120. Bekker PJ, Gay CV. Biochemical characterization of an electrogenic vacuolar proton pump in purified chicken osteoclast plasma membrane vesicles. *J Bone Miner Res* 1990;5:569–79.

121. Gluck S, Caldwell J. Proton-translocating ATPase from bovine kidney medulla: Partial purification and reconstitution. *Am J Physiol* 1988;254:F71–9.

122. Tuukkanen J, Vaananen HK. Omeprazole, a specific inhibitor of H^+-K^+-ATPase, inhibits bone resorption in vitro. *Calcif Tissue Int* 1986;38:123–5.

123. Andersen RE, Woodbury DM, Jee WSS. Humoral and ionic regulation of osteoclast acidity. *Calcif Tissue Int* 1986;39:252–8.

124. Baron R. Polarity and membrane transport in osteoclasts. *Connect Tissue Res* 1989;20:109–20.

125. Akisaka T, Gay CV. Ultracytochemical evidence for a proton-pump adenosine triphosphatase in chick osteoclasts. *Cell Tissue Res* 1986;245:507–12.

126. Bekker PJ, Gay CV. Characterization of a Ca^{2+}-ATPase in osteoclast plasma membrane. *J Bone Miner Res* 1990;5:557–67.

127. Vaananen HK. Immunohistochemical localization of carbonic anhydrase isoenzymes I and II in human bone, cartilage and giant cell tumor. *Histochemistry* 1985;81:485–7.

128. Cao H, Gay CV. Effects of parathyroid hormone and calcitonin on carbonic anhydrase location in osteoclasts of cultured embryonic chick bone. *Experientia* 1985;41:1472–4.

129. Silverton SF, Dodgson SJ, Fallon MD, Forster RE. Carbonic anhydrase activity of chick osteoclasts is increased by parathyroid hormone. *Am J Physiol* 1987;253:E670–4.

130. Teti A, Blair HC, Teitelbaum SL, et al. Cytoplasmic pH regulation and chloride/bicarbonate exchange in avian osteoclasts. *J Clin Invest* 1989;83:227.

131. Hall TJ, Chambers TJ. Optimal bone resorption by isolated rat osteoclasts require chloride/bicarbonate exchange. *Calcif Tissue Int* 1989;45:378–80.

132. Teti A, Blair HC, Teitelbaum SL, Kahn JA, Carano A, Grano M, Santacroce G, Schlesinger P, Zambonin-Zallone A. Cytoplasmic pH is regulated in isolated avian osteoclasts by a Cl-/HCO3-exchanger. *Boll Soc Ital Biol Sper* 1989;65:589–95.

133. Hall TJ, Chambers TJ. Na^+/H^+ antiporter is the primary proton transport system used by osteoclasts during bone resorption. *J Cell Physiol* 1990;142:420–4.

134. Akisaka T, Subita GP, Kawaguchi H, et al. Different tartrate sensitivity and pH optimum for two isoenzymes of acid phosphatase in osteoclasts. An electron-microscopic enzyme-cytochemical study. *Cell Tissue Res* 1989;255:69–76.

135. Teti A, Grano M, Teitelbaum SL, Hruska KA, Colucci S, Zambonin-Zallone A. Regulation of podosomes by intracellular pH in avian osteoclasts. *Boll Soc Ital Biol Sper* 1989;65:597–601.

136. Teti A, Grano M, Teitelbaum SL, Hruska KA, Colucci S, Zambonin-Zallone A. Intracellular acidification induces decrease of

cytosolic calcium in isolated osteoclasts. *Boll Soc Ital Biol Sper* 1989;65:689–93.

137. Baron R, Neff L, Van PT, Nefussi J-R, Vignery A. Kinetic and cytochemical identification of osteoclast precursors and their differentiation into multinucleated osteoclasts. *Am J Pathol* 1986;122:363–78.

138. van de Wijngaert FP, Burger EH. Demonstration of tartrate-resistant acid phosphate in un-decalcified, glycolmethacrylate-embedded mouse bone: a possible marker for (pre) osteoclast identification. *J Histochem Cytochem* 1986;34:1317–23.

139. Anderson TR, Toverud SU. Purification and characterization of purple acid phosphatase from developing rat bone. *Arch Biochem Biophys* 1986;247:131–9.

140. Clark SA, Ambrose WW, Anderson TR, et al. Ultrastructural localization of tartrate-resistant, purple acid phosphatase in rat osteoclasts by histochemistry and immunocytochemistry. *J Bone Miner Res* 1989;4:399–405.

141. Andersson G, Lindunger A, Ek-Rylander B. Isolation and characterization of skeletal acid ATPase—a new osteoclast marker? *Connect Tissue Res* 1989;20:151–8.

142. Palle S, Chappard D, Vico L, Riffat G, Alexandre C. Evaluation of the osteoclastic population in iliac crest biopsies from 36 normal subjects: a histoenzymologic and histomorphometric study. *J Bone Miner Res* 1989;4:501–6.

143. Efstratiadis T, Moss DW. Tartrate-resistant acid phosphatase of human lung: apparent identity with osteoclastic acid phosphatase. *Enzyme* 1985;33:34–40.

144. Miller SC. The rapid appearance of acid phosphatase activity at the developing ruffled border of parathyroid hormone activated medullary bone osteoclasts. *Calcif Tissue Int* 1985;37:526–9.

145. Chambers TJ, Fuller K, Darby JA. Hormonal regulation of acid phosphatase release by osteoclasts disaggregated from neonatal rat bone. *J Cell Physiol* 1987;132:90–6.

146. Eilon G, Raisz LG. Comparison of the effects of stimulators and inhibitors of resorption on the release of lysosomal enzymes and radioactive calcium from fetal bone in organ culture. *Endocrinology* 1978;103:1969–75.

147. Baron R, Neff L, Brown W, Courtoy PJ, Louvard D, Farquhar MG. Polarized secretion of lysosomal enzymes: co-distribution of cation-independent mannose-6-phosphate receptors and lysosomal enzymes along the osteoclast exocytic pathway. *J Cell Biol* 1988;106:1863–72.

148. Blair HC, Teitelbaum SL, Schmike PA, Konsek JD, Koziol CM, Schlesinger PH. Receptor-mediated uptake of a mannose-6-phosphate bearing glycoprotein by isolated chicken osteoclasts. *J Cell Physiol* 1988;137:476–82.

149. Garrett IR, Boyce BF, Oreffo RO, Bonewald L, Poser J, Mundy GR. Oxygen-derived free radicals stimulate osteoclastic bone resorption in rodent bone in vitro and in vivo. *J Clin Invest* 1990;85:632–9.

150. Key LL Jr, Ries WL, Taylor RG, Hays BD, Pitzer BL. Oxygen derived free radicals in osteoclasts: the specificity and location of the nitroblue tetrazolium reaction. *Bone* 1990;11:115–9.

151. Oursler MJ, Li L, Osdoby P. Characterization of an osteoclast membrane protein related to superoxide dismutase. *J Bone Miner Res* 1989;4(Suppl 1):591A.

152. Beard CJ, Key L, Newburger PE, Ezekowitz RAB, Arceci R, Miller B, Proto P, Ryan T, Anast C, Simons ER. Neutrophil defect associated with malignant infantile osteopetrosis. *J Lab Clin Med* 1986;108:498–505.

153. Ferrier J, Ward A, Kanehisa J, Heersche JNM. Electrophysiological responses of osteoclasts to hormones. *J Cell Physiol* 1986;128:23–26.

154. Sims SM, Dixon SJ. Inwardly rectifying K⁺ current in osteoclasts. *Am J Physiol* 1989;256:C1277–82.

155. Ravesloot JH, Ypey DL, Vrijheid-Lammers T, Nijweide PJ. Voltage-activated K⁺ conductances in freshly isolated embryonic chicken osteoclasts. *Proc Natl Acad Sci USA* 1989;86:6821–5.

156. Zaidi M, Datta HK, Patchell A, Moonga B, MacIntyre I. "Calcium-activated" intracellular calcium elevation: a novel mechanism of osteoclast regulation. *Biochem Biophys Res Commun* 1989;163:1461–5.

157. Datta HK, MacIntyre I, Zaidi M. The effect of extracellular cal-

158. Christoffersen J. Dissolution of calcium hydroxyapatite. *Calcif Tissue Int* 1981;33:557–60.

159. Teti A, Grano M, Colucci S, Argentino L, Barattolo R, Miyauchi A, Teitelbaum SL, Hruska KA, Zambonin-Zallone A. Voltage dependent calcium channel expression in isolated osteoclasts. *Boll Soc Ital Biol Sper* 1989;65:1115–8.

160. Luben RA, Goggins JF, Raisz LG. Stimulation by parathyroid hormone of bone hyaluronate synthesis in organ culture. *Endocrinology* 1974;94:737–45.

161. Luben RA, Cohn DV. Effects of parathormone and calcitonin on citrate and hyaluronate metabolism in cultured bone. *Endocrinology* 1976;98:413.

162. Lowik CWGM, van Leeuwen JPTM, van der Meer JM, van Zeeland JK, Scheven BAA, Hermann-Erlee MPM. A two-receptor model for the action of parathyroid hormone on osteoblasts: a role for intracellular free calcium and cAMP. *Cell Calcium* 1985;6:311–26.

163. Yamaguchi DT, Hahn TJ, Iida-Klein A, Kleeman CR, Muallem S. Parathyroid hormone-activated calcium channels in an osteoblast-like clonal osteosarcoma cell line. cAMP-dependent and cAMP-independent calcium channels. *J Biol Chem* 1987;262:7711–8.

164. Reid IR, Civitelli R, Halstead LR, Avioli LV, Hruska KA. Parathyroid hormone acutely elevates intracellular calcium in osteoblast-like cells. *Am J Physiol* 1987;253:E45–51.

165. Fritsch J, Edelman A, Balsan S. Early effects of parathyroid hormone on membrane potential of rat osteoblasts in culture: role of cAMP and Ca²⁺. *J Bone Miner Res* 1988;3:547–54.

166. Cosman F, Morrow B, Kopal M, et al. Stimulation of inositol phosphate formation in ROS 17/2.8 cell membranes by guanine nucleotide, calcium, and parathyroid hormone. *J Bone Miner Res* 1989;4:413–20.

167. Civitelli R, Reid IR, Westbrook S, Avioli LV, Hruska KA. PTH elevates inositol polyphosphates and diacylglycerol in a rat osteoblast-like cell line. *Am J Physiol* 1988;255:E660–7.

168. Ferrier J, Ward-Kesthely A, Homble F, Ross S. Further analysis of spontaneous membrane potential activity and the hyperpolarizing response to parathyroid hormone in osteoblast-like cells. *J Cell Physiol* 1987;130:344–51.

169. Stern PH, Stathopoulos VM, Shankar G, Fenton JW II. Second messengers in thrombin-stimulated bone resorption. *J Bone Miner Res* 1990;5:443–9.

170. Lorenzo JA, Raisz LG, Hock JM. DNA synthesis is not necessary for osteoclastic responses to parathyroid hormone in cultured fetal rat long bones. *J Clin Invest* 1983;72(6):1924–29.

171. Lorenzo JA, Quinton J, Sousa S, Raisz LG. Effects of DNA and prostaglandin synthesis inhibitors on the stimulation of bone resorption by epidermal growth factor in fetal rat long-bone cultures. *J Clin Invest* 1986;77:1897–1902.

172. Lorenzo JA, Sousa SL, Centrella M. Interleukin-1 in combination with transforming growth factor-α produces enhanced bone resorption in vitro. *Endocrinology* 1988;123:2194–200.

173. Shoukri KC, Woodiel FN, Raisz LG. Role of DNA synthesis in prostaglandin E₂ mediated bone resorption. *J Bone Miner Res* 1990;5(Suppl 2):Abstract 309.

174. Lorenzo JA, Sousa S. Phorbol esters stimulate bone resorption in fetal rat long bone cultures by mechanisms independent of prostaglandin synthesis. *J Bone Miner Res* 1988;3:63–8.

175. Vargas SJ, Feyen JHM, Raisz LG. Effects of pertussis toxin on resorption of 19-day-old fetal rat long bones. *Endocrinology* 1989;124:2159–65.

176. Ransjo M, Kerner UH. Inhibitory action of pertussis toxin on parathyroid hormone and prostaglandin E₂-stimulated bone resorption in cultured neonatal mouse calvaria. *Acta Physiol Scand* 1987;131:315–7.

177. Thesingh CW. Formation sites and distribution of osteoclast progenitor cells during the ontogeny of the mouse. *Dev Biol* 1986;117:127–34.

178. Ries WL, Gong JK, Gunsolley JC. The distribution and kinetics of nuclei in rat osteoclasts. *Cell Tissue Kinet* 1987;20:1–14.

179. Chambers TJ, Fuller K, McSheehy PMJ, Pringle JAS. The effects

of calcium regulating hormones on bone resorption by isolated human osteoclastoma cells. *J Pathol* 1985;145:297–305.

180. Ito MB, Schraer H, Gay CV. The effects of calcitonin, parathyroid hormone and prostaglandin E$_2$ on cyclic AMP levels of isolated osteoclasts. *Comp Biochem Physiol [A]* 1985;81:653–7.

181. Nicholson GC, Moseley JM, Yates AJP, Martin TJ. Control of cyclic adenosine 3′,5′-Monophosphate production in osteoclasts: calcitonin-induced persistent activation and homologous desensitization of adenylate cyclase. *Endocrinology* 1987;120:1902–8.

182. Ransjo M, Lerner UH, Heersche JNM. Calcitonin-like effects of forskolin and choleratoxin on surface area and motility of isolated rabbit osteoclasts. *J Bone Miner Res* 1988;3:611–9.

183. McLeod JF, Raisz LG. Comparison of inhibition of bone resorption and escape with calcitonin and dibutyryl 3′,5′ cyclic adenosine monophosphate. *Endocr Res Commun* 1981;8:49–59.

184. Lorenzo JA, Sousa S, Quinton J. Forskolin has both stimulatory and inhibitory effects on bone resorption in fetal rat long bone cultures. *J Bone Miner Res* 1986;1:313–8.

185. Ransjo M, Lerner UH. Effects of cholera toxin on cyclic AMP accumulation bone resorption in cultured mouse calvaria. *Biochim Biophys Acta* 1987;930:378–91.

186. Klein RF, Nissenson RA, Strewler GJ. Forskolin mimics the effects of calcitonin but not parathyroid hormone on bone resorption in vitro. *Bone Miner* 1988;4:247–56.

187. Krieger NS, Stern PH. Effects of forskolin on bone in organ culture. *Am J Physiol* 1987;252(1):E44–8.

188. Lerner UH, Ransjo M, Fredholm BB. Comparative study of the effects of cyclic nucleotide phosphodiesterase inhibitors on bone resorption and cyclic AMP formation in vitro. *Biochem Pharm* 1986;352:4177–89.

189. Lerner UH, Ransjo M, Klaushofer K, Horander H, Hoffman O, Czerwenka E, Koller K, Peterlik M. Comparison between the effects of forskolin and calcitonin on bone resorption and osteoclast morphology in vitro. *Bone* 1990;10:377–88.

190. Lerner UH, Sahlberg K, Fredholm BB. Characterization of adenosine receptors in bone. Studies on the effect of adenosine analogues on cyclic AMP formation and bone resorption in cultured mouse calvaria. *Acta Physiol Scand* 1987;131:287–96.

191. Lerner UH, Ransjo M, Sahlberg K, et al. Forskolin sensitizes parathyroid hormone-induced cyclic AMP response, but not the bone resorptive effect, in mouse calvarial bones. *Bone Miner* 1989;5:169–81.

192. Conaway HH, Diez LF, Raisz LG. Effects of prostacyclin and prostaglandin E$_1$ (PGE$_1$) on bone resorption in the presence and absence of parathyroid hormone. *Calcif Tissue Int* 1986;38:130–4.

193. Lerner UH, Ransjo M, Ljunngren O. Prostaglandin E$_2$ causes a transient inhibition of mineral mobilization, matrix degradation, and lysosomal enzyme release from mouse calvaria bones in vitro. *Calcif Tissue Int* 1987;40:323–31.

194. Nicholson GC, Livesey SA, Moseley JM, Martin TJ. Actions of calcitonin, parathyroid hormone, and prostaglandin E$_2$ on cyclic AMP formation in chicken and rat osteoblasts. *J Cell Biochem* 1986;31:229–41.

195. Arnett TR, Dempster DW. A comparative study of disaggregated chick and rat osteoclasts in vitro: effects of calcitonin and prostaglandins. *Endocrinology* 1987;120:602–8.

196. De Vernejoul M-C, Horowitz M, Demignon J, Neff L, Baron R. Bone resorption by isolated chick osteoclasts in culture is stimulated by murine spleen cell supernatant fluids (osteoclast-activating factor) and inhibited by calcitonin and prostaglandin E$_2$. *J Bone Miner Res* 1988;3:69–80.

197. Yamamoto T, Gay CV. Ultrastructural localization of adenylate cyclase in chicken bone cells. *J Histochem Cytochem* 1989;37:1705–9.

198. Holtrop ME, Raisz LG, Simmons HA. The effects of parathyroid hormone, colchicine, and calcitonin on the ultrastructure and the activity of osteoclasts in organ culture. *J Cell Biol* 1974;60:346–55.

199. Chambers TJ, Chambers JC, Symonds J, Darby JA. The effect of human calcitonin on the cytoplasmic spreading of rat osteoclasts. *J Clin Endocrinol Metab* 1986;63:1080–5.

200. King GJ, Holtrop ME, Raisz LG. The relation of ultrastructural changes in osteoclasts to resorption in bone cultures stimulated with parathyroid hormone. *Metab Bone Dis Rel Res* 1978;1:67–74.

201. Raisz LG, Nuki K, Alander C, Craig RG. Interactions between bacterial endotoxin and other stimulators of bone resorption in organ culture. *J Periodont Res* 1981;16:1–7.

202. Dewhirst FE, Ago JM, Peros WJ, Stashenko P. Synergism between parathyroid hormone and interleukin 1 in stimulating bone resorption in organ culture. *J Bone Miner Res* 1987;2:127–34.

203. Sato K, Fujii Y, Kasono K, Ozawa M, Imamura H, Kanaji Y, Kurosawa H, Tsushima T, Shizume K. Parathyroid hormone-related protein and interleukin-1α synergistically stimulate bone resorption in vitro and increase the serum calcium concentration in mice in vivo. *Endocrinology* 1989;124:2172–8.

204. Stashenko P, Dewhirst FE, Peros WJ, Kent RL, Ago JM. Synergistic interactions between interleukin 1, tumor necrosis factor, and lymphotoxin in bone resorption. *J Immunol* 1987;138:1464–8.

205. Tatakis DN, Schneeberger G, Dziak R. Recombinant interleukin-1 stimulates prostaglandin E$_2$ production by osteoblastic cells: synergy with parathyroid hormone. *Calcif Tissue Int* 1988;42:358–62.

206. Hurley MM, Fall P, Harrison JR, Petersen DN, Kream BE, Raisz LG. Effects of transforming growth factor α and interleukin-1 on DNA synthesis, collagen synthesis, procollagen mRNA levels, and prostaglandin E$_2$ production in cultured fetal rat calvaria. *J Bone Miner Res* 1989;4:731–6.

207. Marusic A, Kalinowski JF, Harrison JR, Centrella M, Lorenzo JA. Synergistic effects of transforming growth factor beta and interleukin 1 alpha on prostaglandin E2 synthesis in bone cells. *J Bone Miner Res* 1990;5(Suppl 1):Abstract 312.

208. Harrison JR, Simmons HA, Lorenzo JA, Kream BE, Raisz LG. Stimulation of prostaglandin E$_2$ production by interleukin-1α and transforming growth factor-α in MC3T3-E1 cells is associated with increased prostaglandin H synthase mRNA levels. *J Bone Miner Res* 1989;4(Suppl 1):Abstract 664.

209. Dominguez JH, Raisz LG. Effect of ACTH on PTH-stimulated bone resorption in vitro. *Calcif Tissue Int* 1980;30:205–8.

210. Bergmann PJ, Simmons HA, Vizet A, Raisz LG. Cationized serum albumin enhances response of cultured fetal rat long bones to parathyroid hormone. *Endocrinology* 1984;116:1729–33.

211. Feyen JHM, van der Wilt G, Moonen P, et al. Stimulation of arachidonic acid metabolism in primary cultures of osteoblast-like cells by hormones and drugs. *Prostaglandins* 1984;28:769–81.

212. Raisz LG, Simmons HA. Effects of parathyroid hormone and cortisol on prostaglandin production by neonatal rat calvaria in vitro. *Endocr Res* 1985;11:59–74.

213. Yang CY, Gonnerman WA, Taylor L, Nimberg RB, Polgar PR. Synthetic human parathyroid hormone fragment stimulates prostaglandin E$_2$ synthesis by chick calvariae. *Endocrinology* 1987;120:63–70.

214. Klein Nulend J, Aaron JN, Harrison JR, Simmons HA, Raisz LG. Comparison of the effects of parathyroid hormone and interleukin-1 on resorption, prostaglandin production, and PGH synthase mRNA levels in cultured mouse calvariae. *J Bone Miner Res* 1989;4(Suppl 1):Abstract 660.

215. Ljunngren O, Lerner UH. Parathyroid hormone stimulates prostanoid formation in mouse calvarial bones. *Acta Endocrinol* 1989;120:357–61.

216. Feyen JHM, Elford P, Di Padova FE, Trechsel U. Interleukin-6 is produced by bone and modulated by parathyroid hormone. *J Bone Miner Res* 1989;4:633–8.

217. Garrett IR, Black KS, Mundy GR. Interactions between interleukin-6 and interleukin-1 in osteoclastic bone resorption in neonatal mouse calvariae. *Calcif Tissue Int* 1990;46:Abstract 140.

218. Orloff JJ, Wu TL, Stewart AF. Parathyroid hormone-like proteins—biochemical responses and receptor interactions. *Endocr Rev* 1990;10:476–95.

219. Kemp BE, Moseley JM, Rodda CP, Ebeling PR, Wettenhall REH, Stapleton D, Diefenbach-Jagger H, Ure F, Michelangeli VP, Simmons HA, Raisz LG, Martin TJ. Parathyroid hormone-related protein of malignancy: active synthetic fragments. *Science* 1987;238:1568–70.

220. Yates AJP, Gutierrez GE, Smolens P, Travis PS, Katz MS, Aufdemorte TB, Boyce BF, Hymer TK, Poser JW, Mundy GR. Effects of a synthetic peptide of a parathyroid hormone related protein on calcium, resorption, and bone metabolism in vivo and in vitro in rodents. *J Clin Invest* 1988;81:932–8.

221. Stewart AF, Mangin M, Wu T, Goumas D, Insogna KL, Burtis WJ, Broadus AE. Synthetic human parathyroid hormone-like protein stimulates bone resorption and causes hypercalcemia in rats. *J Clin Invest* 1988;81:596–600.

222. Thompson DD, Seedor G, Fisher JE, Rosenblatt M, Rodan GA. Direct action of the parathyroid hormone-like human hypercalcemic factor on bone. *Proc Natl Acad Sci USA* 1988;85:5673–7.

223. Fukayama S, Bosma TJ, Goad DL, Voelkel EF, Tashjian AH. Human parathyroid hormone (PTH)-related protein and human PTH: comparative biological activities on human bone cells and bone resorption. *Endocrinology* 1988;123:2841–8.

224. Raisz LG, Simmons HA, Vargas SJ, Kemp BE, Martin TJ. Comparison of the effects of amino-terminal synthetic parathyroid hormone-related peptide (PTHrP) of malignancy and parathyroid hormone on resorption of cultured fetal rat long bones. *Calcif Tissue Int* 1990;46:233–8.

225. Klein-Nulend J, Fall PM, Raisz LG. Comparison of the effects of synthetic human parathyroid hormone (PTH)-(1-34)-related peptide of malignancy and bovine PTH-(1-34) on bone formation and resorption in organ culture. *Endocrinology* 1990;126:223–7.

226. Akatsu T, Takahashi N, Ugadawa N, et al. Parathyroid hormone (PTH)-related protein is a potent stimulator of osteoclast-like multinucleated cell formation to the same extent as PTH in mouse marrow cultures. *Endocrinology* 1989;125:20–7.

227. Alander CB, Pilbeam CC, Simmons HA, Raisz LG. Comparison of the effects of various forms of synthetic human parathyroid hormone-related peptide of malignancy on bone resorption and formation in organ culture. *J Bone Miner Res* 1990;5(Suppl 2):Abstract 475.

228. Raisz LG. Direct effects of vitamin D and its metabolites on skeletal tissue. *Clin Endocrinol Metab* 1980;9:27–41.

229. Stern PH. The D vitamins and bone. *Pharmacol Rev* 1980;32:47–80.

230. Stern PH, Hamstra AJ, DeLuca HF, Bell NH. Bioassay capable of measuring 1 picogram of 1,25-dihydroxyvitamin D_3. *J Clin Endocrinol Metab* 1978;46:891.

231. Weinstein RS, Underwood JL, Hutson MS, DeLuca HF. Bone histomorphometry in vitamin D-deficient rats infused with calcium and phosphorus. *Am J Physiol* 1984;246:E499–505.

232. Paulson SK, Perlman K, DeLuca HF, Stern PH. 24- and 26-homo-1,25-dihydroxyvitamin D_3 analogs: potencies on in vitro bone resorption differ from those reported for cell differentiation. *J Bone Miner Res* 1990;5:201–6.

233. Perlman K, Kutner A, Prahl J, Smith C, Inaba M, Schnoes HK, DeLuca HF. 24-Homologated 1,25-dihydroxyvitamin D_3 compounds: separation of calcium and cell differentiation activities. *Biochemistry* 1990;29:190–5.

234. Raisz LG, Martin TJ. Prostaglandins in bone and mineral metabolism. *Bone Miner Res* 1983;2:286–310.

235. Harvey W, Bennett A. *Prostaglandins in bone resorption.* Boca Raton, FL: CRC Press, 1988;134.

236. Yamasaki K, Miura F, Suda T. Prostaglandin as a mediator of bone resorption induced by experimental tooth movement in rats. *J Dent Res* 1980;59:1635–42.

237. Murray DW, Rushton N. The effect of strain on bone cell prostaglandin E_2 release. *Calcif Tissue Int* 1990;47:35–9.

238. Klein-Nulend J, Veldhuijzen JP, Vanstrien ME, Dejong M, Burger EH. Inhibition of osteoclastic bone resorption by mechanical stimulation in vitro. *Arthritis Rheum* 1990;33:66–72.

239. Burger EH, Veldhuijzen JP, Nulend JK, Van Loon JJ. Osteoclastic invasion and mineral resorption of fetal mouse long bone rudiments are inhibited by culture under intermittent compressive force. *Connect Tissue Res* 1989;20:131–41.

240. Raisz LG, Vanderhoek JY, Simmons HA, Kream BE, Nicolaou KC. Prostaglandin synthesis by fetal rat bone in vitro: evidence for a role of prostacyclin. *Prostaglandins* 1979;7:903–14.

241. Voelkel EF, Tashjian AH Jr, Levine L. Cyclo-oxygenase products of arachidonic acid metabolism by mouse bone in organ culture. *Biochim Biophys Acta* 1980;620:418–28.

242. Raisz LG, Alander CB, Simmons HA. Effects of prostaglandin-E_3 and eicosapentaenoic acid on rat bone in organ culture. *Prostaglandins* 1989;37:615–25.

243. Raisz LG, Woodiel FN. Effect of alterations in the cyclopentane ring on bone resorptive activity of prostaglandin. *Prostaglandins* 1989;37:229–36.

244. Tashjian AH, Bosma TJ, Levine L. Use of minoxidil to demonstrate that prostacyclin is not the mediator of bone resorption stimulated by growth factors in mouse calvariae. *Endocrinology* 1988;123:969–74.

245. Raisz LG, Alander CB, Fall PM, Simmons HA. Effects of prostaglandin $F_{2\alpha}$ on bone formation and resorption in cultured neonatal mouse calvariae: role of prostaglandin E_2 production. *Endocrinology* 1990;126:1076–79.

246. Meghji S, Sandy JR, Scutt AM, Harvey W, Harris M. Stimulation of bone resorption by lipoxygenase metabolites of arachidonic acid. *Prostaglandins* 1988;36:139–49.

247. Hayward MA, Howard GA, Neuman RG. Prostaglandins in inflammatory bone pathology: mechanism and therapeutic benefit of etodolac. *Agents Actions* 1989;26:310–8.

248. Williams RC, Jeffcoat MK, Howell TH, Reddy MS, Johnson HG, Hall CM, Goldhaber P. Ibuprofen—an inhibitor of alveolar bone resorption in beagles. *J Periodont Res* 1988;23:225–9.

249. Hoffman O, Klaushofer K, Koller K, Peterlik M. Prostaglandin-related bone resorption in cultured neonatal mouse calvaria—evaluation of biopotency of nonsteroidal anti-inflammatory drugs. *Prostaglandins* 1985;30:857–66.

250. Williams RC, Jeffcoat MK, Howell TH, Rolla A, Stubbs D, Teoh KW, Reddy MS, Goldhaber P. Altering the progression of human alveolar bone loss with the non-steroidal anti-inflammatory drug flurbiprofen. *J Periodontol* 1989;60:485–490.

251. Raisz LG, Simmons HA, Fall PM. Biphasic effects of nonsteroidal anti-inflammatory drugs on prostaglandin production by cultured rat calvariae. *Prostaglandins* 1989;37:559–565.

252. Tashjian AH Jr, Voelkel EF, Lazzaro M, Goad D, Bosma T, Levine L. Tumor necrosis factor-α (cachectin) stimulates bone resorption in mouse calvaria via a prostaglandin-mediated mechanism. *Endocrinology* 1987;120:2029–36.

253. Tashjian AH Jr, Voelkel EF, Lazzaro M, Singer FR, Roberts AB, Derynck R, Winkler ME, Levine L. α and β human transforming growth factors stimulate prostaglandin production and bone resorption in cultured mouse calvaria. *Proc Natl Acad Sci USA* 1985;82:4535–8.

254. Tashjian AH Jr, Levine L. Epidermal growth factor stimulates prostaglandin production and bone resorption in cultured mouse calvaria. *Biochem Biophys Res Commun* 1978;85:966–75.

255. Suzuki Y, Morita I, Yamane Y, et al. Cadmium stimulates prostaglandin E_2 production and bone resorption in cultured fetal mouse calvaria. *Biochem Biophys Res Commun* 1989;158:508–13.

256. Horton JE, Raisz LG, Simmons HA, Oppenheim JJ, Mergenhagen SE. Bone resorbing activity in supernatant fluid from cultured human peripheral blood leukocytes. *Science* 1972;177:793–5.

257. Raisz LG, Luben RA, Mundy GR, Dietrich JW, Horton JE, Trummel CL. Effect of osteoclast activating factor from human leukocytes on bone metabolism. *J Clin Invest* 1975;56:408–13.

258. Dewhirst FE, Stashenko PP, Mole JE, Tsurumachi T. Purification and partial sequence of human osteoclast-activating factor: identity with interleukin 1β. *J Immunol* 1985;135:2562–8.

259. Lorenzo JA, Sousa SL, Alander C, Raisz LG, Dinarello CA. Comparison of the bone-resorbing activity in the supernatants from phytohemagglutinin-stimulated human peripheral blood mononuclear cells with that of cytokines through the use of an antiserum to interleukin 1. *Endocrinology* 1987;121:1164–70.

260. Bertolini DR, Nedwin GE, Bringman TS, Smith DD, Mundy GR. Stimulation of bone resorption and inhibition of bone formation in vitro by human tumour necrosis factors. *Nature* 1986;319:516–8.

261. Thomson BM, Mundy GR, Chambers TJ. Tumor necrosis factors α and β induce osteoblastic cells to stimulate osteoclastic bone resorption. *J Immunol* 1987;138:775–9.

262. Gowen M, Mundy GR. Actions of recombinant interleukin 1, interleukin 2, and interferon-gamma on bone resorption in vitro. *J Immunol* 1986;136:2478–82.

263. Sato K, Fujii Y, Kasono K, Saji M, Tsushima T, Shizume K. Stimulation of prostaglandin-E₂ and bone resorption by recombinant human interleukin-1 alpha in fetal mouse bones. *Biochem Biophys Res Commun* 1986;138:618–24.

264. Garrett IR, Mundy GR. Relationship between interleukin-1 and prostaglandin in resorbing neonatal calvaria. *J Bone Miner Res* 1989;4:789.

265. Gowen M, Chapman K, Littlewood A, Hughes D, Evans D, Russell G. Production of tumor necrosis factor by human osteoblasts is modulated by other cytokines, but not by osteotropic hormones. *Endocrinology* 1990;126:1250–5.

266. Lorenzo JA, Sousa SL, Van Den Brink-Webb SE, Korn JH. Production of both interleukin-1α and β by newborn mouse calvarial cultures. *J Bone Miner Res* 1990;5:77–83.

267. Abe E, Ishimi Y, Takahashi N, et al. A differentiation-inducing factor produced by the osteoblastic cell line MC3T3-E1 stimulates bone resorption by promoting osteoclastic formation. *J Bone Miner Res* 1988;3:635–45.

268. Reid IR, Lowe C, Cornish J, Skinner SJM, Hilton DJ, Wilson TA, Gearing DP, Martin TJ. Leukemia inhibitory factor: a novel bone-active cytokine. *Endocrinology* 1990;126:1416–20.

269. Lorenzo JA, Sousa SL, Leahy CL. Leukemia inhibitory factor (LIF) inhibits basal bone resorption in fetal rat long bone cultures. *Cytokines* 1990;in press.

270. Shiina-Ishimi Y, Abe E, Tanaka H, Suda T. Synthesis of colony-stimulating factor (CSF) and differentiation-inducing factor (D-factor) by osteoblastic cells, clone MC3T3-E1. *Biochem Biophys Res Commun* 1986;134:400–6.

271. Felix R, Elford PR, Stoerckle C, Cecchini M, Witterwald A, Trechsel U, Fleische H, Stadler BM. Production of hemopoietic growth factors by bone tissue and bone cells in culture. *J Bone Miner Res* 1988;3:27–36.

272. Horowitz MC, Coleman DL, Ryaby JT, Einhorn TA. Osteotropic agents induce the differential secretion of granulocyte-macrophage colony-stimulation factor by the osteoblast cell line MC3T3-E1. *J Bone Miner Res* 1990;4:911–22.

273. Sato K, Kasono K, Fujii Y, Kawakami M, Tsusima T, Shiqume K. Tumor necrosis factor type α (cachectin) stimulates mouse osteoblast-like cells (MC3T3-E1) to produce macrophage-colony stimulating activity and prostaglandin E₂. *Biochem Biophys Res Commun* 1987;145:323–9.

274. Felix R, Fleisch H, Elford PR. Bone-resorbing cytokines enhance release of macrophage colony-stimulating activity by the osteoblastic cell MC3T3-E1. *Calcif Tissue Int* 1989;44:356–60.

275. Shinar DM, Sato M, Rodan GA. The effect of hemopoietic growth factors on the generation of osteoclast-like cells in mouse bone marrow culture. *Endocrinology* 1990;126:1728–35.

276. Hattersley G, Dorey E, Horton MA, Chambers TJ. Human macrophage colony-stimulating factor inhibits bone resorption by osteoclasts disaggregated from rat bone. *J Cell Physiol* 1988;137:199–203.

277. Lorenzo JA, Sousa SL, Fonseca JM, Hock JM, Medlock ES. Colony-stimulating factors regulate the development of multinucleated osteoclasts from recently replicated cells in vitro. *J Clin Invest* 1987;80:160–4.

278. Mundy GR, Shapiro JL, Bandelin JG, Canalis EM, Raisz LG. Direct stimulation of bone resorption by thyroid hormones. *J Clin Invest* 1976;58:529–34.

279. Klaushofer K, Hoffman O, Gleispach H, et al. Bone-resorbing activity of thyroid hormones is regulated to prostaglandin production in cultured neonatal mouse calvaria. *J Bone Miner Res* 1989;4:305–12.

280. Hoffman O, Klaushofer K, Koller K, Peterlik M, Mavreas T, Stern P. Indomethacin inhibits thrombin-, but not thyroxin-stimulated resorption of fetal rat limb bones. *Prostaglandins* 1986;31:601–8.

281. Fell HB, Mellanby E. The effect of hypervitaminosis A on embryonic limb-bones cultivated in vitro. *J Physiol* 1952;116:320.

282. Trechsel U, Stutzer A, Fleisch H. Hypercalcemia induced with an arotinoid in thyroparathyroidectomized rats—new model to study bone resorption in vivo. *J Clin Invest* 1987;80:1679–86.

283. Miyaura C, Segawa A, Nagasawa H, Abe E, Suda T. Effects of retinoic acid on the activation and fusion of mouse alveolar macrophages induced by 1α,25-dihydroxyvitamin D₃. *J Bone Miner Res* 1986;1:359–68.

284. Scheven BAA, Hamilton NJ. Retinoic acid and 1,25-dihydroxyvitamin D₃ stimulate osteoclast formation by different mechanisms. *Bone* 1990;11:53–9.

285. Oreffo ROC, Teti A, Triffitt JT, Francis MJO, Carano A, Zambonin Zallone A. Effects of vitamin A on bone resorption: evidence for direct stimulation of isolated chicken osteoclasts by retinol and retinoic acid. *J Bone Miner Res* 1988;3:203–10.

286. Raisz LG, Simmons HA, Sandberg AL, Canalis E. Direct stimulation of bone resorption by epidermal growth factor. *Endocrinology* 1980;107:270–3.

287. Stern PH, Krieger NS, Nissenson RA, Williams RD, Winkler ME, Derynck R, Strewler GJ. Human transforming growth factor-alpha stimulates bone resorption in vitro. *J Clin Invest* 1985;76:2016–19.

288. Ibbotson KJ, Harrod J, Gowen M, D'Souza S, Smith DD, Winkler ME, Derynck R, Mundy GR. Human recombinant transforming growth factor α stimulates bone resorption and inhibits formation in vitro. *Proc Natl Acad Sci USA* 1986;83:2228–32.

289. Feyen JHM, Kuntzelmann GMM, Mackie EJ. Basic and acidic fibroblast growth factor stimulate prostaglandin production and bone resorption in neonatal mouse calvaria. *Calcif Tissue Int* 1990;46:Abstract 135.

290. Shen V, Kohler G, Huang J, Huang SS, Peck WA. An acidic fibroblast growth factor stimulates DNA synthesis, inhibits collagen and alkaline phosphatase synthase and induces resorption in bone. *Bone Miner* 1990;7:205–20.

291. Simmons HA, Raisz LG. Effects of heparin and acidic fibroblast growth factor on resorption of cultured fetal rat long bones. *J Bone Miner Res* 1989;4:Abstract 659.

292. Goldhaber P. Heparin enhancement of factors stimulating bone resorption in tissue culture. *Science* 1965;147:407–8.

293. Hauschka PV, Mavrakos AE, Iafrati MD, Doleman SE, Klagsbrun M. Growth factors in bone matrix. Isolation of multiple types by affinity chromatography on heparin-sepharose. *J Biol Chem* 1986;261:12665–74.

294. Globus RK, Plouet J, Gospodarowicz D. Cultured bovine cells synthesize basic fibroblast growth factor and store it in their extracellular matrix. *Endocrinology* 1989;124:1539–47.

295. Tashjian AH Jr, Voelkel EF, Lloyd W, Derynck R, Winkler ME, Levine L. Actions of growth factors on plasma calcium—epidermal growth factor and human transforming growth factor-alpha cause elevation of plasma calcium in mice. *J Clin Invest* 1986;78:1405–9.

296. Marie PJ, Hott M, Perheentupa J. Effects of epidermal growth factor on bone formation and resorption in vivo. *Am J Physiol* 1990;258:E275–81.

297. Murrills RJ, Shane E, Lindsay R, et al. Bone resorption by isolated human osteoclasts in vitro: effects of calcitonin. *J Bone Miner Res* 1989;4:259–268.

298. Kanehisa J. Time course of "escape" from calcitonin-induced inhibition of motility and resorption of disaggregated osteoclasts. *Bone* 1989;10:125–30.

299. Wener JA, Gorton SJ, Raisz LG. Escape from inhibition of resorption in cultures of fetal bone treated with calcitonin and parathyroid hormone. *Endocrinology* 1972;90:752–9.

300. Nakamura T, Toyofuku F, Kanda S. Whole-body irradiation inhibits the escape phenomenon of osteoclasts in bones of calcitonin-treated rats. *Calcif Tissue Int* 1985;37:42–5.

301. Findlay DM, Michelangeli VP, Robinson PJ. Protein kinase-C-induced down-regulation of calcitonin receptors and calcitonin-activated adenylate cyclase in T47D and BEN cells. *Endocrinology* 1989;125:2656–63.

302. Eliam MC, Basle M, Bouizar Z, Bielakoff J, Moukhtar M, de Vernejoul MC. Influence of blood calcium on calcitonin receptors in isolated chick osteoclasts. *J Endocrinol* 1988;119:243–8.

303. Fischer JA, Born W. Calcitonin gene products: evolution, expression and biological targets. *Bone Miner* 1987;2:347–59.

304. Zaidi M, Mone X, Chambers TJ, Bevis Y, Beacham TJ, Beacham PJR, Gaines Das JL, Iain RE, MacIntyre I. Effects of peptides

from the calcitonin genes on bone and bone cells. *Q J Exp Physiol* 1988;73:471–86.

305. MacIntyre I. Amylinamide, bone conservation, and pancreatic beta cells. *Lancet* 1989;2:1026–7.

306. Datta HK, Zaidi M, et al. In vivo and in vitro effects of amylin and amylin-amide on calcium metabolism in the rat and rabbit. *Biochem Biophys Res Commun* 1989;162:876–81.

307. Michelangeli VP, Fletcher AE, Allan EH, et al. Effects of calcitonin gene-related peptide on cyclic AMP formation in chicken, rat and mouse bone cells. *J Bone Miner Res* 1989;4:269–72.

308. Yasumura S. Effect of adrenal steroids on bone resorption in rats. *Am J Physiol* 1976;230:90–3.

309. Raisz LG, Trummel CL, Wener JA, Simmons H. Effect of glucocorticoids on bone resorption in tissue culture. *Endocrinology* 1972;90:961–7.

310. Tobias J, Chambers TJ. Glucocorticoids impair bone resorptive activity and viability of osteoclasts disaggregated from neonatal rat long bones. *Endocrinology* 1989;125:1290–5.

311. Reid IR, Katz JM, Ibbertson HK, Gray DH. The effects of hydrocortisone, parathyroid hormone and the bisphosphonate, APD, on bone resorption in neonatal mouse calvaria. *Calcif Tissue Int* 1985;38:38–43.

312. Gronowicz G, McCarthy MB, Raisz LG. Glucocorticoids stimulate resorption in fetal rat prenatal bones in vitro. *J Bone Miner Res* 1990;in press.

313. Lukert BP, Raisz LG. Glucocorticoid-induced osteoporosis: pathogenesis and management. *Ann Intern Med* 1990;112:352–64.

314. Ishikawa H, Tanaka H, Iwato K, Tanabe O, Asaoku H, Nobuyoshi M, Yamamoto I, Kawano M, Kuramoto A. Effect of glucocorticoids on the biologic activities of myeloma cells: inhibition of interleukin-1 beta osteoclast activating factor-induced bone resorption. *Blood* 1990;75:715–20.

315. Caputo CB, Meadows D, Raisz LG. Failure of estrogens and androgens to inhibit bone resorption in tissue culture. *Endocrinology* 1976;98:1065–8.

316. Takano-Yamamoto T, Rodan GA. Direct effects of 17-beta-estradiol on trabecular bone in ovariectomized rats. *Proc Natl Acad Sci USA* 1990;87:2172–6.

317. Fukayama H, Tashjian AH Jr. Direct modulation by androgens of the response of human bone cells (SaOS-2) to human parathyroid hormone (PTH) and PTH-related protein. *Endocrinology* 1989;125:1789–94.

318. Fukayama S, Tashjian AH. Direct modulation by estradiol of the response of human bone cells (SaOS-2) to human parathyroid hormone (PTH) and PTH-related protein. *Endocrinology* 1989;124:397–401.

319. Pilbeam CC, Klein-Nulend J, Raisz LG. Inhibition by 17β-estradiol of PTH stimulated resorption and prostaglandin production in cultured neonatal mouse calvariae. *Biochem Biophys Res Commun* 1989;183:1319–24.

320. Feyen JHM, Raisz LG. Prostaglandin production by calvariae from Sham operated and oophorectomized rats: effect of 17β-estradiol in vivo. *Endocrinology* 1987;121:819–21.

321. Ernst M, Heath JK, et al. Estradiol effects on proliferation, messenger ribonucleic acid for collagen and insulin-like growth factor-1, and parathyroid hormone-stimulated adenylate cyclase activity in osteoblastic cells from calvariae and long bone. *Endocrinology* 1989;125:825–33.

322. Keeting PE, Bonewald LF, Colvard DS, Spelsberg TC, Mundy GR, Riggs BL. Estrogen-mediated release of transforming growth factor-beta by normal human osteoblast-like cells. *J Bone Miner Res* 1989;4:Abstract 655.

323. Pacifici R, Rifas L, McCracken R, et al. Ovarian steroid treatment blocks a postmenopausal increase in blood monocyte interleukin-1 release. *Proc Natl Acad Sci USA* 1989;86:2398–402.

324. Pacifici R, Brown C, Rifas L, Avioli LV. TNFα and GM-CSF secretion from blood monocytes in normal and osteoporotic women: a preliminary study on the effect of menopause and estrogen/progesterone treatment. *Calcif Tissue Int* 1990;46:Abstract 217.

325. Jones SJ, Ali NN, Boyde A. Survival and resorptive activity of chick osteoclasts in culture. *Anat Embryol* 1986;174:265–75.

326. Marks SC Jr, Seifert MF. The lifespan of osteoclasts: experimen-

tal studies using the giant granule cytoplasmic marker characteristic of Beige mice. *Bone* 1985;6:451–5.

327. Parfitt AM. Trabecular bone architecture in the pathogenesis and prevention of fracture. *Am J Med* 1987;92:68–72.

328. Takahashi N, Mundy GR, Roodman GD. Recombinant human interferon-γ inhibits formation of human osteoclast-like cells. *J Immunol* 1986;137:3544–9.

329. Peterlik M, Hoffman O, Swetly P, Klaushofer K, Koller K. Recombinant γ-interferon inhibits prostaglandin-mediated and parathyroid hormone-induced resorption in cultured neonatal mouse calvaria. *FEBS Lett* 1985;185:287–90.

330. Hoffman O, Klaushofer K, Gleispach H, Leis HJ, Luger T, Koller K, Peterlik M. τInterferon inhibits basal and interleukin 1-induced prostaglandin production and bone resorption in neonatal mouse calvaria. *Biochem Biophys Res Commun* 1987;143:38–43.

331. Klaushofer K, Horandner H, Hoffmann O, Czerwenka E, Konig U, Koller K, Peterlik M. Interferon gamma and calcitonin induce differential changes in cellular kinetics and morphology of osteoclasts in cultured neonatal mouse calvaria. *J Bone Miner Res* 1989;4:585–606.

332. Vignery A, Niven-Fairchild T, Shepard MH. Recombinant murine interferon-γ inhibits the fusion of mouse alveolar macrophages in vitro but stimulates the formation of osteoclastlike cells on implanted syngeneic bone particles in mice in vivo. *J Bone Miner Res* 1990;5:637–44.

333. Bonewald LF, Mundy GR. Role of transforming growth factor-beta in bone remodeling. *Clin Orthop* 1990;250:261–76.

334. Pfielschifter J, Seyedin SM, Mundy GR. Transforming growth factor-beta inhibits bone resorption in fetal rat long bone cultures. *J Clin Invest* 1988;82:680–5.

335. Chenu C, Pfeilschifter J, Mundy GR, Roodman GD. Transforming growth factor-β inhibits formation of osteoclast-like cells in long-term human marrow cultures. *Proc Natl Acad Sci USA* 1988;85:5683–7.

336. Pfeilschifter J, Mundy GR. Modulation of type β transforming growth factor activity in bone cultures by osteotropic hormones. *Proc Natl Acad Sci USA* 1987;84:2024–8.

337. Centrella M, McCarthy TL, Canalis E. Parathyroid hormone modulates transforming growth factor β activity and binding in osteoblast-enriched cell cultures from fetal rat parietal bone. *Proc Natl Acad Sci USA* 1988;85:5889–93.

338. Oreffo ROC, Mundy GR, Seyedin SM, et al. Activation of the bone-derived latent TGFβ complex by isolated osteoclasts. *Biochem Biophys Res Commun* 1989;158:817–23.

339. Pfeilschifter J, Bonewald L, Mundy GR. Characterization of the latent transforming growth factor beta complex in bone. *J Bone Miner Res* 1990;5:49–58.

340. Oreffo ROC, Bonewald L, Kukita A, Garrett IR, Seyedin SM, Rosen D, Mundy GR. Inhibitory effects of the bone-derived growth factors osteoinductive factor and transforming growth factor-β on isolated osteoclasts. *Endocrinology* 1990;126:3069–75.

341. Shinar DM, Rodan GA. Biphasic effects of transforming growth factor-β on the production of osteoclast-like cells in mouse bone marrow cultures: the role of prostaglandins in the generation of these cells. *Endocrinology* 1990;126:3153–8.

342. Nefussi J-R, Baron R. PGE₂ stimulates both resorption and formation of bone in vitro: differential responses of the periosteum and the endosteum in fetal rat long bone cultures. *Anat Rec* 1985;211:9–16.

343. Arend WP, Joslin FG, Thompson RC, Hannum CH. An IL-1 inhibitor from human monocytes. Production and characterization of biologic properties. *J Immunol* 1989;143:1851–8.

344. Seckinger P, Klein-Nulend J, Alander C, Thompson RC, Dayer J-M, Raisz LG. Natural and recombinant human interleukin-1 receptor antagonists block the effects of interleukin-1 on bone resorption and prostaglandin production. *J Immunol* 1990;in press.

345. Lorenzo JA, Raisz LG. Divalent cation ionophores stimulate resorption and inhibit DNA synthesis in cultured fetal rat bone. *Science* 1981;212:1157–9.

346. Lorenzo JA, Sousa S. Phorbol esters stimulates bone resorption

in fetal rat long-bone cultures by mechanisms independent of prostaglandin synthesis. *J Bone Miner* 1988;3:63–7.

347. Segre GV, Rosenblatt M, Tully GL III, Laugharn J, Reit B, Potts JT Jr. Evaluation of an in vitro parathyroid hormone antagonist in vivo in dogs. *Endocrinology* 1985;116:1024–9.

348. Doppelt SH, Neer RM, Nussbaum SR, Federico P, Potts JT Jr, Rosenblatt M. Inhibition of the in vivo parathyroid hormone-mediated calcemic response in rats by a synthetic hormone antagonist. *Proc Natl Acad Sci USA* 1986;83:7557–60.

349. Goldman ME, Chorev M, Reagen JE, Nutt RF, Levy JJ, Rosenblatt M. Evaluation of novel parathyroid hormone analogs using a bovine renal membrane receptor binding assay. *Endocrinology* 1988;123:1468–75.

350. D'Santos CS, Nicholson GC, Moseley M, Evans T, Martin TJ, Kemp BE. Biologically active, derivatizable salmon calcitonin analog: design, synthesis, and applications. *Endocrinology* 1988;123:1483–8.

351. Epand RM, Epand RF, Stafford AR, Orlowski RC. Deletion sequences of salmon calcitonin that retain the essential biological and conformational features of the intact molecule. *J Med Chem* 1988;31:1595–8.

352. Roos BA, Fischer JA, Pignant W, Alander CB, Raisz LG. Evaluation of the in vivo and in vitro calcium-regulating actions of noncalcitonin peptides produced via calcitonin gene expression. *Endocrinology* 1986;118:46–51.

353. Reichel H, Keoffler P, Norman AW. The role of the vitamin D endocrine system in health and disease. *N Engl J Med* 1989;320:980–91.

354. Lorenzo JA, Holtrop ME, Raisz LG. Effects of phosphate on calcium release, lysosomal enzyme activity in the medium, and osteoclast morphometry in cultured fetal rat bones. *Metab Bone Dis Relat Res* 1984;5:187–90.

355. Sutuzer A, Fleisch H, Trechsel U. Short- and long-term effects of a single dose of biphosphonates on retinoid-inducing bone resorption in thyroparathyroidectomized rats. *Calcif Tissue Int* 1988;43:294–9.

356. van Rooijen N, Kors N. Effects of intracellular diphosphonates on cells of the mononuclear phagocyte system: in vivo effects of liposome-encapsulated diphosphonates on different macrophage subpopulations in the spleen. *Calcif Tissue Int* 1989;45:153–6.

357. Sato M, Grasser W. Effects of bisphosphonates on isolated rat osteoclasts as examined by reflected light microscopy. *J Bone Miner Res* 1990;5:31–40.

358. Carano A, Teitelbaum SL, Konsek JD, Schlesinger PH, Blair HC. Bisphosphonates directly inhibit the bone resorption activity of isolated avian osteoclasts in vitro. *J Clin Invest* 1990;85:456–61.

359. Cecchini MG, Felix R, Fleisch H, Cooper PH. Effect of bisphosphonates on proliferation and viability of mouse bone marrow-derived macrophages. *J Bone Miner Res* 1987;2:135–42.

360. Hughes DE, Macdonald BR, Russell RGG, et al. Inhibition of osteoclast-like cell formation by bisphosphonates in long-term cultures of human bone marrow. *J Clin Invest* 1989;83:1930–5.

361. Lowik CWGM, Van der Pluijm G, Van der Wee-Pals LJA, Van Treslong-De Groot HB, Bijvoet OLM. Migration and phenotypic transforming of osteoclast precursors into mature osteoclasts: the effect of a bisphosphonate. *J Bone Miner Res* 1988;3:185–92.

362. Marshall MJ, Wilson AS, Davie MWJ. Effects of (3-amino-1-hydroxypropylidene)-1,1-bisphosphonate on mouse osteoclasts. *J Bone Miner Res* 1990;5:955–62.

363. Gaffar A, Alander CB, Raisz LG. Direct inhibition of bone resorption and inactivation of stimulators of resorption by potassium peroxydiphosphate. *J Bone Miner Res* 1990;in press.

364. Delaisse J-M, Eeckhout Y, Sear C, Galloway A, McCullagh K, Vaes G. A new synthetic inhibitor of mammalian tissue collagenase inhibits bone resorption in culture. *Biochem Biophys Res Commun* 1985;133:483–90.

365. Everts V, Beertsen W, Schroder R. Effects of the proteinase inhibitors leupeptin and E-64 on osteoclastic bone resorption. *Calcif Tissue Int* 1988;43:172–8.

366. Lerner UH, Gustafson GT. Inhibition of bone resorption in vitro by serine-esterase inhibitors. *Biochim Biophys Acta* 1988; 964:129–36.

367. Vargas SJ, Jones TG, Hurley MM, Raisz LG. Comparison of the effects of auranofin, gold sodium thiomalate, and penicillamine

on resorption of cultured fetal rat long bones. *J Bone Miner Res* 1987;2:183–9.

368. Katz JM, Gray DH. The in vitro effect of gold complexes on bone resorption. *J Orthop Res* 1986;4:188–93.

369. Klaushofer K, Hoffman O, et al. Effect of auranofin on resorption, prostaglandin synthesis and ultrastructure of bone cells in cultured mouse calvaria. *J Rheumatol* 1989;16:749–56.

370. Delaisse J-M, Eeckhout Y, Vaes G. Inhibition of bone resorption in culture by (+)-catechin. *Biochem Pharmacol* 1986;35:3091–4.

371. Zaidi M, Moonga B, Moss DW, et al. Inhibition of osteoclastic acid phosphatase abolishes bone resorption. *Biochem Biophys Res Commun* 1989;159:68–71.

372. Tsuda M, Kitazaki T, Ito T, Fujita T. The effect of ipriflavone (TC-80) on bone resorption in tissue culture. *J Bone Miner Res* 1986;1:207–11.

373. Krieger NS, Kim SG. Dichlorbenzamin inhibits stimulated bone resorption in vitro. *Endocrinology* 1988;122:415–20.

374. Eilon G, Raisz LG. Chloroquine, hydroxystilbamidine, and dapsone inhibit resorption of fetal rat bone in organ culture. *Calcif Tissue Int* 1982;34:506–9.

375. Johannesson AJ, Raisz LG. Effects of ammonium chloride on resorption of fetal rat bones in organ culture. *Am J Physiol* 1984;246:E516–8.

376. Krieger NS, Stathopoulos VM, Stern PH. Does amrinone inhibition of stimulated bone resorption involve Na^+–Ca^{++} exchange? *Circulation* 1986;73:59–64.

377. Lerner U, Fredholm BB, Hanstrom L. Diphenylhydantoin inhibits parathyroid hormone and prostaglandin E_2-stimulated bone resorption in mouse calvaria without affecting cyclic AMP formation. *J Oral Pathol* 1985;14:644–53.

378. Ly SY, Rebut-Bonneton C, Miravet L. Effects of the calcium antagonist, diltiazem, on in vitro and in vivo/in vitro bone resorption. *Horm Metab Res* 1985;17:152–5.

379. Waite LC, Volkert WA, Kenny AD. Inhibition of bone resorption by acetazolamide in the rat. *Endocrinology* 1970;87:1129–39.

380. Raisz LG, Simmons HA, Thompson WJ, Shepard KL, Anderson PS, Rodan GA. Effects of a potent carbonic anhydrase inhibitor on bone resorption in organ culture. *Endocrinology* 1988; 122:1083–6.

381. Lemann J Jr, Gray RW, Maierhofer WJ, Cheung HS. Hydrochlorothiazide inhibits bone resorption in men despite experimentally elevated serum 1,25-dihydroxyvitamin D concentrations. *Kidney Int* 1985;28:951–8.

382. Klein-Nulend J, Raisz LG. Effects of two inhibitors of anion transport on bone resorption in organ culture. *Endocrinology* 1989;125:1019–24.

383. Warrell RP, Alcock NW, Bockman RS. Gallium nitrate inhibits accelerated bone turnover in patients with bone metastases. *J Clin Oncol* 1987;5:292–8.

384. Cournot-Witmer G, Bourdeau A, Lieberherr M, Thil CL, Plachot JJ, Enault G, Bourdon R, Balsan S. Bone modeling in gallium nitrate-treated rats. *Calcif Tissue Int* 1987;40:270–5.

385. Shaker JL, Fallon MD, Goldfarb S, Farber J, Attie MF. WR-2721 reduces bone loss after hindlimb tenotomy in rats. *J Bone Miner Res* 1990;4:885–90.

386. Hirschel-Scholz S, Caverzasio J, Rizzoli R, Bonjour J-Ph. Normalization of hypercalcemia associated with a decrease in renal calcium reabsorption in Leydig cell tumor-bearing rats treating with WR-2721. *J Clin Invest* 1986;78:319–22.

387. Stewart PJ, Stern PH. Cyclosporines: correlation of immunosuppressive activity and inhibition of bone resorption. *Calcif Tissue Int* 1989;45:222–6.

388. Stewart PJ, Green OC, Stern PH. Cyclosporine A inhibits calcemic hormone-induced bone resorption in vitro. *J Bone Miner Res* 1986;1:285–91.

389. Orcel P, Bielakoff J, Modrowski D, et al. Cyclosporin A induces in vivo inhibition of resorption and stimulation of formation in rat bone. *J Bone Miner Res* 1989;4:387–91.

390. Movsowitz C, Epstein S, Ismail F, et al. Cyclosporin A in the oophorectomized rat: unexpected severe bone resorption. *J Bone Miner Res* 1989;4:393–8.

391. Lloyd W, Fang VS, Wells H, Tashjian AH Jr. 2-Thiophenecarboxylic acid: a hypoglycemic, antilipolytic agent with hypocalce-

mic and hypophosphatemic effects in rats. *Endocrinology* 1969;85:763.

392. Raisz LG, Alander C, Onkelinx C, Rodan GA. Effects of thionaphthene 2-carboxylic acid and related compounds on bone resorption in organ culture. *Calcif Tissue Int* 1985;37:556–9.

393. Decker JE, Morrison NE, Lorenzo JA, Samour CM, McCarron BA, Raisz LG. The effects of thionaphthene-2-carboxylic acid-lysine on the hypercalcemia of malignancy in the rat. *Calcif Tissue Int* 1989;44:61–4.

394. Hausmann E, Raisz LG, Miller WA. Endotoxin: stimulation of bone resorption in tissue culture. *Science* 1970;168:862–4.

395. Hausmann E, Luderitz O, Knox K, Weinfeld N. Structural requirements for bone resorption by endotoxin and lipoteichoic acid. *J Dent Res* 1975;54:B94–9.

396. Raisz LG, Alander C, Eilon G, Whitehead SP, Nuki K. Effects of two bacterial products, muramyl dipeptide and endotoxin, on bone resorption in organ culture. *Calcif Tissue Int* 1982;34:365–9.

397. Millar SJ, Goldstein EG, Levine MJ, Hausmann E. Lipoprotein: a gram-negative cell wall component that stimulates bone resorption. *J Periodont Res* 1986;21:256–9.

398. Umezu A, Kaneko N, Toyama Y, Watanabe Y, Itoh H. Appearance of osteoclasts by injections of lipopolysaccharides in rat periodontal tissue. *J Periodont Res* 1989;24:378–83.

399. Bom-van Noorloos AA, van Steenbergen TJM, Burger EH. Direct and immune-cell-mediated effects of bacteroides gingivalis on bone metabolism in vitro. *J Clin Periodontol* 1989;16:412–8.

400. Sismey-Durrant HJ, Atkinson SJ, Hopps RM, et al. The effect of lipopolysaccharide from bacteroides gingivalis and muramyl dipeptide on osteoblast collagenase release. *Calcif Tissue Int* 1989;44:361–3.

401. Williams RC. Periodontal disease. *N Engl J Med* 1990;322:373–82.

402. Taylor ML, Boyde A, Jones SJ. The effect of fluoride on the patterns of adherence of osteoclasts cultured on and resorbing dentine: a 3-D assessment of vinculin-labelled cells using confocal optical microscopy. *Anat Embryol Berl* 1989;180:427–35.

403. Lindskog S, Flores ME, Lilja E, Hammarstrom L. Effect of a high dose of fluoride on resorbing osteoclasts in vivo. *Scand J Dent Res* 1989;97:483–7.

404. Riggs BL, Hodgson SF, O'Fallon WM, Chao EYS, Wahner HW, Muhs JM, Cedel SL, Melton LJ III. Effect of fluoride treatment on the fracture rate in postmenopausal women with osteoporosis. *N Engl J Med* 1990;322:802–9.

405. Sprague SM, Bushinsky DA. Mechanism of aluminum-induced calcium efflux from cultured neonatal mouse calvariae. *Am J Physiol* 1990;258:F583–8.

406. Rodriguez M, Felsenfeld AJ, Llach F. The role of aluminum in the development of hypercalcemia in the rat. *Kidney Int* 1987;31:766–71.

407. Bhattacharyya MH, Whelton BD, Stern PH, Peterson DP. Cadmium accelerates bone loss in ovariectomized mice and fetal rat limb bones in culture. *Proc Natl Acad Sci USA* 1988;85:8761–5.

408. Nogawa K, Tsuritani I, Kido T, Honda R, Yamada Y, Ishizaki M. Mechanism for bone disease found in inhabitants environmentally exposed to cadmium: decreased serum 1,25-dihydroxyvitamin D level. *Int Arch Occup Environ Health* 1987;59:21–30.

409. Zaidi M, Patchell A, Datta HK, MacIntyre I. Uncoupling of receptor-mediated cellular responses by ionic lithium. *J Endocrinol* 1989;123:R5–7.

410. Holak HM, Raisz LG. Effect of lithium on bone metabolism in organ culture. *Endocrinology* 1979;104:908.

411. Lazarus JH, Davies CJ, Woodhead JS, Walker DA, Owen GM. Effect of lithium on the metabolic response to parathyroid hormone. *Miner Electrolyte Metab* 1987;13:63–6.

412. McIntosh WB, Horn EH, Mathieson LM, Sumner D. The prevalence, mechanism and clinical significance of lithium-induced hypercalcaemia. *Med Lab Sci* 1987;44:115–8.

Disorders of Bone and Mineral Metabolism,
edited by Fredric L. Coe and Murray J. Favus,
© 1992 by Raven Press, Ltd. All rights reserved.

CHAPTER 14

The Biology, Chemistry, and Biochemistry of the Mammalian Growth Plate

David S. Howell and David D. Dean

In this chapter we discuss selected aspects of the anatomy, cell biology, physiology, and biochemistry of the growth plate. Particular emphasis is placed on the postnatal mammalian growth plate, although other examples will be used when appropriate. The chapter has been constructed as a reference source for those who are students, academic clinicians, or basic scientists working in the field of cartilage research. Each section surveys a specific research area. General reviews and papers on specific topics are cited. The chapter bypasses a detailed discussion of various dysplasias (1–3), cartilage embryology (4–6), biomechanical–electrical forces (7), and fracture healing (8). For this information the reader should consult the references cited. For discussions of early historical developments, older reviews are recommended. Definition of various terms appear in the text. Some older terminology, such as *spongiosa,* has been retained since it serves a purpose in understanding structure. To simplify discussion, the terms *calcification* and *mineralization* have not been distinguished.

GROWTH PLATE FUNCTION AND CLASSIFICATION

Role of the Growth Plate in Determining Bone Growth

The growth plate is a specialized tissue located at the distal and proximal ends of long bones in mammals. It is responsible for regulating longitudinal bone growth and

D. S. Howell: U.S. Veterans Administration Medical Center, Miami, Florida 33125 and Department of Medicine, University of Miami School of Medicine, Miami, Florida 33101
D. D. Dean: U.S. Veterans Administration Medical Center, Miami, Florida 33125 and Departments of Medicine and Biochemistry–Molecular Biology, University of Miami School of Medicine, Miami, Florida 33101.

is under the control of many local and systemic factors (9).

Knowledge of these factors has increased over the last three decades but is still incomplete. Precise synchronization of bone growth throughout the entire skeleton is achieved in response to physical forces and endocrine, paracrine, and autocrine factors (10). The effect of prolonged absence of specific hormones critical to growth plate regulation leads to reduced function and phenotypically presents as dwarfism.

Complex controls exist for regulating growth at a precise locus independent of growth at other sites: for example, the "catch-up" growth of a limb after immobilization. Some of this control must be vested in the cells themselves, since examples of different rates and types of mineralization can be found in mammals (as discussed here) as well as in shark cartilage and deer antler (11,12).

Thus the growth plate must accomplish some rather remarkable functions. Any derangement would be likely to result in clinically significant disease, such as gigantism, dwarfism, or various bony deformities where one segment of growth plate differentiation is omitted (1). Well-known genetic disorders affecting growth plate function are reviewed elsewhere (1–3).

Prenatal Bone Formation

The formation of cartilage and bone during embryonic development is quite different from that found postnatally (4,6). Differences are noticeable in both control and sequence. In the embryo, tubular bone is formed from a cartilaginous anlage that defines the outer limits of the first marrow cavity. In this case, the cartilage provides a scaffold for new membranous bone as well as a "message" system for the proper placement of marrow and vascular elements. In late embryonic development coarse-weave (woven) bone forms a coating on calcified cartilage as studied in bovine cartilages. Once this "first bone" is formed postnatally, growth center function and enchondral bone formation can begin.

Postnatal Bone Formation; Enchondral Calcification

Postnatal epiphyseal cartilage derives from embryological cartilage and remains functioning into adolescence. It participates in the growth and lengthening of long bones until the time of growth plate closure. The organ operates through a highly complex and synchronous mechanism of continuous cell proliferation, cell enlargement, and removal of enlarged cells by capillary invasion (9).

This sequence is highly ordered to promote bone growth along the appropriate axis. At the epiphyseal end of the growth plate, progenitor cells of chondrogenic potential are formed continuously. These cells mature and are invaded by metaphyseal blood vessels prior to formation of metaphyseal bone. The cartilage of the growth plate remains at approximately the same thickness, with the metaphyseal front advancing at the same rate as new cartilage cells form and enlarge at the epiphyseal front (1). The diaphysis increases in length by remodeling of secondary spongiosa. In longitudinal bone growth, new bone is always laid down on a framework of calcified cartilage matrix called primary spongiosa. (See section on "Tissue Organization at the Ends of Bones," below.)

Bone Growth in Fracture Repair Sites; Ectopic Growth Centers

Interestingly, the early stages of immobilized fracture repair resemble the events described for enchondral growth plates (8). Histologically, the chondrocytes enlarge or hypertrophy, adjacent septa calcify, and then become replaced with bone. In many respects, the cellular and biochemical composition of these tissues duplicate the normal enchondral process. One matter of controversy concerns whether rapid cartilage lysis and replacement by trabecular bone in the presence of chondrogenic stimulating agents more closely resembles postnatal bone spicule formation or prenatal spicule formation. Repair in the adult is distinctly different from that in the embryo since adult (i.e., postnatal) tissues contain a different profile of paracrine and autocrine factors active in directing cartilage growth (4). The identity and function of these factors in matrix repair is only beginning to be elucidated (13,14).

An area of current research interest involves the study of ectopic growth centers that can be induced at various sites. For example, when demineralized bone matrix is implanted subcutaneously, the combination of differentiation and chemotactic factors found in the matrix can attract and induce differentiation of progenitor cells (9,10,13–17). The cells subsequently mature into hypertrophic chondrocytes; this is followed by calcification of the matrix. Capillary invasion is then followed by the formation of coarse-weave (woven) bone on top of the calcified cartilage, as well as a complete complement of bone marrow cells and circulation derived from the new marrow (13,14). As mentioned for fracture healing, the sequence mimics in almost every detail the functioning of a normal growth plate and the formation of metaphyseal bone. Detailed studies over the course of 30 days have shown the appearance of characteristic biochemical markers for each stage and a single protein that can initiate these events (10,13–17).

ANATOMY AND HISTOLOGY OF THE GROWTH PLATE

Tissue Organization at the Ends of Long Bones

The distal and proximal ends of long bones (sometimes called tubular bones) are exquisitely designed for controlled bone lengthening as well as structural support and load bearing. Several terms are used to describe the constituent regions found at the ends of long bones (Fig. 1). A brief description follows.

The *growth plate* is a transverse disc of cartilage lodged between epiphyseal and metaphyseal bone that functions as a primary growth center to provide for longitudinal bone growth (1). The term *epiphysis* includes the entire end of the bone beyond the growth plate. The *bony island* or *epiphyseal bone* forms from a secondary growth center and provides structure and shape to the articulation as well as the blood supply for the metabolically active growth plate. The term *physis* is interchangeable with growth plate, although some find this cumbersome and confusing (1). Adult remodeling of bone after growth plate closure (see below) depends on the reopening of focal growth centers in subchondral cartilage.* Modified, reopened focal growth centers are also found in pathological conditions such as osteoarthritis (18,19). In these examples of bone lengthening or remodeling, mineral deposition occurs through enchondral ossification (9). Lateral growth of bone, as discussed in Chapter 10, occurs through membranous ossification in a direction perpendicular to that produced by growth centers. The layer of new bone directly under the growth plate is in a region called the *metaphysis*. This area extends deep into the central space directly below the growth plate. It contains an array of capillaries that penetrate the growth plate per se, as well as the calcified cartilage septae which are being replaced by newly evolving bone (1,9).

Extensions of the circulatory system called *cartilage canals* can be found to penetrate directly varying dis-

---

* Ch. 15 also discussed remodeling—*Ed.*

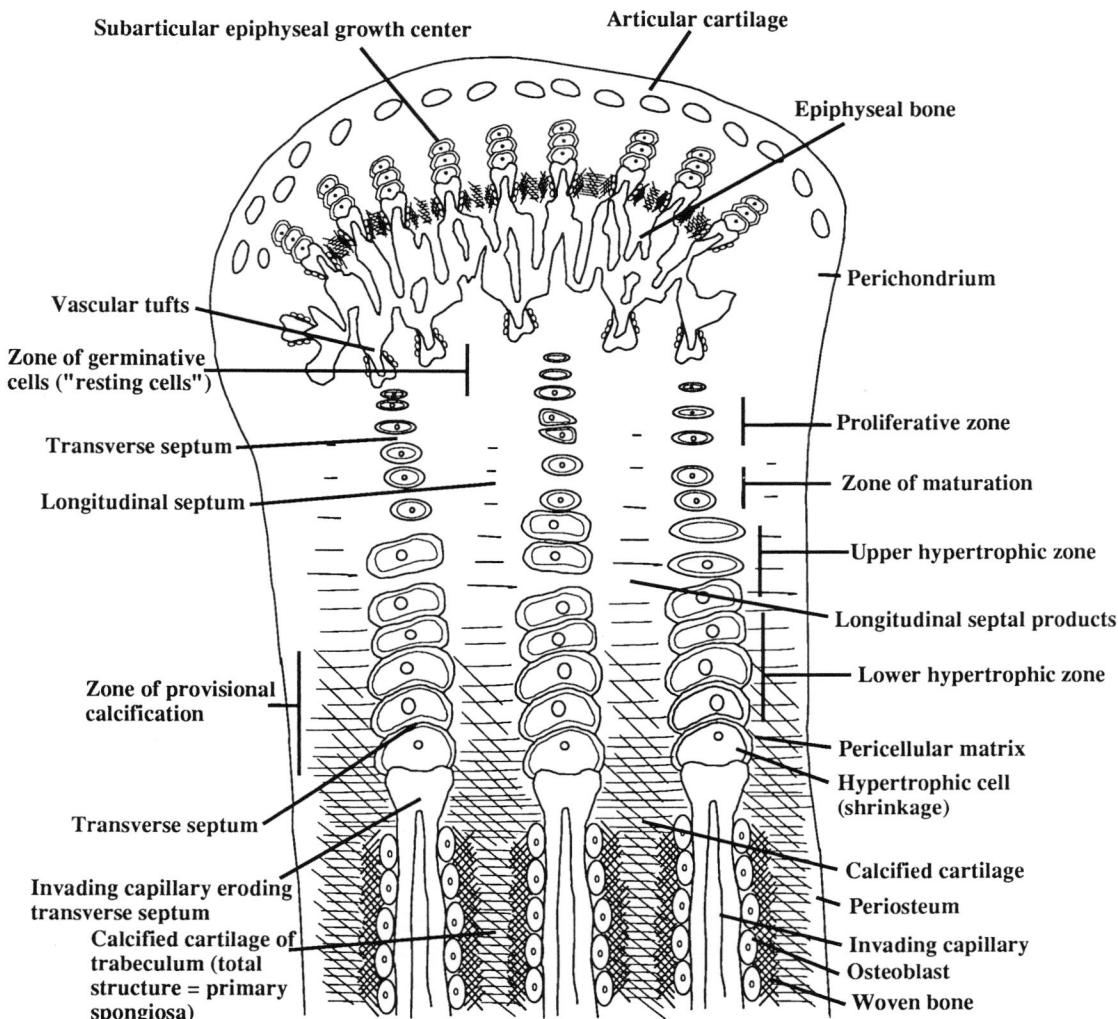

FIG. 1. Artist's rendering of the postnatal mammalian growth plate showing the articular cartilage, subarticular growth center, epiphyseal bone, growth plate per se, and metaphyseal bone. The direction of bone elongation is toward the top of the page and occurs due to new chondrocyte formation. The chondrocytes divide, elaborate matrix, expand (hypertrophy), and are eventually invaded by capillaries from below. As hypertrophic cells are invaded, approximately 60% of the residual calcified septae are retained and coated with woven bone.

tances into avian growth centers. In mammals, these canals are distinctly different and can be found along the circumference of the growth plate connecting the epiphysis to the metaphysis. The role of these canals in avian growth plates is extremely significant since this is the region where mineralization begins (20,21). In mammalian growth plates, however, mineralization does not seem to be controlled by the presence of these canals, although a similar circulatory unit is quite possible (22).

Shortly after puberty in humans, the growth plate undergoes a process called *closure*. At a time that is specific for each growth plate, capillaries migrate through the cartilage and lay down trabecular bone and marrow elements (1). This process has been observed in most mammals, as well; in rodents, however, growth plates remain permanently open.

The growth plate is surrounded by a fibrous collagenous tissue called the *perichondrium*. Part of this tissue, the sheath of LeBlond, is thickened and layered in such a manner as to suggest that it functions in protecting the growth plate from osmotic swelling forces (23). The *groove of Ranvier* is a circumferential sulcus that contains blood vessels (9,23). It is believed that this groove may have a role in cartilage lateral growth regulation since mesenchymal cells from the perichondrium migrate into this region and become the progenitors of growth plate chondrocytes.

Morphology of the Growth Plate

As mentioned above, long bones extend their length by a complex sequence of events that are largely controlled by the growth plate. When viewed in cross section under a light microscope (Figs. 2 and 3), the plate can be seen to consist of an orderly grouping of cells into four well-defined morphological zones: (1) the zone of resting cartilage or germinal cell zone; (2) the zone of proliferating cartilage, which contains the zone of maturation at its lower end; (3) the upper zone of hypertrophic cell cartilage; and (4) the lower zone of hypertrophic cell cartilage, which includes the zone of calcified cartilage (24–27).

At the metaphyseal border of the calcified cartilage zone a parallel array of longitudinally oriented capillary loops invade the hypertrophic cell columns in the area known as the *metaphyseal junction* (Fig. 3). It is here that chondroclasts and mononuclear macrophages congregate (21). Osteogenic cells differentiate and deposit a layer of osteoid on the longitudinal bars of calcified cartilage. This newly mineralized structure is then termed *primary* spongiosa (1). Following extensive remodeling, the spongiosa is termed *secondary*.

Description of the Upper Cell Zones in the Growth Plate

The uppermost region of the growth plate contains chondrocytes of moderate size scattered irregularly throughout the matrix. The cells in the central region are believed to originate from epiphyseal vascular tufts,

whereas those in the peripheral areas may originate from the perichondrium. The collagen matrix in this region consists of randomly oriented fibers that serve to anchor the growth plate to the bony epiphysis and perichondrium. As the cells mature, they form small aggregates and become columnated; the mechanism of this process is poorly understood (24–27).

The chondrocytes in the proliferative zone are plate-like or polyspheroid in shape (25). In sagittal section, these cells have been described as having a triangular outline. Matrix is produced at a rapid rate in this region. The cells divide rapidly and form well-oriented columns lying in the longitudinal axis of the bone (26). The random collagenous matrix found in the resting cell zone becomes more ordered, forming longitudinal septa, and by the end of the proliferating zone the predominant fiber direction is longitudinal (27).

Description of the Lower Cell Zones in the Growth Plate

In the hypertrophic cell zone, the chondrocytes maintain their columnar orientation while undergoing a tremendous expansion in size (24–35). As the cells mature in this zone, their expansion (over a distance of just a few cells in the longitudinal direction) can be as much as 500% (24,25,27,33,34). During this process, the cells lose much of their spherical shape and become super ellipses

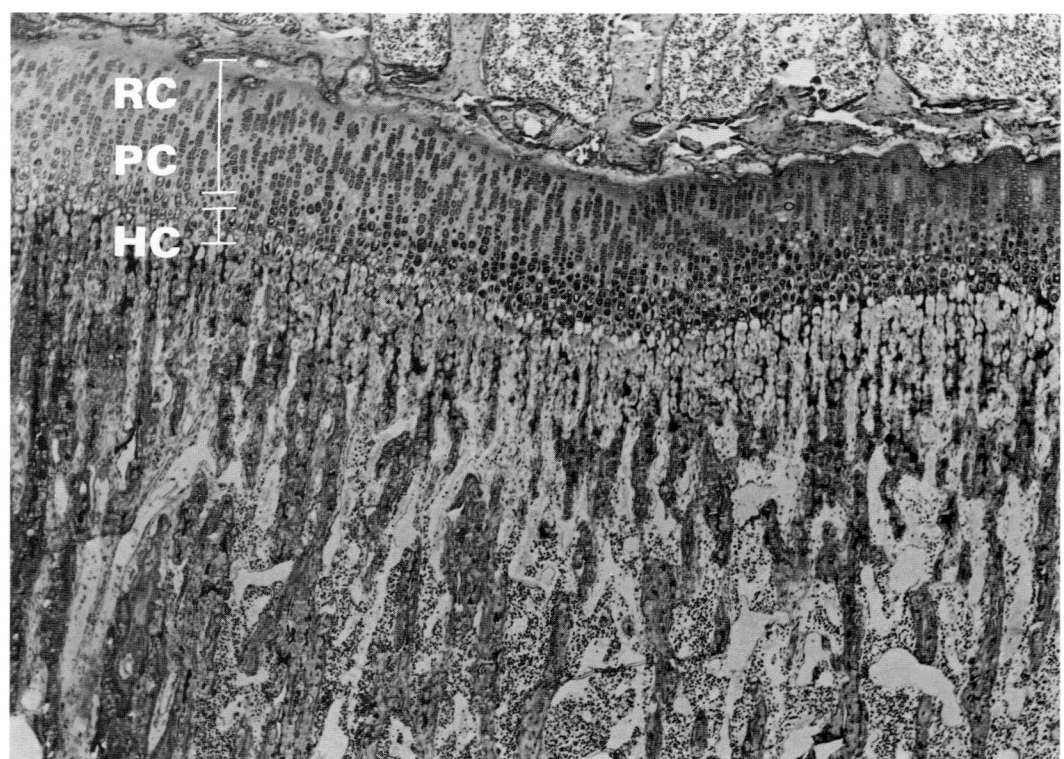

FIG. 2. Light micrograph of the upper tibial rat growth plate (×100). (Provided from unpublished materials by Dr. Isaac Atkin.) Histological zones of: RC, resting cell; PC, proliferating cells; HC, hypertrophic cells.

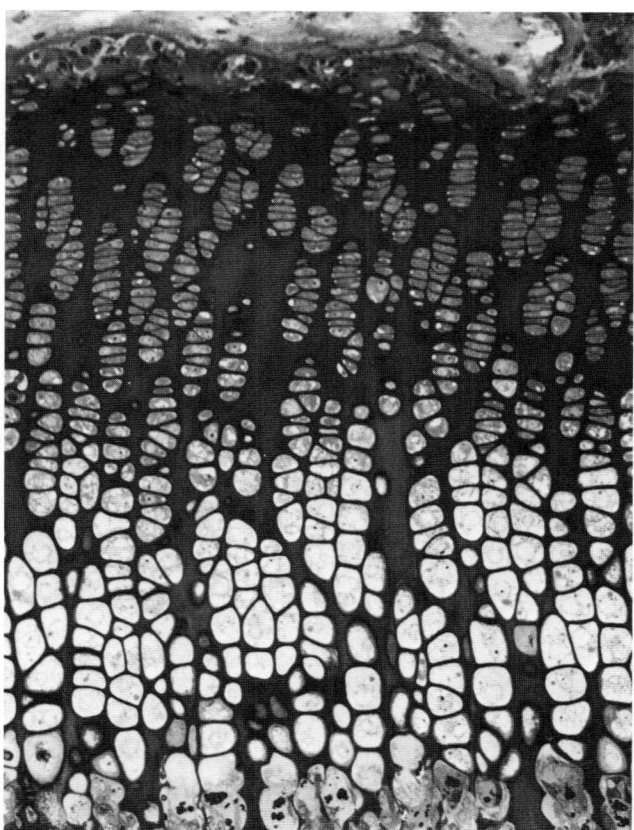
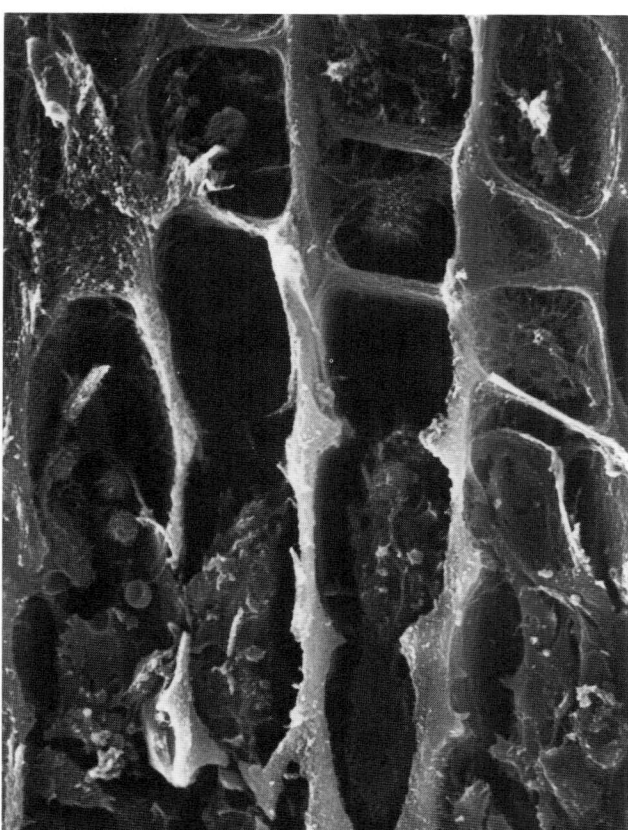

A   B

FIG. 3. A: Light micrograph of the rat growth plate (×240). Fixation of the tissue in the presence of ruthenium hexamine trichloride (RHT) permits rapid and homogeneous penetration of the fixative and stain. Chondrocytes are thereby preserved in their expanded state. Preservation of the extracellular matrix and lack of lacunar spaces should also be noted. (Photograph provided by Dr. E. Hunziker from unpublished work.) **B:** Scanning electron micrograph of the metaphyseal–hypertrophic cell zone (HCZ) junction of a normal rat. Notice that the columns of HCZ cells are separated by longitudinal septae. Capillaries (note the intraluminal disclike red blood cells) can be seen to penetrate the hypertrophic chondrocytes vertically and the transverse septae from below. Each "tube" is composed of septal walls extending as primary spongiosa (×20,000). (Photograph provided by Dr. E. Hunziker from unpublished work.)

with their long axis parallel with the longitudinal septa (25). The cytoplasm, endoplasmic reticulum, cisternae, Golgi, and mitochondria also become greatly expanded (27). Transverse expansion of the lacunae occurs at the expense of narrowing the longitudinal septa adjacent to the cells. At the light microscopic level, the mineral content of the calcifying septae can be seen to increase near the last three to four cells of the lower hypertrophic cell zone (28). In contrast, focal mineralization can rarely be seen by x-ray elemental analysis in the late proliferative cell zone (28).

In the zone of calcified cartilage, cell expansion is complete and provisional calcification of the matrix has occurred. At the lower border of the calcified cartilage, the last horizontal septum is degraded by one or more resorptive mechanisms. In cross section, each cell column appears as a tube with walls composed of calcified cartilage. Capillary loops, followed by chondroclasts and mononuclear macrophages, are found in this region (21,35). About 75% of the calcified tubes coated with bone (primary spongiosa) are resorbed by these phagocytic cells; the remaining 25% are destined to become secondary spongiosa (1). This region, where the growth plate and metaphysis are joined, is stabilized not only by the perichondrium (as mentioned above) but also by the primary spongiosa.

Osteogenic cells are believed to arise from either progenitor cells in the marrow or hypertrophic chondrocytes (30–33). The osteogenic cells differentiate into osteoblasts and then congregate on the longitudinal tubes of calcified cartilage and deposit a thin layer of osteoid. Longitudinal bone growth can proceed in this fashion as long as the growth plate is able to supply the necessary amount of calcified septa for spongy bone apposition.

Role of the Vasculature in Growth Plate Calcification and Nutrition

The growth plate is served by two main arteries. One approaches from the epiphyseal side and supplies nutrients to the bony island of the epiphysis as well as feeding the capillary tufts that enter the growth plate. The other blood supply approaches from the metaphysis and feeds into the capillary loops that invade the growth plate from the metaphyseal side (23,36).

It has been appreciated for some time that the metaphyseal–growth plate border is an area of intense remodeling. Metaphyseal capillary loops synchronously penetrate the last transverse septum of the hypertrophic cell zone at a ratio of one loop per cell across the entire growth plate (23,36). This loop, along with one or two mononuclear cells and a few adjacent chondroclasts, has been termed the *invading capillary complex* (35).

The relative role of each of these blood supplies in nourishing the growth plate was explored by Trueta and Amato (36). In one study, an incision was made so that the capillary tufts in the resting cell zone were separated from the circulation in the epiphyseal bone. This blockage resulted in death of the entire growth plate apparatus, presumably due to nutritional insufficiency. If a similar incision was made so that part of the metaphyseal circulation was destroyed, the columns of cartilage cells opposite the injury continued to grow, but no calcification occurred. Thus the lesion interfered with the ingrowth of blood vessels and calcification, but nutrition was adequate for growth plate survival. Similar experiments have been performed with rat, rabbit, dog, and even human growth plates, indicating a common function for the two blood supplies in various species. Other observations are also relevant to these findings.

Studies in the authors' laboratory with rat growth plates have shown that ligating the metaphyseal circulation in vivo drops the normal alkaline pH of the micropuncture fluid (extracellular fluid obtained by aspiration) and blocks calcification but allows for growth plate survival (D. S. Howell, unpublished observation). In dyschondroplasias, the capillary invasion apparatus is interrupted in such a way that calcification and bone growth are arrested (1). A similar failure can be observed after chemical or metabolic interference. For example, in rats fed a diet deficient in vitamin D and phosphate or calcium, a rachitic syndrome is produced that results in the persistence of the lower hypertrophic cells and failure of bone growth (1,9). Administration of certain metallic ions (e.g., aluminum, beryllium, manganese, strontium, thallium) that appear to bind to various components of the mineral-forming apparatus can also induce rachitic syndromes similar to vitamin D deficiency (1,9,37).

The growth plate apparatus and its associated blood supply undergo continuous and concurrent cartilage formation and resorption. The rate of these processes is strictly controlled so that the linear accretion of mineral is balanced with the generation of new primary and secondary spongiosa. In the postnatal rat, the linear rate of growth is approximately 30 μm every 3 h; this requires the generation of an entire new growth plate roughly every 48 h (38–40).

PHYSIOLOGY OF NORMAL GROWTH PLATES

Introduction to Physiologic Functions of the Growth Plate

As discussed above, the primary role of the growth plate is to extrude calcified tubes at precisely controlled rates. The process must be engineered carefully so that the tubes are evenly distributed across the entire growth plate. New trabecular bone must arrive at the growing trabecular and cortical bone compartments concordant with funnelization so that shaping of the external margins of the metaphysis can occur properly.

For this to happen at the rates actually observed in vivo, high levels of energy must be consumed by the chondrocytes for synthesis of the organic and mineral constituents. In addition, special structural and adhesive proteins must be synthesized to provide a compact and dense matrix capable of binding high concentrations of mineral. Control of these factors probably depends on more complex pathways than those that simply regulate cell proliferation and steady-state synthetic rates. Much control seems vested in the terminal hypertrophic chondrocyte as well as the organic matrix, which can mineralize at different rates under various conditions.

The basis for the suggestion that mineralization imposes unique requirements on the tissues involved can be found by comparing membranous and enchondral bone formation. Membranous bone forms at a rate of 3–5 μm/day, whereas that of enchondral bone is usually on the order of 200 μm (or more) per day, involving synthesis of coarse weave rather than lamellar bone (38–40).

Difficulties in Studying Mineralized Tissues

By their very nature mineralized tissues are difficult to study because the organic and cellular constituents are intimately associated (in fact, entrapped) with the mineral phase. As a result, it has been difficult, using ordinary methodologies, to ascertain the organization of these elements and their physiologic function.

Over the last 10 years, considerable progress has been made in the ability to study cells of mineralized tissues. For example, low-temperature, high-pressure anhydrous embedding techniques, together with ruthenium hexamine trichloride staining of cartilage (Fig. 3A), have allowed updated stereological methods to be applied to the study of growth plate (24). By mathematical treatment of the cellular constituents and their matrix, our understanding of cell size and shape has increased dramatically. As examples of these powerful techniques, hypertrophic cell enlargement rates have been assessed, the absolute size of ultrastructural particles within cells and the numbers and size of matrix vesicles determined, and the relative proportions of interterritorial and territorial matrix derived (25–27). Antibodies are now readily available so that the tissue and/or cellular localization of special proteins can be determined. In situ hybridization methods are able to pinpoint the location of mRNA for specific proteins, while Northern analyses can estimate quantities of similar mRNA species. These technical advances have enriched our approach to the study of mineralized tissues. Some examples worth mentioning are cited in the following paragraphs.

In the older literature, the term *zone of cellular degeneration* was used frequently. This usage should probably be discontinued since much information shows that the cells in this zone are alive and very vigorous in synthetic capacity until the terminal cell disappears (30–33). The term *lacunar space* should be used with caution because the most recent fixation and embedding techniques fail to show these spaces. Furthermore, mitochondria and rough endoplasmic reticulum (rER) that were thought to be blebbing or fractured are, in fact, artifacts of tissue preparation (25).

Evidence for cellular secretion into the matrix through specialized channels has been found in articular cartilage (41). These structures, described as canaliculi at the electron microscopic level, include collagen fiber orientations that are different from the adjacent interterritorial matrix. If such a mechanism can be found and confirmed to operate in growth plate cartilage, it would account for nutrient transport and some vesicle transport phenomena now thought to be due to filopodia budding directly from the plasma membranes of lower proliferative cell zone chondrocytes (41).

Much attention has focused on defining the apparatus responsible for initiating the onset of new mineral formation. The most widely studied of these structures is the matrix vesicle (42–51). These subcellular organelles are particles surrounded by a trilaminar membrane found in the longitudinal septae of the lower proliferating cell zone and upper hypertrophic cell zone of the growth plate. Their appearance under a variety of circumstances at sites of initial mineralization support their proposed function (42,43), although recent studies have found them in large numbers in the resting cell zone where no mineral is formed (50,51). One group has hypothesized that they distribute themselves along the vertical axis (near longitudinal septae) and when mineralization begins, their numbers decrease substantially. These events are not singular but occur in concert with other changes. Immunolocalization studies with antibodies to the C-propeptide of type II collagen (chondrocalcin), link protein, and proteoglycan monomer have also been used in an effort to determine which changes are critical for the initiation of mineralization and their relationship to matrix vesicles (52–55). We discuss these events further later.

Kinetics of Chondrocyte Proliferation and Hypertrophy and Its Relation to Mineralization

The growth plate is continuously undergoing cartilage formation on one side and cartilage resorption on the other. Both processes are balanced so that long bone linear accretion is precisely controlled. Cartilage resorption starts at the primary and secondary spongiosa and ends up in the diaphyseal trabecular bone. In the postnatal rat, the linear rate of growth can be approximately 20 to 30 μm every 3 h, with the entire growth plate being renewed every 48 h (40). When one considers the half-life of collagen (almost infinity) and proteoglycan (beyond 100 days) in articular cartilage, the synthetic capacity of this tissue can be fully appreciated. In a recent study of long bone growth it was found that between 25 and 35 days of age rats exhibited a period of accelerated bone growth followed by a period of decelerated growth (56). During the time of rapid growth, the diameter of the growth plate remained relatively constant while the rate of bone lengthening increased. Stereologic analysis revealed that the linear growth rate change was due to a change in the rate of hypertrophic cell enlargement (i.e., lengthening) rather than a change in the cell proliferation rate (56).

The fate of the terminal hypertrophic chondrocyte is also being scrutinized by stereological methods. The new techniques suggest that these cells may undergo shrinkage or apoptosis, possibly due to programed death by monocyte mediated cytotoxicity (31). A high potassium concentration inside the terminal hypertrophic chondrocyte would indicate that these cells remain viable until the vascular events are well under way (32). These findings favor the hypothesis that hypertrophic chondrocytes remain active in coordinating vascular invasion and provisional calcification.

The kinetics of cell turnover are also affected by diurnal variation. In the normal rat growth plate, cell proliferation and matrix synthesis are greatest at midday and lowest during nighttime (57). This cycle can be changed to some extent by the feeding schedule and by altering light and dark cycles. Parathyroid hormone, vitamin D, and growth hormone have diurnal effects on matrix synthesis and cell proliferation, as well (58). Therefore, it can be seen that the kinetics of growth plate function are determined not only by cell proliferation, as once thought, but by a host of other complex factors.

Oxygenation and Energetics of the Growth Plate

It is well known that articular cartilage can satisfy many of its nutritional requirements through contact with the synovial fluid (59). The mechanical effect of compression and decompression plays a minor role in distributing various nutrients throughout the interstitial spaces of the cartilage, while diffusion is responsible for meeting most of the oxygen and other nutrient requirements. The same pattern of fluid flow induced by compression can be hypothesized to occur in the growth plate, but most investigators believe that this contribution to total growth plate nutrition is minor, since the rigid walls surrounding the growth plate limit distortion of the tissue during weight bearing. Thus other mechanisms have been sought to explain how the needs of this metabolically active tissue are met.

In the 1970s, Brighton and Heppenstall studied oxygen tension in the growth plate by use of platinum electrodes (60). It was found that a high oxygen tension was associated with the proliferating cell zone, a region where cell division and matrix synthesis were high. The extensive energy requirements for this region were assumed to be met by aerobic metabolism through the Krebs cycle and electron transport chain. The hypertrophic cell zone, by contrast, had a lower oxygen tension. This observation correlated well with the much lower rates of proteoglycan and collagen synthesis measured in this region. It was also thought that anaerobic glycolysis was the predominant source of metabolic energy under these conditions, since the level of glycolytic and Krebs cycle enzymes were consistent with this viewpoint (61–63). Loss of calcium and phosphate from the mitochondria at the same time that mineralization was beginning in the cartilage septae led to intensive study of these organelles.

The hypertrophic chondrocyte mitochondrion has been implicated in mineralization for several decades. In the early 1960s, active transport of calcium was observed in isolated kidney cell mitochondria (64). Intracellular calcium homeostasis requires maintenance of micromolar levels of this cation in the cytosol, and there is firm evidence that mitochondria play an important role in this function. Lehninger has postulated that mitochondria may serve as a way of overcoming the energy barrier necessary for the formation of new calcium–phosphate mineral at calcifying sites (65). Martin and Matthews demonstrated mineral deposition in growth plate mitochondria in vivo as well as mitochondrial granules in cells adjacent to calcifying septa (66). Brighton and Hunt, using potassium pyroantimonate stain, showed that calcium in the mitochondria was shifted out and "reappeared" in matrix vesicles at calcifying sites (67). Because of the low oxygen tension measured in this region (see below), Brighton hypothesized that this might be the trigger for the observed calcium movement and

the onset of calcification. Arsenis performed some subcellular fractionations and separated mitochondria rich in mineral from those lacking mineral (68). The latter predominated in cartilage prior to calcification, whereas the former predominated in cartilage after calcification had begun. A more specific demonstration of calcium-phosphate mineral in the granules of such cartilage cells was shown in microprobe analyses by Sutfin et al. (69). This was later confirmed and extended by Hargest et al. (70), who showed a similar pattern of calcium uptake and release by mitochondria using quantitative microprobe x-ray analysis on freeze-dried and embedded sections of growth plate.

Another approach used to study these observed changes has focused on the energy status of the chondrocytes in relation to calcification. Kakuta et al. have described some aspects of this process by measuring the NADH and NAD content of normal and rachitic growth cartilage (71). In precalcified regions, the reduced pyridine nucleotide content of the cells and the NADH/NAD ratio was low. The cells showed an increase in this ratio and accumulation of NADH as the cells became hypertrophic. It was suggested that the oxygen tension in the hypertrophic cell zone was lower than that found in the proliferating cell zone. Indeed, Brighton and Heppenstahl (60) had shown that the top half of the growth plate had an oxygen tension of 57 mmHg, while the bottom half had only 24 mmHg. This could be due to a poor blood supply or increased utilization. It was likely that reduced levels of nutrients (and thus energy) were getting to the chondrocytes. Low cellular levels of nucleotides have also been found in the precalcifying zones (72).

Further data concerning the relative oxidative activity of these two zones of chondrocytes have been described by Yamamoto and Gay (73). Histochemical detection of cytochrome oxidase activity in chicken growth plates revealed positive staining throughout the tissue. This indicated that at least some of the chondrocytes were involved in aerobic metabolism. The absolute number of cells was difficult to quantitate, but appeared elevated in the lower zone. Stereological analysis determined that the mitochondrial mass in the hypertrophic cell zone was three times that of the proliferating cell zone, suggesting that the region was geared for aerobic activity (27). This was further substantiated by finding an increased surface area of plasma, rough endoplasmic reticulum (ER), and Golgi membranes (25,27). The inference to be drawn from these findings is that the process of cell enlargement, involving synthesis and degradation of pericellular matrix and the possible uptake of amino acids, requires extensive amounts of energy (27,74).

An amendment to the cell hypoxia hypothesis has been proposed to reconcile some of the differences in oxygenation between the two zones: namely, could metabolism be very high in the distal hypertrophic cell zone due to its proximity to the circulation? In this case, could the apparent oxygen tension be low due to rapid utilization rather than lack of availability?

Shapiro et al. (75), using a new high-resolution technique for studying oxidative metabolism, have begun dissecting the complex metabolism of each zone of the avian growth plate. In early hypertrophic zones, the chondrocytes distant from the nutrient canals have high fluorescent signals, indicating elevated amounts of NADH. The perivascular cells, conversely, were more oxidized. An oxidized region 30–60 μm wide was found that was sufficient to contain one or more rows of chondrocytes. Shapiro et al. extended these results by hypothesizing that new mineral formation occurs in a basic architectural unit of active cells surrounding the perivascular elements. They noted several examples of similar design in nature, such as haversian bone. By this

view, mineralization would be accelerated in areas where capillaries are able to oxygenate the cells, allowing aerobic metabolism to proceed at a rapid rate. This would provide the speed required of the nutrient system, although evidence for this in mammals is still lacking. In addition, it can be reconciled with Brighton's observations since it is possible that some phases of the mineralization process are more energetically favorable under one set of oxygen tension than another. This possibility may be important in calcium ion flux (76,77).

Data supporting the suggestion of rapid oxygen utilization were obtained by studying interstitial fluid aspirated by micropuncture techniques from the hypertrophic cell zone (78). The chemistry of this fluid, as well as plasma taken from the same animals, was studied (Table 1). The only notable differences between the chemistry of this fluid and the plasma were with respect to high

TABLE 1. *Micropuncture fluid from hypertrophic cell zone cartilage septa[a]*

Parameter	Serum	Cartilage fluid, C_{fl}	Units	Interpretation
1. Na	142	140	mM/L	1–4: Profile of electrolytes assures an extracellular fluid phase (78,178)
2. K	4.0	4.5	mM/L	
3. Mg	1.33	0.6	mM/L	
4. Calcium	2.34	1.80	mM/L	
5. Phosphate	0.71	1.58	mM/L	5: High ratio of C_{fl}/serum phosphate in −VDP rickets; a booster mechanism for inorganic phosphate production may be revealed in these samples (78)
6. pH	7.3–7.4	7.6–7.7		6: Increased alkalinity would accelerate mineral deposition in normal rachitic and healing rachitic samples (79)
7. HCO$_3$	23	35.6	mM/L	7: Presence of high HCO$_3$ concentrations may have an effect of mineral deposition (79)
8. Alkaline phosphatase	100	275	pM/min/μL	8,9: Phosphohydrolytic enzymes in the fluid phase may generate inorganic phosphate (220)
9. ATPase	20	118	pM/min/μL	
10. Nucleotide	0.5	1.0	mg/mL	10: Possible source of organic phosphate for hydrolysis (78)
11. Acid-resistant mineral promoter	—	++		11: Structures with appearance of membranes under TEM presence of phospholipids and calcium in mineral-inducing fraction after ultracentrifugation of C_{fl} (220,221,246)
12. Proteoglycan inhibitor of mineralization	—	9.6	mg/mL	12: Mineral formation blocked in the presence of proteoglycan aggregates measured by ultracentrifugation (147,277,280)

[a] Fluid (10–30 mL) found in extracellular spaces bathing ~2000 chondrocytes, including spaces destined to calcify. Changes in fluid versus serum have been interpreted to favor calcification. Site of pipette placement has been determined by injection of a fluorescent dye through a double-barreled pipette (277). Although many of the mineralizing factors may not be susceptible to aspiration in C_{fl}, the presence of a nucleating factor for mineral, an inhibitor of mineral production, and other factors indicate the presence of a unique compartment. Tests for hemoglobin and various serum proteins were negative on C_{fl} samples.

protein content, high levels of proteoglycan containing large amounts of complexed calcium, and high pH being found in the cartilage fluid (78–80). From the data accumulated it was calculated that the bicarbonate level in the cartilage fluid was approaching 35 mM. This indicated the existence of an extremely effective mechanism for removing hydrogen ions while hydroxyapatite was forming. The only pathway capable of handling this amount of hydrogen ions and still maintaining the physiologic balance found in the cartilage fluid would have to be the circulatory system. To confirm that this was the case, the partial pressure of carbon dioxide in the cartilage fluid was measured under a column of mercury (to assure no loss of carbon dioxide). It was found that the cartilage fluid had a normal partial pressure of carbon dioxide (40 mmHg) and confirmed the high bicarbonate level and alkaline pH reported earlier (78). This indicated that at sites undergoing calcification, rapid equilibrium between cartilage fluid and the circulation must be occurring.

The enigma that remained concerned the fact that there was no evidence for any system capable of performing such rapid removal of hydrogen ion. Presumably, if the septae were blocked with mineral, communication would have to occur through the intercellular spaces between the chondrocytes. Could there be a chloride for bicarbonate exchange mechanism in the chondrocytes? Alternatively, could the endothelial cells per se secrete bicarbonate in exchange for hydrogen ion? Carbonic anhydrase was detected by specific antibodies and tritiated acetazolamide binding in hypertrophic chondrocytes (81; H. K. Vanaanan, personal communication). A high pH value was confirmed by Wuthier (82).

Culture studies have also sought to describe the energetics of mineralization. Cartilage slices of whole growth plate and those dissected into various cell zones have been incubated for 18 h under conditions simulating normal cartilage lymph (i.e., cartilage fluid). Despite positive staining, little mineral was found in the septa, even when supplemented with various growth factors (D. S. Howell, unpublished observation). Thomas et al. have found that cartilage slices greater than 1.0 mm thick, and incubated under conditions favorable for calcification, fail to mineralize (83). It was concluded that diffusion of calcium and phosphate through the matrix was impeded to such an extent that a positive line test was unobtainable. The pH of growth plate cartilage fluid falls from 7.6 to 7.3 in 15 min after explantation (78; D. S. Howell, unpublished observation). The loss of bicarbonate secretion is one of probably many functions that are lost after being removed from the vasculature of the animal. Other studies indicate that normal mineralization requires both living chondrocytes and a "free" calcium-phosphate product of at least 50 mg^2% (84). More complete mineralization can be obtained by incubation of cartilage in the presence of small organic phosphate molecules such as ATP or glycerol phosphate, in which inorganic phosphate is generated at high levels (85).

In conclusion, the hypertrophic chondrocyte must make a continuous and very important contribution to the environmental conditions required for normal calcification to occur. None of the conditions created in vitro are able to duplicate completely the speed and quantity of mineralization seen in vivo. Future studies should continue to examine the many new proteins and factors being discovered in growth cartilage so that our understanding of this process will continue to increase.

BIOCHEMISTRY OF STRUCTURAL MACROMOLECULES IN THE GROWTH PLATE

Collagens

Functional Role of Collagens in the Growth Plate

Collagens are one of the most abundant proteins in vertebrates. They are generally characterized by their fibrillar structure and a tensile strength which often approaches that of steel cables. The protein contains a high amount of proline, hydroxyproline, and glycine and forms a superhelix with a unique quaternary structure that makes it very resistant to proteolytic degradation (see chs. 10, 12). The collagens are found in virtually all tissues but are particularly abundant in bone, cartilage, and other tissues of the skeletal system. In general, the turnover of this molecule is measured in months or years, but where rapid remodeling is occurring, this time may be considerably reduced.

The structural integrity of the growth plate is largely dependent on its collagenous matrix. Each zone contains a unique mixture of various collagen types at different concentrations. This is sometimes reflected in dry weight measurements. For example, the total collagen content of the resting-proliferating cell zone in bovine growth plate is about 40–50% of the dry weight (86). This drops to a value of 23–25% in the hypertrophic cell zone (86,87). The decrease from one zone to the other is probably due to the decrease in amount of extracellular matrix per unit volume (from approximately 70% to 40%) found across these two zones (27). The extracellular matrix is also a permissive factor in differentiation and may thus enhance and/or stabilize the chondrocytic phenotype.

Collagens in the growth plate are formed and resorbed rapidly due to the large amount of remodeling that occurs in this tissue (88). Collagenase, a metalloproteinase with the unique capability of cleaving collagen under physiologic conditions, is responsible for much of this remodeling. Collagens are believed to determine the shape of the perichondrial sheath (1) and the size, shape, and in conjunction with proteoglycans, elasticity of the territorial (pericellular) and interterritorial matrices. In the territorial matrix, it is possible that so-called "minor collagens" may be partially responsible for inhibiting or accelerating the deposition of mineral. The association of type X collagen with areas of cartilage calcification in the hypertrophic cell zone is one example where a unique collagen type may be found, but its function remains unknown (89,90).

In addition to different collagen types, the degree of collagen network integrity can also be variable. This parameter is probably due to a varying combination of complex factors but can be measured empirically by submersion of the tissue in physiologic saline (0.9% NaCl) for varying periods of time and then weighing (91). The rationale of the method is based on the fact that in the absence of an intact (and therefore "loose") network, proteoglycans will take on water, swell, and tissue weight will increase. Evidence from studies of Maroudas and Urban suggest that a tight collagen network will prevent increases of greater than 10% (91). When samples of resting and proliferating cell zone cartilage have been studied, increases of only 10–15% were found. A somewhat looser network was found in the hypertrophic cell zone with 20–30% increases in weight (D. D. Dean, unpublished observation). But the magnitude of this increase is small compared with the 100–130% increases found with the cartilage-like nucleus pulposus (91) or 50–60% increases with osteoarthritic cartilage (91–93). Taken together, these findings suggest that the collagen network in the growth plate is largely intact compared with the nucleus pulposus, but not as tight as that found in articular cartilage, which shows only 5–10% increases in weight (92). This conclusion is further supported by the observation of increased extractability of proteoglycans from the hypertrophic cell zone compared to articular cartilage (94).

Teleologically, an intact collagen would seem necessary since the growth plate is bounded by the bony end plates of the metaphysis and epiphysis and the fibrous perichondrial structures along the margins. By itself, this architectural design would be unable to withstand the high osmotic pressures transmitted through the growth plate or maintain the shape of the tissue; therefore, it must require the strength imparted by the collagen.

The mechanisms involved in stabilizing the collagen network are variable and include hydrogen bonding, covalent bonding, and hydrophobic interactions. In certain pathological situations, involving derangements of only one or a few of these stabilizing forces, molecular defects can be tied to changes in tissue organization. For example, lysine residues may not be properly hydroxylated and covalent cross-link formation impaired as recently suggested in vitamin B_6 deficiency (95). In experimental rickets, the hypertrophic cell zone expands greatly due to lack of vitamin D and phosphate or other causes (50,51). In this case, mineralization of osteoid matrix is inhibited and collagen cross-link levels are somewhat elevated (96).

It must be emphasized that the collagen, by itself, cannot maintain the shape and overall integrity of the growth plate. Many other factors are involved. For example, several noncollagenous proteins in cartilage have been discussed (97). Various functions, including the role of "cellular glue" or fiber–fiber adhesion, have been suggested. Binding of these proteins to collagen and cells could depend on intact divalent cation associations. Hypothetically, such binding might explain the phenomena observed when growth cartilage is incubated with 0.05 M EDTA or EGTA, resulting in 200–300% increases in volume (98). When examined microscopically, the EDTA-treated cartilage matrix in the hypertrophic zone was significantly more disrupted than that of the resting and proliferating zone. The possibility that this resulted from protease action seemed less likely since EDTA is inhibitory to the metalloproteases under the experimental conditions used. There are several types of noncollagenous proteins in cartilage that bind calcium. The exact role of these proteins in growth plate is entirely hypothetical.

Genetically Distinct Collagen Types in the Growth Plate

As might be surmised from the list of functions ascribed to the collagens, the heterogeneity of this group of macromolecules is extensive (99). To date, 13 genetically distinct collagens have been described with gene sequences located on 18 different chromosomes (100). For classification purposes, each collagen type will be denoted by a Roman numeral; each of the chains that make up the triple helix may or may not have a unique amino acid sequence and will be denoted by an α with an Arabic subscript for each different chain. For example, the designation for type I collagen is $\alpha_1(I)$, $\alpha_2(I)$, indicating two genetically distinct chains, with one of the "one" variety and "two" of the two variety (99–101). The collagens found in the growth plate belong to two major subgroups of the collagen family (Table 2). One group of growth plate collagens is composed of the class 1, or fibril-forming, collagens; the second group belongs to the class 2, or short helix, collagens.

Approximately 70% of the total collagen found in the growth plate is type II. It forms narrow, cross-striated fibrils that are heavily glycosylated and virtually unique to cartilaginous tissues. The relatively low content of type II collagen in growth plate compared to articular cartilage is probably due to its favorable anatomical position for transmitting compressive rather than tensile loads. A second significant difference is the increased amount of minor collagens found in the growth plate: this may be due to the increased cellularity found in this tissue.

Whereas most investigators agree that types II, IX, X, and XI collagens are present in the growth plate (100–103), the close juxtaposition of the metaphysis with the adherent osteoid matrix makes it difficult to distinguish

TABLE 2. *Collagen types found in growth plate cartilage*

| Collagen type | Molecular characteristics | | Locations in growth plate |
	Chains[a]	Class[b]	
I	α_1(I), α_2(I)	1	Perichondrium, metaphyseal junction; last two to three hypertrophic cells?
II	α_1(II)	1	Throughout cartilage matrix
V (AB collagen)	α_1(V), α_2(V), α_3(V)	1	Pericellular, near metaphyseal junction?
IX	α_1(IX), α_2(IX), α_3(IX)	3	Throughout cartilage matrix; cross-linked to type II collagen
X	α_1(X)	3	In hypertrophic cell zone at calcifying sites; only collagen specific for growth plate
XI	α_1(XI), α_2(XI), α_3(XI)	1	Pericellular; cartilage equivalent of type V?

[a] Three chains of these types organize themselves as homo- or heteropolymers.

[b] Collagens can be grouped into three major classes. Class 1 collagens form 67-nm banded fibrils and contain at least 290 nm of uninterrupted helix. Class 2 collagens are not found in cartilage. Class 3 collagens form variable polymeric structures and are much shorter than 290 nm in uninterrupted helix length.

clearly the presence of types I and III collagen at the distal end of the growth plate. Epitopes for types I and III collagens have been found around chondrocytes in this region, but in situ hybridization for the mRNAs corresponding to these collagens have not been done. Types V and XI collagens appear to be a subclass of the class I fibril-forming collagens (103). Type V collagen codistributes with type I and consistently appears at a concentration of about 3% of that found for type I. Type XI, a close relative of type V, codistributes in a similar manner but with type II collagen. Another similarity that these two collagens share is that they are both found in the extracellular matrix with their *N*-propeptide regions still intact. In the next four sections we describe briefly what is known about the four collagens (types II, IX, X, and XI) found in growth plate cartilage.

Type II Collagen

This collagen type predominates in hyaline cartilages and in growth plate may constitute at least half of the tissue dry weight (102). In many respects it is very similar to type I collagen, but the fibrils formed by type II collagen are much thinner (101). In the tissue, this collagen is found in a matrix containing the so-called large proteoglycans aggregated on the surface of long filaments of hyaluronic acid. The mechanical stresses and strains borne by this tissue are much less than expected of articular cartilage, while the turnover of collagen in the growth plate is greatly increased.

Fibril formation is a poorly understood process. The structural differences between type I and type II collagen do not seem large enough to account for the vast differences in their fibrils. The only way, to date, of accounting for these differences in quaternary structure depends on the matrix in which a given collagen is found and such factors as the extent of glycosylation of the collagen per se. Small single- or double-chained dermatan sulfate proteoglycans have been found to affect fibril size dra-

matically (104). The effect seems to depend on the core protein, not on glycosaminoglycan side-chains (105). At present, some controversy exists about whether these small proteoglycans are present in growth plate (106,107).

Type IX Collagen

This collagen has been found in growth plate at a relative concentration of 10–12% of the total collagen level (102). It is a fibril-associated collagen with an interrupted helix formed from three genetically distinct chains (103,108–113). The molecule contains seven regions along its length (Fig. 4); three helices (Col 1 to Col 3) are separated by four nonhelical domains (NC1 to NC4). The NC4 domain is visualized as a small knob at one end of the molecule, with the NC3 domain acting as a hinge. In between is a small collagenous domain called Col 3. The NC1 domain is not easily visualized by rotary shadowing, and the NC2 domain does not appear to have a kink in its structure. This last observation is a little unusual since the overall length of type IX collagen corresponds to the length of its three collagenous domains (Col 1 to Col 3).

Of the three genetically distinct chains, the α_1(IX) chain contains a large amino terminal globular domain. The second chain, α_2(IX), contains an attachment site for a dermatan or chondroitin sulfate chain within the nontriple helical domain mentioned above (NC3) which separates the amino terminal and central triple helical domains and contains a flexible hinge. It has been postulated that this arrangement allows type IX collagen, as it is positioned on the type II collagen molecule through lysine-derived cross-links, to project a large amino terminal globular domain from the surface of the fibril into the surrounding matrix (103,114,115). These projections, then, could be possible attachment sites for proteoglycans or adhesive proteins and serve to generate and maintain the three-dimensional structure of the matrix

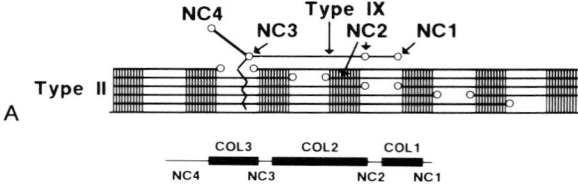

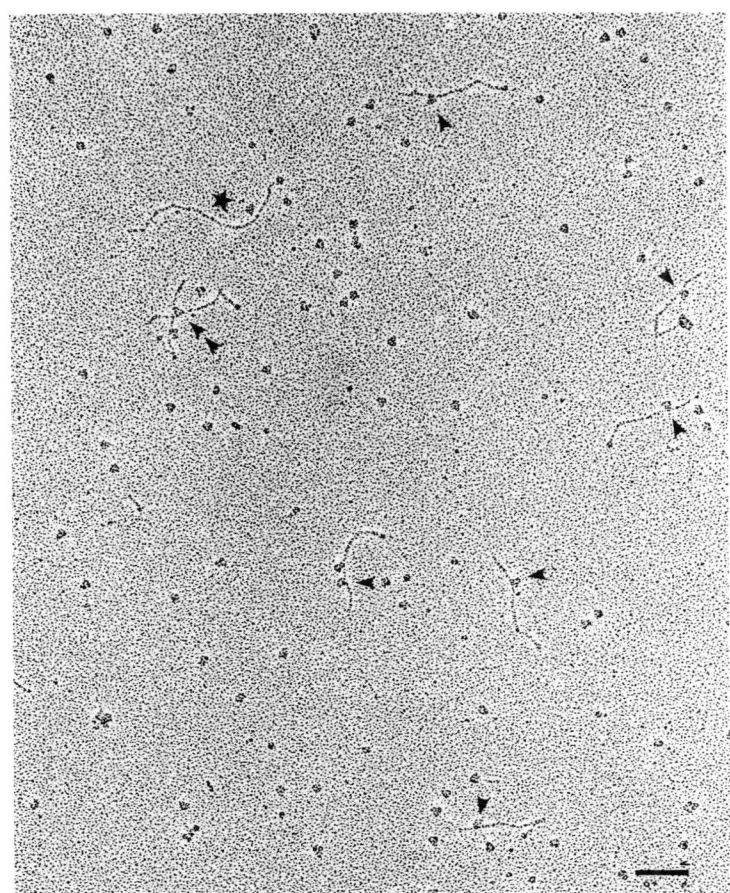

FIG. 4. A: Collagen fibrils. Model for the structural domains of type IX collagen and its postulated interaction with type II collagen. The numbering of the collagenous (Col 1 to Col 3) and noncollagenous (NC1 to NC4) domains begins at the carboxyl end of the protein. Type IX collagen has been shown by two independent groups to be cross-linked to type II collagen and contain a proteoglycan extension at the hinge region. [Adapted and reproduced with permission from M. Van der Rest, R. Mayne, and Academic Press (108).] **B:** Immunoelectron micrograph of collagens secreted by embryonic chick chondrocytes. Collagens were rotary shadowed in the presence of monoclonal antibody 2C2, which is specific for type IX collagen. A *double arrow* shows two type IX molecules that have been cross-linked by the antibody. The *asterisk* indicates the location of type II collagen. *Bar* = 100 nm. [Reproduced with permission of R. Mayne, M. Irwin, and Raven Press (103).]

required for mineralization. In addition, type IX may also be responsible for maintaining a tight collagen network (112). This could occur at sites where fibrils cross in the matrix, although this has not been proven (100).

Type X Collagen

A third collagen found in the growth plate (Fig. 5), type X collagen, is virtually synthesized only by hypertrophic chondrocytes (116–119). It is a short collagen molecule composed of three identical chains, with each chain having an M_r of 59,000 and an overall length of 138 nm (103). The thermal stability of this collagen is greater than that found in the interstitial collagens, with a melting temperature of 47°C. The molecule is susceptible to digestion by vertebrate collagenase, producing two fragments where only one is produced upon digestion of type I collagen (116). Pepsin digestion produces a chain of 45,000 molecular weight, and rotary shadowing of intact type X reveals a noncollagenous domain at one end (120). A genomic clone, encoding the entire amino acid sequence of type X, demonstrated that this noncollagenous domain was at the carboxyl end of the molecule (121).

Whereas types II, IX and XI collagens are distributed throughout the cartilage matrix, type X is restricted to those sites undergoing calcification and may account for up to 45% of the total collagen synthesized by hypertrophic chondrocytes (102,117,121,122). During embryonic development of long bones, deposition of type X precedes invasion of hypertrophic chondrocytes by marrow elements or calcification per se (123). Type X persists into adulthood in the calcified cartilage just below the tidemark (124). Despite strong indications that the molecule contains a hydrophobic transmembrane region and is found associated with matrix vesicles, no intimate membrane association has been found with chondrocytes or matrix vesicles (125). The collagen seems to exist as a fine filamentous macromolecular aggregate, which is distinct from the small-diameter fibrils produced by type II collagen. Attempts to show nucleation of mineral or inhibition of mineral growth by type X collagen have failed (see below).

Type XI Collagen

Like types IX and X collagen, type XI collagen is found in hyaline and growth cartilage. Its concentration in one study of growth plate has been surprisingly high and approached 30% of the level found for type II collagen (102). This extremely high level may have to do with the rapid remodeling and high cellular content of the

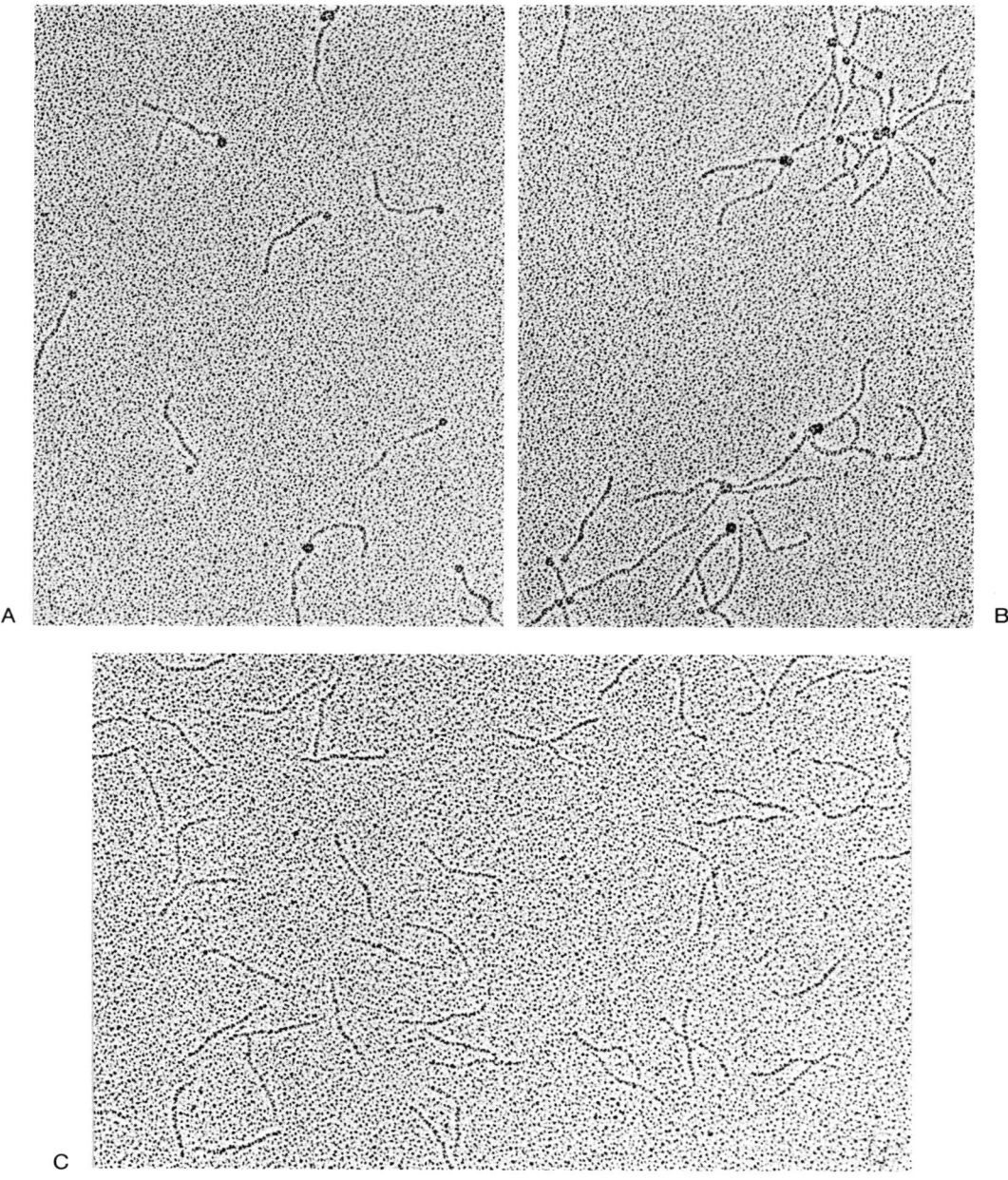

FIG. 5. Rotary shadowed preparations of type X collagen. **A:** *and* **B:** Micrographs of the intact molecule (59-kD chains). **C:** The pepsin resistant form of type X collagen (45-kD chains). This collagen is specifically localized to the hypertrophic cell zone and subarticular calcified cartilage (see the text). [Reproduced by permission from T. Schmid et al. and Academic Press (120).]

growth plate compared to articular cartilage, which has only 10% of the type XI level found in the growth plate. Lack of well-characterized antibodies has hampered progress in understanding the structure and localization of this collagen. Most available evidence indicates that it consists of a single molecule of chain composition: $\alpha_1(XI)$, $\alpha_2(XI)$, $\alpha_3(XI)$. The first two chains have strong similarities with $\alpha_1(V)$ and $\alpha_2(V)$ chains of type V collagen, as reviewed elsewhere (126). The amounts present in tissues is small. Interactions with proteoglycans have been demonstrated and a role for type XI in regulating fibril formation like type V collagen has been postulated (127).

Proteoglycans

Function of Proteoglycans in the Growth Plate

The growth plate contains another major class of extracellular matrix macromolecules called proteoglycans.

These molecules are required to maintain the elastic properties of the tissue, modulate cellular differentiation, and may regulate mineralization. They interact with other macromolecules such as collagens and other noncollagenous proteins. They profoundly influence the characteristics of the matrix in which they are found and are ubiquitous throughout the various regions of the growth plate (128).

Proteoglycans participate in performing a structural function in conjunction with collagen. The combination of these two macromolecules are responsible for imparting an elastic, yet tough property to the tissue in the noncalcified regions. The load-bearing properties of the growth plate are largely due to the osmotic properties of the proteoglycans confined within the collagen network. They also form a region on which mineralization can begin. Evidence has also implicated proteoglycans in inhibiting the overexpansion of crystal formation and might conversely participate in mineral formation.

The osmotic swelling of the matrix is due to the proteoglycans immobilized within the collagen network and is capable of exerting at least 3 atm of pressure. This physical property is due largely to the enormous anionic charge concentrated within a small space (94).

Structure and Organization of Proteoglycans

Proteoglycans are probably the most complex macromolecules known to date. They are characterized by their content of covalently attached glycosaminoglycan (GAG) chains to a central protein core (Fig. 6). Four classes of GAGs are known and they are distinguished by their chemical structure and content of repeating disaccharide backbones. The most common ones include chondroitin sulfate (CS) and its modified form dermatan sulfate, keratan sulfate (KS), heparin sulfate and hepa-

rin, and hyaluronic acid (HA). Recent research has found that each tissue may have a unique complement of GAGs that characterize it. For example, articular cartilage contains up to 90% chondroitin-6-sulfate and keratan sulfate, while the mammalian growth plate contains a much higher proportion of chondroitin-4-sulfate. A small dermatan sulfate proteoglycan found in articular cartilage in increasing amounts with aging is virtually absent in growth plate cartilage, despite a recent report concerning the presence of small proteoglycans (e.g., biglycan and decorin) in growth plate and their potential involvement in regulating collagen fibril formation (107). A large number of genetically distinct protein cores representing over six gene families have been described. In cartilage, the large aggregating proteoglycan is the only one of universally accepted importance. It contains both KS and CS attached to a long, centrally located core protein.

Figure 6 shows a schematic model of the cartilage proteoglycan (PG) subunit. The central HA filament forms a backbone upon which the PG subunit can bind; additional stabilization is provided by link glycoprotein. Recent studies have delineated the chemical nature of the distinct sites required for aggregate stability. These include (1) a unique site on the PG subunit which binds to HA called the HA binding region, (2) a site on the PG subunit as well as on the link protein (LP) that interact with each other, and (3) the site on the LP that binds to the HA (129–134).

Figure 7 is an electron micrograph of proteoglycan aggregates prepared from fetal calf growth plates (135,136). A central thread of hyaluronic acid can be seen that contains PG subunits attached along its entire length. The PG subunits appear like bristles on a brush, and small condensations of the GAG side chains can be seen periodically along the PG subunit. With rotary

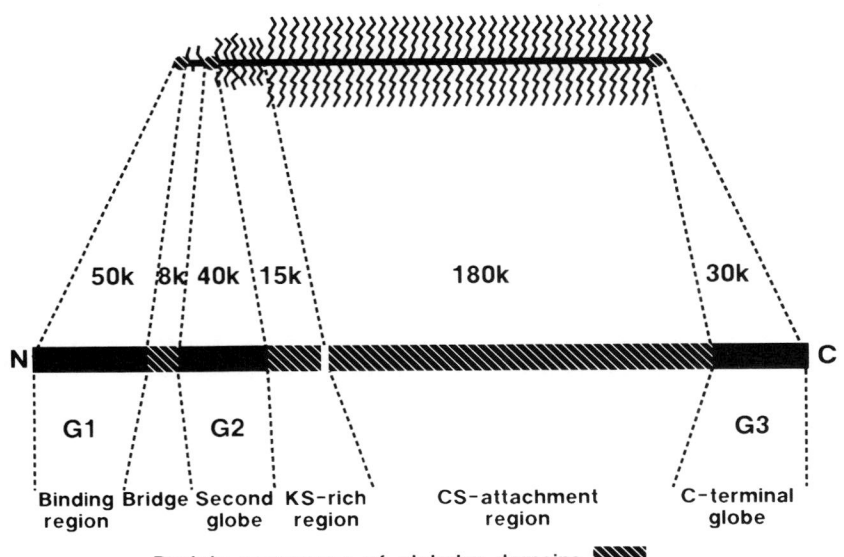

FIG. 6. Domain structure of the core protein of the aggregating proteoglycan subunit. The three globular regions (G1 to G3) were identified by rotary shadowing electron microscopy. (Reproduced from T. Hardingham et al., Cartilage proteoglycans, in: *Functions of the proteoglycans,* 1986, Ciba Foundation, with permission.)

shadowing techniques, several regions along the protein core can be distinguished (137). At the C terminus is a 30-kD globular domain designated G3 (Fig. 6); a function for this region is not currently known, but it may be involved in intracellular processing during biosynthesis (128,137). Moving toward the N terminus, a region of 180 kD is found that is associated with the attachment of chondroitin sulfate. Keratan sulfate attachment occurs in the next region of the core protein structure. This region has a molecular weight of 15 kD. A second globular domain is found on the carboxyl side of the KS attachment region. This region is designated G2 and is believed to be involved in providing a site for interaction with other matrix proteins or in regulating aggregate forma-

tion. A small region of molecular weight 8 kD separates G2 from the last region of the core protein molecule, globular domain G1. This N-terminal region has been characterized extensively and clearly functions in aggregation by binding to hyaluronic acid (128–134).

Recently, the complete reading frame for PG subunit has been reported and its complete amino acid sequence deduced (138). The tentative amino acid composition of LP has also been deduced from its cDNA (139–143). Interestingly, a close homology has been found between the sequence of the PG subunit HA binding region and LP (144). The cDNA for the G3 globular region has shown high sequence homology with a hepatic lectin and other vertebrate carbohydrate binding proteins

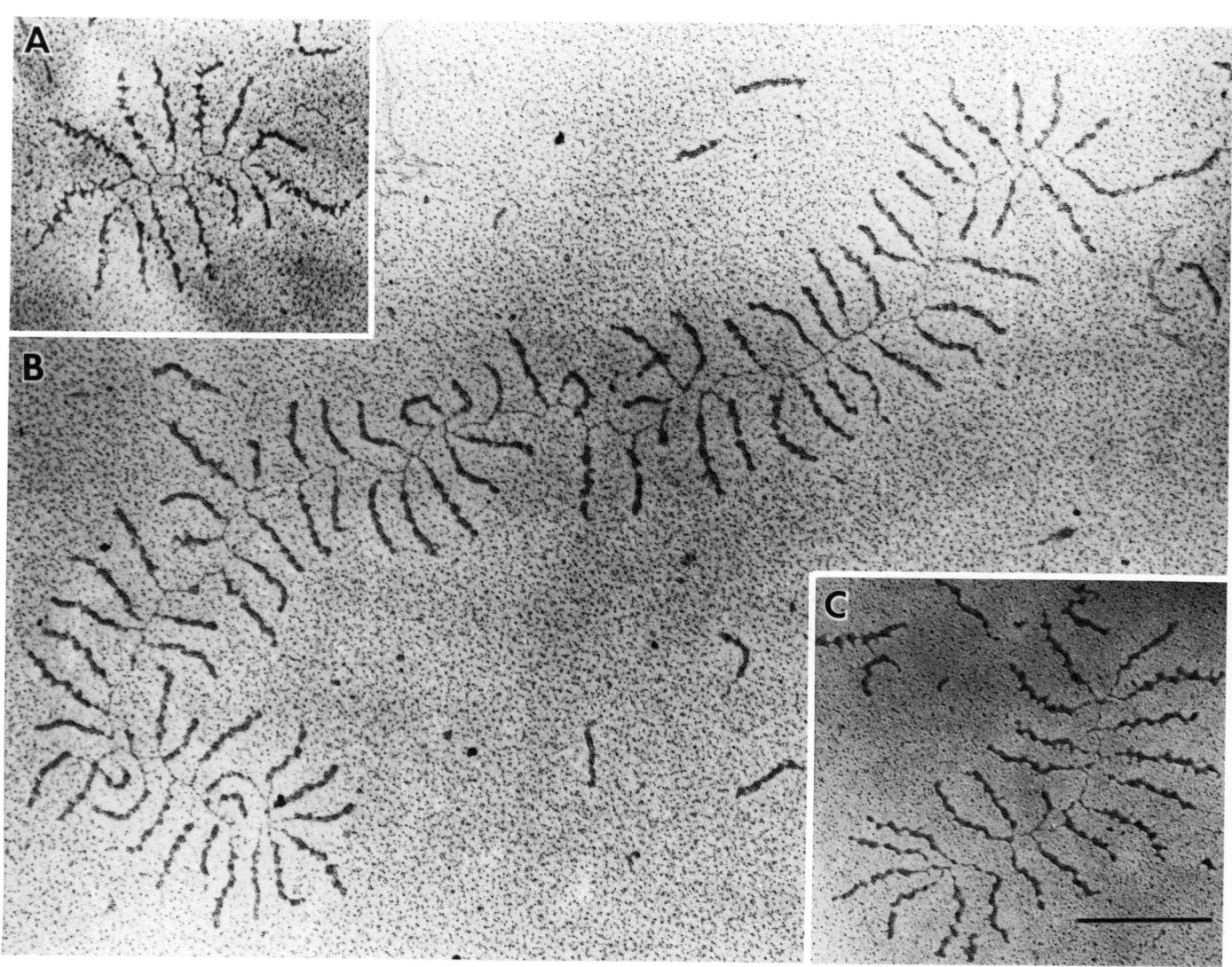

FIG. 7. Electron micrographs of proteoglycan aggregates from fetal calf growth plates (proliferative and hypertrophic cell zones) after extraction under different conditions. **A:** Small proteoglycan aggregate extracted under dissociative conditions (4 *M* guanidine). **B:** Large proteoglycan aggregate extracted under dissociative conditions. **C:** Proteoglycan aggregate extracted under associative conditions. *Bar* = 500 nm. [Reproduced with permission of J. Buckwalter. L. Rosenberg, and Raven Press (267).]

(145,146). When expressed in the rat, this protein showed a predilection for galactose and fructose ligands (142). Therefore, in addition to the potential function ascribed to G3 (above), this protein may also serve an organizational role by interacting with carbohydrate moieties on cartilage matrix proteins and/or cell surface proteins (128).

Interaction of Proteoglycans with Themselves and Other Macromolecules

Detailed studies of proteoglycans by growth cartilage zone suggest that 70–80% are found in aggregate form prior to calcification (147; D. Manicourt and D. S. Howell, unpublished observations). With refined staining methods, Hunziker and Schenk have shown a close relationship between collagen and proteoglycan aggregates (148). Hyaluronic acid (HA) was found to span the spaces between collagen fibers, stabilize the proteoglycan subunits on the HA filaments, and prevent losses during mechanical stress. In addition, proteoglycan aggregates have been shown to better resist compressive forces than subunits alone (149,150). The organization of proteoglycans into closely packed, geometrically organized groups with parallel arrays of negatively charged GAG chains results in a high charge density. This arrangement would not only seem optimal for containment of osmotic swelling, but also for shielding and prevention of mineral growth.

In normal growth plates, where 90% or more of the cartilage is comprised of resting and proliferating cell zone, the collagen network is found to be intact. The significance of this finding is that the osmotic pressure of the tissue (due to the proteoglycans) can probably be contained without any change in shape. By contrast, the hypertrophic cell zone collagen network may be partially loosened (88; D. D. Dean, unpublished observation). This would fit the ultrastructural findings of longitudinally arranged collagen fibrils in the longitudinal septa, the presence of a high cell content, and the absence of randomly arranged collagen fibrils that typify a tight network. (A further explanation of these phenomena is given later in this chapter under "Collagens."

Structure and Function of Noncollagenous Proteins

Role of Noncollagenous Proteins in the Growth Plate

Although the classification and function of various noncollagenous proteins in the growth plate is still incomplete, the existence of these molecules is of great interest and the subject of two recent reviews (97,151). Many events occurring in the growth plate would seem to require components capable of binding cells and matrix together, organizing the collagenous matrix "basket weave," as well as influencing cell differentiation and mediating matrix mineralization. These are all functions that cannot be explained solely on the basis of collagen and proteoglycan interactions. The cellular events involving proliferation and hypertrophy, as an example, probably depend on each cell interacting with a local matrix that must change through degradation and/or resynthesis to accommodate either new cells or cells that are in the process of expanding (88,152). As the hypertrophic cells mature, the organic matrix must also change from a nonmineralizable to mineralizable form. A more local function of these proteins might involve regulating discrete sites of matrix degradation on one side of the cell and pericellular matrix synthesis on the other. Without this capability, it would be impossible to explain how enlarging hypertrophic chondrocytes can excavate space for their expansion and, at the same time, deposit new matrix molecules like type X collagen.

Anchorin CII

One of the most interesting new molecules to be described in the growth plate is anchorin CII (153). Anchorin CII is a 34-kD glycoprotein that was originally isolated from purified membrane proteins of embryonic chick chondrocytes by affinity chromatography on type II collagen (154). Recently, chondrocyte membranes from adult chick xiphoid cartilage have been used (155). The protein's name is derived from its ability to anchor type II collagen in the chondrocyte cell membrane. The original studies were performed in the presence of detergent and binding appeared weaker than would be expected. After reconstitution into lecithin liposomes, significant increases in anchorin CII binding to type II collagen were observed: types I, III, V, IX, and XI collagen all displayed binding that was only 20% of that seen with type II collagen. Binding was dependent on the native, triple helical structure of the collagen molecule and was probably through the N-telopeptide region (156).

At the cellular level, anchorin CII has been immunolocalized in sections of chick tibial and sternal cartilage and on the surface of chondrocytes in culture (154). In tissue sections, the protein was found in the pericellular area. In cultured chondrocytes, the pericellular matrix of type II collagen contained a punctate pattern of positive staining. In other culture studies, antibodies to anchorin CII reduced the ability of chondrocytes to attach to the plastic culture flasks.

It is possible that anchorin CII serves to anchor the cell in the extracellular matrix by interacting with both collagen and cytoskeletal elements. A similar arrangement has been described for fibronectin, which is connected to actin via a structure called a fibronexus (157). Anchorin CII has also been hypothesized to serve as a nucleation site for the assembly of extracellular collagen fibrils (153).

Other Noncollagenous Proteins in Cartilage

The fact that antibodies to anchorin CII cannot completely block the binding of cells to collagen implies the existence of other molecules that must function in a similar capacity. One such protein is fibronectin, but this molecule only mediates the adhesion of fibroblasts, not chondrocytes, to collagen. It is found to a very small extent in growth cartilage and at much higher levels in osteoarthritic cartilage (158).

Chondronectin is an adhesive protein of 150 kD that mediates the binding of chondrocytes to type II collagen (159). It does not bind to collagen directly, but does so in the presence of chondroitin sulfate. Although first discovered in serum, it has also been found to be produced by chondrocytes (160).

Additional proteins such as the cartilage matrix protein described by Fife (97) and collagens (153) have been reported in cartilage. Recently, osteonectin has been found at calcifying sites in growth cartilage (161,162). Chondrocalcin, also known as the C-propeptide of type II collagen, may also play a role in the growth plate (53–55). It appears to be intimately associated with the mineral phase as well as with proteoglycan. Chondrocalcin is also a calcium-binding protein that is distributed with proteoglycan in regions undergoing active calcification (53–55). A recent review has reported on the presence of several cartilage proteins including thrombospondin, fibromodulin, a 148-kD protein, cartilage oligomeric high-molecular-weight protein (COMP), and a 21-kD protein in cartilage (97,163).

The combination of collagens, proteoglycans, and noncollagenous proteins described in this section are part of an assembly required for normal growth, differentiation, and mineralization of this tissue. The interaction of type IX collagen with type II as well as proteoglycans, the cation binding studies of Campo using EDTA and EGTA, the ability of anchorin CII to bind chondrocyte membranes and type II collagen, and the discovery of chondrocalcin (C-propeptide of type II collagen) in sites undergoing active calcification are examples of the complexity of the interactions involved (55,98, 153,164,165).

MECHANISMS OF GROWTH PLATE MINERALIZATION

Elemental Analysis of the Mineral Phase Found in the Growth Plate

In the 1950s to early 1970s, several comprehensive studies were performed that laid the baseline for our understanding of the major organic and inorganic substituents in the growth plate (see Chapter 12 and Refs. 9, 23, 166, and 167). Cross-sectional analysis of growth plate cartilage revealed that collagen and proteoglycan were the major organic components of the matrix; this ex-

tended and confirmed prior studies (9,23,167). It has been shown that proteoglycans constitute the major anion in cartilage and that sodium is the major cation (86,87,168). Details of other monovalent and divalent ions in the tissue are discussed here.

Attempts to localize and quantitate calcium and phosphate in the growth plate have been reported. Increases in both have been found at the end of the growth plate (86,87,168). The storage of calcium in organic complexes, however, could not be adequately discerned. This was due to deficiencies in technique since no reliable distinction could be made between organic or ionic forms of phosphate and the intracellular versus extracellular location of this anion. These problems aside, the entire population of anions and cations was found to be remarkably balanced in each zone. Since organic cations were not measured, the data may be slightly erroneous, as several cationic proteins, such as lysozyme, have been detected in cartilage (169).

Recent studies utilizing high-resolution technology have collectively reported on the levels of calcium, phosphorus, sulfur, sodium, potassium, and magnesium in various regions (170–177). Some of the data have been consistent with increases in the ratio of calcium to phosphorus in the extracellular matrix. Calcium storage appears to be confined to the mitochondrion in nonmineralizing regions; the concentration of this ion increases in regions populated by matrix vesicles in sites beginning to calcify. Shepperd and Mitchell have used a dye-binding method to show an association between calcium signals in septal matrix and a high content of proteoglycans (174).

Arsenault and Otismeyer have reported increased sulfur levels in regions of high proteoglycan content (175). Interestingly, Howell and Carlson in their early x-ray elemental studies reported increases in sulfur adjacent to these same regions but failed to comment on this in the discussion of the results (28). Magnesium has also been reported in association with mitochondrial granules, matrix vesicles, and mineral nodules. It is believed that this element may be responsible for reducing the degree of crystallinity in mineralized structures (70).

High potassium levels have been found in stereotactically isolated terminal hypertrophic chondrocytes (176). This implies that the chondrocytes must be viable and healthy. In the studies of Hargest et al. (70), as well as those of Wroblewski et al. (177), a high content of potassium was found in the extracellular matrix prior to calcification. The level of sodium was also surprisingly high inside the chondrocytes at the lower edge of the hypertrophic cell zone (70). Recent studies on micropuncture extracellular fluid from rat growth plates have failed to reveal elevated levels of potassium by use of helium glow photometry or electron probe analysis (178). This is in contrast to Wuthier, who found high levels of potassium in the fluid phase after compression of bovine growth cartilage (49). Crushing of cells by the high pressure seemed unlikely since nucleotide levels were low. The function of high potassium levels in growth plate septa is unknown at present, but is reminiscent of finding high potassium levels in bone matrix (179).

Nature of the Mineral Phase In Vivo

Our understanding of the initial mineral phase in cartilage has undergone a series of changes as more refined physical methods and high-resolution microscopy have become available. To trace the increasing sophistication of the methods used in this area, several other papers are recommended (180,181). It should be noted that some investigators believe that these initial transformations will be very difficult, if not impossible, to detect in cartilage since the initial changes into hydroxyapatite are very rapid (Ref. 182, and see below).

Recent analyses of calcified cartilage have been performed with the aid of infrared Fourier transform spectroscopy (183). Poorly crystallized carbonate apatite has been identified and mineral crystals found in clusters of varying size. A large proportion of the mineral has been observed in spaces between collagen fibers. Its alignment along (or within) the fibers has been difficult to demonstrate and very different from those crystals found within type I collagen of bone matrix and calcifying tendon (see Chapter 12 and Refs. 184–188). The presence of this mineral species is consistent with the secretion of bicarbonate mentioned above and with the high pH found in growth cartilage fluid (78–82). In contrast, the mineral phases found in matrix vesicles in vitro were reported to be octacalcium phosphate and hydroxyapatite (189). These mineral species, however, have not been detected in mineralizing sites in vivo, even though our knowledge of mineral formation, from in vitro studies, would suggest that they might be found (181,187,190–193).

By use of x-ray microradiography and x-ray spectrophotometry, Hjertquist was able to quantitate mineral versus organic phases in growth plate septae. The experimental apparatus was able to focus on the entire width of a cartilage septum or the length of one or two cells, providing a physiologically significant compartment (194). In contrast to bone matrix, where the mineral content may be more than 60% of tissue dry weight (195), the growth plate septa could be as much as 85% mineral (194). The water content in cross-sectional slices of uncalcified growth cartilage has been estimated to be as much as 75–80%.

Studies by Howell and co-workers of calf costal cartilage using x-ray spectrophotometry have supported these estimates. Phosphorus, sulfur, and total mass were measured in the septa opposite the first, second, and third cells of the calcified cartilage. A rough estimate of mineral content was 76% of dry mass. Based on an 80% water content of the organic phase and a 2.1 g/cm^3 mineral density, a rough calculation estimated a 50% water content opposite the third cell of the lower hypertrophic cell zone, where there was 76% mineralization (28,29). Unlike compact bone studied by Robinson, where water content was only 5–10% (195), the time required for crystal formation in the growth plate is so short as to mitigate against a very low total water content.

Rates of Mineral Formation In Vitro versus In Vivo

The numerous constituents required for mineral formation in vivo have been elucidated slowly over many years. The successful in vitro simulation of these events has been elusive, since neither the quality of the mineral formed, nor the rate at which it forms, has been observed.

Boskey has recently reported on a system designed to simulate the in vivo situation more closely (196). An apparatus was designed to provide two infinitely large, circulating sources of calcium and phosphate ions which could diffuse from opposite sides into a mineralizing gel. The concentration of ions reaching the gel was determined by the diffusion coefficient and actual predetermined ion levels in the two reservoirs. In one case, a calcium phosphate product of 5–7 mM^2 was used, but the 10% gelatin matrix remained unmineralized after 5 days. When the calcium-phosphate product was raised to 37 mM^2 and a cross-linked collagen gel used, reasonable mineral deposition occurred. By using this system, Boskey was able to show that proteoglycans inhibited mineralization, while phospholipids were stimulatory. This was probably the most advanced demonstration of the effects of these two classes of compounds on the kinetics of mineralization. In addition, this study showed that keeping the ion concentration product high, while mineralization was proceeding, accelerated the mineralization process by at least an order of magnitude. Even with this accomplishment, the rate was still unable to approach the one believed to occur in vivo. The system, however, answered many of the questions posed by the work of earlier authors. A high concentration of nucleation material (i.e., calcium phospholipid phosphate complex and control hydroxyapatite) and the ability to monitor the pH and to provide an adequate supply of ions were improved features over earlier studies. It is the authors' contention that the current theories of mineralization are not complete enough to explain the high rate of mineralization seen in growth plate septae.

Matrix Vesicle Hypothesis

Structure of Matrix Vesicles

Matrix vesicles are trilaminar membrane-enclosed structures that have been detected in the extracellular matrix of mineralizing growth cartilage and other tissues (Fig. 8; 42–52, 85, 197). Since their discovery over two

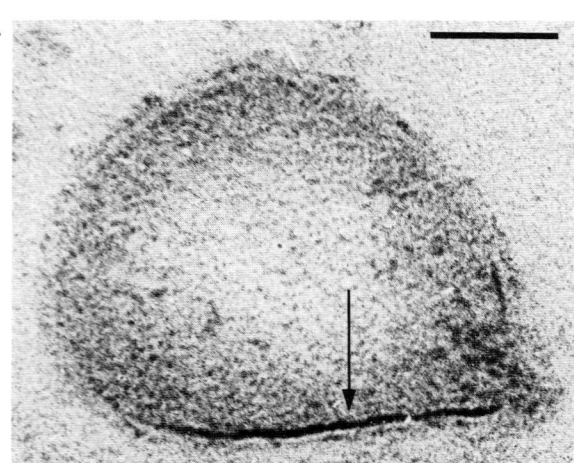

FIG. 8. A: Matrix vesicle in the growth plate of a rachitic rat as seen in the early stage of mineralization. The *arrow* indicates a rigid precipitate of electron-dense calcium phosphate mineral deposited at the inner leaflet of the matrix vesicle trilaminar membrane (×400,000). *Bar* = 0.1 µm. (Unpublished work provided by H. C. Anderson.) **B:** Matrix vesicles produced by rabbit mandibular condylar chondrocytes in culture. Cells were cultured in DMEM containing 10% FBS and antibiotics at 37°C in 5% CO_2 and 100% humidity. Post-confluent cultures form calcifying nodules that resemble the ultrastructural morphology of the growth plate. Matrix vesicles are embedded in a collagen-rich extracellular matrix and contain hydroxyapatite-like crystals. Stained with uranyl acetate and lead citrate. Print magnification: ×18,000. (Micrograph is courtesy of L. D. Swain, F. Engel, Z. Schwartz, and B. D. Boyan, the University of Texas Health Science Center at San Antonio, 1990.)

decades ago (42,43), they have been studied intensely from cell biological and biochemical standpoints in an effort to characterize their ultrastructural organization and function in the extracellular matrix (48,49). Although some investigators have postulated that they originate in the resting cell zone as detritus and migrate to the longitudinal septa (51,52), many others would agree that their major function is to participate in the initial deposition of calcium phosphate mineral in the septa.

A variety of sophisticated fixation and embedding techniques, as well as high-resolution probes for elemental analysis, have been applied to the study of these particles. With only a few exceptions (198,199), much evidence favors the idea that these vesicles in growth cartilage septae accumulate organically bound calcium and phosphate (42–49), in addition to mineral per se, either within or on the vesicle membrane (47,48). Some studies have suggested the presence and proliferation of hydroxyapatite-like crystals on the inner membrane surface of the vesicles and outgrowth of these crystals as mineral volume increases in the lower hypertrophic cell zone septae (200,201). Mineral has also been found inside vesicles in the lower proliferating and upper hypertrophic cell zones in advance of extracellular mineral deposition (201). Arsenault, using advanced tissue preservation and high-resolution techniques, also obtained data suggesting the presence of poorly crystallized material inside matrix vesicles (202); Hunziker et al., in collaboration with Arsenault, have commented on the various limitations of these methods and results (203).

Freeze-fracture studies have shown that some hypertrophic cells have microvillar projections extending into the extracellular matrix (204,205). These structures have been found in both tissues and cell cultures and have been postulated to be the principal mechanism for matrix vesicle formation in vivo (204,205). They are not simple extensions of the chondrocyte membrane, though, since they are enriched in phosphatidyl serine, sphingomyelin, lysophospholipids, and free cholesterol and depleted in phosphatidyl choline (205,206). Similar membrane phospholipid and protein compositions have been found in matrix vesicles from several calcifying tissues, indicating that a unifying chemistry may characterize these subcellular particles (47–49).

Calcium and Phosphate Ions in Matrix Vesicles

When matrix vesicles are isolated from tissues by collagenase digestion or other separatory methods, they are found to contain substantial amounts of calcium and phosphate (47–49,207,208). This characteristic has been retained across different species. Results of both electron probe analysis and electron spatial imaging on vesicles in vivo are consistent with the high elemental content found in vitro (201,202). Wuthier has estimated the concentration of calcium and phosphate in vesicles from in vitro data (49,209). Protein- or lipid-bound calcium was calculated to be in the range 30–40 mM, while the amount of free ion was 1–2 µM. Phosphate levels, under similar conditions, were 20 mM bound to protein, 2 mM

bound to lipid, and 25 m*M* free. Electron micrographs of freshly isolated vesicles have shown little evidence of crystalline mineral. Sauer and Wuthier hypothesized that within matrix vesicles, there is an initial formation of octacalcium phosphate that gradually transforms into hydroxyapatite (189). Electrolyte profiles indicate that sodium is present at higher levels than potassium, a reversal of the normal potassium to sodium distribution found in cells (49,209).

Generation of Inorganic Phosphate by Enzymes

Matrix vesicles also contain a number of enzymes, such as alkaline phosphatase (210,211), nucleotide triphosphate (NTP) pyrophosphohydrolase (212,213), peptidases (214), and proteases (215; also see below). Ali and Evans (216), as well as Hsu and Anderson (217), have shown that isolated matrix vesicles can cause mineral deposition from metastable solutions of calcium and phosphate. In their studies, two requirements had to be satisfied: alkaline phosphatase as well as an organophosphate such as ATP or AMP were necessary for mineral formation to occur.

Morris et al. were able to localize alkaline phosphatase on the inner leaflet of the vesicle membrane (218). Although the monoclonal antibody and immunoelectron microscopic techniques they used were sensitive, it was impossible to exclude extensions to the outside. Immunolocalization and amino acid composition studies of de Bernard et al. (219) on bovine scapular growth plate and isolated matrix vesicles led to the hypothesis that a calcium-binding alkaline phosphatase may be released from vesicles and bind to the matrix at mineral forming sites.

Some evidence from past work is consistent with the idea of ecto-phosphatases (enzymes on the outer surface of chondrocyte or matrix vesicle membranes) functioning on chondrocyte or matrix vesicle membranes to generate extracellular inorganic phosphate. Micropuncture fluid from calcifying sites in rachitic growth plates consistently had a high 260/280 *ratio, indicating a nucleotide content approaching 1 m*M* (78). Whether this assessment reflects the presence of ATP, AMP, or some other nucleotide is unknown, but this family of molecules could still comprise a source of organic phosphate groups. In contrast to the micropuncture fluid data, studies by Wuthier on fluid from compressed calf costal cartilage containing hypertrophic cells fail to confirm a high content of nucleotides (49). Perhaps, there is rapid turnover. Alternatively, there could be other phosphorylated substrates present, such as phosphoethanolamine, pyridoxal phosphate, or pyrophosphate.

Micropuncture fluid analyses reveal further information on phosphate in growth plate calcifying sites (Table 1). A higher level of inorganic phosphate was found in rachitic rat micropuncture fluid than in serum from the

same animals. Howell hypothesized that although phosphate generation from organic sources was slow in the rachitic cartilage, it was demonstrable due to the expanded zone of calcifying cartilage. In normal, and healing rachitic, growth plates, increased levels of free inorganic phosphate were absent. Failure to obtain samples in the focal mineralizing sites (undiluted with fluid from noncalcifying sites) or rapid uptake of mineral ions on new mineral crystals may account for this result (78). Alkaline phosphatase activity in rat and rabbit growth plate micropuncture fluid was three times higher than found in plasma (220). Vesicle membrane fragments were tentatively identified in this fluid as well as other substances with the properties of a mineral-forming agent (221). Another study showed that ATP, in the presence of micropuncture fluid in vitro, was rapidly hydrolyzed (220). The failure of mineralization seen in hypophosphatasia could be attributed to the lack of sufficient phosphate generation by the mechanism just described (222).

Immediately after matrix vesicles rupture and extrude mineral into the extracellular matrix, other enzymatic regulators of crystal proliferation may be present (48,49). Alkaline phosphatase has been reported to bind to calcium as well as matrix in regions adjacent to matrix vesicle mineralization (219). Based on his finding of alkaline phosphatase binding to collagen, Wuthier postulates that this enzyme may function in extending the mineral phase by secondary nucleation (see Chapter 12 for other viewpoints).

Nonenzymatic Routes to Phosphate Production

Despite some of the appealing aspects of the enzymatic pathways just described, other equally strong hypotheses have been advanced. It has been shown that matrix vesicle-enriched microsomes can form mineral in the absence of alkaline phosphatase substrates (223). Furthermore, considerable evidence has accrued that mineral forms inside matrix vesicles from ions already stored within the vesicles (48,49). This idea has been developed and matured by Eanes and Hailer in a model system (224). His group has shown that physiologic concentrations of potassium phosphate can be encapsulated within liposomes. When these are incubated in solutions of calcium, sodium, and a calcium ionophore (e.g., X-537A), calcium phosphate mineral is produced. The sodium-to-potassium gradient, as well as the ionophore, induce rapid entrance of calcium into the phosphate-rich lumen. A loss of magnesium has been postulated to permit the conversion of early mineral clusters into apatite (225). This model, then, suggests that high cytosolic levels of phosphate, magnesium, and potassium in chondrocytes at the time of matrix vesicle formation could "prime" the newly formed vesicles for subsequent mineral formation. The finding of a sodium-potassium-dependent ATPase (49), a hydrogen-ion porter, proteolipid (226), and a calcium-dependent ATPase (227) all favor the ion diffusion mechanism just described.

Another explanation for the presence of a poorly formed crystalline mineral phase in the lumen of matrix vesicles has been advanced (228). According to this idea, intracellular mineral could be encapsulated in vesicles when they are formed. Mitochondria during the latter stages of chondrocyte hypertrophy could release calcium in the vicinity of the plasma membrane. This event, coupled with high cytosolic levels of phosphate and extensive hydrolysis of ATP, might cause local precipitation of mineral in this region and promote vesiculation (or membrane blebbing) as seen in red blood cells. Poorly crystalline calcium phosphates have been shown to be potent membrane fusigens and may be a prerequisite for matrix vesicle formation in this process. It has been extremely difficult, however, to establish this hypothesis firmly.

Role of Membrane Phospholipids in Mineralization

A large amount of research has been devoted to the study of phospholipids and proteolipid complexes and their potential role in mineralization (48,49,229–233). In matrix vesicles, for example, there is an especially high content of phosphatidyl serine, phosphatidyl inositol, and an apoprotein (49,229–233). The acidic phospholipids are localized predominately on the interior lamina of the matrix vesicle membrane and have a high affinity for calcium and phosphate. It is believed that in vivo these complexes form spontaneously; this association of ions and phospholipids has been termed a *calcium phosphate–phospholipid complex* (CPLX) (234–236). When functional, these complexes induce de novo mineral formation in the absence of alkaline phosphatase (229,230).

The formation of mineral by way of phospholipids can also be found outside the animal kingdom (237). The bacterium *Bacterionema matruchotii* contains a CPLX-like molecule linked to an apoprotein similar in composition to that found in mammals (237–239). In this instance a layer of hydroxyapatite forms across the inner layer of the bacterial membrane at the same site where these complexes are found. In the remainder of this section we discuss the role of CPLX or proteolipid in mammalian systems (240).

In 1968, Irving showed that Sudan black was a very sensitive histological stain for phospholipids in a variety of tissues, including growth plate (241). Matrix vesicles and their disintegrating membranes were subsequently observed to contain positive staining inclusions with this technique. By association, either inside or outside the matrix vesicle membrane, these molecules seemed to have a fundamental role in the generation of mineral. The mineral-forming capacity of CPLX and proteolipids

has been demonstrated by implanting Millipore chambers under the skin of rats (242). Changes in proteolipid composition in rachitic chicks, when compared to normal, and the reversal of this profile by treatment of rachitic chicks with vitamin D have been presented as further evidence for their involvement in mineralization (243). Rats have also been found to show similar changes in proteolipid composition, but vitamin D was not as stringent a requirement for them as for the chick (244–246).

Other evidence for the involvement of CPLX in generating mineral in vivo comes from micropuncture studies of Howell and Boyan (246). Fluid aspirated from the upper tibial growth plate of rachitic rats has been shown to contain a factor capable of nucleating mineral. The characteristics of this factor suggested that it was a phospholipid. The following findings led the authors to this conclusion: (1) the factor was found in the lowest density fraction after ultracentrifugation: (2) the factor bound calcium and induced hydroxyapatite formation in 3–5 h in vitro; and (3) the factor resisted acidification at pH 5.8 and therefore was not an hydroxyapatite seed crystal. Furthermore, the factor was soluble in chloroform–methanol, resistant to phospholipase D, and degraded by phospholipase C. Analysis of the phospholipids in this fluid indicated a composition similar to that of matrix vesicles, containing phosphatidyl serine, phosphatidyl inositol, phosphatidyl ethanolamine, phosphatidyl choline, and sphingomyelin (246).

The Chondrocalcin Hypothesis

Some Original Observations

Stimulated by controversies surrounding the matrix vesicle hypothesis, Poole et al. in 1984 sought alternative mechanisms to explain calcification of growth cartilage septae. In serial sections it was noted that the earliest particles of calcification per se appeared somewhat dissociated from the presence of matrix vesicles (55). They went on to describe the discrete focal sites adjacent to matrix vesicles where calcification was occurring. The region contained the *large proteoglycans,* which bind hyaluronic acid and have chondroitin sulfate chains attached to core protein, as well as a previously undetectable molecule which they named *chondrocalcin* (247,248). Both proteoglycan and chondrocalcin coexisted in the same microenvironment with matrix vesicles, although the vesicles seemed distinct and separate and stained for alkaline phosphatase. The investigators also pointed out that the concentration of matrix vesicles decreased in the lower hypertrophic cell zone; this was reminiscent of Reinholt's earlier observation and in direct contrast to what would have been expected if these particles functioned as nucleation centers (50,51). The concentration of chondrocalcin, on the other hand, increased in direct proportion to the amount of calcification (Fig. 9; 247,248). According to this view, then, chondrocalcin would be a generator of mineral while the matrix vesicle would be important as a source of inorganic phosphate.

Chondrocalcin

This 35-kD protein was originally described in fetal bovine epiphyseal cartilage around areas of intense calcification (53–55). The protein was purified and antibodies prepared so that its chemical nature and immunolocalization in the tissue could be studied. The immune localization studies revealed that this protein was present throughout the growth plate but at increased levels in the lower hypertrophic cell zone. Protein sequencing studies (249) ultimately demonstrated that it was identical to the C-propeptide region of type II collagen (i.e., CPII). Numerous other studies have confirmed that the protein binds tightly to hydroxyapatite as well as calcium.

The synthesis of chondrocalcin is dependent on vitamin D metabolites. The 24,25 isomer is required for normal synthesis of chondrocalcin and subsequent calcification (250). This was demonstrated in cultures of growth plates from rachitic rats. The normal (vitamin D replete) rat requires both isomers of vitamin D (1,25 and 24,25) to maintain maximal synthesis of chondrocalcin as well as maximal calcification. Interestingly, the 24,25 isomer is also required for normal synthesis of alkaline phosphatase by growth plate chondrocytes (251). Thus a coordinate regulatory pathway may exist to facilitate matrix calcification.

The original observations that associated chondrocalcin with regions undergoing calcification employed relatively low resolution immunoelectron microscopic techniques (55). Confirmation of these earlier findings has been provided with new colloidal gold methods. Lee et al. have shown the endoplasmic reticulum of hypertrophic chondrocytes to be enlarged and to contain type II collagen with its C-propeptide intact (247). This localization has never been observed in proliferating cells, where collagen synthesis is occurring at a high rate. The accumulation of type II collagen in the endoplasmic reticulum of hypertrophic cells appears to be a storage form of the protein so that it can be released at the time of matrix calcification (247). Calcium is also stored in the mitochondria of these cells. Since chondrocalcin is a calcium-binding protein, Poole and his colleagues have hypothesized that calcium may be redistributed to chondrocalcin (still a part of the type II procollagen molecule) at intracellular sites immediately before secretion into the extracellular matrix. Once in the matrix, chondrocalcin would be cleaved off the type II procollagen molecule; the ensuing matrix reorganization that would occur involves chondrocalcin and the large aggregating proteogly-

can (see below). Poole et al. have hypothesized that one facet of these complex events may involve the redistribution of chondrocalcin from the collagen fibrils to nucleation sites (248).

Proteoglycans, Glycosaminoglycans, and the Poole–Hunter Ion-Exchange Hypothesis for Storage and Release of Calcium in the Matrix

Large aggregating proteoglycans have a presumed role in matrix calcification, but the exact changes that occur in this molecule have been difficult to determine. In the lower hypertrophic cell zone, some investigators have reported a loss of proteoglycan based on biochemical measurements, while other investigators have seen no such changes (see below). By elemental analysis, no significant loss of sulfur has been found around the first three cells in the calcified cartilage (27). Poole et al. have shown the presence of large aggregating proteoglycans in both proliferating and hypertrophic cell zone cartilage, with no change in aggregatability or reduction in size. Several other workers have observed the opposite, with lower concentrations of aggregates in the calcified zone and monomer size remaining unchanged.

Although the meaning of these observations has been debated extensively, most investigators would agree that calcification can occur only after the proteoglycans are altered in a complex way. Shepard and Mitchell have identified small regions of concentrated proteoglycan in mineralizing sites with dye binding and elemental analyses (174,252). Arsenault and Ottensmeyer were able to demonstrate similar findings based on elevated levels of sulfur and calcium around proteoglycans before calcification, while phosphorus was present as well after calcification had occurred (175).

Calcium levels are also relevant to this discussion. The ability of calcium to bind proteoglycan and its possible role in mineral-forming complexes has been studied (252–254). It has been found at elevated levels in various articular cartilages (202) and, probably, bound to proteoglycans. Boyd and Neuman attempted to obtain evidence for this by equilibrating columns containing chondroitin sulfate with either calcium chloride or sodium chloride and then determining the relevant dissociation constants as a function of pH (255). Synthetic lymphs, containing known amounts of calcium, were then loaded onto the columns; this was then followed by a solution containing phosphate. Precipitates of calcium phosphate formed, appearing as small spheres (255). This ion-exchange concept has been further studied by Hunter (256–258).

The total calcium content in rat cartilage fluid was found by Howell et al. to be 1.46 mM. In studies of bovine costal cartilage that excluded the zone of calcification, the calcium content was found to be 15 mM per kilogram of wet weight (86). Thus it could be estimated

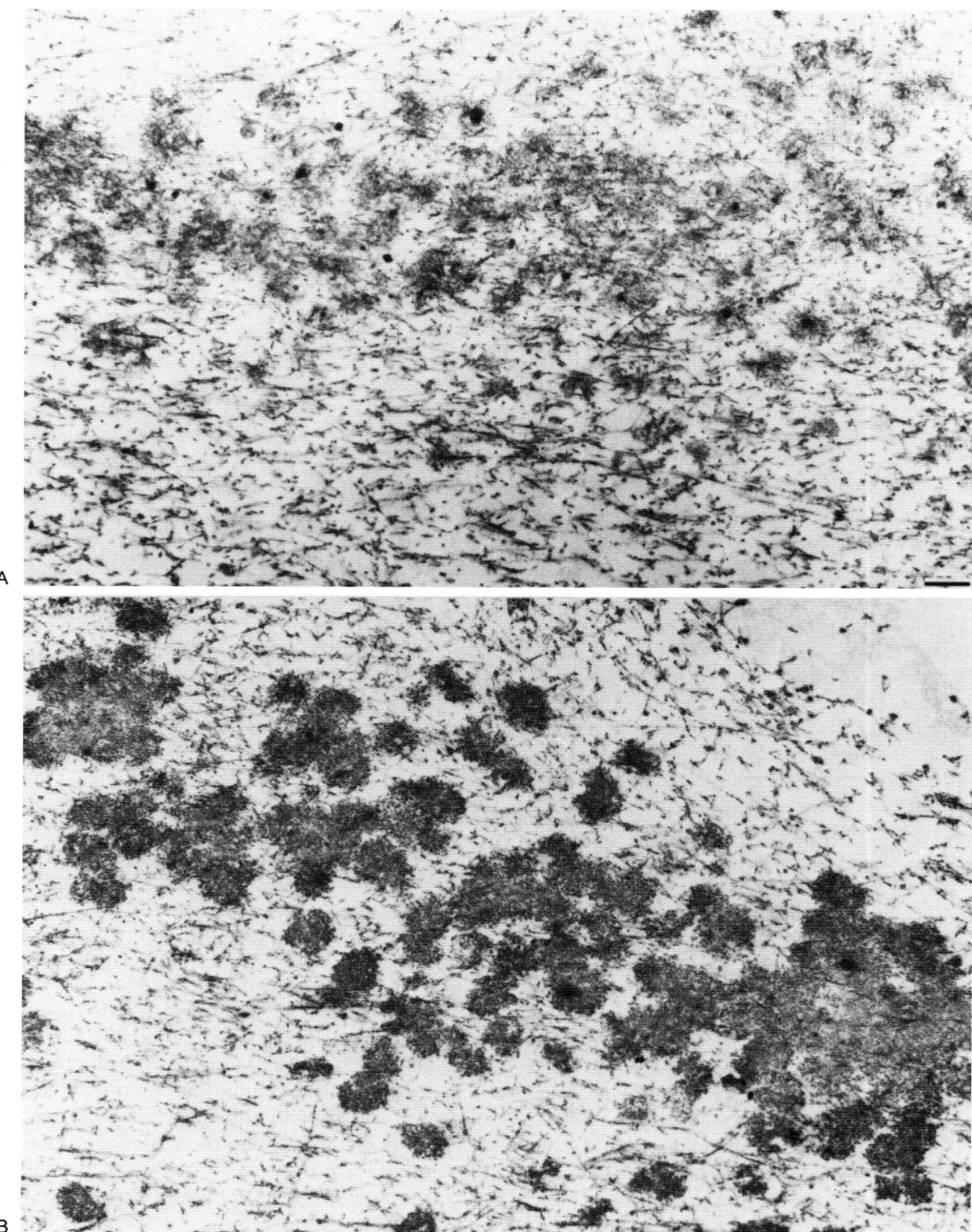

FIG. 9. Electron micrographs showing a close association between mineral and chondrocalcin in the lower hypertrophic cell zone of bovine fetal growth plate. **A:** Tissue treated with nonimmune immunoglobulin, showing only mineral deposits. **B:** Tissue stained with antibody to chondrocalcin using the peroxidase technique. *Bar* = 500 nm. [Reproduced with permission of A. R. Poole, L. Rosenberg, and Academic Press (247).]

that 6- to 10-fold higher levels of calcium are bound to the matrix than in the fluid itself. Studies by Wuthier have confirmed these estimates (87). Eichelberger and Roma have shown a rise in total calcium, independent of phosphate, in calcifying puppy cartilage (168). Calcium, therefore, appears to be mobile in the cartilage and could possibly build to high levels in the matrix (258). It should be noted that these whole-tissue profiles fail to show the histological location of calcium. Most electron probe studies, however, show signals strong enough to indicate that septal levels of this ion are severalfold higher than that found in the cartilage fluid.

Nevertheless, these observations suggest that calcium rearrangements must occur prior to calcification and that proteoglycans might serve as a minor storage site for calcium (259). Hunter has reported that chondroitin sulfate can function in this manner and that phosphate can displace calcium from proteoglycans (258). Therefore, an increase in local phosphate levels (possibly due to

alkaline phosphatase?) could be the localizing factor that causes the release of calcium from proteoglycans and subsequent mineral formation. This ion-exchange theory elaborated on by Hunter (258) fits conveniently into the Poole hypothesis (247,248; also see below).

Poole has described the primary nucleation sites presumably composed of proteoglycan, link protein, chondrocalcin, and other, as yet, unidentified substances. If growth plates are incubated in the presence of chelators and protease inhibitors at 4°C, proteoglycans and various ions are extracted (247,248). The remaining insoluble material is immunoreactive with antibodies to proteoglycan at specific focal sites. The sites are 100–300 nm in diameter and very similar in size and location to those of the primary nucleation sites found in the hypertrophic cell zone. These sites have been named *proteoglycan condensation sites* by Poole and colleagues; they are never found in cartilages destined not to calcify.

Poole has suggested that the mechanism of in vivo

TABLE 3. *Mechanisms and essential features of six discrete theories of cartilage septal calcification, evolved over 3 decades.*

I	II	III	IV	V	VI
Down regulation of mitochondrial metabolism	Matrix vesicles begin budding from late PCZ and HCZ zone	Chondrocalcin synthesized and accumulates in hypertrophic cell ER	Calcium storage on proteoglycan	Mineral generation; involvement of type II collagen and/or phosphoproteins, osteonectin degraded membrane proteolipid, Ca–alkaline–phosphatase, etc.	Mineral generation may occur after enzymatic removal of systemic or local inhibitors of mineral formation such as pyrophosphate or citrate
Accumulation of calcium and phosphate within mitochondria (as an amorphous mineral phase?)	Uptake of calcium and phosphate into matrix vesicles via transmembrane channels from extracellular sites; uptake of calcium from mitochondria uptake of phosphate ions from proteins–phospholipids; proteolipids, etc.[a]	Mitochondrial calcium binds to chondrocalcin intracellularly	Cell or vesicle alkaline phosphatases hydrolyzes various organic phosphate substrates		
Shift of calcium ions from mitochondria to calcifying extracellularly sites accompanied by changes in energy metabolism (compatible with views II–V)	Maturing matrix vesicles in extracellular sites accumulate stores of calcium and phosphate; efflux of H⁺ ions[b]	Chondrocalcin secreted extracellularly into septal matrix	Inorganic phosphate levels increase		
	Crystal aggregates accumulate	Chondrocalcin–proteoglycan–calcium complexes accumulate in matrix	Calcium ions shift off proteoglycans		
		Calcium precipitates with phosphate	Calcium precipitates with phosphate		

[a] Several candidate proteins demonstrated in matrix vesicles (e.g., calpactin II, calbindin, etc.).
[b] Important possible role in regulation of mineral formation by zinc, magnesium, vitamin D, etc. (See the text for specific references).
[c] PCZ, proliferating cell zone; HCZ, hypertrophic cell zone; ER, endoplasmic reticulum.

calcification can be described by combining certain aspects of the matrix vesicle, ion exchange, and chondrocalcin hypotheses. Although proteoglycans may be inhibitory in vitro, this does not necessarily mean that they behave as such in vivo. It is possible that some rearrangement occurs prior to calcification and that, later, proteoglycans directly participate in the local deposition of mineral at focal sites in the hypertrophic cell zone (as mentioned above). Examples of various changes that may occur in the proteoglycan structure include cleavage of hyaluronic acid and/or proteoglycan monomers to allow collapse of the proteoglycan aggregates as well as the redistribution of calcium (247,248).

According to this hypothesis, after mineral nucleation begins, mineral growth is supported by the continued production of chondrocalcin by hypertrophic cells. Local calcium levels can be increased substantially by release from proteoglycans and mitochondrial stores. At the same time, inorganic phosphate can be mobilized by the action of alkaline phosphatase in (or on?) matrix vesicles, resulting in accelerated mineral deposition. Table 3 summarizes many of the current ideas discussed in this section on mineralization.

Whether involving matrix vesicles, chondrocalcin, or phospholipids, this sequence of events must be under tight regulation. Autocrine, endocrine, and paracrine factors, in addition to streaming potentials and the direct effect of physical forces, probably control the sequence and intensity of this process. Capillary invasion, chondrocyte proliferation, and hypertrophy are just a few of the many events that need to be strictly regulated.

INHIBITION OF MINERAL GROWTH

One of the most amazing events occurring in the growth plate is the localized deposition of mineral in some regions, but not in others. During longitudinal septum mineralization of murine growth plates, transverse septae, and pericellular matrix remain uncalcified. These areas appear as sharp zones in transmission electron micrographs and, by inference, must contain inhibitors that prevent the deposition of mineral. In contrast, the border between unmineralized and mineralized cartilage along the advancing calcification front is not sharply demarcated, although inhibitors must also be present here since mineralization is occurring at a consistent height across the entire distal end of the growth plate.

The pericellular matrix must enlarge, while the interterritorial matrix is degraded, to make room for the hypertrophying chondrocytes. The matrix must have holes to allow for microvillar extensions into adjacent areas. When probed with thin micropuncture pipettes, the pericellular matrix has been found to be tough and impenetrable. This would make sense teleologically, since the cells must be protected from the high osmotic pressures developed in the presence of the proteoglycans. This per-

icellular matrix therefore not only regulates (i.e., inhibits) mineral deposition, but may also protect the chondrocyte from osmotic forces.

These tissues have other mechanisms for regulating mineral deposition. One proposed mechanism might involve micro-ions such as pyrophosphate. The discovery of NTP-pyrophosphohydrolase on chondrocyte membranes, as well as matrix vesicles, suggest a regulatory system where the addition of pyrophosphate to the matrix through nucleotide triphosphate hydrolysis, for example, could inhibit crystal proliferation (213).

Role of Proteoglycans in Mineral Formation

Several alternative hypotheses have been advanced over the last two decades to explain how proteoglycans might regulate mineralization. Proteoglycan aggregates, more than monomers, have been found to retard the formation of mineral from solutions of calcium and phosphate (259–262). Chen and Boskey have shown with well-characterized preparations that mineralization was inhibited in the presence of aggregate and hypothesized that this effect was due to binding of calcium ion, sequestering of small mineral clusters, shielding ion transfer, and lengthening the diffusion path of the ions by the proteoglycans (263–265). They concluded that these effects were facilitated by the large size and elaborate structure of the proteoglycans (265).

Many investigators have held the opinion that proteoglycan aggregates must be altered for mineralization to occur in the lower hypertrophic cell zone (135). Proteolytic degradation of the proteoglycan core protein is one way this could happen, although other mechanisms have been described (266–270). Alternatively, aggregates could be disrupted by a disaggregating agent such as lysozyme (169) or condensed into specific foci in the longitudinal septae with loss of hyaluronate (247,248). Theoretically, combinations of these hypotheses are possible.

Electron microscopic studies of Buckwalter and Rosenberg have examined proteoglycan aggregates from bovine growth plate and metaphysis (267). In earlier work it was shown that the aggregating monomers were not decreased in size and might be associated with mineralization. It was not clear whether mineralization might have accompanied a decrease in aggregate size or whether any changes had occurred in the nonaggregating monomers. These changes have been followed in more detail and changes with respect to zone studied. The results suggested that those proteoglycan monomers retained in the aggregate state were not degraded prior to mineralization (268). Further, in the lower proliferative and hypertrophic cell zones, the size of proteoglycan aggregates decreased sharply and the percent of nonaggregating monomers increased. The results were consistent with the view that large proteoglycan aggregates establish and maintain a densely packed distribution of monomers (i.e., subunits) in the matrix and prevent displacement of the monomers (268). This organization allows for a malleable matrix in the upper zones of the growth plate that inhibits mineralization, while in the lower zone there is a loss of monomers from the aggregates that decreases the capacity of the proteoglycans to inhibit mineralization.

Buckwalter et al. has shown an absolute increase in the population of nonaggregating monomers in the lower hypertrophic cell zone (268). The length of these monomers clustered into two subpopulations. In one, a length of 300 nm was observed. This was the size observed when monomer was cleaved by neutral metalloproteinase in vitro and corresponded to a loss of the hyaluronic acid–binding region. The second population contained monomers of 150 nm in length. This size was also obtainable after metalloproteinase digestion and represented cleavage of the monomer in the chondroitin sulfate-binding region (269). This was highly suggestive of proteolysis being responsible for these events. Even so, only reduced levels of proteoglycan aggregates have been found in cartilage after calcification (270–272). But this does not interdict the role of proteoglycans in regulating mineralization in confined, focal sites. Both Tyler (273) and Ratcliffe et al. (274) have shown selective cleavage of proteoglycan core protein, loss of nonaggregated monomers, and a decrease in the number of monomers per aggregate in articular cartilage explant cultures after stimulation with interleukin-1. As first studied by Sandy et al. in 1978, the phenomenon of proteoglycan cleavage resulting in diffusion of monomers from the cartilage has been well documented (275) and perhaps occurs by facilitated diffusion (276) in growth plate cartilage septae in the early stages of calcification, where rapid diffusion of ions into the matrix would seem essential. Could the postulated conversion of aggregated proteoglycans into chondrocalcin complexes cause a reduction of measurable aggregates?

These results are consistent with results using micropuncture to obtain a reproducible fluid phase from calcifying sites in growth plates of normal and rachitic rats (277). Samples of fluid containing proteoglycans were analyzed by transport ultracentrifugation techniques. As found in tissue samples from rachitic rats, the fluid in calcifying sites of these same rachitic animals contained proteoglycan aggregates prior to calcification (278–280). During reversal of rickets (i.e., healing), the aggregates disappeared as mineral formation proceeded (147). In isolated micropuncture fluids from healing rats, it was observed that in vitro mineral formation was spontaneous (281). Moreover, in normal and rachitic cartilage fluids mineralization could be induced in vitro by prior treatment of the fluid with leech hyaluronidase, trypsin, or cartilage neutral metalloproteinase (278; and D. S. Howell, unpublished observations). It was concluded that proteoglycans were an important inhibitor of mineral deposition in this system.

Degradation of Proteoglycans by Proteases

Inasmuch as mineralization is accompanied by changes in proteoglycan structure, some investigators have sought evidence for proteases that might degrade these macromolecules. Lysosomal proteases were originally hypothesized to function in this capacity. In this group are cathepsin D, cathepsin B, aryl sulfatase, endopolysaccharidases, chondrosulfatases, N-acetylgalactosaminidases, and acid phosphatase. Acid hydrolase activity has been shown to increase in the transition from proliferating to hypertrophic cell zones and, in some cases, localize to matrix vesicles (185,228,282–286).

Since all of these enzymes have acid pH optima and the pH of the extracellular matrix where mineralization is to occur is near neutrality, it seemed logical to look for enzymes with optimal activity at more physiologic pH values. Neutral proteases that degrade proteoglycans have been found in culture media conditioned by rat costal cartilage (287), rabbit articular cartilage (288), and human growth cartilage (289). Similar, but low levels of enzyme have been extracted from rabbit growth plates (290); it had many of the same properties as described by Sapolsky et al. (291) and Woessner and Selzer (292) for human articular cartilage neutral metalloproteinase. Recently, Ehrlich et al. have reported that growth plates contain stromelysin based on antibody reactivity and substrate specificity (293–295). Enzyme activity has been found in the tissue at calcifying sites and in matrix vesicles derived from cultures, suggesting a role in removing proteoglycan from these areas (296,297).

Proteoglycan Disaggregation with Lysozyme

Since the protease hypothesis has yielded equivocal findings, other methods for the removal and/or dissociation of proteoglycans have been sought. One way to dissociate proteoglycan aggregates might involve lysozyme. At present, lysozyme's action is not fully understood, but it was originally thought to function by releasing proteoglycan monomers from aggregates. This would increase the accessibility of these macromolecules to various degradative enzymes, such as proteases or hyaluronidase. At present, though, this is only conjecture. The characteristics of cartilage lysozyme have been reviewed in detail by Kuettner (169).

EFFECTS OF HORMONES AND GROWTH FACTORS ON THE GROWTH PLATE

Growth Hormone and Insulin-like Growth Factors

Effects of Growth Hormone on Skeletal Growth

Many hormones and growth factors have been described that affect skeletal growth and development; of the many examples that could be cited, the circulating hormones produced by the thyroid, adrenals, gonads, and pituitary are of well-known importance (298). The only recognized hormone, however, that can stimulate dose-dependent longitudinal bone growth over a wide range of doses is growth hormone (299,300). Many other biological effects have been attributed to this hormone. The reader is referred to several other excellent reviews for information on growth hormone–dependent effects on lipid and carbohydrate metabolism (301–303).

The effect of growth hormone on bone is believed to be mediated through its effect on germinative cells in the perichondrial margins and epiphyseal growth plate. It has been proposed that growth hormone directly promotes the differentiation of these cells and that during maturation these cells produce, and become sensitive to, insulin-like growth factor-1, IGF-1 (304,305). This increase in cell differentiation and proliferation leads to a continuous supply of cells entering the growth plate (306).

Somatomedins and Insulin-like Growth Factors (IGFs)

Salmon and Daughaday were the first to show an effect of growth hormone on costal chondrocyte cultures (307). In their studies, the addition of serum from hypophysectomized rats had little effect on sulfation rate when compared to that of normal rat serum or serum from hypophysectomized rats that had been treated with growth hormone. It was later discovered that the general stimulatory effect of growth hormone was mediated through circulating peptides (known as "sulfation factors") produced in response to growth hormone (308). Eventually, the term *somatomedin* became the accepted name for this group of poorly described peptides (309).

Three peptides were ultimately recognized. One, a neutral peptide, was named somatomedin A (310,311); a second factor was found to be basic and named somatomedin C (312). Another form was acidic and identified as somatomedin B, although this was eventually found to be identical with epidermal growth factor (313). The relationship of these proteins to each other was finally clarified in 1978 when the purification and primary structure of each was reported (314,315). Insulin-like growth factor-1 (IGF-1), formerly somatomedin C, was found to be a single-chain, basic peptide, containing 70 amino acids and having a molecular weight of 7650 D (314,316). The gene for this protein in humans has been localized to the long arm of chromosome 12 and its sequence determined (317–322). IGF-2, sometimes called *multiplication stimulating activity* (MSA) and believed to be the rat analog of human IGF-2, was reported to be very similar to IgF-1, although it was slightly acidic and had a molecular weight of 7470 D (315,323). The gene for this protein in humans has been localized to the short arm of chromosome 11 and its sequence determined (317,318,324–326).

Some early work demonstrated that hepatic cells, after stimulation with growth hormone, were a potential source of circulating IGFs. This suggestion was confirmed by further studies in rats that had undergone partial hepatectomy (327). Studies on catheterized dogs showed an arteriovenous difference in IGF-1 concentrations across the liver (328). Other tissues have been shown to make a contribution to systemic levels as well. For example, it has been shown that after growth hormone treatment, a rise in tissue IGF-1 levels precedes the rise in serum levels by several hours (329). Of the skeletal tissues examined, epiphyseal growth plates and fetal rat tibial bones were found to be sources of IGF-1 after growth hormone treatment (330,331). In the case of growth plate, exogenous IGF-1 by itself caused definitive changes (332).

Despite these characterizations, the physiologic role of IGFs remain uncertain. IGF-1 levels are low during fetal life, increase to a peak during puberty, and then decline progressively with increasing age (333). In contrast, IGF-2 levels are high in the embryo and do not show any increase during adolescence (334). IGF-2 is present at three to four times the level of IGF-1 in human adults. IGF-1 levels also seem more growth hormone regulated and dependent on nutritional status than IGF-2 (334).

Assigning relative roles for each of the IGFs are particularly difficult because of species differences and differing sensitivities of various tissues. For example, rats have IGF-1 levels that are 40 times higher than IGF-2 (334). IGF-1 and IGF-2 are known to have potent growth-stimulating effects on many different cell types in culture; examples include fetal limb buds, brain cells, pituitary tumor cells, certain blood cell lines, smooth muscle cells, lens epithelium, fetal liver cells, granulosa cells, Sertoli cells, fibroblasts, and chondrocytes (335,336). In addition, effects on differentiation have also been observed. IGF-1 has been reported to induce differentiation of myotubes into myoblasts and osteoblast precursor cells into osteoblasts (337,338).

IGF-1 has been shown to be the major factor in fetal calf serum responsible for increased levels of proteoglycan synthesis in cartilage. In one study IGF-1 at 10–20 ng/mL was the only factor necessary for the maintenance of steady-state proteoglycan synthesis. IGF-2 was also effective in this system, but not to the same extent as IGF-1. In older bovine cartilage explants, IGF-1 had no effect on cell proliferation, while growth plate tissue from the same species was stimulated to divide (339,340).

IGF-1 Binding Proteins

Once IGF-1 is secreted, as much as 99% of the circulating growth factor is bound to plasma carrier proteins. Two proteins with this capacity have been isolated; one is a small protein of 35 kD molecular weight, the other is relatively large and has a molecular weight of 150 kD.

The physiologic role of these two proteins is unclear at present (341–344).

Receptors for the IGFs have been described (345,346). Two subtypes of the human receptor have been identified based on their deduced primary structures (347–349). Although no absolute specificity for either receptor subtype has been found, there is preferential binding of IGF-1 to the type 1 receptor and IGF-2 to the type 2 receptor. Insulin can also bind to the type 1 receptor, but with low affinity (350,351). Like the insulin receptor, the IGF-1 receptor consists of two α and two β subunits connected by disulfide bonds. Ligand binding occurs at the α subunit, while the β subunit spans the cell membrane and has intracellular, tyrosine-specific protein kinase activity. The type 2 receptor has little or no affinity for insulin and consists of a single-chain glycoprotein that spans the cell membrane. It exhibits no kinase activity and may be identical to the mannose-6-phosphate receptor (349).

Growth Regulation and IGF-1

A number of studies using natural and recombinant sources of IGF-1 have clearly demonstrated increases in body length, organ growth, and sulfate uptake by cartilage. One unexpected finding was the observation that growth hormone alone stimulated more bone growth than an equivalent amount of IGF-1. Originally, this was thought to be due to a lack of IGF-binding proteins which might be produced in response to growth hormone. However, studies have found no potentiating effect of growth hormone on the production of IGF-1 binding proteins (352). Altogether, it would seem that growth hormone has a greater effect on bone than IGF-1.

Several investigators have explored the idea that local IGF production could be stimulated by circulating growth hormone. This paracrine/autocrine phenomenon would then explain some of the foregoing observations. Still, the classic somatomedin hypothesis would argue against such action, since growth hormone is supposed to function by stimulating liver production of IGFs, which then act on peripheral target tissues. It may be that the original hypothesis will be modified; recent data support the paracrine–autocrine hypothesis. When growth hormone was injected directly into the growth plate of hypophysectomized rats, unilateral bone growth was stimulated (353,354). This indicated a direct effect of growth hormone on growth plate chondrocytes. Local synthesis of IGF-1 has also been found in cartilage in response to growth hormone based on the presence of IGF-1 immunoreactive protein. Furthermore, the stimulatory effect of locally administered growth hormone could be abolished if antibodies to IGF-1 were coinfused with growth hormone (355). Other evidence has accrued to show that the mRNA for IGF-1 is elevated in skeletal muscle in response to growth hormone, just as has been shown in growth plate (356). Thus a dual effector theory

may more adequately describe growth hormone and IGF-1 function.

Some weaknesses in this theory exist. For example, it has been shown that the mRNA for IGF-1 is found in the perichondrium, not the chondrocytes, of human fetal growth plate (357). In contrast, the mRNA for IGF-1 has been found in chondrocytes of postnatal rat growth plates (330,358). It remains to be seen whether these differences can be explained on the basis of fetal versus postnatal tissues.

Vitamin D and Parathyroid Hormone

Previtamin D_3 is produced by a photochemical reaction in skin from 7-dehydrocholesterol and over a period of several days undergoes a temperature-dependent isomerization to vitamin D_3. The vitamin can then be hydroxylated in the liver to form 25(OH)-vitamin D_3. Further hydroxylation in the kidney results in production of the two major active metabolites of vitamin D: $1,25(OH)_2D_3$ and $24,25(OH)_2D_3$. (See Ch. 7.) There is firm evidence that the vitamin D–endocrine system is important not only in regulation of bone and mineral metabolism but also in modulation of other systems, such as those found in the growth plate (359–362).

$1,25(OH)_2D_3$ has proven biological activity in relation to mineral metabolism. It facilitates intestinal absorption of calcium and phosphorus, enhances renal mineral reabsorption, stimulates osteoclastic bone resorption, and promotes deposition of mineral in epiphyseal cartilage and newly formed bone. (See Chs. 1–3, 11, 12.) Some evidence suggests that it may be responsible for inducing cell differentiation in myeloid leukemia cells in vitro (362), for inducing interleukin-1 production in monocyte/macrophages (363), and for maintaining calcium in mitochondria and crystals in matrix vesicles in vitro (364). Differential responsiveness of isolated matrix vesicles and plasma membranes from resting-proliferating and hypertrophic chondrocytes to vitamin D metabolites by production of phospholipase A_2 and/or alkaline phosphatase has also been observed (365–369). In addition, $1,25(OH)_2D_3$ coordinately regulates, with parathyroid hormone (PTH), the release of calcium from bone in the control of plasma calcium levels (see below). Deficiency of vitamin D in a growing animal causes rickets, hypocalcemia, and secondary hyperparathyroidism.

On the other hand, the biological role of $24,25(OH)_2D_3$ is less well understood. Some investigators have postulated that this metabolite plays a crucial role in bone formation (370–373), while others consider it to be a catabolic by-product without any significant biological function (374). Despite this controversy, it is clear that both metabolites have substantially different effects on growth plate cartilage histology (371) and biochemistry; in particular, chondrocalcin levels are clearly influenced by vitamin D metabolites (375) as well as matrix vesicle and plasma membrane enzymes (365–369: see above). Receptors have been postulated by autoradiography for both metabolites (372). (See Ch. 8) Receptors for $24,25(OH)_2D_3$ were localized to the proliferating cells in the growth plate, while those for $1,25(OH)_2D_3$ were found in osteoprogenitor cells and osteoblasts. Further evidence for both metabolites being required in normal mineralization (and hence two different target cells?) has been deduced from studies of rachitic rats in which normal plasma levels of $1,25(OH)_2D_3$ were retained during the first week on rachitogenic diet but mild rachitic lesions formed anyway (376). In addition, in vitro studies show $24,25(OH)_2D_3$ to be responsible for cytoplasmic deposition of calcium granules, while most matrix vesicles were devoid of crystals (364). Thus the target cells for both metabolites appear different, implying a distinct biological function for each. It is possible that the main action of $1,25(OH)_2D_3$ is to maintain circulating levels of calcium as well as mineral homeostasis, while $24,25(OH)_2D_3$ is probably important for maturation of growth plate cartilage. Some of the controversy surrounding the function of these two metabolites deserves additional comment.

DeLuca and his colleagues have shown that virtually vitamin D–free rats, showing signs of hypocalcemia, could have normal bone growth and mineralization rates restored by simple infusion of calcium and phosphate. Further, the rats were found to acquire more mineral under these conditions than if vitamin D was infused by itself. This elegant experiment would seem to indicate decisively that rats require only calcium and phosphate for normal enchondral ossification and membranous bone formation (377–379). On the other hand, Lund has shown that rats fed a low-phosphate, vitamin D–deficient diet respond to $1,25(OH)_2D_3$, but not $24,25(OH)_2D_3$, with elevated x-ray healing indices (380). Boskey et al. has reported similar results with $1,25(OH)_2D_3$ in a model of calcium and vitamin D deficiency (381). Thus there is adequate evidence that vitamin D metabolites have some function in the rat, but it appears that they are not absolutely necessary for mineralization to proceed. The central question raised by these results remains: How essential is vitamin D?

In the authors' opinion, a variety of circumstances may have led to more subtle regulatory mechanisms whereby bone and cartilage cells became adapted to respond to these metabolites. In some instances, as in the fetus, vitamin D is not an essential regulator (382). Postnatally, during periods of nutritional or environmental stress, a transient calcium and/or phosphate deficiency may occur; at this time, the function of these metabolites may have evolved for a fine tuning role. During other times, the metabolites may have been somewhat superfluous. But this is only conjecture.

PTH works in conjunction with $1,25(OH)_2D_3$ in regulating calcium homeostasis (383–386). (See Ch. 4–6) Both hormones mobilize calcium from bone, with PTH

also acting in the kidney to increase calcium reabsorption as well as the synthesis of $1,25(OH)_2D_3$ by inducing the enzyme 25-hydroxylase. The resultant increase in plasma calcium decreases the secretion of PTH and subsequently the production of $1,25(OH)_2D_3$. The two calcium-regulating hormones thus influence each other's biosynthesis, although some evidence suggests that the two regulators may function independently as well (387). (See Ch. 17) Recent studies have suggested that $1,25(OH)_2D_3$ regulates PTH synthesis at the level of gene transcription (383,384,388). Sites of PTH binding, presumably due to receptors, have been found by use of radiolabeled PTH and its analogs (389,390). Binding was found in liver and kidney, as well as around osteoblasts, but not osteoclasts of bone. Differential response of various tissues to different forms of PTH have been used for a cytochemical bioassay (391).

Calcifying cartilage is also influenced by PTH in vitro (392,393). In embryonic cartilaginous bones, normal deposition of mineral between the central hypertrophic chondrocytes has been observed to occur. In the presence of PTH, this process was inhibited. The authors hypothesized that PTH not only mobilizes calcium from bone, but also prevents mineral deposition as well. This is consistent with Howell's unpublished observation that capillaries invade the growth plate cartilage without calcification after PTH stimulation in vivo. Barley and Bibby have observed binding of PTH to hypertrophic chondrocytes before the development of new blood vessels (390). No binding was found in other zones of the growth plate or articular cartilage. Thus some unknown function for PTH must exist that is related to growth plate differentiation and subsequent calcification.

Transforming Growth Factors

Transforming growth factors (TGFs) are homodimeric polypeptides known to function in cell growth and phenotypic expression (394,395). Two major TGFs have been described. TGF-α is a 50-amino acid protein synthesized by transformed cells and not, as yet, isolated from skeletal tissues. TGF-β, on the other hand, has been isolated from these sources at very high levels (sometimes 100 times higher than other tissues) and is a polypeptide of molecular weight 25 kD consisting of two subunits linked by disulfide bonds. Three forms have been identified. Although the effects of TGF-β vary with cell model and conditions of study, it is clear that TGF-β is an essential regulator of cell replication and differentiation.

Initial studies have shown that TGF-β induces rat embryonic muscle cells to express type II collagen and cartilage proteoglycans; both of which are markers for the chondrocyte phenotype (396,397). Growth plate chondrocytes respond to TGF-β by decreasing collagen synthesis and increasing noncollagen protein synthesis (398) as well as DNA synthesis (399). In another study, synthesis of mRNA for TGF-β has been reported to be coupled with type I collagen gene expression during endochondral bone formation (400). Antibody staining for TGF-β in fetal bovine articular cartilage (401), as well as during chondrogenesis in mouse embryos (402), has also been established. Alkaline phosphatase levels have been found to be elevated in matrix vesicle preparations derived from an osteosarcoma cell line, indicating that bone formation and repair may be dependent on TGF-β induced increases in alkaline phosphatase (403). In the growth plate, cell hypertrophy was accompanied by increases in TGF-β synthesis as assessed by a radioreceptor assay (404). Similarly, recent studies by the authors in collaboration with Bolander and Jingushi have shown TGF-β immunostaining in the growth plate (405). At present, it is not entirely clear what specific role TGF-β plays in the growth plate.

The physiologic role of TGF-β is generally uncertain. The regulation of bone TGF-β synthesis by systemic hormones has not been reported, but its release from bone matrix is increased in response to hormones that induce bone resorption such as PTH. It has also been shown that TGF-β stimulates osteoblast replication, but this effect can be blocked by EGF, PDGF, and TNF-α. It is thus clear that the milieu in which a cell finds itself will determine its response to various factors. As examples of this, FGF has been found to increase the amount of TGF-β mRNA in an osteoblast cell line (406), while growth plate chondrocyte responses to TGF-β are enhanced by factors in serum (398,399). Several reviews have recently been published that elaborate on the involvement of TGF-β in skeletal tissue regulation (407–409).

Heparin-Binding Growth Factors and Angiogenesis in the Growth Plate

Early Observations on the Nature of Angiogenesis

The term "angiogenesis" dates back to 1935 when new blood vessels were observed to form in the placenta.

Normal and pathologic capillary growth results from small venule sprouting (410), basement membrane degradation by proteinases (411), movement of endothelial cells toward an angiogenic stimulus, and alignment of endothelial cells to create a solid sprout. Fusion of two hollow sprouts allows blood flow to begin. Excellent reviews of these phenomena have been published (412–414).

Classes of Angiogenic (Growth) Factors and Their Possible Role in Directing Capillary Invasion in the Growth Plate

The development of methods to study angiogenesis resulted in studies searching for factors that would induce directed migration (chemotaxis), proteinase secretion, and proliferation of endothelial cells. The first such factors to be isolated were basic fibroblast growth factor (bFGF) from brain (415) and endothelial cell growth factor (ECGF) from hypothalamus (416). Other sources of these factors were also identified. The unique affinity of these factors for heparin formed the basis of a simple technique for isolating them in large quantities. The first such factor to be purified by heparin–Sepharose chromatography was a chondrosarcoma-derived growth factor (417). Later, distinct classes of growth factors were deduced from their relative affinity for heparin–Sepharose. Those factors that bound heparin–Sepharose and eluted with 1.0 M NaCl had pI values between 5 and 7 and molecular weights of 15–18 kD. The group included acidic FGF (aFGF). ECGF, eye-derived growth factor II, and acidic retina-derived growth factor. The second class also bound to heparin–Sepharose, eluted with 1.5 M NaCl, had pI values of 8–10, and had molecular weights of 16–18 kD. This group included bFGF and was more abundant and potent than the aFGF group. A publication that is particularly relevant to growth plate reports on heparin-binding growth factors in bone (418). Interestingly, the multiplicity of factors found in bone have

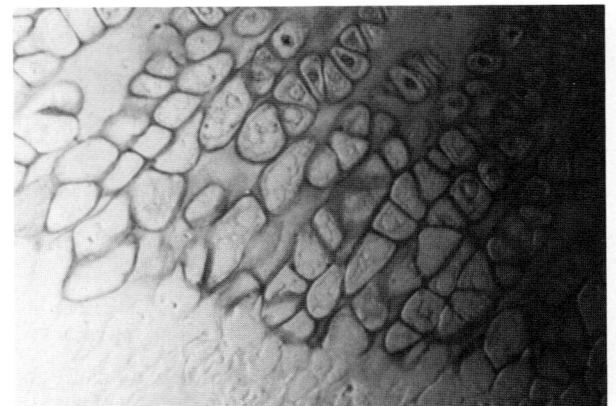
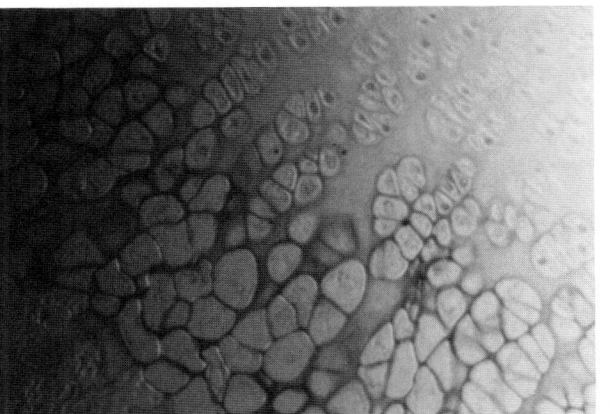

A   B

FIG. 10. Light micrograph (×240) of rat growth plate immunostained with antibodies to **A:** basic fibroblast growth factor (bFGF) and **B:** transforming growth factor (TGF-β₁) (cc), an extracellular form. [Reproduced from work of M. Bolander and S. Jingushi with permission of M. E. Bolander and Elsevier Science Publishers (428)].

also been found in the growth plate of rachitic rats and include aFGF, bFGF, TGF-β, and PDGF (Fig. 10; 405, 419). Several excellent reviews on the distribution, structure, and molecular biology of heparin-binding growth factors have been published (420–422).

Low-Molecular-Weight Angiogenic Factors

The factors described above are only representative of a large group. Other factors have been isolated from wound fluid and monocyte cultures (423,424). A third group includes those factors that are clearly nonproteinaceous and of low molecular weight. Interestingly, these factors display many of the properties expected of true angiogenic agents and have been described by four groups of investigators. One of these, endothelial cell stimulating angiogenic factor (ESAF), has been shown to stimulate capillary endothelial cells in culture and to give positive angiogenic responses in vivo (425). In addition, ESAF activates procollagenase (426) and is able to reactivate collagenase inhibited with tissue inhibitor of metalloproteinases (TIMP). ESAF has also been extracted from tumors, retina, and vitreous and synovial fluid (427). How ESAF and the polypeptide growth factors interact to control capillary invasion in the growth plate is unknown and currently under investigation.

ACKNOWLEDGMENTS

The authors' studies and the time to prepare this chapter were supported by a Medical Investigatorship (DSH) from the U.S. Veterans Administration and NIH Grant AR-08662. The authors greatly appreciate the assistance of Ms. Geneva Jackson in assembling the references.

REFERENCES

1. Rubin P. *Dynamic classification of bone dysplasias.* Chicago: Year Book Medical Publishers, 1964;1–410.
2. McKusick VA. *Mendelian inheritance in man: catalogs of autosomal dominant, autosomal recessive, and X-linked phenotypes,* 7th ed. Baltimore: Johns Hopkins University Press, 1986.
3. Stanescu V, Stanescu R, Maroteaux P. Pathogenic mechanisms in osteochondrodysplasias. *J Bone Joint Surg* 1984;66:817–36.
4. Caplan AI. Bone development. In: Evered D, Harnett S, eds. *Cell and molecular biology of vertebrate hard tissues.* New York: John Wiley, 1988;3–20.
5. Caplan AI. Cartilage. *Sci Am* 1984;251:84–94.
6. Hall BK. The embryonic development of bone. *Am Sci* 1988;76:174–81.
7. Carter DR. Mechanical loading history and skeletal biology. *J Biomechan* 1987;20:1095–109.
8. McKibbin B. The biology of fracture healing in long bones. *J Bone Joint Surg* 1978;60:149–62.
9. Urist MR. *Fundamental and clinical bone physiology.* Philadelphia: JB Lippencott, 1980.
10. Reddi AH, Sullivan NE. Matrix-induced endochondral bone differentiation: influence of hypophysectomy, growth hormone, and thyroid-stimulating hormone. *Endocrinology* 1980; 107:1291–9.
11. Newbrey JW, Bank WJ. Ultrastructural changes associated with the mineralization of deer antler cartilage. *Am J Anat* 1983;166:1–18.
12. Takagi M, Parmley RT, Denys FR, et al. Ultrastructural cytochemistry of proteoglycans associated with calcification of shark cartilage. *Anat Rec* 1984;208:149–58.
13. Reddi AH. Cell biology and biochemistry of endochondral bone development. *Coll Relat Res* 1981;1:209–26.
14. Sampath TK, Reddi AH. Importance of geometry of the extracellular matrix in endochondral bone differentiation. *J Cell Biol* 1984;98:2192–7.
15. Steinmann BU, Reddi AH. Changes in synthesis of types I and III collagen during matrix-induced endochondral bone differentiation in the rat. *Biochem J* 1980;186:919–24.
16. Myllyla R, Tryggvason K, Kivirikko KI, et al. Changes in intracellular enzymes of collagen biosynthesis during matrix-induced cartilage and bone development. *Biochim Biophys Acta* 1981;674:238–45.
17. Sampath TK, Muthukumaran N, Reddi AH. Isolation of osteogenin, an extracellular matrix-associated, bone-inductive protein, by heparin affinity chromatography. *Proc Natl Acad Sci USA* 1987;84:7109–13.
18. Johnson LC. Kinetics of osteoarthritis. *Lab Invest* 1959;8:1223–38.
19. Lane LB, Bullough PG. Age-related changes in the thickness of the calcified zone and the number of tidemarks in adult human articular cartilage. *J Bone Joint Surg* 1980;62B:372–5.
20. Cole AA, Wezeman FH. Cytochemical localization of tartrate-resistant acid phosphatase, alkaline phosphatase, and nonspecific esterase in perivascular cells of cartilage canals in the developing mouse epiphysis. *Am J Anat* 1987;219:237–42.
21. Schenk RK, Wiener J, Spiro D. Fine structural aspects of vascular invasion of the tibial epiphyseal plate of growing rats. *Acta Anat* 1968;69:1–17.
22. Boyde A, Shapiro IM. Morphological observations concerning the pattern of mineralization of the normal and the rachitic chick growth cartilage. *Anat Embryol* 1987;175:457–66.
23. Cruess RL. *The musculoskeletal system: embryology, biochemistry, and physiology.* New York: Churchill Livingstone, 1982.
24. Hunziker EB, Herrmann W, Schenk RK, et al. Cartilage ultrastructure after high pressure freezing, freeze substitution, and low temperature embedding. I. Chondrocyte ultrastructure: implications for the theories of mineralization and vascularization. *J Cell Biol* 1984;98:267–76.
25. Hunziker EB, Schenk RK, Cruzorive LM. Quantitation of chondrocyte performance in growth plate cartilage during longitudinal bone growth. *J Bone Joint Surg* 1987;69A:162–73.
26. Carlson CS, Hilley HD, Henrikson CK. Ultrastructure of normal epiphyseal cartilage of the articular-epiphyseal cartilage complex in growing swine. *Am J Vet Res* 1985;46:306–13.
27. Buckwalter JA, Mower D, Ungar R, et al. Morphometric analysis of chondrocyte hypertrophy. *J Bone Joint Surg* 1986;68A:243–55.
28. Howell DS, Carlson L. Alterations in the composition of growth cartilage septa during calcification studied by microscopic x-ray elemental analysis. *Exp Cell Res* 1968;51:185–95.
29. Woessner JF, Howell DS. Hydrolytic enzymes in cartilage. In: Maroudas A, Holborow EJ, eds. *Studies in joint disease,* vol 2. London: Pitman Medical, 1981;106–52.
30. Holtrop ME. The ultrastructure of the epiphyseal plate. II. The hypertrophic chondrocyte. *Calcif Tissue Res* 1972;9:140–51.
31. Farnum CE, Wilsman NJ. Morphologic stages of the terminal hypertrophic chondrocyte of growth plate cartilage. *Anat Rec* 1987;219:221–32.
32. Boyde A, Shapiro IM. Is there life after calcification? Microdissection analysis of normal and rachitic tibial growth cartilage. *Calcif Tissue Int* 1983;35:638.
33. Howlett CR. The fine structure of the proximal growth plate and metaphysis of the avian tibia: endochondral osteogenesis. *J Anat* 1980;130:745–68.
34. Eggli PS, Herrmann W, Hunziker EB, et al. Matrix compartments in the growth plate of the proximal tibia of rats. *Anat Rec* 1985;211:246–57.
35. Anderson CE, Parker J. Invasion and resorption in enchondral ossification. *J Bone Joint Surg* 1966;48A:899–915.

36. Trueta J, Amato VP. The vascular contribution to osteogenesis. III. Changes in the growth cartilage caused by experimentally induced ischemia. *J Bone Joint Surg* 1960;42B:571–87.

37. Reinholt FP, Engfeldt B, Heinegard D, et al. Proteoglycans and glycosaminoglycans of normal and strontium rachitic epiphyseal cartilage. *Coll Relat Res* 1985;5:41–54.

38. Walker KVR, Kember NF. Cell kinetics of growth cartilage in the rat tibia. II. Measurements during aging. *Cell Tissue Kinet* 1972;5:409–19.

39. Kember NF. Cell kinetics in cartilage. In: Hall BK, ed. *Cartilage,* vol 1. New York: Academic Press, 1983;149–80.

40. Kember NF, Walker KVR. Control of bone growth in rats. *Nature* 1971;229:428–9.

41. Poole CA, Flint MH, Beaumont BW. Morphological and functional interrelationships of articular cartilage matrices. *J Anat* 1984;138:113–38.

42. Anderson HC. Vesicles associated with calcification in the matrix of epiphyseal cartilage. *J Cell Biol* 1969;41:59–72.

43. Bonnucci E. Fine structure of early cartilage calcification. *J Ultrastruct Res* 1967;20:33–50.

44. Ali SY, Sajdera SW, Anderson HC. Isolation and characterization of calcifying matrix vesicles from epiphyseal cartilage. *Proc Natl Acad Sci USA* 1970;67:1513–20.

45. Anderson HC, Howell DS, eds. First international conference on matrix vesicle calcification. *Fed Proc* 1976;35:105–71.

46. Ascenzi A, Bonucci B, de Bernard B, eds. *Matrix vesicles: proceedings of the 3rd international conference on matrix vesicles.* Milan: Wichtig Editore, 1981.

47. Ali SY, ed. *Cell mediated calcification and matrix vesicles: proceedings of the 4th international conference on matrix vesicles.* Amsterdam: Excerpta Medica, 1986.

48. Anderson HC. Biology of disease: mechanism of mineral formation in bone. *Lab Invest* 1989;60:320–30.

49. Wuthier RE. Mechanism of matrix vesicle-mediated mineralization of cartilage. *ISI Atlas Sci Biochem* 1988;231–41.

50. Reinholt FP, Hjerpe A, Jansson K, et al. Stereological studies on the epiphyseal growth plate in low phosphate, vitamin D-deficiency rickets with special reference to the distribution of matrix vesicles. *Calcif Tissue Int* 1984;36:94–101.

51. Reinholdt FP, Engfeldt B, Hjerpe A, et al. Stereological studies on the epiphyseal growth plate with special reference to the distribution of matrix vesicles. *J Ultrastruct Res* 1982;80:270–9.

52. Poole AR, Pidoux I, Rosenberg L. Role of proteoglycans in endochondral ossification: immunofluorescent localization of link protein and proteoglycan monomer in bovine fetal epiphyseal growth plate. *J Cell Biol* 1982;92:249–60.

53. Choi HU, Tang TL, Johnson S, et al. Isolation and characterization of a 35,000 molecular weight subunit fetal cartilage matrix protein. *J Biol Chem* 1983;258:655–61.

54. Poole AR, Pidoux I, Reiner A, et al. Kniest dysplasia is characterized by an abnormal processing of the C-propeptide of type II collagen resulting in imperfect fibril assembly. *J Clin Invest* 1988;81:579–89.

55. Poole AR, Pidoux I, Reiner A, et al. Association of an extracellular protein (chondrocalcin) with the calcification of cartilage in endochondral bone formation. *J Cell Biol* 1984;98:54–65.

56. Hunziker EB, Schenk RK. Physiological mechanisms adopted by chondrocytes in regulating longitudinal bone growth in rats. *J Physiol* 1989;414:55–71.

57. Simmons DJ, Arsenis C, Whitson SW, et al. Mineralization of rat epiphyseal cartilage: a circadian rhythm. *Miner Electrolyte Metab* 1983;9:28–37.

58. Russell JE, Walker WV, Simmons DJ. Adrenal/parathyroid regulation of DNA, collagen and protein synthesis in rat epiphyseal cartilage and bone. *J Endocrinol (Lond)* 1984;103:49–57.

59. Hodge JA, McKibbin B. The nutrition of mature and immature cartilage in rabbits. *J Bone Joint Surg* 1969;51B:140–8.

60. Brighton CT, Heppenstall RB. Oxygen tension in zones of the epiphyseal plate, the metaphysis and diaphysis: an in vitro and in vivo study in rats and rabbits. *J Bone Joint Surg* 1971;53A:719–28.

61. Kuhlman RE. A microchemical study of the developing epiphyseal plate. *J Bone Joint Surg* 1960;42A:457–66.

62. Kunin AS, Krane SM. The effect of dietary phosphorous on the intermediary metabolism of epiphyseal cartilage from rachitic rats. *Biochim Biophys Acta* 1965;107:203–14.

63. Kunin AS, Krane SM. Utilization of citrate by epiphyseal cartilage of rachitic and normal rats. *Biochim Biophys Acta* 1965;111:32–9.

64. Vasington FD, Murphy JV. Calcium uptake by rat kidney mitochondria and its dependence on respiration and phosphorylation. *J Biol Chem* 1962;237:2670–7.

65. Lehninger AL, Vercesi A, Bababunmi EA. Regulation of calcium release from mitochondria by the oxidation–reduction state of pyridine nucleotides. *Proc Natl Acad Sci USA* 1978;75:1690–4.

66. Martin JH, Matthews JL. Mitochondrial granules in chondrocytes. *Calcif Tissue Res* 1969;3:184–93.

67. Brighton CT, Hunt RM. Electron microscopic pyroantimonate studies of matrix vesicles and mitochondria in the rachitic growth plate. *Metab Bone Dis Relat Res* 1978;1:199–204.

68. Arsenis C. Role of mitochondria in calcification: mitochondrial activity distribution in the epiphyseal plate and accumulation of calcium and phosphate ions by chondrocyte mitochondria. *Biochem Biophys Res Commun* 1972;46:1928–35.

69. Sutfin LV, Holtrop ME, Ogilvie RE. Microanalysis of individual mitochondrial granules with diameters less than 1000 angstroms. *Science* 1971;174:947–9.

70. Hargest TE, Gay CV, Schraer H, et al. Vertical distribution of elements in cells and matrix of epiphyseal growth plate cartilage determined by quantitative electron probe analysis. *J Histochem Cytochem* 1985;33:275–86.

71. Kakuta S, Golub EE, Hasselgrove JHC, et al. Redox studies of the epiphyseal growth cartilage: pyridine nucleotide metabolism and the development of mineralization. *J Bone Miner Res* 1986;1:433–40.

72. Matsumoto H, DeBolt K, Shapiro IM. Adenine, guanine and inosine nucleotides of chick growth cartilage: relationship between energy status and the mineralization process. *J Bone Miner Res* 1988;3:347–52.

73. Yamamoto T, Gay CV. Ultrastructural analysis of cytochrome oxidase in chick epiphyseal growth plate cartilage. *J Histochem Cytochem* 1988;36:1161–6.

74. Ishikawa Y, Chin JE, Hubbard HL, et al. Utilization and formation of amino acids by chicken epiphyseal chondrocytes: comparative studies with cultured cells and native cartilage tissue. *J Cell Physiol* 1985;123:79–88.

75. Shapiro IM, Golub EE, Chance B, et al. Linkage between energy status of perivascular cells and mineralization of the chick growth cartilage. *Dev Biol* 1988;129:372–9.

76. Iannotti JP, Brighton CT, Iannotti V. The mechanism of action of parathyroid hormone induced proteoglycan synthesis in the growth plate. *Trans Orthop Res Soc* 1988;13:291.

77. Iannotti JP, Brighton CT, Iannotti V. The effects of a plasma derived serum factor on intracellular ionized calcium in the growth plate chondrocyte. *Trans Orthop Res Soc* 1988;13:269.

78. Howell DS, Pita JC, Marquez JF, et al. Partition of calcium, phosphate, and protein in the fluid phase aspirated by micropuncture at calcifying sites in epiphyseal cartilage. *J Clin Invest* 1968;47:1121–32.

79. Pita JC. Potentiometric determination of carbon dioxide partial pressure and pH in ultramicro volumes of biological fluids. *Anal Chem* 1969;41:273–8.

80. Cuervo LA, Pita JC, Howell DS. Ultramicroanalysis of pH, P_{CO_2} and carbonic anhydrase activity at calcifying sites in cartilage. *Calcif Tissue Res* 1971;7:220–31.

81. Gay CV, Anderson RE, Schraer H, et al. Identification of carbonic anhydrase in chick growth plate cartilage. *J Histochem Cytochem* 1982;30:391–4.

82. Wuthier RE. Electrolytes of isolated epiphyseal chondrocytes, matrix vesicles, and extracellular fluid. *Calcif Tissue Res* 1977;23:125–34.

83. Thomas WC, Connor TB, Howard JE. Some physico-chemical aspects of calcification in vitro. *Bull Johns Hopkins Hosp* 1956;99:287–95.

84. Sobel AE, Burger M, Nobel S. Mechanisms of nuclei formation in mineralizing tissues. *Clin Orthop* 1960;17:103–23.

85. Hsu HHT, Anderson HC. A simple and defined method to study calcification by isolated matrix vesicles: effect of ATP and vesicle phosphatase. *Biochim Biophys Acta* 1977;500:162–72.

86. Howell DS, Delchamps EE, Reimer W, et al. A profile of electrolytes in the cartilaginous plate of growing ribs. *J Clin Invest* 1960;39:919–29.

87. Wuthier RE. Zonal analysis of electrolytes in epiphyseal cartilage of bone of normal and rachitic chickens and pigs. *Calcif Tissue Res* 1971;8:24–35.

88. Dean DD, Muniz OE, Berman I, et al. Localization of collagenase in the growth plate of rachitic rats. *J Clin Invest* 1985;76:716–22.

89. Schmid TM, Conrad HE. A unique low molecular weight collagen secreted by cultured chick embryo chondrocytes. *J Biol Chem* 1982;257:12451–7.

90. Gannon JM, Fischer M, Hofmeister R, et al. Localization of type X collagen in fetal canine growth plate and adult canine articular cartilage. *Trans Orthop Res Soc* 1989;14:59.

91. Urban JPG, Maroudas A. Swelling of the invertebral disc in vitro. *Connect Tissue Res* 1981;9:1–10.

92. Maroudas A, Urban JPG. Swelling pressures of cartilaginous tissues. In: Maroudas A, Holborow EJ, eds. *Studies in joint disease*, vol 1. London: Pitman Medical, 1980;87–116.

93. Altman RD, Tenenbaum J, Latta L, et al. Biomechanical and biochemical properties of dog cartilage. *Ann Rheum Dis* 1984;43:83–90.

94. Buckwalter JA, Rosenberg LC, Ungar R. Changes in proteoglycan aggregates during cartilage mineralization. *Calcif Tissue Int* 1987;41:228–36.

95. Masse P, Cashin CH, Weiser H. Bone metabolic disturbances induced by lack of vitamin B-6. *J Bone Miner Res* 1989;4(suppl 1):S157.

96. Mechanic G, Banes A, Yamauchi MHM. Possible collagen structural control of mineralization. In: Butler WT, ed. *The chemistry and biology of mineralized tissues*. Birmingham, AL: Ebsco Media, 1985;98–106.

97. Heinegard D, Oldberg A. Structure and biology of cartilage and bone matrix noncollagenous macromolecules. *FASEB J* 1989;3:2042–51.

98. Campo RD. Effects of cations on cartilage structure: swelling of growth plate and degradation of proteoglycans induced by chelators of divalent cations. *Calcif Tissue Int* 1988;43:108–21.

99. Mayne R, Burgeson RE. *Structure and function of collagen types*. New York: Academic Press, 1987.

100. Eyre DR. Collagens of the disc. In: Ghosh P, ed. *The biology of the invertebral disc*. Boca Raton, FL: CRC Press, 1988;171–88.

101. Miller EJ. The structure of fibril-forming collagens. *Ann NY Acad Sci* 1985;460:1–13.

102. Wu JJ, Eyre DR, Dean DD, et al. Quantitative studies on the collagen composition of the growth plate in the rachitic rat. *Trans Orthop Res Soc* 1989;14:58.

103. Mayne R, Irwin MH. Collagen types in cartilage. In: Kuettner K, Schleyerbach R, Hascall VC, eds. *Articular cartilage biochemistry*. New York: Raven Press, 1986;23–38.

104. Vogel K, Trotter JA. The effect of proteoglycans on the morphology of collagen fibrils formed in vitro. *Coll Relat Res* 1987;7:105–14.

105. Vogel K, Paulsson M, Heinegard D. Specific inhibition of type I and type II collagen fibrillogenesis by the small proteoglycan of tendon. *Biochem J* 1984;223:587–97.

106. Poole AR, Webber I, Pidoux H, et al. Localization of a dermatan sulfate proteoglycan (DS-PGII) in cartilage and the presence of an immunologically related species in other tissues. *J Histochem Cytochem* 1986;34:619–25.

107. Bianco P, Fisher LW, Young MF, et al. Differential expression of small proteoglycans I and II (Biglycan and Decorin) in human developing bone and non-bone tissues as revealed by immunolocalization and in situ hybridization. *J Bone Miner Res* 1989;4(suppl 1):S321.

108. van der Rest M, Mayne R. Type IX collagen. In: Mayne R, Burgeson RE, eds. *Structure and function of collagen types*. New York: Academic Press, 1987;195–221.

109. Ninomiya Y, Olsen BR. Synthesis and characterization of cDNA encoding a cartilage specific short collagen. *Proc Natl Acad Sci USA* 1984;81:3014–8.

110. Ninomiya Y, van der Rest M, Mayne R, et al. Construction and characterization of cDNA encoding the alpha-2 chain of chicken type IX collagen. *Biochemistry* 1985;24:4223–9.

111. van der Rest M, Mayne R, Ninomiya Y, et al. The structure of type IX collagen. *J Biol Chem* 1985;260:220–5.

112. Bruckner P, Vaughan L, Winterhalter KH. Type IX collagen from sternal cartilage of chicken embryo contains covalently bound glycosaminoglycans. *Proc Natl Acad Sci USA* 1985;82:2608–12.

113. Noro A, Kimata K, Oike Y, et al. Isolation and characterization of third proteoglycan (PG-Lt) from chick embryo cartilage which contains a disulfide-bonded collagenous peptide. *J Biol Chem* 1983;258:9323–31.

114. Eyre DR, Apone S, Wu JJ, et al. Collagen type IX: evidence for covalent linkages to type II collagen in cartilage. *FEBS Lett* 1987;220:337–41.

115. van der Rest M, Mayne R. Type IX collagen proteoglycan from cartilage is covalently cross-linked to type II collagen. *J Biol Chem* 1988;263:1615–8.

116. Schmid TM, Conrad HE. A unique low molecular weight collagen secreted by cultured chick embryo chondrocytes. *J Biol Chem* 1982;257:12444–50.

117. Grant WT, Sussman MD, Balian G. A disulfide-bonded short chain collagen synthesized by degenerative and calcifying zones of bovine growth plate cartilage. *J Biol Chem* 1985;260:3798–803.

118. Kielty CM, Kwan APL, Holmes DF, et al. Type X collagen, a product of hypertrophic chondrocytes. *Biochem J* 1985;27:545–54.

119. Jimenez SA, Yankowski R, Reginato AM. Quantitative analysis of type X collagen biosynthesis by embryonic chick sternal cartilage. *Biochem J* 1986;233:357–67.

120. Schmid TM, Mayne R, Bruns RR, et al. Molecular structure of short-chain (sc) cartilage collagen by electron microscopy. *J Ultrastruct Res* 1984;86:186–91.

121. Ninomiya Y, Gordon M, van der Rest M, et al. The developmentally regulated type X collagen gene contains a long open reading frame without introns. *J Biol Chem* 1986;261:5041–50.

122. Schmid TM, Linsenmayer TF. Immunohistochemical localization of short chain cartilage collagen (type X) in avian tissues. *Dev Biol* 1985;107:373–81.

123. Schmid TM, Linsenmayer TF. Developmental acquisition of type X collagen in the embryonic chick tibiotarsus. *J Cell Biol* 1985;100:598–605.

124. Gannon JM, Fischer M, Hofmeister F, et al. Localization of type X collagen in fetal canine growth plate and adult canine articular cartilage. *Trans Orthop Res Soc* 1989;14:59.

125. Habuchi H, Conrad HE, Glaser JH. Coordinate regulation of collagen and alkaline phosphatase levels in chick embryo chondrocytes. *J Biol Chem* 1985;260:13029–34.

126. Eyre DR, Wu JJ. Type XI collagen. In: Mayne R, Burgeson RE, eds. *Structure and function of collagen types*. Orlando, FL: Academic Press, 1987;261–81.

127. Poole AR. Proteoglycans in health and disease: structures and functions. *Biochem J* 1986;236:1–14.

128. Hascall VC. Proteoglycans: the chondroitin sulfate/keratin sulfate proteoglycan of cartilage. *ISI Atlas Sci Biochem* 1988;189–98.

129. Hardingham TE, Muir H. The specific interaction of hyaluronic acid with cartilage proteoglycans. *Biochim Biophys Acta* 1972;279:401–5.

130. Hardingham TE, Muir H. Binding of oligosaccharides of hyaluronic acid to proteoglycans. *Biochem J* 1973;135:905–8.

131. Hascall VC, Heinegard D. Aggregation of cartilage proteoglycans: oligosaccharide competitors of the proteoglycan–hyaluronic acid interaction. *J Biol Chem* 1974;249:4242–9.

132. Christner JM, Brown M, Dziewiatkowski DD. Interaction of cartilage proteoglycans with hyaluronic acid: the role of the hyaluronic acid carboxyl groups. *Biochem J* 1977;167:711–6.

133. Tengblad A. A comparative study of the binding of cartilage link protein and the hyaluronate binding region of the cartilage proteoglycan to hyaluronate-substituted Sepharose gel. *Biochem J* 1981;199:297–305.

134. Faltz LL, Caputo CB, Kimura JH, et al. Structure of the complex between hyaluronic acid, the hyaluronic acid–binding region, and the link protein of proteoglycan aggregates from the Swarm rat chondrosarcoma. *J Biol Chem* 1979;254:1381–7.

135. Buckwalter JA. Proteoglycan structure in calcifying cartilage. *Clin Orthop* 1983;172:207–32.
136. Buckwalter JA, Rosenberg LC. Electron microscopic studies of cartilage proteoglycans. *Electron Microsc Rev* 1988;1:87–112.
137. Weidemann JA, Paulsson M, Timpl R, et al. Domain structure of cartilage proteoglycans revealed by rotary shadowing of intact and fragmented molecules. *Biochem J* 1984;224:331–3.
138. Doege K, Sasaki M, Horigan E, et al. Complete primary structure of the rat cartilage proteoglycan core protein deduced from cDNA clones. *J Biol Chem* 1987;262:17757–67.
139. Neame PJ, Christner JE, Baker JR. The primary structure of link protein from rat chondrosarcoma proteoglycan aggregate. *J Biol Chem* 1986;261:3519–35.
140. Doege K, Hassell JR, Caterson B, et al. Link protein cDNA sequence reveals a tandemly repeated protein structure. *Proc Natl Acad Sci USA* 1986;83:3761–5.
141. Deak F, Kiss I, Sparks KJ, et al. Complete amino acid sequence of chicken cartilage link protein deduced from cDNA clones. *Proc Natl Acad Sci USA* 1986;83:3766–70.
142. Perin J-P, Bonnet F, Thurieau C, et al. Link protein interactions with hyaluronate and proteoglycans: characterization of two distinct domains in bovine cartilage link proteins. *J Biol Chem* 1987;262:13269–72.
143. Goetinck PF, Stirpe NS, Tsonis PA, et al. The tandemly repeated sequences of cartilage link protein contain the sites for interaction with hyaluronic acid. *J Cell Biol* 1987;105:2403–8.
144. Neame PJ, Christner JE, Baker JR. Cartilage proteoglycan aggregates: the link protein and proteoglycan amino-terminal globular domains have similar structures. *J Biol Chem* 1987;262:17768–78.
145. Halberg DF, Proulx G, Doege K, et al. A segment of the cartilage proteoglycan core protein has lectin-like activity. *J Biol Chem* 1988;263:9486–90.
146. Doege K, Fernandez P, Hassell JR, et al. Partial cDNA sequence encoding a globular domain at the C-terminus of the rat cartilage proteoglycan. *J Biol Chem* 1986;261:8108–11.
147. Pita JC, Muller FJ, Howell DS. Structural changes of sulfated proteoglycans of rat growth cartilage during endochondral calcification. In: Gregory J, Jeanloz RW, eds. *Proceedings of the 4th international symposium on glycoconjugate research.* New York: Academic Press, 1979;743–6.
148. Hunziker EB, Schenk RK. Structural organization of proteoglycans in cartilage. In: Wight TN, Meachim RP, eds. *Biology of proteoglycans.* New York: Academic Press, 1987;155–85.
149. Mow VC, Mak AF, Lai WM, et al. Viscoelastic properties of proteoglycan subunits and aggregates in varying solution concentrations. *J Biomechan* 1984;17:325–38.
150. Hardingham TE, Muir H, Kwan MK, et al. Viscoelastic properties of proteoglycan solutions with varying proportions present as aggregates. *J Orthop Res* 1987;5:36–46.
151. Boskey AL. Noncollagenous matrix proteins and their role in mineralization: a mini-review. *Bone and Miner* 1989;6:111–123.
152. Dean DD, Muniz OE, Howell DS. Association of collagenase and tissue inhibitor of metalloproteinases (TIMP) with hypertrophic cell enlargement in the growth plate. *Matrix* 1989b;9:366–375.
153. von der Mark K, Mollenhauer J, Pfaffle M, et al. Role of anchorin CII in the interaction of chondrocytes with extracellular collagen. In: Kuettner K, Schleyerbach R, Hascall VC, eds. *Articular cartilage biochemistry.* New York: Raven Press, 1986;125–42.
154. Mollenhauer J, Bee JA, Lizarbe MA, et al. Role of anchorin CII, a 31,000 molecular weight membrane protein, in the interaction of chondrocytes with type II collagen. *J Cell Biol* 1984;98:1572–9.
155. Mollenhauer J, von der Mark K. Isolation and characterization of a collagen binding glycoprotein from chondrocyte membranes. *EMBO J* 1983;2:45–50.
156. von der Mark K, Mollenhauer J, Muller PK, et al. Anchorin CII: a Type II collagen-binding glycoprotein from chondrocyte membranes. *Ann NY Acad Sci* 1985;460:214–23.
157. Singer II. The fibronexus: a transmembrane association of microfilaments in hamster and human fibroblasts. *Cell* 1979;16:675–85.
158. Lust G, Burton-Wurster N, Leipold H. Fibronectin as a marker for osteoarthritis. *J Rheumatol* 1987;14:28–9.
159. Hewitt AT, Kleinmann HR, Pennypacker JP, et al. Identification of an adhesion factor for chondrocytes. *Proc Natl Acad Sci USA* 1980;77:385–8.
160. Hewitt AT, Varner HH, Silver MH, et al. The isolation and partial characterization of chondronectin, an attachment factor for chondrocytes. *J Biol Chem* 1982;257:2330–4.
161. Romberg RW, Werness PG, Lollar B, et al. Isolation and characterization of native adult osteonectin. *J Biol Chem* 1985;260:2728–36.
162. LeBoy PS, Shapiro IM, Ushmann BD, et al. Gene expression in mineralizing chick epiphyseal cartilage. *J Biol Chem* 1986;263:8515–20.
163. Miller RR, McDevitt CA. Thrombospondin in articular cartilage. *Trans Orthop Res Soc* 1989;14:154.
164. Eyre DR, Apone JJ, Wu JJ, et al. Cartilage type IX collagen: direct evidence for covalent intermolecular crosslinks to type II collagen. *Trans Orthop Res Soc* 1988;13:118.
165. van der Rest M, Mayne R. Identification and localization of a lysine-derived crosslink between cartilage type IX and type II collagens. *Trans Orthop Res Soc* 1988;13:119.
166. Neuman WF, Neuman MW. *The chemical dynamics of bone and mineral.* Chicago: University of Chicago Press, 1958.
167. McLean FC, Urist MR. *Bone: fundamentals of the physiology of skeletal tissue,* 3rd ed. Chicago: University of Chicago Press, 1968.
168. Eichelberger L, Roma M. Effects of age on the histochemical characterization of costal cartilage. *Am J Physiol* 1954;178:296–304.
169. Kuettner K, Sorgente N, Croxen R, et al. Lysozyme in preosseous cartilage. VII. Evidence for a physiological role of lysozyme in normal endochondral calcification. *Biochim Biophys Acta* 1974;372:335–44.
170. Krefting ER, Barkhaus RH, Hohling HJ, et al. Electronprobe x-ray microanalysis in hard tissue research. In: *Electron microscopy: 10th international congress on electron microscopy. (Deutsche Gessellschaft fur elecktronmikrospie e V),* vol 3. Hamburg: Paul Hartung, 1982;387–8.
171. Shapiro IM, Boyde A. Microdissection–elemental analysis of the mineralizing growth cartilage of the normal and rachitic chick. *Metab Bone Dis Rel Res* 1984;5:317–26.
172. Althoff J, Quint P, Krefting ER, et al. Morphological studies on the epiphyseal growth plate combined with biochemical and x-ray microprobe analyses. *Histochemistry* 1982;74:541–52.
173. Davis WL, Jones RG, Knight JP, et al. Cartilage calcification: an ultrastructural, histochemical and analytical x-ray microprobe study of the zone of calcification in the normal avian epiphyseal growth plate. *J Histochem Cytochem* 1982;30:221–34.
174. Shepard N, Mitchell N. Ultrastructural modifications of proteoglycans coincident with mineralization in local regions of rat growth plate. *J Bone Joint Surg* 1985;67A:455–64.
175. Arsenault AL, Ottensmeyer FP. Quantitative spatial distribution of calcium, phosphorous, and sulfur in calcifying epiphysis by high resolution electron spectroscopic imaging. *Proc Natl Acad Sci USA* 1983;80:1322–6.
176. Boyde A, Shapiro IM. Energy dispersive x-ray elemental analysis of isolated epiphyseal growth plate chondrocyte fragments. *Histochemistry* 1980;69:85–94.
177. Wroblewski J, Roomans GM, Madsen K, et al. X-ray microanalysis of cultured chondrocytes. *Scanning Electron Microsc* 1983;2:777–84.
178. Larsson PA, Howell DS, Pita JC, et al. Aspiration and characterization of predentin fluid in developing rat teeth by means of a micropuncture and micro-analytical technique. *J Dent Res* 1988;67:870–5.
179. Triffitt JT, Terepka AR, Neuman WF. A comparative study of the exchange in vivo of major constituents of bone mineral. *Calcif Tissue Res* 1968;2:165–76.
180. Grynpas MD, Pritzker KPH, Hancock RGV. Neutron activation analysis of bulk and selected trace elements in bones using low flux SLOWPOKE reactor. *Biol Trace Elem Res* 1987;13:333–44.
181. Roufosse AH, Awe WP, Glimcher MJ, et al. An investigation of the mineral phases of bone by solid state ^{31}P magic and sample spinning NMR. *Biochemistry* 1984;23:6115–20.
182. Cheng P-T. Formation of octacalcium phosphate and subsequent

transformation to hydroxyapatite at low supersaturation: a model for cartilage calcification. *Calcif Tissue Int* 1987;40:339–43.

183. Mendelsohn R, Hassankhani A, DiCarlo E, et al. FT-IR microscopy of endochondral ossification at 20 micron spatial resolution. *Calcif Tissue Int* 1989;44:20–24.

184. Glimcher MJ. Molecular biology of mineralized tissues with particular reference to bone. *Rev Mod Phys* 1959;31:359–93.

185. Glimcher MJ. Composition, structure, and organization of bone and other mineralized tissues and the mechanism of calcification. In: Geiger SR, ed. *Handbook of physiology and endocrinology*, vol 7, *The parathyroid gland.* Baltimore: Williams & Wilkins, 1976;25–116.

186. Glimcher MJ, Kossiva D, Roufosse A. Identification of phosphopeptides and γ-carboxyglutamic acid-containing peptides in epiphyseal growth plate cartilage. *Calcif Tissue Int* 1979;27:187–91.

187. Grynpas MD, Bonar LC, Glimcher MJ. Failure to detect an amorphous calcium phosphate phase in bone mineral. *Calcif Tissue Int* 1984;36:291–301.

188. Endo A, Glimcher MJ. The potential role of phosphoproteins in the in vitro calcification of bone collagen. *Trans Orthop Res Soc* 1986;11:221.

189. Sauer GR, Wuthier RE. Fourier transform infrared characterization by mineral phases formed during induction of mineralization by collagenase-released matrix vesicles in vitro. *J Biol Chem* 1988;263:13718–24.

190. Termine JD, Peckhauskas RA, Posner AS. Calcium phosphate formation in vitro. II. Effects of environment on amorphous-crystalline transformation. *Arch Biochem Biophys* 1970; 140:318–25.

191. Boskey AL, Posner AS. Formation of hydroxyapatite at low supersaturation. *J Phys Chem* 1976;80:40–5.

192. Brown WE, Schroeder LRW, Ferris JS. Interlayering of crystalline octacalcium phosphate and hydroxyapatite. *J Phys Chem* 1979;83:1385–8.

193. Nancollas GH. Phase transformation during precipitation of calcium salts. In: Nancollas GH, ed. *Biological mineralization and demineralization.* Berlin: Springer-Verlag, 1982;79–99.

194. Hjertquist SO. Biophysical studies of epiphyseal growth zones and adjacent compact bone tissue in normal and rachitic dogs and rats. *Acta Soc Med Ups* 1961;66:202–16.

195. Robinson RA. Crystal–collagen–water relationships in bone matrix. *Clin Orthop* 1960;17:69–76.

196. Boskey AL. Hydroxyapatite formation in a dynamic collagen gel system: effects of type I collagen, lipids, and proteoglycans. *J Phys Chem* 1989;93:1628–33.

197. Ali SY. Analysis of matrix vesicles and their role in the calcification process. *Fed Proc* 1976;35:135–42.

198. Landis WJ, Paine ML, Glimcher MJ. Electron microscopic observations of bone tissue prepared anhydrously in organic solvents. *J Ultrastruct Res* 1977;59:1–30.

199. Landis WJ, Glimcher MJ. Electron optical and analytical observations of rat growth plate cartilage by ultramicrotomy. *J Ultrastruct Res* 1982;78:227–68.

200. Morris DC, Vaananen HK, Anderson HC, et al. Matrix vesicle calcification in rat epiphyseal growth plate cartilage prepared anhydrously for electron microscopy. *Metab Bone Dis Relat Res* 1983;5:131–7.

201. Akisaka T, Kawaguchi H, Subita GP, et al. Ultrastructure of matrix vesicles in chick growth plate as revealed by quick freezing and freeze substitution. *Calcif Tissue Int* 1988;42:383–93.

202. Arsenault AL, Ottensmeyer FP, Heath IB. An electron microscopic and spectroscopic study of murine epiphyseal cartilage: analysis of fine structure and matrix vesicles preserved by slam freezing and freeze substitution. *J Ultrastruct Res* 1988;98:32–47.

203. Hunziker E, Herrmann W, Cruz-Orive LM, et al. Image analysis of electron micrographs relating to mineralization in calcifying cartilage: theoretical considerations. *J Electron Microsc Tech* 1989;11:9–15.

204. Cecil RNA, Anderson HC. Freeze-fracture studies of matrix vesicle calcification in epiphyseal growth plate. *Metab Bone Dis Relat Res* 1978;1:89–96.

205. Hale JE, Wuthier RE. The mechanism of matrix vesicle formation: studies on the composition of chondrocyte microvilli and on the effects of microfilament-perturbing agents on cellular vesiculation. *J Biol Chem* 1987;262:1916–25.

206. Majeska RJ, Holwerda DL, Wuthier RE. Localization of phosphatidylserine in isolated chick epiphyseal cartilage matrix vesicles with trinitrobenzene sulfonate. *Calcif Tissue Int* 1979; 27:41–6.

207. Watkins EL, Stillo JV, Wuthier RE. Subcellular fraction of epiphyseal cartilage: isolation of matrix vesicles and profiles of enzymes, phospholipids, calcium and phosphate. *Biochim Biophys Acta* 1980;631:289–304.

208. Wuthier RE. Electrolytes of isolated epiphyseal chondrocytes, matrix vesicles and extracellular fluid. *Calcif Tissue Res* 1977;23:125–33.

209. Wuthier RE, Gore ST. Partition of inorganic ions and phospholipids in isolated cell membrane and matrix vesicle fractions: evidence for calcium-phosphate–acidic phospholipid complexes. *Calcif Tissue Res* 1977;24:163–71.

210. Robison R. The possible significance of hexose phosphoric esters in ossification. *Biochem J* 1923;17:286–93.

211. McLean FM, Keller PJ, Genge BR, et al. Disposition of preformed mineral in matrix vesicles: internal localization and association with alkaline phosphatase. *J Biol Chem* 1987;262: 10481–8.

212. Hsu HHT. Purification and partial characterization of ATP pyrophosphohydrolase from fetal bovine epiphyseal cartilage. *J Biol Chem* 1983;258:3486–8.

213. Caswell AM, Ali SY, Russell RGG. Nucleoside triphosphate pyrophosphatase in skeletal tissues. In: Ali SY, ed. *Cell mediated calcification and matrix vesicles.* Amsterdam: Excerpta Medica, 1986;101–6.

214. Hirschman A, Deutsch D, Hirschman M, et al. Neutral peptidase activities in matrix vesicles from bovine fetal alveolar bone and dog osteosarcoma. *Calcif Tissue Int* 1983;35:791–7.

215. Katsura N, Yamada K. Isolation and characterization of a metalloprotease associated with chicken epiphyseal cartilage matrix vesicles. *Bone* 1986;7:137–43.

216. Ali SY, Evans L. The uptake of calcium ions by matrix vesicles isolated from calcifying cartilage. *Biochem J* 1973;134:647–50.

217. Hsu HHT, Anderson HC. The deposition of calcium pyrophosphate and phosphate by matrix vesicles isolated from fetal bovine epiphyseal cartilage. *Calcif Tissue Int* 1984;36:615–21.

218. Morris DC, Vaananen HK, Munoz P, et al. Light and electron microscopic immunolocalization of alkaline phosphatase in bovine growth plate cartilage. In: Ali SY, ed. *Cell mediated calcification and matrix vesicles: proceedings of the 4th international conference on matrix vesicles.* Amsterdam: Excerpta Medica, 1986;21–6.

219. de Bernard B, Gheranediut GGC, Lunazzic M, et al. Role of calcium binding alkaline phosphatase in the mechanism of calcification. In: Ali SY, ed. *Cell mediated calcification and matrix vesicles: proceedings of the 4th international conference on matrix vesicles.* Amsterdam: Excerpta Medica, 1986;95–100.

220. Howell DS, Blanco LN, Pita JC, et al. Further characterization of a nucleational agent in hypertrophic cell extracellular cartilage fluid. *Metab Bone Dis Relat Res* 1978;1:155–60.

221. Howell DS, Pita JC, Alvarez J. Possible role of matrix vesicles in initial calcification of healing rickets. *Fed Proc* 1976;35:122–6.

222. Frazer D. Hypophosphatasia. *Am J Med* 1957;22:730–46.

223. Eanes ED. Dynamic aspects of apatite phases of mineralized tissues: model studies. In: Butler WT, ed. *Chemistry and biology of mineralized tissues.* Birmingham, AL: Ebsco Media, 1985;213–20.

224. Eanes ED, Hailer EW. Liposome mediated calcium-phosphate formation in metastable solutions. *Calcif Tissue Int* 1985; 37:390–4.

225. Eanes ED, Rattner SL. The effect of magnesium on apatite formation in seeded supersaturated solutions at pH 7.4. *J Dent Res* 1981;60:1719–23.

226. Swain LD, Boyan BD. Ion translocating properties of calcifiable proteolipids. *J Dent Res* 1988;67:526–30.

227. Akisaka T, Gay C. Maturational changes in the ultrastructural distribution of calcium-ATPase in epiphyseal growth plate. In: Ali SY, ed. *Cell mediated calcification and matrix vesicles: pro-*

ceedings of the 4th international conference on matrix vesicles. Amsterdam: Excerpta Medica, 1986;63–7.

228. Wuthier RE. A review of the primary mechanism of endochondral calcification with special emphasis on the role of cells, mitochondria and matrix vesicles. *Clin Orthop Relat Res* 1982;169:219–42.

229. Boskey A. Phospholipids and biological calcification. In: Veis A, ed. *The chemistry and biology of mineralized connective tissues.* New York: Elsevier/North-Holland, 1982;531–5.

230. Boyan-Salyers B. A role for proteolipid in membrane-initiated calcification. In: Vies A, ed. *The chemistry and biology of mineralized connective tissues.* New York: Elsevier/North-Holland, 1981;539–42.

231. Boskey A. Overview of cellular elements and macromolecules implicated in the initiation of mineralization. In: Butler WT, ed. *The chemistry and biology of mineralized tissues.* Birmingham, AL: Ebsco Media, 1985;334–44.

232. Boyan BD. Proteolipid-dependent calcification. In: Butler WT, ed. *The chemistry and biology of mineralized tissues.* Birmingham, AL: Ebsco Media, 1985;125–31.

233. Boyan BD, Schwartz Z, Swain LD, et al. The role of lipids in calcification of cartilage. *Anat Rec* 1989;224:211–9.

234. Boskey AL, Posner A. The role of synthetic and bone extracted calcium–phospholipid–phosphate complexes in hydroxyapatite formation. *Calcif Tissue Res* 1977;23:251–8.

235. Boskey AL, Timchak DM, Lane JM, et al. Phospholipid changes during fracture healing. *Proc Soc Exp Biol Med* 1980;165:368–73.

236. Boskey A, Posner A. Effect of magnesium on lipid-induced calcification: an in vitro model for bone mineralization. *Calcif Tissue Int* 1980;32:139–43.

237. Ennever J, Vogel J, Rider L, et al. Nucleation of microbiologic calcification by proteolipid. *Proc Soc Exp Biol Med* 1976;152:147–50.

238. Ennever J, Boyan-Salyers B, Riggan L. Proteolipid and bone matrix calcification in vitro. *J Dent Res* 1977;56:967–70.

239. Boyan-Salyers B, Boskey A. Relationship between proteolipids and calcium phospholipid–phosphate complexes in *Bacterionema matruchotii*. *Calcif Tissue Int* 1980;30:167–74.

240. Boyan B, Boskey A. Co-isolation of proteolipids and calcium–phospholipid–phosphate complexes. *Calcif Tissue Int* 1984;36:214–8.

241. Irving JT. A histological stain for newly calcified tissues. *Nature (Lond)* 1958;181:704–5.

242. Raggio CL, Boyan BD, Boskey AL. In vivo hydroxyapatite formation induced by lipids. *J Bone Miner Res* 1986;1:409–15.

243. Boyan BD, Ritter NM. Proteolipid–lipid relationships in normal and vitamin D–deficient chick cartilage. *Calcif Tissue Int* 1984;36:328–33.

244. Boskey AL, Weintraub S. The effect of vitamin D deficiency on rat bone lipid composition. *Bone* 1986;7:277–81.

245. Boyan BD, Schwartz Z, Swain LD, et al. Differential expression of phenotype by resting zone and growth region costochondral chondrocytes in vitro. *Bone* 1988;9:185–94.

246. Cieslak S, Howell DS, Boyan B. Microanalysis of phospholipids in epiphyseal cartilage extracellular fluid *J Dental Res* 1986;65A:323.

247. Lee ER, Yasumoto M, Poole AR. Immunochemical and immunocytochemical studies of the C-propeptide of type II procollagen in chondrocytes of the growth plate. *J Histochem Cytochem* 1990;38:659–673.

248. Poole AR, Matsui Y, Hinek A, et al. Cartilage macromolecules and the calcification of cartilage matrix. *Anat Rec* 1989;224:167–79.

249. van der Rest M, Rosenberg LC, Olsen BR, et al. Chondrocalcin is identical to C-propeptide of type II collagen. *Biochem J* 1986;237:923–5.

250. Hinek A, Poole AR. The influence of vitamin D metabolites on the calcification of cartilage matrix and the C-propeptide of type II collagen (chondrocalcin). *J Bone Miner Res* 1988;3:421–9.

251. Hale LV, Kemick MLS, Wuthier RE. Effect of vitamin D metabolites on the expression of alkaline phosphatase activity by hypertrophic chondrocytes in primary cell culture. *J Bone Miner Res* 1986;1:489–95.

252. Mitchell N, Shepard N, Harrod J. The measurement of proteoglycan in the mineralizing region of the rat growth plate: an electron microscopic and x-ray microanalytical study. *J Bone Joint Surg* 1982;64:32–8.

253. Dunstone J. Ion-exchange reactions between cartilage and various cations. *Biochem J* 1960;77:164–70.

254. Bowness J, Lee K. Effects of chondroitin sulfates on mineralization in vitro. *Biochem J* 1967;103:382–90.

255. Boyd E, Neuman W. The surface chemistry of bone. V. The ion-binding properties of cartilage. *J Biol Chem* 1951;193:243–51.

256. Hunter GK, Nyburg SC, Pritzker KPH. Hydroxyapatite formation in collagen, gelatin, and agarose gels. *Coll Relat Res* 1986;6:229–38.

257. Hunter GK. Chondroitin sulfate–derivatized agarose beads: a new system for studying cation binding to glycosaminoglycans. *Anal Biochem* 1987;165:435–41.

258. Hunter GK. An ion exchange mechanism of cartilage calcification. *Connect Tissue Res* 1987;16:111–20.

259. Blumenthal NC. Mechanism of proteoglycan inhibition of hydroxyapatite formation. *Dev Biochem* 1981;22:509–15.

260. Posner AS, Blumenthal NC. The role of proteoglycans in tissue mineralization. In: Ascenzi A, Bonucci B, deBernard B, eds. *Matrix vesicles: proceedings of the 3rd international conference on matrix vesicles.* Milan: Wichtig Editore, 1981;143–7.

261. Cuervo LA, Pita JC, Howell DS. Inhibition of calcium phosphate mineral growth by proteoglycan aggregate fractions in a synthetic lymph. *Calcif Tissue Res* 1973;13:1–10.

262. Dziewiatkowski DD, Majznerski LL. Role of proteoglycans in endochondral ossification: inhibition of calcification. *Calcif Tissue Int* 1985;37:560–4.

263. Chen CC, Boskey AL, Rosenberg LC. The inhibitory effect of cartilage proteoglycans on hydroxyapatite growth. *Calcif Tissue Int* 1984;36:285–90.

264. Chen CC, Boskey AL. Mechanisms of proteoglycan inhibition of hydroxyapatite growth. *Calcif Tissue Int* 1985;37:395–400.

265. Chen CC, Boskey AL. The effects of proteoglycans from different cartilage types on in vitro hydroxyapatite proliferation. *Calcif Tissue Int* 1986;39:324–7.

266. Campo RD, Dziewiatkowski DD. Turnover of the organic matrix of cartilage and bone as visualized by autoradiography. *J Cell Biol* 1963;18:19–29.

267. Buckwalter JA, Rosenberg L. Structural changes in reassembled growth plate aggregates. *J Orthop Res* 1986;4:1–9.

268. Buckwalter JA, Rosenberg LC, Ungar R. Changes in proteoglycan aggregates during cartilage mineralization. *Calcif Tissue Int* 1987;41:228–36.

269. Buckwalter JA, Ehrlich MG, Armstrong AL, et al. Electron microscopic analysis of articular cartilage proteoglycan degradation by growth plate enzymes. *J Orthop Res* 1987;5:128–32.

270. Lohmander S, Hjerpe A. Proteoglycans of mineralizing rib and epiphyseal cartilage. *Biochim Biophys Acta* 1975;404:93–109.

271. Axelsson I, Berman I, Pita JC. Proteoglycans from rabbit articular and growth plate cartilage: ultracentrifugation, gel chromatography, and electron microscopy. *J Biol Chem* 1983;258:8915–21.

272. Campo RD, Romano JE. Changes in cartilage proteoglycans associated with calcification. *Calcif Tissue Int* 1986;39:175–84.

273. Tyler JA. Chondrocyte-mediated depletion of articular cartilage proteoglycans in vitro. *Biochem J* 1985;225:493–507.

274. Ratcliffe A, Billingham MEJ, Muir H, et al. Experimental canine osteoarthritis and cartilage explant culture: increased release of specific proteoglycan components. *Biochem J* 1986;238:571–80.

275. Sandy JD, Brown HLG, Lowther DA. Degradation of proteoglycan in articular cartilage. *Biochim Biophys Acta* 1978;543:536–44.

276. Cumming GJ, Handley CJ, Preston BN. Permeability of composite chondrocyte-culture-Millipore membranes to solutes of varying size and shape. *Biochem J* 1979;181:257–66.

277. Howell DS, Pita JC. Calcification of growth plate cartilage with special reference to studies on micropuncture fluids. *Clin Orthop* 1976;118:208–29.

278. Howell DS, Pita JC, Marquez JF, et al. Demonstration of macromolecular inhibitor(s) of calcification and nucleating factor(s) in fluid from calcifying sites in cartilage. *J Clin Invest* 1969;48:630–41.

279. Pita JC, Cuervo LA, Madruga JE, et al. Evidence for a role of protein polysaccharides in regulation of mineral phase separation in calcifying cartilage. *J Clin Invest* 1970;49:2188–97.

280. Howell DS, Muniz OE, Blanco LN, et al. A micropuncture study of growth cartilage in phosphonate-induced rickets. *Calcif Tissue Int* 1980;30:35–42.

281. Pita JC, Muller F, Howell DS. Disaggregation of proteoglycan aggregate during endochondral calcification: physiological role of cartilage lysozyme. In: Burleigh PMC, Poole AR, eds. *Dynamics of connective tissue macromolecules.* Amsterdam: North-Holland, 1974;247–58.

282. Thyberg J, Friberg U. The lysosomal system in endochondral growth. *Prog Histochem Cytochem* 1978;10:1–46.

283. Hirschman A, Hirschman M. Soluble sulfatase in growing bone of rats. *Science* 1969;164:834–5.

284. Granda JL, Posner AS. Distribution of four hydrolases in the epiphyseal plate. *Clin Orthop Relat Res* 1971;74:269–72.

285. Ingmar B, Wasteson A. Sequential degradation of a chondroitin sulphate trisaccharide by lysosomal enzymes from embryonic chick epiphyseal cartilage. *Biochem J* 1979;179:7–13.

286. Arsenis C, Eisenstein R, Soble LW, Kuettner KE. Enzyme activities in chick embryonic cartilage: their subcellular distribution in isolated chondrocytes. *J Cell Biol* 1971;49:459–67.

287. Wasteson A, Lindahl U, Hallen A. Mode of degradation of the chondroitin sulphate proteoglycan in rat costal cartilage. *Biochem J* 1972;130:729–38.

288. Sandy JD, Brown HLG, Lowther DA. Degradation of proteoglycan in articular cartilage. *Biochim Biophys Acta* 1978;543:536–44.

289. Ehrlich MG, Mankin HJ, Davis MW. Human epiphyseal plate proteoglycans and degradation patterns. *Trans Orthop Res Soc* 1979;4:139.

290. Woessner JF, Howell DS. Hydrolytic enzymes in cartilage. In: Maroudas A, Holborow EJ, eds. *Studies in joint disease,* vol 2. London: Pitman Medical, 1983;106–52.

291. Sapolsky AI, Keiser H, Howell DS, et al. Metalloproteases of human articular cartilage that digest cartilage proteoglycans at neutral and acid pH. *J Clin Invest* 1976;58:1030–41.

292. Woessner JF, Selzer MG. Two latent metalloproteinases of human articular cartilage that digest proteoglycan. *J Biol Chem* 1984;259:3633–8.

293. Ehrlich MG, Armstrong AL, Neuman RG, et al. Patterns of proteoglycan degradation by a neutral protease from human growth plate epiphyseal cartilage. *J Bone Joint Surg* 1982;64A:1350–4.

294. Ehrlich MG, Tebor GB, Armstrong AL, et al. Comparative study of neutral proteoglycanase activity by growth plate zone. *J Orthop Res* 1985;3:269–76.

295. Ehrlich MG, Armstrong AL, Zaleske DJ, et al. The discovery and characterization of physeal stromelysin. *Trans Orthop Res Soc* 1989;14:111.

296. Katsura N, Yamada K. Further characterization of matrix vesicle protease. In: Ali SY, ed. *Cell mediated calcification and matrix vesicles.* Amsterdam: Elsevier, 1986;89–94.

297. Einhorn TA, Hirschman A, Gordon SL, et al. Enzymes associated with matrix vesicles isolated from osteoarthritic cartilage. In: Ali SY, ed. *Cell mediated calcification and matrix vesicles.* Amsterdam: Elsevier, 1986;359–64.

298. Sissons HA. The growth of bone. In: Bourne GH, ed. *The biochemistry and physiology of bone.* New York: Academic Press, 1971;443–74.

299. Cheek DB, Hill DE. Effect of growth hormone on cell and somatic growth. In: Knobil E, Sawyer WH, eds. *Handbook of physiology,* vol 4 (part 2). Washington, DC: American Physiological Society, 1974;159–85.

300. Simpson ME, Asling CW, Evans HM. Some endocrine influences on skeletal growth and differentiation. *Yale J Biol Med* 1950;23:1–27.

301. Altszuler N. Actions of growth hormone on carbohydrate metabolism. In: Knobil E, Sawyer WH, eds. *Handbook of physiology,* vol 4 (part 2). Washington, DC: American Physiological Society, 1974;233–52.

302. Davidson MB. Effect of growth hormone on carbohydrate and lipid metabolism. *Endocr Rev* 1987;8:115–31.

303. Goodman HM, Schwartz J. Growth hormone and lipid metabolism. In: Knobil E, Sawyer WH, eds. *Handbook of physiology,* vol 4 (part 2). Washington, DC: American Physiological Society, 1974;211–31.

304. Isaksson OGP, Lindahl A, Nilsson A, et al. Mechanism of the stimulatory effect of growth hormone on longitudinal bone growth. *Endocr Rev* 1987;8:426–38.

305. Nilsson A, Isgaard J, Lindahl A, et al. Effects of unilateral arterial infusion of GH and IGF-1 on tibial longitudinal bone growth in hypophysectomized rats. *Calcif Tissue Int* 1987;40:91–6.

306. Kember NF. Cell kinetics of cartilage. In: Hall BK, ed. *Cartilage,* vol 1. New York: Academic Press, 1983;149–77.

307. Salmon WD, Daughaday WH. A hormonally controlled serum factor which stimulates sulfate incorporation by cartilage in vitro. *J Lab Clin Med* 1957;49:825–36.

308. Phillips LS, Vassilopoulou-Sellin R. Somatomedins. *N Engl J Med* 1980;302:371–80.

309. Daughaday WH, Hall K, Raben MS, Salmon WD, Van den Brande JL, Van Wyk JJ. Somatomedin: proposed designation for sulphation factor. *Nature* 1972;235:107.

310. Hall K. Human somatomedin: determination, occurrence, biological activity and purification. *Acta Endocrinol (Copenh)* 1972;70(suppl 163):1–45.

311. Uthne K. Human somatomedins: purification and studies of their biological actions. *Acta Endocrinol (Copenh)* 1973;73(suppl 175):1–35.

312. van Wyk JJ, Underwood LE, Hintz RE, et al. The somatomedins: a family of insulin-like growth factors under growth hormone control. *Recent Prog Horm Res* 1974;30:259–318.

313. Heldin CH, Wasteson A, Fryklund L, et al. Somatomedin B: mitogenic activity derived from contaminant epidermal growth factor. *Science* 1981;213:1122–3.

314. Rinderknecht E, Humbel RE. The amino acid sequence of human insulin-like growth factor-1 and its structural homology with proinsulin. *J Biol Chem* 1978;253:2769–76.

315. Rinderknecht E, Humbel RE. Primary structure of human insulin-like growth factor-2. *FEBS Lett* 1978;89:283–6.

316. Klapper DG, Svoboda ME, Van Wyk JJ. Sequence analysis of somatomedin C: confirmation of identity with insulin-like growth factor-1. *Endocrinology* 1983;112:2215–7.

317. Brissenden JE, Ullrich A, Francke U. Human chromosomal mapping of genes for insulin-like growth factors 1 and 2 and epidermal growth factor. *Nature* 1984;310:781–4.

318. Tricoli JV, Rall LB, Scott J, et al. Localization of insulin-like growth factor genes to human chromosomes 11 and 12. *Nature* 1984;310:784–6.

319. Hoppener JWM, de Pagter-Holthuizen P, Geurts van Kessel AHM, et al. The human gene encoding insulin-like growth factor 1 is located on chromosome 12. *Hum Genet* 1985;69:157–60.

320. Ullrich A, Berman CH, Dull TJ, et al. Isolation of the human insulin-like growth factor-1 gene using a single synthetic DNA probe. *EMBO J* 1984;3:361–4.

321. Bell GI, Gerhard DS, Fong NM, et al. Isolation of the human insulin-like growth factor genes: insulin-like growth factor-2 and insulin genes are contiguous. *Proc Natl Acad Sci USA* 1985;82:6450–4.

322. Rotwein P, Pollock KM, Didler KM, et al. Organization and sequence of the human insulin-like growth factor-1 gene. *J Biol Chem* 1986;261:4828–32.

323. Marquardt H, Todaro GJ. Purification and primary structure of a polypeptide with multiplication-stimulating activity from rat liver cell cultures: homology with human insulin-like growth factor-2. *J Biol Chem* 1981;256:6859–65.

324. de Pagter-Holthuizen P, Hoppener JWM, Jansen M, et al. Chromosomal localization and preliminary characterization of the human gene encoding insulin-like growth factor-2. *Human Genet* 1985;69:170–3.

325. de Pagter-Holthuizen P, van Schalk FMA, Verduijn GM, et al. Organization of the human genes for insulin-like growth factors 1 and 2. *FEBS Lett* 1986;195:179–84.

326. de Pagter-Holthuizen P, Jansen M, van Schalk FMA, et al. The human insulin-like growth factor-2 gene contains two development-specific promoters. *FEBS Lett* 1987;214:259–64.

327. Uthne K, Uthne T. Influence of liver resection and regeneration on somatomedin (sulphation factor): activity in sera from nor-

mal and hypophysectomized rats. *Acta Endocrinol (Copenh)* 1972;71:255–64.

328. Schimpff RM, Donnadieu M, Glasinovic JC, et al. The liver as a source of somatomedin: an in vivo study in the dog. *Acta Endocrinol (Copenh)* 1976;83:365–72.

329. D'Ercole AJ, Stiles AD, Underwood LE. Tissue concentrations of somatomedin C: further evidence for multiple sites of synthesis and paracrine or autocrine mechanisms of action. *Proc Natl Acad Sci USA* 1984;81:935–9.

330. Nilsson A, Isgaard J, Lindahl A, et al. Regulation by growth hormone of number of chondrocytes containing IGF-1 in rat growth plate. *Science* 1986;233:571–4.

331. Stracke H, Schulz A, Moeller D, et al. Effect of growth hormone on osteoblasts and demonstration of somatomedin C/IGF-1 in bone organ culture. *Acta Endocrinol (Copenh)* 1984;107:16–24.

332. Trippel SB, Corvol MT, Dumontier MF, et al. Effect of somatomedin-C/insulin-like growth factor-1 and growth hormone on cultured growth plate and articular chondrocytes. *Pediatr Res* 1989;25:76–82.

333. Bala RM, Lopatka J, Leung A, et al. Serum immunoreactive somatomedin levels in normal adults, pregnant women at term, children at various ages, and children with constitutionally delayed growth. *J Clin Endocrinol Metab* 1981;52:508–12.

334. van Wyk JJ. The different roles of IGF-1 and IGF-2 in growth and differentiation. In: Imura K, ed. *Progress in Endocrinology 1988.* Amsterdam: Elsevier, 1988;947–55.

335. Clemmons DR, van Wyk JJ. Somatomedin C and platelet-derived growth factor stimulate human fibroblast replication. *J Cell Physiol* 1981;106:361–7.

336. van Wyk JJ. The somatomedins: biological actions and physiological control mechanisms. In: Li CH, ed. *Hormonal proteins and peptides.* New York: Academic Press, 1984;81–125.

337. Ewton DZ, Florini JR. Effects of the somatomedins and insulin on myoblast differentiation in vitro. *Dev Biol* 1981;86:31–9.

338. Schmid C, Steiner T, Froesch ER. Insulin-like growth factor-1 supports differentiation of cultured osteoblast-like cells. *FEBS Lett* 1984;173:48–51.

339. McQuillan DJ, Handley CJ, Campbell MA, et al. Stimulation of proteoglycan biosynthesis by serum and insulin-like growth factor-1 in cultured bovine articular cartilage. *Biochem J* 1986;240:423–30.

340. Luyten FP, Hascall VC, Nissley SP, et al. Insulin-like growth factors maintain steady state metabolism of proteoglycans in bovine articular cartilage explants. *Arch Biochem Biophys* 1988;267:416–25.

341. Hintz RL, Liu F. Demonstration of specific plasma protein binding sites for somatomedin. *J Clin Endocrinol Metab* 1977; 45:988–95.

342. Kaufmann U, Zapf J, Torretti B, et al. Demonstration of a specific serum carrier protein of nonsuppressible insulin-like activity in vivo. *J Clin Endocrinol Metab* 1977;44:160–6.

343. Kaufmann U, Zapf J, Froesch ER. Growth hormone dependence of non-suppressible insulin-like activity (NSILA) and of NSILA-carrier protein in rats. *Acta Endocrinol (Copenh)* 1978;87:716–27.

344. Ooi GT, Herington AC. The biological and structural characterization of specific serum binding proteins for the insulin-like growth factors. *J Endocrinol* 1988;118:7–18.

345. Trippel SB, van Wyk JJ, Foster MB, et al. Characterization of a specific somatomedin-C receptor on isolated bovine growth plate chondrocytes. *Endocrinology* 1983;112:2128–36.

346. Trippel SB, van Wyk JJ, Mankin HJ. Localization of somatomedin C binding to bovine growth plate chondrocytes in situ. *J Bone Joint Surg* 1986;68A:897–903.

347. Ullrich A, Gray A, Tam AW, et al. Insulin-like growth factor-1 receptor primary structure: comparison with insulin receptor suggests structural determinants that define functional specificity. *EMBO J* 1986;5:2503–12.

348. Morgan DO, Edman JC, Standring DN, et al. Insulin-like growth factor-2 receptor as a multifunctional binding protein. *Nature* 1987;329:301–7.

349. MacDonald RG, Pfeffer SR, Coussens L, et al. A single receptor binds both insulin-like growth factor-2 and mannose-6-phosphate. *Science* 1988;239:1134–7.

350. Rosenfeld RG. Insulin-like growth factor receptors: binding and function. In: Imura K, ed. *Progress in endocrinology 1988.* Amsterdam: Elsevier, 1988;957–63.

351. Trippel SB, Chernausek SD, van Wyk JJ, et al. Demonstration of type I and type II somatomedin receptors on bovine growth plate chondrocytes. *J Orthop Res* 1988;6:817–26.

352. Skottner A, Clark RG, Robinson ICAF, et al. Recombinant human insulin-like growth factor: testing the somatomedin hypothesis in hypophysectomized rats. *J Endocrinol* 1987;112:123–32.

353. Isaksson OGP, Jansson J-O, Gause IAM. Growth hormone stimulates longitudinal bone growth directly. *Science* 1982;216:1237–9.

354. Russell SM, Spencer EM. Local injections of human or rat growth hormone or of purified human somatomedin C stimulate unilateral tibial epiphyseal growth in hypophysectomized rats. *Endocrinology* 1985;116:2563–7.

355. Schlechter NL, Russell SM, Spencer EM, et al. Evidence suggesting that the direct growth-promoting effect of growth hormone on cartilage in vivo is mediated by local production of somatomedin. *Proc Natl Acad Sci USA* 1986;83:7932–4.

356. Murphy WJ, Bell GI, Friesen HG. Tissue distribution of insulin-like growth factor 1 and 2 messenger ribonucleic acid in the adult rat. *Endocrinology* 1987;120:1279–82.

357. Han VKM, D'Ercole AJ, Lund PK. Cellular localization of somatomedin (insulin-like growth factor) messenger RNA in the human fetus. *Science* 1987;236:193–7.

358. Wroblewski J, Engstrom M, Skottner A, et al. Subcellular location of IGF-1 in chondrocytes from rat rib growth plate. *Acta Endocrinol (Copenh)* 1987;115:37–43.

359. DeLuca HF, Schnoes HK. Vitamin D: recent advances. *Ann Rev Biochem* 1983;52:411–39.

360. Bell NH. Vitamin D-endocrine system. *J Clin Invest* 1985; 76:1–6.

361. DeLuca HF. The metabolism and functions of vitamin D. In: Norman AW, Schaefer K, Grigoleit H-G, Herrath DV, eds. *Vitamin D: chemical, biochemical and clinical update.* New York: Walter de Gruyter, 1985;361–75.

362. DeLuca HF. The vitamin D story: a collaborative effort of basic science and clinical medicine. *FASEB J* 1988;2:224–36.

363. Bhalla AK, Amento EP, Krane SM. Differential effects of 1,25-dihydroxyvitamin D_3 on human lymphocytes and monocyte/macrophages: inhibition of interleukin-2 and augmentation of interleukin-1 production. *Cell Immunol* 1986;98:311–22.

364. Plachot JJ, Bailly Du Bois M, Halpern S, et al. In vitro action of 1,25-dihydroxycholecalciferol and 24,25-dihydroxycholecalciferol on matrix organization and mineral distribution in rabbit growth plate. *Metab Bone Dis Relat Res* 1982;4:135–42.

365. Schwartz Z, Knight G, Swain LD, et al. Localization of vitamin D_3-responsive alkaline phosphatase in cultured chondrocytes. *J Biol Chem* 1988;263:6023–6.

366. Boyan BD, Schwartz Z, Carnes DL, et al. The effects of vitamin D metabolites on the plasma and matrix vesicle membranes of growth and resting cartilage cells in vitro. *Endocrinology* 1988;122:2851–60.

367. Schwartz Z, Schlader DL, Swain LD, et al. Direct effects of 1,25-dihydroxyvitamin D_3 and 24,25-dihydroxyvitamin D_3 on growth zone and resting zone chondrocyte membrane alkaline phosphatase and phospholipase-A_2 specific activities. *Endocrinology* 1988;123:2878–84.

368. Schwartz Z, Boyan BD. The effects of vitamin D metabolites on phospholipase A_2 activity of growth zone and resting zone cartilage cells in vitro. *Endocrinology* 1988;122:2191–8.

369. Boyan BD, Schwartz Z, Swain LD, et al. Differential expression of phenotype by resting zone and growth region costochondral chondrocytes in vitro. *Bone* 1988;9:185–94.

370. Ornoy A, Goodwin D, Noff D, et al. 24,25-Dihydroxyvitamin D is a metabolite of vitamin D essential for bone formation. *Nature* 1978;276:517–9.

371. Atkin I, Pita JC, Ornoy A, et al. Effects of vitamin D metabolites on healing of low phosphate, vitamin D deficient induced rickets in rats. *Bone* 1985;6:113–23.

372. Fine N, Binderman I, Somjen D, et al. Autoradiographic localization of 24R,25-dihydroxyvitamin D_3 in epiphyseal cartilage. *Bone* 1985;6:99–104.

373. Tam CS, Heersche JNM, Jones G, et al. The effect of vitamin D on bone in vivo. *Endocrinology* 1986;118:2217–24.

374. Parfitt AM, Mathews CHE, Brommage R, et al. Calcitriol but no other metabolite of vitamin D is essential for normal bone growth and development in the rat. *J Clin Invest* 1984;73:576–86.

375. Hinek A, Poole AR. The influence of vitamin D metabolites on the calcification of cartilage matrix and the C-propeptide of type II collagen (chondrocalcin). *J Bone Miner Res* 1988;3:421–9.

376. Harrison JE, Hitchman JW, Jones G, et al. Plasma vitamin D metabolite levels in phosphorous deficient rats during the development of vitamin D deficient rickets. *Metabolism* 1982; 31:1121–7.

377. Underwood JL, DeLuca HF. Vitamin D in not directly necessary for bone growth and mineralization. *Am J Physiol* 1984;246(Endocrinol Metab 9):E493–8.

378. Weinstein RS, Underwood JL, Hutson MS, et al. Bone histomorphometry in vitamin D–deficient rats infused with calcium and phosphorous. *Am J Physiol* 1984;246(Endocrinol Metab 9):E499–505.

379. Brommage R, Jarnagin K, DeLuca HF, et al. 1- but not 24-hydroxylation of vitamin D is required for skeletal mineralization in rats. *Am J Physiol* 1983;244(Endocrinol Metab 7):E298–304.

380. Lund B, Charles P, Egsmose C, et al. Changes in vitamin D metabolites and bone histology in rats during recovery from rickets. *Calcif Tissue Int* 1985;37:478–83.

381. Boskey AL, DiCarlo EF, Gilder H, et al. The effect of short-term treatment with vitamin D metabolites on bone lipid and mineral composition in healing vitamin D–deficient rats. *Bone* 1988;9:309–18.

382. Miller SC, Halloran BP, DeLuca HF, et al. Studies on the role of vitamin D in early skeletal development, mineralization, and growth in rats. *Calcif Tissue Int* 1983;35:455–60.

383. Silver J, Russell J, Sherwood LM. Regulation by vitamin D metabolites of messenger ribonucleic acid for preproparathyroid hormone in isolated bovine parathyroid cells. *Proc Natl Acad Sci USA* 1985;82:4270–3.

384. Okazaki T, Igarashi T, Kronenberg HM. 5'-Flanking region of the parathyroid hormone gene mediates negative regulation by 1,25-(OH)$_2$ vitamin D$_3$. *J Biol Chem* 1988;263:2203–8.

385. Reeve J, Zanelli JM. Parathyroid hormone and bone. *Clin Sci* 1986;71:231–8.

386. Cantley LK, Russell JB, Lettieri DS, et al. Effects of vitamin D$_3$, 25-hydroxyvitamin D$_3$, and 24,25-dihydroxyvitamin D$_3$ on parathyroid hormone secretion. *Calcif Tissue Int* 1987;41:48–51.

387. Bushinsky DA, Riera GS, Favus MJ, et al. Evidence that blood ionized calcium can regulate serum 1,25(OH)$_2$D$_3$ independently of parathyroid hormone and phosphorous in the rat. *J Clin Invest* 1985;76:1599–604.

388. Silver J, Naveh-Many T, Mayer H, et al. Regulation by vitamin D metabolites of parathyroid hormone gene transcription in vivo in the rat. *J Clin Invest* 1986;78:1296–301.

389. Rouleau MF, Warshawsky H, Goltzman D. Parathyroid hormone binding in vivo to renal, hepatic, and skeletal tissues of the rat using a radioautographic approach. *Endocrinology* 1986; 118:919–31.

390. Barling PM, Bibby NJ. Study of the localization of H^3-bovine parathyroid hormone in bone by light microscope autoradiography. *Calcif Tissue Int* 1985;37:441–6.

391. Dunham J, Chayen J. An effect of parathyroid hormone on the epiphyseal plate and osteoblasts: studies towards a cytochemical bioassay. *J Immunoassay* 1983;4:329–38.

392. Burger EH, Gaillard PJ. Structural and ultrastructural responses of calcifying cartilage to parathyroid hormone in vitro. *Calcif Tissue Res* 1976;21:75–80.

393. Burch WM, Lebovitz HE. Parathyroid hormone stimulates growth of embryonic chick pelvic cartilage in vitro. *Calcif Tissue Int* 1983;35:526–32.

394. Roberts AB, Flanders KC, Kondaiah P, et al. Transforming growth factor-β: biochemistry and roles in embryogenesis, tissue repair, remodelling, and carcinogenesis. *Recent Prog Horm Res* 1988;44:157–97.

395. Rosen DM, Stempien SA, Thompson AY, et al. Transforming growth factor-β modulates the expression of osteoblast and chondroblast phenotypes in vitro. *J Cell Physiol* 1988;134:337–46.

396. Seyedin SM, Thomas TC, Thompson AC, et al. Purification and characterization of two cartilage-inducing factors from bovine demineralized bone. *Proc Natl Acad Sci USA* 1984;82:2267–71.

397. Seyedin SM, Thompson AY, Bentz H, et al. Cartilage-inducing factor A: apparent identity to transforming growth factor-β. *J Biol Chem* 1985;261:5693–5.

398. O'Keefe RJ, Puzas JE, Brand JS, et al. Effects of transforming growth factor-β on matrix synthesis by chick growth plate chondrocytes. *Endocrinology* 1988;122:2953–61.

399. O'Keefe RJ, Puzas JE, Brand JS, et al. Effect of transforming growth factor-β on DNA synthesis by growth plate chondrocytes: modulation by factors present in serum. *Calcif Tissue Int* 1988;43:352–8.

400. Bortell R, Barone L, Tassinari M, et al. Coupling of transforming growth factor-β and type I collagen gene expression during endochondral bone formation. *J Bone Miner Res* 1989;4(suppl 1):S245.

401. Ellingsworth LR, Brennan JE, Fok K, et al. Antibodies to the N-terminal portion of cartilage-inducing factor A and transforming growth factor-β. *J Biol Chem* 1986;261:12365–7.

402. Heine UI, Munoz EF, Flanders KC, et al. Role of transforming growth factor-β in the development of the mouse embryo. *J Cell Biol* 1987;105:2861–76.

403. Bonewald L, Schwartz Z, Swain L, et al. More TGF-β responsive alkaline phosphatase is localized to matrix vesicles than plasma membranes in ROS 17/2.8 osteosarcoma cells. *J Bone Miner Res* 1989;4(suppl 1):S154.

404. Rosier RN, Gelb D, Landesberg RL, et al. Transforming growth factor beta synthesis in endochondral ossification. *J Bone Miner Res* 1989;4(suppl 1):S325.

405. Jingushi S, Joyce M, Roberts A, et al. Distribution of acidic fibroblast growth factor, basic fibroblast growth factor, and transforming growth factor β-1 in rat growth plate. *J Bone Miner Res* 1989;4(suppl 1):S325.

406. Noda M, Vogel R. Transcriptional regulation of transforming growth factor-β gene expression in osteoblast-like cells by fibroblast growth factor. *J Bone Miner Res* 1989;4(suppl 1):S326.

407. Sporn MB, Roberts AB. Peptide growth factors are multifunctional. *Nature* 1988;332:217–9.

408. Centrella M, McCarthy TL, Canalis E. Skeletal tissue and transforming growth factor-β. *FASEB J* 1988;2:3066–73.

409. Canalis E, McCarthy T, Centrella M. Growth factors and the regulation of bone remodelling. *J Clin Invest* 1988;81:277–81.

410. Ausprunk D, Folkman J. Migration and proliferation of endothelial cells in preformed and newly formed blood vessels during tumor angiogenesis. *Microvasc Res* 1977;14:53–65.

411. Gross J, Moscatelli D, Rifkin DB. Increased capillary endothelial cell protease activity in response to angiogenic stimuli in vitro. *Proc Natl Acad Sci USA* 1983;80:2623–7.

412. D'Amore P, Thompson RW. Mechanisms of angiogenesis. *Annu Rev Physiol* 1987;49:453–64.

413. Folkman J. Tumor angiogenesis. *Adv Cancer Res* 1985;43:175–203.

414. Joseph-Silverstein J, Rifkin D. Endothelial cell growth factors and the vessel wall. *Semin Thromb Hemost* 1987;13:504–13.

415. Gospodarowicz D, Bialecki H, Greenburg G. Purification of the fibroblast growth factor activity from bovine brain. *J Biol Chem* 1978;253:3736–43.

416. Maciag T, Cerundolo I, Kelley P, et al. An endothelial cell growth factor from bovine hypothalamus: identification and partial characterization. *Proc Natl Acad Sci USA* 1979;76:5674–8.

417. Shing Y, Folkman J, Sullivan R, et al. Heparin affinity: purification of a tumor-derived capillary endothelial cell growth factor. *Science* 1984;223:1296–9.

418. Hauschka P, Mavrakos A, Iafrati M, et al. Growth factors in bone matrix: isolation of multiple types by affinity chromatography on heparin Sepharose. *J Biol Chem* 1986;261:12665–74.

419. Howell DS, Dean DD, Muniz OE, et al. Hypertrophic cell zone growth cartilage contains heparin-binding growth factors. *Trans Orthop Res Soc* 1989;14:525.

420. Gospodarowicz D, Neufeld G, Schweigerer L. Molecular and biological characterization of fibroblast growth factor, an angiogenic factor which also controls the proliferation and differentiation of

mesoderm and neuroectoderm derived cells. *Cell Differ* 1986;19:1–17.

421. Schweigerer L. Basic fibroblast growth factor and its relation to angiogenesis in normal and neoplastic tissue. *Klin Wochenschr* 1988;66:340–5.

422. Thomas KA. Fibroblast growth factors. *FASEB J* 1987;1:434–40.

423. Hockel M, Sasse J, Wissler JH. Purified monocyte-derived angiogenic substance (angiotropin) stimulates migration, phenotypic changes, and "tube formation" but not proliferation of capillary endothelial cells in vitro. *J Cell Physiol* 1987;133:1–13.

424. Koch AE, Cho M, Burrows, et al. Inhibition of production of macrophage-derived angiogenic activity by the anti-rheumatic agents gold sodium thiomalate and auranofin. *Biochem Biophys Res Commun* 1988;154:205–12.

425. Brown RA, Taylor C, McLaughlin B, et al. Epiphyseal growth plate cartilage and chondrocytes in mineralising cultures produce a low molecular mass angiogenic procollagenase activator. *Bone Miner* 1987;3:143–58.

426. Weiss JB, Hill CR, McLaughlin B, et al. Potentiating effect of heparin in the activation of procollagenase by a low-M_r angiogenesis factor. *FEBS Lett* 1983;163:62–5.

427. Brown RA, Tomlinson IW, Hill CR, et al. Relationship of angiogenesis factor to various joint diseases. *Ann Rheum Dis* 1983;42:301–7.

428. Jingushi S, Joyce ME, Flanders KC, et al. Distribution of acidic fibroblast growth, basic fibroblast growth factor, and transforming growth factor 1 in rat growth plate. In: Cohn DV, Glorieux FH, Martin TJ, eds. *Calcium Regulation Bone Metabolism.* Amsterdam: Excerpta Medica, 1990, pp. 298–303.

Disorders of Bone and Mineral Metabolism,
edited by Fredric L. Coe and Murray J. Favus,
© 1992 by Raven Press, Ltd. All rights reserved.

CHAPTER 15

Bone Remodeling

David W. Dempster

Bone remodeling is clearly an important aspect of skeletal biology in large animals. Much of the cellular activity in bone—at least that of the osteoclasts and osteoblasts, and possibly also of the osteocytes—is directed toward this process. The purpose of this chapter is to outline how remodeling is achieved, why it occurs in the first place, and how remodeling activity varies as a function of age, sex, skeletal site, and species. This text focuses on remodeling as it pertains to the healthy, adult animal. Changes in remodeling activity in specific disease states are dealt with elsewhere in the volume.

DEFINITION OF REMODELING AND HISTORICAL PERSPECTIVE

The general term *bone remodeling* has been used ambiguously to describe various aspects of bone behavior. Some writers (e.g., Refs. 1 and 2) use the phrase *adaptive remodeling* to characterize a reactive response of bone to an external stimulus. These adaptive responses occur both on the surface of bones, in which case they are referred to as *external remodeling* and usually result in a change in the shape or size of a bone, and within the bone, where they are referred to as *internal remodeling.* Others (e.g., Refs. 3 and 4) employ the term *external remodeling* to describe the process that maintains the characteristic shape of each bone throughout the growth phase. Frost (5), on the other hand, defines remodeling, without an adjective, as the continuous process whereby old, lamellar bone matrix is replaced by new, with little or no net change in the mass or shape of the bones. It is this process, which occurs primarily in humans and other large animals, that is the focus of the present review.

D. W. Dempster: College of Physicians and Surgeons, Columbia University, New York, New York 10032; Regional Bone Center, Helen Hayes Hospital, West Haverstraw, New York 10993

The historical aspects of bone remodeling are nicely covered in Martin and Burr's book (6); the highlights of this fascinating story are as follows. The study of remodeling began with the morphological observations of Antonie van Leeuwenhoek (7,8) and Clopton Havers (9), both of whom described the presence of a network of canals (including Haversian canals) in cortical bone. The Haversian system, or secondary osteon, was named after Havers, but ironically, he probably never observed one himself. The first vague description of this structure was provided by van Leeuwenhoek in 1693 (8), but it took another 150 years before Haversian systems, cement lines, and interstitial bone were properly characterized (10) (Fig. 1). The notion that bone is remodeled continuously throughout life was first perceived about 200 years ago; Alexander Monro, a Scottish pathologist whose work on bone was published posthumously in 1776 (11), clearly understood this when he wrote the following prescient passages, quoted from Martin and Burr (6):

> There is a perpetual waste and renewal of the particles which compose the solid fibres of bone; addition from the fluids exceeding the waste during the growth of the bones; the renewal and waste keeping pretty near par in adult middle age; and the waste exceeding the supply from the liquors in old age; as is demonstrable from their weight . . . the bones of old people are thinner and firmer in their sides, and have larger cavities than those of young persons.

The microanatomic basis of cortical bone remodeling was established in the first half of the nineteenth century. In 1816, Howship (12) recognized that interstitial bone could be "absorbed," resulting in an increase in the diameter of the Haversian canals. He also realized that the bone surface surrounding these enlarged canals was crenated (Howship's lacunae). However, Howship apparently considered bone removal in this manner to be a pathological process (6). Forty years later, Tomes and DeMorgan (13) appreciated that this was a physiological occurrence and they further proposed that the creation

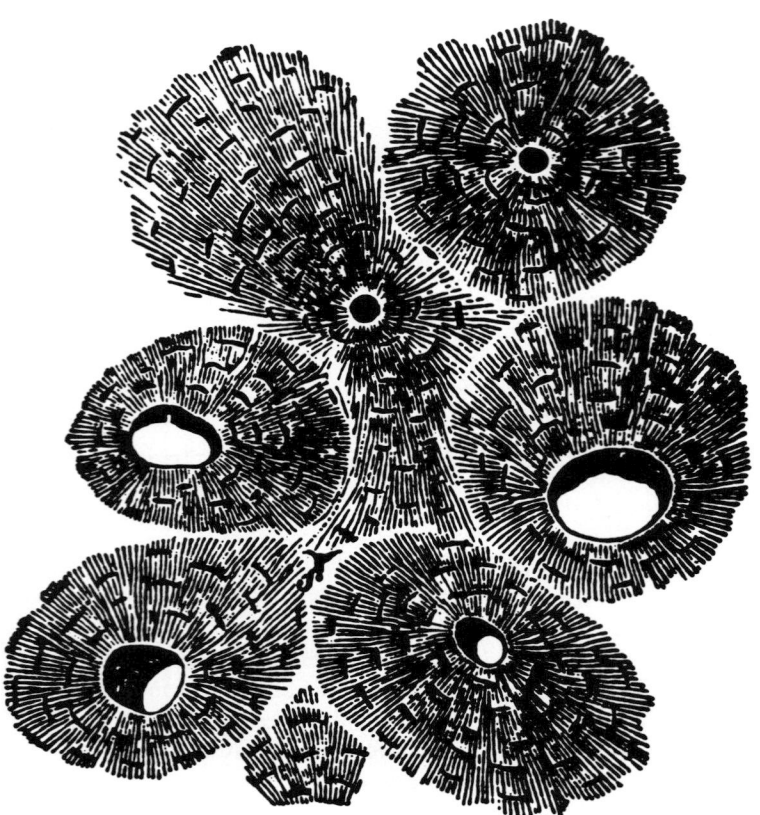

FIG. 1. Todd and Bowman's depiction of secondary osteons published in 1845. (Reproduced with permission from Ref. 6.)

of resorption spaces preceded the formation of new osteons, thus establishing themselves as the fathers of bone remodeling theory (4). They knew that Haversian systems replaced older bone, that interstitial bone was the remainder of old Haversian systems, and that remodeling activity was influenced by age and various diseases. Thereafter, important contributions on the mechanism and function of remodeling were made by von Ebner (14) and Amprino and Bairati (15–17). In the mid-1930s there was considerable debate but no consensus as to what constituted the functional unit of bone (6,18,19). Frost (20,21) resurrected this concept in the early 1960s, identifying the osteon as the functional unit and building on the observations of those above and his own extensive studies of undecalcified bone sections, he developed the current "quantum theory" of bone remodeling which holds that bone matrix is sequentially removed and replaced in discrete osteonal units or "packets," with destruction and formation being linked not only spatially, but also temporally.

CELLULAR MECHANISM OF BONE REMODELING

Bone remodeling is achieved by the concerted action of groups of bone cells, termed either *basic multicellular units* (BMUs) (5) or *bone remodeling units* (BRUs) (22); the latter term will be used here. Although the three-dimensional geometry of the completed osteons differs between cortical and cancellous bone (Fig. 2), the BRUs in each of these two skeletal compartments behave in a fundamentally similar fashion. The work done by each BRU is divided into four distinct phases: activation, resorption, reversal, formation (5,19,23) (Figs. 3 and 4).

Activation

The term *activation* is used to describe the initiating event that converts a resting bone surface into a remodeling surface. In the normal adult skeleton, a new BRU is activated about once every 10 s (22). Activation involves recruitment of mononucleated osteoclast precursors of hemopoietic origin, penetration of the bone lining cells, and fusion of the precursor cells to form functional osteoclasts in contact with mineralized bone matrix. These events have been demonstrated elegantly by Tran Van and his colleagues in studies of the bone remodeling sequence associated with tooth egression in the rat (24,25). The fact that the receptors for most, if not all, humoral agents act to stimulate bone remodeling reside in osteoblasts rather than osteoclasts led to speculation that bone lining cells, which are derived from osteoblasts, may play

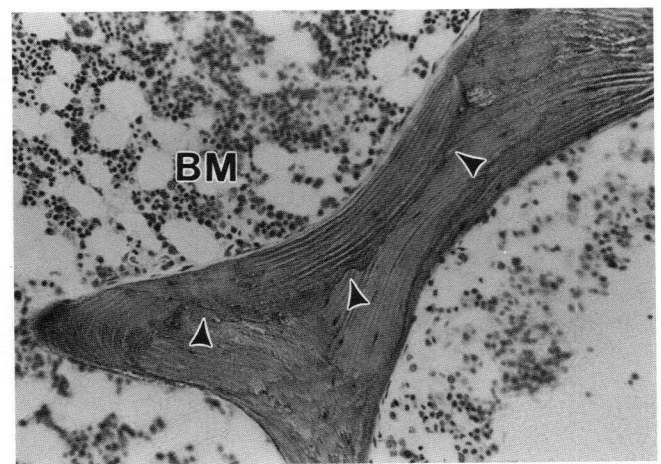

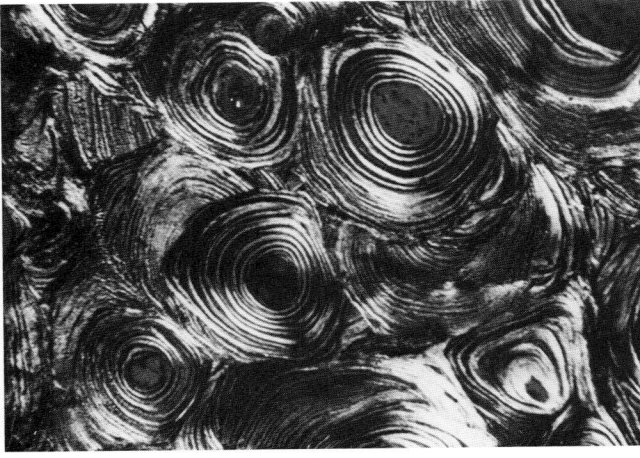

FIG. 2. Photomicrographs of basic structural units in human cancellous (**A**) and cortical bone (**B**). In cancellous bone, the packet is roughly saucer-shaped and extends from the scalloped reversal line (*arrowheads*) to the trabecular surface apposed to bone marrow (BM). Note the lamellar structure of the packet. Parts of other packets are visible on the opposite side and end of this trabecular plate. In the cortical bone sample, the cylindrical Haversian systems are seen in cross section. They are composed of concentric lamellae surrounding the central Haversian canal. Remnants of older Haversian systems that have been partially replaced are clearly visible.

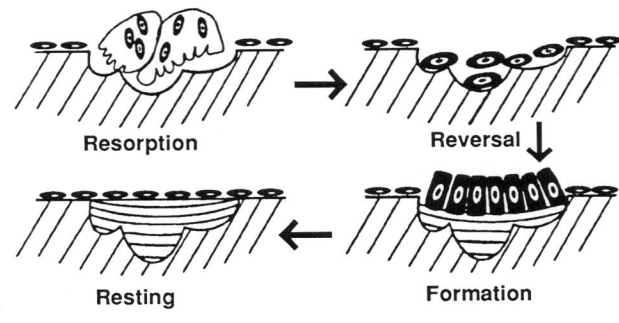

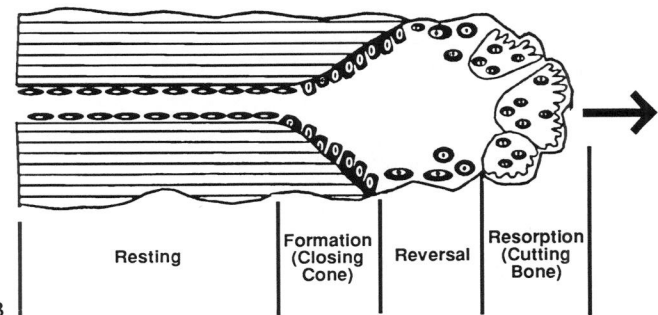

FIG. 3. Principal phases of the adult bone remodeling cycle in cancellous (**A**) and cortical (**B**) bone. Details of the activity and duration of each phase are given in the text. See also Figs. 4 to 7. (Modified from Ref. 23.)

an important role in activation (26). There is growing evidence to support this view. Parathyroid hormone, for example, induces shrinkage of the lining cells, opening up gaps in the lining cell layer that would allow its penetration by osteoclasts precursors (27–29). In addition, osteoblasts are stimulated by bone resorbing factors to digest the thin layer of unmineralized matrix that lines all free bone surfaces and is resistant to osteoclastic resorption (30–35). This could serve the dual function of allowing osteoclasts access to mineralized bone matrix and, at the same time, releasing factors from the matrix, such as bone Gla protein (osteocalcin), which are chemotactic for osteoclasts or their precursors (36–39).

The factors that determine why a particular bit of bone is "chosen" for remodeling are not clear. Remodeling can be classified as either random, redundant, or selective, with the former being the most common type of activity in humans (6,40). Johnson (41) noted the presence of isolated Howship's lacunae at intervals along the Haversian canal walls and proposed that they represented the activity of "test" osteoclasts probing for suitable sites to initiate remodeling. Only in the case of selective remodeling does one need to invoke the concept of a local signal from bone that stimulates activation. There are a number of obvious candidates for such a signal. A change in the mechanical properties of aging bone could influence bone cell behavior either directly (42,43) or indirectly, via localized changes in stress-generated electrical potentials (streaming potentials) in the bone matrix (2,6,44,45). Deterioration of the bone matrix could also prompt the release of paracrine or autocrine factors from the bone cells, nearby immune cells, or the bone matrix itself (46). Each of these mechanical, electrical, or chemical signals has the potential to attract osteoclasts or their precursors into the region in need of remodeling. One of the most attractive of the current hypotheses, whose origins date back to the earlier part of the twentieth century (47,48), is that the osteocyte may be involved in activation (5,31,49,50). Despite the fact that the osteocyte is the most numerous of the bone cell types and that osteocyte death presages bone death, the func-

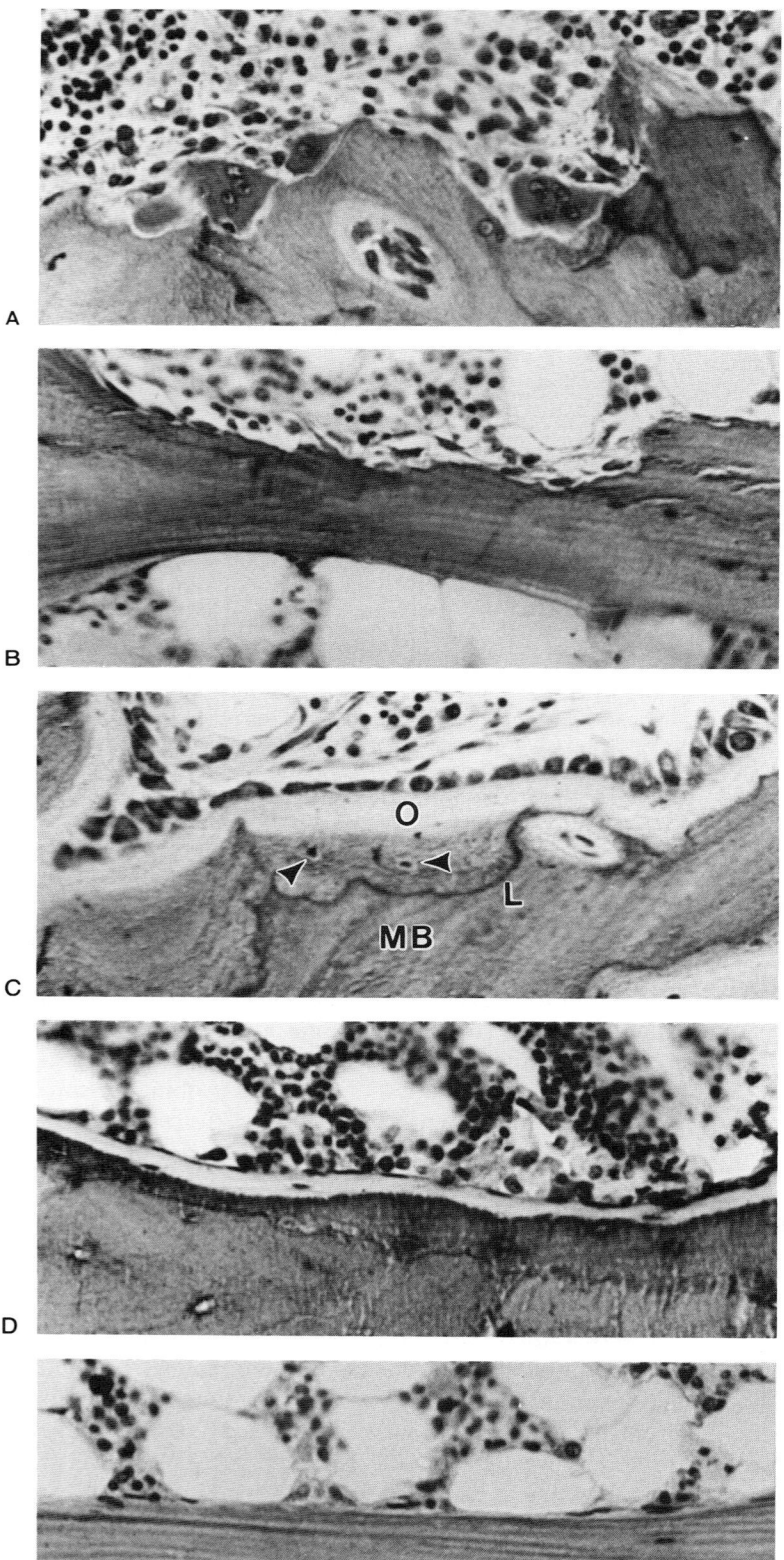

A

B

C

D

E

FIG. 4. Light micrographs of human iliac crest biopsies reconstructing the principal phases of the remodeling cycle in cancellous bone. **A:** *Resorption:* several multinucleated osteoclasts are seen in the process of excavating a Howship's lacuna. **B:** *Reversal:* the Howship's lacuna no longer contains osteoclasts but, instead, small mononucleated cells in contact with the scalloped surface. **C, D:** *Formation:* In C, a sheet of plump osteoblasts is seen depositing osteoid (O) on top of mineralized bone (MB). Note the reversal line (L) and osteocyte lacunae (*arrowheads*) in the mineralized matrix. D represents a later stage in formation in which the osteoblasts have been replaced by flattened lining cells. Matrix production has ceased but a thin layer of osteoid still remains to be mineralized. **E:** *Resting:* no remodeling activity in progress but note the layer of attenuated cells lining the surface.

tion of this cell is somewhat of an enigma. Osteocytes form a complex three-dimensional network in bone, communicating with each other and with the cells lining the bone surface. This places them in an ideal situation for sensing changes in stress and strain in, or damage to, the bone matrix and for communicating this to the bone lining cells, which, as described above, could prompt BRU activation. Interestingly, Lanyon and his team (50–52) have reported that mechanical loading, both in vivo and in vitro, increases tritiated uridine uptake and glucose 6-phosphate dehydrogenase activity in osteocytes.

Resorption

The newly formed squad of osteoclasts work in a concerted fashion, removing both the mineral and organic components of bone matrix and creating Howship's lacunae in cancellous bone and "cutting cones" in cortical bone (Figs. 4A and 5 to 7). In cancellous bone, the result of their labors is a roughly saucer-shaped cavity some 50 μm in depth toward its center. In cortical bone, the osteoclasts drill through the matrix in a direction that is approximately parallel with the long axis of the bone, creating a cylindrical tunnel about 2.5 mm long and 200 μm in diameter. Eriksen (53) performed a detailed histomorphometric analysis of this phase of the remodeling cycle in human iliac cancellous bone, allowing him to reconstruct the sequence of events at the resorptive sites. The data would suggest that although resorption is initiated by multinucleated osteoclasts, they are responsible for removing only the first one- to two-thirds of the bone, with the remainder being excavated by mononuclear

cells. The fate of the osteoclast once it has completed its task is unknown (54), but it is possible that at least some of the mononucleated, resorbing cells described by Eriksen (53) are derived from osteoclasts. Evidence for fission of osteoclasts in experimental animals has been obtained both in vivo (55,56) and in vitro (57), and fission of a human osteoclast in vitro has been observed in the author's laboratory (R. J. Murrills and D. W. Dempster, 1987, unpublished observations) (Fig. 8).

Reversal

The reversal phase lasts from 7 to 14 days and heralds the switchover from destruction to repair. The resorption bays are now devoid of osteoclasts and are, instead, occupied by a group of mononucleated cells which at the light microscope level are rather nondescript (Figs. 4B and 7). However, the transmission electron microscope has revealed the presence of at least three different cell types: osteocytes that have been liberated from the matrix, macrophage-like mononuclear cells, perhaps derived from the osteoclast, which apparently smooth off the resorbed surface and deposit the collagen-deficient, cement-like substance that will bind the new bone to the old, and farther out from the surface, preosteoblasts (58).

It is during the reversal phase that the all-important coupling of bone formation to bone resorption occurs. The mechanism by which osteoblasts are summoned into the reversal lacuna is uncertain, but it is probable that a paracrine factor or, more likely, a number of such factors produced in or around the remodeling site are involved. These "coupling factors" could be elaborated by cells involved in the activation of resorption (e.g., lin-

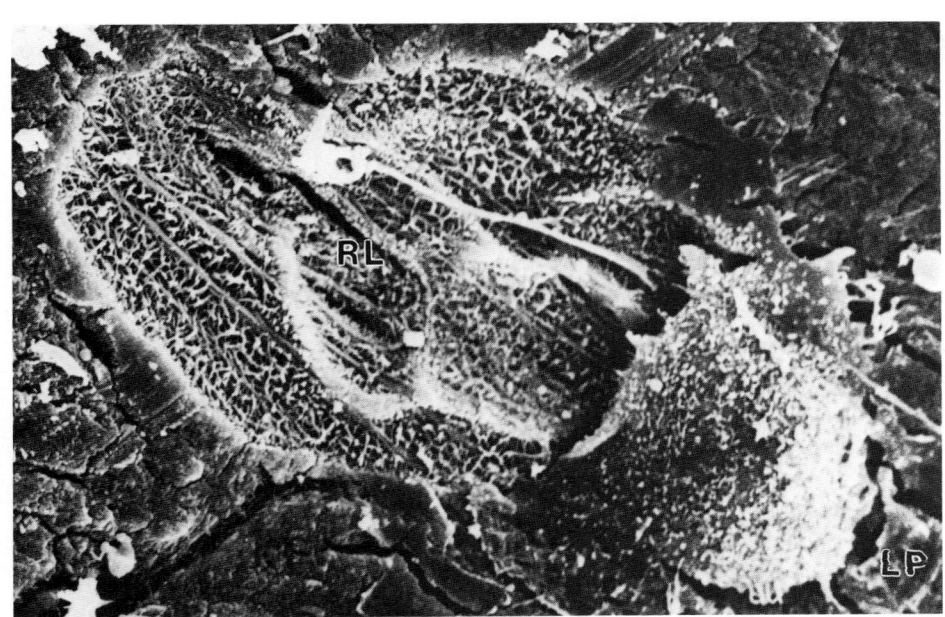

FIG. 5. Scanning electron micrograph of a human osteoclast following a 24-h incubation on a slice of cortical bone. The cell has created a characteristic resorption lacuna (RL) by removing both mineralized and organic components of the matrix. Note exposed collagen fibrils on the base of the lacuna and the osteoclast's lamellipodia (LP), which indicate that the cell was moving toward the bottom right of the field. (Reproduced from Ref. 217 with permission.)

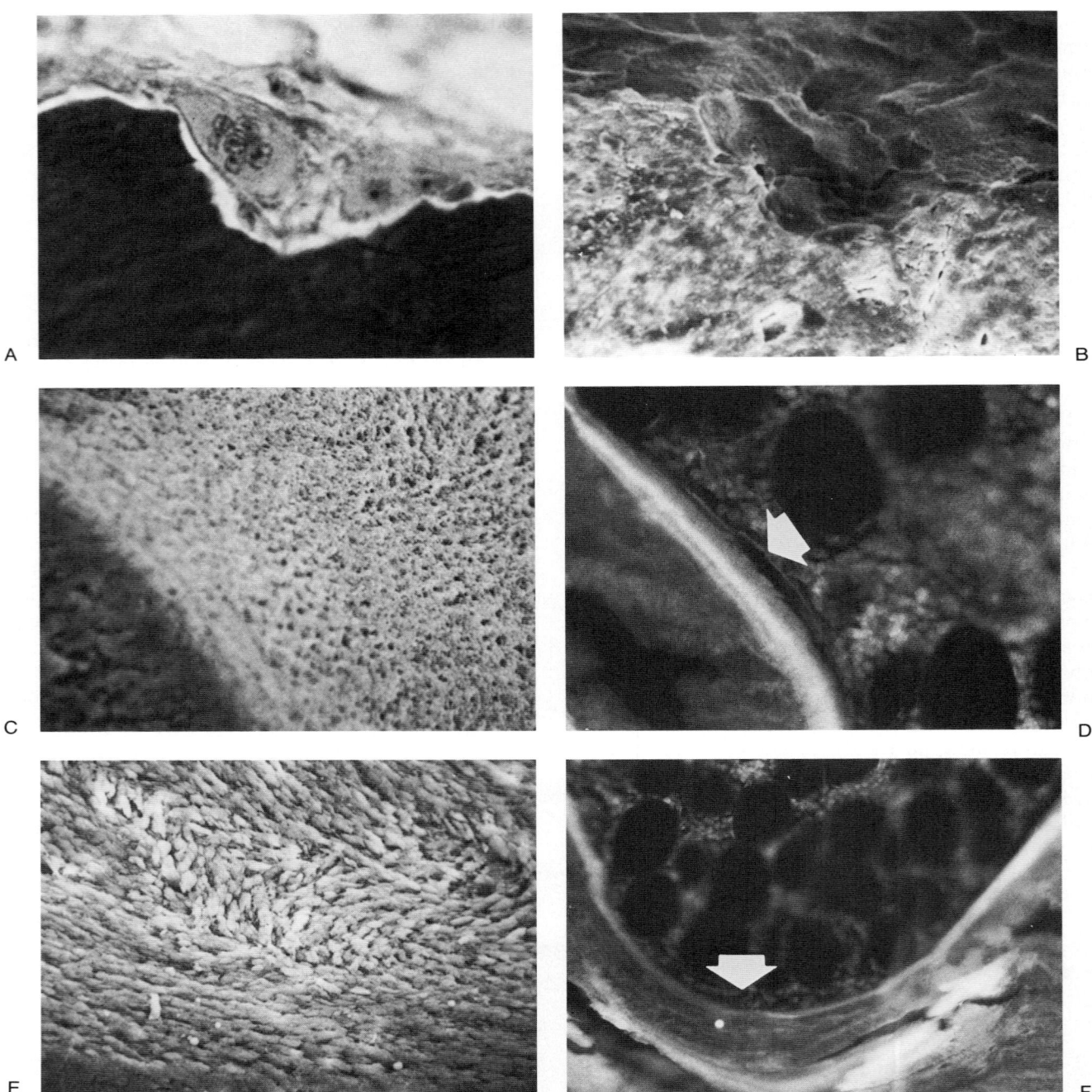

FIG. 6. Correlative light and scanning electron micrographs of the resorptive and formative phases of the remodeling cycle in human iliac bone. **A:** An osteoclast-containing Howship's lacuna in thin section. **B:** The same lacuna following removal of the cells to reveal the surface topography and extent of the resorbed bone. **C:** The mineralization front as seen in the scanning electron microscope. The surface is composed of countless, tiny mineral particles. Active mineralization is confirmed by the presence of double tetracycline labels (**D**, *arrow*). **E:** A later stage of mineralization consisting of rows of larger mineral nodules. In contrast to C, the orientation of the collagen fibers within which these nodules were embedded can now be clearly seen. There was no visible uptake of tetracycline at this site (**F**, *arrow*). (Reproduced from Ref. 218 with permission.)

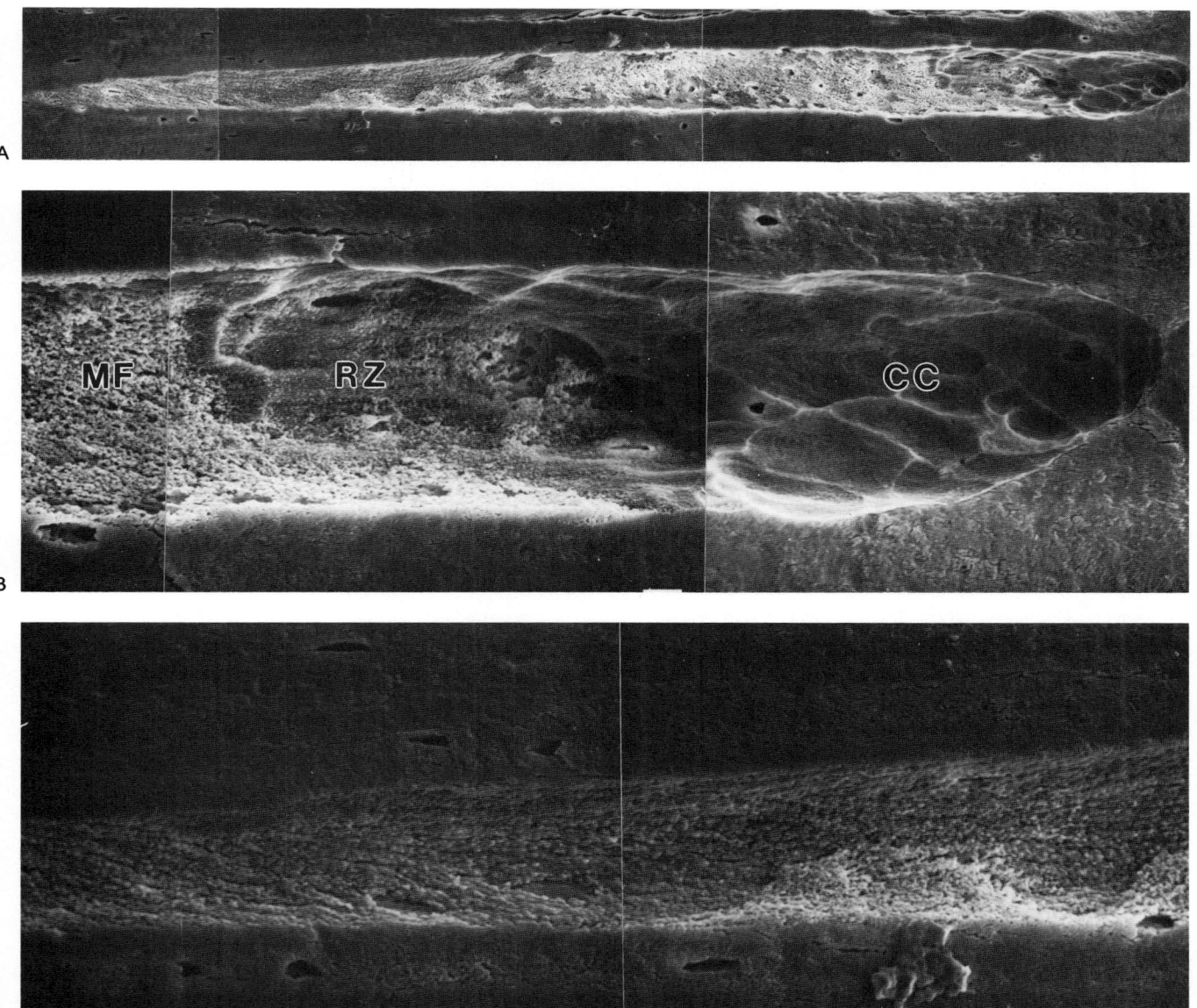

FIG. 7. A: Scanning electron micrograph of an evolving Haversian system in the cortex of a dog radius. The cells and organic component of the matrix have been removed by treatment with sodium hypochlorite. The system, which is 1.1 mm in length, was moving toward the right of this page. **B:** A higher power view of the leading edge showing the cutting cone (CC), the reversal zone (RZ), and the mineralization front (MF) in the closing cone. **C:** A higher power view of the tail end of the system. Bone formation is still in progress as indicated by the rows of mineral nodules, which in this anorganic preparation, represent partially calcified collagen fibers (218, 219). Bar = 10 μm (*B* and *C*). The bone sample was kindly supplied by G. V. B. Cochran and V. Palmieri. See Fig. 3B.

ing cells), or second, by the osteoclasts themselves or other cell types present in the resorption and reversal lacunae, or third, could be released from bone matrix during the resorption phase (46) (Fig. 9). There are a number of possible candidates for such coupling factors, several of which are intrinsic to bone and which are known to stimulate osteoblast replication and/or differentiation. Skeletal growth factor (SGF), which was the

first to be discovered and has been extensively studied by Baylink and colleagues, is an osteoblast mitogen present in demineralized bone matrix and presumably, therefore, an osteoblast product (59,60). A similar, perhaps identical osteoblast growth factor, is produced by resorbing chicken bones in organ culture (61). Resorption, stimulated by parathyroid hormone, is paralleled by release of this osteoblast-derived peptide, making it an at-

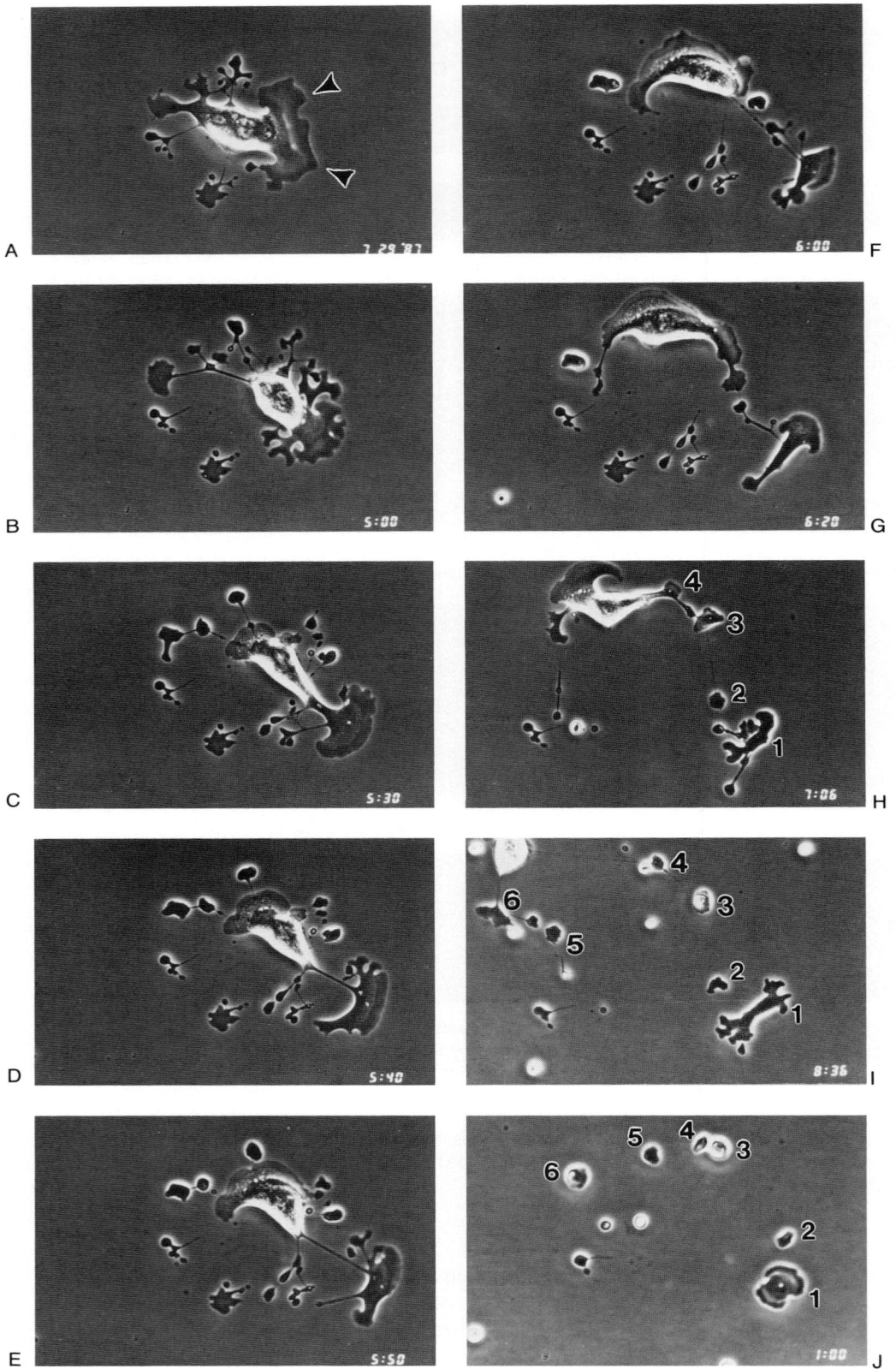

FIG. 8. Time-lapse sequence of a human osteoclast filmed on a plastic substrate. Frame **A** was taken at 4.30 P.M. and the time of subsequent shots is indicated in the lower right-hand corner. The cell was highly motile as indicated by the extended lamellipodia with phase-dense edges (*arrows*). In the 10 min between frames **C** and **D** the cell began to split into two parts, with complete separation occurring approximately 1 h and 20 min later in frame **H.** Here a large cell (#1) and a small cell (#2) ("post-osteoclasts"?) derived from the original osteoclast can be seen and the osteoclast is in the process of shedding two more cells (#3 and #4). In frame **H,** the main body of the original cell moved upward and to the left (frame **I**) and eventually wandered out of the field of view, leaving behind two more daughter cells (#5 and #6). Four and a half hours later (frame **J**) all of these cells derived from the original osteoclast were still alive and highly motile and they remained so for at least an additional 7.5 h. It should be noted that human calcitonin (1 ng/mL) was added to the preparation 5 min after frame **G** was taken. Whether the amount of cell fission that subsequently occurred is related to the presence of calcitonin is unknown, although clearly the cell had begun to split up prior to the calcitonin treatment. For details of how the cells were isolated and filmed, see Ref. 217.

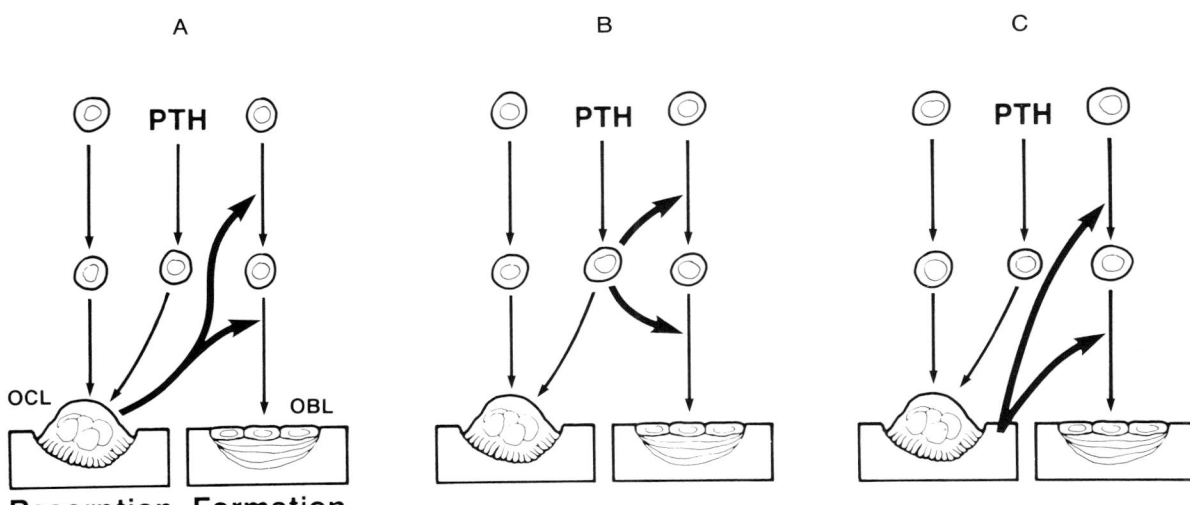

FIG. 9. Three possible mechanisms to explain the tight coupling of bone formation to resorption. Current evidence suggests that agents which stimulate bone resorption [e.g., parathyroid hormone (PTH), 1,25-dihydroxyvitamin D, interleukin-1] do not act directly on the osteoclast (OCL) itself but, rather, communicate with it through an intermediary cell [possibly the osteoblast (OBL) or bone lining cell], which in turn activates the osteoclast. This gives rise to three possible sources of the putative coupling factor, which summons osteoblast precursors into the Howship's lacuna: (**A**) the osteoclast itself, (**B**) the intermediary cell that transmits the activation signal to the osteoclast, and (**C**) the bone matrix that is being resorbed. It is possible that some one or more of these mechanisms is involved in coupling. (Reproduced with permission from Ref. 46.)

tractive candidate. SGF was originally described as a high-molecular-weight polypeptide (ca. 83,000), but more recent work has indicated the existence of lower-molecular-weight forms, one of which has recently been shown to be identical to insulin-like growth factor II (IGF-II) (62). Canalis and colleagues have isolated another growth factor from bone matrix and calvarial cultures. Originally referred to as bone-derived growth factor (BDGF), this has recently been identified as β_2-microglobulin, a polypeptide with a molecular weight of 11,800 (63). β_2-Microglobulin enhances both DNA and bone collagen synthesis in calvarial cultures. Transforming growth factor β is another strong candidate for the role of coupling factor (64). It is present in latent form in bone matrix and may be activated by the low pH in the osteoclastic resorbing zone. It also has been shown to stimulate cell replication in the osteoprogenitor zone of intact rat calvaria (65) and in osteoblast-enriched cultures of fetal bovine bone (66); to regulate alkaline phosphatase activity and matrix production by osteoblast-like cells (67,68); to stimulate bone formation in vivo (69); and to inhibit bone resorption by decreasing osteoclast recruitment (70,71). Other putative coupling factors include platelet-derived growth factor (72), interleukin-1 (73,74), insulin-like growth factor I (somatomedin C) (75–77), macrophage-derived growth factor (78), and osteoinductive factor (79,80). The latter has similar actions to TGF-β in that it inhibits osteoclast and stimulates osteoblast function. More detailed information on

local bone growth factors can be found in reviews (81–83). Clearly, at this point we do not know for certain if any or all of these factors are involved in the coupling process. However, this is an important area of skeletal research, with clear-cut clinical implications, and with the present modern techniques for purification and synthesis of large quantities of peptides it is likely that our understanding of this process will increase significantly over the next decade.

The notion that an active principal, such as TGF-β, released from the matrix during resorption serves as a coupling factor is intellectually satisfying, as one can then readily imagine a quantitative mechanism whereby the number of osteoblasts assembled in the reversal lacuna would be related directly to the volume of bone removed. In this way the bone balance at the BRU level could be maintained. According to Parfitt (40), the local elaboration of osteoblast mitogens may be sufficient to explain the recruitment of osteoblasts into the general area of the remodeling site but cannot account for the highly ordered and polarized manner in which they deploy themselves along the cement line. This is particularly true in cancellous bone, where, in contrast to cortical bone, the local microcirculation is part of an open network, which would tend to convey such factors away from the precise location in which bone formation should begin. Accordingly, the existence of chemotactic factors contained in the cement substance itself has been proposed (54,84).

Formation

Although we cannot fully comprehend the coupling mechanism at this time, it does work. Osteoblasts and their precursors assemble in the right place at the right time, and in the appropriate numbers required to refill the resorption cavity (Figs. 4C and D, and 6C and D). Bone matrix formation is a two-stage process beginning with the deposition by the osteoblasts of osteoid, an organic matrix consisting primarily of type I collagen and various other components, including proteoglycans, carbohydrates, lipids, and noncollagenous proteins, such as bone Gla protein (osteocalcin), matrix Gla protein, and osteonectin (85,86). In normal, adult bone—both cancellous and cortical—osteoid is laid down in discrete layers or lamellae some 3 μm thick. Within each lamella, the orientation of the collagen fibers is relatively consistent, but the fiber orientation changes direction from one lamella to the next. In cancellous bone, the lamellae are deposited in gently curved sheets that follow the contours of the trabeculum. Whereas in cortical bone, osteoblasts, accompanied by blood vessels, follow the osteoclasts through the tunnel in a structure referred to as the *closing cone* and lay down successive, concentric lamellae, starting from the walls of the tunnel and moving toward its center until, eventually, only a narrow central canal containing the blood vessels is left open.

The second stage in bone formation is mineralization of the organic matrix, which occurs after a delay of about 20 days called the *mineralization lag time.* During this time the osteoid undergoes a variety of biochemical changes that render it mineralizeable. After the mineralization process is triggered, the mineral content of the matrix increases rapidly over the first few days to 75% of the final mineral content (primary mineralization), but it may take as much as a year for the matrix to reach its maximum mineral content (secondary mineralization) (87). The principal component of the mature mineral phase is a microcrystalline, nonstoichiometric analog of the naturally occurring mineral hydroxyapatite, $Ca_{10}(PO_4)_6(OH)_2$ (88). Working at linear matrix apposition rates, which in the early stages of the formation phase may be as high as 3 μm per day, it takes the osteoblasts about 150 days to refill the resorption cavity in cancellous bone (53).

The completed piece of new bone is termed either a basic structural unit or a bone structural unit (BSU) (Fig. 2). In cancellous bone the BSU is most commonly called a *packet,* and, occasionally, a *trabecular* or *cancellous osteon.* In cortical bone, the commonly used terms for the BSU are the *secondary osteon* and the *Haversian system.* Cancellous bone packets are conveniently thought of as being saucer-shaped, although this is a little idealized. In reality, the packets vary considerably in shape and this tends to be determined by the overall shape of the trabecula and the location of the BSU within the trabecula. Cortical BSUs, on the other hand, are uniformly cylindrical in shape and are about 2.5 mm in length and 200 μm in diameter. A detailed account of the ultrastructural aspects of bone remodeling is given elsewhere.

FUNCTIONAL SIGNIFICANCE OF REMODELING

Bone remodeling has been proposed to subserve two principal functions: (1) to renew the fabric of the skeleton continuously so that its biomechanical properties are not compromised by daily wear and tear, and (2) to play a role in mineral homeostasis by transferring calcium and other ions into and out of the skeletal reservoir (4,5,22). The relative merits of these two explanations of why remodeling occurs has been the topic of considerable debate. Each is discussed in turn.

Remodeling and Biomechanical Competence

It is known that when subjected to loads applied either in vivo (19,89–92) or in vitro (93–97), cortical bone matrix accumulates microdamage, consisting of prefailure planes and microcracks, which if allowed to grow past a critical size could result in fatigue failure of the whole bone (Figs. 10 to 12). There are many proponents of the view that remodeling prevents or delays this fatigue failure by repairing the microdamage (49,90,94–96,98–103). Frost (19) argues that in bone and other fibrous tissues, complete cessation of remodeling activity would result in total mechanical failure of the tissue within 2 years. This may explain why remodeling is primarily restricted to large, long-lived animals. In rodents and other small animals, remodeling is not necessary (see below). Circumstantial evidence to support the concept that suppression of remodeling activity leads to gross mechanical failure comes from the observation that in diseases in which fractures are commonplace, the bone biopsy frequently reveals depressed remodeling activity (104). Moreover, administration of antiremodeling agents, such as bisphosphonates or sodium fluoride, to humans and experimental animals may lead to spontaneous fractures (19,105). Conversely, if remodeling serves to repair microdamage, one might expect that in situations where the damage is inflicted more rapidly than the remodeling system can cope with, structural failure would result. Indeed, this seems to be the case in overzealous athletes and in soldiers given heavy marching duty (104). In ad-

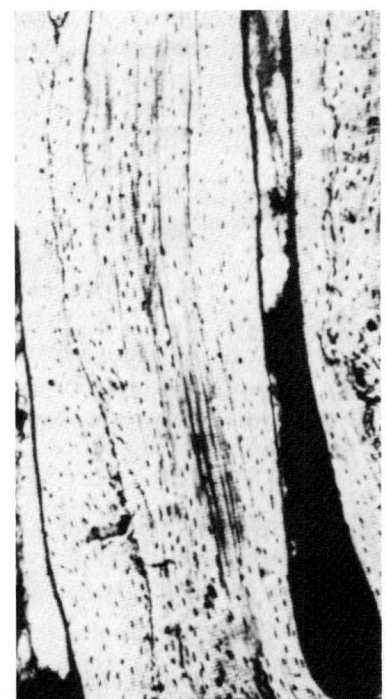
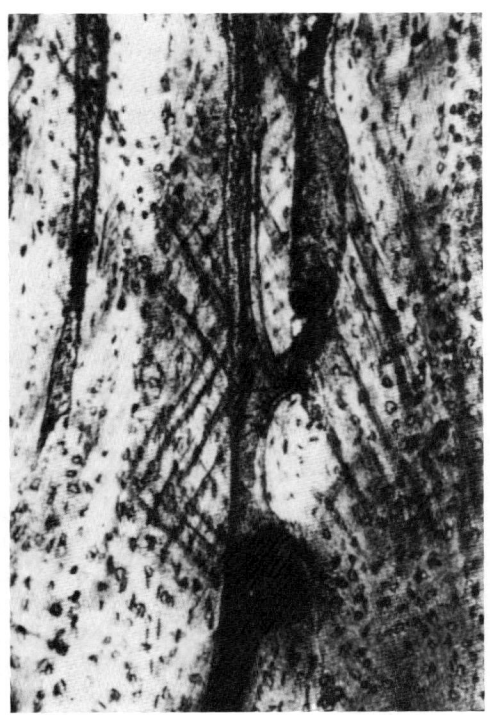

A

B

FIG. 10. Histological demonstration of microdamage in bone. **A:** Both pre-failure planes and microcracks can be seen as dark, fuchsin-stained lines running vertically in this section of bone from a patient with severe genu varum. **B:** Similar preparation showing pre-failure planes in a bone sample that was subjected to a shear test ex vivo. (Reprinted with permission from Ref. 19.)

dition to replacing effete bone with new, stronger material, the remodeling process may also act to limit the extent of microdamage because of the way in which it compartmentalizes the bone matrix. This is best visualized in cortical bone where a crack propagating along cement lines or interlamellar boundaries may be arrested or "trapped" by individual osteons (96,106) (Figs. 11 and 12A). This damage-containment mechanism is thought to be important primarily in regions of bone undergoing tensile stress, whereas in compression, microcracks may penetrate several osteons without becoming trapped (Fig. 12B). Both of these situations will result in a reduction in stress and strain in the wall of the "debonded" osteons, creating a localized disuse state; Martin and Burr (6,106) have hypothesized that this will in turn activate new bone remodeling units to interrupt and repair the crack (Fig. 12C and D).

In the foregoing paragraph, remodeling was presented as being primarily a reparative process, serving to replace bone matrix that has already accumulated microdamage. However, there is also evidence that there may be a predictive element to remodeling. For instance, Lanyon et al. (1) found that new bone deposited on the cortex of sheep radius in response to increased strain was intensively remodeled within weeks of its formation (i.e., long before one would have expected significant fatigue damage to have occurred under the prevailing loading conditions). This implies that the strain experienced in a particular region of bone influences its remodeling behavior. In this way potential damage could be avoided before it occurs.

It should be noted here that not all bone biologists were or are convinced that the primary function of remodeling is to maintain the biomechanical competence of the skeleton. Amprino and Bairati (15) reasoned that if remodeling were solely a response to the mechanical demands on the skeleton, one would not expect to see such a large interindividual variability in remodeling activity. It has been clearly demonstrated that remodeled bone with secondary Haversian systems is in almost all respects mechanically inferior to primary, fibrolamellar bone (102,107–113). The work of Evans and Bang (109,110) on the relationship between the mechanical properties and microstructure of human cortical bone indicated that the presence of osteons and their fragments decreased the tensile strength and modulus of bone, while interstitial lamellae increased these indices. They proposed that the weak points in secondary bone were the cement lines surrounding the Haversian systems, a view that was supported by the experiments of Dempster and Coleman (114) and others (96,115,116). The implication of these findings is that the progressive remodeling of bone that occurs throughout life leads to a decrease in the mechanical strength of the skeleton (113). However, this, in itself, does not argue strongly against the reparative role of remodeling as new Haversian bone is still stronger than damaged primary bone and remodeling is the only feasible mechanism for renewing bone, be it primary or secondary. Currey (2) has challenged the importance of remodeling as a means of removing microcracks. While he concedes that bone remodeling activity increases in response to increased

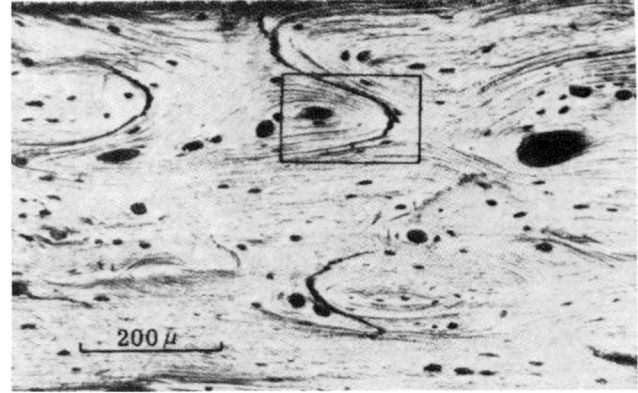

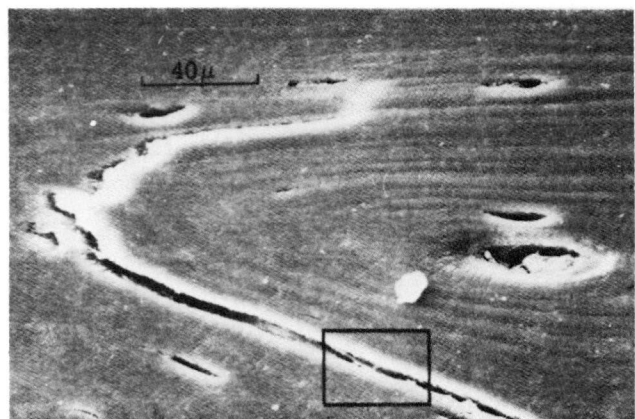

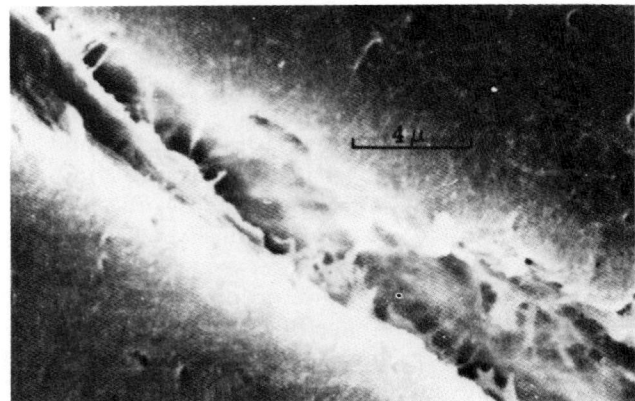

FIG. 11. Reflected light photomicrograph (**A**) and scanning electron micrographs (**B** and **C**) showing progressively higher-power views of a microcrack in bovine cortical bone. The sample had been subjected to flexural fatigue to a point where the mechanical properties of the bone were significantly altered, but a complete fatigue fracture had not yet occurred. The micrographs were taken from the side of the specimen that was under tension. The crack has propagated along the cement line and has been trapped by the osteon. See Figure 12. (Reproduced with permission from Ref. 96.)

loading of bone (3,108,117,118), he points out that the spatial distribution of the remodeling that occurs in this situation is inconsistent with the microcrack repair hypothesis. In the experiments of Hert et al. (108), for example, in which rabbit tibiae were loaded in bending, the remodeling did not take place in the subperiosteal area, which experiences the greatest stress under bending conditions, but rather it occurred deeper in, toward the center of the cortex. Moreover, bone remodeling tends to occur symmetrically in contralateral limbs (2,119) (Fig. 13), which implies either that microdamage also occurs symmetrically—an unlikely scenario according to Currey (2)—or that remodeling is programmed by other factors. Burr et al. (120) found that when bone was experimentally fatigued in vivo, microcracks were associated with resorption cavities 44 times as often as would be predicted by chance alone. This certainly argues for a causal relationship between fatigue and remodeling. However, when the microdamage burden was increased, a concomitant increase in resorption sites did not occur, leaving open the possibility that the microcracks had appeared where there were preexisting resorption spaces, not vice versa (6). Another point arguing against a simple relationship between mechanical stress and remodeling is that whereas increasing the mechanical forces on bone certainly increases the activation frequency of remodeling units in some circumstances, so does decreasing it, as in immobilization or weightlessness (see Ref. 121 for a review of this topic). Furthermore, increased mechanical loading does not always lead to increased remodeling. Frost (122) points out that in adults, vigorous mechanical usage tends to depress recruitment of bone remodeling units—at least in bone adjoining marrow—a response that will have the appropriate effect of conserving bone mass at these sites. These kinds of observation have led to the development of the view that there may be a wide range of physiological strain levels within which changes in strain will have no effect on remodeling activity (19,123–126). Strain levels above and below the normal physiological range will trigger an adaptive remodeling response involving not only replacement of existing bone but a compensatory change in bone mass. The reader is referred to Currey (2), Frost (125,126), and Martin and Burr (6) for a discussion of the role of remodeling in mechanical adaptation.

What other functions could remodeling serve in addition to, or perhaps instead of, repairing microcracks? One notion is that Haversian remodeling allows a reorientation of the grain of the bone in order to strengthen it (2). While primary bone is generally stronger than secondary bone, badly oriented primary bone is weaker than well-oriented Haversian bone. This is likely to be an important function in localized regions of bone, for example, under muscle insertions and during fracture repair (127,128). However, this process accounts for only a small proportion of the total remodeling activity, as, very often, remodeling occurs in perfectly well-oriented regions of bone and many new Haversian systems simply replace others of similar orientation (129). Two other roles that have been ascribed to remodeling are removal of dead bone and improving the blood supply of bone (130). The latter seems untenable because secondary

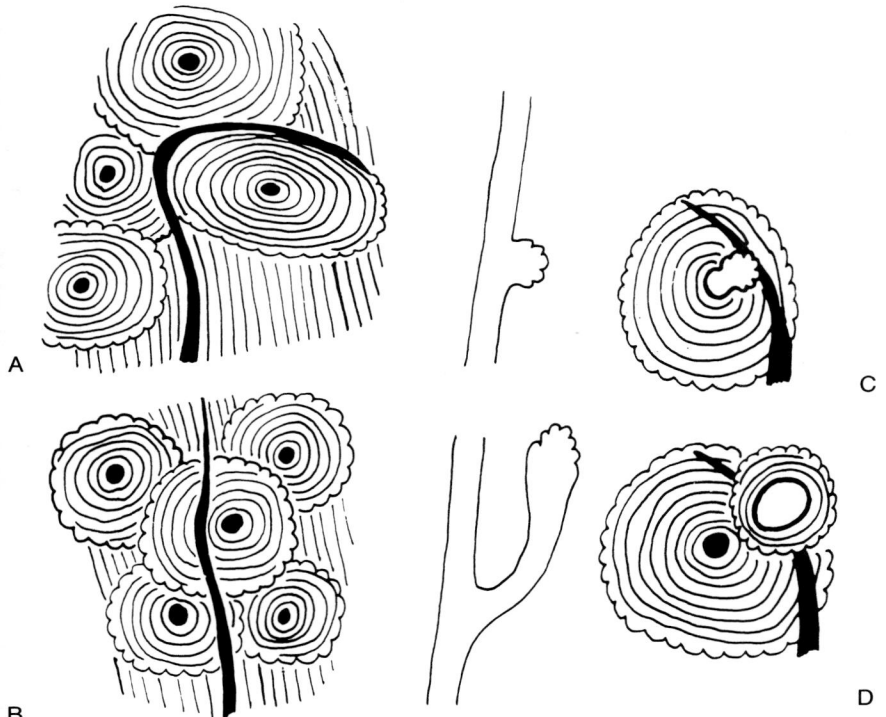

FIG. 12. Diagram illustrating how microcracks tend to be trapped by osteons in regions of bone under tension (**A**) and traverse osteons in compressed areas (**B**). **C** and **D** show, in both longitudinal and transverse section, how a new bone remodeling unit, activated by the debonding of the osteon, could interrupt and repair part of the crack. (Reproduced with permission from *J. Biomech* 15, R. B. Martin and D. B. Burr, A hypothetical model for the stimulation of osteonal remodeling by fatigue damage, 1982, Pergamon Press.)

bone is actually less vascular than primary bone, the average distance between an osteocyte and the nearest blood vessel therefore being greater in secondary bone (131), and as few blood vessels or osteocyte canaliculi penetrate the cement line, creation of new osteons essentially cuts off the blood supply to interstitial bone. Replacement of dead bone by new Haversian systems does appear to occur (130) but probably only to a limited extent, and as for the microcrack repair theory, the spatial distribution of remodeling activity cannot be accounted for solely by removal of dead bone (2).

Thus the evidence that the phenomenon of bone remodeling can be explained solely on the basis of main-taining the biomechanical integrity of bone seems less than compelling. Which brings us to the other main contender for remodeling's *raison d'être,* which was originally proposed by Amprino and Bairati (15): namely, its role in mineral metabolism.

Remodeling and Mineral Homeostasis

The adult skeleton contains approximately 99% of the body's total calcium content, as well as 35% of its sodium, 80% of its carbonate, 80% of its citrate, and 60% of its magnesium (132). Access to this skeletal ionic reservoir, via the bone remodeling units, is clearly of vital

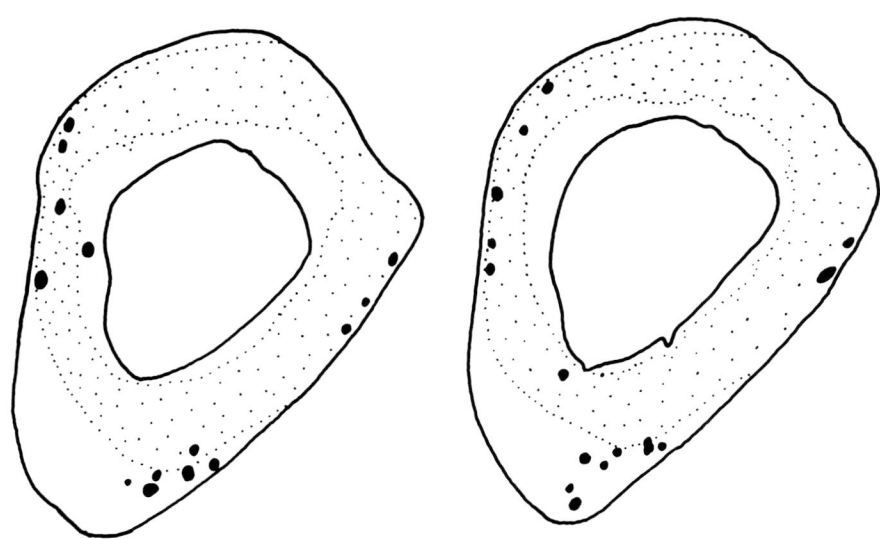

FIG. 13. Sketches of cross sections of the paired ulnae of a cat. The fine stippling delineates the area of Haversian bone and the dark dots indicate forming Haversian systems. Note the striking symmetry of both remodeled and remodeling bone. (Reproduced with permission from John Currey, *The mechanical adaptations of bones,* copyright 1984 by Princeton University Press.)

importance in disease states, for example, in nutritional vitamin D deficiency with secondary hyperparathyroidism, where calcium is transferred from bone to blood, and in metabolic acidosis, where the same is true for bicarbonate. However, in the present discussion we address the question of whether bone remodeling plays a significant role in mineral homeostasis under normal physiological conditions. On choosing to live on land as opposed to the oceans, animals left behind an abundant source of calcium and were forced to evolve effective mechanisms for dealing with the constant threat of calcium deficiency. As illustrated in Fig. 14, any tendency for the plasma calcium concentration to fall will be compensated by an increased secretion of parathyroid hormone, which will act to mobilize calcium by three mechanisms: increased tubular reabsorption in the kidney, increased absorption from the gut (via 1,25-dihydroxyvitamin D), and increased activation of new bone remodeling units. The renal response is the most sensitive and most rapid and the skeletal response is less sensitive and slower (132,133). Thus, on a minute-to-minute basis the kidney is probably the main regulator, with the skeleton being more important for long-term homeostasis. However, because of its independence from dietary habits,

the skeleton is a much more reliable source of calcium than the gut and its capacity is, to all intents and purposes, unlimited. In this context the concept of a reversible mineral deficit in bone is important (134,135). Despite the fact that bone remodeling, because it involves both resorption and formation, does not result in net transfer of mineral to the blood in the long run, an increase in remodeling rate can, in the short term, mobilize significant amounts of mineral. This is so because of the temporal relationship between resorption and formation and the fact that mature, highly mineralized matrix may be removed within a matter of days to be replaced over the ensuing weeks by osteoid, which after a delay of some 20 days is mineralized gradually, perhaps taking as much as a year to reach the same mineral content as the matrix that was removed. To use a common analogy, when calcium is needed it may be withdrawn fairly rapidly from the skeletal bank and then paid back gradually later. In this way the skeleton can participate in calcium homeostasis without permanently compromising its structural integrity.

A similar mechanism can be proposed for skeletal involvement in phosphate homeostasis. A fall in the plasma phosphate concentration will stimulate 1,25-di-

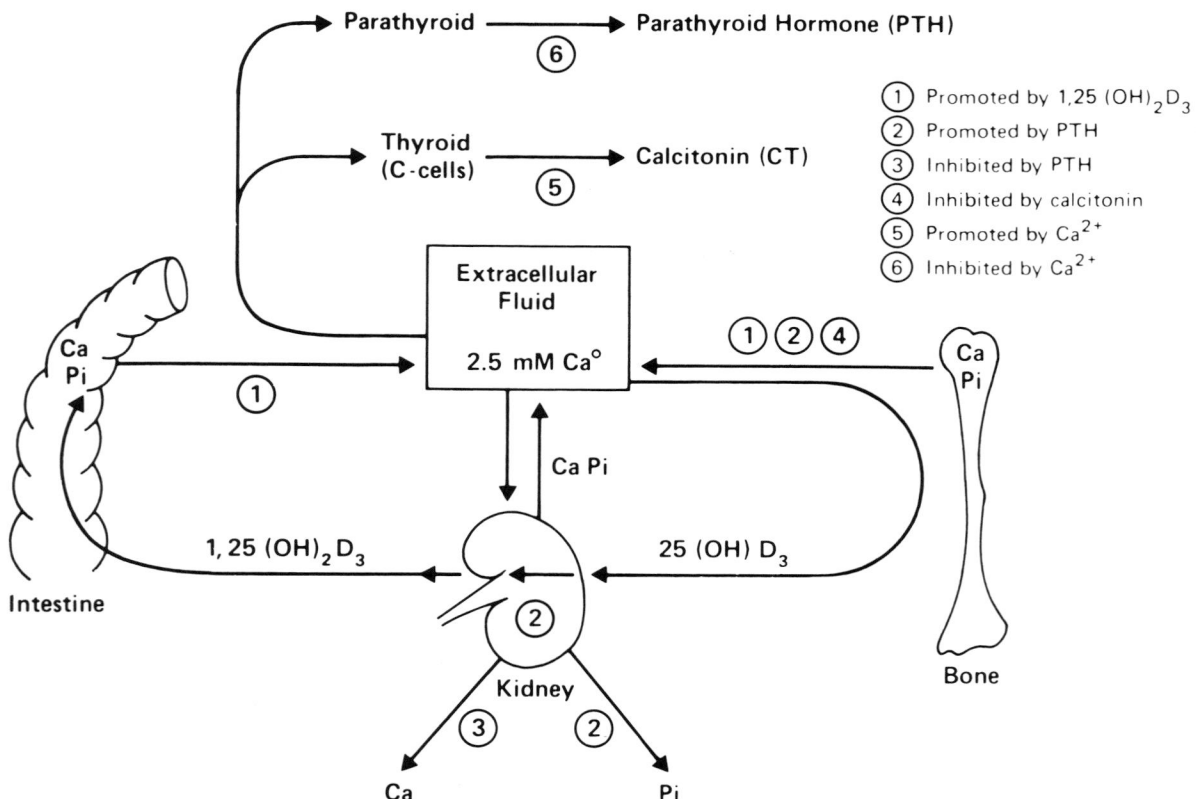

FIG. 14. Diagram illustrating the main elements in the homeostatic control of plasma calcium concentration. Parathyroid hormone secreted by the parathyroid gland in response to a lowering of plasma calcium acts directly, or indirectly through activation of vitamin D, on kidney, gut, and bone to increase the flow of calcium into the blood. See the text for further details. (Reproduced with permission from Ref. 132.)

hydroxyvitamin D production in the kidney, which, in addition to its positive effects on phosphate absorption from the gut, will activate new bone remodeling units and, in so doing, mobilize phosphate from the skeleton. It is apparent that phosphate cannot be withdrawn from the skeleton without calcium, and vice versa. However, this can be compensated at the level of the kidney. In the case of a hypophosphatemic stimulus to bone remodeling, parathyroid hormone levels will be suppressed by the excess calcium from bone and gut and therefore renal calcium excretion will be elevated. Whereas in the event of a hypocalcemic stimulus, parathyroid hormone will be elevated and therefore renal phosphate excretion will be enhanced.

The participation of bone remodeling in mineral homeostasis is most clearly evident at times of calcium stress. Birds deposit significant amounts of cancellous bone in the medullary cavities shortly before the commencement of egg-lay and then draw on this store for the large quantities of calcium required for shell formation (136,137). Although, within the confines of this chapter, this process cannot really be considered as remodeling. A more pertinent example is the deer, in which increased bone turnover occurs during antler formation (138) (Fig. 15). Enhanced remodeling has been proposed as a likely mechanism for increasing the calcium supply during pregnancy and lactation in mammals (134). This has been demonstrated in rats (139) and dogs (140), and recently, a reversible mineral deficit has been observed in the spine during human pregnancy and lactation (141). Interestingly, in the latter study, several of the women had significantly higher bone density at the end of lactation than they had before becoming pregnant. There is also an increase in cortical remodeling during the prepubertal growth spurt in humans (142,143). Although not generally appreciated, when calcium is required to fulfill a physiological need in large animals, it is preferentially withdrawn from cortical rather than cancellous bone. By this means, a large amount of calcium may be obtained with minimum impact, even if it is only temporary, on the structural integrity of the skeleton (40,135).

It is worth noting that there are two other mechanisms, in addition to bone remodeling, that allow the skeleton to participate in the regulation of plasma mineral levels. These are the blood-bone barrier, maintained by the bone lining cells, and the percolation of bone extracellular fluid through the osteocyte lacunocanalicular network. These will not be expanded upon here but are discussed in detail by Frost (19) and Parfitt (144,145).

The two most likely explanations of why bones remodel have been presented separately for the purpose of clarity. However, in reality the two are very much entangled. There is evidence to ascribe both a mechanical and a metabolic function to remodeling and it is likely that neither is dominant all of the time. Rather, depending on the ambient conditions, each will assume priority at

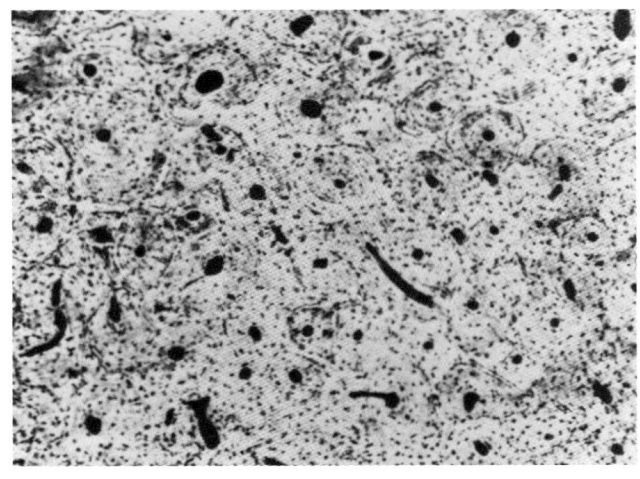

A

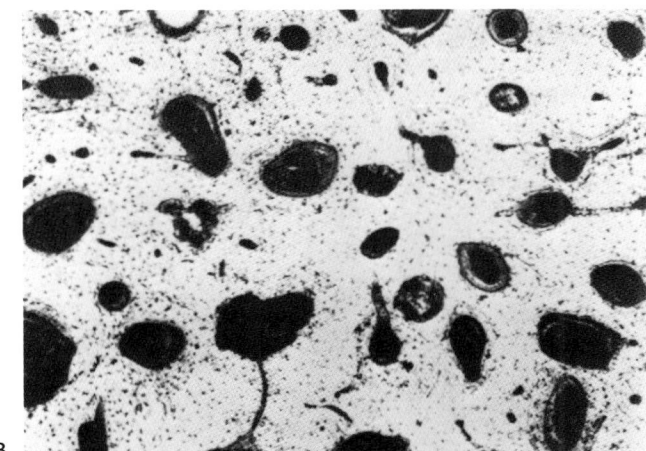

B

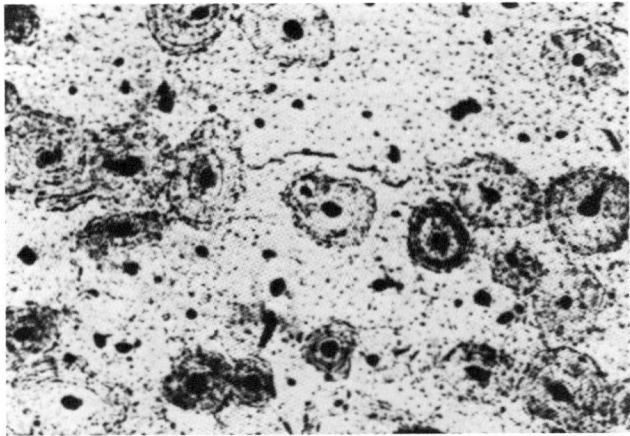

C

FIG. 15. Sections of cortical bone from the ribs of a Rocky Mountain mule deer before (**A**), during (**B**), and after (**C**) the antler growth period. Note the reversible mineral deficit in B, where there is a dramatic increase in remodeling activity. This occurred despite the provision of an unrestricted diet that was rich in calcium and phosphorus. (Reproduced with permission from Ref. 138.)

different times and at different skeletal sites in a complex interplay that we do not yet fully understand. It is also possible that remodeling serves some other function of which we are at present completely unaware (2).

EFFECTS OF AGE, SEX, AND RACE ON BONE REMODELING

Bone remodeling occurs throughout the entire human lifespan. Haversian systems have been observed in children as young as 2 years of age (16), and there at least two reports of the occurrence of remodeling in the human fetus (146,147). The most recent of these papers documents the presence of secondary osteons in the humerus, ulna, radius, femur, tibia, fibula, and sixth and seventh ribs as early as week 24 of gestation. The activation frequency of bone remodeling units is very high in children —at least in the rib—and declines during the teens and 20s to a nadir in the mid-30s (21). Aging is associated with significant changes in bone remodeling, the most

obvious effect of which is a reduction in cancellous and cortical bone mass accompanied by a modest increase in remodeling activation with age in both men and women. The latter has been demonstrated by biochemical (148–151), histological (21,151,152), and radiokinetic (151,153) techniques. Cancellous bone loss occurs in both men and women, but the pattern, mechanism, and magnitude of loss differs between the sexes. In both sexes, cancellous bone is lost by a combination of trabecular thinning and trabecular plate removal; in men the former mechanism predominates, whereas the latter is the most important in women (154–157) (Fig. 16). In men, there is a linear reduction in cancellous bone volume with age, and a similar trend occurs in women until around age 55, when there is a marked acceleration in the rate of bone loss, the onset of which is associated with menopause (Fig. 17). After a period of 5–10 years the rate of loss slows down again to the premenopausal level.

Accompanying this accelerated bone loss there is a marked increase in bone turnover rate, over and above the gradual, age-related increase mentioned above. This

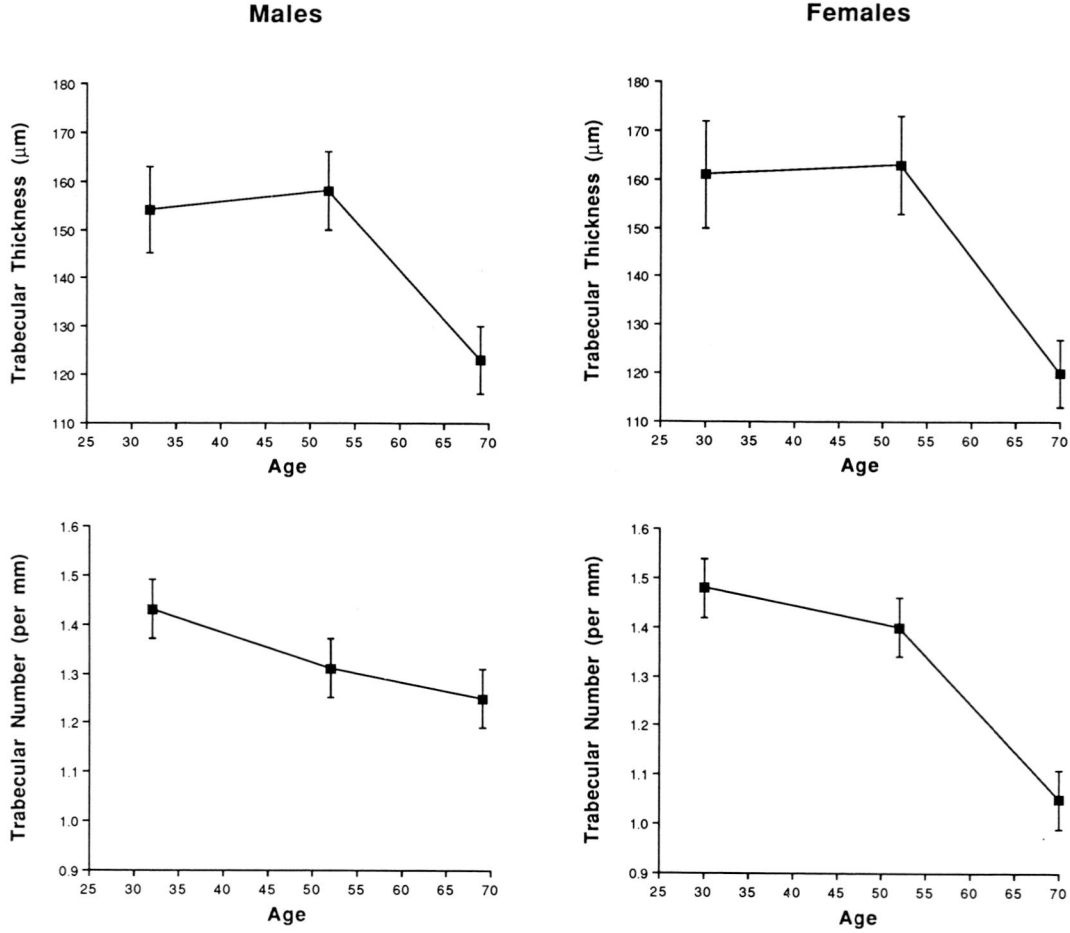

FIG. 16. Changes in trabecular thickness and number with age in men (**left**) and women (**right**). The reduction in trabecular thickness was statistically significant in males but not in females, whereas the reverse was the case for trabecular number. (Drawn from data given in Ref. 157.)

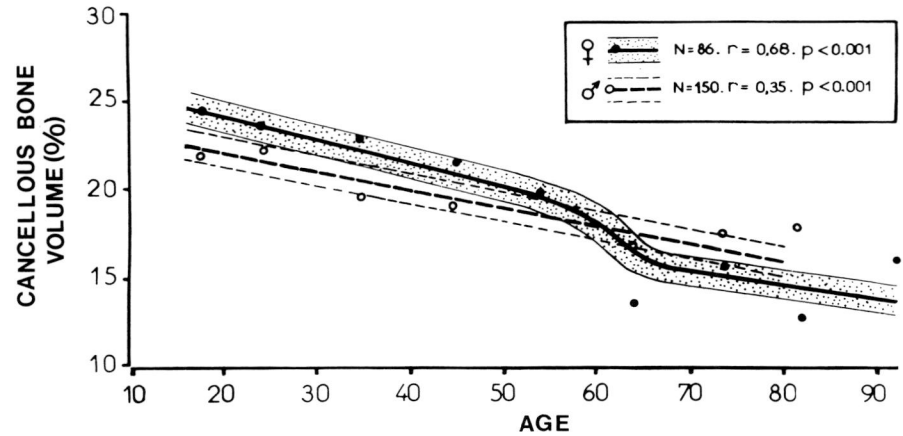

FIG. 17. Cancellous bone volume in the iliac crest as a function of age in men and women. Note the sharp acceleration of bone loss in women following the menopause. (Reproduced with permission from Ref. 158.)

too has been confirmed in biochemical (148,149,159), calcium kinetic (160), and histomorphometric studies (40), and is reversed by estrogen replacement (161–165). The gradual bone loss that occurs in both sexes is partly caused by an age-related reduction in the completed wall thickness of the cancellous bone packets (166,167) (Fig. 18,19). Reduction in wall thickness is accompanied by a decrease in mineral appositional rate and an increase in the formation period (40,168,169) indicating a generalized decline in osteoblast activity with age. This could be due to a reduction in the synthetic capacity of individual osteoblasts, or a decreased recruitment of osteoblasts during the reversal phase of the remodeling cycle, or a combination of the two (40). The negative effect of the age-related decrease in wall thickness on cancellous bone volume is partially offset by a simultaneous reduction in the depth of the resorption cavities (53,170,171).

Rapid, postmenopausal bone loss is not caused by thinning of trabeculae but by their complete removal

(155,169,172). The cellular mechanism underlying this process is largely a matter of speculation at the present time, as longitudinal studies of rapid bone loss over the period in question have not been conducted. One of the most plausible theories is that the trabeculae are removed by hyperactive osteoclasts that penetrate too deeply into the trabecular plates and perforate them (Figs. 19 and 20). This could occur by a plate being simultaneously resorbed on both sides or by unusually aggressive resorption occurring on one side of a thinner than normal plate (173). This theory is consistent with the rate of loss and the architecture of cancellous bone *after* the period of rapid loss; increases in resorption cavity depth have been noted in women, but not men, in the fifth decade (174) and in animal models of rapid bone loss (175–177). The deleterious effects of the penetrating osteoclasts will be exacerbated by the enhanced remodeling activation due to decreased estrogen levels. The two models of cancellous bone loss—trabecular thinning

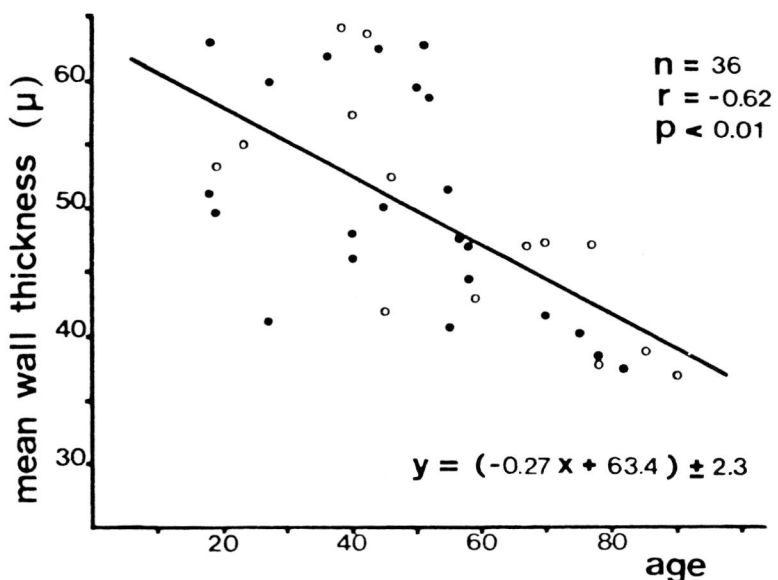

$$y = (-0.27\,x + 63.4) \pm 2.3$$

n = 36
r = -0.62
p < 0.01

FIG. 18. Relationship between the wall thickness of cancellous bone packets and age in men (*closed circles*) and women (*open circles*). See Fig. 2. (Reproduced with permission from Ref. 166.)

RAPID LOSS   SLOW LOSS

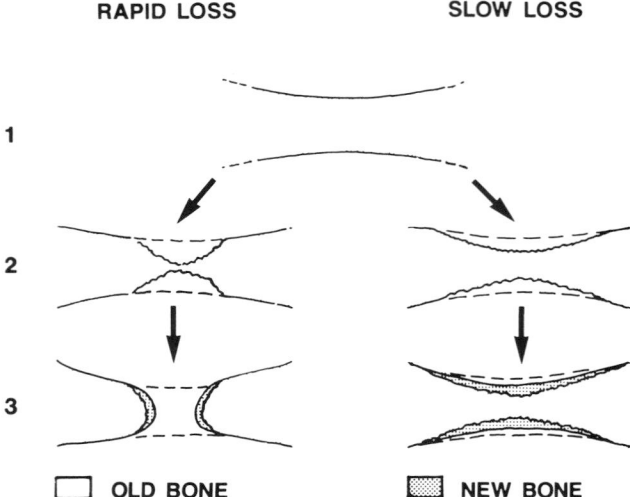

☐ OLD BONE   ▨ NEW BONE

FIG. 19. Two mechanisms of cancellous bone loss. Rapid loss is caused by overenthusiastic osteoclastic activity leading to perforation and, ultimately, loss of the whole trabecula (see Fig. 20). Slow loss is caused by a deficit in osteoblast function that results in reduced thickness of individual packets and gradual thinning of the trabecular plates. (Reproduced with permission from Ref. 40.)

and trabecular removal—are not of course mutually exclusive. It is possible that prior thinning of the selected plates predisposes them to osteoclastic perforation and removal (173). The fact that the remaining plates are of normal thickness in a biopsy taken several years after-

ward does not preclude this possibility. Appreciation of the relative contribution of trabecular thinning versus removal to the overall cancellous bone loss in women awaits longitudinal data.

An increase in osteoclast resorption cavity depth on the endocortical surface is also the primary mechanism underlying cortical bone loss with age (40,84). This imbalance ultimately leads to the creation of large voids on the endosteal surface which are continuous with the marrow space, so that ultimately the inner third of the cortex resembles cancellous bone in structure (Fig. 21). In the cortex itself, aging is associated with a reduction in the area occupied by circumferential lamellar bone and an increase in the number of Haversian systems and their fragments, indicating the progressive nature of the remodeling that occurs throughout life (178–181). These findings are so consistent that Kerley (179) concluded that cortical bone structure may be used to predict the age of a subject with an accuracy of ±10 years in 95 of 100 cases. Other changes in cortical remodeling with age include a decrease in the radial rate of closure of osteons (152), an increase in Haversian canal diameter, a decrease in osteon wall thickness, and an increase in the number of resorption cavities that are abandoned in the reversal phase and remain unfilled (183–186). Each of these contributes to increased cortical porosity, and as for the slow-loss phenomenon in cancellous bone, can be accounted for by an age-related decline in osteoblast recruitment and vigor. With advancing age there is also an increase in the proportion of cortical osteons in which

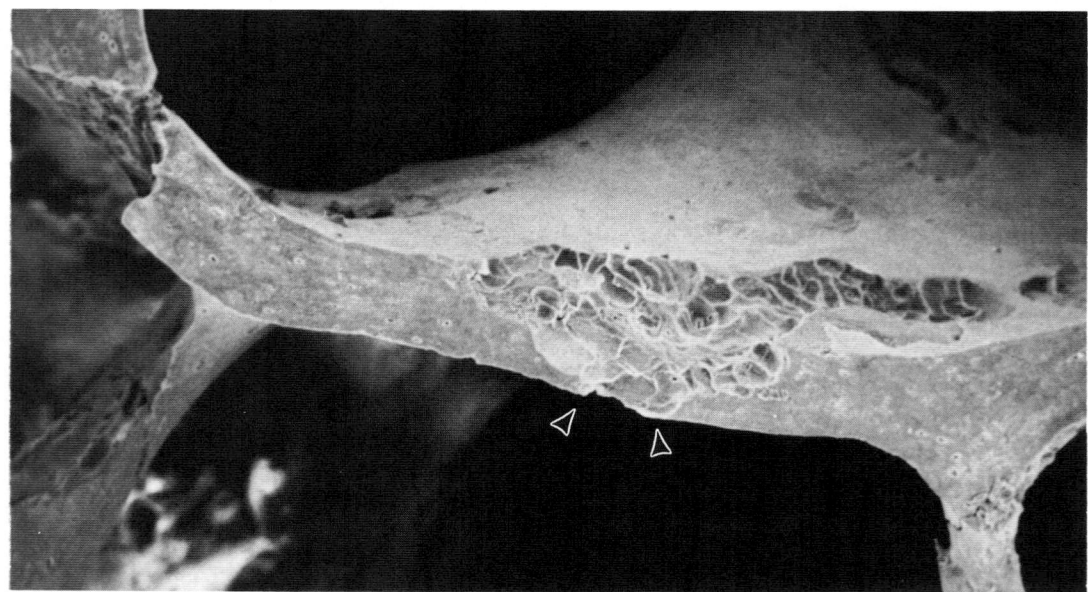

FIG. 20. Scanning electron micrograph of a trabecular plate that has been perforated (*arrow*) by intense osteoclastic resorption. The characteristic imprints of the osteoclasts show that they have penetrated deep into the plate over a large area. Another breach of the same plate from the opposite side can be seen in the upper left of the field. The sample was from iliac crest of a 74-year-old woman.

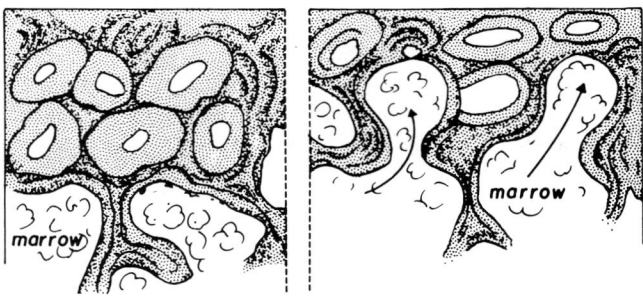

FIG. 21. Trabecularization of the endosteal surface of cortical bone with aging (**left** to **right**). The Haversian canals enlarge due to osteoblast insufficiency and increased resorption cavity depth on the endocortical surface allows the invasion of marrow. (Reproduced with permission from Ref. 220.)

matrix synthesis has been completed but which fail to reach their maximum mineral content (182,187).

Very little work has been done on racial differences in bone remodeling. Weinstein and Bell (188) have reported that the bone formation rate in a group of 12 normal American black subjects was only 35% of that in a group of age- and weight-matched whites, a finding that was consistent with earlier biochemical studies (189) and which the authors concluded was due to a lower bone remodeling rate in blacks. This difference in remodeling rate may help explain the characteristically higher skeletal mass, and lower incidence of osteoporosis, in black people (190–193). However, low bone turnover in blacks may not be universal. South African blacks have higher cancellous bone volumes than their white counterparts but have increased remodeling rates, at least when assessed by static histomorphometric parameters (194), and suffer far fewer fractures than do American blacks (195). Studies of racial differences in bone remod-

eling may provide important insight into the role of remodeling in preserving the mechanical properties of bone.

REMODELING IN DIFFERENT SKELETAL ENVELOPES AND VARIATION THROUGHOUT THE SKELETON

The bone turnover rate varies considerably both within and among the different bones of the skeleton. Within individual bones, there is a striking difference in turnover rate between the cancellous and cortical compartments. Averaged over the entire skeleton, approximately 12 BRUs are activated each minute in cancellous bone and the annual turnover rate is of the order of 25% (22). The activation frequency of cortical BRU, by contrast, is roughly three per minute with only 2–3% of the total volume being turned over per year. The higher remodeling rate in cancellous bone is generally attributed to the higher surface-to-volume ratio compared to cortical bone. All of the surface of cancellous bone is in contact with bone marrow, which contains the precursors of osteoclasts, and cancellous bone is also more vascularized than cortical bone. The net difference between the volume of bone removed and that replaced by each BRU depends on their anatomical location within the bone. It is customary to think in terms of four distinct surfaces or "envelopes" (19): periosteal, Haversian, cortical–endosteal, and trabecular (Fig. 22). In the Haversian envelope the net bone balance is slightly negative, particularly in the inner half of the cortex. In the periosteal envelope, each BRU deposits a bit more bone than it removes. Conversely, in the cortical-endosteal envelope less bone is laid down than is resorbed, and the deficit here is

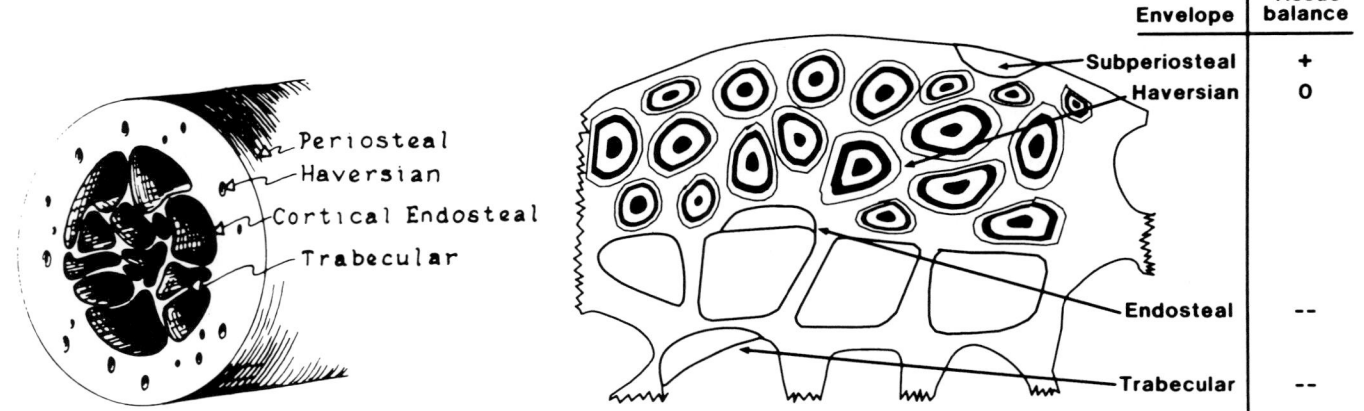

A

B

FIG. 22. **A:** Location of the four skeletal envelopes and the tissue balance of each bone remodeling units in each envelope (**B**). See the text for further details. [(**A**) Reprinted with permission from Ref. 19. (**B**) From Ref. 221.]

greater than the slight positive balance in the periosteal envelope. As discussed previously, in the trabecular envelope there is a shortfall in the amount of bone replaced compared to that removed. With aging the effects of these small increments or decrements of bone mass will accumulate. This provides a BRU-based explanation for the following, long-established facts concerning the changes that occur in the three-dimensional geometry of bones as a function of age (19). Both the periosteal and the cortical-endosteal surfaces increase in circumference, with the latter moving outward at a greater rate than the former, with a consequent reduction in cortical thickness. The cortical porosity increases by 1–2% in the outer half and by 5–10% in the inner half, and the cancellous bone volume decreases (Fig. 23). The BRU-based mechanisms underlying the negative balance on the cortical-endosteal and trabecular envelopes are discussed above.

There have been relatively few assessments of the regional variation in bone remodeling and turnover throughout the skeleton, and most of these have focused on cancellous bone. In particular, the relationship between the standard iliac crest biopsy site and other skeletal sites has received some attention (196). The histomorphometrically determined turnover rate in the iliac crest is about 40% per year, a value approximately double that in the vertebral bodies (22). Based on measurements of osteoid and osteoblast-covered surfaces, Krempien et al. (197) revealed a marked disparity between four different skeletal sites, with an implied rank order of remodeling rate as follows: iliac crest > lumbar vertebra > femoral head > distal femur. The most reliable way to assess regional differences in remodeling rate (i.e., histomorphometric analysis of tetracycline-labeled bone samples) is obviously not practical for human studies (some animal data will be discussed below), although there is one reported case (198) of an elderly osteoporotic woman who died suddenly before a scheduled bone biopsy for which she had been prelabeled with tetracycline. Twenty-four skeletal sites were sampled at autopsy and the calculated bone formation rates were found to vary widely from a high of 37% per year (iliac crest) to a low of <2% per year (tenth thoracic vertebra). There were also significant variations between bones within fairly localized regions of the skeleton (e.g., from one vertebra to the next, or between the right and left iliac crest). The tetracycline-based bone formation rate in cortical bone of the rib, a once-favored biopsy site, is 3–4% per year, which is about twice that in cortical bone elsewhere in the skeleton (22).

The reasons for the high intersite variation in turnover rates are unclear; probably, multiple biomechanical and metabolic factors are at play (see above). If, however, one makes the assumption that a substantial proportion of bone remodeling occurs randomly with all cancellous

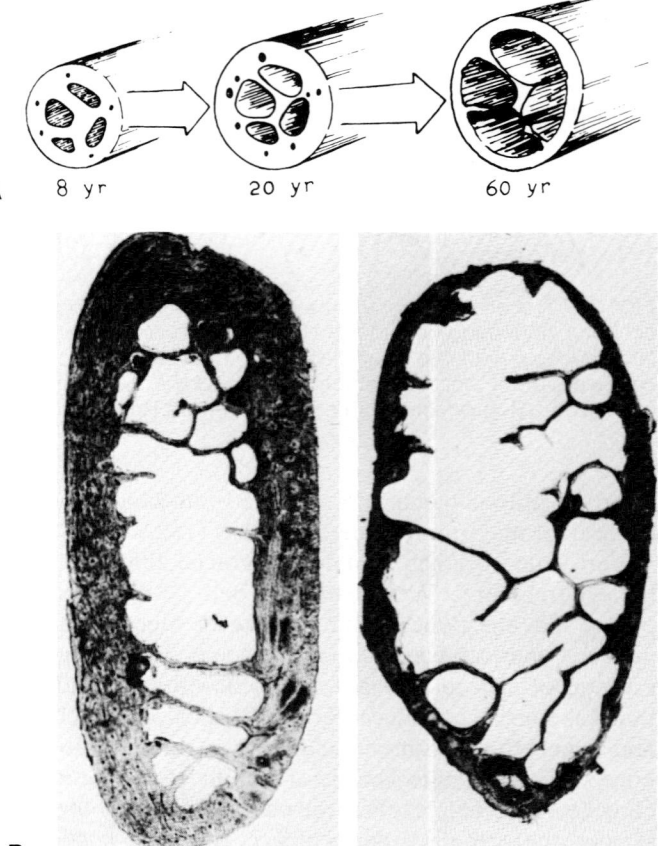

FIG. 23. Changes in bone with age. Diagrammatic representation (**A**) and histological demonstration (**B**) of the cumulative effects over time of the small imbalances between resorption and formation in each of the four skeletal envelopes. Panel B shows transverse sections of the middle of the sixth rib from two women aged 25 years (**left**) and 65 years (**right**). Note the slightly greater horizontal diameter of the periosteum and the markedly increased marrow cavity diameter of the bone from the older woman. The cortex and the trabeculae are also thinner in this sample, but the cortical porosity is similar to that in the bone from the 25-year-old. [(**A**) reprinted with permission from Ref. 19 and (**B**) from H. M. Frost, *Bone remodeling and its relation to metabolic bone disease*, Charles C Thomas, Springfield, IL, 1973.]

bone surfaces having an equal probability of undergoing activation, and then further assumes that there is a constant turnover rate per unit surface, the turnover rate at different skeletal sites would be proportional to their surface-to-volume ratio (19,22,40).

BONE REMODELING IN ANIMALS

There is little Haversian remodeling in the lower vertebrates with the exception of the dinosaurs, early amphibia, and a few of the reptiles, such as turtles and crocodilians (2,199). In the birds and mammals, the general rule is the larger the bone, the more extensive the remodeling. Small birds have very thin cortices which are not remodeled, but domestic fowl and ostriches, for example, have numerous Haversian systems (2,200,201). In most modern fish—the advanced teleosts—the bone is acellular, so no remodeling takes place; in the lower teleosts and lungfish, bone tends to be replaced by cartilage (2). Within the mammals the most extensive remodeling is seen in the primates, carnivores, and artiodactyls, with relatively little occurring in the smaller species (5,202). However, in situations of calcium stress something akin to remodeling is known to occur in rodents. Ruth (203) induced the appearance of Haversian systems in rat long bones by feeding lactating mothers a calcium-free diet for 3 weeks and then replacing it for a further month with a normal diet. Moreover, Baron and colleagues (204) have presented histomorphometric evidence of coupled bone remodeling in the secondary spongiosa of rat tail vertebrae. This has led to a resurgence in the use of the rat as an experimental model for at least some aspects of human bone biology (e.g., Refs. 205–209). The reclassification of the rabbit from a rodent to a lagomorph makes sense at least from a skeletal point of view as the rabbit bone is quite unlike that of rodents, with significant amounts of Haversian remodeling occurring under normal conditions (182,185,202).

Remodeling activity in the dog has been quite well characterized (210). Marotti (211) gathered detailed information on tetracycline-based bone formation rates in 21 mongrels, ranging in age from 2 to 72 months. There was a fairly broad range in bone formation rates throughout the skeleton, but in general the pattern was similar in all animals, regardless of age, breed, and size. The bone formation rate was higher in the vertebrae, mandibles, and ribs than in the shafts of the long bones. In the long bones themselves, the highest values were recorded in the ulna and the lowest in the humerus and femur with intermediate values in the radius, third metacarpal and metatarsal, and tibia (Fig. 24). Norrdin et al. (212) measured the activation frequency of bone remodeling units in various bones of beagles and produced data that complemented Marotti's findings well. The activation frequency was very low in the humerus and femur, slightly higher in the mandible and highest in the ribs. The higher activation frequencies in the ribs and mandible were attributed to mechanical stimuli associated with respiration and mastication. This is supported by the observation that monkeys fed a hard diet show more intense remodeling of their mandibles than do those maintained on soft food (118). Jee et al. (210) cite evidence for a generalized decline in remodeling activity with aging in

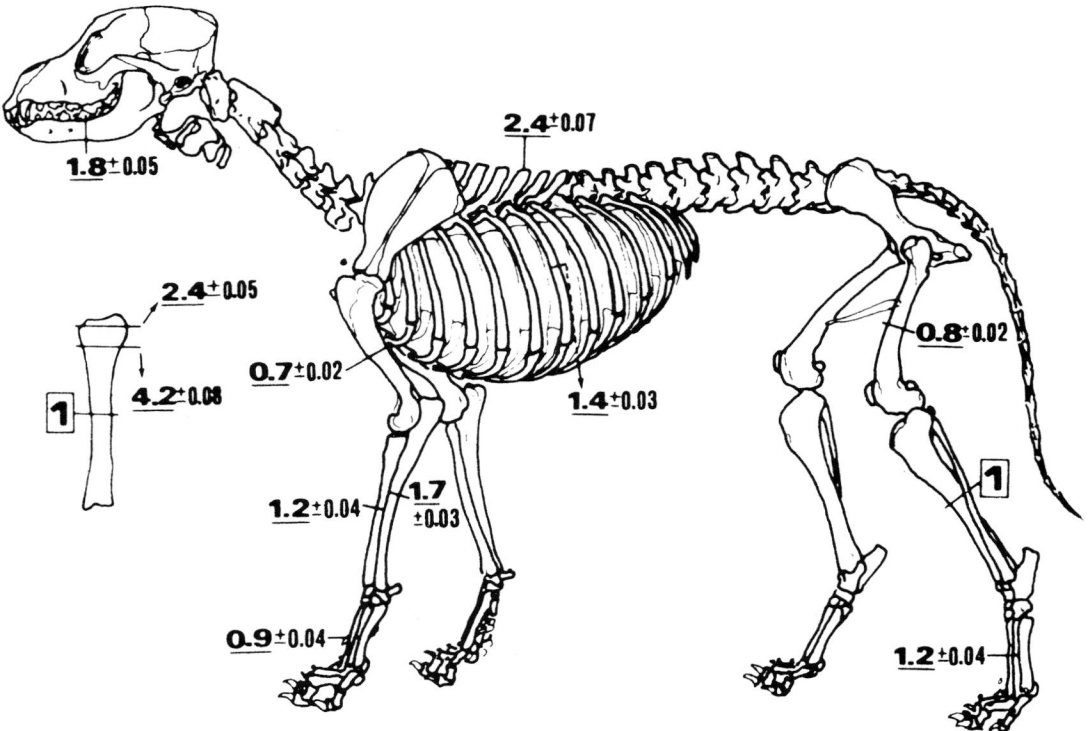

FIG. 24. Comparison of tetracycline-based bone formation rates throughout the skeleton of the dog. The values represent the formation rate at each site relative to that in the mid-diaphysis of the tibia, which was arbitrarily assigned a value of 1. The inset diagram of the single bone gives the average epiphysis/diaphysis and metaphysis/diaphysis ratios for bone formation rate in the long bones. (Reprinted with permission from Ref. 211.)

the dog. In their own study, a reduction in the remodeling rate of 5.5% per year was observed in the lumbar vertebrae of beagle dogs between the ages of 1.3 and 5.1 years. Both Marotti's (211) and Norrdin et al.'s (212) studies confirmed the age-related reduction in remodeling activity, a phenomenon that was also noted in Baron et al.'s (204) study in the rat. In this respect, the animal data would appear to be inconsistent with the human studies mentioned above.

Jowsey (185) compared the diameter of cortical osteons in the rat, rabbit, cat, dog, monkey, cow, and humans as well as in samples from *Diadactes* and *Iguanodon*. The average cement-line diameter ranged from 72 to 246 μm. In general, the smaller the animal, the smaller the diameter of the osteon and its canal. However, there appears to be an upper limit for osteon size in that osteons from the cow and the dinosaurs were not significantly larger than human ones. This upper limit may be imposed by the maximum distance over which adequate transport of fluid through the canalicular system can be sustained (182). The dimensions of the cutting and closing cones and the duration of each stage of the remodeling cycle are broadly similar in dog, monkey, and humans (22). The resorption period is shortest in the dog at 8 days, compared to 13 and 15 days in the monkey and humans, respectively. On the other hand, the formation period in the dog (63 days) is closer to that in humans (76 days) than is the monkey (55 days). Since canine and human bone remodeling activity are comparable in many respects, the dog has been used quite extensively as a laboratory model of skeletal disease (e.g., Refs. 213–215). Among animals that remodel their skeletons, there are considerable interspecific differences in the intensity of remodeling activity. Cows and deer, for example, represent an exception to the general rule that remodeling activity is proportional to body size for their long bones retain their primary, laminar structure throughout life with only small amounts of remodeling occurring around areas of muscle insertions (2,113,216). By contrast, human bones are extensively, in fact almost completely, remodeled (J. C. Currey, 1989, personal communication). There is no unifying concept to explain these differences other than to reiterate that from one species to another there are presumably differences in the mechanical, metabolic, and other unspecified forces that govern remodeling activity.

In conclusion, modern investigative techniques, particularly bone histomorphometry, have significantly improved our understanding of the cellular mechanisms involved in bone remodeling. However, a number of important questions remain to be answered with regard to the signals that activate new remodeling units, the coupling mechanism that tethers formation to resorption, and perhaps most intriguing of all, the function of remodeling and why it occurs to such a significant extent in human beings.

ACKNOWLEDGMENTS

This work was supported in part by National Institutes of Health Grants AR35647 and AR39191. The author is indebted to Wendy Horbert and Michelle Schnitzer, who provided expert technical assistance, and to Stephanie Roberts, Brian Yarborough, and Lester Ferguson for help with the illustrations.

REFERENCES

1. Lanyon LE, Goodship AE, Rye CJ, MacFie JH. Mechanically adaptive bone remodeling. *J Biomech* 1982;15:141–54.
2. Currey JC. *The mechanical adaptation of bones.* Princeton, NJ: Princeton University Press, 1984.
3. Enlow DH. *Principles of bone remodeling.* Springfield, IL: Charles C Thomas, 1963.
4. Lacroix P. The internal remodeling of bones. In: Bourne GH, ed. *The biochemistry and physiology of bone,* vol 3. New York: Academic Press, 1971;119.
5. Frost HM. *Bone remodeling and its relationship to metabolic bone disease,* Springfield, IL: Charles C Thomas, 1973.
6. Martin RB, Burr DB. *Structure, function and adaptation of compact bone.* New York: Raven Press, 1989.
7. Leeuwenhoek A. Microscopical observations on the structure of teeth and other bones. *Philos Trans R Soc Lond* 1678;12:1002–3.
8. Leeuwenhoek A. Several observations on the texture of bone of animals, compared with that of wood: on the bark of trees, on the little scales found on the cuticula, etc. *Philos Trans R Soc Lond* 1693;17:828–43.
9. Havers C. *Osteologia nova.* London: Samuel Smith, 1691.
10. Todd RB, Bowman W. *The physiological anatomy and physiology of man.* Philadelphia: Blanchard and Lea, 1845.
11. Monro A. *The anatomy of the human bones, nerves and lacteal sac and duct.* Dublin: unknown publisher, 1776.
12. Howship J. Microscopical observations on the structure of bone. *Medico-chirurgical transactions.* London: Longman, Hurst, Reese, Orme & Bro, 1815–1819.
13. Tomes J, DeMorgan C. Observations on the structure and development of bone. *Philos Trans R Soc Lond* 1853;143:109–39.
14. von Ebner V. Uber den feineren bau der knochensubstanz. *Sitzungsber Deutsch Akad Wiss Berlin,* 1875;72:49–138.
15. Amprino R, Bairati A. Contributo allo stùdio del valóre funzionale dela struttura della sostanza compatta della ossa. *Chir Organi Mov* 1936;20:527–41.
16. Amprino R, Bairati A. Procèssi di ricostruzióne e di riassorbimento della sostanzea compatta delle ossa dell'uomo. *Z Zellforsch* 1936;24:439–511.
17. Amprino R. A contribution to the functional meaning of the substitution of primary by secondary bone tissue. *Acta Anat* 1948;5:291–300.
18. Murray PDF. *Bones.* Cambridge: University Press, 1936.
19. Frost HM. *Intermediary organization of the skeleton.* Boca Raton, FL: CRC Press, 1986.
20. Frost HM. *Bone remodeling dynamics.* Springfield, IL: Charles C Thomas, 1963.
21. Frost HM. *The laws of bone structure.* Springfield, IL: Charles C Thomas, 1964.
22. Parfitt AM. The physiological and clinical significance of bone histomorphometric data. In: Recker RR, ed. *Bone histomorphometry: techniques and interpretation.* Boca Raton, FL: CRC Press, 1983;143–223.
23. Baron R. Importance of the intermediate phases between resorption and formation in the measurement and understanding of the bone remodeling sequence. In: Meunier PJ, ed. *Bone histomorphometry: proceedings of the 2nd international workshop.* Toulouse: Société de la Nouvelle Imprimerie Fournie, 1977;179–83.
24. Tran Van P, Vignery A, Baron R. An electron microscopic study

of the bone-remodeling sequence in the rat. *Cell Tissue Res* 1982;225:283–92.

25. Tran Van P, Vignery A, Zaron R. Cellular kinetics of the bone remodeling sequence in the rat. *Anat Rec* 1982;202:441–51.

26. Rodan GA, Martin TJ. Role of osteoblasts in hormonal control of bone resorption: a hypothesis. *Calcif Tissue Int* 1981;33:349–52.

27. Miller SS, Wolf AM, Arnaud CD. Bone cells in culture: morphologic transformation by hormones. *Science* 1976;192:1340–3.

28. Jones SJ, Boyde A. Experimental study of changes in osteoblastic shape induced by calcitonin and parathyroid extract in an organ culture system. *Cell Tissue Res* 1976;169:449–65.

29. Jones SJ, Boyde A. Scanning electron microscopy of bone cells in culture. In: Copp DH, Talmage RV, eds. *Endocrinology of calcium metabolism.* Amsterdam: Excerpta Medica, 1978;97–114.

30. Heath JK, Atkinson SJ, Meikle MC, Reynolds JJ. Mouse osteoblasts synthesize collagenase in response to bone resorbing agents. *Biochim Biophys Acta* 1984;802:151.

31. Chambers TJ. The pathobiology of the osteoclast. *J Clin Pathol* 1985;38:241–52.

32. Chambers TJ, Fuller K. Bone cells predispose bone surfaces to resorption by exposure of mineral to osteoclastic contact. *J Cell Sci* 1985;76:155.

33. Sakamoto S, Sakamoto S. Bone collagenase, osteoblasts and cell-mediated bone resorption. In: Peck WA, ed. *Bone and mineral research,* vol 4. Amsterdam: Elsevier, 1986;49–102.

34. Partridge NC, Jeffrey JJ, Ehlich LS, et al. Hormonal regulation of the production of collagenase and of a collagenase inhibitor activity by rat osteogenic sarcoma cells. *Endocrinology* 1987; 120:1956.

35. Delaisse JM, Eeckhout Y, Vaes G. Bone-resorbing agents affect the production and distribution of procollagenase as well as the activity of collagenase in bone tissue. *Endocrinology* 1988; 123:264–76.

36. Malone JD, Teitelbaum SL, Griffin GL, Senior RM, Kahn AJ. Recruitment of osteoclast precursors by purified bone matrix constituents. *J Cell Biol* 1982;92:227.

37. Mundy GR, Poser JW. Chemotactic activity of γ-carboxyglutamic acid containing protein in bone. *Calcif Tissue Int* 1983;15:164.

38. Lian JB, Tassinari M, Glowacki JG. Resorption of implanted bone from normal and warfarin treated rats. *J Clin Invest* 1984;73:1223.

39. Lian JB, Dunn K, Key LL Jr. In vitro degradation of bone particles by human monocytes is decreased with the depletion of the vitamin K–dependent bone protein from the matrix. *Endocrinology* 1986;118:1636.

40. Parfitt AM. Bone remodeling: relationship to the amount and structure of bone, and the pathogenesis and prevention of fractures. In: Riggs BL, Melton LJ III, eds. *Osteoporosis: etiology, diagnosis and management.* New York: Raven Press, 1988;45–93.

41. Johnson LC. The kinetics of skeletal remodeling. *Birth Defects Orig Art Ser* 1966;2:66–142.

42. Somjen D, Binderman I, Berger E, Harell A. Bone remodeling induced by physical stress is prostaglandin E_2 mediated. *Biochim Biophys Acta* 1980;627:91–100.

43. Yeh CK, Rodan GA. Tensile forces enhance prostaglandin E synthesis in osteoblastic cells grown on collagen ribbons. *Calcif Tissue Int* 1984;36:S67–71.

44. Ferrier J, Ross SM, Kanehisa J, Aubin JE. Osteoclasts and osteoblasts migrate in opposite directions in response to a constant electrical field. *J Cell Physiol* 1986;129:283–8.

45. Ferrier J. Electrical modulation of bone cell behaviour. In: Tam CS, Heersche JNM, Murray TM, eds. *Metabolic bone disease: cellular and tissue mechanisms.* Boca Raton, FL: CRC Press, 1989;269–75.

46. Mundy GR, Roodman GD. Osteoclast ontogeny and function. In: Peck WA, ed. *Bone and mineral research,* vol 5. Amsterdam: Elsevier, 1987;209–79.

47. Jores L. Experimentelle untersuchungen uber die einwikung mechanischen druckes auf den knochen. *Beitr Pathol Anat Allg Pathol* 1920;66:433–69.

48. Peterson H. Die organe des skeletsystems. In: Von Mollendorff W, ed. *Handbuch der Mikroskopischen Anatomie des Menschen Herausgegeben.* Berlin: unknown publisher, 1930.

49. Frost HM. Bone dynamics in osteoporosis and osteomalacia. Springfield, IL: Charles C Thomas, 1966.

50. Lanyon LE. Functional strain in bone tissue as an objective and controlling stimulus for adaptive bone remodeling. *J Biomech* 1987;20:1083–93.

51. Lanyon LE, Elhaj A, Minter S, Pead MJ, Skerry TM. Early changes in loading-related functional adaptation in bone tissue. *J Bone Miner Res* 1988;3(suppl 1):194.

52. Skerry TM, Bitensky L, Chayen J, Lanyon LE. Early strain-related changes in enzyme activity in osteocytes following bone loading in vivo. *J Bone Miner Res* 1988;4:783–8.

53. Eriksen EF. Normal and pathological remodeling of human trabecular bone: three-dimensional reconstruction of the remodeling sequence in normals and in metabolic bone disease. *Endocr Rev* 1986;7:379–408.

54. Baron R, Vignery A, Horowitz M. Lymphocytes, macrophages and the regulation of bone remodeling. In: Peck WA, ed. *Bone and mineral research,* vol 2. Amsterdam: Elsevier, 1984;175–245.

55. Baron R, Vignery A. Behaviour of the osteoclasts during a rapid change in their number induced by high doses of parathyroid hormone or calcitonin in intact rats. *Metab Bone Dis Relat Res* 1981;2:339–46.

56. Zambonin-Zallone A, Teti A. The osteoclasts of hen medullary bone under hypocalcemic conditions. *Anat Embryol* 1981; 162:379–92.

57. Zambonin-Zallone A, Teti A, Primavera MV. Isolated osteoclasts in primary culture: first observations on structure and survival in culture media. *Anat Embryol* 1982;165:405–13.

58. Baron R, Vignery A, Tran Van P. The significance of lacunar erosion without osteoclasts: studies on the reversal phase of the remodeling sequence. *Metab Bone Dis Relat Res* 1980;2S:35–40.

59. Farley JR, Baylink DJ. Purification of a skeletal growth factor from human bone. *Biochemistry* 1982;21:3502–7.

60. Mohan S, Jennings J, Linkhart T, Taylor A, Baylink DJ. Purification and characterization of a small molecular weight human skeletal growth factor (hSGF). *J Bone Miner Res* 1986;1:60.

61. Howard GA, Bottenmiller BL, Turner RT, Rader JI, Baylink DJ. Parathyroid hormone stimulates bone formation and resorption in organ culture: evidence for a coupling mechanism. *Proc Natl Acad Sci (USA)* 1981;78:3024–8.

62. Mohan S, Jennings JC, Linkhart TA, Wergedal JE, Baylink DJ. Primary structure of human skeletal growth factor (SGF): homology with IGF-II. *J Bone Miner Res* 1988;3(suppl 1):218.

63. Canalis E, McCarthy T, Centrella M. A bone-derived growth factor isolated from rat calvaria is β_2 microglobulin. *Endocrinology* 1987;121:1198–2000.

64. Mundy GR. Identifying mechanisms for increasing bone mass. *J Natl Inst Health Res* 1989;1:65–8.

65. Hock JM, Centrella M, Canalis E. Transforming growth factor beta (TGF-β-1) stimulates bone matrix apposition and bone cell replication in cultured rat calvaria. *Calcif Tissue Int* 1988;42:A32.

66. Gehron Robey P, Young MF, Flanders KC, et al. Osteoblasts synthesize and respond to transforming growth factor β (TGF-β) in vitro. *J Cell Biol* 1987;105:457–63.

67. Noda M, Rodan G. Type β transforming growth factor inhibits proliferation and expression of alkaline phosphatase in murine osteoblast-like cells. *Biochem Biophys Res Commun* 1986;140:56–65.

68. Pfeilschifter J, D'Souza SM, Mundy GR. Effects of transforming growth factor-β on osteoblastic osteosarcoma cells. *Endocrinology* 1987;121:212–8.

69. Noda M, Camilliere JJ. In vivo stimulation of bone formation by transforming growth factor-β. *Endocrinology* 1989;124:2991–4.

70. Pfeilschifter J, Seyedin SM, Mundy GR. Transforming growth factor-β inhibits bone resorption in rat long bone cultures. *J Clin Invest* 1988;82:680.

71. Chenu C, Pfeilschifter J, Mundy GR, Roodman GD. Transforming growth factor beta inhibits formation of osteoclast-like cells in long-term human marrow cultures. *Proc Natl Acad Sci USA* 1988;85:5683–7.

72. Centrella M, McCarthy TL, Canalis E. Platelet-derived growth

factor enhances deoxyribonucleic acid and collagen synthesis in osteoblast-enriched cultures from fetal rat parietal bone. *Endocrinology* 1989;125:13–9.

73. Gowen M, Wood DD, Russell RGG. Stimulation of the proliferation of human bone cells in vitro by human monocyte production with interleukin-1 activity. *J Clin Invest* 1985;75:1223–9.

74. Canalis E. Interleukin-1 has independent effects on DNA and collagen synthesis in cultures of rat calvariae. *Endocrinology* 1986;118:74–81.

75. Canalis E. Effect of insulin-like growth factor I on DNA and protein synthesis in cultured rat calvariae. *J Clin Invest* 1980;66:709–19.

76. Canalis E, McCarthy T, Centrella M. Isolation and characterization of insulin-like growth factor I (somatomedin-C) from cultures of fetal rat calvariae. *Endocrinology* 1988;122:22–7.

77. Chenu C, Valentin-Opran A, Delmas P, et al. Growth hormone and somatomedin C activity on human osteoblasts in short term cultures. *J Bone Miner Res* 1986;1(suppl 1):154.

78. Rifas L, Shen V, Mitchell K, Peck WA. Macrophage-derived growth factor for osteoblast like cells and chondrocytes. *Proc Natl Acad Sci (USA)* 1984;81:4558–62.

79. Rosen DM, Stempien SA, Segarini PR, Dasch J, Bentz H, Seyedin SM. Osteoinductive factor (OIF) and transforming growth factor-β (TGF-β) differentially modulate the expression of osteoblastic markers by a murine bone marrow stromal cell line. *J Bone Miner Res* 1989;4(suppl 1):S325.

80. Oreffo ROC, Bonewald L, Seyedin D, Rosen D, Mundy GR. Inhibition of osteoclastic bone resorption by bone growth factors. *J Bone Miner Res* 1989;4(suppl 1):S154.

81. Peck WA. The cells of bone. In: Riggs BL, Melton LJ III, eds. *Osteoporosis: etiology, diagnosis and management.* New York: Raven Press, 1988;1–44.

82. Canalis E, McCarthy T, Centrella M. Growth factors and the regulation of bone remodeling. *J Clin Invest* 1988;81:277–81.

83. Canalis E. The regulation of bone formation by local growth factors. In Peck WA, ed. *Bone and mineral research,* vol 6. Amsterdam: Elsevier, 1989;27–56.

84. Parfitt AM. The cellular basis of bone remodeling: the quantum concept re-examined in the light of recent advances in cell biology. *Calcif Tissue Int* 1984;36:537–45.

85. Tracey RP, Stenner DD, Mintz KP, et al. Components of compact bone: the noncollagenous proteins. In: Cohn DV, Martin TJ, Meunier PJ, eds. *Calcium regulation and bone metabolism: basic and clinical aspects.* Amsterdam: Elsevier, 1987;401–8.

86. Robey PG, Fisher LW, Young MF, Termine JD. The biochemistry of bone. In: Riggs BL, Melton LJ III, eds. *Osteoporosis: etiology, diagnosis and management.* New York: Raven Press, 1988;95–109.

87. Amprino R, Engstrom A. Studies on x-ray absorption and diffraction of bone tissue. *Acta Anat* 1952;15:1–22.

88. Posner AS. Bone mineral and the mineralization process. In: Peck WA, ed. *Bone and mineral research,* vol 5. New York: Elsevier, 1987;65–116.

89. Frost HL. Presence of microscopic cracks in vivo in bone. *Henry Ford Hosp Med Bull* 1960;8:27–35.

90. Tschantz P, Rutishauser E. La surcharge mécanique de los vivant. *Ann Anat Pathol* 1967;12:223–48.

91. Devas MB. *Stress fractures.* London: Churchill Livingstone, 1975.

92. Carter DR. The relationship between in vivo strains and cortical bone remodeling. *CRC Crit Rev Biomech Eng* 1981;8:1–28.

93. Chamay A. Mechanical and morphological aspects of experimental overload and fatigue in bone. *J Biomech* 1970;3:263–70.

94. Wright TM, Hayes WC. The fracture mechanics of fatigue crack propagation in compact bone. *J Biomed Mater Res Symp* 1976;7:637–48.

95. Carter DR, Hayes WC. Compact bone fatigue damage. I. Residual strength and stiffness. *J Biomech* 1977;10:325–37.

96. Carter DR, Hayes WC. Compact bone fatigue damage: a microscopic examination. *Clin Orthop* 1977;127:265–74.

97. Carter DR, Caler WE. Uniaxial fatigue of human cortical bone: the influence of tissue physical characteristics. *J Biomech* 1981;14:461–70.

98. Currey JD. Stress concentrations in bone. *Q J Microsc Sci* 1962;103:111–33.

99. Swanson SAV, Freeman MAR, Daw W II. The fatigue properties of human cortical bone. *Med Biol Eng* 1971;9:23–32.

100. Baker J, Frankel VH, Burstein A. Fatigue fractures: biomechanical considerations. *J Bone Joint Surg* 1972;54A:1345–6.

101. Chamay A, Tschantz P. Mechanical influences in bone remodeling: experimental research on Wolff's law. *J Biomech* 1972;5:173–80.

102. Carter DR, Hayes WC. Fatigue life of compact bone. I. Effects of stress amplitude, temperature and density. *J Biomech* 1976;9:27–34.

103. Piekarski K. Morphology of fracture of bone. *4th international conference on fracture,* vol 1. Waterloo: University of Waterloo, 1976;607–42.

104. Frost HM. Mechanical microdamage, bone remodeling and osteoporosis: a review. In: DeLuca HF, Frost HM, Jee WSS, Johnston CC Jr, Parfitt AM, eds. *Osteoporosis.* Baltimore: University Park Press, 1981;185–90.

105. Flora L, Hassing GS, Parfitt AM, Villaneuva AR. Comparative skeletal effects of two diphosphonate drugs. In: DeLuca HF, Frost HM, Jee WSS, Johnston CC Jr, Parfitt AM, eds. *Osteoporosis.* Baltimore: University Park Press, 1981:389–407.

106. Martin RB, Burr DB. A hypothetical model for the stimulation of osteonal remodeling by fatigue damage. *J Biomech* 1982;15:137–9.

107. Smith JW, Walmsley R. Elastic after-effect, plasticity and fatigue in bone. *J Anat* 1957;91:603.

108. Hert J, Pribylova E, Liskova M. Microstructure of compact bone after intermittent loading. *Acta Anat* 1972;82:218–30.

109. Evans FG, Bang S. Physical and histological differences between human fibular and femoral compact bone. In: Evans FG, ed. *Studies on the anatomy and function of bone and joints.* New York: Springer-Verlag, 1966;142–55.

110. Evans FG, Bang FG. Differences and relationships between the physical properties and microscopic structure of human femoral, tibial and fibular bone. *Am J Anat* 1967;120:79.

111. Currey JD. The effect of strain rate, reconstruction, and mineral content on some mechanical properties of bovine bone. *J Biomech* 1975;8:81–6.

112. Carter DR, Hayes WC, Schurman DJ. Fatigue life of compact bone. II. Effects of microstructure and density. *J Biomech* 1976;9:211–8.

113. Carter DR, Spengler DM. Mechanical properties of cortical bone. *Clin Orthop Rel Res* 1978;135:192–217.

114. Dempster WT, Coleman RF. Tensile strength of bone along and across the grain. *J Appl Physiol* 1960;16:355.

115. Piekarski K. Fracture of bone. *J Appl Physiol* 1970;41:215.

116. Pope MH, Outwater JO. Mechanical properties of bone as a function of position and orientation. *J Biomech* 1974;7:61.

117. Churches AE, Howlett CR. The response of mature cortical bone to controlled time varying loading. In: Cowin SC, ed. *Mechanical properties of bone,* AMD vol 45. New York: American Society of Mechanical Engineers, 1981;69–80.

118. Bouvier M, Hylander WL. Effect of bone strain on cortical bone structure in macaques (*Macaca mulatta*). *J Morphol* 1981;167:1–12.

119. Marotti G. Number and arrangement of osteons in corresponding regions of homotypic long bones. *Nature* 1961;191:1400–1.

120. Burr DB, Martin RB, Schaffler MB, Radin EL. Bone remodeling in response to in vivo fatigue microdamage. *J Biomech* 1985;18:189–200.

121. Smith EL, Gilligan C. Mechanical forces and bone. In: Peck WA, ed. *Bone and mineral research,* vol 6. Amsterdam: Elsevier, 1989;139–73.

122. Frost HM. Mechanical usage, bone mass, bone fragility: a brief overview. In: Kleerekoper M, Krane SM, eds. *Clinical disorders of bone and mineral metabolism.* New York: Mary Ann Liebert, 1989;15–40.

123. Cowin SC. Mechanical modeling of the stress adaptation process in bone. *Calcif Tissue Int* 1984;36:S98–103.

124. Carter DR, Harris WH, Vasu R, Caler WE. The mechanical and biological response of cortical bone to in vivo strain histories. In: Cowin SC, ed. *Mechanical properties of bone.* New York: American Society of Mechanical Engineers, 1981.

125. Frost HM. Vital biomechanics: proposed general concepts for

skeletal adaptations to mechanical usage. *Calcif Tissue Int* 1987;42:145–56.

126. Frost HM. Structural adaptations to mechanical usage: a proposed "3-way rule" for bone remodeling. Parts I and II. *Vet Comp Orthop Traumatol* 1988;1:7–17 and 2:80–5.

127. Vasciaveo F, Bartoli E. Vascular channels and resorption cavities in the long bone cortex: the bovine bone. *Acta Anat* 1961;47:1–33.

128. Enlow DH. *A handbook of facial growth.* Philadelphia: WB Saunders, 1975.

129. Cohen J, Harris WH. The three dimensional anatomy of Haversian systems. *J Bone Joint Surg* 1958;40A:419–34.

130. Currey JD. Differences in the blood supply of bone of different histological types. *Q J of Microsc Sci* 1960;101:351–70.

131. Dempster WT, Enlow DH. Patterns of vascular channels in the cortex of the human mandible. *Anat Rec* 1959;135:189–205.

132. Martin TJ, Raisz LG, Rodan G. Calcium regulation and bone metabolism. In: Martin TJ, Raisz LG, eds. *Clinical endocrinology of calcium metabolism.* New York: Marcel Dekker, 1987;1–52.

133. Rasmussen H. Parathyroid hormone: nature and mechanism of action. *Am J Med* 1961;30:112–28.

134. Parfitt AM. Morphological basis of bone mineral measurements: transient and steady state effects of treatment in osteoporosis. *Miner Electrolyte Metab* 1980;4:273–87.

135. Parfitt AM. The integration of skeletal and mineral homeostasis. In: DeLuca HF, Frost HM, Jee WSS, Johnston CC Jr, Parfitt AM, eds. *Osteoporosis: recent advances in pathogenesis and treatment.* Baltimore: University Park Press, 1981;115–26.

136. Dacke CG. *Calcium regulation in sub-mammalian vertebrates.* London: Academic Press, 1979.

137. Feinblatt JD. The comparative physiology of calcium regulation in sub-mammalian vertebrates. *Adv Physiol Biochem* 1982;8:73–110.

138. Banks WJ, Epling GP, Kainer RA, Davio RW. Antler growth and osteoporosis. I. Morphological and morphometric changes in the costal compacta during the antler growth cycle. *Anat Rec* 1968;162:387–98.

139. Miller SC, Shupe JG, Redd EH, Miller MA, Omura TH. Changes in bone formation rates during pregnancy and lactation in rats. *Bone* 1986;7:283–7.

140. Miller MA, Omura TH, Miller SC. Increased cancellous bone remodeling during lactation in beagles. *Bone* 1989;10:237–41.

141. Cann CE. Pregnancy and lactation cause reversible trabecular bone loss in humans. *J Bone Miner Res* 1989;4(suppl 1):S384.

142. Wilson JS, Genant HK. In vivo assessment of bone metabolism using the cortical striation index. *Invest Radiol* 1979;14:131–6.

143. Parfitt AM. Cortical porosity in the pathogenesis of postmenopausal and adolescent wrist fractures. In: Uhthoff H, Jaworski ZFG, eds. *Bone fragility in orthopedics and medicine.* New York: Springer-Verlag, 1987;167–72.

144. Parfitt AM. Bone and plasma calcium homeostasis. *Bone* 1987;8(suppl 1):51–8.

145. Parfitt AM. Plasma calcium control at quiescent bone surfaces: a new approach to the homeostatic function of bone lining cells. *Bone* 1989;10:87–8.

146. Goret-Nicaise M, Dhem A. The mandibular body of the human fetus: histological analysis of the basilar part. *Anat Embryol* 1984;169:231–6.

147. Burton P, Nyssen-Behets C, Dhem A. Haversian bone remodelling in the human fetus. *Acta Anat* 1989;135:171–5.

148. Delmas PD, Stenner D, Wahner HW, Mann KG, Riggs BL. Increase in serum bone γ-carboxyglutamic acid protein with aging in women: implications for the mechanism of age-related bone loss. *J Clin Invest* 1983;71:1316–21.

149. Epstein S, Poser J, McClintock R, Johnston CC Jr, Bryce G, Hui S. Difference in serum bone gla protein with age and sex. *Lancet* 1984;i:307–10.

150. Duda RJ Jr, O'Brien JF, Katzmann JA, Peterson JM, Mann K, Riggs BL. Concurrent assays of circulating bone Gla-protein and bone alkaline phosphatase: effects of sex, age, and metabolic bone disease. *J Clin Endocrinol Metab* 1980;66:951–7.

151. Eastell R, Delmas PD, Hodgson SF, Eriksen EF, Mann KG, Riggs BL. Bone formation rate in older normal women: concurrent assessment with bone histomorphometry, calcium kinetics,

and biochemical markers. *J Clin Endocrinol Metab* 1988; 67:741–8.

152. Frost HM. Tetracycline-based histological analysis of bone remodeling. *Calcif Tissue Res* 1969;3:211–37.

153. Recker RR, Heaney RP. Effects of age, sex, and race on bone remodeling. In: Kleerekoper M, Krane S, eds. *Clinical disorders of bone and mineral metabolism.* New York: Mary Ann Liebert, 1989;59–70.

154. Wakamatsu E, Sissons HA. The cancellous bone of the iliac crest. *Calcif Tissue Res* 1969;4:147–61.

155. Parfitt AM, Matthews CHE, Villanueva AR, Kleerekoper M, Frame B, Rao DS. Relationships between surface, volume, and thickness of iliac trabecular bone in aging and in osteoporosis: implications for the microanatomic and cellular mechanisms of bone. *J Clin Invest* 1983;72:1396–1409.

156. Aaron JE, Makins NB, Sagreiya K. The microanatomy of trabecular bone loss in normal and aging men and women. *Clin Orthop Rel Res* 1987;215:260–71.

157. Mellish RWE, Garrahan NJ, Compston JE. Age-related changes in trabecular width and spacing in human iliac crest bone biopsies. *Bone Miner* 1989;6:331–8.

158. Meunier PJ, Courpron P, Edouard C, Bernard J, Bringuier J, Vignon G. Physiological senile involution and pathological rarefaction of bone: quantitative and comparative histological data. *Clin Endocrinol Metab* 1973;2:239–56.

159. Fogelman I, Poser JW, Smith ML, Hart DM, Bevan JA. Alterations in skeletal metabolism following oophorectomy. In: Christiansen C, Arnaud CD, Nordin BEC, Parfitt AM, Peck WA, Riggs BL, eds. *Osteoporosis: Proceedings Copenhagen international symposium on osteoporosis.* Glostrup, Denmark: Aalborg Stiftsbogtrykkeri, 1984;519–21.

160. Heaney RP, Recker RR, Saville PD. Menopausal changes in bone remodeling. *J Lab Clin Invest* 1978;92:964–70.

161. Riggs BL, Jowsey J, Kelly PJ, Jones JD, Maher FT. Effect of sex hormones on bone in primary osteoporosis. *J Clin Invest* 1969;48:1065–72.

162. Lindsay R, Aitken JM, Anderson JB, Hart DM, MacDonald EB, Clark AC. Long-term prevention of postmenopausal osteoporosis by oestrogen. *Lancet* 1976;i:1038–41.

163. Horsman A, Gallagher JC, Simpson M, Nordin BEC. Prospective trial of estrogen and calcium in postmenopausal women. *Br Med J* 1977;2:789–92.

164. Lindsay R, Hart DM, Forrest C, Baird C. Prevention of spinal osteoporosis in oophorectomized women. *Lancet* 1980;ii:1151–4.

165. Melsen F, Mosekilde L, Eriksen EF, Charles P, Steinicke T. In vivo hormonal effects on trabecular bone remodeling osteoid mineralization and skeletal turnover. In: Kleerekoper M, Krane S, eds. *Clinical disorders of bone and mineral metabolism.* New York: Mary Ann Liebert, 1989;73–86.

166. Lips P, Courpron P, Meunier PJ. Mean wall thickness of trabecular bone packets in the human iliac crest: changes with age. *Calcif Tissue Res* 1978;26:13–7.

167. Kragstrup J, Melsen F, Mosekilde L. Thickness of bone formed at remodeling sites in normal human iliac trabecular bone: variations with age and sex. *Metab Bone Dis Relat Res* 1983;5:17–21.

168. Parfitt AM, Mathews CHE, Villanueva AR, et al. Microstructural and cellular basis of age related bone loss and osteoporosis. In: Frame B, Potts JT Jr, eds. *Clinical disorders of bone and mineral metabolism,* Amsterdam: Excerpta Medica, 1983;328–32.

169. Recker RR, Kimmel DB, Parfitt AM, Davies M, Keshawarz N, Hinders S. Static and tetracycline-based bone histomorphometric data from 34 normal postmenopausal females. *J Bone Miner Res* 1988;3:133–44.

170. Courpron P, Lepine P, Arlot M, Lips P, Meunier P. Mechanisms underlying the reduction with age of the mean wall thickness of the trabecular basic structural units (BSU) in human iliac bone. In: Jee WSS, Parfitt AM, eds. *Bone histomorphometry: 3rd international workshop.* Paris: Armour Montagu, 1981:323.

171. Croucher PT, Mellish REW, Vedi S, Garrahan J, Compston JE. The relationship between resorption depth and mean interstitial bone thickness: age-related changes in man. *Calcif Tissue Int* 1989;45:15–9.

172. Parfitt AM. Trabecular bone architecture in the pathogenesis and prevention of fracture. *Am J Med* 1987;82(suppl 1B):68–72.

173. Reeve J. Bone turnover and trabecular plate survival after artificial menopause. *Br Med J* 1987;295:757–60.
174. Eriksen EF, Melsen F, Mosekilde L. Reconstruction of the resorptive site in iliac trabecular bone: a kinetic model for bone resorption in 20 normal individuals. *Metab Bone Dis Relat Res* 1984;5:235–42.
175. Jaworski ZFG, Liskova-Kiar M, Uhthoff HK. Effect of long-term immobilization on the pattern of bone loss in older dogs. *J Bone Joint Surg* 1980;62B:104–19.
176. Matthews CHE, Aswani SP, Parfitt AM. Hypogravitational effects of hypodynamics on bone cell function and the dynamics of bone remodeling. In: *A 14-day ground-based hypokinesia study in non-human primates: a compilation of results.* NASA Technical Memorandum 81268, April 1981.
177. Parfitt AM, Duncan H. Metabolic bone disease affecting the spine. In: Rothman R, Simcone F, eds. *The spine,* 2nd ed. Philadelphia: WB Saunders, 1982;775–905.
178. Currey JD. Some effects of ageing in human Haversian systems. *J Anat (London),* 1964;98:69–75.
179. Kerley ER. The microscopic determinates of age in human bone. *Am J Phys Anthropol* 1976;23:149.
180. Evans FG. Age changes in mechanical properties and histology of human compact bone. *Yearb Phys Anthropol* 1977;20:57–72.
181. Stout S, Simmons DJ. Use of histology in ancient bone research. *Yearb Phys Anthropol* 1979;22:228–49.
182. Jowsey J. Age and species differences in bone. *Cornell Vet* 1968;58(suppl):74–94.
183. Martin RB, Picket JC, Zinaich S. Studies of skeletal remodeling in aging men. *Clin Orthop Relat Res* 1980;149:268–82.
184. Arnold JS, Bartley MH, Tont SA, Jenkins DP. Skeletal changes in aging and disease. *Clin Orthop Relat Res* 1966;49:17–38.
185. Jowsey J. Studies of Haversian systems in man and some animals. *J Anat* 1966;100:857–64.
186. Jaworski ZFG, Meunier P, Frost HM. Observations on 2 types of resorption cavities in human lamellar cortical bone. *Clin Orthop* 1972;83:279.
187. Ortner DJ. Aging effects on osteon remodeling. *Calcif Tissue Res* 1975;18:27–36.
188. Weinstein RS, Bell NJ. Diminished rates of bone formation in normal black adults. *N Engl J Med* 1988;319:1698–701.
189. Bell NH, Greene A, Epstein S, Oexmann MJ, Shaw S, Shary J. Evidence for alteration of the vitamin D–endocrine system in blacks. *J Clin Invest* 1985;75:470–3.
190. Trotter M, Broman GE, Peterson RR. Densities of bones of White and Negro skeletons. *J Bone Joint Surg* 1960;42A:50–8.
191. Smith RW Jr, Rizek J. Epidemiologic studies of osteoporosis in women of Puerto Rico and Southeastern Michigan with special reference to age, national origin and to other related or associated findings. *Clin Orthop* 1966;45:31–48.
192. Cohn SH, Abesamis C, Yasumura S, Aloia JF, Zanzi I, Ellis KJ. Comparative skeletal mass and radial bone mineral content in black and white women. *Metabolism* 1977;26:171–8.
193. Garn SM. The phenomenon of bone formation and bone loss. In: DeLuca HF, Frost HM, Jee WSS, Johnstone CC, Parfitt AM, eds. *Osteoporosis: recent advances in pathogenesis and treatment.* Baltimore: University Park Press, 1981.
194. Schnitzler CM, Pettifor JM, Mesquita JM, Bird MDT, Schnaid E, Smyth AE. Bone loss in blacks and whites: a unifying concept. *J Bone Miner Res* 1989;4(suppl 1):S414.
195. Parfitt AM. Overview: bone remodeling. In: Kleerekoper M, Krane S, eds. *Clinical disorders of bone and mineral metabolism.* New York: Mary Ann Liebert, 1989;45–8.
196. Dempster DW. The relationship between iliac crest bone biopsy and other skeletal sites. In: Kleerekoper M, Krane S, eds. *Clinical disorders of bone and mineral metabolism.* New York: Mary Ann Liebert, 1988.
197. Krempien B, Lemminger FM, Ritz E, Weber E. The reaction of different skeletal sites to metabolic bone disease: a micromorphometric study. *Klin Wochenschr* 1987;T56:755–9.
198. Podenphant J, Engel U. Regional variations in histomorphometric bone dynamics from the skeleton of an osteoporotic woman. *Calcif Tissue Int* 1987;40:184–8.

199. Enlow DH. The bone of reptiles. In Gans C, ed. *Biology of the reptilia.* New York: Academic Press, 1969;45–80.
200. Rubin CT, Lanyon LE. Regulation of bone mass by mechanical strain magnitude. *Calcif Tissue Int* 1988;37:411–7.
201. Belanger LF, Copp DH. The skeletal effects of prolonged calcitonin administration in birds, under various conditions. In: Talmage RV, Munson PL, eds. *Calcium, parathyroid hormone, and the calcitonins.* Amsterdam: Excerpta Medica, 1972;41–50.
202. Enlow DH, Brown SO. A comparative histological study of fossil and recent bone tissues. *Texas J Sci* Part 1, 1956;8:405–43. Part 2, 1957;9:186–214. Part 3, 1958;10:187–230.
203. Ruth EB. Bone studies. II. An experimental study of the Haversian-type vascular channels. *Am J Anat* 1953;93:429–55.
204. Baron R, Tross R, Vignery A. Evidence of sequential remodeling in rat trabecular bone: morphology, dynamic, histomorphometry and changes during skeletal maturation. *Anat Rec* 1984;208:137–45.
205. Faugere MC, Okamoto S, DeLuca HF, Malluche HH. Calcitriol corrects bone loss induced by oophorectomy in rats. *Am J Physiol* 1986;250:E35.
206. Wronski TJ, Cintron M, Dann LM. Temporal relationship between bone loss and increased bone turnover in ovariectomized rats. *Calcif Tissue Int* 1988;43:179–83.
207. Turner RT, Wakley GK, Hannon KS, Bell NH. Tamoxifen inhibits osteoclast-mediated resorption of trabecular bone in ovarian hormone-deficient rats. *Endocrinology* 1988;122:1146–50.
208. Thompson DD, Rodan GA. Indomethacin inhibition of tenotomy-induced bone resorption in rats. *J Bone Miner Res* 1988;3:409–14.
209. Kalu DN, Liu CC, Hardin RR, Hollis BW. The aged rat model of ovarian hormone deficiency bone loss. *Endocrinology* 1989;124:7–16.
210. Jee WSS, Bartley MH, Cooper RR, Dockum NL. Bone structure. In: Anderson AC, ed. *The beagle as an experimental dog.* Ames: The Iowa State University Press, 1970;162–88.
211. Marotti G. Map of bone formation rate values recorded throughout the skeleton of the dog. In: Jaworski ZFG, Zlosevych S, Cameron E, eds. *Proc. first workshop on bone morphometry.* Ottowa: University of Ottowa Press, 1976;202–7.
212. Norrin RW, Villafane FA, Lopresti CA. Haversian remodeling activity in various bones of beagles and the effect of chronic renal failure. In: Meunier P, ed. *Bone histomorphometry: 2nd international workshop.* Toulouse: Société de la Nouvelle Imprimirie, 1977;171–8.
213. Jaworski ZFG, Liskova-Kiar M, Uhtoff HK. Effect of long-term immobilization on the pattern of bone loss in older dogs. *J Bone Joint Surg* 1980;62B(1):104–10.
214. Malluche HH, Faugere MC, Friedler RM, Mathews C, Fanti P. Calcitriol, parathyroid hormone, and accumulation of aluminum in bone in dogs with renal failure. *J Clin Invest* 1987;79:754–61.
215. Malluche HH, Faugere MC, Friedler RM, Fauti P. 1,25-dihydroxyvitamin D_3 corrects bone loss but suppresses bone remodeling in ovariehysterectomized beagle dogs. *Endocrinology* 1988;122:1988–2006.
216. Currey JD. Differences in the tensile strength of bone of different histological types. *J Anat* 1959;93:87–95.
217. Murrills RJ, Shane E, Lindsay R, Dempster DW. Bone resorption by isolated human osteoclasts in vitro: effects of calcitonin. *J Bone Miner Res* 1989;4:259–68.
218. Dempster DW, Shane ES, Horbert W, Lindsay R. A simple method for correlative light and scanning electron microscopy of human iliac crest bone biopsies: qualitative observations in normal and osteoporotic subjects. *J Bone Miner Res* 1986;1:15–21.
219. Dempster DW, Elder HY, Smith DA. Scanning electron microscopy of rachitic rat bone. *Scanning Electron Microsc II* 1979;513–20.
220. Rasmussen H, Bordier P. *The physiology and cellular basis of metabolic bone disease.* Baltimore: Williams & Wilkins, 1974.
221. Dempster DW. Adult bone remodeling. In: Canfield REC, ed. *The pathophysiological basis of metabolic bone diseases and their therapies.* New York: Columbia University Press, 1985:13–29.

PART III

Mineral Metabolism During the Human Life Cycle

Disorders of Bone and Mineral Metabolism,
edited by Fredric L. Coe and Murray J. Favus,
© 1992 by Raven Press, Ltd. All rights reserved.

CHAPTER 16

Mineral Metabolism During Pregnancy and Lactation

Russell W. Chesney, Bonny L. Specker, Francis Mimouni, and Charles P. McKay

GESTATION

An increased need for calcium and phosphorus prevails during pregnancy to meet the requirements for fetal bone mineral accretion and to maintain normal serum concentrations of these divalent minerals in the mother. The transfer of calcium and phosphorus from the mother to the fetus is the major event in mineral metabolism during pregnancy. The endocrine and nutritional process which maintains maternal serum calcium and phosphorus concentrations in the face of massive significant mineral transfer interests both reproductive physiologists and scholars who study disorders of bone and mineral metabolism. This chapter examines the normal physiology of mineral metabolism during pregnancy, emphasizing and examining separately the three components of the maternal–placental–fetal unit and during lactation to indicate how an interplay among the three components permits normal mineral balance and mineralization of fetal bone.

The Mother

Skeletal Changes During Pregnancy

The maternal skeleton is a potential source of mineral for the fetus during pregnancy. Fetal calcium accumulation during human pregnancy reaches approximately 25 g at term, with the greatest transfer to the fetus occurring after 35–36 weeks of gestation (1). Estimates of total maternal calcium accumulation approach 30 g at term, and thus a "cushion" of 5 g or more is evident (2). However,

because most calcium accumulated in pregnancy is absorbed by the fetus and because fetal calcium is derived only from maternal intestinal calcium absorption or maternal bone mineral, the maternal skeleton is at potential risk for demineralization, although the effect of pregnancy on maternal bone mineral status is uncertain.

First, the amount of calcium and phosphorus accumulation during pregnancy only amounts to 2.5% and 3.5%, respectively, of total human maternal body content (2). Thus, any method of measuring maternal bone status needs to be precise to reveal more than small differences. Second, maternal mineral accumulation occurs earlier (20–24 weeks of pregnancy) than the period of significant fetal skeletal accretion (3). Third, bone mineral status during pregnancy shows interspecies differences. For example, rats appear to store calcium in bone during pregnancy (4) or have no change in bone calcium content from the nonpregnant state as late as 18 or 20 days gestation, just prior to delivery (5). In sheep, bone mineral resorption begins after day 65 of gestation (normal pregnancy is 140 days), at which time the rate of mineral transfer from the ewe to the fetus accelerates (6). These differences may be related to certain properties of the rodent and ovine skeleton, since bone mineral accretion occurs throughout the lifetime of the rat, mouse, or guinea pig, whereas the ovine, lagomorph, and human skeleton reach peak bone mass at the time of epiphyseal closure (7).

In some species, dietary calcium has been shown to influence maternal bone mineral status. A calcium-deficient diet fed to a pregnant rat reduces the ash content of the maternal long bones (8,9). Near term, when the metacarpal and metatarsal bones were examined in goats ingesting a low-calcium diet, significant bone demineralization was evident (10). Thus, when calcium intake is inadequate, fetal demands may outstrip the calcium

R. W. Chesney and C. P. McKay: Department of Pediatrics, University of Tennessee, Memphis College of Medicine, Memphis, Tennessee 38103.
B. L. Specker, and F. Mimouni: Department of Pediatrics, College of Medicine, University of Cincinnati Medical Center, Cincinnati, Ohio, 45267–0541.

available from intestinal absorption, forcing the reservoir of the maternal skeleton to be utilized.

Changes in Mineral Metabolism During Pregnancy

Because pregnant animals transfer substantial amounts of calcium via the placenta, changes in mineral metabolism are required to meet fetal demands. Calcium absorption from the intestine increases during pregnancy in many mammalian species by an increase in the efficiency of calcium active transport (2). Although the mechanisms of this augmentation in calcium uptake are discussed later, the influence on maternal serum calcium and phosphorus concentration are noteworthy. Human maternal serum calcium concentration falls during pregnancy, reaching a nadir at 30–34 weeks (11,12). Thereafter, serum calcium rises slightly until term (40 weeks). Since serum albumin concentration also falls in pregnancy because of the increase in plasma volume attendant with this state, it is noteworthy that the pattern of the change in serum calcium concentration parallels serum albumin (12). The decline in serum calcium during pregnancy is in the protein-bound fraction, and the ionized fraction remains normal during pregnancy (13). This same decline in protein-bound calcium late in pregnancy occurs in both rats (14) and rabbits (10).

Plasma phosphate concentration falls in the third trimester in human (11), rabbit (10), and ovine (2) pregnancy. Because a diurnal variation in serum phosphate concentration exists and diet affects the concentration of phosphate in plasma, studies of serum phosphate may be difficult to interpret.

Integration of Mineral Metabolism During Pregnancy

Role of Kidney in the Control of Mineral Metabolism

The plasma concentrations of both calcium and phosphate, as well as total body pool size, can be regulated in part by urinary excretion. (The mechanisms of renal calcium and phosphate handling are described elsewhere in this volume.) Urinary calcium excretion is determined by the amount of calcium absorbed by the intestine, the filtered calcium load (which depends on the ionized and bound level in plasma), and the circulating concentrations of parathyroid hormone and calcitonin. An increase in circulating 1α-25-dihydroxyvitamin D_3 [$1,25(OH)_2D_3$] and in the rate of intestinal calcium absorption have been observed in some mammalian pregnancies (2). These changes have been regarded as a compensatory mechanism to meet fetal mineral needs. An alternate possibility is that these adjustments anticipate third-trimester fetal demands (13). From recent data in humans, circulating $1,25(OH)_2D_3$ values are elevated throughout pregnancy (i.e., in each trimester), and uri-

nary calcium excretion is also increased throughout pregnancy. In the Gertner et al. (13) study, an oral calcium tolerance test was followed by a hypercalciuric response after a standard calcium load, which supports absorptive (or hyperabsorption of calcium in the intestine, which leads to hypercalcemia) hypercalciuria. These findings are consistent with normal pregnancy being a state of physiologic absorptive hypercalciuria wherein 24-h calcium excretion levels are found to range widely between 50 and 700 mg/24 h (13).

Urinary calcium excretion is also increased in rats from the second week of pregnancy (14,15) and is also higher in ovine pregnancy (2); however, the latter situation is less clear than in humans or the rodent.

Urinary calcium excretion in women with preeclampsia is only 15–25% of that found in normal control pregnant subjects. In pregnant women with preeclampsia, hypocalciuria is probably due to increased tubular reabsorption of calcium; plasma concentrations of $1,25(OH)_2D_3$, calcium, and phosphate are not different between normal and preeclamptic women (16).

Urine phosphate excretion appears to be slightly higher during human pregnancy than during nonpregnancy, because in the former the renal threshold is lower (from 3.8 ± 0.1 to 3.2 ± 0.2 mg/dL) (13); however, since plasma phosphate concentrations are lower in the former than in the latter, overt phosphaturia is not evident.

Role of the Intestine

Intestinal hyperabsorption of calcium during pregnancy is found in many mammalian species, with the greatest increase in absorption occurring late in pregnancy (2). While ingesting a low-calcium diet, both rats and ewes have increased absorption. Using a combination of isotope absorption techniques and balance studies, calcium absorption was increased only in the last 3 days before term in rats (15) but was increased throughout pregnancy in ewes (6). When the everted gut-sacs technique is used to measure calcium transfer, a marked increase in duodenal and proximal jejunal uptake is noted (17,18). Similar results were evident using an in vivo perfusion technique (19) in humans in which the stable isotope ^{48}Ca was used in pregnant women; a twofold increase in calcium absorption was noted at 20–24 weeks and remained elevated throughout the remainder of pregnancy.

When the levels of the intestinal vitamin-D-dependent protein, calbindin, were measured in pregnant rats, they were elevated (20,21). This increase in calbindin in rat intestine appears to occur between days 17.5 and 19.5 of pregnancy (20). Calbindin is also a calcium-binding protein that appears to be involved in active calcium transport in the intestine.

Hormones Regulating Mineral Homeostasis

Because plasma calcium concentrations are regulated by the vitamin D endocrine system, it is necessary to understand the influence of pregnancy on several hormones, such as parathyroid hormone (PTH), calcitonin (CT), and the vitamin D metabolite, $1,25(OH)_2D_3$.

PTH

Human pregnancy is associated with increased serum concentrations of PTH during the latter half of pregnancy (22). Pitkin (23) observed that increased PTH secretion is the appropriate maternal response to expansion of the extracellular fluid space, increased urinary calcium excretion, and transfer of this divalent mineral across the placenta. Several groups reported an increase in circulating PTH values, but some groups reported this finding only in the third trimester (24) while other groups reported either no change or a reduction (2). Although these discrepant results may represent differences in the PTH antibody used, many of these studies are performed without regard to dietary calcium intake, parity, or other factors that theoretically could influence hormone secretion.

Studies indicate an abrupt rise in PTH values in pregnant cows at the time of parturition (25), as discussed below. Hyporesponsiveness of the parathyroid gland may play an important role in parturient paresis in dairy cows that have an enormous increase in calcium demands as a result of lactational needs (2). The plasma concentration of PTH in other animals, including deer (26) and rats (27), also rises in the third trimester.

Thyroparathyroidectomy of pregnant rats results in a decline in serum calcium of 2.7 mg/dL, with tetanic death in 40% of experimental animals at the onset of fetal ossification (17.5 days). Other evidence of an increased need for PTH in late pregnancy is the increased parathyroid gland size found in several mammalian species (2). Thyroparathyroidectomy of pregnant rats also reduces circulating $1,25(OH)_2D_3$ concentrations by 50% and reduces intestinal calbindin values, thus supporting the importance of PTH in pregnancy (29). During human pregnancy, both the plasma concentrations of PTH and of free (non-protein-bound) $1,25(OH)_2D_3$ appear to rise simultaneously between weeks 36 and 40 of gestation (2). Maternal bone ash content does not appear to be reduced after thyroparathyroidectomy in rats (30).

Vitamin D

Because of the role of $1,25(OH)_2D_3$ in the maintenance of calcium and phosphorus homeostasis and because of its pivotal position in the vitamin D endocrine system (2), the importance of this "vitamin" during pregnancy is obvious. As recognized previously, pregnancy places a demand on maternal calcium and phosphorus metabolism because of fetal bone mineral accretion. The mother meets this demand by an augmentation of intestinal calcium absorption, which probably depends on the action of circulating $1,25(OH)_2D_3$ on intestinal receptors.

Pregnancy seems to have little influence on the circulating values of 25-hydroxyvitamin D_3 [$25(OH)D_3$] as noted by Reynolds et al. (30). Maternal plasma $1,25(OH)_2D_3$ concentrations are elevated during pregnancy in humans and other mammalian species (31–43). The concentrations of $1,25(OH)_2D_3$ double to the 75- to 125-pg/mL range during pregnancy as noted above, but factors regulating this increase in hormone synthesis are uncertain. A host of possible factors include PTH, prolactin, growth hormone, and estrogen, although none of these have been shown unequivocally to regulate $1,25(OH)_2D_3$ synthesis during pregnancy (2,30). Finally, as shown below, the placenta of humans and other species is capable of synthesizing $1,25(OH)_2D_3$ by a process whose regulation is incompletely understood.

Plasma concentrations of $24,25(OH)_2D_3$ are reduced in pregnancy in both humans (44) and rodents (45), but the significance of these changes is unclear.

All molecular forms of vitamin D are transported in blood by a 58-kD globulin called "vitamin-D-binding protein" (DBP). The concentration of DBP increases during pregnancy (46). Hence, total $1,25(OH)_2D_3$ concentrations in plasma reflect, in part, this increased availability of its binding protein. Because $1,25(OH)_2D_3$ can exist in blood bound to DBP or free, the circulating value for free hormone depends on the concentration of DBP. During pregnancy in humans, the greatest increase in DBP occurs between weeks 10 and 20; in addition, the free $1,25(OH)_2D_3$:DBP index [$1,25(OH)_2D_3$:DBP ratio] remains constant up to 35 weeks of pregnancy (46). After this time, the free $1,25(OH)_2D_3$ index increases (38,46). A major determinant of $1,25(OH)_2D_3$ concentration is the activity of maternal kidney $25(OH)D-1\alpha$-hydroxylase, which is above that found in nongravid kidney (47). No study to date in humans has measured the influence of maternal kidney production of $1,25(OH)_2D_3$ in relation to this increase in its plasma concentrations.

Placental $25(OH)D-1\alpha$-hydroxylase activity has been detected in a number of species, including rat (48), guinea pig (47), and human (49). Fetal kidney can also produce the $1,25(OH)_2D_3$. Fetal $25(OH)D-1\alpha$-hydroxylase activity has been found in rabbit (50), guinea pig (47), rat (51), and pig (52). Hence, the source of the increase in circulating concentrations of $1,25(OH)_2D_3$ could arise from at least three sites. Which source of hormone is dominant is unclear. The human fetus is clearly capable of $1,25(OH)_2D_3$ synthesis, because umbilical arterial values for the hormone are greater than those from umbilical venous sampling (35).

In utero fetal nephrectomy in sheep also reduces

plasma 1,25(OH)$_2$D$_3$ concentrations (41). A simultaneously integrated overview of the rates of 25(OH)D-1α-hydroxylase activity in maternal kidney, placenta, and fetal kidney has been conducted only in guinea pig (47) and rat (52). Activity of 25(OH)D-1α-hydroxylase is greater in all three sites during pregnancy than in the nonpregnant adult guinea-pig kidney (47). In rat studies in which a cell culture system of maternal and fetal kidney and placenta were used, placental tissue appeared to have the greatest activity (52).

The physiological necessity for the availability of vitamin D has been evaluated using the vitamin-D-deficient rat model (53,54). Vitamin-D-deficient animals fed a conventional calcium and phosphorus diet were capable of reproduction, but their fertility rate was reduced by 75% and litter size by 30%. Although these rat mothers were completely vitamin-D-deficient and had nondetectable serum vitamin D levels, intestinal calcium absorption increased during pregnancy when compared to that in the nongravid state (18). It has been postulated that pregnancy-related intestinal hypertrophy may be responsible for this augmentation in calcium transport.

The increase in intestinal calcium transport in normal pregnancy depends on 1,25(OH)$_2$D$_3$, but some vitamin-D-independent factors are important in the vitamin-D-deficient rat (54).

Vitamin-D-deficient pregnant rats can maintain normal serum calcium levels. Indeed, the level actually rose from 5.5 to 6.7 mg/dL during the first 17 days of pregnancy, in contrast to the slight decline in vitamin-D-repleted animals (54). As anticipated serum PTH concentrations were elevated in these vitamin-D-deficient rats, but the precise mechanism of these increases in serum calcium concentration is unclear.

A histomorphometric examination of bones from vitamin-D-deficient pregnant rats demonstrates metaphyseal hypomineralization and epiphyseal size reduction (55). Femoral diaphyseal hypomineralization, as evidence of alterations in cortical bone mineral content, is also evident. Presumably the increase in serum calcium reported by Tuan (56) is related to bone resorption as demonstrated in this histomorphometric study (55).

In a recent study, urinary calcium excretion (Fig. 1) was not different in a group of healthy women when examined in third-trimester pregnancy and during lactation (57). The elevation of circulating 1,25(OH)$_2$D$_3$ concentrations (Fig. 2) and endogenous creatinine clearance (Fig. 3) was evident in the third trimester of pregnancy, as noted by others (2,10). An important finding of this study is that the positive correlation between fasting urinary calcium:creatinine ratio (assumed to be indicative of bone resorption in normal humans and hypoparathyroid subjects) and plasma 1,25(OH)$_2$D$_3$ concentrations was not found during pregnancy but was evident during lactation. Hence, it was speculated that during

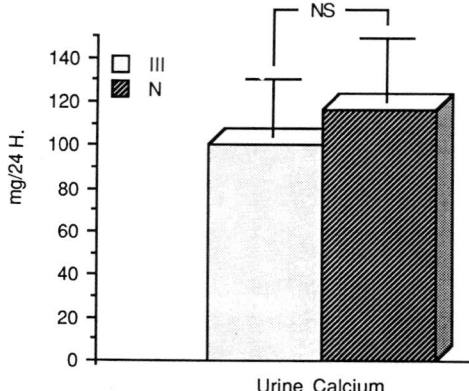

FIG. 1. Urinary calcium excretion in 13 healthy women during the third trimester of pregnancy (III) and during 6 weeks after delivery when they are nursing (N). [Data derived from Bruns et al. (66).]

pregnancy the maternal skeleton is protected against the high serum 1,25(OH)$_2$D$_3$ values.

To conclude, in terms of vitamin D metabolism, an increase in 1,25(OH)$_2$D$_3$ in plasma, arising possibly from the maternal kidney and the placenta, leads to increased intestinal calcium absorption. The higher degree of calcium absorption results in the availability of calcium needed to maintain maternal skeleton and plasma mineral concentration and to meet fetal calcium needs.

Calcitonin (CT)

Theoretically, pregnancy should be associated with an increase in serum CT values so as to protect the maternal skeleton against bone resorption (23). Several groups (2,23,58) have reported elevated CT values during human pregnancy, whereas others (23) have reported that values remain unchanged. The jugular venous plasma CT values in pregnant ewes are higher in the last 2 months of gestation (59); CT values are the highest in ewes bearing triplets, in whom the rate of placental calcium transfer is quite high. CT values are high in the third trimester of rats (60) and are elevated throughout pregnancy in deer (26).

A study examining hormonal responsiveness (i.e., a change from baseline after an EDTA challenge) in pregnant rhesus monkeys showed reduced PTH responsiveness and increased CT response in the pregnant state as compared to control monkeys (30). This situation clearly favors preservation of the maternal skeleton under conditions of hypocalcemia, while permitting skeletal calcium storage when hypercalcemia is evident. In a separate study, bone is demineralized in CT-deficient pregnant goats whether fed a normal or high-calcium diet (10,59). In these goats, both plasma and urinary calcium concentrations are elevated, as is the degree of fecal

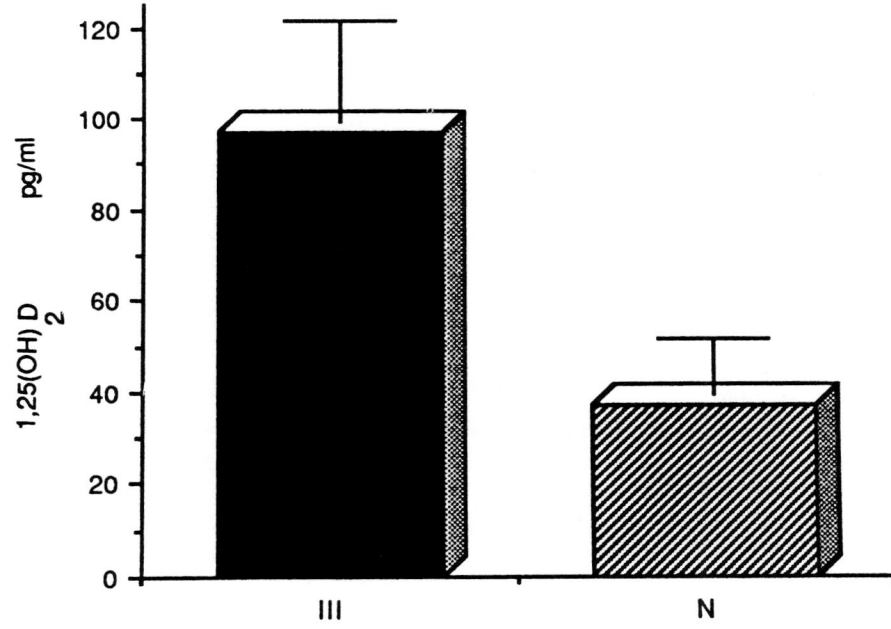

FIG. 2. Serum 1,25(OH)D$_2$ concentration in 13 healthy women during the third trimester of pregnancy (III) and 6 weeks after delivery when they are nursing (N). [Data derived from Bruns et al. (66).]

calcium excretion, supporting the role of CT during pregnancy.

The Placenta

The precise mechanisms of placental calcium transport and their regulation have been the object of extensive research in the past 20 years. Because of the relative inaccessibility of the placenta and the fetus during human pregnancy, most studies in vivo have been done using various animal models; that is, the rat, guinea pig, sheep, or the rhesus monkey. In all these species, net maternofetal transfer of Ca increases dramatically in the last third of pregnancy (61,62). From studying the body composition of the human fetus, it was found that about

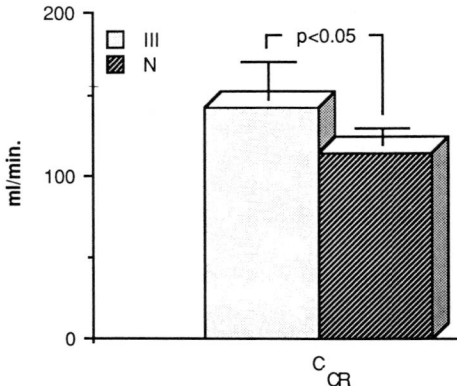

FIG. 3. Creatinine clearance in 13 healthy women during the third trimester of pregnancy (III) and while they are nursing (N) [Data derived from Bruns et al. (66).]

two-thirds of the average 28 g of calcium accreted by the fetus in a term pregnancy are accumulated during the third trimester of pregnancy (61). In the following subsections we summarize the evidence indicating that (a) placental transport of calcium is active, (b) bidirectional fluxes of calcium travel through the placenta, and (c) a calcium-binding protein and an ATPase might be involved; in addition, we review the possible mechanisms of placental calcium transport regulation.

Placental Transport of Calcium Is Active

In humans and animals, from midpregnancy, fetal serum calcium concentrations are elevated above maternal concentrations (63). Maternal–fetal transport, in this circumstance, would not be through passive transport mechanism. From studies of placental calcium transport in situ in the rat, it appears that the maternal–fetal clearance of radiolabeled calcium is significantly higher than that of molecules such as sucrose, which, because of its inert, electrically neutral, and hydrophilic properties, is believed to cross the placenta by passive diffusion through water-filled channels (64). Furthermore, metabolic inhibitors such as dinitrophenol or cyanide, known to inhibit active transport mechanisms, significantly decrease placental calcium transport (64).

Bidirectional Fluxes of Calcium Travel Across the Placenta

From studies using radioactive calcium tracers, it appears that part of the calcium crossing the placenta towards the fetus will "back flow" to the mother (65). However, the magnitude of this backflow is considerably different from one species to another: This backflow is approximately 5% of the calcium transported to the fetus in the sheep but is approximately 80% in the rhesus monkey (65).

Involvement of a Calcium-Binding Protein and ATPases

A calcium-binding protein (CaBP) has been isolated in the rat (20,66), mouse (67), and human placenta (56). A role for the involvement of the CaBP in placental calcium transport has been suggested from experiments, showing that uptake of calcium by human placental microsomal membrane vesicles is inhibited by antihuman CaBP antibodies (56). In the rat, the placental CaBP has the same immunological properties as the intestinal one (66). However, in contrast to that of the intestinal CaBP, the regulation of placental CaBP synthesis by 1,25-dihydroxyvitamin D [1,25(OH)$_2$D] is less certain (29,67).

Several ATPases have been localized in various subcellular fractions of the placenta: There is a Ca^{2+},Mg^{2+}-dependent, a Ca^{2+}-dependent, and an Na$^+$,K$^+$-dependent ATPase (68,69). Their relative role in placental calcium transport is unclear and is the object of extensive investigations. Nevertheless, these enzymes could play a determining role in the provision of energy required for the active transport of calcium (69).

Regulation of Placental Calcium Transport

Uteroplacental Blood Flow

Neonatal bone mineral content is low in infants who are small for their gestational age (SGA), as compared to infants of appropriate weight for the time of gestation (70). These infants are believed to have suffered from relative "placental insufficiency." In the Wigglesworth rat model, in which uterine arteries are ligated on day 17 of gestation, net placental calcium transport in situ is significantly reduced by day 20–21 of gestation (71). It could be concluded from the above that changes in uterine blood flow may regulate placental calcium transport, but it is also possible that in both SGA infants and Wigglesworth rats, chronic placental energy deprivation (i.e., deprivation of substrates such as glucose, or O$_2$ deprivation) may impair the active mechanism of placental calcium transport, regardless of the changes in uteroplacental blood flow (71).

Maternal Serum Calcium Concentration

In human pregnancy, infants born to hypercalcemic mothers suffer neonatal hypocalcemia due to transient fetal and neonatal hypoparathyroidism (72). Furthermore, infants born to hypocalcemic mothers may suffer significant bone loss due to the development of transient fetal and neonatal hyperparathyroidism (73). From the above situations, it is generally assumed that the fetus of the hypercalcemic mother is probably hypercalcemic in

utero, and the fetus of the hypocalcemic mother is probably hypocalcemic as well. The effects of acute or chronic changes of maternal serum calcium concentrations on maternal–fetal calcium transport have been studied in various species and have led to conflicting results: In some species, maternal changes of serum calcium led to parallel changes of fetal calcium whereas in others (such as the rat) there was very little or no effect of maternal changes in serum calcium on placental calcium transport (74–79). These species variations remain to be explained.

Hormonal Regulation

From animal experiments, 1,25(OH)$_2$D, PTH, and CT have all been suggested as hormonal regulators of placental calcium transport. 1,25(OH)$_2$D has been studied both by experiments of maternal pharmacological administration of 1,25(OH)$_2$D (80) and by experiments involving maternal vitamin D deficiency (81,82) or fetal nephrectomy (41,83). Results are conflicting, and there is no conclusive evidence that 1,25(OH)$_2$D increases placental calcium transport. Furthermore, the observation that placental CaBP concentration is increased by 1,25(OH)$_2$D administration has not been confirmed in the majority by investigators (20,29).

A role for fetal PTH has been suggested by studies that show a reduction of placenta calcium transport across the placentas of rat fetuses parathyroidectomized by decapitation (84). This reduction is partly corrected by PTH administration to the fetus as well as by an adenylate activator (i.e., forskolin) (84). Some investigators also suggested that the PTH-related peptide, a PTH-like substance secreted by some tumors, might be secreted by the fetus (85) and might increase placental calcium transport (86).

The Fetus

Serum concentrations of minerals and calciotropic hormones exhibit a pattern which is unique to the fetus and which seems to be directed toward a single goal: enhancing mineral accretion in bone. Indeed, human cord blood (presumed to give an accurate picture of the intrauterine milieu) contains very high concentrations of calcium and phosphate as compared to maternal values (87); bone resorptive hormones [i.e., PTH and 1,25(OH)$_2$D] have relatively low cord blood concentrations as compared to maternal concentrations (32,88,89); and CT, known to oppose PTH action at the bone, has relatively high cord blood concentrations (90,91). In addition, serum 24,25(OH)$_2$D concentrations are relatively high at birth (92), and this vitamin D metabolite theoretically might also have anabolic actions on bone growth (93). This unique biological milieu, combined with the active transport of calcium across the placenta, might explain the massive rate of net calcium accretion observed in the third trimester of pregnancy, estimated to be up to 150 mg/kg of fetal weight per day in the human (61).

PARTURITION

Changes in Mother and Mineral Balance

At parturition, the greatest demand for calcium comes from the stress of lactation (8). This is especially true in cows, all of which become transiently hypocalcemic. Certain cows remain hypocalcemic and develop the disorder known as "parturient paresis." This transient hypocalcemia can also be seen in goats (10) and mares. The reasons for parturient paresis are still uncertain, because bovine intestinal calcium absorption is increased (94), increased PTH secretion is evident (95), and abnormalities in calcitonin secretion are not evident (2). The serum concentrations of $1,25(OH)_2D_3$ concentrations rise (96). The idea that diminished bone resorption may account for paresis has arisen as a result of the finding that low-calcium diets, which stimulate PTH secretion and $1,25(OH)_2D_3$ synthesis, appear to substantially protect against paresis (97). A greater dependence on skeletal calcium mobilization rather than on intestinal calcium absorption may be the reason that low-calcium diets prevent paresis. Conversely, a high-calcium diet suppressed both PTH secretion and bone resorption (98,99).

LACTATION

Hormonal Changes During Lactation

Maternal losses of calcium and phosphorus through breast milk during 9 months of lactation are four times greater than during 9 months of pregnancy (100). The mother, therefore, theoretically may adapt to these increased calcium losses, apparently through increased intestinal calcium absorption, decreased renal calcium excretion, and increased mobilization of calcium from bone. Under normal circumstances, the active metabolite of vitamin D (1,25-dihydroxyvitamin D [$1,25(OH)_2D$]) increases the efficiency of intestinal absorption of calcium and phosphorus, appears to cause renal retention of these elements, and, in concert with PTH, mobilizes calcium from bone; hence, elevations of $1,25(OH)_2D$ are thought to be the prime calcium-related adaptive response during lactation.

Serum $1,25(OH)_2D$ and PTH concentrations have been previously reported to be elevated during lactation in rats (45,101). A lower serum calcium concentration also is observed (45) and is thought to be related to the efflux of calcium out of blood and into milk. This drain on the blood's calcium pool theoretically might cause an increase in PTH secretion and subsequent stimulation of the renal 1α-hydroxylase activity, resulting in an increase in serum $1,25(OH)_2D$ concentrations. However, this cascade of events appears insufficient to maintain serum calcium concentrations in the lactating rat at the same level as in nonlactating rats; furthermore, when injections of high doses of PTH are given to lactating rats, no increase in serum calcium concentration has been observed (102).

Increased CT secretion during lactation has been suggested to be responsible for the decreased serum calcium concentrations during this period. Toverud et al. (102) found that when PTH was administered to both lactating and nonlactating thyroparathyroidectomized (and thus, CT-deficient) rats, serum calcium concentrations were markedly increased. Their data support the hypothesis that the hypocalcemia observed in lactating rats is not due to PTH unresponsiveness or PTH insufficiency, but that CT has a major influence on maintaining low serum calcium concentrations. It therefore appears that a major stimulus to increased PTH and $1,25(OH)_2D$ production in lactation is reduced serum calcium: The cause of this reduction may be related to increased CT production, since serum CT concentrations after feeding are higher, and the postprandial CT increase greater, in lactating rats than in nonlactating rats (102). However, this increase in CT appears to be insufficient to protect the animal from the bone loss observed during lactation. In thyroidectomized lactating rats (who are CT-deficient), the decrease in bone weight is of magnitude similar to that among nonmated thyroidectomized rats, supporting the concept that CT does not play a special role in bone preservation during lactation (103).

The calcium loss per kilogram of body weight in lactating rats is approximately 60 times that of lactating women (39), and changes observed in the calcitropic hormones during rat lactation are not consistently observed during human lactation. Serum calcium concentrations are not decreased during human lactation and have even been found to be elevated in women nursing twins (104). Human data on serum $1,25(OH)_2D$ concentrations during lactation also are conflicting. In a longitudinal study of 18 women, Greer et al. (105) found only slight increases in serum $1,25(OH)_2D$ after 6 months of lactation. In this study, since serum PTH concentrations actually decreased during lactation, PTH was presumably not the stimulus causing increased serum $1,25(OH)_2D$ concentrations. In another study, no differences in serum $1,25(OH)_2D$ concentrations at 6 weeks postpartum were observed in 28 lactating women when compared to 20 nonlactating women (106).

Cundy et al. (107) studied a hypoparathyroid woman during lactation and found that serum $1,25(OH)_2D$ and calcium concentrations were maintained within the normal range without exogenous $1,25(OH)_2D$ treatment, as long as lactation was maintained. A negative correlation between exogenous 1,25(OH)$_2$D requirement and serum prolactin concentrations was observed, and the researchers speculated that the lactation-associated increase in serum 1,25(OH)$_2$D results from a PTH-independent mechanism, possibly from prolactin stimulating the 1α-hydroxylase. Human data on PTH concentrations during lactation also are conflicting. Although PTH concentrations are elevated during lactation in rats and have been thought to represent a state of physiological hyperparathyroidism in humans (108), most studies of women nursing single infants have found either no (39,106,109) or only a slight (110) increase. In Greer et al.'s (105) longitudinal study, as mentioned, serum PTH concentrations actually decreased.

Serum CT concentrations have not been found to be increased during lactation in most human studies (105,106). However, Greer et al. (104) reported increases in 1,25(OH)$_2$D, PTH, and CT concentrations in women nursing twins when compared with women nursing single infants. In women nursing single infants, daily calcium losses are estimated to be approximately 220–340 mg, and the losses theoretically are double in women nursing twins. Thus, it appears that given enough "stress," in the form of calcium losses, several calcium regulatory hormone responses in humans during lactation become apparent.

Calcium Absorption During Lactation

One reason for discrepancies in human studies could be variations in maternal diet. In none of these previous studies was the relationship between dietary intake and calcitropic hormones investigated. Restriction of dietary calcium in lactating rats results in a large increase in serum PTH concentrations (111). Intestinal absorption of calcium during lactation also appears to be increased in rats (18,112); however, 1,25(OH)$_2$D does not seem to be responsible for this increase in absorption in rats. Boass et al. (112) found intestinal calcium absorption in the vitamin-D-depleted and vitamin-D-repleted lactating rats to be similar to one another, and both conditions had higher calcium absorption than did the vitamin-D-repleted nonlactating rat. Both intestinal and serum 1,25(OH)$_2$D concentrations were higher in vitamin-D-repleted lactating rats compared to either vitamin-D-depleted lactating or vitamin-D-repleted nonlactating rats. It has been suggested that prolactin may be responsible for the increase in calcium absorption observed in rat lactation (113).

In humans, results from a recent cross-sectional study indicate that lactating women who consume a strict vegetarian diet with low calcium intake have elevated serum 1,25(OH)$_2$D concentrations when compared to lactating women consuming an omnivorous diet (110). Maternal dietary calcium, therefore, might modify the hormonal response to lactation. In this study, however, no effect of diet on serum PTH concentrations was observed. It is unclear how these changes in the calciotropic hormones will influence the calcium balance of the human mother. The role of prolactin on calcium absorption during human lactation also is not clear. In studies with patients who have hyperprolactinemia, intestinal absorption of calcium, using dual isotopes, has been found to be similar to that of control patients who do not have hyperprolactinemia (114).

Urinary Calcium Excretion During Lactation

Urinary calcium loss in lactating rats is small (1%) relative to the amount lost daily in milk. In the human, however, the amount of calcium lost in urine daily is approximately the same as that lost in milk; therefore, small changes in urinary calcium excretion can result in significant changes in the net calcium balance. 1,25(OH)$_2$D and PTH may increase renal reabsorption of calcium. A lower urinary loss of calcium has been observed in lactating rats when compared with nonlactating rats (115); urinary calcium loss was lower in lactating rats on a low-calcium diet than in lactating rats on a high-calcium diet. Based on preliminary findings, a similar effect of decreased urinary calcium excretion has been observed in lactating humans (116).

Bone Calcium During Lactation

Lactating rats that receive an adequate amount of calcium intake have a reduction in bone mass of 15–35% of their skeletal mineral, with the percent of loss of ultradistal (trabecular) bone being greater than that of cortical bone (55). In rats fed diets exceedingly low in calcium, up to 50% of skeletal mineral is lost during lactation. During lactation, the amounts of bone mineral lost by vitamin-D-deficient rats are similar to the amounts lost by vitamin-D-repleted rats, suggesting that 1,25(OH)$_2$D does not protect against mineral loss in the lactating rat. Brommage and DeLuca (117) observed that the decreased bone mineral content in adrenalectomized or oophorectomized lactating rats was similar to that in intact lactating rats, suggesting that lactation-induced bone loss in the rat is not caused by an adrenal or ovarian factor. Findings from a study by Pahuja and DeLuca (118) indicate that prolactin may act independently of vitamin D and PTH in stimulating the release of calcium and phosphorus from bone.

Bone loss studied in lactating women has resulted in conflicting findings. No effect has been observed in the mid-forearm bone mass of women nursing single infants for 6 months (119,120). Wardlaw and Pike (121), however, observed a loss of ultradistal (trabecular) bone after long-term (average of 11 months) lactation. Chan et al.

(120) also reported a decrease in midshaft bone mineral content of lactating adolescents, who are theoretically at increased nutritional demand for their own growth and maturation.

In summary, our understanding of calcium homeostasis during lactation is not complete and appears to involve many hormonal controls. There are differences between animals and humans in calcium losses per body weight, in calcitropic hormonal responses, and perhaps in different effects of prolactin on calcium metabolism. Further investigations of calcium metabolism during human lactation might help clarify some of the apparent discrepancies.

ACKNOWLEDGMENTS

This work was supported, in part, by: NIH grant DK37223-06; Le Bonheur Chair of Excellence in Pediatrics funds from the Department of Pediatrics, the University of Tennessee, Memphis; and the Perinatal Research Institute.

REFERENCES

1. Givens MH, Macy IG. The chemical composition of the human fetus. *J Biol Chem* 1933;102:7–17.
2. Garel JM. Hormonal control of calcium metabolism during the reproductive cycle in mammals. *Physiol Rev* 1987;67:1–66.
3. Heaney RP, Skillman TG. Calcium metabolism in normal human pregnancy. *J Clin Endocrinol Metab* 1971;33:661–70.
4. Ellinger GM, Duckworth J, Dalgarno AC, Quenouille MH. Skeletal changes during pregnancy and lactation in the rats: effect of different levels of dietary calcium. *Br J Nutr* 1952;6:235–53.
5. Halloran BP, DeLuca HF. Skeletal changes during pregnancy and lactation: the role of vitamin D. *Endocrinology* 1980; 107:1923–9.
6. Braithwaite GD, Glascock RF, Riazuddin S. Calcium metabolism in pregnant ewes. *Br J Nutr* 1970;24:661–70.
7. Gilsanz V, Roe TF, Gibbens DT, Schultz EE, Carlson ME, Gonalez O, Boechat MI. Effect of sex steroids on peak bone density of growing rabbits. *Am J Physiol* 1988;255:E416–21.
8. Rasmussen P. Calcium deficiency, pregnancy, and lactation in rats. *Calcif Tissue Res* 1977;23:87–94.
9. Bawden JW, McIver FT. Distribution of Ca^{45} during pregnancy under conditions of calcium deficiency in rats. *J Dent Res* 1964;43:563–7.
10. Barlet JP. Role physiologique de la calcitonine chez la chevre gestante ou allaitante. *Ann Biol Anim Biochim Biophys* 1974;14:447–57.
11. Pitkin RM. Calcium metabolism in pregnancy: a review. *Am J Obstet Gynecol* 1975;121:724–37.
12. Pitkin RM. Calcium metabolism during pregnancy and its effects on the fetus and newborn. In: Laron Z, ed. *The influence of maternal hormones on the fetus and newborn. Pediatric adolescent endocrinology*, vol 5. Basel: Karger, 1979;67–87.
13. Gertner JM, Coustan DR, Kliger AS, Mallette LS, Raven M, Broadus AE. Pregnancy state of physiologic absorptive hypercalciuria. *Am J Med* 1986;81:451–6.
14. Pic P. Evolution de la calcemie foetale du rat en fin de gestation. *C R Seances Soc Biol Fil* 1969;163:1033–8.
15. Chef R. Metabolisme du calcium chez la ratte en gestation. Etude ceinetique par le ^{45}Ca. *C R Seances Soc Biol Fil* 1969;163:541–5.
16. Taufield PA, Ales KL, Resnick LM, Druzin ML, Gertner JM, Laragh JH. Hypocalciuria in preeclampsia. *N Engl J Med* 1987;316:715–8.
17. Wrobel J, Nagel B. Diurnal variations of active calcium transport in the intestine of pregnant and lactating rats. *Biomedicine* 1980;33:143–5.
18. Halloran BP, DeLuca HF. Calcium transport in small intestine during pregnancy and lactation. *Am J Physiol* 1980;239(*Endocrinol Metab* 2):E64–8.
19. Toraason M. Calcium flux in vivo in the rat duodenum and ileum during pregnancy and lactation. *Am J Physiol* 1983;245(*Gastrointest Liver Physiol* 8):G624–7.
20. Delorme A, Marche P, Garel JM. Vitamin D-dependent calcium-binding protein. Changes during gestation, prenatal and postnatal development in rats. *J Dev Physiol* 1979;1:181–94.
21. Bruns MEH, Vollmer S, Bruns DE. Vitamin D-dependent calcium-binding protein. Immunochemical studies and synthesis by placental tissue in vitro. *J Biol Chem* 1981;256:4649–53.
22. Cushard WG, Creditor MA, Canterbury JM, Reiss E. Physiologic hyperparathyroidism in pregnancy. *J Clin Endocrinol Metab* 1972;34:767–71.
23. Pitkin RM. Calcium metabolism in pregnancy and the perinatal period: a review. *Am J Obstet Gynecol* 1985;151:99–109.
24. Bouillon R, DeMoor P. Pathophysiological data obtained with a radioimmunoassay for human parathyroid hormone. *Ann Endocrinol* 1973;34:657–67.
25. Kichura TS, Horst RL, Beitz DC, Littledyke ETL. Relationship between prepartal dietary calcium and phosphorus, vitamin D metabolism and parturient paresis in dairy cows. *J Nutr* 1982;112:480–7.
26. Chao CC, Brown RD, Deftos LJ. Metabolism of calcium and phosphorus during pregnancy and lactation in white-tailed deer. *Acta Endocrinol* 1985;109:269–75.
27. Garel JM. Parathyroid hormone, calcitonin and the mineral metabolism in the mammalian fetus and neonate. In: Holic MF, Anast CS, Gray TK, eds. *Perinatal calcium and phosphorus metabolism*. Amsterdam: Elsevier, 1983;71–104.
28. Garel JM, Gilbert M, Besnard P. Fetal growth and 1,25-dihydroxyvitamin D$_2$ injections into thyroparathyroidectomized pregnant rats. *Reprod Nutr Dev* 1981;21:961–8.
29. Garel JM, Delorme AC, Marche P, Nguyen TM, Garabedian M. Vitamin D$_2$ metabolite injections to thyroparathyroidectomized pregnant rats: effects on calcium-binding proteins of maternal duodenum and of feto-placental unit. *Endocrinology* 1981; 109:284.
30. Reynolds WA, Williams GA, Pitkin RM. Calcitropic hormone responsiveness during pregnancy. *Am J Obstet Gynecol* 1981;139:855–62.
31. Kumar R, Cohen WR, Silva P, Epstein FH. Elevated 1,25-dihydroxyvitamin D plasma levels in normal human pregnancy and lactation. *J Clin Invest* 1979;64:342.
32. Steichen JJ, Tsang RC, Gratton TL, Hamstra A, DeLuca HF. Vitamin D homeostasis in the perinatal period. *N Engl J Med* 1980;302:315.
33. Fleischman AR, Rosen JF, Cole J, Smith CM, DeLuca HF. Maternal and fetal serum 1,25-dihydroxyvitamin D levels at term. *J Pediatr* 1980;97:640.
34. Gertner JM, Glassman MS, Coustan DR, Goodman DBP. Feto-maternal vitamin D relationships at term. *J Pediatr* 1980;97:637.
35. Wieland P, Fischer JA, Trechsel U, Roth HR, Vetter K, Schneider H, Fuch A. Perinatal parathyroid hormone, vitamin D metabolites and calcitonin in man. *Am J Physiol* 1980;239:E385.
36. Delvin EE, Glorieux FH, Salle BL, Varenne JP. Control of vitamin D metabolism in preterm infants: fetal–maternal relationships. *Arch Dis Child* 1982;57:754.
37. Reddy GS, Normal AW, Willis DM, Goltzman D, Guyda H, Soloman S, Phillips D, Bishop JE, Mayer E. Regulation of vitamin D metabolism in normal human pregnancy. *J Clin Endocrinol Metab* 1983;56:363.
38. Bikle DD, Gee E, Halloran B, Haddad JG. Free 1,25-dihydroxyvitamin D levels in serum from normal subjects, pregnant subjects, and subjects with liver disease. *J Clin Invest* 1984;74:1966.
39. Pike JW, Packer JB, Haussler MR, Boass A, Toverud SV. Dynamic changes in the circulating 1,25-dihydroxyvitamin D during reproduction in rats. *Science* 1979;204:1427.
40. Halloran BP, Barthell EN, DeLuca HF. Vitamin D metabolism during pregnancy and lactation in the rat. *Proc Natl Acad Sci USA* 1979;76:5549.
41. Ross R, Care AD, Robinson JS, Pickard DW, Weatherley AJ. Perinatal 1,25-dihydroxycholecalciferol in the sheep and its role

in the maintenance of the transplacental Ca gradient. *J Endocrinol* 1980;87:17P–18P.

42. Kubota M, Ohno J, Shuna Y, Suda T. Vitamin D metabolism in pregnant rabbits: differences between the maternal and fetal response to administration of large amounts of vitamin D. *Endocrinology* 1982;110:1950.

43. Paulson SK, DeLuca HF, Battaglia FC. Vitamin D metabolite levels in the pregnant ewe and its fetus. *Proc Soc Exp Biol Med* 1987;185:267.

44. Hillman LS, Slatopolsky E, Haddad JG. Perinatal vitamin D metabolism. IV. Maternal and cord serum 24,25-dihydroxyvitamin D concentrations. *J Clin Endocrinol Metab* 1978;47:1073–7.

45. Halloran BP, Barthell EN, DeLuca HF. Vitamin D metabolism during pregnancy and lactation in the rat. *Proc Natl Acad Sci USA* 1979;76:5549–53.

46. Bouillon R, Van Baelen H, DeMoor P. 25-hydroxyvitamin D and its binding protein in maternal and cord serum. *J Clin Endocrinol Metab* 1977;45:679–84.

47. Fenton E, Brillon HG. 25-hydroxycholecalciferol 1 alpha-hydroxylase activity in the kidney of the fetal, neonatal and adult guinea pig. *Biol Neonate* 1980;37:254–61.

48. Tanaka Y, Halloran B, Schnoes HK, DeLuca HF. In vitro production of 1,25-dihydroxyvitamin D_3 by rat placental tissue. *Proc Natl Acad Sci USA* 1979;76:5033–6.

49. Whitsett JA, Ho M, Tsang RC, Norman EJ, Adams KG. Synthesis of 1,25-dihydroxyvitamin D by human placenta in vitro. *J Clin Endocrinol Metab* 1981;53:484–8.

50. Sunaga S, Noruichi N, Takahashi N, Okuyama K, Suda T. The site of 1,25-dihydroxyvitamin D_3 production in pregnancy. *Biochem Biophys Res Commun* 1979;90:948–58.

51. Grey TK, Lester GE. Vitamin D metabolism in the pregnant rat. In: Cohn DV, Talmage RV, Matthews JL, eds. *Hormonal control of Ca metabolism.* Amsterdam: Excerpta Medica, 1981;236–42.

52. Sommerville BA, Fox J, Care AD. The in vitro metabolism of 25-hydroxycholecalciferol by kidney: effect of low dietary levels of Ca and P. *Br J Nutr* 1978;40:159–66.

53. Halloran BP, DeLuca HFL. Effect of vitamin D-deficiency on fertility and reproductive capacity in the female rat. *J Nutr* 1980;110:1573–80.

54. Halloran BP, DeLuca HF. Calcium transport in small intestine during pregnancy and lactation. *Am J Physiol* 1980;239(*Endocrinol Metab* 2):E64–8.

55. Miller SC, Halloran BP, DeLuca HF, Jee WSS. Role of vitamin D in maternal skeletal changes during pregnancy and lactation: a histomorphometric study. *Calcif Tissue Int* 1982;34:245–52.

56. Tuan RS. Ca^{2+}-binding protein of the human placenta. *Biochem J* 1985;227:317–26.

57. Nolten W, Chesney RW, Viosca S, DeLuca HF, Slatopolsky E. Urinary calcium excretion in relation to circulating vitamin D metabolite values in the third trimester of pregnancy and lactation. *Clin Res* 1989;37:61A.

58. Samaan N, Hill CS, Beceiro JR, Schutz PN. Immunoreactive calcitonin in medullary carcinoma of the thyroid and in maternal and cord serum. *J Lab Clin Med* 1973;81:671–81.

59. Barlet JP, Garel JM. Physiological role of calcitonin in pregnant goats and ewes. In: Talmage RV, Owen M, Parsons JA, eds. *Calcium-regulating hormones.* Amsterdam: Excerpta Medica, 1975;119–21.

60. Garel JM, Jullienne A. Plasma calcitonin levels in pregnant and newborn rats. *J Endocrinol* 1977;75:373–82.

61. Widdowson EM, Spray CM. Chemical development in utero. *Arch Dis Child* 1951;26:205–14.

62. Comar CL. Radiocalcium studies in pregnancy. *Ann NY Acad Sci* 1956;64:281–98.

63. Schauberger CW, Pitkin RM. Maternal–perinatal calcium relationships. *Obstet Gynecol* 1979;53:74–6.

64. Stulc J, Stulcova B. Transport of calcium by the placenta of the rat. *J Physiol* 1986;371:1–16.

65. Ramberg CF, Delivoria-Papadopoulos M, Crandall ED, Kronfield DS. Kinetic analysis of calcium transport across the placenta. *J Appl Physiol* 1973;35:662–88.

66. Bruns MEH, Fausto A, Avioli LV. Placental calcium binding protein in rats. Apparent identity with vitamin D-dependent calcium binding protein from the rat intestine. *J Biol Chem* 1978;253:3186–90.

67. Bruns MEH, Wallshein V, Bruns DE. Regulation of calcium-binding protein in mouse placenta and intestine. *Am J Physiol* 1982;242:E47–52.

68. Miller RK, Brent WO. Evidence for Mg^{2+}-dependent (Na^+ + K^+)-activated ATPase and Ca^{2+}-ATPase in the human placenta. *Proc Soc Exp Biol Med* 1973;143:118–22.

69. Whitsett JA, Tsang RC. Calcium uptake and binding by membrane fractions of the human placenta. *Pediatr Res* 1973;14:118–22.

70. Minton SD, Steichen JJ, Tsang RC. Decreased bone mineral content in small-for-gestational-age infants compared with appropriate-for-gestational-age infants: normal serum 25-hydroxyvitamin D and decreasing parathyroid hormone. *Pediatrics* 1983;71:383–8.

71. Mughal MZ, Ross R, Tsang RC. Clearance of calcium across in-situ perfused placentas of intrauterine growth retarded rat fetuses. *Pediatr Res* 1989;25:420–2.

72. Croom RD, Thomas CG. Primary hyperparathyroidism in pregnancy. *Surgery* 1984;96:1109–16.

73. Loughead JL, Mughal Z, Mimouni F, Tsang, Oestreich AE. The spectrum and natural history of congenital hyperparathyroidism secondary to maternal hypocalcemia. *Am J Perinatol* 1990; 4:350–5.

74. Graham RW, Porter GP. Fetal maternal plasma calcium relationships in the rabbit. *Q J Exp Physiol* 1971;56:160.

75. Durand D, Dalle M, Barlet JP. Plasma calcium homeostasis in the guinea pig during the perinatal period. *Biol Neonate* 1982;42:120–6.

76. Care AD, Ross R, Pickard DW, Weatherley X, Garel JM, Manning RM, Allgrove J, Papapoulous S, Oriodran JLH. Calcium homeostasis in the fetal pig. *J Dev Physiol* 1982;4:85–106.

77. Bawden JW, Wolkoff AS. Fetal blood calcium responses to maternal calcium infusion in sheep. *Am J Obstet Gynecol* 1967;99:55–60.

78. Barlet JP, Davicco MJ, LeFaivre J, Carillo BJ. Fetal blood calcium response to maternal hypercalcemia induced in the cow by calcium infusion or by Solanium glaucophyllum ingestion. *Horm Metab Res* 1979;11:57–60.

79. Chalon S, Garel JM. Plasma calcium control in the rat fetus. III. Influence of alterations in maternal plasma calcium on fetal plasma calcium levels. *Biol Neonate* 1985;48:329–35.

80. Durand D, Barlet JP, Braithwaite GD. The influence of 1,25-dihydroxycalciferol on the mineral content of fetal guinea pigs. *Reprod Nutr Dev* 1983;23:235–44.

81. Brommage R, DeLuca HF. Placental transport of calcium and phosphorus is not regulated by vitamin D. *Am J Physiol* 1984;246:F526–9.

82. Mughal MZ, Robinson NR, Sibley CP. Materno-fetal calcium (Ca) transfer across the in situ perfused rat placenta: relation to maternal 1,25-dihydroxyvitamin D (1,25D) administration. *Pediatr Res* 1987;433A.

83. Moore ES, Langman CB, Favus MJ, Coe FL. Role of fetal 1,25-dihydroxyvitamin D production in intrauterine phosphorus and calcium metabolism. *Pediatr Res* 1985;19:566–9.

84. Robinson NR, Sibley CP, Mughal MZ, Boyd RDH. Fetal control of calcium transport across the rat placenta. *Pediatr Res* 1989;26:109–15.

85. Abbas SK, Caple IW, Care AD, Loveridge N, Martin TJ, Pickard DW, Rodda C. The role of the parathyroid glands in fetal calcium homeostasis in the sheep. *J Physiol (Lond)* 1987;386:27.

86. Rodda CP, Kubota M, Heath JA, Ebeling PR, Moseley JM, Care AD, Caple IU, Martin TJ. Evidence for a novel parathyroid hormone-related protein in fetal lamb parathyroid glands and sheep placenta: comparisons with a similar protein implicated in humoral hypercalcaemia of malignancy. *J Endocrinol* 1988; 117:261–71.

87. Torn CM, Raman A. Maternal–fetal calcium relationships in man. *Q J Exp Physiol* 1972;57:56–9.

88. David L, Anast C. Calcium metabolism in newborn infants: The interrelationship of parathyroid function and calcium, magnesium, and phosphorus metabolism in normal, sick and hypocalcemic newborns. *J Clin Invest* 1974;54:287.

89. Tsang RC, Chen IW, Freidman MA, Chen I. Neonatal parathyroid function: role of gestational age and postnatal age. *J Pediatr* 1973;83:728–33.

90. Hillman LS, Rojanasathit S, Slatopolsky E, Haddad JG. Serial measurements of serum calcium, magnesium, parathyroid hormone, calcitonin and 25-hydroxyvitamin D in premature and term infants during the first week of life. *Pediatr Res* 1977;11:739.

91. Bergman L. Studies on early neonatal hypocalcemia. *Acta Paediatr Scand (Suppl)* 1974;248:1–25.

92. Hollis BW, Pittard WB. Evaluation of the total fetomaternal vitamin D relationships at term: evidence for racial differences. *J Clin Endocrinol Metab* 1984;59(4):652–7.

93. Ornoy A, Goodwin D, Noff D, Edelstein S. 24,25-Dihydroxyvitamin D is a metabolite of vitamin D essential for bone formation. *Nature* 1978;276:517–9.

94. Garel JM, Martin-Rosset W, Barlet JP. Plasma immunoreactive calcitonin levels in pregnant mares and newborn foals. *Horm Metab Res* 1975;7:429–32.

95. Mayer GP, Rambert CF, Kronfeld DS, Buckle RM, Sherwood LM, Aurbach GD, Potts JT. Plasma parathyroid hormone concentration in hypocalcemic parturient cows. *Am J Vet Res* 1969;30:1587–97.

96. Hollis BW, Draper HH, Burton JH, Etches RJ. A hormonal assessment of bovine parturient paresis: evidence for a role of estrogen. *J Endocrinol* 1981;88:161–71.

97. Wrobel J, Nagel B. Diurnal variations of active calcium transport in the intestine of pregnant and lactating rats. *Biomedicine* 1980;33:143–5.

98. Black HE, Capen CC, Arnaud CD. Ultrastructure of parathyroid glands and plasma immunoreactive parathyroid hormone in pregnant cows fed normal and high calcium diets. *Lab Invest* 1973;29:173–85.

99. Black HE, Capen CC, Yarrington JT, Rowland GN. Effect of a high calcium prepartal diet on calcium homeostatic mechanisms in thyroid glands, bone, and intestine of cows. *Lab Invest* 1973;29:437–48.

100. Albright F, Reifenstein EC. *The parathyroid glands and metabolic bone disease. Selected studies.* Baltimore: Williams & Wilkins, 1948.

101. Toverud SU, Boass A, Haussler MR, Pike JW. Circulating levels and function of 1,25(OH)₂D in lactation. *J Steroid Biochem* 1983;19:505–10.

102. Toverud SU, Cooper CW, Munson PL. Calcium metabolism during lactation: elevated blood levels of calcitonin. *Endocrinology* 1978;103:472.

103. Hirsch PF, Hagaman JR. Reduced bone mass in calcitonin-deficient rats whether lactating or not. *J Bone Miner Res* 1986; 1:200–6.

104. Greer FR, Lane J, Ho M. Elevated serum parathyroid hormone, calcitonin, and 1,25(OH)₂D in lactating women nursing twins. *Am J Clin Nutr* 1984;40:562–8.

105. Greer FR, Tsang RC, Searcy JE, Levin RS, Steichen JJ. Mineral homeostasis during lactation: relationship to serum 1,25-dihydroxyvitamin D, 25-hydroxyvitamin D, parathyroid hormone, and calcitonin. *Am J Clin Nutr* 1982;36:431–7.

106. Hillman L, Sateesha S, Haussler M, Wiest W, Slatopolsky E, Haddad J. Control of mineral homeostasis during lactation: interrelationships of 25-hydroxyvitamin D, 24,25-dihydroxyvitamin D, 1,25-dihydroxyvitamin D, parathyroid hormone, calcitonin, prolactin, and estradiol. *Am J Obstet Gynecol* 1981;139:471–6.

107. Cundy T, Haining SA, Guilland-Cumming DF, Butler J, Kanis JA. Remission of hypoparathyroidism during lactation: evidence for a physiological role for prolactin in the regulation of vitamin D metabolism. *Clin Endocrinol* 1987;26:667–74.

108. Retallack RW, Jeffried M, Kent GN, Hitchcock NE, Gutteridge DH. Physiological hyperparathyroidism in human lactation. *Calcif Tissue Res* 1977;22(Suppl):142–6.

109. Cushard WG Jr, Creditor MA, Canterbury JM, Reiss E. Physiologic hyperparathyroidism in pregnancy. *J Clin Endocrinol Metab* 1972;34:767–71.

110. Specker BL, Tsang RC, Ho ML, Miller D. Effect of vegetarian diet on serum 1,25-dihydroxyvitamin D concentrations during lactation. *Obstet Gynecol* 1987;70:870–4.

111. Garner SC, Peng T-C, Hirsch PF, Boass A, Toverud SU. Increase in serum parathyroid hormone concentration in the lactating rat: effects of dietary calcium and lactational intensity. *J Bone Miner Res* 1987;2:347–52.

112. Boass A, Toverud SU, Pike JW, Haussler MR. Calcium metabolism during lactation: enhanced intestinal calcium absorption in vitamin D-deprived, hypocalcemic rats. *Endocrinology* 1981; 109:900–7.

113. Mainoya JR. Effects of bovine growth hormone, human placental lactogen and ovine prolactin on intestinal fluid and ion transport in the rat. *Endocrinology* 1975;96:1165–70.

114. Kumar R, Abboud CF, Riggs BL. The effect of elevated prolactin levels on plasma 1,25-dihydroxyvitamin D and intestinal absorption of calcium. *Mayo Clin Proc* 1980;55:51–3.

115. Fournier P, Susbiele H. Les echanges de calcium chez le rat au cours de la gestation de la lactation et du sevrage. I. Influence d'un regime riche en calcium. II. Influence d'un regime pauvre en calcium. *J Physiol* 1952;44:123:575.

116. Specker BL, Yergey A, Vieira N, Heubi J, Ho M, Tsang RC. Effect of lactation and diet on calcium metabolism: stable isotope studies. *J Am Coll Nutr* 1987;6:432(Abs.)

117. Brommage R, DeLuca HF. Regulation of bone mineral loss during lactation. *Am J Physiol* 1985;248:E182–7.

118. Pahuja DN, DeLuca HF. Stimulation of intestinal calcium transport and bone calcium mobilization by prolactin in vitamin D-deficient rats. *Science* 1979;204:1427–9.

119. Lamke B, Brundin J, Moberg P. Changes of bone mineral content during pregnancy and lactation. *Acta Obstet Gynecol Scand* 1977;56:217.

120. Chan GM, Roberts CC, Folland D, Jackson R. Growth and bone mineralization of normal breast-fed infants and the effects of lactation on maternal bone mineral status. *Am J Clin Nutr* 1982;36:438–43.

121. Wardlaw GM, Pike AM. The effect of lactation on peak adult shaft and ultra-distal forearm bone mass in women. *Am J Clin Nutr* 1986;44:283–6.

CHAPTER 17

Mineral Metabolism During Childhood

Charles P. McKay, Bonny L. Specker, Reginald C. Tsang,
and Russell W. Chesney

During childhood, the skeleton undergoes a series of changes that influence the mineral metabolism system. It is during this period that mature adult stature is reached. For adult stature to occur there must be coordination of many factors, including provision of appropriate minerals and organic compounds in the extracellular fluid, proper handling of these substances by the kidneys, bone, and intestine, and regulation of these processes by complex hormonal control. These processes are necessary for growth to achieve normal adult stature as well as normal adult bone density (1). The importance of bone mass achieved during childhood and adolescence in the prevention of osteoporosis later in life was recognized at a Consensus Conference conducted recently at the National Institutes of Health (2).

GROWTH AND MINERAL METABOLISM

Skeletal Changes with Growth

Growth is defined simply as an increase in size (3). It occurs through three processes: (1) hyperplasia or an increase in cell number, (2) hypertrophy or an increase in cell or organ size, and (3) storage of organic or inorganic materials within or among the cells. The growth of the skeleton requires the coordinated participation of all three of these processes.

C. P. McKay: Department of Pediatrics, University of Tennessee, Memphis College of Medicine, Memphis, Tennessee, 38103.
B. L. Specker: Department of Pediatrics, University of Cincinnati College of Medicine, Cincinnati, Ohio 45267.
R. C. Tsang: Department of Pediatrics, University of Cincinnati College of Medicine, Cincinnati, Ohio 45267.
R. W. Chesney, Department of Pediatrics, University of Tennessee Memphis College of Medicine, Memphis, Tennessee 38103.

Humans have an interesting growth pattern and share common growth characteristics with other primates (4). During fetal life there is very rapid growth, which then decelerates during the neonatal period and infancy. Between the second and third years of life, a steady rate of growth is attained which continues until adolescence—when a characteristic growth spurt occurs, followed by the cessation of growth when the epiphyseal plates of the long bones close (5). These phases are reflected in a varying rate of growth per annum: 20–25 cm in the first year, 10 cm in the second, 5–8 cm/year until puberty when the rate returns to 10 cm/year, and finally ceasing about 4 years after puberty (6).

The biology of bone growth is covered in detail in the section "Bone Structure and Biology," but in brief, bone grows through two major processes: intramembranous and endochondral ossification (7). *Intramembranous ossification,* characteristic of flat bones, is an appositional process. During fetal life mesenchymal cells accumulate at the site of the forming bone. The mesenchymal cells differentiate into osteoblasts, which lay down immature "woven collagen," which is then mineralized. This immature bone is later resorbed and replaced by mature lamellar bone. Growth of the flat bones occurs by the formation of bone by osteoblasts that compose the inner surface of the periosteum. Expansion of these surfaces ceases at the time of the closure of the epiphyseal plates of the long bones. *Endochondral ossification* is the process by which long bones grow and is characterized by growth of the cartilagenous epiphyseal growth plates. These sites contain successive zones in which chondrocytes proliferate, hypertrophy, and then disintegrate. The cartilage remnants are mineralized to form the primary spongiosa, which is later replaced by bony secondary spongiosa. Cartilage of the growth plate expands and then undergoes mineralization. Subsequent replacement of the mineralized cartilage by bone then results in longitudinal growth of the long bones. The ultimate width of the long bones depends on appositional growth along the periosteal surfaces.

Bone undergoes four processes: growth, modeling, remodeling, and repair (8). Remodeling and repair occur in both adults and children, whereas growth and modeling occur only in the growing skeleton of the child. As described above, growth is the process by which bone increases in size. Modeling is the process by which bone is sculptured into its adult shape. Bone formed at the wide epiphyseal plate is shaped to fit the thinner shaft by resorption at the epiphyseal surface and bone formation at the endosteal surface. Remodeling is the process by which bone is constantly being resorbed by osteoclasts and replaced by osteoblasts. It was originally thought to be important in maintaining mineral homeostasis but now is considered to be more important for skeletal integrity (9). Finally, bone repair is the mechanism by which callus formation results in the healing of fractures.

Challenges of Growth for Mineral Metabolism

Growth presents a formidable challenge for the maintenance of mineral homeostasis. A mathematical model for the changes in the calcium regulatory system induced by growth has recently been developed (9). This model describes two major perturbations for mineral homeostasis during growth: volume expansion of the entire carcass and rapid growth of the skeleton. In humans total body weight will increase from 3.5 kg to 70 kg in males, whereas the skeletal weight will increase from approximately 100 g to 3600 g (10). In general, males will achieve greater skeletal weights than females, and blacks will have heavier skeletons than whites. The process of growth therefore requires that the organism accumulate large amounts of calcium and phosphorus via intestinal absorption and transfer them to the growing skeleton while maintaining extracellular concentrations of calcium and phosphorus in the normal range.

INTEGRATION AND CONTROL OF MINERAL METABOLISM DURING GROWTH

Role of the Kidney in the Control of Mineral Metabolism during Growth

The high serum phosphorus demonstrated in infants and children is due, in part, to the ability of the kidney to conserve phosphorus (11). Early studies by Dean and McCance (12) and McCrory et al. (13) on the relationship between serum phosphate, glomerular filtration rate (GFR), and phosphate excretion suggested that the glomerular filtration rate determined the serum phosphate level in infants. McCrory et al. (13) hypothesized that low glomerular filtration rates of immature kidneys,

rather than a relatively high tubular reabsorption of phosphate, resulted in high serum phosphate in infants. Another study in both infants and children comparing phosphate to inulin clearances demonstrated tubular reabsorption of 82.6% in newborn infants, 74.7% in older infants, and 87.7% in children and adolescents. These results were interpreted to indicate the immaturity of renal function in infants (14). A more recent study in 51 infants and 143 children showed that the fractional tubular reabsorption of phosphate was higher in infants than in older children (15). Moreover, infants have higher serum phosphate concentrations at each increment of tubular reabsorption of phosphate. The high serum phosphate during infancy was therefore thought to be due to high phosphate reabsorption as well as possibly lower glomerular filtration rates. Three other studies in children have also demonstrated lower phosphate excretion as compared to adults (16–18). Thalassinos et al. (16) studied 55 children and found higher serum phosphate levels and a lower phosphate excretion index $[PEI = C_p/C_{cr} - (S_p - 1)/20]$ than in adults. In the study by Kruse et al., 546 school children between 6 and 17.9 years were found to have $TmPO_4/GFR$ values that correlated with age in both boys and girls and were significantly higher than adult values (17). Similar findings were reported by Stark et al. in 26 children (18).

The mechanisms by which renal phosphate excretion is decreased in developing animals has been extensively investigated with clearance studies. Growing rats were shown to have greater maximal net phosphate reabsorption per volume glomerular filtration rate than adult rats (19–21) (Fig. 1). Greater phosphate reabsorption in young as compared to adult rats was evident with phosphate deprivation as well (19). In fact, Caverzasio et al. (20) found that this difference was amplified by short-

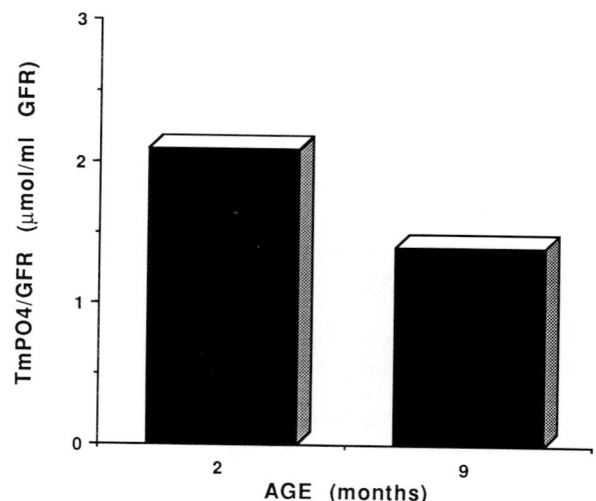

FIG. 1. Effect of age on maximal net tubular phosphate reabsorption per volume glomerular filtration rate in rats. (From Ref. 11.)

term phosphate deprivation and was not abolished by thyroparathyroidectomy. Greater maximal net phosphate reabsorption in young rats occurred despite no difference in the amount of cyclic AMP (cAMP) excretion per unit glomerular filtration rate between young and adult rats (20). Short-term administration of growth hormone to adult rats in dosages sufficient to promote growth also did not abolish this age-related difference (20). Webster and Haramati (21) also found a disassociation between cAMP excretion and phosphaturia in young versus old rats that were thyroparathyroidectomized and subsequently treated with exogenous parathyroid hormone. Further studies by this group confirmed that the mechanism by which young growing rats have a greater capacity to reabsorb phosphate is parathyroid hormone independent (22). Studies of the characteristics of the Na^+-dependent phosphate transport in brush border vesicles isolated from adult and growing rat kidneys demonstrated greater transport in vesicles from young versus adult rats. This was evident in rats fed low-phosphate diets but not those fed normal-phosphate diets, suggesting that mechanisms other than the Na^+-dependent phosphate transport were responsible for the high tubular phosphate transport in growing rats (23). Similar results demonstrating enhanced renal phosphate reabsorption have been found in the guinea pig (24–26). Whole kidney studies of newborn versus adult guinea pigs demonstrate higher phosphate reabsorption in the newborn kidneys at all filtered loads and that the maximal tubular reabsorption of phosphate per unit of glomerular filtration rate was significantly higher as well (24) (Fig. 2). Parathyroid hormone increased reabsorption of calcium and excretion of phosphate and cAMP in

the adult kidney. In the newborn kidney, PTH only increased calcium reabsorption, despite augmentation of urinary cAMP excretion (24). The site of this phenomenon was shown to be the proximal tubule (25) and possibly a more distal site. Studies of the Na^+-dependent phosphate transport in brush border vesicles from guinea pig kidneys demonstrated a higher V_{max} value of phosphate transport in vesicles from newborn versus adult kidneys (26). Furthermore, there was a lesser degree of adaptability to changes in dietary phosphate in the neonatal kidneys, which explained the greater degree of change in serum phosphate concentration in neonatal versus adult animals in response to high and low dietary phosphate in these animals (26).

Role of the Intestine in the Control of Mineral Metabolism during Growth

Few studies have examined the role of the gastrointestinal tract in the control of mineral metabolism during human development. There is a large amount of data in animal models, especially the rat, which have been recently reviewed (27). Knapp (28) showed an increase in urinary calcium with age as dietary calcium intake is increased, but this may well be due in part to extraintestinal handling of calcium and not increased absorption. Further studies in the rat have examined calcium absorption during different stages of development. The rat undergoes several stages of maturation: suckling (2 weeks old), weanling (3 weeks old), adolescent (6 weeks old), and adult. In one of the earliest studies of calcium absorption in a developing animal, Batt and Shachter (29) demonstrated that newborn animals absorb calcium in all segments of the gastrointestinal tract, whereas animals at the time of weaning have a selective increase in duodenal calcium absorption. Similar results were obtained in perfusion studies comparing calcium absorption in proximal and distal small intestine and colon from suckling, weanling, and adolescent rats (30,31). A linear relationship between calcium concentration in the intestinal lumen and calcium transport, consistent with a passive mechanism of calcium transport, was demonstrated in all segments in the suckling rats, whereas the weanling rats demonstrated a curvilinear relationship in all segments. The more mature adolescent rats demonstrated a curvilinear relationship in the more proximal gut segments representing active calcium transport, but a linear relationship in the more distal segments (30). These data are consistent with those of Batt and Shachter (29) and suggest passive mechanisms of calcium absorption in the immature rat with the development of active transport in the proximal bowel at the time of weaning. Halloran and DeLuca did not observe active calcium uptake in rats at 3 and 14 days of age but did in rats 25 days of age (32). Pansu et al. found a saturable compo-

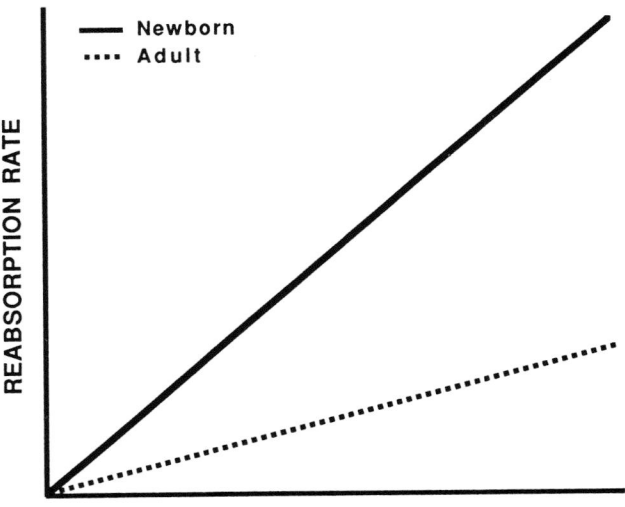

FIG. 2. Relationship between renal tubular phosphate reabsorption and filtered load in newborn and adult guinea pigs. From Ref. 11.

nent of calcium uptake developed between 19 and 24 days (33), whereas Dostal and Toverud detected a saturable component between 18 and 26 days (34). These studies are consistent with a passive process being responsible for calcium absorption until the time of weaning in the rat (at about 3 weeks), at which point there is the development of active calcium absorption. After weaning, the passive calcium absorption declines but is still present until at least sexual maturity (33). The active process also has been shown to peak at about 35 days of age when maximum growth is occurring, after which it, too, decreases (33).

Recent studies of the cellular mechanisms of calcium absorption have examined brush border (35) and basolateral membrane transport (36), as well as mitochondrial calcium transport (37). There was evidence of a saturable calcium absorption in brush border vesicles from both suckling and adolescent rats, but with maturation there is an increase in both K_m and V_{max} in this transport system (35). Studies of basolateral calcium exit from the cells also show a maturational change from suckling to adolescence, with an increase in both K_m and V_{max} values consistent with the greater active transport with age (36). Finally, adolescent rats display greater mitochondrial calcium uptake that is linked to greater ATP hydrolysis compared to the younger suckling rats (37). Therefore, the maturational increase in active calcium transport is linked to increased transport at the brush border, mitochondrial, and basolateral steps of calcium transport.

Active duodenal calcium transport in adolescent rats has been shown to be a vitamin D–dependent phenomenon (32–34). Although vitamin D in young suckling rats will raise serum calcium, presumably by promoting release of calcium from bone (28), calcium absorption in these animals is insensitive to vitamin D (32–34). Significant concentrations of intestinal receptors for 1,25-dihydroxyvitamin D$_3$ [1,25(OH)$_2$D$_3$] appear between ages 18 and 28 days in the rat (38,39). The timing of the appearance of this receptor may be under glucocorticoid regulation. Glucocorticoids have been shown to increase 1,25(OH)$_2$D$_3$ specific binding activity (40,41) and calcium absorption (42). Several groups have studied the appearance of the calcium-binding protein during development in the rat (32,43–47). Bruns et al. have described a 74-fold increase in calcium-binding protein between birth and 38 days, with the majority of this increase occurring at the time of weaning (43), which was similar to the findings of Delorme et al. (44) and Gleason and Lankford (47). Bruns et al. (43) found that 1,25(OH)$_2$D$_3$ caused a premature rise as early as 15 days. By contrast, Ueng et al. (45) found a 1,25(OH)$_2$D$_3$-dependent rise by 12 days of age. The importance of the development of the calcium-binding protein to calcium absorption is illustrated by the parallel increase in calcium-binding content and active calcium absorption, which are both de-

pendent on the action of 1,25(OH)$_2$D$_3$ (28,33). The role of 1,25(OH)$_2$D$_3$ on calcium absorption during development is further demonstrated by a 1,25(OH)$_2$D$_3$-induced increase in the V_{max} of calcium transport across both the brush border and basolateral membranes from suckling and adolescent rats (48). Finally, the role of lactose in the enhancement of calcium absorption has been described in adult rats. In studies with growing rats, lactose increased calcium uptake in adolescent but not in suckling rats (49).

Less is known about phosphorus handling by the maturing gastrointestinal tract. In the mature rat, phosphate transport occurs as an active process in the small intestine, particularly the jejunum. Phosphate transport across the jejunal brush border consists of a saturable, electroneutral sodium-dependent process as well as an unsaturable sodium-independent process. Recent studies of phosphate transport in rat jejunal brush border membrane vesicles indicate that immature suckling rats have a more active sodium-dependent uptake of phosphate than do adult rats (50). These studies indicate that the transport in the suckling animals displays not only a higher K_m value but also a much higher V_{max} value for phosphate than do adult animals. So despite having carriers with greater affinity for phosphate, adult animals may have many fewer carriers than in the young. Moreover, there is also evidence of greater passive uptake of phosphate in the immature jejunum as well. A decline in duodenal and jejunal phosphate uptake with maturation has also been demonstrated by Armbrecht (51). This author also showed that 1,25(OH)$_2$D$_3$ and a low-calcium diet stimulates the phosphate uptake in immature animals more than in adult animals. The transcellular process by which phosphate absorption occurs may involve an ATP-dependent uptake into the endoplasmic reticulum that is greater in suckling than in older rats (52). In addition, developmental maturation of jejunal mitochondrial transport with a ATP-dependent component that is regulated by 1,25(OH)$_2$D may occur (53).

Hormonal Control of Mineral Metabolism during Growth

Parathyroid Hormone

The concentrations of parathyroid hormone (PTH) seen in children were reported in two early studies (54,55). The normal inverse relationship between ionized calcium and PTH was demonstrated, and an age-dependent change in serum PTH was noted with values highest in the youngest children, a nadir at ages between 7 and 9 years, and finally a moderate rise to a plateau during adolescence (54). There were no difference between boys and girls, but the nadir in boys occurred later than that in girls (54). Other investigators have reported the levels of PTH in children to be both lower than (56), and higher than (57), adult levels. One study has indicated that both PTH and urinary cAMP concentrations were lower in children than in adults (58). While other investigators have also reported values for urinary cAMP excretion in children (59–62), the significance of these data are questionable since total cAMP excretion was reported and not the calculated nephrogenous component, which best correlates with parathyroid function (63,64). A variety of studies have described the response to the infusion of PTH in normal children and those with bone diseases (65–72). In one of the studies, parathyroid extract was administered to a group of 18 children aged 5–17 years. The children responded with a rise in their urinary cAMP excretion from 2.5 to 107 nmol/min per square meter and a fall in their tubular reabsorption of phosphate from 92% to 81% (71). A similar degree of PTH-dependent augmentation of urinary cAMP was demonstrated in a study of 50 healthy infants and children from 9 to 468 nmol/kg per hour (72). The response of PTH secretion to a hypocalcemic stimulus (73), and following intravenous calcium to raise plasma calcium values (74), has also been correlated with urinary cyclic AMP excretion. Studies in animals on the effect of PTH on cAMP production from renal cortical slices show similar rises in cAMP from young as compared to adult animals but greater potentiation of cAMP concentrations in younger animals after treatment with phosphodiesterase inhibitors (75).

Vitamin D Metabolism

Multiple studies have examined the circulating values of the different vitamin D metabolites in healthy children (76–86). The concentrations of 25-hydroxyvitamin D [25(OH)D] in children after the newborn period are essentially the same as adult values (81,83) and there are no differences with increasing age during childhood and adolescence (83). Evidence for sex differences in metabolite values is lacking (82). Studies have looked at seasonal differences and have found significantly higher concentrations in the summer than in winter (75,79,83); moreover, this difference is even greater when one compares the D_2 versus D_3 derivatives. The concentrations of $25(OH)D_3$ in summer were twice the levels they were in winter, whereas the concentrations of $25(OH)D_2$ were unchanged (75). The concentrations of $1,25(OH)_2D$ has been reported to be the same as, or greater than, adult values (76,77,80,81). Some studies have reported no change with age (79,81), whereas others have noted that older children have greater concentrations (77) or that higher concentrations correlate with growth velocity (80). At least one study has reported no effect of gender on concentrations of $1,25(OH)_2D$ (82). Unlike 25(OH)D, which increases in summer, there is no evidence for seasonal variation in $1,25(OH)_2D$ concentrations despite rises in its precursor 25(OH)D (79,82). One interesting observation is the variability of $1,25(OH)_2D$ values in childhood (76), which may relate to the observation that, at least in Caucasian children, the production of $1,25(OH)_2D$ is less tightly regulated than in adults (87,88). In this study vitamin D supplementation increased not only 25(OH)D levels but also increased $1,25(OH)_2D$ concentrations in children but not adults. Studies of $24,25(OH)_2D$ concentrations in children have shown that there is a seasonal variation paralleling 25(OH)D concentrations and that there is no age-related difference in $24,25(OH)_2D$ values (79,81,83,85). The metabolic conversion of 25(OH)D to $1,25(OH)_2D$ has been studied directly in the rat; young rats have increased conversion of 25(OH)D to $1,25(OH)_2D$ compared to adult rats (89).

An interesting debate has been over a physiologic role for $24,25(OH)_2D$ during development. This metabolite was suggested to play a role in the mineralization of bone in the chick in conjunction with $1,25(OH)_2D_3$ (90). Further studies described the ability of $24,25(OH)_2D$ to stimulate sulfation of cultured growth plates (91) and the presence of receptors for $24,25(OH)_2D_3$ in newborn-rat long bones (92). More sophisticated studies have used a difluorinated metabolite of $25(OH)D_3$ which is biologically active but cannot be converted by 24-hydroxylation in the kidney to $24,25(OH)_2D_3$ (93). These studies show that difluorinated metabolites are active in calcium and phosphorus homeostasis and allow normal growth and mineralization in young rats (92,94,95). These conclusions strongly suggest that $24,25(OH)_2D_3$ does not play an essential physiological role.

Calcitonin Metabolism

The physiologic role of calcitonin is unknown, but there has been speculation that it may participate in the mineralization of bone (96). Thus it could possibly be important in the growing child whose skeleton is rapidly growing and undergoing mineralization. Two different studies have suggested that serum calcitonin concentrations are very high in human infants and fall with age but remain higher than adult values throughout childhood (97,98). Klein et al. found a direct correlation between serum calcitonin and serum concentrations of bone Gla-protein concentrations, a measure of osteoblastic activity (98). These results are in direct contrast to those of Shainkin-Kerstenbaum et al. (99), who reported that in normal children between ages 6 and 12 years calcitonin concentrations rose with age and did not correlate with alkaline phosphatase levels. Silva et al. measured urine calcitonin excretion and found a decrease in excretion until age 13 years, at which time excretion was not different from adult values (100). This decline in urine calcitonin with age has been confirmed in Japanese children as well (101). Studies in rats have shown that serum calcitonin concentrations rise in baby rats after suckling and appear to prevent marked increases in blood calcium concentration associated with intestinal calcium absorption (102). Therefore, calcitonin may be important in the development of the growing skeleton, but more studies are needed.

Growth Hormone

Growth hormone as its name implies is one of the pivotal hormonal modulators of linear growth (103). A complete discussion of growth hormone is beyond the scope of this chapter and has been covered elsewhere, as has the role of somatomedins or insulin-like growth factors in bone growth (102,104–106). We will address the mechanisms by which growth hormone and somatomedins directly affect mineral metabolism. These mechanisms are probably essential to the development of a normal skeleton in children and may explain some of the differences in mineral metabolism between growing children and adolescents as compared to adults.

Over 30 years ago it was shown that administration of human growth hormone to a pituitary dwarf resulted in elevated serum phosphate concentration and alkaline phosphatase activity as well as statural growth (107). A direct effect of growth hormone on bone in children was suggested by the presence of osteopenia in growth hormone–deficient children (108). The degree of osteopenia is greater than can be accounted for by delayed bone maturation in these children. Further evidence of deficient bone formation in growth hormone–deficient children is demonstrated by the low serum levels of bone Gla protein, which returns to normal with growth hormone treatment (109). Studies in animals have indicated that growth hormone in dogs augments bone mass by increasing endosteal new bone formation as well as increasing calcium incorporation into bone by activating intestinal absorption and inhibiting urinary excretion of calcium (110,111).

Many of the effects of growth hormone on mineral metabolism may be manifested by its effects on the kidney. One of the first recognized effects of human growth hormone was a reduction in urinary phosphorus excretion (112–114). Studies in adult volunteers demonstrated that growth hormone can raise serum phosphate by increasing the maximal reabsorption of phosphate (115). This is in agreement with findings in untreated acromegalics who manifest high serum phosphate and decreased phosphate excretion (116–118). Corvilain and Abramow reported that pituitary dwarfs have serum phosphate and renal phosphate threshold concentration (TmPO$_4$/GFR) values that are not significantly different from those in normal children (118). Later studies by Gertner and co-workers (119,120) have demonstrated that growth hormone treatment of growth hormone–deficient children resulted in significant increases in serum phosphate and TmPO$_4$/GFR and that the TmPO$_4$/GFR

values correlated with serum somatomedin concentrations. Thus there is evidence in humans for an effect of growth hormone on renal phosphate handling. There is also evidence of hypercalciuria in acromegalics (117) as well as in children treated with growth hormone (121), although these results have not been consistently confirmed in other studies (119,120).

Animal studies have suggested an effect of growth hormone on phosphate handling by the kidney. In normal and parathyroidectomized dogs, Corvilain showed that human growth hormone increased TmPO$_4$ regardless of the parathyroid status (122). This increase was seen after 8 days of therapy, whereas a single dose of growth hormone did not increase TmPO$_4$, suggesting a possible role of somatomedin (123). The cellular mechanism of growth hormone–induced renal hyper-reabsorption of phosphate was shown by Hammerman et al. (124) to be increased phosphate transport across brush border membranes via the Na$^+$-stimulated phosphate transport mechanism. At least two studies have examined the effect of hypophysectomy on in vivo adaptation of renal phosphate reabsorption in phosphate-depleted rats. Phosphate depletion in intact animals leads to conservation of phosphate by the proximal renal tubule and enhanced generation of 1,25(OH)$_2$D. It has been hypothesized that growth hormone may play a key role in this phenomenon. Hypophysectomized rats given ACTH and thyroxine replacement and then deprived of phosphate were found to increase their TmPO$_4$/GFR but to a lesser extent than in intact rats (125,126). Further studies on the effect of hypophysectomy on the renal adaptive response to phosphate deprivation indicate that the hypophysectomized rat starts with a lower initial transport, but both the intact and hypophysectomized rat demonstrate approximately a twofold increase in Na$^+$-dependent phosphate transport (127). These studies suggest that growth hormone does not play a direct role in the renal adaptation to phosphate deprivation, but rather a secondary role.

The effect of growth hormone on parathyroid hormone secretion has been questioned. Some patients with acromegaly have hyperparathyroidism (117). However, in another study the serum parathyroid hormone concentrations were not raised and did not change after pituitary adenomectomy (128). Three studies in growth hormone–deficient children treated with growth hormone indicate no significant change in parathyroid hormone (119,120,129). In a fourth study there was no acute change in nephrogenous cAMP nor response of parathyroid hormone secretion to a hypocalcemic challenge (130). In contrast, a study of the effect of excess growth hormone on parathyroid hormone secretion in rats demonstrated a significant rise in blood parathyroid hormone concentrations after growth hormone secretion (131). Similarly, hypophysectomy in rats resulted in decreased parathyroid hormone secretion (132), decreased growth of parathyroid glands (133), and prevention of the hypertrophy of parathyroid glands in response to a low-calcium, vitamin D–deficient diet (134). These conflicting studies provide no consistent insight into a role for growth hormone in controlling parathyroid hormone secretion. However, it is possible that a high pharmacologic dose may have different effects than the physiologic doses given in replacement therapy.

The influence of growth hormone on vitamin D metabolism is suggested by the demonstration in acromegalics of increased plasma concentrations of $1,25(OH)_2D$ which were corrected after pituitary adenomectomy (128,135). In children receiving growth hormone replacement therapy there exist conflicting data as to the effect of growth hormone on plasma $1,25(OH)_2D$ concentrations. An acute infusion of growth hormone was shown to have no effect on plasma $1,25(OH)_2D$ concentrations (120), whereas therapy for 1 week was reported to result in a significant rise in plasma $1,25(OH)_2D$ concentrations followed by a return to baseline by 1 month (130). Other studies have shown that after 3 months of growth hormone treatment there was no change in plasma $1,25(OH)_2D$ concentrations from baseline (119), and after 5–14 months there was a decrease in plasma $1,25(OH)_2D$ concentrations from baseline (129).

Studies in rats have shown that hypophysectomy results in decreased plasma $1,25(OH)_2D$ concentrations (132,136–138); decreased conversion of $25(OH)D$ to $1,25(OH)_2D$ (133,134,139); decreased $1,25(OH)_2D$ bound to the intestinal mucosa (136,139); and increased conversion of $25(OH)D$ to $24,25(OH)_2D$ (133,136,137). Treatment of these animals resulted in at least partial restoration of metabolism of $25(OH)D$ to $1,25(OH)_2D$ (132–134,136–138) and reduction in the formation of $24,25(OH)_2D$ (133,136,137). Whereas hypophysectomy prevented the rise in plasma $1,25(OH)_2D$ in response to phosphate deprivation in rats, growth hormone restored this well-known response (127,140). Direct measurements of 1α-hydroxylase activity from rat kidneys demonstrate that hypophysectomy abolished the activation seen following phosphate deprivation and that growth hormone restored this activity (141). Further studies from this same group suggest that somatomedin C may be required for the increase in $1,25(OH)_2D$ formation with phosphate depletion (142), a finding that has been confirmed by others (143). In contrast, studies in chicks demonstrated stimulation of $1,25(OH)_2D$ production by prolactin, but not by growth hormone (144).

Increased calcium absorption may occur in patients with acromegaly (128,145), as well as in patients treated with growth hormone (129,145). Studies in rats show that hypophysectomy initially increased but then decreased calcium absorption by inverted gut sacs (146). This effect could be reproduced with prolactin but not by other pituitary hormones. Krawitt et al. (147) found that in immature rats, calcium absorption expressed in terms of intestinal wet weight actually increased with hypophysectomy. Aloia and Yeh (148) treated intact rats with growth hormone and found that growth hormone increased calcium absorption by vitamin D–independent mechanisms. When these investigators performed hypophysectomy on their rats they found that serum $1,25(OH)_2D$ concentrations fell, and in contrast to Krawitt et al. (147), they found that calcium absorption was unchanged when expressed per unit of intestinal wet weight (149). Furthermore, when growth hormone was administered, active and passive calcium transport increased and $1,25(OH)_2D$ increased calcium absorption in both intact and hypophysectomized rats (149). These investigators also have presented evidence that hypophysectomy affects calcium transport by a mechanism other than the levels of $1,25(OH)_2D$ or its receptors (150). There is very little known about the effect of growth hormone on intestinal phosphorus absorption, but in one study in rats hypophysectomy decreased phosphorus absorption in part by decreasing mucous mass and passive transport. Treatment with growth hormone did not correct these abnormalities (151).

Sex Steroids

One of the phases of growth in childhood, adolescence, is partially characterized by marked hormonal changes (152). These hormonal changes are important to normal growth during adolescence (153). Trabecular bone density increases during adolescence and reaches a plateau between the ages of 14 and 19 (154). Between late adolescence and the fourth decade, peak bone density is obtained (1,2). Therefore, the factors relating to bone development during adolescence, including the sex hormones, have lifelong significance. The importance of sex steroids to the normal development of the skeleton is illustrated by the abnormally low bone density in estrogen-deficient patients with Turner syndrome (155), in amenorrheic female athletes (156–158), and in women with amenorrhea secondary to hyperprolactinemia (159,160). Androgens and estrogens have been shown to have independent and additive functions on the attainment of peak trabecular bone density in women aged 18–22 (161). Detailed discussion of these problems as well as postmenopausal osteoporosis are beyond the scope of this chapter; they are considered in detail in Chapter 37, "Primary Osteoporosis."

In humans as well as in other animals, both estrogen and testosterone have been shown to increase bone mass (162). Estrogens in mice promoted differentiation of osteoblasts (163), which occurred despite the absence of estrogen receptors in bone cells (164). Canalis and Raisz (165) demonstrated with fetal rat calvarial cultures that estrogen and androgens have very little effect on bone formation, but progesterone seems to be inhibitory. Studies of intramembranous bone formation can be contrasted to studies examining endochondral bone formation which show progesterone in combination with estradiol to be stimulatory in bone formation and mineralization (166). An age-dependent sulfation of rabbit cartilage cells by testosterone, dihydrotestosterone, and estradiol has also been found (167). Estrogens may also modulate the way in which bone responds to other calcium-regulating hormones. Estrogen may inhibit PTH-induced bone resorption (168), but this may occur by a toxic effect (169). In contrast, in intact male rats there is even evidence that estradiol may inhibit the effect of calcitonin and potentiate the effect of parathyroid hormone on bone (170). Finally, in vivo evidence indicates that bone growth in the female rat is cyclical and involves coupling with PTH and estrogen (171). These studies suggest that even though an important role for estrogen in the development and maintenance of bone probably exists, the exact mechanism of this effect is still uncertain.

Initial reports of alterations in the circulating concentrations of calciotropic hormones over the menstrual cycle suggested that there was an increase in parathyroid hormone during the periovulatory period (172) and increased $1,25(OH)_2D$ levels on day 15 of the ovulatory cycle (173), but later studies have not shown any significant changes in the levels of PTH, $1,25(OH)_2D$, or calcitonin (174,175). More direct studies of the effect of estradiol and progesterone on PTH secretion demonstrate that both hormones stimulate PTH secretion from bovine parathyroid cells that was not blocked by the estrogen receptor antagonist tamoxifen (176). In addition, these hormones stimulate PTH secretion from abnormal human parathyroid tissue in vitro (177).

The effect of estrogens on vitamin D metabolism has been studied in humans and rats, but most of the studies have been in chicks. Estrogen treatment of tall pubertal girls increased plasma $1,25(OH)_2D$ values and the level of vitamin D–binding protein, which results in unchanged concentration of free $1,25(OH)_2D$ (178). Whereas ovariectomy inhibits conversion of $25(OH)D$ to $1,25(OH)_2D$ in the rat, estradiol augments this conversion, an event that is inhibited by parathyroidectomy (179). In studies in birds, estradiol increased the 1-hydroxylase and suppressed 24-hydroxylase in quail kidney homogenates (180–182), whereas progesterone increased $24,25(OH)_2D$ formation (180). Pike et al. demonstrated that short-term treatment of estrogen (but not progesterone or testosterone) increased conversion of $25(OH)D$ to $1,25(OH)_2D$, and furthermore, chronic estrogen allowed testosterone and progesterone to increase $1,25(OH)_2D$ formation (183). Tanaka et al. reported a similar synergism among estrogen, progesterone, and testosterone (184). The addition of estradiol and $25(OH)D$ in a chick kidney cell culture system decreased rather than increased $1,25(OH)_2D$ formation, suggesting that the increase in $1,25(OH)_2D$ formation demonstrated in vivo is the result of an extrarenal effect

(185,186). Further support for no direct effect of estrogen on $1,25(OH)_2D$ formation comes from a third study using chick kidney cell cultures (187). More recent studies of estrogen's effect in vivo showed activation of $25(OH)D_3$-1-hydroxylase in embryonic but suppression of enzyme activity in mature avian kidneys (188). A study of the effect of androgens on a osteoblastic cell culture demonstrated that members of this class of agents promoted cell proliferation and differentiation (189). In conclusion, the exact role of sex steroids in controlling $1,25(OH)_2D$ is not currently clear but probably involves the interaction of other factors not yet defined.

Testosterone deficiency in hypogonadal males is associated with decreased bone mass (190,191) which has been hypothesized to reflect abnormal bone development possibly related to low serum $1,25(OH)_2D$ concentrations in these patients during puberty (192). In tall boys treated with testosterone an increase in bone density was noted (193). Excess endogenous androgen production in young women have also increased bone density (194). In a study of teenage boys there was no change in levels of vitamin D metabolites across puberty and no relationship between serum concentrations of vitamin D metabolites and either testosterone or stages of puberty (195). In many tissues, formation of dihydrotestosterone occurs at the site of action where it is the active metabolite; such a transformation has been identified in human bone, including that from children (196). Studies in rats suggest a coupled mechanism and have shown that male rats have higher $1,25(OH)_2D$ levels which may relate to their greater growth and need for calcium (197). Opposing effects of testosterone and stomatostatin on bone formation in the mouse demonstrates the physiologic role of growth hormone and testosterone on the bone formation unit (198). There is evidence in rats that testosterone does not stimulate bone growth directly, but rather by modulating hypothalamopituitary function (199). The effect of testosterone and dihydrotestosterone in rats seems to be dependent on length and timing of treatment (200). Thus testosterone and its metabolite dihydrotestosterone seem to enhance bone formation in a manner that may relate to the control of growth of the animal, which is ultimately controlled by growth hormone, but also affects $1,25(OH)_2D$ formation and, thereby, intestinal calcium absorption and availability of calcium for bone growth.

SEXUAL MATURATION AND ATTAINMENT OF PEAK BONE MASS

Adolescence is the period of life during which sexual maturity occurs and statural growth ceases after closure of the epiphyses. It is also during this period that the most rapid gain in the weight of the skeleton occurs (201). Although bone density continues to increase until the fourth decade of life, important increases in bone mass and density occur during the adolescent growth spurt (1,2,202,203). This growth spurt occurs at different ages according to gender, with the maximum growth velocity occurring at age 14 years in boys and 2 years earlier in girls (153). Similarly, reproductive changes occur with puberty at approximately age 10.5 years in girls and 11.5 years in boys with completion approximately 4 years later (153). There are complicated serum hormonal changes of sex steroids during the adolescent growth spurt whose specific effects on mineral metabolism have been covered above under "Hormonal Control of Mineral Metabolism During Growth."

During puberty the greatest increase in bone density is after the growth spurt has slowed and in boys is associated with high concentrations of serum testosterone (204). In states associated with low levels of testosterone such as delayed puberty, neither the growth spurt nor the increase in mineralization are seen (200). Similarly, Gilsanz et al. have demonstrated with quantitative computerized tomography the increase in bone density and an increase in trabecular bone density during puberty (154). Their study differed in that they found no difference in cortical or trabecular bone density between boys and girls, suggesting that osteoporosis is not caused by a differential augmentation of bone density between males and females at puberty (154). Increased mineralization during puberty has been associated with high serum phosphate and high Ca × P solubility products which could potentially provide the needed calcium and phosphorus for mineralization (205). In a study of the relative timing of these events, the rise in serum phosphorus occurred 4 months before the peak of the growth spurt and a peak in serum alkaline phosphatase levels occurred simultaneously with the peak of the growth spurt (206,207). In males when phosphorus and alkaline phosphatase and bone mineral content are related to the pubic hair stages and peak height velocity, one finds that bone mineral content rises progressively from pubic hair stages PH_2 to PH_4 which is around the time of the peak height velocity (208). A similar study comparing alkaline phosphatase concentrations to "sexual maturity ratings (SMR)" found the highest mean alkaline phosphatase levels to occur at SMR 2 in girls and SMR 3 in boys (209). Serum alkaline phosphatase concentrations rise during early adolescence, but the degree of rate of rise slackens at the time of peak height velocity (203). In fact, a fall in alkaline phosphatase concentrations has been reported as peak bone density is achieved in late adolescence (210). The rise in alkaline phosphatase that precedes the maximal increase in bone mineral content is paralleled by a rise in bone Gla protein (211). Studies in males of the role of testosterone in these changes have demonstrated that the maximal serum concentrations of testosterone and not the adrenal androgens is achieved concurrently with the maximal rise in alkaline phosphatase and bone Gla protein (212). Furthermore, this level of testosterone precedes the maximal rise in bone mineral content by 5–10 months (204,205). The plasma con-

centrations of $1,25(OH)_2D$ were found to peak at stage 3 of puberty in both boys and girls with a decrease between stages 4 and 5 in one study (213) but not in another (195). The difference in findings of these two studies may relate to the fact that Asknes and Aarskog included 191 patients in their positive study (213), whereas Krabbe et al. included only 20 patients in their negative study (195). Thus studies of mineral metabolism during puberty demonstrate a significant increase in bone mineral content, which increases after statural growth ceases. Changes in mineral metabolism precede the greatest changes in growth velocity and bone density, providing the necessary materials for bone growth. The stimulus for these changes in boys involves the surge in testosterone at puberty. In the absence of these pubertal changes deficient mineralization occurs, which has important implications in later life.

ROLE OF NUTRITION IN MINERAL METABOLISM DURING GROWTH

Recent attention has been paid to the importance adequate dietary calcium to later development of osteoporosis. Specifically, it is thought that inadequate intake in the second and third decades of life may predispose women to worsened bone loss later in life (214,215). For adequate formation of bone there must be provision of adequate amounts of calcium, phosphorus, and vitamin D as well as other nutrients (Table 1).

Calcium Requirements

The diet must provide sufficient calcium to allow accretion of the approximately 1200 g of calcium found in an average 70-kg adult. Calcium absorption varies greatly: Whereas adults generally absorb less than 50%, children during active growth may absorb as much as 75% of calcium intake. The amount absorbed also varies greatly with source and intake. Whereas a breast-fed in-

TABLE 1. *Recommended daily intake of calcium, phosphorus, magnesium and vitamin D*

Calcium	
Infants	60 mg/kg
Children	800 mg/day
Adolescents	1200 mg/day
Phosphorus	
Infants	60 mg/kg
Children	800 mg/day
Adolescents	1200 mg/day
Magnesium	
Young infants	50 mg/day
Older infants	70 mg/day
Children 1–3 years	150 mg/day
Children 4–6 years	200 mg/day
Children 7–10 years	250 mg/day
Female adolescents	300 mg/day
Male adolescents	350 mg/day
Vitamin D	400 IU/day

fant ingests about 60 mg of calcium per kilogram of body weight but retains about 70% of this amount, a cow milk fed infant may take in 170 mg of calcium per kilogram of body weight but retains only 25–30% (216). Also, certain substances, such as lactose, enhance absorption (49), whereas oxalate- and phytate-containing foods reduce gastrointestinal calcium absorption. The ninth edition of the Recommended Dietary Allowances suggests that the calcium intake for children between the ages of 1 and 10 years be at least 800 mg/day (216), which relates per unit weight to an intake of as much as four times the allowance for adults. With the growth spurt during preadolescence and adolescence an intake of 1200 mg/day is recommended. The basis for the development of these figures comes from the position of the National Academy of Science to allow adequate calcium intake for the fastest-growing child (216). This approach is most evident in adolescence, when allowances are made to cover both the timing and magnitude of the adolescent growth spurt (216). These allowances are significantly higher, therefore, than those of the World Health Organization, which recommends 400–500 g of calcium per day in children and 600–700 g/day in adolescents (217,218), which is similar to the requirements recommended in the United Kingdom (219). During the first decade of childhood, skeletal growth requires 150 mg/day, so an intake of 800 mg/day should be more than adequate. During the adolescent growth spurt, incorporation of from 275 to 500 mg/day should be easily satisfied by the recommendation of 1200 mg/day (220). One of the compounding factors in the confusion regarding the requirements for calcium during childhood is the varying level of retention of dietary calcium intake (221,222). Studies have indicated that there is a decrease in retention with age so that younger children can absorb and maintain sufficient supplies of calcium for growth (222,223). In contrast to the high recommendations listed above, there is evidence that an intake of only 200 mg/day can result in positive calcium balance in preschool children accustomed to such a diet (224). Despite evidence of considerable adaptation to low calcium intakes, there has been a report of an endemic form of rickets ascribed to extremely low calcium intakes in rural South Africa (225), which has been confirmed by a report from Belgium (226). Thus the exact amount of calcium needed during childhood and adolescence has not been established, but the present recommendations are set to provide more than sufficient calcium for adequate bone growth during periods of need, such as the peak growth spurt in male adolescents.

Phosphorus Requirements

Despite the rare occurrence of phosphate depletion in humans after the neonatal period, the importance of this condition is illustrated by studies in growing animals (227–231). Phosphorus is needed for development of the skeleton as well as for soft tissues, where it is essential for formation of high-energy bonds. The total accretion of phosphorus into the skeleton is about one-half the amount of calcium. Phosphorus is absorbed from the diet more efficiently than calcium (60–70%), contributing to the rarity of dietary phosphorus deficiency with a normal Western diet. The recommended intake for phosphorus after infancy is said to be the same as calcium (216). Human milk provides calcium and phosphorus in the ratio of 2:1, whereas cow milk has a Ca/P ratio of 1.2:1. It is therefore suggested that the Ca/P ratio be 1.5:1 until 1 year of age, at which time a ratio of 1:1 is recommended (216).

Vitamin D Requirements

Vitamin D plays an important role in the regulation of calcium and phosphorus absorption and skeletal mineralization. Deficiency of vitamin D causes rickets in growing children and osteomalacia in adults (see Chapter 37). There are two forms of vitamin D: vitamin D_2 (ergocalciferol) and vitamin D_3 (cholecalciferol). These two forms are essentially biologically equivalent, but whereas vitamin D_2 arises from irradiation of the plant sterol, ergosterol, vitamin D_3 arises in the skin by irradiation of 7-dehydrocholesterol (232). Photoproduction of vitamin D is sufficient near the equator, but at higher latitudes and during winter, dietary supplementation becomes increasingly important (233,234). There is evidence that even during winter in northern latitudes, photoproduction of vitamin D is more important as a contributor to the circulating level of 25(OH)D than dietary intake. Vitamin D is usually expressed in terms of international units, which is the amount of activity contained in 0.025 μg of cholecalciferol. Whereas 100 IU of vitamin D is usually sufficient to support calcium absorption and can prevent rickets, 400 IU seems to be slightly superior and is the recommended daily allowance for infants, children, and adolescents given limited amounts of sunshine exposure (216). The recommended allowance is decreased to 300 IU during the ages 19–22 and to 200 IU thereafter (216). The needs during gestation and in premature infants is a more complicated matter and is covered in Chapter 15. Prolonged vitamin D intake in great excess to the recommended allowance is potentially hazardous and should be avoided (235).

Magnesium and Trace Minerals

Magnesium deficiency produces a variety of abnormalities of mineral homeostasis, including rickets (236), impaired release of PTH (237), impaired peripheral responsiveness to PTH (238), low serum $1,25(OH)_2D$ concentrations (239), and skeletal resistance to $1,25(OH)_2D$ (240). Primary dietary deficiency of magnesium is fortunately rare and requirements are easily provided in a normal diet. During infancy, the magnesium content of milk ranges from 40 mg/L in human milk up to 120 mg/L in cow milk and appears to be quite adequate (216). Therefore, a recommended allowance of 50 mg/day has been set for young infants and 70 mg/day for older infants, with increases to 150 mg/day in children ages 1–3 years, 200 mg/day in children ages 4–6, 250 mg/day in children 7–10, and finally, 350 mg/day in males and 300 mg/day in females thereafter (216).

Certain trace elements are particularly important in the structure and function of the skeleton (241). Zinc is required for normal collagen metabolism (241). Zinc deficiency has resulted in reduced bone size and strength (242,243), as well as deficient bone mineralization (244). The effect of zinc deprivation may be due to deficient endochondral bone formation (245) or deficient alkaline phosphatase activity (246). A syndrome of zinc deficiency and radiologic rickets has been described in children with thalassemia major treated with deferoxamine (247). A variety of metabolic studies have led to the recommendation of a daily allowance for zinc of 3 mg during the first 6 months of life, 5 mg in the second 6 months, 10 mg in preadolescent children, and 15 mg during adolescence (216). Copper deficiency has also been associated with osteoporosis and metaphyseal abnormalities (241). Similar to other trace metals, copper deficiency is rare with normal diets but has occurred with states of malnutrition. The suggested daily requirement for infants and children is 0.08 mg/kg, with higher intakes suggested for premature infants (216). Manganese is required for normal formation of bone and cartilage because of its role as a cofactor for glycosyl transferases and other metalloproteins (248). Manganese deficiency has resulted in abnormally developed bone and cartilage (241). A negative balance for manganese is common in the first 6 months of life when the intake is 0.01–0.294 mg/day and is without signs of deficiency (216). In older children and adolescents an intake of 1.4–2.18 mg/day is common and felt to be sufficient (216). The importance of fluoride for the development of bones and especially teeth is well recognized (249), as are the ill effects of chronic fluoride toxicity or fluorosis (250) and will not be covered in depth here. Fluoride intake varies greatly depending on the fluoride content of drinking water. Suggested intakes of 0.1–1.0 mg/day during the first year of life followed by 0.5–1.5 mg/day during the next two years and then an intake up to 2.5 mg/day until adulthood are suggested (216). The addition of 1 mg/L to public water supplies has led to a reduced incidence of tooth decay of as much as 50% without ill effects (251).

RACIAL DIFFERENCES IN MINERAL METABOLISM

Race Differences in Bone Mineralization

Black infants appear to be at increased risk of rickets (252), which is commonly thought to be due to an increased risk for vitamin D deficiency, yet several studies have shown higher bone density in blacks compared to whites in adolescence and adulthood. Black adults (253,254) have higher total body calcium and phospho-

rus, as measured by neutron activation, than do sex- and age-matched white adults of similar height. In addition, lean body mass is significantly higher in black adults compared to white adults (255). Greater body mass, resulting in increased physical strain on bone, has been thought to be protective against the development of osteoporosis (256). Black women are at a lower risk of developing osteoporosis compared to white women, which is thought to be related to the higher bone mineral mass of black versus white women. A higher bone density in black adolescent females compared to white females has been observed with no difference in body mass as measured by subscapular skinfold thicknesses and body weight (253).

Peak bone mass achieved at the end of the second decade of life may be predictive of future development of osteoporosis (162). The rate of decrease of bone mass and total body calcium with age is similar between white and black adults (257). Studies with tetracycline labeling have shown a lower bone formation rate among black adults, and it was suggested that there was a reduction in the rate of bone matrix synthesis (258). The paradox of increased bone mass with lower rate of bone formation in black adults could be explained by increased bone formation earlier in life but lower bone turnover later in life (258).

Race Differences in Parameters of Calcium Metabolism

Dark skin allows less transmission of UV radiation compared to light skin. Black infants are thought to be at increased risk for vitamin D–deficiency rickets due to increased skin pigmentation. However, results of in vitro studies completed by Holick and co-workers (259) indicate that skin pigmentation may influence vitamin D production only when UV exposure is minimal.

In a study investigating the effect of sunshine exposure on vitamin D status in exclusively breast-fed infants not receiving vitamin supplements, black infants were observed to have lower serum 25(OH)D concentrations than those of white infants. However, infant serum 25(OH)D was also correlated with maternal 25(OH)D and infant sunshine exposure; black mothers had a lower serum 25(OH)D concentrations and black infants had significantly less sunshine exposure than white infants, and thus no significant race differences were evident when maternal serum 25(OH)D and sunshine exposure were taken into account statistically (260). No race difference in serum 25(OH)D concentrations has been observed in formula-fed infants (261), presumably related to the effect of a significant amount of vitamin D in formula (400 IU/L).

The relationship between maternal and infant vitamin D status therefore could be related to transfer of vitamin D of 25(OH)D either by the placenta in utero or in milk. Race differences in human milk vitamin D concentrations (262) have been observed with black women having lower vitamin D activity than white women. In addition, human milk vitamin D concentrations correlate with maternal serum 25(OH)D concentrations (262). Thus maternal vitamin D status appears to be decreased in black women and theoretically may result in an increased risk of vitamin D deficiency in the infant.

In a cross-sectional study of 198 infants less than 18 months of age, black infants had lower serum phosphorus and higher serum $1,25(OH)_2D$ concentrations than white infants despite *similar* serum 25(OH)D concentrations within the normal range (261,263). One possible explanation for reduced serum phosphorus could be a difference in dietary intake of phosphorus. However, a tendency for similar race differences in serum phosphorus also was observed in the subgroup of infants fed human milk and race differences in human milk mineral content have not been reported.

In adults, higher serum $1,25(OH)_2D$, serum PTH, and urinary cyclic adenosine $3',5'$-monophosphate concentrations, with a lower urinary calcium and phosphorus excretion have been observed among blacks compared to whites (264). It was suggested that alterations in the vitamin D-endocrine system were a result of secondary hyperparathyroidism among blacks and that the greater muscle mass observed in blacks causes an increased strain on the skeleton, resulting in increased bone formation. However, serum concentrations of bone Gla protein were lower in black adults than in white adults, and as mentioned, a recent study has shown that bone formation, using tetracycline labeling, is actually lower in black adults than in white adults (258). Calcitonin (CT) concentrations were not measured, and lower urinary phosphate excretion among blacks is inconsistent with hyperparathyroidism. The black adults had a mean serum 25(OH)D well below the normal limit of 25(OH)D, and significantly less than the mean for white adults; this low vitamin D status by itself theoretically could have resulted in alterations in calcium metabolism, including hyperparathyroidism in that study.

Serum CT concentrations have been found to be higher in black than in white adults and in males compared to females, with blacks having approximately twice the serum concentrations of whites of the same sex (265). However, studies in infants have not found a significant race difference in serum CT. A higher CT concentration in adult blacks theoretically could explain the higher bone mineral content that has been observed, since CT is thought to protect bone from PTH-induced resorption (266).

STUDY OF MINERAL METABOLISM IN CHILDHOOD

Methodology for the Study of Mineral Metabolism in Children

Use of Stable Isotopes in the Study of Mineral Absorption in Children

Standard nonisotopic balance measurements are incapable of measuring fecal calcium loss arising from endog-

enous sources or differentiating this source from unabsorbed calcium. In addition, sample collection is extensive. The use of stable isotopes of calcium, coupled with mass spectrometric measurements of their concentration, permits the accurate and direct measurement of many of the physiologically important parameters, such as the rate of absorption, fecal excretion, urinary excretion, and bone turnover. Moreover, the use of two isotopes administered simultaneously, one as an intravenous tracer and the other as an oral dose, simplifies sampling requirements that are needed if only one isotope is administered and allows for determination of endogenous intestinal secretion of calcium (267). The use of isotopes also reduces dependence on the quantitative collection necessitated in classical calcium balance studies.

Study of Renal Handling of Minerals in Children

Calcium excretion in children has received much attention recently in light of the importance of idiopathic hypercalciuria and its association with hematuria and urolithiasis in children (268–270). An early study of calcium excretion in normal subjects, including children, found that the mean calcium excretion was 2 mg/kg per day at all ages of childhood and varied little with intake (271). A later study using 24-h urine collections to measure calcium excretion similarly reported a daily normal mean calcium excretion of 2.38 mg/kg with an upper limit of normal of 4 mg/kg (272). These investigators found a good correlation of the ratio of calcium to creatinine of the second voided urine specimen in the morning and the 24-h urinary calcium. The mean urinary calcium/creatinine (mg/mg) was found to be 0.14, with an upper limit of normal of 0.25 mg/mg. These investigators also reported the 24-h magnesium excretion to be 2.82 mg/kg and a normal magnesium-to-creatinine ratio of 0.21 mg/mg.

Measurement of urinary calcium/creatinine before and after a calcium load in adult patients who have been on a low-calcium diet for 7 days has been suggested as a means to determine whether hypercalciuria arises from a renal leak or elevated gastrointestinal absorption (273). Such a protocol has been evaluated in 48 normal children, and fasting mean urine calcium/creatinine values of 0.09 mg/mg and postload values of 0.12 mg/mg were found (274). The authors placed their patients on a milk-free diet for at least 5 days prior to the calcium load and stopped all vitamins or medications. On the evening prior to the challenge, the children fasted after their evening meal except for 240 mL of tap water at 21.00 h and midnight. At 07.00 h the bladder was emptied and another 240 mL of tap water consumed and the fasting urine sample was collected from 07.00 to 09.00 h. At 09.00 h, 1.0 g of calcium glubionate per 1.73 m^2 of body surface area (Neo-Calglucon) was given, with a standardized breakfast containing 300 cal, 25 mEq of sodium, 100 mg of calcium, and 100 mg of phosphorus. Urine is analyzed for calcium and creatinine. A similar study is described by Kruse et al. (275) in 236 healthy children. Despite the appeal of such studies it has recently been suggested that they offer little in the diagnosis of hypercalciuria in children over a standard 24-h urine collection for calcium performed after a proper low-calcium diet (276); further, a 24-h urinary calcium excretion after 3 days on a normal calcium diet (containing 700–800 mg/day of calcium, 100–130 mg/day of protein, and about 150 mg/day of sodium) or a low-calcium diet (same intake except calcium content of 400–600 mg/day) was found in another study in children (277) to be superior to the calcium load test of Pak et al. (273).

Phosphate excretion in children has been well studied over the past century (12–16). The most reliable and meaningful way to express renal phosphate handling is the renal phosphate threshold concentration (278) and is calculated by the maximal rate of tubular phosphate reabsorption divided by the glomerular filtration rate (Tm_p/GFR). Tedious studies requiring phosphate loading and timed urine collections have been replaced clinically in adults with the use of a nomogram developed by Walton and Bijvoet (279) which has been evaluated in children (17,18,280). In children, direct use of the nomogram of Walton and Bijvoet may result in Tm_p/GFR values (17) that are falsely elevated compared to direct studies of Tm_p/GFR (18,269). Stark et al. (18) and Brodehl et al. (280) have found that measurement of creatinine and phosphate in untimed urine and blood samples can be used to calculate Tm_p/GFR with the formula

$$\frac{Tm_p}{GFR} = P_p - \frac{U_p \times P_{creat}}{U_{creat}}$$

The Walton and Bijvoet nomogram has been found to be useful in children only when the clearance of phosphate (C_p) corrected for GFR was less than 0.2 (280). This is because infants and children lack the splay of the renal tubular phosphate handling built into the Walton and Bijvoet nomogram (279).

Study of Calcium-Regulating Hormones in Children

Several studies have reported serum concentrations of PTH in children (54,55,58). Parathyroid hormone is secreted in response to low-serum calcium concentrations, and thus a better measure of PTH secretion may be the level of maximal secretion in response to a hypocalcemic stimulus (73,281). The infusion of disodium edetate (EDTA) to induce hypocalcemia may reveal insufficient PTH secretion not revealed by normal testing (282). After placement of intravenous catheters and promethazine hydrochloride given to provide analgesia for the test, EDTA (50 mg/kg to a maximum of 2.5 g) is placed in 10 mL/kg of D5 0.2% sodium chloride plus 2% lidocaine (0.3 mL/kg) for analgesia. This solution is infused over 1 h and blood for total and ionized calcium and PTH were drawn at 0, 30, 60, 90, and 120 min (73). Newly available PTH assays are ideal for such a provocative test, but blood should be measured at much shorter

intervals: 0, 2, 5, 10, 15, 20, 30, 45, and 60 min (283). Another provocative test for patients with hypocalcemia is the PTH infusion test to evaluate for peripheral resistance to PTH as seen in pseudohypoparathyroidism (66–71). Whereas a parathyroid extract was available previously from Eli Lilly Co., Indianapolis, Indiana, it has been taken off the market, but there is a 1-38 human PTH fragment available that represents the active region of PTH and can be used in infusion tests (72). This peptide has recently been available from Bissendorf Peptide, D-3002 Wedemark 2, Federal Republic of Germany. To evaluate for responsiveness to PTH (72), patients are evaluated after an overnight fast and their bladders emptied at 06.00 h and they are given 200–300 mL of tap water. At 08.00 h a 2-h urine sample is collected for the baseline sample and an intravenous cannula is placed for infusion of 0.5 μg per kilogram of weight of 1-38 hPTH diluted in 20 mL of 0.9% NaCl to be given over 1–2 min. Blood is withdrawn from the cannula at 0, 5, 10, and 30 min for phosphate, creatinine, and cAMP, and urine is collected at 30 and 60 min for phosphate, creatinine, and cAMP. Urinary cAMP is expressed per unit GFR using the formula

$$\text{urinary cAMP} = \frac{UcAMP \times Vol}{\text{creatinine clearance} \times 100}$$

Tubular reabsorption of phosphate is expressed by the formula

%TRP

$$= 100 \times \left(\frac{\text{1-urine phosphate}}{\text{serum phosphate}} \times \frac{\text{serum creatinine}}{\text{urine creatinine}} \right)$$

Normal Values for Mineral Metabolism in Childhood

Serum Calcium, Phosphorus, and Magnesium

After the neonatal period, the normal values for total serum calcium are slightly higher than those in adults (82). Arnaud et al. reported that children 6 months to 2 years of age had the highest serum total calcium level (10.2 mg/dL), which fell to a plateau by 6–8 years and reached the adult value (9.6 mg/dL) by ages 16–20 years (54). Ionized calcium values fell from 4.48 mg/dL at ages 6–16 years to an adult value of 4.22 mg/dL by 16–20 years (54). Similar results were reported by Bergman and Isaksson, who found children after the first of life to have higher total serum calcium values than adults because of higher ultrafilterable calcium (284). Serum phosphate values are also significantly higher in early childhood and fall with age (Fig. 3A) (285,286). The degree of change with age has been found to be greatest during the ages 0.5–4 years and 12–16 years (54). Another interesting finding is the large circadian fluctuation in serum phosphate during adolescence as compared to adults (3.0 mg/dL versus 1.2 mg/dL) (287). In contrast, serum magnesium concentrations in children do not differ from adult values despite one report of slightly higher magnesium levels in children younger than 2 years (54,263).

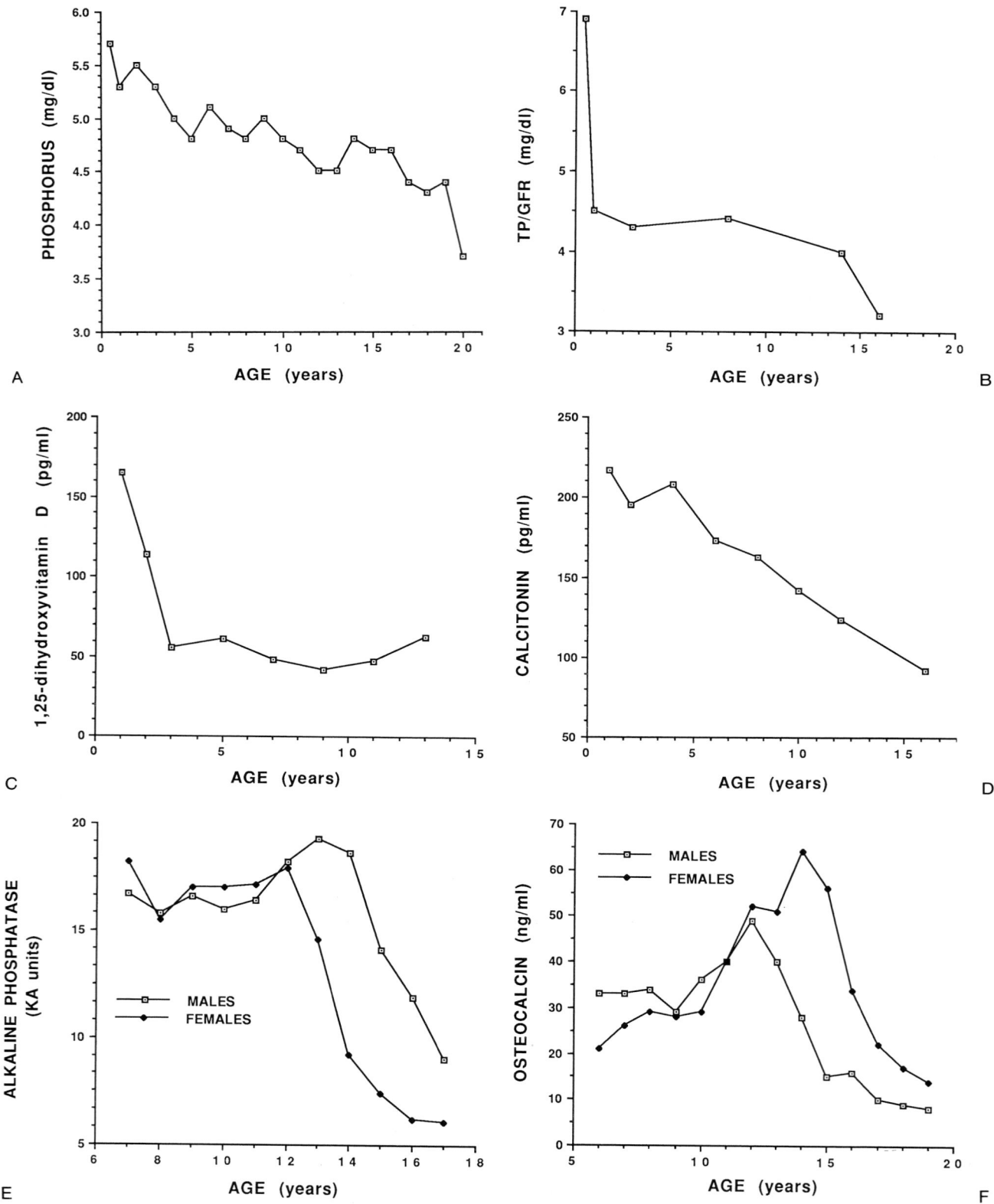

FIG. 3. Normal values for mineral metabolism in childhood. Pediatric age appropriate normal values for (**A**) serum phosphorus concentrations (285); (**B**) maximal renal tubular phosphate reabsorption per unit glomerular filtration rate (18); (**C**) serum 1,25(OH)$_2$D concentrations (81); (**D**) serum calcitonin concentrations (288); (**E**) serum alkaline phosphatase concentrations (286); (**F**) serum osteocalcin concentrations (298).

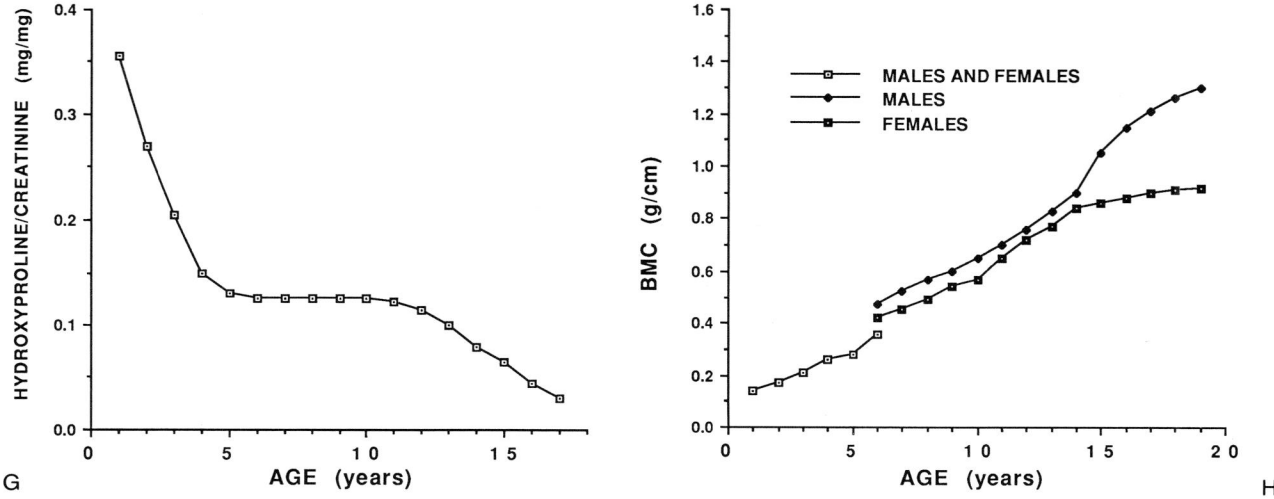

FIG. 3 continued: (G) urinary hydroxyproline excretion per milligram of creatinine (304); **(H)** bone mineral content (315, 316).

Parathyroid Hormone

The determination of PTH in the blood is greatly dependent on the method used (see Chapter 4) and should be evaluated in comparison with the level of serum calcium. The serum concentrations of PTH in children have been reported to be the same as or modestly different from the levels in adults (54–57). Therefore, age-related normals for PTH are not available.

Vitamin D Metabolites

There is no significant difference between children and young adults for serum concentrations of 25(OH)D and 24,25(OH)$_2$D (76,80,82,84–86). In contrast, several studies have suggested that 1,25(OH)$_2$D concentrations are higher in children than in adults (Fig. 3C) (77–79,81). Two of these studies found that levels fell from early childhood (79,81) and two found a rise with adolescence. A seasonal increase has been reported for 25(OH)D (75,80,82,84) but not 1,25(OH)$_2$D (79,81). Any seasonal variation for 24,25(OH)$_2$D is controversial (80,84,85).

Calcitonin

Serum calcitonin falls from birth until adulthood (Fig. 3D) (97,98,288) as does urinary calcitonin (100,101).

Alkaline Phosphatase and Acid Phosphatase

Alkaline phosphatase has long been used as a measure of bone cell activity and a sign of metabolic bone disease (289). Serum concentrations in children are higher than in adults (290,291) and are characterized by peak levels in infancy that fall during childhood with a second peak during adolescence (Fig. 3E) (286,287). Different alkaline phosphatase isoenzymes arise from bone and liver and it is the bone isoenzyme that is elevated in childhood

and adolescence (289,292). Whereas alkaline phosphatase is produced by osteoblasts and therefore correlates with osteoblastic activity, tartrate-resistant acid phosphatase is produced by osteoclasts and may be a valuable marker of osteoclastic activity. Similar to alkaline phosphatase, tartrate-resistant acid phosphatase is higher in children than in adults (293,294).

Osteocalcin

Osteocalcin is a vitamin K dependent protein synthesized in bone whose serum concentrations reflect osteoblast activity (295,296). Osteocalcin has been shown to be higher in children than in adults and to peak during the adolescent growth spurt (Fig. 3F) (297–299). During adolescence osteocalcin levels correlate with serum alkaline phosphatase, serum somatomedin C, and urinary hydroxyproline levels (296,297). A significant circadian rhythm has been demonstrated in adults with a nadir around noon and a peak around 0400 h, suggesting the importance of obtaining osteocalcin levels at a standardized time (300).

Urinary Hydroxyproline

Many studies have evaluated the excretion of hydroxyproline in children as a marker of bone turnover (301–308). Absolute hydroxyproline excretion is higher in children than in adults (302) and peaks during adolescence (303). When normalized to creatinine excretion, urinary hydroxyproline excretion falls after the first month of life, with a secondary peak often seen during puberty (Fig. 3G) (304–308).

Bone Density

As noted above, the skeleton during childhood and adolescence will increase from 10 g to 3600 g. The amount and density of bone mineral can be determined by many methods (309), but single photon absorptiometry has been the most widely used since its conception (310). Photon absorptiometry was shown to be superior to radiographic morphometry in determining bone mineral content in children (Fig. 3H) (311,312). These early studies suggested that bone mineral content increased at about 10.5% annually between the ages of 6 and 14 years (311,312). Interestingly, twin studies suggest there is a significant genetic component determining bone density (313). Normative data now exist for children (314–316). These studies demonstrate bone mineral content to be similar in boys and girls until after puberty, when boys demonstrate a marked increase in bone density (315). Other published normal bone density values for children include those for photon absorptiometry of the os calcis (317), dual photon absorptiometry (318), and gamma absorptiometry of the forearm (319).

ACKNOWLEDGMENTS

From LeBonheur Children's Medical Center and the University of Tennessee, Memphis, we wish to acknowledge support of Grants RR-00211-26 and DK37223 from the National Institutes of Health. From the Perinatal Research Institute, Children's Hospital Medical Center and University of Cincinnati Medical Center, Departments of Pediatrics and Obstetrics and Gynecology, we wish to acknowledge support from Grants (PPG) HD-11725 and (PERC) HD-20748 from the National Institutes of Health.

REFERENCES

1. Heaney RP, Gallagher JC, Johnston CC. Calcium and bone health in the elderly. *Am J Clin Nutr* 1982;36:986–1013.
2. Peck WA, Riggs BL, Bell NH, et al. Research directions in osteoporosis. *Am J Med* 1988;84:275–82.
3. Roche AF. Bone growth and maturation. In: Falkner F, Tanner JM, eds. *Human growth,* 2nd ed., vol II. New York: Plenum Press, 1986.
4. Rimion DL, Horton WA. Short stature. Part I. *J Pediatr* 1978;92:523–8.
5. Sissons HA. The growth of bone. In: Bourne GH, ed. *The biochemistry and physiology of bone,* 2nd ed., vol III. *Development and growth.* New York: Academic Press, 1971.
6. Royer P. Growth and development of bony tissues. In: Davis JA, Dobbing J, eds. *Scientific foundations of paediatrics,* 2nd ed. Baltimore: University Park Press, 1981.
7. Vaughan J. *The physiology of bone,* 3rd ed. Oxford: Clarendon Press, 1981.
8. Avioli LV. Childhood renal osteodystrophy. *Kidney Int* 1978;14:355–60.
9. Hurwitz S, Fishman S, Talpaz H. Model of plasma calcium regulation: system oscillations induced by growth. *Am J Physiol* 1987;252:R1173–81.
10. Trotter M, Peterson RR. Weight of the skeleton during postnatal development. *Am J Phys Anthropol* 1970;33:313–23.
11. Spitzer A, Kaskel FJ, Feld L, et al. Renal regulation of phosphate homeostasis during growth. *Semin Nephrol* 1983;3:87–93.
12. Dean RFA, McCance RA. Phosphate excretion in infants and adults. *J Physiol* 1948;107:182–6.
13. McCrory WM, Foreman CW, McNamara H, Barnett HL. Renal excretion of inorganic phosphate in newborn infants. *J Clin Invest* 1952;31:357–66.
14. Richmond JB, Kravitz H, Segar W, Waisman HA. Renal clearance of endogenous phosphate in infants and children. *Proc Soc Exp Biol Med* 1951;77:83–7.
15. Brodehl J, Gellison K, Weber H-P. Postnatal development of tubular phosphate reabsorption. *Clin Nephrol* 1982;17:163–71.
16. Thalassinos NC, Lesse B, Latham SC, Joplin GF. Urinary excretion of phosphate in normal children. *Arch Dis Child* 1970;45:269–72.
17. Kruse K, Kracht U, Gopert G. Renal threshold phosphate concentration (TmPO4/GFR). *Arch Dis Child* 1982;57:217–23.
18. Stark H, Eisenstein B, Tieder M, Rachmel A, Alpert G. Direct measurement of TP/GFR: a simple and reliable parameter of renal phosphate handling. *Nephron* 1986;44:125–8.
19. Armbrecht HJ, Zenser TV, Gross CJ, Davis BB. Adaptation to dietary calcium and phosphorus restriction changes with age in the rat. *Am J Physiol* 1980;239:E322–7.
20. Caverzasio J, Bonjour J-P, Fleisch H. Tubular handling of Pi in young growing and adult rats. *Am J Physiol* 1982;242:F705–10.
21. Webster SK, Haramati A. Developmental changes in the phosphaturic response to parathyroid hormone in the rat. *Am J Physiol* 1985;249:F251–5.
22. Haramati A, Mulroney SE, Webster SK. Developmental changes in the tubular capacity for phosphate reabsorption in the rat. *Am J Physiol* 1988;255:F287–91.
23. Caverzasio J, Murer H, Fleisch H, Bonjour J-P. Phosphate transport in brush border membrane vesicles isolated from renal cortex of young growing and adult rats. *Pflugers Arch* 1982;394:217–21.
24. Johnson V, Spitzer A. Renal reabsorption of phosphate during development: whole kidney events. *Am J Physiol* 1986;251:F251–6.
25. Kaskel FJ, Kumar AM, Feld LG, Spitzer A. Renal reabsorption of phosphate during development: tubular events. *Pediatr Nephrol* 1988;2:129–34.
26. Neiberger RE, Barac-Nieto M, Spitzer A. Renal reabsorption of phosphate during development: transport kinetics in BBMV. *Am J Physiol* 1989;257:F268–74.
27. Toverud SU, Dostal LA. Calcium absorption during development: experimental studies of the rat small intestine. *J Pediatr Gastroenterol Nutr* 1986;5:688–95.
28. Knapp EL. Factors influencing the urinary excretion of calcium. *J Clin Invest* 1947;26:182–202.
29. Batt ER, Schachter D. Developmental pattern of some intestinal transport mechanisms in newborn rats and mice. *Am J Physiol* 1969;216:1064–8.
30. Ghishan FK, Jenkins JT, Younoszai MK. Maturation of calcium transport in the rat small and large intestine. *J Nutr* 1980;110:1622–8.
31. Ghishan FK, Parker P, Nichols S, Hoyumpa A. Kinetics of intestinal calcium transport during maturation in rats. *Pediatr Res* 1984;18:235–9.
32. Halloran BP, DeLuca HF. Calcium transport during early development: role of vitamin D. *Am J Physiol* 1980;239:G473–9.
33. Pansu D, Bellaton C, Bronner F. Developmental changes in the mechanisms of duodenal calcium transport in the rat. *Am J Physiol* 1983;244:G20–6.
34. Dostal LA, Toverud SU. Effect of vitamin D3 on duodenal calcium absorption in vivo during early development. *Am J Physiol* 1984;246:G528–34.
35. Ghishan FK, Arab N. Developmental maturation of calcium transport by rat brush border membrane vesicles. *Pediatr Res* 1987;22:173–6.
36. Ghishan FK, Dannan G, Arab G, Kikuchi K. Intestinal maturation: calcium transport by basolateral membranes. *Pediatr Res* 1987;21:257–60.
37. Kikuchi T, Kikuchi K, Arab N, Ghishan FK. Intestinal maturation: characterization of mitochondrial calcium transport in the rat. *Pediatr Res* 1989;25:107–13.
38. Halloran BP, DeLuca HF. Appearance of the intestinal cytosolic receptor for 1,25-dihydroxyvitamin D3 during neonatal development in the rat. *J Biol Chem* 1981;256:7338–42.
39. Pierce EA, DeLuca HF. Regulation of the intestinal 1,25-dihy-

droxyvitamin D$_3$ receptor during neonatal development in the rat. *Arch Biochem Biophys* 1988;261:241–9.

40. Massaro ER, Simpson RU, DeLuca HF. Glucocorticoids and appearance of 1,25-dihydroxyvitamin D$_3$ receptor in rat intestine. *Am J Physiol* 1983;244:E230–5.

41. Massaro ER, Simpson RU, DeLuca HF. Stimulation of specific 1,25-dihydroxyvitamin D$_3$ binding protein in cultured postnatal rat intestine by hydroxycortisone. *J Biol Chem* 1982;257:13736–9.

42. Ghishan FK, Meneely RL. Intestinal maturation: the effect of glucocorticoids on in vivo net magnesium and calcium transport in the rat. *Life Sci* 1982;31:133–8.

43. Bruns MEH, Bruns DE, Avioli LV. Vitamin D–dependent calcium-binding protein of rat intestine: changes during postnatal development and sensitivity to 1,25-dihydroxycholecalciferol. *Endocrinology* 1979;105:934–8.

44. Delorme AC, Marche P, Garel JM. Vitamin D-dependent calcium-binding protein: changes during gestation, prenatal and postnatal development in rats. *J Dev Physiol* 1979;1:181–94.

45. Ueng T-H, Golug EE, Bronner F. The effect of age and 1,25-dihydroxyvitamin D$_3$ treatment on the intestinal calcium-binding protein of suckling rats. *Arch Biochem Biophys* 1979;196:624–9.

46. Armbrecht HJ, Zenser TV, Bruns MEH, Davis BB. Effect of age on intestinal calcium absorption and adaptation to dietary calcium. *Am J Physiol* 1979;236:E769–74.

47. Gleason WA, Lankford GL. Intestinal calcium-binding protein in the developing rat duodenum. *Pediatr Res* 1982;16:403–6.

48. Ghishan FK, Leonard D, Pietsch J. Calcium transport by plasma membranes of enterocytes during development: role of 1,25-(OH)$_2$ vitamin D$_3$. *Pediatr Res* 1988;24:338–41.

49. Ghishan FK, Stroop S, Meneely R. The effect of lactose on the intestinal absorption of calcium and zinc in the rat during maturation. *Pediatr Res* 1982;16:566–8.

50. Borowitz SM, Ghishan FK. Maturation of jejunal phosphate transport by rat brush border membrane vesicles. *Pediatr Res* 1985;19:1308–12.

51. Armbrecht HJ. Age-related changes in calcium and phosphorus uptake by rat small intestine. *Biochim Biophys Acta* 1986;882:281–6.

52. Ghishan FK, Arab N. Phosphate transport by intestinal endoplasmic reticulum during maturation. *Pediatr Res* 1988;23:612–5.

53. Kikuchi T, Arab NL, Kikuchi K, Ghishan FK. Intestinal maturation: characterization of mitochondrial phosphate transport in the rat and its regulation by 1,25-(OH)$_2$ vitamin D$_3$. *Pediatr Res* 1989;25:605–11.

54. Arnaud SB, Goldsmith RS, Stickler GB, McCall JT, Arnaud CD. Serum parathyroid hormone and blood minerals: interrelationships in normal children. *Pediatr Res* 1973;7:485–93.

55. Root A, Gruskin A, Reber RM, Stopa A, Duckett G. Serum concentrations of parathyroid hormone in infants, children, and adolescents. *J Pediatr* 1974;85:329–36.

56. Fairney A, Jackson D, Clayton BE. Measurement of serum parathyroid hormone, with particular reference to some infants with hypocalcemia. *Arch Dis Child* 1973;48:419–24.

57. Root BS, Gordan GS, Goldman L, Piel CF. Berson and Yalow's radioimmunoassay for parathyroid hormone (PTH): a clinical progress report. *Mt Sinai J Med* 1973;40:433–47.

58. Stark H, Eisenstein B, Davidovits M. Parameters for evaluation and correlation of renal phosphate handling and of parathyroid function in children. *Nephron* 1989;51:478–81.

59. August GP, Hung W. The urinary excretion of adenosine 3′,5′-monophosphate on children and adolescents. *J Clin Endocrinol Metab* 1973;37:476–9.

60. Murad F, Moss WW, Johanson AJ, Selden RF. Urinary excretion of adenosine 3′,5′-monophosphate in normal children and those with cystic fibrosis. *J Clin Endocrinol Metab* 1975;40:552–9.

61. Vitek V, Lang DJ. Urinary excretion of cyclic adenosine 3′,5′-monophosphate in children of different ages. *J Clin Endocrinol Metab* 1976;42:781–4.

62. Kruse K, Kracht U. Urinary adenosine 3′,5′-monophosphate excretion in childhood. *J Clin Endocrinol Metab* 1981;53:1251–5.

63. Drezner MK, Neelon FA, Curtis HB, Lebovitz HE. Renal cyclic adenosine monophosphate: an accurate index of parathyroid function. *Metabolism* 1976;25:1103–12.

64. Broadus AE, Mahaffey JE, Bartter FC, Neer RM. Nephrogenous cyclic adenosine monophosphate as a parathyroid function test. *J Clin Invest* 1977;60:771–83.

65. Connelly JP, Crawford JD, Watson J. Studies of neonatal hyperphosphatemia. *Pediatrics* 1962;30:425–32.

66. Evanson JM. The response to the infusion of parathyroid extract in hypocalcemic states. *Clin Sci* 1966;31:63–75.

67. Werder EA, Fischer JA, Illig R, et al. Pseudohypoparathyroidism and idiopathic hypoparathyroidism: relationship between serum calcium and parathyroid hormone levels and urinary cyclic adenosine-3′,5′-monophosphate response to parathyroid extract. *J Clin Endocrinol Metab* 1978;46:872–9.

68. Mallet E, Basuyau J-P, Brunelle P, De Menibus CH. Plasma cyclic nucleotide determination in the investigation of hypocalcemia. *Pediatr Res* 1979;13:647–8.

69. Ishida M, Seino Y, Simotsuji T, et al. Differential diagnosis of hypoparathyroid disorders during childhood. *Calcif Tissue Int* 1980;31:203–7.

70. Suh SM, Firek AF, Kim DH, Ramanathan S. Urinary excretion of cyclic nucleotides and phosphate in response to parathyroid hormone and calcitonin in man. *Pediatr Res* 1981;15:1359–62.

71. Hochberg Z, Moses AM, Richman RA. Parathyroid hormone infusion test in children and adolescents. *Miner Electrolyte Metab* 1984;10:113–116.

72. Kruse K, Kracht U. A simplified diagnostic test in hypoparathyroidism and pseudohypoparathyroidism type I with synthetic 1-38 fragment of human parathyroid hormone. *Eur J Pediatr* 1987;146:373–7.

73. Tsang RC, Chen I-W, McEnery P, Brown DR, Johnson JR, Lesniewkz J. Parathyroid function tests with EDTA infusions in infancy and children. *J Pediatr* 1976;88:250.

74. Kruse K, Kracht U. Effect of intravenous calcium on urinary cyclic adenosine-3′,5′-monophosphate and hydroxyproline in children with hypoparathyroidism. *Acta Endocrinol* 1982;101:217–22.

75. Muschek LD, Hook JB. Changes in adenosine 3′,5′-monophosphate induced by parathyroid hormone and theophylline in the developing rat renal cortex. *Dev Biol* 1973;33:56–61.

76. Arnaud SB, Matthusen M, Gilkinson JB, Goldsmith R. Components of 25-hydroxyvitamin D in serum of young children in upper midwestern United States. *Am J Clin Nutr* 1977;30:1082–6.

77. Scriver CR, Reade TM, DeLuca HF, Hamstra AJ. Serum 1,25-dihydroxyvitamin D levels in normal subjects and in patients with hereditary rickets or bone disease. *N Engl J Med* 1978;299:976–9.

78. Chesney RW, Rosen JF, Hamstra AJ, DeLuca HF. Serum 1,25-dihydroxyvitamin D levels in normal children and in vitamin D disorders. *Am J Dis Child* 1980;134:135–9.

79. Seino Y, Shimotsuji T, Yamaoka K, et al. Plasma 1,25-dihydroxyvitamin D concentrations in cords, newborns, infants, and children. *Calcif Tissue Int* 1980;30:1–3.

80. Taylor AF, Norman ME. Vitamin D metabolite levels in normal children. *Pediatr Res* 1984;18:886–90.

81. Lund B, Clausen N, Lund B, Andersen E, Sorensen OH. Age-dependent variations in serum 1,25-dihydroxyvitamin D in childhood. *Acta Endocrinol* 1980;94:426–9.

82. Fujisawa Y, Kida K, Matsuda H. Role of change in vitamin D metabolism with age in calcium and phosphorus metabolism in normal human subjects. *J Clin Endocrinol Metab* 1984;59:719–26.

83. Chesney RW, Rosen JF, Hamstra AJ, Smith C, Mahaffey K, DeLuca HF. Absence of seasonal variation in serum concentrations of 1,25-dihydroxyvitamin D despite a rise in 25-dihydroxyvitamin D in summer. *J Clin Endocrinol Metab* 1981;53:139–42.

84. Kano K, Yoshida H, Yata J, Suda T. Age and seasonal variations in the serum levels of 25-hydroxyvitamin D and 24,25-hydroxyvitamin D in normal humans. *Endocrinol Jpn* 1980;27:215–21.

85. Chesney RW, Hamstra A, DeLuca HF. Absence of seasonal fluctuation in serum concentration of 24,25(OH)$_2$-vitamin D in childhood. *Calcif Tissue Int* 1982;34:527–30.

86. Nguyen TM, Garabedian M, Mallet E, Balsan S. Serum concentration of 24,25-dihydroxyvitamin D in normal children and in children with rickets. *Pediatr Res* 1979;13:973–6.

87. Stern PH, Taylor AB, Bell NH, Epstein S. Demonstration that

circulating 1,25-dihydroxyvitamin D is loosely regulated in normal children. *J Clin Invest* 1981;68:1374–7.

88. Bell NH, Stern PH, Paulson SK. Tight regulation of circulating 1,25-dihydroxyvitamin D in black children. *N Engl J Med* 1985;313:1418.

89. Armbrecht HJ, Zenser TV, Davis BB. Effect of age on the conversion of 25-hydroxyvitamin D$_3$ to 1,25-dihydroxyvitamin D$_3$ by kidney of rats. *J Clin Invest* 1980;66:1118–23.

90. Ornoy A, Goodwin D, Noff D, Edelstein S. 24,25-dihydroxyvitamin D is a metabolite of vitamin D essential for bone formation. *Nature* 1978;276:517–9.

91. Corvol MT, Dumontier MF, Garabedian M, Rappaport R. Vitamin D and cartilage: biological activity of 24-hydroxycholecalciferol and 24,25-dihydroxycholecalciferol and 1,25-dihydroxycholecalciferol on cultured growth plate chondrocytes. *Endocrinology* 1978;102:1269–74.

92. Somjen D, Somjen GJ, Weisman Y, Binderman I. Evidence for 24,25-dihydroxycholecalciferol receptors in long bones of newborn rats. *Biochem J* 1982;204:31–6.

93. Halloran BP, DeLuca HF, Barthell E, Yamada S, Ohmori M, Takayama H. An examination of the importance of 24-hydroxylation to the function of vitamin D during early development. *Endocrinology* 1981;108:2067–71.

94. Jarnagi K, Brommage R, DeLuca HF, Yamada S, Takayama H. 1- but not 24-hydroxylation of vitamin D is required for growth and reproduction in rats. *Am J Physiol* 1983;244:E290–7.

95. Brommage R, Jarnagin K, DeLuca HF, Yamada S, Takayama H. 1- but not 24-hydroxylation of vitamin D is required for skeletal mineralization in rats. *Am J Physiol* 1983;244:E298–304.

96. Austin LA, Heath H. Calcitonin. *N Engl J Med* 1981;304:269–78.

97. Samaan N, Anderson GD, Adam-Mayne ME. Immunoreactive calcitonin in the mother, neonate, child, and adult. *Am J Obstet Gynecol* 1975;121:622–5.

98. Klein GL, Wallington EL, Collins ED, Catherwood BD, Deftos LJ. Calcitonin levels in sera of infants and children: relation to age and periods of bone growth. *Calcif Tissue Int* 1984;36:635–8.

99. Shainkin-Kerstenbaum R, Funkenstein B, Conforti A, Shani S, Berlyne GM. Serum calcitonin and blood mineral interrelationships in normal children aged six to twelve years. *Pediatr Res* 1977;11:112–6.

100. Silva OL, Becker KL, Snider RH, Moore CF, Lando HM. Urine calcitonin in normal children. *Pediatr Res* 1981;15:1032–5.

101. Morimoto S, Fukuo K, Yamamoto H, et al. Age and sex on urine calcitonin-like immunoreactivity in normal subjects. *Endocrinol Jpn* 1986;33:901–4.

102. Cooper CW, Obie JF, Toverud SU, Munson PL. Elevated serum calcitonin and serum calcium during suckling in the baby rat. *Endocrinology* 1977;101:1657–64.

103. Rechler MM, Nissley SP, Roth J. Hormonal regulation of human growth. *N Engl J Med* 1987;316:941–3.

104. Thorner MO, Vance ML. Growth hormone 1988. *J Clin Invest* 1988;82:745–7.

105. Phillips LS, Vassilopoulou-Sellin R. Somatomedins. *N Engl J Med* 1980;302:371–80, 438–44.

106. Isaksson OGP, Lindahl A, Nilsson A, Isgaard J. Mechanism of stimulatory effect of growth hormone on longitudinal bone growth. *Endocr Rev* 1987;8:426–18.

107. Raben MS. Treatment of a pituitary dwarf with human growth hormone. *J Clin Endocrinol Metab* 1958;18:901–3.

108. Shore RM, Chesney RW, Mazess RB, Rose PG, Bargman GJ. Bone mineral status in growth hormone deficiency. *J Pediatr* 1980;96:393–6.

109. Delmas PD, Chatelain P, Malaval L, Bonne G. Serum bone GLA-protein in growth hormone deficient children. *J Bone Miner Res* 1986;1:333–8.

110. Harris WH, Heaney RP, Jowsey J, et al. Growth hormone: the effect on skeletal renewal in the adult dog. I. Morphometric studies. *Calcif Tissue Res* 1972;10:1–13.

111. Heaney RP, Harris WH, Cockin J, Weinberg EH. Growth hormone: the effect on skeletal renewal in the adult dog. II. Mineral kinetic studies. *Calcif Tissue Res* 1972;10:14–22.

112. Ikkos D, Luft R, Gemzell CA. The effect of growth hormone in man. *Acta Endocrinol* 1959;32:341–61.

113. Henneman PH, Forbes AP, Moldawer M, Dempsey EF, Carroll EL. Effects of growth hormone in man. *J Clin Invest* 1960;39:1223–38.

114. Beck JC, McGarry EE, Dyrenfurth I, Morgen RO, Bird ED, Venning EH. Primate growth hormone studies in man. *Metabolism* 1960;9:699–737.

115. Corvilain J, Abramow M. Some effects of human growth hormone on renal hemodynamics and on tubular phosphate transport in man. *J Clin Invest* 1962;41:1230–5.

116. Camanni F, Massara F, Losama O, Molinatti GM. Increased renal tubular reabsorption of phosphorus in acromegaly. *J Clin Endocrinol* 1968;28:999–1005.

117. Halse J, Haugen HN. Calcium and phosphate metabolism in acromegaly. *Acta Endocrinol* 1980;94:459–67.

118. Corvilain J, Abramow M. Growth and renal control of plasma phosphate. *J Clin Endocrinol* 1972;34:452–9.

119. Gertner JM, Horst RL, Broadus AE, Rasmussen H, Genel M. Parathyroid function and vitamin D metabolism during human growth hormone replacement. *J Clin Endocrinol Metab* 1979;49:185–8.

120. Gertner JM, Tamborlane WV, Hintz RL, Horst RL, Genel M. The effects on mineral metabolism of overnight growth hormone infusion in growth hormone deficiency. *J Clin Endocrinol Metab* 1981;53:818–22.

121. Bryson MF, Forbes GB, Amerhakimi GH, Reina JC. Metabolic response to growth hormone administration, with particular reference to the occurrence of hypercalciuria. *Pediatr Res* 1972;6:743–51.

122. Corvilain J, Abramow M. Effect of growth hormone on tubular transport of phosphate in normal and parathyroidectomized dogs. *J Clin Invest* 1964;43:1608–12.

123. Westby GR, Goldfarb S, Goldberg M, Agus ZS. Acute effects of bovine growth hormone on renal calcium and phosphate excretion. *Metabolism* 1977;26:525–30.

124. Hammerman MR, Karl IE, Hruska KA. Regulation of canine renal vesicle Pi transport by growth hormone and parathyroid hormone. *Biochem Biophys Acta* 1980;603:322–35.

125. Caverzasio J, Faundez R, Fleisch H, Bonjour J-P. Tubular adaptation to Pi restriction in hypophysectomized rats. *Pflugers Arch* 1981;392:17–21.

126. Lee DBN, Brautbar N, Walling MW, et al. Role of growth hormone in experimental phosphorus deprivation in the rat. *Calcif Tissue Int* 1980;32:105–12.

127. Tennenhouse HS, Klugerman AH, Gurd W, Lapoint M, Tannenbaum GS. Pituitary involvement in renal adaptation to phosphate deprivation. *Am J Physiol* 1988;255:R373–8.

128. Takamoto S, Tsuchiya H, Onishi T, et al. Changes in calcium homeostasis in acromegaly treated by pituitary adenomectomy. *J Clin Endocrinol Metab* 1985;61:7–11.

129. Chipman JJ, Zerwekh J, Nicar M, Marks J, Pak CY. Effect of growth hormone administration: reciprocal changes in serum 1α,25-dihydroxyvitamin D and intestinal calcium absorption. *J Clin Endocrinol Metab* 1980;51:321–4.

130. Burstein S, Chen I-W, Tsang RC. Effects of growth hormone replacement therapy on 1,25-dihydroxyvitamin D and calcium metabolism. *J Clin Endocrinol Metab* 1983;56:1246–51.

131. Lancer SR, Bowser EN, Hargis GK, Williams GA. The effect of growth hormone on parathyroid function in rats. *Endocrinology* 1976;98:1289–93.

132. Spanos E, Barrett D, MacIntyre E, Pike JW, Safilian EF, Haussler MR. Effect of growth hormone on vitamin D metabolism. *Nature* 1978;273:246–7.

133. Fontaine O, Pavlovitch H, Balsan S. 25-Hydroxycholcalciferol metabolism in hypophysectomized rats. *Endocrinology* 1978;102:1822–6.

134. Pavlovitch H, Fontaine O, Balsan S. Effect of growth hormone on the metabolism of 25-hydroxycholcalciferol in hypophysectomized rats on a diet without vitamin D and low in calcium. *J Endocrinol* 1978;79:277–81.

135. Brown DJ, Spanos E, MacIntyre I. Role of pituitary hormones in regulating renal vitamin D metabolism in man. *Br Med J* 1980;280:277–8.

136. Yeh JK, Aloia JF. The influence of growth hormone on vitamin D metabolism. *Biochem Med* 1979;21:311–22.

137. Pahuja DN, DeLuca HF. Role of the hypophysis in the regulation of vitamin D metabolism. *Mol Cell Endocrinol* 1981;23:345–50.

138. Gray RW. Control of plasma 1,25-(OH)$_2$-vitamin D concentrations by calcium and phosphorus in the rat: effects of hypophysectomy. *Calcif Tissue Int* 1981;33:485–8.

139. Spencer EM, Tobiassen O. The mechanism of the action of growth hormone on vitamin D metabolism in the rat. *Endocrinology* 1981;108:1064–70.

140. Gray RW, Garthwaite TL, Phillips LS. Growth hormone and triiodothymidine permit an increase in plasma 1,25(OH)$_2$D concentrations in response to dietary phosphate in hypophysectomized rats. *Calcif Tissue Int* 1983;35:100–6.

141. Gray RW, Garthwaite TL. Activation of renal 1,25-dihydroxyvitamin D$_3$ synthesis by phosphate deprivation: evidence for a role for growth hormone. *Endocrinology* 1985;116:189–93.

142. Gray RW. Evidence that somatomedins mediate the effect of hypophosphatemia to increased serum 1,25-dihydroxyvitamin D$_3$ levels in rats. *Endocrinology* 1987;121:504–12.

143. Halloran BP, Spencer EM. Dietary phosphorus and 1,25-dihydroxyvitamin D metabolism: influence of insulin-like growth factor I. *Endocrinology* 1988;123:1225–9.

144. Bikle DD, Spencer EM, Burke WH, Rost CR. Prolactin but not growth hormone stimulates 1,25-dihydroxyvitamin D$_3$ production by chick renal preparations in vitro. *Endocrinology* 1980;107:81–4.

145. Hanna S, Harrison MT, MacIntyre I, Fraser R. Effects of growth hormone on calcium and magnesium metabolism. *Br Med J* 1961;3:12–5.

146. Finkelstein JD, Schachter D. Active transport of calcium by intestine: effects of hypophysectomy and growth hormone. *Am J Physiol* 1962;203:873–80.

147. Krawitt EL, Kunin AS, Sampson HW, Bacon BF. Effect of hypophysectomy on calcium transport by rat duodenum. *Am J Physiol* 1977;232:E229–33.

148. Aloia JF, Yeh JK. Growth hormone and intestinal calcium transport in the rat. *Metab Bone Dis Relat Res* 1980;2:251–5.

149. Yeh JK, Aloia JF. Effect of hypophysectomy and 1,25-dihydroxyvitamin D on duodenal calcium absorption. *Endocrinology* 1984;114:1711–7.

150. Yeh JK, Aloia JF, Vaswani AN, Semla H. Effect of hypophysectomy on the occupied and unoccupied binding sites for 1,25-dihydroxyvitamin D$_3$ in rat intestine. *Bone* 1986;7:49–53.

151. Aloia JF, Yeh JK. Effect of hypophysectomy on intestinal phosphate absorption in rats. *Bone* 1985;6:73–7.

152. Sizonenko PC. Endocrinology in preadolescents and adolescents. I. Hormonal changes during normal puberty. *Am J Dis Child* 1978;132:704–12.

153. Sizonenko PC. Regulation of puberty and pubertal growth. In: Ritzen M, ed. *The biology of normal human growth.* New York: Raven Press, 1981.

154. Gilsanz V, Gibbens DT, Roe TF, et al. Vertebral bone density in children: effect of puberty. *Radiology* 1988;166:847–50.

155. Brown DM, Jowsey J, Bradford DS. Osteoporosis in ovarian dysgenesis. *J Pediatr* 1974;84:816–20.

156. Drinkwater BL, Nilson K, Chestnut CH, Bremner WJ, Shainholtz S, Southworth MB. Bone mineral content of amenorrheic and eumenorrheic athletes. *N Engl J Med* 1984;311:277–81.

157. Cann CE, Martin MC, Genant HK, Jaffe RB. Decreased spinal mineral content in amenorrheic women. *JAMA* 1984;251:626–9.

158. Marcus R, Cann C, Madvig P, et al. Menstrual function and bone mass in elite women distance runners: endocrine and metabolic features. *Ann Intern Med* 1985;102:158–63.

159. Klibanski A, Neer RM, Beitins IZ, Ridgway C, Zervas NT, McArthur JW. Decreased bone density in hyperprolactinemic women. *N Engl J Med* 1980;303:1511–4.

160. Klibanski A, Biller BM, Rosenthal DI, Schoenfeld DA, Saxe V. Effects of prolactin and deficiency in amenorrheic bone loss. *J Clin Endocrinol Metab* 1988;67:124–30.

161. Buchanan JR, Myers C, Lloyd T, Leuenberger P, Demers LM. Determinants of peak trabecular bone density in women: the role of androgens, estrogen, and exercise. *J Bone Miner Res* 1988;3:673–80.

162. Gilsanz V, Roe TF, Gibbens DT, et al. Effect of sex steroids on peak bone density of growing rabbits. *Am J Physiol* 1988; 255:E416–21.

163. Simmons DJ. Collagen formation and endochondral ossification in estrogen treated mice. *Proc Soc Exp Med Biol* 1966;121: 1165–8.

164. van Passen HC, Poortman J, Borgart-Creutzburg IHC, Thijssen JHH, Duursma SA. Oestrogen binding proteins in bone cell cytosol. *Calcif Tissue Res* 1978;25:249–54.

165. Canalis E, Raisz LG. Effect of sex steroids on bone collagen synthesis in vitro. *Calcif Tissue Res* 1978;25:105–10.

166. Burnett CC, Reddi AH. Influence of estrogen and progesterone on matrix-induced endochondral bone formation. *Calcif Tissue Int* 1983;35:609–14.

167. Corvol M-T, Carrascosa A, Tsargris L, Blanchard O, Rappaport R. Evidence for a direct in vitro action of sex steroids on rabbit cartilage cells during skeletal growth: influence of age and sex. *Endocrinology* 1987;120:1422–9.

168. Atkins D, Zanelli JM, Peacock M, Nordin BEC. The effect of oestrogens on the response of bone to parathyroid hormone in vitro. *J Endocrinol* 1972;54:107–17.

169. Liskova M. Influence of estrogens on bone resorption in organ culture. *Calcif Tissue Res* 1976;22:207–18.

170. Shai F, Wallach S. Interactions of estradiol and calcitonin on the rat skeleton. *Endocrinology* 1973;93:1044–51.

171. Whitson SW, Dawson LR, Jee WSS. A tetracycline study of cyclic longitudinal bone growth in the female rat. *Endocrinology* 1978;103:2006–10.

172. Pitkin RM, Reynolds WA, Williams GA, Hargis GK. Calcium regulating hormones during the menstrual cycle. *J Clin Endocrinol Metab* 1978;47:626–32.

173. Gray TK, McAdoo T, Hatley L, Lester GE, Thierry M. Fluctuation of serum concentrations of 1,25-dihydroxyvitamin D$_3$ during the menstrual cycle. *Am J Obstet Gynecol* 1982;144:880.

174. Baran DT, Whyte MP, Haussler MR, Deftos LJ, Slatopolsky E, Avioli LV. Effect of the menstrual cycle on calcium-regulating hormones in the normal young woman. *J Clin Endocrinol Metab* 1980;50:377–9.

175. Muse KN, Manolagas SC, Deftos LJ, Alexander N, Yen SSC. Calcium-regulating hormones across the menstrual cycle. *J Clin Endocrinol Metab* 1986;62:1313–6.

176. Greenberg C, Kukreja SC, Bowser EN, Hargis GK, Henderson WJ, Williams GA. Parathyroid hormone secretion: effect of estradiol and progesterone. *Metabolism* 1987;36:151–4.

177. Duarte B, Hargis GK, Kukreja SC. Effects of estradiol and progesterone on parathyroid hormone secretion from human parathyroid tissue. *J Clin Endocrinol Metab* 1988;66:584–7.

178. Aarskog D, Aksnes L, Markestad T, Rodland O. Effect of estrogen on vitamin D metabolism in tall girls. *J Clin Endocrinol Metab* 1983;57:1155–8.

179. Ash SL, Goldin BR. Effects of age and estrogen on renal vitamin D metabolism in the female rat. *Am J Clin Nutr* 1988;47:694–9.

180. Tanaka Y, Castillo L, DeLuca HF. Control of renal vitamin D hydroxylase in birds by sex hormones. *Proc Natl Acad Sci USA* 1976;73:2701–5.

181. Castillo L, Tanaka Y, DeLuca HF, Sunde ML. The stimulation of 25-hydroxyvitamin D$_3$-1α-hydroxylase by estrogen. *Arch Biochem Biophys* 1977;179:211–7.

182. Baksi SN, Kenny AD. Vitamin D$_3$ metabolism in immature Japanese quail: effects of ovulation hormones *Endocrinology* 1977;101:1216–20.

183. Pike JW, Spanos E, Colston KW, MacIntyre I, Haussler MR. Influence of estrogen on renal vitamin D hydroxylases and serum 1,25-(OH)$_2$D$_3$ in chicks. *Am J Physiol* 1978;235:E338–43.

184. Tanaka Y, Castillo L, Wineland MJ, DeLuca HF. Synergistic effect of progesterone, testosterone, and estradiol in the stimulation of chick renal 25-hydroxyvitamin D$_3$-1α-hydroxylase. *Endocrinology* 1978;103:2035–9.

185. Henry HL. 25(OH)D$_3$ metabolism in kidney cell cultures: lack of a direct effect of estradiol. *Am J Physiol* 1981;240:E119–24.

186. Trechsel U, Bonjour J-P, Fleisch H. Regulation of the metabolism of 25-hydroxyvitamin D$_3$ in primary cultures of chick kidney cells. *J Clin Invest* 1979;64:206–17.

187. Spanos E, Barrett DI, Chong KT, MacIntyre I. Effect of oestrogen and 1,25-dihydroxycholcalciferol on 25-hydroxycholecalciferol

metabolism in primary chick kidney-cell cultures. *Biochem J* 1978;174:231–6.

188. Martz A, Forte LR, Langeluttig SG. Renal cAMP and 1,25(OH)$_2$D$_3$ synthesis in estrogen-treated chick embryos and hens. *Am J Physiol* 1985;249:E626–33.

189. Kasperk CH, Wergedal JE, Farley JR, Linkhart TA, Turner RT, Baylink DJ. Androgens directly stimulate proliferation of bone cells in vitro. *Endocrinology* 1989;124:1576–8.

190. Finkelstein JS, Kliblanski A, Neer RM, Greenspan SL, Rosenthal DI, Crowley WF. Osteoporosis in men with hypogonadotropic hypogonadism. *Ann Intern Med* 1987;106:354–61.

191. Smith DAS, Walker MS. Changes in plasma steroids and bone density in Kleinfelter's syndrome. *Calcif Tissue Res* 1976;22:225–8.

192. Francis RM, Peacock M, Aaron JE. Osteoporosis in hypogonadal men: role of decreased plasma 1,25-dihydroxyvitamin D, calcium absorption and low bone formation. *Bone* 1986;7:261–8.

193. Exner GU, Prader A, Elsasser U, Aniliker M. Effects of high dose oestrogen and testosterone treatment in adolescents upon trabecular and compact bone mass measured by I^{125} computed tomography: a preliminary study. *Acta Endocrinol* 1980;94:126–31.

194. Buchanan JR, Hospodar P, Myers C, Leuenberger P, Demers LM. Effect of excess endogenous androgens on bone density in young women. *J Clin Endocrinol Metab* 1988;67:937–43.

195. Krabbe S, Hummer L, Christiansen C. Serum levels of vitamin D metabolites and testosterone in male puberty. *J Clin Endocrinol Metab* 1986;62:503–7.

196. Schweikert HU, Rulf W, Niederle N, Schafer HE, Keck E, Kruck F. Testosterone metabolism in human bone. *Acta Endocrinol* 1980;95:258–64.

197. Bushinsky DA, Favus MJ, Coe FL. Elevated 1,25(OH)$_2$D$_3$, intestinal absorption, and renal mineral conservation in male rats. *Am J Physiol* 1984;246:F140–5.

198. Marie PJ, Hott M, Durand D. Somatostatin infusion inhibits the stimulatory effect of testosterone on endosteal bone formation in the mouse. *Metabolism* 1988;37:429–35.

199. Jansson J-O, Eden S, Isakssoon O. Sites of action of testosterone and estradiol on longitudinal bone growth. *Am J Physiol* 1983;244:E135–40.

200. Kapur SP, Reddi AH. Influence of testosterone and dihydrotestosterone on bone-matrix induced endochondral bone formation. *Calcif Tissue Int* 1989;44:108–13.

201. Trotter M, Hixon BB. Sequential changes in weight, density, and percentage of ash weight of human skeletons from an early fetal period through old age. *Anat Rec* 1974;179:1–18.

202. Garn SM, Wagner B. The adolescent growth of the skeletal mass and its implications to mineral requirements. In: Heald FP, ed. *Adolescent nutrition and growth.* New York: Appleton-Century-Crofts, 1969.

203. Garn SM. The course of bone gain and the phases of bone loss. *Orthop Clin North Am* 1972;3:503–20.

204. Krabbe S, Christiansen C, Rodbro P, Transbol I. Effect of puberty on rates of bone growth and mineralization. *Arch Dis Child* 1979;54:950–3.

205. Krabbe S, Transbol I, Christiansen C. Bone mineral homeostasis, bone growth, and mineralization during years of pubertal growth: a unifying concept. *Arch Dis Child* 1982;57:359–63.

206. Round JM, Butcher S, Steele R. Changes in plasma inorganic phosphorus and alkaline phosphatase activity during the adolescent growth spurt. *Ann Hum Biol* 1979;6:129–36.

207. Fleisher GA, Eikelberg ES, Elveback LR. Alkaline phosphatase activity in the plasma of children and adolescents. *Clin Chem* 1977;23:469–72.

208. Krabbe S, Christiansen C. Longitudinal study of calcium metabolism in male puberty. I. Bone mineral content, and serum levels of alkaline phosphatase, phosphate and calcium. *Acta Paediatr Scand* 1984;73:745–9.

209. Bennett DL, Ward MS, Daniel WA. The relationship of serum alkaline phosphatase concentrations to sex maturity ratings in adolescents. *J Pediatr* 1976;88:633–6.

210. Krabbe S, Christiansen C, Rodbro P, Transbol I. Pubertal growth as reflected by simultaneous changes in bone mineral content and serum alkaline phosphatase. *Acta Paediatr Scand* 1980;69:49–52.

211. Riis BJ, Krabbe S, Christiansen C, Catherwood BD, Deftos LJ. Bone turnover in male puberty: a longitudinal study. *Calcif Tissue Int* 1985;37:213–7.

212. Krabbe S, Hummer L, Christiansen C. Longitudinal study of calcium metabolism in male puberty. II. Relationship between mineralization and serum testosterone. *Acta Paediatr Scand* 1984;73:750–5.

213. Asknes L, Aarskog D. Plasma concentrations of vitamin D metabolites in puberty: effect of sexual maturation and implications for growth. *J Clin Endocrinol Metab* 1982;55:94–101.

214. Avioli LV. Postmenopausal osteoporosis: prevention versus cure. *Fed Proc* 1981;40:2418–22.

215. Avioli LV. Calcium and osteoporosis. *Annu Rev Nutr* 1984;4:471–91.

216. National Academy of Sciences. *Recommended dietary allowances,* 9th ed. Washington, DC: National Academy of Sciences, 1980.

217. *Calcium requirements: report of an FAO/WHO expert group.* Geneva: World Health Organization, 1962.

218. American Academy of Pediatrics, Committee on Nutrition. Calcium requirements in infancy and childhood. *Pediatrics* 1978;62:826–34.

219. Paterson CR. Calcium requirements in man: a critical review. *Postgrad Med J* 1978;54:244–8.

220. Garn SM. Calcium requirements for bone building and skeletal maintenance. *Am J Clin Nutr* 1970;23:1149–50.

221. Daniels AL, Hutton MK, Knott EM, Wright OE, Forman M. Calcium and phosphorus needs of preschool children. *J Nutr* 1935;10:373–88.

222. Holmes JO. The requirement for calcium during growth. *Nutr Abstr Rev* 1945;14:597–612.

223. Harrison HE. Factors influencing calcium absorption. *Fed Proc* 1959;18:1085–92.

224. Begum A, Pereira SM. Calcium balance studies on children accustomed to low calcium intakes. *Br J Nutr* 1969;23:905–11.

225. Pettifor JM, Ross P, Wang J, Moodley G, Couper-Smith J. Rickets in children of rural origin in South Africa: is low dietary calcium a factor? *J Pediatr* 1978;92:320–4.

226. Leguis E, Proesmans W, Eggermont E, Vandamme-Lombaerts R, Bouillon R, Smet M. Rickets due to dietary calcium deficiency. *Eur J Pediatr* 1989;148:784–5.

227. Day HG, McCollum EV. Mineral metabolism, growth, and symptomatology of rats on a diet extremely deficient in phosphorus. *J Biol Chem* 1939;130:269–83.

228. Freeman D, McLean FC. Experimental rickets. *Arch Pathol* 1941;32:387–408.

229. Baylink DJ, Stauffer M. Formation, mineralization, and resorption of bone in hypophosphatemic rats. *J Clin Invest* 1971;50:2519–30.

230. Cuisinier-Gleizes P, Thomasset M, Sainteny-Debove F, Mathieu H. Phosphorus deficiency, parathyroid hormone and bone resorption in the growing rat. *Calcif Tiss Res* 1976;20:235–49.

231. Brautbar N, Lee DBN, Coburn JW, Kleeman CR. Normophosphatemic phosphate depletion in growing rat. *Am J Physiol* 1979;236:E283–8.

232. Holick MF, MacLaughlin JA, Clark MB, et al. Photosynthesis of previtamin D$_3$ in human skin and the physiologic consequences. *Science* 1980;210:203–5.

233. Webb AR, Holick MF. The role of sunlight in the cutaneous production of vitamin D$_3$. *Annu Rev Med* 1988;8:375–99.

234. Poskitt EME, Cole TJ, Lawson DEM. Diet, sunlight, and 25-hydroxy vitamin D in healthy children and adults. *Br Med J* 1979;1:221–3.

235. American Academy of Pediatrics, Committee on Nutrition. The relation between infantile hypercalcemia and vitamin D–public health implications in North America. *Pediatrics* 1967;40:1050–61.

236. Reddy V, Sivakumar B. Magnesium-dependent vitamin-D-resistant rickets. *Lancet* 1974;1:963–5.

237. Anast CS, Winnacker JL, Forte LR, Burns TW. Impaired release of parathyroid hormone in magnesium deficiency. *J Clin Endocrinol Metab* 1976;43:707–17.

238. Hahn TJ, Chase LR, Avioli LV. Effect of magnesium depletion on responsiveness to parathyroid hormone in parathyroidectomized rats. *J Clin Invest* 1972;51:886–91.

239. Rude RK, Adams JS, Ryzen E, et al. Low serum concentrations of 1,25-dihydroxyvitamin D in human magnesium deficiency. *J Clin Endocrinol Metab* 1985;61:933–40.
240. Carpenter TO, Carnes DL, Anast CS. Effect of magnesium depletion on metabolism of 25-hydroxyvitamin D in rats. *Am J Physiol* 1987;253:E106–13.
241. Tinker D, Rucker RB. Role of selected nutrients in synthesis, accumulation, and chemical modification of connective tissue proteins. *Physiol Rev* 1985;65:607–57.
242. Miller ER, Lueke RW, Ullrey DE, Baltzer BV, Bradley BL, Hoefer JA. Biochemical, skeletal and allometric changes due to zinc deficiency in the baby pig. *J Nutr* 1968;95:278–86.
243. Brown ED, Chan W, Smith JC. Bone mineralization during developing zinc deficiency. *Proc Soc Exp Biol Med* 1978;157:211–14.
244. Leek JC, Keen CL, Vogler JB, et al. Long-term marginal zinc deprivation in rhesus monkeys. IV. Effects on skeletal growth and mineralization. *Am J Clin Nutr* 1988;47:889–95.
245. Leek JC, Vogler JB, Gershwin ME, Golub MS, Hurley LS, Hendrickx AG. Studies of marginal zinc deprivation in rhesus monkeys. V. Fetal and infant skeletal effects. *Am J Clin Nutr* 1984;40:1203–12.
246. Yamaguchi M, Yamaguchi R. Action of zinc on bone metabolism in rats. *Biochem Pharmacol* 1986;35:773–7.
247. De Virgillis S, Congia M, Frau F, et al. Deferoxamine-induced growth retardation in patients with thalassemia major. *J Pediatr* 1988;113:661–9.
248. Leach RM, Muenster A-M, Wien EM. Studies on the role of manganese in bone formation. II. Effect upon chondroitin sulfate synthesis in chick epiphyseal cartilage. *Arch Biochem Biophys* 1969;133:22–8.
249. Sognnaes RF. Fluoride protection of bones and teeth. *Science* 1965;150:989–93.
250. Faccini JM, Teotia SPS. Histopathological assessment of endemic skeletal fluorosis. *Calcif Tissue Res* 1974;16:45–57.
251. American Academy of Pediatrics, Committee on Nutrition. Fluoride as a nutrient. *Pediatrics* 1972;49:456–60.
252. Specker BL, Greer FR, Tsang RC. Vitamin D. In: Tsang, Nichols, eds. *Nutrition: conception to weaning.* Philadelphia: Hanley and Belfus Publishing, 1988;264–76.
253. Wakefield T Jr, Disney GW, Mason RL, Beauchene RE. Relationships among anthropometric indices of growth and creatinine and hydroxyproline excretion in preadolescent black and white girls. *Growth* 1980;44:192–204.
254. Mangaroo J, Glasser JH, Roht LH, Kapadia AS. Prevalence of bone demineralization in the United States. *Bone* 1985;6:135–9.
255. Cohn SH, Abesamis C, Zanzi I, Aloia JF, Yasumura S, Ellis KJ. Body elemental composition: comparison between black and white adults. *Am J Physiol* 1977;234(4):E419–22.
256. Cohn SH, Abesamis C, Yasamura S, Aloia JF, Zanzi I, Ellis EJ. Comparative skeletal mass and radial bone mineral content in black and white women. *Metab Clin Exp* 1977;26:171–8.
257. Trotter M, Broman GE, Peterson PR. Densities of bones of white and negro skeletons. *J Bone Joint Surg* 1970;42A:50–9.
258. Weinstein RS, Bell NH. Diminished rates of bone formation in normal black adults. *New Engl J Med* 1988;319(26):1698–1701.
259. Holick MF, MacLaughlin JA, Doppelt. Regulation of cutaneous previtamin D_3 photosynthesis in man: skin pigment is not an essential regulator. *Science* 1981;211:590–3.
260. Specker BL, Tsang RC, Hollis BW. Effect of race and diet on human-milk vitamin D and 25-hydroxyvitamin D. *Am J Dis Child* 1985;139:1134–7.
261. Lichtenstein P, Specker B, Tsang RC, Mimouni F, Gormley C. Calcium regulating hormones and minerals from birth to 18 months: a cross sectional study. I. Effects of sex, race, age, season, and diet on vitamin D status. *Pediatrics* 1986;77:883–90.
262. Specker BL, Valanis B, Hertzberg V, Edwards N, Tsang RC. Sunshine exposure and serum 25-hydroxyvitamin D concentration in exclusively breast-fed infants. *J Pediatr* 1985;107:372–6.
263. Specker B, Luchtenstein P, Mimouni F, Gormley C, Tsang RC. Calcium regulating hormones and minerals from birth to 18 months: a cross sectional study. II. Effects of sex, race, age, season and diet on serum minerals, parathyroid hormone, and calcitonin. *Pediatrics* 1986;77:891–6.
264. Bell NH, Greene A, Epstein S, Oexmann MJ, Shaw S, Shary J.

Evidence for alteration of the vitamin D–endocrine system in blacks. *J Clin Invest* 1985;76:470–3.
265. Stevenson JC, Myers CH, Ajdukiewicz AB. Racial differences in calcitonin and katacalcin. *Calcif Tissue Int* 1984;36:725–8.
266. Ziegler R, Deutschle U, Raue F. Calcitonin in human pathophysiology. *Horm Res* 1984;20:65–73.
267. Yergey AL, Voiera NE, Covell DG. Direct measurement of dietary fractional absorption using calcium isotopic tracers. *Biomed Environ Mass Spectrom* 1987;14:603–7.
268. Moore ES, Coe FL, McMann BJ, Favus MJ. Idiopathic hypercalciuria in children: prevalence and metabolic characteristics. *J Pediatr* 1978;92:906–10.
269. Stapleton FB, Roy S, Noe N, Jerkins J. Hypercalciuria in children with hematuria. *N Engl J Med* 1984;310:1345–8.
270. Stapleton FB, Noe N, Roy S, Jerkins G. Hypercalciuria in children with urolithiasis. *Am J Dis Child* 1982;136:675–8.
271. Knapp EL. Factors influencing the urinary excretion of calcium. I. In normal persons. *J Clin Invest* 1947;26:182–202.
272. Ghazali S, Barratt TM. Urinary excretion of calcium and magnesium in children. *Arch Dis Child* 1974;49:97–101.
273. Pak CYC, Kaplan R, Bone H, Townsend J, Waters O. A simple test for the diagnosis of absorptive, resorptive and renal hypercalciurias. *N Engl J Med* 1975;292:497–500.
274. Stapleton FB, Noe HN, Jerkins G, Roy S III. Urinary excretion of calcium following an oral calcium loading test in healthy children. *Pediatrics* 1982;69:594–7.
275. Kruse K, Kracht U, Kruse U. Reference values for urinary calcium excretion and screening for hypercalciuria in children and adolescents. *Eur J Pediatr* 1984;143:25–31.
276. Stapleton FB, Southwest Pediatric Nephrology Study Group. Idiopathic hypercalciuria: association with isolated hematuria and risk for urolithiasis in children. *Kidney Int* 1990;37:807–11.
277. Cervera A, Corral MJ, Gomez Campdera FJ, De Lecea AM, Luque A, Lopez Gomez JM. Idiopathic hypercalciuria in children: classification, clinical manifestations and outcome. *Acta Paediatr Scand* 1987;76:271–8.
278. Bijvoet OLM. Kidney function in calcium and phosphate metabolism. In: Avioli LV, Krane SM, eds. *Metabolic bone disease,* vol 1. London: Academic Press, 1977.
279. Walton RJ, Bijvoet OLM. Nomogram for derivation of renal threshold phosphate concentration. *Lancet* 1975;2:309–10.
280. Brodehl J, Krause A, Hoyer PF. Assessment of maximal tubular phosphate reabsorption: comparison of direct measurement with the nomogram of Bijvoet. *Pediatr Nephrol* 1988;2:183–9.
281. Gertner JM, Broadus AE, Anast CS, Grey M, Pearson H, Genel M. Impaired parathyroid response to induced hypocalcemia in thalassemia major. *J Pediatr* 1979;95:210–3.
282. Gidding SS, Manicotti AL, Langman CB. Unmasking of hypoparathyroidism in familial partial DiGeorge syndrome by challenge with disodium edetate. *N Engl J Med* 1988;319:1589–91.
283. McKay CP. Evaluation of the efficacy of IV 1,25(OH)$_2$ vitamin D on secondary hyperparathyroidism in children using the Allegro "INTACT" PTH IRMA assay. *Clin Res* 1990;38:69A.
284. Bergman L, Isaksson B. Plasma calcium fractions in normal subjects from birth to adult ages. *Acta Paediatr Scand* 1971;60:630–6.
285. Bullock JK. The physiologic variations in the inorganic blood phosphorus content at the different age periods. *Am J Dis Child* 1940;40:725–40.
286. Round JM. Plasma calcium, magnesium, phosphorus, and alkaline phosphatase levels in normal British schoolchildren. *Br Med J* 1973;3:137–40.
287. Markowitz ME, Rosen JF, Laxminarayan S, Mizruchi M. Circadian rhythms of blood minerals during adolescence. *Pediatr Res* 1984;18:456–62.
288. Woloszczuk W, Kovarik J, Bohrn E, Swoboda W, Wagner W. Calcitonin in healthy children. *Horm Metab Res* 1981;13:415–6.
289. Bodansky A, Jaffe HL. Phosphatase studies. III. Serum phosphatase in diseases of the bone: interpretation and significance. *Arch Int Med* 1934;54:88–110.
290. Harrison AP, Roderuck C, Lesher M, et al. Nutritional status of children. VIII. Blood serum alkaline phosphatase. *J Am Diet Assoc* 1948;24:503–9.

291. Clark LC, Beck E. Plasma "alkaline" phosphatase activity. I. Normative data for growing children. *J Pediatr* 1950;36:335–41.

292. Schiele F, Henny J, Hiltz J, Petitclerc C, Guegen R, Siest G. Total bone and liver alkaline phosphatase in plasma: biological variations and reference limits. *Clin Chem* 1983;29:634–41.

293. Lam WKW, Eastlund DT, Li C-Y, Yam LT. Biochemical properties of tartrate-resistant acid phosphatase in serum adults and children. *Clin Chem* 1978;24:1105–8.

294. Stepan JJ, Tesarova A, Havranek T, Jodl J, Formankova J, Pacovsky V. Age and sex dependency of the biochemical indices of bone remodeling. *Clin Chim Acta* 1985;151:273–83.

295. Price PA, Nishimoto SK. Radioimmunoassay for the vitamin K-dependent protein of bone and its discovery in plasma. *Proc Natl Acad Sci USA* 1980;77:2234–8.

296. Gundberg CM, Lian JB, Gallop PM. Measurements of γ-carboxyglutamate and circulating osteoclacin in normal children and adults. *Clin Chim Acta* 1983;128:1–8.

297. Johansen JS, Giwercman A, Hartwell D, et al. Serum bone Gla-protein as a marker of bone growth in children and adolescents: correlation with age, height, serum insulin-like growth factor I, and serum testosterone. *J Clin Endocrinol Metab* 1988;67:273–8.

298. Cole DEC, Carpenter TO, Gundberg CM. Serum osteocalcin in children with metabolic bone disease. *J Pediatr* 1985;106:770–6.

299. Kruse K, Kracht U. Evaluation of serum osteocalcin as an index of altered bone metabolism. *Eur J Pediatr* 1986;145:27–33.

300. Gundberg CM, Markowitz ME, Mizruchi M, Rosen JF. Osteocalcin in human serum: a circadian rhythm. *J Clin Endocrinol Metab* 1985;60:736–9.

301. Jasin HE, Fink CW, Wise W, Ziff M. Relationship between urinary hydroxyproline and growth. *J Clin Invest* 1962;41:1928–35.

302. Smiley JD, Ziff M. Urinary hydroxyproline excretion and growth. *Physiol Rev* 1964;44:30–44.

303. Jones CR, Bergman MW, Kittner PJ, Pigman WW. Urinary hydroxyproline excretion in normal children and adolescents. *Proc Soc Exp Biol Med* 1964;115:85–7.

304. Allison DJ, Walker A, Smith QT. Urinary hydroxyproline: creatinine ratio of normal humans at various ages. *Clin Chim Acta* 1966;14:729–34.

305. Younozai MK, Andersen DW, Filer LJ, Fomon SJ. Urinary excretion of endogenous hydroxyproline by normal male infants. *Pediatr Res* 1967;1:266–70.

306. Crowne RS, Wharton BA, McCance RA. Hydroxyproline indices and hydroxyproline/creatinine ratios in older children. *Lancet* 1969;1:395–6.

307. Wharton BA, Gough G, Willians A, Kitts S, Pennock CA. Urinary total hydroxyproline: creatinine ratio: range of normal, and clinical application in British children. *Arch Dis Child* 1972;47:74–9.

308. Clark S, Zorab PA. Hydroxyproline centiles for normal adolescent boys and girls. *Clin Orthop Relat Res* 1978;137:217–26.

309. Health and Policy Committee, American College of Physicians. Bone mineral densitometry. *Ann Intern med* 1987;107:932–6.

310. Cameron JR, Sorenson J. Measurement of bone mineral in vivo: an improved method. *Science* 1963;142:230–32.

311. Mazess RB, Cameron JR. Skeletal growth in school children: maturation and bone mass. *Am J Phys Anthropol* 1971;35:399–408.

312. Mazess RB, Cameron JR. Growth of bone in school children: comparison of radiographic morphometry and photon absorptiometry. *Growth* 1972;36:77–92.

313. Smith DM, Nance WE, Kang KW, Christian JC, Johnston CC. Genetic factors in determining bone mass. *J Clin Invest* 1973;52:2800–8.

314. Chesney RW, Mazess RB, Rose PG. Bone mineral status measured by direct photon absorptiometry in childhood renal disease. *Pediatrics* 1977;60:864–72.

315. Chesney RW, shore RM. The noninvasive determination of bone mineral content by photon absorptiometry. *Am J Dis Child* 1982;136:578–80.

316. Specker BL, Brazerol W, Tsang RC, Levin R, Searcy J, Steichen J. Bone mineral content in children 1 to 6 years of age: detectable sex differences after 4 years of age. *Am J Dis Child* 1987;141:343–4.

317. Klemm T, Banzer DH, Schneider U. Bone mineral content of the growing skeleton. *Am J Roentgenol* 1976;126:1283–4.

318. Christiansen C, Rödbro P, Nielsen T. Bone mineral content and estimated total body calcium in normal children and adolescents. *Scand J Clin Lab Invest* 1975;35:507–10.

319. Landin L, Nilsson BE. Forearm bone mineral content in children. *Acta Paediatr Scand* 1981;70:919–23.

Disorders of Bone and Mineral Metabolism,
edited by Fredric L. Coe and Murray J. Favus,
© 1992 by Raven Press, Ltd. All rights reserved.

CHAPTER **18**

Integration of Calcium Metabolism in the Adult

David A. Bushinsky and Nancy S. Krieger

On a daily basis there is marked variation in dietary mineral and electrolyte ingestion, yet the stable minute to minute regulation of plasma calcium concentration is of vital importance to the maintenance of cellular function. The homeostatic regulation of plasma calcium concentration occurs through a coordinated response of the gastrointestinal tract, kidneys, and bone. In certain diseases, such as metabolic acidosis, the plasma calcium concentration is maintained at the expense of a depletion of bone mineral content. While sufficient mineral content in bone is necessary for ambulation and to contain, support, and protect most organs, maintenance of a stable concentration of plasma calcium must take priority over maintenance of bone mineral content. We will first present a simple mathematical formulation to describe the influences of bone, kidney, and the gastrointestinal tract on extracellular fluid calcium concentration and then use the formulation to understand and predict the homeostatic response to variations in dietary mineral intake and to disease states which impact on calcium metabolism.

DETERMINANTS OF PLASMA CALCIUM CONCENTRATION

The variation in the calcium content in the extracellular fluid (ECF) reflects a change in the difference between the continual input and output of calcium (equation 1) (1).

D. A. Bushinsky: Departments of Medicine and Physiology, University of Rochester School of Medicine and Dentistry; Renal Unit, Strong Memorial Hospital, Rochester, New York 14642.

Nancy S. Krieger: Departments of Medicine and Pharmacology, University of Rochester School of Medicine and Dentistry, Rochester, New York 14642.

$$\Delta ECF_{Ca} = ECF\ input_{Ca} - ECF\ output_{Ca} \quad (1)$$

where ΔECF_{Ca} = the change in the ECF calcium content
$ECF\ input_{Ca}$ = the addition of calcium to the ECF
$ECF\ output_{Ca}$ = the loss of calcium from the ECF

(all in mass per unit time). Over a short period of time (minutes to hours) the ECF volume can be assumed to be constant and the ΔECF_{Ca} will normally be zero as there is an equal input and output of calcium. ΔECF_{Ca} will become positive when the input of calcium to the ECF exceeds the output of calcium from the ECF and negative when the output exceeds the input. An alteration in ΔECF_{Ca} will change the calcium concentration in the ECF by the following relationship:

$$[ECF_{Ca}]_{new} = [(\Delta ECF_{Ca} \times time)/ECF_{volume}]$$
$$+ [ECF_{Ca}]_{old} \quad (2)$$

where $[ECF_{Ca}]_{new}$ = the extracellular fluid volume calcium concentration at the end of the time period

ECF_{volume} = the extracellular fluid volume at the end of the time period

$[ECF_{Ca}]_{old}$ = the extracellular fluid calcium concentration at the beginning of the time period.

In this analysis we are most concerned with plasma calcium concentration. It is understood that the ECF consists not only of the plasma water but the interstitial, transcellular, bone, and connective tissue fluid as well. The equilibrium of calcium between the many ECF fluid compartments, especially the bone fluid, is not well understood. Strictly speaking the bone mineral is defined as part of the ECF; however, for the purposes of this analysis it will be treated as a separate compartment since only approximately 1% of the calcium contained within the bone mineral appears to be rapidly accessible to the ECF (2).

The input of calcium into the ECF can come only from resorption of bone mineral and absorption of gastrointestinal calcium (equation 3).

$$\text{ECF input}_{Ca} = Br_{Ca} + (D_{Ca} \times \alpha_{Ca}) \quad (3)$$

where Br_{Ca} = calcium released into the ECF during bone resorption (mass/time)
D_{Ca} = dietary calcium supply (mass/time)
α_{Ca} = fraction of intestinal calcium absorbed.

α_{Ca} is defined as (equation 4):

$$\alpha_{Ca} = (\text{dietary calcium intake}$$
$$- \text{fecal calcium excretion})/\text{dietary calcium intake} \quad (4)$$

α_{Ca} is overall net calcium absorption, which takes into account not only the calcium absorbed into the ECF but reabsorption of calcium secreted into the intestine. For this analysis it is not necessary to subdivide the absorption of dietary calcium from the reabsorption of secreted calcium. Thus α_{Ca} may be negative, for example during consumption of an extremely low calcium diet when there is little intake of calcium and a portion of the secreted intestinal calcium is lost into the feces (3,4).

The sole avenue for increasing the total body calcium content is through intestinal calcium absorption. As detailed elsewhere calcium may be absorbed in all segments of the intestine (5–9); however, quantitatively most absorption occurs in the duodenum (10) through pericellular diffusion and active transport (11–15). The active transport of calcium is regulated by 1,25(OH)$_2$D$_3$ (calcitriol) and occurs in three distinct steps (16). There is first movement of calcium across the luminal membrane into the intestinal cell. As cellular calcium concentration is in the nanomolar range this step occurs down a steep concentration gradient. The mechanism of this transport may involve a 1,25(OH)$_2$D$_3$-induced carrier protein (17), alterations in the membrane structure itself (18), or opening of a calcium channel (19). Calcium is then transported through the cytosol by binding to a 1,25(OH)$_2$D$_3$-dependent calcium binding protein (20). Lastly, calcium is transported across the basolateral cell membrane against a steep concentration gradient, a step which requires a calcium ATPase, although there appears to be a component of sodium/calcium exchange as well (21,22). Both absorption and secretion of calcium have been demonstrated in the jejunum and ileum and 1,25(OH)$_2$D$_3$ appears to stimulate active calcium transport in both segments of intestine (8). Although net calcium absorption in the colon is limited, at least in rats the cecum is capable of substantial calcium transport (23).

The egress of calcium from the ECF can be either through bone formation or renal calcium excretion (equation 5).

$$\text{ECF output}_{Ca} = Bf_{Ca} + U_{Ca} \quad (5)$$

where Bf_{Ca} = calcium being deposited in the bone (mass/time) and U_{Ca} = the urinary excretion of calcium. U_{Ca} is defined as:

$$U_{Ca} = GFR \times UF_{Ca} \times (1 - fr_{Ca}) \quad (6)$$

where the GFR = glomerular filtration rate (volume/time)
UF_{Ca} = ultrafilterable calcium (mass/volume)
fr_{Ca} = overall renal tubule fractional reabsorption of calcium.

We have excluded from consideration the small losses of calcium in sweat and the large losses of calcium in the milk of lactating females. The former is very difficult to accurately quantify (24,25), while the latter only occurs during relatively short, intermittent periods in the reproductive span of some females (26,27). However, pregnant females are included since bone formation of either the mother or the fetus involves loss of calcium from the ECF. Thus:

$$\Delta ECF_{Ca} = [Br_{Ca} + (D_{Ca} \times \alpha_{Ca})]$$
$$- \{Bf_{Ca} + [GFR \times UF_{Ca} \times (1 - fr_{Ca})]\}. \quad (7)$$

JB_{Ca} is defined as the net flux of calcium from the bone mineral (equation 8):

$$JB_{Ca} = Br_{Ca} - Bf_{Ca} \quad (8)$$

and JB_{Ca} consists of the combination of a net cellular calcium flux and a net physicochemical calcium flux, both in units of mass/time. Since our analysis is written in terms of the ECF calcium concentration, a positive JB_{Ca} indicates movement of calcium from bone into the ECF and a negative JB_{Ca} indicates movement of calcium from the ECF into bone. Since the vast majority of body calcium is contained within bone mineral (28,29), a positive net calcium balance indicates that bone formation is greater than bone resorption which is a negative JB_{Ca}, since the calcium deposited on the bone mineral must be derived from the ECF$_{Ca}$. Negative net calcium balance indicates that bone resorption is greater than bone formation; thus there is addition of calcium to the ECF, a positive JB_{Ca}.

Finally, over a period of time (1)

$$\Delta ECF_{Ca} = JB_{Ca} + (D_{Ca} \times \alpha_{Ca})$$
$$- [GFR \times UF_{Ca} \times (1 - fr_{Ca})] \quad (9)$$

or expressed in terms of JB_{Ca}:

$$JB_{Ca} = \Delta ECF_{Ca} - (D_{Ca} \times \alpha_{Ca})$$
$$+ [GFR \times UF_{Ca} \times (1 - fr_{Ca})]. \quad (10)$$

Thus the change in JB_{Ca} over a period of time is simply the combination of changes in ECF$_{Ca}$, gastrointestinal calcium absorption, and renal calcium excretion (Figure 1). The ECF, especially the plasma, provides the conduit

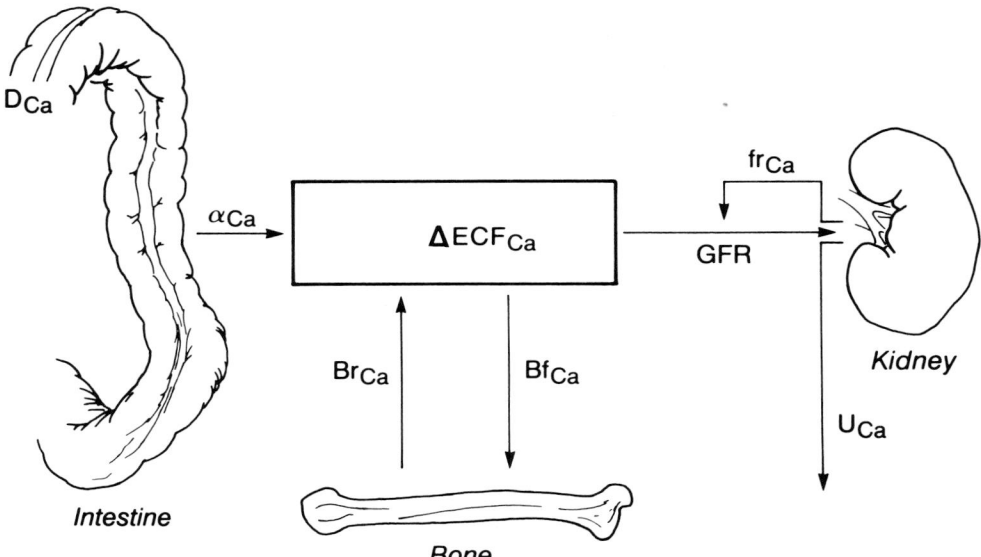

FIG. 1. Determinants of the distribution of calcium between the gastrointestinal tract, bone, kidney, and the extracellular fluid. D_{Ca}, dietary calcium supply (mass/unit time); α_{Ca}, fraction of intestinal calcium absorbed; Br_{Ca}, calcium released during bone resorption (mass/unit time); Bf_{Ca}, calcium being deposited upon bone (mass/unit time); GFR, glomerular filtration rate; fr_{Ca}, renal fractional reabsorption of calcium; U_{Ca}, urinary calcium excretion; ΔECF_{Ca}, change in ECF calcium content (mass/unit time). From Bushinsky and Krieger (1).

to connect the gastrointestinal tract, kidney, and bone, and the daily fluxes of calcium between these organs are often far greater than the total calcium content of the plasma. How the body is able to closely regulate plasma calcium concentration while still allowing for large fluxes between organs is a problem of integrative physiology, which we will explore in the remainder of the chapter.

INTEGRATION OF CALCIUM FLUXES AND POOLS

Large quantities of calcium are transported through the ECF between the gastrointestinal tract, kidney, and bone, yet the concentration of ECF_{Ca}, especially that of plasma water, must be tightly regulated to maintain cellular metabolic processes. The maintenance of a stable concentration of ECF_{Ca} in theory could depend upon (i) absorption of gastrointestinal calcium, (ii) reabsorption of calcium in the glomerular filtrate, or (iii) deposition and release of bone calcium through either cell-mediated or physicochemical mechanisms (30).

Although the gastrointestinal tract provides the only route for the net influx of calcium into the body, the intestine appears to be a poor site for the control of $[ECF_{Ca}]$. Intestinal calcium absorption is critically dependent on dietary calcium, a variable fraction of which is unregulated (8). The regulated component of calcium

absorption occurs through changes in levels of $1,25(OH)_2D_3$, a hormone that is not stored for release and must be synthesized de novo in response to increases in the level of parathyroid hormone (PTH) or decreases in phosphorus or ionized calcium. There is little evidence to suggest that the intestine can respond to the short-term requirements for regulation of $[ECF_{Ca}]$.

One reasonable hypothesis for the regulation of ECF_{Ca} concentration is by alteration in the tubular reabsorption of calcium in the glomerular filtrate (30,31). Approximately 98% of filtered calcium is reabsorbed, and the normal daily reabsorption of ~270 mmoles is large relative to the normal ECF_{Ca} content of ~35 mmoles (see below) indicating that small changes in tubular reabsorption of calcium will have large effects on $[ECF_{Ca}]$. A small increase in the tubular fractional reabsorption of calcium would increase ΔECF_{Ca} and a decrease in tubular reabsorption would decrease ΔECF_{Ca} (equation 9). While alterations in the tubular reabsorption of calcium must have an effect on $[ECF_{Ca}]$, control cannot be solely at the level of the kidney because of three clinical examples: (i) renal failure (32), (ii) hemodialysis, and (iii) pseudohypoparathyroidism (30). During renal failure, when there is little glomerular filtration of calcium, the level of serum calcium is still reasonably well-regulated. Were renal calcium excretion the principal regulator of $[ECF_{Ca}]$, then an acute loss of GFR would lead to the return to the ECF of the entire load of previously excreted calcium. Given an average excretion of approxi-

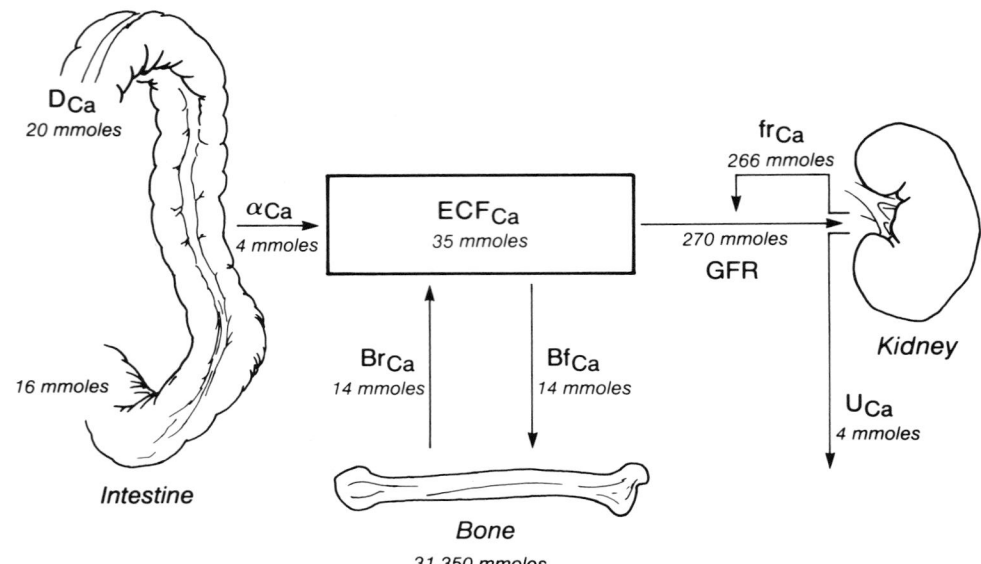

FIG. 2. Flux of calcium between compartments within the body. From Bushinsky and Krieger (1).

mately 1.25 to 7.5 mmoles/day, the [ECF_{Ca}] would steadily increase by ~ 0.1 to 0.5 mmoles each day. This increase in ECF_{Ca} has not been observed. During hemodialysis the calcium concentration of the bath is generally 3.25–3.5 mM (~ 13–14 mg/dL) producing a large calcium gradient relative to the patient's blood (33). As hemodialysis blood flow rates are usually ~ 300 mL/min, over the ~ 4 h of dialysis multiple ECF volumes (~ 0.3 L/min $\times \sim 240$ min = ~ 80 L) are exposed to this high dialysate calcium concentration yet blood calcium concentration rises only initially and then rapidly returns to predialysis levels in the absence of significant renal function (34,35). During the hypocalcemia of pseudohypoparathyroidism, the renal reabsorption of calcium appears to be normal or only slightly impaired, yet the level of serum calcium is maintained below normal (36).

Regulation of ECF_{Ca} at the level of the bone is also an attractive hypothesis (30). Bone formation and resorption are regulated by changes in the physicochemical driving forces for mineralization (37,38) and by alterations in osteoclastic and osteoblastic activity (39). The ECF is markedly supersaturated with respect to apatite, the most abundant phase of the bone mineral (37,40). There appears to be a barrier to the free diffusion of calcium from the ECF into the mineral, which prevents circulating calcium from being readily incorporated into apatite (41–48). The nature of this barrier is not clear but it may be an early phase of the mineral, perhaps $CaHPO_4$ or carbonated apatite or a cellular–organic layer. In vitro bone culture medium is in passive physiochemical equilibrium with carbonated apatite in the bone mineral (37). Lowering the culture medium driving force for crystallization with respect to carbonated apatite induces

TABLE 1. ΔECF_{Ca} and its components under various conditions

Condition	ΔECF_{Ca} =	(Br_{Ca} −	Bf_{Ca})	+ (D_{Ca} ×	α_{Ca})	− [GFR ×	UF_{Ca})	× (1 − fr_{Ca})]
Normal	−	n	n	n	n	n	n	n
Very low calcium diet	↓	↑	↓	↓	↑	n	↓	↓
Excess PTH	↑	↑	↑	n	n − ↑	n	↑	↓
Excess 1,25(OH)$_2$D$_3$	↑	n − ↑	n − ↑	n	↑	n	↑	↑
Metabolic acidosis	−	↑	?	n	n	n − ↓	↑	↑
Respiratory acidosis	↑	n − ↑	?	n	?	n	↑	? − ↓
Renal failure	↓	↑	↑ − n − ↓	n	↓	↓	↓	↑

Source: Bushinsky and Krieger (1).

ΔECF_{Ca}, change in ECF calcium content (mass/unit time, ΔECF_{Ca} is normally zero); Br_{Ca}, calcium released during bone resorption (mass/unit time); Bf_{Ca}, calcium being deposited upon bone (mass/unit time); D_{Ca}, dietary calcium supply (mass/unit time); α_{Ca}, fraction of intestinal calcium absorbed; GFR, glomerular filtration rate; UF_{Ca}, ultrafilterable calcium; fr_{Ca}, renal fractional reabsorption of calcium; n, normal level; ↑, increase; ↓, decrease. For details see text.

loss of bone mineral; increasing the driving force results in an increase in mineral calcium. If these experimental results with cultured bone can be applied to humans this would suggest that a lowered ECF_{Ca} concentration would decrease the driving force for mineralization with respect to an early, relatively unstable phase of the mineral and result in an efflux of calcium from bone to increase ΔECF_{Ca}. Similarly a primary increase in ΔECF_{Ca} would result in movement of calcium from the ECF onto an early phase of the mineral. Thus the changes in the ECF_{Ca} concentration are lessened or "buffered" by calcium influx into or efflux from the bone mineral. Regulation of $[ECF_{Ca}]$ can also occur through hormonal alterations in cell-mediated bone resorption and formation though these processes would probably not be operative over very short periods of time (minutes).

There is a time dependency of the response of different organs to a change in $[ECF_{Ca}]$. Almost certainly the physicochemical response of the bone mineral to alterations in $[ECF_{Ca}]$ occurs most rapidly. Changes in $[ECF_{Ca}]$ alter the filtered load of calcium and induce changes in PTH secretion which subsequently affect renal calcium reabsorption and cell-mediated bone resorption. Finally changes in $[ECF_{Ca}]$ affect $1,25(OH)_2D_3$ levels to alter gastrointestinal calcium absorption and cell-mediated bone formation and resorption. Thus while acute minute-to-minute regulation of $[ECF_{Ca}]$ probably occurs on the surface of the bone mineral, the kidney and gastrointestinal tract are clearly involved in the longer term regulation.

It is instructive to examine clinical examples to illustrate how the integrated response of gastrointestinal tract, bone, and kidney are coordinated to maintain a constant $[ECF_{Ca}]$.

Normal

A 70-kg man has an ECF volume of approximately 14 liters and an $[ECF_{Ca}]$ of approximately 2.5 mM leading to a total ECF calcium content, excluding the bone mineral, of ~35 mmoles or approximately 0.1% of total body calcium (10,29,49) (Figure 2).

The vast majority of total body calcium is contained within the bone mineral (28,29). Through cadaveric chemical analysis and neutron activation analysis it is estimated that bone contains ~31,350 mmoles of the total body calcium content of ~31,500 mmoles; thus in excess of 99.5% of total body calcium resides within the bone (10,29,49). Much of the calcium contained within the mineral is inaccessible to the ECF, at least over the short term, but it is estimated that approximately 1% of total body calcium is freely exchangeable between the bone and the ECF (2). By neutron activation analysis total body calcium is greater in normal men than in nor-

mal women at all ages (49). Based on measurements of single and dual photon absorptiometry, bone mass appears maximal at approximately age 25 (50). In normal females there is continuous loss of vertebral mass from early adulthood although appendicular skeletal bone mass does not begin to decrease until approximately age 50, while in normal males there is minimal bone loss with age (50). The onset of menopause is associated with an increased rate of mineral loss in many women (51–54). In studies of monozygotic and dizygotic twins bone mass was found to have significant genetic determinants (55).

The normal American daily diet contains approximately 20 mmoles of calcium of which approximately 16 mmoles are excreted in the feces, indicating that the fraction of calcium absorbed, α_{Ca}, equals ~0.20 (3,10,16,56). The intestinal absorption of calcium varies with dietary calcium intake (Figure 3) (3,31,57–61). When dietary calcium is less than ~5 mmoles, fecal calcium excretion exceeds calcium intake, resulting in negative α_{Ca}. As dietary calcium intake increases net intestinal calcium absorption increases at a decreasing rate, stabilizing at intakes greater than ~25 mmole/day. Increasing serum $1,25(OH)_2D_3$ increases net intestinal calcium absorption (57,59,61) and at any level of $1,25(OH)_2D_3$ increasing dietary calcium will result in a greater net intestinal calcium absorption (Figure 4). When additional calcium is needed, for example during periods of rapid growth or during pregnancy and lactation, there is an increase in intestinal calcium absorption due to increased $1,25(OH)_2D_3$ (62,63).

As discussed in detail elsewhere renal calcium excretion represents the difference between the filtered load of calcium and its subsequent tubular reabsorption (equation 6). To date there is no evidence for net secretion of calcium by the kidney (16). The filtered load of calcium equals the GFR (~180 L/day in normals) × the ultrafilterable calcium concentration. The ultrafilterable calcium concentration equals ~0.6% of total $[ECF_{Ca}]$ of 2.5 mM or 1.5 mM. Thus the filtered load of calcium equals 180 L/day × 1.5 mmoles/L = 270 mmoles/day.

Eating a typical American diet containing 20 mmoles of calcium, the average urinary calcium excretion (U_{Ca}) in healthy adults ranges from approximately 1 to 7.5 mmole/day, averaging ~4 mmoles/day, indicating that normally over 98% of the filtered load of calcium is reabsorbed; thus $(1 - fr_{Ca})$ is approximately 0.015 (4,16,64,65). U_{Ca} varies directly, but not linearly, with the intake and serum level of calcium, as well as with the intake of sodium and protein and inversely with phosphorus intake (Fig. 5) (4,66). U_{Ca} will fall within several days of instituting a low calcium diet; however, urine calcium can never be totally eliminated, minimal excretion rates are at least 0.5 mmole/day (4). U_{Ca} must be tightly regulated as the flux of calcium through the nor-

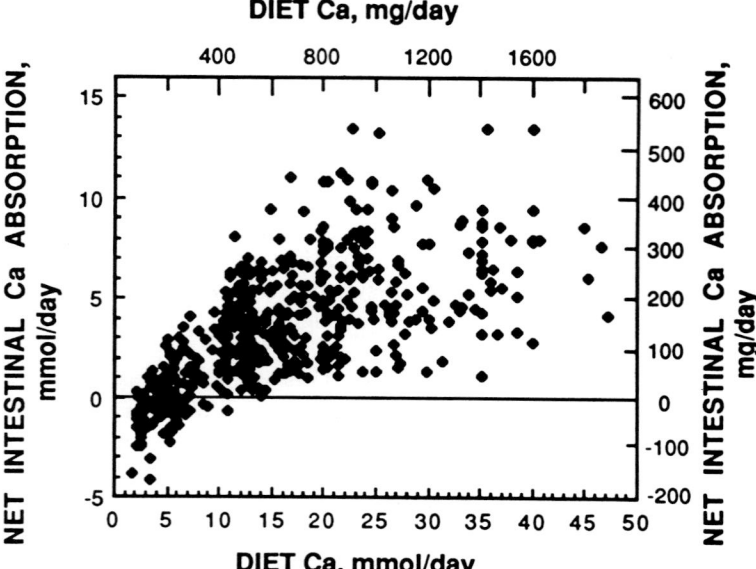

FIG. 3. Effect of dietary calcium intake on net intestinal calcium absorption. From Lemann (3).

mal kidney of 270 mmoles/day is far greater than the concentration of circulating calcium in the ECF of 35 mmoles.

In the normal adult ingesting a diet adequate in calcium, there is no appreciable net bone formation or resorption, i.e., $JB_{Ca} = 0$ over the course of a day. Thus, for the normal adult on a daily basis, the input of calcium from the gastrointestinal tract is balanced by the U_{Ca}, as shown by substituting into equation 9. Ideally there is no net change in ΔECF_{Ca} over this period of time and $[ECF_{Ca}]_{new}$ will not differ from $[ECF_{Ca}]_{old}$.

$$\Delta ECF_{Ca} = JB_{Ca} + (D_{Ca} \times \alpha_{Ca})$$
$$- [GFR \times UF_{Ca} \times (1 - fr_{Ca})] \quad (9)$$

$$0 = 0 + (20 \text{ mmoles/day} \times 0.20)$$
$$- (180 \text{ L/day} \times 1.5 \text{ mmoles/L} \times 0.015).$$

However, there are generally daily alterations in D_{Ca}, and U_{Ca} varies—for example, due to changes in acid–base status, sodium excretion, or renal function, PTH may change in disease and vitamin D may change with alterations in intake or renal function. It is often difficult to understand changes of each component of this integrated system in health; however, variations in dietary calcium intake and clinical disorders can be utilized to shed light on the physiologic response of this homeostatic system.

Very Low Calcium Diet

The ingestion of diet with a very low calcium content provokes a coordinated physiological response aimed at overall calcium conservation and maintaining $[ECF_{Ca}]_{new}$ as close to $[ECF_{Ca}]_{old}$ as possible. When adults are fed ~ 3.5 mmoles/day of calcium, compared to the normal diet of ~ 20 mmoles/day, there is a decreased $[ECF_{Ca}]_{new}$ (67) indicating that ΔECF_{Ca} is negative. The lower $[ECF_{Ca}]_{new}$ will stimulate physicochemical bone dissolution, with release of mineral calcium into the ECF (37). In addition, the lower $[ECF_{Ca}]_{new}$ will cause some fall in the ionized component of blood calcium (Ca^{2+}) leading to an increase in PTH secretion and $1,25(OH)_2D_3$ production, the latter a consequence of the increased PTH and decreased $[Ca^{2+}]$ (Fig. 6) (68,69). The increase in $1,25(OH)_2D_3$ will directly increase α_{Ca} and the increase in PTH will increase fr_{Ca}; however, the fall in $[ECF_{Ca}]_{new}$ will lead to a decrease in UF_{Ca}. The increase in PTH will also increase cell-mediated bone turnover but the net

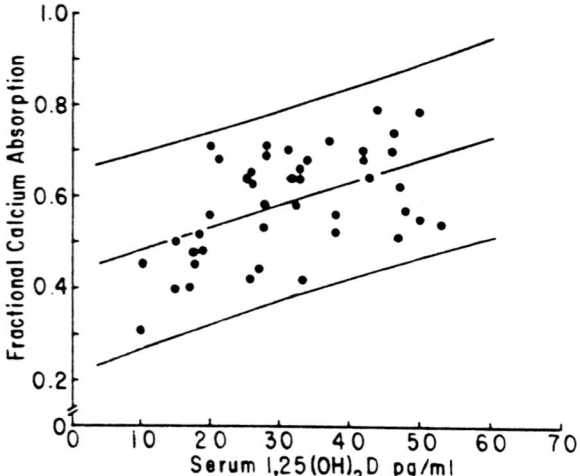

FIG. 4. Fractional calcium absorption plotted as a function of the level of serum $1,25(OH)_2D_3$ in normal subjects. From Gallagher et al. (57).

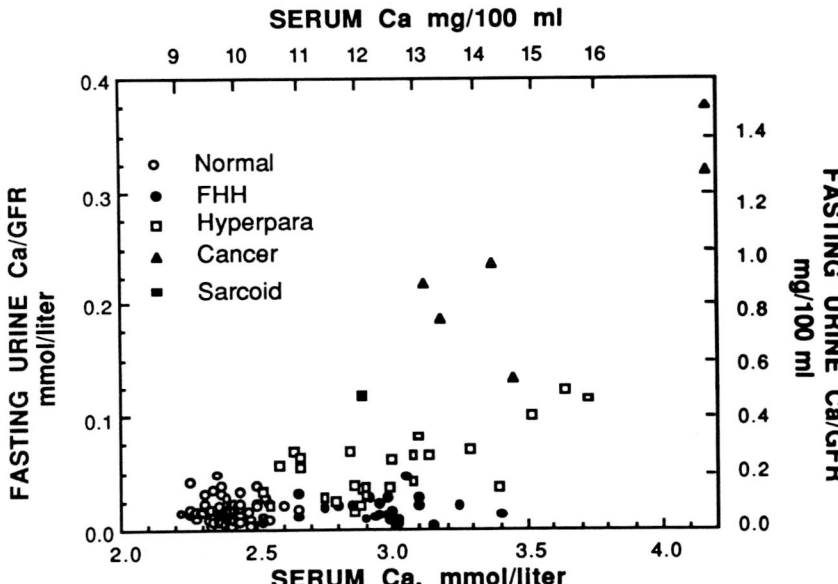

FIG. 5. Urinary calcium excretion as a function of total serum calcium concentration. (O), normal subjects; (●) patients with familial hypocalciuric hypercalcemia; and (□), patients with primary hyperparathyroidism. From Lemann (4).

effect of a low calcium diet on JB_{Ca} is dependent upon the level of D_{Ca}. At a D_{Ca} of 5 mmoles/day there is still positive net calcium retention in many patients (70), indicating that Bf_{Ca} remains positive and greater than or equal to Br_{Ca}. However, when dietary calcium falls further, below ~3.5 mmoles/day, there is continued U_{Ca}

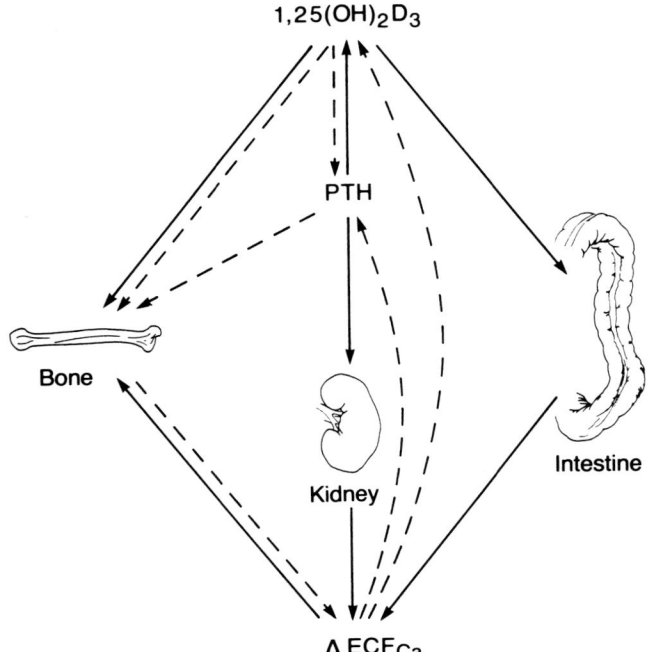

FIG. 6. Schematic diagram of the regulation of parathyroid hormone (PTH), 1,25-dihydroxyvitamin D_3 [1,25(OH)$_2$D$_3$], and calcium (Ca) in relation to bone, kidney, and intestine. Solid arrows indicate up regulation, bone formation, enhanced renal calcium reabsorption, or intestinal calcium absorption. Dashed lines indicate down-regulation, bone mineral dissolution, or enhanced renal calcium excretion.

which exceeds the product of $D_{Ca} \times \alpha_{Ca}$ in spite of the 1,25(OH)$_2$D$_3$-induced increase in α_{Ca}. At this level of calcium intake there is simply not enough D_{Ca} that can be absorbed to equal U_{Ca}. The capacity of ECF with respect to calcium is limited; so to prevent a marked fall in [ECF$_{Ca}$]$_{new}$ there must be net bone resorption, greater Br_{Ca} than Bf_{Ca}, resulting in an increased JB_{Ca}. In the absence of calcium intake (zero D_{Ca}), because renal reabsorption of calcium can never be complete (fr$_{Ca}$ < 1), U_{Ca} must be equivalent to the release of bone calcium, positive JB_{Ca}, or [ECF$_{Ca}$]$_{new}$ will continue to fall. The positive JB_{Ca} is a function of a low [ECF$_{Ca}$]$_{new}$ producing low [Ca^{2+}], which promotes physicochemical bone mineral dissolution and stimulates secretion of PTH and 1,25(OH)$_2$D$_3$ leading to enhanced cell-mediated bone mineral resorption (Fig. 6). [ECF$_{Ca}$]$_{new}$ can then be maintained within a range adequate to support physiologic functions at the expense of the mass of bone mineral.

Excess Parathyroid Hormone

Chronic excess PTH, as present in primary hyperparathyroidism, leads to predictable physiologic responses. The excess PTH results in increased renal tubule fractional reabsorption of calcium (fr$_{Ca}$), leading to a positive ΔECF$_{Ca}$ and an increase in [ECF$_{Ca}$]$_{new}$ (Fig. 6) (71–74). While the increase in ΔECF$_{Ca}$ tends to increase bone formation, positive Bf_{Ca}, by physicochemical mechanisms, the marked PTH-induced increase in bone turnover favors osteoclastic bone resorption, Br_{Ca} greater than Bf_{Ca}, as indicated by radiographic evidence of bone mineral depletion, leading to a positive JB_{Ca} (38,75–78). With a continued large excess of PTH, there is a continued positive ΔECF$_{Ca}$ and increasing [ECF$_{Ca}$]$_{new}$. [Ca^{2+}] and UF$_{Ca}$ will increase to such an extent that the elevated

UF_{Ca} exceeds the increase in fr_{Ca}, leading to an absolute increase in urinary calcium excretion, U_{Ca} (72). In many patients the excess PTH stimulates an increase in $1,25(OH)_2D_3$ production (79) and the increased serum levels of $1,25(OH)_2D_3$ lead to an increase in α_{Ca} and the product of $D_{Ca} \times \alpha_{Ca}$ (80,81). This further increases ΔECF_{Ca}, $[ECF_{Ca}]_{new}$, and UF_{Ca}, resulting in greater urinary calcium excretion (72). $1,25(OH)_2D_3$ does not increase in all patients, perhaps due to the rise in $[Ca^{2+}]$, which has been shown to directly suppress the level of serum $1,25(OH)_2D_3$ (82–88). ΔECF_{Ca} continues to increase leading to a further increase in $[ECF_{Ca}]_{new}$, whose ultimate level is a function of the elevation of serum PTH.

Excess $1,25(OH)_2D_3$

The administration of excess $1,25(OH)_2D_3$ will have a primary effect of increasing α_{Ca} leading to an increase in the product of $D_{Ca} \times \alpha_{Ca}$ (80,81). ΔECF_{Ca} will be positive, leading to an increase in $[ECF_{Ca}]_{new}$ and UF_{Ca} and thus in the product of $GFR \times UF_{Ca}$. $[Ca^{2+}]$ will also increase, causing a fall in PTH (89) and thus a subsequent fall in fr_{Ca} (72) and a rise in $(1 - fr_{Ca})$ and in $GFR \times UF_{Ca} \times (1 - fr_{Ca})$ (Fig. 6). There is no consistent evidence that $1,25(OH)_2D_3$ itself will alter fr_{Ca} independently of PTH (68). U_{Ca} will increase markedly under the influence of an increased UF_{Ca} and decreased fr_{Ca} (68). In vitro $1,25(OH)_2D_3$ causes marked cell-mediated resorption of the bone mineral (90) while an increase in medium calcium causes physicochemically induced calcium deposition in bone (37). In vivo, the net effect of $1,25(OH)_2D_3$ on bone is critically dependent on D_{Ca} (91). When normal rats are injected with $1,25(OH)_2D_3$, a high-calcium diet will protect their bone mineral stores (91). However, when normal adults were fed a low calcium diet (2 mmoles/day) and injected with $1,25(OH)_2D_3$, net intestinal calcium absorption ($D_{Ca} \times \alpha_{Ca}$) was also approximately 2 mmoles/day, yet U_{Ca} [$GFR \times UF_{Ca} \times (1 - fr_{Ca})$] rose to 6–10 mmoles/day, indicating negative calcium balance (70). The source of this additional U_{Ca} could only have been bone mineral, indicating that Br_{Ca} was greater than Bf_{Ca}. Since ΔECF_{Ca} was positive and $[Ca^{2+}]$ rose, physicochemical forces would actually favor bone formation. This indicates that $1,25(OH)_2D_3$-induced cell-mediated bone resorption must account for the enhanced U_{Ca} during a low calcium diet.

Metabolic Acidosis

A lowered systemic pH will increase the displacement of albumin bound calcium, increasing $[Ca^{2+}]$ and UF_{Ca} (92). ΔECF_{Ca} is not altered since acidosis does not increase the total calcium concentration (82). Acidosis will also decrease fr_{Ca} through a direct effect of lowered bicarbonate on renal tubular calcium reabsorption (93,94). Decreased pH independent of decreased $[HCO_3^-]$ will not decrease calcium reabsorption (95). The net result of an increased UF_{Ca} and decreased fr_{Ca}, in spite of some fall in GFR (93), is a marked increase in U_{Ca} (82,83,96–98).

The effect of acidosis on the serum levels of PTH and $1,25(OH)_2D_3$ has been studied in detail in animals (82,83) and in man (98,99). In the rat there is impaired conversion of ^3H-$25(OH)D_3$ to ^3H-$1,25(OH)_2D_3$ during metabolic acidosis (100) and impaired production of $1,25(OH)_2D_3$ in the isolated perfused kidney obtained from rats with metabolic acidosis (101). The basal serum levels of PTH and $1,25(OH)_2D_3$ are unaltered by acidosis in the rat (68,82); however, during acidosis $1,25(OH)_2D_3$ does not rise in response to a low calcium diet (82) except with concomitant phosphate depletion (102). The arterial blood $[Ca^{2+}]$, which increases with acidosis, appears to regulate the level of $1,25(OH)_2D_3$ in both the nonacidemic and acidemic rat (Fig. 7) (82,83,86). In man serum PTH and $1,25(OH)_2D_3$ are not directly increased by acidosis (98,99) in spite of the increased urinary calcium excretion and negative calcium balance. However, during acidosis the infusion of PTH will increase serum $1,25(OH)_2D_3$ (103). α_{Ca} does not appear to be significantly altered in man during acidosis (93,98,104).

The effect of metabolic acidosis on bone calcium has been studied in detail both in vitro and in vivo. In vitro studies support the assertion that bone is involved in the systemic response to metabolic acidosis. Neuman and Neuman found that a reduction of medium pH produced a marked increase in hydroxyapatite solubility (40) and Dominguez and Raisz (105) determined that an acid medium induced movement of prelabeled ^{45}Ca from bone. Cultured neonatal mouse calvariae exhibit proton-dependent calcium flux during both acute (3 h) and more chronic (24–99 h) incubations (1,37,38,69,75,90,106–108). During acute incubations there is calcium efflux from the calvariae when medium pH was below the physiologic normal of 7.40, no net flux at 7.40, and an influx of calcium into bone when pH was above 7.40 (108). During acute incubations bone cells contributed a constant, pH-independent efflux of calcium from the mineral; thus the calcium release was the result of physicochemical dissolution and not cell-mediated resorption (38). However, during chronic (99 h) studies there was calcium efflux only from live bone cultured in acidic medium indicating that bone cell function is necessary for calcium release during chronic acidosis (106).

The calcium efflux from bone is critically dependent upon both the decrement in pH and $[HCO_3^-]$. In acute studies there is greater calcium efflux during culture in reduced $[HCO_3^-]$ medium (a model of metabolic acidosis) than during culture in medium acidified to the same

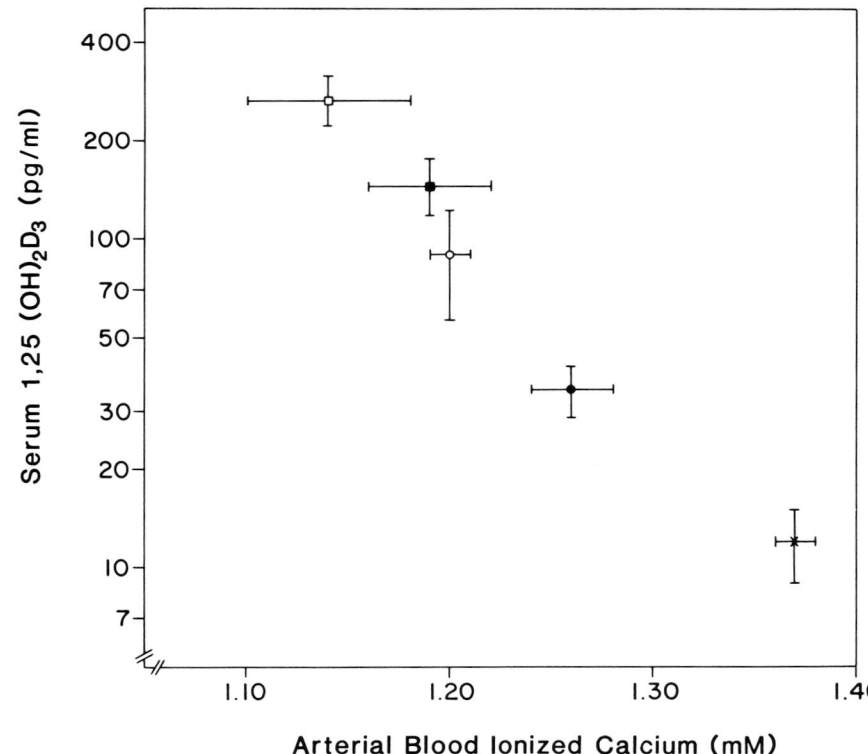

FIG. 7. Effect of arterial blood ionized calcium on serum 1,25(OH)₂D₃ in the rat. Values are mean ± SE. Rats were infused for 24 h with NaCl alone at 0.4 ml/h (●, n = 10); 10 μm/kg/h synthetic bovine PTH 1–34 (x, n = 11); PTH and 0.67 μm/min EGTA (○, n = 7); PTH and 1.00 μm/min EGTA (■, n = 6); or PTH and 1.33 μm/min EGTA (□, n = 7). For all data included, log serum 1,25(OH)₂D₃ was correlated inversely with arterial blood ionized calcium (r = −0.667, n = 41, p < 0.001). From Bushinsky et al. (84).

pH with an increase in PCO₂ (a model of respiratory acidosis) (107). During chronic (99 h) studies there is calcium efflux only from bone incubated in medium of reduced [HCO₃⁻] and not from bones incubated in the presence of an increased PCO₂ (106). A decrement in both pH and [HCO₃⁻] is also necessary for the additional hydrogen ions to be buffered during acidosis. Cultured calvariae buffer the increase in [H⁺] only when the medium is acidified by decreasing the [HCO₃⁻] as in metabolic acidosis, but not when the medium is acidified by increasing the PCO₂, as in respiratory acidosis (75,107).

Direct dissolution of bone mineral surface by an acid pH should lead to either a ratio of 5 nEq of protons to 3 nEq of calcium if hydroxyapatite is dissolved or a ratio of 1:1 if brushite or calcium carbonate is dissolved (109,110). However, for every 16–21 nEq of protons that enters bone only 1 nEq of calcium leaves (108). This suggests that sodium and/or salts of carbonate or phosphate may participate in proton for sodium and/or potassium exchange (1,37,69,90,108). Indeed in addition to a loss of bone carbonate (37) high-resolution scanning ion microprobe analysis of bone reveals a reduction in the surface sodium and potassium during acidosis (90).

During in vivo acute metabolic acidosis, ∼60% of the administered protons are buffered outside of the extracellular fluid (111) by soft tissues (112–114) and by bone (37,69,75,107,108). The in vivo evidence that bone acutely buffers protons and in the process releases calcium derives principally from the loss of bone sodium

(111,115–117) and carbonate (37,117,118) and the increase in serum calcium (119) observed during acute acidosis. Bone sodium loss implies proton for sodium exchange and carbonate loss suggests consumption of this buffer by the administered protons. As the vast majority of body calcium is contained within bone (28) the increase in serum calcium is likely to derive from these mineral stores. Chronic metabolic acidosis, found in patients with renal insufficiency (120,121) and renal tubular acidosis (120,122) increases U_Ca (68,83,96), generally without an increase in α_Ca (98,99), resulting in a negative calcium balance (82,93) which appears to reflect proton-mediated dissolution of bone mineral (37,38,68,69,75, 90,93,96,97,106–108). Indeed, chronic metabolic acidosis appears to decrease mineral content in most in vivo studies (82,93,102,117,123–125).

Respiratory Acidosis

In contrast to metabolic acidosis, in vivo respiratory acidosis may (126) or may not (127–129) produce a significant increase in U_Ca. However [ECF_Ca] generally increases implying an increase in fr_Ca or α_Ca, or that Br_Ca has become greater than Bf_Ca (126–128,130). Although D_Ca will not necessarily change, little is known about the affect of respiratory acidosis on the serum level of 1,25(OH)₂D₃ or α_Ca.

In vitro respiratory acidosis induces physicochemical dissolution of the bone mineral that is quantitatively less than that induced by metabolic acidosis for the same reduction in pH (106,107). While the reason for less calcium release is not known, it may be due to excess carbon dioxide increasing the driving force for the formation of carbonated apatite, the bone mineral in equilibrium with the culture medium (37). Cell-mediated bone resorption does not appear to increase with respiratory acidosis (106). Again the reason for the lack of a cellular response is not known, but may relate to the presence of a chloride/bicarbonate exchanger on the basolateral membrane of the osteoclast (131,132). In metabolic acidosis the low medium [HCO_3^-] will promote the egress of cellular bicarbonate, leading to enhanced proton secretion by the osteoclast and greater cell-mediated bone resorption. In respiratory acidosis the medium [HCO_3^-] is not lowered, the gradient for bicarbonate is not increased and thus cell-mediated bone resorption may not be stimulated.

Renal Failure

Elevated levels of PTH are consistently found in patients with renal failure and the greater the impairment of renal function the higher the level of PTH (133–135) (Fig. 8). The secretion of PTH is increased principally due to the decline in the circulating level of arterial blood [Ca^{2+}] and the fall in $1,25(OH)_2D_3$ (89). The factors responsible for the low [Ca^{2+}] are multiple and the importance of each is controversial. Phosphate retention, decreased levels of serum $1,25(OH)_2D_3$ with the conse-

quent reduction of α_{Ca} and alteration in the set point for PTH secretion and impaired degradation of PTH may all contribute to the increase in the serum levels of PTH. The excess PTH and the acidemia produced by the failure to excrete endogenous acids will promote bone mineral resorption in many patients with renal failure (Fig. 9).

It is clear that phosphate retention will increase PTH levels in humans (136) and experimental animals (137) with no impairment in renal function. In patients with renal insufficiency (138) and in animals with renal failure (139,140) the restriction of dietary phosphate will lower elevated PTH levels and the levels of PTH correlate with the serum levels of phosphate (141). The mechanism by which phosphate retention increases PTH secretion is not completely known. There is no evidence for a direct effect of phosphate on PTH secretion; rather the increased secretion appears due to a fall in blood [Ca^{2+}]. Blood [Ca^{2+}] may fall because increased phosphate will increase the physicochemical driving forces for bone mineral formation (37) and favor ectopic precipitation of calcium phosphate complexes (142). Alternatively, phosphate retention could directly decrease serum $1,25(OH)_2D_3$ leading to a fall in α_{Ca}, a negative ΔECF_{Ca}, and a decrease in [Ca^{2+}] (143).

The enzyme responsible for the conversion of $25(OH)D_3$ to $1,25(OH)_2D_3$ 25-hydroxycholecalciferol-1α-hydroxylase is located in the proximal tubule (144–146). A decrement in the functional renal mass will decrease the conversion and thus the serum levels

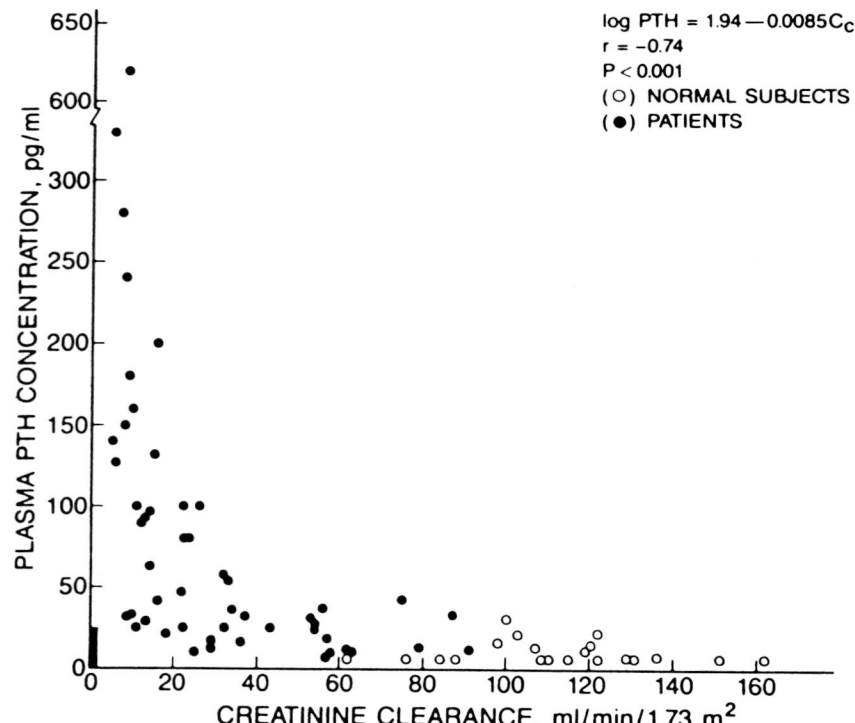

log PTH = 1.94 − 0.0085C_{cr}
r = −0.74
P < 0.001
(○) NORMAL SUBJECTS
(●) PATIENTS

FIG. 8. The correlation between plasma PTH concentration and endogenous creatinine clearance in normal subjects (○) and patients with renal insufficiency (●). From Pitts et al. (135).

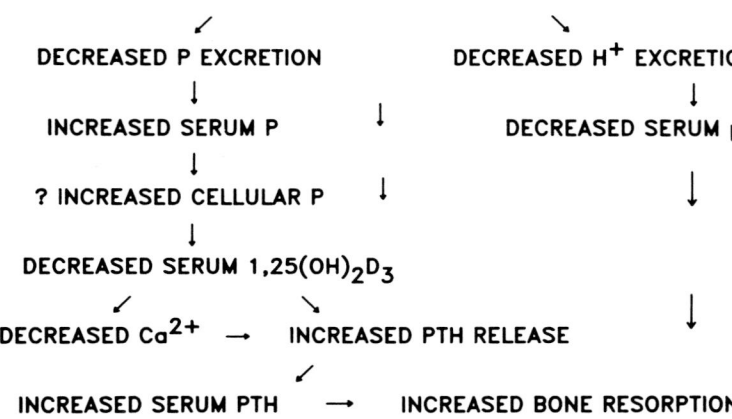

FIG. 9. Schematic diagram of the mechanisms leading to increased bone turnover during renal failure. Ca^{2+}, arterial blood ionized calcium concentration; Pi, concentration of blood phosphorus; PTH, parathyroid hormone; and $1,25(OH)_2D_3$, concentration of 1,25-dihydroxyvitamin D_3. From Bushinsky and Krieger (1).

of $1,25(OH)_2D_3$ (135) (Fig. 10). The decrease in $1,25(OH)_2D_3$ leads to an increase in PTH through at least two distinct mechanisms; (i) the fall in intestinal calcium absorption and subsequent negative ΔECF_{Ca} leading to a fall in $[ECF_{Ca}]_{new}$ and $[Ca^{2+}]$ and (ii) the direct effect of $1,25(OH)_2D_3$ to suppress PTH secretion.

During renal insufficiency, the serum levels of $1,25(OH)_2D_3$ appear to be relatively normal until the GFR falls below approximately 50 mL/min (135,137). With a further decline in GFR, levels of $1,25(OH)_2D_3$ fall further and are extremely low and often undetectable in patients on hemodialysis in spite of the usual elevations in PTH (147–150). The lack of $1,25(OH)_2D_3$ results in depressed α_{Ca}. Calcium balance has been shown to be negative with fecal excretion exceeding dietary intake (151–154), implying a negative α_{Ca}.

The relative lack of $1,25(OH)_2D_3$ also directly leads to enhanced PTH secretion (155–160). Parathyroid cells have specific receptors for $1,25(OH)_2D_3$ (161–163) and

$1,25(OH)_2D_3$ suppresses PTH gene expression and the secretion of PTH (155–160). In addition, during renal failure there appears to be decreased $1,25(OH)_2D_3$ binding to the parathyroid cells (164). Thus, during renal failure the combination of decreased levels of $1,25(OH)_2D_3$ and decreased binding of the available $1,25(OH)_2D_3$ to the parathyroid cells results in a marked increase in secretion of PTH at all levels of $[Ca^{2+}]$. This so-called "altered set point" for PTH secretion can be reversed by the administration of intravenous $1,25(OH)_2D_3$ (165,166) or a noncalcemic analogue of vitamin D, 22-oxocalcitriol (167). Parathyroid hormone is degraded principally in the liver and the kidney into carboxy-terminal fragments and these fragments are catabolized by the kidney (168–170). With renal failure there is accumulation of PTH fragments in the serum, some of which are biologically active (171).

Despite some evidence for the skeletal resistance to the actions of PTH on bone during renal failure, excess PTH

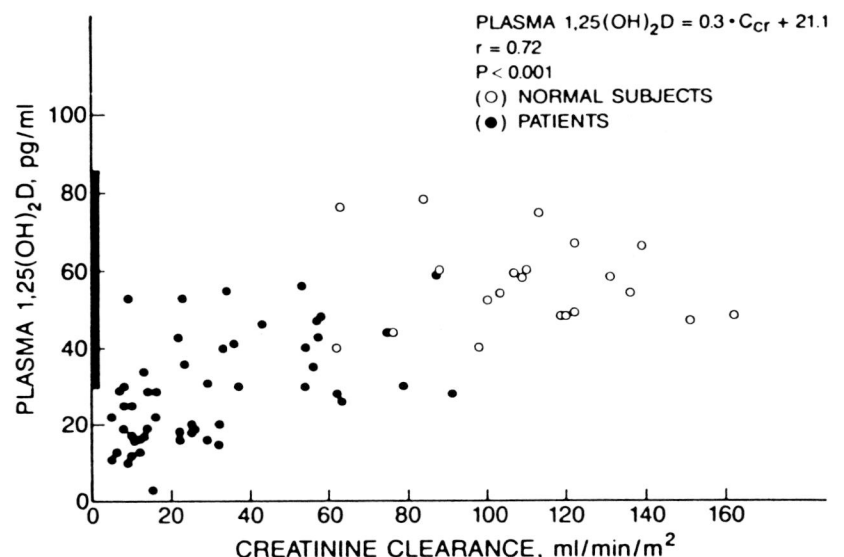

FIG. 10. The correlation between plasma $1,25(OH)_2D_3$ concentration and endogenous creatinine clearance in normal subjects (○) and patients with renal insufficiency (●). From Pitts et al. (135).

promotes resorption of bone mineral in uremia leading to increased Br_{Ca} and JB_{Ca} (138,172–175). However, in some patients with renal failure there is an accumulation of aluminum which is currently the best available agent to bind intestinal phosphate. In patients with aluminum accumulation in bone, osteomalacia, which represents defective mineralization of osteoid, is frequently observed (176–181). Aluminum has been found to inhibit osteoblastic activity (178–180) and to enhance osteoclastic bone resorption (182), both leading to an increase in Br_{Ca}.

Thus in renal failure ΔECF_{Ca} is negative due to a decrease in the product of $D_{Ca} \times \alpha_{Ca}$ in spite of a decrease in the U_{Ca} due to a lowered GFR and a PTH-induced increase in Br_{Ca}. When $1,25(OH)_2D_3$ is administered there is an increase in α_{Ca}, often leading to a positive ΔECF_{Ca} and frank hypercalcemia (165–167).

ACKNOWLEDGMENTS

This work was supported by National Institutes of Health grants AM-33949 and AR-39906. The expert secretarial assistance of Marilyn Walkowicz is gratefully acknowledged.

REFERENCES

1. Bushinsky DA, NS Krieger. Role of the skeleton in calcium homeostasis. In: Seldin DW, Giebisch G, eds. *The kidney: physiology and pathophysiology.* New York: Raven Press, 1991.
2. Heaney RP. Calcium kinetics in plasma: as they apply to the measurements of bone formation and resorption rates. In: Bourne GH, ed. *The biochemistry and physiology of bone, vol IV, Calcification and physiology.* New York: Academic Press, 1976;106–33.
3. Lemann J Jr. Intestinal absorption of calcium, magnesium and phosphorus. In: Favus MJ, ed. *Primer on the metabolic bone diseases and disorders of mineral metabolism.* Kelseyville, CA: American Society for Bone and Mineral Research, 1990;32–6.
4. Lemann J Jr. The urinary excretion of calcium, magnesium and phosphorus. In: Favus MJ, ed. *Primer on the metabolic bone diseases and disorders of mineral metabolism.* Kelseyville, CA: American Society for Bone and Mineral Research, 1990;36–9.
5. Karbach U. Mechanism of intestinal calcium transport and clinical aspects of disturbed calcium absorption. *Dig Dis* 1989;7:1–18.
6. Wasserman RH, CS Fullmer. On the molecular mechanism of intestinal calcium transport. *Adv Exp Med Biol* 1989;249:45–65.
7. Bronner F. Intestinal calcium absorption: mechanisms and applications. *J Nutr* 1987;117:1347–52.
8. Favus MJ. Factors that influence absorption and secretion of calcium in the small intestine and colon. *Am J Physiol (Gastroint and Liver Physiol 11)* 1985;248:G147–57.
9. Bronner F, Pansu D, Stein WD. An analysis of intestinal calcium transport across the rat intestine. *Am J Physiol (Gastroint and Liver Physiol 13)* 1986;250:G561–9.
10. Parfitt AM, Kleerekoper M. The divalent ion homeostatic system-physiology and metabolism of calcium, phosphorus, magnesium, and bone. In: Maxwell MH, Kleeman CR, Narins RG, eds. *Clinical disorders of fluid and electrolyte metabolism.* New York: McGraw-Hill, 1980;947–1151.
11. Bronner F. Intestinal calcium absorption and transport. In: Carafoli E, ed. *Membrane transport of calcium.* New York: Academic Press, 1982;237.
12. Levine BS, Walling MW, Coburn JW. Intestinal absorption of calcium: its assessment, normal physiology, and alterations in various disease states. In: Bronner F, Coburn JW, eds. *Disorders of mineral metabolism, vol II, Calcium physiology.* New York: Academic Press, 1982;103–88.
13. Wasserman RH, CS Fullmer. Calcium transport proteins, calcium absorption, and vitamin D. *Annu Rev Physiol* 1983;45:375–90.
14. Wasserman RH. Intestinal absorption of calcium and phosphorus. *Fed Proc* 1981;40:68–72.
15. Pak CY, Poindexter J, Finlayson B. A model system for assessing physicochemical factors affecting calcium absorbability from the intestinal tract. *J Bone Miner Res* 1989;4:119–27.
16. Marx ST, Bourdeau JE. Calcium metabolism. In: Maxwell MH, Kleeman CR, Narins RG, eds. *Clinical disorders of fluid and electrolyte metabolism.* New York: McGraw-Hill, 1990;207–44.
17. Kowarski S, Schachter D. Intestinal membrane calcium-binding protein. Vitamin D-dependent membrane component of the intestinal calcium transport mechanism. *J Biol Chem* 1980; 255:10834–40.
18. Rasmussen H, Matsumoto T, Fontaine O, Goodman DB. Role of changes in membrane lipid structure in the action of 1,25-dihydroxyvitamin D_3. *Fed Proc* 1982;41:72–7.
19. Miller A III, Li ST, Bronner F. Characterization of calcium binding to brush-border membranes of rat duodenum. *Biochem J* 1982;208:773–81.
20. Feher JJ. Facilitated calcium diffusion by intestinal calcium-binding protein. *Am J Physiol (Cell Physiology 13)* 1983; 244:C303–7.
21. Ghijsen WE, De Jong MD, Van Os CH. Kinetic properties of Na^+Ca^{2+} exchange in basolateral plasma membranes of rat small intestine. *Biochem Biophys Acta* 1983;730:85–94.
22. Ghijsen WE, De Jong MD, Van Os CH. ATP-dependent calcium transport and its correlation with Ca^{2+}-ATPase activity in basolateral plasma membranes of rat duodenum. *Biochem Biophys Acta* 1982;689:327–36.
23. Favus MJ, Kathpalia SC, Coe FL, Mond AE. Effects of diet calcium and 1,25-dihydroxyvitamin D_3 on colon calcium active transport. *Am J Physiol (Gastroint and Liver Physiol 1)* 1980;238:G75–8.
24. Isaksson B, Lindholm B, Sjogren B. A critical evaluation of the calcium balance technic. II. Dermal calcium losses. *Metabolism* 1967;16:303–13.
25. Charles P, Jensen FT, Mosekilde L, Hansen HH. Calcium metabolism evaluated by ^{47}Ca kinetics: estimation of dermal calcium loss. *Clin Science* 1983;65:415–22.
26. Paterson CR. Calcium requirements in man: a critical review. *Postgrad Med J* 1978;54:244–8.
27. Walker AR. Calcium balance in pregnancy. *Lancet* 1975;1:107.
28. Widdowson EM, McCance RA, Spray CM. The chemical composition of the human body. *Clin Sci* 1951;10:113–25.
29. Widdowson EM, Dickerson JWT. Chemical composition of the body. In: Comar CL, Bronner F, eds. *Mineral metabolism.* New York: Academic Press, 1964;1–247.
30. Parfitt AM. Bone and plasma calcium homeostasis. *Bone* 1987;8(Suppl 1):S1–8.
31. Nordin BEC. Plasma calcium and plasma magnesium homeostasis. In: Nordin BEC, ed. *Calcium, phosphate and magnesium metabolism.* Edinburgh: Churchill Livingstone, 1976.
32. Frame B, Parfitt AM. The syndromes of parathyroid hormone resistance. *Clin Aspects Metabolic Bone Dis* 1973;454–64.
33. Slatopolsky E, Weerts C, Norwood K, et al. Long-term effects of calcium carbonate and 2.5 mEq/liter calcium dialysate on mineral metabolism. *Kidney Int* 1989;36:897–903.
34. Goldsmith RS, Furszyfer J, Johnson WJ, Beeler GW Jr, Taylor WF. Calcium flux during hemodialysis. *Nephron* 1978;20:132–40.
35. Raman A, Chong YK, Sreenevasan GA. Effects of varying dialysate calcium concentrations on the plasma calcium fractions in patients on dialysis. *Nephron* 1976;16:181–7.
36. Parfitt AM. Target cell resistance in pseudohypoparathyroidism single or multiple? In: Norman AW, ed. *Vitamin D: basic research and its clinical application.* Berlin: Walter de Gruyter, 1979;949–50.

37. Bushinsky DA, Lechleider RJ. Mechanism of proton-induced bone calcium release: calcium carbonate dissolution. *Am J Physiol (Renal Fluid Electrolyte Physiol 22)* 1987;253:F998–1005.

38. Bushinsky DA, Goldring JM, Coe FL. Cellular contribution to pH mediated calcium flux in neonatal mouse calvariae. *Am J Physiol (Renal Fluid Electrolyte Physiol 17)* 1985;248:F785–9.

39. Heersche JNM. Bone cells and bone turnover. In Tam CS, Heersche JNM, Murray TM, eds. *Metabolic bone disease: cellular and tissue mechanisms*. Boca Raton, FL: CRC Press, 1989;1–17.

40. Neuman WF, Neuman MW. *The chemical dynamics of bone mineral*. Chicago: University of Chicago Press, 1958.

41. Bushinsky DA, Chabala J, Levi-Setti R. Ion microprobe analysis of mouse calvariae in vitro: evidence for a "bone membrane." *Am J Physiol (Endocrinol Metab 19)* 1989;256:E152–8.

42. Ramp WK. Cellular control of calcium movements in bone: interrelationships of the bone membrane, parathyroid hormone and alkaline phosphatase. *Clin Orthop* 1975;106:311–22.

43. Peterson DR, Heideger WJ, Beach KW. Calcium homeostasis: the effect of parathyroid hormone on bone membrane electrical potential difference. *Calcif Tissue Int* 1985;37:307–11.

44. McGrath KM, Heideger WJ, Beach KW. Calcium homeostasis. III. The bone membrane potential and mineral dissolution. *Calcif Tissue Int* 1986;39:279–83.

45. Canas F, Terepka AR, Neuman WF. Potassium and milieu interieur of bone. *Am J Physiol* 1969;217:117–20.

46. Levinskas GJ, Neuman WF. The solubility of bone mineral. I. Solubility studies of synthetic hydroxyapatite. *J Phys Chem* 1955;59:164–8.

47. Triffitt JT, Terepka AR, Neuman WF. A comparative study of the exchange in vivo of major constituents of bone mineral. *Calcif Tissue Res* 1968;2:165–76.

48. Neuman WF. The milieu interieur of bone: Claude Bernard revisited. *Fed Proc* 1969;28:1846–50.

49. Cohn SH, Vaswani A, Zanzi I, Aloia JF, Roginsky MS, Ellis KJ. Changes in body chemical composition with age measured by total-body neutron activation. *Metabolism* 1976;25:85–96.

50. Riggs BL, Wahner HW, Dunn WL, Mazess RB, Offord KP, Melton LJ III. Differential changes in bone mineral density of the appendicular and axial skeleton with aging: relationship to spinal osteoporosis. *J Clin Invest* 1981;67:328–35.

51. Horsman A, Marshall DH, Nordin BEC, Crilly RG, Simpson M. The relation between bone loss and calcium balance in women. *Clin Science* 1990;59:137–42.

52. Gotfredsen A, Hadberg A, Nilas L, Christiansen C. Total body bone mineral in healthy adults. *J Lab Clin Med* 1987;110:362–8.

53. Heaney RP, Recker RR, Saville PD. Menopausal changes in calcium balance performance. *J Lab Clin Med* 1978;92:953–63.

54. Heaney RP, Recker RR, Saville PD. Calcium balance and calcium requirements in middle-aged women. *Am J Clin Nutr* 1977;30:1603–10.

55. Smith DM, Nance WE, Kang KW, Christian JC, Johnston CC Jr. Genetic factors in determining bone mass. *J Clin Invest* 1973;52:2800–8.

56. Heaney RP, Recker RR, Stegman MR, Moy AJ. Calcium absorption in women: relationships to calcium intake, estrogen status, and age. *J Bone, Miner Res* 1989;4:469–75.

57. Gallagher JC, Riggs L, Eisman J, Hamstra A, Arnaud SB, DeLuca HF. Intestinal calcium absorption and serum vitamin D metabolites in normal subjects and osteoporotic patients. *J Clin Invest* 1979;64:729–36.

58. Alpers DH. Absorption of vitamins and divalent minerals. In: Sleisenger MH, Fordtran JS, eds. *Gastrointestinal disease*. Philadelphia: WB Saunders, 1989.

59. Kaplan RA, Haussler MR, Deftos LJ, Bone H, Pak CYC. The role of 1α-25-dihydroxyvitamin D_3 in the mediation of intestinal hyperabsorption of calcium in primary hyperparathyroidism and absorptive hypercalciuria. *J Clin Invest* 1977;59:756.

60. Sheikh MS, Ramirez A, Emmett M. Role of vitamin D-dependent and vitamin D-independent mechanisms in absorption of food calcium. *J Clin Invest* 1988;81:126–32.

61. Wilz DR, Gray RW, Dominguez JH, Lemann J Jr. Plasma 1,25-$(OH)_2$-vitamin D_3 concentrations and net intestinal calcium, phosphate and magnesium absorption in humans. *Am J Clin Nutr* 1979;32:2052–60.

62. Wilson SG, Retallack RW, Kent JC, Worth GK, Gutteridge DH. Serum free 1,25-dihydroxyvitamin D and the free 1,25-dihydroxyvitamin D index during a longitudinal study of human pregnancy and lactation. *Clin Endocrinol* 1990;32:613–22.

63. Norman AW. Intestinal calcium absorption: a vitamin D-hormone-mediated adaptive response. *Am J Clin Nutr* 1990;51:290–300.

64. Lemann J. Idiopathic hypercalciuria, in nephrolithiasis. In: Coe FL, Brenner BM, Stein JH, eds. *Contemporary issues in nephrology*. New York: Churchill Livingstone, 1980;86–135.

65. Epstein FH. Calcium and the kidney. *Am J Med* 1968;45:700–14.

66. Nordin BEC, Peacock M. Role of kidney in regulation of plasma-calcium. *Lancet* 1969;2:1280–3.

67. Coe FL, Favus MJ, Crockett T, et al. Effects of low-calcium diet on urine calcium excretion, parathyroid function and serum 1,25$(OH)_2D_3$ levels in patients with idiopathic hypercalciuria and in normal subjects. *Am J Med* 1982;72:25–32.

68. Coe FL, Bushinsky DA. Pathophysiology of hypercalciuria. *Am J Physiol (Renal Fluid Electrolyte Physiol 16)* 1984;247:F1–13.

69. Bushinsky DA. Internal exchanges of hydrogen ions: bone. In: Seldin DW, Giebisch G, eds. *The regulation of acid-base balance*. New York: Raven Press, 1989;69–88.

70. Maierhofer WJ, Gray RW, Cheung HS, Lemann J Jr. Bone resorption stimulated by elevated serum 1,25-$(OH)_2$-vitamin D_3 concentrations in healthy men. *Kidney Int* 1983;24:555–60.

71. Chen PS Jr, Neuman WF. Renal excretion of calcium by the dog. *Am J Physiol* 1955;180:623–31.

72. Peacock M, Robertson WG, Nordin BEC. Relation between serum and urinary calcium with particular reference to parathyroid activity. *Lancet* 1969;1:384–6.

73. Poulos PP. The renal tubular reabsorption and urinary excretion of calcium by the dog. *J Lab Clin Med* 1957;49:253–7.

74. Peacock M, Nordin BEC. Tubular reabsorption of calcium in normal and hypercalciuric subjects. *J Clin Path* 1968;21:353–8.

75. Bushinsky DA. Effects of parathyroid hormone on net proton flux from neonatal mouse calvariae. *Am J Physiol (Renal Fluid Electrolyte Physiol 21)* 1987;252:F585–9.

76. Richardson ML, Pozzi-Mucelli RS, Kanter AS, Kolb FO, Ettinger B, Genant HK. Bone mineral changes in primary hyperparathyroidism. *Skeletal Radiol* 1986;15:85–95.

77. Silverberg SJ, Shane E, de la Cruz L, et al. Skeletal disease in primary hyperparathyroidism. *J Bone Miner Res* 1989;4:283–91.

78. Seeman E, Wahner H, Offord K, Kumar R, Johnson W, Riggs B. Differential effects of endocrine dysfunction on the axial and the appendicular skeleton. *J Clin Invest* 1982;69:1302–9.

79. Eisman JA, Wark JD, Prince RL, Moseley JM. Modulation of plasma 1,25-dihydroxyvitamin D_3 in man by stimulation and suppression tests. *Lancet* 1979;2:931–3.

80. Murer H, Hildmann B. Transcellular transport of calcium and inorganic phosphate in the small intestinal epithelium. *Am J Physiol (Gastrointest Liver Physiol 3)* 1981;240:G409–16.

81. Krejs GJ, Nicar MJ, Zerwekh JE, Norman DA, Kane MG, Pak CYC. Effect of 1,25-dihydroxyvitamin D_3 on calcium and magnesium absorption in the healthy human jejunum and ileum. *Am J Med* 1983;75:973–6.

82. Bushinsky DA, Favus MJ, Schneider AB, Sen PK, Sherwood LM, Coe FL. Effects of metabolic acidosis on PTH and 1,25$(OH)_2D_3$ response to low calcium diet. *Am J Physiol (Renal Fluid Electrolyte Physiol 12)* 1982;243:F570–5.

83. Bushinsky DA, Riera GS, Favus MJ, Coe FL. Response of serum 1,25$(OH)_2D_3$ to variation of ionized calcium during chronic acidosis. *Am J Physiol (Renal Fluid Electrolyte Physiol 18)* 1985;249:F361–5.

84. Bushinsky DA, Riera G, Favus MJ, Coe FL. Evidence that blood ionized calcium can regulate serum 1,25$(OH)_2D_3$ independently of PTH and phosphorus in the rat. *J Clin Invest* 1985;76:1599–604.

85. Bushinsky DA, Favus MJ. Mechanism of hypercalciuria in genetic hypercalciuric rats: inherited defect in intestinal calcium transport. *J Clin Invest* 1988;82:1585–91.

86. Weisinger JR, Favus MJ, Langman C, Bushinsky DA. Regulation of 1,25-dihydroxyvitamin D_3 by calcium in the parathyroid-

ectomized parathyroid hormone replete rat. *J Bone Miner Res* 1989;4:929–35.

87. Bushinsky DA, Nalbantian-Brandt C, Favus MJ. Elevated Ca^{++} does not inhibit the 1,25(OH)$_2$D$_3$ response to phosphorus restriction. *Am J Physiol (Renal Fluid Electrolyte Physiol 25)* 1989;256:F285–9.

88. Bushinsky DA, Kittaka MK, Weisinger JR, Langman CB, Favus MJ. Effects of chronic metabolic alkalosis on Ca^{++}, PTH and 1,25(OH)$_2$D$_3$ in the rat. *Am J Physiol (Endocrinol Met Physiol 20)* 1989;257:E579–82.

89. Brown EM. PTH secretion in vivo and in vitro. Regulation by calcium and other secretagogues. *Miner Electrolyte Metab* 1982;8:130–50.

90. Bushinsky DA, Levi-Setti R, Coe FL. Ion microprobe determination of bone surface elements: effects of reduced medium pH. *Am J Physiol (Renal Fluid Electrolyte Physiol 19)* 1986;250:F1090–7.

91. Bushinsky DA, Favus MJ, Coe FL. Mechanism of chronic hypocalciuria with chlorthalidone: reduced calcium absorption. *Am J Physiol (Renal Fluid Electrolyte Physiol 16)* 1984;247:F746–52.

92. Moore F. Ionized calcium in normal serum, ultrafiltrates and whole blood determined by ion-exchange electrodes. *J Clin Invest* 1970;49:318–34.

93. Lemann J Jr, Litzow JR, Lennon EJ. The effects of chronic acid loads in normal man: further evidence for the participation of bone mineral in the defense against chronic metabolic acidosis. *J Clin Invest* 1966;45:1608–14.

94. Sutton RAL, Wong NLM, Dirks JH. Effects of metabolic acidosis and alkalosis on sodium and calcium transport in the dog kidney. *Kidney Int* 1979;15:520–33.

95. Peraino RA, Suki WN. Urine HCO$_3$ augments renal Ca^{2+} absorption independent of systemic acid-base changes. *Am J Physiol (Renal Fluid Electrolyte Physiol 7)* 1980;238:F394–8.

96. Lemann J Jr, Adams ND, Gray RW. Urinary calcium excretion in human beings. *N Engl J Med* 1979;301:535–41.

97. Litzow JR, Lemann J Jr, Lennon EJ. The effect of treatment of acidosis on calcium balance in patients with chronic azotemic renal disease. *J Clin Invest* 1967;46:280–6.

98. Adams ND, Gray RW, Lemann J Jr. The calciuria of increased fixed acid production in humans: evidence against a role for parathyroid hormone and 1,25(OH)2-vitamin D. *Calcif Tissue Int* 1979;28:233–8.

99. Weber HP, Gray RW, Dominguez JH, Lemann J Jr. The lack of effect of chronic metabolic acidosis on 25-OH vitamin D$_3$ metabolism and serum parathyroid hormone in humans. *J Clin Endocrinol Metab* 1976;43:1047–55.

100. Lee SW, Russell J, Avioli LV. 25-Hydroxycholecalciferol to 1,25-dihydroxycholecalciferol: conversion impaired by systemic metabolic acidosis. *Science* 1977;195:994–6.

101. Reddy GS, Jones G, Kooh SW, Fraser D. Inhibition of 25-hyroxyvitamin D$_3$ 1-hydroxylase by chronic metabolic acidosis. *Am J Physiol* 1982;243:E265–71.

102. Kraut JA, Mishler DR, Singer FR, Goodman WG. The effects of metabolic acidosis on bone formation and bone resorption in the rat. *Kidney Int* 1986;30:694–700.

103. Kraut JA, Gordon EM, Ransom JC, et al. Effect of chronic metabolic acidosis in vitamin D metabolism in humans. *Kidney Int* 1983;24:644–8.

104. Greenberg AJ, McNamara H, McCrory WW. Metabolic balance studies in primary renal tubular acidosis: effects of acidosis on external calcium and phosphorus balances. *J Pediatr* 1966;69:610–8.

105. Dominguez JH, Raisz LG. Effects of changing hydrogen ion, carbonic acid, and bicarbonate concentrations on bone resorption in vitro. *Calcif Tissue Int* 1979;29:7–13.

106. Bushinsky DA. Net calcium efflux from live bone during chronic metabolic, but not respiratory acidosis. *Am J Physiol (Renal Fluid Electrolyte Physiol 25)* 1989;256:F836–42.

107. Bushinsky DA. Net proton influx into bone during metabolic, but not respiratory, acidosis. *Am J Physiol (Renal Fluid Electrolyte Physiol 23)* 1988;254:F306–10.

108. Bushinsky DA, Krieger NS, Geisser DI, Grossman EB, Coe FL. Effects of pH on bone calcium and proton fluxes in vitro. *Am J Physiol (Renal Fluid Electrolyte Physiol 14)* 1983;245:F204–9.

109. Glimcher MJ. The nature of the mineral component of bone and the mechanism of calcification. *Instr Course Lect* 1987;36:49–69.

110. Glimcher MJ. Composition, structure and organization of bone and other mineralized tissues, and the mechanism of calcification. In: Greep RO, Astwood EB, Aurbach GD, eds. *Handbook of physiology, endocrinology.* Washington, DC: American Physiological Society, 1976;25–116.

111. Swan RC, Pitts RF. Neutralization of infused acid by nephrectomized dogs. *J Clin Invest* 1955;34:205–12.

112. Levitt MF, Turner LB, Sweet AY, Pandiri D. The response of bone, connective tissue, and muscle to acute acidosis. *J Clin Invest* 1956;35:98–105.

113. Adler S, Roy A, Relman AS. Intracellular acid-base regulation. I. The response of muscle cells to changes in CO$_2$ tension or extracellular bicarbonate concentration. *J Clin Invest* 1965;44:8–20.

114. Poole-Wilson PA, Cameron IR. Intracellular pH and K$^+$ of cardiac and skeletal muscle in acidosis and alkalosis. *Am J Physiol* 1975;229:1305–10.

115. Bergstrom WH, Ruva FD. Changes in bone sodium during acute acidosis in the rat. *Am J Physiol* 1960;198:1126–8.

116. Bettice JA, Gamble JL Jr. Skeletal buffering of acute metabolic acidosis. *Am J Physiol* 1975;229:1618–24.

117. Burnell JM. Changes in bone sodium and carbonate in metabolic acidosis and alkalosis in the dog. *J Clin Invest* 1971;50:327–31.

118. Bettice JA. 1984. Skeletal carbon dioxide stores during metabolic acidosis. *Am J Physiol (Renal Fluid Electrolyte Physiol 16)* 1984;247:F326–30.

119. Kraut JA, Mishler DR, Kurokawa K. Effect of colchicine and calcitonin on calcemic response to metabolic acidosis. *Kidney Int* 1984;25:608–12.

120. Bushinsky DA. Metabolic acidosis. In: Jacobson HR, Striker GE, Klahr S, eds. *The principles and practice of nephrology.* Philadelphia: BC Decker, 1990;62–70.

121. Madias NE, Kraut JA. Uremic acidosis. In: Seldin DW, Giebisch G, eds. *The regulation of acid-base balance.* New York: Raven Press, 1989;285–317.

122. Batlle DC. Renal tubular acidosis. In: Seldin DW, Giebisch G, eds. *The regulation of acid-base balance.* New York: Raven Press, 1989;353–90.

123. Irving L, Chute AL. The participation of carbonates of bone in the neutralization of ingested acid. *J Cell Com Physiol* 1932;2:157–76.

124. Biltz RM, Pellegrino ED, Letteri JM. Skeletal carbonates and acid-base regulation. *Miner Electrolyte Metab* 1981;5:1–7.

125. Lemann J Jr, Litzow JR, Lennon EJ. Studies of the mechanism by which chronic metabolic acidosis augments urinary calcium excretion in man. *J Clin Invest* 1967;46:1318–28.

126. Canzanello VJ, Bodvarsson M, Kraut JA, Johns CA, Slatopolsky E, Madias N. Effect of chronic respiratory acidosis on urinary calcium excretion in the dog. *Kidney Int* 1990;38:409–16.

127. Lau K, Rodriguez, Nichols F, Tannen RL. Renal excretion of divalent ions in response to chronic acidosis: evidence that systemic pH is not the controlling variable. *J Lab Clin Med* 1987;109:27–33.

128. Schaefer KE, Pasquale S, Messier AA, Shea M. Phasic changes in bone CO$_2$ fractions, calcium, and phosphorus during chronic hypercapnia. *J Appl Physiol* 1980;48:802–11.

129. Schaefer KE, Nichols G Jr, Carey CR. Calcium phosphorus metabolism in man during acclimatization to carbon dioxide. *J Appl Physiol* 1963;18:1079–84.

130. Schaefer KE. Effects of increased ambient CO$_2$ levels on human and animal health. *Experientia (Basel)* 1982;38:1163–8.

131. Hall TJ, Chambers TJ. Optimal bone resorption by isolated rat osteoclasts requires chloride/bicarbonate exchange. *Calcif Tissue Int* 1989;45:378–80.

132. Teti A, Blair HC, Teitelbaum SL, et al. Cytoplasmic pH regulation and chloride/bicarbonate exchange in avian osteoclasts. *J Clin Invest* 1989;83:227–33.

133. Reiss E, Canterbury JM, Egdahl RH. Experience with a radioimmunoassay of parathyroid hormone in human sera. *Trans Assoc Am Physicians* 1968;81:104–15.

134. Arnaud CD. Hyperparathyroidism and renal failure. *Kidney Int* 1973;4:89–94.

135. Pitts TO, Piraino BH, Mitro R, et al. Hyperparathyroidism and 1,25-dihydroxyvitamin D deficiency in mild, moderate and severe renal failure. *J Clin Endocrinol Metab* 1988;67:876–81.
136. Reiss E, Canterbury JM, Bercovitz MA, Kaplan EL. The role of phosphate in the secretion of parathyroid hormone in man. *J Clin Invest* 1970;49:2146–9.
137. Slatopolsky E, Caglar S, Pennell JP, et al. On the pathogenesis of hyperparathyroidism in chronic experimental insufficiency in the dog. *J Clin Invest* 1971;50:492–9.
138. Llach F, Massry SG, Singer FR, Kurokawa K, Kaye JH, Coburn JW. Skeletal resistance of endogenous parathyroid hormone in patients with early renal failure: a possible cause for secondary hyperparathyroidism. *J Clin Endocrinol Metab* 1975;41:339–45.
139. Rutherford WE, Bordier P, Marie P, et al. Phosphate control and 25-hydroxycholecalciferol administration in preventing experimental renal osteodystrophy in the dog. *J Clin Invest* 1977;60:332–41.
140. Slatopolsky E, Caglar S, Gradowska L, Canterbury J, Reiss E, Bricker NS. On the prevention of secondary hyperparathyroidism in experimental chronic renal disease using "proportional reduction" of dietary phosphorus intake. *Kidney Int* 1972;2:147–51.
141. Slatopolsky E, Rutherford WE, Hruska K, Martin K, Klahr S. How important is phosphate in the pathogenesis of renal osteodystrophy? *Arch Intern Med* 1978;138:848–52.
142. Parfitt AM. Soft tissue calcification in uremia. *Arch Intern Med* 1969;124:544–56.
143. Tanaka Y, DeLuca HF. The control of 25-hydroxyvitamin D_3 metabolism by inorganic phosphorus. *Arch Biochem Biophys* 1973;154:566–74.
144. Brunette MG, Chan M, Ferriere C, Roberts KD. Site of 1,25-$(OH)_2$ vitamin D_3 synthesis in the kidney. *Nature* 1978;276:287–9.
145. Kawashima H, Torikai S, Kurokawa K. Localization of 25-hydroxyvitamin D_3-1 α-hydroxylase and 24-hydroxylase along the rat nephron. *Proc Natl Acad Sci USA* 1981;78:1199–203.
146. Akiba T, Endou H, Koseki C, Sakai F. Localization of 25-hydroxyvitamin D_3 1α-hydroxylase activity in the mammalian kidney. *Biochem Biophys Res Commun* 1980;94:313–8.
147. Slatopolsky E, Gray R, Adams N, et al. The pathogenesis of secondary hyperparathyroidism in early renal failure. In: Norman AW, ed. *Vitamin D basic research and its clinical application.* New York: Walter de Gruyter, 1979;1209–15.
148. Mawer EB, Taylor CM, Backhouse J, Lumb GA, Stanbury SW. Failure of formation of 1,25-dihydroxycholecalciferol in chronic renal insufficiency. *Lancet* 1973;1:626–8.
149. Schaefer KE, von Herrath D, Stratz R. Metabolism of 1,2-^{3}H-4-^{14}C-cholecalciferol in normal, uremic and anephric subjects. *Isr J Med Sci* 1972;8:80–3.
150. Christiansen C, Christensen MS, Melsen F, Rodbro P, DeLuca HF. Mineral metabolism in chronic renal failure with special reference to serum concentrations of $1,25(OH)_2D_3$ and $24,25(OH)_2D_3$. *Clin Nephrol* 1965;66:535.
151. Malluche HH, Werner E, Ritz E. Intestinal absorption of calcium and whole body calcium retention in incipient and advanced renal failure. *Miner Electrolyte Metab* 1978;1:263–70.
152. Coburn JW, Koppel MH, Brickman AS, Massry SG. Study of intestinal absorption of calcium in patients with renal failure. *Kidney Int* 1973;3:264–72.
153. Parker TF, Vergne-Marini P, Hull AR, Pak CYC, Fordtran JS. Jejunal absorption and secretion of calcium in patients with chronic renal disease on hemodialysis. *J Clin Invest* 1974;54:358–65.
154. Kaye M, Silverman M. Calcium metabolism in chronic renal failure. *J Lab Clin Med* 1965;66:535–48.
155. Silver J, Russell J, Sherwood LM. Regulation by vitamin D metabolites of messenger ribonucleic acid for pre-proparathyroid hormone in isolated bovine parathyroid cells. *Proc Natl Acad Sci USA* 1985;82:4270–3.
156. Russell J, Lettieri D, Sherwood LM. Suppression by 1,25-$(OH)_2D_3$ of transcription of the parathyroid hormone gene. *Endocrinology* 1986;119:2864–6.
157. Cantley LK, Russell J, Lettieri D, Sherwood LM. 1,25-Dihydroxyvitamin D_3 suppresses parathyroid hormone secretion from bovine parathyroid cells in tissue culture. *Endocrinology* 1985;117:2114–9.
158. Chan YL, McKay C, Dye E, Slatopolsky E. The effect of 1,25-dihydroxycholecalciferol on parathyroid cells. *Calcif Tissue Int* 1986;38:27–32.
159. Oldham SB, Smith R, Hartenbower DL, Henry HL, Norman AW, Coburn JW. The acute effects of 1,25-dihydroxycholecalciferol on serum immunoreactive parathyroid hormone in the dog. *Endocrinology* 1979;104:248–54.
160. Chertow BS, Baylink DJ, Wergedal JE, Su MH, Norman AW. Decrease in serum immunoreactive parathyroid hormone in rats and in parathyroid hormone secretion in vitro by 1,25-dihydroxycholecalciferol. *J Clin Invest* 1975;56:668–75.
161. Hughes MR, Haussler MR. 1,25-Dihydroxyvitamin D_3 receptors in parathyroid glands. *J Biol Chem* 1978;253:1065–73.
162. Henry HL, Norman AW. Studies on the mechanism of action of calciferol. VII. Localization of 1,25-dihydroxyvitamin D_3 in chick parathyroid glands. *Biochem Biophys Res Commun* 1975;62:781–8.
163. Brumbaugh PF, Hughes MR, Haussler MR. Cytoplasmic and nuclear binding components for the 1α,25-dihydroxyvitamin D_3 in chick parathyroid glands. *Proc Natl Acad Sci USA* 1975;72:4871–5.
164. Korker AB. Reduced binding of [^{3}H]-1,25-dihydroxyvitamin D_3 parathyroid glands of patients with renal failure. *N Engl J Med* 1987;316:1573–7.
165. Slatopolsky E, Weerts C, Thielan J, Horst R, Harter H, Martin KJ. Marked suppression of secondary hyperparathyroidism by intravenous administration of 1,25-dihydroxycholecalciferol in uremic patients. *J Clin Invest* 1984;74:2136–43.
166. Andress DL, Norris KC, Coburn JW, Slatopolsky EA, Sherrard DJ. Intravenous calcitriol in the treatment of refractory osteitis fibrosa of chronic renal failure. *N Engl J Med* 1989;321:274–9.
167. Brown AJ, Ritter CR, Finch JL, et al. The noncalcemic analogue of vitamin D, 22-oxocalcitriol, suppresses parathyroid hormone synthesis and secretion. *J Clin Invest* 1989;84:728–32.
168. Martin KJ, Hruska KA, Freitag JJ, Klahr S, Slatopolsky E. The peripheral metabolism of parathyroid hormone. *N Engl J Med* 1979;301:1092–8.
169. Martin K, Hruska K, Greenwalt A, Klahr S, Slatopolsky E. Selective uptake of intact parathyroid hormone in the liver: differences between hepatic and renal uptake. *J Clin Invest* 1976;58:781–8.
170. Martin KJ, Hruska KA, Lewis J, Anderson C, Slatopolsky E. The renal handling of parathyroid hormone: role of peritubular uptake and glomerular filtration. *J Clin Invest* 1977;60:808–14.
171. Goltzman D, Henderson B, Loveridge N. Cytochemical bioassay of parathyroid hormone: characteristics of assay and analysis of circulating hormonal forms. *J Clin Invest* 1980;65:1309–17.
172. Massry SG, Arieff AI, Coburn JW, Palmieri G, Klefman CR. Divalent ion metabolism in patients with acute renal failure. Studies on the mechanism of hypocalciuria. *Kidney Int* 1974;5:437–45.
173. Massry SG, Coburn JW, Lee DBW, Jowsey J, Kleeman CHR. Skeletal resistance to parathyroid hormone in renal failure: studies in 105 human subjects. *Ann Int Med* 1973;78:357–64.
174. Galceran T, Martin KJ, Morrissey JJ, Slatopolsky E. Role of 1,25-dihydroxyvitamin D on the skeletal resistance to parathyroid hormone. *Kidney Int* 1987;32:801–7.
175. Massry SG, Stein R, Garty J, et al. Skeletal resistance to the calcemic action of parathyroid hormone in uremia: role of $1,25(OH)_2D_3$. *Kidney Int* 1976;9:467–74.
176. Cournot-Witmer G, Zingraff J, Plachot JJ, et al. Aluminum localization in bone from hemodialyzed patients: relationship to matrix mineralization. *Kidney Int* 1981;20:375–8.
177. Hodsman AB, Sherrard DJ, Wong EGC, et al. Vitamin-D-resistant osteomalacia in hemodialysis patients lacking secondary hyperparathyroidism. *Ann Intern Med* 1981;94:629–37.
178. Parisien M, Charhon SA, Arlot M, et al. Evidence for a toxic effect of aluminum on osteoblasts: a histomorphometric study in hemodialysis patients with aplastic bone disease. *J Bone Miner Res* 1988;3:259–67.
179. Dunstan CR, Evans RA, Hills E, Wong SY, Alfrey AC. Effect of

aluminum and parathyroid hormone on osteoblasts and bone mineralization in chronic renal failure. *Calcif Tissue Int* 1984;36:133–8.

180. Plachot JJ, Cournot-Witmer G, Halpern S, et al. Bone ultrastructure and x-ray microanalysis of aluminum-intoxicated hemodialysis patients. *Kidney Int* 1984;25:796–803.

181. Talwar HS, Reddi AH, Menczel J, Thomas WC Jr, Meyer JL. Influence of aluminum on mineralization during matrix-induced bone development. *Kidney Int* 1986;29:1038–42.

182. Sprague SM, Bushinsky DA. Mechanism of aluminum-induced calcium efflux from cultured neonatal mouse calvariae. *Am J Physiol (Renal Fluid Electrolyte Physiol 27)* 1990;258:F583–8.

PART IV

Introduction to Clinical Mineral Disorders

Disorders of Bone and Mineral Metabolism,
edited by Fredric L. Coe and Murray J. Favus,
© 1992 by Raven Press, Ltd. All rights reserved.

CHAPTER 19

Clinical and Laboratory Approach to the Patient with Disorders of Bone and Mineral Metabolism

Fredric L. Coe and Murray J. Favus

As in many areas of medicine, patients with mineral disorders do not present themselves with isolated symptoms or physical findings, but rather with clusters of such findings, clusters that have long been known about and are often referred to as syndromes. We can identify at least nine such syndromes in our field, each rather old and well recognized. Given one part of a syndrome, most physicians look for the rest, attempt to confirm the syndrome using routine laboratory measures, and then proceed to a more analytical inquiry to find the disease that is the cause, and the object of treatment. This entire volume offers itself as a guide to practice, so in this chapter we will outline a reasonable way to use this text, listing the diseases conveniently and identifying where this information can be found. We have omitted references from this chapter as our aim is an introduction to clinical disorders, not a comprehensive evaluation of each disorder.

THE SYNDROMES

Our nine syndromes (Table 1) range from complex clinicopathological entities such as osteomalacia, to the broad notion of disorders that have in common only abnormal serum mineral levels; even so, we believe that doctors usually practice by recognizing syndromes such as these, and proceeding from them to detailed work. The nine syndromes are not trivial to define (Table 2).

Rickets is defined clinically, and the gold standard is osseous deformities in a child whose radiographs also are abnormal in a special way: expansion of the epiphyseal regions and bowing. Bone biopsy is not required, and

usually is omitted, even though biopsy can reveal a characteristic slowing of mineralization. *Osteomalacia* is a disease of adults, whose epiphyses have closed, but is related to rickets in that bones soften and bend or fracture, and biopsy shows slowing of mineralization. Unlike rickets, biopsy always is the gold standard for rigorous diagnosis of osteomalacia.

Osteoporosis is purely clinical in diagnosis, and requires proof of reduced bone mass with at least one fracture not accounted for by appropriate trauma, and exclusion of specific non-osteoporotic bone diseases such as osteomalacia, or hyperparathyroidism. A measurement of bone mineral content is necessary for diagnosis; biopsy may be needed for exclusion of other causes. Osteoporosis can be a primary disorder, or secondary to many diseases (see Chapters 37 and 38).

Uremic Osteodystrophy occurs only as a consequence of chronic renal failure, with or without dialysis. This syndrome requires that renal failure be present, evidence for chronicity such as serial measurements of serum creatine or small kidneys as well as evidence of bone disease such as fractures, bone pain, or elevated alkaline phosphatase. The definition of bone involvement depends on at least one certain evidence of bone disease, otherwise unexplained, in the presence of chronic renal failure. Biopsy is often needed, more to dissect the various components of the disease, that include osteomalacia, rickets in some children, hyperparathyroidism, and bony sclerosis, than to establish the presence of the disease.

Nephrolithiasis is defined by the passage, radiographic visualization, or removal of a stone, a microcrystalline aggregate containing calcium salts, uric acid, amino acids such as cystine, struvite, drugs such as triampterine, or proteins such as β_2-microglobulin. Almost all stones are made up of calcium oxalate, uric acid, cystine, or struvite (magnesium ammonium phosphate).

Abnormal serum mineral levels include all of the possible combinations of high or low serum calcium, phospho-

---

F. L. Coe: Departments of Medicine and Physiology, Nephrology Program, University of Chicago, Pritzker School of Medicine, Chicago, Illinois 60637.

M. J. Favus: Departments of Medicine, Endocrinology Section, and Nephrology Program, University of Chicago, Pritzker School of Medicine, Chicago, Illinois 60637.

TABLE 1. *Main syndromes of bone and mineral disorders*

Rickets (R)
Osteomalacia (OM)
Pathologic calcification (PC)
Osteoporosis (OP)
Uremic osteodystrophy (UOD)
Nephrolithiasis and nephrocalcinosis (NL)
Abnormal serum mineral levels (ASML)
Pathological fractures (PF)
Primary radiographic bone abnormalities (RBA)

TABLE 2. *Definitions of syndromes*

Syndrome	Definition
R	Typical osseous deformities and radiographic abnormalities
OM	Documented reduced mineralization rate by biopsy
PC	Radiographic visualization of abnormal calcification
OP	Reduced bone mass and at least one PF otherwise unexplained
UOD	Chronic renal failure and any of reduced mineralization rate, increased resorption, sclerosis
NL	Passage, radiographic visualization, or removal of a stone
ASML	Documented abnormal level
PF	Documented fracture without appropriate trauma
RBA	Specific lesion documented by radiograph

Abbreviations are defined in Table 1.

rus, or magnesium levels, the three materials we usually mean when we refer to minerals. Abnormal levels always reflect some underlying disease process, but many patients present themselves with only abnormal serum mineral levels as overt abnormalities and require analytical investigation to discover their cause; that is why the syndrome is useful, if only as a beginning for the clinical process. For example, primary hyperparathyroidism presents itself far more often as unexplained hypercalcemia than as stone passage or bone disease. This syndrome may be among the most common reasons for consultation.

Pathological fracture, which means a fracture that occurred in the absence of appropriate trauma, occurs in osteomalacia and osteoporosis, but also may be a primary presenting problem of its own. This can occur when the cause is obscure, such as osteogenesis imperfecta, or simply uncertain, such as osteomalacia. Why include this entity? Simply because fractures of unknown cause are an important clinical presentation by patients, a major way in which bone disease presents itself. When bone mineral loss is obvious, the fracture becomes part of a putative osteoporosis syndrome but many times fracture is the starting point for clinical evaluation.

Pathological calcification in soft tissue can reflect any of several diseases, and occasionally is the starting place for clinical inquiry. The calcifications can be single and large as in myositis ossificans, or multiple and small as in renal failure or primary hyperoxaluria. The syndrome is established radiographically.

Primary radiographic bone abnormality means an osseous abnormality not known to be due to a specific disease, and occurring in the absence of any of the other syndromes. For example, radiographs may be incidental, or done for symptoms of gait problems, bone pain, or any other symptom, an abnormal bone region is found and none of the other syndromes exists. Tumors, cysts, and hereditary malformations all may present this way.

RECOGNITION OF SYNDROMES

Clinical Findings

We comment on some (Tables 3 and 4) findings most doctors encounter less often than ourselves, leaving the rest to common knowledge.

Bone Pain

Acute bone pain from vertebral collapse, common in osteoporosis, may begin suddenly as a severe "paralysing" pain or sometimes a gripping spasm, occurring in the back but not necessarily localized and often associated with bending, lifting, stooping, or routine housework, that persists for one to up to six months. Some fracture without symptoms, while others can fracture with chronic aching as a symptom, often misunderstood because the pain is not acute or associated with physical effort. Osteomalacia produces an aching bone pain, often in the ribs or pelvis and legs, worse at night because of the pressure while lying down. Paget's disease causes a constant aching pain, localized to affected areas, usually long bones and pelvis. Bowing and distortion of limbs may cause secondary degenerative arthritis with concomitant pain of its own.

Renal Colic

Pain from stone passage follows the time course of urinary tract and renal distension from obstruction. The pain begins as a sudden but usually mild discomfort in one flank, that mounts to a plateau of severity over 30 to 60 minutes and then remains steady and unaffected by posture or activity. The pain has a boring or piercing character, like an extreme toothache. With stone movement downward, the pain moves forward from the flank to the anterior abdomen and downward, following the general path of open fingers laid upon the abdomen pointing downwards, with the thumb hooked behind the lowest rib. The pain vanishes magically with stone passage, leaving little or no residual. At the ureterovesicle junction, stones cause dysuria, frequency, and urgency that mimic cystitis, and often is mistaken as such. The legendary severity of colic demands narcotic treatment, usually in hospital or emergency room settings.

TABLE 3. *Symptoms that suggest the presence of bone and mineral disorders*

Symptom	R	OM	PC	OP	UOD	NL	ASML	PF	RBA
Bone pain	C	C	—	—	C	—	C	O	C
Flank pain	—	—	—	—	—	C	—	—	—
Listlessness and lethargy	O	O	—	—	C	—	O	—	—
Coma	—	—	—	—	—	—	O	—	—
Weakness	C	O	—	—	C	—	C	—	—
Delayed growth or development	C	—	—	—	C	—	—	—	O
Difficulty walking	C	C	—	O	C	—	O	O	O
Mental retardation	—	—	—	—	—	—	O	—	—
Low back pain	—	O	—	C	O	O	—	O	O
Hematuria	—	—	—	—	—	C	—	—	—
Stone passage	—	—	—	—	—	P	—	—	—
Dysuria	—	—	—	—	—	C	—	—	—
Polyuria	—	—	—	—	—	—	C	—	—
Tetany and neuromuscular irritability	C	C	—	—	C	—	O	—	—
Seizure	O	O	—	—	O	—	O	—	—
Bone fracture	O	O	—	C	C	—	—	N	O
Loss of height	—	—	—	C	—	—	—	O	—

Abbreviations are defined in Table 1.
O, Occurs; C, Common; P, Pathognomonic; N, Necessary for diagnosis.

Muscle Weakness

The weakness of mineral disorders like osteomalacia, hypercalcemia, and hypophosphatemia mainly involves proximal muscles, causing an inability to arise from a low chair, climb stairs, comb or dry long hair. The weakness alters gait to a wobbling "waddling" sort. The same occurs with hyperthyroid myopathy, in the absence of mineral disorders.

Low Back Pain

By the phrase low back pain we mean the pain of musculoskeletal derangements, osteoarthritis, nerve root compression, and distorted skeletal anatomy. The pain can be confused with renal colic, but need not be, as it is chronic though punctuated by acute episodes, and episodes of pain lack the special time course of colic. Exercise worsens and some postures improve the pain, unlike renal colic, and disappearance of pain never is magical. It can resemble the chronic pain from vertebral collapse, but never arises from osteoporosis itself in the absence of fracture. It also shares in common with osteomalacia a chronic character, but not its location, being predominantly axial and radicular.

Polyuria

Polyuria requires only the comment that dysuria and frequency can imply a non-existent polyuria, and true polyuria can go unnoticed for some time until nocturia

TABLE 4. *Physical findings that suggest disorders of bone and minerals*

Physical findings	R	OM	PC	OP	UOD	NL	ASML	PF	RBA
Rachitic deformities	N				C		O		O
Short stature	N	C			O		O	O	C
Abnormal gait	C	C		O	O		O	O	C
Kyphosis				C	O			O	O
Scoliosis		O	O	O	O				O
Bowing of long bones	C	C			O		O	O	O
Subcutaneous hard mass			C				O		O
Cafe-au-lait spots									C
Skin ulcers/trophic changes			C		O		O		O
Bank keratopathy							O		
Blue sclera				C[a]				C[a]	C[a]
Bone tenderness	C	C			O		O		
Flank tenderness						C	O		C
Hyporeflexia	O	O					O	O	
Axial weakness	C	C					O	C	O
Chvostek/Trousseau sign	O	O			O		O	C	O
Altered mental status					C		O		

Abbreviations are defined in Tables 1 and 3.
[a] Specific for osteogenesis imperfecta.

becomes a problem. Asking about the volume of frequent voidings usually makes the distinction.

Tetany and Neuromuscular Irritability

Numbness and tingling, of the finger tips, toes, and about the mouth dominate the history and antedate dramatic events like carpo-pedal spasms. In fact, experienced patients recognize these early symptoms and take calcium orally, knowing what will soon follow. Difficulty walking or standing, and falling spells, may reflect leg muscle spasms, instead of carpo-pedal spasms involving the hands and feet. Right upper quadrant pain from biliary tree spasm can mimic cholecystitis.

Rickets

Few of us see patients affected with childhood rickets, but typical findings include growth retardation, bone pain and irritability, genu valgum (knock knees), which means a rotation of the knees towards one another from bending of the femurs, genu varum, which means bowleggedness, frontal bossing—a prominence of the frontal bone with elongation of the head in the anteroposterior plane—the "rosary" of beadlike proliferations along the costal chondral junctions of the ribs.

Kyphosis

Kyphosis means a bowing forward centered at about the mid thoracic spine, usually from wedge compression fractures from osteoporosis. Kyphosis must be distinguished from mere forward displacement of the head from muscle weakness, or from arthritis that fixes the spine downward so patients cannot straighten up. Ankylosing spondylitis, which curves the spine forward, angles forward from the lumbosacral junction not the mid thoracic spine. Patients with either kyphosis or ankylosing spondylitis, however, must hold their heads thrown back at the neck to see straight ahead. In kyphosis, the ribs lie lower and more over the abdomen than normal, causing protrusion, a "potbelly" appearance, and early satiety. The traditional waist disappears, having been obliterated by the closure of the normal space between the ribs and pelvis. Patients complain about clothes no longer fitting, and the loss of a waistline. Naturally, height is lost because of the collapses and the bowing, the loss being not in the legs, or neck, but in the chest.

Axial Weakness

Axial weakness is a way of saying proximal weakness, because large antigravity muscles when weak causes instability of gait and posture.

Chvosteks and Trousseaus Signs

Chvostek's sign is a twitching of the face upon percussion of the preauricular area in its lower half, or at the corner of the mouth. Trousseau's sign is contractions of the forearm from a blood pressure cuff left inflated for 2 minutes. Because flexors predominate in strength, the Trousseau sign is flexion of the fingers, adduction of the thumb, and flexion at the wrist. The wrist flexion and thumb adduction make the fingers extend about their small joints, though they flex at the metacarpophalangeal joints.

Band Keratopathy

Band keratopathy is a white, incomplete curving border about the limbus of the eyes, most prominent between the open lids. Not shining, as one might expect, but rather drab, granular up close, and chalky, which depicts its true character as a calcium salt deposit of weak crystallinity. Arcus senilis differs, being circumferentially continuous, and softer and smoother in appearance.

Blue Sclera

The sclerae range from deep blue to blue gray, and our patients with it do not seem to know about the finding themselves so much as from physicians. Infants normally have blue sclera, so anyone who wishes can see the finding in any nursery. Important for its extreme association with osteogenesis imperfecta.

TABLE 5. *Routine laboratory findings that suggest bone and mineral disorders*

Finding	R	OM	PC	OP	UOD	NL	ASML	PF	RBA
Anemia	O	O			C		O	O	
Abnormal leukocytes							O	O	
Abnormal urinalysis					C	C			
CO$_2$ content	L				L	L	H		
Chloride	H					H	H/L		
Calcium	L/N	L/N	H/N		N/L	H/N	H/N/L	H/N	
Phosphorus	L/N	L	H/N		H/N		H/N/L	H/N/L	
Magnesium	N/L	N/L			N/H		H/L/N		
Alkaline phosphatase	H	H			H/N	H/N	H/N	N/H	
BUN/Creatinine					H		H/N	H/N	

Abbreviations are defined in Tables 1 and 3. H, N, and L are high, normal, and low, respectively.

TABLE 6. *Specialized tests needed to establish syndromes*

Type of data	R	OM	PC	OP	UOD	NL	ASML	PF	RBA
Bone biopsy	O	N		O	C		O	O	O
Abdominal flatplate					C	N		O	
Serum 25(OH) vitamin D	N	N		C			O	C	O
Serum 1,25 (OH)$_2$D	N	N	N	C	C	N	C	C	O
Serum PTH	C	C	O	O	N	C	C	O	O
Renal Ultrasound						N			
Intravenous Pyelogram						N			
Bone Radiographs	N	N		N	C	O	O	C	C
Wrists	N				O		O	O	O
Lateral Spine			N		C		O	O	C
Suspected Fracture Site	N	N	N	N	N			N	N
Tissue Biopsy			N	O	C		O	O	O

Abbreviations are defined in Table 1. N, necessary; C, common; and O, occasional.

TABLE 7. *Disorders of bone and mineral metabolism*

Disease	Ch	R	OM	PC	OP	NL	ASML	PF	RBA
Vitamin D deficiency	41	+	+				+	+	+
Phosphate deficiency	28, 41	+	+				+	+	+
Malabsorption states/celiac sprue/inflammatory bowel disease	41	+	+				+LC, LMg	+	+
Hypophosphatasia	42	+					+	+	+
Primary biliary cirrhosis	41	+	+				+	+	+
Biliary atresia	41	+					+	+	+
Fanconi's syndrome	34, 40	+	+				+	+	+
Pancreatic insufficiency, cystic fibrosis	41	+	+				+	+	+
Vitamin D dependent rickets, type I	40	+					+	+	+
Vitamin D dependent rickets, type II	40	+					+	+	+
X-linked hypophosphatemic rickets	40	+	+				+	+	+
Hereditary hypophosphatemic rickets with hypercalciuria	40		+						
Renal tubular acidosis II	34, 40	+						+	+
Total parenteral nutrition	23, 41	+	+				+	+	+
Axial osteomalacia	42		+				+	+	+
Drug induced osteomalacia	38, 41		+		+		+	+	+
Tumor associated osteomalacia	25, 40		+				+	+	+
Post-gastrectomy	41		+				+	+	+
Neurofibromatosis	42		+						
Fibrogenesis imperfecta ossium	42		+				+	+	+
Tumoral calcinosis	42			+			+		+
Myositis ossificans	42			+			+		+
Humoral hypercalcemia of malignancy	25								
Primary hyperparathyroidism	23, 24, 41			+	+	+	+	+	+
Sarcoidosis/other granulomatous diseases	26			+		+	+		+
Vitamin D intoxication	23			+		+	+		
Milk alkali syndrome	23			+		+	+		
Hypoparathyroidism	27, 42			+		+	+		
Postmenopausal osteoporosis	37				+			+	+
Juvenile osteoporosis	38				+			+	+
Regional osteoporosis	38				+			+	+
Steroid induced osteoporosis	38				+	+		+	+
Male hypogonadism	38				+			+	+
Mastocytosis	38				+			+	+
Immobilization	38				+	+		+	+
Multiple myeloma	25				+		+	+	+
Heparin	38				+			+	+
Osteogenesis imperfecta	42				+			+	+
Hyperphosphatasia	42				+				
Idiopathic hypercalciuria	32				+	+			

TABLE 7. *Continued.*

Disease	Ch	R	OM	PC	OP	NL	ASML	PF	RBA
Hyperthyroidism	23, 38				+	+		+	
Renal tubular acidosis I	34					+			
Paget's disease	43					+	+	+	+
Primary hyperoxaluria	33					+			
Enteric hyperoxaluria	33					+			
Hyperuricosuria	35					+			
Low urine citrate	35					+			
Non-calcium stones	36					+			
Malignant tumors	23, 25						+HC	+	+
Thiazide diuretics	23						+HC		
Lithium carbonate	23						+HC		
Vitamin A intoxication	23, 38						+HC		
Familial hypocalciuric hypercalcemia	23						+HC		
William's syndrome	26						+HC		
Pheochromocytoma	23						+HC		
VIPoma	23						+HC		
Addison's disease	23						+HC		
Hypomagnesemia	27, 28						+LC		
Osteoblastic tumor metastases	25						+LC	+	+
Neonatal hypocalcemia	17						+LC		
Post-renal transplantation	39								
Chronic renal failure	39						+HP		
Acute renal failure	39						+HP		
Alcohol bone disease/chronic abuse	28						+LP		
Iatrogenic magnesium excess	28						+HMg		
Cisplatin, amphotericin, cyclosporine and aminoglycoside nephropathies	28						+LMg		
Lasix, thiazide, ethacrynic acid	28						+LMg		
Primary aldosteronism	28						+LMg		
Osteopetrosis	42						+LC	+	+
Carbonic anhydrase II deficiency	42			+				+	+
Pseudohypophosphatasia	42								
Fibrous dysplasia and hyperostosis syndromes	42, 44							+	+
Bone cysts	44							+	+
Benign bone tumors	44							+	+
Malignant bone tumors	44							+	+

Abbreviations are defined in Table 1. Ch, chapter(s); +, present as part of the disease; L, low; H, hyper-; C, calcium; Mg, magnesium; and P, phosphorus.

Flank Tenderness

Real flank tenderness from urinary infection, a distended kidney, renal infarction, and bone fractures, needs no heavy pounding for diagnosis, only a soft palpation that usually shows some muscle spasm. Pain occurs with a very modest compression or tap. Heavy pounding makes anybody wince.

Loss of Height

With age and bone diseases, the part of the body that shrinks is above the hips, not the long bones unless they have curved or fractured. So in most cases, loss of "height" means deformity, a loss of torso height in relation to leg length, whether from fractures, kyphosis, diffuse loss of intervertebral disk thickness, muscle weakness, or some combination. The loss of torso length obliterates the waist, creating a barrel shape or at best a cylindrical shape.

Cafe-au-lait Spots

Cafe-au-lait spots are hyperpigmented macules that may be found on the trunk or extremities. Cafe-au-lait spots with rough border (coast of Maine) are found in polyostotic fibrous dysplasia, the McCune-Albright syndrome. A smooth border (coast of California) characterizes the lesions found in neurofibromatosis, first noted in childhood as axillary freckles.

Routine Laboratory Findings

Table 5 is a good data base for the field, and a subset of the standard screening blood panel, so every screening test offers an opportunity to detect mineral disorders. Interpretation of abnormalities is implicit in the syndromes, and their definitions.

ESTABLISHMENT OF SYNDROMES

We would almost rewrite this volume giving all details of clinical evaluation. Table 6 summarizes testing useful for determining if one of the main syndromes exists in a patient, and treatment is implied by the definition of each syndrome. Skin biopsy in osteogenesis imperfecta, and the particular radiographs most useful for the different syndromes may not be entirely obvious, and are in the table. By tissue biopsy, we mean lesions associated with pathological fractures, which usually are suspected tumors.

ANALYSIS OF THE SYNDROMES

Table 7 represents a compendium of all recognized disorders, collated by their presenting syndromes. As a labor of love, we have listed the chapters presenting material for each disease. The rest, their use in cases, we leave to the readers of this book.

Disorders of Bone and Mineral Metabolism,
edited by Fredric L. Coe and Murray J. Favus,
© 1992 by Raven Press, Ltd. All rights reserved.

CHAPTER 20

The Imaging and Quantitation of Bone by Radiographic and Scanning Methodologies

Charles H. Chesnut III

Radiographic techniques are of major importance in the clinical evaluation and management of mineral metabolism disorders. Radiography, bone densitometry, and radionuclide bone imaging are the three radiographic modalities currently used in the field of metabolic bone disease. All utilize ionizing radiation to provide diagnostic information, but there the similarity ends: each utilizes a different mechanism, and provides a unique type of information. For instance, x-ray radiography may be characterized as a *descriptive* discipline, in which the diagnosis of metabolic bone disease is made by assessing morphology (structure and form) on a visual, radiographic image. This image is produced from the differing absorption coefficients of various tissues for x-rays. Bone densitometry is characterized more as an *analytical* discipline, in which numerical data derived from the attenuation of ionizing radiation (x-rays or gamma rays) by bone is used to predict skeletal fracture risk, and to monitor response to therapy. Radionuclide bone imaging (the bone scan) may be thought of as combining qualities of both *descriptive* and *analytical* disciplines, in that it diagnoses the presence of disease via a visual image, and also (at least putatively) may assess bone remodeling parameters by quantitating radionuclide uptake throughout the skeleton. The bone scan utilizes metabolic/physiologic change, or changes in bone vascularity, to delineate abnormality, rather than assessing morphological change as occurs in radiography.

These three techniques can be utilized efficaciously, alone or together, in evaluating mineral metabolism disorders. In addition, ultrasonography may also be utilized

in metabolic bone disease, to quantitate and possibly to qualitate bone mass, and to delineate parathyroid abnormalities such as adenomas. These techniques, with their various assets and liabilities, will be discussed individually.

RADIOGRAPHY

The radiograph assesses morphological patterns and appearances of certain diseases. A number of metabolic bone diseases possess morphological patterns specific to each (1). The physical mechanisms by which diagnostic images are obtained (the passage of x-rays through various tissues) are described in standard radiology textbooks.

Parathyroid Disorders

Primary Hyperparathyroidism (Fig. 1)

The most frequent radiographic finding in primary hyperparathyroidism is subperiosteal resorption, particularly of the phalanges, although cortical and trabecular bone resorption elsewhere may also be seen. Demineralization of cortical and trabecular bone may also be present, although, as will be seen, the radiograph is a very insensitive measurement of osteopenia (bone mass loss or demineralization). Destructive cystic lesions ("brown" tumors), osteitis fibrosa cystica, occasional vertebral body sclerosis, and renal calculi on IVP or KUB, are additional x-ray findings. It should be remembered that patients with primary hyperparathyroidism may show few radiographic finding of osteoporosis such as vertebral compression fractures (2).

C. H. Chesnut III: Departments of Medicine, Radiology, Nutritional Sciences, and Orthopaedics, Osteoporosis Research Center, University of Washington Medical Center, Seattle, WA 98195.

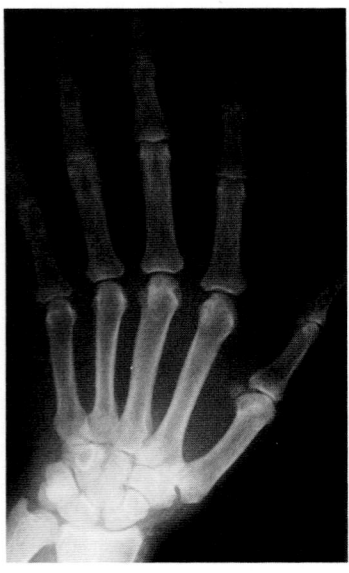 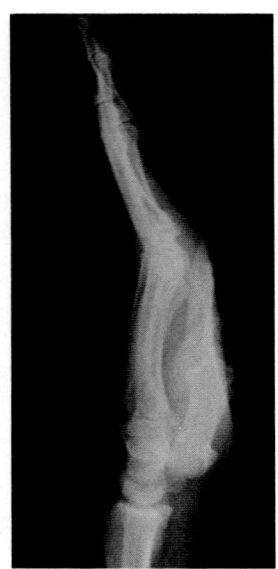

FIG. 1. Periosteal bone resorption, cortical erosions of the phalangeal tufts, and cystic changes in the hands of a subject with primary hyperparathyroidism. Courtesy of Dr. Thurmond Gillespie, University of Washington Medical Center, Seattle, Washington.

Hypoparathyroidism

Radiographic findings of either idiopathic or acquired hypoparathyroidism include an increased bone density, but (as previously noted) the radiograph is an insensitive method for determining bone mineralization.

Pseudohypoparathyroidism, Pseudo-Pseudohypoparathyroidism

In this disorder, radiographic findings of skeletal anomalies include shortened metacarpals or metatarsals, and soft tissue calcification.

In general, the diagnosis of parathyroid disorders, including primary hyperparathyroidism, will be obtained by assessing such serum parameters as calcium, phosphorus, and immunoreactive parathyroid hormone, rather than by the x-ray alone. The x-ray will provide confirmatory evidence of hyperparathyroidism.

Rickets and Osteomalacia

Demineralization, thickening of trabeculae producing coarse striations on the radiograph, and pseudofractures are radiographic findings seen in both rickets and osteomalacia. The pseudofractures are particularly characteristic of osteomalacia (and, to a lesser extent, of Paget's disease), and appear as areas of decreased density, typically perpendicular to the cortex, extending *partially* across the bone. A marginal sclerosis may be seen at the pseudofracture.

As with primary hyperparathyroidism, the usual diagnosis of rickets or osteomalacia will be made with various blood parameters, but also with the additional histological diagnostic information provided by the iliac crest bone biopsy. The radiographic finding of pseudo-

fractures, however, may be most helpful in establishing this diagnosis.

Renal Osteodystrophy

Renal osteodystrophy's radiographic appearance (3) includes components of radiographic rickets and osteomalacia (due to calcitriol deficiency), of secondary hyperparathyroidism (due to excess parathyroid hormone), as well as of osteoporosis and osteosclerosis. It will also be affected by such therapeutic manipulations as dialysis, renal transplantation, etc.

Rickets/Osteomalacia

Radiographic changes in this variant of renal osteodystrophy will be indistinguishable from those of rickets/osteomalacia secondary to other causes, and include demineralization, a generalized decrease in radiolucency, increased coarsening and haziness of the trabecular pattern, and the presence of pseudofractures. These appear indistinguishable from those found in other forms of osteomalacia.

Secondary Hyperparathyroidism

Here, the radiographic changes are primarily those of osteitis fibrosa cystica. In addition to subperiosteal resorption, generalized demineralization, and thinning cortices, there also will be seen multiple, well-demarcated cystic lucent areas of bone destruction ("brown" tumors) throughout the skeleton.

Osteopenia/Osteoporosis

There is occasionally radiographic demineralization, progressing to compression fractures, possibly due to chronic renal failure superimposed upon an underlying osteoporotic process.

Osteosclerosis

This radiographic finding may appear at various sites throughout the skeleton, particularly in the vertebrae, pelvis, ribs, skull, and long bones (in the spine, alternating bands of sclerosis are characterized as a "rugger jersey" appearance).

Ectopic Calcification

Extensive ectopic and dystrophic calcification, particularly in the soft tissues, may be seen in untreated renal osteodystrophy. There may also be aseptic necrosis of the femoral head.

In renal osteodystrophy, the radiograph may display components of all of the above findings. The diagnosis of significant renal osteodystrophy will be made with serum parameters in combination with the x-ray.

Paget's Disease of Bone

Osteoporosis/Osteosclerosis

Early Paget's disease may present radiographically as osteoporosis, or later in its development as sclerosis. Classically, the osteoporotic presentation is seen in the skull, where it is termed "osteoporosis circumscripta," and is characterized by radiolucencies, poor bone detail, and generalized demineralization. In the more frequently observed sclerotic form, the cortex and trabeculae are thickened, with occasional severe osteosclerosis of much of the bone area (Fig. 2). Pseudofractures may occur, usually in the long bones.

Cortical thickening, coarse and dense trabeculae, and focal sclerosis, all combined with areas of demineralization and radiolucency, may be indicative of evolving Paget's disease.

Chondrosarcoma/Osteogenic Sarcoma

It should be remembered that chondrosarcoma and osteogenic sarcoma may develop in a small number of patients with Paget's disease, with consequent characteristic radiographic appearance of these malignancies.

Paget's Disease Activity and the X-Ray

The radiograph in Paget's disease may not mirror the *current* metabolic and clinical activity of the disease. It is quite possible that inactive Paget's disease may demonstrate a most striking radiographic appearance. The x-ray of course is recording the residue of changes that may have taken place at an earlier time, and the disease may currently be quiescent. The metabolic and clinical activity of Paget's is more sensitively assessed with blood and

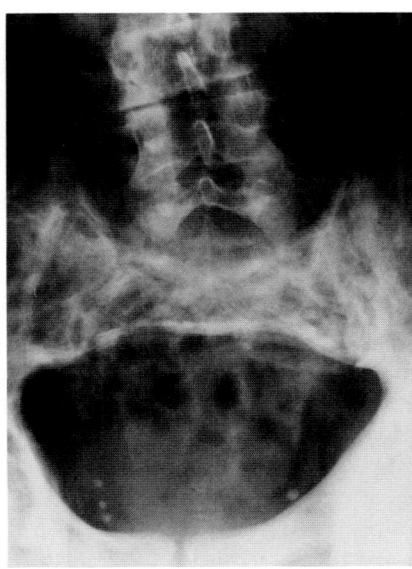

FIG. 2. Sclerosis, trabecular thickening, and demineralization in the pelvis of a subject with Paget's disease. Courtesy of Dr. Thurmond Gillespie, University of Washington Medical Center, Seattle, Washington.

urine tests, and, most specifically, with the radionuclide bone scan (see below).

Osteoporosis

Usage of the X-ray in Osteoporosis

The clinical usefulness of radiography in osteoporosis is to diagnose the presence of fracture, most frequently in the spine (vertebral compression fractures), hip, or wrist (Colles' fracture), as well as at other sites such as the ribs and long bones (i.e., the humerus). To a lesser extent, it may also be used to follow response to therapy; i.e., a new vertebral compression fracture twelve months after therapy commences indicates failure of treatment. However, the x-ray may not be used to predict future fracture risk, since the x-ray is a very insensitive technique for assessing demineralization: perhaps 50% of bone mass must be lost before radiographic demineralization is detected (4).

The x-ray cannot, therefore, be used to screen individuals at risk for osteoporosis (fracture), but, rather, can be used to diagnose the presence of the disease. Also, as will be seen, the bone mass measuring techniques have a greater sensitivity for monitoring response to treatment (by evaluating changes in bone mass). A methodology determining a specific therapy's efficacy is clearly of greater value if it can precisely and accurately measure such efficacy (such as a change in bone mass) before the osteoporotic fracture occurs, rather than after fracture occurrence, as with the x-ray.

Defining a Spinal Fracture

A lack of consensus as to what constitutes a vertebral fracture limits x-ray usage for other than the diagnoses of osteoporosis-associated fracture. While a 25% or greater reduction in anterior, middle, and posterior vertebral height usually indicates a compressed vertebral "crush" fracture, the definition of a clinically significant wedged vertebral "deformity" is as yet unstandardized. Is it a 15%, 20%, or 25% reduction in anterior height—alone— as compared to posterior height—and is such a deformity a significant predictor of future progression to a "completed" vertebral fracture? What is the significance of Schmorl's nodes, endplate disruption without vertebral height loss, etc.? This lack of standardization in vertebral fractures particularly compromises clinical research trials attempting to define the efficacy of various therapies in preventing spinal compression fractures. A universally accepted standardized classification of spinal deformity and fracture is acutely needed (5).

BONE DENSITOMETRY (6–12)

Since bone mass is the primary, although not the sole, determinant of bone fracture, noninvasive bone mass measurements would be of value in metabolic bone diseases associated with osteopenia (loss of bone mass) such as the parathyroid disorders associated with excess parathyroid hormone, and particularly in the metabolic skeletal disorder osteoporosis (loss of bone mass with fracture). Such noninvasive measurements, providing analytical numerical data, could be used in predicting the risk of fracture and in following response to treatment. As previously noted, spine radiographs are relatively insensitive in quantitating bone mass (4). Other techniques for quantitating bone mass more sensitively are required. Over the past 25 years, a number of noninvasive procedures have been developed to accomplish this aim. These currently include single and dual photon absorptiometry (SPA and DPA), dual energy x-ray absorptiometry (DEXA), and computerized tomography (CT). Such noninvasive techniques provide quantitation of bone mass at those axial and appendicular sites which are the principal areas (i.e., spine, wrist, and hip) usually involved in those metabolic diseases (such as osteoporosis) in which bone loss is a primary feature. In addition, it is now also possible to quantitate bone mass at the os calcis (with SPA), and at practically any site throughout the entire skeleton (with DEXA).

Basic Principles of Bone Mass Quantitation

Bone attenuates (absorbs) ionizing radiation. An exponential relationship exists between bone mass and radiation attenuation: the greater the amount of bone present, the greater the attenuation of ionizing radiation and the less radiation is quantified in a radiation detector (Fig. 3). Such attenuation is the basic principle behind the majority of the noninvasive bone mass measurement techniques (SPA, DPA, DEXA, and CT). In SPA and DPA, the radionuclides iodine 125 and gadolinium 153 are the source of this radiation; in DEXA and CT, x-rays are the source.

The Ideal Noninvasive Techniques for Assessing Bone Mass

The ideal noninvasive techniques quantitate primarily trabecular bone, as this is metabolically more active than cortical bone, and may be preferentially affected by metabolic bone diseases such as osteoporosis. Trabecular bone is also the bone type most affected by medications currently utilized in osteoporosis therapy, including calcitonin, sodium fluoride, bisphosphonates, and estrogen. However, cortical bone mass measurements at the wrist, hip, and possibly other sites (such as the femoral shaft) may be of value in monitoring a possible differential effect of osteoporosis and of a number of its therapies (i.e., fluoride, parathyroid hormone fragments) on trabecular and cortical bone, and in such diseases as primary hyperparathyroidism, renal osteodystrophy, and cortisone-induced osteopenia (which may affect cortical as well as trabecular bone).

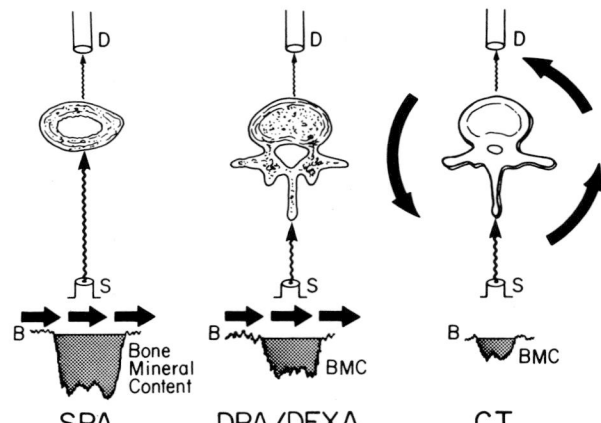

FIG. 3. Principles of single photon absorptiometry (SPA), dual photon absorptiometry (DPA), dual energy x-ray absorptiometry (DEXA), and computerized tomography (CT). D, detector; S, source of ionizing radiation (see text); →, direction of scan (CT, rotary); B, baseline count rate; BMC, bone mineral content. A scan across the radius (SPA) or vertebra (DPA/DEXA, CT) results in the absorption profile noted, utilizing an exponential relationship between bone mass and radiation attenuation. Computer integration of the area below the baseline is performed, and the results are compared with calibration standards, providing units of bone mass and/or linear, areal, or formatted volumetric density [grams, grams/centimeter, grams/centimeter^2, milligrams/cc [CT]. From Chesnut (6).

As spine and hip fractures are associated with the greatest osteoporosis morbidity, these are the sites most usefully measured by these ideal techniques. Such techniques should also be capable of predicting an individual's risk for osteoporotic fracture and be readily applicable to assessing therapeutic response. They should be reasonably precise and accurate, logistically acceptable (i.e., not require excessive patient time nor cause patient discomfort), be relatively inexpensive, and be safe (i.e., not associated with significant radiation exposure). The techniques previously mentioned satisfy these criteria to varying degrees (Table 1).

Specific Techniques

Single Photon Absorptiometry

Single photon absorptiometry (SPA) measurements are most frequently performed at the wrist, but may also be obtained at the os calcis. SPA wrist measurements, usually at "ultra distal," distal, and/or proximal forearm sites, are quantitated in analytical units of grams per centimeter (linear density) and grams per centimeter square (areal density). These measurements are usually compared to laboratory/diagnostic center referent populations to determine bone mass surplus or deficit. The distal and proximal wrist sites measure primarily cortical bone mass; the ultra distal wrist and the os calcis sites measure primarily trabecular bone. As previously noted, cortical bone at the wrist is neither the type nor site most frequently involved in osteoporosis, but may be representative of the type of bone affected in other metabolic bone diseases, including primary hyperparathyroidism and renal osteodystrophy. While it is accepted that SPA (as measured at either the wrist or heel) can predict fracture risk (11), not only at the wrist but also at other skeletal sites, there is no definitive evidence indicating that a measurement of bone mass at the wrist will predict bone mass, or bone mass change, with clinically acceptable accuracy at the spine or hip.

Cortical SPA is therefore of limited value as a screening technique for osteoporosis, although it may be of value in other metabolic diseases affecting both cortical and trabecular bone, such as hyperthyroidism, hyperparathyroidism, renal osteodystrophy, and certain pediatric clinical situations. It may also be of value in following response to therapies affecting cortical as well as trabecular bone, such as cortisone and estrogen. In addition, SPA may be of value in monitoring cortical sites in patients being treated with sodium fluoride or the parathyroid hormone fragment (amino acid) 1-34, each of which may have a differential effect on cortical and trabecular bone (i.e., a positive effect on trabecular and a negative effect on cortical bone). While the SPA ultra distal wrist site, and the os calcis site, do assess primarily trabecular bone, they do so at sites subject to mechanical stresses, local hormonal interactions, and loading forces quite different from those occurring at spine and hip sites. Although these latter sites may have value in predicting future fracture risk, in general trabecular bone as measured at the spine with DPA, DEXA, or CT is a more meaningful and specific predictor.

As seen in Table 1, SPA's assets include a reasonable cost, acceptable precision, logistical simplicity, and low radiation exposure. Whether these assets balance the liabilities noted above is problematic.

Dual Photon Absorptiometry (DPA) and Dual Energy X-Ray Absorptiometry (DEXA)

The history of bone densitometry began in the late 1960s, with SPA the first available technique. At its inception about 10 years ago, DPA represented a major breakthrough in the evaluation of the individual with metabolic bone disease, particularly osteoporosis: for the first time, a measurement of primarily trabecular bone at spine and hip was possible. As seen in Table 1, DPA demonstrates precision and accuracy (acceptable at the time the technique was introduced), and can be used to predict risk of future fracture as well as to follow response to treatment. However, for reasons discussed below, DPA in 1991 has largely been replaced in most research laboratories and clinical centers by DEXA. However, it should be noted that while DEXA offers many advantages over DPA, the biological information (i.e., an analytical assessment of bone mass) provided by both machines is similar, and data obtained by DPA remain quite useful in the clinical management of patients at risk for or with osteoporosis.

As noted in Table 1, DEXA offers a number of advances compared to DPA. DEXA's usage of an x-ray tube to replace DPA's radionuclide (gadolinium 153) as a source of ionizing radiation provides a greater photon flux; this change, combined with DEXA's improved detector configuration and data analysis, results in an improved precision (1–1.5% at spine and hip), resolution, and scan time (7–10 minutes) as compared to DPA. The radiation exposure (5–10 mrem) is acceptable and the cost of the scan to the patient may be priced below DPA, due to a shorter scan time and a lower maintenance cost. Finally, as shown in Table 1, total and multiple skeletal sites of bone mass may be easily examined with DEXA. Also, DEXA will undoubtedly prove acceptable for predicting future fracture and monitoring response to treatment. DEXA's greater precision (~1%), which permits identification of significant change in bone mass over time with a smaller bone mass change than would be necessary with DPA (precision 3–5%), may permit a more definitive assessment of therapy. Both DPA and DEXA measure primarily trabecular bone as bone mineral content in grams and bone mineral density (areal density) in grams per centimeter square at the spine (Fig.

TABLE 1. *Noninvasive techniques for measuring bone mass*

Technique	Site measured	Cortical/trabecular bone (%)	Precision/accuracy (%, ±)	Risk prediction	Response to therapy	Radiation dose (in mrem)	Duration of procedure (minutes)	Cost in U.S. $
SPA	Radius/ulna							
	Distal	80–95/20–5	±2–4/±3–4%	+	±[a]	10	10–15	75–125
	Ultradistal	25/75	±2–4/?	?	?	10	10–15	75–125
	Os calcis	20/80	±2–4/?	+	?	10	10–15	75–125
DPA	Spine L1–4[b]	35/65	±3–5/±2–4%	+	+	10	20–30	150–200
	Femur-neck	75/25	±3–5/?	?	+[a]	10	20–30	75
	Trochanter	50/50	±3–5/?	?	?	10	20–30	—
DEXA	Spine L1–4[b]	35/65	±1–1.5%/?	+[c]	+[c]	<10	10	150
	Femur							
	Neck	75/25	±1.5/?	?	+[c]	<10	10	75
	Trochanter	50/50	±1.5/?	?	?	<10	10	—
	Total skeleton	80/20	±1/?	?	?	<5	5–10	?
	Radius-ulna[d]	80–95/20–5	±1.2/?	+[c]	±[a]	<10	6	?
	Lateral spine[d,e]	35/65	±4/?	?	?	<10	20	?
CT	Single energy							
	Spine T12–L3[f]	5/95	±3.5/6–8%	+	+	300–750	30	150
	Dual energy							
	Spine T12–L3[f]	5/95	±5–8/5%	+[c]	+[c]	750	30	150
US	Patella[d]	?5/95	2–3/?	+	?	—	5	35–50[g]
	Os calcis[d]	20/80	2–3/?	?	?	—	5	35–50[g]

Source: From Chesnut (6).
[a] ?Estrogens.
[b] *Total* vertebral body including spinous processes, aortic calcification.
[c] Unproven—but probable.
[d] Experimental.
[e] Lateral decubitus (excludes posterior spinous processes, aortic calcification, etc.).
[f] Centrum—area of interest *within* vertebral body.
[g] Projected.

4), hip (Fig. 5), and—in grams only—total skeleton (Fig. 6). These values are automatically compared to age- and sex-matched normal referent databases, and to young normal databases (each unique to each manufacturer's machine). The resultant bone mass deficit or surplus is quantitated as a percentage or standard deviation (Z scores) above or below age-matched or young normal means.

The DEXA lateral scan, developed over the past two years, theoretically provides increased accuracy, as it deletes the posterior spinous processes, aortic calcification, and severe osteophytes, which the standard A-P DPA and DEXA scans assess as bone. In addition, the DEXA lateral view may provide an area-of-interest measurement *within* the vertebral body, a measurement of primarily trabecular bone similar to that obtained with the CT centrum measurement (see below), a measurement that at least putatively could be of increased importance in predicting future fracture risk. However, imprecision due to variation in soft tissue lateral to the spine, patient positioning problems, and inaccuracy caused by ribs and iliac crest overlapping the vertebral bodies, have to date been a source of concern; the lateral scan therefore remains a research technique.

Measurement of bone mass at the wrist is also possible with DEXA at distal, ultradistal, and mid-shaft radius and ulna sites. The shortened scan time of 5–6 minutes and improved precision of 1.2% (as compared to SPA's 2–4%) will undoubtedly result in DEXA wrist scans replacing SPA-radionuclide scans at some time in the near future.

Lastly, DEXA's total skeleton bone mass measurements can provide an overall assessment of bone mass

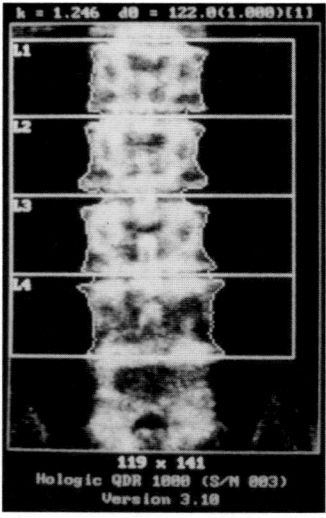

FIG. 4. Measurement of bone mass at the lumbar spine (L1–4) with the DEXA technique. Courtesy of Hologic, Inc., Waltham, Massachusetts.

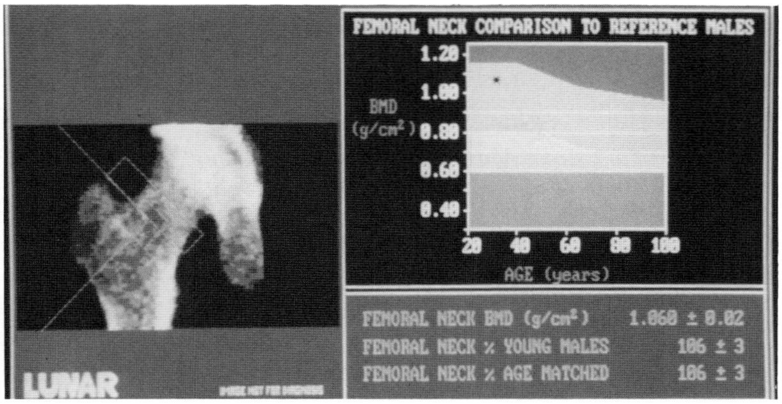

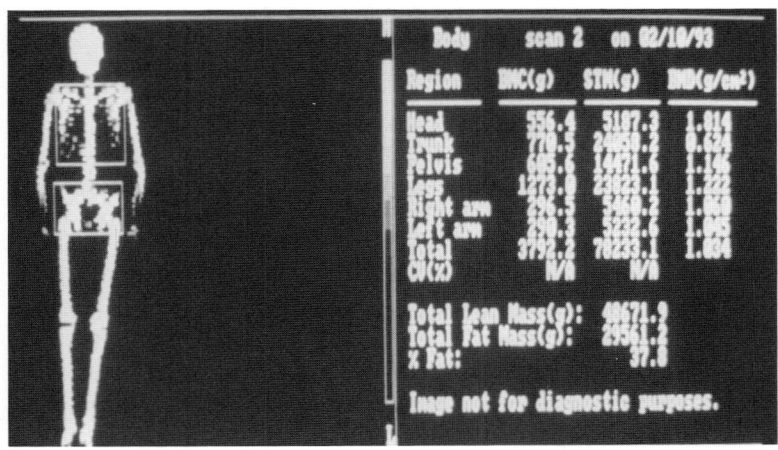

FIG. 5. Measurement of bone mass at the hip with the DEXA technique. Courtesy of Lunar, Inc., Madison, Wisconsin.

throughout the skeleton, and of various components of the skeleton. Repetitive total-skeletal measurements track changes throughout the skeletal areas, and might be used to identify differential responses to therapy (i.e., a gain in bone mass at one site at the expense of another site). However, overall the total skeleton measurement remains primarily a research tool. Analyses of body composition, including lean body mass, fat composition, etc., are also available with a number of DEXA machines (currently for investigational use only). Such measurements are theoretically of value in assessing body composition in cases of anorexia nervosa, etc.

There are currently three major DEXA vendors in the United States: Hologic in Waltham, MA; Lunar in Madison, WI; and Norland in Ft. Atkinson, WI. The machines cost, on average, about $75,000–$95,000.

Computerized Tomography

Computerized tomography (CT) was developed almost concurrently with DPA about 10 years ago. This technique provides an analytical quantitation of bone mass (usually at the spine), as a formatted, three-dimensional volumetric slice of vertebral bone mass quantitated in mg/cc. A CT image provides either a "centrum" measurement of primarily trabecular bone within the

vertebral body, or an "integral" measurement of the entire vertebral body, including the transverse processes and posterior elements (a mixture of trabecular and cortical bone). The centrum measurement, and the region-of-interest measurement on the lateral DEXA, are unique among all currently available bone mass assessing techniques in their measurement of almost exclusively trabecular bone within the vertebral body (Table 1). Such measurements of primarily trabecular bone mass may *hypothetically* provide a more accurate assessment of fracture risk than measurements of the entire vertebral body, such as are obtained with the integral CT, DPA, and DEXA. This potential asset of the centrum CT measurement must be balanced against a number of liabilities: problems with accuracy and quality assurance, and high radiation dosage (Table 1).

First, accuracy with single energy CT continues to be a problem, in spite of advances in software and hardware. The technique is particularly vulnerable to errors occasioned by marrow fat. As noted in Table 1, dual energy CT may reduce this error, but at the expense of reduced precision and increased radiation exposure. As with DPA and DEXA, CT's accuracy may be adversely affected by scoliosis and kyphosis, pre-existing compressed vertebral fractures, and vertebral sclerosis.

FIG. 6. Measurement of bone mass throughout the skeleton with the DEXA technique. Courtesy of Norland, Inc., Ft. Atkinson, Wisconsin.

Second, quality assurance is suspect for CT procedures performed in hospitals, offices, and laboratories not involved on a day-to-day basis with CT to quantitate bone mass. Difficulties with patient positioning, compliance in phantom standardization, centering of the CT "slice" through the vertebral body, etc., may worsen CT's precision and accuracy in these settings.

Third, significant radiation exposure occurs with CT measurements, particularly as compared to DPA and DEXA.

Therefore, while research labs with dedicated CT scanners may provide the most acceptable spinal bone mass measurement, CT seems less useful in comparison to DEXA in terms of precision, accuracy, radiation exposure, quality assurance, and day to day logistical ease of operation, particularly in a clinical practice setting.

Bone Mass Quantitation and Fracture

Quantitation versus Qualitation

DEXA, DPA, CT, and SPA quantitate bone mass. Can a measurement of bone quantity alone accurately predict future fracture risk, or must other variables such as bone quality be utilized? In 1991, extensive data indicate that bone mass quantitation alone can indeed predict the risk of fracture. A significant relationship between bone mineral density (BMD) and bone strength exists (13), and BMD accounts for perhaps 75% of the variance in bone strength (14). Most importantly, a significant correlation also exists between BMD and fracture risk: an increase in fracture risk is associated with a lower bone mass (15–17). Fracture risk can be stratified according to bone mass levels, and bone mass measurements of the hip, spine, or wrist can predict fracture risk at these sites.

Discrimination Between Normal and Osteporotic Groups

However, it should be noted that bone mass quantitation alone may not discriminate between osteoporotic and normal subjects of the same age and sex. Bone mass measurements in normal and osteoporotic groups will reveal significant overlaps in bone mass at the hip, spine and wrist, as measured by any of the above techniques (18). This lack of discrimination may lie in the fact that bone mass is not the only determinant of fracture risk: bone quality and microarchitecture, propensity to fall, lack of neuromuscular coordination, etc., will also contribute to fracture occurrence, particularly in the elderly. Such a lack of discrimination should not be seen as a shortcoming of the bone mass measuring techniques; discriminatory ability assesses the techniques' value in diagnosing the presence of osteoporotic fracture. Spinal x-rays can sensitively diagnose the presence of fracture,

therefore, bone densitometry techniques should not be utilized in fracture diagnosis. They are more properly utilized in predicting fracture risk.

Can Bone Mass Measurements at One Site Predict Bone Mass and Fracture Risk at Another Site?

There are concerns regarding the relative amounts of bone mass present, and the relative changes in bone mass, at different skeletal sites. Significant correlations do exist between the amount of bone mass present at the spine, wrist, and hip; however, there are 10–20% standard errors in such correlations, a degree of inaccuracy which prevents the clinical prediction of bone mass at one site from a bone mass measurement at another site (19). Also, no correlation exists between changes in bone mass among the various sites (20). While the risk of fracture at multiple sites may be predicted by a bone mass measurement at a single site, fracture risk at a specific site (such as the hip) is more accurately assessed with a measurement at that site. To determine bone mass, bone mass change, and fracture risk at one site with an acceptable and clinically useful accuracy, one should measure bone at that site.

The Value of Risk Factors in Assessing Fracture Risk

Risk factors such as estrogen depletion, lack of activity, leanness, alcohol and smoking history, etc., are important in the development of metabolic bone diseases, particularly osteoporosis. How important are they in determining fracture risk? The usage of risk factors to determine fracture risk is unfortunately not supported by available data (21). Risk factors for bone loss cannot reliably predict bone mass loss, or subsequent fracture risk, at least not in individual patients. The use of such risk factors as substitutes for bone mass assessment to determine fracture risk, and the need for therapy, is therefore inappropriate. On the other hand, risk factors assessed *in combination with* bone mass measurements may more fully define an individual's risk.

Clinical Indications for Bone Mass Assessment

General

The noninvasive bone mass measuring techniques are extremely useful in clinically evaluating conditions characterized by osteopenia or osteoporosis; e.g., postmenopausal osteoporosis or hyperparathyroidism. In which clinical situations should these techniques specifically be utilized? Recently, a National Osteoporosis Foundation task force defined a number of clinical indications for bone mass measurements (9). The following represent an adaptation of this information:

Specific Indications

1. In estrogen-deficient women, to diagnose significantly low bone mass in order to make decisions regarding hormone replacement therapy (HRT), or alternatives to HRT. For such an indication, the methodology should be safe, inexpensive, and logistically simple for both the operator and the patient. Most importantly, the measurements obtained should relate to risk for future fracture. The newer techniques, particularly DEXA, satisfy the majority of these requirements.

2. In patients with radiographically detected vertebral abnormalities, "demineralization," or "osteopenia," to diagnose the presence of significant bone loss in order to make clinical decisions regarding further diagnostic and/or therapeutic evaluations. As has been mentioned previously, the radiograph is an insensitive screen of significant bone loss. If a radiograph describes "demineralization," this should be an indication for a more definitive assessment.

3. In patients receiving long-term glucocorticoid therapy, to diagnose low bone mass. This indication might be widened to include assessment of significant bone loss in a number of other conditions in which osteopenia is an accompanying manifestation, such as anorexia nervosa, bulimia, athletic amenorrhea, premature menopause, Turner's syndrome, medically managed hyperparathyroidism, etc.

4. In patients on osteoporosis therapy, to monitor the efficacy of such therapy. This indication requires measurement techniques of high precision and reproducibility, and DEXA's 1–1.5% precision satisfies this requirement.

5. The use of the above techniques for screening *all* women after the menopause remains controversial, and is not indicated at this time.

Other Clinical Questions

The practitioner in the metabolic bone disease field is also faced with numerous additional clinical questions regarding the noninvasive techniques:

1. Which site (spine, wrist, hip, etc.) and which bone type (cortical or trabecular) should be measured to assess fracture risk? As discussed earlier, in individual patients each of the above sites seems to provide some information defining risk for future fracture. However, an accurate assessment of risk is relatively site-specific. Overall, the spine seems to be the most reasonable site for measurement, at least through age 65–70. After age 70, bone mass measurements at the spine *and* hip may be of clinical value. Finally, in metabolic bone diseases such as primary hyperparathyroidism and renal osteodystrophy, measurements of cortical bone may be indicated.

2. Which site should be measured to assess therapeutic efficacy? For following response to treatment of

various metabolic bone diseases, the spine again appears to be the most significant site. However, as noted previously, certain osteoporosis medications (such as sodium fluoride, estrogen, parathyroid hormone analogs, and cortisone) may affect cortical as well as trabecular bone, and a measurement of cortical bone (usually performed at the forearm) may be indicated as well. Generally, measurements at 1 to 2 year intervals appear reasonable in order to assess response to treatment.

For such measurements, DEXA appears to be the technique of choice in 1991, due to its ease of measurement, improved precision, low radiation exposure, and excellent quality control.

3. A problem for the patient undergoing bone mass evaluation in 1991 is the reimbursement policy of third-party health care carriers (Medicare/Medicaid, private insurers, etc.) who do not uniformly reimburse the costs for these procedures. Given the clinical value of these techniques, such a position seems inappropriate. It is hoped that reimbursement will be uniformly available in the future.

Conclusions Regarding Bone Densitometry

The risk of fracture increases as bone mass decreases. Techniques are available that can precisely and accurately quantitate bone mass, and predict fracture risk. These techniques can and should be utilized in evaluating patients at risk for, and with, the metabolic diseases associated with bone loss.

RADIONUCLIDE BONE IMAGING

Radionuclide bone imaging may be used descriptively and analytically to define the presence of disease and to monitor response to treatment.

Basic Principles of Radionuclide Bone Imaging

The Bone Scan (8,22)

Radionuclide bone scanning utilizes γ photon images derived from an intravenously injected diphosphonate radiolabeled with technetium 99m; such a radionuclide combination is deposited in newly formed bone. Areas of abnormality on the bone scan are defined as "hot spots" (areas of increased radionuclide accretion), or as "cold spots" (photon deficient areas of decreased radionuclide accretion). The pathogenesis of these abnormalities is typically an initial increase in bone resorption (an increase secondary to tumor, metabolic bone disease such as hyperparathyroidism, etc.), coupled with a compensatory increase in bone formation, which incorporates the technetium 99m-labeled diphosphonate into the newly formed bone. Increased vascularity in such conditions as osteomyelitis, Paget's disease, etc., may also contribute to increased radionuclide concentration in areas of skeletal abnormality. The pathogenesis of "cold spots" is presumably replacement of bone-forming elements (presumably the osteoblasts) by tumor, with the bone then unable to increase formation in response to increased reabsorption. A decrease in vascular supply (sickle cell disease in crisis with vascular sludging, avascular necrosis, etc.) may also result in photon-deficient lesions.

Diphosphonate Retention (23)

The basic principle of "diphosphonate retention" to assess bone remodeling lies in the fact that in individuals with high or low bone turnover ("high or low bone remodeling") there is an increase or decrease in bone formation; as above, most frequently secondary to an initial increase or decrease in bone resorption. With this change in bone formation, there will be a greater or lesser retention of technetium 99m, with more or less excreted in the urine (the primary route of diphosphonate elimination). Quantitating the degree of retention is performed by assessing radioactivity in the urine, or by assessing the amount of radioactivity remaining in the skeleton at a specified time after injection.

Radionuclide versus X-Ray

It should be remembered that the disciplines of radionuclide bone imaging and diphosphonate retention dynamically assess bone physiology and metabolism, as compared to the x-ray, which is a static measurement of bone morphology and structure.

Clinical Indications for Radionuclide Bone Imaging

Metabolic Bone Disease

In Paget's disease the radionuclide bone scan is used primarily to assess the current activity of the disease. Since the x-ray provides a static measurement of morphology rather than a dynamic assessment of bone turnover and vascularity, it cannot be used for disease activity monitoring. The bone scan may also be used to localize and define the extent of active skeletal involvement (such diagnostic information is, again, unique to the bone scan and cannot be obtained from such diagnostic parameters as urinary hydroxyproline or skeletal alkaline phosphatase assays). Lastly, the bone scan may be used (Fig. 7) to monitor response to treatment of Paget's disease.

The bone scan may also be of occasional interest in defining the presence of such diseases as primary and secondary hyperparathyroidism (particularly renal osteodystrophy). Frequently seen in hyperparathyroidism is the "superscan" (22), with increased radionuclide uptake at the trabecular ends of the long bones, secondary

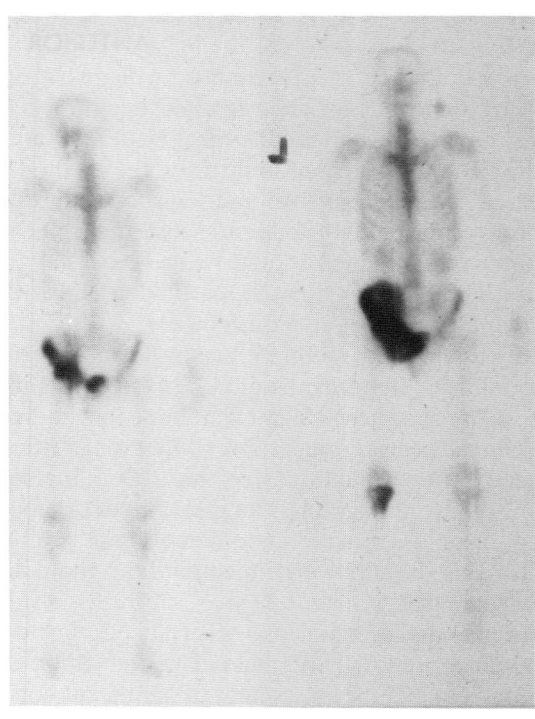

FIG. 7. Technetium 99m diphosphonate bone scan of a subject with Paget's disease of bone. The image on the right demonstrates active Paget's disease in the left pelvis and proximal tibia; the image on the left demonstrates marked improvement after mithramycin therapy (8).

to parathyroid hormone stimulated bone resorption, and a compensatory increase in bone formation. However, the overall clinical value of the bone scan in the management of parathyroid hormone disorders is unproven.

The bone scan may be used to identify incipient vertebral compression fractures in osteoporosis (24). Presumably, microfractures may occur in vertebral bodies before a full macrofracture occurs, and these microfractures may appear as "hot spots" on the scan, similar in appearance to stress fractures elsewhere. The bone scan may also be used to evaluate back pain in osteoporotic patients, in that a positive scan indicates incipient, current, or healing compression fractures as a cause of pain, while a negative scan will indicate a non-skeletal cause, such as paraspinous muscle spasm.

Diphosphonate retention technique can presumably be used to identify osteoporotic individuals with high bone remodeling (resorption and formation). Such individuals would presumably respond well to anti-bone resorbing therapeutic agents. However, whether diphosphonate retention is more sensitive (and more cost-effective) than urinary hydroxyproline or other blood and urine remodeling markers is unproven.

Radionuclide Imaging of Parathyroids

Of importance in the radiographic assessment of metabolic bone disease is the imaging of abnormal parathyroid tissue (such as parathyroid adenomas) with combined thallium 201-technetium 99m pertechnetate scans. The basic principle involves the concentration of thallium 201 in parathyroid and thyroid tissue, and the concentration of technetium 99m pertechnetate only in the thyroid. A subtraction technique may be performed, leaving the thallium 201 localized parathyroid adenoma as a "hot" area (25,26). This technique is particularly useful in locating ectopic parathyroid adenomas. It is generally noninvasive, logistically acceptable to the patient, safe, and entails minimal radiation exposure. Whether it is superior to ultrasound localization is unclear at this time (see below).

Ultrasound

The basic principle of ultrasound (US) measurement of the skeleton is that the speed at which US propagates in bone is determined by the mass density, and by the "elastic modulus" (inherent material quality) of the bone. The higher the mass density and the elastic modulus, the higher the speed of US. Presumably, bone exhibiting high US velocity is high in strength, and will resist fracture when force is applied; whereas bone with low US velocity will deform more with force, and consequently will be less able to resist fracture.

Ultrasound has been evaluated in recently completed clinical trials (27,28) as a measuring technique for assessing bone quantity and, presumably, bone quality, at the patella and os calcis. As shown in Table 1, at both these sites the bone is primarily trabecular, precision is acceptable with current techniques, and there is of course no radiation exposure. In studies to date, discrimination between normal and osteoporotic women is equivalent to that of SPA, DPA/DEXA, and CT. US measurements at the patella also seem to have some utility in predicting fracture risk. Whether these techniques can be used to follow response to treatment has not been assessed.

The primary advantage of US is a theoretical one: it measures not only bone quantity, but also bone quality. Associated with this advantage would be a putatively improved fracture risk assessment in the individual patient. As the measurement requires only 3–5 minutes of patient time, and could be much less expensive than other techniques (potentially, $25–$50 for examination of the patella), US could be an acceptable screening parameter even if its discriminatory and risk predicting abilities are no better than that of other techniques which only quantitate bone mass. However, US remains an experimental technique; more work on this interesting procedure is indicated.

In addition to its usage in assessing bone mass quality and quantity, high-resolution real-time US may also play a role in localizing parathyroid adenomas in patients with hyperparathyroidism. In this role, US is safe, logistically acceptable to the patient, and relatively inexpensive. US provides a morphological assessment of a parathyroid abnormality, whereas thallium 201-technetium 99m radionuclide images provide anatomical and vascularity/metabolism information on the parathyroid gland. The advantages of one technique over the other remain unclear (29,30).

REFERENCES

1. Teplick JG, Haskin ME, Schimert AP. *Roentgenologic diagnosis. A complement in radiology to the Beeson and McDermott textbook of medicine,* vol 2. Philadelphia: WB Saunders, 1967.
2. Wilson RJ, Rao S, Ellis B, Kleerekoper M, Parfitt AM. Mild asymptomatic primary hyperparathyroidism is not a risk factor for vertebral fractures. *Ann Intern Med* 1988;109:959–62.
3. Parfitt AM. Clinical and radiographic manifestations of renal osteodystrophy. In: David DS, ed. *Calcium metabolism in renal failure and nephrolithiasis.* New York: John Wiley, 1977.
4. Lachman E. Osteoporosis: the potentialities and limitations of its roentgenologic diagnosis. *Am J Roent* 1955;74:712–5.
5. Eastell R, Cedel SL, Wahner HW, Riggs BL, Melton LJ. Classification of vertebral fractures. *J Bone Miner Res* 1991;6:207–15.
6. Chesnut CH. Noninvasive methods for bone mass measurement. In: Avioli LV, ed. *The osteoporotic syndrome,* 3rd ed. New York: Grune & Stratton, 1991.
7. Chesnut CH. Methods and role of bone densitometry in the estrogen-deficient woman. In: Swartz DP, ed. *Hormone replacement therapy in the ovarian deficient woman.* Williams & Wilkins, 1991.
8. Chesnut CH. Bone imaging techniques. In: Becker KL, ed. *Principles and practice of endocrinology and metabolism.* Philadelphia: JB Lippincott, 1990;480–4.
9. Johnston CC Jr, Melton LJ III, Lindsay R, Eddy D. Clinical indication for bone mass measurement. *J Bone Miner Res* 1989; 4(Suppl 2).
10. Consensus Development Conference. Prophylaxis and treatment of osteoporosis. *Am J Med* 1991;90:107–10.
11. Johnston CC, Melton LJ. Bone density measurement in the management of osteoporosis. *Primer on metabolic bone diseases and disorders of mineral metabolism.* American Society of Bone and Mineral Research, 1990;93–100.
12. *Physician's Resource Manual.* National Osteoporosis Foundation, 1991.
13. Hayes WC, Gerhart TN. Biomechanics of bone: applications for assessment of bone strength. In: Peck WA, ed. *Bone and mineral research/3.* Elsevier Science Publishers B.V., 1985;259–94.
14. Melton LJ, Chao EYS, Lane J. Biomechanical aspects of fractures. In: Riggs BL, Melton LJ, eds. *Osteoporosis: etiology, diagnosis, and management.* New York: Raven Press, 1988;111–31.
15. Hui SL, Slemenda CW, Johnston CC Jr. Age and bone mass as predictors of fracture in a prospective study. *J Clin Invest* 1988;81:1804–9.
16. Wasnich RD, Ross PD, Heilbrun LK, Vogel JM. Selection of the optimal site for fracture risk prediction. *Clin Orthop* 1987;216:262–8.
17. Ross PD, Wasnich RD, Vogel JM. Detection of prefracture spinal osteoporosis using bone mineral absorptiometry. *J Bone Miner Res* 1988;3:1–11.
18. Ott SM, Kilcoyne RF, Chesnut CH. Ability of four different techniques of measuring bone mass to diagnose vertebral fractures in osteoporotic women. *J Bone Miner Res* 1987;2:201–10.
19. Ott SM, Kilcoyne RF, Chesnut CH. Comparisons among methods of measuring bone mass and relationship to severity of vertebral fractures in osteoporosis. *J Clin Endocrinol Metab* 1987; 366:501–7.
20. Ott SM, Kilcoyne RF, Chesnut CH. Longitudinal changes in bone mass after one year as measured by different techniques in patients with osteoporosis. *Calcif Tissue Int* 1986;39:133–8.
21. Wasnich RD, Ross PD, Vogel JM, MacLean CJ. The relative strength of osteoporotic risk factors in a prospective study of postmenopausal osteoporosis. *J Clin Bone Miner Res* 1987;2(Suppl 1):343.
22. Chesnut CH, Larson SM. Bone and parathyroid imaging. In:

Rothfeld B, ed. *Nuclear medicine: endocrinology.* Philadelphia: JB Lippincott, 1977;252–69.

23. Civitelli R, Gonnelli S, Zacchi F, et al. Bone turnover in postmenopausal osteoporosis. Effect of calcitonin treatment. *J Clin Invest* 1988;82:1268–74.

24. Chesnut CH, Nelp WB, Lewellen TK. Nuclear medicine techniques in the evaluation of postmenopausal osteoporosis (abstract). *J Nucl Med* 1976;17:526.

25. MacFarlane SD, Hanelin LG, Taft DA, et al. Localization of abnormal parathyroid glands using thallium-201. *Am J Surg* 1984;148:7+.

26. Young AE, Gaunt JI, Croft DW, et al. Localization of parathyroid adenomas by thallium-201 and technetium-99ᵐ subtraction scanning. *Br Med J* 1983;286:1384.

27. Heaney RP, Avioli LV, Chesnut CH, Lappe J, Recker RR, Brandenburger GH. Osteoporotic bone fragility: detection by ultrasound transmission velocity. *JAMA* 1989;261:2986–90.

28. Agren M, Karellas A, Leahey D, Marks S, Baran D. Ultrasound attenuation of the calcaneous: a sensitive and specific discrimination of osteopenia in postmenopausal women. *Calcif Tissue Int* 1991;48:240–4.

29. Butch RJ, Simeone JF, Mueller PR. Thyroid and parathyroid ultrasonography. *Radiol Clin North Am* 1985;23:57.

30. Winzelberg GC, Hydovitz JD, O'Hara XR, et al. Parathyroid adenomas evaluated by thallium-201 and technetium-99ᵐ pertechnetate subtraction scintigraphy and high-resolution ultrasonography. *Radiology* 1985;155:231.

Disorders of Bone and Mineral Metabolism,
edited by Fredric L. Coe and Murray J. Favus,
© 1992 by Raven Press, Ltd. All rights reserved.

CHAPTER 21

Clinical Use of Bone Biopsy

Robert S. Weinstein

The quantitative histological analysis of percutaneous transileal bone biopsy specimens has become an indispensable part of the evaluation of metabolic disorders of the skeleton. In 1954, Nordin and Bordier pioneered the use of the bone needles and trocars necessary to perform an outpatient bone biopsy with minimal trauma (1). With the advent of plastic embedding and sledge microtomes, undecalcified bone specimens could be examined so that mineralized bone and osteoid could be definitively distinguished (2,3). In 1961, Frost applied quantitative analysis to tetracycline-labeled bone, which allowed direct dynamic measurement of bone formation (4). Today, the use of computers, digitizing tablets, video enhancement, and image analysis contribute precision and accuracy to the histomorphometric examination of bone viewed with bright-field, epifluorescence, polarized light, phase-contrast, and differential interference contrast microscopy. To increase communication in this rapidly expanding field, the nomenclature, symbols, and units used in bone histomorphometry have been standardized (5).

In this chapter we emphasize the clinical use and diagnostic significance of bone biopsy measurements. Eighteen illustrations in color are used to illustrate the use of the bone biopsy and the expected histomorphometric findings in the major metabolic disorders of the skeleton.

REQUIREMENTS FOR A BONE BIOPSY

When to Do a Bone Biopsy

A specimen for microscopic examination is removed from a living patient for the purpose of precise diagnosis, to estimate the severity and reversibility of disease, for

R. S. Weinstein: The Metabolic Bone Disease Laboratory, Section of Metabolic and Endocrine Disease, Department of Medicine, Medical College of Georgia, Augusta, Georgia 30912.

the confirmation of normal conditions, or to assess the response to therapy. As a diagnostic tool, bone biopsy is usually required to recognize subtle osteomalacia (6) and to distinguish between the various forms of renal osteodystrophy (7). Bone biopsy may also be indispensable in the evaluation of a patient with unusually painful disease or rapidly progressive loss of bone mass, particularly when the results of the physical examination, radiographs, and biochemical findings are ambiguous. Biopsy may be indicated in patients with unexplained hypophosphatemia or hyperphosphatasemia. In osteoporotic states, bone biopsy is the only method that reveals the trabecular architecture, so that the clinician can determine whether the bone loss is due to trabecular atrophy, interruption of trabecular continuity, or both (8). If treatment successfully increases bone mass, only biopsy can show if the new bone has merely augmented the trabecular width or has actually helped restore trabecular connectivity and resistance to fracture (9). Bone biopsy can also help explain treatment failures and suggest alternative regimens.

Limitations of Bone Biopsy

There are four limitations to the clinical utility of bone biopsy. The most restrictive of these is that bone biopsy samples only a single skeletal site, and disorders such as postmenopausal osteoporosis and renal osteodystrophy show considerable regional variation. The variation is, however, usually in the severity of the findings. All bones usually show at least some involvement that may be recognized by biopsy. Large regional variations in the rate of bone formation have, nevertheless, been documented. In one 74-year-old woman with osteoporosis who received two courses of oral tetracycline before she died, the bone formation rate was much lower in the spine than at the standard biopsy site (10). This was primarily a result of variation in the mineralizing perimeter rather than differences in the mineral appositional rate.

The second limitation occurs when the primary pathophysiology that caused the loss of bone mass has abated or ceased and the present rate of bone remodeling is within normal limits. Even in this circumstance, bone histomorphometry based on the interstitial bone, contour of the cement lines, trabecular architecture, and shape of the resorption cavities may allow some deductions about the original process (11,11a). The third limitation is that convincing evidence of clinical benefit of bone biopsy in therapeutic decisions can only be presented in occult osteomalacia and in renal osteodystrophy (6,7). At the present time, classification of osteoporosis into groups with normal, elevated, and low bone turnover based on bone biopsy has not helped predict the response to therapy (12).

The fourth limitation is the difficulty in estimating the rate of bone resorption by histomorphometry. However, because bone formation and bone resorption are closely coupled, the rate of bone formation is an index of skeletal turnover (13). Under most circumstances, the error incurred by assuming that the rates of bone resorption and formation are equal is about 10% and is less than the error of the histomorphometric measurements (5). Eriksen has, however, developed a new method for the calculation of the bone resorption rate, based on direct measurement of the resorption depth and the tetracycline-based bone formation rate (14).

Bone Biopsy Arrangements

Once it has been determined that a bone biopsy is needed, several arrangements must be carefully made. Foremost is the requirement to find a physician experienced in obtaining bone biopsy specimens with large-diameter trocars. Next, a pathologist must be recruited to help with proper fixation of the bone core and processing of the necessary paperwork. Unless the pathologist is familiar with plastic embedding and sectioning, the specimen will have to be referred to a specialist in histomorphometry. Often the best solution is to refer the patient to the histomorphometry center for biopsy. This ensures satisfactory communication between the clinician, operator, and pathologist and is the best insurance against the incomplete, broken, or fragmented cores obtained by inexperienced operators.

Arrangements must begin as soon as possible since the procedure must be delayed for 24 days while the patient receives the double tetracycline labels (Table 1). The labeling regimen should be explained graphically to the patient to help ensure compliance with the instructions. A picture of the rings in a tree stump is a valuable visual aid.

TABLE 1. *Advice for patients needing a metabolic bone biopsy*

1. Take the tetracycline capsules EXACTLY as ordered: one capsule three or four times a day for 3 days, _____ , then 2 weeks without any tetracycline, and then one capsule three or four times a day for 3 more days, _____ . Please notify Dr. _____ if you have recently taken any other tetracycline: Achromycin, Tetracyn, Panmycin, Sumycin, Aureomycin, Terramycin, Declomycin, Rondomycin, Mysteclin, Vibramycin, or Minocin.
2. Mark the days on your calendar!
3. On the two 3-day periods that you take the tetracycline, you must avoid dairy products (especially milk), antacids (such as Maalox, Amphojel, Rolaids), calcium supplements, and iron-containing medications. During the 2-week interval without any tetracycline, you may take any food or medication that you used previously.
4. On the morning of the bone biopsy, have only a very light breakfast.
5. Come to the outpatient clinic room at 8:30 A.M. on _____ .
6. You will be ready to return home before noon. Have someone ready to take you back home just in case the biopsy anesthetic medication has made you sleepy.
7. Call Dr. _____ , (____) ____-_____ , if you have any problems or questions or if you are sensitive or allergic to Demerol, Valium, Novacaine, Betadine, or adhesive gauze pads.
8. After the biopsy, the area must stay dry and covered with a gauze pad for 2 days. The sutures should be removed in 1 week. You may return to your normal daily activities as soon as you feel up to it. Results from the microscopic evaluation will be available in about 4 weeks.

Several special situations may arise. The specimen may occasionally be obtained in the operating room at the time of an unrelated procedure, during an osteotomy, or in children under 12 or 13 years of age, in whom it is not reasonable to attempt the procedure with local anesthesia. If at all possible in these cases, the clinician should go to the operating room to ensure that an adequate specimen is obtained and that it is properly fixed. Once obtained, a core for undecalcified quantitative histological analysis should not be let out of sight until it is handed to the histomorphometry lab receiving area. Remember that routine bone samples from the operating room are usually cut into small pieces and decalcified as soon as they are logged in at the regular surgical pathology office. Surgical bone specimens are sometimes obtained from a fracture site, but these specimens are of little or no value in the evaluation of metabolic disorders.

Some patients refuse meperidine before the biopsy, and patients with epilepsy should not receive meperidine since it lowers the seizure threshold. In these situations, the procedure can comfortably be done with only diazepam and local lidocaine. Patients with severe diarrhea or malabsorption must receive 2 or 3 g of tetracycline each day of their labeling regimen to ensure that an adequate mark is made in the bone. If there is a convincing history of allergy to tetracycline, doxycycline may be used, but the pale green fluorescent labels that result require epifluorescence with a xenon or mercury light source for adequate visualization. When the patient has recently received several courses of tetracycline for prostatitis, bronchitis, or bacterial intestinal overgrowth, the bone labeling regimen must use a different tetracycline that gives a contrasting fluorescence. With epifluorescence and plan-neofluar lenses, a 75-W xenon light source, a 20-nm band exciter filter centered at 485 nm, a barrier filter set at 520 nm, and a BG-18 heat filter, demeclocycline appears orange yellow, doxycycline pale green, oxytetracycline leaf green, and tetracycline golden yellow. The exact appearance of the tetracycline labels depends on the fluorescent system used. Even with the use of different tetracyclines, the labels may be difficult to distinguish and multiple fluorescent rings in the specimen may complicate measurement of the rates of bone formation and mineralization.

With the closed needle transileal bone biopsy procedure described below, it is not necessary to reschedule hemodialysis periods or attempt to normalize the bleeding time. It is, however, a good idea to avoid aspirin for several days before and after a biopsy. Coumadin therapy must be interrupted. Coagulation studies should be monitored in patients with known bleeding disorders.

Despite all possible precautions, there are times when a specimen is broken or otherwise damaged. A qualitative analysis can, of course, still be done, but measurements of the cancellous bone area, trabecular spacing, and cortical width may be impossible. In fragmented cores, the bone perimeter may be too disrupted for measurements of the osteoid, osteoblast, osteoclast, and reversal perimeters. However, even in severely damaged cores, the osteoid area/bone area, osteoid width, trabecular width, and mineral appositional rate can often still be obtained.

Transileal Closed Needle Bone Biopsy

Percutaneous transileal bone biopsy is a simple procedure that can be learned after observing the procedure and then practicing on a cadaver. Orthopedic surgeons may offer to do the biopsy but are usually unfamiliar with the biopsy trocars used for the investigation of metabolic disorders of the skeleton and are unaware of the need to gently obtain an intact specimen from the standard location. Experience with at least 25–30 patients is necessary before the operator can reliably obtain bone cores with both cortices and the intervening cancellous bone tissue intact for a quantitative histological analysis. Since about 0.5 mm of the cylindrical bone biopsy core diameter is damaged by the teeth of the cutting trocar, the internal diameter of the trocar must be 7.0–8.0 mm

to obtain an undamaged core of 6.0–7.0 mm diameter. These large-bore trocars are required to get a specimen suitable for measurement of the trabecular microarchitecture. Patients who have had a 5-mm transileal bone biopsy followed a year later by a 7.5-mm biopsy report no difference in the acceptability of the procedure. Biopsies acquired by other procedures may give less ideal specimens. Vertical iliac crest biopsies have only one cortex, a distorted distal end, and are usually only 3–4 mm in diameter. Specimens obtained with an electric drill have as much as 1.0 mm damage at their circumference and contain smashed bone and bone powder at their proximal and distal margins. If the drill gets stuck, the resulting heat may severely damage the core. Wedge sections of the iliac crest are absolutely contraindicated. They are difficult to fix adequately and cause pain at the biopsy site for over a year. Rib biopsies are also contraindicated in metabolic diseases of the skeleton because of the paucity of cancellous bone tissue in the specimen and the significant risk of pneumothorax. The author has used the following outpatient transileal closed needle bone biopsy technique for more than 12 years. The procedure is safe, the anterior–superior ilium is easy to anesthetize, and there are normal data from this site.

Several other techniques have been described (1,3,6,15–18), but it is apparent that closed needle biopsy procedures have the lowest rate of complications (15,17). About 5% of patients may develop a small superficial ecchymosis. After just a light breakfast, the patient gives a signed informed consent and is premedicated with 50–75 mg intramuscularly (IM) of meperidine and 10–15 mg IM of diazepam about 30 min before the procedure. An examination table with foot pedal controls is desirable. The patient must be supine with legs outstretched, elbows touching the table, and hands folded over the chest. The appropriate hip is elevated on three to four folded sheets placed well under the buttock. A skin-marking pen is used to indicate a point 2.5-cm posterior and inferior to the anterior–superior iliac spine and clearly below the external lip of the iliac crest. A second point is marked 2–3 cm medial to the crest of the ilium in a line with the first point and the opposite elbow. After a povidone–iodine or hexachlorophene detergent cleanser scrub, drapes are applied and a skin wheal is made at both points with 0.5% lidocaine without epinephrine and a $\frac{3}{4}$-in. 25-gauge needle on a 3-mL syringe. The subcutaneous tissue, fascia, and lateral iliac periosteum is anesthetized with 5–10 mL of 0.5% lidocaine and a $1\frac{1}{2}$-in. 18-gauge needle on a 10-mL syringe. With a 10-mL three-finger control syringe and a 5-in. 20-gauge anesthesia needle inserted at the second point, the medial iliac periosteum is explored, and if there is no blood return, anesthetized with an additional 5 mL of lidocaine. Next, with a No. 3 knife handle and No. 15 blade, a 1.5-cm incision is made parallel to the iliac crest at the first point. After incising the superficial fascia, a single stab incision is made and extended down to the lateral periosteum. Enough lidocaine should be used so that the patient is unable to feel pain during this part of the procedure. The outer sleeve of the biopsy needle is placed over the large trocar and delivered to the lateral periosteum with a gentle twisting motion until the sleeve's teeth rest on the ilium. The trocar is then withdrawn and the outer sleeve is aimed toward the contralateral elbow and anchored to the lateral ilium by a few taps with the large trocar's handle.

The patient is told, "You will hear a knock, like a knock at a door, but it will not hurt." With the sleeve held down firmly to act as a guide for the trephine, the cutting trephine is slowly inserted with a gentle to-and-fro rotary motion until it has transfixed the inner cortex and the hub of the trephine meets the top of the outer sleeve. Heavy pressure on the trephine must be avoided! If the medial iliac periosteum has not been completely anesthetized, the patient will feel a momentary pain at the time the inner cortex is penetrated. Excessive penetration is prevented by the hub of the trephine. The trephine is then rotated 360 degrees several times to separate the specimen from the underlying tissue. With the operator's thumb held tightly over the distal opening of the trephine, the instrument is slowly withdrawn 1–2 mm at a time with a gentle to-and-fro rotary motion.

The long, thin, blunt trocar is used to very gently push the bone core out of the trephine and into the cold fixative. If the specimen does not come out of the trephine easily, a few gentle taps with the handle of the large trocar will suffice to expel it. If the core does not have both cortices or is otherwise inadequate, a second try should be made through the same incision. A $\frac{1}{2} \times 3$ in. piece of absorbable hemostat gauze (oxidized regenerated cellulose) is placed into the biopsy hole with the small trocar and then the small trocar and outer sleeve are withdrawn. The wound is closed with one or two 3-0 nylon sutures, and after application of benzoin, a pressure dressing is made with fluffed gauze and an elastic bandage. The procedure takes about 30 to 45 min. Blood loss is usually less than 1 mL. The patient is instructed to turn over and lie on the pressure dressing for about 1 h, after which the dressing is removed, a small adhesive gauze pad applied, and the patient may go home. The wound should not be allowed to get wet for 48 h and the sutures should be removed in 1 week. Most patients do not require more than 2–3 days of acetaminophen for analgesia and readily agree to a second biopsy. A repeat biopsy to evaluate the response to therapy or to reveal the natural course of a disorder must be done on the opposite side. The first side should not be reused for at least 1 year.

Examination Plan for a Bone Biopsy Specimen

Optimal clinical use of a bone biopsy requires a methodical plan for the examination of the specimen. A checklist or inventory of features is helpful (Table 2). Diagnostic interpretation of the histomorphometry should only follow a complete qualitative and quantitative assessment.

After embedding and before any sections have been obtained, the bone mineral density of the biopsy core can be measured in a water bath with single photon absorptiometry (19). When compared with the subsequent histomorphometry, this procedure reveals differences between the quantity and quality of the bone tissue. In

TABLE 2. *Examination list for the evaluation of a bone biopsy*

  I. Adequacy of the specimen
   A. Number of cortices
   B. Condition of the core
   C. Diameter of the core
   D. Obliquity of the core
   E. Condition of the slides
 II. Examination under polarized light
   A. Woven versus lamellar collagen architecture
   B. Confirmation of resorption bays
III. Examination with phase contrast microscopy
   A. Wall width and cement lines
   B. Interstitial width
   C. Verify osteoid area
 IV. Subperiosteal borders
   A. Contour
   B. Resorption bays and osteoclasts
   C. Subperiosteal osteoid
  V. Cortical bone tissue
   A. Porosity
   B. Width
   C. Intracortical resorption
   D. Intracortical osteoid
 VI. Endocortical borders
   A. Cortical-cancellous junction
   B. Cancellization of cortical bone
VII. Cancellous bone tissue
   A. Central versus total bone area
   B. Trabecular architecture
   C. Osteoid
      1. Area; buried osteoid
      2. Surface
      3. Width
      4. Osteoblasts
   D. Resorption
      1. Shape of resorption cavities
      2. Osteoclasts
      3. Intraosseous resorption
   E. Reversal perimeter
   F. Peritrabecular fibrosis
   G. Iron and aluminum staining
   H. Marrow
      1. Fat
      2. Mast cells
      3. Granulomata
      4. Myeloma and other dysplastic marrows
      5. Metastases
   I. Examination with fluorescent light
      1. Label number and character
      2. Distance between double labels
      3. Woven bone fluorescence
      4. Buried tetracycline

osteoporosis, the bone core density and the mineralized area are directly related ($r = 0.921$, $p < 0.001$), but in renal osteodystrophy, the relationship is not significant (19). Bone biopsy core density determinations help the clinician appreciate the contributions of partly mineralized osteoid and incompletely mineralized bone to the specimen. This help is most useful in patients with renal osteodystrophy, partly treated osteomalacia, or X-linked hypophosphatemia.

With a magnifying glass or low-power ocular loupe, the sections should be appraised for adequacy by itemizing the number of cortices present, the presence of fracture, compression, or hemorrhage artifacts and the diameter of the core versus the useful, readable diameter. Longitudinal sections of a bone core from the ilium taken at the correct location and in the correct direction will usually resemble a rectangle or parallelogram (Fig. 1) (see color pages). A trapezoid configuration may indicate inordinate obliquity that limits the cancellous bone tissue available for analysis. Under higher magnification ($\times 100$), the sections should be examined for folds or wrinkles, retraction of the marrow from the endocortical and cancellous bone, and cracks in the bone that may mimic marrow islands. All potential obstacles to accurate quantitative analysis should be recorded.

Next, examination of a few decalcified sections under polarized light establishes if the bone is made of normal lamellar collagen (Fig. 2) or woven collagen architecture (Fig. 3), a sign of pathology in the adult. Furthermore, polarized light can be used as needed throughout the rest of the examination to verify the presence of osteoid seams and ensure that the measured seams are more than one birefringent lamella wide. In addition, the number of lamellae in an osteoid seam is a good measure of the seam width that overcomes the problem of accidental tangential sectioning, which can exaggerate seam width (Fig. 4) (20). Therefore, the calculated or measured seam width should always be verified by polarized light. Polarized light can also confirm the presence of disrupted collagen lamellae at individual erosion sites so as to distinguish an empty, shallow resorption bay or reversal perimeter from a quiescent perimeter.

At this point, examination of unstained slides with phase contrast microscopy permits measurement of the wall width. A wide-band green interference filter enhances the contrast of the cement lines. The cement lines should be classified as smooth, scalloped, or mosaic. Direct measurement of the interstitial width can also be made. An orthogonal grid helps make these measurements rapidly and without bias. While the bone is examined with phase contrast, the reader can estimate the osteoid area and thereby eliminate the possibility of an error from staining mishaps that can underestimate the amount of osteoid present (Fig. 5). Osteoid is also dramatically revealed with Nomarski differential interference contrast microscopy (Fig. 6). Discrepancies between the extent of osteoid revealed by the modified Masson stain and the von Kossa procedure may unpredictably occur in specimens from patients with hypophosphatemic osteomalacia and those with oncogenic osteomalacia (21,22). Phase contrast and differential interference contrast microscopy help eliminate diagnostic errors from such staining problems.

The subperiosteal margins of a transileal specimen may be distorted by muscle attachments but are usually smooth and subperiosteal osteoclasts are absent. A serrated or dentated subperiosteal margin should be noted and prompt a search for subperiosteal erosion bays and fibrosis (Fig. 7). In adults, subperiosteal osteoid seams more than 10 μm wide are seen only in severe osteoidosis.

Cortical bone tissue should be assessed for width and porosity. The cortical width of transileal specimens is normally quite variable (990–1500 μm), but cortical porosity is always less than 9% (13). It is important that these determinations are made from the mean of measurements taken from both cortices of the transileal specimen, since the medial or inner cortex of the core is often thinner than the lateral or outer cortex (Fig. 1). The presence of more than one intracortical osteoclast should be noted since these cells are normally rare in the cortical tissue of a transileal specimen.

The endocortical borders should be examined separately from the rest of the cortical and cancellous bone tissue. Endocortical erosion cavities may become deep and coalesce until the previously solid cortical bone becomes whittled into broad new trabeculae, a process known as cancellization of cortical bone. These more recent trabeculae must be measured separately from the central cancellous bone tissue to avoid an upward bias in the trabecular width. The normal junction between cortical and cancellous bone is sharply demarcated (Fig. 1). Disruption of this junction is typically found in renal osteodystrophy (Figs. 8 and 9).

In cancellous bone tissue, measurements should therefore be confined to the central cancellous bone tissue to appraise the original cancellous bone. A simple rule is to sidestep the endocortical borders by about 500 μm on either side. The trabecular microarchitecture should always be evaluated since it discloses information about the pathogenesis of bone loss, the degree of skeletal fragility, and the possibility of recovery (9). Furthermore, the microarchitecture can easily be calculated from the cancellous bone area and perimeter (23) or, more precisely, measured directly at orthogonal intersections (8). If a low-power, flat-field lense is used, the measurement of the trabecular spacing of the entire cancellous tissue area is facilitated.

Osteoid area, perimeter, and seam width must be measured. This requires that a decision be made about the inclusion of the osteoid buried deep within mineralized bone. If included, the osteoid area will be more accurate, but the seam width calculated from osteoid area and perimeter will become progressively more inaccurate.

Seam width is best measured directly, since it is such a valuable diagnostic feature of osteomalacia (11). The endosteal membrane, a 1-μm-wide layer of loosely textured collagen fibers devoid of mineral that lines cancellous bone, should not be counted as osteoid. This is easily avoided by the requirement that measured osteoid seams contain more than one birefringent lamina (see above). The osteoblast perimeter, composed of only the plump, cuboidal osteoblasts (Fig. 10), should be distinguished from the flat, pavement-like cells that line quiescent perimeters.

Bone resorption should be measured precisely as the osteoclast perimeter, which requires magnification at ×160 to 250 for accurate recognition. Enough detail should be supplied so that the measurement could be calculated with different referents, since some histomorphometry laboratories express the osteoclast perimeter per cancellous perimeter, while others prefer the referent to be the nonosteoid cancellous perimeter or mineralized perimeter (11). Osteoclasts may also be counted per millimeter of cancellous perimeter or per square millimeter of cancellous bone tissue (5). Resorption cavities with unusual shapes should be noted (24). Hook resorption (Fig. 7) is characteristic of hyperparathyroidism. Tunneling resorption is seen with osteoid perimeter values of 60–80%, as is typical of specimens taken from patients with severe renal hyperparathyroidism (24). The reversal perimeter should, however, never be included in the measurements of bone resorption, since it clearly marks a different and independently changeable phase of bone turnover (25). Peritrabecular marrow fibrosis should be noted as a characteristic feature of severe hyperparathyroidism.

The aluminon reagent is used to evaluate the bone aluminum burden in renal osteodystrophy. This reagent also detects chromium, beryllium, cadmium, and iron (26). Dialysis patients who receive frequent transfusions may have high tissue iron loads that must not be mistaken for aluminum. The measurement of the bone aluminum burden must be accompanied by an examination of the sections with potassium ferrocyanide to look for the Prussian blue stain of bone iron. If bone iron is found, a positive stain with the aluminon reagent cannot be interpreted with confidence as representative of aluminum.

The marrow fat content is normally about 35–50% of the marrow space and increases with age (27). Both increased marrow fat and abundant mast cells have been noted in osteoporosis (28,29). The marrow should also be examined for dysplastic changes and metastases. In some situations the slides should be reviewed with a hematologist or pathologist using oil immersion. The accelerated bone turnover that accompanies persistent erythroid hyperplasia can be revealed with histomorphometric analysis of iron and tetracycline staining (30). Sarcoidosis, a chronic granulomatous disease, can cause osteopenia or osteosclerosis, and peritrabecular granulomas may be recognizable in a biopsy (31,32). Oxalate crystals can be demonstrated in bone biopsies taken from patients with primary hyperoxaluria and may be of diagnostic significance (33). However, detection of the doubly refractile calcium oxalate crystals requires that the bone specimen be fixed in absolute ethanol.

Examination under epifluorescent light is usually the last step before making a diagnostic impression. The percentages of the cancellous bone boundary that have single labels, double labels, diffuse or unclear labels, and no labels should be recorded. This can be done at ×100 with high-numerical-aperture neofluar lenses and a high-intensity light source such as xenon or mercury. However, with routine tungsten–halogen epifluorescent light and plain achromat lenses, tetracycline labels may be poorly resolved at ×100 magnification and are better visualized at 250 to ×400. The distance between the midpoints of the double tetracycline labels is best measured at ×250, and if high-numerical-aperture lenses are used, problems with the section thickness are minimized or eliminated. Unusual tetracycline patterns, such as the diffuse fluorescence typical of abnormal mineralization (Fig. 11) or deeply buried old tetracycline, should be noted.

Normal Values for Bone Histomorphometry

Normal values are required for evaluation of the findings in individual patients with skeletal disorders. Racial, climatic, cultural, and geographical differences in bone metabolism emphasize the need for each histomorphometry laboratory to collect normal data from the same population that is examined for disease. In addition, methodological differences may compromise evaluations based on historical controls or those obtained from different laboratories. Periods of focal osteoblast inactivity may vary with different diseases. The tetracycline regimen must, therefore, be identical in the patients and controls, or else changes in the interval between the two courses of tetracycline will result in considerable variation in the mineral appositional rate and mineralized perimeter (34).

If normal values for the dynamic histomorphometry are taken from the literature, it is important to realize that bone fluorescence is subject to several influences that are hard to control (35). The intensity and color of the tetracycline depends on the excitation and emission filters, the light source, the use of transmission or epifluorescence, and the aperture and glass used in the objectives. Small changes in the histological processing may alter visibility of the tetracycline. Furthermore, 20-μm-thick sections show significantly lower values for mineral appositional rate and double-labeled mineralizing perimeter than that found on 5-μm sections (36). The best solution to these problems is accomplished when the histomorphometry laboratory that will analyze the pathological specimens obtains its own tetracycline-labeled control biopsies.

Normal, healthy subjects should be recruited for establishing bone histomorphometry control values. The

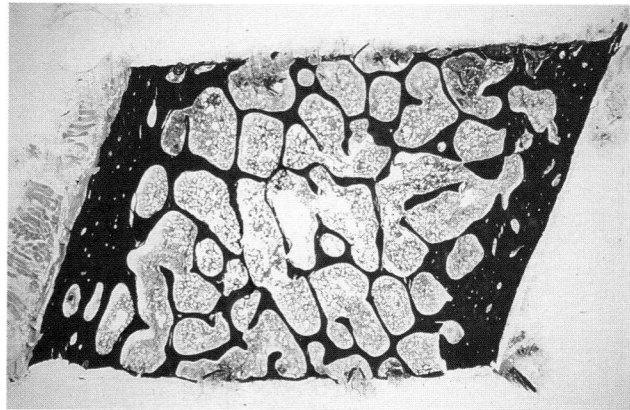

FIG. 1. *Normal Bone Biopsy.* This transileal specimen, taken from a healthy 30-year-old Black woman, shows the typical parallelogram appearance of a longitudinal section. The cancellous bone area is 25.5% and is composed primarily of a continuous network of curved trabecular plates. Note that the junction between cortical and cancellous bone is sharply demarcated and that the medial cortex is thinner than the lateral cortex. (Modified Masson stain, planachromat ×1 objective.)

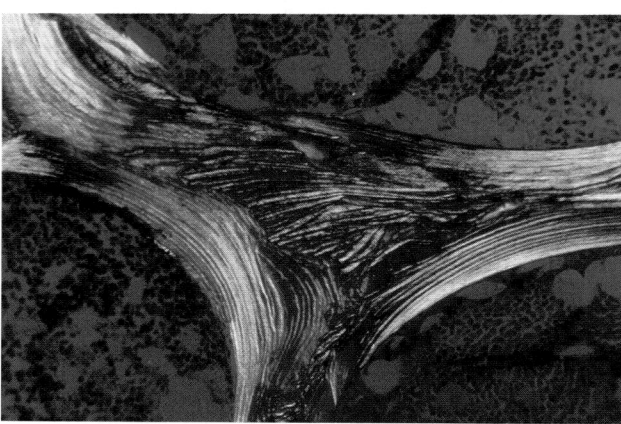

FIG. 2. *Lamellar Bone.* The collagen fibers form an orderly pattern like the grain of wood. The older interstitial bone is clearly seen between the surrounding new bone remodeling units. (Weigert's H & E stain, achromat ×25 objective, polarized light with a rose quartz plate.)

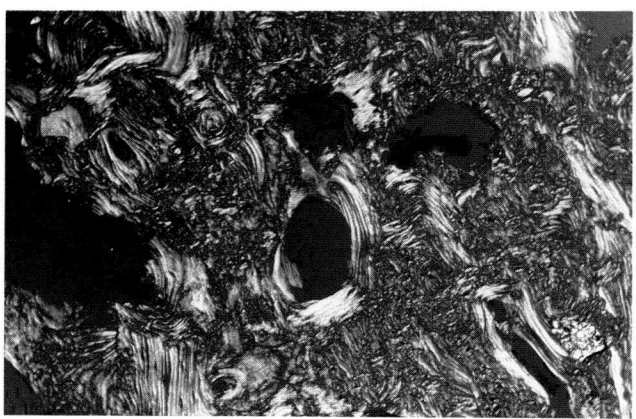

FIG. 3. *Woven Bone.* The patchwork quilt appearance of this haphazard collagen architecture is evident in this specimen taken from a dialysis patient with severe secondary hyperparathyroidism. (Weigert's H & E stain, achromat ×20 objective, polarized light with a rose quartz plate.)

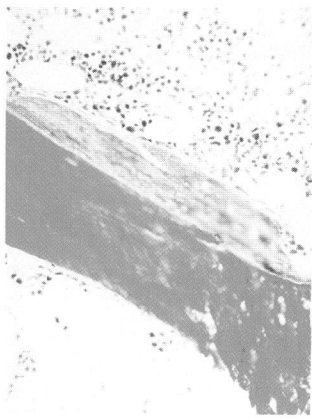
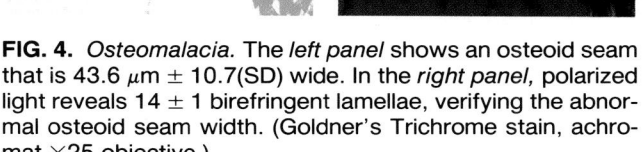

FIG. 4. *Osteomalacia.* The *left panel* shows an osteoid seam that is 43.6 μm $\pm$ 10.7(SD) wide. In the *right panel,* polarized light reveals 14 $\pm$ 1 birefringent lamellae, verifying the abnormal osteoid seam width. (Goldner's Trichrome stain, achromat ×25 objective.)

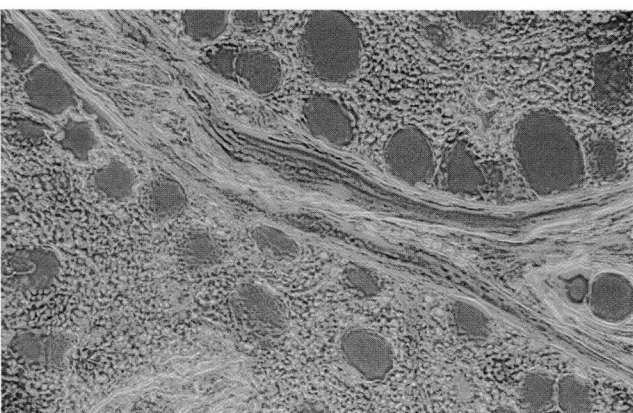

FIG. 5. *Osteomalacia.* Wide osteoid seams can be easily recognized on unstained specimens, thus avoiding staining artifacts. (unstained, planachromat ×16 phase II objective, wide band green interference filter, phase contrast microscopy.)

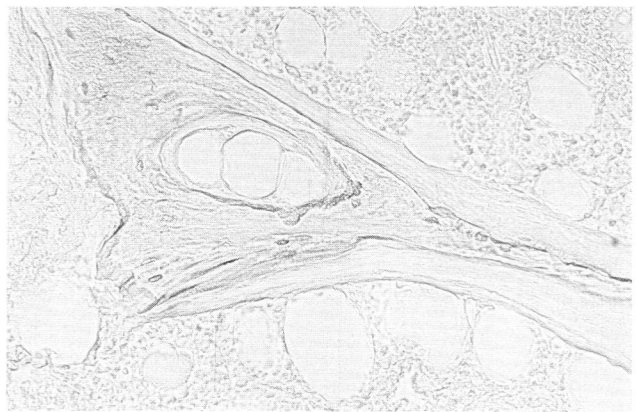

FIG. 6. *Osteomalacia.* Osteoid seams and the boundary between mineralized bone and osteoid are clear on this unstained specimen. (unstained, planachromat ×20 objective, dydidium filter, differential interference contrast microscopy.)

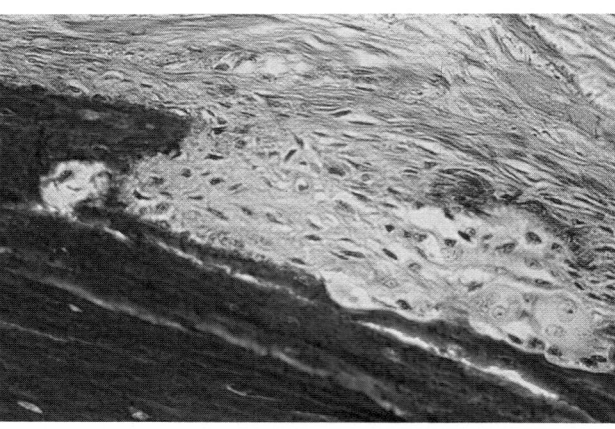

FIG. 7. *Subperiosteal Erosion.* A large hook-shaped resorption cavity beneath the periosteum contains multinucleated osteoclasts and a loose fibrous stroma. (Modified Masson stain, achromat ×40 objective.)

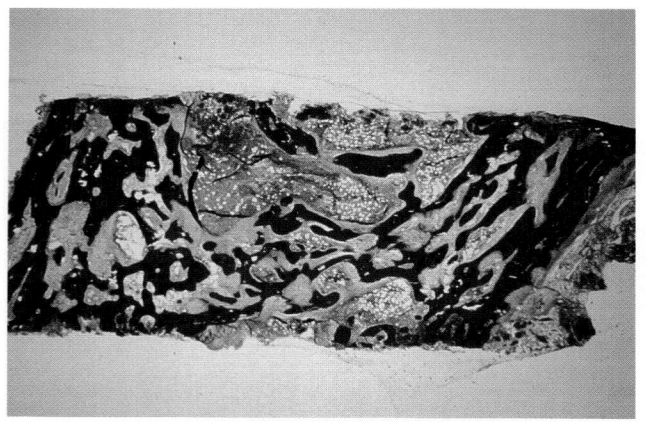

FIG. 8. *Osteitis Fibrosa.* This panoramic photomicrograph shows the subperiosteal erosions, thin and porous cortical bone, disrupted junction between cortical and cancellous bone, and prominent peritrabecular marrow fibrosis found in a patient receiving long term dialysis therapy. (Modified Masson stain, planachromat ×1 objective.)

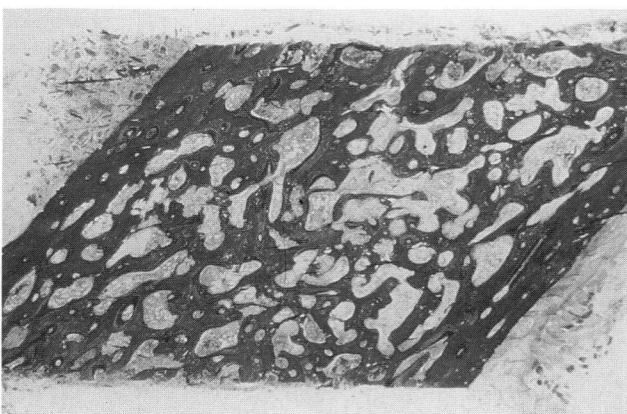

FIG. 9. *Osteosclerosis.* Cortical thinning and increased porosity with cancellous bone augmentation has completely obscured the junction between cortical and cancellous bone. The central cancellous bone area is increased to 58.1%, albeit by contributions of excessive osteoid (osteoid area is 29.6%) and poorly mineralized woven bone. (Modified Masson stain, planachromat ×1 objective.)

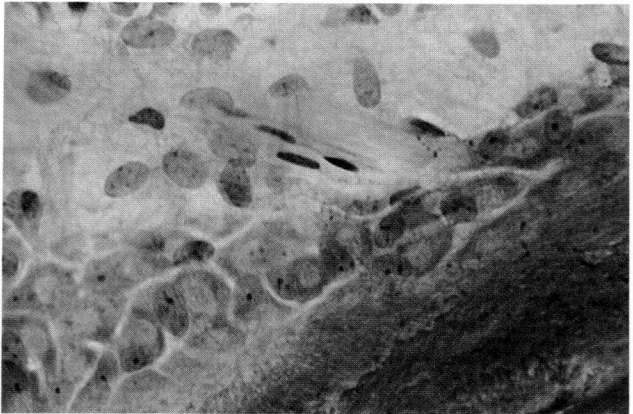

FIG. 10. *Osteoblast Perimeter.* Palisades of plump, cuboidal osteoblasts are lining a partly mineralized osteoid seam in a patient with renal osteodystrophy. Note the perinuclear halo of the prominent Golgi apparatus. (Modified Masson stain, plan-neofluar ×63 objective.)

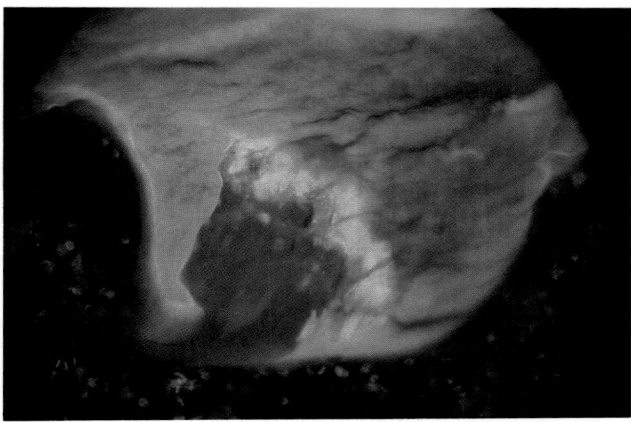

FIG. 11. *Diffuse Fluorescence.* An abnormal spread of the tetracycline labels indicated delayed or defective mineralization. This example is from a patient with hypophosphatasia. (unstained, neofluar×25 objective, xenon epifluorescent light.)

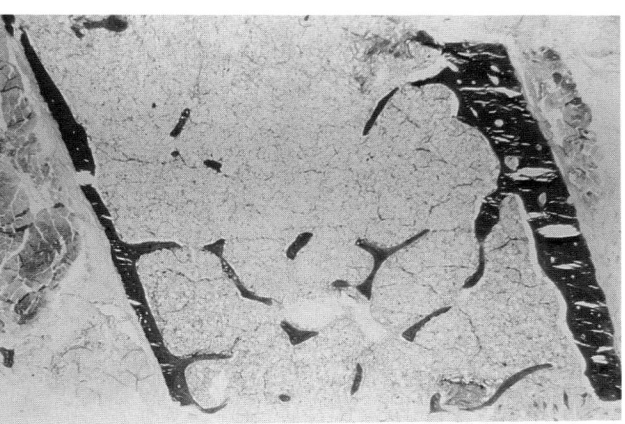

FIG. 12. *Osteoporosis.* In this postmenopausal woman with vertebral fractures, cancellous bone area is only 4.2%. The cancellous bone has been transformed into a discontinuous array of thin struts (trabecular width is 85.4 μm $\pm$ 27.6(SD), trabecular spacing 1656 μm $\pm$ 553 and trabecular number 0.49 per mn; see Table 3 for normal values). Cortical bone width is only 387 μm but cortical porosity is 3.21%, a normal value. (Modified Masson stain, planachromat ×1 objective.)

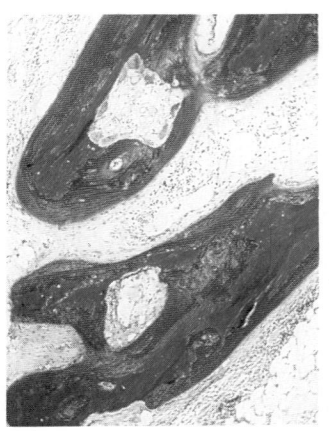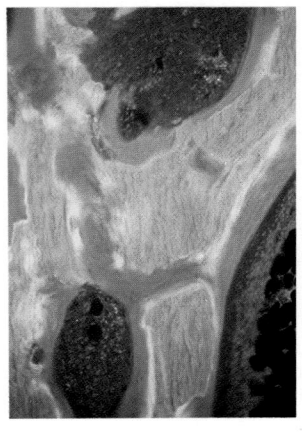

FIG. 13. *Osteomalacia.* Osteomalacia in patients with chronic renal failure often has spectacular accumulations of osteoid and absence of double tetracycline labels. In the left panel note the osteoclasts on the osteoid perimeter of the intratrabecular erosion cavity. (*left panel:* Modified Masson stain, neofluar ×10 objective; *right panel:* unstained, neofluar ×25 objective, xenon epifluorescent light.)

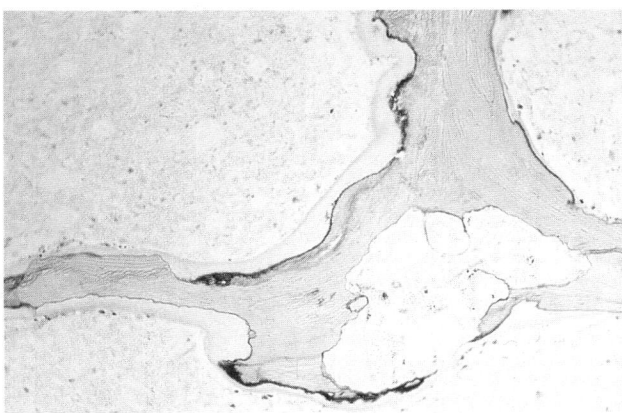

FIG. 14. *Bone Aluminum.* Aluminum deposition is seen at the boundary between osteoid and mineralized bone, in cement lines and on the quiescent perimeter. (Aluminon stain, achromat ×10 objective.)

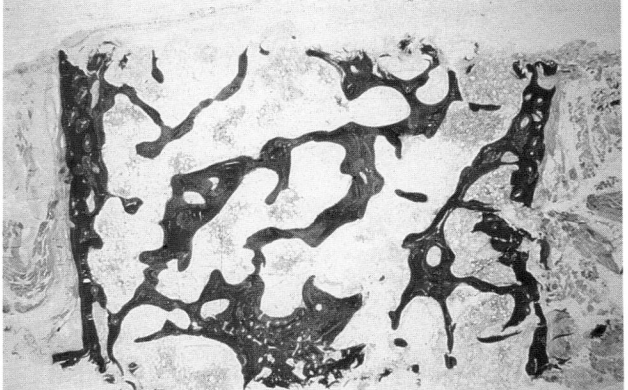

FIG.15. *Osteomalacia.* This transileal specimen shows a cancellous bone area of 45.3%, osteoid area 79.5%, osteoid perimeter 98.0%, and mean osteoid width 165.8 μm. Double tetracycline labels were absent. (Modified Masson stain, planachromat ×1 objective.)

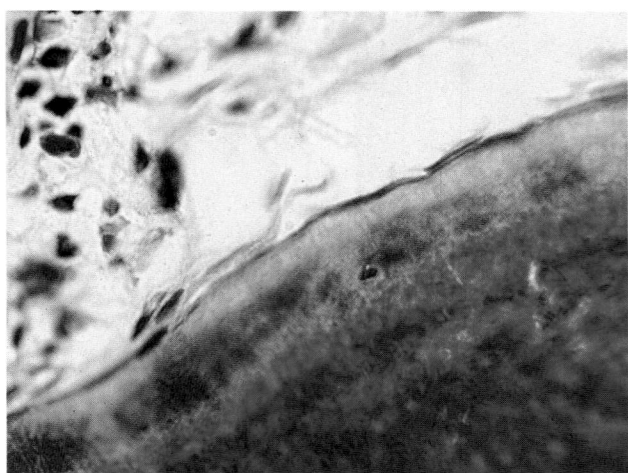

FIG. 16. *Osteomalacia.* The osteoblasts that line this osteoid seam are flattened and resemble cobblestone pavement. The seam is 16.3 μm $\pm$ 2.4(SD) wide and contains 4 to 5 birefringent lamellae. (Modified Masson stain, neofluar $\times$40 objective.)

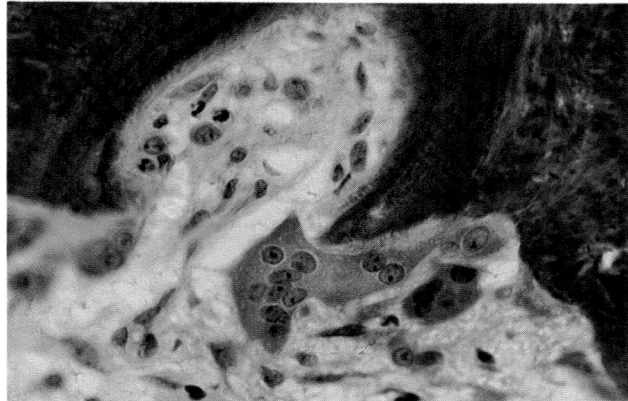

FIG. 17. *Osteomalacia.* Osteoclastic erosion of osteroid juxtaposed to scalloped resorption bays is clearly demonstrated in this specimen taken from a patient with X-linked hypophosphatemic rickets and phosphate therapy-induced hyperparathyroidism. (Modified Masson stain, plan-neofluar $\times$40 objective.)

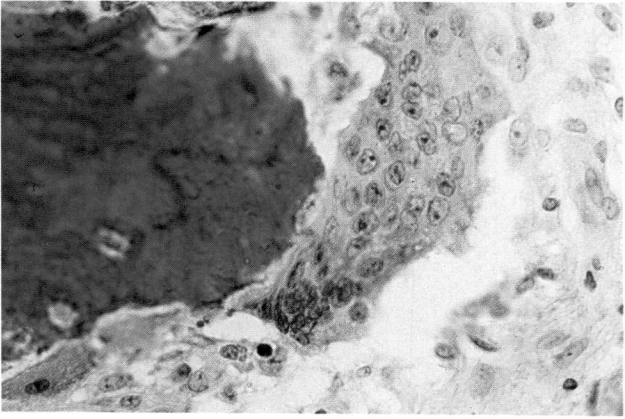

FIG. 18. *Paget's Disease.* This giant osteoclast with more than 40 nuclei is pathognomonic of Paget's disease of bones. (Modified Masson stain, plan-neofluar $\times$63 objective.)

biopsy should be obtained after tetracycline labeling and done at the standard skeletal site. Postmortem series have two problems: tetracycline double labels are absent and preexisting disorders and diseases (especially alcoholism) cannot be completely excluded. Tetracycline-labeled specimens obtained during an apparently unrelated surgical procedure may be compromised by prior changes in ambulation, diet, and solar exposure.

It is, however, usually necessary to use published normal ranges until the laboratory has accumulated its own controls, and therefore the workers should use the same techniques as the reference laboratory (37). Age, sex, and race must also be considered (38; and see Chapter 14). Reader variation will add an additional nuance to the interpretation of the published data (39). Although this variation may be only about 10%, it will be difficult to be certain. Variation differs according to the diagnosis and the histological feature. In osteoporosis, the intersample

variations in bone area, osteoid area and perimeter, and eroded perimeter are large, reflecting the low mean values for these features. In osteomalacia, mean values for osteoid area, perimeter, and width are high and show less intersample variation. In renal osteodystrophy, variation is the lowest since most histological features are abundant (39). Therefore, renal osteodystrophy represents a "best case" situation in measurement precision. The greatest variance is usually in the analysis of bone lining cells and in the mineralizing perimeter (40). The coefficient of variation of multiple determinations of the osteoclast perimeter in renal osteodystrophy is 25%. Variation in the mineral appositional rate is, however, less than 12% (40).

The normal histomorphometric values in Tables 3 and 4 are for young white and black adults (13). Recker et al. have reported a detailed account of the normal values for postmenopausal white females (41). For the

TABLE 3. *Static bone histomorphometry: normal values*[a]

	Median	Mean	SD	SEM	Percentile 25th	Percentile 75th	Range
Bone biopsy core[b]							
BM (g/cm)	0.284	0.285	0.078	0.0159	0.227	0.341	
BW (cm)	1.088	1.072	0.230	0.0469	0.869	1.261	
BMD (g/cm²)	0.263	0.269	0.061	0.0124	0.227	0.316	0.20–0.34
Cortical bone tissue							
Ct.Wi (μm)	1173	1202	314	63	992	1533	990–1500
Ct.Po (%)	4.22	4.64	1.95	0.39	3.21	6.85	3.2–7.0
Cancellous bone tissue							
B.Ar/T.Ar (%)	21.9	21.56	4.52	0.90	18.52	25.87	13.0–28.0
W.Wi (μm)	58.8	59.0	7.3	1.4	54.0	64.8	45.0–71.0
It.Wi[c] (μm)	38.4	38.6	27.4	5.7	12.9	61.3	neg–61[d]
Tb.Wi (μm)	155.2	152.7	30.6	6.1	127.5	171.9	100–225
Tb.Sp[c] (μm)	1030	1072	172	35	961	1157	800–1500
Tb.N (mm⁻¹)	1.42	1.44	0.28	0.06	1.27	1.59	1.0–1.8
O.Ar/B.Ar (%)	1.83	2.21	1.40	0.28	1.21	3.13	0.4–4.0
O.Wi (μm)	7.3	7.6	1.9	0.4	6.2	9.2	4.3–12.0
O.Pm/B.Pm[c] (%)	14.53	16.50	8.22	1.64	11.1	19.13	4.0–39.0
Ob.Pm/B.Pm[e,c] (%)	1.86	2.17	1.70	0.34	1.18	2.65	0.08–7.26
Oc.Pm/B.Pm[e] (%)	0.70	0.97	0.83	0.17	0.40	1.41	0–3.1
Oc.N/mm	0.11	0.13	0.10	0.02	0.05	0.22	0–0.4
Rv.Pm/B.Pm[e] (%)	7.80	7.35	2.53	0.51	5.16	9.15	3.5–12.0

[a] Static measurements from 25 healthy subjects, aged 19–46 years old. The measurements were made on 5-μm-thick methyl methacrylate embedded sections stained with a modification of Masson's trichrome (13,77). A stage micrometer was used to calibrate the digitizer tablet and image analysis computer (8). Width and spacing measurements were guided by orthogonal intersections. Wall width was determined on unstained sections viewed with phase contrast and a wide-band green interference filter (13). The cancellous measurements were confined to the central cancellous bone.

[b] Determined on 7-mm intact, embedded, transileal cores by Norland single-photon absorptiometry in a water bath (18,32).

[c] Kurtotic.

[d] It.Wi may be a negative number in 8% of normal biopsies.

[e] The referent is the cancellous bone perimeter.

BM, bone mineral; BW, bone width; BMD, bone mineral density; Ct.Wi, cortical width; Ct.Po, cortical porosity; B.Ar/T.Ar, bone area per tissue area; W.Wi, wall width; It.Wi, interstitial width; Tb.Wi, trabecular width; Tb.Sp, trabecular spacing; Tb.N, trabecular number; O.Ar/B.Ar, osteoid area per bone area; O.Wi, osteoid width; O.Pm/B.Pm, osteoid perimeter per bone perimeter; Ob.Pm/B.Pm, osteoblast perimeter per bone perimeter; Oc.Pm/B.Pm, osteoclast perimeter per bone perimeter; Oc.N/mm, osteoclast number per mm bone perimeter; Rv.Pm/B.Pm, reversal perimeter per bone perimeter.

TABLE 4. *Race-specific normal values for dynamic histomorphometry*[a]

	Median	Mean	SD	SEM	Percentile 25th	Percentile 75th	Range
					White adults (n = 13)		
M.Pm/B.Pm (%)[b]	9.29	10.60	5.15	1.43	7.62	16.67	5–20
M.Pm/O.Pm (%)[c]	82.53	71.44	28.16	7.81	55.90	100	50–100
MAR (μm/day)	0.929	0.904	0.109	0.030	0.829	0.976	0.83–0.98
Aj.AR (μm/day)	0.656	0.639	0.260	0.072	0.521	0.882	0.52–0.90
Mlt (days)[d]	11				9	20	8–25
BFR/B.Pm[e]	0.078	0.095	0.044	0.012	0.067	0.145	0.07–0.15
BFR/BV[e]	7.86	9.29	4.97	1.38	6.08	13.96	6–14
BFR/TV[e]	1.74	2.16	1.39	0.39	1.24	3.06	1.2–3.0
FP (days)[d]	81				73	119	75–120
					Black adults (n = 12)		
M.Pm/B.Pm (%)[b]	4.66	4.67	2.43	0.70	2.868	6.759	1.0–9.2
M.Pm/O.Pm (%)[c]	29.13	31.48	14.80	4.27	23.50	44.10	4.5–56.4
MAR (μm/day)	0.697	0.630	0.206	0.060	0.470	0.806	0.22–0.89
Aj.AR (μm/day)	0.169	0.206	0.137	0.039	0.110	0.356	0.02–0.44
Mlt (days)[d]	37				28	65	22–447
BFR/B.Pm[e]	0.031	0.033	0.023	0.007	0.015	0.056	0.01–0.07
BFR/BV[e]	3.767	4.222	3.287	0.949	1.374	7.868	0.03–9.63
BFR/TV[e]	0.617	0.957	0.901	0.260	0.240	1.749	0.07–2.67
FP (days)[d]	395				171	768	124–3102

[a] Each subject received 1 g of oral tetracycline HCl per day, 23, 22, 21, 6, 5, and 4 days before the biopsy (13). A drawing tube and digitizer tablet were used to make the measurements on 5-μm-thick sections viewed by epifluorescence at ×100 and ×250 magnification with Zeiss plan-neofluar objectives. The exciter was a 20-nm band centered at 485 nm, the barrier 520 nm, and the light source 75-W xenon with a BG-18 heat filter.

[b] Includes all the double-labeled plus half the single-labeled cancellous perimeter.

[c] The referent is the osteoid perimeter.

[d] Kurtotic.

[e] The units for the BFR/B.Pm are μm^2/μm/day, BFR/BV %/yr, and BFR/TV %/yr.

M.Pm/B.Pm, mineralizing perimeter per bone perimeter; M.Pm/O.Pm, mineralizing perimeter per osteoid perimeter; MAR, mineral appositional rate; Aj.AR, adjusted appositional rate; Mlt, mineralizing lag time; BFR/B.Pm, bone formation rate per bone perimeter; BFR/BV, bone formation rate per bone volume; BFR/TV, bone formation rate per tissue volume; FP, formation period.

histomorphometric interpretation of individual bone biopsies, the expected range of normal values may be of greater clinical utility than the mean values and their statistical variation. This is particularly important when the normal range includes zero, as with the osteoclast perimeter and number measurements, or when the range normally includes negative values, as with the calculation of interstitial width from the trabecular width minus twice the wall width. The latter problem is a result of the theoretical modeling of the cancellous architecture into the average parallel plate.

The clinician who must read and understand the histomorphometry report from the laboratory must be alert to a number of potential pitfalls. The biopsy report should be based on the random assessment of at least 20–30 mm^2 of tissue to avoid focal variations in the histological features. This is facilitated by the examination of sections taken from multiple regions of the biopsy core. In the report, the terminology should be unmistakably clear as to what was measured (5). Misleading terms, such as *active, inactive, formation surfaces* and *resorption surfaces,* do not tell the reader whether or not the

measurement included the use of tetracycline markers or bone cells. The clinician must also be wary of an excessive number of variables derived from a single histological feature expressed with several different denominators. These multiple expressions may help support a particular interpretation but, in themselves, supply no additional information. The histomorphometry report should use only two-dimensional or only three-dimensional terminology. Although the actual values are the same for volume and area or for surface and perimeter, the calculation used to convert measured widths in two dimensions to thickness in three dimensions must be clearly explained in the report (5).

There are, in addition, differences between direct and indirect measurements that the clinician should appreciate. Osteoid seam width may increase from acceleration of the rates of matrix and mineral apposition, as occurs in hyperparathyroidism secondary to chronic renal failure, or from a prolongation of the mineralization lag time, as occurs in osteomalacia (42). The importance of the osteoid width in the diagnosis of osteomalacia demands that the measurement be made directly (11). Vedi and Compston have shown that when osteoid width is calculated from the relative osteoid area divided by the osteoid perimeter, the ratio variably overestimates the directly measured osteoid width in normals and may be unreliable in osteoidosis (43). Greater variance with the indirect methods compared with the direct measurement of osteoid width has also been demonstrated by Quarles and Lobaugh (44). The inaccuracy of the ratio is due, at least in part, to the interrelationship of the osteoid area and mineralized area. A decrease in mineralized area alone results in an increase in osteoid area/bone area. When direct measurements are made at orthogonal intersections (Table 3), normal osteoid width is 7.6 μm ± 1.9 SD and ranges from 4.3 to 12.0 μm. Mean values greater than 15 μm indicate pathology and require concomitant tetracycline markers for confident interpretation. The direct method is not only more precise but also provides the frequency distribution of the individual values, information that is not provided by the indirect method.

Calculated and directly measured trabecular width and spacing also show significant differences (8,45). These differences may become clinically important when the bone area of the biopsy specimen is low and unevenly distributed in the tissue area, as occurs with severe osteoporosis (45).

SUMMARY OF THE EXPECTED HISTOMORPHOMETRIC FINDINGS IN CLINICAL DISORDERS

Primary Hyperparathyroidism (24,46–58)

Although the individual variation is great and rare patients may show normal values, most have characteristic findings (Table 5). Some woven collagen architecture may be present, but today, most patients are identified before the skeletal disease is clinically evident and, in them, woven bone is usually absent. In cortical bone tissue, the width tends to be low-normal or subnormal and the porosity is usually increased. Subperiosteal osteoclastosis and fibrosis are occasionally noted (Fig. 5). Intracortical and endocortical erosions may be prominent. The cancellous bone area is usually within normal limits, although rare patients have increased cancellous area. If the cancellous area is subnormal, the hyperparathyroidism is probably not to blame and another explanation should be sought. Wall width is slightly reduced, but trabecular width is usually well maintained. Osteoid is abundant. The increase in osteoid is due to an increase in the osteoid perimeter rather than to augmentation of the osteoid seam width. Numerous osteoblasts, osteoclasts, and at least, some peritrabecular marrow fibrosis are expected. Hook-shaped resorption cavities may be noted. The mineralizing surface, mineral appositional rate, and mineralization lag time are usually within the normal limits.

TABLE 5. *Expected bone histomorphometry in primary hyperparathyroidism*[a]

	Mean (SD)	
	Patients	Controls
Cortical bone tissue		
Cortical width (μm)	850 (169)	1202 (314)
Cortical porosity (%)	10.3 (4.4)	4.6 (2.0)
Cancellous bone tissue		
Bone area/tissue area (%)	24.0 (4.0)	21.6 (4.5)
Trabecular width (μm)	152 (44)	153 (31)
Wall width (μm)	51 (5)	59 (7)
Osteoid area/bone area (%)	4.2 (3.8)	2.2 (1.4)
Osteoid width (μm)	10 (3)	8 (2)
Osteoid perimeter (%)	20.0 (11.0)	16.5 (8.2)
Osteoblast perimeter (%)	7.6 (7.6)	2.2 (1.7)
Osteoclast perimeter (%)	3.0 (2.8)	0.97 (.83)
Dynamic measurements		
Mineralizing perimeter (%)[b]	73.5 (29.1)	71.4 (28.2)
Mineral appositional rate (μm/day)	0.68 (.13)	0.90 (.11)

Source: Medical College of Georgia.
[a] n = 10 white adults.
[b] The referent is the osteoid perimeter.

Bone biopsy in primary hyperparathyroidism may be done to estimate the amount of potential gain in bone density that would result from mineralization of the excess osteoid, to predict the severity of the hungry bones syndrome, to provide diagnostic information in borderline cases with decreased bone mass on radiographs or by densitometry, and rarely, to distinguish hyperparathyroidism from the hypercalcemia of malignancy. In the hypercalcemia of malignancy, osteoid and osteoblasts are rare (54).

The histomorphometric appearance of the biopsy specimen and the clinical presentation may be altered dramatically in patients with primary hyperparathyroidism and concurrent vitamin D deficiency (56). Double tetracycline labels may be absent and osteoid area may be as high as 29–80% of the cancellous bone area and osteoid perimeter 90–98% of the cancellous bone perimeter (57). When a bone biopsy is obtained after parathyroid surgery, even if the parathyroid hormone level is still elevated but has been reduced from the preoperative level, there are striking changes in the remodeling activity. The osteoclast perimeter has been found to decrease within a few hours. The osteoid perimeter and osteoblast perimeter expand to cover most of the cancellous perimeter by about 2 weeks after surgery and then decline back to normal (58).

Acromegaly (59–63)

Transileal bone biopsies from patients with acromegaly have been well studied by the group from Aarhus,

Denmark. In contrast to previous reports that described osteoporosis in acromegaly, the Danish workers found a significant increase in both cortical width (1517 μm ± 415 SD) and cancellous bone area (26.4% ± 5.2) in patients with active acromegaly. Osteoid perimeter was also increased (27.8% ± 12.2), while the mineralizing perimeter per cancellous bone perimeter and mineral appositional rate were high-normal to elevated (23.1% ± 7.7 versus 11.2 ± 5.8 and 0.87 μm/day ± 0.30 versus 0.60 ± 0.11). Abundant osteoblasts and osteoclasts were noted. In a hypercalcemic patient with acromegaly, however, bone biopsy is of less clinical benefit than measurement of the intact parathyroid hormone concentration.

Glucocorticoids (64–69)

In glucocorticoid-induced osteopenia, a marked reduction in cancellous bone is typical, with values often below 11–12%. Cortical bone also shows significantly reduced values for width, whereas porosity often remains within normal limits. Diminished wall width is to be expected with glucocorticoid excess and the wall width decreases with the cancellous bone area. Several investigators have described abundant osteoid but only with osteoid seams of low-normal width. The osteoidosis is usually modest, with osteoid areas of only about 3–4% and osteoid perimeters of 18–25%. The osteoblast perimeter is usually unremarkable but may be subnormal. Elevated measurements of osteoclast perimeter and osteoclast number are expected, but are rarely more than about twice the normal mean values. Decreased mineralizing cancellous perimeter and closely spaced double tetracycline labels are the rule. An absence of double labels may occur, a finding that is never seen in normal volunteers (13,41). The adjusted appositional rate, or the rate of bone formation averaged over the entire osteoid perimeter, is reduced significantly. This index of osteoblast vigor reveals the profound inhibitory effects of glucocorticoid excess on bone formation. In any single biopsy specimen from a patient with hypercortisolism, the findings will be dependent on the underlying disease, glucocorticoid type and dose, duration of treatment, and age and sex of the patient. Recent reductions in the dose of glucocorticoids or after the treatment of Cushing's disease, may markedly increase the rate of bone formation. Therefore, interpretation of the bone specimen depends on a complete historical examination and medication review.

Anticonvulsant Drug-Induced Bone Disease (70,71)

Patients receiving long-term anticonvulsant drug treatment may show osteoidosis on bone biopsy examination, but double-tetracycline-labeled histomorphome-

tric studies have revealed that in ambulatory adults with epilepsy, a mineralization defect is absent. Osteomalacia can occur, however, in patients treated with anticonvulsant drugs when the patients are institutionalized or otherwise have limited access to solar exposure and dietary sources of vitamin D. Bone biopsy may be indicated in patients receiving anticonvulsant drug treatment when osteopenia or skeletal fragility are noted and the role of the anticonvulsant drugs as an accelerating factor in the loss of bone mass is uncertain.

In cortical bone tissue, the cortical width is reduced and porosity increased. The values are similar to those found in primary hyperparathyroidism (71), probably because they are the result of secondary hyperparathyroidism. In cancellous bone, the bone area is typically normal but the osteoid area is increased (5.2% ± 1.1 SEM). The increased osteoid is due to an increase in the osteoid perimeter (22.8% ± 2.8) and not to significant augmentation of the osteoid width (11.7 μm ± 0.9). Osteoblast and osteoclast perimeters are generally within normal limits. The mineralizing perimeter is high-normal (85.2% ± 4.3), the mineral appositional rate is normal (0.80 μm/day ± 0.04), and the mineralization lag time is normal (18.5 days ± 2.2). Although woven bone and peritrabecular marrow fibrosis are usually absent, the probable explanation for the occasional appearance of these findings is secondary hyperparathyroidism instead of osteomalacia.

Immobilization (72–76)

Bone biopsy may sometimes be indicated when an immobilized patient sustains a fracture with trivial trauma or becomes hypercalcemic and the results of the parathyroid hormone studies are not clear. In these cases it is clinically useful to know the expected histomorphometric findings in long-term immobilization. In cortical bone tissue, the width may be reduced by 50%. In cancellous bone tissue, the bone area is diminished to values of about 10–12%. However, even after years of immobilization, lower values are unanticipated. A recent study suggests that the decreased cancellous bone is characterized by reduced trabecular width and augmented trabecular spacing. Osteoid area may be less than 0.1% but is more often in the low-normal range. Osteoclast perimeter and number may be unchanged or modestly increased by about 15–25%. Tetracycline labels are absent in 25% of patients. When double labels are seen, they are closely spaced. In any individual patient, however, the histomorphometry will reflect the original condition that caused immobilization, prior treatment with glucocorticoids, disodium etidronate that may have been used to prevent heterotopic ossification, calcitonin or hyperalimentation, and renal status. The combined effects may seriously complicate assessment of the biopsy.

Mastocytosis (29,77–85)

Systemic mastocytosis may masquerade as idiopathic osteoporosis, and therefore bone biopsy specimens obtained for the evaluation of low bone mass should be processed with metachromatic staining (toluidine blue and Geimsa techniques) to recognize mast cell accumulations and the characteristic spindle-shaped granulomata. The metachromatic staining quality can be precluded by decalcification. The expected bone histomorphometric findings in mastocytosis are distinct from those found in postmenopausal osteoporosis. Accelerated bone turnover is found in mastocytosis with increased numbers of plump osteoblasts (osteoblast perimeter 3.1–6.4%), osteoclasts (osteoclast perimeter 0.3–1.0%), peritrabecular marrow fibrosis (4–44%), and osteoidosis (osteoid area 3.9–9.0%). Osteoid seams are normal in width. In patients with increased radiolucency, cancellous bone area may be less than 10%. However, some patients have radiographic osteosclerosis, increased cancellous area, and woven collagen architecture. Mineral appositional rate and bone formation rates may be further increased in those patients with mastocytosis and osteosclerosis. It is important to note that increased numbers of scattered mast cells have been described in women with postmenopausal osteoporosis and in patients with renal hyperparathyroidism. In these situations the numbers of mast cells are about twice that found in normal women (up to 7 mast cells per square millimeter versus less than 4 per square millimeter in normal women) and there are no significant relationships between the mast cell numbers and the bone histomorphometry. In mastocytosis, the mean number of mast cells is 40–60 times greater than in postmenopausal osteoporosis and the typical granulomata are present.

Postmenopausal Osteoporosis (9,23,25,27,28,86–94)

Histomorphometric analysis of transileal bone specimens taken from untreated women with postmenopausal osteoporosis reveals that the disorder is not uniform (86), but the heterogeneity may be no greater than that found in primary hyperparathyroidism. Although there is considerable overlap in the determination of cancellous bone between groups with and without vertebral fractures, cancellous bone area in patients with compression fractures is usually below the normal range (<13%, Table 3) (Fig. 12). The cancellous area also shows a significant correlation with the percentage of the marrow area composed of hematopoietic cells (27). Subnormal cancellous area is usually accompanied by increased marrow fat (28). There is, however, a stronger relationship between the presence of vertebral fractures and the trabecular microstructure. Patients with vertebral compression fractures due to postmenopausal osteo-

porosis were compared with a control group of women without fractures matched for age, race, menopausal status, bone mineral content at the proximal radius, and transileal cancellous bone area (9). In the fracture group, trabecular number was significantly lower and trabecular separation significantly greater than in the control group. Even the thicker trabecular plates in the fracture group failed to compensate for the disruption of connections between trabeculae and the resultant increase in trabecular separation. It is not uncommon to observe these perforations and disconnections in the biopsy specimen. Parts of the cancellous network can be noted to breakup and become disengaged, like strings of islands leading away from a mainland (Fig. 12).

Transileal cortical width is often subnormal, but this cortical osteopenia is usually accompanied by normal cortical porosity. Cancellization of the endocortical border is often present. The endocortical bone may show more osteoid, osteoclasts, and mineralizing perimeter than the cortical or cancellous bone tissue (87). Except at the endocortical borders, osteoclastosis is an unexpected finding in postmenopausal osteoporosis and should prompt a search for subtle hyperparathyroidism or thyrotoxicosis. Empty Howship's lacunae may, however, be abundant. These empty lacunae are not equivalent to the so-called "inactive resorption surface" and have been shown to vary independently from the osteoclastic surface (25). The abnormal accumulation of these empty Howship's lacunae represent the abortive reversal perimeter and may indicate delayed or defective coupling. Small increases in the percentages of the osteoid area and perimeter are often seen, but these findings are merely the result of the diminished mineralized bone area. Osteoid width, wall width, and mineralizing perimeter are usually decreased.

In more than two-thirds of biopsy specimens from patients with vertebral fractures and postmenopausal osteoporosis, bone formation rates are low (89,90), although not all investigators agree on this point. Increased proportions of patients with high turnover osteoporosis have also been reported (87,88). These differences may possibly reflect geographical decreases in vitamin D intake and solar exposure that result in compensatory secondary hyperparathyroidism and an increase in bone turnover. Differences in the proportion of patients with high turnover may also be due to the inclusion of elderly women with decreased creatinine clearance.

Many patients with postmenopausal osteoporosis receive some form of therapy for osteoporosis before bone biopsy, and therefore the potential effects on the bone histology brought about by the therapy must be appreciated. Calcium supplementation is the most commonly applied treatment but has little or no effect on cancellous bone area, wall width, or bone formation rate (91). A subtle decrease in osteoid perimeter and width may be noted, however. Any potential benefit of calcium treatment on cortical bone tissue is not likely to be evident in a transileal bone biopsy. With estrogen therapy, the activation frequency in cancellous bone tissue decreases by about 50% (91). Osteoid and mineralizing perimeters are diminished, but there is no change in seam width, adjusted mineralization rate, mineralization lag time, wall width, or bone area. The primary effect of estrogen therapy is thus a reduction in the activation frequency of new bone remodeling units and a resultant fall in bone turnover. Calcitonin treatment also reduces the activation frequency. The osteoclast perimeter declines to a variable extent without any consistent effects on cortical or cancellous bone area, osteoid, or mineralization (92). The effects of long-term sodium fluoride therapy (40–60 mg/day) on cortical bone tissue in osteoporotic patients include a 50–75% increase in cortical porosity without a change in cortical width, increased osteoid-covered osteons with a decrease in mineralizing osteons, and prolongation of the mineralization lag time (93). In cancellous bone tissue, an increase in the bone area/tissue area, wall width, seam width, and osteoid perimeter may be found in about two-thirds of treated patients. However, trabecular connectivity remains interrupted (94). Decreased mineralizing perimeter and increased mineralization lag time may develop with fluoride treatment despite supplementation with calcium and vitamin D. If the serum fluoride concentration becomes too high, as can happen when the patient has subtle renal insufficiency, the mineralization defect may be more pronounced, resulting in generalized osteomalacia. The osteomalacia may also be focal with fluoride treatment, in that a spotty increase in osteoid seam width may develop without elevated mean values for the osteoid area or perimeter (95).

Renal Osteodystrophy (7,19,40,95–114)

Although more bone biopsies are probably done in patients with end-stage renal disease than in any other clinical situation, the explanation for the extraordinarily wide spectrum of histological findings remains unclear. Reports of normal bone histology may be due to problems with fixation and staining, inappropriate use of normal data from other laboratories, or to differences in the patient population studied (106). The wide range of histological features usually found results, at least in part, from differences in the degree and duration of renal failure, duration and type of dialysis, dialysate calcium concentration, water supply and filtration, geographical location, exposure to glucocorticoids and drugs used to prevent rejection of a renal transplant, past history of diabetes (104), nephrectomy or intestinal resection, extent of ambulation, history of severe infections, strict long-term control of the serum phosphorus concentration (102), and prior treatment with vitamin D metabo-

lites or parathyroid surgery (40,105). These differences often hinder efforts to discover the underlying mechanisms of renal osteodystrophy. Furthermore, the spectrum of histological features in renal osteodystrophy is often subdivided without clear clinical meaning. Terms such as "pure" osteitis fibrosa, "low turnover" osteomalacia, and "aplastic bone disease" are misnomers (7). Low bone turnover is characteristic of all forms of osteomalacia and there is no good reason for restricting this term to renal bone disease (107). Furthermore, there is no condition of "high-turnover" osteomalacia. The histological specimens usually contain more bone cells than normal samples and rarely show all the classical findings of one particular end of the broad histological spectrum (96). Osteitis fibrosa with accelerated rates of mineral apposition and bone formation is the most frequent form of renal osteodystrophy (7,97), but the point at which it merges into osteoidosis with subnormal bone turnover defies rigorous subset classification. In this spectrum of findings, stainable aluminum may be found in about 30% of specimens with accelerated bone turnover (7). In these patients, single and double tetracycline labels are sometimes recognized at sites that stained positively for aluminum (96,99). Aluminum is found in most but not all patients with osteoidosis and subnormal bone turnover, but from the observations in the patients with accelerated bone turnover, aluminum bone disease cannot be viewed as a discrete disorder (101–103). Aluminum staining may be found without osteomalacia, cause focal or atypical osteomalacia, induce osteoblast defects without osteomalacia or low turnover, or cause any combination of these lesions (95). Moreover, in the absence of aluminum exposure, dialysis patients may still develop an adynamic bone disease associated with a relative hypoparathyroidism (108).

Osteitis fibrosa in the cortical bone tissue of a transileal bone biopsy specimen taken from a patient with severe secondary hyperparathyroidism is characterized by reduced cortical width, increased cortical porosity, and prominent intracortical osteoid and intraosseous erosions (24) (Fig. 8 and Table 6). Subperiosteal cortical erosions containing osteoclasts, osteoid, and a loose fibrous stroma are often present (Fig. 7). Under polarized light, the bone contains abundant woven collagen architecture (100). Woven bone is most evident in severe osteitis fibrosa (Fig. 3) and appears to represent a qualitative defect due to the high levels of parathyroid hormone and inorganic phosphorus. The normally sharp junction between cortical and cancellous bone is obscured by both deep, coalescent, endocortical resorption bays and augmentation of the cancellous bone area. Specimens with a cancellous bone area greater than the upper limits of normal are typically found in patients with osteosclerosis and the "rugger-jersey sign" on standard radiographs of the thoracolumbar spine (Fig. 9). Bone biopsy core density is, however, usually below the normal range

TABLE 6. *Bone histomorphometry in a 30-year-old black man on hemodialysis for 7 years: typical osteitis fibrosa in renal osteodystrophy[a]*

	Patient	Normal range
Bone biopsy core		
Mineral density (g/cm^2)	0.198	0.20–0.34
Cortical bone tissue		
Cortical width (μm)	880	990–1500
Cortical porosity (%)	10.4	3.2–7.0
Cancellous bone tissue		
Bone area/tissue area (%)	36.1	13.0–28.0
Trabecular width (μm)	158.9	100–225
Trabecular number (mm^{-1})	2.28	1.00–1.80
Trabecular spacing (μm)	951.5	800–1500
Osteoid area/bone area (%)	14.9	0.4–4.0
Osteoid width (μm)	17.8	4.3–12.0
Osteoid perimeter (%)[b]	78.0	4.0–39.0
Osteoblast perimeter (%)[b]	8.1	0.1–7.3
Osteoclast perimeter (%)[b]	7.9	<3.0
Reversal perimeter (%)[b]	2.8	3.5–12.0
Fibrous perimeter (%)[b]	10.6	None
Aluminum boundary (%)[c]	25.4	None
Iron boundary (%)[c]	0.0	None
Dynamic measurements		
Mineralizing perimeter (%)[d]	57.5	4.5–56.4
Mineral appositional rate (μm/day)	1.31	0.22–0.89
Adjusted appositional rate (μm/day)	0.75	0.02–0.44
Mineralization lag time (days)	23.6	22–447
Bone formation rate (μm^2/μm/day)[b]	0.59	0.01–0.07

[a] Bone biopsy was done because of progressively increasing serum alkaline phosphatase activity: ionized calcium was 4.91 mg/dL (n = 4.73–5.21), phosphorus 5.35 mg/dL (n = 2.20–3.90), alkaline phosphatase 81 rising to 369 mu/mL (n = 25–100), and intact parathyroid hormone 200 pg/mL (n = 10–66).
[b] The referent is the cancellous bone perimeter.
[c] The referent is the cancellous bone boundary.
[d] The referent is the osteoid perimeter.

(Table 6). Osteosclerosis indicates severe secondary hyperparathyroidism (19). Renal osteodystrophy is the only disorder in which trabecular number is typically increased. Osteoid area, perimeter, and width are amplified, but the mineralization lag time is either normal or else not as prolonged as in vitamin D deficiency. The augmented seam width is probably from discordance between the increased matrix appositional rate and the mineral appositional rate during the early part of the osteoid seam lifespan, a phenomenon that may be due to the high parathyroid hormone levels and hyperphosphatemia. Plump, cuboidal osteoblasts in palisades (Fig. 10) and osteoclasts with 8–10 nuclei are more evident than in any other metabolic bone disease (except Paget's disease). Tunneling, intratrabecular, and hook resorption cavities are common (24). Osteoclastic resorption of

osteoid is usually evident with severe secondary hyperparathyroidism (98). Reversal perimeter may be subnormal, reflecting a decrease in the time necessary for teams of osteoblasts to appear in the previously resorbed cavities. The marrow space may be obliterated by fibrous tissue and contain foci of hemosiderin-laden macrophages. Positive aluminum staining may be seen despite abundant tetracycline uptake. Tetracycline labels are often widely separated. Entire osteons and cancellous packets may fluoresce diffusely. Race-specific normal values are required to appreciate the spectacular acceleration of bone formation that may be found in specimens taken from black dialysis patients (Table 6).

In patients with subnormal bone turnover, some have only scant osteoid, but these patients usually have a complicated past history of transplant rejections, multiple infections, diabetes mellitus, surgical procedures, and drug regimens. When low bone turnover is found in patients without these confounding problems, osteoid may be exceptionally increased and osteoid seam width may be more than 30 to 50 μm (Fig. 13 and Table 7). The

TABLE 7. *Bone histomorphometry in a 40-year-old white man on hemodialysis for 2 years: typical osteomalacia in renal osteodystrophy[a]*

	Patient	Normal range
Bone biopsy core		
Mineral density (g/cm^2)	0.219	0.20–0.34
Cortical bone tissue		
Cortical width (μm)	691	990–1500
Cortical porosity (%)	8.5	3.2–7.0
Cancellous bone tissue		
Bone area/tissue area (%)	16.0	13.0–28.0
Trabecular width (μm)	102.2	100–225
Trabecular number (mm^{-1})	1.6	1.00–1.80
Trabecular spacing (μm)	1178	800–1500
Osteoid area/bone area (%)	11.7	0.4–4.0
Osteoid width (μm)	33.2	4.3–12.0
Osteoid perimeter (%)[b]	32.3	4.0–39.0
Osteoblast perimeter (%)[b]	2.7	0.1–7.3
Osteoclast perimeter (%)[b]	4.3	<3.0
Reversal perimeter (%)[b]	14.2	3.5–12.0
Fibrous perimeter (%)[b]	3.7	None
Aluminum boundary (%)[c]	0.0	None
Iron boundary (%)[c]	0.0	None
Dynamic measurements		
Mineralizing perimeter (%)[d]	4.3	50–100
Mineral appositional rate (μm/day)	0.0	0.83–0.98

[a] Bone biopsy was done because of hypercalcemia: serum total calcium was 11.0 mg/dL (n = 9.2–10.4), phosphorus 7.4 mg/dL (n = 2.3–4.5), alkaline phosphatase 84 mg/mL (n = 25–100, and C-terminal parathyroid hormone 300 mEq/mL (n < 60).
[b] The referent is the cancellous bone perimeter.
[c] The referent is the cancellous bone boundary.
[d] The referent is the osteoid perimeter.

typical clinical presentation is hypercalcemia rather than bone pain, fractures, or encephalopathy, which have become quite rare. In some patients, the osteoidosis is only focal, with high-normal values for the osteoid perimeter, whereas in other patients the osteoid perimeter approaches 100%. Cortical width is usually reduced and cortical porosity increased. Lamellar collagen is predominant. When compared with the specimens obtained from patients with osteitis fibrosa, there is a relative paucity of osteoblasts and osteoclasts (101), but the osteoclast perimeter is often greater than that found in normal subjects (96). The reversal perimeter may accumulate, indicating a defect or delay in the coupling of bone resorption and bone formation. Peritrabecular marrow fibrosis is usually rare or absent. Aluminum staining is detectable in many but not all of these patients (Fig. 14). Assurance that the staining is due to aluminum requires a negative result for bone iron staining. Single tetracycline labels prevail, and double labels are often absent.

Treatment of hemodialysis patients with vitamin D metabolites to decrease the degree of hyperparathyroidism results in a reduction in the osteoblast, osteoclast, and fibrous perimeters, a decrease in osteoid area, and a decline in the bone formation rate toward the upper limit of the normal range (112). The decrease in bone turnover is accompanied by a slight increase in the stainable bone aluminum.

Bone histomorphometry in patients after renal transplantation reflects the severity of the renal osteodystrophy before transplantation, the immunosuppressive drug regimen, and hypophosphatemia (109–110). Both cortical and cancellous bone are reduced compared to normal controls. Osteoid area and perimeter are slightly increased. Bone formation rate is decreased and mineralization lag time prolonged.

After parathyroidectomy in hemodialysis patients, the bone shows reduced osteoblast and osteoclast perimeters, scant peritrabecular fibrosis, and a decreased bone formation rate (40,111). Osteoid area/bone area, osteoid perimeter, and osteoid width are often excessive, but osteoid area/tissue area is similar to that found in dialysis patients without prior parathyroidectomy. Lamellar osteoid is, however, more abundant. These findings result from the preoperative renal osteodystrophy altered by the decline in parathyroid hormone concentrations and the reduction in the calcium × phosphate product. After parathyroid surgery in dialysis patients, aluminum deposition may be enhanced as a result of the osteoidosis and low bone turnover (111).

Bone biopsies taken from dialysis patients after long-term treatment with deferoxamine reveal that the stainable aluminum boundary decreases by 50–70%, but the percentage of aluminum in cement lines may increase (113,114). This apparent translocation of the bone aluminum burden has been associated with a doubling of the osteoblast and osteoclast perimeters. The increase in double-labeled tetracycline boundary and mineral appositional rate may result in up to a fivefold increase in bone formation rate. In patients with prior parathyroid surgery, the decrease in stainable aluminum may be only modest and the osteoblast perimeter and bone formation rate may not change.

Metabolic Bone Disease Associated with Gastrointestinal Diseases (11,115–118)

Among the best known late complications of gastrointestinal disease or surgery is osteomalacia. The prevalence of osteomalacia 5–15 years after gastrectomy, intestinal bypass surgery, small bowel resection, or chronic malabsorption is, however, only about 5–30%. Therefore, a search for osteomalacia may be indicated, but only a few patients will have it. Clues that suggest osteomalacia include diffuse skeletal tenderness, proximal myopathy, decreased urinary calcium excretion, ionized hypocalcemia, hypophosphatemia, and elevated serum alkaline phosphatase activity (11,117). Since the majority, however, will have osteoporosis, bone biopsy may be necessary for definitive diagnosis. In the absence of osteomalacia, the typical histomorphometric features include a reduced cancellous bone area with narrow and widely spaced trabeculae, rare osteoclasts and osteoblasts, an accumulation of empty Howship's lacunae (reversal perimeter), diminished wall width, decreased rates of mineral apposition, and bone formation and prolongation of the mineralization lag time. Low or negative values for interstitial width may be found. The significant impairment of osteoblast function that is present may be due to the malabsorption of some unidentified nutrient required for normal osteoblast vigor. The bone loss in these quasi-nutritional situations appears to result from a transient increase in bone resorption and a sustained decrease in bone formation. Treatment with vitamin D may decrease the amount of osteoid in the specimen but in many patients, the improvement is negligible (11). Osteoidosis may persist even with the use of 1-hydroxylated metabolites (118).

Thyrotoxicosis (119–126)

Untreated thyrotoxic patients are seldom subjected to bone biopsy for clinical reasons. Reports of bone loss caused by mild overmedication with exogenous thyroid hormone have, however, resulted in the need to recognize the impact of thyroid hormone replacement in bone biopsies taken from patients with otherwise idiopathic osteoporosis.

All investigators agree that the histology of thyrotoxic bone shows reduced amounts of cortical and cancellous tissue, osteoidosis, osteoclastosis, and increased bone remodeling. Hyperthyroidism is a model of high-turnover bone loss. Meunier et al. have made an excellent summary of the classical histological findings in thyrotoxicosis (124). In cortical bone tissue, the cortical width is low-normal or normal, but cortical porosity may be more than three times greater than the normal mean values. This "worm-eaten" appearance of the cortical bone tissue is due to intraosseous resorption cavities. Intracortical osteoclasts and osteoblasts are abundant. The presence of intracortical fibrosis without peritrabecular marrow fibrosis helps distinguish the findings in thyrotoxicosis from those in hyperparathyroidism. Another diagnostic point is that in thyrotoxicosis, the subperiosteal borders show no evidence of osteoclastic erosion. Endocortical osteoclastosis may, however, be conspicuous.

In cancellous bone tissue, the bone area is reduced and may be as low as 10%, although more typical values are 12–14%. Wall width is normal. Osteoid area is slightly increased. The increase in osteoid is from a small increase in the osteoid perimeter (about 17–24%) rather than to augmentation of the seam width. Osteoid width may be less than the normal mean value. Plump, cuboidal osteoblasts are abundant. Osteoclast perimeter is increased but less than that seen in hyperparathyroidism.

The mineralizing perimeter may be 95–100%, and double labels are generally abundant. The mineral appositional rate is often greater than 1 μm/day. Bone formation rates are increased and mineralization lag time is decreased.

Osteomalacia (11,117,127,128)

Osteomalacia is a generic term that indicates the clinical consequences of defective mineralization of the organic lamellar matrix of bone. Although characteristic clinical, radiographic, and biochemical findings may suggest osteomalacia, the absence of these findings cannot exclude the diagnosis. Quantitative histological examination of undecalcified bone is, therefore, usually required to establish the unequivocal presence of osteomalacia and has become one of the major indications for a tetracycline-labeled bone biopsy (117). Rigorous kinetic criteria for the histological recognition of osteomalacia are necessary to preserve the traditional clinical, biochemical, and therapeutic connotations of the term (11) (Fig. 15). The histomorphometric diagnosis of osteomalacia requires the simultaneous presence of excessive osteoid (osteoid area greater than 10%), augmentation of the osteoid seam width (osteoid width more than 15 μm) (Fig. 16), and prolongation of the mineralization lag time (to more than 100 days) (11). In the first requirement, an increase in osteoid can occur with merely a decrease in trabecular width or in states of increased bone turnover, such as hyperparathyroidism, Paget's disease of bones, and thyrotoxicosis (117). In the second requirement, wide osteoid seams may be seen in

bone specimens obtained from patients with severe secondary hyperparathyroidism, such as those on maintenance hemodialysis therapy. In the third requirement, reduced mineral appositional rate, decreased mineralizing perimeter, diminished bone formation, and increased mineralization lag time are nonspecific indices of impaired matrix synthesis by osteoblasts, as is often found in patients with postmenopausal osteoporosis. Only when all three requirements are fulfilled is the diagnosis of osteomalacia irrefutable. Recently, Reid et al. reported that in patients with X-linked hypophosphatemia, bone pain was significantly more common, with osteoid area values greater than 25% (127). Osteomalacic bone pain has been shown to be significantly more prevalent in patients in whom the rigorous histological diagnosis of osteomalacia has been proven (11). The cause of this bone pain remains unknown, since the cortical width and mineralized cancellous bone area in osteomalacia may be within normal limits. Bone cells in osteomalacia are often scarce. The osteoblasts that line the osteoid perimeter may appear flattened (Fig. 16). The osteoclast perimeter/bone perimeter is usually less than 4%, but when the referent is the mineralized perimeter instead of the entire cancellous perimeter, osteoclasts may be increased 10- to 20-fold due to the decreased nonosteoid perimeter (5). Unusual types of resorption cavities may be seen in osteomalacia. Tunneling, intraosseous, and hook resorption are likely to be observed when the osteoid perimeter reaches values above 60% (24). Examples of osteoclastic erosion of osteoid can be observed (Fig. 17). Osteoclasts resorbing osteoid contain more nuclei per profile than do osteoclasts resorbing mineralized bone (98).

Paget's Disease of Bones (129–134)

Bone biopsy is rarely required for the diagnosis of Paget's disease of bones. Occasionally, neoplasia may masquerade as Paget's disease or putative Paget's disease may present in an unusual location, conditions that may indicate the need for biopsy. These events are, however, quite rare at the ilium. The investigators from Lyon have accumulated the largest morphometric experience with transileal biopsies from Pagetic bone (129). Cortical and cancellous bone may be increased more than twofold above the mean normal values (cancellous bone area, 42% ± 15 SD) with wide, irregular trabeculae and a poorly defined junction between cortical and cancellous bone. The increased bone area is composed of a mosaic of smaller bone packets, some of which are woven and others lamellar in collagen organization. Scalloped cement lines are prominent. Osteoclastosis and fibrosis are marked. The differentiating features of the histological changes involve the qualitatively and quantitatively abnormal osteoclasts. The osteoclast number may be 10 times normal, with the cells over 100 μm wide and containing 20 to 100 nuclei (130) (Fig. 18). These giant multinucleated osteoclasts are unique to Paget's disease of bones. Osteoclasts of normal dimensions are, however, also present. Similarly, the osteoblast perimeter is increased and the cells are plump and cuboidal, with prominent perinuclear clear zones (the Golgi apparatus). Osteoid area may be moderately excessive, with typical values about fourfold more than the normal mean values. Osteoid perimeter is also increased (50% ± 12) and seam width may be augmented. Mineral appositional rate is accelerated (1.36 μm/day ± 0.27) and the mineralizing perimeter may be up to 80%, with more than three-fourths constructed from double labels. Peritrabecular and marrow fibrosis is prevalent near osteoclasts. The number of blood vessels in the marrow is increased and hemorrhage may be noted.

If the response to drug treatment of Paget's disease is less than that expected or if diagnosis remains doubtful, bone biopsy specimens may occasionally be obtained after the treatment of Paget's disease. Histological changes after calcitonin therapy include a decrease in osteoclast perimeter of about 40% (131). Furthermore, there may be a decrease in osteoclast size and a reduction in the number of nuclei per osteoclast. Lamellar instead of woven bone becomes more evident. Once these diagnostic features are eliminated, only the mosaic architecture may remain to indicate the Pagetic bone. The differential diagnosis includes hyperparathyroidism, fibrous dysplasia, a healing fracture, idiopathic bone necrosis, osteomyelitis, and osteoblastic metastases. Histomorphometric changes after etidronate in the treatment of Paget's disease are time and dose related (132). There is a reduction in the osteoclast perimeter and in marrow fibrosis, but these findings are accompanied by a decrease in the mineral appositional rate. With 20 mg/kg per day for 6 months, osteoid seam width is augmented and the mineralization lag time is prolonged over 100 days. This defect in mineralization may be focal, with osteoid width increased to a relatively greater extent than osteoid perimeter (95,133,134). Even with low-dose therapy, a patchy increase in osteoid width may be found.

Hypophosphatasia (135–138)

Although a few patients with hypophosphatasemia, premature loss of adult teeth, and mild or absent skeletal symptoms will have normal bone histomorphometry, nondecalcified sections of bone from symptomatic patients reveal defective mineralization. The excess osteoid may be dramatic, with osteoid area values as high as 40–75%, osteoid perimeters 70–90%, and seam width 20–57 μm. Cancellous bone area is usually quantitatively normal, but this results from the extensive contribution of the unmineralized bone matrix. Osteoblast pe-

rimeters are low-normal and often undetectable. Osteoclast numbers range from undetectable to slightly elevated. A few patients have unexplained small amounts of peritrabecular marrow fibrosis. Tetracycline fluorescence is typically absent or scarce and the few labels seen are diffuse and single (Fig. 11). The mineralizing perimeter/osteoid perimeter is usually less than 15%.

Osteogenesis Imperfecta (139–146)

Occasionally, a patient with multiple fractures and a family history of skeletal fragility may have a bone biopsy to determine if osteogenesis imperfecta is present. Diagnosis of this group of disorders of collagen formation is, however, more effectively reached with a skin biopsy and quantitative collagen studies. If normal control data are available, electron microscopy or bone samples may demonstrate the thin collagen bundles described in osteogenesis imperfecta. With the light microscope, the bone histomorphometric findings, although characteristic, are not, in themselves, diagnostic and vary according to the age and mobility of the patient. Typical findings include reduced cortical bone width, decreased cancellous bone area (adults often less than 11%), decreased trabecular width, increased osteoid area due to an increase in the osteoid perimeter with maintenance of a normal osteoid seam width, increased osteoblast perimeter, and normal osteoclast perimeter. Although controversial, most previously untreated, ambulatory patients have accelerated rates of bone formation. The osteocyte compaction defect that has been described in osteogenesis imperfecta may result from the presence of woven bone found in specimens taken from adolescent patients with the disease. Another explanation for the more closely packed osteocytes is that a reduced amount of bone matrix is made by each osteoblast.

Alcoholism (147–152)

The clear evidence of a significant relationship between alcohol abuse and skeletal fragility usually preempts the value of bone biopsy in this situation. Rarely, if ever, will a precise diagnosis of alcohol-induced bone disease have a clinical impact on the patient. In this regard, the most promising new information about the bone histomorphometry in alcoholics is that the damage appears to be less severe in abstainers. All reports agree that the cancellous bone area is significantly reduced in heavy drinkers. Wall width is decreased. Osteoid area, perimeter, and width are diminished and osteoblasts and osteoclasts are rare. Bone formation rate is dramatically reduced and may be unmeasurable, due to the absence of double tetracycline labels.

Hepatic Osteodystrophy (153–157)

There is now widespread concurrence that in chronic cholestatic liver disease, primary biliary cirrhosis, sclerosing cholangitis, and alcoholic cirrhosis, osteomalacia is absent and the most frequent skeletal disease is osteoporosis, which occurs in only about 20–40% of patients. In some patients with early or mild liver disease, the bone histomorphometry may be essentially normal. However, with severe disease and particularly in long-standing primary biliary cirrhosis, bone loss and skeletal fragility may be a serious clinical problem. Hepatic osteodystrophy has no pathognomonic features, but in patients with skeletal fragility, the osteoid area/bone area, mineralizing perimeter, adjusted mineral appositional rate, and bone formation rate are subnormal. Osteoblast perimeter is often below the mean values found in healthy control subjects and double-labeled mineralizing perimeter may be absent. The osteoblast dysfunction has been related to the degree of hepatic impairment (157).

Atypical Insufficiency Fractures and Transileal Bone Biopsy (117,158–160)

Bilateral nonhealing pseudofractures in bones that are normal except for decreased radiodensity have been regarded as the radiographic hallmark of osteomalacia. These symmetrical radiolucent bands are 2–4 mm wide and run perpendicular to the bone surface in the femoral neck, ischial and pubic rami, ribs, or axillary border of the scapula and are associated with little or no trauma. Similar bands have, however, been reported in patients in the absence of histological evidence of osteomalacia. Lack of awareness of this fact may lead to unnecessary and potentially dangerous treatment with vitamin D. Patients in whom these bands are found without histological osteomalacia usually have radiographic evidence of at least some callus formation and marginal sclerosis around the bands. Furthermore, pseudofractures that herald treatable osteomalacia are almost always accompanied by ionized hypocalcemia, hypophosphatemia, increased alkaline phosphatase activity, diffuse skeletal tenderness, and proximal muscle weakness. These fractures may show focal intense uptake of radionuclides on bone scans and prompt an unwarranted search for metastatic disease. If the radiographic, biochemical, and clinical features of the patient presenting with bilateral pseudofractures remains uncertain, a tetracycline-labeled transileal bone biopsy is indicated. In patients in whom biopsies have been done and osteomalacia was excluded, histomorphometric findings have revealed that cancellous bone area may be from 6 to 27%, osteoid area 0.6 to 8.9%, osteoid width 5.5 to 12.8 μm, mineralizing perimeter 10 to 100%, and bone formation rates undetectable to elevated. These atypical insufficiency fractures seem to occur in bone that cannot repair the stresses of normal activity. Predisposing conditions for some of these fractures includes osteoporosis, corticosteroid drugs, and prior irradiation. When a history of irradiation is associated with the atypical fractures, the bone scan may be unremarkable.

ACKNOWLEDGMENTS

I thank A. Michael Parfitt for his advice on this manuscript. The expert technical assistance of Marion Hutson, Linda J. Sappington, and Kathy New is gratefully appreciated.

REFERENCES

1. Hodgkinson A, Knowles CF. Laboratory methods. In: Nordin BEC, ed. *Calcium, phosphate and magnesium metabolism: clinical physiology and diagnostic procedures.* New York: Churchill Livingstone, 1976;516–24.
2. Merz WA, Schenk RK. Quantitative structural analysis of human cancellous bone. *Acta Anat* 1970;75:54–66.
3. Jowsey J. *The bone biopsy.* New York: Plenum Press, 1977;59–89.
4. Frost HM. *Bone remodeling and its relationship to metabolic bone diseases.* Springfield, IL: Charles C Thomas, 1973.
5. Parfitt AM, Drezner MK, Glorieux FH, et al. Bone histomorphometry: standardization of nomenclature, symbols, and units. *J Bone Miner Res* 1987;2:595–610.
6. Byers PD. The diagnostic value of bone biopsies. In: Avioli LV, Krane SM, eds. *Metabolic bone diseases,* vol 1. New York: Academic Press, 1977;183–236.
7. Malluche HH, Faugere MC. Renal osteodystrophy. *N Engl J Med* 1989;321:317–8.
8. Weinstein RS, Hutson MS. Decreased trabecular width and increased trabecular spacing contribute to bone loss with aging. *Bone* 1987;8:137–42.
9. Kleerekoper M, Villanueva AR, Stanciu J, Sudhaker Rao D, Parfitt AM. The role of three-dimensional trabecular microstructure in the pathogenesis of vertebral compression fractures. *Calcif Tissue Int* 1985;37:594–7.
10. Podenphant J, Engel U. Regional variations in histomorphometric bone dynamics from the skeleton of an osteoporotic woman. *Calcif Tissue Int* 1987;40:184–8.
11. Parfitt AM, Podenphant J, Villanueva AR, Frame B. Metabolic bone disease with and without osteomalacia after intestinal bypass surgery: a bone histomorphometric study. *Bone* 1985;6:211–20.
11a. Parfitt AM, Foldes J. The ambiguity of interstitial bone thickness; a new approach to the mechanism of trabecular thinning. *Bone* 1991;12:119–22.
12. Kleerekoper M, Frame B, Villanueva AR, et al. Treatment of osteoporosis with sodium fluoride alternating with calcium and vitamin D. In: DeLuca HF, Frost HM, Jee WSS, Johnston CC, Parfitt AM, eds. *Osteoporosis: recent advances in pathogenesis and treatment.* Baltimore: University Park Press, 1981;441–8.
13. Weinstein RS, Bell NH. Diminished rates of bone formation in normal black adults. *N Engl J Med* 1988;319:1698–1701.
14. Eriksen EF. Normal and pathological remodeling of human trabecular bone: three dimensional reconstruction of the remodeling sequence in normals and in metabolic bone disease. *Endocr Rev* 1986;7:379–408.
15. Rao DS. Practical approach to bone biopsy. In: Recker RR, ed. *Bone histomorphometry: techniques and interpretation.* Boca Raton, FL: CRC Press, 1983;3–11.
16. Rasmussen H, Bordier P. *The physiological and cellular basis of metabolic bone disease.* Baltimore: Williams & Wilkins, 1974;57–69.
17. Hodgson SF, Johnson KA, Muhs JM, Lufkin EG, McCarthy JT.

Outpatient percutaneous biopsy of the iliac crest: methods, morbidity and patient acceptance. *Mayo Clin Proc* 1986;61:28–33.

18. Recker RR, ed. *Bone histomorphometry: techniques and interpretation.* Boca Raton, FL: CRC Press, 1983.

19. Weinstein RS, Sappington LJ. Qualitative bone defect in uremic osteosclerosis. *Metabolism* 1982;31:805–11.

20. Woods CG, Morgan DB, Paterson CR, Gossman HH. Measurement of osteoid in bone biopsy. *J Pathol Bacteriol* 1968;95:441–7.

21. Whyte MP, Kim GS, Bergfeld MA, Murphy WA, Teitelbaum SL. Marked discrepancy between modified Masson and von Kossa stains for osteoid in selected cases of hypophosphatemic osteomalacia. *J Bone Miner Res* 1986;1S:81.

22. Taylor HC, Santa-Cruz D, Teitelbaum SL, Bergfeld MA, Whyte MP. Assessment of calcitriol and inorganic phosphate therapy before cure of oncogenic osteomalacia by resection of a mixed mesenchymal tumor. *Bone* 1988;9:37–43.

23. Parfitt AM, Mathews CHE, Villanueva AR, Frame B, Rao DS. Relationship between surface, volume and thickness of iliac trabecular bone in aging and in osteoporosis: implications for the microanatomic and cellular mechanisms of bone loss. *J Clin Invest* 1983;72:1396–1409.

24. Sato K, Byers P. Quantitative study of tunneling and hook resorption in metabolic bone disease. *Calcif Tissue Int* 1981;33:459–66.

25. Baron R, Vignery A, Lang R. Reversal phase and osteopenia: defective coupling of resorption to formation in the pathogenesis of osteoporosis. In: DeLuca HF, Frost HM, Jee WSS, Johnston CC, Parfitt AM, eds. *Osteoporosis: recent advances in pathogenesis and treatment.* Baltimore: University Park Press, 1981:311–20.

26. Windholz M, Budavari S, Strumtsos LY, Fertig MN, eds. *The Merck index.* Rahway, NJ: Merck & Co., 1976;44.

27. Burkhardt R, Kettner G, Bohm W, et al. Changes in trabecular bone, hematopoiesis and bone marrow vessels in aplastic anemia, primary osteoporosis, and old age: a comparative histomorphometric study. *Bone* 1987;8:157–64.

28. Meunier P, Aaron J, Edouard C, Vignon G. Osteoporosis and the replacement of cell populations of the marrow by adipose tissue. *Clin Orthop Rel Res* 1971;80:147–54.

29. Frame B, Nixon RK. Bone-marrow mast cells in osteoporosis of aging. *N Engl J Med* 1968;279:626–30.

30. Weinstein RS, Lutcher CL. Chronic erythroid hyperplasia and accelerated bone turnover. *Metab Bone Dis Relat Res* 1983;5:7–12.

31. Fallon MD, Perry HM, Teitelbaum SL. Skeletal sarcoidosis with osteopenia. *Metab Bone Dis Rel Res* 1981;3:171–4.

32. DeSimone DP, Brilliant HL, Basile J, Bell NH. Granulomatous infiltration of the talus and abnormal vitamin D and calcium metabolism in a patient with sarcoidosis: successful treatment with hydroxychloroquine. *Am J Med* 1989;87:694–6.

33. Mathews M, Stauffer M, Cameron EC, Maloney N, Sherrard DJ. Bone biopsy to diagnose hyperoxaluria in patients with renal failure. *Ann Intern Med* 1979;90:777–9.

34. Tam CS, Harrison JE, Heersche JNM, et al. Short term variation in the rate of apposition of mineralized bone matrix in small animals. *Metab Bone Dis Relat Res.* 1980;2S:159–66.

35. Rahn BA. Polychrome fluorescence labeling of bone formation. *Zeiss-Information No. 85,* 1978.

36. Birkenhager-Frenkel DH, Birkenhager JC. Bone appositional rate and percentage of doubly and singly labeled surfaces: comparison of data from 5 and 20 μm sections. *Bone* 1987;8:7–12.

37. Chavassieux PM, Arlot ME, Meunier PJ. Intermethod variation in bone histomorphometry: comparison between manual and computerized methods applied to iliac bone biopsies. *Bone* 1985;6:221–9.

38. Recker RR, Heaney RP. Effects of age, sex, and race on bone remodeling. In: Kleerekoper M, Krane SM, eds. *Clinical disorders of bone and mineral metabolism.* New York: Mary Ann Liebert, 1989;59–70.

39. Chavassieux PM, Arlot ME, Meunier PJ. Intersample variation on bone histomorphometry: comparison between parameter values measured on two contiguous transiliac bone biopsies. *Calcif Tissue Int* 1985;37:345–50.

40. Weinstein RS. Decreased mineralization in hemodialysis patients after subtotal parathyroidectomy. *Calcif Tissue Int* 1982;34:16–20.

41. Recker RR, Kimmel DB, Parfitt AM, Davies KM, Keshawarz N, Hinders S. Static and tetracycline-based bone histomorphometric data from 34 normal postmenopausal females. *J Bone Miner Res* 1988;3:133–44.

42. Parfitt AM. The cellular mechanisms of osteoid accumulation in metabolic bone disease. In: *Mineral metabolism research in Italy,* vol 4. Milan: Wichtig Editore, 1984;3–9.

43. Vedi S, Compston JE. Direct and indirect measurements of osteoid seam width in human iliac crest trabecular bone. *Metab Bone Dis Relat Res* 1984;5:269–74.

44. Quarles LD, Lobaugh B. Equivalency of various methods for estimating osteoid seam width. *J Bone Miner Res* 1989;4:671–7.

45. Birkenhager-Frenkel DH, Courpron P, Hupscher EA, et al. Age-related changes in cancellous bone structure. *Bone Miner* 1988;4:197–216.

46. Lalor BC, Freemont AJJ, Laite R, Mawer EB, Bogle S, Adams PH. The determinants of trabecular bone mass in primary hyperparathyroidism. *Bone* 1986;7:310.

47. Charhon SA, Edouard CM, Arlot ME, Meunier PJ. Effects of parathyroid hormone on remodeling of iliac trabecular bone packets in patients with primary hyperparathyroidism. *Clin Orthop Rel Res* 1980;162:255–63.

48. Bordier PJ, Arnaud C, Hawker C, Tun Chot S, Hioco D. Relationship between serum immunoreactive parathyroid hormone, osteoclastic and osteocytic bone resorptions and serum calcium in primary hyperparathyroidism and osteomalacia. In: Frame B, Parfitt AM, Duncan H, eds. *Clinical aspects of metabolic bone disease.* Amsterdam: Excerpta Medica, 1973;222–8.

49. Wilde CD, Jaworski ZF, Villanueva AR, Frost HM. Quantitative histological measurements of bone turnover in primary hyperparathyroidism. *Calcif Tissue Res* 1973;12:137–42.

50. Rasmussen H, Bordier P. *The physiological and cellular basis of metabolic bone disease.* Baltimore: Waverly Press, 1974.

51. Tam CS, Bayley A, Cross EG, Murray TM, Harrison JE. Increased bone apposition in primary hyperparathyroidism: measurements based on short interval tetracycline labeling of bone. *Metabolism* 1982;31:759–65.

52. Melsen F, Mosekilde L. Trabecular bone mineralization lag time determined by tetracycline double-labeling in normal and certain pathological conditions. *Acta Pathol Microbiol Scand* 1980;88:83–8.

53. Silverberg SJ, Shane E, De La Cruz L, et al. Skeletal disease in primary hyperparathyroidism. *J Bone Miner Res* 1989;4:283–91.

54. Stewart AF, Vignery A, Silverglate A, et al. Quantitative bone histomorphometry in humoral hypercalcemia if malignancy: uncoupling of bone cell activity. *J Clin Endocrinol Metab* 1982;55:219–27.

55. Parisien M, Silverberg SJ, Shane E, et al. Preservation of trabecular plates in primary hyperparathyroidism. *J Bone Miner Res* 1989;4S:307.

56. Weinstein RS, Harris RL. Hypercalcemic hyperparathyroidism and hypophosphatemic osteomalacia complicating neurofibromatosis. *Calcif Tissue Int* 1990;46:361–6.

57. Coen G, Bondatti F, de Matteis A, et al. Severe vitamin D deficiency in a case of primary hyperparathyroidism caused by parathyroid lipoadenoma, effect of 250HD₃ treatment. *Miner Electrolyte Metab* 1989;15:332–7.

58. Merz WA, Olah AT, Schenk RK, Dambacher MA, Guncaga J, Haas HG. Bone remodeling in primary hyperparathyroidism. *Israel J Med Sci* 1971;7:494.

59. Ramser JR, Frost HM, Smith R. Tetracycline-based measurement of the tissue and cell dynamics in rib of a 25-year-old man with active acromegaly. *Clin Orthop* 1966;49:169–72.

60. Riggs L, Randall R, Wahner H, Jowsey J, Kelly P, Singh M. The nature of the metabolic bone disorder in acromegaly. *J Clin Endocrinol Metab* 1971;34:911–8.

61. Aloia JF, Roginsky MS, Jowsey J, Dombrowski CS, Shukla KK, Cohn SH. Skeletal metabolism and body composition in acromegaly. *J Clin Endocrinol Metab* 1972;35:543–51.

62. Villanueva A, Frost H, Ilnicki L, Frame B, Smith R, Arnstein R.

Cortical bone dynamics measured by means of tetracycline labeling in 21 cases of osteoporosis. *J Lab Clin Med* 1966;68:599–616.

63. Halse J, Melsen F, Mosekilde L. Iliac crest bone mass and remodeling in acromegaly. *Acta Endocrinol* 1981;97:18–22.

64. Cascio VL, Bonucci E, Imbimbo B, et al. Bone loss after glucocorticoid therapy. *Calcif Tissue Int* 1984;36:435–8.

65. Bressot C, Meunier PJ, Chapuy MC, Lejeune E, Edouard C, Darby AJ. Histomorphometric profile, pathophysiology and reversibility of corticosteroid-induced osteoporosis. *Metab Bone Dis Relat Res* 1979;1:303–11.

66. Hahn TJ, Halstead LR, Teitelbaum SL, Hahn BH. Altered mineral metabolism in glucocorticoid-induced osteopenia. *J Clin Invest* 1979;64:655–65.

67. Dempster DW, Arlot MA, Meunier PJ. Mean wall thickness and formation periods of trabecular bone packets in corticosteroid-induced osteoporosis. *Calcif Tissue Int* 1983;35:410–17.

68. Klein M, Villanueva AR, Frost HM. A quantitative histological study of rib from 18 patients treated with adrenal cortical steroids. *Acta Orthop Scand* 1965;35:171–84.

69. Dempster DW. Bone histomorphometry in glucocorticoid-induced osteoporosis. *J Bone Miner Res* 1989;4:137–41.

70. Melsen F, Mosekilde L. Dynamic studies of trabecular bone formation and osteoid maturation in normal and certain pathological conditions. *Metab Bone Dis Relat Res* 1978;1:45–8.

71. Weinstein RS, Bryce GF, Sappington LJ, King DW, Gallagher BB. Decreased serum ionized calcium and normal vitamin D metabolite levels with anticonvulsant drug treatment. *J Clin Endocrinol Metab* 1984;58:1003–9.

72. Evans RA, Bridgeman M, Hills E, Dunstan CR. Immobilization hypercalcemia. *Miner Electrolyte Metab* 1984;10:244–8.

73. Vico L, Chappard D, Alexandre C, et al. Effects of a 120 day period of bed-rest on bone mass and bone cell activities in man: attempts at countermeasure. *Bone Miner* 1987;2:383–94.

74. Minaire P, Meunier P, Edouard C, Bernard J, Courpron P, Bourret J. Quantitative histological data on disuse osteoporosis. *Calcif Tissue Res* 1974;17:57–73.

75. Stout S. The effects of long-term immobilization on the histomorphology of human cortical bone. *Calcif Tissue Int* 1982;34:337–42.

76. Judge DM, Schneider V, LeBlanc A. Disuse osteoporosis. *J Bone Miner Res* 1989;4S:238.

77. Fallon MD, Whyte MP, Craig RB, Teitelbaum SL. Mast-cell proliferation in postmenopausal osteoporosis. *Calcif Tissue Int* 1983;35:29–31.

78. Peart KM, Ellis HA. Quantitative observations on iliac bone marrow mast cells in chronic renal failure. *J Clin Pathol* 1975;28:947–55.

79. Fallon MD, Whyte MP, Teitelbaum SL. Systemic mastocytosis associated with generalized osteopenia. *Hum Pathol* 1981;12:813–20.

80. Korenblat PE, Wedner HJ, Whyte MP, Frankel S, Avioli LV. Systemic mastocytosis. *Arch Intern Med* 1984;144:2249–53.

81. Cundy T, Beneton MNC, Darby AJ, Marshall WJ, Kanis JA. Osteopenia in systemic mastocytosis: natural history and responses to treatment with inhibitors of bone resorption. *Bone* 1987;8:149–55.

82. Hills E, Dunstan CR, Evans RA. Bone metabolism in systemic mastocytosis. *J Bone Joint Surg* 1981;63-A:665–9.

83. Cryer PE, Kissane JM. Osteopenia. *Am J Med* 1980;69:915–22.

84. te Velde J, Vismans FJFE, Leenheers-Binnendijk L, Vos CJ, Smeenk D, Bijvoet OLM. The eosinophilic fibrohistiocytic lesion of the bone marrow. *Virchows Arch A Path Anat Histol* 1978;377:277–85.

85. Rywlin AM, Hoffman EP, Ortega RS. Eosinophilic fibrohistiocytic lesion of bone marrow: a distinctive new morphologic finding, probably related to drug hypersensitivity. *Blood* 1972;40:464–72.

86. Whyte MP, Bergfeld MA, Murphy WA, Avioli AV, Teitelbaum SL. Postmenopausal osteoporosis, a heterogeneous disorder as assessed by histomorphometric analysis of iliac crest bone from untreated patients. *Am J Med* 1982;72:193–202.

87. Brown JP, Delmas PD, Arlot M, Meunier PJ. Active bone turnover of the cortico-endosteal envelope in postmenopausal osteoporosis. *J Clin Endocrinol Metab* 1987;64:954–9.

88. Eastell R, Delmas PD, Hodgson SF, Eriksen EF, Mann KG, Riggs BL. Bone formation rate in older women: concurrent assessment with bone histomorphometry, calcium kinetics, and biochemical markers. *J Clin Endocrinol Metab* 1988;67:741–8.

89. Carasco MG, de Vernejoul MC, Sterkers Y, Morieux C, Kuntz D, Miravet L. Decreased bone formation in osteoporotic patients compared with age-matched controls. *Calcif Tissue Int* 1989;44:173–5.

90. Marie PJ, Sabbagh A, de Vernejoul MC, Lomri A. Osteocalcin and deoxyribonucleic acid synthesis in vitro and histomorphometric indices of bone formation in postmenopausal osteoporosis. *J Clin Endocrinol Metab* 1989;69:272–9.

91. Steiniche T, Hasling C, Charles P, Eriksen EF, Mosekilde L, Melsen F. A randomized study on the effects of estrogen/gestagen or high dose oral calcium on trabecular bone remodeling in postmenopausal osteoporosis. *Bone* 1989;10:313–20.

92. McDermott MT, Kidd GS. The role of calcitonin in the development and treatment of osteoporosis. *Endocr Rev* 1987;8:377–90.

93. Kragstrup J, Shijie Z, Mosekilde L, Melsen F. Effects of sodium fluoride, vitamin D, and calcium on cortical bone remodeling in osteoporotic patients. *Calcif Tissue Int* 1989;45:337–41.

94. Eriksen EF, Mosekilde L, Melsen F. Effect of sodium fluoride, calcium, phosphate, and vitamin D_2 on trabecular bone balance and remodeling in osteoporotics. *Bone* 1985;6:381–9.

95. Parfitt AM. The localization of aluminum in bone: implications for the mechanism of fixation and for the pathogenesis of aluminum-related bone disease. *Int J Artif Organs* 1988;11:79–90.

96. Gundberg CM, Weinstein RS. Multiple immunoreactive forms of osteocalcin in uremic serum. *J Clin Invest* 1986;77:1762–7.

97. Andress DL, Norris KC, Coburn JW, Slatopolsky EA, Sherrard DJ. Intravenous calcitriol in the treatment of refractory osteitis fibrosa of chronic renal failure. *N Engl J Med* 1989;321:274–9.

98. Qiu M-C, Mathews C, Parfitt AM. Osteoclastic resorption of osteoid in secondary hyperparathyroidism. In: Frame B, Potts JT Jr, eds. *Clinical disorders of bone and mineral metabolism.* Amsterdam: Excerpta Medica, 1983;209–12.

99. Maloney NA, Ott SM, Alfrey AC, Miller NL, Coburn JW, Sherrard DJ. Histological quantitation of aluminum in iliac bone from patients with renal failure. *J Lab Clin Med* 1982;99:206–16.

100. Malluche HH, Ritz E, Lange HP, et al. Bone histology in incipient and advanced renal failure. *Kidney Int* 1976;9:355–62.

101. deVernejoul MC, Kuntz D, Miravet L, Gueris J, Bielakoff J, Ryckewaert A. Bone histomorphometry in hemodialysis patients. *Metab Bone Dis Relat Res* 1981;3:175–9.

102. Delmez JA, Fallon MD, Harter HR, Hruska KA, Slatopolsky E, Teitelbaum S. Does strict phosphorus control precipitate renal osteomalacia? *J Clin Endocrinol Metab* 1986;62:747–52.

103. McCarthy JT, Kurtz SB, McCall JT. Elevated bone aluminum content in dialysis patients without osteomalacia. *Mayo Clin Proc* 1985;60:315–20.

104. Aubia J, Serrano S, Marinoso LL, et al. Osteodystrophy of diabetes in chronic dialysis: a histomorphometric study. *Calcif Tissue Int* 1988;42:297–301.

105. Quarles LD, Gitelman HJ, Drezner MK. Aluminum-associated bone disease: what's in a name? *J Bone Miner Res* 1986;1:389–90.

106. Malluche HH, Faugere MC. *Atlas of mineralized bone histology.* Basel: S Karger, 1986.

107. Parfitt AM, Rao D, Stanciu J, Villanueva AR. Comparison of aluminum related with vitamin D related osteomalacia by tetracycline based bone histomorphometry. In: Massry SG, Olmer M, Ritz E, eds. Phosphate and mineral homeostasis. *Adv Exp Biol Med* 1986;208:283–7.

108. Moriniere P, Cohen-Solal M, Belbrik S, et al. Disappearance of aluminic bone disease in a long term asymptomatic dialysis population restricting Al(OH)₃ intake: emergence of an idiopathic adynamic bone disease not related to aluminum. *Nephron* 1989;53:93–101.

109. Melsen F, Mosekilde L, Kragstrup J. Metabolic bone diseases as evaluated by bone histomorphometry. In: Recker RR, ed. *Bone histomorphometry: techniques and interpretation.* Boca Raton, FL: CRC Press, 1983;280–1.

110. Nielsen HE, Melsen F, Christensen MS. Spontaneous fractures

following renal transplantation. *Miner Electrolyte Metab* 1979;2:323–30.

111. Andress DL, Ott SM, Maloney NA, Sherrard DJ. Effect of parathyroidectomy on bone aluminum accumulation in chronic renal failure. *N Engl J Med* 1985;312:468–73.

112. Dunstan CR, Hills E, Norman AW, et al. Treatment of hemodialysis bone disease with 24,25-(OH)$_2$D$_3$ and 1,25-(OH)$_2$D$_3$ alone or in combination. *Miner Electrolyte Metab* 1985;11:358–68.

113. Malluche HM, Smith AJ, Abreo K, Faugere M-C. The use of deferoxamine in the management of aluminum accumulations in bone in patients with renal failure. *N Engl J Med* 1984;311:140–4.

114. Andress DL, Nebeker HG, Ott SM, et al. Bone histologic response to deferoxamine in aluminum-related bone disease. *Kidney Int* 1987;31:1344–50.

115. Parfitt AM, Miller MJ, Frame B, et al. Metabolic bone disease after intestinal bypass for treatment of obesity. *Ann Intern Med* 1978;89:193–9.

116. Garrick R, Ireland AW, Posen S. Bone abnormalities after gastric surgery. *Ann Intern Med* 1971;75:221–5.

117. Weinstein RS. Osteomalacia. In: Hurst JW, ed. *Medicine for the practicing physician,* 2nd ed. Boston: Butterworth, 1988;552–7.

118. Compston JE, Horton LWL, Laker MF, Woodhead JS, Gazet JC, Pilkington TRE. Treatment of bone disease after jejunoileal bypass for obesity with oral 1-hydroxyvitamin D$_3$. *Gut* 1980;21:669–74.

119. Coindre J, David J, Riviere L, et al. Bone loss in hypothyroidism with hormone replacement. *Arch Intern Med* 1986;146:48–53.

120. Fallon MD, Perry HM, Bergfeld M, Droke D, Teitelbaum SL, Avioli LV. Exogenous hyperthyroidism with osteoporosis. *Arch Intern Med* 1983;143:442–4.

121. Eriksen EF, Mosekilde L, Melsen F. Trabecular bone remodeling and bone balance in hyperthyroidism. *Bone* 1985;6:421–8.

122. Eriksen EF, Mosekilde L, Melsen F. Kinetics of trabecular bone resorption and formation in hypothyroidism: evidence for a positive balance per remodeling cycle. *Bone* 1986;7:101–8.

123. Melsen F, Mosekilde L. Morphometric and dynamic studies of bone changes in hyperthyroidism. *Acta Pathol Microbiol Scand* 1977;85:141–50.

124. Meunier PJ, Bianchi GS, Edouard CM, Bernard JC, Courpron P, Vignon GE. Bony manifestations of thyrotoxicosis. *Orthop Clin N Am* 1972;3:745–74.

125. Kragstrup J, Melsen F, Mosekilde L. Effects of thyroid hormone(s) on mean wall thickness of trabecular bone packets. *Metab Bone Dis Relat Res* 1981;3:181–5.

126. Melsen F, Mosekilde L, Eriksen EF, Charles P, Steinicke T. In vivo hormonal effects on trabecular bone remodeling, osteoid mineralization, and skeletal turnover. In: Kleerekoper M, Krane SM, eds. *Clinical disorders of bone and mineral metabolism.* New York: Mary Ann Liebert, 1989;73–87.

127. Reid IR, Hardy DC, Murphy WA, Teitelbaum SL, Bergfeld MA, Whyte MP. X-linked hypophosphatemia: a clinical, biochemical, and histological assessment of morbidity in adults. *Medicine* 1989;68:336–52.

128. Parfitt AM, Kleerekoper M. Diagnostic value of bone histomorphometry and comparison of histologic measurements and biochemical indices of bone remodeling. In: Christiansen C, Arnaud CD, Nordin BEC, Parfitt AM, Peck WA, Riggs BL, eds. *Osteoporosis.* Glostrup, Denmark: Aalborg Stiftsbogtrykkeri, 1984;111–9.

129. Meunier PJ, Coindre JM, Edouard CM, Arlot ME. Bone histomorphometry in Paget's disease. *Arthritis Rheum* 1980;23:1095–103.

130. Singer FR. *Paget's disease of bone.* New York: Plenum Press, 1977.

131. Fornasier VL, Stapleton K, Williams CC. Histological changes in Paget's disease treated with calcitonin. *Hum Pathol* 1978;9:455–61.

132. Johnston CC, Khaira MRA, Meunier PJ. Use of etidronate (EHDP) in Paget's disease of bone. *Arthritis Rheum* 1980;23:1172–6.

133. Weinstein RS. Focal mineralization defect during disodium etidronate treatment of calcinosis. *Calcif Tissue Int* 1982;34:224–8.

134. Boyce BF, Smith L, Fogelman I, Johnston E, Ralston S, Boyle IT. Focal osteomalacia due to low-dose diphosphonate therapy in Paget's disease. *Lancet* 1984;1:821–4.

135. Weinstein RS, Whyte MP. Heterogeneity of adult hypophosphatasia. *Arch Intern Med* 1981;141:727–31.

136. Fallon MD, Teitelbaum SL, Weinstein RS, Goldfischer S, Brown DM, Whyte MP. Hypophosphatasia: clinicopathologic comparison of the infantile, childhood, and adult forms. *Medicine* 1984;63:12–24.

137. Whyte MP, Teitelbaum SL, Murphy WA, Bergfeld MA, Avioli LV. Adult hypophosphatasia. *Medicine* 1979;58:329–47.

138. Whyte MP. Hypophosphatasia. In: Scriver CR, Beaudet AL, Sly WS, Valle D, eds. *The metabolic basis of inherited disease,* 6th ed. New York: McGraw-Hill, 1989;2843–56.

139. Teitelbaum SL, Kraft WJ, Lang R, Avioli LV. Bone collagen aggregation abnormalities in osteogenesis imperfecta. *Calcif Tissue Res* 1974;17:75–9.

140. Doty SB, Mathews RS. Electron microscopic and histochemical investigation of osteogenesis imperfecta tarda. *Clin Orthop Relat Res.* 1971;80:191–201.

141. Riley FC, Brown DM. Morphological and biochemical studies in osteogenesis imperfecta. *J Lab Clin Med* 1971;78:1000.

142. Weinstein RS. Osteogenesis imperfecta: histomorphometric investigation of a family. *Clin Res* 1978;26:792A.

143. Villanueva AR, Frost HM. Bone formation in human osteogenesis imperfecta, measured by tetracycline bone labeling. *Acta Orthop Scand* 1970;41:531–8.

144. Ramser JR, Villanueva AR, Pirok D, Frost HM. Tetracycline-based measurement of bone dynamics in 3 women with osteogenesis imperfecta. *Clin Orthop* 1966;49:151–62.

145. Falvo KA, Bullough PG. Osteogenesis imperfecta: a histometric analysis. *J Bone Joint Surg* 1973;55-A:275–86.

146. Jett S, Ramser JR, Frost HM, Villanueva AR. Bone turnover and osteogenesis imperfecta. *Arch Pathol* 1966;81:112–6.

147. Spencer H, Rubio N, Rubio E, Indreika M, Seitam A. Chronic alcoholism: frequently overlooked cause of osteoporosis in men. *Am J Med* 1986;80:393–7.

148. Feitelberg S, Epstein S, Ismail F, D'Amanda C. Deranged bone mineral metabolism in chronic alcoholism. *Metabolism* 1987;36:322–6.

149. Diamond T, Stiel D, Lunzer M, Wilkinson M, Posen S. Ethanol reduces bone formation and may cause osteoporosis. *Am J Med* 1989;86:282–8.

150. Crilly RG, Anderson C, Hogan D, Delaquerriere-Richardson L. Bone histomorphometry, bone mass, and related parameters in alcoholic males. *Calcif Tissue Int* 1988;43:269–76.

151. Bikle DD, Genant HK, Cann C, Recker RR, Halloran BP, Strewler GJ. Bone disease in alcohol abuse. *Ann Intern Med* 1985;103:42–8.

152. Lalor B, Davies M, Adams PH, Counihan TB. Aetiology of osteoporosis in heavy drinkers. In: Norman AW, Schaefer K, Grigoleit H-G, von Herrath D, eds. *Vitamin D, chemical, biochemical and clinical update.* Berlin: Walter de Gruyter, 1985;1012.

153. Stellon AJ, Webb A, Compston J, Williams R. Lack of osteomalacia in chronic cholestatic liver disease. *Bone* 1986;7:181–5.

154. Shih M, Anderson C. Does "hepatic osteodystrophy" differ from peri- and postmenopausal osteoporosis? A histomorphometric study. *Calcif Tissue Int* 1987;41:187–91.

155. Hodgson SF, Dickson ER, Wahner HW, Johnson KA, Mann KG, Riggs BL. Bone loss and reduced osteoblast function in primary biliary cirrhosis. *Ann Intern Med* 1985;103:855–60.

156. Herlong HF, Recker RR, Maddrey WC. Bone disease in primary biliary cirrhosis: histologic features and responses to 25-hydroxyvitamin D. *Gastroenterology* 1982;83:103–8.

157. Diamond TH, Stiel D, Lunzer M, McDowall D, Eckstein RP, Posen S. Hepatic osteodystrophy: static and dynamic bone histomorphometry and serum bone Gla-protein in 80 patients with chronic liver disease. *Gastroenterology* 1989;96:213–21.

158. Perry HM, Weinstein RS, Teitelbaum ST, Avioli LV, Fallon MD. Pseudofractures in the absence of osteomalacia. *Skeletal Radiol* 1982;8:17–9.

159. McKenna MJ, Kleerekoper M, Ellis BI, Rao DS, Parfitt AM, Frame B. Atypical insufficiency fractures confused with looser zones of osteomalacia. *Bone* 1987;8:71–8.

160. Hauge MD, Cooper KL, Litin SC. Insufficiency fractures of the pelvis that stimulate metastatic disease. *Mayo Clin Proc* 1988;63:807–12.

Disorders of Bone and Mineral Metabolism,
edited by Fredric L. Coe and Murray J. Favus,
© 1992 by Raven Press, Ltd. All rights reserved.

CHAPTER **22**

The Physiologic and Pathogenetic Significance of Bone Histomorphometric Data

A. M. Parfitt

In Chapter 21, Weinstein describes how a bone biopsy can help to distinguish between various forms of metabolic bone disease, to select appropriate treatment, and to monitor its effects, whether beneficial or harmful. In the present chapter I relate the results of measurements made on a bone biopsy obtained after double tetracycline labeling to the underlying cellular mechanisms, both physiologic and pathologic. The purpose is partly to explain how disordered bone remodeling may have contributed to the clinical problem of an individual patient, but more particularly to promote insight into the pathogenesis of disease and the mode of action of different forms of treatment. Dynamic bone histomorphometry is unable to identify the primary target of any skeletally active agent, whether endogenously produced or exogenously administered. Nevertheless, at present it is the only way to determine the cumulative summation of all effects of an agent on bone cell function and bone remodeling, whether primary or secondary, direct or indirect, immediate or remote.

CONCEPTS OF BONE REMODELING

The discussion assumes reasonable familiarity with the contents of Chapters 10 to 14, and detailed knowledge of Chapter 15, but I will summarize the most salient points from my own perspective. Bone is remodeled in temporally discrete episodes that occur at spatially discrete sites, each episode comprising the erosion and refilling of a cavity on a bone surface by an organized group of cells, the basic multicellular unit (BMU) (1–3). Included in the BMU are not only osteoclasts, osteoblasts,

A. M. Parfitt: Bone and Mineral Research Laboratory, Henry Ford Hospital, 2799 West Grand Boulevard, E&R 7092, Detroit, Michigan 48202

and their precursors, but capillaries, autonomic nerve fibers, and loose connective tissue. Depending on whether the cavity is overfilled, exactly filled, or underfilled, the outcome of each episode is a net gain, no change, or a net loss of bone, but once completed, the transaction is irrevocable. The summation of all such transactions determines the direction and magnitude of bone balance on a particular surface over a particular period of time. All physiologic, pathologic, and pharmacologic influences on the amount and structure of bone are mediated by the cellular mechanisms that underlie the net outcome of each remodeling episode and the frequency with which the episodes occur.

Analogy between the Remodeling Cycle and the Cell Cycle

All bone remodeling begins with the event of activation that initiates the conversion of a small region of surface from remodeling quiescence to remodeling activity. The beginning of a new cycle of remodeling is often referred to erroneously as *activation of osteoclasts,* but initially no osteoclasts are present on the surface, only lining cells. The quiescent surface is analogous to the G_0 period of the cell cycle in tissues with low turnover, and activation of the surface is analogous to the transition from G_0 to G_1 that occurs in some cells when an increase in the supply of cells is needed. Activation is followed by recruitment of precursor cells, proliferation of new blood vessels, and preparation of the bone surface to allow the mononuclear precursors access, attraction, and adhesion to the surface, which is followed by their fusion into multinucleated osteoclasts (4). These processes are analogous to the events during G_1 that prepare for the onset of DNA synthesis. To continue the analogy, resorption corresponds to S phase, reversal to G_2, and formation to

M. Three aspects of this analogy are important: First, both cell cycle and remodeling cycle are initiated by a trigger out of a resting state. Second, both cycles comprise two periods of execution, always in the same order, each preceded by a period of preparation. Finally, once started, both cycles proceed to completion without the need for further intervention.

Relationship between Remodeling Cycles and Periods

In the human ilium the average duration of the quiescent period between successive cyclic episodes of remodeling at the same location is about 30 months, much longer than the duration of each episode (the remodeling period), which is about 4–6 months. The average duration between successive activation events—the total remodeling cycle period, including the remodeling and quiescent periods—is about 3 years. The duration of quiescence varies widely between subjects and between locations as an inverse function of the frequency of remodeling activation, which is the reciprocal of the total cycle period. Each location on a bone surface has its own remodeling history, which can be depicted as shown in Fig. 1. Several important points are apparent: First, there is a random component to remodeling that is inevitably associated with large sampling variation. Second, at any instant, every time point in the remodeling cycle is represented at multiple locations in the skeleton, because remodeling is incoherent, in the sense used by physicists for electromagnetic radiation. Consequently, a bone biopsy represents a sample in time as well as in space (2). Third, the cumulative effect of remodeling over a period of time depends both on the number of cycles that occurred in that time and on the events within each cycle (3; Fig. 2A and B). These two determinants can vary independently, and their relative contributions cannot be revealed by any biochemical or kinetic indices of bone turnover (2,4).

Three Levels of Organization of Bone Remodeling

Crucial to the understanding of bone remodeling is the distinction between recruitment of new, partly differentiated, immature precursor cells, and the expression of the differentiated function of existing mature cells. Remodeling and its outcome are regulated mainly by cell recruitment rather than by cell function (5). Few of the innumerable short-term changes in cell activity that can be induced experimentally have been shown to affect the quantity of work that is ultimately carried out. The four stages of the remodeling cycle represent in succession the recruitment of pre-osteoclasts, the expression of osteoclast function, the recruitment of preosteoblasts, and the

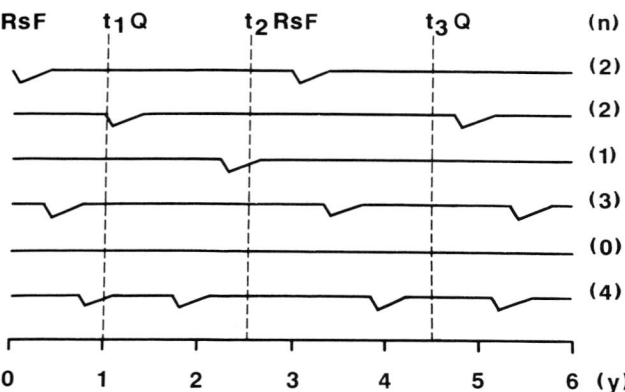

FIG. 1. Relationship between remodeling cycles and periods. The histories of six individual bone surface locations over a 6-year period are depicted diagrammatically to show successive periods of resorption (Rs—down), formation (F—up), and quiescence (Q—horizontal). It is assumed that final resorption depth and final wall thickness in each cycle are equal, so that bone balance is preserved. n = number of cycles at each location, which ranges from 0 to 4 with a mean of 2, corresponding to an activation frequency of 0.33 per year, assumed not to change over the period of observation. Biopsies at different times (t_1, t_2, and t_3) would intercept the six locations at different stages, and the different remodeling activities would be found in different proportions, with average values of 5.5% for Rs (1/18), 11% for F (2/18), and 83.5% for Q (15/18).

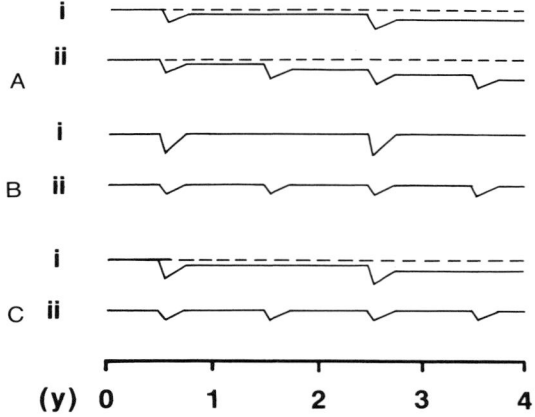

FIG. 2. Some implications of quantal remodeling theory. Each line represents the remodeling history of an individual bone surface location, as explained in the legend to Fig. 1. In Ai and Aii, with a constant deficit per remodeling cycle, the amount of bone lost from a surface (the difference between the final locations of the interrupted line and the solid line) increases with the rate of remodeling activation. In Bi and Bii, the same total rates of resorption and formation can be the result of fewer cycles with deeper cavities or of more cycles with shallower cavities. These two situations would have identical effects on biochemical and kinetic indices of remodeling, but arise from different cellular mechanisms. In Ci and Cii, if the number of osteoblasts that can be recruited per activation event is limited, for example by the availability of precursor cells, fewer but deeper cavities will lead to bone loss, whereas more but shallower cavities may allow maintenance of bone balance.

expression of osteoblast function. Because remodeling is incoherent, all four processes are going on all the time. The distinction between cell number and cell activity is fundamental, but because of the quantal nature of remodeling, there are not just two, but three levels at which the process must be examined: the birthrate of new teams of cells, the number of members in each team, and the total work capacity of each team member.

The concept of a team was developed to express the notion of a group of cells brought together at the same time and place to cooperate in carrying out a common task (5). A team of osteoclasts and a subsequent team of osteoblasts are each a subset (or component) of a BMU, as defined previously. The collective work of the team reflects the number of cells recruited, the rate at which each cell works, and its active lifespan, which together determine the total amount of work it can perform, and the manner in which the work of each cell is coordinated with that of its neighbors. The resorption of a small number of large cavities and a large number of small cavities could have different outcomes even if the total number of new osteoclasts were the same (Fig. 2c). Large cavities could outstrip the local capacity for osteoblast recruitment within a short window of time and produce irreversible structural changes such as trabecular plate perforation, leaving no surface upon which osteoblasts can build (6). On the other hand, the same total number of osteoblasts could lead to bone gain if concentrated in a small number of cavities, but to bone loss if distributed over a larger number (5,7). It is the focal balance between the total work of successive teams of osteoclasts and osteoblasts at the same location that determines the outcome of the remodeling transaction. Expressed another way, the osteoclast team determines the nature and magnitude of the task that must be completed by the osteo-

blast team if bone volume and structure are to be maintained (5).

Remodeling Cycle in Detail

In cortical bone, evolution of the remodeling process in three dimensions can be inferred from a combination of both longitudinal and transverse sections, although several points remain unclear (8). In cancellous bone, very little is known about the three-dimensional aspects of either resorption or formation, but the unfolding of these processes at a single location can be reconstructed using the number of eroded lamellae as a marker of time during resorption (9) and distance from the cement line as a marker of time during formation (9,10). In this analysis, distances and rates are measured in a perpendicular or vertical sense, as the bone surface retreats away from and advances toward its initial location, corresponding to resorption depth and wall thickness, respectively.

During the first 10 days of resorption, about two-thirds of the final depth of the cavity is eroded by multinucleated osteoclasts at a rate of 3–4 μm/day. During the next 20 days the remaining one-third is apparently eroded by mononuclear cells of uncertain nature at a rate of 0.5–0.7 μm/day. The transition between cell types and between rates is presumably gradual rather than abrupt. The origin and fate of the mononuclear resorbing cells remain unknown; since fission of human osteoclasts has been observed in vitro (Chapter 15) they could be disaggregated osteoclasts, but proof of this is lacking. The floor of the cavity is made smoother and then covered with a thin layer of cement substance, corresponding to the cement line in two-dimensional sections (11), in which the matrix contains less collagen and more sul-

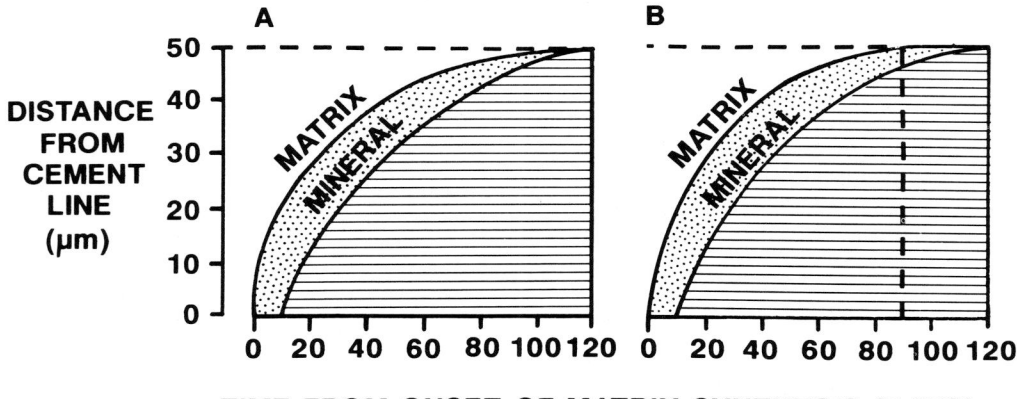

FIG. 3. Alternative models of bone formation. The graphs depict movement of the bone (osteoid) surface (*upper curve,* matrix apposition), and the osteoid–bone interface (*lower curve,* mineral apposition) as functions of time since the beginning of bone formation at an individual bone surface location. *Linear shading,* mineralized bone; *dotted shading,* osteoid. **A:** Matrix synthesis and mineralization continue throughout and terminate together. **B:** Matrix apposition ceases at 90 days (*vertical dashed line*), after which mineralization continues slowly until its completion.

fur, and which is less highly mineralized, but with a higher calcium/phosphorus ratio than in the adjacent bone (12). These reversal period activities are presumably carried out by the adjacent mononuclear cells, but the nature of these cells and their relationship to the mononuclear resorbing cells is unknown (11).

The osteoblasts that assemble on the cement surface are columnar and densely packed and begin immediately to deposit matrix at the rate of 2–3 μm/day; after 10–15 days the osteoid seam reaches a maximum thickness of about 20 μm and mineralization begins. The osteoblasts and their nuclei become progressively broader and flatter, and there is a steady fall in the rates of both matrix and mineral apposition (9,10). The osteoid seam declines in thickness, and after about 4–5 months it disappears, to be replaced by the endosteal membrane, and the cells on the surface complete their transformation to lining cells (2,3). There is some uncertainty about the latter stages of this process. According to one model (Fig. 3A), matrix apposition and mineralization continue throughout and terminate together (8–10); an alternative view (Fig. 3B) is that matrix apposition ceases first and mineralization continues slowly until its completion (5,13).

PRINCIPLES OF INTERPRETATION

Before particular histomorphometric measurements are considered, some general principles will be discussed. These each relate in some way to the central fact that the histologic features in a biopsy represent a series of events and processes existing in time that are randomly intercepted at different stages of their life history.

Relationship between Space and Time

The fundamental theorem of bone histomorphometry is that fractions of space are equivalent to fractions of time (8), provided that the bone is in a steady state, that remodeling activity is randomly distributed over the surface, and that a statistically adequate sample has been examined. For example, if a bone surface is subdivided according to the characteristics of different stages in remodeling, the fraction of the surface occupied by each subdivision is equal to the average fraction of time for which the corresponding remodeling activity is in progress, regardless of the rate at which the activity is carried out. The same principle applies to the fraction of bone volume occupied by osteoid, which is equivalent to the fraction of its total lifespan during which each moiety of bone is unmineralized. Consequently, a change in the relative extent of different histologic features usually reflects a change in their relative durations. For example, a disproportionate increase in the extent of eroded surface relative to osteoclast covered surface is due either to a

longer reversal period between resorption and formation, or to aborted remodeling with arrested resorption and absence of formation, as indicated in Chapter 21.

Birthrate and Lifespan

In cortical bone, osteoid seams and resorption cavities can be treated as individual members of a population whose size depends on both birthrate and lifespan. In cancellous bone, individual BMUs are less easy to study, and it is more convenient to express the same concept as

$$prevalence = incidence \times duration$$

For example, if the fractional surface extent of osteoid is 0.15 and the mean duration of an osteoid seam (formation period) is 150 days, then

$$0.15 = 1/1000 \text{ days} \times 150 \text{ days}$$

The observed prevalence and duration imply that at every point on the surface, a new moiety of osteoid appears once every 1000 days, which is an alternative expression of the activation frequency per unit of bone surface. It is evident that an increase in the surface extent of any histologic feature can result from either an increase in activation frequency or an increase in the time required to complete the corresponding remodeling activity. Generally, this is the result of a retardation in the rate of the relevant activity (8) but can also reflect an increase in the amount of work to be performed.

The same kind of analysis can be applied to the volume of osteoid. For example, if the fractional volume extent of osteoid is 0.02 and the mean osteoid tissue lifespan (equivalent to the mean mineralization lag time) is 40 days, then

$$0.02 = 1/2000 \times 40$$

In other words, the observed prevalence and duration of osteoid imply that on the average, each moiety of bone is replaced by osteoid once every 2000 days, equivalent to a volume-based bone formation rate, or bone turnover rate, of about 18% per year. An increase in osteoid volume can result from an increase either in activation frequency or in lag time; this and other relationships of similar form will be explored in more detail in a later section.

Transient States and Steady States

For bone remodeling to be in a steady state there should have been no significant perturbation, either in activation frequency or in individual cell function, for a time equal to about twice the total remodeling period (8). For example, if there has been a recent increase in activation frequency, there will be an increase in the number of resorption sites without a corresponding increase in the number of formation sites, a disproportion that may erroneously be taken as evidence for so-called "uncoupling." Similarly, a biopsy taken a few months after beginning treatment of osteomalacia may show a very high bone formation rate; this is not a reflection of current activation frequency but of the more or less simultaneous resumption of mineralization over most of the extended osteoid surface. Transient effects can also occur with measurements that change during the life history of an individual osteoid seam (Figs. 3 and 4). For example, if activation frequency increased only 1–2 months ago, there would be a higher than usual proportion of osteoblasts in their period of maximum vigor, and the mean apposition rate and mean osteoid thickness would be increased, even if the function of each individual cell was normal.

Individual Values and Mean Values

The transient effect of an increase in activation frequency on appositional rate is a specific example of the importance of considering individual measurements as well as mean values. As bone histomorphometry is currently practiced on cancellous bone, this distinction applies only to measurements of distance rather than of perimeter and area (14), since remodeling sites are not characterized as individual structures. As well as a change in the age distribution of distance measurements due to a change in activation frequency, mean values may conceal other important differences. For example, treatment with sodium fluoride may create two populations of measurements, one derived from the bone that was present before treatment and the other from the new bone formed in response to treatment. Focal defects in mineralization from any cause (15) may produce two populations of osteoid width measurements, one higher and one lower than normal, with a normal mean value. The existence of two populations may be obvious to an experienced observer but can also be demonstrated by probit analysis of the individual values (8), one of the several advantages of direct rather than indirect measurements of distance (14). A more subtle example is the possibility of bias due to differential loss of individual

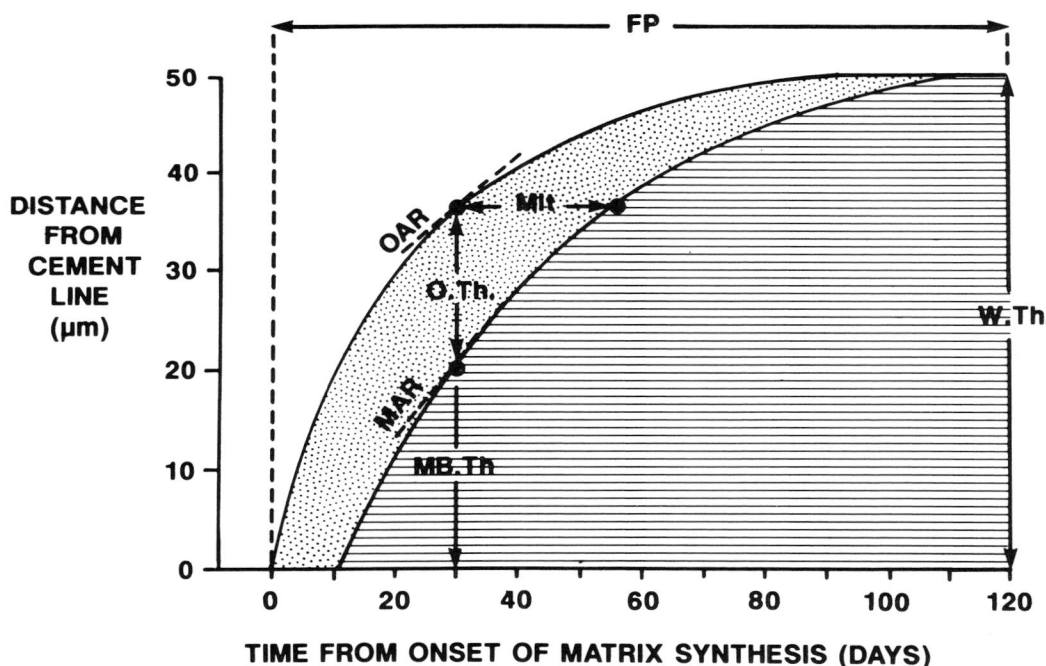

FIG. 4. Model of bone formation, with growth curves showing distances from cement line as functions of time. At any distance from the cement line, the horizontal distance between the lines is the instantaneous mineralization lag time at that distance. At any time, the vertical distance between the lines is the instantaneous osteoid thickness at that time. At any point the slopes of the lines (tangents) represent instantaneous apposition rates. For example, at $t = 30$ days, the instantaneous values are 20 μm for mineralized bone thickness, 16 μm for osteoid thickness, 0.5 μm/day for osteoid apposition rate, and 0.8 μm/day for mineral apposition rate; the matrix deposited at that time will have a mineralization lag time of 26 days. Formation period (FP) is counted from the onset of matrix synthesis to the completion of mineralization, and in this example is 120 days, at which time completed wall thickness (W.Th) equals 50 μm. It is evident that the total area between the curves is given by FP $\times$ $\overline{\text{O.Th}}$ and by W.Th $\times$ $\overline{\text{Mlt}}$, where the bar indicates a value averaged throughout the lifespan of the osteoid seam at a single location, so that these expressions are equal. Furthermore, it follows that $\overline{\text{O.Th}} = \overline{\text{Mlt}} \times \overline{\text{OAR}}$.

trabeculae with different initial characteristics (6). For example, selective removal of trabeculae with higher values for wall thickness could result in an apparent fall in mean wall thickness with age, even though wall thickness at all surviving locations had not changed (5). Finally, detailed analysis of individual distance measurements is the basis for complete remodeling sequence reconstruction (9,10), indicating how the thicknesses of osteoid, mineralized bone and total matrix, and the matrix and mineral apposition rates, change as functions of time (Figs. 3 and 4).

SIGNIFICANCE OF PARTICULAR MEASUREMENTS

The clinical significance of a measurement depends on its validity as a basis for diagnosis or treatment, but its pathophysiologic significance rests on understanding its relationship to disordered structure and function. Every measurable characteristic of a bone biopsy must ultimately be explicable in terms of the function of cells, considered as members of a hierarchy of intermediary mechanisms (1,16) rather than as isolated individuals.

Geometric and Topological Aspects of Bone Structure

It is customary to divide the skeleton into cortical and cancellous compartments, but the differences between cortical and cancellous bone are primarily geometric rather than biologic. For example, Haversian systems are the outcome of remodeling of bone that is inaccessible from the surface (17) and may be absent in the very thin cortices of the vertebral bodies and present at the confluence of thick trabeculae (18). A more fundamental division of the skeleton is into axial and appendicular components, which differ in their principal types of hard and soft tissue and in patterns of biomechanical loading (19). In the appendicular skeleton, the amount of cancellous tissue contracts rather than expands with age, the bone marrow is fatty rather than hematopoietic, and turnover is low rather than high (19). Unfortunately, no part of the appendicular skeleton is convenient for bone biopsy, and it must be remembered that cortical bone in the ilium is probably not representative of cortical bone throughout the skeleton.

The void volume/tissue volume ratio, or porosity, of typical cortical bone is about 3–6% and of typical cancellous bone about 70–80%, corresponding to bone volume/tissue volume ratios (BV/TV) of 94–97% and 20–30% respectively. The bone surface/bone volume ratio (BS/BV) of typical cortical bone is about 2–4 mm²/mm³ for internal voids and about 4–6 mm²/mm³, including periosteal and endocortical surfaces, but the BS/BV of typical cancellous bone is about 12–16 mm²/mm³ (8). At the junction of cortical and cancellous bone is a transi-

tional zone, intermediate in its geometric properties, that increases in width with advancing age (20); the eventual cancellization of the inner third of the cortex accounts for the expansion of cancellous tissue volume with age. The product of BV/TV and BS/BV gives the bone surface/tissue volume ratio (BS/TV), which shows a curvilinear relationship to porosity, with a peak value at a porosity of about 40% (8). In the ilium BV/TV is about four times higher, and BS/BV about four times lower in cortical than in cancellous bone, so that their product is about the same, and in healthy premenopausal women BS/TV is about 3–4 mm²/mm³ in both cortical and cancellous bone tissue. Finally, since a full-thickness transilial biopsy, including both inner and outer cortices, represents the whole bone as an organ in vivo, bone surface and bone volume can be related to the volume of the entire biopsy core (BS/CV and BV/CV), which allows the separate contributions of cortical and cancellous bone to be compared (14).

These geometric features have an important bearing on the interpretation of histomorphometric data and their relationship to other indices of bone remodeling. For example, the activation frequency is essentially the same on the intracortical, endocortical, and cancellous surfaces (21). At least in the axial skeleton, the lower bone turnover of cortical than cancellous bone is entirely a consequence of its difference in geometry and does not reflect any biological difference in the response of its internal surfaces to hormonal and mechanical signals. Indirect evidence suggests that the same is true also for the appendicular skeleton (22). As bone is lost, BS/TV and BS/CV both tend to increase in cortical bone, because of increased number and size of its voids, but to decrease in cancellous bone, because some trabeculae are completely removed (19). Consequently, with advancing age the relative contribution of cortical bone to total remodeling increases and that of cancellous bone decreases, a trend that is accentuated in patients with vertebral fracture (19). A final example of the importance of geometry is the greater wall thickness in cortical than in cancellous bone, which can be explained by the relationship between initial extent of surface available for formation and final volume of bone formed, assuming the same initial density and bone-forming capacity of osteoblasts (5,21). Consequently, surface-based bone formation rate (BFR/BS) is higher on the intracortical than on the cancellous surface in the ilium, even though activation frequency is similar.

Topology is the study of spatial relationships that do not depend on measurement, picturesquely referred to as "rubber sheet geometry" (23). From this standpoint, all the marrow spaces and cortical voids, apparently separated in two-dimensional sections, form a single connected three-dimensional cavity, and the cancellous, endocortical, and intracortical surfaces form a single connected boundary—the endosteal envelope—that separates marrow inside from bone outside (19). One determinant of the strength of cancellous bone is its three-dimensional connectedness (or connectivity), which is difficult to study in two-dimensional sections. The partitioning of cancellous bone volume into trabecular number and thickness, assuming a parallel-plate model (24), was a useful start but is subject to many limitations. Another two-dimensional approach is to skeletonize the trabecular network and determine the number of nodes and termini and their relationships (25). A closer approach to three-dimensional reality is the separate estimation of star volume for marrow and for bone using new stereologic methods (26); there is a significant correlation between measurements of marrow star volume made separately in the ilium and in the lumbar vertebrae (27). The most direct approach is high-resolution microcomputed tomography, which demonstrated a significant correlation between Euler number/tissue volume, a measure of three-dimensional connectivity, and the simpler two-dimensional measures of trabecular number and separation (28). Each of these new methods has confirmed the original observation that some trabeculae are completely removed (6), so that spacing between the remaining trabeculae is increased and bone strength is disproportionately reduced (29).

Tetracycline Labeling and Indices of Bone Formation

In all its forms, tetracycline chelates calcium and binds reversibly to all bone surfaces, but after its administration is stopped it diffuses back into the circulation, except where it is trapped by new mineral deposition (8). The particular advantages of tetracycline as a bone labeling agent and the factors underlying the choice of labeling regimen are discussed elsewhere (30), and practical details are given in Chapter 21. A double band of fluorescence establishes unequivocally that bone formation occurred at a specific site during the relevant time period and enables the mineral apposition rate (MAR) to be measured. Since mineralization cannot occur unless matrix is available, and the volumes of matrix and mineralized bone formed are always the same, except in osteomalacia, the mean rates of mineral apposition and matrix apposition averaged over the lifespan of the osteoid seam are identical, even though (as indicated earlier) their instantaneous rates are systematically out of step (Fig. 4). Furthermore, a reduction in MAR much more commonly reflects reduced matrix production by osteoblasts than impairment of mineralization (5,14). Mean MAR has a natural lower limit of about 0.25 μm/day, with average values two to three times as great (31).

The total length of the band of fluorescence (or label) is an estimate of the extent of surface where mineralization was in progress [mineralizing surface (MS), or mineralization front] during the period of administration. An alternative method of estimating this quantity is the extent of the band of dark granules stainable with toluidine blue, and in both normal subjects and in patients with osteoporosis, the two methods agree quite well (32). The length of label increases with the dose of tetracycline (33), and varies with the type of tetracycline, being greater with declomycin than with oxytetracycline (13). This suggests that there is a threshold for detection of fluorescence that depends mainly on the number of tetracycline molecules retained, which will be affected by the blood levels achieved, the affinity for bone mineral, and the thickness of the mineral barrier preventing escape (8). Other factors that may alter the detection threshold include the relevant physical properties of the particular tetracycline given, the method of preparation and thickness of the section, the method used for exciting fluorescence, the optical characteristics of the microscope by which the fluorescence is observed, and the visual accuracy of the observer, points covered in detail in Chapter 21. Consequently, it should not be assumed that the absence of detectable fluorescence at a particular location necessarily indicates cessation of mineralization at that location. Indeed, it is likely that the length of label often underestimates the true extent of MS (13). Nevertheless, because of the large spatial and temporal variation in bone turnover (8), MS has a natural lower limit of zero (31).

If mineralization was continuous, once it had started at a particular location, the proportion of osteoid surface labeled (MS/OS) would be at least 85%, but in normal healthy young women this quantity averages only 70% and values as low as 40% can be observed (5). One possible explanation for unlabeled osteoid is that mineralization temporarily ceases and subsequently resumes (34), but when three labels were given, absence of the middle label was never observed (35). Unlabeled osteoid occurs preferentially at the end of the osteoid seam lifespan when mineralization is much slower (9,10; Fig. 4), and an alternative explanation is that too few tetracycline molecules are retained to exceed the threshold discussed earlier. Such terminal seams must eventually mineralize; otherwise, within a few years the entire surface would be covered by osteoid, but do so by a mechanism that escapes detection by the tetracycline method as currently used. Since wall thickness averages about 50 μm, and terminal mineralization reduces seam thickness from about 5 μm to zero, bone formation rate is underestimated by about 10% (13). Until there is a sounder basis for choice between the two models in Fig. 3, it seems reasonable to continue to calculate the Aj.AR, adjusted apposition rate (Aj.AR = MAR × MS/OS) as an estimate of the matrix apposition rate averaged over the entire osteoid seam lifespan. In the absence of osteomalacia, this can be referred to as the *osteoid apposition rate* (OAR).

Two important indices are derived from the osteoid apposition rate. The FP, formation period (FP = W.Th/

OAR), which is considered here, and Mlt, mineralization lag time (Mlt = O.Th/OAR), which is considered in a later section. (O.Th is osteoid thickness.) Wall thickness is the average distance between the cement line and the bone surface, and osteoid apposition rate is the average rate at which the distance is traveled. Consequently, formation period is the average time required to complete the travel (in a perpendicular or vertical sense, as explained elsewhere) from the beginning of matrix synthesis to the end of mineralization, at any point on a bone surface (Fig. 4). Formation period is the key quantity needed for calculation of all temporal subdivisions of the remodeling sequence (8,9,14). For example, the total cycle period = FP × BS/OS, and activation frequency, which is the reciprocal of the total period, = 1/FP × OS/BS. Formation period is related to, but is generally shorter than, the total lifespan of the osteoblast team—sigma, in Frost's terminology (1,16)—since the BMU is organized in three dimensions and involves coordinated movement along the axis of cortical bone or across the surface of cancellous bone (2). In this extended sense, sigma cannot be measured in two-dimensional histologic sections, so that the formation period as defined is the closest practical approach to a natural time unit for the remodeling system.

Wall thickness is an index of the amount of matrix synthesized by a team of osteoblasts and can be regarded as determined by the initial number of osteoblasts assembled per unit area of cement surface (initial cell density), and the average total volume of matrix synthesized by one osteoblast during its lifespan (matrix capacity) (5). A fall in cell density alone would be expected to reduce wall thickness and osteoid apposition rate in the same proportion with no change in formation period, and a fall in matrix capacity alone would be expected to reduce wall thickness and formation period in the same proportion with no change in osteoid apposition rate. Since a reduction in formation period occurs only when apposition rate is increased (9,10), it seems likely that variation in osteoblast team performance is more often due to changes in initial cell density than in matrix capacity; this is part of the evidence for the previous assertion that the number of cells recruited is more important than individual cell function. Based on this conclusion, three measurable aspects of osteoblast team performance—work, rate and time—can provisionally be related to two primary variables—cell number and cell vigor—as shown in Fig. 5. An index of cell vigor is given by the reciprocal of formation period, which expresses the proportion of its total work capacity that an osteoblast can carry out in one day (5,31), with the advantage over formation period that a lower limit of zero is more convenient to scale than an upper limit of infinity.

Another key quantity derived from the primary measurements is the surface-based bone formation rate, the product of mineral apposition rate, and mineralizing

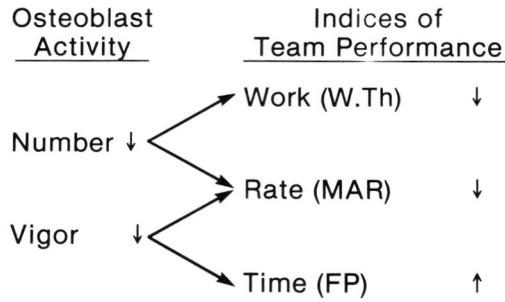

FIG. 5. Relationship between histomorphometric indices of osteoblast team performance and primary variables reflecting osteoblast activity. For further explanation, see the text.

surface as a fraction of bone surface (BFR/BS = MAR × MS/BS). From the definition of activation frequency (Ac.f.) earlier, it can be shown that BFR/BS = Ac.f. × W.Th., where W.Th is wall thickness. Since activation frequency is the probability that bone formation will begin at any point on a surface in a given time period, and wall thickness is an estimate of the average quantity of bone made at each point after each activation event, it is reasonable that the product of these quantities would be the total amount of bone formed in the same time period. Since the coefficient of variation is much smaller for wall thickness than for activation frequency, variation in activation frequency is the main determinant of variation in bone formation rate (2–5). Bone remodeling is essentially a surface phenomenon, so that surface-based formation rate and activation frequency both reflect the interaction and summation of all the stimuli that influence bone remodeling, whether biomechanical signals, systemic hormones, or local cytokines or growth factors (4,19).

Each of the surface-to-volume ratios based on the different referents described earlier (BS/BV, BS/TV, and BS/CV) can be used to convert BFR/BS into a volume-based bone formation rate. Expression per unit of bone volume (BFR/BV) is equivalent to the rate of bone turnover, which determines bone age and various age-dependent properties of bone (2). For example, if the turnover rate is 20% per year, the average lifespan of bone is 5 years (100/20), and in a steady state, and if every moiety of bone had the same lifespan, the mean age of the bone would be 2.5 years. Volume-based formation rate is also useful for considering bone loss in a global sense, since the difference between the volume-based resorption and formation rates is an expression of the fractional rate of bone loss. A more detailed approach to bone age and bone loss is considered in the next section. Bone formation rate per unit of tissue volume (BFR/TV) is most appropriate when considering the relationship between histologic and biochemical markers of bone remodeling, since the entire tissue is perfused and contributes its products to the circulation (36,37). If formation rate is measured in the entire biopsy specimen, including all three subdivisions of the endosteal envelope, the tissue volume referent is the core volume, representing the sum of cortical and cancellous bone tissue (14). The core volume referent has the advantage that the separate contributions of intracortical, endocortical, and cancellous bone surfaces to total remodeling activity can be compared.

Resorption Depth, Wall Thickness, Bone Balance, and Bone Age

The outcome of a remodeling transaction can be considered separately for each point on the surface and is determined by the relationship at that point between resorption depth (Rs.De), which is an index of the amount of bone resorbed by an osteoclast team, and wall thickness (W.Th), which is an index of the amount of bone formed by an osteoblast team. It is both a necessary and a sufficient condition for bone loss that W.Th < Rs.De, and for bone gain that W.Th > Rs.De. This is so for modeling as well as for remodeling (Chapter 15), since if either resorption or formation are absent, they effectively take values of zero. The net rate of change in the location of a point on a bone surface relative to some fixed landmark (ΔBS/t), such that positive values indicate bone gain and negative values bone loss, is determined by the extent of focal remodeling imbalance as just defined and by the activation frequency, which is the probability of initiating a cycle of remodeling at any point on the surface per unit of time (19). This relationship can be written as

$$\Delta BS/t(\mu m/yr) = (W.Th - Rs.De)(\mu m) \times Ac.f(yr^{-1}) \quad [1]$$

If mean values, rather than particular individual values, are used for W.Th and Rs.De, this equation defines the average rate of movement of the entire relevant surface, outward movement being positive and inward movement negative. This is also true if instead of actual mean values for W.Th and Rs.De, deviations from control or other reference values are used.

Application of this relationship to the study of bone loss is hampered by the problems associated with determining bone balance at the histologic level. One possibility is to assume that bone volume changes in proportion to some noninvasive local or whole-body measurement of bone mineral (38). Another is to estimate the change in bone volume from sequential bone biopsies (39), but because of sampling variation this is applicable only to groups of subjects rather than to individuals. Nevertheless, some insight is provided by applying Eq. (1) to cross-sectional data for bone surface location as a function of age or disease duration. A change in location for the cancellous surface is given by one-half the change in trabecular thickness (since loss or gain can occur from

either side of a trabecular plate), for the endocortical surface by changes in cortical thickness, and for the intracortical surface by changes in osteonal canal radius (19). In each case, the relevant value can be obtained indirectly from measurement of area combined with either perimeter or number, which gives only the mean, or direct measurement at multiple locations, which also gives the frequency distribution (14). The results can only be approximate, since the effect of local surface curvature is disregarded.

As an example of this approach, cross-sectional data indicate that in normal subjects trabecular thickness declines by about 1 μm per year after the onset of bone loss at about age 35 (40,41). The average value for activation frequency is about 0.3 per year (21), so that the average difference between resorption depth and wall thickness on the cancellous surface during the period of skeletal involution is about 1.7 μm (= 0.5/0.3), or 3%. Since wall thickness falls by about 25 μm between the ages of 40 and 80 years (42), resorption depth must fall by almost the same amount. Consequently, the fall in trabecular thickness is fully explained by a decline in the amount of work performed by the average osteoblast team (43), and most of this decline could be regarded as an adaptive response to the fall in resorption depth (44,45). These conclusions apply only to the trabeculae that remain, not to those that have been completely removed, a process that needs separate discussion. A second example concerns the cellular mechanisms of cortical bone loss. In primary hyperparathyroidism, with an assumed disease duration of 20 years, ΔBS/t for the endocortical surface can be estimated as -21 μm/yr (19,46). Combining this with the measured value for activation frequency of 0.84 per year and the measured reduction in wall thickness of 2.6 μm, the estimated increase in resorption depth over the duration of the disease derived from Eq. (1) was 22 μm. Only trivial changes in resorption depth were evident on the cancellous and intracortical surface. Consequently, the major mechanism of cortical bone loss in hyperparathyroidism is an increase in the amount of work performed by the average osteoclast team, and the same probably applies also to age-related cortical thinning in the metacarpal and to thinning of iliac cortical bone in osteoporosis (19,46).

In cancellous bone, resorption depth and wall thickness can be related not only to trabecular thickness but also to interstitial bone thickness (Ir.B.Th), which is the distance between the cement lines closest to the surface on opposite sides of a trabecula. Mean Ir.B.Th is given by

$$\text{mean Tb.Th} - 2 \times \text{mean W.Th}$$

but it is more accurate to measure Ir.B.Th directly at multiple locations in order to obtain a frequency distribution as well as a mean value. A change in interstitial bone thickness has previously been assumed to be the cumulative result of a converse change in resorption depth (47,48), but if trabecular thickness is changing, the point from which resorption begins is also changing. Consequently, the assumption is valid only if interstitial bone thickness is changing in the opposition direction to trabecular thickness (49). It is convenient to relate cement line location as well as bone surface location to the midline of a trabecula (Fig. 6). In the example shown, wall thickness is abruptly reduced by 2 μm and resorption depth by 1 μm, without further change. After 10 successive cycles of remodeling at the same location, half trabecular thickness will have fallen by 10 μm and half interstitial bone thickness, after a transient increase, will have fallen by 8 μm. Thus if both interstitial bone thickness and trabecular thickness fall together, no inference is possible concerning a change in resorption depth, unless the history of the bone surface is reconstructed in accordance with Eq. (1), for which must be known the number of successive remodeling cycles corresponding to the observed changes in structure.

Equation (1) could also be used to predict changes in bone balance from measurements of resorption depth. The change in surface location is equivalent to the difference between surface-based formation and resorption rates, so that Eq. (1) can be rewritten

$$(\text{BFR/BS} - \text{BRs.R/BS})(\mu m^3/\mu m^2/yr)$$

$$= (\text{W.Th} - \text{Rs.De})(\mu m) \times \text{Ac.f}(yr^{-1})$$

Consequently, from simultaneous measurements of formation rate, wall thickness, and resorption depth, both resorption rate and bone balance could be calculated (50). Furthermore, using the various surface/volume ratios defined previously, resorption rate could be expressed in terms of a bone volume, tissue volume, or core volume referent. Wall thickness as usually measured is an index of the activity of previous osteoblast teams averaged over the total cycle period, but there is no way of making comparable measurements of previous resorption depth as an index of the activity of previous osteoclast teams. Nevertheless, measurement of current resorption depth can be based on the number of eroded lamellae, and measurement of current wall thickness on the distance between the thinnest terminal seams and the cement line (9,50). A potential pitfall is the assumption that resorption always continues until pre-osteoblast-like cells are observed; if this were not so, the method would be biased in favor of the deepest regions of the lacunae and would provide an estimate of maximum resorption depth rather than mean resorption depth, in which case inferences concerning pathogenesis (51) would be invalid.

There is now general agreement that complete removal of some trabeculae is a major component of age-related loss of cancellous bone, and that the process is initiated by perforation of trabecular plates (6,9,24–26,40,41), but the mechanism of perforation is controversial (Chapter 15). A generalized reduction in trabecular thickness is probably not a prerequisite for perforation (24), but in some instances perforation could be preceded by rapidly progressive focal thinning (40,41). Increased resorption depth has been demonstrated on the endocortical surface (19) and provides a reasonable explanation for rapid loss of cancellous bone in early menopause, but evidence for such a mechanism is suggestive rather than conclusive (9). Like thieves in the night, the osteoclasts that cause perforation work quickly and can rarely be observed directly, so that their activities must generally be inferred from what has been removed. A stochastic model, based on the frequency distributions of resorption depth and trabecular thickness, can account for an increase in the probability of perforation as a result of more frequent remodeling activation, with no change in mean resorption depth (52),

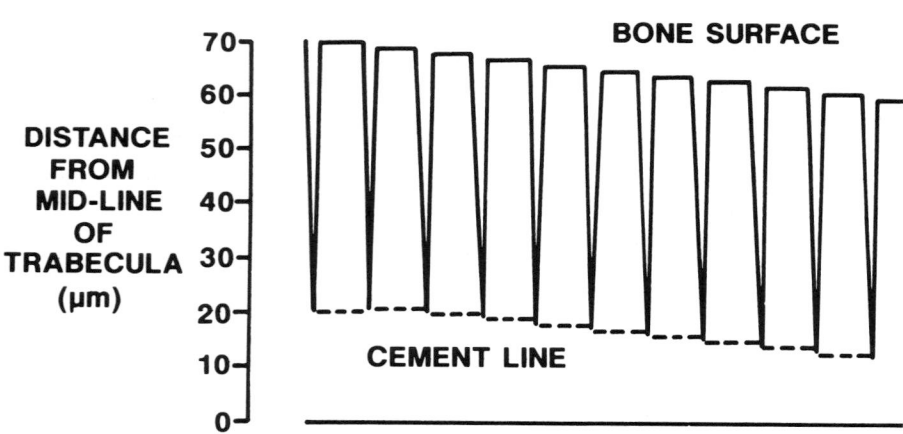

FIG. 6. Interpretation of interstitial bone thickness. Diagrammatic representation of movement of bone surface and cement line in relation to the midline of a trabecula as a result of successive cycles of remodeling. The distance from the cement line (stepped dashed line) to the midline (solid line at zero) represents half interstitial bone thickness, and the distance from the bone surface (stepped solid line) to the midline represents half trabecular thickness. In the first cycle, both resorption depth and wall thickness are equal at 50 μm, but in the second and subsequent cycles resorption depth is reduced to 49 μm and wall thickness to 48 μm. For further explanation and discussion, see the text.

but there is no evidence for increased perforation in primary hyperparathyroidism (19) and only agents that decrease resorption depth as well as activation frequency, such as calcitonin (48) and bisphosphonates (53), are effective substitutes for estrogen in preventing cancellous bone loss (54,55). Consequently, the available data remain consistent with the view that complete removal of trabeculae is a manifestation of rapid osteoclast-mediated bone loss, and thinning of residual trabeculae a manifestation of slow osteoblast-mediated bone loss (2).

A final illustration of the interaction between geometry and remodeling is their joint relationship to bone age. As bone becomes older it becomes more highly mineralized and more brittle, it accumulates more fatigue damage and its osteocytes are more likely to die (56,57). A stochastic model of bone age, based on the frequency distributions of resorption depth and trabecular thickness (the same data as for the stochastic model of perforation), relates the probability of remodeling of a moiety of bone to the frequency of activation and to the distance of the moiety from the surface (57). Within 30 μm of the surface activation frequency is the main determinant of bone age, but beyond 50 μm, distance from the surface becomes increasingly important, and beyond 80 μm the interstitial bone is essentially isolated from surface remodeling, regardless of the activation frequency, and would have an age approaching the years of life of the subject since skeletal maturity (57). Any trabecular element in the central zone that remained within reach of the deeper resorption cavities would have a significant likelihood of being completely removed as a consequence of perforation, so that a very low probability of remodeling of interstitial bone may be a necessary condition for its survival (57). Thus even in healthy subjects a significant fraction of bone is old enough for osteocyte death to be a plausible consequence, although its occurrence has not yet been demonstrated.

Kinetics of Osteoid Accumulation

Osteoid is bone matrix that has not yet become mineralized, and its existence in measurable amounts is a consequence of the delay between the synthesis of matrix and the onset of its mineralization. In cross sections of cortical bone, individual osteoid seam profiles are readily identified as annuli surrounding large Haversian canals. In cancellous bone, osteoid seam profiles are crescents of length between 250 and 750 μm, but it is customary to ignore their individuality and to determine three indices of osteoid accumulation: surface, thickness, and volume. Osteoid surface is usually expressed as a fraction or a percentage of bone surface (OS/BS) but can also be related to any of the volume referents mentioned earlier if multiplied by the appropriate surface/volume ratio. With the core volume referent (OS/CV), the separate

contributions of the different subdivisions of the endosteal surface can be compared. Osteoid thickness (O.Th) can be calculated indirectly from volume and surface (58), but is more accurately measured directly at multiple sites, giving a standard deviation as well as a mean value. Osteoid volume is usually expressed as a fraction of bone volume (OV/BV), but tissue volume and core volume referents can also be used.

If the length of the seam is measured equidistant between the bone surface and the osteoid bone interface, then (in terms of the primary osteoid measurements) area = length $\times$ mean width. In cancellous bone, with a mixture of both convex and concave surfaces, perimeters measured on the surface can be used as an index of length with minimal error, but in cortical bone, where the surfaces are all concave, the error would be greater. Consequently, the following analysis is applicable mainly to cancellous bone. Based on the foregoing, the three osteoid indices are related as follows (59):

$$OV/BV(\%) = O.Th(\mu m) \times OS/BS(\%)$$
$$\times BS/BV(\mu m^2/\mu m^3)$$

The decline in trabecular thickness that occurs with age (and is exaggerated in some patients with osteoporosis) is associated with an increase in BS/BV. Consequently, there can be an increase in OV/BV even if thickness and surface of osteoid are unchanged. To examine changes in osteoid volume that are independent of changes in bone structure, OV/BV can be corrected to a representative value for BS/BV in healthy young adults, but ignoring this refinement will generally lead only to trivial error.

Each osteoid index is separately related to the kinetic indices of bone remodeling discussed previously (5,59). Mean osteoid thickness is the average amount of bone matrix remaining to be mineralized at any point on an osteoid seam, and osteoid thickness divided by osteoid apposition rate is an estimate of the average time between the deposition of any infinitesimal volume of matrix and the onset of its mineralization, which is the mineralization lag time (Mlt). At the initiation of a particular osteoid seam (Fig. 4), the lag time is synonymous with the osteoid maturation time (Omt), which is the time required for the structural and biochemical changes that must occur in bone matrix after its deposition to enable mineralization to begin (60). Because OAR has a lower limit of zero (31), Mlt and Omt (like FP) have upper limits of infinity. This drawback can be circumvented by using osteoid mineralization rate (OMR) as the reciprocal of Mlt, and osteoid maturation rate (OmR) as the reciprocal of Omt, quantities which express the fraction of osteoid thickness that mineralizes in 1 day.

The mineralization lag time averaged throughout the lifespan of the seam is invariably longer than the initial maturation time (Fig. 4), whether the latter is estimated as O.Th/MAR (14), or measured from the proportion of

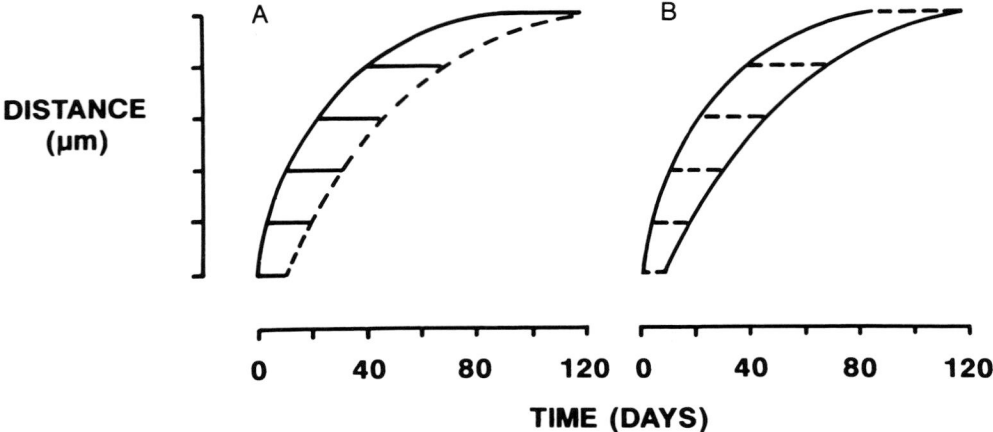

FIG. 7. Two models of the relationship between matrix apposition, mineral apposition and mineralization lag time. **A:** Mineral apposition rate and mineralization lag time are separately and independently regulated as functions of osteoblast age, and the rate of mineral apposition changes as an automatic consequence. **B:** The rates of matrix and mineral apposition are separately and independently regulated as functions of time and the lag time changes as an automatic consequence. In both cases, the genuine independent variables are depicted by solid lines and the automatically determined variables by dashed lines.

surface with no mineralized bone between osteoid and cement line (9). This could be because the time required for matrix maturation increases with the age of the osteoblast, and changes in matrix apposition rate and lag time together would determine the progress of mineralization (Fig. 7A); in this case, lag time would be a genuine independent variable, but changes in mineral apposition rate would follow automatically. Alternatively, the rates of matrix and mineral apposition could be separately and independently regulated, in which case lag time would not be a genuine independent variable but would automatically follow changes in the other variables (Fig. 7B). It is also possible that each of these mutually exclusive relationships could be true in different disease states. Fortunately, the uncertainty in the pathophysiologic significance of the lag time does not detract from its usefulness in the understanding of histomorphometric data and of the mechanisms of osteoid accumulation.

The kinetic interpretation of osteoid surface and volume in terms of birthrate and lifespan was mentioned earlier. In a steady state the rate at which osteoid newly appears at any point on the surface is the same as the frequency of remodeling activation, and the average lifespan of the osteoid seam at any point on the surface is the same as the formation period, so that $OS/BS(\%) = Ac.f(yr^{-1}) \times FP(yr) \times 100$. In a similar manner, the rate at which osteoid newly appears in any volume of bone is the same as the volume-based bone formation rate, and the average lifespan of each volume moiety of osteoid is the same as the mineralization lag time, so that $OV/BV(\%) = BFR/BV(\%/yr) \times Mlt(yr)$, where $BFR/BV = Ac.f(yr^{-1}) \times W.Th(\mu m) \times BS/BV(\mu m^2/\mu m^3) \times 100$. Since wall thickness and bone surface/volume ratio

show little variation, the relationships between the static indices of osteoid accumulation and the kinetic indices of bone formation is as summarized in Fig. 8. Note in particular that osteoid volume is independent of osteoid apposition rate; this is inversely related to formation period, and in a steady state affects osteoid surface and thickness in opposite directions, and to a reciprocal extent.

In normal subjects, and in every metabolic bone disease except osteomalacia, there is a significant positive correlation between mean osteoid thickness and mean osteoid apposition rate, with broadly similar slopes (b) and intercepts (a) of the regression lines (15,59). Although such a relationship is to be expected, it has an unanticipated consequence for the interpretation of the mineralization lag time, since we can write

$$O.Th = b(OAR) + a$$

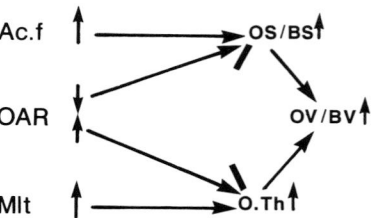

FIG. 8. Relationship between kinetic indices of bone formation and static indices of osteoid accumulation. The bars indicate an absence of effect of OAR on OV/BV, since OS/BS and O.Th are affected in opposite directions by changes in OAR.

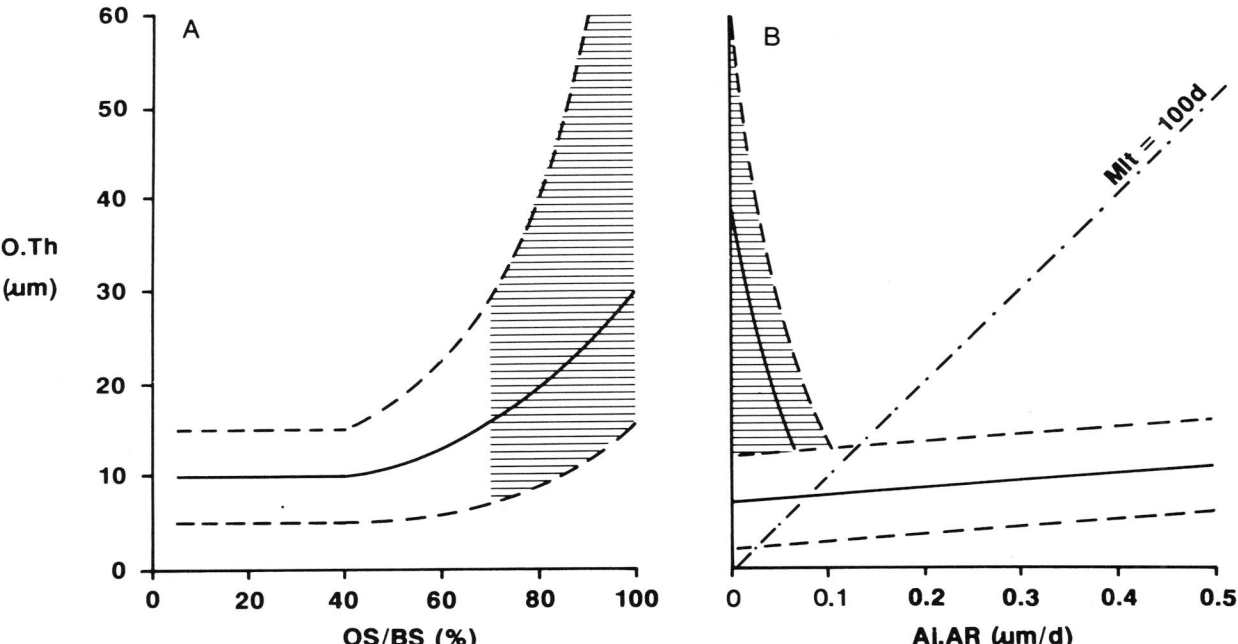

FIG. 9. Relationship of osteoid thickness to osteoid surface (**A**) and adjusted apposition rate (**B**). In normal subjects and in patients with osteoporosis there is no relationship between osteoid thickness and surface (**A**), but there is a significant positive relationship between osteoid thickness and adjusted apposition rate (**B**). During the development of osteomalacia there is a direct hyperbolic relationship between osteoid thickness and surface (**A**) and an inverse hyperbolic relationship between osteoid thickness and adjusted apposition rate (**B**); the usual ranges of values in established osteomalacia are shaded. The oblique line through the origin in (**B**) corresponds to a mineralization lag time of 100 days. (Modified from Ref. 15 and 61.)

If this is combined with the previously given relationship between mineralization lag time and osteoid apposition rate, the following equation is obtained:

$$Mlt = b + a/OAR \qquad [2]$$

Because of this relationship, which defines a rectangular hyperbola, when the osteoid or adjusted apposition rate falls, the mineralization lag time increases (59). Since a prolonged lag time is an inevitable consequence of a fall in osteoid apposition rate, it does not by itself indicate defective mineralization. Another way of arriving at the same conclusion is to consider the effect of prolongation of FP, which is also an inevitable consequence of a reduction in osteoid apposition rate. As indicated in the legend to Fig. 4, FP × O.Th = Mlt × W.Th. Since O.Th has a minimum value [the intercept in Eq. (2)] and W.Th is constant, at least in the short term, an increase in FP must be accompanied by an increase in Mlt.

There is no relationship between osteoid thickness and surface in normal subjects or in patients with osteoporosis, but there is a hyperbolic relationship between these variables in vitamin D–related bone disease (Fig. 9A). During the evolution of osteomalacia, osteoid surface increases first as a result of an increase in Ac.f due to secondary hyperparathyroidism (61; Chapter 21) and osteoid thickness increases only slightly until OS/BS ex-

ceeds 60–70%, after which a further increase in osteoid volume is due mainly to increasing thickness. In the same patients, osteoid thickness shows a more complex relationship to adjusted apposition rate. When above approximately 0.1 μm/day there is the usual positive relationship between these variables, but below approximately 0.1 μm/day further decrements in Aj.AR are associated, not with a fall in osteoid thickness as in all other situations, but with a progressive increase (Fig. 9B), limited only by the normal thickness of new matrix, or wall thickness (62). The reversal of the relationship between osteoid thickness and adjusted apposition rate is the cardinal kinetic characteristic of defective mineralization, which consequently cannot be defined on the basis of kinetic data alone, without reference to osteoid thickness (15).

REFERENCES

1. Frost HM. *Bone remodeling dynamics.* Springfield, IL: Charles C. Thomas, 1964.
2. Parfitt AM. Bone remodeling: relationship to the amount and structure of bone and the pathogenesis and prevention of fractures. In: Riggs BL, Melton LJ, eds. *Osteoporosis: etiology, diagnosis and management.* New York: Raven Press, 1988.
3. Melsen F, Mosekilde L. Calcified tissues: cellular dynamics. In: Nordin BEC, ed. *Calcium in human biology.* Berlin: Springer-Verlag, 1988;187–208.

4. Parfitt AM. Pharmacologic manipulation of bone remodelling and calcium homeostasis. In: Kanis JA, ed. *Calcium metabolism progressive basic and clinical pharmacology*, vol 4. Basel. S. Karger, 1990;1–27.

5. Parfitt AM. Bone forming cells in clinical disorders. In: Hall BK, ed. *Bone: a treatise*, vol 1, *The osteoblast and osteocyte*. New Jersey: Telford Press, 1990;351–429.

6. Parfitt AM. Trabecular bone architecture in the pathogenesis and prevention of fracture. *Am J Med* 1987;82(suppl 1B):68–72.

7. Beyer HS, Parfitt AM, Shih M-S, Heath H. Idiopathic acquired diffuse osteosclerosis in a young woman. *J Bone Miner Res* [in press].

8. Parfitt AM. The physiologic and clinical significance of bone histomorphometric data. In: Recker RB, ed. *Bone Histomorphometry: techniques and interpretations*. Boca Raton, FL: CRC Press, 1983;143–223.

9. Eriksen EF. Normal and pathological remodeling of human trabecular bone: three dimensional reconstruction of the remodeling sequence in normals and in metabolic bone disease. *Endocr Rev* 1986;7:379–408.

10. Parfitt AM, Villanueva AR, Mathews CHE, Aswani JA. Kinetics of matrix and mineral apposition in osteoporosis and renal osteodystrophy: relationship to rate of turnover and to cell morphology. In: Jee WSS, Parfitt AM, eds. *Bone histomorphometry: 3rd international workshop*. Paris: Armour-Montagu, 1981;213–9.

11. Baron R, Vignery A, Horowitz M. Lymphocytes, macrophages and the regulation of bone remodeling. In: Peck W, ed. *Bone and Mineral Research*, Vol 2. Amsterdam: Elsevier, 1984;175–245.

12. Schaffler MB, Burr DB, Frederickson RG. Morphology of the osteonal cement line in human bone. *Anat Rec* 1987;217:223–8.

13. Parfitt AM, Foldes J, Villanueva AR, Shih M-S. The difference in label length between demethylchlortetracycline and oxytetracycline: implications for the interpretation of histomorphometric data. *Calc Tissue Int* [in press].

14. Parfitt AM, Drezner MK, Glorieux FH, et al. Bone histomorphometry nomenclature, symbols and units: report of the ASBMR histomorphometry nomenclature committee. *J Bone Miner Res* 1987;2:595–610.

15. Parfitt AM. Osteomalacia and related disorders. In: Avioli LV, Krane SM, eds. *Metabolic bone disease*, 2nd ed. Philadelphia: Saunders, 1990;329–396.

16. Frost HM. *Intermediary organization of the skeleton*, vol 1. Boca Raton, FL: CRC Press, 1986.

17. Ham AW. Some histophysiological problems peculiar to calcified tissues. *J Bone Joint Surg* 1952;34-A:701–28.

18. Sato K, Wakamatsu E, Sato T, Honma T, Kotake H, Byers PD. Histomorphometric study of trabecular channels in normal iliac bone. *Calcif Tissue Int* 1986;39:2–7.

19. Parfitt AM. Surface specific bone remodeling in health and disease. In: Kleerekoper M, Krane S, eds. *Clinical disorders of bone and mineral metabolism*. New York: Mary Ann Liebert, 1989;7–14.

20. Keshawarz NM, Recker RB. Expansion of the medullary cavity at the expense of cortex in postmenopausal osteoporosis. *Metab Bone Dis Relat Res* 1984;5:223–8.

21. Parfitt AM, Villanueva AR, Rao DS. Surface differences in iliac bone remodelling; contribution of geometric and biologic factors and effect of menopause. *J Bone Miner Res* 1988;3(suppl 1):S215.

22. Parfitt AM, Rao DS, Stanciu J, Villanueva AR, Kleerekoper M, Frame B. Irreversible bone loss in osteomalacia: comparison of radial photon absorptiometry with iliac bone histomorphometry during treatment. *J Clin Invest* 1985;76:2403–2412.

23. Kasner E, Newman J. *Mathematics and the imagination*. London: G Bell, 1949.

24. Parfitt AM, Mathews CHE, Villanueva AR, Kleerekoper M, Frame B, Rao DS. Relationship between surface, volume and thickness of iliac trabecular bone in aging and in osteoporosis: implications for the microanatomic and cellular mechanism of bone loss. *J Clin Invest* 1983;72:1396–1409.

25. Compston JE, Mellish RWE, Garrahan NJ. Age-related changes in iliac crest trabecular microanatomic bone structure in man. *Bone* 1987;8:289–92.

26. Vesterby A, Gundersen HJG, Melsen F. Star volume of marrow space and trabeculae of the first lumbar vertebra: sampling efficiency and biological variation. *Bone* 1989;10:7–13.

27. Vesterby A. Star volume of marrow space and trabeculae in iliac crest: sampling procedure and correlation to star volume of first lumbar vertebra. *Bone* 1990;11;149–55.

28. Feldkamp LA, Goldstein SA, Parfitt AM, Lesion G, Kleerekoper M. The direct examination of three dimensional bone architecture in vitro by computed tomography. *J Bone Miner Res* 1989;4:3–11.

29. Kleerekoper M, Villanueva AR, Stanciu J, Rao DS, Parfitt AM. The role of three dimensional trabecular microstructure in the pathogenesis of vertebral compression fractures. *Calcif Tissue Int* 1985;37:594–7.

30. Frost HM. Bone histomorphometry: choice of marking agent and labeling schedule. In: Recker RR, ed. *Bone histomorphometry: techniques and interpretation*. Boca Raton, FL: CRC Press, 1983.

31. Foldes J, Shih M-S, Parfitt AM. Frequency distributions of tetracycline based measurements: implications for the interpretation of bone formation indices in the absence of double labelled surfaces. 1989. *J Bone Miner Res* 1990;5:1063–1067.

32. Villanueva AR, Kujawa M, Mathews CHE, Parfitt AM. Identification of the mineralization front: comparison of a modified toluidine blue stain with tetracycline fluorescence. *Metab Bone Dis Relat Res* 1983;5:41–5.

33. Hattner RS, Ilnicki LP, Hodge HC. The dose-response relationship of tetracycline to the detectability of labeled osteons by fluorescence microscopy. In: Norman AW, Schaefer K, Coburn JW, et al., eds. *Vitamin D, biochemical, chemical and clinical aspects related to calcium metabolism*. New York: Walter deGruyter, 1977;377–80.

34. Martin RB. Label escape theory revisited: the effects of resting periods and section thickness. *Bone* 1989;10:255–64.

35. Ott SM. Bone formation fails to show "on-off" pattern in postmenopausal osteoporosis. *J Bone Miner Res* 1989;4(suppl 1):S415.

36. Parfitt AM, Kleerekoper M. Diagnostic value of bone histomorphometry and comparison of histologic measurements and biochemical indices of bone remodeling. In: Christiansen C, Arnaud CD, Nordin BEC, Parfitt AM, Peck WA, Riggs BL, eds. *Osteoporosis: Proceedings of the Copenhagen international symposium on osteoporosis*, June 3–8, 1984. Glostrup, Denmark; Aalborg Stiftsbogtrykkeri, 1984;111–20.

37. Parfitt AM, Simon LS, Villanueva AR, Krane SM. Procollagen type I carboxyterminal extension peptide in serum as a marker of collagen biosynthesis in bone: correlation with iliac bone formation rates and comparison with total alkaline phosphatase. *J Bone Miner Res* 1987;2:427–36.

38. Gruber HE, Ivey JL, Thompson ER, Chesnut CH III, Baylink DJ. Osteoblast and osteoclast cell number and cell activity in postmenopausal osteoporosis. *Miner Electrolyte Metab* 1986;12:246–54.

39. Frost HM. Bone histomorphometry: analysis of trabecular bone dynamics. In: Recker R, ed. *Bone histomorphometry: techniques and interpretation*. Boca Raton, FL: CRC Press, 1983;109–31.

40. Weinstein RS, Hutson MS. Decreased trabecular width and increased trabecular spacing contribute to bone loss with aging. *Bone* 1987;8:137–42.

41. Mellish RWE, Garrahan NJ, Compston JE. Age-related changes in trabecular width and spacing in human iliac crest biopsies. *Bone Miner* 1989;6:331–8.

42. Lips P, Courpron P, Meunier PJ. Mean wall thickness of trabecular bone packets in the human iliac crest: changes with age. *Calcif Tissue Res* 1978;26:13–7.

43. Courpron P. Bone tissue mechanisms underlying osteoporoses. *Orthop Clin North Am* 1981;12:513–43.

44. Recker RR, Kimmel DB, Parfitt AM, Davies KM, Keshawarz N, Hinders S. Static and tetracycline-based bone histomorphometric data from 34 normal postmenopausal females. *J Bone Miner Res* 1988;2:133–44.

45. Parfitt AM. ADFR, or coherence therapy, for osteoporosis. In: DeLuca HF, Mazess R, eds. *Osteoporosis: physiological basis, assessment, and treatment*. New York: Elsevier, 1990;315–20.

46. Parfitt AM, Villanueva AR, Rao D, Kleerekoper M. Remodeling mechanisms that contribute to bone loss and fracture. In Takahashi H, ed. *Bone morphometry: proceedings of the fifth international congress*. Niigata, Nishimura, 1990;346–354.

47. Parfitt AM, Podenphant J, Villanueva AR, Frame B. Metabolic

bone disease with and without osteomalacia after intestinal bypass surgery: a bone histomorphometric study. *Bone* 1985;6:211–20.

48. Marie PJ, Caulin F. Mechanisms underlying the effects of phosphate and calcitonin on bone histology in postmenopausal osteoporosis. *Bone* 1986;7:17–22.

49. Croucher PI, Mellish RWE, Vedi S, Garrahan NJ, Compston JE. The relationship between resorption depth and mean interstitial bone thickness: age-related changes in man. *Calcif Tissue Int* 1989;45:15–9.

50. Charles P, Eriksen EF, Mosekilde L, Melsen F, Jensen FT. Bone turnover and balance evaluated by a combined calcium balance and ^{47}calcium kinetic study and dynamic histomorphometry. *Metabolism* 1987;36:1118–24.

51. Eriksen EF, Hodgson SF, Eastell R, Cesel SL, O'Fallon WM, Riggs BL. Cancellous bone remodeling in type I (postmenopausal) osteoporosis: quantitative assessment of rates of formation, resorption, and bone loss at tissue and cellular levels. *J Bone Miner Res* 1990;5:311–319.

52. Reeve J. Bone turnover and trabecular plate survival after artificial menopause. *Br Med J* 1987;295:757–60.

53. Boyce RW, Eriksen EF, Franks AF, Stokes CL, Jankowsky ML. Effect of NE-58095 on trabecular bone remodeling: 3-D reconstruction of the remodeling site. *J Bone Miner Res* 1989;4(suppl 1):S194.

54. Overgaard K, Riis BJ, Christiansen C, Hansen MA. Effect of salca-

tonin given intranasally on early postmenopausal bone loss. *Br Med J* 1989;299:477–9.

55. Reginster JY, Lecart MP, Deroisy R, et al. Prevention of postmenopausal bone loss by tiludronate. *Lancet* 1989;1469–71.

56. Frost HM. The pathomechanics of osteoporoses. *Clin Orthop Rel Res* 1985;200:198–225.

57. Parfitt AM, Kleerekoper M, Villanueva AR. Increased bone age: mechanisms and consequences. In: Christiansen C, Johansen C, Riis BJ, eds. *Osteoporosis* Copenhagen: Osteopress Aps, 1987;301–8.

58. Quarles LD, Lobaugh B. Equivalency of various methods for estimating osteoid seam width. *J Bone Miner Res* 1989;4:671–7.

59. Parfitt AM. The cellular mechanisms of osteoid accumulation in metabolic bone disease. In: *Mineral metabolism research in Italy,* vol 4. Milan: Wichtig Editore, 1984;3–9.

60. Baylink DJ, Morey EM, Ivey JL, Stauffer ME. Vitamin D and bone. In: Norman AW, ed. *Vitamin D molecular biology and clinical nutrition.* New York: Marcel Dekker, 1980.

61. Rao DS. Metabolic bone disease in gastrointestinal and biliary disorders. In: Farus M, ed. *Primer on the metabolic bone diseases of mineral metabolism.* Kelseyville, American Society for Bone and Mineral Research, 1990;175–178.

62. Meunier PJ, Van Linthoudt D, Edouard C, Charhon S, Arlot M. Histologic analysis of the mechanisms underlying pathogenesis and healing of osteomalacia. *Calcif Tissue Int* 1981;33(suppl):771–4.

PART V

Disorders of Serum Mineral Levels

Disorders of Bone and Mineral Metabolism,
edited by Fredric L. Coe and Murray J. Favus,
© 1992 by Raven Press, Ltd. All rights reserved.

CHAPTER 23

Hypercalcemic States

Their Differential Diagnosis and Acute Management

John P. Bilezikian

Hypercalcemia is a relatively common medical problem. The clinical spectrum ranges from emergent life-threatening hypercalcemia that requires immediate attention to a larger number of patients whose hypercalcemia is more mild and frequently asymptomatic. Widespread use of the multichannel screening test has been responsible for a shift away from seeing hypercalcemia as a medical emergency to less urgent presentations. Increased recognition of less severe aspects of hypercalcemia has presented problems in differential diagnosis and management that are more difficult to address when compared to the time when hypercalcemia was virtually always symptomatic and the diagnosis was usually quickly apparent.

Irrespective of the severity of the hypercalcemia and the presence or absence of symptoms, the approach to the patient requires an appreciation of the principles of calcium homeostasis, knowledge of its differential diagnosis and associated pathophysiologies, and the clinical judgment to know when and how to administer appropriate therapy. Thus the approach is a multifaceted one. To cover the subject completely, this chapter has to take into consideration a number of issues that are dealt with in detail in other chapters. For example, most of the etiologies of hypercalcemia are treated separately elsewhere. In this chapter, however, these etiologies are presented in the context of the differential diagnosis of hypercalcemia and thus are reviewed with a different perspective. Also considered are the symptomatology of hypercalcemia, risk of potential target organ involvement, and therapeu-

tics. It focuses the evaluation of the hypercalcemic patient in a way that is both expedient and accurate.

GENERAL PRINCIPLES OF CALCIUM HOMEOSTASIS

Detailed basic physiological and biochemical information about the regulation of calcium homeostasis is given in Parts I–III of this book. Only a brief summary of the general principles of calcium homeostasis is covered here.

The serum calcium is controlled within very narrow limits by parathyroid hormone and 1,25-dihydroxyvitamin D [$1,25(OH)_2D$]. Stimulated directly by hypocalcemia, parathyroid hormone mobilizes calcium from bone and conserves calcium in the kidney. These actions serve to restore the serum calcium to normal. Of the large number of potential stimulators of parathyroid hormone secretion, the most important one is the signal generated by the reduction in the circulating calcium concentration. The most important inhibitor of parathyroid hormone is an elevation in the serum calcium. If the hypercalcemia is not due to excessive secretion of parathyroid hormone, parathyroid hormone output will be inhibited rapidly by hypercalcemia. This is a key physiological point that provides a fundamental operating principle when considering the differential diagnosis of hypercalcemia. The recent demonstration that $1,25(OH)_2D$ can also inhibit parathyroid hormone secretion (1) is of interest, particularly in the context of the mutual regulation of each of these two calcium-regulating hormones by the other. However, $1,25(OH)_2D$ does not enjoy the prominence of calcium as a major regulator of parathyroid hormone. Very recent observations suggest that the mechanism by which $1,25(OH)_2D$ regulates parathyroid

J. P. Bilezikian: Departments of Medicine and Pharmacology, College of Physicians and Surgeons, Columbia University, New York, New York 10032

hormone secretion may be through an effect to raise intracellular calcium (2).

1,25(OH)$_2$D, the other hormone that regulates the circulating serum calcium concentration within narrow normal limits, is the metabolic product of sequential hydroxylation steps of vitamin D in the liver and the kidney (3–6). The final conversion step, due to activation of a renal 1α-hydroxylase, is stimulated by hypophosphatemia and parathyroid hormone (7). Enhanced production of 1,25 (OH)$_2$D by hypocalcemia is believed to occur through the secondary stimulation of parathyroid hormone. Thus parathyroid hormone shares with 1,25(OH)$_2$D a regulatory function on the expression of each other. 1,25(OH)$_2$D mobilizes calcium from bone in a manner similar to parathyroid hormone but differs from parathyroid hormone by acting directly in the gastrointestinal tract to facilitate calcium absorption. In concert with parathyroid hormone, therefore, 1,25(OH)$_2$D helps to restore calcium levels to normal. In contrast to parathyroid hormone, calcium is not believed to have a major direct inhibitory action on 1,25(OH)$_2$D production, although recent information has revived this idea (8). Another important action of 1,25(OH)$_2$D is facilitation of phosphate absorption in the gastrointestinal tract. This is a useful point because in hypercalcemic conditions associated with excess 1,25(OH)$_2$D production or enhanced sensitivity, the serum phosphate may be elevated. In contrast to conditions associated with elevations in parathyroid hormone, the serum phosphate in vitamin D–sensitive states would not be expected to be low or in the low-normal range. Hyperphosphatemia is a direct major inhibitor of 1,25(OH)$_2$D production.

Understanding the differential diagnosis of hypercalcemia is facilitated by understanding these features of calcium control under normal conditions. Specific examples will follow when each of the diagnostic possibilities is considered. In general, however, in cases of parathyroid hormone dependent hypercalcemia, a clinically useful radioimmunoassay for parathyroid hormone will indicate an elevation. On the other hand, if the hypercalcemia is not due to excess parathyroid hormone, the parathyroid glands should be suppressed by the hypercalcemia and the circulating level is low or undetectable. As will be appreciated, the ability to rely on a useful clinical assay for parathyroid hormone in order to distinguish between parathyroid hormone dependent (the hyperparathyroid states) and parathyroid hormone independent hypercalcemia has simplified, to a great extent, the evaluation of hypercalcemia.

DIFFERENTIAL DIAGNOSIS OF HYPERCALCEMIA

A consideration of the differential diagnosis of hypercalcemia accommodates those individuals who like short lists as well as those who like long lists (Table 1). For despite the fact that there are many potential causes for hypercalcemia, the overwhelming majority of hypercalcemic patients will be shown to have either primary hyperparathyroidism or a malignancy. These two etiologies constitute over 90% of the hypercalcemic population in this country. Thus the most simple and direct differential diagnosis of hypercalcemia is a distinction between these two most common causes. For those who like long lists, the remaining 10% of the hypercalcemic population is scattered among a great variety of other potential etiologies. This is not just for academic discussion because, in the occasional patient, one must search diligently beyond the short list of causes to a consideration of the many other possible etiologies of hypercalcemia. It is important to bear these other disorders in mind, especially in the patient who becomes a diagnostic problem. This section covers the entire differential diagnosis of hypercalcemia, emphasizing the features that are helpful in distinguishing one from another.

Primary Hyperparathyroidism

Depending on the nature of the clinical setting, primary hyperparathyroidism is either the most common or the second most common cause of hypercalcemia. In

TABLE 1. *Causes of hypercalcemia*

Primary hyperparathyroidism
Malignancy
    Lytic bone metastases
    Humoral peptide of malignancy
    Ectopic production of 1,25-dihydroxyvitamin D
    Other factor(s) produced ectopically
Nonparathyroid endocrine disorders
    Thyrotoxicosis
    Pheochromocytoma
    Adrenal insufficiency
    VIPoma
Vitamin D
    Vitamin D toxicity
    Granulomatous diseases
        Sarcoidosis
        Tuberculosis
        Histoplasmosis
        Coccidioidomycosis
        Leprosy
    Lymphoma
Medications
    Thiazide diuretics
    Lithium
    Estrogens/antiestrogens
    Milk-alkali syndrome
    Vitamin A toxicity
    Vitamin D toxicity
Familial hypocalciuric hypercalcemia
Immobilization
Parenteral nutrition
Acute and chronic renal disease

the outpatient setting, it ranks first, whereas in hospitalized patients it is usually second to malignancy. When primary hyperparathyroidism is considered among the endocrine disorders, here again it surfaces frequently with estimates of incidence ranging from 1 in 500 to 1 in 1000 (9). Primary hyperparathyroidism has become a common endocrine disorder, in comparison to its relatively rare status 50 years ago, as a result of the widespread use of the multichannel analyzer (10). The serum calcium is now routinely available on patients who are being evaluated for complaints that are completely unrelated to hypercalcemia. A few generations ago, hypercalcemia would have to be suspected before a serum calcium measurement would be ordered. Now the serum calcium is as routinely found in a patient's record as the glucose, BUN, and cholesterol. It is evident that the multichannel analyzer is responsible for the incidence of primary hyperparathyroidism (known cases of primary hyperparathyroidism) now reaching its prevalence (true number of cases) in the population. Primary hyperparathyroidism is likely to have been a common endocrine disorder well before it was recognized to be one. It occurs with a peak incidence in the sixth decade of life but can occur at all ages. Women are affected more commonly

than men by a 3:2 ratio, and the disorder is rather unusual in children.

Signs and Symptoms

The most common sign of primary hyperparathyroidism, indeed its sine qua non, is hypercalcemia (see below). Independent of the hypercalcemia is a set of characteristic signs and symptoms. The skeleton and the kidneys are the two major sites for potential involvement. These two organ systems are responsible for the appellation given the disease as one of "bones and stones."

Bone Involvement

Subperiosteal resorption of the distal phalanges (11), a "salt and pepper" appearance of the skull, tapering of the distal clavicles, bone cysts, and brown tumors are all classic radiographic signs of parathyroid bone disease, osteitis fibrosa cystica (Fig. 1). We are used to remembering a time when osteitis fibrosa cystica was more commonly seen in primary hyperparathyroidism, but it never comprised more than 10–15% of the hyperparathyroid population. Radiological evident bone disease is

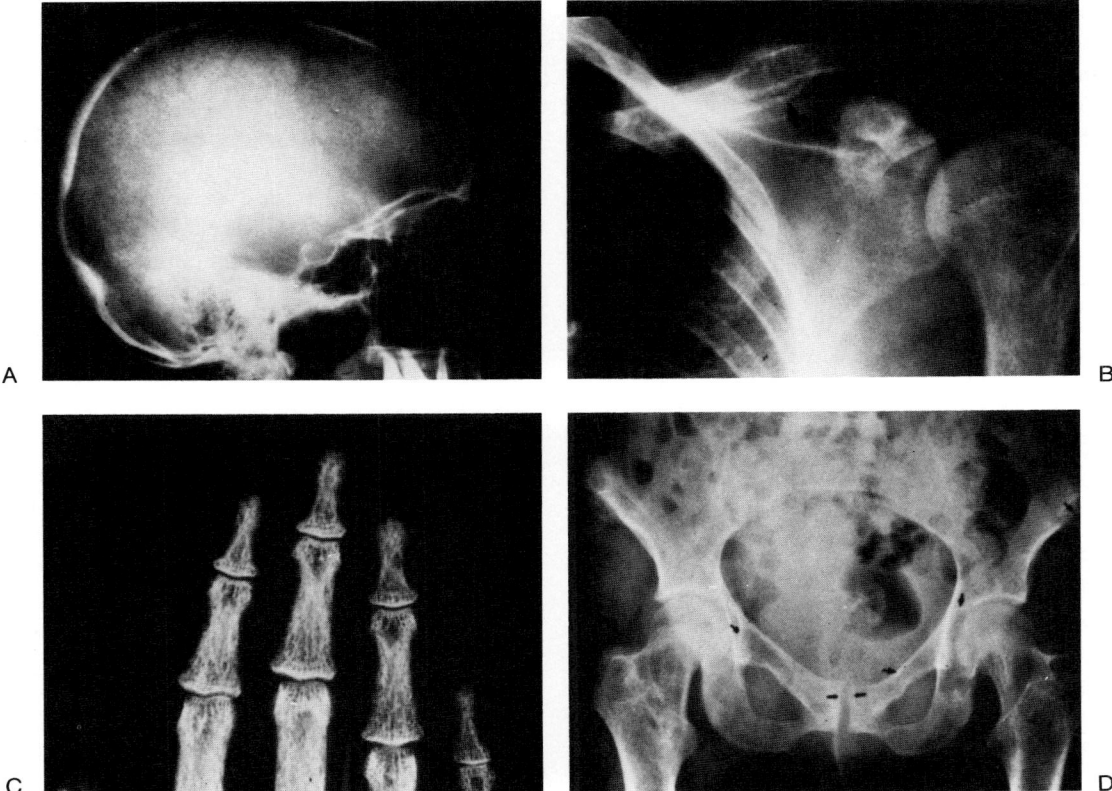

FIG. 1. Radiographic bone disease in primary hyperparathyroidism: **A:** salt-and-pepper erosions of the skull; **B:** subperiosteal bone resorption of the distal phalanges; **C:** cortical erosion of the distal femur; **D:** confluent cystic disease of the pelvis.

now even more uncommon in primary hyperparathyroidism. In a recent experience, no patient could be shown to have radiologically specific features of parathyroid bone disease (12). This point is important in the differential diagnosis of hypercalcemia because a set of skeletal films is rarely helpful in pointing to a diagnosis of primary hyperparathyroidism.

Even though specific radiographic signs of primary hyperparathyroidism have become distinctly unusual, assessment of bone mineral density, a much more sensitive technique, is indicating a pattern of skeletal demineralization among many asymptomatic patients with primary hyperparathyroidism (13,14). The particular distribution of reduced bone mineral density in primary hyperparathyroidism appears to be preferential to cortical bone (long bones) as compared to cancellous bone (spine) (12) (Fig. 2). Involvement of cortical bone with preservation of cancellous bone is compatible with the physiological actions of parathyroid hormone. One can take advantage of this observation in terms of management questions. In the absence of overt skeletal disease, reduced cortical bone density by bone densitometry can be an important consideration in terms of making a therapeutic decision.

Subclinical involvement of cortical bone in primary hyperparathyroidism is confirmed with even greater sensitivity by histomorphometric analysis of the percutaneous bone biopsy. In a recent study of 27 biopsy specimens obtained from the iliac crest of patients with primary hyperparathyroidism, the histomorphometric analysis reflected a disorder of bone turnover, in that osteoid surface, osteoid volume, eroded surface, mineralizing surfaces, and bone formation rates at the tissue level were all elevated (15,16). Structural parameters

showed a decrease in cortical thickness with preservation of trabecular connectivity. The latter two points are of particular note because they indicate a disorder with selective effects on bone. Other indices of bone structure support the view that primary hyperparathyroidism leads to preservation of cancellous bone and loss of cortical bone. For example, trabecular number is increased without any significant change in trabecular thickness leading to an increase in cancellous bone volume. These results are remarkable in that they were obtained from patients the majority of whom were asymptomatic. They call attention furthermore to the fact that the physiological actions of parathyroid hormone on cortical bone can be appreciated even in the modern-day setting of asymptomatic disease (Fig. 3).

These observations raise important new issues of management that have yet to be resolved. Are these changes indicative of a disease process that is progressive or merely a reflection of parathyroid hormone activity (if one can distinguish between the supraphysiological actions of parathyroid hormone from a disease process). Another key question raised by these observations relates to the postmenopausal woman who is at risk for the development of osteoporosis. Is primary hyperparathyroidism protective of trabecular bone mineral density and thus a beneficial feature in women predisposed to loss of vertebral bone in the postmenopausal years? On the other hand, is the preferential loss of cortical bone placing this type of person at further risk for fractures associated with age-related bone loss of the hip and wrist?

Although it is becoming clear by accumulating experience with bone mineral densitometry and histomorphometry that evidence for excessive parathyroid hormone activity on bone is relatively common, it is not clear whether this information is going to be helpful in predicting or selecting those patients who are destined to experience important skeletal complications of the disease.

Renal Involvement

The status of the kidney in primary hyperparathyroidism has always been a key consideration when assessments are made of complications of the disease. Stone disease is the most apparent manifestation of hyperparathyroid renal involvement. Despite the fact that the incidence of stone disease in primary hyperparathyroidism is lower now than it used to be (17), 15–20% of patients in most series will have had evidence for kidney stones (12). This subject is covered in greater detail in Chapter 31. Hypercalciuria, another renal manifestation of primary hyperparathyroidism, is also still relatively common. Our recent experience places the mean urinary calcium excretion in women at 237 ± 23 mg (normal, <250) and in men at 320 ± 33 mg (normal, <300). Although such relatively high figures for urinary calcium

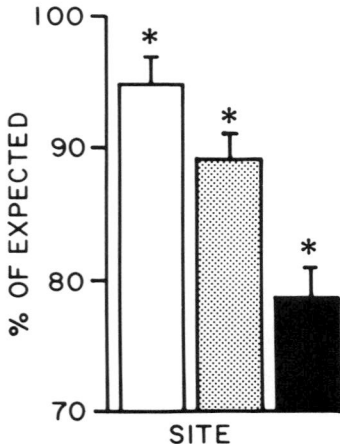

FIG. 2. Bone densitometry in primary hyperparathyroidism. Three different sites—radius (*solid black*), femoral neck (*gray*), and lumbar spine (*white*)—are shown in comparison to expected values for age-, sex-, and ethnicity-matched normal subjects. Divergence from expected values is different at each site (*p* = 0.0001). (Reproduced with permission from Ref. 12.)

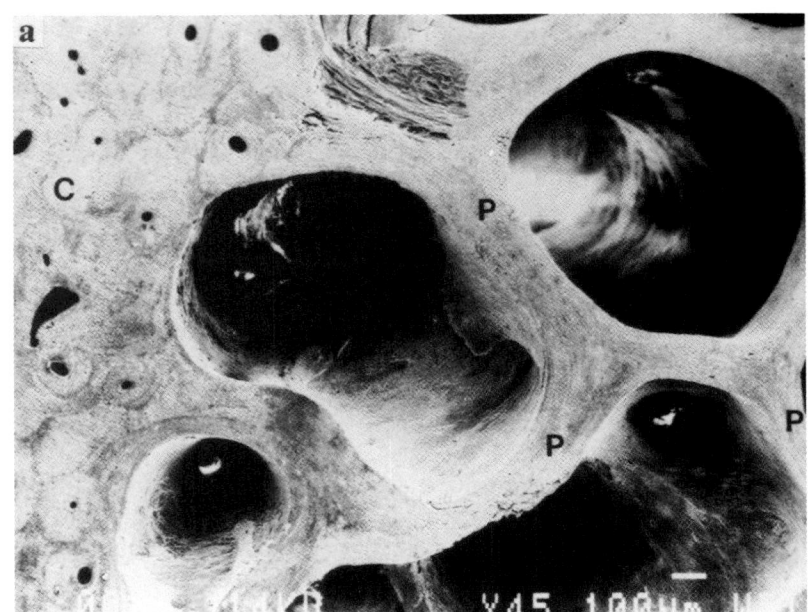

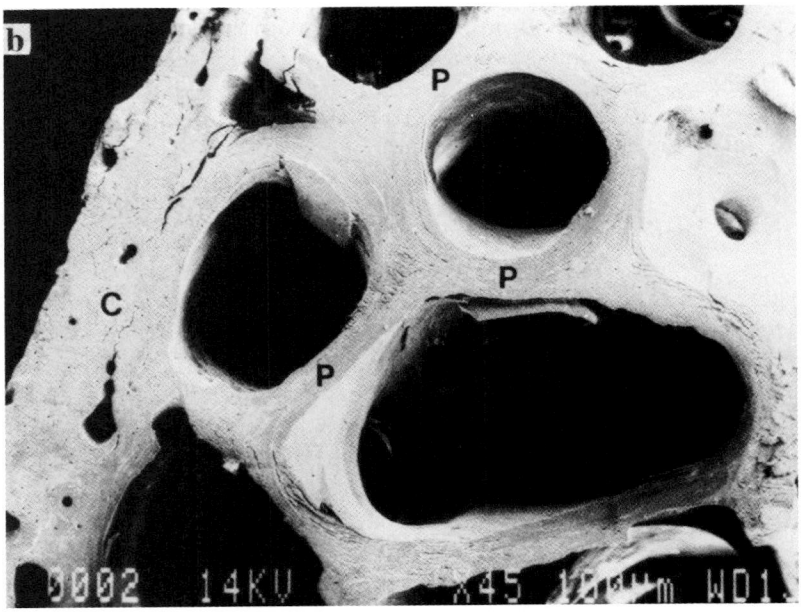

FIG. 3. Scanning electron micrographs of bone biopsy specimens from normal (**A**) and hyperparathyroid (**B**) subjects. Each micrograph is shown at the same magnification, ×45. The field width is 2.4 mm in each case. Loss of cortical thickness (C) with preservation of trabecular plates (P) can be seen in the hyperparathyroid subject (**B**). (Reproduced with permission from Ref. 12.)

excretion in primary hyperparathyroidism might seem to be paradoxical, considering the physiological property of parathyroid hormone to conserve renal calcium, it is accounted for by the greater filtered load of calcium among these patients. Patients who have normal urinary calcium excretion and no history of renal stone disease may nevertheless show a subtle renal manifestation of hyperparathyroid renal involvement by a reduction in the creatinine clearance. In the absence of any other definable cause for impaired renal function, one sometimes must attribute this rather nonspecific abnormality to primary hyperparathyroidism.

The clinical spectrum of primary hyperparathyroid-ism includes other elements besides "bones and stones." Neuromuscular involvement with histologically verifiable type II muscle fiber atrophy may well account for the easy fatigability that used to be a very common, albeit rather nonspecific, complaint among patients (18). Easy fatigability continues to be regularly reported in primary hyperparathyroidism, but in contrast to an older experience, patients now typically do not show by neuromuscular examination muscle weakness or atrophy (19).

A myriad of other associations is purported to be integral aspects of the hyperparathyroid syndrome. These include peptic ulcer disease, pancreatitis (20), hypertension (21), gout and pseudogout (22), anemia (23), and depression (24,25). In addition, a sense of "slowing down" may be volunteered by the middle-aged patient with primary hyperparathyroidism. It is not clear whether any of these associations are clearly related in a pathophysiological context to the state of hyperparathyroidism.

Clinical Forms of Primary Hyperparathyroidism

Asymptomatic Primary Hyperparathyroidism

Asymptomatic primary hyperparathyroidism is covered separately in Chapter 24. This is the most common of several different presentations of the disorder. It is characterized by mild but persistent hypercalcemia, usually no more than 1 mg/dL above the upper limits of normal. It is this form of primary hyperparathyroidism that is associated with few, if any, signs and symptoms of the disease. As a result, management decisions vis-à-vis therapy (conservative versus surgery) are often not clear.

Although asymptomatic primary hyperparathyroidism dominates the clinical presentation of the disease, it is important to bear in mind that there are many other ways in which the disease can appear (Table 2). This is a particularly important point because hypercalcemia can be erroneously attributed to other etiologies if one assumes that primary hyperparathyroidism is a consideration only when the serum calcium is minimally elevated.

Acute Primary Hyperparathyroidism

The differential diagnosis of life-threatening hypercalcemia includes the entity *acute primary hyperparathyroidism* (also referred to as *parathyroid crisis* or *parathyroid poisoning*). Acute primary hyperparathyroidism has been associated with the highest recorded serum calcium levels. In contrast to the asymptomatic form of the disease, virtually all patients are symptomatic of hypercalcemia (see symptoms) and many have evidence for both bone and stone disease (26). Approximately 25% of these patients have a previous history of mild, asymptomatic hypercalcemia. Among patients with life-threatening hypercalcemia, acute primary hyperparathyroidism continues to be an important consideration in the differential diagnosis. Acute primary hyperparathyroidism is a curable disease and rapid action should be taken to confirm or deny the diagnosis (see the section on evaluation and diagnosis).

Extremely high levels of parathyroid hormone in acute primary hyperparathyroidism suggest that parathyroid hormone secretion is completely autonomous. Against a background of mild hypercalcemia and only moderate elevations in parathyroid hormone, it is possible that an intercurrent illness with immobilization and dehydration, a common history in these patients, could contribute to rapidly worsening hypercalcemia. It is also possible, but only theoretical, that the parathyroid gland itself has been insulted by hemorrhage, infarction, or rupture of a cystic element. Extraordinary increases in circulating hormone levels could result from any of these events. As symptoms begin to ensue, hypercalcemia can rapidly worsen as dehydration and compromised renal function set up a vicious cycle of further worsening hypercalcemia and symptomatology.

Parathyroid Carcinoma

Parathyroid carcinoma is a pathological diagnosis and can only be suspected clinically. It is a rare presentation seen in fewer than 1% of patients who present with primary hyperparathyroidism (27). Clinically, these patients are most similar to those with acute primary hyperparathyroidism. Features, which are noted in Table 3, include moderate-to-severe hypercalcemia (>14 mg/dL), very high levels of parathyroid hormone, and involvement of the bones and kidneys. Clues to the possibility of parathyroid carcinoma at the time of operation include large size, dense fibrous capsule, attachment to contiguous structures, gross infiltration of thyroid, nerve, and muscles, or obvious lymph node metastases. These gross features, however, may be absent when parathyroid carcinoma is present.

The diagnosis rests on pathological examination of tissue. However, histological distinction between benign and malignant parathyroid tissue can also be difficult. If any of the following features are noted, the diagnosis becomes more secure: (1) trabecular, lobulated pattern of uniform sheets of cells separated by thick fibrous bands; (2) mitoses within the parenchymal cells; and (3) capsular or vascular invasion (28). Electron microscopy may show nuclear and mitochondrial anomalies, increased cellular activity, and basement membrane modifications (29–32). Despite these pathological guidelines, the diagnosis of parathyroid carcinoma may sometimes be made only in retrospect when recurrent hypercalcemia and obvious metastases become evident.

Distinctions between Primary Hyperparathyroidism, Acute Primary Hyperparathyroidism, and Parathyroid Carcinoma

The distinction between "routine" primary hyperparathyroidism and acute primary hyperparathyroidism or

TABLE 2. *Clinical presentations of primary hyperparathyroidism*

Asymptomatic hypercalcemia
Bone or stone disease
Other recognized complications (neuromuscular, gastrointestinal, articular, hematologic, central nervous system)
Acute primary hyperparathyroidism
Parathyroid carcinoma
Familial primary hyperparathyroidism
Familial cystic parathyroid adenomatosis
Neonatal hyperparathyroidism
Multiple endocrine neoplasia, type I or II

parathyroid carcinoma is fairly readily determined. On the one hand, hypercalcemia is mild (primary hyperparathyroidism); on the other hand, hypercalcemia is moderate to life-threatening (acute primary hyperparathyroidism or parathyroid carcinoma). Whereas in primary hyperparathyroidism, renal and bone involvement at the clinical level is not common, involvement of both the kidneys and the skeleton is seen frequently in the two more severe disorders (27). The parathyroid hormone level in acute primary hyperparathyroidism is approximately 20 times the upper limit of normal, another point distinguishing acute primary hyperparathyroidism from asymptomatic disease, in which levels of parathyroid hormone are usually not more than twice normal. Further comparisons are shown in Table 3.

Familial Forms of Primary Hyperparathyroidism

The familial forms of primary hyperparathyroidism occur in conjunction with multiple endocrine neoplasia, type 1 or 2, and with familial primary hyperparathyroidism. Another familial form of primary hyperparathyroidism recently recognized is cystic parathyroid adenomatosis (33). This disorder is characterized by recurrent parathyroid disease over years as glands become sequentially involved. No other endocrine tumors have yet been described in familial cystic adenomatosis, but fibrous maxillary or mandibular tumors have been seen.

Primary Hyperparathyroidism in Pregnancy and in Neonates

Primary hyperparathyroidism may become evident during pregnancy (34,35). Occasionally, the diagnosis is suspected in retrospect after delivery when neonatal hypocalcemia and tetany in the offspring occur. Management of primary hyperparathyroidism during pregnancy is controversial because of the risks of surgery during the pregnancy, on the one hand, and the risks of chronic hypercalcemia to the fetus, on the other hand. Some individuals believe, in addition, there to be an increased incidence of fetal demise when hyperparathyroidism is present during pregnancy.

Neonatal primary hyperparathyroidism is a condition of life-threatening hypercalcemia discovered soon after birth (36). These children display a characteristic hypotonia and can be managed only by emergency parathyroidectomy. At operation, all four glands are involved in a hyperplastic process. Of great interest is the fact that kindreds of families with neonatal primary hyperparathyroidism have been described in which familial cystic adenomatosis and/or familial hypocalciuric hypercalcemia are also present (36,37).

Other Clinical Presentations of Primary Hyperparathyroidism

Occasionally, primary hyperparathyroidism will be discovered in a person whose initial presentation is precipitated by a kidney stone. Although only about 5% of patients presenting with a kidney stone will be shown ultimately to have primary hyperparathyroidism, this possibility should always be considered in the course of an evaluation for the cause of nephrolithiasis.

Hypercalcemia is a virtual *sine qua non* of primary hyperparathyroidism, but it is possible for a patient with primary hyperparathyroidism to have a normal serum calcium. The entity "normocalcemic primary hyperparathyroidism," (38) however, more accurately describes the temporary excursion of the serum calcium into the normal range in a patient with primary hyperparathyroidism. It is distinctly unusual for the serum calcium not to return to elevated levels within 6–12 months. The diagnosis of primary hyperparathyroidism in a person whose serum calcium is always normal is extremely rare. The only other example of normocalcemic hyperparathyroidism occurs in patients who suffer with another disorder that predisposes them to hypocalcemia. For example, patients with malabsorption syndromes may not show evidence of primary hyperparathyroidism until the malabsorption syndrome (or vitamin D deficiency state) is corrected (39). These rare patients are shown to harbor an adenoma arguing against an autonomous hyperparathyroidism developing after long-standing secondary stimulation to all parathyroid glands. More likely, they had primary hyperparathyroidism upon which a malabsorption syndrome was superimposed, giving rise to the apparent normal or frankly low serum calcium level and the subsequent unmasking of the primary hyperparathyroidism after appropriate therapy for the malabsorption.

TABLE 3. *Primary hyperparathyroidism versus parathyroid carcinoma versus acute primary hyperparathyroidism*

	Primary hyperparathyroidism	Parathyroid carcinoma	Acute primary hyperparathyroidism
Period of review	1974–1976	1968–1981	1974–1984
Number of cases	51	62	48
Female/male ratio	2.5:1.0	1.2:1.0	1.1:1.0
Average age (years)	62	48	55
Serum calcium (mg/dL)	10.8	15.5	17.5
Renal involvement	2 (4%)	37 (60%)	20/29 (69%)
Skeletal involvement	4 (8%)	34 (55%)	19/36 (53%)
No symptoms	26 (51%)	1 (2%)	0

Source: Reproduced with permission from Ref. 26.

Clinical Spectrum of Primary Hyperparathyroidism

The clinical spectrum of primary hyperparathyroidism thus encompasses a wide variety of presentations. Because the emphasis is now on the mild, asymptomatic form of the disease, it is well to bear in mind the fact that primary hyperparathyroidism can show other clinical formats as reviewed in this section. It can appear as the "old-fashioned" disease with gross skeletal changes, especially among patients whose access to regular medical care is deficient. It can appear among those with life-threatening hypercalcemia. It is seen in the young and in the old. It may or may not be seen in conjunction with a familial syndrome. A useful caveat is that one should never rule out the possibility of primary hyperparathyroidism on the basis of the degree to which the serum calcium level is elevated. It can be seen among the highest levels of serum calcium and among those whose serum calcium is sometimes within normal limits.

Evaluation and Diagnosis of Primary Hyperparathyroidism

The historical elements of the patient who is being evaluated for primary hyperparathyroidism usually do not contain information pointing to specific involvement of the skeleton, the kidneys, or any of the other potential complicating features of primary hyperparathyroidism. The most typical history is that of the incidental discovery of hypercalcemia in the course of an evaluation for some other set of complaints (10,40). A careful history, however, may uncover in some of these patients nonspecific complaints such as weakness and easy fatigability. Typically, the physical examination is also not helpful. Band keratopathy, representing calcium deposition in the cornea, is rarely seen. It is most unusual to palpate an enlarged parathyroid gland unless parathyroid carcinoma is present. Muscle weakness may be observed on detailed examination but is also not appreciated as a rule.

The diagnosis of primary hyperparathyroidism depends on laboratory tests. Hypercalcemia is the cardinal chemical feature of primary hyperparathyroidism. It is virtually always present. The serum phosphorus is usually in the lower range of normal, but in approximately one-third of patients, it may be frankly low. If the serum alkaline phosphatase is elevated in the absence of concurrent liver disease, bone disease is usually present. Elevated serum concentrations of osteocalcin, another marker of osteoblastic activity, may be a more sensitive index of bone turnover in primary hyperparathyroidism, and this marker is more likely to be elevated than the alkaline phosphatase (41). If the serum alkaline phosphatase or osteocalcin is above normal, the urinary hydroxyproline excretion, an index more directly reflective of bone resorption, will also be elevated. The actions of parathyroid hormone to alter acid-base handling in the kidney sometimes leads to a mild hyperchloremia and metabolic acidosis. Urinary calcium excretion will be elevated in approximately one-fourth of all patients. Phosphaturia, a major physiological action of parathyroid hormone, may also be demonstrated in some patients. Characteristic biochemical indices are shown in Table 4.

The most useful test for the diagnosis of primary hyperparathyroidism is the parathyroid hormone measurement per se (42–44). Our thoughts about the usefulness of the radioimmunoassay for parathyroid hormone have changed in light of newer assays that provide a clear measure of discrimination from other causes of hypercalcemia. The most useful assays are those that measure the intact hormone or fragments with specificity for mid- or carboxy-terminal regions of parathyroid hormone (42,44). These assays show frank elevations in parathyroid hormone in well over 90% of patients with surgically

TABLE 4. *Biochemical indices in 52 patients with primary hyperparathyroidism*

Indices	Mean ± SEM	Normal range
Serum		
Calcium	2.8 ± 0.03 mmol/L	2.2–2.7
Phosphorus	0.9 ± 0.03 mmol/L	0.8–1.5
Albumin	44 ± 1 g/L	35–50
Alkaline phosphatase	114 ± 6 IU/L	80–110
N-PTH	36 ± 3 pg/mL	8–24
Midmolecule-PTH	835 ± 110 pg/mL	50–330
IRMA-PTH	126 ± 9 pg/mL	10–65
25-Hydroxyvitamin D	20 ± 2 ng/mL	9–52
1,25-Dihydroxyvitamin D	54 ± 3 pg/mL	15–60
Urine		
Calcium	263 ± 20 mg/g Cr	<250
Phosphorus	25 ± 1.5 mmol/day	
Cyclic AMP	475 ± 45 nmol/mmol Cr	441 ± 124
Hydroxyproline	41.2 ± 3.6 mg/day	<40 mg/day

proved primary hyperparathyroidism. Mid-region, carboxy-terminal, and intact assays for parathyroid hormone are more useful than assays that demonstrate exclusive specificity for the N-terminal fragment (Fig. 4). Another way to monitor parathyroid hormone activity in primary hyperparathyroidism is urinary cyclic AMP excretion. In general, total and nephrogenous cyclic AMP levels are elevated (45). However, in view of the substantial overlap of urinary cyclic AMP values among normal subjects and those with primary hyperparathyroidism and the greatly improved diagnostic usefulness of the radioimmunoassays for parathyroid hormone, urinary cyclic AMP rarely adds much to the diagnostic evaluation.

Another important reason why the radioimmunoassay for parathyroid hormone has become so useful relates to our better understanding of some of the other etiologies of hypercalcemia. In malignant disease, for example, parathyroid hormone levels are not elevated. Even in those malignant disorders associated with the ectopic production of a parathyroid hormone-like molecule, the parathyroid hormone level will be suppressed (44,46). By far, the most likely explanation for an elevated parathyroid hormone level in the face of hypercalcemia and reasonably normal renal function is primary hyperparathyroidism. Virtually all other causes of hypercalcemia are associated with suppressed levels of the hormone. Two noteworthy exceptions to this rule are the

hypercalcemias associated with the use of lithium and thiazide diuretics. The history usually points out these two possibilities fairly readily.

The $1,25(OH)_2D$ level may be elevated in primary hyperparathyroidism. Some investigators feel that this index is a useful means by which subgroups of patients with primary hyperparathyroidism can be distinguished from each other. Those patients with elevated $1,25(OH)_2D$ are believed by some to absorb calcium excessively from the gastrointestinal tract and to be at greater risk for the development of renal stones (47). On the other hand, the wide range of $1,25(OH)_2D$ values among patients with primary hyperparathyroidism may be more a function of the availability of the precursor, $25(OH)D$ than different pathophysiological processes. In this regard it has been reported that patients with primary hyperparathyroidism, in contrast to normal subjects, do not regulate the amount of $1,25(OH)_2D$ produced in the kidney (48). This observation suggests that the level of $1,25(OH)_2D$ in primary hyperparathyroidism is related more directly to the amount of $25(OH)D$ than to any specific pathophysiological subgrouping.

It should also be noted that an elevated level of $1,25(OH)_2D$ is not specific for primary hyperparathyroidism. It is seen in a number of other conditions associated with hypercalcemia, such as sarcoidosis, other granulomatous diseases, certain lymphomas, and vitamin D toxicity (49). It is helpful, however, in the specific differen-

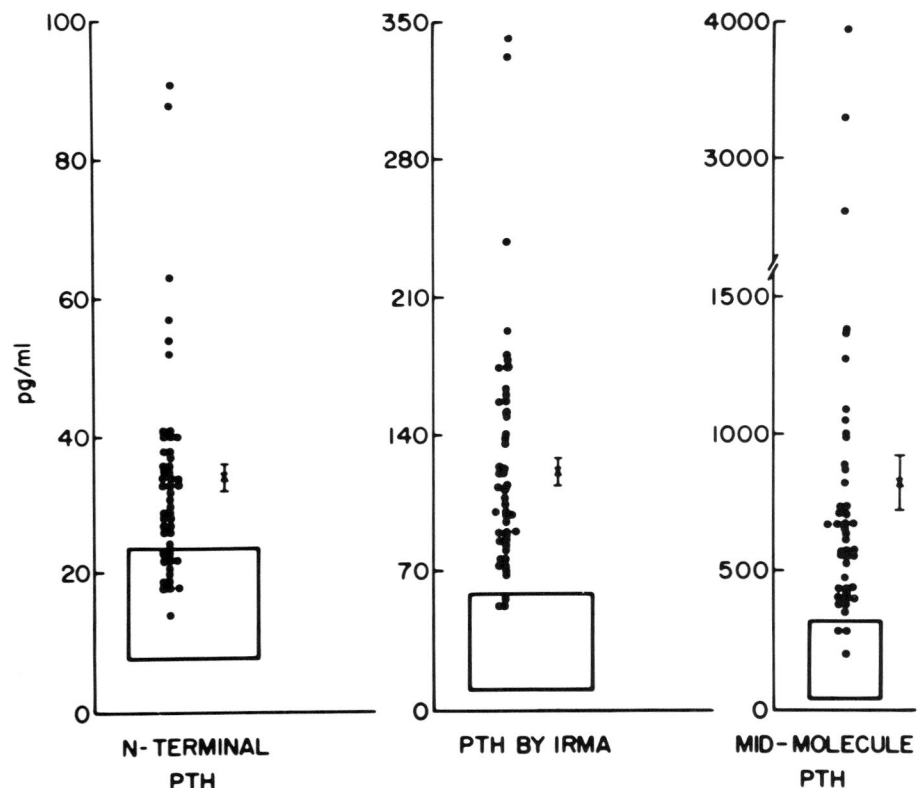

FIG. 4. Parathyroid hormone concentrations in primary hyperparathyroidism as measured in three different assays. Radioimmunoassays with specificities for N-terminal and midmolecular aspects of parathyroid hormone and the immunoradiometric assay were used on identical serum samples. For each assay, *rectangular area* is the normal range. Also shown in each panel is the mean ± SEM for the values. (Reproduced with permission from Ref. 12.)

tial diagnosis between primary hyperparathyroidism and the hypercalcemia of malignancy, the latter more often showing a depressed level of 1,25(OH)$_2$D.

Other aspects of the diagnostic evaluation for primary hyperparathyroidism include a consideration of several classical tests and newer approaches. Before the radioimmunoassay became established as the most useful test in the differential diagnosis of hypercalcemia, it was common to measure the tubular reabsorption of phosphate, the chloride/phosphate ratio, and in some cases to perform a prednisone suppression test (50–52). The first two tests reflect the action of parathyroid hormone to cause phosphaturia and to induce a mild renal tubular acidosis. The prednisone suppression test was considered to be useful because the hypercalcemia of primary hyperparathyroidism, in general, is not ameliorated by glucocorticoids, a point of differentiation from other hypercalcemic states associated with multiple myeloma, vitamin D toxicity, some granulomatous diseases, and breast cancer. None of these maneuvers was ever of great diagnostic value and should not be relied upon to establish the diagnosis of primary hyperparathyroidism.

More problematical in the current presentation of primary hyperparathyroidism are issues related to the patient with very mild hypercalcemia in whom sometimes it is hard to establish the diagnosis unequivocally. In these patients the serum calcium is virtually at the upper limit of normal and the parathyroid hormone level is minimally elevated. An oral calcium challenge test with measurement of parathyroid hormone by an assay that measures intact or biologically active fragments has been reported to be a promising means by which the diagnosis can be established. After an oral calcium load, normal subjects show a rapid suppression of parathyroid hormone, whereas patients with primary hyperparathyroidism show, at most, only a 20% reduction (53).

Hypercalcemia Associated with Malignancy

The two most common causes of hypercalcemia are primary hyperparathyroidism and malignancy. Together, they constitute the vast majority of patients with hypercalcemia (54). Exactly which one is more common depends on the clinical setting. The inpatient setting is more likely to see malignancy-associated hypercalcemia, whereas the outpatient setting tends to emphasize primary hyperparathyroidism. These two disorders are being considered at length in this chapter because they are the practical differential diagnosis of hypercalcemia. The diagnostic evaluation is focused on these two possibilities before pursuing the much longer list of etiologies. Malignancy-associated hypercalcemia is considered separately in Chapter 25.

The first major point to make when these two common causes of hypercalcemia are considered is that the distinction between them is usually fairly easy. The patient's clinical state often provides initial clues to suspect one or the other. The asymptomatic patient whose hypercalcemia is discovered incidentally is more likely to be shown to have primary hyperparathyroidism; the patient who harbors a malignancy is more likely to have a set of worrisome complaints that has initiated the medical attention. In addition, the malignancy is usually readily apparent. When hypercalcemia surfaces in a patient already known to have a malignancy, what has to be ascertained is that the hypercalcemia is caused by it and not due to a concurrent condition. Rarely, hypercalcemia is discovered in a relatively asymptomatic individual in whom the malignancy does not become apparent for a matter of months.

The laboratory provides additional help in making the distinction between malignancy and primary hyperparathyroidism. The most important distinguishing feature between these two conditions is the measurement of parathyroid hormone. In malignancy and other nonparathyroid causes of hypercalcemia, parathyroid glandular activity is inhibited, a normal physiologic response of parathyroid tissue. Thus a good assay for parathyroid hormone will not be able to detect parathyroid hormone in the circulation in patients with malignancy (44) (Fig. 5). If the parathyroid hormone level is suppressed when hypercalcemia is present, the diagnosis of primary hyperparathyroidism becomes extremely unlikely. Practically, it is excluded. However, although suppressed parathyroid hormone levels in hypercalcemia rules out primary hyperparathyroidism, it does not rule in malignancy because a great many other causes of hypercalcemia are associated with suppression of parathyroid gland activity. Having ruled out primary hyperparathyroidism, one focuses more intently upon malignancy in view of the statistical likelihood that it is by far the most common cause of parathyroid hormone–independent hypercalcemia. The many other potential causes of hypercalcemia are considered only after malignancy has been ruled out, unless the history or physical examination suggests that another explanation for the hypercalcemia is likely.

There are a host of different pathophysiological mechanisms for the hypercalcemias of malignancy (55–57). Most of the attention has focused on excessive mobilization of calcium from bone. The cell in bone responsible for bone breakdown, the osteoclast, appears to be activated by a variety of mechanisms. Direct invasion of the skeleton by the tumor may lead to local release of factors that lead to osteoclast activation, excavation of bone, and release of excessive calcium into the circulation (58,59). The metastatic malignant cell thus is believed to secrete factor(s) that in turn activate lymphocytes and/or monocytes in bone to secrete lymphokines or monokines that then, in a concerted manner, act on the osteoclast. In this case, the direct activator of the osteoclast is secreted by the normal host cell(s) stimulated by the neo-

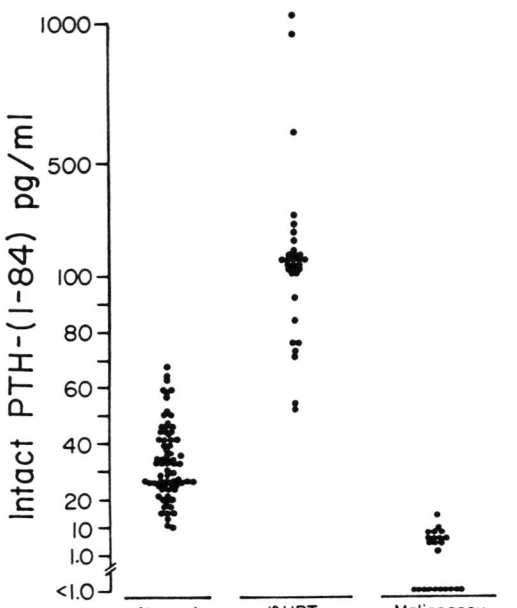

FIG. 5. Utility of parathyroid hormone determination in the diagnosis of primary hyperparathyroidism. Patients with surgically proven primary hyperparathyroidism show elevations (greater than 65 pg/mL) in virtually all cases. Patients with malignancy show levels that are below or at the lower limit of normal (10 pg/mL). Shown here is the immunoradiometric assay for parathyroid hormone. (Reproduced from Ref. 44 with permission.)

plastic cell. Some of the leading local osteoclast activating factors are tumor necrosis factor α, tumor necrosis factor β (lymphotoxin), interleukin-1, and prostaglandin E_2 (60–62). Multiple myeloma and breast cancer are most often believed to utilize this local mechanism of bone destruction, but actually any tumor that metastases directly to bone can cause hypercalcemia in a similar manner.

Humoral Hypercalcemia of Malignancy

In the absence of skeletal metastases, malignant cells can induce osteoclastic bone resorption by producing a factor that circulates to bone. Tumors most commonly associated with humoral hypercalcemia of malignancy (HHM) are squamous cell carcinomas (lung, esophagus, head and neck), renal and bladder tumors, and ovarian cancer. Patients with these diseases typically present with the combination of hypercalcemia and hypophosphatemia seen in primary hyperparathyroidism (63). In fact, like the disease it seems to mimic in chemical terms, primary hyperparathyroidism, urinary cyclic AMP is also usually elevated (64). Skeletal survey does not reveal the presence of metastatic bone disease (63). The idea that these tumors might be producing parathyroid hormone is an old one, first raised by Fuller Albright in the 1940s (65).

A decade of intensive work has led to elucidation of a peptide responsible for the hypercalcemia of malignancy (66–75). The details of this discovery and the peptide itself are covered in Chapter 39. In some respects the structure of the parathyroid hormone related peptide of malignancy (PTHrP), which has limited chemical similarity to parathyroid hormone, explains why the available radioimmunoassays for parathyroid hormone do not detect it in the circulation. The only area of homology between PTHrP and parathyroid hormone is the first 13 amino acids, where great homology exists. Thereafter, PTHrP diverges extensively from parathyroid hormone. The rest of the 84-amino acid polypeptide of parathyroid hormone and the 141-amino acid polypeptide of PTHrP are completely divergent from each other. The available radioimmunoassays for parathyroid hormone, even the ones with amino-terminal specificity, recognize epitopes of the parathyroid hormone molecule that are carboxyterminal to the first 13 amino acids. Thus they do not detect PTHrP in the circulation but register the normal suppression of native parathyroid hormone.

An area of intense current interest is the attempt to develop a clinically useful assay for PTHrP. If one were available, the distinction between humoral hypercalcemia of malignancy, other malignancy-associated hypercalcemias, and primary hyperparathyroidism might become even more definitive. A useful assay for PTHrP would also allow one to address important questions, such as how many patients with the HHM syndrome have circulating levels of PTHrP, are other malignant conditions not associated with hypercalcemia also associated with elevated levels of PTHrP (i.e., is it also a nonspecific tumor marker), and more fundamentally, is PTHrP a circulating factor? Very early observations suggest that PTHrP is elevated in some patients with the hypercalcemia of malignancy syndrome. Experience at this time is too limited to be able to reach any conclusions about some of these key points (76–78a).

Besides the radioimmunoassay for PTH that helps to distinguish primary hyperparathyroidism from hypercalcemia associated with malignancy, several other contrasting features are noteworthy. Suppressed levels of $1,25(OH)_2D$ have been used as a differentiating point because in primary hyperparathyroidism, $1,25(OH)_2D$ tends to be elevated (57,65). Why levels of $1,25(OH)_2D$ should be suppressed in the humoral hypercalcemia of malignancy syndrome is not clear. Actually, it is not universally seen, some patients showing clearly detectable levels. Second, if PTHrP is infused into nude mice, $1,25(OH)_2D$ levels rise dramatically. Third, PTHrP in vitro is a direct stimulator of $1,25(OH)_2D$ production. Some investigators feel that the extent of hypercalcemia in hypercalcemia of malignancy, which would tend to decrease $1,25(OH)_2D$, counteracts the effect of PTHrP to stimulate $1,25(OH)_2D$. Recently, it has been reported that at least one tumor associated with humoral hypercalcemia of malignancy may produce an inhibitor of $1,25(OH)_2D$ production. Whatever the ultimate explanation for these anomalous observations, one must be circumspect in using the $1,25(OH)_2D$ assay to distinguish between the HHM syndrome and primary hyperparathyroidism.

Issues related to fractional urinary calcium excretion as a differentiating feature between primary hyperparathyroidism and hypercalcemia of malignancy are obscure at this point. It is clear that one major mechanism of hypercalcemia in primary hyperparathyroidism is parathyroid hormone–mediated enhanced renal tubular reabsorption of calcium. Some investigators believe that renal tubular mechanisms may, under certain circumstances, also be very important in the pathophysiological mechanisms leading to hypercalcemia in malignancy. The issue is obscured somewhat by the fact that renal handling of calcium is influenced by volume depletion that by itself will enhance renal tubular reabsorption of calcium. If such patients are volume depleted, a not unlikely situation in the hypercalcemic patient, renal tubular reabsorption will appear to be enhanced. However, when measures are taken to maintain plasma volume, reabsorption of calcium is still increased in the rat Leydig cell tumor model. Furthermore, studies with PTHrP in vivo have shown that renal tubular calcium reabsorption is enhanced. Finally, Ralston argues that hypercalcemia in malignancy can occur before significant skeletal changes are detected, invoking the renal mechanism as important in the early stages of hypercalcemia-associated malignancy. It is fair to conclude that in both primary hyperparathyroidism and in hypercalcemia of malignancy, renal mechanisms probably play a role in contributing to the hypercalcemia. It is unlikely, however, to be a pivotal pathophysiological feature for either disease but should be taken into account when considering mechanisms and therapy. One cannot look to renal mechanisms to distinguish between these two common causes of hypercalcemia.

Another point that is believed to be useful in distinguishing primary hyperparathyroidism from humoral hypercalcemia of malignancy is revealed by bone biopsy. Whereas in both situations, evidence for active bone resorption is readily detected, in humoral hypercalcemia of malignancy there is evidence for more vigorous osteoclastic bone resorption than primary hyperparathyroidism. Perhaps more revealing as a differentiating feature is the relative paucity of bone formation in humoral hypercalcemia of malignancy. One could use this point as potentially useful in distinguishing primary hyperparathyroidism from HHM, but usually the distinction is clear before resorting to the bone biopsy (83).

Other Agents Responsible for Humoral Hypercalcemia of Malignancy

The current explosion of interest and knowledge concerning factors that can stimulate bone resorption makes

it likely that factors besides PTHrP are going to be implicated in the syndrome of hypercalcemia of malignancy (59,84). Already, transforming growth factors α and β (TGF-α and TGF-β) are known to possess in vitro bone resorbing properties. TGF-like molecules have also been extracted from tumors associated with this syndrome. The other candidates, such as tumor necrosis factor, lymphotoxin, and interleukin-1, have been mentioned.

Already discussed is the curious suppression of $1,25(OH)_2D$ levels in the HHM syndrome. In contrast, the ectopic production of $1,25(OH)_2D$ has been reported in association with some malignant lymphomas (85–87). In histiocytic lymphoma, elevated levels of $1,25(OH)_2D$ have been measured in the circulation (88). The mechanism by which this occurs appears to be similar to the means by which granulomatous diseases such as sarcoidosis may be responsible for hypercalcemia. The malignant tissue appears to have acquired the capability to convert $25(OH)D$ to $1,25(OH)_2D$. The hypercalcemia associated with human T-lymphotropic virus type I (HTLV-I) is sometimes seen in association with elevated $1,25(OH)_2D$ levels (89,90). Other HTLV-I associated hypercalcemic states have not been shown to have elevated levels (90,91).

An important diagnostic principle emphasized is that in the differential diagnosis between the two most common causes of hypercalcemia, primary hyperparathyroidism and malignancy, the immunoassay (radioimmunoassay on immunoradiometric) for parathyroid hormone is extremely useful. We now believe that when malignancies are associated with the biochemical markers of primary hyperparathyroidism, they are producing PTHrP or conceivably other factors that mimic PTH. They do not produce authentic parathyroid hormone. If the parathyroid hormone level is elevated in association with malignancy, one must think of the possibility of coexistent primary hyperparathyroidism. The original hypothesis that malignant tissue can produce native parathyroid hormone has been virtually discounted by the discovery of PTHrP in these malignant tissues and by the inability to detect native parathyroid hormone in the tissue or in the circulation. Lest one become too dogmatic about this point, a well-studied report has appeared that demonstrates the presence of authentic parathyroid hormone in the circulation, in the primary and in the liver metastases of a man who died from small-cell lung cancer and hypercalcemia (92). The material migrated with parathyroid hormone on gel chromatography showed parallelism in the radioimmunoassay for PTH, was registered as PTH by assays with N-terminal, midmolecule, and carboxyterminal specificities, and was consistent with parathyroid hormone by Northern and Southern blot analysis. In addition, the parathyroid glands were recovered and found to be normal. This is the best studied recent case and adds support to two other cases suggesting the ectopic production of native parathyroid hormone in malignancy (56,93). This information is provided not to discount the operating principle that tumors do not produce native parathyroid hormone ectopically but to indicate that this is a field in which information is gathering rapidly, that hypotheses are continually being reevaluated, and that we will not have a clear picture of the spectrum of humors produced by tumors for several more years.

Other Causes of Hypercalcemia

The algorithm for the diagnostic evaluation of hypercalcemia so far has been relatively uncomplicated. The index of clinical suspicion is usually directed toward one of the two etiologies described above, and the evaluation invariably permits one to come to a diagnosis. When does one consider the longer list of causes for hypercalcemia? The answer is simply, at the time the patient is being evaluated for primary hyperparathyroidism and/or malignancy. For example, the history and physical examination should always provide information about medications (thiazides, lithium, vitamin A or D) or thyrotoxicosis. As an operational point, when one first embarks on an evaluation of hypercalcemia, the entire differential diagnosis of hypercalcemia enters into the evaluation. The complete approach to the patient considers these other etiologies but rather quickly either rules them out or deems them to be extremely unlikely. The more unusual causes of hypercalcemia become important to bear in mind when the initial approaches do not provide a clear diagnosis.

Hypercalcemia Due to Nonparathyroid Endocrine Disorders

Thyrotoxicosis

Thyrotoxicosis is readily apparent in most patients by the history, physical examination, and initial thyroid function tests. Because hyperthyroidism is associated relatively commonly with hypercalcemia (5–10%) and because it can present among the elderly with few signs and symptoms, routine thyroid function tests are always part of the evaluation of the hypercalcemic patient. The hypercalcemia is usually mild, rarely exceeding 11.5 mg/dL. Accelerated bone turnover as opposed to excessive gastrointestinal absorption of calcium is responsible for the mild hypercalcemia (94). Normal calcium levels return rapidly following successful therapy for the hyperthyroidism. As expected for a hypercalcemic condition believed to be independent of parathyroid hormone, parathyroid hormone levels in thyrotoxicosis are not elevated. A recent study, in fact, has shown an inverse relationship between the T_3 level and the parathyroid hormone concentration in hyperthyroidism (95). It is believed that this observation reflects the direct actions of thyroid hormone on bone with release of ionized calcium and subsequent inhibition of parathyroid hormone secretion.

Pheochromocytoma

The diagnosis of pheochromocytoma is one of the more treacherous possibilities in the hypercalcemic patient whose workup is elusive. It is unusual that the patient has signs and symptoms that immediately call attention to this etiology. Nevertheless, hypercalcemia has been seen, rarely, in association with a pheochromocytoma. In view of the disastrous consequences that can follow if the diagnosis is not made, one should always have at least considered this possibility. Hypercalcemia is seen most often in pheochromocytoma in connection with multiple endocrine neoplasia, type II, in which both primary hyperparathyroidism and the adrenal gland tumor coexist (96,97). Because catecholamines are known to stimulate secretion of parathyroid hormone, in vitro, the apparent multiglandular syndrome could be due to the pheochromocytoma alone (98). Occasionally, hypercalcemia is seen without evidence for the multiglandular syndrome and the hypercalcemia remits following successful removal of the pheochromocytoma. Another conceivable mechanism is analogous to the syndrome of humoral hypercalcemia of malignancy, in which the adrenal gland is secreting a factor that induces bone resorption (99). Alternatively, the catecholamines per se could be responsible for osteoclast-activated bone resorption. Even if coexistent primary hyperparathyroidism is suspected in the patient with a pheochromocytoma, the proper therapeutic decision is to remove the adrenal tumor first. This approach properly eliminates the dangerous situation of performing neck surgery on a patient with a pheochromocytoma and also takes into consideration the possibility that the calcium could return to normal following adrenal surgery.

Another rare endocrine cause of hypercalcemia is the islet cell tumor that secretes vasoactive intestinal polypeptide (VIP), the so-called VIPoma. The hypercalcemia can be severe (102). VIPomas can occur as part of a multiple endocrine neoplasia syndrome, type I, and thus seen in association with coexisting primary hyperparathyroidism. However, similar to some pheochromocytomas, patients are described in whom the hypercalcemia remits after surgical removal of the pancreatic tumor.

Causes of Hypercalcemia Due to Vitamin D

Vitamin D–associated hypercalcemia constitutes a family of rather disparate disorders. They include the toxic ingestion of excessive amounts of any of the vitamin D preparations (either via misguided faddist health diets or in the course of therapeutic administration), granulomatous diseases, and lymphoproliferative malignancies. In some instances, especially when the history of excessive vitamin D ingestion is not obtained, the diagnosis can be quite difficult to make. In other cases, the malignancy or the granulomatous disease is quite apparent.

Vitamin D Toxicity

Excessive vitamin D can cause marked and prolonged hypercalcemia. It occurs in the course of therapy for the hypoparathyroid states and in those who ingest excessive quantities of the vitamin. The course of the hypercalcemia depends, in part, on which vitamin D preparation is responsible for the hypercalcemia. The parent compound, vitamin D, causes hypercalcemia that can persist for months because it is stored in fat tissues. Release of the inactive vitamin D and conversion ultimately to $1,25(OH)_2D$ can be continuous until fat depots are finally depleted. Patients treated for months or years on a given dose of vitamin D with good control can rather suddenly become hypercalcemic, an observation that calls for regular monitoring of the serum calcium on all patients treated with vitamin D regardless of how well they are controlled.

Vitamin D toxicity can also occur with overingestion of the other forms of vitamin D that are widely available. $25(OH)D$ and $1,25(OH)_2D$ are more water soluble and thus are not stored as much in fat as the parent vitamin. When overdosage occurs, therefore, the duration of hypercalcemia tends to be shorter. This is particularly true for the highly polar compound, $1,25(OH)_2D$, which is not appreciably stored at all in fat.

The hypercalcemia of vitamin D toxicity can usually be suspected on clinical grounds, as noted above, as well as by a biochemical profile that is different from primary hyperparathyroidism and malignancy-associated hypercalcemia. Instead of a low serum phosphate and lower urinary calcium excretion than expected for the degree of hypercalcemia, patients with vitamin D toxicity tend to show an elevated serum phosphate and marked hypercalciuria. Maintenance or elevation of the serum phosphate is due to the combined actions of vitamin D to facilitate gastrointestinal absorption of phosphate and to mobilize phosphate from bone. The hypercalciuria is due to suppression or lack of parathyroid hormone, leading to greater urinary calcium excretion than expected for the degree of hypercalcemia. Prolonged elevations of calcium and phosphate due to hypervitaminosis D can lead to nephrocalcinosis and renal dysfunction.

If the history suggests the possibility of vitamin D toxicity, it can readily be confirmed by measuring the circulating levels of vitamin D. If toxicity is due to vitamin D, the $25(OH)D$ is markedly elevated and the $1,25(OH)_2D$ level is only minimally so. This is due to the ability of the liver to convert vast quantities of vitamin D to $25(OH)D$ whereas renal conversion is tightly regulated, permitting only a small fraction of excess $25(OH)D$ to be converted to the active metabolite (103). Similar to the situation with excessive vitamin D, when $25(OH)D$ is responsible for the toxicity, this metabolite is markedly elevated and the $1,25(OH)_2D$ is only minimally so. For toxicities due to vitamin D or $25(OH)D$ ingestion, pharmacological quantities of the relatively weak compound $25(OH)D$ are responsible for the hypercalcemia.

The most widely used therapeutic form of vitamin D is its active metabolite, $1,25(OH)_2D$. $1,25(OH)_2D$ does not depend for activation on hepatic and renal conversion steps and thus is useful for virtually all causes of hypocalcemia, including those associated with impaired hepatic or renal function. Another reason why $1,25(OH)_2D$ has become popular is because hypercalcemia, should it occur in the course of therapy, is more readily reversible. Different from the other ingested forms of vitamin D, when vitamin D toxicity is due to $1,25(OH)_2D$, levels of the active metabolite are elevated and the $25(OH)D$ concentration is not.

The diagnosis of excessive ingestion of vitamin D can be made with confidence if the history and the laboratory features described above are compatible with the diagnosis. If the history cannot be obtained but the level of $25(OH)D$ is high, one can be reasonably certain that excessive exogenous ingestion is responsible for the hypercalcemia. No other hypercalcemic disorder associated with a vitamin D mechanism is likely to be associated with elevations in this metabolite. This is not the case when the hypercalcemia is accompanied by elevated levels of $1,25(OH)_2D$. In this instance, the elevated $1,25(OH)_2D$ level could be due to primary hyperparathyroidism (especially if the parathyroid hormone level is elevated), or any of vitamin D–associated hypercalcemias to be described below. One must thus rely heavily on the history and/or exclusion of other vitamin D states before concluding that excessive ingestion of $1,25(OH)D$ is responsible for the hypercalcemia.

Granulomatous Diseases

Hypercalcemia has been associated with a long list of granulomatous diseases, including sarcoidosis, tuberculosis, histoplasmosis, coccidiodomycosis, leprosy, berylliosis, candidiasis, eosinophilic granuloma, and silicone implantation (104–107). In each case, the granulomatous tissue is believed to be the site of uncontrolled production of $1,25(OH)_2D$. This mechanism has been elucidated best in sarcoidosis, the classical vitamin D sensitivity state. Pulmonary alveolar macrophages and lymphoid homogenates from patients with sarcoidosis are capable of synthesizing $1,25(OH)_2D$ (108,109). Moreover, elevated circulating levels of $1,25(OH)_2D$ levels have been detected in an anephric patient with sarcoidosis and hypercalcemia (110). In this fortuitous experiment of nature, the kidney, the only natural endogenous source of $1,25(OH)_2D$—excepting placenta—was completely excluded as a site of production. The extrarenal source of $1,25(OH)_2D$ in sarcoidosis may be accompanied by exquisite sensitivity to exogenous substrates. Marked hypercalcemia after mere sunlight exposure has been reported in patients with sarcoidosis. It would appear that extrarenal sites of 1,25(OH)$_2$D formation may not be under the same kind of tight regulatory control as is found in the kidney. Similar to all examples of vitamin D toxicity or sensitivity in which parathyroid hormone levels are suppressed, sarcoidosis is typically associated with hypercalciuria.

Malignancy-Associated 1,25-Dihydroxyvitamin D Production

Vitamin D–associated hypercalcemia can be due to a malignancy as described (85–87,111). One might include in this category the rarely reported cases of hypercalcemia with acquired immunodeficiency syndrome, although the hypercalcemia in these cases may relate more directly to the granulomatous and malignant lymphomatous processes to which these patients are predisposed (112).

A Practical Approach to the Vitamin D–Associated Hypercalcemias

Whether the hypercalcemia associated with vitamin D is due to excessive ingestion of any of the vitamin D preparations or to extrarenal synthesis in connection with granulomatous or malignant disease, the parathyroid hormone level is not elevated. An evaluation directed to the possibility of a vitamin D–related hypercalcemic state thus is unnecessary if parathyroid hormone levels are elevated. In this instance the elevated 1,25(OH)$_2$D level is best attributed to the primary hyperparathyroid state. If the parathyroid hormone level is suppressed, the differential diagnosis is readily focused upon the vitamin D–associated hypercalcemias. An elevated 25(OH)D level points the diagnostic workup in the direction of an exogenous source of the vitamin. If the 1,25(OH)$_2$D level is elevated, the hypercalcemia may be due either to therapeutic overadministration of the active metabolite or to any of the granulomatous or malignant conditions discussed. It is also obvious that the demonstration of elevated vitamin D levels does not establish a specific diagnosis but rather, directs the diagnostic evaluation toward a smaller set of diagnostic possibilities.

If the 25(OH)D level is not elevated, one can exclude with reasonable certainty a source of exogenous vitamin D or 25(OH)D. If the 1,25(OH)$_2$D level is not elevated, a source of exogenous 1,25(OH)$_2$D can also be excluded. A caveat to this kind of algorithm, however, is that the granulomatous and malignant disorders that have been seen in association with elevated levels of the active vitamin D metabolite cannot readily be dismissed if the 1,25(OH)$_2$D level is not elevated. Similarly, in the syndrome of humoral hypercalcemia of malignancy, in which it is common to find suppressed levels of 1,25(OH)$_2$D, one cannot rule it out simply because the 1,25(OH)$_2$D level is readily detectable. One thus uses the circulating levels of the vitamin D metabolites along with the other diagnostic features of the workup to seek those causes of hypercalcemia that are not readily apparent.

Medication-Induced Hypercalcemia

It goes without saying that the history is as important a part of the evaluation for hypercalcemia as it is for any other presenting abnormality in endocrinology. A complete and reliable medication history will help enormously in considering the etiologies of hypercalcemia in a given patient. This is particularly true for patients whose history includes the use of thiazides or lithium because the differential diagnosis between these two medication-associated hypercalcemias and primary hyperparathyroidism can be perplexing.

Thiazide Diuretics

Thiazide diuretics may cause hypercalcemia by reducing plasma volume, increasing proximal tubular reabsorption of calcium, and perhaps also by enhancing sensitivity of target tissues to parathyroid hormone. There may be no intrinsic abnormality in calcium metabolism (113). Thiazide-induced hypercalcemia is one of those unusual situations in which hypercalcemia and elevated levels of parathyroid hormone may be due to a nonparathyroid etiology. The hypercalcemia in a substantial number of patients will remit after withdrawal of the thiazide. What is confusing is that some patients who develop hypercalcemia in the setting of thiazide use will not revert to normal after the medication is withdrawn. The diagnosis of primary hyperparathyroidism is eventually made. In these patients it is almost as if the thiazide medication unmasks the primary hyperparathyroidism. At the time the patient is first seen, however, one cannot know whether the hypercalcemia is due to the thiazide or to primary hyperparathyroidism. The correct diagnosis is made only when the calcium and parathyroid hormone levels are reevaluated 2–3 months after the diuretic is discontinued. If the hypercalcemia and elevated parathyroid hormone levels persist, the diagnosis of primary hyperparathyroidism can be made.

Lithium

Similar to thiazide diuretic use, administration of lithium carbonate has been associated with hypercalcemia in a manner that is compatible with a hyperparathyroid state (114). In keeping with a medication-induced hyperparathyroidism, anecdotal reports have described reversal of the apparent hyperparathyroidism after discontinuance of lithium. How lithium mimics a condition similar to primary hyperparathyroidism is not clear. The effect of lithium on parathyroid hormone secretion in normal volunteers showed no differences in serum calcium, parathyroid hormone level, and nephrogenous cyclic AMP measurements (115). These observations do not rule out the possibility of a longer-term effect of lithium on the set point of the parathyroid glands for calcium. In fact, in vitro studies indicate that lithium may alter the set point of the parathyroid cell to calcium (116). In a recent study by Mallette et al., the effects of short-term versus long-term administration of lithium were addressed (117). In subjects treated for an average of 1.7 months, serum ionized calcium increased without any change in parathyroid hormone levels. These observations are consistent with an alteration in the set point for parathyroid hormone release. In subjects treated for longer periods of time (average of 103 months), lithium was associated with the same increase in calcium, but now the circulating parathyroid hormone level was significantly increased, by 30–60%. It is noteworthy that no patient treated long term showed an elevation of serum calcium out of the normal range. Consistent with an increase in biologically active parathyroid hormone, the serum chloride was higher, the serum phosphate was lower, and the $1,25(OH)_2D$ level was higher than control subjects. Interestingly, these investigators showed an increase in parathyroid glandular volume as determined by ultrasonography. In practical terms, the diagnosis of primary hyperparathyroidism cannot be made with certainty when the patient is receiving lithium. One would like to withdraw the medication and to reevaluate several months later to ascertain whether or not the patient has primary hyperparathyroidism. This is a particularly difficult issue because it may not be possible to withdraw the medication safely in a patient whose psychiatric illness requires continued administration of lithium. Further compounding the dilemma is the possibility that the depression for which the patient may be receiving lithium may be more difficult to control *because* of the primary hyperparathyroidism.

Estrogens and Antiestrogens

The hypercalcemia associated with estrogen and antiestrogen (Tamoxifen) therapy is a special situation and not usually mistaken for other causes of hypercalcemia. These patients have known breast cancer (118). Patients most likely to develop hypercalcemia in the wake of either of these therapies have known extensive skeletal metastases. They appear to have a better long-term prognosis than that of patients who do not develop hypercalcemia, an observation that may relate to the cytotoxic effects of the therapy on the skeletal metastases. This is a situational hypercalcemia following within the time course of therapy and therefore not often confused with malignancy-associated hypercalcemia.

Milk–Alkali Syndrome

Milk–alkali syndrome is an old-fashioned etiology of hypercalcemia that used to occur when absorbable alkali and large amounts of calcium (milk) were used for peptic ulcer disease. The biochemical hallmarks are metabolic alkalosis, a tendency toward hyperphosphatemia, nephrocalcinosis, and progressive renal insufficiency (119,120). These patients typically do not have hypercalciuria. Although an uncommon presentation of hypercalcemia now, it is worth recalling, especially as calcium carbonate preparations are becoming more widely used as a supplemental nutrient. Reports still appear descriptive of this syndrome (121). Prodigious amounts of elemental calcium have to be absorbed, on the order of 3–6 g daily, together with large amounts of alkali. A variant of this syndrome was recently described in which a severely ill patient with anorexia nervosa developed marked hypercalcemia by a massive intake of cheese, equivalent to 16 g of elemental calcium daily. Alkalosis in this case was due not to the intake of alkali but to the use of a thiazide diuretic and to induced vomiting (122). If this syndrome is recognized early, the attendant renal insufficiency is reversible, but prolonged exposure of the kidneys to this kind of hypercalcemia can lead to irreversibly compromised renal function.

Vitamin A and Vitamin D Toxicity

Vitamin D toxicity, already discussed in detail (see above), is the much more common cause of vitamin use–associated hypercalcemia. It is well to bear in mind, however, vitamin A toxicity, an extremely rare cause of hypercalcemia (123). Because some cases in the literature have not clearly ruled out vitamin D toxicity, the examples of pure vitamin A–associated hypercalcemia are few and far between. Nevertheless, a few well-documented examples exist. When vitamin A is responsible for the hypercalcemia, it is usually associated with more classical features of hypervitaminosis A, such as hepatic dysfunction, dermatitis, and dementia. The vitamin A apparently can cause accelerated bone resorption. A fairly classical radiographic sign is seen in the periosteum of long bones. By the time hypercalcemia becomes apparent, patients have ingested very large amounts of vitamin A for rather long periods. These patients tend to be extremely ill and unable to give a history of vitamin A ingestion. The diagnosis of vitamin A toxicity is usually entertained by the sharp clinician who recognizes the clinical constellation of vitamin A toxicity or who, in desperation, resorts to a consideration of the most unusual etiologies for obscure hypercalcemia. Although total vitamin A levels tend to be elevated, the best way to establish the diagnosis is to detect an excess of retinyl esters as a percentage of circulating vitamin A (123).

Familial Hypocalciuric Hypercalcemia

Familial hypocalciuric hypercalcemia (FHH) is an important consideration in the differential diagnosis of asymptomatic primary hyperparathyroidism (124,125). It is covered in Chapter 24. Like primary hyperparathyroidism, patients with FHH do not tend to have bone disease or stone disease. Other well-known features of primary hyperparathyroidism are also absent. The distinction between this disease and primary hyperparathyroidism resides in several features besides the family history, which, when available, will give an autosomal dominant pattern of transmission (124–126). In keeping with the working premise that parathyroid hormone levels are not elevated in hypercalcemic conditions not associated with primary hyperparathyroidism, the parathyroid hormone level usually is normal in this syndrome. The biochemical distinction that tends to single out FHH from primary hyperparathyroidism and a host of other hypercalcemias is the urinary calcium excretion, which is low. The ratio of renal calcium clearance to creatinine clearance tends to be less than 0.01.

Despite the clinical similarities between FHH and primary hyperparathyroidism, the pathophysiology of the two disorders are completely different. FHH is not a disorder of the parathyroid glands. Those few examples of parathyroidectomy in FHH have ascertained the glands to be normal. In contrast to the blunted responsiveness of the parathyroid cell to calcium in primary hyperparathyroidism, the cellular basis for FHH is proposed to be due to a global defect in cellular calcium (127). Recent studies along these lines have not confirmed this impression (128). Despite the fact that FHH and primary hyperparathyroidism appear to be completely different hypercalcemic disorders, a clear genetic distinction between them is obscured by the presence in single kindreds of both severe neonatal primary hyperparathyroidism and FHH (37,129).

Immobilization Hypercalcemia

It is commonly believed that prolonged bed rest can lead to hypercalcemia. This belief is based on the well-known fact that negative calcium balance ensues regularly in any individual subjected to prolonged immobilization. The negative calcium balance is precipitated by the loss of weightbearing. Levels of parathyroid hormone, nephrogenous cyclic AMP, and 1,25(OH)$_2$D are all suppressed (130). The bone biopsy shows enhanced osteoclastic activity and diminished osteoblastic function (131). The patient with otherwise normal homeostatic control mechanisms for calcium will compensate for these triggered events and not become hypercalcemic. The development of hypercalcemia requires an underlying acceleration in bone turnover rate among the immobilized. Thus, in Paget disease, in malignancies with skeletal involvement, and in the very young, hypercalcemia can certainly develop in the setting of immobilization (130–132). Otherwise, hypercalcemia due exclusively to immobilization is rare among middle-aged and older individuals whose bone metabolism is normal. One should bear in mind that underlying hypercalcemic conditions such as primary hyperparathyroidism can rap-

idly be worsened by immobilization transforming the mild hypercalcemia of primary hyperparathyroidism into a life-threatening parathyroid crisis.

Hypercalcemia with Parenteral Nutrition

The hypercalcemia that used to be seen in patients receiving parenteral nutrition was easily explained when the amount of calcium administered in the infusate was greater than 300 mg/day. It was readily reversed when the infusate calcium was reduced or withdrawn. However, hypercalcemia, not explainable by the amount of calcium in the infusate, still is seen in the setting of parenteral nutrition (133,134). In these patients an aluminum toxicity is seen by a distinctive osteomalacia on bone biopsy (135). The conclusion that aluminum toxicity is responsible for the osteomalacia was reasonable when the casein hydrolysate used in the preparation of the supplemental nutrients contained measurable amounts of aluminum. However, newer methods of casein hydrolysis have been developed that are not accompanied by appreciable amounts of aluminum and the syndrome still develops sometimes. The explanation for this form of hypercalcemia is thus obscure.

Hypercalcemia in Acute and Chronic Renal Disease

The hypercalcemia that develops in the recovery phase of *acute renal failure* is not mistaken for other etiologies because the situation is so well defined. The cause, however, is not known. Transiently elevated levels of parathyroid hormone and 1,25(OH)$_2$D, induced by the hypocalcemia of acute renal failure, could lead to enhanced physiological actions. Hypercalcemia may also occur after *renal transplantation,* perhaps due to excessive production of 1,25(OH)$_2$D by the new kidney. In *chronic renal failure,* hypercalcemia may be a consequence of uncontrolled secondary hyperparathyroidism. The secondary hyperparathyroidism has a complicated and somewhat obscure pathophysiology. Elevations in the serum phosphate, deficient 1,25(OH)$_2$D formation, and malabsorption of calcium are all important factors. The hyperparathyroid state, however, is not primary and the serum calcium is not elevated. If the secondary hyperparathyroidism of renal insufficiency is not controlled by adequate diet, phosphate binding gels, judicious use of vitamin D, or dialysis, the parathyroid glands can become relatively autonomous, leading to frank hypercalcemia. This condition is dubbed *tertiary hyperparathyroidism.* The mild-to-moderate hypercalcemia is associated typically with markedly elevated levels of parathyroid hormone (over 20–30 times normal). A radioimmunoassay that detects metabolic fragments of parathyroid hormone will show even greater elevations than an assay that is more specific for biologic active fragments or intact hormone because inactive fragments of parathyroid hormone accumulate in renal insufficiency.

Multiple Causes of Hypercalcemia in the Same Person

In this section we have concentrated on the practical differential diagnosis of hypercalcemia. The working impression is that when an obvious cause of hypercalcemia is apparent, it is usually responsible for the hypercalcemia. Unfortunately, the clinical situation is not always as straightforward as one would like it to be. Two potential causes of hypercalcemia may be identified in the same person. A known malignancy in a hypercalcemic patient does not necessarily link the hypercalcemia to the malignancy. A patient with sarcoidosis may also develop hypercalcemia for other reasons. Clinical features of the patient and the diagnostic evaluation usually permits an assignment of the hypercalcemia to the correct etiology.

CLINICAL FEATURES OF HYPERCALCEMIA

It is important to consider the clinical features of hypercalcemia apart from its etiology because they help to determine decisions regarding immediate therapy for the hypercalcemia per se as well as therapeutic approaches to the underlying disorder. The signs and symptoms of the patient's underlying disorder should not be confused with those related to hypercalcemia. If these two points are not distinguished from each other, measures to reduce the serum calcium may not necessarily be indicated and the patient's overall condition may not be improved. It is true that hypercalcemia is not always associated with a compelling set of clinical features that dictate whether or not the patient is symptomatic. In fact, more commonly, rather general, nonspecific complaints such as weakness and lethargy challenge our ability to pinpoint the specific cause of the symptomatology. Nevertheless, the attempt is made to address the extent to which signs and symptoms may be present in a given patient. In some cases it is not possible to be certain, and empiric but judicious therapy for the hypercalcemia is instituted.

One usually makes the assumption that the total serum calcium level reflects the physiologically active ionized form. If the serum albumin is normal and there is no derangement of acid-base status, this assumption is generally valid. Rarely, the patient with multiple myeloma will display an elevated total serum calcium concentration because of a circulating calcium-binding myeloma protein (136,137). The clue to this unusual situation is a very high calcium value in a patient who is completely asymptomatic. The ionized calcium in such a patient would be normal.

Symptoms of hypercalcemia are only grossly related to the actual level of the serum calcium. Calcium values greater than 15 mg/dL are more likely to be associated with symptoms than calcium values that are only minimally elevated. Several variables, besides ascertaining that the total calcium is an accurate representation of the ionized calcium, modulate the clinical expression of hypercalcemia. The rate of rise of the serum calcium, for example, is an important determinant. For a given hypercalcemic level, symptoms are much more likely to be present if the serum calcium has risen rapidly. In contrast, if the serum calcium has increased slowly over a matter of months, adaptive changes may permit the patient to adjust and to be relatively asymptomatic. It is distinctly possible for a patient with a very high serum calcium to be less symptomatic than a patient with more moderate hypercalcemia. Age is another important variable. The older patient is more likely to become symptomatic of hypercalcemia than the younger patient. The older patient unfortunately is also more susceptible to somatic changes that may mimic hypercalcemia confounding our ability to attribute the symptoms to the hypercalcemia. Individual variability is perhaps the most important factor that leads to more symptoms in one and fewer symptoms in another. The important point is that the actual serum calcium level is only one determinant of many that are collectively responsible for the symptomatology of hypercalcemia.

Symptomatic hypercalcemia affects many major organs, giving rise to a constellation of signs and symptoms (Table 5). The gastrointestinal tract is affected early, with anorexia and constipation perhaps being the earliest manifestations. Nausea and vomiting may follow. Hypercalcemia impairs the ability of the kidney to concentrate the urine so that a nephrogenic diabetes insipidus is a manifestation of symptomatic hypercalcemia. However, the urine volumes are not typical for the more classical states of diabetes insipidus. More important than the urine volume is the polyuria and polydipsia, which are manifestations of this defect in renal concentrating ability. In fact, polyuria and polydipsia may mimic diabetes mellitus.

The combination of polyuria and anorexia is ominous and may lead to a cycle that culminates in rapidly worsening hypercalcemia. The need to compensate for excessive urinary fluid losses cannot be met if anorexia is present, leading to dehydration and intravascular volume depletion. Dehydration leads to even higher serum calcium levels, which, in turn, lead to worsening polyuria. At some point, dehydration will also lead to a reduction in the glomerular filtration rate, which initiates a more serious problem. When the kidney can no longer clear the circulating calcium, hypercalcemia may become rapidly worse. Prolonged hypercalcemia can lead to crystallization of calcium salts in the kidney with frank renal stone formation (nephrolithiasis), or more generalized precipitation of calcium salts (nephrocalcinosis).

Perhaps the most difficult consideration of the symptoms of hypercalcemia relate to effects on the central nervous system. Hypercalcemia has the capability to suppress mentation and the level of consciousness. The level of consciousness can be affected minimally as ex-

TABLE 5. *Clinical features of hypercalcemia*

General
  Weakness
  Dehydration
  Metastatic calcification
Central nervous system
  Impaired concentration
  Increased sleep requirement
  Altered states of consciousness (confusion,
    lethargy, stupor, coma)
Gastrointestinal tract
  Polydipsia
  Anorexia
  Nausea
  Vomiting
  Constipation
  Pancreatitis
  Peptic ulcer
Renal
  Polyuria
  Decreased function
  Decreased concentrating ability
  Nephrolithiasis
  Nephrocalcinosis
Cardiovascular
  Hypertension
  Electrocardiographic changes (shortened QT
    interval)
  Increased sensitivity to digitalis

pressed by apathy and drowsiness or maximally as seen in a depressed sensorium, obtundation, and coma. It is difficult to assign any of these changes to the hypercalcemia per se because the associated dehydration invariably contributes to these central nervous system features, especially in older people. The older person presents a particularly difficult clinical problem if any of these features is present when hypercalcemia is mild. The obtunded octogenarian whose serum calcium is only 11.5 mg/dL may or may not be symptomatic in this way because of the hypercalcemia. It is incumbent on the physician to seek other etiological factors before concluding that the mild hypercalcemia is responsible for the symptoms. It is all too easy to focus on the hypercalcemia to the exclusion of other, more important but perhaps obscure explanations. On the other hand, if this same set of symptoms is present in the patient with more severe hypercalcemia, it is reasonable to draw the conclusion that the two are related. Empiric therapy in this situation would certainly be indicated. If the central nervous system is affected by the hypercalcemia, the most dramatic example being frank coma, it will reverse itself upon correction.

One usually does not dwell upon the cardiovascular manifestations of hypercalcemia when indications for therapy are sought. The systolic blood pressure is only grossly related to the level of the serum calcium. Thus, if the calcium is markedly elevated, the blood pressure may be higher than normal for the patient. On the other hand, other clinical features of marked hypercalcemia,

such as dehydration, wasting, and general debilitation, could tend to lower the blood pressure. Classically, the QT interval on the electrocardiogram is shortened. However, this sign is not reliably seen in patients who have experienced hypercalcemia for a long period of time. The patient whose hypercalcemia has appeared rather quickly is more likely to show this electrocardiographic manifestation of hypercalcemia. Finally, patients with hypercalcemia may demonstrate enhanced sensitivity to the cardiac glycosides.

THERAPY OF HYPERCALCEMIA

Hypercalcemia is a treatable disorder but it is not always treated. It sometimes heralds the diagnosis of a treatable underlying disorder, which is given more initial attention than the hypercalcemia. On the other hand, hypercalcemia may present as a life-threatening disorder that demands emergent therapy independent of the underlying disorder that may or may not be known. The logic of therapy relates importantly to two elements: the underlying etiology and the hypercalcemia per se. Under nonemergent conditions (i.e., when the serum calcium is not life threatening), the underlying disorder is properly given the center stage of attention. The best example of the latter point is the modern-day presentation of primary hyperparathyroidism. In contrast, under emergent conditions, when the serum calcium is over 15 mg/dL, the hypercalcemia is treated first. It is well to bear in mind the fact that if the etiology of the marked hypercalcemia is an incurable, widely disseminated malignancy, sometimes the better part of valor is not to treat the hypercalcemia at all.

Treatment of Primary Hyperparathyroidism

Indications for Surgery

Surgery is the only way to cure primary hyperparathyroidism. The case for parathyroid surgery is relatively straightforward when obvious signs and symptoms of primary hyperparathyroidism are present. In the typically asymptomatic patient, however, it is often not clear that parathyroidectomy is the best course. If we knew who among asymptomatic patients are at definable risk for the development of complications of hyperparathyroidism, the process of decision making would be easier. Unfortunately, we do not know who among the asymptomatic are at risk. We do not even know who among the asymptomatic are truly asymptomatic. Reasons for uncertain therapeutic guidelines include lack of sufficient long-term experience with the asymptomatic form of primary hyperparathyroidism, the need to apply more sensitive approaches to evaluating the skeleton in asymptomatic patients, and incomplete knowledge regarding reversibility of findings that may have become apparent only by sensitive skeletal testing.

In the absence of this kind of necessary information, we use a set of admittedly imperfect guidelines to help us decide who are candidates for surgery: serum calcium greater than 1 mg/dL above the upper limits of normal; any complications of primary hyperparathyroidism (e.g., overt bone disease, nephrolithiasis); an episode of acute hyperparathyroidism; hypercalciuria; relative youthfulness (138,139). In the asymptomatic patient, these guidelines do not help and it is usually the bias of the physician that influences the outcome most. Some physicians feel that parathyroidectomy is indicated in all patients, whether or not they meet the guidelines above. Their point is that all patients with primary hyperparathyroidism are at risk for its complications. Because the operation is relatively straightforward, not presenting any major concerns in the otherwise healthy person, patients should be encouraged to have their presumed adenoma removed when the diagnosis is made. Other physicians feel that in the absence of overt complications, the patient is best advised to be followed conservatively. They point to lack of evidence that asymptomatic primary hyperparathyroidism is a progressive disease. It is of interest in this regard that Rao has reported that even among patients with primary hyperparathyroidism who had diminished cortical bone mineral density at the time of initial evaluation, there was no evidence for progression over an average follow-up of 46 months (140). Another point that is becoming recognized is the fact that the typical profile of bone mineral density in primary hyperparathyroidism shows preservation of cancellous bone at the expense of cortical bone (15,16). In the postmenopausal women at risk for cancellous bone loss (i.e., vertebral bone) the state of parathyroid hormone excess could conceivably be protective. Of course, this point should be balanced against the possibility of cortical bone loss that could become more evident over time.

Issues related to the surgical approach to the patient with primary hyperparathyroidism also have to consider the patient's personal viewpoint. Even if parathyroidectomy is indicated by the presence of overt bone or stone disease, some will refuse surgery. Others with coexisting medical problems may not wish to face greater risks associated with surgery. On the other hand, some patients who appear to be completely asymptomatic prefer surgery to facing the unknown consequences of long-term primary hyperparathyroidism. A last group of patients may, in fact, be the most difficult: namely, those who have had previous unsuccessful neck surgery. In these patients, preoperative localization procedures are indicated. If an adenoma is visualized, the surgeon is more confident of finding the elusive gland. If the adenoma is not visualized, surgery, which may still be indicated, is likely to be more difficult.

Surgery

The principles of parathyroid surgery are relatively straightforward. The surgeon experienced in the nuances of the procedure usually correctly identifies and removes the parathyroid adenoma. It is customary to identify all other parathyroid glands and to ascertain that they are normal. If the parathyroid gland on the same side as the adenoma is normal, some surgeons will not explore the other side of the neck because the likelihood is that the other glands will also be normal. Multiple parathyroid adenomas are uncommon. The surgical approach to the less common presentation of primary hyperparathyroidism as a multiglandular, hyperplastic disease is different. In this case all parathyroid tissue is identified and approximately seven-eights of the total parathyroid tissue (three glands) is removed, leaving the equivalent of half a parathyroid gland in situ. Another acceptable approach is to remove all tissue and to transplant slices of parathyroid tissue in the patient's forearm. Autotransplantation is reserved for primary hyperparathyroidism due to four-gland hyperplasia. Adenomatous tissue is not transplanted as a general rule.

Postoperatively, the patient will recover normal parathyroid function, although there may be a brief period of mild, transient hypocalcemia. The interval between parathyroidectomy and recovery of parathyroid function is a matter of only a few days (141). If the patient has preoperative evidence for overt skeletal disease, a period of more prolonged hypocalcemia may ensue. It is due to rapid deposition of calcium into bone (hungry bone syndrome) as the skeleton experiences a sudden reversal of the negative state of calcium balance and accretes new bone (142).

Permanent hypoparathyroidism can be a complication of parathyroid surgery in the patient who has had previous neck surgery. Removal of some parathyroid tissue at previous operations is usually responsible for lack of return of parathyroid function. It is best documented by parathyroid hormone levels that do not increase postoperatively (141). Hypoparathyroidism may not develop sometimes until years following surgery perhaps because the remaining parathyroid tissue is left with a marginal vascular supply and finally becomes critically compromised with age. Another permanent complication of parathyroid surgery is damage to the recurrent laryngeal nerve. Hoarseness and loss of voice volume result. This unusual event is also more likely to occur in the patient who has had previous neck surgery.

Preoperative Localization of Parathyroid Adenomas

Preoperative localization of abnormal parathyroid tissue in primary hyperparathyroidism can be extremely useful for patients who have had previous neck surgery. Distortion of anatomical landmarks and difficulties entering a previously explored operative field make the preoperative identification of the parathyroid adenoma desirable. It is much less important in the patient with no previous neck surgery in whom the experienced surgeon will be successful well over 90% of the time (143).

Noninvasive approaches to localization include ultrasonography, computed tomography, magnetic resonance imaging, and scintigraphy (144,146). None of these noninvasive approaches has yet achieved the requisite degree of resolution to recommend one over another. In fact, none has yet enjoyed a reliably successful record. Imaging with a combination of technetium 99m and thallium 201 has generated some recent enthusiasm. With apparent preferential accumulation of thallium 201 in parathyroid tissue, computer subtraction techniques remove the more general image created by the technetium 99m (Fig. 6). Promising results so far must still be regarded with cautious optimism (146,147). Already a number of false negatives and false positives have been experienced by those using the technique.

Invasive approaches depend on arteriography and selective venous catheterization (148). While arteriography can provide anatomical localization, selective venous catheterization of the draining thyroid veins (through which the parathyroid gland vasculature drains) with measurement of parathyroid hormone concentration in the venous effluent can localize the site(s) of excessive parathyroid hormone production (149,150). When arteriography and selective venous catheterization are used together, both anatomic and functional identification of adenomatous tissue is possible (151,152). Unfortunately, arteriography and selective venous catheterization are time consuming, tedious, expensive, and operative-dependent procedures. They are not routinely performed in most medical centers.

Medical Management of Primary Hyperparathyroidism

Uncertainty regarding the indications for surgery among the large number of patients with asymptomatic primary hyperparathyroidism leads to a consideration of the more conservative approach to the patient. There are a number of general recommendations, which are not necessarily exclusive of surgery. While the issue of definitive surgery is being evaluated, general and specific management of the hypercalcemia may be indicated. The importance of adequate hydration and mobility are emphasized in primary hyperparathyroidism as for any other condition associated with hypercalcemia. Thiazide diuretics are avoided.

Calcium intake should be moderate. There is no good reason to recommend high-or low-calcium diets. It is said that they do not influence the serum calcium concentration in primary hyperparathyroidism. The only situation in which a change in dietary calcium could conceivably be reflected in a change in the circulating serum calcium would be in those patients with elevated levels of $1,25(OH)_2D$. In this case, low dietary calcium could lead to lower serum calcium levels. This point, however, has not been systematically investigated. The only way a high-calcium diet could be helpful would be if the serum calcium were to rise further and perhaps suppress parathyroid glandular activity. Since one is sensitive to the actual level of calcium in asymptomatic primary hyperparathyroidism, most physicians would rather not attempt to achieve control of parathyroid hormone secretion by raising the serum calcium even further. If low dietary calcium were to be associated with a reduction in the serum calcium, an unlikely event, it could theoretically lead to further stimulation of parathyroid hormone

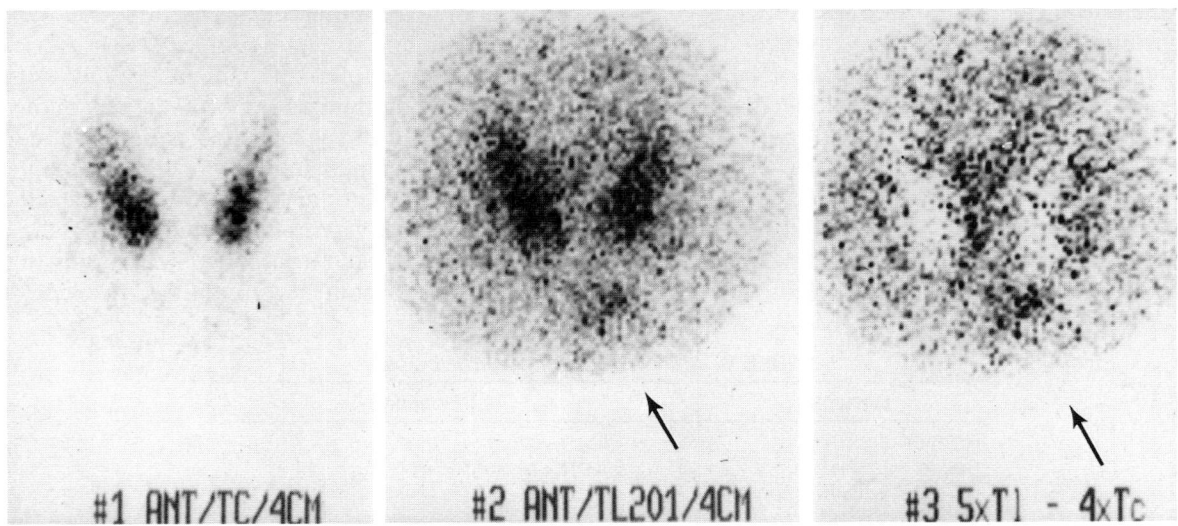

FIG. 6. Localization of a parathyroid adenoma by ^{99}Tc (**left**) and ^{201}Tll (**middle**) imaging. The increase in uptake at the left lower pole of the thyroid is seen better after "subtraction" of the thyroid image (**right**, see *arrows*). At operation, the adenoma was located at this site. (Reproduced with permission from Ref. 144.)

secretion, another undesirable consequence. Most physicians thus recommend a moderate calcium intake.

Specific approaches to the conservative management of primary hyperparathyroidism include attempts to inhibit parathyroid hormone secretion. Beta-adrenergic or H_2 receptor antagonists have not been successful in clinical studies, although they each have in vitro actions to inhibit parathyroid hormone secretion (153). Oral phosphate in doses of 1–2 g daily generally lowers the serum calcium by 0.5–1.0 mg/dL in most patients. Phosphate has several different mechanisms of action, including inhibition of gastrointestinal calcium absorption, inhibition of $1,25(OH)_2D$ formation, and inhibition of skeleton calcium mobilization. Phosphate, however, is not used widely in primary hyperparathyroidism. A realistic concern of metastatic calcification in soft tissues, and a further increase in parathyroid hormone levels keep enthusiasm for this approach modest at best (154).

One might consider estrogens to be an attractive therapy in postmenopausal women with primary hyperparathyroidism. The rather impressive incidence of primary hyperparathyroidism among women who are within 10 years of the menopause implicates estrogen deficiency, at least circumstantially, in the appearance of primary hyperparathyroidism. Another rationale for estrogen use is based on the known antagonism by estrogen of parathyroid hormone–mediated bone resorption. Published work is limited, but several studies have shown a reduction in the serum calcium by approximately 1 mg/dL with estrogen use (155,156). As expected with estrogens, however, parathyroid hormone levels do not decrease and phosphate levels fall even further.

A promising class of antiresorbing agents, the bisphosphonates, may in the future become another medical approach to primary hyperparathyroidism. They have reduced the serum calcium in several studies (157,158). The agent emphasized in the early studies, dichloromethylene diphosphonate, is no longer available in the United States, but newer diphosphonate agents are being developed and may prove to be useful (159,160).

Specific Therapy for Other Causes of Hypercalcemia

Knowledge of the underlying cause of the hypercalcemia provides guidance as to whether specific therapy for the disease process is indicated or possible. Along with the approach to hypercalcemia per se, one should always bear in mind the possibility of treating the cause of the hypercalcemia. Reviewed above are the therapeutic options for the patient with primary hyperparathyroidism. Other etiologies of hypercalcemia are somewhat more straightforward. The hypercalcemia of thyrotoxicosis is best treated by rendering the patient euthyroid. The hypercalcemia of familial hypocalciuric hypercalcemia is not treated. Hypercalcemia due to granulomatous disease has its own distinctive therapeutic approach. If the hypercalcemia is due to a malignancy, therapy for the malignancy may be indicated. Severe hypercalcemia in the patient with incurable malignant disease is sometimes best left untreated. The concept of treating the underlying cause of the hypercalcemia is an important one. It provides a key rational therapeutic framework.

Therapeutic Principles of Hypercalcemia

Quite apart from consideration of the underlying cause of the hypercalcemia is the issue of treating the hypercalcemia itself. The decision to treat is not difficult when the serum calcium is clearly elevated (i.e., >13 mg/dL). On the other hand, more mild hypercalcemia, especially if believed to be chronic, may not necessarily be treated, beyond conservative, general measures to be described. Clinical judgment is important because the individual patient may or may not be symptomatic when the serum calcium is only moderately elevated. The decision to treat with specific measures must thus be given careful consideration in each case.

General Measures

A set of general measures is useful for all hypercalcemias that require attention (Table 6) (161). In view of the fact that the symptomatic patient is likely to be dehydrated, rehydration is an important aspect of the general approach to the hypercalcemic patient. Saline is used because the ensuing saliuresis will be accompanied by an obligatory loss of urinary calcium (162). The older literature tended to overemphasize the use of saline to the point where the patient with marginal cardiovascular tolerance could become overhydrated. In older subjects,

TABLE 6. *Management of hypercalcemia*

General	Specific
Rehydration	Plicamycin
Saline administration	Bisphosphonates
Diuresis with furosemide	Calcitonin
Dialysis	Phosphate
Mobilization	WR2721 (not generally available)
	Gallium nitrate (not generally available)
	Glucocorticoids
	Therapy for underlying etiology

overvigorous hydration can lead to congestive heart failure. To minimize this concern, a loop diuretic, such as furosemide, can be useful. Furosemide can guard against overhydration by facilitating urinary salt and water loss. A concomitant benefit is the more effective loss of urinary calcium.

An important point regarding the use of furosemide in the context of hypercalcemia is to rehydrate the patient first. If furosemide is used before the patient is rehydrated, dehydration can become worse. One should titrate the need for furosemide to the extent of the hypercalcemia, the adequacy of renal function, and the patient's cardiovascular tolerance. It is not always necessary to resort to a loop diuretic as a general measure for hypercalcemia. Thiazides are obviously never used instead of furosemide because hypercalcemia can actually worsen.

A general measure in the severely hypercalcemic individual is hemodialysis or peritoneal dialysis. Dialysis will rapidly lower the serum calcium in patients whose hypercalcemia is refractory to all other approaches.

Another useful general measure is to mobilize the patient as soon as possible. Immobilization can worsen the hypercalcemia by inducing even further negative calcium balance. Although it is not always possible to ambulate the patient, this simple step should be taken as soon as is clinically feasible.

Specific Measures

Specific therapy of hypercalcemia is designed to address the pathophysiological basis of the hypercalcemia (Table 6). Agents that inhibit bone resorption are popular because the most common pathophysiological basis of hypercalcemia is accelerated bone resorption. In cases of vitamin D–associated hypercalcemia, an agent that interferes with the skeletal and gastrointestinal manifestations of vitamin D is indicated. Medication-associated hypercalcemia is best approached by monitoring the patient off therapy.

Agents That Inhibit Bone Resorption

Mithramycin (Plicamycin)

Mithramycin has been the principal specific therapy for acute hypercalcemia for many years. Its action to inhibit osteoclast function and thereby to dramatically reduce, albeit temporarily, the accelerated osteoclast-mediated bone resorption that characterizes most hypercalcemias places mithramycin among the top therapeutic choices (162,163). Since accelerated bone resorption is usually associated with most life-threatening hypercalcemias, mithramycin is the drug of choice when the serum calcium is very high. It can rather quickly control a very difficult situation. When the diagnosis of the underlying disease is not known, mithramycin can establish a level of management while the diagnostic evaluation is initiated.

Mithramycin is administered parenterally, 15–25 μg/kg, as a single, daily dose. It is given for up to 4 days, but in some cases a 7-day course has been used. The serum calcium will begin to fall within 24–48 h. Although the initial response to mithramycin is fairly predictable, the extent to which the calcium will fall and the duration of control are not. If bone resorption is ongoing at a very aggressive pace, the effect of mithramycin will be relatively short-lived. On the other hand, in certain situations such as acute primary hyperparathyroidism, mithramycin can effectively break the pathophysiological cycle and return the serum calcium to premorbid levels (Fig. 7).

A major drawback to mithramycin is that it cannot be used repeatedly to control chronic, recurrent severe hypercalcemia. Adverse side effects associated with continued use of mithramycin include elevated transaminase levels, proteinuria, azotemia, bone marrow suppression, and impaired platelet aggregation. These side effects are rarely seen when mithramycin is used for the first time. However, if there is known underlying liver or renal dysfunction, the dose of mithramycin can be lowered to 12.5 μg/kg.

Bisphosphonates

The bisphosphonates represent another class of agents that inhibit osteoclast activity. Available worldwide are ethane hydroxy-1,1-diphosphonic acid (EHDP) (Fig. 8), dichloromethylene diphosphonate (Cl_2MDP), and aminohydroxypropylidene diphosphonate (APD). Only EDHP is currently available in the United States (164). Parenteral Cl_2MDP, EHDP, and APD are effective calcium-lowering agents (165–168). They are used like mithramycin, as a daily parenteral dose. Also similar to mithramycin, long-term control of hypercalcemia depends on the aggressiveness of the underlying bone resorptive process. Early data suggest that in some cases, after intravenous EHDP has reduced the serum calcium to more manageable levels, use of the oral form may help to maintain reduced calcium levels. A potential adverse long-term effect of EHDP, impaired bone formation, is not a concern when it is used in this limited fashion.

Calcitonin

Among the "antiresorbers," calcitonin belongs in any discussion of the therapy of hypercalcemia. Theoretically, it is an ideal anticalcemic drug because it not only inhibits osteoclast-mediated bone resorption but also increases the urinary excretion of calcium. In this respect it is different from mithramycin and the bisphosphonates. The parenteral dose of calcitonin is 4 IU/kg every 12 h. Despite the theoretical advantages of using an agent like calcitonin that has two mechanisms of action, it does not

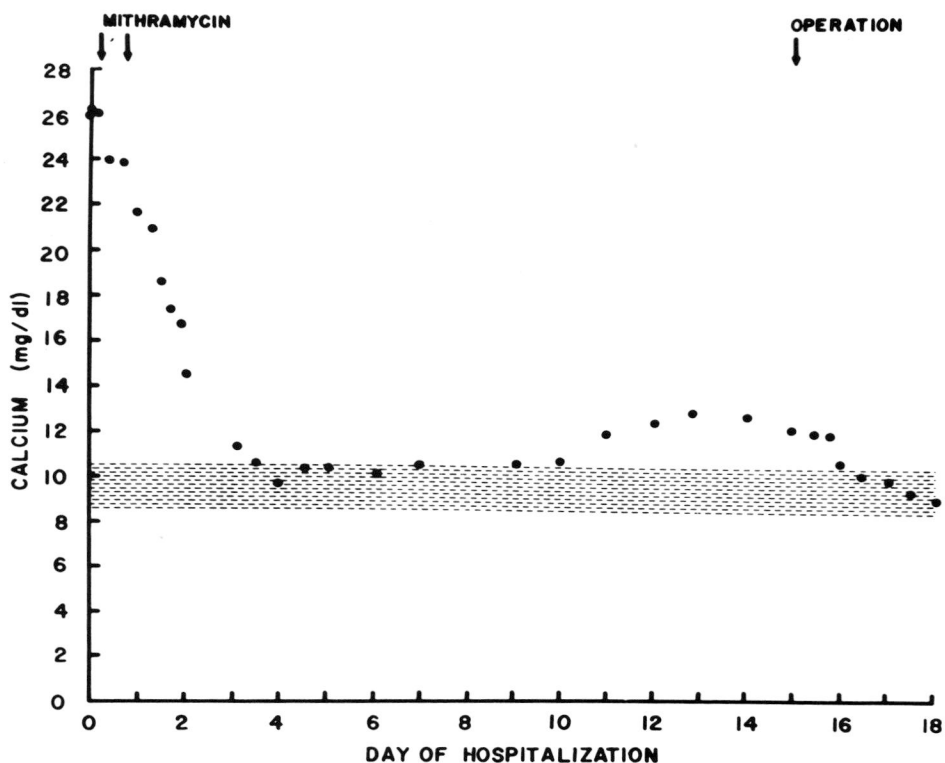

FIG. 7. Therapy of life-threatening hypercalcemia with mithramycin. The patient received two doses of mithramycin (25 µg/kg) 12 h apart on the first day of admission. The calcium descended into the normal range and remained without a return to life-threatening levels until the patient underwent successful parathyroidectomy. (Reproduced with permission from Ref. 26.)

appear to be as effective an anticalcemic drug as mithramycin or the bisphosphonates. One does not usually see dramatic reductions in the serum calcium but rather, a more modest fall of 1–2 mg/dL. On the other hand, calcitonin acts more rapidly to lower the serum calcium than does plicamycin or the bisphosphonates. A limited experience with combination therapy has suggested that calcitonin and glucocorticoids may be more effective than either agent alone (169). Combined bisphosphonate and calcitonin therapy has also been reported to be efficacious (170).

Phosphate

Besides its action to inhibit bone resorption, phosphate has several additional mechanisms by which it lowers the serum calcium. Phosphate interferes with gastrointestinal absorption of calcium and inhibits the formation of $1,25(OH)_2D$. Another mechanism by which phosphate may lower the serum calcium is also a potential side effect of concern: that is, ectopic deposition of calcium phosphate salts in soft tissues. The extremely rapid action of intravenous phosphate to reduce hypercalcemia may be due to ectopic calcium phosphate deposition. It is an undesirable consequence that may lead to acute pulmonary and renal dysfunction. Intravenous

phosphate should be reserved for those rare, life-threatening hypercalcemias refractory to all other modalities.

In contrast to intravenous phosphate, oral phosphate is relatively ineffective in acute situations. One concern is whether the patient can tolerate the oral route of administration, a potential problem when gastrointestinal symptoms of hypercalcemia are present. Another limitation is the dose, which, to prevent the onset of diarrhea, usually cannot exceed 2–3 g daily. A third point is that oral phosphate is relatively ineffective in the emergency management of acute hypercalcemia. It is usually reserved for settings of mild-to-moderate hypercalcemia associated with levels of serum phosphate that are in the lower range of normal. The best rationale for its use is found in situations like the mild hypercalcemia of primary hyperparathyroidism (see above).

Prostaglandin Inhibitors

Prostaglandins are believed to be important local mediators of osteolysis associated with hypercalcemia of cancer. It is rational, therefore, to consider the use of prostaglandin inhibitors to treat the hypercalcemia of malignancy. However, prostaglandin synthetase inhibitors such as aspirin and indomethacin have been disappointing when used to treat hypercalcemia (171).

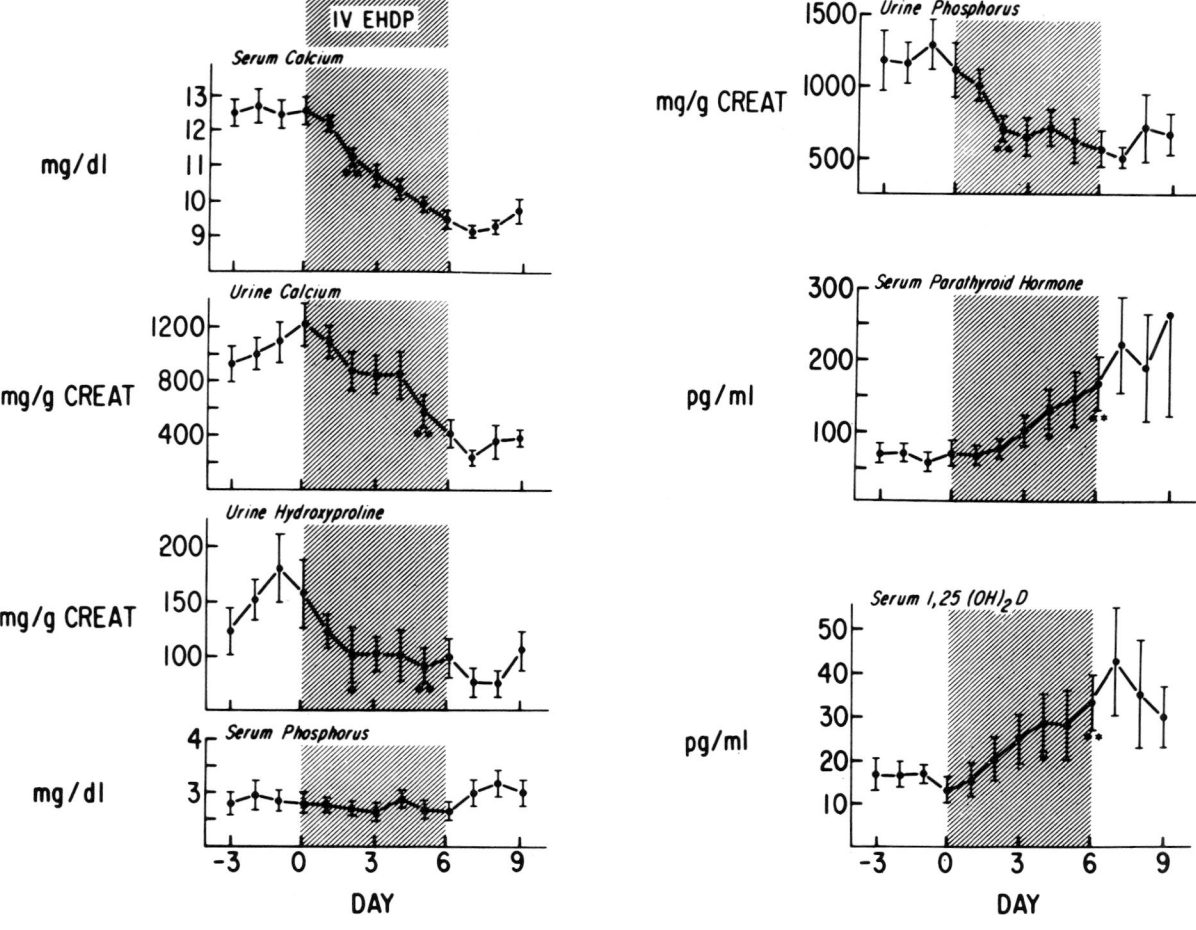

FIG. 8. Biochemical response to intravenous etidronate (EHDP). Mean responses ± SEM are illustrated for serum and urinary indices. Shaded areas represent the period during which EHDP was administered. Significance between pretreatment mean data is noted with single ($p < 0.05$) or double ($p < 0.01$) asterisks. (Reproduced with permission from Ref. 167.)

Other Inhibitors of Bone Resorption

WR2721 is a chemoprotective agent that has shown promise as a therapy for hypercalcemia. It inhibits both bone resorption and parathyroid hormone secretion (172). WR2721 also appears to facilitate urinary calcium excretion. It is thus the only known agent that has all three key sites of action to reduce the serum calcium. However, since the initial report on the experience of WR2721 in hypercalcemic situations, further observations have been extremely limited. It is still very much an experimental agent. Potential side effects have not been extensively investigated such as the possibility that WR2721 may also inhibit many other endocrine secretions besides parathyroid hormone.

Another experimental agent that has shown promise in the treatment of hypercalcemia is gallium nitrate. Similar to the other agents discussed, gallium nitrate appears to inhibit osteoclast-mediated bone resorption. It will reduce hypercalcemia caused by a wide variety of malig-

nancies (173–175). Side effects appear to be minimal. It is still an investigational drug.

Therapy to Reduce Hypercalcemia Due to Excessive Gastrointestinal Absorption of Calcium

Under certain defined circumstances, the gastrointestinal tract can contribute to the hypercalcemic state. It is rare that excessive absorption of calcium, independent of a vitamin D mechanism, will be solely responsible for hypercalcemia, a possible exception being the hypercalcemia associated with milk-alkali syndrome.

When the gastrointestinal tract does play a major role in the pathophysiology of hypercalcemia, a condition associated with excessive presence, production, or sensitivity to vitamin D exists (sarcoidosis, granulomatous diseases, lymphomas, other malignancies, vitamin D toxicity). Even in situations like vitamin D toxicity and lymphoma, however, a component of bone resorption is likely to be important in the development of hypercalcemia. Nevertheless, therapy for this group of hypercalcemic disorders can include reduction of the amount of calcium in the diet. Reducing the availability of calcium for absorption can help to limit absorption by a gastrointestinal tract sensitized to vitamin D.

Another useful approach is to limit the amount of active metabolite, $1,25(OH)_2D$, in these patients. This point can be addressed by treating the underlying cause of the excess production, such as treating the tuberculosis or other granulomatous disease. In patients with sarcoidosis, limiting the patient's exposure to sunlight may be helpful.

Glucocorticoids are an excellent specific therapeutic approach to disorders associated with excessive production of vitamin D. By antagonizing the absorptive effects of vitamin D on calcium in the gastrointestinal tract, they can be particularly effective. Although the glucocorticoids are considered to be "anti-vitamin D," their mechanism of anticalcemic action is not simply a competitive inhibition of the mechanisms involved in vitamin D–associated calcium absorption. It is considerably more complex. In the liver, glucocorticoids may induce the formation of inactive metabolites in the liver diverting precursor compounds from the classical pathway leading to the renal production of $1,25(OH)_2D$. In addition to effects on pathways of vitamin D synthesis and action, the glucocorticoids may also directly limit accelerated bone resorption. The actions of glucocorticoids on bone helps to explain why they are effective in malignant conditions such as multiple myeloma and metastatic breast cancer. Yet another mechanism of glucocorticoid action is their antitumor effects. If the malignancy is responsive to steroid hormones, anticalcemic actions could be explained by their direct effects on the tumor. Doses employed are in the range of 20 mg of prednisone or its equivalent three times daily. Direct therapeutic effects on the underlying malignant process can lead to prolonged control of the hypercalcemic state.

REFERENCES

1. Slatopolsky E, Weerts C, Thielan J, Horst R, Harter H, Martin KJ. Marked suppression of secondary hyperparathyroidism by intravenous administration of 1,25-dihydroxycholecalciferol in uremic patients. *J Clin Invest* 1984;74:2136–43.
2. Sugimoto T, Ritter C, Ried I, Morrissey J, Slatopolsky E. Effect of 1,25-dihydroxyvitamin D₃ on cytosolic calcium in dispersed parathyroid cells. *Kidney Int* 1988;33:850–4.
3. Deluca HF. The vitamin D story: a collaborative effort of basic science and clinical medicine. *FASEB J* 1988;10:224–36.
4. Holick MF. Vitamin D: photobiology, metabolism, and clinical application. In: Arias IM, Jakoby WB, Popper H, Schachter D, Shafritz DA, eds. *The liver: biology and pathobiology.* New York: Raven Press, 1988;475–93.
5. DeLuca HF. The vitamin D–calcium axis—1983. In: Rubin RP, Weiss GB, eds. *Calcium in biological systems.* New York: Plenum Press, 1985;491–511.
6. Tanaka Y, Lorenc RS, DeLuca HF. The role of 1,25-dihydroxyvitamin D₃ and parathyroid hormone in the regulation of renal 25-hydroxyvitamin D₃-24-hydroxylase. *Arch Biochem Biophys* 1975;171:521.
7. Garabedian M, Holick MF, DeLuca HF, Boyle IT. Control of 25-hydroxycholecalciferol metabolism by parathyroid glands. *Proc Natl Acad Sci USA* 1972;69:1973–6.
8. Wortsman J, Haddad JB, Posillico JT, Brown EM. Primary hyperparathyroidism with low serum 1,25-dihydroxyvitamin D levels. *J Clin Endocrinol Metab* 1986;62:1305–8.
9. Bilezikian JP. Hyperparathyroidism. In: Stein JH, ed. *Internal Medicine,* 3rd ed. Boston: Little Brown, 1990:2372–8.
10. Heath H III, Hodgson SF, Kennedy MA. Primary hyperparathyroidism: incidence, morbidity, and potential economic impact in a community. *N Engl J Med* 1980;302:189.
11. Bilezikian JP. Clinical disorders of the parathyroid glands. In: Raisz LG, Martin TJ, eds. *Clinical endocrinology of calcium metabolism.* New York: Marcel Dekker, 1987;53–97.
12. Silverberg SJ, Shane E, De La Cruz L, et al. Skeletal disease in primary hyperparathyroidism. *J Bone Miner Res* 1989;4:283–91.
13. Seeman E, Wahner W, Offord P, Kumar R, Johnson WJ, Riggs BL. Differential effects of endocrine dysfunction on the axial and appendicular skeleton. *J Clin Invest* 1982;69:1302.
14. Parfitt AM, Kleerekoper M, Rao D, Stanciu J, Villanueva AR. Cellular mechanisms of cortical thinning in primary hyperparathyroidism. *J Bone Miner Res* 1987;2(suppl):384A.
15. Parisien M, Dempster DW, Shane E, Silverberg SJ, Lindsay R, Bilezikian JP. Structural parameters of iliac bone biopsies in primary hyperparathyroidism. In Takahashi HE, ed. *Bone morphometry.* Nishimura, 1990:228–31.
16. Parisien MV, Silverberg SJ, Shane E, et al. The histomorphometry of bone in primary hyperparathyroidism: preservation of cancellous bone. *J Clin Endocrinol Metab* 1989. [Submitted].
17. Mallette LE, Bilezikian JP, Heath DA, Aurbach GD. Hyperparathyroidism: a review of 52 cases. *Medicine* 1974;53:127.
18. Patten BM, Bilezikian JP, Mallette LE, Prince A, Engle WK, Aurbach GD. The neuromuscular disease of primary hyperparathyroidism. *Ann Intern Med* 1974;80:182–94.
19. Turken S, Cafferty M, Silverberg SJ, de la Cruz L, Bilezikian JP. Neuromuscular involvement in mild, asymptomatic primary hyperparathyroidism. *J Bone Miner Res* 1988;3:S88 (abstr).
20. Linos DA, VanHeerden JA, Abboad CF, Edis AJ. Primary hyperparathyroidism and peptic ulcer disease. *Arch Surg* 1978;113:384.
21. Scholz DA. Hypertension and hyperparathyroidism. *Arch Intern Med* 1977;137:1123.
22. Bilezikian JP, Aurbach GD, Connor TB, et al. Pseudogout following parathyroidectomy. *Lancet* 1973;1:445.
23. Mallette LE. Anemia in hypercalcemic hyperparathyroidism: renewed interest in an old observation. *Arch Intern Med* 1977;137:572.
24. Reinfrank RF. Primary hyperparathyroidism with depression. *Arch Intern Med* 1961;108:162.
25. Ljunghall S, Joborn C, Palmer M, Rastad J, G Averstram. Primary hyperparathyroidism: the surgically cured patient. In: Kleerekoper M, Krane S, eds. *Clinical disorders of bone and mineral metabolism* (New York): Mary Ann Liebert 1989;353–8.
26. Fitzpatrick LA, Bilezikian JP. Acute primary hyperparathyroidism. *Am J Med* 1987;82:275.
27. Shane E, Bilezikian JP. Parathyroid carcinoma. In: Williams CJ, Krikorian JG, Green MR, Ragavan E, eds. *Textbook of uncommon cancer.* New York: John Wiley, 1988;763–71.
28. Schantz A, Castleman B. Parathyroid carcinoma: a study of 70 cases. *Cancer* 1973;31:600.
29. Holck S, Pedersen NT. Carcinoma of the parathyroid gland: a light and electron microscopic study. *Acta Pathol Microbiol Scand.,* 1981.
30. de la Garza S, de la Garza EF, Batres FH. Functional parathyroid carcinoma: cytology, histology and ultrastructure of a case. *Diag Cytopathol* 1985;1:232.
31. Smith JF, Coombs RRH. Histological diagnosis of carcinoma of the parathyroid gland. *J Clin Pathol* 1984;37:1370.
32. Obara T, Fujimoto Y, Yamaguchi K, Takanashi R, Kino I, Sasaki Y. Parathyroid carcinoma of the oxyphil cell type: a report of two cases, light and electron microscopic study. *Cancer* 1985;55:1482.

33. Mallette LE, Malini S, Rappaport, Kirkland JL. Familial cystic parathyroid adenomatosis. *Ann Intern Med* 1987;107:54.

34. Shangold MM, Dor N, Welt SI, Fleischman AR, Crenshaw CM Jr. Hyperparathyroidism and pregnancy: a review. *Obstet Gynecol Surg* 1982;37:217.

35. Kristoffersson A, Dahlgren S, Lithner F, Jarhult J. Primary hyperparathyroidism in pregnancy. *Surgery* 1985;97:326.

36. Cooper L, Wertheimer J, Levey R, et al. Severe primary hyperparathyroidism in a neonate with two hypercalcemic parents: management with parathyroidectomy and heterotopic autotransplantation. *Pediatrics* 1986;78:263–8.

37. Marx SJ, Attie MF, Spiegel AM, Levine MA, Lasker RD, Fox M. An association between neonatal severe primary hyperparathyroidism and familial hypocalciuric hypercalcemia in three kindreds. *N Engl J Med* 1982;306:257.

38. Wills MR, Pak CYC, Hammond WG, Bartter FC. Normocalcemic primary hyperparathyroidism. *Am J Med* 1969;47:384–91.

39. Keynes WM, Caird FI. Hypocalcemic primary hyperparathyroidism. *Br Med J* 1970;1:208–11.

40. Mundy GR, Cove DH, Fisken R. Primary hyperparathyroidism: changes in the pattern of clinical presentation. *Lancet* 1980;1:1317–20.

41. Delmas PD, Demiaux B, Malaval L, Chapuy MC, Edward C, Menuier PJ. Serum bone gamma carboxyglutamic acid-containing protein in primary hyperparathyroidism and in malignant hypercalcemia. *J Clin Invest* 1986;77:983.

42. Mallette LE, Tumna SN, Berger RE, Kirkland JL. Radioimmunoassay for the middle region of human parathyroid hormone using an homologous antiserum with a carboxy-terminal fragment of bovine parathyroid hormone as radioligand. *J Clin Endocrinol Metab* 1982;54:1017.

43. Segre GV. Amino-terminal radioimmunoassay for human parathyroid hormone, In: Frame B, Potts JT Jr, eds. *Clinical disorders of bone and mineral metabolism*. Amsterdam: Excerpta Medica, 1983;14.

44. Nussbaum SR, Zahradnik RJ, Lavigne JR, et al. Highly sensitive two-site immunoradiometric assay of parathyrin and its clinical utility in evaluating patients with hypercalcemia. *Clin Chem* 1987;33:1364–7.

45. Broadus AE. Nephrogenous cyclic AMP as a parathyroid function test. *Nephron* 1979;23:136.

46. Lufkin EG, Kao PC, Heath H III. Comparison of parathyroid hormone radioimmunoassays in the differential diagnosis of hypercalcemia due to primary hyperparathyroidism or malignancy. *Ann Intern Med* 1987;106:559.

47. Broadus AE, Horst RL, Lang R, Littledike ET, Rasmussen H. The importance of circulating 1,25-dihydroxyvitamin D in the pathogenesis of hypercalciuria and renal stone formation in primary hyperparathyroidism. *N Engl J Med* 1980;302:421.

48. Locascio V, Adami S, Galvanni G, Ferrari M, Cominacini L, Tartarotti D. Substrate–product relation of 1-hydroxylase activity in primary hyperparathyroidism. *N Engl J Med* 1985;313:1123–5.

49. Reichel H, Koeffler HP, Norman AW. The role of the vitamin D endocrine system in health and disease. *N Engl J Med* 1989;320:980–91.

50. Dent CE, Watson L. The hydrocortisone test in primary and tertiary hyperparathyroidism. *Lancet* 1968;ii:662–4.

51. Reeves CD, Palmer F, Bacchus H, Longerbeam JK. Differential diagnosis of hypercalcemia by the chloride/phosphate ratio. *Am J Surg* 1975;130:166–71.

52. Breslau NA, Zerwekh JE, Nicar MJ, Pak CYC. Effects of short term glucocorticoid administration in primary hyperparathyroidism: comparison to sarcoidosis. *J Clin Endocrinol Metab* 1982;54:824–30.

53. Tohme JF, Bilezikian JP, Clemens TL, Silverberg SJ, Shane E, Lindsay R. Suppression of parathyroid hormone secretion with oral calcium in normal subjects and in patients with primary hypoparathyroidism. *J Clin Endocrinol Metab* 1990;70:951–6.

54. Mundy GR, Martin TJ. Hypercalcemia of malignancy: pathogenesis and treatment. *Metabolism* 1982;31:1247.

55. Mundy GR. Pathogenesis of hypercalcaemia of malignancy. *Clin Endocrinol* 1985;23:705.

56. Mundy GR, Ibbotson KJ, D'Souza SM. Tumor products and the humoral hypercalcemia of malignancy. *J Clin Invest* 1985;76:391.

57. Godsall JL, Burtis WJ, Insogna KL, Broadus AE, Stewart AF. Nephrogenous cyclic AMP, adenylate cyclase-stimulating activity and the humoral hypercalcemia of malignancy. *Recent Prog Horm Res* 1986;40:705.

58. Mundy GR, Raisz LG, Cooper RA, Schecter G, Salmon SE. Evidence for the secretion of an osteoclast stimulating factor in myeloma. *N Engl J Med* 1974;291:1041.

59. Mundy GR. Hypercalcemia of malignancy revisited. *J Clin Invest* 1988;82:1–6.

60. Gowen M, Wood OD, Ehrie EJ, McGuire MKB, Russell RGG. An interleukin 1 like factor stimulates bone resorption in vitro. *Nature (Lond)* 1983;306:378–80.

61. Mundy GR, Ibbotson KJ, D'Souza SM, Simpson EL, Jacobs JW, Martin TJ. The hypercalcemia of malignancy: clinical implications and pathogenic mechanisms. *N Engl J Med* 1984;310:1718.

62. Garrett IR, Durie BGM, Nedwin GE, et al. Production of lymphotoxin, a bone-resorbing cytokine by cultured human myeloma cells. *N Engl J Med* 1987;317:527.

63. Lafferty FW. Pseudohyperparathyroidism. *Medicine* 1966; 45:247–60.

64. Stewart AF, Horst R, Deftos LJ, Cadman EC, Lang R, Broadus AE. Biochemical evaluation of patients with cancer-associated hypercalcemia: evidence for humoral and non-humoral groups. *N Engl J Med* 1980;303:1377.

65. Albright F. Case records of the Massachusetts General Hospital. *N Engl J Med* 1941;255:789.

66. Insogna KL, Broadus AE. Hypercalcemia of malignancy. *Annu Rev Med* 1987;38:241–56.

67. Simpson EL, Mundy GR, D'Souza SM, Ibbotson KJ, Bockman R, Jacobs JW. Absence of parathyroid hormone messenger RNA in nonparathyroid tumors associated with hypercalcemia. *N Engl J Med* 1983;309:325.

68. Strewler GJ, Williams RD, Nissenson RA. Human renal carcinoma cells produce hypercalcemia in the nude mouse and a novel protein recognized by parathyroid hormone receptors. *J Clin Invest* 1983;71:769–74.

69. Moseley JM, Kubota M, Diefenbach-Jagger H, et al. Parathyroid hormone-related protein purified from a human lung cancer cell line. *Proc Natl Acad Sci USA* 1987;84:5048–52.

70. Stewart AF, Wu T, Goumas D, Burtis WJ, Broadus AE. N-terminal amino acid sequence of two novel tumor-derived adenylate cyclase stimulating proteins: identification of parathyroid hormone-like and parathyroid hormone-unlike domains. *Biochem Biophys Res Commun* 1987;146:672–8.

71. Strewler GJ, Stern PH, Jacobs JW, et al. Parathyroid hormone-like protein from human renal carcinoma cells: structural and functional homology with parathyroid hormone. *J Clin Invest* 1987;80:1803–7.

72. Suva LJ, Winslow GA, Wettenhall REH, et al. A parathyroid hormone-related protein implicated in malignant hypercalcemia: cloning and expression. *Science* 1987;237:893–6.

73. Mangin M, Wegg AC, Dreyer BE, et al. Identification of a cDNA encoding a parathyroid hormone-like peptide from a human tumor associated with a humoral hypercalcemia of malignancy. *Proc Natl Acad Sci USA* 1988;85:597–601.

74. Kemp BE, Moseley JM, Rodda CP, et al. Parathyroid hormone-related protein of malignancy: active synthetic fragments. *Science* 1987;238:1568–70.

75. Weir EC, Insogna KL, Brownstein DG, Banelis NH, Broadus AE. In vitro-adenylate cyclase-stimulating activity predicts the occurrence of humoral hypercalcemia of malignancy in nude mice. *J Clin Invest* 1988;81:818–82.

76. Burtis WJ, Brady TG, Orloff JJ, et al. Immunohistochemical characterization of circulating parathyroid hormone-related protein in patients with humoral hypercalcemia of cancer. *N Engl J Med* 1990;322:1106–12.

77. Budayr AA. Nissenson RA, Klein RF, et al. Increased serum levels of a parathyroid hormone-like protein in malignancy-associated hypercalcemia. *Ann Intern Med* 1989;111:807–12.

78. Henderson JE, Shustik C, Kremer R, Rabbani SA, Hendy ON, Goltzman D. Circulating concentrations of parathyroid

hormone-like peptide in malignancy and in hyperparathyroidism. *J Bone Miner Res* 1990;5:105–13.

78a.Bilezikian JP. Parathyroid hormone-related peptide in sickness and in health. *N Eng J Med* 1990;322:1151–3.

79. Fukumoto S, Matsumoto T, Yamoto H, et al. Suppression of serum 1,25-dihydroxyvitamin D in humoral hypercalcemia of malignancy is caused by elaboration of a factor that inhibits renal 1,25-dihydroxyvitamin D_3 production. *Endocrinology* 1989;124:2057–62.

80. Hirschel-Scholz S, Caverzasio J, Rizzoli R, Bonjour JP. Normalization of hypercalcemia associated with a decrease in renal calcium reabsorption in Leydig cell tumor-bearing rats treated with WR-2721. *J Clin Invest* 1986;78:319–22.

81. Rodan SB, Insogna KL, Vignery AMC, et al. Factors associated with humoral hypercalcemia of malignancy stimulate adenylate cyclase in osteoblastic cells. *J Clin Invest* 1983;72:1511–5.

82. Ralston SH, Boyce BF, Cowan RA, Gardner MD, Fraser WD, Boyle IT. Contrasting mechanisms of hypercalcemia in early and advanced humoral hypercalcemia of malignancy. *Calcif Tissue Int* 1988;42(suppl):181.

83. Stewart AF, Vignery A, Silvergate A, et al. Quantitative bone histomorphometry in humoral hypercalcemia of malignancy: uncoupling of bone cell activity. *J Clin Endocrinol Metab* 1982;55:219.

84. Mundy GR, Ibbotson KJ, D'Souza SM. Tumor products and the humoral hypercalcemia of malignancy. *J Clin Invest* 1985;76:391.

85. Breslau NA, McGuire JL, Zerwekh JE, Frenkel EP, Pak CYC. Hypercalcemia associated with increased serum calcitriol levels in three patients with lymphoma. *Ann Intern Med* 1984;100:1.

86. Davies M, Hayes ME, Mawer EB, Lumb GA. Abnormal vitamin D metabolism in Hodgkin's lymphoma. *Lancet* 1985;1:1186–8.

87. Rosenthal ND, Insogna KL, Godsall JW, Smaldone L, Waldron JW, Stewart AF. 1,25-dihydroxyvitamin D-mediated humoral hypercalcemia in malignant lymphoma. *J Clin Endocrinol Metab* 1985;60:29.

88. Mudde AH, van den Berg H, Boshuis PG, et al. Ectopic production of 1,25-dihydroxyvitamin D by B-cell lymphoma as a cause of hypercalcemia. *Cancer* 1987;59:1543–6.

89. Fetchik DA, Bertolini DR, Sarin PS, Weintraub ST, Mundy GR, Dunn JF. Production of 1,25-dihydroxyvitamin D_3 by human T cell lymphotropic virus-I-transformed lymphocytes. *J Clin Invest* 1986;78:592–6.

90. Reichel H, Koeffler HP, Norman AW. 25-Hydroxyvitamin D_3 metabolism by human T-lymphotropic virus-transformed lymphocytes. *J Clin Endocrinol Metab* 1987;65:519–26.

91. Dodd RC, Winkler CR, Williams ME, Bunn PA, Gray TK. Calcitriol levels in hypercalcemic patients with adult T-cell lymphoma. *Arch Intern Med* 1986;146:1971–2.

92. Yoshimoto K, Yamasaki R, Sakai H, et al. Ectopic production of parathyroid hormone by small cell lung cancer in a patient with hypercalcemia. *J Clin Endocrinol Metab* 1989;68:976–81.

93. Schmelzer HJ, Hesch RD, Mayer H. Parathyroid hormone and PTH mRNA in a human small cell lung cancer. In: Havemann K, Sorenson G, Gropp C, eds. *Peptide hormones in lung cancer* Berlin: Springer-Verlag, 1985;83–93. See also Ref. 84, pp. 391–4.

94. Peerenboom H, Keck E, Kruskeniper HL, Strohmeyer G. The defect in intestinal calcium transport in hyperthyroidism and its response to therapy. *J Clin Endocrinol Metab* 1984;59:936.

95. Ross DS, Nussbaum SR. Reciprocal changes in parathyroid hormone and thyroid function after radioiodine treatment of hyperthyroidism. *J Clin Endocrinol Metab* 1989;68:1216–9.

96. Brandi ML, Marx SJ, Aurbach GD, Fitzpatrick LA. Familial multiple endocrine neoplasia type I: a new look at pathophysiology. *Endocr Rev* 1987;8:391.

97. Miller SS, Sizemore GW, Sheps SG, Tyce GM. Parathyroid function in patients with pheochromocytoma. *Ann Intern Med* 1975;82:372.

98. Williams GA, Hargis GK, Bowser EN, Henderson WJ, Martinez NJ. Evidence for a role of adenosine 3',5'-monophosphate in parathyroid hormone release. *Endocrinology* 1973;92:687.

99. Stewart AF, Hoecker J, Segre GV, Mallette LE, Amatruda T, Vignery A. Hypercalcemia in pheochromocytoma: evidence for a novel mechanism. *Ann Intern Med* 1985;102:776.

100. Pederson KOK. Hypercalcemia in Addison's disease. *Acta Med Scand* 1967;181:691.

101. Muls E, Bouillon R, Boelart J, et al. Etiology of hypercalcemia in a patient with Addison's disease. *Calcif Tissue Int* 1982;34:523.

102. Verner JV, Morrison AB. Endocrine pancreatic islet disease with diarrhea. *Arch Intern Med* 1974;133:429.

103. Hughes MR, Baylink DJ, Jones PG, Haussler MR. Radioligand receptor assay for 25-hydroxyvitamin D_2/D_3 application to hypervitaminosis D. *J Clin Invest* 1976;58:61.

104. Gkonos PJ, London R, Hendler ED. Hypercalcemia and elevated 1,25(OH)$_2$D levels in a patient with end stage renal disease and active tuberculosis. *N Engl J Med* 1984;311:1683.

105. Murray JJ, Heim DR. Hypercalcemia in disseminated histoplasmosis. *Am J Med* 1985;78:881.

106. Kozemy GA, Barbato AL, Bansal VK, Vertuno LL, Hano JE. Hypercalcemia associated with silicone-induced granulomas. *N Engl J Med* 1984;311:1103.

107. Ryzen E, Tea TH, Singer FR. Hypercalcemia and abnormal 1,25-dihydroxyvitamin D concentrations in leprosy. *Am J Med* 1988;84:325–9.

108. Mason RS. Extra-renal production of 1,25(OH)$_2$D$_3$, the metabolism of vitamin D by non-traditional tissues. In: Norman AW, Schaefer K, Grigoleit HG, Herrath DV, eds. *Vitamin D: chemical, biochemical and clinical update.* New York: Walter de Gruyter, 1985;23–32.

109. Adams JS, Singer FR, Gacad MA, et al. Isolation and structural identification of 1,25-dihydroxyvitamin D_3 produced by cultured alveolar macrophages in sarcoidosis. *J Clin Endocrinol Metab* 1985;60:960–6.

110. Barbour GL, Coburn JW, Slatopolsky E, Norman AW, Horst RL. Hypercalcemia in an anephric patient with sarcoidosis, evidence for extrarenal generation of 1,25-dihydroxyvitamin D. *N Engl J Med* 1981;305:440–3.

111. Mudde AH, van den Berg H, Boshius PG, et al. Ectopic production of 1,25-dihydroxyvitamin D by B-cell lymphoma as a cause of hypercalcemia. *Cancer* 1987;59:1543–6.

112. Blayney DW, Jaffee ES, Fisher RI, et al. Human T-cell leukemia/lymphoma virus, lymphoma, lytic bone lesions, and hypercalcemia. *Ann Intern Med* 1983;98:144.

113. Porter RH, Cox BG, Heaney D, Hostetter TH, Stinebaugh BJ, Suki WN. Treatment of hypoparathyroid patients with chlorthalidone. *N Engl J Med* 1978;298:577.

114. Christiansen C, Baastrup P, Transbol I. Development of primary hyperparathyroidism during lithium therapy: longitudinal study. *Neuropsychobiology* 1980;6:280.

115. Spiegel AM, Rudorfer M, Marx SJ, Linnoila M. The effect of short term lithium administration on suppressibility of parathyroid hormone secretion by calcium in vitro. *J Clin Endocrinol Metab* 1984;59:354.

116. Brown E. Lithium induces abnormal calcium-regulated PTH release in dispersed bovine parathyroid glands. *J Clin Endocrinol Metab* 1981;52:1046.

117. Mallette LE, Khouri K, Zengotita H, Hollis B, Malini S. Lithium treatment increases intact and midregion parathyroid hormone and parathyroid volume. *J Clin Endocrinol Metab* 1989;68:654–60.

118. Leha SS, Powell K, Buzdar AR, Blumenschein GR. Tamoxifen-induced hypercalcemia in breast cancer. *Cancer* 1981;47:2803.

119. McMillan DE, Freeman RB. The milk alkali syndrome: a study of the acute disorder with comments on the development of the chronic condition. *Medicine* 1965;44:485.

120. Orwoll ES. The milk-alkali syndrome: current concepts. *Ann Intern Med* 1982;97:242.

121. Roberts RW, Tuthill SW. Milk-alkali syndrome: unusual today but not forgotten. *J La State Med Soc* 1984;136:42–3.

122. Kallner G, Karlsson H. Recurrent factitious hypercalcemia. *Am J Med* 1987;82:536–8.

123. Ragavan VV, Smith JE, Bilezikian JP. Vitamin A toxicity and hypercalcemia. *Am J Med Sci* 1982;283:161.

124. Marx SJ, Attie MF, Levine MA, Spiegel AM, Downs RW Jr, Lasker RD. The hypocalciuric or benign variant of familial hypercalcemia: clinical and biochemical features of fifteen kindreds. *Medicine* 1981;60:397.

125. Law WM Jr, Heath H III. Familial benign hypercalcemia (hypocalciuric hypercalcemia)-clinical and pathogenetic studies in 21 families. *Ann Intern Med* 1985;102:511.

126. Rajala MM, Heath HH III. Distribution of serum calcium values in patients with familial benign hypercalcemia (hypocalciuric hy-

percalcemia): evidence for a discrete genetic defect. *J Clin Endocrinol Metab* 1987;65:1039–41.

127. Hoare SF, Paterson CR. Familial benign hypercalcemia: a possible abnormality in calcium transport by erythrocytes. *Eur J Clin Invest* 1984;14:428.

128. Donahue HJ, Penniston JT, Heath H III. Kinetics of erythrocyte plasma membrane (Ca^{2+}, Mg^{2+}) ATPase in familial benign hypercalcemia. *J Clin Endocrinol Metab* 1989;68:893–8.

129. Sopwith AM, Burns C, Grant DB, Taylor GW, Wolf E, Besser GM. Familial hypocalciuric hypercalcemia: association with neonatal primary hyperparathyroidism, and possible linkage with HLA haplotype. *Clin Endocrinol* 1984;21:57–64.

130. Stewart AF, Alder M, Byers CM, Segre GV, Broadus AE. Calcium homeostasis in immobilization: an example of resorptive hypercalciuria. *N Engl J Med* 1982;306:1136.

131. Minaine P, Meunier P, Edouard C, Bernard J, Courpron P, Bourrett J. Quantitative histological data on disuse osteoporosis. *Calcif Tissue Res* 1974;17:57.

132. Bergstrom WH. Hypercalciuria and hypercalcemia complicating immobilization. *Am J Dis Child* 1978;132:553.

133. Klein GL, Horst RL, Norman AW, Ament ME, Slatopolsky E, Coburn JW. Reduced serum 1,25-dihydroxyvitamin D during long-term total parenteral nutrition. *Ann Intern Med* 1981;94:638.

134. Shike M, Sturtridge WC, Tam CS, et al. A possible role of vitamin D in the genesis of parenteral-nutrition-induced metabolic bone disease. *Ann Intern Med* 1981;95:560.

135. Ott SM, Maloney NA, Klein GL, et al. Aluminum is associated with low bone formation in patients receiving chronic parenteral nutrition. *Ann Intern Med* 1983;98:910.

136. Merlini G, Fitzpatrick LA, Siris ES, et al. A human myeloma immunoglobulin G binding four moles of calcium associated with asymptomatic hypercalcemia. *J Clin Immunol* 1984;4:185.

137. Jaffe JP, Mosher DF. Calcium binding by a myeloma protein. *Am J Med* 1979;67:343–6.

138. Bilezikian JP. The medical management of primary hyperparathyroidism. *Ann Intern Med* 1982;96:198.

139. Bilezikian JP. Surgery or no surgery for primary hyperparathyroidism. *Ann Intern Med* 1985;102:402.

140. Rao DS, Wilson RJ, Kleerekoper M, Parfitt M. Lack of biochemical progression or continuation of accelerated bone loss in mild asymptomatic primary hyperparathyroidism: evidence for biphasic disease course. *J Clin Endocrinol Metab* 1988;67:1294–8.

141. Brasier AR, Wang C, Nussbaum SR. Recovery of parathyroid hormone secretion after parathyroid adenomectomy. *J Clin Endocrinol Metab* 1988;61:495–500.

142. Brasier AR, Nussbaum SR. Hungry bone syndrome: clinical and biochemical predictors of its occurrence after parathyroid surgery. *Am J Med* 1988;84:654–60.

143. Rossi RL, ReMine SG, Clerkin EP. Hyperparathyroidism. *Surg Clin North Am* 1985;65:187.

144. Winzelberg GG. Parathyroid imaging. *Ann Intern Med* 1987;107:64.

145. Stark DD, Clark OH, Moss AA. Magnetic resonance imaging of the thyroid, thymus, and parathyroid glands. *Surgery* 1984;96:1083–91.

146. Young AE, Gaunt JI, Croft DN, Collins REC, Wells CP, Coakley AJ. Location of parathyroid adenomas by thallium-201 and technetium-99m subtraction scanning. *Br Med J* 1983;286:1384–6.

147. Brecht-Krauss D, Kusmiereck J, Hellwig D, Adam WE. Quantitative bone scintigraphy in patients with hyperparathyroidism. *J Nucl Med* 1987;28:458–61.

148. Eisenberg H, Pallotta J, Sherwood LM. Selective arteriography, venography and venous hormone assay in diagnosis and localization of parathyroid lesions. *Am J Med* 1974;56:810–20.

149. Powell D, Shimkin PM, Doppman JL, et al. Primary hyperparathyroidism: preoperative tumor localization and differentiation between adenomas and hyperplasia. *N Engl J Med* 1972;286:1169–75.

150. Bilezikian JP, Doppman JL, Shimkin PM, et al. Preoperative localization of abnormal parathyroid tissue: cumulative experience with venous sampling and arteriography. *Am J Med* 1973;55:505–14.

151. Bilezikian JP, Pearson KD, Powell D, Ketcham AS, Doppman

JL, Aurbach GD. Selective venous catheterization of the neck: localization of a parathyroid adenoma with anomalous drainage by non-thyroidal veins. *J Clin Endocrinol Metab* 1973;36:826–9.

152. Mallette LE, Gomez L, Fisher RG. Parathyroid angiography: a review of current knowledge and guidelines for clinical application. *Endocr Rev* 1981;2:124.

153. Heath H III. Biogenic amines and the secretion of parathyroid hormone and calcitonin. *Endocr Rev* 1980;1:319–37.

154. Broadus AE, Magee JSI, Mallette LE, et al. A detailed evaluation of oral phosphate therapy in selected patients with primary hyperparathyroidism. *J Clin Endocrinol Metab* 1983;56:953.

155. Marcus R, Madvig P, Crim M, Pont A, Kosek J. Conjugated estrogens in the treatment of postmenopausal women with hyperparathyroidism. *Ann Intern Med* 1984;100:633.

156. Selby PL, Peacock M. Ethinyl estradiol and norethindrone in the treatment of primary hyperparathyroidism in postmenopausal women. *N Engl J Med* 1986;314:1481.

157. Shane E, Baquiran DC, Bilezikian JP. Effects of dichloromethylene diphosphonate on serum and urine calcium in primary hyperparathyroidism. *Ann Intern Med* 1981;95:23.

158. Douglas DL, Duckworth T, Kanis JA, et al. Effect of dichloromethylene diphosphonate in Paget's disease of bone and in hypercalcemia due to primary hyperparathyroidism or malignant disease. *Lancet* 1980;i:1043–7.

159. Douglas DL, Kanis JA, Paterson AD, et al. Drug treatment of primary hyperparathyroidism: use of clodronate disodium. *Clin Res* 1983;286:587–90.

160. Frijlink WB, Bijvoet OLM, Te Velde J, Heynen G. Treatment of Paget's disease with (3-amino-1-hydroxy propylidene)-1,1-biphosphonate (APD). *Lancet* 1979;i:799–803.

161. Bilezikian JP. Hypercalcemia. *Dis-Mon* 1988;12:739–99.

162. Stewart AF. Therapy of malignancy-associated hypercalcemia. *Am J Med* 1983;74:475.

163. Perlia CP, Gubisch NJ, Cootter J, Edelberg D, Dederick MM, Taylor SG. Mithramycin treatment of hypercalcemia. *Cancer* 1970;25:389.

164. Siris ES, Canfield RC. Paget's disease of bone. In: Rakel RE, ed. *Conn's current therapy*. Philadelphia: WB Saunders, 1987;476–9.

165. Jacobs TP, Siris ES, Bilezikian JP, Baquiran DC, Shane E, Canfield RC. Hypercalcemia of malignancy: treatment with intravenous dichloromethylene diphosphonate. *Ann Intern Med* 1981;94:312.

166. Canfield RC. Rationale for diphosphonate therapy in hypercalcemia of malignancy. *Am J Med* 1987;82(suppl 2A):1.

167. Jacobs TP, Gordon AC, Silverberg SJ, et al. Neoplastic hypercalcemia: physiologic response to intravenous etidronate disodium. *Am J Med* 1987;82(suppl 2A):42.

168. Thiebaud D, Portmann L, Jaeger PH, Jacquet AF, Burckhardt P. Oral versus intravenous AHPBP (APD) in the treatment of hypercalcemia of malignancy. *Bone* 1986;7:247–53.

169. Binstock ML, Mundy GR. Effect of calcitonin and glucocorticoids in combination on the hypercalcemia of malignancy. *Ann Intern Med* 1980;93:269.

170. Ralston SH, Alzaid AA, Gardner MD, Boyle IT. Treatment of cancer associated hypercalcemia with combined aminohydroxypropylidene diphosphonate and calcitonin. *Br Med J* 1986;292:1549–50.

171. Brenner DE, Harvey HA, Lipton A, Demers L. A study of prostaglandin E_2, parathormone and response to indomethacin in patients with hypercalcemia of malignancy. *Cancer* 1982;49:556.

172. Glover DJ, Riley L, Carmichael K, et al. Hypocalcemia and inhibition of parathyroid hormone secretion after administration of WR 2721. *N Engl J Med* 1983;309:1137–41.

173. Warrell RP Jr, Bockman RS, Coonley CJ, Isaacs M, Stasewski H. Gallium nitrate inhibits calcium resorption from bone and is effective treatment for cancer-related hypercalcemia. *J Clin Invest* 1984;73:1487.

174. Warrell RP Jr, Skelos A, Alcock NW, Bockman RS. Gallium nitrate for acute treatment of cancer-related hypercalcemia: clinicopharmacological and dose response analysis. *Cancer Res* 1986;46:4208–12.

175. Warrell RP, Israel R, Frisone M, Snyder T, Gaynor JJ, Bockman RS. Gallium nitrate for acute treatment of cancer-related hypercalcemia. *Ann Intern Med* 1988;108:669–74.

Disorders of Bone and Mineral Metabolism,
edited by Fredric L. Coe and Murray J. Favus,
© 1992 by Raven Press, Ltd. All rights reserved.

CHAPTER 24

Asymptomatic Primary Hyperparathyroidism

Neil A. Breslau and Charles Y. C. Pak

Initially in the mid-1920s, primary hyperparathyroidism (PHPT) was regarded as a rare and severe disease of bone, osteitis fibrosa cystica (1). Subsequently, in the 1940s and 1950s, Albright's group recognized a different clinical presentation of PHPT in patients with renal stones but without evidence of overt bone disease (2,3). It soon became clear that renal stones were a far more frequent complication of PHPT than overt osteitis, being the presenting complaint in as many as 50% of patients in some series (4). In recent years, routine screening of serum Ca by automated clinical chemistry techniques has contributed to an increased rate of detection of PHPT in the population. For example, introduction of multichannel screening at the Mayo Clinic resulted in a fourfold increase in the diagnosis of PHPT among local residents (4). It is currently estimated that the prevalence of PHPT is approximately one case per thousand population or about 0.1% of the American population (5). For the middle-aged, the annual incidence rate is 100–200 cases per 100,000 (higher in women), representing 60,000 new cases of PHPT occurring each year in the United States (6).

In association with widespread chemical screening, the typical presentation of PHPT in the 1970s and 1980s had become more subtle. Bone disease was now rare (<10%), and even the incidence of kidney stones had diminished. For example, at the Mayo Clinic, the frequency of urolithiasis in patients with PHPT declined from 51% to 4% after Ca screening began (4). The proportion of patients with no symptoms or objective adverse effects of PHPT rose from 18% to 51%. Other series, as well, have confirmed that over half the cases of PHPT currently diagnosed are totally asymptomatic (7). What to do with the increasing number of patients pre-

senting with mild asymptomatic PHPT is a pressing but as yet unresolved problem. A review of studies attempting to grapple with the question of which is more dangerous—parathyroidectomy or the untreated disease—is the basis of this chapter. Chapters 23 and 31 complement the discussion in this chapter.

CASE FOR MEDICAL MANAGEMENT

Perhaps the earliest, serious study of asymptomatic PHPT was that performed at the Mayo Clinic by Scholz and Purnell (8). This was a 10-year prospective study, started in 1968, that involved 142 patients with asymptomatic PHPT. Patients were enrolled in this study if they did not meet any of the criteria for surgical treatment as shown in Table 1.

During the course of follow-up, approximately 20% of the patients developed surgical indications within the first 5 years, and a total of nearly 25% of the patients required surgery by the end of 10 years. The indications for surgery that occurred are shown in Table 2.

Thus 75% of patients with PHPT who presented asymptomatically did not develop a surgical indication over a 10-year period. Unfortunately, it was not possible to predict from the initial presentation which patients would ultimately require surgery and which would not. Also, a sizable portion of the initial patient group (15–20%) stopped coming for follow-up. For these reasons and because of concern about insidious spinal bone mineral loss (6,9) or progressive renal impairment (which was believed to occur in up to 5% of patients) (10), some investigators had suggested that perhaps all patients in whom the diagnosis of PHPT is made should be operated upon.

Another early contribution to the assessment of patients with asymptomatic PHPT compared 6 patients with asymptomatic PHPT to 7 hyperparathyroid patients with bone disease or nephrolithiasis (11). It was found that both groups of patients demonstrated evi-

N. A. Breslau and C. Y. C. Pak: Mineral Metabolism Section, Department of Medicine, University of Texas Southwestern Medical Center at Dallas, 5323 Harry Hines Boulevard, Dallas, Texas 75235

TABLE 1. *Criteria for surgical treatment in primary hyperparathyroidism*

1. Mean serum calcium >11.0 mg/dL
2. Roentgenographic evidence of bone disease
   a. Subperiosteal resorption of phalanges, distal clavicles, or other bones
   b. Fraying, distal phalangeal tufts
   c. Bone cyst (brown tumor)
   d. Granular demineralization of skull
   e. Osteoporosis with vertebral compression or other bone disease
3. Decreased renal function
4. Metabolically active or infected renal lithiasis
5. Prolonged observation impractical
   a. Patient cooperation unsatisfactory
   b. Geographic remoteness
   c. Psychiatric complications
6. Gastrointestinal complications
   a. Peptic ulcer not controlled by medical management
   b. Recurrent or chronic pancreatitis

Source: Modified with permission from Ref. 8.

TABLE 3. *Features of asymptomatic PHPT without physiologic derangement (n = 10)*

	Patients	Normal
Serum Ca (mg/dL)	11.1	<10.5
Serum P (mg/dL)	2.8	>2.5
Serum Mg (mg/dL)	2.0	1.7–2.4
Serum PTH (μL-eQ/mL)	65	<40
Urine cyclic AMP (nmol/100 mL gfr)	7.26	<5.40
24-h urine Ca (mg/day)	142	<200
Fasting urine Ca (mg/mg creatinine)	0.07	<0.11
Bone density, fractional change	+0.01	0.0
Intestinal ^{47}Ca absorption, fraction	0.55	<0.61

dence of the sequelae of PTH excess, including low radial bone density by ^{125}I-photon absorption, hypercalciuria (urinary Ca > 200 mg/day on an intake of 400 mg/day), negative Ca balance (absorbed Ca less than urinary Ca), elevated fasting urinary Ca (greater than 0.11 mg/mg creatinine), and decreased renal function (creatinine clearance of less than 65 mL/min). Following parathyroidectomy, most of these deleterious effects were reversed commensurate with the return of serum PTH, serum Ca, and urinary cyclic AMP toward normal. Parathyroidectomy was felt to be indicated in this subgroup of patients with asymptomatic PHPT who had underlying physiologic derangements because these abnormalities could herald the eventual development of overt symptoms (stones and bones) and were corrected by parathyroid surgery. However, another group of patients with asymptomatic PHPT were detected who did not have any underlying physiologic derangements (Table 3).

The need for parathyroid exploration in the asymptomatic patients without physiologic derangements has

not been established. Preliminary data in six of these patients showed a lack of progression of the disease over 4–6 years of follow-up (unpublished observation). Assessment of bone histomorphometry revealed that only about 10% of these patients had abnormalities of bone (increased resorption surface, increased bone turnover) compared to 75% of those with physiologic derangements. Further characterization and long-term follow-up will be required before it is known whether the asymptomatic hyperparathyroid patients without physiologic derangements represent an early stage of the disease or a pathogenetically unique subset characterized by skeletal resistance to PTH and an exaggerated renal tubular reabsorption of Ca. This group, which comprises up to 10% of patients with PHPT, probably does not have familial hypocalciuric hypercalcemia (see later), since there was no hypermagnesemia or family history of hypercalcemia.

Based on our past work, we have classified patients with PHPT as shown in Fig. 1. For those patients with overt symptoms (stones, bones, ulcers, symptomatic hypercalcemia) we have recommended surgery. For those patients that have been asymptomatic but who manifest underlying physiologic abnormalities, we have also recommended parathyroidectomy, or in some cases, medical therapy (see later). However, for the group with asymptomatic PHPT in the absence of physiologic derangements, our management has been conservative (serial observation). Although this approach to asymptomatic PHPT appears reasonable, it can be validated only by comparing the outcome for each subset over time with and without intervention.

Meanwhile, several other longitudinal studies reported from Australia (12) and England (13,14) provided more support for a conservative approach to asymptomatic PHPT. For example, Rohl et al. reported the follow-up over 3 years of 15 patients with negative cervical exploration or no fall in serum Ca postoperatively (12). There was no deterioration in serum Ca or creatinine levels or progression in parathyroid hormone levels. Seven patients with repeat abdominal radiography showed either no stones or no increase in the size of

TABLE 2. *Indications for surgery in patients with initial asymptomatic PHPT followed 10 years (n = 142)*

Indication	Number of patients	%
Increased serum calcium	8	6
Decreased renal function	6	4
Active stone disease	5	4
Psychologic	4	3
Bone disease	4	3
Unknown	4	3
Prophylactic	1	1
Renal colic	1	1
	33	23

Source: Modified with permission from Ref. 8.

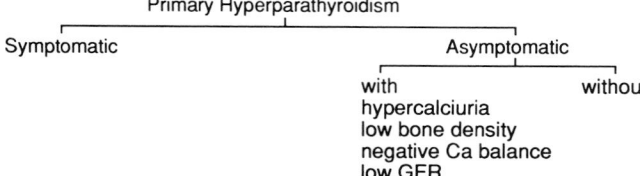

FIG. 1. Patients with PHPT may be divided into those with overt symptoms (stones, fractures, ulcers) and those who are asymptomatic. The asymptomatic group may be further subdivided into those with and without physiologic derangements. The authors have recommended parathyroidectomy only in patients who were symptomatic or had underlying physiologic abnormalities.

stones already present. They also followed 30 patients with PHPT who avoided operation because of age, lack of symptoms, or other pathology. These were followed for 89 patient years and showed no hypercalcemic crisis, no significant new symptoms, and no deterioration in renal function, even in the presence of stones. Twenty-one patients had abdominal radiography at presentation and on follow-up, 17 were normal, 3 showed no increase in the size of the stones already present, and in 1 patient the stones were said to have increased slightly. Vant Hoff et al. studied 32 patients with mild PHPT for a mean of 4.2 years (13). One patient required an operation because of a rise in plasma calcium concentration. There was no significant change in the mean plasma Ca and creatinine concentrations or in blood pressure during the period of follow-up. The progress of these patients who were managed medically was compared with that of a group of 60 patients who had had successful operations for PHPT. There was no significant change in mean plasma creatinine concentration or in blood pressure in the group who had operations during a mean follow-up period of 5.9 years. This would suggest that hypertension which occurs in up to 50% of patients with PHPT (compared to 20% of U.S. adults in general) generally does not respond to parathyroidectomy and should not be considered an indication for surgery in patients with asymptomatic PHPT (15). In another British study, Adams followed up 31 patients with mild PHPT for a mean of 4 years (14). There was no significant change in the mean serum creatinine concentration during the period of observation, and only 1 patient required an operation because of a rise in serum Ca concentration.

Two large retrospective studies have provided similar results. In one study, 160 patients found to have hypercalcemia on routine multiphasic chemistry screening were compared to an age-matched control group, with a mean follow-up of 8.5 years (16). There were no significant differences in symptomatology or renal function between patients and matched controls. For the controls, the mean initial serum creatinine was 1.00 ± 0.22 mg/dL, and the final value was 0.94 ± 0.21 mg/dL. In

the patients, the mean initial value was 1.03 ± 0.21 mg/dL and 0.94 ± 0.22 was the final value. Another retrospective survey was performed on 265 patients with PHPT who had received three forms of treatment on a nonrandomized basis (17). Successful surgery was carried out on 142 patients, unsuccessful surgery on 33, and no surgery on 90. The mean duration of follow-up was 8, 7, and 5 years, respectively. At the time of follow-up, the prevalence of hypertension, renal impairment, and vertebral crush fractures was similar in all three groups, although the "successfully" operated group (normalization of serum Ca) had a higher forearm bone density. It was concluded that untreated PHPT is compatible with long survival and a lack of demonstrable deleterious effects on kidney and bone. However, it must be noted that 13/90 (14%) of the patients who were initially not operated on were later felt to require surgery (6 because of hypercalcemia, 1 because of renal calculi, and 6 because of pressure from patients or colleagues).

Although the aforementioned studies may be faulted for rather imprecise descriptions of the "mild" PHPT groups and did not distinguish patients with and without physiologic derangements, in the aggregate they make a strong case for conservative management of mild asymptomatic PHPT (12–17). Collectively, these studies involved 391 nonoperated patients studied over a mean period of 3–8 years, and except for a rare patient, there was no change in serum Ca or creatinine (Fig. 2). Nor was there development of other parathyroid-related

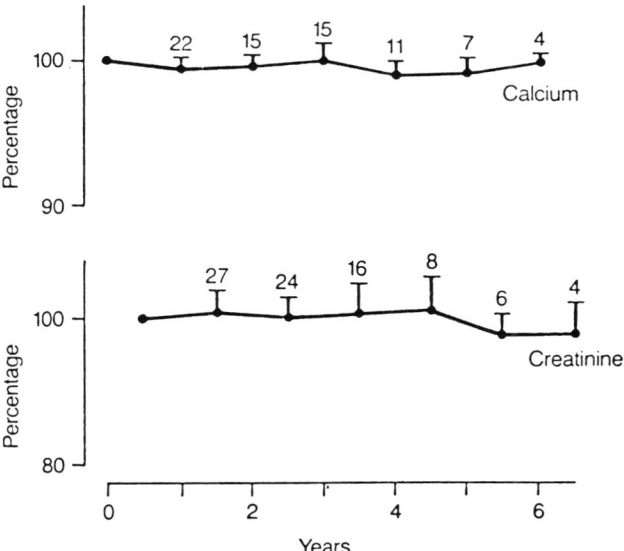

FIG. 2. Sequential changes in the serum calcium and creatinine concentrations in asymptomatic PHPT. Serum calcium is expressed as a percentage of initial value; serum creatinine is the average value for each year expressed as a percentage of the mean value of the first year. Numbers represent number of patients in each group. Mean and SE are shown. (By permission from Ref. 14.)

problems. Isolated case reports of patients with PHPT of 25–30 years' duration (18,19), who showed no or minimal morbidity, lend additional credence to the idea that PHPT may follow a benign course over a long duration.

Thus the natural history of mild asymptomatic PHPT is probably different from and better than that of the type of PHPT that was usually seen before the advent of routine chemical screening. The type of PHPT that we are seeing now may be at one end of the range of PHPT that was rarely detected before the advent of routine chemical screening and that may not require operation. Although most patients with asymptomatic PHPT seem to be at little risk of severe hypercalcemia or progressive renal impairment, there has been nagging concern about the long-term effect of sustained hyperparathyroidism on the skeleton, particularly in postmenopausal women (6,9). Based on bone mineral density measurements of the radius, a more sensitive index than skeletal x-ray, it has been known for some time that many patients with PHPT have less bone than normal for their age (20,21), a deficiency that becomes more apparent after the menopause (22). In contrast to cortical bone, there has been controversy as to whether excessive PTH secretion causes increased loss of trabecular bone (spine). Seeman et al. reported that trabecular bone is reduced preferentially in PHPT (9), and the Mayo Clinic group has also described vertebral crush fractures occurring as an unemphasized mode of presentation of PHPT (6,23). Convincing recent work from Bilezikian and co-workers at Columbia (24) and Parfitt's group in Detroit (25), which will now be described, has lessened concern about the development of spinal osteoporosis in patients with asymptomatic PHPT.

Bilezikian's group investigated 52 patients with PHPT (24). They had mild hypercalcemia (Ca 11.1 ± 0.1 mg/dL) and no symptoms or specific radiologic signs of skeletal involvement. Although they were asymptomatic with respect to bone disease, 20% of the patients did give a history of nephrolithiasis. The purpose of the study was to determine whether skeletal involvement could be appreciated when more sensitive techniques such as bone densitometry and bone biopsy were utilized. A major subset of this population, 31 patients, had completed densitometric studies of three skeletal sites that correspond principally to cortical bone (diaphyseal radius), cancellous bone (lumbar spine), or a combination of both (femoral neck). The bone density at each site in comparison to expected values for age-, sex-, and ethnic-matched normal subjects is shown in Fig. 3. At the lumbar spine, the average bone mineral density was 1.07 ± 0.03 g/cm², which is within 5% of the expected mean for matched normal subjects. At the femoral neck, the hyperparathyroid population began to diverge from normal with a mean value of 0.78 ± 0.14 g/cm², 89 ± 2% of the expected value. The radius showed the greatest difference from normal. Mean bone density at this site was

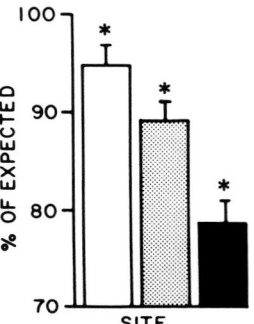

FIG. 3. Densitometric measurements at three skeletal sites (*white*, lumber; *gray*, femoral; *black*, radius) in 31 patients with PHPT who did not have any symptoms or radiologic signs of skeletal disease. The bone density at each site is shown as a percentage of values for age-, sex-, and race-matched normal subjects. (By permission from Ref. 24.)

0.54 ± 0.10 g/cm², only 79 ± 2% of the expected mean. The three sites were significantly different from each other in the extent of their divergence from their expected normal value ($p < 0.0001$). Bone density of the spine did not differ significantly from normal, whereas bone density of the radius showed the greatest reduction.

Another way of showing that sites comprised primarily of cortical bone were the most frequently affected in PHPT was to assess the percentage of bone density measurements at each site with a value less than 80% of the age- and sex-matched control value (24). Thus defined, the percentage of low bone density values at the lumbar, femoral neck, and radial sites were 13, 23, and 58%, respectively. The extent to which bone mineral density was reduced did not correlate significantly with the level of the serum or urinary Ca, the serum PTH concentration, or any other biochemical index of PHPT.

Twenty of Bilezikian's patients had histomorphometric analysis of bone obtained by percutaneous transiliac biopsy (24). Mean cortical width and cancellous bone volume are shown in Figs. 4 and 5, respectively. Most patients (84%) with PHPT had cortical width below the control mean, consistent with the data obtained by single-photon absorptiometry showing decreased radial bone mineral density. In contrast to the relative decrease in mean cortical width, cancellous bone volume was preserved. Representative scanning electron micrographs of bone biopsy specimens from normal (Fig. 6A) and hyperparathyroid (Fig. 6B) subjects show loss of cortical bone and preservation of cancellous bone in PHPT (24).

Compared to control subjects, 85% of PHPT patients had greater than average values for cancellous bone volume (Fig. 5). Preservation of cancellous bone, as determined by histomorphometric analysis, was consistent with normal bone mineral density of trabecular sites (lumbar spine) as determined by dual-photon absorptiometry. There were no significant correlations between cortical width or cancellous bone volume and serum or urinary Ca, PTH level, or bone density at any site.

One may conclude from Bilezikian's studies that the majority of patients with asymptomatic PHPT have evidence by bone densitometry and bone biopsy for cortical bone disease. The significance of this pervasive but sub-

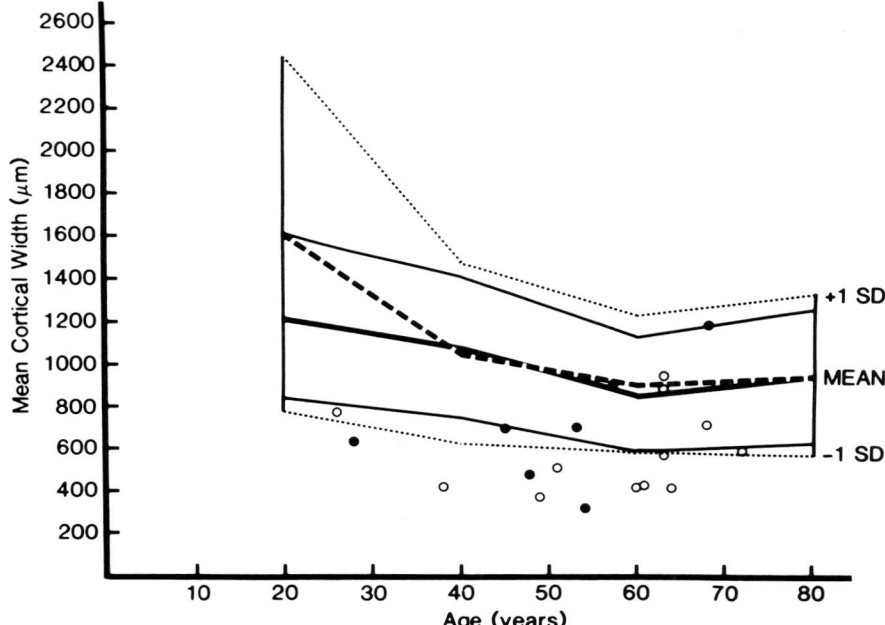

FIG. 4. Mean cortical width of bone obtained by transiliac biopsy in patients with PHPT compared to normal control subjects. Values for hyperparathyroid men are shown in *solid circles* and those for women in *open circles*. The *solid lines* depict mean ± SD values for control men and the *dashed lines* for control women. (By permission from Ref. 24.)

tle cortical bone loss in patients with "asymptomatic" PHPT with respect to potential increase in fracture incidence at the radius or at the femoral neck (a site of mixed cortical and cancellous bone) must await the results of ongoing longitudinal follow-up. The good news in Bilezikian's report is that the mild hyperparathyroid state may be protective of cancellous bone. Most reports that have measured cancellous bone volume confirm its pres-

ervation in PHPT (26,27). Preliminary data from Parfitt et al. have suggested that in PHPT, osteoclast resorptive activity is increased on the endocortical but not on the trabecular surfaces of bone (28). It has been speculated that the endocortical surface of bone gradually becomes "trabecularized" with maintenance of total bone volume at the expense of the cortical elements. The important clinical implication of these data is that postmeno-

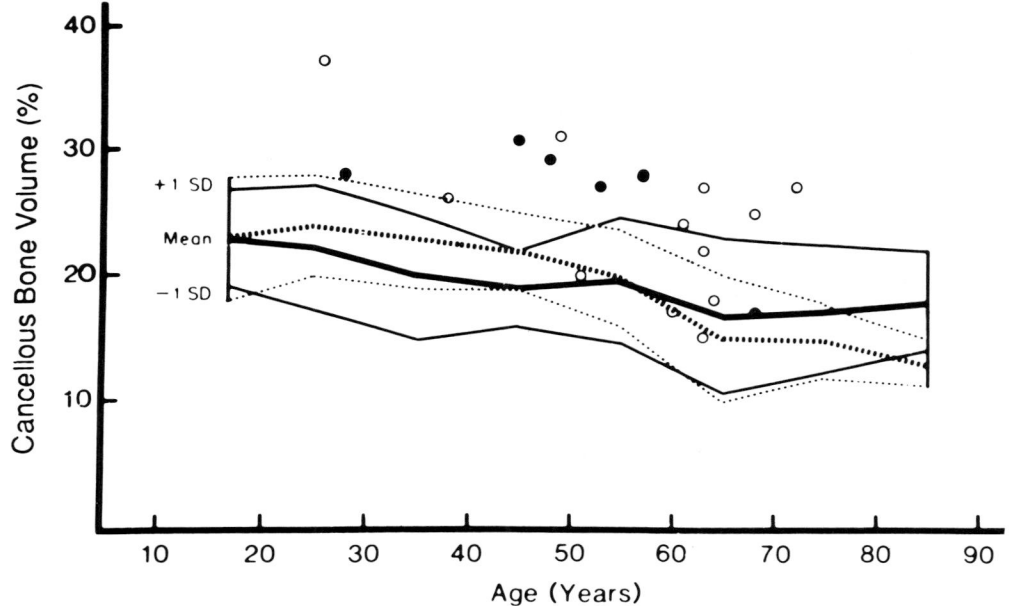

FIG. 5. Cancellous bone volume in transiliac biopsy specimens from patients with PHPT compared to normal control subjects. Values for hyperparathyroid men are shown in solid circles and those for women in open circles. The solid lines depict mean ± SD values for control men and the dashed lines for control women. (By permission from Ref. 24.)

pausal women with asymptomatic PHPT have preservation of cancellous bone and may actually be protected against spinal osteoporosis. It is conceivable that the increased level of PTH in these patients is actually helping to preserve cancellous bone. In this regard, treatment of osteoporosis with low-dose PTH has led to an increase in cancellous bone mass (29,30).

Parfitt's group has provided additional evidence for protection of the trabecular skeleton in the postmenopausal woman with asymptomatic PHPT. The prevalence of vertebral fractures in 174 patients (mean age 62 years) with mild asymptomatic PHPT was 1.7%; in a subset of white women, the prevalence was 2.8% (25). These rates were not higher than those found in a retrospective control group or in a historical control group of similar age, and may even be lower. Parfitt's group concluded that the risk for vertebral fractures was not increased in patients with mild asymptomatic PHPT and that concern about this risk should not constitute a reason to recommend surgical intervention in these patients. The increased rates of vertebral fractures reported in previous series (6,9,23) were attributed to inappropriate control groups, the influence of referral or selection bias (e.g., patients referred to Mayo Clinic with coexistent osteoporosis), the inclusion of patients with severe disease, and the effect of geographic differences in vitamin D nutrition on the expression of disease.

The Detroit group has also recently summarized a set

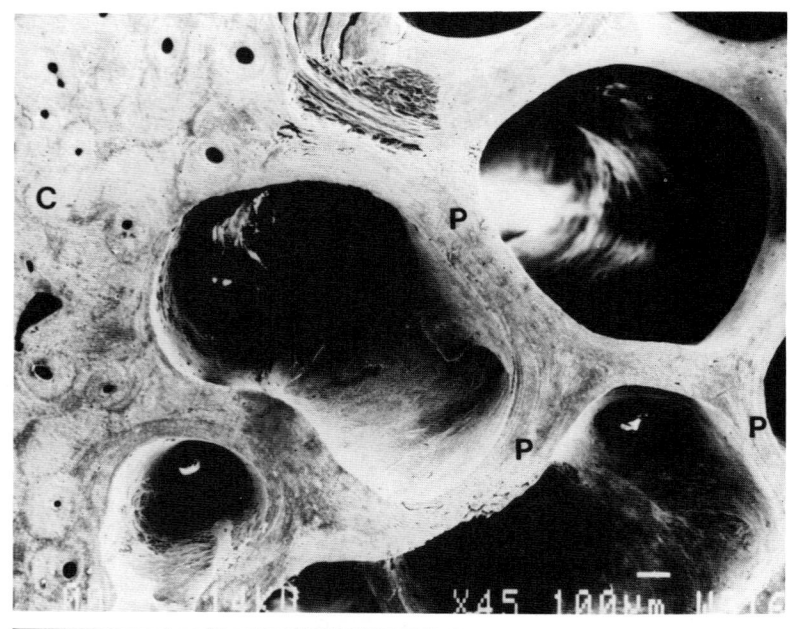

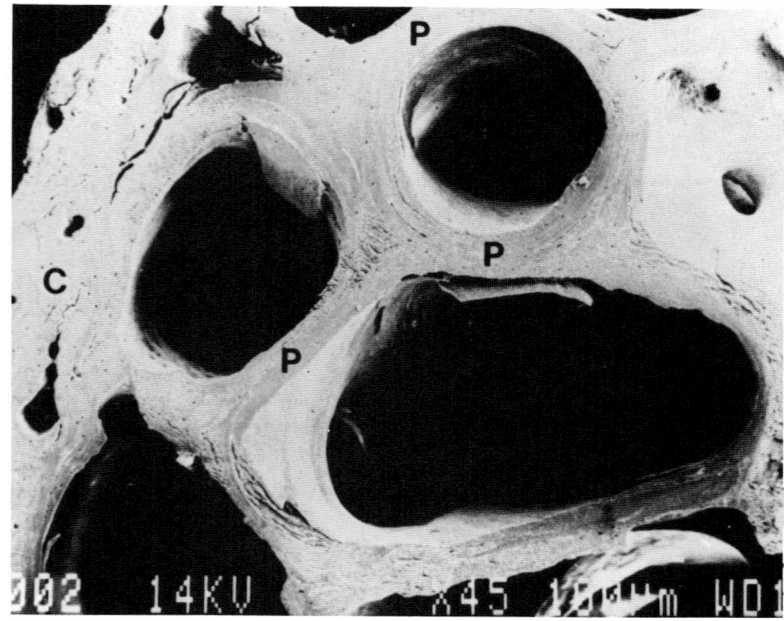

FIG. 6. Representative scanning electron micrographs of bone biopsy specimens from a normal (**A**) and a hyperparathyroid (**B**) subject. Loss of cortical bone thickness (C) with preservation of trabecular plates (P) can be seen in the hyperparathyroid subject (**B**). (By permission from Ref. 24.)

TABLE 4. *Biochemical measurements in patients with PHPT[a]*

Measurement	n	Initial	Final
Serum calcium (mmol/L)	80	2.77 ± 0.09	2.77 ± 0.11
Serum phosphate (mmol/L)	80	0.87 ± 0.14	0.87 ± 0.13
Serum creatinine (μmol/L)	80	87.5 ± 17.7	87.5 ± 20.3
Serum alkaline phosphatase (μkat/L)	76	1.7 ± 0.7	1.9 ± 0.9
Serum PTH (ng/L; C-terminal assay)	49	1110 ± 640	1040 ± 570
Serum PTH (ng/L; midregion assay)	13	2360 ± 1090	2160 ± 1770
NcAMP/GFR (nmol/L)	42	3.98 ± 1.48	4.19 ± 1.63
TmP/GFR (mmol/L)	42	0.76 ± 0.17	0.77 ± 0.19
Urinary calcium (mmol/day)	42	6.5 ± 3.3	6.1 ± 3.3
Creatinine clearance (mL/min)	42	82 ± 26	85 ± 27

Source: Modified with permission from Ref. 31.
[a] Values are the mean ± SD. None of the differences is significant.

of very complete data on the natural history of asymptomatic PHPT (31). They selected patients in whom the disease was discovered fortuitously by multichannel biochemical screening and whom they elected to follow conservatively because they met the following criteria: asymptomatic, no renal stone disease, no radiographic osteitis fibrosa, serum Ca below 12 mg/dL, serum creatinine below 133 μmol/L, and forearm bone density not more than 2.5 SD below the mean expected for age, sex, and race. Thus they had a well-defined group of patients with asymptomatic PHPT, although the patients were not divided into those with and without physiologic derangements. One hundred and seventy-four patients met their criteria during a 10-year period from 1976 to 1985, of whom 80 (mean age, 61 years) had adequate follow-up. These 80 patients were followed for 1–11 years (mean, 46 months; median, 38 months), during which there was no change, mean or individual, in any index of PTH secretion or any of its biochemical effects (Table 4)

and no decline in forearm bone density apart from that expected from increased age (Table 5).

The report from Parfitt's group (31) is particularly relevant because of concern over the potential risk with conservative management of persistent cortical bone loss. As already noted, patients with asymptomatic PHPT have a disproportionate loss of appendicular cortical bone by the time of diagnosis. Increased cortical bone loss would be expected to increase the risk of long bone fractures in general and hip fractures in particular, and it would be unwise to withhold surgery in patients losing cortical bone more rapidly than normal. But Parfitt's data suggest that mild asymptomatic PHPT follows a biphasic course, with a short period of disease progression (accounting for the initial biochemical and bone density presentation), followed by a long period of disease stability. In Table 5, note that for proximal BM/BW there was no change in z score (number of SDs below normal mean) indicating that bone density fell at the rate expected for age. Distal BM/BW actually showed an increase in z score, indicating slower than expected loss at this site, consistent with a beneficial effect of mild asymptomatic PHPT on cancellous bone. During the course of the 4-year study, one 80-year-old woman sustained a traumatic hip fracture, which healed uneventfully, but no nontraumatic fractures occurred. There were no episodes of temporary worsening of hypercalcemia or hypercalcemic crisis, no changes in renal function, and no symptoms attributable to renal stone disease. In no patient were the initial criteria for surgery satisfied. Therefore, the data appeared to support the decision to withhold surgical intervention in patients with mild asymptomatic PHPT, but the Detroit group recognized that a larger, controlled clinical trial would be necessary before definitive recommendations could be made.

THE CASE FOR SURGICAL INTERVENTION

Although a growing body of evidence favors the view that patients with mild asymptomatic PHPT may be followed safely without the need for immediate surgical intervention, this approach remains controversial. There

TABLE 5. *Changes in forearm bone densitometry measured by single-photon absorpiometry in patients with PHPT[a]*

	Proximal		Distal	
	Initial	Final	Initial	Final
Bone mineral (g/cm)	0.843 ± 0.108	0.815 ± 0.198[b]	0.839 ± 0.199	0.831 ± 0.192
Bone width (cm)	1.288 ± 0.166	1.287 ± 0.156	1.814 ± 0.242	1.781 ± 0.191
BM/BW (g/cm²)	0.657 ± 0.107	0.631 ± 0.112[b]	0.466 ± 0.079	0.464 ± 0.083
z Score	−0.929 ± 0.891	−0.987 ± 0.944	−1.305 ± 1.223	−1.059 ± 1.263[c]

Source: By permission from Ref. 31.
[a] Values are the mean ± SD. Comparisons are between initial and final values.
[b] $p < 0.001$.
[c] $p < 0.05$.

TABLE 6. *Symptoms elicited by questioning 17 "asymptomatic" patients undergoing parathyroidectomy whose hypercalcemia was an unexpected finding on routine blood testing and 17 patients undergoing operation for otherwise symptomless thyroid swellings*

Group		Gastrointestinal	Urological	Psychiatric	Lethargy	Bone pain	Neurological	Total
"Asymptomatic" hyperparathyroid patients	Elicited	12	11	3	9	4	5	44
	Improved/ cured	9	6	2	8	3	5	33 (=75%)
Symptomless thyroid patients	Elicited	4	6	2	4	3	13	32
	Improved/ cured	0	1	0	0	0	2	3 (=9%)

Source: Modified by permission from Ref. 34.

are a number of clinicians who would still maintain that once the diagnosis of PHPT is made, a parathyroidectomy should be performed. The case for surgical intervention will be summarized in the following 10 points.

1. *Insidious nature of "asymptomatic" PHPT.* Some patients who are truly symptomatic may be unaware of their disease until surgery relieves their symptoms (32). These symptoms are often very vague and include weakness, fatigue, arthralgia, and personality changes. In one series of 289 patients operated on for PHPT, 35% were picked up by routine chemical screening and were considered asymptomatic (33). On specific, careful questioning, most admitted to various symptoms that disappeared following surgery: malaise, fatigue, and muscular weakness disappeared in 79%, upper abdominal pains in 66%, constipation in 63%, pains in the extremities in 51%, and depression in 65%. In another series involving 17 patients with so-called asymptomatic PHPT, 75% of symptoms elicited by more careful probing improved following surgery (Table 6) (34). In contrast, a similar group of "asymptomatic" patients undergoing operations for thyroid nodules had only a 9% improvement in elicited symptoms. It was gratifying to the surgeons that most patients with asymptomatic PHPT showed subjective improvement in symptoms that had not seemed remarkable to them before their operation.

2. *Underlying physiologic derangements.* As noted earlier, if evaluated carefully, many patients with asymptomatic PHPT will be found to have important, though subtle physiologic derangements (hypercalciuria, reduced bone density, negative Ca balance, decreased creatinine clearance) (11). Although not yet proven, these abnormalities may herald potential target organ damage (kidney, bone). There is persistent concern about progressive bone loss and increased fracture incidence, especially in those predisposed to osteopenia (patients with diabetes, those taking steroids, the immobilized, postmenopausal women). It is noteworthy that following parathyroidectomy there is a partial improvement in radial bone density (20,21).

3. *Relatively high complication rate in some longitudinal studies.* In some longitudinal studies, an unacceptably high number of patients with asymptomatic PHPT eventually developed overt symptoms requiring surgical intervention or even more serious complications (8,35). It will be recalled that in Scholz and Purnell's study at the Mayo Clinic, 25% of patients with asymptomatic PHPT developed surgical indications (hypercalcemia, decreased renal function, stones, bone disease) during the 10-year follow-up (Table 2) (8). In another study, Corlew et al. followed 47 patients with PHPT for at least 5 years and for an average of $8\frac{1}{2}$ years (35). Although there was no progressive increase in serum Ca or PTH, 16 of the 47 patients (34%) experienced a complication usually associated with PHPT: peptic ulcer disease (8 patients), decreased renal function (5 patients), renal stone (1 patient), hypercalcemic crisis (1 patient), and ventricular conduction defect (1 patient). Four deaths were attributed to these complications (Table 7). None of the pa-

TABLE 7. *Deaths attributable to a complication of untreated primary hyperparathyroidism in 47 patients during long-term follow-up*

Type	Age (yr)	Sex	Associated condition
Hypercalcemic crisis	70	M	Hypertension, diabetes
Progressive renal failure	85	F	Hypertension, gout
Ventricular arrhythmia	78	F	Hypertension, IHSS[a]
Gastrointestinal hemorrhage	74	F	Duodenal ulcer

Source: Modified with permission from Ref. 35.
[a] IHSS, idiopathic hypertrophic subaortic stenosis.

TABLE 8. *Safety and efficacy of parathyroidectomy at major centers*

Center	n	Successful	Recurrent laryngeal nerve	Hypopara	Other[a]	Mortality
Gaz and Wang (MGH)	242	238 (98%)	0	1 (0.4%)	6 (2.5%)	0
Russell and Edis (Mayo Clinic)	500	461 (92%)	1 (0.2%)	10 (2%)	17 (3.4%)	1 (0.2%)

Source: Derived from Refs. 36 and 37.

[a] Includes miscellaneous transient complications such as wound hematoma, stitch abscess, gouty attack, thrombophlebitis, wound infection, and atrial fibrillation.

rameters studied offered an accurate prediction of the likelihood of progression or severity of complications in a given patient. This study did not, however, involve typical patients with mild, asymptomatic PHPT, but rather, any patients who were unwilling or unable to have parathyroidectomy. Many of these patients had serum Ca greater than 11.5 mg/dL and up to 12.9 mg/dL. Moreover, as shown in Table 7, some of the deaths could easily have been explained by causes unrelated to PHPT (e.g., renal failure in an 85-year-old woman with hypertension and gout or ventricular arrhythmia in a 78-year-old woman with hypertension and IHSS). Nevertheless, the risks associated with long-term nonoperative management of asymptomatic PHPT are considerable in some series and exceed the morbidity and mortality rates resulting from neck exploration (see the next section).

4. *High success rate, low complication rate of parathyroidectomy.* When performed by skilled, experienced neck surgeons, the cure rate for PHPT (asymptomatic or overt) consistently exceeds 90%, and the morbidity and mortality rate is very low (Table 8) (36,37).

The criteria used by the MGH surgeons for surgical intervention in asymptomatic PHPT were similar to the approach taken in Dallas (11,36). They operated on those patients with physiologic derangements and followed the others "expectantly." But they also utilized a serum Ca rising above 11 mg/dL as an indication to operate. In their series of 242 patients with asymptomatic PHPT, 98% had confirmation of parathyroid disease and were treated successfully. The pathologic diagnosis was similar to that seen in patients with overt parathyroid disease (i.e., 83% had a single adenoma, 16% had hyperplasia, and 1% had normal glands). None of the patients had parathyroid carcinoma.

In contrast, the surgeons at the Mayo Clinic favored operating on all patients with a bona fide diagnosis of PHPT (37). Their results in patients with asymptomatic or "biochemical" PHPT compared to patients with symptomatic PHPT are shown in Table 9. In both groups, they achieved greater than a 90% success rate, although there was a higher incidence of negative neck exploration in the asymptomatic group (perhaps some

were normal subjects at the high range of serum Ca or patients with familial hypocalciuric hypercalcemia—see below). In any event, they argued that cervical exploration in patients with asymptomatic PHPT was safe (no deaths, no permanent cord paralysis, only 2 patients with hypoparathyroidism among 84 patients) and effective (92% cure rate). In contrast to some series of prolonged clinical observation, morbidity and mortality were negligible.

5. *Noninvasive parathyroid localization tests may facilitate the decision for surgical intervention.* Preoperative confirmation and localization of enlarged parathyroid glands may facilitate the decision for surgical intervention in asymptomatic PHPT (38–40). Current noninvasive parathyroid localization techniques include thallium–technetium subtraction imaging, computerized tomography, ultrasound, and magnetic resonance imaging. These techniques have an overall 80% sensitivity and 65–75% true positivity (specificity) in localizing abnormal parathyroid glands (Table 10) (40). A combination of any two techniques was just as sensitive in localizing parathyroid adenomas but was more specific (Table 11) (40). That is, if it was required that the lesion suspected of being a parathyroid adenoma had to be confirmed by two localization tests, there was much less error due to artifact, and the true-positive ratio as con-

TABLE 9. *Comparison of surgical outcomes for patients with asymptomatic PHPT and symptomatic PHPT*

Outcome	Asymptomatic PHPT (n = 84)		Symptomatic PHPT (n = 311)	
	No.	%	No.	%
Cured	77	91.7	291	93.6
Four normal glands, no disease found	7	8.3[a]	9	2.9[a]
Vocal cord paralysis	0	0	0	0
Protracted hypoparathyroidism	2	2.4	7	2.2

Source: Modified with permission from Ref. 37.

[a] Significant difference between groups (p < 0.025).

TABLE 10. *Comparison of parathyroid localization tests in 26 consecutive patients with confirmed parathyroid adenomas*

Test	Sensitivity (%)	True-positive ratio (%)
Thallium–technetium scan	65	82
Computerized tomography	76	64
Ultrasonography	77	71
Magnetic resonance imaging	81	77

Source: Modified with permission from Ref. 40.

firmed by surgery rose to 86%. As the usefulness of non-invasive localization tests continues to improve, it could have bearing on the approach to asymptomatic PHPT because of the potential further reduction in surgical risk. In one minor study, the duration of operation and postoperative complications were significantly reduced compared to a retrospective control group when sono-graphic localization was applied (38). There was a higher cure rate of hypercalcemia and a lower incidence of hypo-parathyroidism and recurrent laryngeal nerve damage.

6. *Prolonged observation impractical; high dropout rate.* Many nonoperated PHPT patients are lost to medical follow-up for a variety of reasons: lack of symptoms, expense, inconvenience, mobile society, and so on. In the 10-year prospective study of asymptomatic PHPT conducted at the Mayo Clinic, the dropout rate was 15–20% (8).

7. *Prolonged medical observation is expensive.* It has been calculated that repeated visits and tests obtained during long-term conservative management of asymptomatic PHPT exceeds the cost of surgery after 5 years (4,6).

8. *Changes in health status during prolonged observation may preclude needed surgery.* If surgery is deferred, the patient may acquire independent systemic or vascular disease, jeopardizing or contraindicating neck exploration when complications of PHPT eventually occur (32). Moreover, if other conditions develop, they may be complicated by coexistent PHPT. For example, there may be a risk of severe life-threatening hypercalcemia during periods of dehydration or immobilization. Another example might be the development of congestive heart failure in a patient with PHPT with increased risk of conduction disturbance or arrhythmia during digitalis administration because of hypercalcemia.

9. *Medical therapy of PHPT leaves much to be desired (41).* See the next section.

10. *Young patients with long life expectancy.* Young people with PHPT are not only excellent surgical risks, but if unoperated have a long time to develop complications.

MEDICAL THERAPY OF PHPT

It is not clear that the increasingly large number of patients with only mild hypercalcemia and no other manifestations of parathyroid disease should undergo surgery. It may be difficult for physicians to recommend surgery for these patients, whose mild PHPT could have been discovered as an incidental finding on a routine health screening test. For many of these persons, careful and regular observation may be all that is required. Other patients with asymptomatic PHPT may have significant underlying physiologic derangements but may still be reluctant to undergo parathyroidectomy. Yet one might wish to do something about the postmenopausal woman with negative calcium balance and low bone density, or the young male with intestinal Ca hyperabsorption and marked hypercalciuria. For these patients, nonsurgical approaches to the disease might be considered. Although the current medical management of PHPT is far from ideal (41), there appears to be a role for estrogen and phosphate therapy, and also, perhaps, for some of the newer diphosphonates.

Therapy with Estrogen

Estrogen therapy provides a medical option in postmenopausal women with PHPT. It has been established that estrogens may inhibit the action of parathyroid hormone on bone and lead to a reduction in bone resorption (42–45). The evidence for reduced bone resorption has included reductions in serum and urine Ca as well as in urinary hydroxyproline excretion in postmenopausal women with PHPT who were treated with estrogens. The ability of estrogens to block bone resorption appeared to be a direct effect, and indeed estrogen receptors have been identified in human osteoblast-like cells (46,47).

In addition to blocking bone resorption, estrogen therapy was shown to stimulate the parathyroid–vitamin D axis resulting in an increase in the serum free 1,25-dihydroxyvitamin D [$1,25(OH)_2D$] concentration and in fractional intestinal ^{47}Ca absorption (48). Because of the reduction in urinary Ca excretion combined with the increase in intestinal Ca absorption, estimated Ca balance (absorbed Ca − urinary Ca) improved from -14 ± 68 to $+125 \pm 70$ mg daily in a group of 10 postmeno-

TABLE 11. *Sensitivity and specificity of any combination of parathyroid localization tests*

	Sensitivity (%)	True-positive ratio (%)
Two techniques	79	86
Three techniques	63	92
Four techniques	40	100

Source: Modified with permission from Ref. 40.

pausal women with PHPT during treatment with estrogen (48). The improvements in intestinal Ca absorption and estimated Ca balance persisted over a 24-month period and were accompanied by an increase in radial bone density of 6%. This rise in radial bone density was equivalent to that observed following parathyroidectomy (21).

Although the effects of estrogen on bone in postmenopausal women with PHPT appeared beneficial, several caveats should be considered. The effect of estrogen in preserving radial bone density persisted only for as long as estrogen was given (unpublished observation). Once stopped, radial bone density began to decline. Moreover, in limited studies available, estrogen treatment did not normalize bone histomorphometry (44). In 6 patients who underwent bone biopsies before and after 1 year of treatment, osteoid was still abnormally plentiful. In contrast, bone osteoid content became normal within 6 months of parathyroidectomy in two patients who did not respond to estrogen and who underwent surgery. It was unclear whether the persistent osteoid in the estrogen-treated patients reflected continued high bone turnover or reduced mineralization because of the low serum phosphorus levels that estrogen produced (44). With limited information on the long-term impact of untreated mild PHPT on bone histomorphometry, the benefit of estrogen therapy remains somewhat uncertain. In addition, the potential usefulness of estrogens for reducing bone turnover and protecting cortical bone must be balanced against the risks of using this form of therapy (49). In the author's unpublished experience following 10 postmenopausal women with asymptomatic PHPT who received ethinyl estradiol 50 μg daily over a 2-year period, one developed significant hypertension, one developed hypertriglyceridemia causing pancreatitis, and one suffered a cerebrovascular accident.

Therapy with Phosphate

For patients with PHPT who have enhanced intestinal Ca absorption and hypercalciuria, phosphate therapy may help prevent the development of kidney stones (50,51). Although it is still not known exactly how phosphate therapy lowers the serum Ca, one hypothesis is that an increase in the calcium–phosphate product promotes Ca deposition into bone, and perhaps into soft tissues as well (41). Another mechanism of phosphate action was demonstrated in the subset of hyperparathyroid patients with high Ca absorption and elevated 1,25(OH)$_2$D levels (50). In response to phosphate therapy, these patients showed reductions in 1,25(OH)$_2$D concentration, intestinal Ca absorption as assessed by oral Ca loading, and in urinary Ca excretion (51). Hypercalciuria is also reduced because of direct effects of phosphate treatment to increase renal tubular Ca reabsorption (52,53). Administration of phosphate also protects against kidney stones because it is associated with enhanced urinary excretion of pyrophosphate and phosphocitrate, inhibitors of Ca oxalate, and brushite crystal formation (54).

However, there are several concerns regarding the long-term use of oral phosphate therapy in patients with PHPT. One problem is that of potential ectopic calcification by deposition of calcium phosphate crystals into soft tissues (55). Most cases of massive extraskeletal calcification have occurred when large doses of phosphate were given to severely hypercalcemic patients, often in the presence of moderate renal failure. In a 1-year study of 10 carefully selected patients with PHPT, whose serum Ca was <11.5 mg/dL, serum P < 3.5 mg/dL, and who had normal creatinine clearance, Broadus et al. found no evidence of soft tissue calcification or declining renal function following treatment with oral phosphate (1500 mg of elemental phosphorus daily) (51). This dosage of phosphate was sufficient to reduce 24-h urine Ca excretion from 438 mg to 269 mg daily (on a 1000-mg Ca diet) and to prevent further stone formation. This response, however, was accompanied by an increase in biochemical hyperparathyroidism, as assessed by circulating immunoreactive PTH and nephrogenous cyclic AMP excretion (51). The long-term effects of this excessive PTH secretion on skeletal homeostasis remain unclear. Nevertheless, with careful monitoring, phosphate is a therapeutic alternative for patients with PHPT who are unwilling or unable to have surgery.

Therapy with Diphosphonates

Another class of agents that have been investigated in the medical management of PHPT are the diphosphonates. These compounds are related to an endogenous product of metabolism, pyrophosphate, but the P—O—P bond is replaced by a P—C—P bond, and hence they are not as readily degradable. The diphosphonates have a great affinity for bone and appear to work by impairing the function of the osteoclast, the cell responsible for calcium mobilization (56). Diphosphonates also coat the hydroxyapatite crystal and may inhibit its dissolution and sometimes its growth (57). The first diphosphonate to be investigated in PHPT was ethane hydroxy-1,1-diphosphonate (EHDP) (58). During the first 5 weeks of treatment there was a decrease in urinary Ca and hydroxyproline excretion, suggesting an inhibition of bone resorption. However, the serum Ca level was never reduced, and urine Ca excretion rebounded after 6 months of treatment. It appeared that the beneficial effect of EHDP to impair bone resorption was offset by another effect, to retard bone mineralization. Another diphosphonate, dichloromethylene diphosphonate (Cl$_2$MDP), was evaluated because while it was known to block bone resorption, it had not been shown to affect mineralization when administered in usual therapeutic doses. In a double-blind, placebo-controlled study of 14 patients with PHPT, the serum Ca, urinary Ca, and hydroxyproline excretion were all reduced significantly when Cl_2MDP was administered (59). Unfortunately, a few patients treated with Cl_2MDP developed leukemia, and the drug was removed from further testing. A newer diphosphonate that is currently undergoing evaluation is 3-amino-1-hydroxypropylidine-1,1-diphosphonate (APD). It has thus far proven to be an effective medical therapy for hypercalcemia both in patients with malignancy and in patients with PHPT (60). Like Cl_2MDP, it inhibits bone resorption at doses that do not affect mineralization. Side effects that have been observed with APD therapy include transient fever and mouth ulcerations.

It should be apparent from this brief review that a completely safe and effective medical therapy for PHPT is lacking. Patients who meet accepted surgical guidelines should undergo parathyroidectomy. For the increasingly large number of patients who may not be obvious candidates for surgery, alternative forms of treatment are needed but are still not available.

OCCURRENCE OF ASYMPTOMATIC PHPT IN SPECIAL SITUATIONS

Familial Forms of PHPT

At least three distinct familial syndromes of PHPT have been recognized, accounting for 2–18% of all cases of PHPT (61). These are multiple endocrine neoplasia, types I and II (MEN I and MEN II), and familial hypocalciuric hypercalcemia (FHH). Each of these conditions is inherited as an autosomal dominant trait and each entails particular consideration regarding management of PHPT, which may or may not be asymptomatic.

Multiple Endocrine Neoplasia, Type I (MEN I)

MEN I is characterized by hyperfunction of parathyroid, pancreatic islet, and anterior pituitary cells. Among the patients who express the gene for this disorder, 95% have PHPT, whereas less than a third have either gastrinoma or prolactinoma. The features of PHPT in MEN I are similar to the features of PHPT in the general population except that the average age of onset is earlier (age 20–40) and the sex ratio does not favor females (61). At the time of parathyroid exploration, symmetric hyperplasia of all four glands is typically found. The recurrence rate of PHPT in patients with MEN I who have undergone apparently successful subtotal parathyroidectomy approaches 50% at 10 years after surgery. Recently, Brandi et al. reported that plasma from MEN I patients contains a mitogenic factor for cultured bovine parathyroid cells (62). The average mitogenic activity in MEN I plasma was over 20-fold that in plasma from normal

controls. Isolation and characterization of this mitogenic factor have indicated that it is similar to basic fibroblast growth factor (63). A study of a large MEN I kindred revealed that plasma mitogenic activity may precede the clinical manifestation of parathyroid hyperfunction (64). Although the source of the mitogenic activity is unknown, it persisted for up to 4 years post-total parathyroidectomy (65).

Because of the high rate of recurrence after parathyroidectomy in MEN I, it may be particularly appropriate to delay neck exploration until the first signs of morbidity appear. For example, at the Mayo Clinic, there is reluctance to recommend parathyroidectomy unless significant hypercalcemia (>1.0 mg/dL above the upper limit of normal) or documented renal dysfunction or bone disease is present (66). This view is shared by the mineral metabolism group at the NIH (61) as well as our own group. We are also in agreement with the NIH group regarding the appropriate surgical approach to the parathyroid hyperplasia of MEN I (61). This approach entails deliberate total parathyroidectomy with simultaneous autograft of fresh parathyroid tissue to the forearm muscle bed of the nondominant arm. The likelihood of graft function is close to 100%. The autograft procedure is unlikely to decrease the incidence of recurrent PHPT, but it should be easier to manage hyperfunctioning parathyroid tissue in the forearm than in the neck.

Two other points relating to PHPT in the MEN I syndrome concern screening and monitoring in MEN I kindreds and the relationship between PHPT and the Zollinger–Ellison syndrome. In most MEN I kindreds, PHPT is the commonest and usually the earliest manifestation of the MEN I gene. Although primary hypergastrinemia can cause greater morbidity than PHPT in MEN I, it almost always occurs later and is unlikely to cause serious morbidity without the synergistic effects of PHPT. Thus it is generally recommended that screening for carriers should be based upon detection of PHPT (61). Specifically, first-degree relatives should be screened every 5 years starting at age 15 by measurement of albumin-adjusted serum calcium and PTH. Once carriers of the MEN I gene have been identified, these patients should be monitored more comprehensively, including measurement of serum gastrin, serum prolactin, and pituitary size at 5-year intervals.

Recent recommendations regarding medical management of Zollinger-Ellison syndrome in MEN I patients have suggested a new criterion for parathyroidectomy in the management of this ulcer diathesis (67). Pharmacologic control of primary hypergastrinemia is particularly difficult in the presence of PHPT. This reflects at least two well-characterized effects of hypercalcemia: direct augmentation of gastrin secretion rate and synergism with gastrin in promoting acid production (68,69). A prospective study evaluated the effect of parathyroidectomy in 10 patients with PHPT, Zollinger-Ellison syndrome, and MEN I (70). Nine of 10 patients became normocalcemic postoperatively, and each patient had a lower basal acid output. Six of nine patients no longer had gastric acid hypersecretion. The dose of histamine H_2-receptor antagonists required to control gastric acid secretion was reduced in 60% of the patients. Thus all efforts should be made to treat PHPT once primary hypergastrinemia is recognized in MEN I.

Multiple Endocrine Neoplasia, Type II (MEN II)

MEN II is characterized by hyperfunction of the parathyroids, thyroidal C-cells, and adrenal medullary cells. Actual PHPT occurs in only 20–30% of cases (61). However, parathyroid hyperplasia is a common finding in patients with MEN II at the time of neck exploration for C-cell hyperplasia or C-cell cancer of the thyroid (71,72). Usually, these patients are normocalcemic, although they may show subnormal suppression of PTH secretion in response to calcium infusion (73). The cause of the parathyroid hyperplasia in MEN II remains unclear and no parathyroid mitogenic factor has been detected in plasma from these patients (62). Although only one-fourth of patients with MEN II will develop overt PHPT, some authors have suggested that all patients with MEN II who are having thyroidectomy for medullary carcinoma of the thyroid should have total parathyroidectomy with fresh parathyroid autograft (61). This recommendation is based on the frequency of parathyroid hyperplasia and the risk of permanent hypoparathyroidism from total thyroidectomy. Others have suggested that the operative approach should be individualized, and that in normocalcemic patients with histologically normal parathyroid glands, extirpation of the glands would be unwarranted (66).

Measurement of calcitonin levels following stimulation by pentagastrin or calcium infusion is the most sensitive way to screen for MEN II. Special efforts to monitor for PHPT are not required in carriers of the MEN II gene. Since these carriers must be closely followed for evaluation of C-cell and adrenal medullary function, parathyroid testing can be done at the same time. It should be noted that pheochromocytoma may cause hypercalcemia in the absence of PHPT. This may occur by stimulation of PTH secretion by catecholamines (74) or by production of humoral factors by the pheochromocytoma (75). Therefore, in patients with MEN II, hypercalcemia should be reassessed after removal of the pheochromocytoma. Finally, MEN II B is a variant of the disorder in which affected members show combinations of C-cell hyperfunction, adrenal medullary hyperfunction, and nerve cell hyperfunction (mucosal neuromas, ganglioneuromas of the intestines, and thickened corneal nerves) (76). These patients tend to have a char-

acteristic marfanoid body habitus. PHPT does not occur in MEN II B.

Familial Hypocalciuric Hypercalcemia

Familial hypocalciuric hypercalcemia (FHH) is an autosomal dominant condition characterized by hypercalcemia beginning in childhood but exhibiting a benign course (77,78). In addition to hypercalcemia, the most striking biochemical feature is the relative hypocalciuria. Patients with this disorder tend to be asymptomatic and their level of hypercalcemia remains stable. They typically lack the characteristic manifestations of PHPT such as kidney stones, bone disease, or peptic ulcers. However, most of the evidence suggests that mild hyperparathyroidism is an intrinsic feature of FHH (61,79), although this opinion is controversial (80,81). The evidence for excessive parathyroid function in FHH includes:

1. PTH levels indicated by RIA are inappropriate for the degree of hypercalcemia and are frankly elevated in 10–20% of patients.
2. The parathyroid glands show hyperplasia that is inappropriate in the face of lifelong hypercalcemia.
3. Neonates with double dose of the FHH gene have life-threatening PHPT (82).

The pathogenetic defect in FHH is believed to be an insensitivity to Ca in both the parathyroid glands and the kidneys (61). Because of the disturbance in the process whereby the parathyroid cell recognizes extracellular Ca, there is a shift to the right of the calcium set point (i.e., the Ca concentration at which PTH secretion is suppressed to 50% of maximal). At the kidney there is increased tubular reabsorption of Ca despite the hypercalcemia. This enhanced renal tubular Ca reabsorption is mostly PTH independent (83).

It is generally better not to treat FHH because of its benign course and because the outcome of subtotal parathyroidectomy is usually persistent hypercalcemia (77,78). If total parathyroidectomy is performed, the outcome will be chronic postoperative hypoparathyroidism. The syndrome should be diagnosed so that patients will not be made to undergo unnecessary treatment (81). FHH should be suspected in any asymptomatic hypercalcemic individual, especially if the patient is young (<40 years of age) or if there is a family history of hypercalcemia. A family history of failed neck explorations could be a warning sign. Careful review of old medical records may reveal whether the patient was ever normocalcemic. An elevated serum calcium dating from childhood is helpful. Stigmata of the MEN syndromes should be sought. Regrettably, it is not possible to diagnose with confidence FHH in an isolated individual, although a low 24-h urine Ca < 100 mg, a C_{ca}/C_{cr} ratio < 0.01, and a high serum magnesium level would be very suggestive. For a firm diagnosis, a family screening would be essential. In a given person it may be difficult to separate FHH from mild asymptomatic PHPT. However, since mild PHPT is not very threatening over the short term, in such doubtful cases, close follow-up would be a safe and reasonable alternative to cervical exploration.

Management of Asymptomatic PHPT during Pregnancy

Occasionally, asymptomatic PHPT may first be diagnosed in a mother after her baby has developed neonatal tetany (84). This occurrence of transient neonatal hypoparathyroidism secondary to excessive placental calcium transport from a mother with hyperparathyroidism was first described in 1939 (85) and is well recognized. It is the most common neonatal complication of maternal hyperparathyroidism, reported to occur in up to half the infants born to affected women, although spontaneous abortion and fetal death in late gestation also occur with increased frequency (86). Complications of maternal PHPT also occur in the mother. Hyperemesis gravidarum, generalized weakness, renal calculi, pancreatitis, or psychiatric disturbances have been reported in at least a third of cases (86). Because of the high rate of maternal and neonatal complications, the conclusion of most large series was that parathyroidectomy should be performed in a pregnant woman with PHPT even if she is asymptomatic (87–89). The optimal time should be during the second trimester, after all the fetal systems have developed, but before the third trimester when there is a greater likelihood of preterm labor.

In a report comparing fetal outcome following parathyroidectomy or no surgery in women with PHPT, there was a 26% pregnancy loss (abortion, stillbirth, or neonatal death) and a 33% frequency of neonatal hypocalcemia among 61 patients not operated upon, compared with 6% and 0%, respectively, in 16 women who underwent parathyroidectomy during gestation (89). Although PHPT does not seem to be well tolerated in pregnancy, most of the cases presented in the literature seem to be patients who had overt clinical disease prior to the onset of pregnancy. Conceivably, with recognition of more mild cases of asymptomatic PHPT in the current era, some women may be safely followed throughout pregnancy without need for surgical intervention.

CONCLUSION

With the widespread application of multichannel biochemical screening, the expression of PHPT has changed from a rare disease with serious complications to a common disorder usually discovered incidentally in an asymptomatic patient. Some authorities continue to recommend parathyroidectomy for all of these asymptom-

atic patients, whereas others restrict surgery to those patients with underlying physiologic abnormalities. Increasing numbers of patients are being followed conservatively for as long as they remain free of harmful effects. There is a need for a large-scale, prospective study comparing the natural course of asymptomatic PHPT with and without physiologic derangements. A prospective trial comparing the outcome of withholding therapy to provision of either medical or surgical therapy is also much needed. In the absence of such investigations, the long-term balance of risks and benefits of these alternative approaches will remain uncertain (10,31,90).

ACKNOWLEDGMENTS

The work in this chapter has been supported in part by the following NIH Grants: RO1-HD25860, RO1-AR16061, PO1-AM20543, and MO1-RR00633. The authors also gratefully acknowledge the contributions of the staff of the Dallas General Clinical Research Center and the able secretarial assistance of Betty Bousselot.

REFERENCES

1. Albright F. A page out of the history of hyperparathyroidism. *J Clin Endocrinol Metab* 1948;8:637–57.
2. Axelrod L. Bones, stones and hormones: the contributions of Fuller Albright. *N Engl J Med* 1970;283:964–70.
3. Cope O. The story of hyperparathyroidism at the Massachusetts General Hospital. *N Engl J Med* 1966;274:1174–82.
4. Heath H III, Hodgson SF, Kennedy MA. Primary hyperparathyroidism: incidence, morbidity and potential economic inpact in a community. *N Engl J Med* 1980;302:189–93.
5. Boonstra CE, Jackson CE. Serum calcium survey for hyperparathyroidism: results in 50,000 clinic patients. *Am J Clin Pathol* 1971;55:523–6.
6. Hodgson SF, Heath H III. Asymptomatic primary hyperparathyroidism: treat or follow? *Mayo Clin Proc* 1981;56:521–3.
7. Bone HG III, Snyder WH III, Pak CYC. Diagnosis of hyperparathyroidism. *Annu Rev Med* 1977;28:111–7.
8. Scholz DA, Purnell DC. Asymptomatic primary hyperparathyroidism: 10 year prospective study. *Mayo Clin Proc* 1981;56:473–8.
9. Seeman E, Wahner HW, Offord KP, et al. Differential effects of endocrine dysfunction on the axial and the appendicular skeleton. *J Clin Invest* 1982;69:1302–9.
10. Coe FL, Favus MJ. Does mild, asymptomatic hyperparathyroidism require surgery? *N Engl J Med* 1980;302:224–5.
11. Kaplan RA, Snyder WH, Stewart A, Pak CYC. Metabolic effects of parathyroidectomy in asymptomatic primary hyperparathyroidism. *J Clin Endocrinol Metab* 1976;42:415–26.
12. Rohl PG, Wilkinson M, Clifton-Bligh P, Posen S. Hyperparathyroidism: experiences with treated and untreated patients. *Med J Aust* 1981;1:519–21.
13. Vant Hoff W, Ballardie FW, Bicknell EJ. Primary hyperparathyroidism: the case for medical management. *Br Med J* 1983;287:1605–8.
14. Adams PH. Conservative management of primary hyperparathyroidism. *J R Coll Physicians Lond* 1982;16:184–90.
15. Breslau NA, Pak CYC. Clinical evaluation of parathyroid tumors. In: Thawley SE, Panje WR, Batsakis JG, Lindberg RD, eds. *Comprehensive management of head and neck tumors.* Philadelphia: WB Saunders, 1987;1635–49.
16. Rubinoff H, McCarthy N, Hiatt RA. Hypercalcemia: long-term follow-up with matched controls. *J Chron Dis* 1983;36:859–68.
17. Posen S, Clifton-Bligh P, Reeve TS, Wagstaffe C, Wilkinson M. Is

parathyroidectomy of benefit in primary hyperparathyroidism? *Q J Med* 1985;54:241–51.

18. Arnstein AR, Haubrich WS, Frame B. Primary hyperparathyroidism with hypercalcemia twenty-eight years before treatment. *Henry Ford Hosp Med Bull* 1964;12:327–31.

19. Kosinski D, Roth SI, Chapman EH. Primary hyperparathyroidism with 31 years of hypercalcemia. *JAMA* 1976;236:550–91.

20. Dalen N, Hjern B. Bone mineral content in patients with primary hyperparathyroidism without radiologic evidence of skeletal changes. *Acta Endocrinol* 1974;75:297–304.

21. Leppla DC, Snyder W, Pak CYC. Sequential changes in bone density before and after parathyroidectomy in primary hyperparathyroidism. *Invest Radiol* 1982;17:604–6.

22. Pak CYC, Stewart A, Kaplan R, Bone H, Notz C, Browne R. Photon absorptiometric analysis of bone density in primary hyperparathyroidism. *Lancet* 1975;2:7–8.

23. Dauphine RT, Riggs BL, Scholz DA. Back pain and vertebral crush fractures: an unemphasized mode of presentation for primary hyperparathyroidism. *Ann Intern Med* 1975;83:365–7.

24. Silverberg SJ, Shane E, DeLaCruz L, et al. Skeletal disease in primary hyperparathyroidism. *J Bone Miner Res* 1989;4:283–91.

25. Wilson RJ, Rao S, Ellis B, Kleerekoper M, Parfitt AM. Mild asymptomatic primary hyperparathyroidism is not a risk factor for vertebral fractures. *Ann Intern Med* 1988;109:959–62.

26. Eriksen EF, Mosekilde L, Melsen F. Trabecular bone remodeling and balance in primary hyperparathyroidism. *Bone* 1986;7:213–21.

27. Charhon SA, Edouard CM, Arlot ME, Meunier PJ. Effect of PTH on remodeling of iliac trabecular bone packets in patients with primary hyperparathyroidism. *Clin Orthop* 1982;162:255–63.

28. Parfitt AM, Kleerekoper M, Rao D, Stanciu J, Villanueva AR. Cellular mechanisms of cortical thinning in primary hyperparathyroidism. *J Bone Miner Res* 1987;2(suppl 1):abstr 384.

29. Reeve J, Meunier PJ, Parsons JA, et al. Anabolic effect of human PTH on trabecular bone in involutional osteoporosis. *Br Med J* 1987;280:1340–4.

30. Slovik DM, Rosenthal DC, Coppelt SH, et al. Restoration of spinal bone in osteoporotic men by treatment with human PTH (1–34) and 1,25-$(OH)_2$D. *J Bone Miner Res* 1986;1:377–81.

31. Rao DS, Wilson RJ, Kleerekoper M, Parfitt AM. Lack of biochemical progression or continuation of accelerated bone loss in mild asymptomatic primary hyperparathyroidism: evidence for biphasic disease course. *J Clin Endocrinol Metab* 1988;67:1294–8.

32. Lueg MC. Asymptomatic primary hyperparathyroidism. *Hosp Prac* 1982;17:29–39.

33. Sivula HR, Sivula A. Long-term effect of surgical treatment on the symptoms of primary hyperparathyroidism. *Ann Clin Res* 1985;17:141–7.

34. Thomas JM, Cranston D, Knox AJ. Hyperparathyroidism: patterns of presentation, symptoms, and response to operation. *Ann R Coll Surg Engl* 1985;67:79–82.

35. Corlew DS, Bryda SL, Bradley EL, et al. Observations on the course of untreated primary hyperparathyroidism. *Surgery* 1985;98:1064–70.

36. Gaz RD, Wang C. Management of asymptomatic hyperparathyroidism. *Am J Surg* 1984;147:498–502.

37. Russell CF, Edis AJ. Surgery for primary hyperparathyroidism: experience with 500 consecutive cases and evaluation of the role of surgery in the asymptomatic patient. *Br J Surg* 1982;69:244–7.

38. Mohr R, Graif M, Itzchak Y, et al. Parathyroid localization: sonographic-surgical correlation. *Am Surg* 1985;51:286–90.

39. Winzelberg, GG. Parathyroid imaging. *Ann Intern Med* 1987;107:64–70.

40. Erdman WA, Breslau NA, Weinreb JC, et al. Non-invasive localization of parathyroid adenomas: a comparison of computerized tomography, ultrasound, scintigraphy and MRI. *Magn Reson Imaging* 1989;7:187–94.

41. Bilezikian JP. The medical management of primary hyperparathyroidism. *Ann Intern Med* 1982;96:198–302.

42. Gallagher JC, Nordin BEC. Treatment with estrogens of primary hyperparathyroidism in postmenopausal women. *Lancet* 1972;1:503–7.

43. Gallagher JC, Wilkinson R. The effect of ethinyl estradiol on calcium and phosphorus metabolism of postmenopausal women with primary hyperparathyroidism. *Clin Sci Mol Med* 1973;45:785–802.

44. Marcus R, Madvig P, Crim M, Pont A, Kosek J. Conjugated estrogens in the treatment of postmenopausal women with hyperparathyroidism. *Ann Intern Med* 1984;100:633–40.

45. Selby PL, Peacock M. Ethinyl estradiol and norethindrone in the treatment of primary hyperparathyroidism in postmenopausal women. *N Engl J Med* 1986;314:1481–5.

46. Komm BS, Terpening CM, Benz DJ, et al. Estrogen binding, receptor mRNA, and biologic response in osteoblast-like osteosarcoma cells. *Science* 1988;241:81–4.

47. Eriksen EF, Colvard DS, Berg NJ, et al. Evidence of estrogen receptors in normal human osteoblast-like cells. *Science* 1988;241:84–6.

48. Breslau NA, Zerwekh JE, Pak CYC. Responsiveness to short-term estrogen therapy of postmenopausal women with primary hyperparathyroidism. *67th meeting of the Endocrine Society,* Baltimore, 1985;14(abstr 53).

49. Weiss NS. Risks and benefits of estrogen use. *N Engl J Med* 1975;293:1200–2.

50. Broadus AE, Horst RL, Lang R, et al. The importance of circulating 1,25-$(OH)_2$D in the pathogenesis of hypercalciuria and renal-stone formation in primary hyperparathyroidism. *N Engl J Med* 1980;302:421–6.

51. Broadus AE, Magee JS, Mallette LE, et al. A detailed evaluation of oral phosphate therapy in selected patients with primary hyperparathyroidism. *J Clin Endocrinol Metab* 1983;56:953–61.

52. Coburn JW, Massry SG. Changes in serum and urine calcium during phosphate depletion: studies on mechanisms. *J Clin Invest* 1970;49:1073–87.

53. Goldfarb S, Westby GR, Goldberg M, et al. Renal tubular effects of chronic phosphate depletion. *J Clin Invest* 1977;59:770–9.

54. Thomas WC Jr. Use of phosphates in patients with calcareous renal calculi. *Kidney Int* 1978;13:390–6.

55. Dudley FJ, Blackburn CRB. Extra skeletal calcification complicating oral neutral-phosphate therapy. *Lancet* 1970;2:628–30.

56. Fleisch H, Felix R. Diphosphonates. *Calcif Tissue Int* 1979;27:91–4.

57. Fleisch H, Russel RGG, Francis MD. Diphosphonates inhibit hydroxyapatite dissolution in vitro and bone resorption in tissue culture and in vivo. *Science* 1969;165:1262–4.

58. Kaplan RA, Geho WB, Poindexter C, et al. Metabolic effects of diphosphonate in primary hyperparathyroidism. *J Clin Pharmacol* 1977;17:410–9.

59. Shane E, Baquiran DC, Bilezikian JP. Effects of dichloromethylene diphosphonate on serum and urinary calcium in primary hyperparathyroidism. *Ann Intern Med* 1981;95:23–7.

60. Mundy GR, Wilkinson R, Heath DA. Comparative study of available medical therapy for hypercalcemia of malignancy. *Am J Med* 1983;74:421–32.

61. Marx SJ, Brandi ML. Familial primary hyperparathyroidism. In: Peck WA, ed. *Bone and mineral research* vol 5. Amsterdam: Elsevier, 1987;375–407.

62. Brandi ML, Aurbach GD, Fitzpatrick LA, et al. Parathyroid mitogenic activity in plasma from familial multiple endocrine neoplasia type I. *N Engl J Med* 1986;314:1287–93.

63. Zimering MB, Brandi ML, DeGrande DA, et al. Circulating fibroblast growth factor-like substance in familial multiple endocrine neoplasia type I. *J Clin Endocrinol Metab* 1990;70:149–54.

64. Marx SJ, Sakaguchi K, Green J III, Aurbach GD, Brandi ML. Mitogenic activity on parathyroid cells in plasma from members of a large kindred with multiple endocrine neoplasia type I. *J Clin Endocrinol Metab* 1988;67:149–53.

65. Brandi ML, Marx SJ, Aurbach GD, Fitzpatrick LA. Familial multiple endocrine neoplasia type I: a new look at pathophysiology. *Endocr Rev* 1987;8:391–405.

66. Fitzpatrick LA. Hypercalcemia in the multiple endocrine neoplasia syndromes. *Endocrinol Metab Clin North Am* 1989;18:741–52.

67. Jensen RT, Gardner JD, Raufman JP, Pandol SJ, Doppman JL, Collen MJ. Zollinger-Ellison syndrome: current concepts and management. *Ann Intern Med* 1983;98:59–75.

68. Gogel HK, Buckman MT, Cadieux D, McCarthy DM. Gastric secretion and hormonal interactions in multiple endocrine neoplasia type I. *Arch Intern Med* 1985;145:855–9.

69. Soll AH. Extracellular calcium and cholinergic stimulation of isolated canine parietal cells. *J Clin Invest* 1981;68:270–8.
70. Norton JA, Cornelius MJ, Doppman JL, et al. Effect of parathyroidectomy in patients with hyperparathyroidism, Zollinger-Ellison syndrome, and multiple endocrine neoplasia type I: a prospective study. *Surgery* 1987;102:958–66.
71. Block MA, Jackson CE, Tashjian AH Jr. Management of parathyroid glands in surgery for medullary thyroid carcinomas. *Arch Surg* 1975;110:617–22.
72. Keiser HR, Beaven MA, Doppman J, Wells S Jr, Buja LM. Sipple's syndrome: medullary thyroid carcinoma, pheochromocytoma and parathyroid disease: studies in a large family. *Ann Intern Med* 1973;78:561–79.
73. Heath H III, Sizemore GW, Carney JA. Preoperative diagnosis of occult parathyroid hyperplasia by calcium infusion in patients with multiple endocrine neoplasia, type 2a. *J Clin Endocrinol Metab* 1976;43:428–35.
74. Kukreja SC, Hargis GK, Rosenthal IM, Williams GA. Pheochromocytoma causing excessive parathyroid hormone production and hypercalcemia. *Ann Intern Med* 1973;79:838–40.
75. Stewart AF, Hoecker JL, Mallette LE, Segre GV, Amatruda TT, Vignery A. Hypercalcemia in pheochromocytoma: evidence for a novel mechanism. *Ann Intern Med* 1985;102:776–9.
76. Khairi MRA, Dexter RN, Burzynski NJ, Johnston CC Jr. Mucosal neuroma, pheochromocytoma and medullary thyroid carcinoma: multiple endocrine neoplasia, type 3. *Medicine* 1975;54:89–112.
77. Marx SJ, Attie MF, Levine MA, Spiegel AM, Downs RW Jr, Lasker RD. The hypocalciuric or benign variant of familial hypercalcemia: clinical and biochemical features in fifteen kindreds. *Medicine* 1981;60:397–412.
78. Law WM Jr, Heath H III. Familial benign hypercalcemia (hypocalciuric hypercalcemia): clinical and pathogenetic studies in 21 families. *Ann Intern Med* 1985;102:511–9.
79. Marx SJ, Spiegel AM, Levine MA, et al. Familial hypocalciuric hypercalcemia: the relation to primary parathyroid hyperplasia. *N Engl J Med* 1982;307:416–26.
80. Lau WM Jr, James EM, Charbonneau JW, Purnell DC, Heath H III. High-resolution parathyroid ultrasonography in familial benign hypercalcemia (familial hypocalciuric hypercalcemia). *Mayo Clin Proc* 1984;59:153–5.
81. Heath H III. Familial benign (hypocalciuric) hypercalcemia. A troublesome mimic of mild primary hyperparathyroidism. *Endocrinol Metab Clin North Am* 1989;18:723–40.
82. Marx SJ, Attie MF, Spiegel AM, Levine MA, Lasker RD, Fox M. An association between neonatal severe primary hyperparathyroidism and familial hypocalciuric hypercalcemia. *N Engl J Med* 1982;306:257–64.
83. Attie MF, Gill JR Jr, Stock JL, et al. Urinary calcium excretion in familial hypocalciuric hypercalcemia: persistence of relative hypocalciuria after induction of hypoparathyroidism. *J Clin Invest* 1983;72:667–76.
84. Better OS, Levi J, Greif E, Tuma S, Gellei B, Erlik D. Prolonged neonatal parathyroid suppression: a sequel to asymptomatic maternal hyperparathyroidism. *Arch Surg* 1973;106:722–4.
85. Friedrichsen C. Tetany in a suckling with latent osteitis fibrosa in the mother. *Lancet* 1939;1:85–6.
86. Pitkin RM. Calcium metabolism in pregnancy and the perinatal period: a review. *Am J Obstet Gynecol* 1985;151:99–109.
87. Ludwig GD. Hyperparathyroidism in relation to pregnancy. *N Engl J Med* 1962;267:637–42.
88. Delmonico FL, Neer RM, Cosimi AB, Barnes AB, Russell PS. Hyperparathyroidism during pregnancy. *Am J Surg* 1976;131:328–37.
89. Wilson DT, Martin T, Christensen R, Yee AH, Reynolds C. Hyperparathyroidism in pregnancy: case report and review of the literature. *Can Med Assoc J* 1983;129:986–9.
90. Coe FL, Favus MJ, Parks JH. Is estrogen preferable to surgery for postmenopausal women with primary hyperparathyroidism? *N Engl J Med* 1986;314:1508–9.

CHAPTER 25

Disorders of Serum Minerals Caused by Cancer

John J. Orloff and Andrew F. Stewart

Disorders of mineral homeostasis are particularly common in patients with cancer. Primary bone tumors rarely lead to systemic disorders of mineral homeostasis; in most instances, the neoplasm that disrupts mineral homeostasis is a hematologic neoplasm with extensive bone marrow replacement, an epithelial neoplasm metastatic to the skeleton, or a malignancy that does not involve the skeleton directly but alters skeletal and systemic mineral homeostasis in a "paraneoplastic," "humoral," or endocrine fashion.

In this chapter, attention is focused on three classes of disorders. The first is *malignancy-associated hypercalcemia,* a syndrome that is encountered on occasion by almost all practicing physicians. An explosive growth of information regarding the etiology of this syndrome has occurred over the past decade; this syndrome will be addressed in greatest detail. The second area is *hypocalcemia resulting from cancer or its treatment.* The third syndrome is *hypophosphatemia resulting from cancer.* Mild hypophosphatemia is caused with surprising frequency by certain tumors. More severe hypophosphatemia, together with renal phosphorous wasting and osteomalacia, occur less commonly ("tumor rickets" or "oncogenic osteomalacia") but represent a fascinating, well-described syndrome.

It should be clear that while these disorders are caused *by* cancers or occur *only in the setting* of cancer management, the full spectrum of mineral disorders may be observed in patients with cancer. The complete differential diagnoses of hypercalcemia, hypocalcemia, hyperphosphatemia, and hypophosphatemia are addressed elsewhere in this volume. When patients with cancer are encountered, there is a tendency to ascribe all of their symptoms and problems to their neoplasm. Hypercalce-

mia, for example, when discovered in a patient with cancer, may be reflexly diagnosed as malignancy-associated hypercalcemia. Thoughtful and meticulous attention to the complete differential diagnoses of hypo- and hypercalcemia and of hypophosphatemia cannot be overemphasized, and is essential for thoughtful, rational, and successful therapy.

MALIGNANCY-ASSOCIATED HYPERCALCEMIA

Serum calcium measurements first became available for clinical use in the early 1920s. Hypercalcemia was reported to occur in patients with cancer almost simultaneously (1). Today it is clear that while primary hyperparathyroidism is the most common cause of hypercalcemia among outpatients (2), cancer is the most common cause of hypercalcemia among hospitalized patients (3). Dramatic advances in the understanding of the mechanisms responsible for malignancy-associated hypercalcemia (MAHC) have occurred over the past decade.

Hypercalcemia most often occurs in patients with breast cancer, multiple myeloma, squamous carcinomas, renal carcinoma, lymphomas, and bladder carcinoma, with up to 20–40% of such patients developing hypercalcemia at some point during the course of their disease. In contrast to these tumor types, which are commonly associated with hypercalcemia, hypercalcemia almost never occurs in certain other settings. For example, colon cancer, prostate cancer, and adenocarcinoma of the stomach, despite the frequency with which they occur in the general population, are rarely associated with hypercalcemia. It should also be clear that essentially every type of human malignancy has been reported on occasion to be associated with hypercalcemia.

The signs and symptoms associated with hypercalcemia are discussed in Chapter 23. Patients with MAHC

J. J. Orloff and A. F. Stewart: Department of Medicine, West Haven Veterans Administration Medical Center, West Haven, Connecticut 06516, and Yale University School of Medicine, New Haven, Connecticut 06510

may be asymptomatic or may display a full range of neurologic symptoms ranging from mild drowsiness to frank coma. Polyuria, polydipsia, and constipation are common. Reduction in the glomerular filtration rate is common and results from a combination of hypercalcemia-induced polyuria with inadequate oral fluid intake, nephrocalcinosis, and occasionally, ureteral or urethral obstruction by kidney stones or tumor. Therapy of MAHC is discussed in Chapter 23.

From a mechanistic or pathophysiological standpoint, it is useful to divide MAHC into three categories (Table 1): (1) hypercalcemia resulting from direct skeletal involvement by tumor (local osteolytic hypercalcemia or "LOH"), (2) hypercalcemia due to secretion by tumors of systemic bone-resorbing factors (humoral hypercalcemia of malignancy, or "HHM"), and (3) unusual causes of MAHC. These three mechanistic categories are discussed below.

Local Osteolytic Hypercalcemia

The first collection of patients with hypercalcemia resulting from skeletal metastases was published in 1936 by Gutman et al. (4). Patients in this series primarily had multiple myeloma or breast cancer and had extensive marrow infiltration by tumor (myeloma) or skeletal metastatic disease (breast cancer). Serum phosphorus values were high-normal. Hypercalcemia was presumed to result from direct skeletal destruction by tumor and in turn resulted in parathyroid suppression. Early series suggested that this "local osteolytic hypercalcemia" (LOH) included the vast majority of patients with MAHC (4,5). More recent series, however, suggest that LOH may be responsible for only 20–40% of cases of MAHC (see below). The tumor histologies that have consistently been associated with the LOH scenario are myeloma, breast cancer, lymphoma, and other hematologic malignancies (Table 1) (4–8). Bone scans and/or skeletal radiographs generally display extensive destruction in multiple locations throughout the skeleton,

TABLE 1. *Tumors commonly associated with hypercalcemia*

Local osteolytic hypercalcemia
  Breast cancer
  Multiple myeloma
  Lymphoma/leukemia

Humoral hypercalcemia of malignancy
  Squamous carcinoma (lung, esophagus,
    oropharynx, cervix, vulva, skin)
  Renal carcinoma
  Bladder carcinoma
  HTLV-I lymphoma/leukemia
  Breast cancer

$1,25(OH)_2D$-secreting lymphomas

and pathological fractures are common in affected patients (4–8).

The mechanisms responsible for bone destruction have received considerable attention. Photomicrographs of bone histomorphometry observed in patients with LOH are shown in Fig. 1. Early concepts focusing on direct mechanical destruction of trabecular and cortical bone by malignant cells have lost their appeal for three reasons. First, hypercalcemia does not occur in all patients with extensive skeletal metastases. For example, patients with small-cell carcinoma of the lung and with prostate carcinoma regularly have extensive marrow infiltration by malignant cells, yet these patients rarely develop hypercalcemia (9,10). Thus a "packed marrow" may be *necessary* but is clearly not *sufficient* for the development of hypercalcemia. Second, histological studies in rabbits bearing an osteolytic breast carcinoma line revealed that resorption of trabecular or cortical bone adjacent to skeletal metastases was almost always mediated by osteoclasts (11). Third, studies using cultured malignant plasma cells from patients with hypercalcemia associated with myeloma indicated that while the plasma cells did not directly resorb devitalized bone, they did secrete into their culture medium a factor or factors that stimulate bone resorption (12,13). These *osteoclast activating factors* (or OAFs) have now been characterized in some detail and appear to comprise a mixture of cytokines including prostaglandins of the E series, tumor necrosis factor β (lymphotoxin), tumor necrosis factor α (cachectin), interleukin-1α, interleukin-1β, and transforming growth factors α and β (14–16). In patients with multiple myeloma, evidence for lymphotoxin as the primary OAF has recently appeared (16). A prominent role for PGE_2 has been proposed in breast cancer (17). Finally, while this local endocrine or "paracrine" scenario is accepted as being the most prevalent in patients with LOH, it should be noted that in rare instances, direct phagocytosis of devitalized bone by breast cancer cells has been observed (18).

Approximately one-third of patients with breast cancer and skeletal metastases who receive estrogens or antiestrogens develop a hypercalcemic flare (19,20). The precise cellular events underlying this "flare" are incompletely understood. Valentin-Opran et al. have reported that estrogens accentuate the production of bone-resorbing factors by cultured breast cancer cells (21). Others have suggested that the development of an estrogen flare is a favorable prognostic sign (19,20).

Biochemically, patients with LOH are characterized by hypercalcemia and the expected results of parathyroid hormone suppression (Figs. 2 and 3). Specifically, patients typically display normal serum phosphorus concentrations (6,8,22), suppressed immunoreactive PTH values, and 1,25-dihydroxyvitamin D [$1,25(OH)_2D$] concentrations (6,8), marked hypercalciuria (6,8), normal renal phosphorus thresholds (6,8),

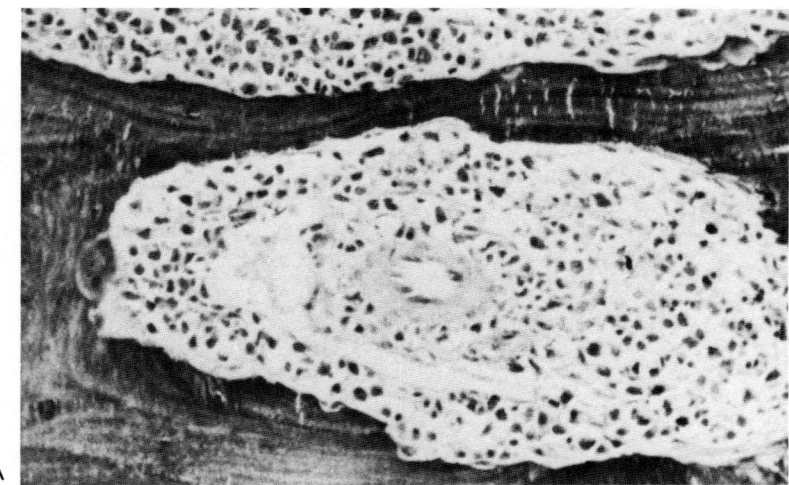

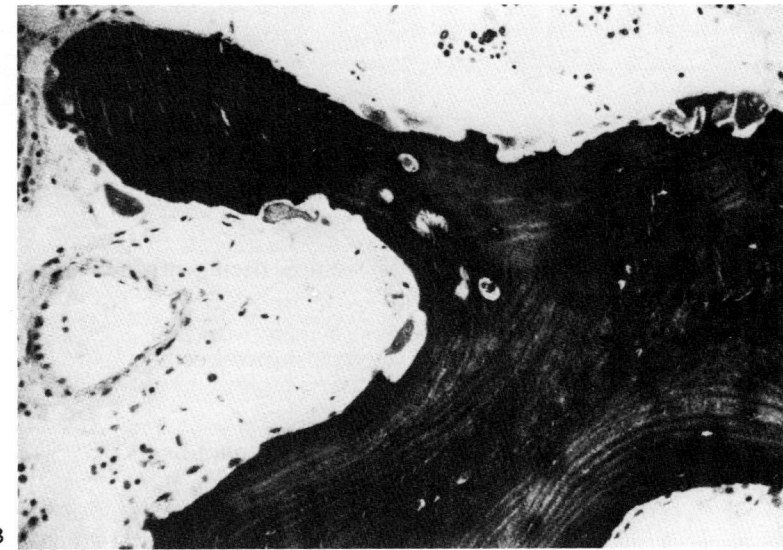

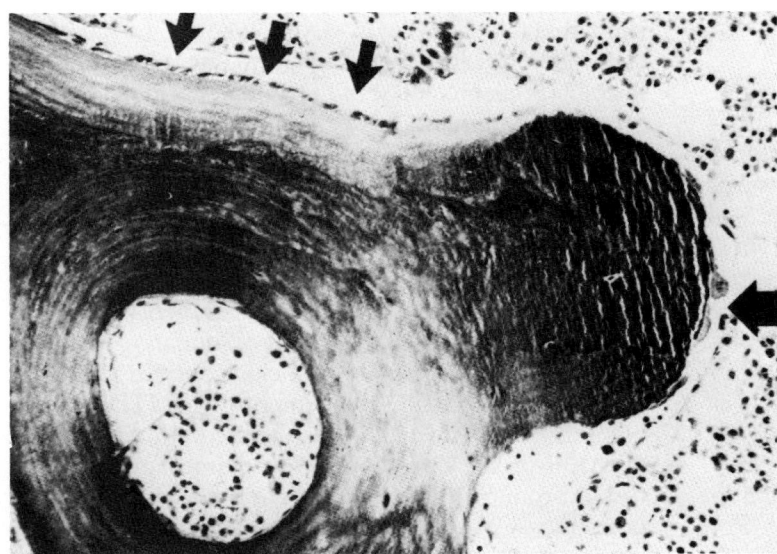

FIG. 1. Bone histology associated with MAHC. **A:** Photomicrograph of a bone biopsy from a patient with leukemia. Note the active osteoclastic bone resorption, the absence of bone formation, and the heavy infiltration of the marrow space with malignant leukemic cells. **B:** From a patient with humoral hypercalcemia of malignancy. Note that the marrow is devoid of malignant cells, that osteoclastic bone resorption is active nevertheless, and that bone formation and osteoblastic activity are absent. **C:** From a patient with primary hyperparathyroidism; demonstrates an increase in osteoclastic activity (*large arrow*) and a coupled increase in osteoblast number and formation of new osteoid (*small arrows*). (Reproduced with permission from Ref. 38.)

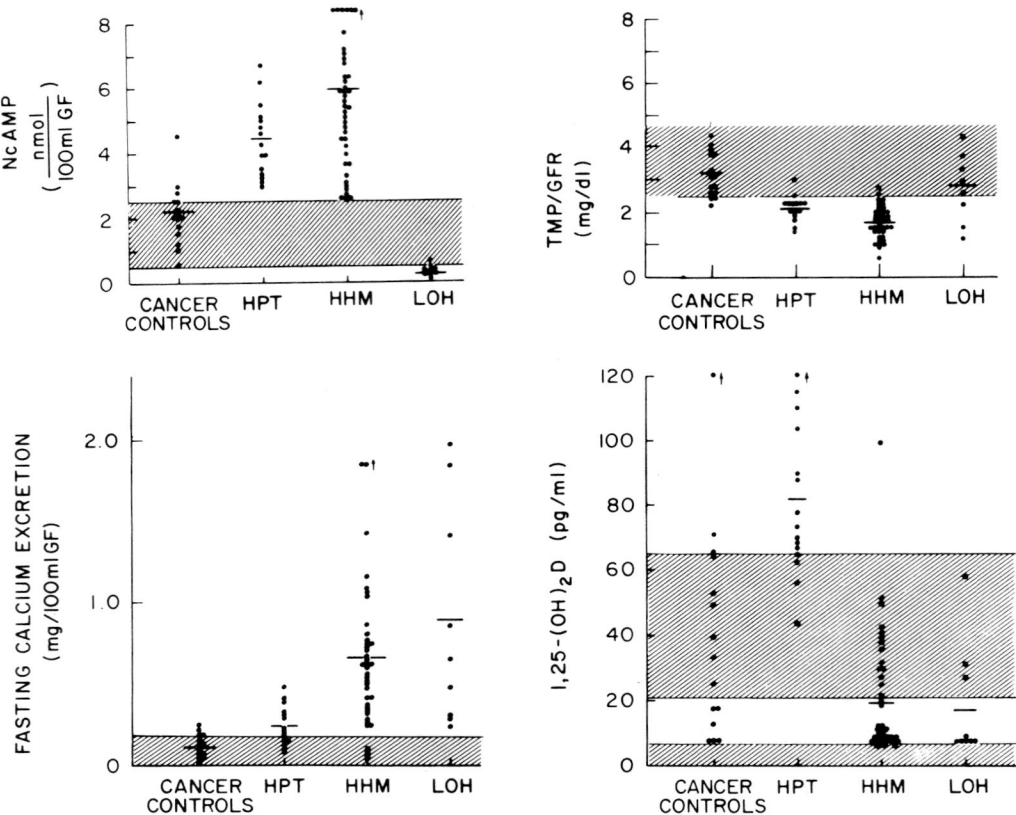

FIG. 2. Biochemical findings in normocalcemic patients with cancer (cancer controls), primary hyperparathyroidism (HPT), humoral hypercalcemia of malignancy (HHM), and local osteolytic hypercalcemia (LOH). NcAMP indicates nephrogenous cyclic AMP excretion. TmP/GFR indicates the renal phosphorus threshold. See the text for details. (Reproduced with permission from Ref. 6.)

and suppressed urinary and nephrogenous cyclic AMP excretion (6,8).

Humoral Hypercalcemia of Malignancy

In 1941, Albright described a patient with a renal carcinoma in whom hypercalcemia and hypophosphatemia developed in the presence of a single skeletal metastasis (23). Reasoning that a solitary skeletal metastasis was inadequate to cause hypercalcemia, and that hyperphosphatemia, not hypophosphatemia, was the expected result of the LOH scenario, Albright proposed that the patient's renal carcinoma was secreting a calcium-mobilizing, phosphaturic substance related to parathyroid hormone. Subsequent series of patients with MAHC occurring in the absence of skeletal metastases and associated with hypophosphatemia appeared in the 1950s (24,25). Documentation that the syndrome was due to ectopic secretion of a humoral calcemic factor was provided by the observation that ablation of tumor in such patients resulted in correction of hypercalcemia and hypophosphatemia (24,25). In the 1960s, terms such as *ectopic hyperparathyroidism* and *pseudohyperparathyroidism* proliferated. In 1966, Lafferty reported the first large series of patients with "pseudohyperparathyroidism," that is, patients with MAHC who had no radiologically demonstrable metastases (26). In contrast to the histologies characteristic of LOH, patients in the Lafferty series had predominantly squamous carcinomas (of any site), renal carcinomas, and bladder carcinomas (Table 1). More recent series (6–8,24,27–29) have corroborated Lafferty's study with respect to the typical tumor histologies and have extended that list: whereas most patients with breast cancer develop hypercalcemia through local osteolytic mechanisms, 30–50% of women with breast cancer have HHM (6,8,22,30,31). Similarly, most patients with lymphoma are best characterized as having LOH (32), but the subset of patients with HTLV-1 lymphomas clearly have HHM as the predominant mechanism (33–35). Anecdotes describing almost every known tumor producing ectopic hyperparathyroidism have appeared (5–8,24–29), but the preponderance of patients remain those described by Lafferty.

With the advent of parathyroid hormone immunoassays in the late 1960s and early 1970s, it came as a sur-

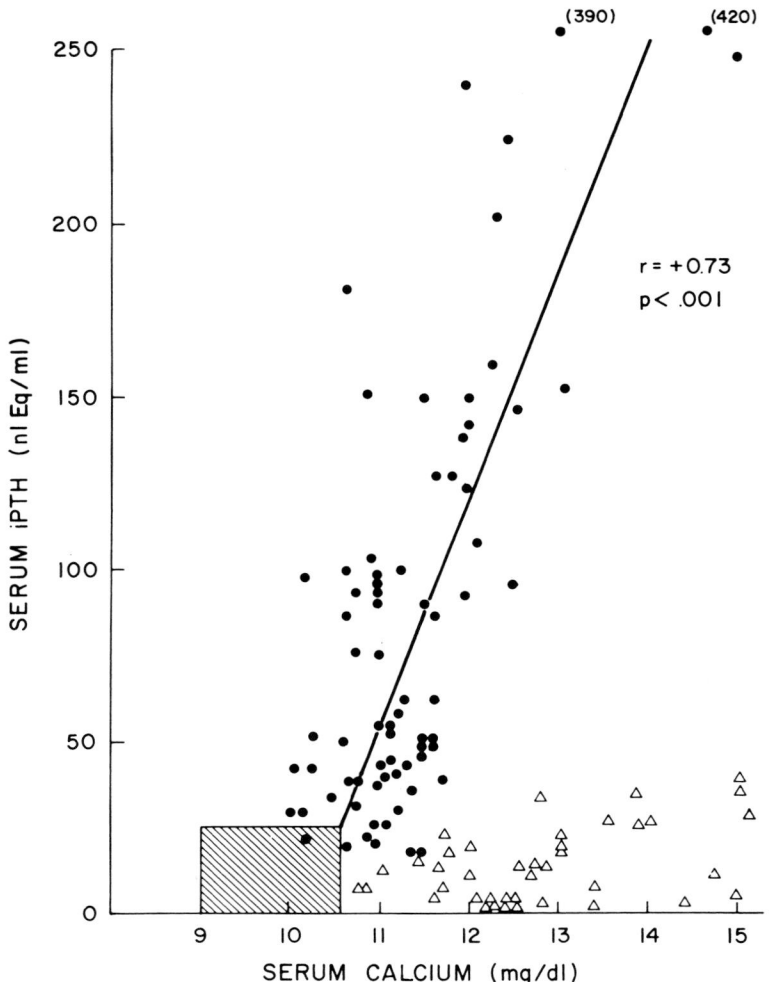

FIG. 3. Relationship between serum calcium concentration and immunoreactive parathyroid hormone concentration in patients with primary hyperparathyroidism (*circles*) and malignancy-associated hypercalcemia (*triangles*). (Reproduced with permission from Ref. 8.)

prise that immunoreactive PTH concentrations were found to be normal or reduced in patients with ectopic hyperparathyroidism, in contrast to the elevated values reported in patients with primary hyperparathyroidism (Fig. 3) (6,8,36,37). In 1980, a comprehensive evaluation of patients with what had been considered "ectopic hyperparathyroidism" appeared (6). This study demonstrated that patients with primary hyperparathyroidism and ectopic hyperparathyroidism resembled one another in that both syndromes were humoral in nature, both were associated with hypercalcemia, hypophosphatemia and phosphaturia, and both groups of patients displayed increases in nephrogenous cyclic AMP excretion (Fig. 2). On the other hand, in patients with ectopic hyperparathyroidism, in contrast to those with primary hyperparathyroidism, renal calcium reabsorption was reduced, circulating 1,25-dihydroxyvitamin D values were reduced, and immunoreactive PTH values were reduced (6). These observations led to the conclusions that (1) "ectopic hyperparathyroidism" and "pseudohyperparathyroidism" are misnomers. *Humoral hypercalcemia of malignancy* or (HHM) was proposed as a more appro-

priate designation; (2) HHM is the most common cause of MAHC, accounting for approximately 80% of such patients; (3) the humoral factor responsible for HHM is not PTH but mimics certain of the actions of PTH; (4) elevated nephrogenous cyclic AMP excretion serves as a marker for the HHM syndrome and can be used clinically to distinguish patients with HHM from those with LOH; and (5) the observed elevations in nephrogenous cyclic AMP excretion suggest that PTH-sensitive renal and bone adenylate cyclase assays might be useful in identifying and purifying the PTH-like protein responsible for HHM.

Skeletal metastases may be present in patients with HHM but in general are not as extensive as are those in patients with LOH (Fig. 4) (6–8,24–29). In representative series of patients with HHM, only 5 of 59 patients studied had extensive skeletal metastases (8). Bone histomorphometry reveals striking changes. Osteoclast number and activity (bone resorption) are markedly increased (Fig. 1) and appear to explain in quantitative terms the hypercalcemia that occurs in patients with HHM (38). Osteoblastic activity (bone formation) is

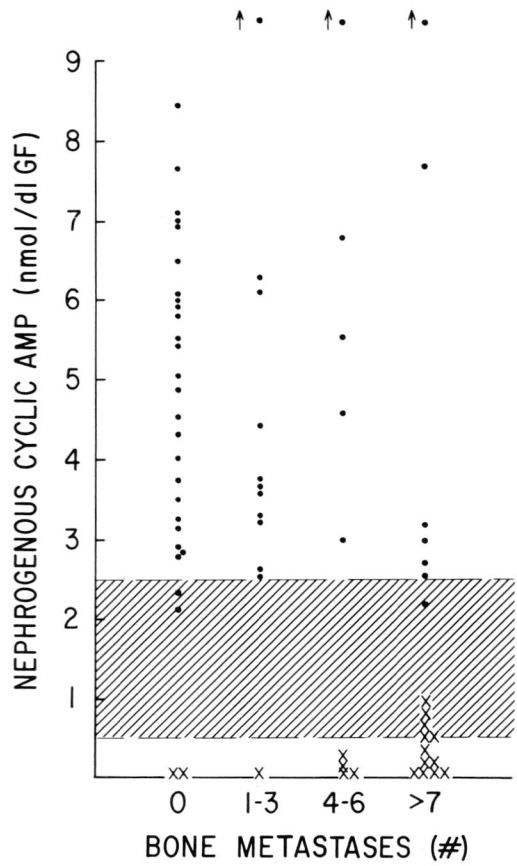

FIG. 4. Number of skeletal metastases in patients with MAHC as a function of nephrogenous cyclic AMP excretion in patients with HHM (*circles*) and LOH (*X's*). Note that the majority of patients with HHM have little or nothing in the way of bone metastases, whereas occasional patients have extensive bone metastases. Conversely, most patients with LOH have widespread skeletal metastases. (Reproduced with permission from Ref. 8.)

markedly reduced (Fig. 1), potentiating the net skeletal mineral losses that occur in patients with HHM (38). This striking "uncoupling" of bone/cell activity has been observed in animal models (39,40) of HHM and differs markedly from primary hyperparathyroidism, in which a coupled increase in both osteoclastic and osteoblastic activities are found (38). Finally, bone biopsies from patients with HHM are devoid of tumor in the marrow space (38) (Fig. 1), emphasizing the humoral nature of the syndrome and the contrast of this syndrome with LOH.

In 1987 and 1988, three laboratories described the purification and N-terminal amino acid sequencing of a novel class of proteins that appear to be responsible for the majority of instances of HHM (41–44). In each report, the putative HHM factor was detected and followed through purification using PTH-sensitive renal or bone adenylate cyclase assays. In each instance, the N-terminal amino acid sequence was used to develop oligonucleotide probes, which in turn were used to isolate three complementary DNAs (cDNAs) encoding these peptides (45–47). Most recently, the structure of the gene has been determined (48–50). The structures of the PTHLP cDNAs are shown in Figs. 5 and 6. The most striking observation from all of these studies is that the HHM-associated adenylate cyclase-stimulating protein displays dramatic amino acid and nucleotide sequence homology to the N-terminal amino acid sequence of parathyroid hormone: Of the first 13 amino acids, eight are identical and three more represent conservative substitutions. Amino acid homology in this region is particularly interesting, for the N terminus of PTH is known to be crucial for the stimulation of adenylate cyclase by PTH (51). Because of the N-terminal amino acid homology with PTH, this novel family of peptides has been

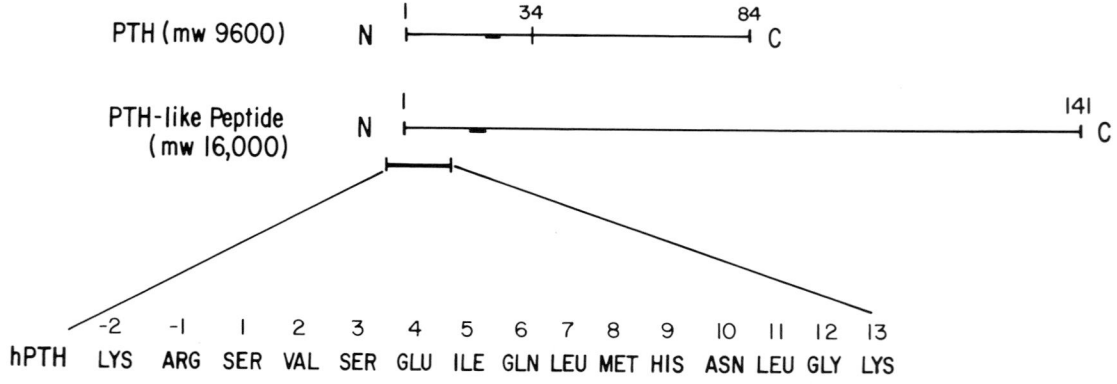

FIG. 5. Comparison of the size and amino acid sequences of parathyroid hormone (PTH) and PTHLP (1–141). See the text for details. (Reproduced with permission from *N Engl J Med* 1988;319:556–63.)

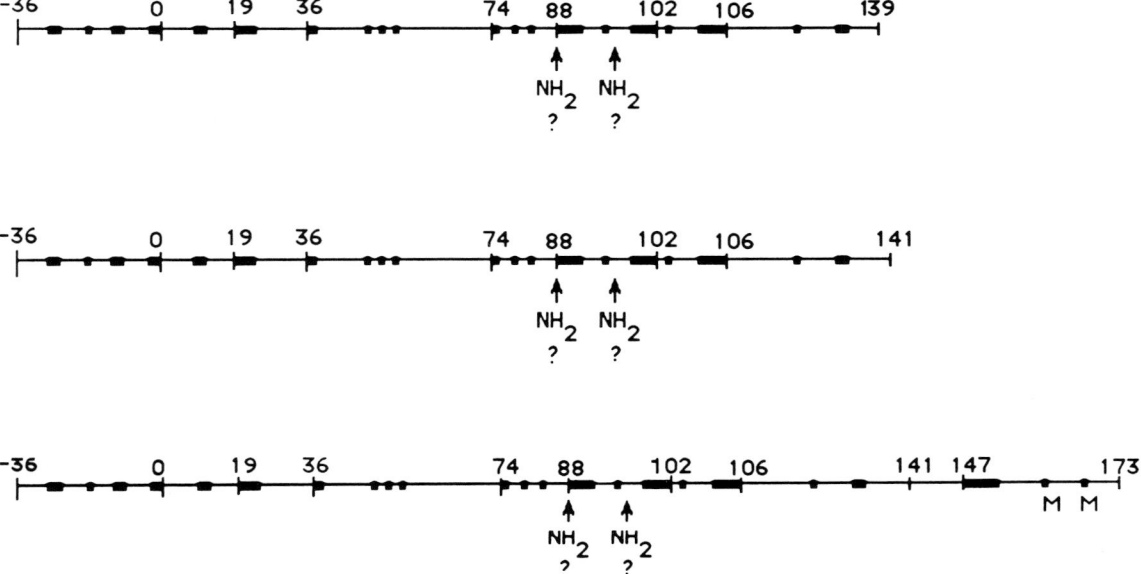

FIG. 6. Structures of the three cDNA-predicted PTHLP forms. Each peptide shares a common −36 to −1 "pre-pro" sequence, as well as identity in the +1 to +139 region. The three peptides differ only in the C-terminus after amino acid +139. The darker portion of the peptides indicate regions that are rich in dibasic amino acids (arginine or lysine) and are presumed to be proteolytic cleavage sites. The NH₂?s indicate presumed cleavage/amidation signals; M, methionine. The actual secretory PTHLP forms are unknown.

referred to as *PTH-like proteins* (PTHLP or PLP) or *PTH-related proteins* (PTHrP).

In contrast to the homology observed prior to amino acid 13, after amino acid 13 the two sequences diverge completely; the remainder of the PTHLP sequence is unique (Fig. 6). These regional homologies and differences may explain why patients with HHM mimic those with primary hyperparathyroidism in some respects but differ in others. For example, PTHLPs are homologous with the regions of PTH required for stimulation of adenylate cyclase but differ in regions recognized by PTH immunoassays. These findings would appear to explain the apparently paradoxical elevation of nephrogenous cyclic cAMP excretion in the presence of normal immunoreactive PTH concentrations observed in patients with HHM. The function of the large region of the PTHLP amino acid sequence that is not homologous to PTH is unknown.

The availability of the cDNA-predicted PTHLP amino and acid sequences has permitted the preparation of synthetic PTHLPs. Because of the known biologic importance of the N-terminal 34 amino acids of the PTH sequence, most synthetic PTHLPs have included the N-terminus. Full-length recombinant PTHLP (1-141) has also been prepared. Synthetic and recombinant PTHLPs have been shown to reproduce both in vitro and in vivo most of the biochemical finding observed in patients with HHM: synthetic and recombinant PTHLPs stimulate renal and skeletal adenylate cyclase (Fig. 7) (52–57),

inhibit renal phosphorus reabsorption (55,56,58,59), stimulate distal tubular calcium reabsorption (55–60), stimulate osteoclastic bone resorption in vitro (52–55), and cause hypercalcemia when infused into experimental animals in vivo (Fig. 8) (52–56).

More recently, PTHLPs have been shown to act in the kidney and bone through PTH receptors. Both PTH and PTHLP bind to the 80,000–85,000 MW renal and skeletal PTH receptor and bind with equivalent affinities (Fig. 9) (56,61–63). In addition to there being receptors for PTH and PTHLPs in bone and kidney, preliminary evidence suggests that PTH/PTHLP receptors exist in vascular smooth muscle (64), heart (65), gastric smooth muscle (66), placenta (67), and brain (64–68).

One of the most enlightening studies was performed using a rat model of HHM. Immunodeficient mice were innoculated with a human HHM-associated tumor (69). The human tumor produced hypercalcemia, hypophosphatemia, and elevated nephrogenous cyclic AMP excretion in the murine host. These biochemical abnormalities were corrected by the infusion into the mice of an antiserum directed against synthetic human PTHLP. These observations, together with the fact that (1) PTHLPs have been identified in HHM-associated tumors but not controls (70,71) and (2) synthetic PTHLPs reproduce the HHM syndrome in vitro and in vivo (52–60) would appear to fulfill Koch's postulates with respect to PTHLPs being responsible for the vast majority of cases of HHM.

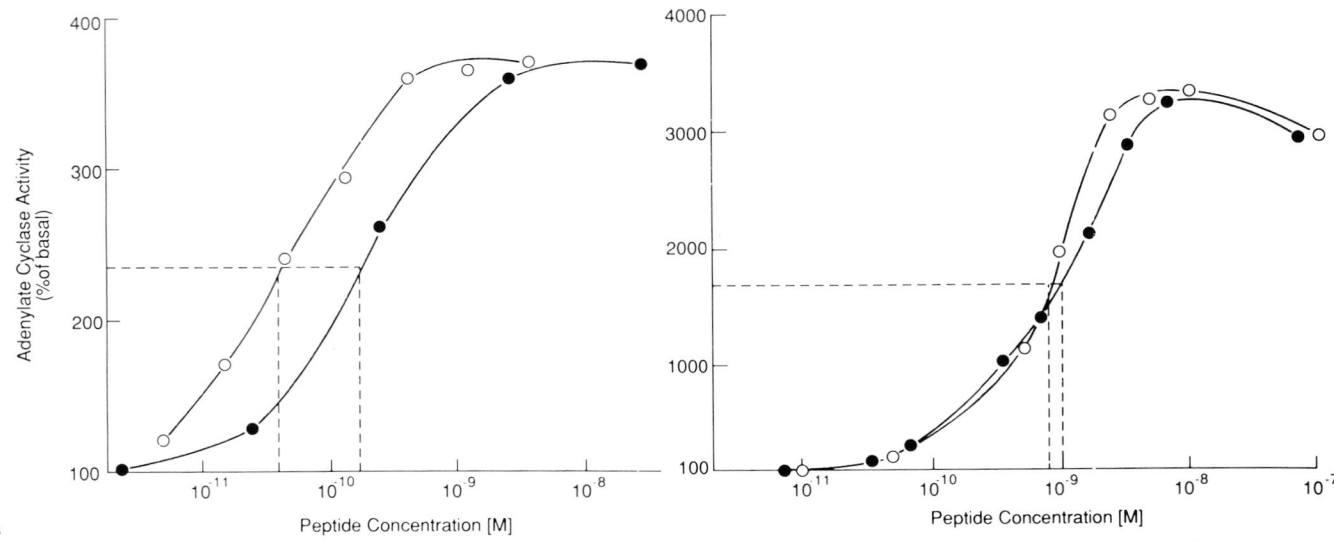

FIG. 7. Effects of bPTH (1–34) (*open circles*) and synthetic PTHLP (1–36) (*closed circles*) on canine renal cortical membrane adenylate cyclase (**A**) and on adenylate cyclase in rat osteosarcoma (ROS 17/2.8) cells (**B**). See the text for details. (Reproduced with permission from Ref. 52.)

At present, information is available describing only genomic and cDNA-predicted PTHLP amino acid sequences. Essentially nothing is known regarding the normal secretory and circulating PTHLP forms. It is likely that extensive post-translational processing and post-secretory cleavage of PTHLP translation products occurs, for the cDNA-predicted PTHLP sequences are rich in presumed proteolytic and processing signals (Fig. 6) (45–47). A number of laboratories are currently using synthetic and recombinant PTHLPs in an effort to develop immunoassays that are capable of reliable measurement of circulating PTHLPs (71–75). Evidence available at present suggests that PTHLPs circulate in 10^{-11} M concentrations in patients with HHM (72–75).

Most of the "ectopic hormones" described to date have proven to be normal secretory products of the parent tissue from which the malignancy in question arose. For example, ACTH and calcitonin are made "ectopi-

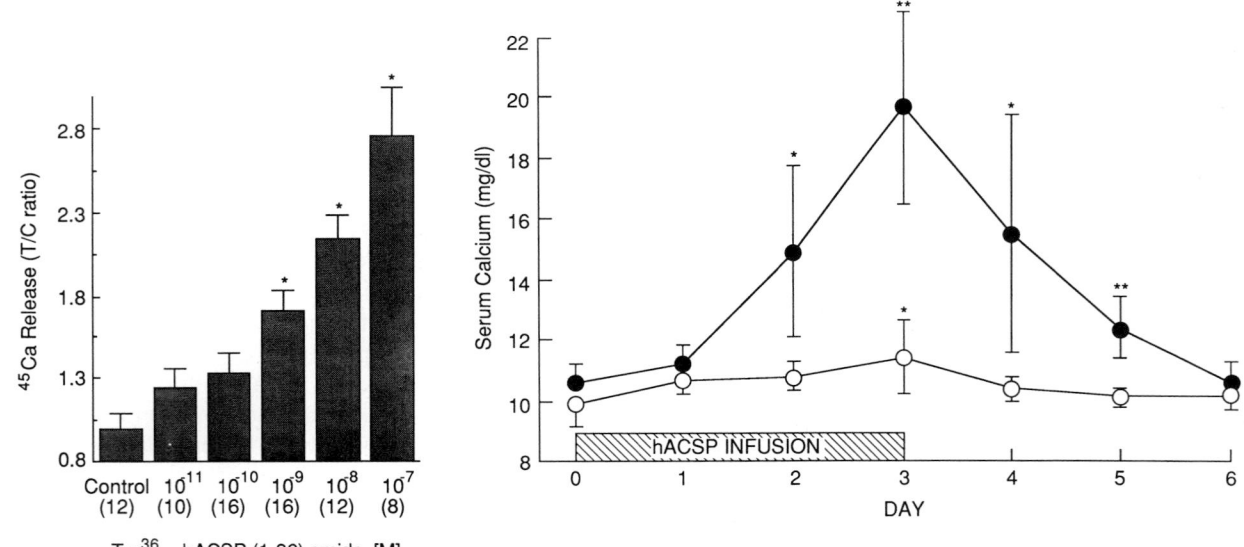

FIG. 8. (**A**): Osteoclastic bone resorption induced by synthetic PTHLP (1–36) as assessed by release of calcium-45 from prelabeled fetal rat long bones. Note that increasing doses of the synthetic peptide lead to progressively more *in vitro* bone resorption. (**B**): Hypercalcemia induced by the infusion of the same synthetic peptide into rats at a dose of 1.4 (*closed circles*) or 0.14 (*open circles*) μg/h over a 3-day period. (Reproduced with permission from Ref. 52.)

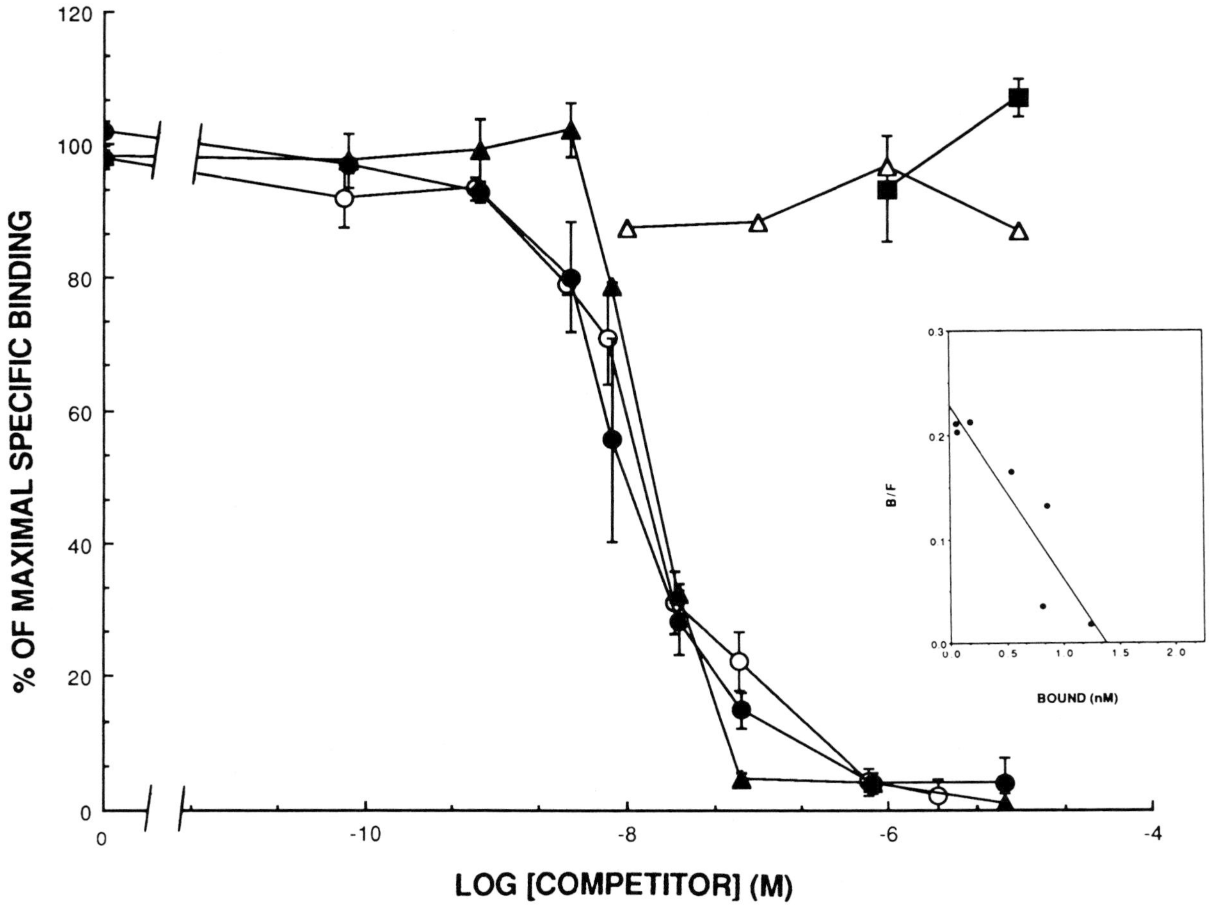

FIG. 9. Binding of ^{125}I-labeled PTHLP (1–36) to the PTH receptor in canine renal cortical membranes. Note that binding is completed equally effectively by PTHLP (1–36) (○), and PTH (1–34) analogs (▲, and ●), but not by control ligands (△ and ■). This indicates that the affinity of synthetic PTHLP (1–36) and PTH for this receptor are equivalent. The inset is a Scatchard plot that demonstrates binding to a single class of receptors. (Reproduced with permission from Ref. 61.)

cally" by bronchial carcinomas, but have also proven to be produced in small amounts in normal bronchial epithelial cells (76,77). Similarly, hCG is produced ectopically by colonic adenocarcinomas but is also produced in small amounts by normal colonic mucosa (78). Thus the designation "ectopic" in most instances is inappropriate. Production of peptide hormones in these instances should be regarded as *eutopic:* abnormal with respect to quantity but not with respect to source.

PTHLPs are no exception to this rule: PTHLPs are encoded by a gene located on chromosome 12 (48–50). This gene is expressed not only by malignant tumors but also by a large variety of nonmalignant tissues. These tissues include the fetal parathyroid gland (67), parathyroid adenomas (79), keratinocytes (46–80), placenta (67), brain (79), lactating (but not other) breast (81) and milk (82), adrenal medulla and cortex (79), fetal liver (79), gastric mucosa (79), and bone cells (79). As with malignant tissues that secrete PTHLPs, the precise secretory and circulating PTHLP forms that are found under

normal circumstances are unknown. Preliminary immunoassay evidence suggests that PTHLPs circulate in far lower concentration in normals than in patients with HHM (72–75). A major focus of interest in a number of laboratories regards the normal role of PTHLPs in nonmalignant tissues. Evidence exists at present to support roles for PTHLPs in the regulation of proliferation and differentiation of keratinocytes and fibroblasts (83–85), in the production of milk in the breast or in the action of milk in the neonate (81,82), in regulation of intestinal and vascular smooth muscle tone (64,65), and in the regulation of mineral transport by the placenta (67).

In summary, HHM appears to result in the vast majority of instances through the systemic production of relatively large quantities of PTHLP. These PTHLPs are the product of a normal gene and presumably serve local paracrine or autocrine roles in a variety of normal tissues. When overexpressed by malignant tumors, PTHLPs interact in a classical endocrine fashion with PTH receptors in kidney and bone, mimic most of the effects of PTH, and thereby lead to a syndrome that resembles hyperparathyroidism. A number of areas are currently under study. These include the regulation of PTHLP gene expression by normal tissues and malignant tumors, the development of clinically useful PTHLP immunoassays for use in the differential diagnosis of hypercalcemia, elucidation of PTHLP secretory and circulating forms, characterization of unique PTHLP receptors, development of specific PTHLP and PTH antagonists, and characterization of the normal functional roles of PTHLPs.

Unusual Causes of Malignancy-Associated Hypercalcemia

The vast majority of patients with malignancy-associated hypercalcemia will fall into one of the two broad mechanistic classes described above. It should be clear, however, that not all patients can be easily "pigeonholed" into one of these mechanistic categories. These patients with unusual causes of malignancy-associated hypercalcemia are discussed in this section.

Lymphomas That Produce 1,25(OH)₂D

Hypercalcemia has been estimated to occur in 5% of patients with lymphoma (32). The majority of these patients have extensive skeletal involvement with tumor and can be considered examples of LOH, although in most instances, the paracrine mediator of the syndrome within the skeleton is uncertain. Patients with HTLV-I lymphomas or leukemias, 90% of whom develop hypercalcemia, generally have little in the way of skeletal metastases (33–35). These patients display the biochemical features of typical HHM, with increases in nephrogenous cyclic AMP excretion (Fig. 10). Malignant lymphocytes from these patients express both PTHLP mRNA and bioactive PTHLP protein. Thus at the time of this writing, HTLV-I lymphomas and leukemias appear to produce hypercalcemia through a prototypical HHM mechanism.

In contrast to these two subgroups of hypercalcemic patients with lymphomas, a third subgroup has been described in whom skeletal metastases are absent or limited and in whom nephrogenous cyclic AMP excretion is reduced (86,87). These unusual patients (seven cases have been described to date) have had a variety of different histologic types of lymphoma but are bound by the common pathophysiological thread of displaying elevated circulating levels of 1,25(OH)₂D (Fig. 11), and in this respect stand in marked contrast to all other groups of patients with MAHC (Fig. 2) (86,87). The increases in circulating 1,25(OH)₂D would appear to result directly from overproduction of 1,25(OH)₂D by the lymphoma, a scenario that represents the "malignant" version of the hypercalcemia that occurs in granulomatous disorders such as sarcoidosis (see Chapter 26).

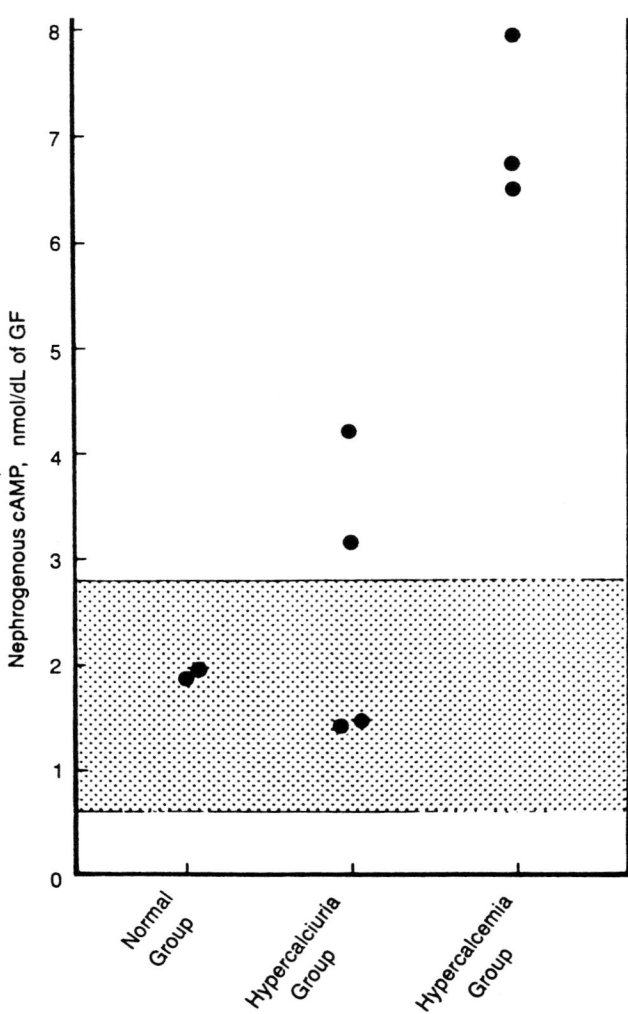

FIG. 10. Nephrogenous cyclic AMP excretion in patients with HTLV-I lymphoma/leukemia who display normal serum and urinary calcium excretion, hypercalciuria but normal serum calcium values, or both hypercalcemia and hypercalciuria. (Reproduced with permission from Ref. 33.)

Like PTHLP overproduction by squamous and breast carcinomas, excessive production of 1,25(OH)₂D by malignant lymphomas and by benign granulomatous disorders appears to represent eutopic production by an abnormal tissue of what is a normal paracrine factor or cytokine. In the case of 1,25(OH)₂D, there is now ample evidence that this vitamin D metabolite is not only a systemically acting regulator of calcium homeostasis, but also a locally acting cytokine that is both produced by and regulates the differentiation of lymphocytes and macrophages (88,89). Finally, it should be emphasized that patients in this category do indeed have a "humoral" form of malignancy-associated hypercalcemia, in that the hypercalcemia results from secretion of a systemic humoral factor [in this case 1,25(OH)₂D] by a tumor that does not involve the skeleton.

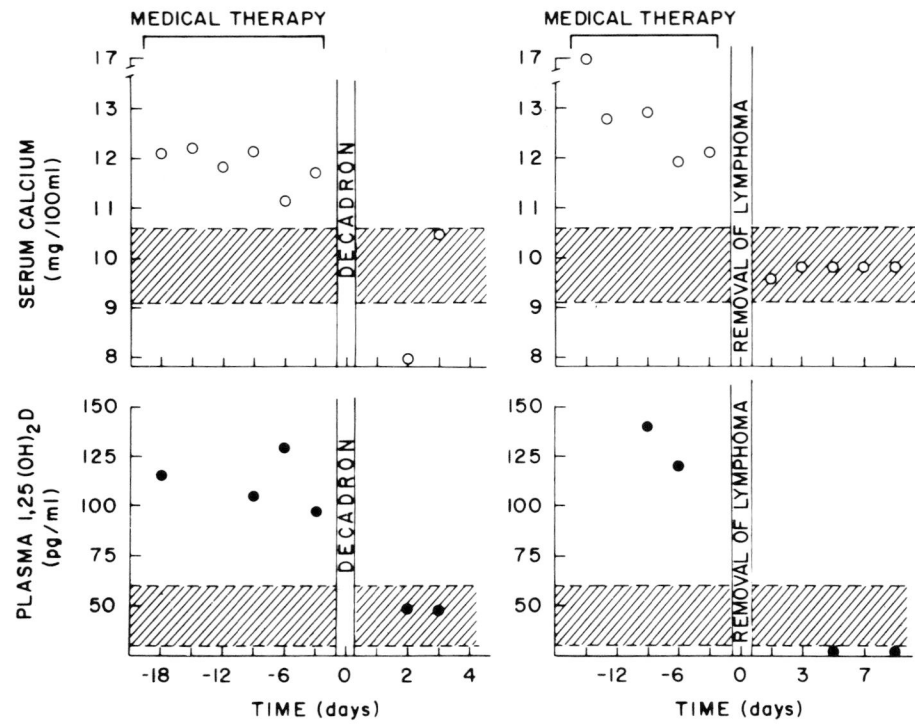

FIG. 11. Serum calcium and plasma 1,25(OH)₂D values in two patients with the lymphoma-1,25(OH)₂D-hypercalcemia syndrome. The patient in the **left** panel had a B-cell immunoblastic sarcoma with widespread cutaneous and nodal involvement. He responded poorly to medical therapy until glucocorticoids were employed. The patient on the **right** panel had a solitary splenic T-cell immunoblastic sarcoma. He also responded poorly to standard medical therapy but promptly became normocalcemic following splenectomy. (Reproduced with permission from Ref. 87.)

Other Humoral Factors

Prostaglandins of the E series have been reported to cause hypercalcemia in laboratory animals and to resorb bone in vitro (90,91). While local production of prostaglandins within the skeleton may modulate bone resorption by osteoclasts, systemic production of prostaglandin by tumors leading to hypercalcemia is now viewed as rare. Clearly, the administration of inhibitors of prostaglandin synthesis to patients with MAHC rarely corrects hypercalcemia in these patients (92). On the other hand, it is also clear that rare patients with MAHC do not fit into any of the categories described thus far, and in some of these, particularly those with renal carcinomas, a humoral mechanism involving production of PGE₂ seems plausible (93).

Bringhurst has described the production of a novel calcemic bone-resorbing factor by a human transitional carcinoma cell line (94). This factor, unlike PTHLP, does not appear to activate PTH-sensitive adenylate cyclase. Attempts to further characterize this factor, to clarify the mechanism through which it causes hypercalcemia, and to delineate the frequency with which it is produced need to be performed. A related factor has been described as occurring in a patient with hypercalcemia resulting from malignant melanoma (95).

Nonmalignant Causes of Hypercalcemia

The differential diagnosis and approach to patients with hypercalcemia is discussed in detail in Chapter 23. It is important to emphasize, in the context of patients in whom the diagnosis of malignancy-associated hypercalcemia is being entertained, that patients with cancer frequently develop hypercalcemia due to causes other than cancer. These patients are important to identify, for hypercalcemia is generally most responsive to therapy when its etiology is nonmalignant.

Primary hyperparathyroidism may occur in patients with cancer. In the author's experience, hyperparathyroidism was responsible for hypercalcemia in 8 of 133 patients presenting with cancer and hypercalcemia (8). Similar results have been reported by others (96). Some authors have even suggested that hyperparathyroidism may occur with greater frequency in patients with cancer than in healthy controls (97). Tuberculosis, sarcoidosis, milk-alkali syndrome, lithium- and thiazide-induced hypercalcemia, vitamin D intoxication, immobilization hypercalcemia, and hyperalimentation-induced hypercalcemia are additional examples of disorders that have been misdiagnosed as malignancy-associated hypercalcemia in the authors' experience. Again, since therapy of hypercalcemia is relatively simple and effective in these patients, and since hypercalcemia due to cancer implies a grave prognosis that may not be warranted, thoughtful attention should be given to *all* causes of hypercalcemia in patients with cancer.

HYPOCALCEMIA DUE TO CANCER

As with hypercalcemia, hypocalcemia may occur in patients with cancer for all of the reasons that it can occur in other patients. The differential diagnosis of and approach to hypocalcemia are discussed in detail in Chapter 27. Several of these disorders, such as hypomagnesemia, pancreatitis, and vitamin D deficiency, perhaps occur with increased frequency in patients with cancer. In particular, hypoalbuminemia occurs with increased frequency in patients with cancer and leads to a reduction in the total but not the ionized portion of serum calcium. Two situations, however, deserve particular emphasis, for they occur only in patients with cancer.

Hypocalcemia Resulting from Osteoblastic Metastases

The occurrence of hypocalcemia in patients with osteoblastic metastases was first described by Sackner et al. in 1960 (98). The largest series of such patients was reported by Raskin et al. (99). The most common neoplasm associated with hypocalcemia is prostate cancer. Adenocarcinoma of the lung and breast cancer have also been implicated. The mean serum calcium in the Raskin series was 7.8 mg/dL, and hypocalcemia occurred in 23 of 75 (31%) patients with prostate cancer and bone metastases. In most patients, extensive osteoblastic bone metastases were present. The serum phosphorus was also reduced (mean 3.1 mg/dL). Serum albumin values averaged 2.5 g/dL in these patients. While ionized serum calcium measurements were not performed, hypoalbu-

minemia did not appear to account for the hypocalcemia observed since there was no correlation between serum albumin and calcium concentrations. Parathyroid hormone and magnesium were not measured in this study.

In a more recent study, Schenkein reported on a patient with profound hypocalcemia (6.4 mg/dL) due to extensive osteoblastic activity (100). This patient had acute monocytic leukemia and was hypophosphatemic (2.8 mg/dL). The serum magnesium concentration was normal. Serum albumin was near normal (3.2 g/dL) and did not account for the hypocalcemia. Immunoreactive PTH was elevated. Bone biopsy revealed thickened trabeculae and increased numbers of active osteoblasts (Fig. 12). Balance measurements indicated that the patient was in markedly positive calcium balance. In this patient there appears to be little doubt that hypocalcemia occurred as the result of increased osteoblastic activity induced by leukemic cells within the marrow.

Pepper et al. have demonstrated similar findings, together with quantitatively increased skeletal uptake of [^{99m}Tc]pyrophosphate, in a patient with breast cancer (101). Smallridge also demonstrated increased skeletal uptake (i.e., positive balance) of calcium in a patient with prostate cancer with extensive skeletal metastases and documented that the skeleton was a "calcium sink" (102). More extensive studies employing modern techniques will need to be performed on patients such as those described by Raskin in order to determine the fre-

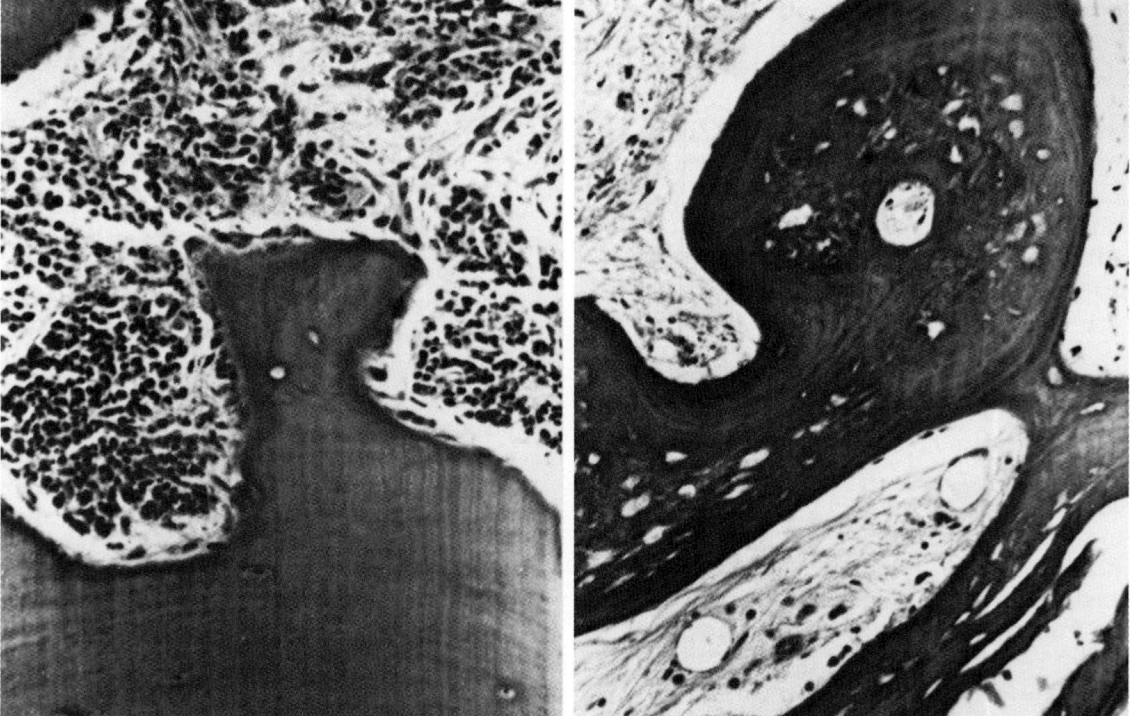

A   B

FIG. 12. Increased osteoblastic activity lining the trabecular bone surface in a patient with leukemia and hypocalcemia prior to therapy (**A**). Note that following chemotherapy (**B**) both the leukemic infiltrate and osteoblastic activity have disappeared. (Reproduced with permission from Ref. 100.)

quency with which this type of hypocalcemia occurs and to clearly define whether hypocalcemia results primarily from osteoblastic metastases, hypoalbuminemia, or from other factors.

Hypocalcemia Due to Hyperphosphatemia and the Tumor-Lysis Syndrome

A second form of hypocalcemia that is unique to patients with cancer is the *tumor-lysis syndrome* (103–

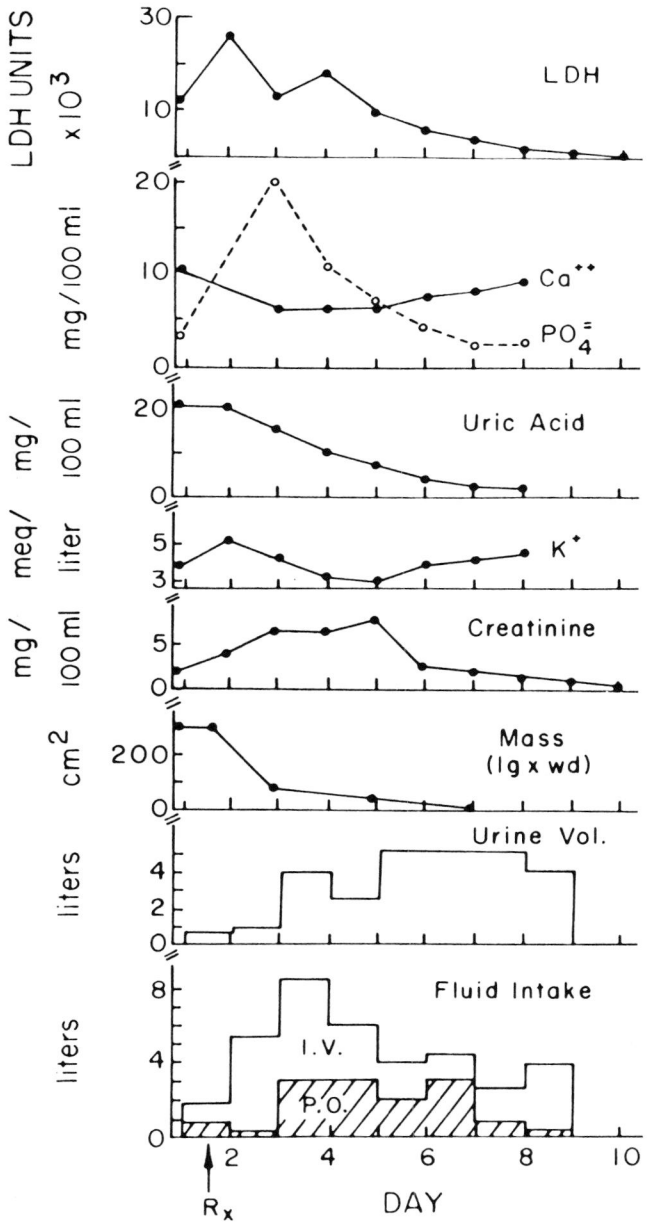

FIG. 13. Sequential changes in serum calcium, phosphorus, creatinine, and other pertinent chemistries following chemotherapy (Rx) in a patient with Burkitt's lymphoma/leukemia and the tumor-lysis syndrome. (Reproduced with permission from Ref. 106.)

107). Typically, patients have rapidly proliferating, chemotherapy-sensitive malignancies such as acute childhood leukemias and Burkitt lymphoma. One to 3 days following administration of chemotherapeutic agents, lethargy, tetany, muscle cramps, and convulsions occur. Hyperkalemia, hyperuricemia, azotemia, and oliguria are common (Fig. 13) and are due to release into the circulation of intracellular contents by dying tumor cells. Hyperphosphatemia is typically severe, ranging from 6 to 35 mg/dL, and appears to result from a combination of tumor cell lysis and from renal failure resulting from hyperuricemia and nephrocalcinosis. Documentation that hyperphosphatemia is due not only to renal failure but also to tumor lysis is provided in an elegant balance study involving children with the syndrome reported by Zussman et al. (104). In this study, urinary phosphorus excretion was shown to increase from normal baseline values of 400 to 600 mg/day to 1600 mg/day following chemotherapy and tumor shrinkage in patients developing the syndrome.

Hypocalcemia may be severe and appears to result from a rise in the serum calcium × phosphorus ion product, leading to precipitation of calcium into soft tissues, including (but not confined to) the kidney (103–107). Secondary hyperparathyroidism has been documented (107).

A report by Dunlay et al. suggests that the hypocalcemia may also be due in part to reduction in circulating concentrations of 1,25(OH)$_2$D, which in turn appear to result from hyperphosphatemia and renal failure (107). The authors of this study suggest that hypocalcemia may persist after reversal of hypophosphatemia, and that recovery of the PTH-1,25(OH)$_2$D axis needs to be complete before hypocalcemia can be corrected.

HYPOPHOSPHATEMIA AND OSTEOMALACIA

Mesenchymal Tumors

Tumor-induced oncogenic or oncogenous osteomalacia is a syndrome that was first described in 1947 by McCance (108). The causal relationship between malignancy and osteomalacia was not recognized until 1959 (109). The syndrome most commonly results from benign, nonendocrine, mesenchymal tumors, although it has been described rarely with malignant mesenchymal neoplasms (110).

Clinical Features

Over 50 patients with oncogenic osteomalacia have now been described in the literature (108–156), but the actual incidence is probably much greater than this would indicate. The bulk of reported cases consists of benign tumors of mesenchymal origin, including sclerosing and cavernous hemangiomas, hemangiopericyto-

TABLE 2. *Oncogenic osteomalacia: tumor types*

Type (percentage)
Hemangioma (59%)
Hemangiopericytoma (21%)
Ossifying mesenchymal (9%)
Osteoblastoma (7%)
Nonossifying fibroma (7%)
Giant cell (7%)
Malignant (9%)

Source: Adapted from Ref. 110.

mas, giant-cell tumors of bone, fibromas and fibroangiomas, ossifying mesenchymomas, osteoblastomas, neuromas, and neurofibromas (Table 2). In a review of 44 patients, 59% of tumors were classified as hemangiomas, frequently hemangiopericytomas (21%) (110). Only four tumors (9%) were considered malignant in this series. Histologically, tumors are characteristically highly vascular with prominent giant cells and spindle cells (Fig. 14). Some of these tumors have been difficult to classify and have been given highly variable designations, depending on a pathologist's preference (157). In one pathological review, approximately 87% of these tumors contained multinucleated giant cells and 80% had a prominent vascular component (157). In a more recent review of 17 mesenchymal tumors documented as causing osteomalacia or rickets, classification into four morphological groups was accomplished (158). The first group was comprised of 10 unique tumors showing mixed connective tissue features together with variable vascular and/or osteoclast-like giant-cell components. With one exception, all tumors of this group occurred in soft tissue and were benign. The remaining three groups

occurred in bone, were benign, and were grouped according to their resemblance to other bone tumors: osteoblastoma-like (four tumors), nonossifying fibroma-like (two tumors), and ossifying fibroma-like (one tumor). Although these tumors were histologically polymorphous, it remains possible that mesenchymal tumors causing oncogenic osteomalacia represent a morphologic spectrum of a unique tumor (157).

Patients with oncogenic osteomalacia typically present with symptoms of severe osteomalacia, including bone pain (93%), muscle weakness (63%), and pseudofractures. Some patients are incapacitated to a degree that prevents walking (39%) (110). The mean age when symptoms first appear is 34 years, while the mean age at diagnosis is 40 years (110). The duration of symptoms before diagnosis ranges from 6 months to 14 years (149). Although the disease usually manifests itself in adult life, 19% of affected patients were 18 years old or less at the time of diagnosis (149). A majority of tumors were located on the lower extremities (44%) or around the head (27%); the upper extremities accounted for 17%. Only 5% involve multiple sites (110). Overall, nearly two-thirds of tumors occurred in the extremities and almost half of these were of osseous origin (110,149). It should be emphasized that tumors are frequently very small and difficult to locate. Consequently, the syndrome may persist for many years before a tumor is detected and removed. Careful physical examination and radiologic evaluation of the head and extremities may be rewarding in this regard.

The biochemical profile in patients with oncogenic osteomalacia includes hypophosphatemia, phosphaturia, normocalcemia, elevated alkaline phosphatase, and subnormal or "inappropriately normal" circulating

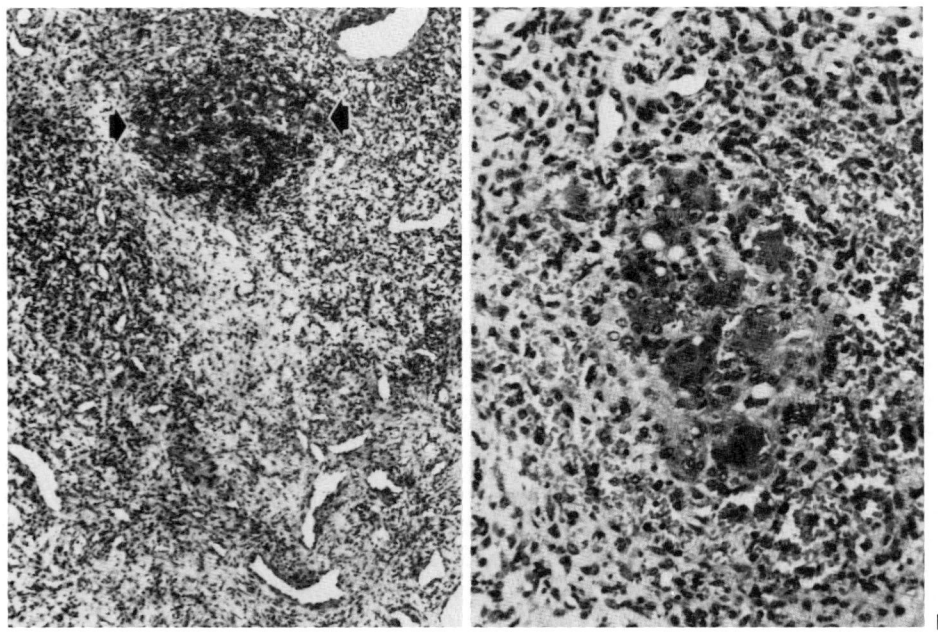

FIG. 14. Mesenchymal tumor: mixed connective tissue variant. **A:** Cellular stroma composed of primitive-appearing stromal cells containing prominent vascularity and a cluster of osteoclast-like giant cells (*arrows*). **B:** Cluster of osteoclast-like giant cells surrounded by hemorrhagic, poorly differentiated stroma composed of small, round to spindle-shaped mesenchymal cells. (Reproduced with permission from Ref. 158.)

1,25(OH)$_2$D levels (110,149). When renal phosphate excretion has been formally assessed, most patients displayed tubular reabsorption of phosphate values in the range of 40–60% (a normal value is greater than 80%) despite severe hypophosphatemia, although rare patients had values as high as 79–94% (110). In others, inadequate renal phosphate reabsorption was documented by a low calculated tubular maximum of phosphate reabsorption/glomerular filtration rate (TmP/GFR). The mean initial serum phosphorus concentration in one series was approximately 1.5 mg/dL (110).

Abnormal vitamin D metabolism is evident in a majority of patients who have been tested. Although circulating concentrations of 25(OH)D are generally normal, indicating adequate vitamin D stores, plasma 1,25(OH)$_2$D levels are often distinctly low or inappropriately normal in the face of severe hypophosphatemia (125,131,135,138). In a recent review, 1,25(OH)$_2$D values were found to be frankly low in 9 of 11 patients in whom it was measured (149). An impairment of 1α-hydroxylation of 25(OH)D has been postulated to account for these abnormalities (125). Gastrointestinal malabsorption of calcium and phosphorus may result from inadequate levels of this vitamin D metabolite.

Aminoaciduria, particularly for glycine, is found in approximately 30% of affected patients. Glycosuria in the absence of hyperglycemia is detected in up to 50% of patients (110,149). A more generalized disorder of proximal renal tubular function (Fanconi syndrome) may also be seen (125,131,146).

Serum parathyroid hormone and calcitonin concentrations are generally normal, but in a minority marginal elevations of iPTH have been found (110,152). The serum calcium level was normal in all of 44 patients recently reviewed (110). Hypocalcemia might be expected in view of the impaired absorption of calcium in association with low levels of 1,25(OH)$_2$D (126,153). Maintenance of serum calcium concentrations may be related to marked renal conservation of calcium despite PTH levels that are not significantly elevated, and to increased osteoclast-mediated bone resorption (153). The coexistence of parathyroid hyperfunction and oncogenic osteomalacia has been documented in at least five cases (115,122,148,153,159). All of these patients had been treated with inorganic phosphate supplements, and it has been suggested that this may have stimulated PTH secretion, ultimately leading to parathyroid autonomy (153,160). Low concentrations of plasma 1,25(OH)$_2$D were observed in one patient despite the presence of both hypophosphatemia and marked hyperparathyroidism (153).

Bone histomorphometry is similar to that encountered in other patients with hypophosphatemic osteomalacia and reveals a reduction in bone formation and accumulation of unmineralized osteoid. Adenomotoid renal lesions in the glomeruli and proximal tubules have been observed in one patient with an angiosarcoma (161,162) and in another with a malignant, nonmesenchymal tumor of the liver (163). It remains to be determined whether renal histologic lesions such as these are noted in the majority of patients with oncogenic osteomalacia, and what relationship, if any, they bear to the proximal renal tubular abnormalities seen in this disorder.

The differential diagnosis of renal phosphate wasting with hypophosphatemia includes hyperparathyroidism, familial X-linked hypophosphatemic rickets, Fanconi syndrome, heavy metal poisoning, idiopathic renal phosphate leaks, diuretics or saline infusion, and calcitonin therapy. Clinical recognition of these disorders is usually straightforward. Severe hypophosphatemia may occur in diabetic ketoacidosis, acute alcoholism, and severe restriction of dietary phosphorus, but in these conditions phosphaturia is not present. Osteomalacia is a feature of a wide spectrum of diseases, the differential diagnosis of which is discussed in Chs. 40 and 41.

Pathogenesis

The pathogenesis of oncogenic osteomalacia is incompletely understood. The observation that surgical removal of a tumor can completely reverse all the clinical and biochemical features of this syndrome suggests that tumors elaborate humoral agents that are causally related to osteomalacia. It has been suggested that the primary renal abnormality is subnormal production of 1,25(OH)$_2$D, which in turn results in a reduced TmP/GFR, and that treatment with this vitamin D metabolite can correct the clinical and biochemical abnormalities (125). However, subsequent reports describe only partial correction of these manifestations with 1,25(OH)$_2$D therapy, which has led to the conclusion that abnormal vitamin D metabolism cannot by itself account for the syndrome (110). The most widely accepted current hypothesis holds that a tumor-derived substance(s) induces a proximal renal tubular defect, resulting in renal phosphate wasting and deficient 1α-hydroxylase activity. The potency of the putative tumor factor(s) in inhibiting 25(OH)D-1α-hydroxylase is illustrated by the finding of low concentrations of plasma 1,25(OH)$_2$D in at least one patient despite the presence of both hypophosphatemia and marked hyperparathyroidism (153). The possibility that this factor may be a physiologic regulator of 1,25(OH)$_2$D production that is produced in excess by these tumors has been raised (153).

Attempts to purify and characterize such a tumor-derived phosphaturic substance have met with modest success. Tumor extracts have been shown by some investigators to produce significant phosphaturia when injected into experimental animals (124,132,142). Aschinberg et al. (124) were able to demonstrate profound phosphaturia following injection of a saline tumor (verrucous epidermal nevi) extract into a puppy, a result that could not be duplicated later. Homogenate of this same tumor grown in culture also failed to induce phosphaturia when injected (124). Two preliminary reports describe a phosphaturic effect of tumor extracts in rat kidney perfusion systems (132,142). In contrast, Yoshikawa et al. (123) were unable to demonstrate a phosphaturic effect when these extracts from a benign osteoblastoma associated with oncogenic osteomalacia were injected into rats. Several investigators have been unable to detect any ultrastructural evidence of secretory granules in the tumors that were studied (123,114,121,126).

Experimental animal models employing transplantation of tumors into mice have succeeded in reproducing the clinical syndrome. A prostate carcinoma associated with oncogenic osteomalacia (see below) was transplanted into immunodeficient mice, and induced phosphaturia, hypophosphatemia, and reduced serum $1,25(OH)_2D$ levels (164). More recently, Miyauchi et al.

(165) have successfully transplanted into mice a hemangiopericytoma which reproduced the clinical syndrome, including phosphaturia, hypophosphatemia, and elevated serum alkaline phosphatase concentrations. Further, tumor extract directly suppressed renal 25(OH)D-1α-hydroxylase activity in a mouse kidney culture system. The inhibitory effect was heat labile, trypsin resistant, and lipid insoluble (165). The tumor extract failed to stimulate cAMP formation in the same primary renal cell culture system (165). On the other hand, stimulation of a PTH-responsive chick renal adenylate cyclase system has been described in tumor extracts from three patients with oncogenic osteomalacia (145). The tumors included a giant-cell tumor of the thigh, an odontogenic fibroma of the mandible, and a hemangiopericytoma of the ethmoid sinus. Competitive inhibition of adenylate cyclase activity was accomplished with $Nle^{8,18}Tyr^{34}$ bovine PTH(3-34) amide, indicating that the extracts stimulated adenylate cyclase through the PTH receptor (145).

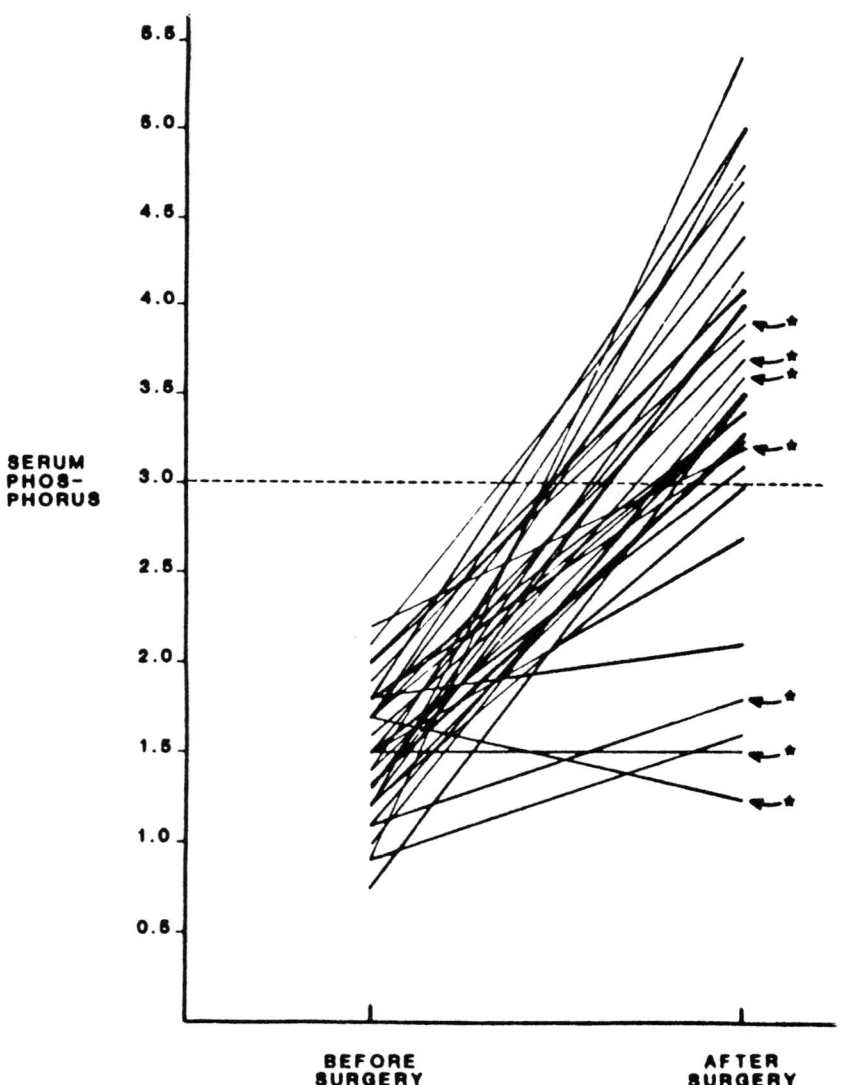

FIG. 15. Response of serum phosphorus to surgical excision of tumor in 35 patients. The arrows identify patients with incomplete resection of tumor. Of the three patients with apparently complete resection of tumor who remained hypophosphatemic postoperatively, one had a clinical remission and the other two showed slight improvement. (Reproduced with permission from Ref. 110.)

None of the tumor extracts contained PTH-like immunoreactivity (145). No other reports of adenylate cyclase–stimulating activity have appeared.

Parathyroid hormone does not appear to be involved in the pathogenesis of oncogenic osteomalacia; serum PTH levels are usually normal, all patients are normocalcemic, nephrogenous cAMP is not elevated, and parathyroidectomy has no beneficial effects (124). Similarly, PTH-like proteins (see the earlier discussion of humoral hypercalcemia of malignancy) are not likely to be involved because of the absence of hypercalcemia, the normal urinary cyclic AMP excretion, and because of the severity of the renal phosphate leak. The humoral factor(s) responsible for the syndrome appears to have properties that are unique. The recent ability to transplant and grow these tumors in nude mice should facilitate future investigation into the nature of this factor (165).

Treatment

Complete operative removal of the responsible tumor is the treatment of choice for oncogenic osteomalacia, since over 90% of these patients will be cured within 3–6 months (110) (Fig. 15). Typically, the results are dramatic, with rapid reversal of severe disability. In tumors that are multiple or in unresectable locations, partial resection is associated with clinical amelioration in nearly 60% of instances (110). The kinetics of serum phosphorus and $1,25(OH)_2D$ recovery following tumor removal were studied in one patient with a benign mesenchymal tumor; serum phosphorus values had become normal by 28 h after tumor excision, while $1,25(OH)_2D$ levels normalized within 48 h (152) (Fig. 16). In other reports, postoperative concentrations of $1,25(OH)_2D$ normalized within 24 h of tumor resection, while serum phosphorus levels lagged slightly behind (135,150,151,156). Failure of the abnormalities to normalize may be caused by residual tumor, and recurrence of the hypophosphatemia and clinical signs may result from recurrent tumor (147,166).

Vitamin D therapy is sometimes effective in patients not cured by surgery. Treatment with vitamin D, usually in combination with oral phosphate supplements, resulted in some clinical improvement in 7 of 22 patients, but complete normalization of serum phosphorus was attained in only two (110). Most of the remaining nonresponders showed a slight rise of serum phosphorus concentration (Fig. 17). Of the 10 patients reported by Ryan et al. (110) who were treated with $1,25(OH)_2D$ or 1α-(OH)D, seven showed significant clinical improvement (Fig. 18). Complete remission with an increase in serum phosphorus to normal was achieved in only one patient (125). Another patient with a benign osteoblastoma associated with oncogenic osteomalacia, hypophosphatemia, and low $1,25(OH)_2D$ levels was treated with 1α-(OH) vitamin D and achieved high-normal levels of

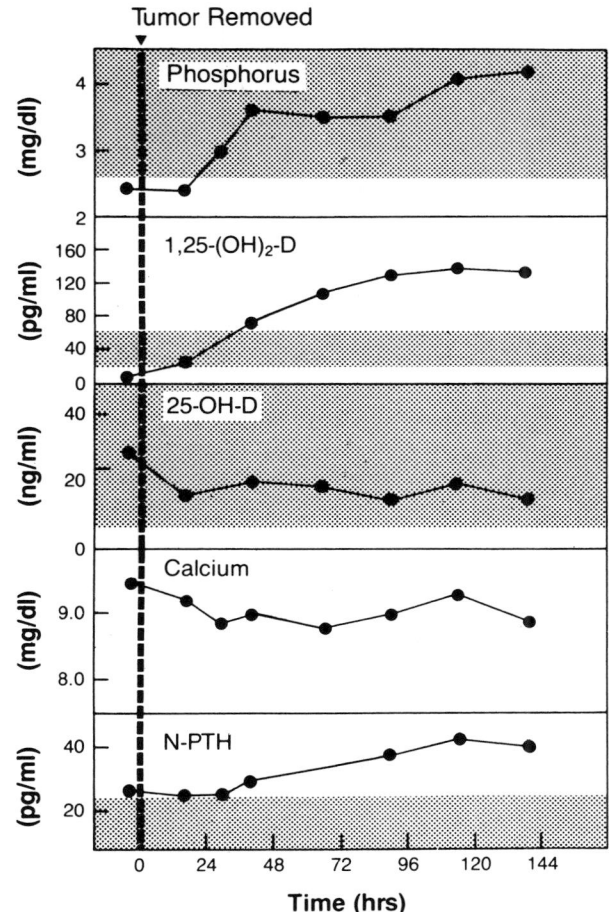

FIG. 16. Changes in indexes of mineral metabolism in response to surgical removal of a mesenchymal tumor in one patient. Shaded areas represent the range of normal values for each assay. (Reproduced with permission from Ref. 152.)

$1,25(OH)_2D$ (131). However, hypophosphatemia and phosphaturia persisted, supporting the concensus that $1,25(OH)_2D$ deficiency is not the sole pathogenetic defect (131). Thus therapy with vitamin D and phosphorus may ameliorate some of the biochemical parameters but rarely results in complete reversal of the clinical syndrome.

Prostate Cancer

Hypophosphatemia is often associated with prostatic carcinoma, occurring in 21% of patients in one large series (167). The association of prostate cancer with hypophosphatemic osteomalacia, however, is rare (167–172). Characteristic findings in these patients include renal phosphate wasting, gastrointestinal malabsorption of calcium and phosphate, normal circulating parathyroid hormone and 25(OH)D concentrations, low $1,25(OH)_2D$ values, and symptoms of bone pain and muscle weakness (167,168,172). These findings are char-

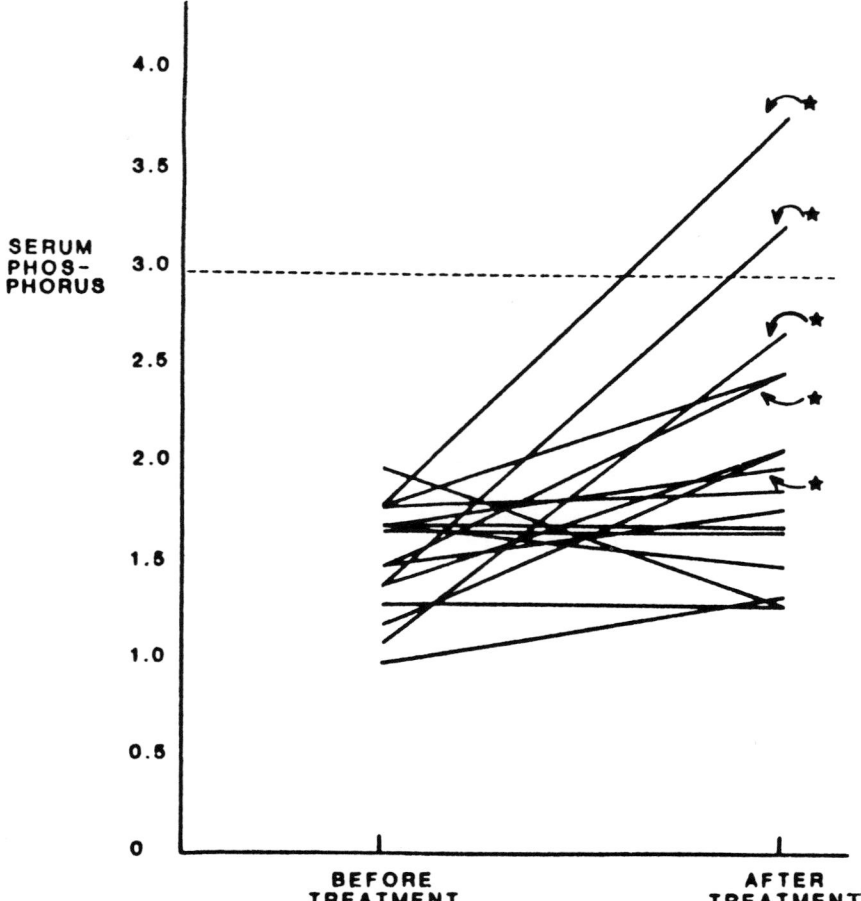

FIG. 17. Response of serum phosphorus to native vitamin D in 16 patients. The arrows identify patients with favorable clinical responses. (Reproduced with permission from Ref. 110.)

acteristic of patients with the classic form of tumor-induced osteomalacia resulting from mesenchymal neoplasms described above. Bone biopsies in affected patients demonstrate the classical findings of osteomalacia: widened osteoid seams with retarded bone mineralization rates (167). Seven of 14 patients with prostate cancer and osteosclerotic bone metastases were shown to have osteomalacia at biopsy in one study (171). Although patients with osteomalacia tended to have lower serum phosphorus and calcium levels than those of control patients with prostate cancer, the only biochemical parameters that were statistically different between the two groups were serum alkaline phosphatase activity, which was higher in affected patients, and plasma urinary calcium excretion, which was lower in the osteomalacia group (171). Plasma 25(OH)D concentrations were not different in the two groups, and 1,25(OH)$_2$D levels were not measured.

It has been suggested in a retrospective analysis of 18 patients with metastatic prostate cancer that long-term, high-dose estrogen therapy can result in renal phosphate wasting with moderate hypophosphatemia and might eventually result in osteomalacia (173). Further, osteoid thickness appears to be increased in estrogen-treated pa-

tients compared with non-estrogen-treated patients (174). It remains to be documented whether conventional-dose estrogen therapy in prostate cancer causes increased phosphaturia or hypophosphatemia (173). Although some of the reports describing the association of prostatic carcinoma with hypophosphatemic osteomalacia have included patients treated with estrogen prior to diagnosis (167,171), at least one report included four patients who had received no prior estrogen therapy (172). Thus estrogen therapy alone appears unlikely to account for all of the cases reported, suggesting that prostate cancer, an endodermal malignancy, is capable of producing a clinical syndrome nearly indistinguishable from the oncogenic osteomalacia associated with mesenchymal tumors. Improvement or remission of the syndrome has been reported with vitamin D therapy (168,170,172).

Miscellaneous Tumors

Hypophosphatemic osteomalacia has been reported sporadically in association with various other tumors, although a definite causal role has not been clearly estab-

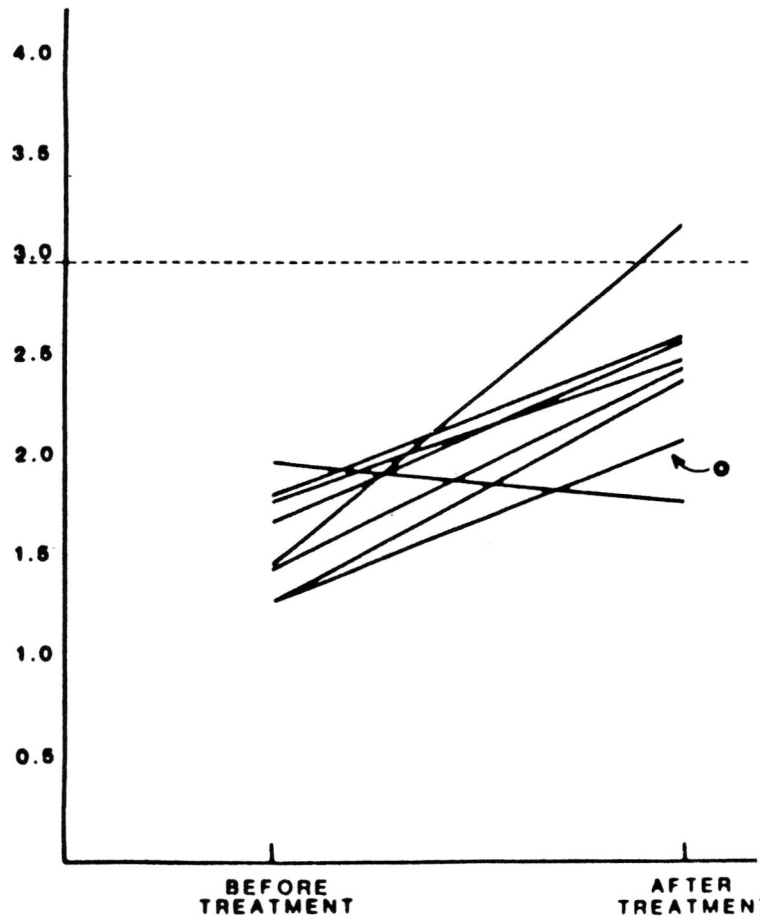

FIG. 18. Response of serum phosphorus to 1,25(OH)₂D or 1α-(OH)D in eight patients, five of whom also received oral phosphate supplements. Arrow identifies patient without clinical improvement. No clinical data are available for the patient in whom the serum phosphorus level decreased. (Reproduced with permission from Ref. 110.)

lished in most instances. The syndrome has been described in one patient with an oat-cell carcinoma of the lung (175). This patient initially displayed the syndrome of inappropriate antidiuretic hormone secretion, and later developed hypophosphatemia, phosphaturia, and reduced plasma 1,25(OH)₂D concentrations in the presence of normal serum calcium and parathyroid hormone values. Aminoaciduria and glycosuria were not present. Osteomalacia was documented on an undecalcified bone biopsy. The patient did not respond to phosphate and calcitriol therapy and died 4 months after presentation. It was concluded that the oat-cell carcinoma in this patient was capable of producing the two distinct paraneoplastic syndromes. This claim has been questioned because of the possibility that a small, asymptomatic, mesenchymal tumor in an obscure location could have escaped detection at autopsy, and reversal of the syndromes following tumor resection was not demonstrated (176). Further, it has been pointed out that since this patient was treated with demeclocycline, renal phosphate wasting and hypophosphatemia could have resulted from selective demeclocycline-induced renal toxity, which had been described previously in a similar patient (177).

The Fanconi syndrome due to light-chain nephropathy in association with multiple myeloma and other hematologic malignancies has been described as another cause of oncogenic osteomalacia. Two well-described patients, one with myeloma and the other with chronic lymphocytic leukemia, displayed reduced renal tubular phosphate reabsorption along with other features of the Fanconi syndrome as a consequence of light-chain nephropathy (178). In both patients serum alkaline phosphatase concentrations were elevated, and in both, osteomalacia was documented by bone biopsy. Plasma 1,25(OH)₂D values were inappropriately low. Complete histologic correction of the osteomalacia was achieved with oral phosphate therapy given alone or in combination with 1,25(OH)₂D. This report (178) also reviews 13 other cases of osteomalacia and Fanconi syndrome associated with light-chain proteinuria, although histologic confirmation of osteomalacia was obtained in only two cases (179,180). Fanconi syndrome with osteomalacia seems to occur only in the small subset of patients with multiple myeloma characterized by an usually benign and slowly progressive course (178,181).

At least four patients with the linear sebaceous nevus syndrome (epidermal nevus syndrome) have been described in whom vitamin D–resistant rickets/osteomalacia developed (124,182,183). In all four patients, rickets was observed at an early age and was associated with muscle weakness and bone pain (182). Clinical and biochemical reversal of the syndrome occurred in one patient following surgical removal of the skin lesions, suggesting that this disorder may be a variant of oncogenic osteomalacia (124). Two patients have been described in whom the skin lesions were so extensively distributed that surgical excision was precluded (182). Both patients demonstrated hypophosphatemia, phosphaturia, elevated alkaline phosphatase activity, normal serum calcium values, reduced plasma 1,25(OH)$_2$D levels, and normal 25(OH)D levels. Administration of 1,25(OH)$_2$D increased plasma 1,25(OH)$_2$D concentrations, serum phosphorus levels, and the TmP/GFR. However, serum phosphorus values and the TmP/GFR were not corrected completely. While clinical improvement was noted, bone histomorphometry improved only partially. It was concluded that the skin lesions in these patients produced a factor that induced another form of tumor-induced osteomalacia. Finally, hypophosphatemic osteomalacia has also been reported in patients with fibrous dysplasia of bone (184,185) and neurofibromatosis (186–189). Many of these patients have responded to pharmacologic vitamin D therapy.

ACKNOWLEDGMENTS

This work was supported by the Veterans Administration, West Haven, CT 06516. We thank Mrs. Ann Blood for her expert secretarial assistance.

REFERENCES

1. Zondek H, Petow H, Siebert W. Die Bedeuting der Calciumbestimmung im Blute für die Diagnose der Niereninsuffizienz. *Z Klin Med* 1924;99:128–38.
2. Heath H III, Hodgson SF, Kennedy MA. Primary hyperparathyroidism: medicine, morbidity and potential economic impact on a community. *N Engl J Med* 1980;302:189–93.
3. Fisken RA, Heath DA, Somers S, Bold AM. Hypercalcemia in hospital patients: clinical and diagnostic aspects. *Lancet* 1981;1:202–7.
4. Gutman AB, Tyson TL, Gutman EB. Serum calcium inorganic phosphorus and phosphatase in hyperparathyroidism, Paget's disease, multiple myeloma, and neoplastic disease of the bones. *Arch Intern Med* 1936;57:379–413.
5. Myers WPL. Hypercalcemia in neoplastic disease. *Arch Surg* 1960;80:308–18.
6. Stewart AF, Horst R, Deftos LJ, Cadman EC, Lang R, Broadus AE. Biochemical evaluation of patients with cancer-associated hypercalcemia: evidence for humoral and nonhumoral groups. *N Engl J Med* 1980;303:1377–83.
7. Rodman JS, Sherwood LM. Disorders of mineral metabolism in malignancy. In: Avioli LV, Krane SM, eds. *Metabolic bone disease,* vol 2. New York: Academic Press, 1978;577–631.
8. Godsall JW, Burtis WJ, Insogna KL, Broadus AE, Stewart AF. Nephrogenous cyclic AMP, adenylate cyclase-stimulating activity, and the humoral hypercalcemia of malignancy. *Recent Prog Horm Res* 1986;40:705–50.
9. Cramer SF, Fried L, Carter KJ. The cellular basis of metabolic bone disease in patients with lung cancer. *Cancer* 1981;48:2649–60.
10. Mehadevia PS, Ramaswami A, Greenwald ES, Wollner DI. Hypercalcemia in prostate cancer. *Arch Intern Med* 1983;143:1339–42.
11. Galasko CSB. Mechanisms of bone destruction in the development of skeletal metastases. *Nature* 1976;263:507–8.
12. Mundy GR, Raisz LG, Cooper RA, Schechter GP, Salmon SE. Evidence for the secretion of an osteoclast stimulating factor in myeloma. *N Engl J Med* 1974;291:1041–6.
13. Mundy GR, Luben RA, Raisz LG, Oppenheim JJ, Buell DN. Bone-resorbing activity in supernatants from lymphoid cell lines. *N Engl J Med* 1974;290:867–71.
14. Mundy GR. Hypercalcemia of malignancy revisited. *J Clin Invest* 1988;82:1–6.
15. Dewhirst FE, Stashenko PP, Mole JE, Tsurumachi T. Purification and partial sequence of human osteoclast-activating factor: identity with interleukin I beta. *J Immunol* 1985;135:2562–8.
16. Garrett IR, Durie BGM, Nedwin GE, et al. Production of the bone-resorbing cytokine lymphotoxin by cultured human myeloma cells. *N Engl J Med* 1987;317:526–32.
17. Powles TJ, Clark SA, Easty DM, Easty GC, Neville AM. The inhibition by aspirin and indomethacin of osteolytic tumour deposits and hypercalcemia in rats with the Walker tumour, and its possible application to human breast cancer. *Br J Cancer* 1973;28:316–21.
18. Eilon G, Mundy GR. Direct resorption of bone by human breast cancer cells in vitro. *Nature* 1978;276:726–8.
19. Villalon AH, Tattersall MHN, Fox RM, Woods RL. Hypercalcemia after tamoxifen for breast cancer: a sign of tumor response? *Br Med J* 1979;4:1329–30.
20. Legha SS, Powell K, Buzdor AU, Blumenschein CR. Tamoxifen-induced hypercalcemia in breast cancer. *Cancer* 1981;47:2803–6.
21. Valentin-Opran A, Eilon G, Saez S, Mundy GR. Estrogens and antiestrogens stimulate release of bone resorbing activity by cultured human breast cancer cells. *J Clin Invest* 1985;75:726–31.
22. Schussler GC, Verso MA, Nemoto T. Phosphaturia in hypercalcemia breast cancer patients. *J Clin Endocrinol Metab* 1972;35:497–504.
23. Case Records of the Massachusetts General Hospital (case 27461). *N Engl J Med* 1941;225:789–91.
24. Plimpton CH, Gelhorn A. Hypercalcemia in malignant disease without evidence of bone destruction. *Am J Med* 1956;21:750–9.
25. Connor TB, Thomas WC Jr, Howard JF. The etiology of hypercalcemia associated with lung carcinoma. *J Clin Invest* 1956;35:697–8.
26. Lafferty FW. Pseudohyperparathyroidism. *Medicine (Baltimore)* 1966;45:247–60.
27. Skrabanek P, McPartlin J, Powell D. Tumor hypercalcemia and ectopic hyperparathyroidism. *Medicine* 1980;58:262–82.
28. Burt ME, Brennan M. Incidence of hypercalcemia and malignant neoplasm. *Arch Surg* 1980;115:704–7.
29. Omenn GS, Roth SI, Baker WH. Hyperparathyroidism associated with malignant tumors of non-parathyroid origin. *Cancer* 1969;24:1004–12.
30. Isales C, Carcangiu ML, Stewart AF. Hypercalcemia in breast cancer: reassessment of the mechanism. *Am J Med* 1987;82:1143–7.
31. Burtis WJ, Wu T, Bunch C, et al. Identification of a novel 17,000-dalton parathyroid hormone-like adenylate cyclase-stimulating protein from a tumor associated with humoral hypercalcemia of malignancy. *J Biol Chem* 1987;262:7151–6.
32. Cannellos GP. Hypercalcemia in malignant lymphoma and leukemia. *Ann NY Acad Sci* 1974;230:240–50.
33. Fukumoto S, Matsumoto T, Ikelada K, et al. Clinical evaluation of calcium metabolism in adult T-cell leukemia/lymphoma. *Arch Intern Med* 1988;148:921–5.
34. Motokura T, Fukumoto S, Takahashi S, et al. Expression of PTH-rP in a human T cell lymphotrophic virus type 1-infected T cell line. *Biochem Biophys Res Commun* 1988;154:1182–8.
35. Fukumoto S, Matsumoto T, Wantabe T, Takahashi H, Mioyoshi J, Ogata E. Secretion of PTH-like activity from human T-cell lymphotrophic virus type-I infected lymphocytes. *Cancer Res* 1989;49:3849–52.

36. Riggs BL, Arnaud CD, Reynolds JC, Smith LH. Immunologic differentiation of primary hyperparathyroidism from hyperparathyroidism due to non-parathyroid cancer. *J Clin Invest* 1971;50:2079–83.

37. Benson RC Jr, Riggs BL, Pickard BM, Arnaud CD. Immunoreactive forms of circulating parathyroid hormone in primary and ectopic hyperparathyroidism. *J Clin Invest* 1974;54:175–81.

38. Stewart AF, Vignery A, Silverglate A, et al. Quantitative bone histomorphometry in humoral hypercalcemia of malignancy: uncoupling of bone cell activity. *J Clin Endocrinol Metab* 1982;55:219–27.

39. Gkonos PJ, Hayes T, Burtis W, et al. Squamous carcinoma model of humoral hypercalcemia of malignancy. *Endocrinology* 1984;115:2384–90.

40. Insogna KL, Stewart AF, Vignery AM-C, et al. Biochemical and histomorphometric characterization of rat model for humoral hypercalcemia of malignancy. *Endocrinology* 1984;114:888–96.

41. Burtis WJ, Wu T, Bunch C, et al. Identification of a novel 17,000-dalton PTH-like adenylate cyclase stimulating protein from a tumor associated with humoral hypercalcemia of malignancy. *J Biol Chem* 1987;262:7151–6.

42. Stewart AF, Wu T, Goumas D, Burtis WJ, Broadus AE. N-terminal amino acid sequence of two novel tumor-derived adenylate cyclase-stimulating proteins: identification of parathyroid hormone-like and parathyroid hormone-unlike domains. *Biochem Biophys Res Commun* 1987;146:672–8.

43. Moseley JM, Kubota M, Diefenbach-Jagger H, et al. Parathyroid hormone-related protein purified from a human lung cancer cell line. *Proc Natl Acad Sci USA* 1987;84:5048–52.

44. Strewler GJ, Stern PH, Jacobs JW, et al. Parathyroid hormone-like protein from human renal carcinoma cells: structural and functional homology with parathyroid hormone. *J Clin Invest* 1987;80:1803–7.

45. Suva LJ, Winslow GA, Wettenhall REH, et al. A parathyroid hormone-related protein implicated in malignant hypercalcemia: cloning and expression. *Science* 1987;237:893–6.

46. Mangin M, Webb AC, Dreyer B, et al. Identification of a cDNA encoding a parathyroid hormone-like peptide from a human tumor associated with humoral hypercalcemia of malignancy. *Proc Natl Acad Sci USA* 1988;85:587–601.

47a. Theide MA, Strewler GJ, Nissenson RA, Rosenblatt M, Rodan GA. Human renal carcinoma expresses two messages encoding a PTH-like peptide: evidence for the alternative splicing of a single copy gene. *Proc Natl Acad Sci USA* 1988;85:4605–9.

47b. Mangin M, Ikeda K, Dryer BE, Milstone L, Broadus AE. Two distinct tumor-derived PTH-like peptides result from alternate RNA splicing. *Mol Endocrinol* 1988;2:1049–55.

48. Mangin M, Ikeda K, Dryer B, Broadus AE. Isolation and characterization of the human PTH-like peptide gene. *Proc Natl Acad Sci USA* 1989;86:1408–2413.

49. Yasuda T, Banville D, Hendy GN, Goltzman D. Characterization of the human PTH-like peptide gene. *J Biol Chem* 1989;264:7720–5.

50. Suva LJ, Matber KA, Gillespie MT, et al. Structure of the 5′ flanking region of the gene encoding PTH-related protein. *Gene* 1989;77:95–105.

51. Habener JF, Rosenblatt M, Potts JT. Parathyroid hormone: biochemical aspects of biosynthesis, secretion, action, and metabolism. *Physiol Rev* 1984;64:985–1054.

52. Stewart AF, Mangin M, Wu T, et al. A synthetic human parathyroid hormone-like protein stimulates bone resorption and causes hypercalcemia in rats. *J Clin Invest* 1988;81:596–600.

53. Stewart AF, Elliot J, Burtis WJ, Wu T, Insogna KL. Synthetic parathyroid hormone-like protein (1-74): biochemical and physiological characterization. *Endocrinology* 1989;124:642–8.

54. Thorikay M, Kramer S, Reynolds F, et al. Synthesis of a gene encoding parathyroid hormone-like protein (1-141): purification and biological characterization of the expressed protein. *Endocrinology* 1989;124:111–8.

55. Kemp BE, Moseley JM, Rodda CP, et al. PTH-related protein of malignancy: active synthetic fragments. *Science* 1988;238:1568–70.

56. Horiuchi N, Caulfield MD, Fisher JE, et al. Similarity of synthetic peptide from human tumor to PTH in vivo and in vitro. *Science* 1988;138:1566–8.

57. Yates AJP, Guttuerez GE, Smolens P, et al. Effects of a synthetic peptide of PTH-related protein on calcium homeostasis, renal tubular calcium reabsorption, and bone metabolism in vivo and in vitro in rodents. *J Clin Invest* 1988;81:932–8.

58. Sartori L, Weir EC, Stewart AF, et al. Synthetic and partially-purified adenylate cyclase-stimulating proteins from tumors associated with humoral hypercalcemia of malignancy inhibit phosphate transport in a PTH-responsive renal cell line. *J Clin Endocrinol Metab* 1988;66:459–61.

59. Pizurki L, Rizzoli R, Moseley J, Martin TJ, Caverzasio J, Bonjour J-P. Effect of synthetic tumoral PTH-related peptide on cAMP production and Na-dependent Pi transport. *Am J Physiol* 1988;255:F957–61.

60. Scheinman SJ, Mitnick MA, Stewart AF. Direct anticalciuretic and natriuretic effects of PTH-like peptides. *Clin Res* 1989;37:501A (abstr).

61. Orloff JJ, Wu TL, Heath HW, Brady TG, Brines ML, Stewart AF. Characterization of canine renal receptors for the parathyroid hormone-like protein associated with humoral hypercalcemia of malignancy. *J Biol Chem* 1989;264:6097.

62. Nissenson RA, Diep D, Strewler GJ. Synthetic peptides comprising the amino-terminal sequence of a PTH-like protein from human malignancies. *J Biol Chem* 1988;263:12866–71.

63. Juppner H, Abou-Samra AB, Uneno S, Gu WX, Potts JT, Segre GV. The PTH-like peptide associated with humoral hypercalcemia of malignancy and parathyroid hormone bind to the same receptor on the plasma membranes of ROS 17/2.8 cells. *J Biol Chem* 1988;263:8557–60.

64. Orloff JJ, Wu T, Stewart AF. PTH-like proteins: biochemical responses and receptor interactions. *Endocr Rev* 1989;10:476–95.

65. Nickols GA, Nana AD, Nickols MA, DiPette DJ, Asimakis GK. Hypotension and cardiac stimulation due to the PTH-related protein, humoral hypercalcemia of malignancy factor. *Endocrinology* 1989;125:834–41.

66. Mok LLS, Ajiwe E, Martin TJ, Thompson JC, Cooper CW. PTH-related protein relaxes rat gastric smooth muscle and shows cross desensitization with PTH. *J Bone Miner Res* 1989;4:433–9.

67. Rodda CP, Kubota M, Heath JA, et al. Evidence for a novel PTH-related protein in fetal lamb parathyroid glands and sheep placenta. *J Endocrinol* 1988;117:261–71.

68. Fraser CL, Sarnacki P, Budayr A. Evidence that PTH-mediated calcium transport in rat brain synaptosomes is independent of cAMP. *J Clin Invest* 1988;81:982–8.

69. Kukreja SC, Shevrin DH, Wimbiscus SA, et al. Antibodies to parathyroid hormone-related protein lower serum calcium in athymic mouse models of malignancy-associated hypercalcemia due to human tumors. *J Clin Invest* 1988;82:1798–1802.

70. Stewart AF, Insogna KL, Burtis WJ, Aminifshar A, Wu T, Broadus AE. Frequency and partial characterization of adenylate cyclase-stimulating activity in tumors associated with humoral hypercalcemia of malignancy. *J Bone Miner Res* 1986;1:267–76.

71. Rodan SB, Insogna KL, Vignery AM-C, et al. Factors associated with humoral hypercalcemia of malignancy stimulate adenylate cyclase in osteoblast cells. *J Clin Invest* 1983;72:1511–5.

72. Budayr AA, Nissenson RA, Klein RF, et al. Increased levels of a PTH-like protein in malignancy-associated hypercalcemia. *Proceedings of the 71st Annual Meeting of the Endocrine Society,* Seattle, WA, 1989; abstr 42.

73. Firek AF, Kao PC, Taylor R, Klee GG, Heath H. Plasma intact PTH and PTH-related protein are elevated in some patients with familial benign hypercalcemia. *J Bone Miner Res* 1989;4(suppl):832A.

74. Henderson JE, Shustik C, Kremer R, Rabbani SA, Hendy GN, Goltzman D. Immunoreactive PTH-like peptide in the plasma of patients with malignancy and with hyperparathyroidism. *J Bone Miner Res* 1989;4(suppl):822A.

75. Burtis WJ, Brady TG, Wu T, Ersback J, Stewart AF. Rapid immunoradiometric assay for PTH-like protein. *J Bone Miner Res* 1989;4(suppl):771A.

76. Yalow RS, Eastridge CE, Higgins G, Wolf J. Plasma and tumor ACTH in carcinoma of the lung. *Cancer* 1979;44:1789–92.

77. Becker KL, Silva DL, Snider RM, Moore CF. Pulmonary immunoreactive calcitonin in the primate; anatomic distribution. *Proceedings of the 63rd annual meeting of the Endocrine Society,* Cincinnati, OH, 1981; abstr 590.

78. Odell WD, Wolfson AR. Humoral syndromes associated with cancer. *Annu Rev Med* 1989;29:379–406.

79. Ikeda K, Weir EC, Mangin M, et al. Expression of messenger ribonucleic acids encoding a parathyroid hormone-like peptide in normal human and animal tissues with abnormal expression in human parathyroid adenomas. *Mol Endocrinol* 1988;2:1230–6.

80. Merendino JJ, Insogna KL, Milstone LM, Broadus AE, Stewart AF. Cultured human keratinocytes produce a parathyroid hormone-like protein. *Science* 1986;231:388–90.

81. Thiede MA, Rodan GA. Expression of a calcium-mobilizing PTH-like peptide in lactating mammary tissue. *Science* 1988;242:161.

82. Budayr AA, Halloran BP, King JC, Diep D, Nissenson RA, Strewler GJ. High levels of a PTH-like protein in milk. *Proc Natl Acad Sci USA* 1989;86:7183–5.

83. Insogna KL, Stewart AF, Centrella M, Ikeda K, Milstone LM. Characterization of a PTH-like peptide secreted by human keratinocytes. *Ann NY Acad Sci* 1988;548:146–59.

84. Holick MF, Nussbaum S, Persons KS. PTH-like humoral hypercalcemia factor of malignancy may be an epidermal differentiation factor. *J Bone Miner Res* 1988;3(suppl):S214(abstr).

85. Wu TL, Insogna KL, Hough L, Milstone LM, Stewart AF. Skin-derived fibroblasts respond to human parathyroid hormone-like adenylate cyclase-stimulating proteins. *J Clin Endocrinol Metab* 1987;65:105–9.

86. Breslau NA, McGuire JL, Zerwekh JR, Frenkel EP, Pak CYC. Hypercalcemia associated with increased serum calcitrion levels in three patients with lymphoma. *Ann Intern Med* 1984;100:1–7.

87. Rosenthal N, Insogna KL, Godsall JW, Smaldone L, Waldron JA, Stewart AF. Elevations in circulating 1,25-dihydroxyvitamin D in three patients with lymphoma-associated hypercalcemia. *J Clin Endocrinol Metab* 1985;60:29–33.

88. Tsoukas CD, Provvedini DM, Manolagas SC. 1,25-Dihydroxyvitamin D: a novel immunoregulatory hormone. *Science* 1984;224:1438–9.

89. Tsoukas CD, Watry D, Escobar SS, et al. Inhibition of interleukin-1 production by 1,25-dihydroxyvitamin D. *Endocrinology* 1989;69:127–33.

90. Klein DC, Raisz LG. Prostaglandins: stimulation of bone resorption in tissue culture. *Endocrinology* 1970;86:1436–40.

91. Seyberth HW, Segre GV, Morgan JL, Sweetman BJ, Potts JT, Oates JA. Prostaglandins as mediators of hypercalcemia associated with certain types of cancer. *N Engl J Med* 1975;293:1278–83.

92. Brenner D, Harvey HA, Lipton A, Demers L. A study of prostaglandin E_2 parathormone, and response to indomethacin in patients with hypercalcemia and malignancy. *Cancer* 1982;49:556–61.

93. Metz SA, McRae JR, Robertson RP. Prostaglandins as mediators of paraneoplastic syndromes: review and update. *Metabolism* 1981;30:299–316.

94. Bringhurst FR, Bierer BE, Godeau F, Neyhard N, Varner V, Segre GV. Humoral hypercalcemia of malignancy: release of a prostaglandin-stimulating bone-resorbing factor in vitro by human transitional-cell carcinoma cells. *J Clin Invest* 1986;77:456–64.

95. Bringhurst FR, Varner V, Segre GV. Cancer-associated hypercalcemia: characterization of a new bone-resorbing factor. *Clin Res* 1982;30:386A.

96. Samaan NA, Hickey RC, Sethi MR, Yang KP, Wallace S. Hypercalcemia in patients with known malignant disease. *Surgery* 1976;80:382–9.

97. Drezner MK, Lebovitz HE. Primary hyperparathyroidism in paraneoplastic hypercalcemia. *Lancet* 1978;1:1004–6.

98. Sackner MA, Spirak AP, Balian LJ. Hypocalcemia in the presence of osteoblastic metastases. *N Engl J Med* 1960;262:173–6.

99. Raskin P, McClain CJ, Medsger TA. Hypocalcemia associated with metastatic bone disease. *Arch Intern Med* 1973;132:539–43.

100. Schenkein DP, O'Neill WC, Shapiro J, Miller KB. Accelerated bone formation causing profound hypocalcemia in acute leukemia. *Ann Intern Med* 1986;105:375–8.

101. Pepper GM, Strashun AM, Goldsmith SJ. Hypocalcemia in metastatic bone disease: metabolic and radionuclide studies of a case. *NY State J Med* 1984;84:41–4.

102. Smallridge RC, Wray HL, Schaaf M. Hypocalcemia in a patient with prostate carcinoma. *Am J Med* 1981;71:184–8.

103. Jaffee N, Paed D, Kim BS, Vawter GF. Hypocalcemia: a complication of childhood leukemia. *Cancer* 1972;29:392–8.

104. Zussman J, Brown DM, Nesbit ME. Hyperphosphatemia, hyperphosphaturia and hypocalcemia in acute lymphoblastic leukemia. *N Engl J Med* 1973;289:1335–40.

105. Brereton HD, Anderson T, Johnson RE, Schein PS. Hyperphosphatemia and hypocalcemia in Burkitt's lymphoma. *Arch Intern Med* 1975;135:307–9.

106. Cadman EC, Lundberg WB, Bertino JR. Hyperphosphatemia and hypocalcemia accompanying rapid cell lysis in a patient with Burkitt's lymphoma and Burkitt cell leukemia. *Am J Med* 1977;62:283–90.

107. Dunlay RW, Camp MA, Allon M, Fanti P, Malluche HH, Llach F. Calcitriol in prolonged hypocalcemia due to tumor lysis syndrome. *Ann Intern Med* 1989;110:162–4.

108. McCance RA. Osteomalacia with Looser's nodes (Milkman's syndrome) due to a raised resistance to vitamin D acquired about the age of 15 years. *Q J Med* 1947;16:33–46.

109. Prader VA, Illig R, Vehlinger E, Stalder G. Rachitis infolge Knochentumors. *Helvetica Paediat Acta* 1959;14:554–65.

110. Ryan EA, Reiss E. Oncogenous osteomalacia: review of the world literature of 42 cases and report of two new cases. *Am J Med* 1984;77:501–12.

111. Yoshikawa S, Kawabata M, Hatsuyama Y, et al. Atypical vitamin-D resistant osteomalacia. *J Bone Joint Surg* 1964;46:998–1007.

112. Case records of the Massachusetts General Hospital. *N Engl J Med* 1965;273:494–504.

113. Salassa RM, Jowsey J, Arnaud CD. Hypophosphatemic osteomalacia associated with "nonendocrine" tumors. *N Engl J Med* 1970;283:65–70.

114. Evans DJ, Azzopardi JG. Distinctive tumours of bone and soft tissue causing acquired vitamin-D-resistant osteomalacia. *Lancet* 1972;1:353–4.

115. Olefsy J, Kempson R, Jones H, Reaven G. "Tertiary" hyperparathyroidism and apparent "cure" of vitamin-D-resistant rickets after removal of an ossifying mesenchymal tumor of the pharynx. *N Engl J Med* 1972;286:740–5.

116. Pollack JA, Schiller AL, Crawford JD. Rickets and myopathy cured by removal of nonossifying fibroma of bone. *Pediatrics* 1973;52:364–71.

117. Moser CR, Fessel WJ. Rheumatic manifestations of hypophosphatemia. *Arch Intern Med* 1974;134:674–8.

118. Willhoite DR. Acquired rickets and solitary bone tumor: the question of a causal relationship. *Clin Orthop* 1975;109:210–1.

119. Renton P, Shaw DG. Hypophosphatemic osteomalacia secondary to vascular tumors of bone and soft tissue. *Skeletal Radiol* 1976;1:21–4.

120. Morita M. A case of adult onset vitamin D resistant osteomalacia associated with soft tissue tumor. *Kotsudaisha (Bone Metab)* 1976;9:286–91.

121. Linovitz RJ, Resnick D, Keissling P, et al. Tumor-induced osteomalacia and rickets: a surgically curable syndrome. Report of two cases. *J Bone Joint Surg* 1976;58:419–23.

122. Wyman AL, Paradinas FJ, Daly JR. Hypophosphatemic osteomalacia associated with a malignant tumor of the tibia: report of a case. *J Clin Pathol* 1977;30:328–35.

123. Yoshikawa S, Nakamura T, Takagi M, et al. Benign osteoblastoma as a cause of osteomalacia. *J Bone Joint Surg* 1977;59:279–86.

124. Aschinberg LC, Solomon LM, Zeis PM, et al. Vitamin D–resistant rickets associated with epidermal nevus syndrome: demonstration of a phosphaturic substance in the dermal lesions. *J Pediatr* 1977;91:56–60.

125. Drezner MK, Feinglos MN. Osteomalacia due to 1,25-dihydroxycholecalciferol deficiency. *J Clin Invest* 1977;60:1046–53.

126. Lejeune E, Bouvier M, Meunier P, et al. L'ostéomalacie des tumeurs mésenchymateuses. *Rev Rhum Mal Osteoartic* 1979;46:187–93.

127. Nortman DF, Coburn JW, Brautbar N, et al. Treatment of mesenchymal tumor associated osteomalacia (MTAO) with $1,25(OH)_2D_3$: report of a case. In: Normal AW, Schaeffer K,

Herrath DV, et al., eds. *Vitamin D, basic research and its clinical application*. Berlin: Walter deGruyter, 1979;1167–8.

128. Wener M, Cohen L, Bar RS, Strottman MP, et al. Regulation of phosphate and calcium metabolism by vitamin D metabolites: studies in a patient with oncogenic osteomalacia. *Arthritis Rheum* 1979;22:672–3.

129. Turner ML, Dalinka MK. Osteomalacia: uncommon causes. *AJR* 1979;133:539–40.

130. Daniels RA, Weisenfeld I. Tumorous phosphaturic osteomalacia. *Am J Med* 1979;67:155–9.

131. Fukumoto Y, Tarui S, Tsukiyama K, et al. Tumor-induced vitamin D–resistant hypophosphatemic osteomalacia associated with proximal renal tubular dysfunction and 1,25-dihydroxyvitamin D deficiency. *J Clin Endocrinol Metab* 1979;49:873–8.

132. Lau K, Stom MC, Goldberg M, et al. Evidence for a humoral phosphaturic factor in oncogenic hypophosphatemic osteomalacia (abstract). *Clin Res* 1979;27:421A.

133. Camus JP, Courzet J, Prier A, et al. Ostéomalacies hypophosphoremiques guèries par l'ablation de tumeurs bénignes du tissu conjonctif. *Ann Med Interne* 1980;131:422–6.

134. Crouzet J, Camus JP, Gatti JM, et al. Ostéomalacie hypophosphoremique et hemangiopéricytome de la voûte du crâne. *Rev Rhum Mal Osteoartic* 1980;47:523–8.

135. Sweet RA, Males JL, Hamstra AJ, DeLuca HF. Vitamin D metabolite levels in oncogenic osteomalacia. *Ann Intern Med* 1980;93:279–80.

136. Chacko V, Joseph B. Osteomalacia associated with haemangiopericytoma. *J Indian Med Assoc* 1981;76:173–5.

137. Nitzan DW, Marmary Y, Azaz B. Mandibular tumor-induced muscular weakness and osteomalacia. *Oral Surg* 1981;52:253–6.

138. Parker MS, Klein I, Haussler MR, Minitz DH. Tumor-induced osteomalacia. *JAMA* 1981;245:492–3.

139. Asnes RS, Berdon WE, Bassett CA. Hypophosphatemic rickets in an adolescent cured by excision of a nonossifying fibroma. *Clin Pediatr* 1981;20:646–8.

140. Hioco J, Chanzy MO, Hioco F, et al. Osteomalacia with mesenchymatous tumors: two new cases (abstr). *Rev Rhum Mal Osteoartic* 1981;special:890.

141. Barcelo P Jr, Asensi E, Paso M, et al. Osteomalacia hipofosforemica secundaria a histiocitoma fibroso vascular (abstr). *Rev Rhum Mal Osteoartic* 1981;special:1352.

142. Popovtzer MM. Tumor-induced hypophosphatemic osteomalacia: evidence for a phosphaturic cyclic AMP–independent action of tumor extract (abstract). *Clin Res* 1981;29:418A.

143. Nomura G, Koshino Y, Morimoto H, et al. Vitamin D resistant hypophosphatemic osteomalacia associated with osteosarcoma of the mandible: report of a case. *Jpn J Med* 1982;21:35–9.

144. Agus ZS. Oncogenic hypophosphatemic osteomalacia. Nephrology Forum, *Kidney Int* 1983;24:113–23.

145. Seshadri MS, Cornish CJ, Mason RS, Posen S. Parathyroid hormone-like bioactivity in tumours from patients with oncogenic osteomalacia. *Clin Endocrinol* 1985;23:689–97.

146. Leehey DJ, Ing TS, Daugirdas JT. Fanconi syndrome associated with a nonossifying fibroma of bone. *Am J Med* 1985;78:708–10.

147. Jefferis AF, Taylor PCA, Walsh-Waring GP. Tumour-associated hypophosphataemic osteomalacia occurring in a patient with an odontogenic tumour of the maxilla. *J Laryngol Otol* 1985;99:1011–7.

148. Firth RG, Grant CS, Riggs BL. Development of hypercalcemic hyperparathyroidism after long-term phosphate supplementation in hypophosphatemic osteomalacia: report of two cases. *Am J Med* 1985;78:669–73.

149. Cotton GE, Van Puffelen P. Hypophosphatemic osteomalacia secondary to neoplasia. *J Bone Joint Surg* 1986;68:129–33.

150. Gitelis S, Ryan WG, Rosenberg AG, Templeton AC. Adult-onset hypophosphatemic osteomalacia secondary to neoplasm. *J Bone Joint Surg* 1986;68:134–8.

151. Ryan WG, Gitelis S, Charters JR. Studies in a patient with tumor-induced hypophosphatemic osteomalacia. *Calcif Tissue Int* 1986;38:358–62.

152. Siris ES, Clemens TL, Dempster DW, et al. Tumor-induced osteomalacia: kinetics of calcium, phosphorus, and vitamin D metabolism and characteristics of bone histomorphometry. *Am J Med* 1987;82:307–12.

153. Reid IR, Teitelbaum SL, Dusso A, Whyte MP. Hypercalcemic hyperparathyroidism complicating oncogenic osteomalacia: effect of successful tumor resection on mineral homeostasis. *Am J Med* 1987;83:350–4.

154. Clinicopathologic conference. Osteomalacia in a 61-year-old man. *Am J Med* 1987;83:509–18.

155. McClure J, Smith PS. Oncogenic osteomalacia. *J Clin Pathol* 1987;40:446–53.

156. Cheng CL, Ma J, Wu PC, et al. Osteomalacia secondary to osteosarcoma: a case report. *J Bone Joint Surg* 1989;71:288–92.

157. Weidner N, Bar RS, Weiss D, Strottman MP. Neoplastic pathology of oncogenic osteomalacia/rickets. *Cancer* 1985;55:1691–1705.

158. Weidner N, Santa Cruz D. Phosphaturic mesenchymal tumors: a polymorphous group causing osteomalacia or rickets. *Cancer* 1987;59:1442–54.

159. Glanville HJ, Bloom R. Case of renal tubular osteomalacia (Dent type 2) with later development of autonomous parathyroid tumors. *Br Med J* 1965;2:26–9.

160. Reiss E, Canterbury JM, Bercovitz MA, Kaplan EL. The role of phosphate in the secretion of parathyroid hormone in man. *J Clin Invest* 1970;49:2146–9.

161. Buyse G, Henry M, Lustman F, Parmentier R. Dysplasie rénale associée a un cancer hépatique métastatique, avec ostéomalacie et phosphaturie. *Eur J Cancer* 1965;1:59–66.

162. Lustman F, Parmentier R, Dustin P. Oncogenic osteomalacia and renal adenomatoid dysplasia (letter). *Ann Intern Med* 1985;102:869–70.

163. Eulderink F. Adenomatoid changes in Bowman's capsule in primary carcinoma of the liver. *J Pathol Bacteriol* 1964;87:251–4.

164. Brazy PC, Lobaugh B, Lyles KW, Drezner MK. The pathogenesis of tumor-induced osteomalacia: a new perspective. In: Frame B, Potts JT, eds. *Clinical disorders of bone and mineral metabolism*. New York: Elsevier, 1983;242.

165. Miyauchi A, Fukase M, Tsutsumi M, Fujita T. Hemangiopericytoma-induced osteomalacia: tumor transplantation in nude mice causes hypophosphatemia and tumor extracts inhibit renal 25-hydroxyvitamin D 1-hydroxylase activity. *J Clin Endocrinol Metab* 1988;67:46–53.

166. Sherwood LM. Hormone production by tumours and multiple endocrine neoplasia. *Med Int* 1981;1:279–84.

167. Lyles KE, Berry WR, Haussler M, et al. Hypophosphatemic osteomalacia: association with prostatic carcinoma. *Ann Intern Med* 1980;93:275–8.

168. Hosking DJ, Chamberlain MJ, Shortland-Webb WR. Osteomalacia and carcinoma of the prostate with major redistribution of skeletal calcium. *Br J Radiol* 1975;48:451–6.

169. Delbarre F, Ghozlan R, Amor B. Métastases osseuses avec ostéomalacie au cours du cancer de la prostate. *Nouv Presse Med* 1975;4:1277–8.

170. Kabadi UM. Osteomalacia associated with prostatic cancer and osteoblastic metastases. *Urology* 1983;21:65–7.

171. Charhon SA, Chapuy MC, Delvin EE, et al. Histomorphometric analysis of sclerotic bone metastases from prostatic carcinoma with special reference to osteomalacia. *Cancer* 1983;51:918–24.

172. Murphy P, Wright G, Rai GS. Hypophosphataemic osteomalacia associated with prostatic carcinoma. *Br Med J* 1985;290:1945.

173. Citrin DL, Elson P, Kies MS, Lind R. Decreased serum phosphate levels after high-dose estrogens in metastatic prostate cancer. *Am J Med* 1984;76:787–93.

174. Valentin-Opran A, Edouard C, Charhon S, Meunier PJ. Histomorphometric analysis of iliac bone metastases of prostatic origin. In: Donatti A, Courvoisier B, eds. *Symposium chemo III: bone and tumors*. Geneve: Medecine et Hygyene, 1980;24–8.

175. Taylor HC, Fallon MD, Velasco ME. Oncogenic osteomalacia and inappropriate antidiuretic hormone secretion due to oat-cell carcinoma. *Ann Intern Med* 1984;101:786–8.

176. Weiss D, Bar RS, Weidner N. Oncogenic osteomalacia (letter). *Ann Intern Med* 1985;102:557.

177. Decaux G, Soupart A, Unger J, Delwiche F. Demeclocycline-induced phosphate diabetes in patients with inappropriate secretion of antidiuretic hormone (letter). *N Engl J Med* 1985;313:1480–1.

178. Rao DS, Parfitt AM, Villanueva AR, et al. Hypophosphatemic osteomalacia and adult Fanconi syndrome due to light-chain ne-

phropathy: another form of oncogenous osteomalacia. *Am J Med* 1987;82:333–8.

179. Harrison JF, Blainey JD. Adult Fanconi syndrome with monoclonal abnormality of immunoglobulin light chain. *J Clin Pathol* 1967;20:42–8.

180. Dedmon RE, West JH, Schwartz TB. The adult Fanconi syndrome: report of two cases, one with multiple myeloma. *Med Clin North Am* 1963;47:191–206.

181. Maldonado JE, Velosa JA, Kyle RA, et al. Fanconi syndrome in adults: a manifestation of a latent form of myeloma. *Am J Med* 1975;58:354–64.

182. Carey DE, Drezner MK, Hamdan JA, et al. Hypophosphatemic rickets/osteomalacia in liner sebaceous nevus syndrome: a variant of tumor-induced osteomalacia. *J Pediatr* 1986;109:994–1000.

183. Moorjani R, Shaw DG. Feuerstein and Mims syndrome with resistant rickets. *Pediatr Radiol* 1976;5:120.

184. Dent CE, Friedman M. Hypophosphataemic osteomalacia with complete recovery. *Br Med J* 1964;1:1676–9.

185. Dent CE, Gertner JM. Hypophosphataemic osteomalacia in fibrous dysplasia. *Q J Med* 1976;45:411–20.

186. Retnam VJ, Ranagnekar DM, Bhandarkar SD. Neurofibromatosis with hypophosphatemic osteomalacia (von Recklinghausen-Hernberg-Edgren-Swann syndrome) (a case report). *J Assoc Physicians India* 1980;28:319–322.

187. Mittal MM, Gupta NC, Sharma ML. Osteomalacia in neurofibromatosis (report of two cases). *J Assoc Physicians India* 1971;19:823–5.

188. Saville PD, Nassim JR, Stevenson FH, et al. Osteomalacia in von Recklinghausen's neurofibromatosis: metabolic study of a case. *Br Med J* 1955;1:1311–3.

189. Hernberg CA, Edgren W. Looser-Milkman's syndrome with neurofibromatosis Recklinghausen and general decalcification of the skeleton. *Acta Med Scand* 1949;136:26–33.

Disorders of Bone and Mineral Metabolism,
edited by Fredric L. Coe and Murray J. Favus,
© 1992 by Raven Press, Ltd. All rights reserved.

CHAPTER 26

Hypercalcemia and Abnormal Vitamin D Metabolism

Daniel P. DeSimone and Norman H. Bell

SARCOIDOSIS

Sarcoidosis is a granulomatous disease that involves multiple organ systems. The disorder occurs most frequently in persons in the middle decades of life. Noncaseating epithelioid granulomas characteristically are found in affected organs, most often lymph nodes, lungs, eyes, and skin, although any tissue may become involved (1,2). The cause of the disease is unknown.

Pathophysiology

Since some 90% of patients with sarcoidosis have intrathoracic lesions that involve the lungs and mediastinal lymph nodes, it is assumed that onset of the disease occurs in the respiratory tract and lymphatic system, possibly as an accumulation of inflammatory cells within the alveolus (3,4). Histologic examination of lung tissue from patients with active sarcoidosis demonstrates large numbers of lymphocytes both on the alveolar surface and within the interstitium (5,6). The granulomas are composed of collections of inflammatory and immune effector cells. During formation of a granuloma, loosely arranged epithelioid cells, which develop from macrophages, are surrounded by a ring of lymphocytes. In older granulomas, large numbers of epithelioid cells occur with giant cells and are surrounded by a few lymphocytes. At the outset of the disease, the number of macrophages, lymphocytes, and monocytes is larger than the number of epithelioid cells, but with maturation of the granuloma, the number of epithelioid cells increases as

the number of macrophages, lymphocytes, and monocytes falls (4). In pulmonary sarcoidosis, almost no granulomas are present when alveolitis is the predominant lesion. On the other hand, when granulomas are the predominant lesion, there is little evidence of alveolitis. Thus alveolitis is believed to be the initial lesion and to precede the development of granulomas.

After granulomas are formed, they either resolve with little or no sequela, or undergo fibrosis. The initial process of fibrosis involves deposition of collagen at the border of the granuloma. This is followed by invasion and eventual destruction of the granuloma and obliteration of the normal architecture of the lung. Pulmonary sarcoidosis either resolves so that little structural damage or impairment of pulmonary function remains, or progresses to fibrosis and development of marked pulmonary insufficiency and cor pulmonale. In general, approximately 80% of patients recover and 20% go on to develop chronic pulmonary disease.

In patients with sarcoidosis and alveolitis, the great majority of lymphocytes within an alveolus are T lymphocytes (5,7), primarily T helper cells (7). During active phases of pulmonary sarcoidosis, there is a marked rise in the number of T lymphocytes (8–11) that is due partly to the synthesis and release of the lymphokine, interleukin-2, a T-lymphocyte growth factor, by the activated T lymphocytes (10,11) and partly to induction by antigen-induced macrophages (11). Antigen-pulsed alveolar macrophages from patients with sarcoidosis were shown to stimulate a greater proliferation of T lymphocytes than similarly pulsed alveolar macrophages from normal subjects. Paradoxically, patients with sarcoidosis have a deficiency of T lymphocytes in the peripheral circulation (5,8). In addition to interleukin-2, a number of other factors are produced by the activated T lymphocytes during active pulmonary sarcoidosis and are thought to

D. P. DeSimone and N. H. Bell: Departments of Orthopaedic Surgery (D.P.D.), Medicine, and Pharmacology (N.H.B.), Medical University of South Carolina, and Veterans Administration Medical Center, Charleston, South Carolina 29403.

be important for the development and the maintenance of the inflammatory process, including macrophage chemotactic factor (12), γ-interferon (13), and leukocyte inhibitory factor (5).

Noncaseating granulomas in sarcoid typically contain multinucleated macrophages. These macrophages are the result of stimulation and fusion of peripheral monocytes by a monocyte chemotactic factor that is released by activated T lymphocytes (12). Monocyte chemotactic factor produced by activated T lymphocytes in the lung attract monocytes from the peripheral circulation. The fact that polymorphonuclear leukocytes are not observed in pulmonary granulomas of sarcoidosis is attributed to leukocyte inhibitory factor that is released by the activated T lymphocytes (5). Serum lysozyme, an enzyme that inhibits neutrophil migration (14), is increased during active sarcoidosis and may contribute to the neutropenia (15).

Hypergammaglobulinemia frequently occurs during active pulmonary sarcoidosis. Enhanced antibody production by pulmonary B lymphocytes is apparently responsible (16). Available evidence indicates that activated T lymphocytes stimulate the differentiation of B lymphocytes into immunoglobulin-producing cells. There is an increase in the number of immunoglobulin-producing B lymphocytes during active pulmonary disease. Further, the percentage of T lymphocytes correlates with the number of IgG-secreting B lymphocytes (17). In contrast, circulating lymphocytes from patients with sarcoidosis were found not to release increased amounts of immunoglobulins even though hypergammaglobulinemia was present in the peripheral circulation (15). It is evident, therefore, that the excess gamma globulin that appears in the circulation is produced by stimulated B lymphocytes in the lung.

Pathogenesis of Abnormal Vitamin D Metabolism

Hypercalcemia sometimes occurs in patients with active pulmonary sarcoidosis and results from increased circulating 1,25-dihydroxyvitamin D[1,25(OH)$_2$D] (18,19) (Table 1). The first indication of an extrarenal source of 1,25(OH)$_2$D was the demonstration of increased circulating 1,25(OH)$_2$D, hypercalcemia, and suppression of serum immunoreactive parathyroid hormone in an anephric patient with sarcoidosis (20). It was later found that cultured alveolar macrophages from the bronchoalveolar lavage of patients with sarcoidosis converted [H^3]25(OH)$_2$D$_3$ to [H^3]1,25(OH)$_2$D$_3$ (21–24). The structure of the 1,25(OH)$_2$D$_3$ that was synthesized by the sarcoid alveolar macrophages was confirmed by mass spectroanalysis (22). Kinetic analysis of synthesis of 1,25(OH)$_2$D by pulmonary alveolar macrophages demonstrated K_m values similar to those obtained with mammalian renal tissue, including mouse kidney homoge-

TABLE 1. *Hypercalcemia and abnormal vitamin D metabolism*

INCREASED CIRCULATING 1,25-DIHYDROXYVITAMIN D

Granulomatous diseases
Sarcoidosis
Tuberculosis
Disseminated candidiasis
Leprosy
Silicone-induced granulomas
Rheumatoid arthritis

Lymphoma and solid tumors
T-cell leukemia
Lymphoma
Histiocytic lymphoma
Plasma cell granuloma
Hodgkins disease
Leiomyoblastoma
Seminoma

Miscellaneous
Hypercalcemia of infancy
Idiopathic
Calcitriol intoxication

INCREASED CIRCULATING 25-HYDROXYVITAMIN D

Calcitriol intoxication

nates (25), mouse renal cells (26), rat renal cortical cells (27), and partially purified 25(OH)D-1α-hydroxylase from rat kidney (28). Production of 1,25(OH)$_2$D in the system was enhanced in a dose-dependent fashion by γ-interferon (23,24). γ-Interferon is produced spontaneously by activated T lymphocytes and alveolar macrophages in active sarcoidosis (13). These findings provide evidence that γ-interferon plays a major role in the pathogenesis of extrarenal synthesis of 1,25(OH)$_2$D.

Whereas synthesis of 1,25(OH)$_2$D by the pulmonary alveolar macrophages and mammalian kidney show some similarities, 25(OH)D-1α-hydroxylase from the sarcoid macrophages differs from the renal enzyme in a number of important respects. In contrast to renal 25(OH)D-24-hydroxylase, 25(OH)D-24-hydroxylase in the alveolar macrophage is stimulated only at very high concentrations of 1,25(OH)$_2$D$_3$ (24). Unlike mammalian renal cells (25–29), little inhibition of 25(OH)D-1α-hydroxylase activity occurs in response to 1,25(OH)$_2$D$_3$ in pulmonary alveolar macrophages (24). Synthesis of the metabolite is markedly diminished by the addition of dexamethasone directly to the in vitro system, and inhibition is dose dependent (23,24). These in vitro studies help to account for the clinical observations that serum 1,25(OH)$_2$D in sarcoid patients is not well regulated and is reduced by glucocorticoids (18–20,30).

Receptors for 1,25(OH)$_2$D are present in activated peripheral T lymphocytes from normal human subjects (31). 1,25(OH)$_2$D was shown to inhibit the proliferation and to suppress interleukin-2 activity (32) and γ-interferon synthesis (33) by phytohemagglutinin-stimulated human peripheral lymphocytes. $1,25(OH)_2D$ was found to inhibit activated T-helper lymphocyte activity from normal human subjects in vitro (34). If receptors for $1,25(OH)_2D$ are present in activated pulmonary lymphocytes and if $1,25(OH)_2D$ inhibits the production of γ-interferon and the proliferation of activated T-cells in granulomas of patients with sarcoidosis, production of $1,25(OH)_2D$ by alveolar macrophages could provide a compensatory mechanism mounted by the immune system to inhibit the inflammatory process.

Pathogenesis of Abnormal Calcium Metabolism

Regardless of the potential role of $1,25(OH)_2D$ in the modulation of inflammation, it is evident that granulomas provide a nonrenal source of $1,25(OH)_2D$. It is this production of $1,25(OH)_2D$ by the sarcoid granuloma that is responsible for the abnormal vitamin D and mineral metabolism that occurs in sarcoidosis (20). Among the changes in calcium metabolism are increases in serum and urinary calcium and enhanced intestinal absorption of calcium, as shown by balance studies and measurement of calcium absorption with radiolabeled calcium (35–38). Patients with active sarcoidosis have marked increases in calcium turnover similar to changes observed in normal subjects and in patients with hypoparathyroidism who were given pharmacologic doses of vitamin D (39,40). Hypercalcemia and hypercalciuria occur spontaneously in patients with active sarcoidosis and are produced by small doses of vitamin D that are without effect in normal subjects (35–37) as well as by brief exposure to ultraviolet light (41). The importance of ultraviolet radiation in the pathogenesis of abnormal vitamin D and mineral metabolism in this disease is underscored by the seasonal incidence of hypercalcemia that usually occurs in the summer (42) and by demonstration that abnormal calcium metabolism is reversed by omission of vitamin D from the diet and prevention of exposure to ultraviolet light (43).

Normocalcemic patients with sarcoidosis also may have abnormal calcium metabolism (44,45). Studies with radiolabeled calcium showed increased intestinal absorption of calcium, and the increases significantly correlated with increased excretion of calcium. Therefore, hypercalciuria may be present in sarcoidosis in the absence of hypercalcemia and results from an increase in calcium absorption via the intestine (44,45). Since increases in urinary hydroxyproline, an index of bone resorption, occur in sarcoidosis (46), some of the excess urinary calcium may originate from the skeleton.

Hypercalciuria is found more frequently in sarcoidosis than hypercalcemia (44,47). Hypercalcemia probably occurs in less than 10% and clinically important hypercalcemia probably occurs in less than 5% of patients with sarcoidosis (42). The true incidence, however, is difficult to establish because seasonal variations of serum and urinary calcium occur even in normal subjects. These changes result from seasonal variation in circulating $25(OH)D$ and $1,25(OH)_2D$ as a result of differences in duration of exposure to sunlight and dermal production of vitamin D_3. In addition, urinary calcium varies with race and body habitus. Normal black subjects, both obese and nonobese, and obese white subjects were found to have secondary hyperparathyroidism with increases in circulating $1,25(OH)_2D$ and urinary cyclic adenosine $3',5'$-monophosphate and decreases in urinary calcium as compared to nonobese white men and women (48–50).

As mentioned previously, enhanced intestinal absorption of calcium, hypercalcemia, and hypercalciuria in sarcoidosis are caused by increased circulating $1,25(OH)_2D$ that is produced by the granuloma (18–20,30,51). Values are either inappropriately increased or at the upper range of normal in hypercalcemic patients, and serum immunoreactive parathyroid hormone is either suppressed or in the low-normal range (18–20,30,51,52).

When normocalcemic patients with sarcoidosis and a previous history of hypercalcemia were administered small doses of vitamin D, 10,000 IU a day for 12 days, both serum $1,25(OH)_2D$ and urinary calcium increased (18). This dose of vitamin D did not alter serum $1,25(OH)_2D$ or urinary calcium in normal subjects or in patients with normal calcium metabolism. Larger doses of vitamin D, 100,000 IU a day for 4 days, increased serum $1,25(OH)_2D$ and serum calcium in normocalcemic patients with sarcoidosis who did not have a history of abnormal calcium metabolism but did not change the serum $1,25(OH)_2D$ or serum calcium in normal subjects (53). This defect in regulation of circulating $1,25(OH)_2D$ in response to vitamin D challenge provides the mechanism for the increased sensitivity to vitamin D that is characteristic of this disorder.

It is now well established that in the northern hemisphere patients with active sarcoidosis develop increases in serum $1,25(OH)_2D$ and hypercalcemia during the summer months (18,19,30). Increases in the dermal production of vitamin D_3 as a result of longer exposure to sunlight accounts for the seasonal variation in serum calcium in these patients (42). This takes place because, as indicated earlier, $1,25(OH)_2D$ production is not regulated in sarcoidosis, so that the concentration of $1,25(OH)_2D$ is more likely to be influenced by the concentration of its precursor, $25(OH)D$. Seasonal variation in serum $25(OH)D$, serum $1,25(OH)_2D$ (54), and urinary calcium (55) occur in normal subjects because of differences in time of exposure to ultraviolet light during the daylight hours.

Abnormal elevation of serum $1,25(OH)_2D$ was found in normocalcemic patients with sarcoidosis (44,45). In these individuals, increased fractional intestinal absorption of calcium was present in association with hypercalciuria (45). In patients with sarcoidosis, hypercalcemia develops when there is some degree of renal insufficiency, specifically when the ability of the kidney to excrete the excess calcium from the increased intestinal absorption or skeletal release of calcium is diminished (18). In sarcoidosis, hypercalcemia varies directly with calcium intake (36,37) and can be prevented or corrected by dietary restriction of calcium.

Clinical Findings

Clinical signs and symptoms caused by abnormal calcium metabolism can be grouped according to organ systems: gastrointestinal tract, kidney, and central nervous system. Anorexia, nausea, and vomiting can lead to dehydration and marked loss of weight. Nephrogenic diabetes insipidus with polydipsia, polyuria, and nocturia can be caused by hypercalcemia and hypercalciuria (56). When abnormal calcium metabolism is corrected, the renal concentrating defect improves. Renal stones may produce renal colic, hematuria, urgency, and frequency. Nephrocalcinosis and nephrolithiasis may lead to pyelonephritis and subsequent impairment of renal function. Hypercalcemia may cause no symptoms or produce malaise, muscle weakness, easy fatigability, lethargy, and if severe and extensive, may cause a variety of mental disturbances leading ultimately to coma. In sarcoidosis, the concentration of the serum calcium rarely exceeds 14 or 15 ng/dL and the elevated serum calcium is almost never associated with hypercalcemic crisis.

Treatment

Patients should be given forced fluids and a low-calcium diet and avoid sunlight. Glucocorticoids regularly reduce circulating $1,25(OH)_2D$ and correct the abnormal calcium metabolism in sarcoidosis (18–20,30,51). The dose required must be determined by trial and error in the individual patient. Prednisone and other drugs appear to act by inhibiting inflammation and the production of γ-interferon and $1,25(OH)_2D$ by granulomas (13,21) and usually are effective within a week or so.

More recently, chloroquine and hydroxychloroquine were shown to be effective in correcting the abnormal vitamin D and mineral metabolism (57–60). In one patient, chloroquine was found to lower the elevated serum $1,25(OH)_2D$ and serum calcium to normal values within 3 weeks (60). Thus these drugs provide an alternative means for treatment of patients in whom glucocorticoids may be contraindicated.

In addition to causing hypertension, diabetes mellitus, and poor wound healing, glucocorticoids are known to cause bone loss. Patients with sarcoidosis may be particularly susceptible in this regard (61). The toxic effect of greatest concern with chloroquine and hydroxychloroquine is loss of central visual acuity with granular pigmentation of the macula and constriction of the retinal artery (59). These complications, however, are related to the total accumulated dose and patients should be followed with periodic ophthalmologic examinations so that the drug can be stopped if retinal changes or alterations in visual acuity develop.

TUBERCULOSIS

Pathogenesis

Hypercalcemia and hypercalciuria are frequently encountered in pulmonary tuberculosis (61–69). Recent studies indicate that from 10 to 28% of patients with tuberculosis have abnormal calcium metabolism. Hypercalcemia and hypercalciuria are associated with suppression of immunoreactive parathyroid hormone. As occurs in sarcoidosis, patients with tuberculosis are sensitive to vitamin D, and hypercalcemia is corrected by glucocorticoids (61,63,67). Hypercalcemia in pulmonary tuberculosis appears to be caused by increasing circulating $1,25(OH)_2D$ (68,70). Further, regulation of serum $1,25(OH)_2D$ is abnormal in normocalcemic patients with pulmonary tuberculosis (71). Modest but significant increases in serum $1,25(OH)_2D$ occurred in 11 patients given vitamin D, 100,000 IU a day for 4 days. No change in the serum $1,25(OH)_2D$ was observed in normal subjects. The findings provide evidence that the abnormalities of vitamin D metabolism and calcium metabolism in pulmonary tuberculosis are similar to those that occur in sarcoidosis.

Despite of the apparent similarity in the pathogenesis of hypercalcemia and hypercalciuria in tuberculosis and sarcoidosis, distinct differences in the presentation, clinical course, and prognosis of aberrant calcium metabolism in the two disorders are evident. In sarcoidosis, hypercalcemia occurs following exposure to ultraviolet light during the summer, and patients are often hypercalcemic at the time of presentation. The hypercalcemia and hypercalciuria may be protracted, require treatment with glucocorticoids, and be associated with complications that included renal lithiasis, nephrocalcinosis, urinary tract infections, and chronic renal failure which eventually may lead to death (18,19,30,51). Thus the prognosis for hypercalcemia associated with sarcoidosis is guarded. In contrast, hypercalcemia in pulmonary tuberculosis usually does not occur until after several months of treatment with antituberculosis drugs. Patients usually respond to hydration, so that treatment with glucocorticoids is not necessary and renal impairment is only transient or minimal. The prognosis for calcium metabolism in these two pulmonary diseases is quite different.

Recent studies showed (1) that the concentration of γ-interferon is increased in fluid from pleural effusions of patients with tuberculous pleuritis, (2) that the capacity of fluid to stimulate synthesis of $1,25(OH)_2D_3$ by cultured pulmonary alveolar macrophages from patients with sarcoidosis varies directly with the concentration of γ-interferon, and (3) that production of $1,25(OH)_2D_3$ in response to the pleural fluid is inhibited by a monoclonal antibody to γ-interferon (72). Further, in patients with tuberculous pleuritis concentrations of $1,25(OH)_2D$ were higher in pleural fluid than in peripheral blood (73). These results support the concept that γ-interferon plays a major, if not sole role in the modulation of enhanced production of $1,25(OH)_2D$ by macrophages from patients with tuberculous pleuritis. Thus the pathogenesis of the abnormal vitamin D and calcium metabolism in sarcoidosis and tuberculosis is quite similar.

Treatment

Hypercalcemia in patients with pulmonary tuberculosis is often mild and can be treated by forcing fluids. If severe, however, it may require treatment with glucocorticoids. Under these circumstances, patients should be given a low-calcium diet.

OTHER GRANULOMATOUS DISEASES

There are a number of diseases that are characterized by the formation of granulomas. These include histoplasmosis (74), disseminated coccidiomycosis (75), disseminated candidiasis (76), leprosy (77), silicone-induced granulomas (78), and berylliosis (79). Patients with disseminated candidiasis, leprosy, and silicone-induced granulomas were found to have hypercalcemia and increased serum $1,25(OH)_2D$. The abnormal vitamin D and calcium metabolism were corrected by treatment with salmon calcitonin, saline, furosemide, and mithramycin in the patient with disseminated candidiasis (76) and by prednisone in the patients with leprosy (77) and silicone-induced granulomas (78). The etiology of the abnormal mineral metabolism in the other granulomatous diseases has not been determined. Hypercalcemia caused by increased circulating $1,25(OH)_2D$ was reported in a patient with a squamous cell carcinoma of the lung surrounded by noncaseating epithelioid granulomas (80). The biochemical abnormalities were corrected by removal of the tumor. In addition to aberrant vitamin D metabolism, there may be other mechanisms for abnormal mineral metabolism. For example, one patient with hypercalcemia and disseminated coccidiomycosis (81) and another patient with hypercalcemia and leprosy (82) were reported with marked

decreases in serum $1,25(OH)_2D$. Hypercalcemia, hypercalciuria, and suppression of serum immunoreactive parathyroid hormone caused by increased circulating $1,25(OH)_2D$ was found in a patient with rheumatoid arthritis (83). In this patient there was lack of regulation of serum $1,25(OH)_2D$ in response to small doses of vitamin D, and the elevated serum calcium and serum $1,25(OH)_2D$ were reduced by prednisone. It is not yet established whether the abnormal metabolism of vitamin D in this patient is related to the rheumatoid arthritis.

LYMPHOMA AND SOLID TUMORS

Hypercalcemia associated with a suppression of the serum immunoreactive parathyroid hormone and increases in serum $1,25(OH)_2D$ was found in patients with T-cell leukemia (84,85), lymphoma (84–86), histiocytic lymphoma (84,86), Hodgkin's disease (85–90), plasma cell granuloma (91), and B-cell lymphoma (85,92,93). The hypercalcemia is reversed by glucocorticoids. Hypercalcemia in one patient with histiocytic lymphoma was associated with hyperabsorption of calcium (84). T-cell lymphoma caused by human T-cell lymphotrophic virus (HTLV-I) is associated with hepatosplenomegaly, hypercalcemia, lymphocytosis, and has a rapidly progressive course (94). One patient with the disease had hypercalcemia caused by increased circulating $1,25(OH)_2D$ (84). Other patients with T-cell leukemia were found to have hypercalcemia and suppressed circulating $1,25-(OH)_2D$ (95). These results indicate that the hypercalcemia in these patients was not caused by abnormal vitamin D metabolism.

Human T-lymphocytes from the cord blood of normal infants infected with HTLV-I by incubation of lymphocytes with lymphoma cells carrying the virus secrete HTLV-I proteins and exhibit morphologic and functional properties of the lymphoma cells (96,97). Lymphocytes from cord blood transformed in such a manner were shown to convert $[^3H]25(OH)D_3$ to $[^3H]1,25-(OH)_2D_3$ (98). The putative $1,25(OH)_2D_3$ caused release of ^{45}Ca from long bones of fetal rats in tissue culture, displaced the $[^3H]1,25(OH)_2D_3$ from receptors of rat osteosarcoma cells and had the same retention time as authentic $1,25(OH)_2D_3$ on high-pressure liquid chromatography in a number of different solvent systems. The specific identity of the metabolite was confirmed as $1,25(OH)_2D_3$ by mass spectroanalysis (98). It remains to be demonstrated, however, that lymphocytes from patients with lymphoma produce $1,25(OH)_2D$.

Hypercalcemia caused by increased serum $1,25-(OH)_2D$ was reported in a patient with metastatic leiomyoblastoma of the jejunum (99). Although no skeletal lesions were detected, moderate renal insufficiency developed and the abnormal vitamin D and calcium metabolism persisted despite a subtotal parathyroidectomy. The hypercalcemia and abnormally elevated 1,25-$(OH)_2D$ were corrected by treatment with prednisone, phenytoin, and phenobarbital. Hypercalcemia and increasing circulating $1,25(OH)_2D$ was reported in a patient with seminoma (100). The abnormal findings were reversed by partial resection of the tumor and chemotherapy.

A metabolite of vitamin D was tentatively identified as $1,24(OH)_2D_3$ and was obtained from extracts of serum from the small cell carcinoma of the lung in a patient with hypercalcemia (101). The steroid comigrated with authentic $1,25(OH)_2D_3$ on high-performance liquid chromatography and displaced tritiated $1,25(OH)_2D_3$ bound to chicken intestinal receptor in a manner quite similar to the authentic sterol. Additionally, the two compounds showed identical biologic activity and produced release of ^{45}Ca from mouse calvarial tissue culture. This information provides direct evidence that hypercalcemia, at least in this particular patient, resulted from increased production of $1,25(OH)_2D_3$. This important finding is the first indication that an endogenously produced sterol other than $1,24(OH)_2D$ may be responsible for the clinically apparent abnormal calcium metabolism.

HYPERCALCEMIA OF INFANCY

The William's syndrome is sometimes associated with hypercalcemia. In this syndrome, infants are found with supravalvular aortic stenosis, mental retardation, elfin-like facies, in association with a number of other congenital defects (102–112). White children with the syndrome have been shown to have an exaggerated increase in serum 25(OH)D after vitamin D challenge when compared to normal children (113). This could be attributed to a decrease in serum $1,25(OH)_2D$ in patients and diminished clearance of circulating 25(OH)D (114,115). Increased serum $1,25-(OH)_2D$ was observed in four infants with hypercalcemia and an associated elfin facies (116). This hypercalcemia was successfully treated with a low-calcium diet. Another child with hypercalcemia demonstrated abnormally low serum $1,25(OH)_2D$ (112), indicating that the hypercalcemia in the syndrome of hypercalcemia of infancy may result not only from an elevation of circulating $1,25(OH)_2D$ but from other causes as well. In infants with abnormal elevation of circulating $1,25(OH)_2D$, the source of the metabolite is unknown. Hydration, glucocorticoid administration, and restriction of calcium intake are all effective means of treating children with hypercalcemia and abnormally low vitamin D metabolism (105,107,116).

VITAMIN D INTOXICATION

Hypercalcemia and hypercalciuria that are corrected by glucocorticoid administration and are associated with suppression of immunoreactive parathyroid hormone and urinary cyclic AMP occur in overdoses of vitamin D (117). In patients with vitamin D intoxication, the abnormal calcium metabolism is caused by excessive circulating 25(OH)D and not $1,25(OH)_2D$. The diagnosis of vitamin D intoxication is made by a history of excessive intake of vitamin D and is confirmed by the finding of a markedly elevated serum 25(OH)D, 200 ng/mL or higher (117,118). Abnormal calcium metabolism can be treated by hydration and glucocorticoids (117).

REFERENCES

1. Sharma OP. *Sarcoidosis: clinical management.* London: Butterworth, 1984;22–124.
2. James DG, Williams WJ. *Sarcoidosis and other granulomatous disorders.* Philadelphia: WB Saunders, 1985;38–162.
3. Takahashi M. Histopathology of sarcoidosis and its immunological basis. *Acta Pathol Jpn* 1970;20:171–82.
4. Rosen Y, Athanassiades TJ, Moon S, et al. Nongranulomatous interstitial pneumonitis in sarcoidosis: relationship to the development of epithelioid granulomas. *Chest* 1978;74:122–5.
5. Hunninghake GW, Fulmer JD, Yound RC, et al. Localization of the immune response in sarcoidosis. *Am Rev Respir Dis* 1979;120:49–57.
6. Weinberger SE, Kelman JA, Elson NA, et al. Bronchoalveolar lavage in interstitial lung disease. *Ann Intern Med* 1978;89:459–66.
7. Hunninghake GW, Crystal RG. Pulmonary sarcoidosis: a disorder mediated by excess helper T-lymphocyte activity at sites of disease activity. *N Engl J Med* 1981;305:429–34.
8. Daniele R, Dauber JH, Rossman MD. Immunologic abnormalities in sarcoidosis. *Ann Intern Med* 1980;92:406–16.
9. Hunninghake GW, Bedell GN, Zavala DC, et al. Role of interleukin-2 release by lung T-cells in active pulmonary sarcoidosis. *Am Rev Respir Dis* 1983;128:634–8.
10. Pinkston P, Bitterman PB, Crystal RG. Spontaneous release of interleukin-2 by lung T-lymphocytes in active pulmonary sarcoidosis. *N Engl J Med* 1983;308:793–800.
11. Venet A, Hance AJ, Saltini C, et al. Enhanced alveolar macrophage-mediated antigen-induced T lymphocyte proliferation in sarcoidosis. *J Clin Invest* 1985;75:293–301.
12. Hunninghake GW, Gadek JE, Young RC Jr. Maintenance of granuloma formation in pulmonary sarcoidosis by T lymphocytes within the lung. *N Engl J Med* 1980;302:594–8.
13. Robinson BWS, McLemore TL, Crystal RG. Gamma interferon is spontaneously released by alveolar macrophages and lung T lymphocytes in patients with pulmonary sarcoidosis. *J Clin Invest* 1985;72:1488–95.
14. Gordton LI, Douglas SD, Kay NE, et al. Modulation of neutrophil function by lysozyme: potential feedback system of inflammation. *J Clin Invest* 1979;64:226–32.
15. Gee JB, Godel PT, Zorn SK, et al. Sarcoidosis and mononuclear phagocytes. *Lung* 1978;155:243–53.
16. Hunninghake GW, Crystal RG. Mechanisms of hypergammaglobulinemia in pulmonary sarcoidosis: site of increased antibody production and role of T lymphocytes. *J Clin Invest* 1981;67:86–92.
17. Katz P, Fauci AS. Inhibition of polyclonal B-cell activation of suppressor monocytes in patients with sarcoidosis. *Clin Exp Immunol* 1978;32:554–62.
18. Bell NH, Stern PH, Pantzer E, et al. Evidence that increased circulating $1\alpha,25$-dihydroxyvitamin D is the probable cause for abnormal calcium metabolism in sarcoidosis. *J Clin Invest* 1979;64:218–25.
19. Papapoulos SE, Clemens TL, Fraher LJ, et al. 1,25-Dihydroxycholecalciferol in the pathogenesis of the hypercalcemia of sarcoid. *Lancet* 1979;1:627–30.
20. Barbour GL, Coburn JW, Slatopolsky E, et al. Hypercalcemia in an anephric patient with sarcoidosis: evidence for extrarenal gen-

eration of 1,25-dihydroxyvitamin D₃. *New Engl J Med* 1981;305:440–3.

21. Adams JS, Sharma OP, Gacad MA, et al. Metabolism of 25-hydroxyvitamin D₃ by cultured pulmonary alveolar macrophages in sarcoidosis. *J Clin Invest* 1983;72:1856–60.

22. Adams JS, Singer FR, Gacad MA, et al. Isolation and structural identification of 1,25-dihydroxyvitamin D₃ produced by cultured alveolar macrophages in sarcoidosis. *J Clin Endocrinol Metab* 1985;60:960–6.

23. Adams JS, Gacad MA. Characterization of 1α-hydroxylation of vitamin D₃ sterols by cultured alveolar macrophages from patients with sarcoidosis. *J Exp Med* 1985;161:755–65.

24. Reichel H, Koeffler HP, Barbers R, Norman AW. Regulation of 1,25-dihydroxyvitamin D₃ production by cultured alveolar macrophages from normal human donors and from patients with pulmonary sarcoidosis. *J Clin Endocrinol Metab* 1987; 65:1201–9.

25. Fukase M, Avioli LV, Birge SJ, et al. Abnormal regulation of 25-hydroxyvitamin D₃-1α-hydroxylase activity by calcium and calcitonin in renal cortex from hypophosphatemic (Hyp) mice. *Endocrinology* 1984;114:1203–7.

26. Fukase MS, Birge SJ Jr, Rifas L, et al. Regulation of 25-hydroxyvitamin D₃-1α-hydroxylase in serum-free monolayer cultures of mouse kidney. *Endocrinology* 1982;110:1073–5.

27. Turner RT, Bottemiller BL, Howard GA, et al. In vitro metabolism of 25-hydroxyvitamin D₃ by isolated rat kidney cells. *Proc Natl Acad Sci USA* 1980;77:1537–40.

28. Warner M. Catalytic activity of partially purified renal 25-hydroxyvitamin D hydroxylases from vitamin D-deficient and vitamin D-replete rats. *J Biol Chem* 1982;257:12995–13000.

29. Omdahl JL. Modulation of kidney 25-hydroxyvitamin D₃ metabolism by 1α,25-dihydroxyvitamin D₃ in thyroparathyroidectomized rats. *Life Sci* 1976;19:1943–8.

30. Koide Y, Kugai N, Kimura S, et al. Increased 1,25-dihydroxycholecalciferol as a cause of abnormal calcium metabolism in sarcoidosis. *J Clin Endocrinol Metab* 1981;52:494–8.

31. Provvedini DM, Tsoukas CD, Deftos LJ, et al. 1,25-Dihydroxyvitamin D₃ receptors in human leukocytes. *Science* 1983; 221:1181–3.

32. Tsoukas CD, Provvedini DM, Monalagas SC. 1,25-Dihydroxyvitamin D₃: a novel immunoregulatory hormone. *Science* 1984;224:1438–40.

33. Reichel H, Koeffler HP, Tobler A, Norman AW. 1α,25-Dihydroxyvitamin D₃ inhibits γ-interferon synthesis by normal human peripheral blood lymphocytes. *Proc Natl Acad Sci USA* 1987;84:3385–9.

34. Lemire JM, Adams JS, Kermani-Arab V, et al. 1,25-Dihydroxyvitamin D₃ suppresses human T helper/inducer lymphocyte activity in vitro. *J Immunol* 1985;134:3032–5.

35. Anderson J, Dent CE, Harper C, Philpott GR. Effect of cortisone on calcium metabolism in sarcoidosis with hypercalcemia, possible antagonistic actions of cortisone and vitamin D. *Lancet* 1954;2:720–4.

36. Henneman PH, Dempsey EF, Carroll EL, Albright F. The cause of hypercalciuria in sarcoid and its treatment with cortisone and sodium phytate. *J Clin Invest* 1956;35:1229–42.

37. Bell NH, Gill JR Jr, Bartter FC. On the abnormal calcium metabolism in sarcoidosis: evidence for increased sensitivity to vitamin D. *Am J Med* 1964;36:500–13.

38. Bell NH, Bartter FC. Studies of ⁴⁷Ca metabolism in sarcoidosis: evidence for increased sensitivity of bone to vitamin D. *Acta Endocrinol* 1967;54:173–80.

39. Bell NH, Bartter, FC. The effect of vitamin D on Ca⁴⁷ metabolism in man. *Trans Assoc Am Physicians* 1963;76:163–75.

40. Bell NH, Bartter FC. Studies of ⁴⁷Ca metabolism in sarcoidosis: evidence for increased sensitivity of bone to vitamin D. *Acta Endocrinol* 1967;54:173–80.

41. Dent CE. Calcium metabolism in sarcoidosis. *Postgrad Med J* 1970;46:471–3.

42. Taylor RL, Lynch HJ, Wysor WG Jr. Seasonal influence of sunlight on the hypercalcemia of sarcoidosis. *Am J Med* 1963;34:221–7.

43. Hendrix JZ. Abnormal skeletal mineral metabolism in sarcoidosis. *Ann Intern Med* 1966;64:797–805.

44. Reiner M, Sigurdsson G, Nunziata MA, et al. Abnormal calcium metabolism in normocalcaemic sarcoidosis. *Br Med J* 1976;2:1473–6.

45. Zerwekh JE, Pak CYC, Kaplan RA, et al. Pathogenetic role of 1α-25-dihydroxyvitamin D in sarcoidosis and absorptive hypercalciuria: different response to prednisolone therapy. *J Clin Endocrinol Metab* 1980;51:381–6.

46. Studdy PR, Bird R, Neville E, et al. Biochemical findings in sarcoidosis. *J Clin Pathol* 1980;33:528–33.

47. Goldstein RA, Israel HL, Becker KL, Moore CF. The infrequency of hypercalcemia in sarcoidosis. *Am J Med* 1971;51:21–30.

48. Bell NH, Greene A, Epstein S, et al. Evidence for alteration of the vitamin D-endocrine system in blacks. *J Clin Invest* 1985; 76:470–3.

49. Bell NH, Epstein S, Greene A, et al. Evidence for alteration of the vitamin D-endocrine system in obese subjects. *J Clin Invest* 1985;76:370–3.

50. Epstein S, Bell NH, Shary J, Shaw S, Greene A, Oexmann MJ. Evidence that obesity does not influence the vitamin D-endocrine system in blacks. *J Bone Miner Res* 1986;1:181–4.

51. Sandler LM, Winearls CG, Fraher LJ, et al. Studies of the hypercalcemia of sarcoidosis: effect of steroids and exogenous vitamin D₃ on the circulating concentration of 1,25-dihydroxyvitamin D. *Q J Med* 1984;210:165–80.

52. Cushard WG Jr, Simon AB, Canterbury JM, et al. Parathyroid function in sarcoidosis. *New Engl J Med* 1972;286:395–8.

53. Stern PH, DeOlazabal J, Bell NH. Evidence for abnormal regulation of circulating 1α,25-dihydroxyvitamin D in patients with sarcoidosis and normal calcium metabolism. *J Clin Invest* 1980;66:852–5.

54. Juttmann JR, Visser TJ, Buurman C, et al. Seasonal fluctuations in serum concentrations of vitamin D metabolites in normal subjects. *Br Med J* 1981;282:1349–52.

55. Morgan DB, Rivlin RS, Davis RH. Seasonal changes in the urinary excretion of calcium. *Am J Clin Nutr* 1972;25:652–4.

56. Gill JR Jr, Bartter FC. On the impairment of renal concentrating ability in prolonged hypercalcemia and hypercalciuria in man. *J Clin Invest* 1961;40:716–21.

57. O'Leary TJ, Jones G, Yip A, et al. The effects of chloroquine on serum 1,25-dihydroxyvitamin D and calcium metabolism in sarcoidosis. *N Engl J Med* 1986;315:727–30.

58. Barre PE, Gascon-Barre M, Meakins JL, Goltzman D. Hydroxychloroquine treatment of hypercalcemia in a patient with sarcoidosis undergoing hemodialysis. *Am J Med* 1987;82:1259–62.

59. DeSimone DP, Brilliant HL, Basile J, Bell NH. Granulomatous infiltration of the talus and abnormal vitamin D and calcium metabolism in a patient with sarcoidosis: successful treatment with hydroxychloroquine. *Am J Med.* 1989;87:694.

60. Adams JS, Diz MM, Sharma OP. Effective reduction in the serum 1,25-dihydroxyvitamin D and calcium concentration in sarcoidosis-associated hypercalcemia with short-course chloroquine therapy. *Ann Intern Med* 1989;111:437–8.

61. Rizzato G, Tosi G, Mella C, et al. Researching osteoporosis in prednisone treated sarcoid patients. *Sarcoidosis* 1987;4:45–8.

62. Shai F, Baker RK, Addrizzo JR, et al. Hypercalcemia in mycobacterial infection. *J Clin Endocrinol Metab* 1972;34:251–6.

63. Bradley GW, Sterling GM. Hypercalcaemia and hypokalaemia in tuberculosis. *Thorax* 1978;33:464–7.

64. Abbasi AA, Chemplavil JK, Farah S, et al. Hypercalcemia in active pulmonary tuberculosis. *Ann Intern Med* 1979;90:324–8.

65. Need AG, Phillips PJ, Chiu FTS, et al. Hypercalcemia associated with tuberculosis. *Br Med J* 1980;1:831.

66. Kitrou MP, Phytou-Pallikari A, Tzannes SE, et al. Hypercalcemia in active pulmonary tuberculosis. *Ann Intern Med* 1982;96:55.

67. Sharma OP, Lamon J, Winsor D. Hypercalcemia and tuberculosis (letter). *JAMA* 1972;222:582.

68. Braman SS, Goldman AL, Schwarz MI. Steroid-responsive hypercalcemia in disseminated bone tuberculosis. *Arch Intern Med* 1973;132:269–71.

69. Bell NH, Shary J, Shaw S, et al. Hypercalcemia associated with increased circulating 1,25-dihydroxyvitamin D in a patient with pulmonary tuberculosis. *Calc Tissue Int* 1985;37:588–91.

70. Gkonos PJ, London R, Hendler ED. Hypercalcemia and elevated 1,25-dihydroxyvitamin D levels in a patient with end-stage renal disease and active tuberculosis. *N Engl J Med* 1984;311:1683–5.

71. Epstein S, Stern PH, Bell NH, et al. Evidence for abnormal regulation of circulating 1α,25-dihydroxyvitamin D in patients with pulmonary tuberculosis and normal calcium metabolism. *Calc Tissue Int* 1984;36:54–554.

72. Adams JS, Modlin RL, Diz MM, Barnes PF. Potentiation of the macrophage 25-hydroxyvitamin D-1-hydroxylation reaction by human tuberculous pleural effusion fluid. *J Clin Endocrinol Metab* 1989;69:457–60.

73. Barnes PF, Modlin RL, Bikle DD, Adams JS. Transpleural gradient of 1,25-dihydroxyvitamin D in tuberculous pleuritis. *J Clin Invest* 1989;83:1527–32.

74. Walker JV, Baran D, Yakub YN, et al. Histoplasmosis with hypercalcemia, renal failure and papillary necrosis. *J Am Med Assoc* 1977;237:1350–2.

75. Lee JC, Cantanzaro A, Parthemore JG, et al. Hypercalcemia in disseminated coccidioidomycosis. *N Engl J Med* 1977;297:431–3.

76. Kantarjian HM, Saad MF, Estey EH, et al. Hypercalcemia in disseminated candidiasis. *Am J Med* 1983;74:721–4.

77. Hoffman VN, Korzeniowski OM. Leprosy, hypercalcemia, and elevated serum calcitriol levels. *Ann Intern Med* 1986;105:890–1.

78. Kozeny GA, Barbato AL, Bansal VK, et al. Hypercalcemia associated with silicone-induced granulomas. *N Engl J Med* 1984;311:1103–5.

79. Stoeckle JD, Hardy HL, Weber AL. Chronic beryllium disease; long-term follow-up of sixty cases and selective review of the literature. *Am J Med* 1969;46:545–61.

80. Akai PS, Wong T, Chang-Poon V, et al. Resectable bronchogenic carcinoma presenting with hypercalcemia: tumor-associated granulomatous reaction and probable production of 1,25-dihydroxyvitamin D. *Clin Invest Med* 1989;12:212–6.

81. Parker MS, Dokoh S, Woolfenden JM, et al. Hypercalcemia in coccidioidomycosis. *Am J Med* 1984;76:341–4.

82. Ryzen E, Singer FR. Hypercalcemia in leprosy. *Arch Intern Med* 1985;145:1305–6.

83. Gates S, Shary J, Turner RT, et al. Abnormal calcium metabolism caused by increased circulating 1,25-dihydroxyvitamin D in a patient with rheumatoid arthritis. *J Bone Miner Res* 1986;1:221–6.

84. Breslau NA, McGuire JL, Zerwekh JE, et al. Hypercalcemia associated with increased serum calcitriol levels in three patients with lymphoma. *Ann Intern Med* 1984;100:1–7.

85. Adams JS, Fernandez M, Gacad MA, et al. Vitamin D metabolite-mediated hypercalcemia and hypercalciuria patients with AIDS- and non-AIDS-associated lymphoma. *Blood* 1989;73:235–9.

86. Rosenthal N, Insogna KL, Godsall JW, et al. Elevations in circulating 1,25-dihydroxyvitamin D in three patients with lymphoma-associated hypercalcemia. *J Clin Endocrinol Metab* 1985;60:29–33.

87. Davies M, Hayes ME, Mawer EB, et al. Abnormal vitamin D metabolism in Hodgkin's lymphoma. *Lancet* 1985;1:186–8.

88. Schaefer K, Saupe J, Pauls A, Von Herrath G. Hypercalcemia and elevated serum 1,25-dihydroxyvitamin D₃ in a patient with Hodgkin's lymphoma. *Klin Wochenschr* 1986;64:89–91.

89. Linde R, Basso L. Hodgkin's disease with hypercalcemia detected by thallium-201 scintigraphy. *J Nucl Med* 1987;28:112–5.

90. Rieke JW, Donaldson SS, Horning SJ. Hypercalcemia and vitamin D metabolism in Hodgkin's disease: is there an underlying immunoregulatory relationship? *Cancer* 1989;63:1700–7.

91. Helikson MA, Havey AD, Zerwekh JE, et al. Plasma-cell granuloma producing calcitriol and hypercalcemia. *Ann Intern Med* 1986;105:379–81.

92. Mudde AH, Van Den Berg H, Boshuis PG, et al. Ectopic production of 1,25-dihydroxyvitamin D by B-cell lymphoma as a cause of hypercalcemia. *Cancer* 1987;59:1543–6.

93. Nakazato P, Esquivel CO, Urbach AH, et al. Lymphoma and hypercalcemia in a pediatric orthotopic liver transplant patient. *Transplantation* 1989;48:1003–6.

94. Sarin PS, Gallo RC. Human T lymphotrophic viruses in adult T-cell leukemia lymphoma and acquired immunodeficiency syndrome. *J Clin Immunol* 1984;4:415–23.

95. Grossman B, Schecter GP, Horton JE, et al. Hypercalcemia associated with T cell lymphoma-leukemia. *Am J Clin Pathol* 1981;75:149–55.

96. Popovic M, Sarin PS, Robert-Guroff M, et al. Isolation and transmission of human retrovirus (human T-cell leukemia virus). *Science* 1983;219:856–9.

97. Broder S, Bunn PA, Jaffe ES, et al. T-cell lymphoproliferative syndrome associated with human T-cell leukemia/lymphoma virus. *Ann Intern Med* 1984;100:543–57.

98. Fetchick DA, Bertolini DR, Sarin PS, et al. Production of 1,25-dihydroxyvitamin D by human T-cell lymphotrophic virus-I transformed lymphocytes. *J Clin Invest* 1986;78:592–6.

99. Maislos M, Sobel R, Shany S. Leiomyoblastoma associated with intractable hypercalcemia and elevated 1,25-dihydroxycholecalciferol levels. *Arch Intern Med* 1985;145:565–7.

100. Grote TH, Hainsworth JD. Hypercalcemia and elevated serum calcitriol in a patient with seminoma. *Arch Intern Med* 1987;147:2212–3.

101. Shigeno C, Yamamoto I, Dokoh S, et al. Identification of 1,24(R)-dihydroxyvitamin D₃-like bone-resorbing lipid in a patient with cancer-associated hypercalcemia. *J Clin Endocrinol Metab* 1985;61:761–8.

102. Stapleton T, MacDonald WB, Lightwood R. Management of "idiopathic" hypercalcaemia of infancy. *Lancet* 1956;1:932–4.

103. Morgan HG, Mitchell RG, Stowers JM, Thomson J. Metabolic studies on two infants with idiopathic hypercalcaemia. *Lancet* 1956;1:925–31.

104. Forfar JO, Balf CL, Maxwell GM, Tompsett SL. Idiopathic hypercalcaemia of infancy: clinical and metabolic studies with special reference to the aetiological role of vitamin D. *Lancet* 1956;1:981–8.

105. Fellers FX, Schwartz R. Etiology of the severe form of idiopathic hypercalcemia of infancy: a defect in vitamin D metabolism. *N Engl J Med* 1958;259:1050–8.

106. Smith DW, Blizzard RM, Harrison HE. Idiopathic hypercalcemia: a case report with assays of vitamin D in the serum. *Pediatrics* 1959;24:258–9.

107. Kenny FM, Aceto T Jr, Purisch M, et al. Metabolic studies in a patient with idiopathic hypercalcemia of infancy. *J Pediatr* 1963;62:531–7.

108. Black JA, Bonham Carter RE. Association between aortic stenosis and facies of severe infantile hypercalcaemia. *Lancet* 1963;2:745–9.

109. Garcia RE, Friedman WF, Kabach MM, Rowe RD. Idiopathic hypercalcemia and supravalvular aortic stenosis: documentation of a new syndrome. *N Engl J Med* 1964;271:117–20.

110. Wiltse HE, Goldbloom RB, Anita AU, et al. Infantile hypercalcemia syndrome in twins. *N Engl J Med* 1966;275:1157–60.

111. Williams JCP, Barratt-Boyes BG, Lowe JB. Supravalvular aortic stenosis. *Circulation* 1961;24:1311–18.

112. Jones KL, Smith DW. The Williams elfin facies syndrome: a new perspective. *J Pediatr* 1975;86:718–23.

113. Taylor AB, Stern PH, Bell NH. Abnormal regulation of circulating 25-hydroxyvitamin D in the Williams syndrome. *N Engl J Med* 1982;306:972–5.

114. Bell NH, Shaw S, Turner RT. Evidence that 1,25-dihydroxyvitamin D₃ inhibits the hepatic production of 25-hydroxyvitamin D in man. *J Clin Invest* 1984;74:1540–4.

115. Halloran BP, Bikle DD, Levens MJ, et al. Chronic 1,25-dihydroxyvitamin D₃ administration in the rat reduces the serum concentration of 25-hydroxyvitamin D by increasing metabolic clearance rate. *J Clin Invest* 1986;78:622–8.

116. Garabedian M, Jacqz E, Guillozo H, et al. Elevated plasma 1,25-dihydroxyvitamin D concentrations in infants with hypercalcemia and an elfin facies. *N Engl J Med* 1985;312:948–52.

117. Streck WF, Waterhouse C, Haddad JG. Glucocorticoid effects in vitamin D intoxication. *Arch Intern Med* 1979;139:974–7.

118. Hughes MR, Baylink DJ, Jones PG, et al. Radioligand receptor assay for 25-hydroxyvitamin D₂/D₃ and 1α,25-dihydroxyvitamin D₂/D₃: application to hypervitaminosis D. *J Clin Invest* 1976;58:61–70.

Disorders of Bone and Mineral Metabolism,
edited by Fredric L. Coe and Murray J. Favus,
© 1992 by Raven Press, Ltd. All rights reserved.

CHAPTER 27

The Hypocalcemic States

Their Differential Diagnosis and Management

Richard Eastell and Hunter Heath III

Hypocalcemia may result from many causes (Table 1); some of these are discussed in chapters 38–41. In this chapter we focus on the mechanisms underlying hypocalcemia, the causes of hypocalcemia that are not discussed elsewhere (hypoparathyroidism, acute illness), the clinical and laboratory evaluation of chronic hypocalcemia, and the management of acute and chronic hypocalcemia.

MECHANISMS OF HYPOCALCEMIA

Calcium Kinetics

To clearly understand the laboratory findings and management of hypocalcemia, it is necessary to consider normal calcium kinetics (Fig. 1). *True calcium absorption* is the calcium absorbed from the diet. Bone also supplies calcium to the extraosseous pool. This calcium flux results from three mechanisms: (1) osteoclast-mediated bone resorption, (2) osteocyte-mediated short-term exchange between blood and bone, and (3) long-term exchange of calcium between the bone crystals and blood. Parathyroid hormone acts by mechanisms 1 and 2; short-term demands are met by mechanism 2 and long-term demands by mechanism 1.

The single calcium pool shown in Fig. 1 is an oversimplification; this pool exchanges with large, low-turnover

R. Eastell: Division of Endocrinology, Metabolism, and Internal Medicine, Mayo Clinic and Mayo Foundation, Rochester, Minnesota 55905
H. Heath III: Division of Endocrinology, Metabolism, and Internal Medicine, Mayo Clinic and Mayo Foundation; Professor of Medicine, Mayo Medical School, Rochester, Minnesota 55905

pools. Dilution of the calcium pool (equivalent to dilutional hyponatremia) is not a cause of true hypocalcemia. (See also Chapter 18.)

Urinary calcium is the 1–2% of filtered calcium that is not reabsorbed in the proximal or distal tubules (1). Endogenous fecal calcium is the calcium present in intestinal secretion that is not reabsorbed by the intestine. Bone formation represents: (1) the calcification of the mineralization front in osteoid (i.e., new bone formation); (2) osteocyte-mediated short-term exchange between blood and bone, and (3) long-term exchange of calcium between bone crystals and blood. In certain disease states, calcium may also be deposited in soft tissues.

Hypocalcemia may result from decreased influx of calcium or increased efflux of calcium from the plasma pool. Decreased calcium absorption may follow lack of or resistance to the action of vitamin D or a malabsorption syndrome. Drugs such as calcitonin and mithramycin may decrease bone resorption. Urinary calcium excretion inappropriate for the level of serum calcium may result from lack of or resistance to the action of parathyroid hormone, or use of drugs such as furosemide. Increased endogenous fecal calcium may result from malabsorptive states such as celiac disease. Increased bone mineralization occurs with healing of parathyroid, thyrotoxic, or osteomalacic osteodystrophy or with osteoblastic metastases from prostate carcinoma. Soft-tissue deposition of calcium may result from hyperphosphatemia or pancreatitis (from the formation of "calcium soaps").

Calcium Homeostasis

The principal mediator of systemic calcium homeostasis is parathyroid hormone (PTH). Hypocalcemia in-

TABLE 1. *Classification of hypocalcemia*

Chronic Hypocalcemia
I. Hypoparathyroidism
  A. Surgically induced
  B. Idiopathic
    1. Early
      a. DiGeorge syndrome (with thymic aplasia)
      b. MEDAC/HAM[a]
      c. Isolated persistent neonatal
    2. Isolated late-onset
  C. Functional
    1. Hypomagnesemia
    2. Neonatal (e.g., maternal hyperparathyroidism)
  D. Infiltrative
    1. Hemosiderosis
    2. Wilson disease
    3. Secondary neoplasia
II. Pseudohypoparathyroidism
III. Osteomalacia
  A. Decreased bioavailability of vitamin D
    1. Decreased UV light
    2. Nutritional
    3. Nephrosis?
    4. Malabsorption
  B. Abnormal metabolism of vitamin D
    1. Chronic renal failure
    2. Vitamin D–dependent rickets type I (aut. rec.)
    3. Anticonvulsants
  C. Abnormal response to vitamin D
    1. Vitamin D–dependent rickets type II
    2. Malabsorption (celiac/Crohn's/short bowel)

Acute/Subacute Hypocalcemia
  A. Severe illness
    1. Septicemia (gram-negative)
    2. Fat embolism
    3. Pancreatitis
    4. Tumor lysis
    5. Rhabdomyolysis
    6. Excess phosphate administration
    7. Toxic shock syndrome
  B. After neck surgery
  C. Osteoblastic metastasis
  D. Drugs (e.g., calcitonin, mithramycin, citrated blood)

[a] MEDAC, multiple Endocrine Deficiency–autoimmune–candidiasis; HAM, juvenile familial endocrinopathy–hypoparathyroidism–Addison disease–moniliasis.

creases secretion of PTH. This results in phosphaturia and thus hypophosphatemia. There is increased synthesis of the active form of vitamin D [$1,25(OH)_2D$] as a result of increased serum PTH and decreased serum calcium and phosphate, and the $1,25(OH)_2D$ increases calcium absorption. Increased PTH also increases calcium reabsorption by the distal renal tubule and hence decreases urinary calcium excretion. Increased PTH also causes increased calcium release from bone by short-term and longer-term mechanisms (see above).

Hypocalcemia would be expected as a result of decreased PTH action or decreased $1,25(OH)_2D$ action. Decreased PTH action results from decreased PTH secretion (hypoparathyroidism) or tissue resistance to

PTH (pseudohypoparathyroidism). Decreased $1,25$-$(OH)_2D$ action could result from decreased production (lack of substrate, 25-hydroxyvitamin D [25(OH)D], or renal 1α-hydroxylase enzyme) or resistance to $1,25(OH)_2D$ [malabsorption syndrome, $1,25(OH)_2D$ receptor defect]. These defects may be relative rather than absolute. For example, mild hypoparathyroidism may only be manifest in the presence of increased calcium excretion (e.g., furosemide therapy) (2).

The hypocalcemia of hypoparathyroidism results mainly from decreased renal tubular reabsorption of calcium (1), and this defect is worsened by $1,25(OH)_2D$ deficiency (3). There are less important contributions from decreased $1,25(OH)_2D$ and calcium absorption (4) and decreased net bone resorption (resulting in net bone gain) (5). Patients with hypoparathyroidism adapt poorly to acute hypocalcemia (e.g., infusion of EDTA; see below) and chronic calcium deprivation (e.g., low-calcium diet) (6). Indeed, this sensitivity to EDTA has been used by Parfitt (7) to grade the severity of hypocalcemia in hypoparathyroid states:

Grade 1 Eucalcemia, abnormal EDTA response
Grade 2 Transient hypocalcemia, abnormal EDTA response
Grade 3 $7.5 \le Ca < 8.5$ mg/dL
Grade 4 $6.5 \le Ca < 7.5$ mg/dL
Grade 5 $Ca < 6.5$ mg/dL

The divalent cation-binding agent, sodium cellulose phosphate, may also be used to diagnose latent (grades 1 and 2) hypoparathyroidism (8). Such a classification may be helpful in determining prognosis; for example, grade 3 surgical hypoparathyroidism commonly remits.

PTH deficiency has biochemical effects other than hypocalcemia. The serum phosphorus level tends to increase because of an increased renal threshold for phosphorus (TmP/GFR). This finding is not as constant as

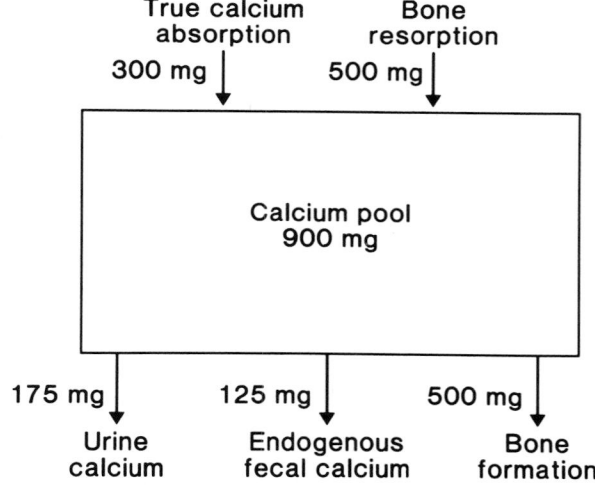

FIG. 1. Calcium kinetics in healthy normal subjects.

hypocalcemia, because less PTH is required to produce this effect than to maintain eucalcemia, and because intestinal phosphorus absorption and bone resorption are decreased variably in hypoparathyroidism (6). The serum magnesium level tends to decrease by about 15% (9) as a result of decreased intestinal absorption of magnesium and decreased renal tubular reabsorption of magnesium (10). There may be a metabolic alkalosis because of decreased renal tubular excretion of bicarbonate. There is also increased sensitivity of the respiratory center to CO_2, elevating plasma pH (11).

CAUSES OF HYPOCALCEMIA

Some of the causes of hypocalcemia have been discussed elsewhere: hypomagnesemia (Chapter 28), neonatal hypocalcemia (Chapter 16), osteomalacia (Chapters 40 and 41), and chronic renal failure (Chapter 39). Also, the pathogenesis of resistance to parathyroid hormone has been described elsewhere (Chapter 6). Here we discuss the clinical syndromes of hypoparathyroidism, pseudohypoparathyroidism, and acute hypocalcemia (Table 1).

Surgically Induced Hypoparathyroidism (11)

Hypocalcemia may follow thyroid and parathyroid gland operations. It is more common following surgery for thyrotoxic goiter than for euthyroid goiter (12) and more common with total thyroidectomy than with hemithyroidectomy (13). It is more common if the surgeon performs the operation infrequently, and after reoperation. Symptoms of hypocalcemia may occur in two-thirds of patients following partial thyroidectomy for Graves' disease, but permanent hypoparathyroidism (i.e., more than 1 year) occurs in less than 10% of cases. It is more common after surgery for parathyroid hyperplasia than for adenoma (14) and more common with adenoma if all three remaining glands are biopsied (15).

Postoperative hypocalcemia may result from hypoparathyroidism or from recalcification tetany. The hypoparathyroidism may result from previous chronic hypercalcemia. In thyrotoxicosis, serum calcium may be slightly elevated, with chronic parathyroid gland suppression. In primary hyperparathyroidism due to adenoma, the remaining three glands are suppressed. Alternatively, the parathyroid glands (which are supplied by a single artery that is a branch of the inferior thyroid artery) may become ischemic. Inadvertent removal of all parathyroid tissue is an unusual cause. It has also been reported that calcitonin levels increase for 24–48 h after thyroidectomy, and this may also contribute to the hypocalcemia (16).

Recalcification tetany or *hungry bone syndrome* refers to the bone repair that takes place postoperatively. Thy-rotoxicosis and hyperparathyroidism are both associated with increased bone remodeling, and once the disease is cured by surgery, bone formation exceeds bone resorption to fill in the *remodeling space*. The plasma concentrations of magnesium and phosphorus may also decrease during bone healing.

Hypoparathyroidism is characterized by increased serum phosphorus, usually occurring 2–6 days postoperatively. Recalcification tetany may occur within the first 10 hours postoperatively and is usually associated with low serum phosphorus and raised parathyroid hormone levels.

Idiopathic Hypoparathyroidism

Idiopathic hypoparathyroidism (6) is a rare condition, with onset of symptoms in childhood. The average duration of symptoms prior to diagnosis is 5 years. These patients are usually aparathyroid and have serum calcium levels in the range 5.4–7.7 mg/dL.

Isolated persistent neonatal hypoparathyroidism usually signifies congenital aplasia of the parathyroids and may be inherited as an X-linked recessive (17). Di-George syndrome results from defective migration of neural crest mesenchyme to the third and fourth branchial clefts and results in decreased cell-mediated immunity and hypoparathyroidism. The latter may be so mild that it can only be diagnosed by EDTA infusion (18).

Some hypoparathyroid patients, especially those presenting in early childhood (mean age 8 years), have autoimmune polyglandular syndrome, type I (Table 2). This condition is probably inherited as an autosomal recessive trait, so siblings may not be affected. It is not linked to the HLA locus. Parathyroid autoantibodies are present in one-third of cases (20). It usually presents with *Candida* infection of toenails and mouth, with later development of hypocalcemic symptoms. Addison disease may be diagnosed later in childhood, and other endocrine abnormalities may be found (Table 2). There is associated abnormal delayed hypersensitivity and T-cell abnormalities. These patients have longstanding hypocalcemia and develop many complications, including cataracts, basal ganglion calcification, and steatorrhea.

TABLE 2. *Autoimmune polyglandular syndrome type I*

Hypoparathyroidism
Addison's disease
Moniliasis
Chronic active hepatitis (13%)
Steatorrhea (22%)
Primary hypogonadism (17%)
Primary hypothyroidism (11%)
Vitiligo
Alopecia (32%)
Pernicious anemia (13%)

Source: After Eisenbarth (19).

Fat malabsorption occurs in 25% of cases, more commonly than in hypoparathyroidism of other causes. It may result from decreased duodenal secretion of cholecystokinin, which, in turn, results in decreased gallbladder contraction and pancreatic secretion (21).

Isolated late-onset hypoparathyroidism is an ill-defined entity with onset at any age; it is usually sporadic, but may be inherited as an autosomal dominant (22) or autosomal recessive. It may present in association with ophthalmoplegia, retinitis pigmentosa, and heart block (Kearns-Sayre syndrome) (23) or with growth retardation and long-bone medullary stenosis (Kenny-Caffey syndrome). The latter syndrome may result from secretion of abnormal PTH (24). The etiology of isolated late-onset hypoparathyroidism is uncertain. Molecular biology studies of 23 affected individuals with the autosomal dominant form showed apparently normal PTH gene structure, but in 2 families (out of 8), linkage analysis showed concordance between the inheritance of hypoparathyroidism and specific PTH alleles, suggesting that in those families, hypoparathyroidism may be due to an alteration in or near the PTH structural gene (25). At autopsy, the glands show atrophic changes with fatty infiltration and fibrosis.

Other Forms of Hypoparathyroidism

Hypomagnesemia results in functional hypoparathyroidism (see Chapters 4, 28). Infiltrative disease of the parathyroid is common in carcinomatosis (12%) (26), hemochromatosis, thalassemia [related to number of transfusions (27)], amyloidosis, syphilis, and tuberculosis, but hypocalcemia is uncommon. Hypoparathyroidism resulting from copper deposition may occur in Wilson's disease (28) and from sarcoid infiltration (29). Aluminum deposition in the parathyroid glands impairs hormone secretion and may contribute to the pathogenesis of aluminum-induced renal osteodystrophy (30). The chemotherapeutic agents asparaginase, doxorubicin, and cytosine arabinoside may also cause hypoparathyroidism. The chemoprotective agent WR-2721 results in hypoparathyroidism by reversible inhibition of PTH secretion (31).

External radiotherapy to the neck does not result in hypoparathyroidism, although it may cause late hyperparathyroidism. A few patients treated with ^{131}I have subsequently developed hypoparathyroidism, but this is a rare event (11). Even more rarely, Reidel's thyroiditis may cause hypoparathyroidism, and this may be reversible by partial thyroidectomy (32).

Pseudohypoparathyroidism (33)

The pathogenesis of this disorder has been reviewed (33,34). Here we summarize the pathogenesis and outline the clinical features.

Pseudohypoparathyroidism is a state of hormonal resistance that may be inherited in autosomally dominant, autosomally recessive, or X-linked dominant forms. The phosphaturic response to exogenous PTH is absent and serum PTH levels are elevated. Most patients have absent or decreased cyclic AMP (35) responses to exogenous PTH (type I); a few have normal cyclic AMP but absent phosphaturic responses (type II) (36). Other manifestations of PTH resistance include reduced hypocalciuric effect (37) of PTH, decreased bone mobilization response to PTH (38), and decreased serum 1,25(OH)$_2$D levels (39) [due to decreased production of cyclic nucleotides (40)]. One important difference from idiopathic hypoparathyroidism is the response of bone cells. A few patients with pseudohypoparathyroidism develop osteitis fibrosa cystica, a manifestation of hyperparathyroid bone disease (41,42). However, when studied as a group (38), patients with pseudohypoparathyroidism have decreased radius bone mineral content and increased urinary hydroxyproline (a marker of bone resorption). In contrast to what had been believed, it is likely that bone cell responsiveness to PTH is normal in pseudohypoparathyroidism. In support of this, Bradbeer et al. (43) reported that PTH bioactivity in pseudohypoparathyroidism was greater in a metatarsal bioassay than in a renal bioassay system.

Some cases of pseudohypoparathyroidism with impaired renal cAMP response to PTH (type I) have a characteristic phenotype (Albright's hereditary osteodystrophy), and they have decreased levels of stimulatory guanine nucleotide-binding regulatory protein in cells (Gs). This protein mediates receptor-induced adenylate cyclase activity. These patients are classified as type Ia, to distinguish them from patients with abnormal cAMP response but normal Gs levels. In patients with type Ia pseudohypoparathyroidism, decreased cellular content of Gs levels has been reported for red blood cells (44–46), platelets (47), kidney (48,49), fibroblasts (50), and transformed lymphoblasts (51). The Gs protein also mediates the adenylate cyclase response of other hormones, and

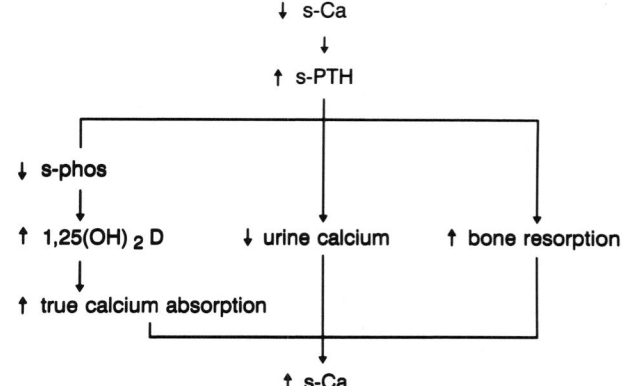

FIG. 2. Calcium homeostatic response to hypocalcemia.

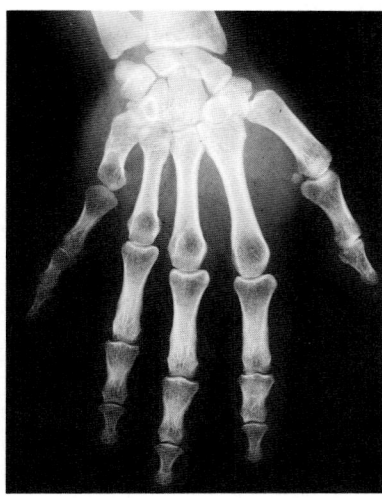 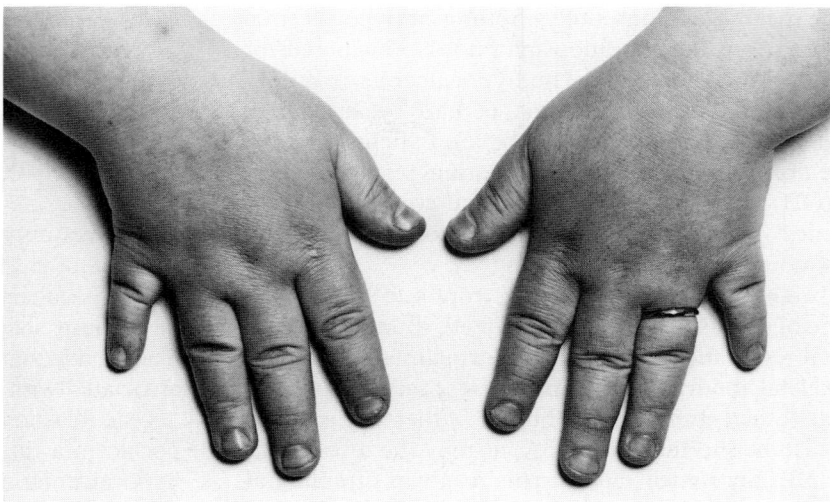

FIG. 3A. Shortened metacarpals are a characteristic finding in pseudohypoparathyroidism. Any metacarpal may be shortened, the least common being the second and the most common, the fourth. In this example, there is shortening of the fifth metacarpal.

abnormal responses to β-adrenergic agonists (52), glucagon, and TSH (53,54) have been reported. Patients with pseudohypoparathyroidism type Ia therefore may have other endocrine disorders resulting from decreased Gs activity. These may include mild primary hypothyroidism and hypergonadotropic hypogonadism presenting as oligomenorrhea (33). Recent studies indicate specific mutations in the α-subunit of the G_s protein $G_{s\alpha}$ in small numbers of patients with pseudohypoparathyroidism.

There are likely to be other causes for pseudohypo-parathyroidism. For example, PTH structure may be abnormal (55,56), with decreased activity in the cytochemical bioassay (57). PTH acts in part via the inositol triphosphate/protein kinase C pathway, and this may be defective. Indeed, the rare type II pseudohypoparathyroidism (normal cAMP response, decreased phosphaturic response to PTH) may be due to an abnormality of this pathway (33). Some cases may represent vitamin D deficiency, a state that may be associated with PTH resistance (33,58).

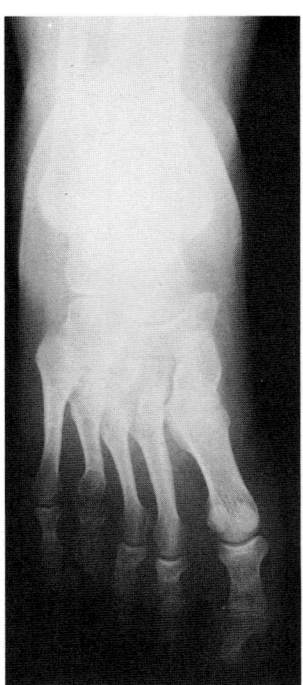 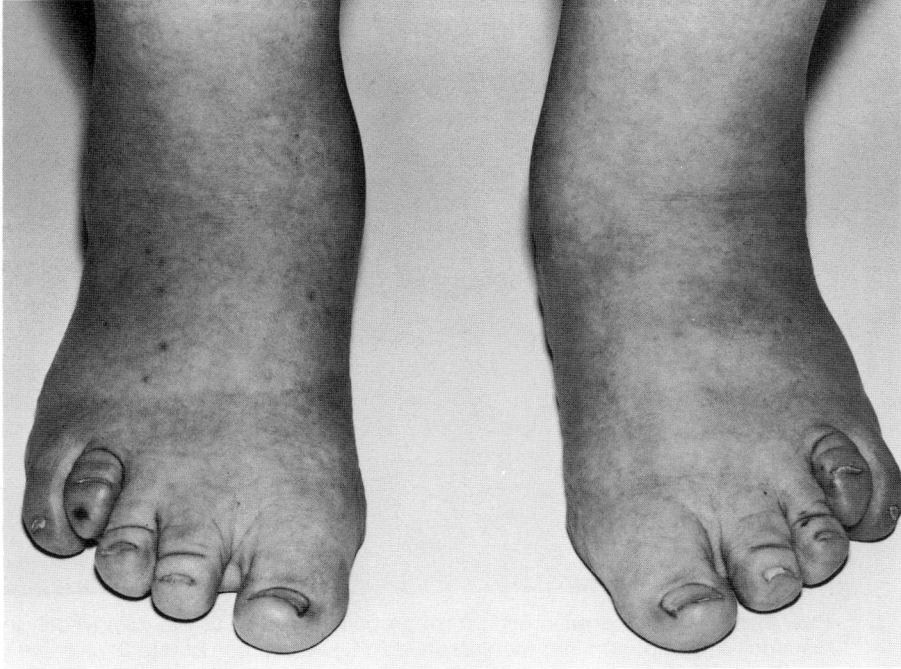

FIG. 3B. Brachydactyly may also affect the feet. In this case there is bilateral shortening of the fourth metatarsal.

The mean age of onset of symptoms of hypocalcemia is 8 years, but the condition may not be diagnosed for another 8–10 years (33). The hypocalcemia is milder than in idiopathic hypocalcemia, perhaps because of the intact bone cell response (see above). Patients who become normocalcemic may have normal serum levels of 1,25(OH)$_2$D (59). The symptoms and complications of chronic hypocalcemia are the same as for idiopathic and surgical hyperparathyroidism (Fig. 2).

Albright's hereditary osteodystrophy (60) is a syndrome of short stature (less than 5 feet), round face, mild mental retardation, and bony abnormalities. The classical skeletal abnormality is shortening of the fourth metacarpal (brachymetacarpia), but the other metacarpals may also be shortened (Fig. 3A) as may the metatarsals (Fig. 3B). Shortened metacarpals result in dimpling at the metacarpophalangeal joints when a fist is made. A shortened fourth metacarpal may be confirmed radiologically as Archibald's sign—a line drawn from the fifth to the fourth metacarpal head should not intersect the third metacarpal, and if it does, it should not be by more than 2 mm. The abnormality results from premature fusion of the epiphysis (Fig. 4). Other skeletal abnormalities include thickening of the calvarium, short phalanges, radius curvus, and abnormal angles of the elbows, hips, and knees. Ectopic ossification may occur. This phenotype may occur with normal cAMP and phosphaturic responses and is then referred to as pseudopseudohypoparathyroidism. Brachymetacarpia also may occur in Turner's syndrome and as an isolated finding, so it is not

pathognomonic of pseudohypoparathyroidism. Some cases of pseudohypoparathyroidism show osteitis fibrosa cystica (Fig. 5).

Acute Hypocalcemia

Pancreatitis may be associated with hypocalcemia in 25–50% of cases between days 3 and 11 of illness (61). The hypocalcemia may result partly from the formation of calcium soaps in the peritoneum (9,61) and partly from inadequate parathyroid response (62). It may be associated with hypomagnesemia.

Osteoblastic metastasis of the breast may produce hypocalcemia due to increased bone mineralization; the hypocalcemia may be worsened by diminished parathyroid reserve resulting from tumorous infiltration of the parathyroid glands (63). Carcinoma of the prostate accounted for one-third of cases in one series (64), and estrogen treatment of these tumors causes a further decrease in serum calcium due to inhibition of bone resorption (65).

Acute hyperphosphatemia may result from oral, intravenous, or rectal (66) administration of phosphate, particularly in the presence of renal failure, increased cellular release of phosphates such as after crush injuries or successful treatment of leukemia, lymphoma (67), or medulloblastoma (68). The hypocalcemia results from increased soft-tissue deposition of calcium phosphate due to increased serum calcium–phosphate product.

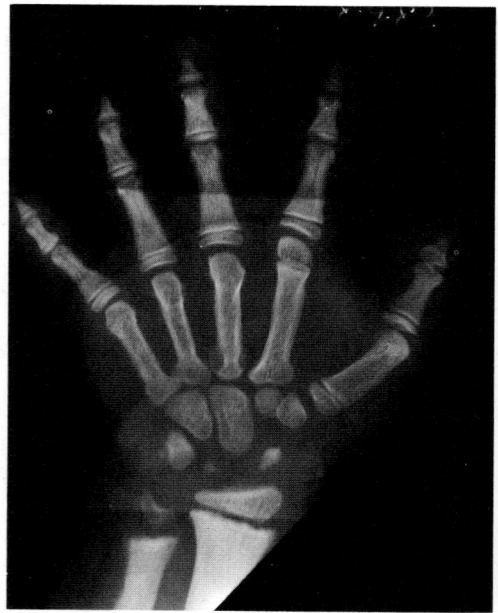 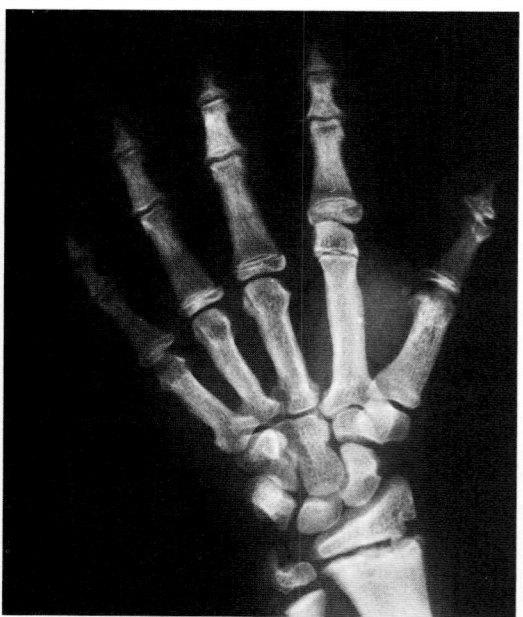

FIG. 4. Short metacarpals result from premature fusion of the epiphyseal growth plate. **A:** Fusion of distal third, fourth, and fifth metacarpal epiphyses in a boy at age 2 years 10 months (normally fuse at age 9 years). **B:** Hand x-ray taken 5 months later. Note also the resorption and sclerosis of the distal metaphyses of the radius and ulna, and the subperiosteal resorption of the phalanges.

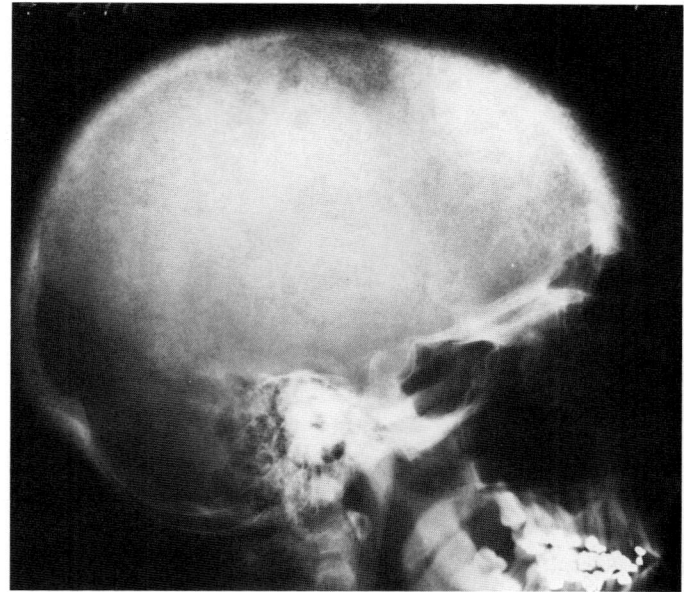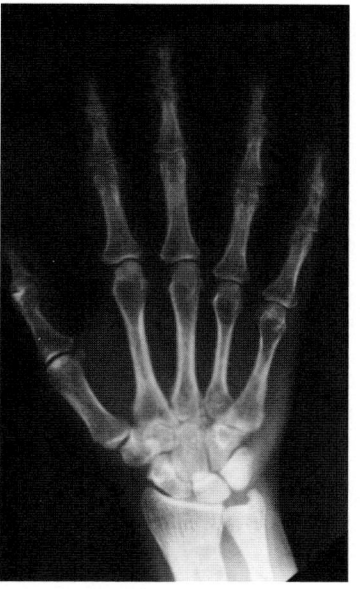

FIG. 5. Osteitis fibrosa cystica in pseudohypoparathyroidism in a 23-year-old woman. **A:** Skull x-rays showing "pepper-pot" appearance. **B:** Hand x-ray showing subperiosteal resorption of the phalanges and brown tumor of the radius.

Out-of-hospital cardiac arrest has been associated with hypocalcemia, which was most marked in association with metabolic/respiratory acidosis (69). Toxic shock syndrome (70), gram-negative septicemia, and measles (71) have been associated with hypocalcemia, but the mechanism is uncertain.

Low serum-ionized calcium level in a critical illness is associated with a poor prognosis (72). The hypocalcemia may result from a combination of increased free fatty acids that increase the affinity of albumin for calcium (73), and acquired PTH resistance (72).

Overzealous use of mithramycin to treat the hypercalcemia of malignancy, or calcitonin, used to treat a high-turnover state such as Paget disease of bone, may cause hypocalcemia. The concurrent use of pentamidine (for pneumocystis cavinii pneumonia) and Foscarnet (for cytomegalovirus pneumonia) in AIDS patients has been associated with severe hypocalcemia that is reversible, but the mechanism is unknown (74). Administration of citrated blood, particularly in the presence of hepatic impairment, may result in hypocalcemia that can be prevented by administering 150 mg of calcium for each unit of blood. Another factor contributing to the hypocalcemia of hemorrhagic shock is parathyroid hormone resistance (75).

CLINICAL APPROACH TO HYPOCALCEMIA

Paresthesias around the mouth and of the extremities indicate mild hypocalcemia. As hypocalcemia progresses, there may be muscle spasm, laryngeal stridor,

seizures, cardiac arrhythmias, cardiac failure, and coma. A careful history is taken to determine the cause of hypocalcemia. In particular, inquire about previous neck surgery, use of anticonvulsant drugs, alcohol, cis-platinum, gentamicin, diuretics (causing hypomagnesemia), lack of sunshine exposure, weight loss, and diarrhea (malabsorption syndrome). Any family history of autoimmune disease, seizures, or short stature may be relevant.

The cardinal signs of latent tetany are the Chvostek's sign and the Trousseau's test. The Chvostek's sign is elicited by tapping with three fingers anterior to the external auditory meatus to test for excitability of the facial nerve (Fig. 6). Twitching of the side of the mouth may be observed in 8% of normal subjects, but movement of the nasolabial fold and outer canthus of the eye are definitely abnormal (76). The Chvostek's sign may be graded as follows:

Grade 1 Twitching of lip at angle of mouth
Grade 2 Twitching of ala nasi, in addition
Grade 3 Twitching of lateral angle of eye, in addition
Grade 4 Twitching of all ipsilateral facial muscles

The Trousseau sign is elicited by use of a sphygmomanometer cuff inflated to 20 mmHg above systolic blood pressure for 5 min. The time to spasm is noted. Specifically, the metacarpophalangeal joints flex, the interphalangeal joints extend, and the thumb adducts (Fig. 7). Spasm that may be overcome by the examiner will occur in 1–4% of normal subjects (6,76). Tetany (overt or latent) usually results from hypocalcemia but may on oc-

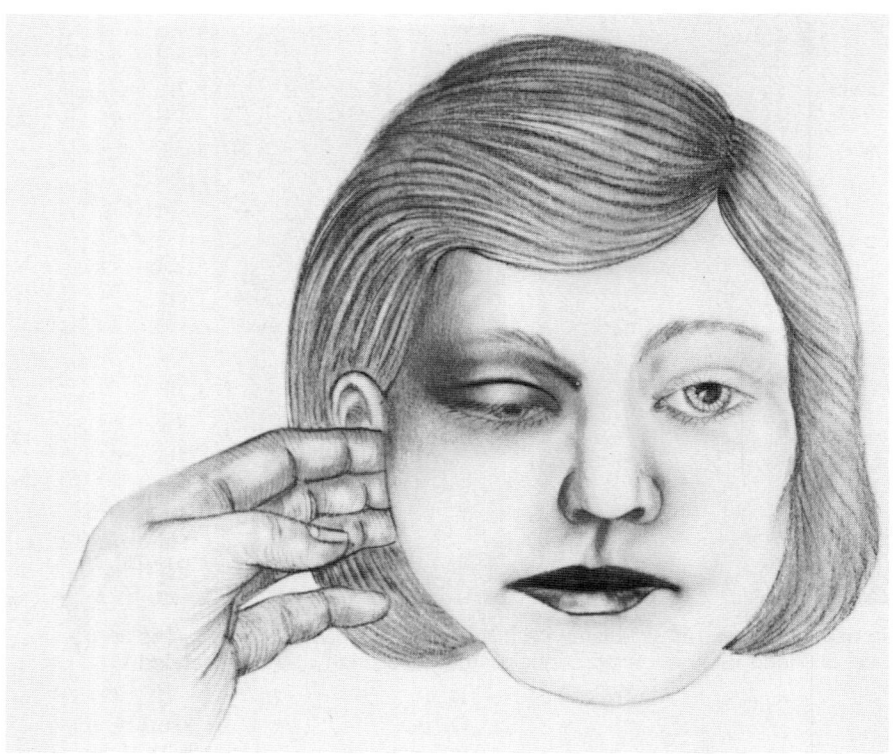

FIG. 6. Chvostek's sign is elicited by tapping with three fingers anterior to the external auditory meatus. This is an example of grade 3 Chvostek with twitching of the lip, ala nasi, and eye.

casion be due to metabolic alkalosis, hypokalemia, hypomagnesemia, or "normocalcemic tetany." Metabolic alkalosis may be present in hypoparathyroidism (see above) and its contribution to tetany is additive with that of hypocalcemia (77). Normocalcemic tetany may result from a primary neuromuscular abnormality and may

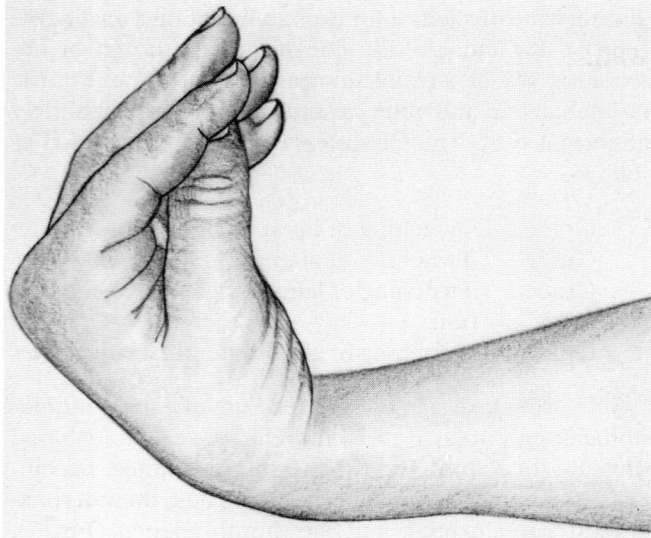

FIG. 7. Trousseau's sign is elicited by use of a sphygmomanometer cuff inflated to 20 mmHg above systolic blood pressure. Time to spasm (main d'accoucheur) is noted.

have a genetic basis (78). Signs of latent tetany may be masked by administration of the anticonvulsants diphenylhydantoin and phenobarbital (76).

Smooth muscle may be affected by hypocalcemia with resultant dysphagia (esophagus), abdominal pain (small intestine), biliary colic (sphincter of Oddi), and wheezing and dyspnea (bronchi). Uterine muscle excitability may be increased by hypocalcemia. In a case seen by one of the authors (79), two second-trimester abortions occurred before the diagnosis of idiopathic hypoparathyroidism was made. Treatment with 1α-hydroxyvitamin D resulted in eucalcemia, allowing a term pregnancy. Other case reports indicate that grade 4 and 5 hypocalcemia, in which serum calcium < 7.5 mg/dL, is associated with onset of labor between 18 and 27 weeks, whereas grades 2 and 3 are associated with full-term pregnancies (79).

The cardiovascular effects of hypocalcemia may be direct and indirect, in the form of arrhythmia, hypotension, or cardiac failure. They may result, in part, from abnormal cardiac conduction [increased Q-aT_c interval (80)] and decreased aldosterone secretion in response to angiotensin II and adrenocorticotrophin (81). The abnormalities may be reversed by correcting the hypocalcemia (82,83). Creatine kinase may be elevated in hypocalcemia (84), but this is the skeletal muscle (MM) rather than the cardiac muscle isoenzyme. Hypertension is present in one-half of cases with pseudohypoparathyroidism. Although it is associated with obesity it differs from obesity-related hypertension in that plasma renin activity is low (85).

Monilia of nails may be found in idiopathic hypoparathyroidism. In chronic hypoparathyroidism the skin may be dry and scaling, the nails brittle and fissured longitudinally, and the hair coarse (6). Specific skin diseases may be associated with hypocalcemia. For example, pustular psoriasis of von Zumbusch may remit with treatment of hypocalcemia (86). Cataracts may be found from all causes of chronic hypocalcemia; the lens opacities are punctate and take at least 5 years to develop (87). Alopecia may be present in type II vitamin D–dependent rickets.

The fists should be examined for brachymetacarpia (Fig. 3A) and the feet for brachymetatarsia (Fig. 3B). Hypocalcemia in childhood may result in delayed dentition, dental caries, or enamel hypoplasia. Enamel hypoplasia is present if hypocalcemia developed before the age of 5 years (88). If hypocalcemia was present during growth, "bone-in-bone" appearance may be present, especially in the vertebrae (89). About half of patients with hypoparathyroidism also have paravertebral ligamentous ossification (90). Antalgic gait or waddling gait may result from osteomalacic pseudofractures and myopathy, respectively.

Hypoparathyroidism is commonly associated with calcification of the basal ganglia [shown by CT scan in most cases (91)], cerebral cortex, and cerebellum, and there may be extrapyramidal neurological syndromes and papilledema. Preexisting epilepsy may be worsened or generalized tetany ("cerebral tetany") may occur (6,11). Occasionally, there may also be depression.

LABORATORY APPROACH TO HYPOCALCEMIA

Total serum calcium may be measured by atomic absorption spectroscopy or by colorimetric methods (e.g.,

by an automated analyzer). Its level is closely related to that of serum albumin because about 50% of calcium is bound to albumin. Hypoalbuminemia is one of the commonest causes of apparent hypocalcemia, particularly in the acutely ill. The effect of albumin may be corrected for by various formulas. An example of such a formula is (92):

$$\text{Adjusted sCa (mg/dL)} = \text{sCa} + 0.8(4 - \text{salb})$$

where sCa is the measured serum calcium and salb is the serum albumin.

However, the slope of the regression line in this equation varies greatly between individuals and within an individual during acute illness, and the equation may be misleading (93). It is preferable to measure ionized calcium (94). Problems with this measurement include the need to collect the blood under anaerobic conditions and the relative scarcity of laboratories that do the test well, although a new generation of ion-selective electrodes makes the measurements more reliable (94).

The level of hypocalcemia may be graded by the system of Parfitt (7; see above). For idiopathic hypoparathyroidism there is a clear demarcation in serum calcium levels between normal and abnormal. Patients with pseudohypoparathyroidism and surgical hypoparathyroidism often have less severe hypocalcemia. Having established the presence of hypocalcemia, the algorithm in Fig. 8 may be used.

Parathyroid hormone may be measured by radioimmunoassay. Normal or low values are found in hypoparathyroidism and hypomagnesemia; normal or high values are found in pseudohypoparathyroidism and vitamin D–deficient states. The new two-site assays for intact PTH, immunoradiometric (IRMA) and immunochemiluminometric, are far more specific than older assays at separating out these disorders. For example, in a study by Blind et al. (95), 23 out of 25 patients with hypopara-

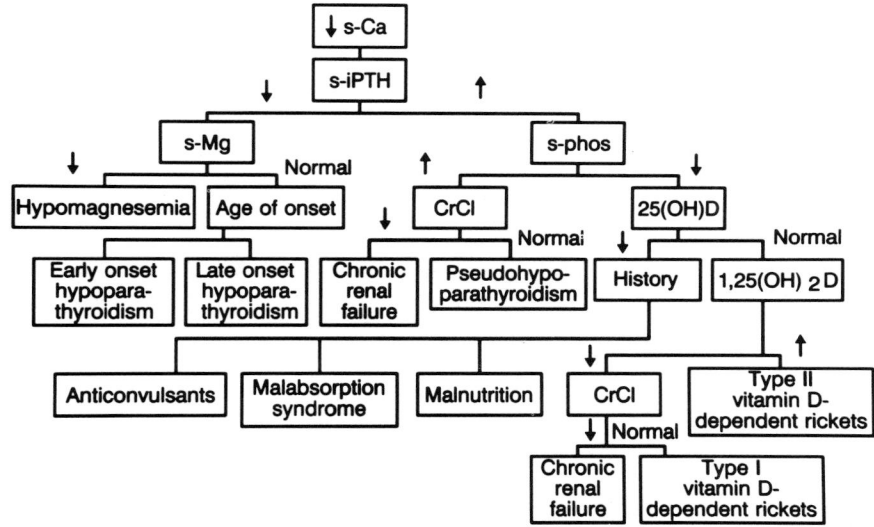

FIG. 8. Diagnostic algorithm for chronic hypocalcemia.

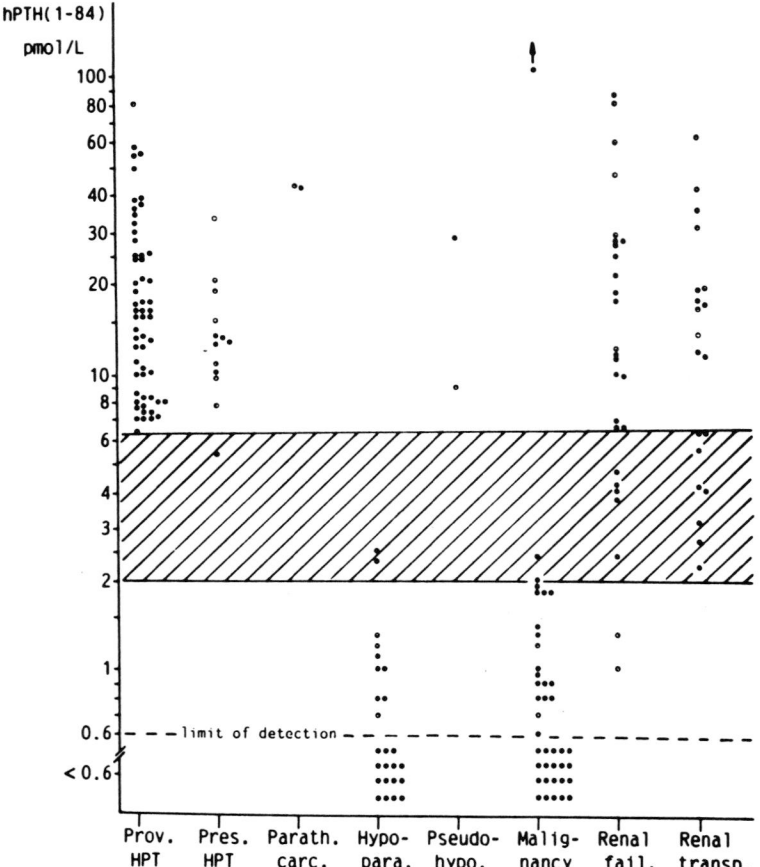

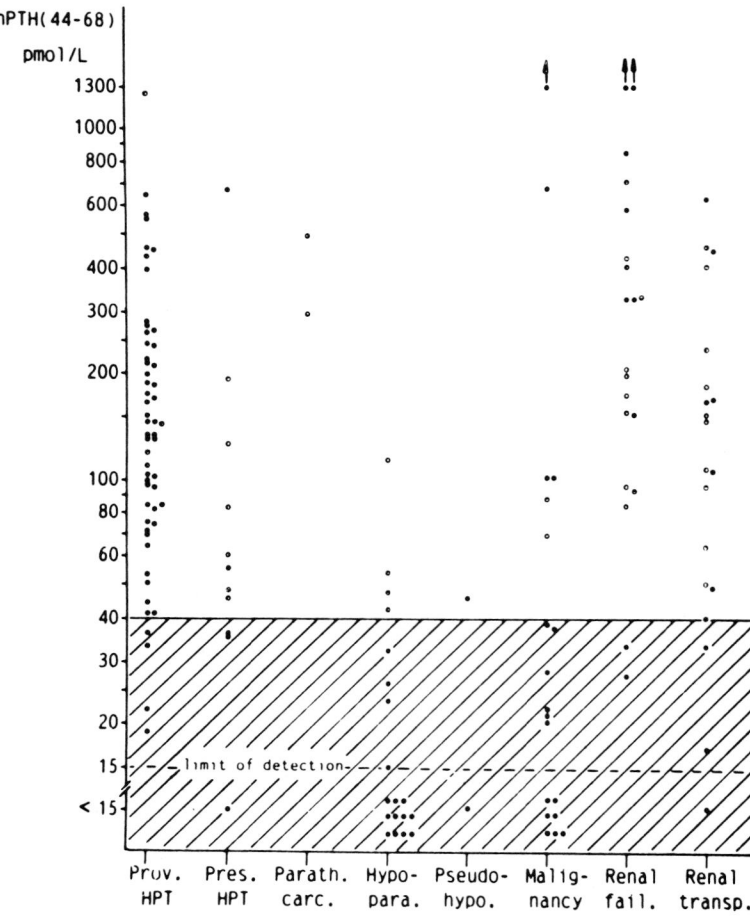

FIG. 9. Parathyroid hormone levels measured by immunoradiometric assay (**A**) and mid-region RIA (**B**) in 25 patients with hypoparathyroidism (hypopara) as compared to 52 normal subjects (hatched areas indicate normal ranges). The IRMA assay, unlike the RIA, distinguishes between normal and subnormal PTH levels. [From Blind, et al. (95)]

thyroidism had low serum PTH levels as measured by IRMA but were indistinguishable from normal when measured by conventional RIA (Fig. 9). Even the most sensitive RIAs are unable to measure low values of PTH (96). Serum magnesium levels are usually below 0.5 mmol/L (or 1 mEq/L) if this is the cause of hypocalcemia.

Fasting serum phosphate is high in the hypoparathyroid state and in end-stage renal disease, but low in vitamin D–deficiency states. The theoretical renal threshold for phosphorus may be calculated (TmP/GFR) from a 2-h fasting urine specimen and simultaneous blood sample. The fractional excretion of phosphorus (FEP) is calculated as

$$FEP = \frac{u\text{-phos}}{s\text{-phos}} \times \frac{s\text{-Cr}}{u\text{-Cr}}$$

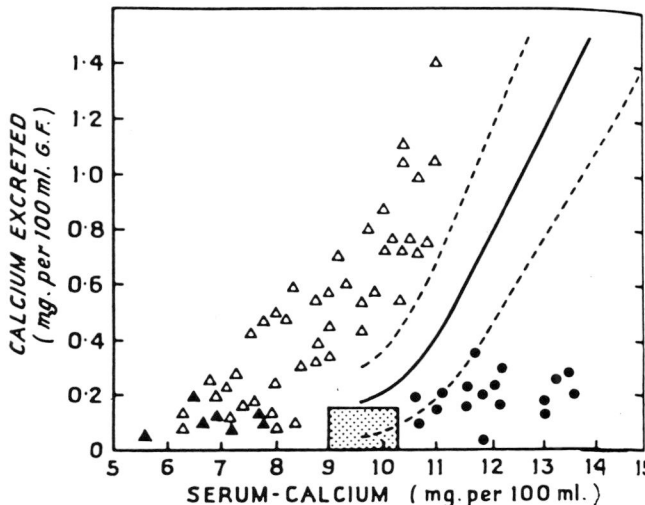

FIG. 11. Relationship between serum and urinary calcium in hypoparathyroid (△), hyperparathyroid (●), and normal subjects (– –, mean ± SD). Shaded area represents basal range in euparathyroid individuals. [From Nordin and Peacock (1).]

where u-phos is urinary phosphorus; s-phos is serum phosphorus; s-Cr is serum creatinine; and u-Cr is urinary creatinine (all in mg/dL), and the TmP/GFR is read from a nomogram (97). The normal range for TmP/GFR is 2.5–4.2 mg/dL, and all cases of hypoparathyroidism with grade 4 or 5 hypocalcemia have values above this range (6).

Plasma 25(OH)D reflects vitamin D nutrition and may be low in malabsorption syndromes and in nutritional and anticonvulsant osteomalacia. Plasma 1,25(OH)$_2$D is the active metabolite; its level is decreased in end-stage renal disease and type I vitamin D–dependent rickets. 1,25(OH)$_2$D levels may be normal in nutritional osteomalacia and thus may be misleading.

The renal responsiveness to parathyroid hormone may be tested using a modification of the Ellsworth–Howard test (98). A 1-34 fragment of human PTH is now available (teriparatide acetate), and after giving the PTH intravenously, the urinary cyclic AMP excretion is measured in a 30-min urine collection (and expressed as a function of creatinine clearance), and the TmP/GFR is calculated from urine collected over the first 60 min (as described above). In response to PTH, normal subjects have increased urinary cAMP and decreased TmP/GFR (Fig. 10). In pseudohypoparathyroidism, there is little change in either measure, although in a few patients (type II) there may be increased cAMP excretion without phosphaturia.

Absolute urinary calcium excretion is low in hypoparathyroidism because of the low filtered load. However, for a given level of plasma calcium, urinary calcium excretion expressed per deciliter of glomerular filtrate is increased because of impaired renal tubular calcium reabsorption (1) (Fig. 11).

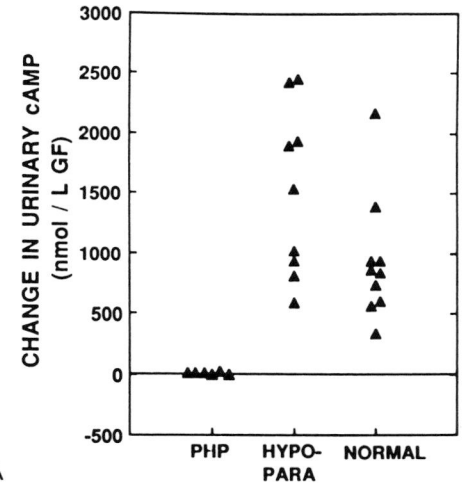

A

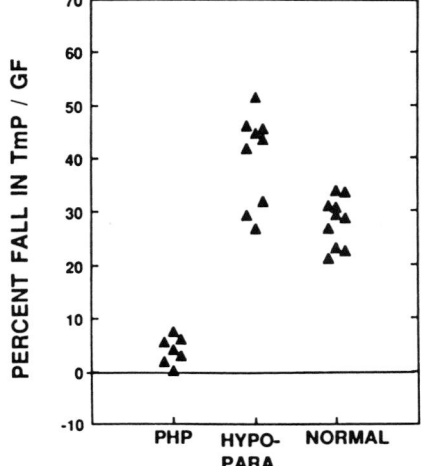

B

FIG. 10. **A:** Increase in cAMP excretion during the first 30 min after infusion of PTH(1-34) in pseudohypoparathyroid (PHP), hypoparathyroid (hypopara), and normal subjects. **B:** Decrease in TmP/GFR from its baseline value in the first hour after PTH(1-34) infusion. [From Mallette et al. (98).]

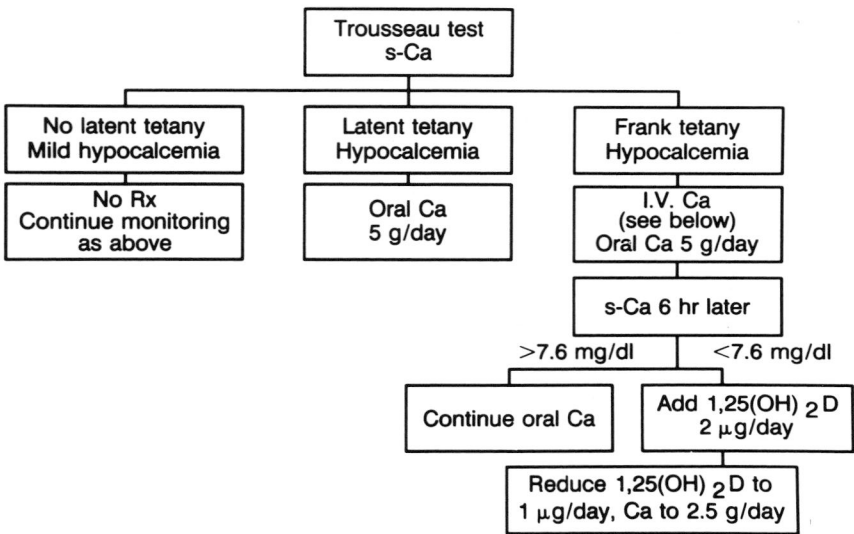

FIG. 12. Algorithm for immediate treatment of hypocalcemia.

IMMEDIATE TREATMENT OF HYPOCALCEMIA

Acute postoperative hypocalcemia may result in laryngeal spasm or seizures and should be treated promptly. An algorithm for treatment of hypocalcemia is shown in Fig. 12. The Trousseau test is an inexpensive and effective approach to monitoring, as it allows an assessment of the biological effect of the hypocalcemia as well as frequent measurements. The time to spasm is noted (the Trousseau time) and plotted on the patient's chart. It must be remembered that the Trousseau sign will be present for up to 4 hours after normalization of serum calcium.

Latent tetany usually responds to oral calcium alone. However, frank tetany requires intravenous calcium and may necessitate the use of the active metabolite of vitamin D, $1,25(OH)_2D$. The aim of treatment is to maintain serum calcium in the range 7.5–9.0 mg/dL without latent tetany.

Following hospital dismissal, serum calcium should be checked at weekly and then 2-weekly intervals if $1,25(OH)_2D$ is required. This is stopped after 3 months and the serum calcium is checked 3 weeks later.

Patients with recalcification tetany may develop hypomagnesemia, and this must be corrected in order to correct the hypocalcemia (Chapter 28). Recalcification tetany may be distinguished from hypoparathyroidism by the early onset, low or normal serum phosphorus, and elevated serum PTH.

LONG-TERM TREATMENT OF HYPOCALCEMIA

The dose, duration of action, and approximate cost of four vitamin D analogs are shown in Table 3. The principal advantages of $1,25(OH)_2D$ (and 1α-hydroxyvitamin D) are the rapid onset and short duration of action, and the latter minimizes the duration of hypercalcemia if overdosage occurs (100–102). However, this agent is 5–10 times the cost of vitamin D_2, and the shorter duration of action can be a disadvantage. Also, in some cases of hypoparathyroidism, there may be resistance even to the 1α-hydroxylated metabolites (103). Dihydrotachysterol and $25(OH)D$ are less expensive than $1,25(OH)_2D$ and so may provide a satisfactory compromise. 25-Hydroxyvitamin D probably acts directly on the vitamin D receptor, but with an affinity three orders of magnitude lower than that of $1,25(OH)_2D$. The dose required is 3–4 μg/kg per day, about 30 times that required for treating vitamin D deficiency states (104). Its serum concentra-

TABLE 3. *Characteristics of available vitamin D preparations*[a]

	D_2	DHT	$25(OH)D$	$1,25(OH)_2D$
Physiologic dose daily	2.5–10 μg	25–100 μg	1–5 μg	0.25–0.5 μg
Pharmacologic dose daily	0.625–6.25 mg	375–750 μg	20–200 μg	0.75–3 μg
Duration of action	1–3 months	1–4 weeks	2–6 weeks	2–5 days
Cost	$0.11/1.25 mg	$0.42/0.4 mg	$0.51/50 μg	$1.50/0.5 μg

. *Source:* Modified from Bikle (99).
[a] D_2, ergocalciferol (calciferol drops 200 μg/mL, tablets 1.25 mg, oil injection 12.5 mg/mL); DHT, dihydrotachysterol (DHT tablets 0.125, 0.2, 0.4 mg; Intensol drops, 0.2 mg/mL); $25(OH)D$, calcifediol (Calderol capsules, 20 and 50 μg); $1,25(OH)_2D$, calcitriol (Rocaltrol capsules, 0.25 and 0.5 μg).

tion may be monitored and used to predict hyper- or hypocalcemic episodes and to monitor patient compliance (105).

Calcium may be administered as the gluconate (9% calcium), chloride (27% calcium), carbonate (40% calcium), citrate (24% calcium), or phosphate (38% calcium) salts. The insoluble salts (carbonate, phosphate) are poorly absorbed by achlorhydric patients unless given along with food (106). Calcium carbonate may cause metabolic alkalosis, and calcium chloride causes gastric irritation. Given along with vitamin D, 1–2 g/day elemental calcium will suffice; the dose is adjusted according to serum calcium (8–9.5 mg/dL) and urinary calcium (<250 mg/day). The treatment response depends on the glomerular filtration rate and tubular reabsorption of calcium. Patients with grade 3 hypocalcemia may respond to calcium alone.

In some cases, eucalcemia cannot be achieved because of hyperphosphatemia. These patients may respond better to vitamin D after giving a phosphate binder, such as aluminum hydroxide (Alucaps). A lower dose of vitamin D or calcium alone may be used if a thiazide diuretic (e.g., chlorthalidone) (107) is administered to promote renal tubular reabsorption of calcium. However, a diuretic is effective only if combined with dietary sodium restriction.

Long-term treatment may be associated with episodes of hypercalcemia: such episodes may be precipitated by administering a thiazide diuretic (108), withdrawing estrogen therapy, the postpartum state, or even excessive sun exposure (109). In pseudohypoparathyroidism, estrogen therapy may decrease serum calcium as a result of decreased bone resorption (110). Chronic hypercalciuria may result in renal calculi or impaired renal function.

Parathyroid allotransplantation has been attempted, but the tissue is usually rejected. However, the operation was successful in a patient who had undergone renal allotransplantation and who was therefore receiving immunosuppressant therapy (111).

REFERENCES

1. Nordin BEC, Peacock M. Role of kidney in regulation of plasma-calcium. *Lancet* 1969;2:1280–3.
2. Bashey A, MacNee W. Tetany induced by furosemide in latent hypoparathyroidism. *Br Med J* 1987;295:960–1.
3. Santos F, Chan JCM. Idiopathic hypoparathyroidism: a case study on the interactions between exogenous parathyroid hormone infusion and 1,25-dihydroxyvitamin D. *Pediatrics* 1986; 78:1139–41.
4. Nolten WE, Chesney RW, Dabbagh S, et al. Moderate hypocalcemia due to normal serum 1,25-dihydroxyvitamin D levels in an asymptomatic kindred with familial hypoparathyroidism. *Am J Med* 1987;82:1157–66.
5. Seeman E, Wahner HW, Offord KP, Kumar R, Johnson WJ, Riggs BL. Differential effects of endocrine dysfunction on the axial and appendicular skeleton. *J Clin Invest* 1982;69:1302–9.
6. Parfitt AM. Surgical, idiopathic, and other varieties of parathyroid hormone-deficient hypoparathyroidism. In: DeGroot LJ, ed.

Endocrinology, 2nd ed. Philadelphia: WB Saunders, 1989;1049–64.
7. Parfitt AM. The spectrum of hypoparathyroidism. *J Clin Endocrinol Metab* 1972;34:152–8.
8. Parfitt AM. Effect of cellulose phosphate on calcium and magnesium homeostasis: studies in normal subjects and patients with latent hypoparathyroidism. *Clin Sci Mol Biol* 1975;49:83–90.
9. Stewart AF, Longo W, Kreulter D, Jacob R, Burtis WJ. Hypocalcemia associated with calcium-soap formation in a patient with a pancreatic fistula. *N Engl J Med* 1986;315:496–8.
10. Stanbury SW. Magnesium metabolism in hypoparathyroidism: a role for calcium in regulating the renal tubular reabsorption of magnesium. In: *Magnesium deficiency: physiopathology and treatment implications. Proceedings of the first European congress on magnesium.* Basel: S Karger, 1984.
11. Nagant de Deuxchaisnes C, Krane SM. Hypoparathyroidism. In: Avioli LV, Krane SM, eds. *Metabolic bone disease*, vol 2. New York: Academic Press, 1978.
12. Michie W, Stowers JM, Duncan T, et al. Mechanism of hypocalcemia after thyroidectomy for thyrotoxicosis. *Lancet* 1971; 1:508–14.
13. Falk SA, Birken EA, Baran DT. Temporary postthyroidectomy hypocalcemia. *Arch Otolaryngol Head Neck Surg* 1988;114:168–74.
14. Rizzoli R, Green J III, Marx SJ. Primary hyperparathyroidism in familial multiple endocrine neoplasia type I: long-term follow-up of serum calcium levels after parathyroidectomy. *Am J Med* 1985;78:467–74.
15. Kaplan EL, Bartlett S, Sugimoto J, Fredland A. Relation of postoperative hypocalcemia to operative techniques: deleterious effect of excessive use of parathyroid biopsy. *Surgery* 1982;92:827–34.
16. Watson CG, Steed DL, Robinson AG, Deftos LJ. The role of calcitonin and parathyroid hormone in the pathogenesis of postthyroidectomy hypocalcemia. *Metabolism* 1981;30:588–9.
17. Tsang RC, Donovan EF, Steichen JJ. Calcium physiology and pathology in the neonate. *Pediatr Clin North Am* 1976;23:611–26.
18. Gidding SS, Minciotti AL, Langman CG. Unmasking of hypoparathyroidism in familial partial DiGeorge syndrome by challenge with disodium edetate. *N Engl J Med* 1988;319:1589–91.
19. Eisenbarth GS. The immunoendocrinopathy syndromes. In: Wilson JD, Foster DW, eds. *Williams textbook of endocrinology*, 7th ed. Philadelphia: WB Saunders, 1985;1290–1300.
20. Blizzard RM, Chee D, Davis W. The incidence of parathyroid and other antibodies in the sera of patients with idiopathic hypoparathyroidism. *Clin Exp Immunol* 1986;1:119–28.
21. Heubi JE, Partin JC, Schubert WK. Hypocalcemia and steatorrhea: clues to etiology. *Dig Dis Sci* 1983;28:124–8.
22. Barr DGD, Prader A, Esper U, Rampini S, Mavrian VJ, Forfar JO. Chronic hypoparathyroidism in two generations. *Helv Pediatr Acta* 1971;26:507–21.
23. Scully RE, Mark EJ, McNeely WF, McNeely BU. Case records of the Massachusetts General Hospital: Case 34-1987. *N Engl J Med* 1987;317:493–501.
24. Fanconi S, Fischer JA, Wieland P, et al. Kenny syndrome: evidence for idiopathic hypoparathyroidism in two patients and for abnormal parathyroid hormone in one. *J Pediatr* 1986;109:469–75.
25. Ahn TG, Antonarakis SE, Kronenberg HM, Igarashi T, Levine, MA. Familial isolated hypoparathyroidism: a molecular genetic analysis of 8 families with 23 affected persons. *Medicine* 1986;65:73–81.
26. Horowitz CA, Myers WPL, Foote FW. Secondary malignant tumors of the parathyroid glands: report of two cases with associated hypoparathyroidism. *Medicine* 1972;52:797–808.
27. Brezin M, Shaler O, Leibel B, Dagan I, Ben-Ishay D. The spectrum of parathyroid function in thalanaemia subjects with transfusional iron overload. *Miner Electrolyte Metab* 1982;8:307–13.
28. Carpenter TO, Carnes DL, Anast CS. Hypoparathyroidism in Wilson's disease. *N Engl J Med* 1983;309:873–7.
29. Dill, JE. Hypoparathyroidism in sarcoidosis. *South Med J* 1983;76:414.
30. Andress D, Felsenfeld AJ, Voigts A, Llach F. Parathyroid hor-

mone response to hypocalcemia in hemodialysis patients with osteomalacia. *Kidney Int* 1983;24:364–70.

31. Glover D, Riley L, Carmichael K, et al. Hypocalcemia and inhibition of parathyroid hormone secretion after administration of WR-2721 (a radioprotective and chemoprotective agent). *N Engl J Med* 1983;309:1137–41.

32. Chopra D, Wool MS, Crosson A, Sawin CT. Reidel's struma associated with subacute thyroiditis, hypothyroidism and hypoparathyroidism. *J Clin Endocrinol Metab* 1978;46:869–71.

33. Levine MA, Aurbach GD. Pseudohypoparathyroidism. In: DeGroot LJ, ed. *Endocrinology*, 2nd ed. Philadelphia: WB Saunders, 1989;1065–79.

34. Van Dop C, Bourne HR. Pseudohypoparathyroidism. *Annu Rev Med* 1983;34:259–66.

35. Chase LR, Melson L, Aurabach GD. Pseudohypoparathyroidism: defective excretion of 3′, 5′-AMP in response to parathyroid hormone. *J Clin Invest* 1969;48:1832–44.

36. Drezner M, Neelon FA, Lebovitz HE. Pseudohypoparathyroidism type II: a possible defect of the reception of the cyclic AMP signal. *N Engl J Med* 1973;289:1056–60.

37. Moses AM, Breslau N, Coulson R. Renal responses to PTH in patients with hormone-resistant (pseudo)hypoparathyroidism. *Am J Med* 1976;61:184–9.

38. Breslau NA, Moses AM, Pak CYC. Evidence for bone remodeling but lack of calcium mobilization response to parathyroid hormone in pseudohypoparathyroidism. *J Clin Endocrinol Metab* 1983;57:638–44.

39. Drezner MK, Neelon FA, Haussler M, McPherson HT, Lebovitz HE. 1,25-Dihydroxycholecalciferol deficiency: the probable cause of hypocalcemia and metabolic bone disease in pseudohypoparathyroidism. *J Clin Endocrinol Metab* 1976;42:621–8.

40. Yamaoka K, Seino Y, Ishida M, et al. Effect of dibutyryl adenosine 3′, 5′-monophosphate administration on plasma concentrations of 1,25-dihydroxyvitamin D in pseudohypoparathyroidism type I. *J Clin Endocrinol Metab* 1981;53:1096–1100.

41. Dabbagh S, Chesney RW, Langer LO, DeLuca HF, Gilbert EF, DeWeerd JH. Renal-nonresponsive, bone-responsive pseudohypoparathyroidism: a case with normal vitamin D metabolite levels and clinical features of rickets. *Am J Dis Child* 1984; 138:1030–3.

42. Kolb FO, Steinbach HL. Pseudohypoparathyroidism with secondary hyperparathyroidism and osteitis fibrosa. *J Clin Endocrinol Metab* 1962;22:59–70.

43. Bradbeer JN, Dunham J, Fischer JA, Nagant de Deuxchaisnes CL, Overidge N. The metatarsal cytochemical bioassay of parathyroid hormone: validation, specificity, and application to the study of pseudohypoparathyroidism type I. *J Clin Endocrinol Metab* 1988;67:1237–43.

44. Downs RW, Sekura RD, Levine MA, Spiegel AM. The inhibitory adenylate cyclase coupling protein in pseudohypoparathyroidism. *J Clin Endocrinol Metab* 1985;61:351–4.

45. Farfel Z, Brickman AS, Kaslow HR, Brothers VM, Bourne HR. Defect of receptor-cyclase coupling protein in pseudohypoparathyroidism. *N Engl J Med* 1980;303:237–42.

46. Levine MA, Downs RW, Singer M, Marx SJ, Aurbach GD, Spiegel AM. Deficient activity of guanine nucleotide regulatory protein in erythrocytes from patients with pseudohypoparathyroidism. *Biochem Biophys Res Commun* 1980;94:1319–24.

47. Farfel Z, Bourne HR. Deficient activity of receptor-cyclase coupling protein in platelets of patients with pseudohypoparathyroidism. *J Clin Endocrinol Metab* 1980;51:1202–4.

48. Downs RW, Levine MA, Drezner MK, Burch WM, Spiegel AM. Deficient adenylate cyclase regulating protein in renal membranes from a patient with pseudohypoparathyroidism. *J Clin Invest* 1983;71:231–5.

49. Drezner MK, Burch WM. Altered activity of the nucleotide regulating site in the parathyroid hormone-sensitive adenylate cyclase from the renal cortex of a patient with pseudohypoparathyroidism. *J Clin Invest* 1978;62:1222–7.

50. Levine MA, Eil C, Downs RW, Spiegel AM. Deficient guanine nucleotide regulatory unit activity in cultured fibroblast membranes from patients with pseudohypoparathyroidism type I: a cause for impaired synthesis of 3′, 5′ -cyclic AMP by intact and broken cells. *J Clin Invest* 1983;72:316–24.

51. Farfel Z, Abood ME, Brickman AS, Bourne HR. Deficient activity of receptor-cyclase coupling protein in transformed lymphoblasts of patients with pseudohypoparathyroidism, type I. *J Clin Endocrinol Metab* 1982;55:113–7.

52. Heinsimer JA, Davies AO, Downs RW, et al. Impaired formation of β-adrenergic receptor–nucleotide regulatory protein complexes in pseudohypoparathyroidism. *J Clin Invest* 1984; 73:1335–43.

53. Levine MA, Downs RW, Moses AM, et al. Resistance to multiple hormones in patients with pseudohypoparathyroidism: association with deficient activity of guanine nucleotide regulatory protein. *Am J Med* 1983;74:545–56.

54. Mallet E, Carayon P, Amr S, et al. Coupling defect of thyrotropin receptor and adenylate cyclase in a pseudohypoparathyroid patient. *J Clin Endocrinol Metab* 1982;54:1028–32.

55. Werder EA, Fischer JA, Illig R, et al. Pseudohypoparathyroidism and idiopathic hypoparathyroidism: relationship between serum calcium and parathyroid hormone levels and urinary cyclic adenosine-3′, 5′-monophosphate response to parathyroid extract. *J Clin Endocrinol Metab* 1978;46:872–9.

56. Mitchell J, Goltzman D. Examination of circulating parathyroid hormone in pseudohypoparathyroidism. *J Clin Endocrinol Metab* 1985;61:328–34.

57. Nagant de Deuxchaisnes C, Fischer JA, Dambacher MA, et al. Dissociation of parathyroid hormone bioactivity and immunoreactivity in pseudohypoparathyroidism type I. *J Clin Endocrinol Metab* 1981;53:1105–9.

58. Rao DS, Parfitt AM, Kleerekoper M, Pumo BS, Frame B. Dissociation between the effects of endogenous parathyroid hormone on adenosine 3′, 5′-monophosphate generation and phosphate reabsorption in hypocalcemia due to vitamin D depletion: an acquired disorder resembling pseudohypoparathyroidism type II. *J Clin Endocrinol Metab* 1985;61:285–90.

59. Drezner MK, Haussler MR. Normocalcemic pseudohypoparathyroidism: association with normal vitamin D₃ metabolism. *Am J Med* 1979;66:503–8.

60. Albright F, Burnett CH, Smith PH, Parson W. Pseudohypoparathyroidism: an example of "Seabright-bantam syndrome": report of three cases. *Endocrinology* 1942;30:922–32.

61. Edmondson HA, Fields IA. Relation of calcium and lipids to acute pancreatic necrosis. *Arch Intern Med* 1942;69:177–90.

62. Robertson GM, Moore EW, Switz DM, Sizemore GW, Estep HL. Inadequate parathyroid response in acute pancreatitis. *N Engl J Med* 1976;294:512–6.

63. Hermus A, Beex L, van Liessum P, Pieters G, Smedts F, Smals A. Hypocalcemia due to osteoblastic metastases and diminished parathyroid reserve in a patient with advanced breast cancer. *Klin Wochenschr* 1988;66:643–6.

64. Raskin P, McClain CJ, Medsger TA. Hypocalcemia associated with metastatic bone disease. *Arch Intern Med* 1973;132:539–43.

65. Vogelgesang SA, McMillin JM. Hypocalcemia associated with estrogen therapy for metastatic adenocarcinoma of the prostate. *J Urol* 1988;140:1025–7.

66. Biberstein M, Parker BA. Enema-induced hyperphosphatemia. *Am J Med* 1985;79:645–6.

67. Cadman EC, Lundberg WB, Bertino JR. Hyperphosphatemia and hypocalcemia accompanying rapid cell lysis in a patient with Burkitt's lymphoma and Burkitt cell leukemia. *Am J Med* 1977;62:283–90.

68. Tomlinson GC, Solberg LA. Acute tumor lysis syndrome with metastatic medulloblastoma. *Cancer* 1984;53:1783–5.

69. Urban P, Scheidegger D, Buchmann B, Barth D. Cardiac arrest and blood ionized calcium levels. *Ann Intern Med* 1988; 109:110–3.

70. Chesney RW, McCarron DM, Haddad JG, et al. Pathogenic mechanisms of the hypocalcemia of the staphylococcal toxic-shock syndrome. *J Lab Clin Med* 1983;101:576–85.

71. Sobel R, Einhorn S, Maislos M, Shainkin-Kestenbaum R, Shany S, Horowitz J. Transitory hypocalcemia complicating measles. *Arch Intern Med* 1985;145:2043–4.

72. Zaloga GP, Chernow B. The multifactorial basis for hypocalcemia during sepsis: studies of the parathyroid–vitamin D axis. *Ann Intern Med* 1987;107:36–41.

73. Zaloga GP, Willey S, Tomasic P, Chernow B. Free fatty acids alter

calcium binding: a cause for misinterpretation of serum calcium values and hypocalcemia in critical illness. *J Clin Endocrinol Metab* 1987;64:1010–4.

74. Youle MS, Clarbour J, Gazzard B, Chanas A. Severe hypocalcemia in AIDS patients treated with foscarnet and pentamidine. *Lancet* 1988;1:1455–6.

75. Lucas CE, Sennish JC, Ledgerwood AM, Harrigan C. Parathyroid response to hypocalcemia after treatment of hemorrhagic shock. *Surgery* 1984;96:711–6.

76. Schaaf M, Payne CA. Effect of diphenylhydantoin and phenobarbital on overt and latent tetany. *N Engl J Med* 1966;174:1228–33.

77. Edmondson JW, Brashear RE, Li TK. Tetany: quantitative interrelationships between calcium and alkalosis. *Am J Physiol* 1975;228:1082–6.

78. Isgreen WP. Normocalcemic tetany: a problem of erethism. *Neurology* 1976;26:825–34.

79. Eastell R, Edmonds CJ, Chazal RCS, McFadyen IR. Prolonged hypoparathyroidism presenting eventually as second trimester abortion. *Br Med J* 1985;291:955–6.

80. Nierenberg DW, Ransil BJ. Q-aT$_c$ interval as a clinical indicator of hypercalcemia. *Am J Cardiol* 1979;44:243–8.

81. Brickman AS, Trujillo AL, Gutin MS, Tuck ML. Diminished aldosterone responses to angiotensin II and adrenocorticotropin in hypocalcemia subjects: restoration of responsiveness with normocalcemia. *J Clin Endocrinol Metab* 1987;64:297–303.

82. Connor TB, Rosen BL, Blaustein MP, Applefeld MM, Doyle LA. Hypocalcemia precipitating congestive cardiac failure. *N Engl J Med* 1982;307:869–72.

83. Levine SN, Rheams CN. Hypocalcemic heart failure. *Am J Med* 1985;78:1033–5.

84. Timms P, Bold AM, Rothe P, Lau E. Severe hypocalcemia and increased serum creatine kinase activity. *Br Med J* 1985;291:937–8.

85. Brickman AS, Stern N, Sowers JR. Hypertension in pseudohypoparathyroidism type I. *Am J Med* 1988;85:785–92.

86. Stewart AF, Battaglini-Sabetta J, Millstone L. Hypocalcemia-induced pustular psoriasis of von Zumbusch. *Ann Intern Med* 1984;100:677–80.

87. Ireland AW, Hornbrook JW, Neale FC, Posen S. The crystalline lens in chronic surgical hypoparathyroidism. *Arch Intern Med* 1968;122:408–11.

88. Nikiforuk G, Fraser D. Etiology of enamel hypoplasia and interglobular dentin: the roles of hypocalcemia and hypophosphatemia. *Metab Bone Dis Rel Res* 1979;2:17–23.

89. Rosen RA, Deshmukh SM. Growth arrest recovery lines in hypoparathyroidism. *Radiology* 1985;155:61–2.

90. Okazaki T, Takuwa Y, Yamamoto M, et al. Ossification of the paravertebral ligaments: a frequent complication of hypoparathyroidism. *Metabolism* 1984;33:710–3.

91. Illum F, Dupont E. Prevalences of LT-detected calcification in the basal ganglia in idiopathic hypoparathyroidism and pseudohypoparathyroidism. *Neuroradiology* 1985;27:32–7.

92. Editorial. Serum calcium. *Lancet* 1979;1:858–9.

93. Zaloga GP, Chernow B, Cook D, Snyder R, Clapper M, O'Brian JT. Assessment of calcium homeostasis in the critically ill surgical patient: the diagnostic pitfalls of the McLean-Hastings nomogram. *Ann Surg* 1985;202:587–94.

94. Bowers GN, Brassard C, Sena SF. Measurement of ionized calcium in serum with ion-selective electrodes: a mature technology that can meet the daily service needs. *Clin Chem* 1986;32:1437–47.

95. Blind H, Schmidt-Gayle H, Scharla S, et al. Two-site assay of intact parathyroid hormone in the investigation of primary hyperparathyroidism and other disorders of calcium metabolism compared with a midregion assay. *J Clin Endocrinol Metab* 1988;67:353–60.

96. Mallette LE, Wilson DP, Kirkland JL. Evaluation of hypocalcemia with a highly sensitive, homologous radioimmunoassay for the midregion of parathyroid hormone. *Pediatrics* 1983;71:64–9.

97. Bijvoet OLM. Kidney function in calcium and phosphate metabolism. In: Avioli LV, Krane SM, eds. *Metabolic bone disease.* New York: Academic Press, 1977;50–141.

98. Mallette LE, Kirkland JL, Gagel RF, Law WM, Heath H III. Synthetic human parathyroid hormone-(1-34) for the study of pseudohypoparathyroidism. *J Clin Endocrinol Metab* 1988;67:964–72.

99. Bikle DD. Osteomalacia and rickets. In: Wyngaarden JB, Smith LH Jr, eds. *Cecil textbook of medicine,* 18th ed. Philadelphia: WB Saunders, 1988;1479–85.

100. Markowitz ME, Rosen JF, Smith C, DeLuca HF. 1,25-Dihydroxyvitamin D$_3$–treated hypoparathyroidism: 35 patient years in 10 children. *J Clin Endocrinol Metab* 1982;55:727–33.

101. Lewin IG, Papapoulos SE, O'Riordan JLH. 1α-Hydroxyvitamin D$_3$ in the long-term management of hypoparathyroidism and pseudohypoparathyroidism. *Clin Endocrinol* 1977;7(suppl):203s–7s.

102. Kanis J, Russell RGG. Rate of reversal of hypercalcaemia and hypercalciuria induced by vitamin D and its 1α-hydroxylated derivatives. *Br Med J* 1977;1:78–81.

103. Chesney RW. Resistance to 1,25-dihydroxyvitamin D in hypoparathyroidism: an enigma. *NY State J Med* 1984;84:226–7.

104. Kooh SW, Fraser D, DeLuca HF, et al. Treatment of hypoparathyroidism and pseudohypoparathyroidism with metabolites of vitamin D: evidence for impaired conversion of 25-hydroxyvitamin D to 1α,25-dihydroxyvitamin D. *N Engl J Med* 1975;293:840–4.

105. Mason RS, Posen S. The relevance of 25-hydroxycalciferol measurements in the treatment of hypoparathyroidism. *Clin Endocrinol* 1979;10:265–9.

106. Recker R. Calcium absorption and achlorhydria. *N Engl J Med* 1985;313:70–3.

107. Porter RH, Cox BG, Heaney D, Hostetter TH, Stinebaugh BJ, Suki WN. Treatment of hypoparathyroid patients with chlorthalidone. *N Engl J Med* 1978;298:577–81.

108. Parfitt AM. Thiazide-induced hypercalcemia in vitamin D–treated hypoparathyroidism. *Ann Intern Med* 1972;77:557–63.

109. Cundy T, Haining SA, Guilland-Cumming GF, Butler J, Kanis JA. Remission of hypoparathyroidism during lactation: evidence for a physiological role for prolactin in the regulation of vitamin D metabolism. *Clin Endocrinol* 1987;26:667–74.

110. Breslau NA, Zerwekh JE. Relationship of estrogen and pregnancy to calcium homeostasis in pseudohypoparathyroidism. *J Clin Endocrinol Metab* 1986;62:45–51.

111. Duarte B, Mozes MF, Eunice J, Aronson I, Pollak R, Jonasson O. Parathyroid allotransplantation in the treatment of complicated idiopathic primary hypoparathyroidism. *Surgery* 1985;98:1072–6.

CHAPTER **28**

Disorders of Phosphate and Magnesium Metabolism

Moshe Levi, Robert E. Cronin, and James P. Knochel

PHOSPHATE DISORDERS

A 70-kg adult contains about 700 g of phosphorus; 85% of this quantity is in bone, 14% is in soft tissues, and the remainder is equally distributed between the teeth, blood, and extravascular fluids. The extracellular fluid pool of phosphorus is only about 600 mg.

In extracellular fluid, phosphorus is present predominately in the inorganic form. In serum, phosphorus exists mainly as $H_2PO_4^-$ and $H_2PO_4^{2-}$, their ratio depending upon pH. At 37°C and the ionic strength of plasma, the pK_a for phosphorus is 6.8. Using the Henderson–Hasselbalch equation, the ratio of HPO_4^{2-}/HPO_4^- under these conditions is about 4:1. Less than 15% of phosphorus is protein-bound. The bulk of the intracellular phosphorus is composed of organic compounds, such as sugar phosphate. Only a small fraction of the cytosolic phosphorus is inorganic. Phosphorus is an integral and critical part of all body cells. Key intracellular organic-phosphorus-containing compounds include adenosine triphosphate (ATP), guanosine triphosphate (GTP), cyclic adenosine monophosphate (cAMP), cyclic guanine adenosine monophosphate (cGMP), and nicotine adenosine dinucleotide (NAD). 2,3-Disphosphoglycerate (2,3-DPG) is found only in erythrocytes. Other important phosphorus compounds include phospholipids, phosphoproteins, and nucleic acids. Although the concentration of inorganic phosphorus in the cell is very

low, it is very important, since it provides the source of phosphorus for synthesis of ATP and it also regulates key intracellular enzymes, including hexokinase, phosphofructokinase, glutaminase, 25-OH-cholecalciferol 1-hydroxylase, and 5′ nucleotidase.

Hypophosphatemia

Definition

Hypophosphatemia is defined as an abnormally low concentration of inorganic phosphorus in serum or plasma. It often indicates phosphorus deficiency. However, hypophosphatemia may also occur under a variety of circumstances in which total body phosphorus stores are normal. Moderate hypophosphatemia may be defined as a serum phosphorus concentration between 2.5 and 1.0 mg/dL; it is common, yet it is not usually associated with signs and symptoms of phosphate deficiency. Severe hypophosphatemia is defined as serum phosphorus levels below 1.0 mg/dL, and patients with severe hypophosphatemia usually display signs and symptoms that require therapy. Phosphorus deficiency is defined as an abnormally low content of total body phosphorus, reflected by a low phosphorus-to-nitrogen ratio by tissue analysis. Phosphorus deficiency may exist in the absence of hypophosphatemia.

Incidence

In several independent studies the prevalence of moderate hypophosphatemia, defined as serum phosphorus levels less than 2.5 mg/dL, has been found to be 2% of hospital admissions (1–4). The prevalence of severe hypophosphatemia, defined as serum phosphorus levels less than 1.0 mg/dL, has been found to be 0.1–0.25% of consecutively hospitalized patients (1–4).

M. Levi and R. E. Cronin: Departments of Internal Medicine and Nephrology, The University of Texas Southwestern Medical Center at Dallas and Veterans Affairs Medical Center, Dallas, Texas 75216.

J. P. Knochel: Department of Internal Medicine, University of Texas Southwestern Medical Center at Dallas, Dallas, Texas 75216; and Department of Internal Medicine, Presbyterian Hospital of Dallas, Dallas, Texas 75231.

Causes of Hypophosphatemia

As discussed earlier, more than 99% of the total body phosphorus is found in soft tissues and bone, and only approximately 0.6% of the total body phosphorus is in the blood and extravascular fluids. Therefore, rapid removal of phosphorus from the blood due to transcellular shift, as occurs in acute hyperventilation and nutrient infusion (Table 1), can result in acute and marked decreases in serum phosphorus concentration. On the other hand, chronic and gradual phosphorus losses caused by impaired intestinal absorption or renal reabsorption (Tables 2 and 3) do not necessarily result in a significant decrease in serum phosphorus concentration, since the large intracellular phosphorus stores can easily compensate for these losses and maintain the serum phosphorus concentration within a normal range. In clinical situations, moderate hypophosphatemia usually results from one or a combination of the following factors: (a) redistribution of phosphorus from the extracellular to the intracellular space (Table 1), (b) decreased gastrointestinal absorption of phosphorus (Table 2), or (c) decreased renal tubular reabsorption of phosphorus (Table 3).

Sometimes some of these factors, especially when they occur in combination, may result in severe hypophosphatemia (1–6) and may require the immediate attention of the clinician (Table 4). Some of these causes of severe hypophosphatemia will be discussed briefly, since they are the most common causes of hospital-acquired hypophosphatemia.

TABLE 1. *Causes of hypophosphatemia: redistribution*

Respiratory alkalosis
Sepsis
Heat stroke
Hepatic coma
Salicylate poisoning
Gout
Interleukin-2
Recovery from hypothermia
Hormonal effects
Insulin
Glucagon
β-Catecholamine agonists
Androgens
Nutrient effects
Glucose
Fructose
Glycerol
Lactate
Amino acids
Xylitol
Acute leukemia and lymphoma
Osteoblastic metastases
Prostate
Breast
Hungry bone syndrome
Post-parathyroidectomy

TABLE 2. *Causes of hypophosphatemia: decreased gastrointestinal absorption*

Decreased dietary intake
Decreased intestinal absorption
Vitamin D deficiency
Malabsorption
Steatorrhea
Secretory diarrhea
Vomiting
Phosphate-binding antacids
Alcohol abuse
Glucocorticoids
Increased intestinal secretion
Draining fistulae
Intrinsic disorders of intestinal phosphate absorption
Familial hypophosphatemic rickets
Aging

Respiratory Alkalosis

Several clinical conditions, such as fever, sepsis, alcohol withdrawal, salicylate poisoning, central nervous system disorders, and some hypoxic pulmonary diseases, induce hyperventilation, which results in respiratory alkalosis. In addition to the decrease in extracellular fluid (ECF) P_{CO_2} and the increase in ECF pH, there is a similar decrease in intracellular P_{CO_2} and an increase in intracellular pH. The glycolytic pathway, and specifically phosphofructokinase, a key rate-limiting enzyme for glycolysis, is stimulated during intracellular alkalosis (7). This increases formation of sugar phosphates and, in turn, induces intracellular entry of phosphorus, resulting in hypophosphatemia. Urinary phosphorus excretion

TABLE 3. *Causes of hypophosphatemia: decreased renal tubular reabsorption*

Primary tubular disorders
Fanconi syndrome
Familial hypophosphatemic rickets
Hypophosphatemia associated with tumors
Vitamin D-deficient rickets
Vitamin D-dependent rickets
Idiopathic hypercalciuria
Secondary or acquired tubular disorders
Parathyroid hormone excess
Glucagon excess
Glucocorticoid administration
Diuretic phase of acute tubular necrosis
Postobstructive diuresis
Postrenal transplantation
Glycosuria
Volume expansion
Diuretics
Metabolic acidosis
Metabolic alkalosis
Respiratory acidosis
Hypercalcemia
Hypokalemia
Alcohol

TABLE 4. *Causes of severe hypophosphatemia*

Respiratory alkalosis
Hyperalimentation
Dietary deficiency and phosphate-binding antacids
Chronic alcoholism and alcohol withdrawal
Recovery from diabetic ketoacidosis
Nutritional recovery syndrome
Leukemia
Severe thermal burns
Postrenal transplantation
Neuroleptic malignant syndrome

during acute respiratory alkalosis is minimal, thus confirming the notion that the hypophosphatemia is the result of redistribution of ECF phosphorus (8–10). When acute respiratory alkalosis occurs in a previously healthy subject, the resultant hypophosphatemia is usually quite mild and transient. However, voluntary forced hyperventilation in healthy volunteers has been observed to reduce serum phosphorus to levels as low as 0.3 mg/dL. Similarly, if acute respiratory alkalosis occurs in the setting of previous phosphorus depletion, such as in chronically ill and malnourished patients, then the resultant hypophosphatemia can be quite severe and persistent. This is especially true if the same chronically ill and malnourished patients are also receiving hyperalimentation, because the two have additive effects.

In recent studies, hypophosphatemia has increasingly been recognized to occur during the treatment of acute severe asthma and chronic obstructive pulmonary disease (COPD) (11–14). In one study, 12 of 23 patients (52%) with acute severe asthma developed moderate hypophosphatemia (serum phosphorus less than 2.5 mg/dL) during bronchodilator therapy. Since these patients had a parallel decrease in urinary phosphorus excretion, the underlying mechanism appears to be phosphorus shift from the extracellular to the intracellular space (11). In a study of 158 patients with COPD, moderate hypophosphatemia occurred in 34 patients (22%); in 31 of these 34 patients (91%) there was an impairment in renal tubular resorption of phosphorus as well (TmPO$_4$/GFR). Thus, in addition to redistribution, use of drugs such as corticosteroids, β_2-adrenergic vasodilators, xanthine derivatives, and loop diuretics may also cause renal tubular wasting of phosphorus, thereby resulting in a negative phosphorus balance. In fact, in this study in muscle samples obtained by quadriceps femoris needle biopsy from 14 COPD patients with hypophosphatemia, there was a significant reduction in muscle phosphorus content (14).

Hyperalimentation

Infusion of glucose, fructose, and other metabolizable nutrients requiring phosphorylation during the glycolytic cycle induces intracellular entry of phosphorus and

causes hypophosphatemia. Indeed, when given to healthy animals, infusion of glucose is associated with increases in muscle-cell total phosphorus, ATP, and glucose-6-phosphate (10). Infusion of certain amino acids also causes a similar response. Since both glucose and amino acids induce insulin release, insulin may play a significant role in promoting intracellular shifts of extracellular phosphorus. When this phenomenon occurs in previously healthy subjects or animals, the resultant hypophosphatemia is mild and transient, since the phosphorylated intracellular compounds release the phosphorus, which is then used for other intracellular metabolic pathways. Hyperalimentation, however, is usually utilized to treat patients with malnutrition, increased catabolism, cachexia, or severe burns. Total phosphorus stores in these patients is often marginal, and as hyperalimentation induces tissue regeneration and repair, phosphorus is incorporated into the new cells. These patients, therefore, can develop progressively severe and persistent hypophosphatemia (15–18). The recognition of this fact has resulted in the inclusion of phosphorus in hyperalimentation formulae and elimination of this potentially important cause of severe phosphatemia. It should be recognized that severe hypophosphatemia can also occur following institution of enteral feedings, because in a recent study of 25 patients receiving postoperative enteral support in the surgical intensive care unit, the initial serum phosphorus levels ranging from 2.4 to 4.8 mg/dL decreased to 0.5–1.2 mg/dL within 2–5 days (19). Since patients with high metabolic demand may have a higher daily requirement for phosphorus than is available in routine isotonic enteral formulas, serum phosphorus in these patients needs to be carefully monitored; if necessary, oral supplementation of phosphorus should be provided accordingly.

Phosphate-Binding Antacids

Most of the present-day antacids contain aluminum hydroxide (or aluminum carbonate) and magnesium hydroxide (or magnesium carbonate). Both aluminum and magnesium ions form complexes with phosphorus in the gastrointestinal tract, resulting in decreased phosphorus absorption. In addition, other agents which are commonly used to treat peptic ulcer disease (including Tums) and which contain calcium carbonate and sucralfate also bind phosphorus and result in reduced phosphorus absorption. Although the kidney is able to adapt to decreased gastrointestinal phosphorus absorption by reabsorbing most of the filtered phosphorus, because of ongoing obligatory gastrointestinal secretion of phosphorus in digestive juices, a negative phosphorus balance can gradually develop. Antacid-induced hypophosphatemia may, therefore, become an important factor when it occurs in patients with hyperventilation who are also receiving hyperalimentation, or in patients with uncontrolled diabetes mellitus and chronic alcoholism, as will be discussed next.

Chronic Alcoholism and Alcohol Withdrawal

The chronic alcoholic patient has several reasons for phosphorus depletion, not necessarily accompanied by hypophosphatemia (i.e., reduction in serum phosphorus concentration) (Table 5). Most of the chronic alcoholics have decreased gastrointestinal absorption of phosphorus because of their poor intake of food, antacid ingestion for symptoms of gastritis, and sometimes abnormally low 1,25-dihydroxyvitamin D_3 [1,25(OH)$_2$D$_3$] levels. In addition, they may also have increased urinary excretion of phosphorus because of direct effects of alcohol, and sometimes the use of diuretics in patients with cirrhosis and ascites results in decreased renal tubular reabsorption of phosphorus (20–27). These factors are compounded in the alcoholic patient who presents to the hospital with either alcohol withdrawal or alcoholic ketoacidosis. In experimental chronic alcoholic intoxication, a major reduction of muscle phosphorus content occurs despite abundant dietary phosphorus and the lack of hypophosphatemia (22). Typically, the serum phosphorus concentration is normal on admission to the hospital, although sometimes it may be low or even high. However, the serum phosphorus concentration almost always falls rapidly during the first few hospital days.

In the patient with alcohol withdrawal (delirium tremens), hyperventilation (resulting in respiratory alkalosis) and the administration of intravenous fluids containing dextrose cause redistribution of phosphorus to the intracellular compartment. In addition, the use of antacids causes a decrease in the gastrointestinal absorption of phosphorus, altogether resulting in severe hypophosphatemia.

TABLE 5. *Causes of hypophosphatemia in the alcoholic patient*

Redistribution
Respiratory alkalosis
Intravenous hydration with dextrose-containing solutions
Decreased gastrointestinal absorption
Poor intake of food
Reduced absorption due to the use of antacids, diarrhea, and vomiting
Impaired 1,25(OH)$_2$D$_3$[a] metabolism
Increased calcitonin secretion
Nasogastric suction
Decreased renal tubular reabsorption
Metabolic acidosis
Magnesium deficiency
Potassium deficiency
Increased ethanol levels
Decreased 1,25(OH)$_2$D$_3$ levels
Increased calcitonin secretion
Diuretic administration

[a] 1,25(OH)$_2$D$_3$ stands for 1,25-dihydroxyvitamin D$_3$.

In the patient with alcoholic ketoacidosis, the nausea and vomiting and the use of antacids and nasogastric suction cause a further decrease in gastrointestinal absorption of phosphorus. The ketoacids also cause a decrease in renal tubular reabsorption of phosphorus.

The phosphorus depletion in the alcoholic patient may further accentuate the direct dose-dependent toxic effect of alcohol on striated muscle and worsen the alcoholic myopathy and cardiomyopathy (28).

Diabetic Ketoacidosis

In the diabetic patient with ketoacidosis, the resultant glycosuria, ketonuria, osmotic diuresis, and ketoacidosis all decrease renal tubular reabsorption of phosphorus. The presence of nausea and vomiting also result in decreased intake of food and phosphorus. In addition, an insulin-dependent diabetic with a long history of poorly controlled diabetes may also have abnormal 1,25(OH)$_2$D$_3$ metabolism, which causes impairment in gastrointestinal and renal tubular transport of phosphorus. Experimentally, acute metabolic acidosis sharply reduces synthesis of 1,25(OH)$_2$D$_3$.

When the patient with diabetic ketoacidosis first presents to the hospital, the serum phosphorus concentration is usually increased or normal (29); however, once insulin therapy is started, hypophosphatemia may occur within 12–48 h (30), because insulin causes a shift of phosphorus from the extracellular fluid to the intracellular compartment. The hypophosphatemia occurs at a time when the initially increased urinary phosphorus excretion becomes markedly reduced.

The great majority of patients with diabetic ketoacidosis who have been ill for a short period of time are not seriously phosphorus-deficient. Characteristically, these patients have had vomiting for a few days at most and simply have not had sufficient time to become frankly depleted. On the other hand, some patients show severe hypophosphatemia when first admitted to the hospital despite coexistent volume depletion and metabolic acidosis, factors that usually cause elevations of serum phosphorus. The usual setting in this latter group of patients is characterized by a long prodrome, lasting a week or more, of marked polyuria, polydipsia, and the absence of vomiting. The lack of vomiting permits a greater fluid intake, a larger urine volume, and a greater opportunity to become profoundly phosphorus-depleted. Most of these patients are young, type I diabetics. Serum potassium concentrations also tend to be low in this group despite acidosis. In such patients, hypophosphatemia becomes very severe during the subsequent hospital course and could be associated with severe morbidity.

Nutritional Recovery Syndrome

The nutritional recovery of refeeding syndrome represents a constellation of findings, consisting of heart failure and a variety of electrolyte derangements observed during treatment of patients with severe protein calorie malnutrition of starvation. In contrast to hyperalimentation, hypophosphatemia may occur during administration of calories in normal quantities (17). Anthropometric measurements may predict the patients at risk for developing the nutritional recovery syndrome, since a recent study showed that anthropometric measurements of arm circumference and arm muscle circumference were below the 5th percentile in all patients developing hypophosphatemia (31). This syndrome can be reproduced in experimental animals and is commonly seen during overzealous feeding of patients who have lost marked quantities of weight as a result of food fadism or anorexia nervosa. On the basis of clinical descriptions, such patients present with many of the complications that were observed in starved prisoners after World War II. In addition to hypophosphatemia provoked by nutrients, most of these patients show other serious disturbances such as hypokalemia, hypomagnesemia, and severe glucose intolerance. The observation that feeding with small quantities of skim milk rather than pure carbohydrates caused less morbidity is very likely ascribable to the reduced calories and the higher phosphorus and potassium contents of skim milk.

Leukemia

Leukemia in a markedly proliferative phase ("blast crisis") with total white blood cell counts in excess of 100,000 μL has been associated with severe hypophosphatemia (32–34). It appears to result from phosphorus uptake by rapidly proliferating cells, and the hypophosphatemia responds to chemotherapy. Since leukemia patients are usually immunocompromised, and since hypophosphatemia may result in development of leukocyte dysfunction, the leukemic patients with hypophosphatemia may be especially susceptible to opportunistic infections.

Severe Thermal Burns

Patients with severe third-degree burns whose kidney function remains intact often become hypophosphatemic 2–10 days after the injury. Hypophosphatemia may become very severe. According to most observers, as serum phosphorus declines, phosphorus excretion into the urine usually falls to very low levels. Most patients with burns hyperventilate, and consequently respiratory alkalosis may be responsible for the hypophosphatemia. On the other hand, it has been suggested that additional factors, including renal tubular injury, volume expansion as a result of fluid administration, mobilization of retained salt and water from injured tissue, and the resulting diuresis, could also be responsible for the declining serum phosphorus levels.

In a series of 33 patients with severe thermal burns, the lowest values of serum phosphorus occurred in seven patients who died (35). Simultaneous reduction of urinary phosphorus excretion indicated that the depletion of phosphorus was mainly the result of extrarenal mechanisms. However, since fractional excretion of phosphorus still increased, renal losses may also have contributed to the hypophosphatemia. An interesting finding was that these patients showed marked increases in serum calcitonin and catecholamine levels, which may have played a role in the hypophosphatemia (35).

Hypophosphatemia in burns has potentially important connotations, because it can be implicated as a contributing factor in burn-wound sepsis and also because of the effects of hypophosphatemia on white cell function, which will be discussed later.

Renal Transplantation

Hypophosphatemia is very commonly seen in patients following successful renal transplantation and is of concern because it may play a role in the pathogenesis of severe osteomalacia in some of these patients (36–49). The causes of the hypophosphatemia are multifactorial. In the immediate post-transplantation period, intravascular volume expansion and osmotic diuresis cause marked phosphaturia. The hypophosphatemia in the ensuing several days after a successful renal transplantation may result from a combination of factors: (a) administration of glucocorticoids, which inhibit renal phosphorus transport and may also inhibit gastrointestinal absorption of phosphorus; (b) ingestion of antacids such as aluminum/magnesium/calcium carbonate, which form complexes with gut phosphorus and inhibit its absorption; (c) persistently elevated parathyroid hormone (PTH) levels, especially in patients with previously severe secondary hyperparathyroidism; and (d) an intrinsic renal tubular defect for phosphorus reabsorption which is independent of all other hormonal/metabolic factors and which may become further exacerbated during periods of rejection. Sometimes the hypophosphatemia can be severe and may require phosphate replacement therapy. Of note, $1,25(OH)_2D_3$ levels are within the normal range in most of these patients; however, some patients with severe hypophosphatemia following renal transplantation may benefit from short periods of $1,25(OH)_2D_3$ therapy to enhance gastrointestinal and renal tubular phosphorus transport.

Clinical Consequences of Severe Hypophosphatemia

When severe hypophosphatemia is associated with phosphorus deficiency, it can result in multiorgan dysfunction (50–60) (Table 6). In some tissues the cellular effects on phosphorus deficiency are caused by its effects on 2,3-DPG and on adenosine nucleotides such as ATP, and in others they are caused by secondary electrical disturbances in excitatory tissue. 2,3-DPG levels are de-

TABLE 6. *Consequences of severe hypophosphatemia*

Cardiopulmonary
Decreased cardiac output, cardiac arrhythmia, hypotension
Decreased vital capacity, impaired diaphragmatic
 contractility, respiratory muscle weakness, hypoxia
Neurologic
Anorexia, irritability, confusion, dysarthria, seizures, coma
Musculoskeletal
Muscle weakness, decreased transmembrane resting
 potential, rhabdomyolysis
Bone pain, pseudofractures, rickets, or osteomalacia
Hematologic
Impaired function of erythrocytes, platelets, and leukocytes
Endocrine/metabolic
Hyperinsulinemia, insulin resistance, decreased glucose
 metabolism
Decreased parathyroid hormone levels, increased
 $1,25(OH)_2D_3$ levels
Renal
Decreased glomerular filtration rate, decreased T_m for
 bicarbonate, decreased titratable acid excretion,
 hypercalciuria, hypermagnesemia

creased in the red blood cells, resulting in an increase in the affinity of hemoglobin for oxygen. This leads to impaired oxygen delivery to the organs or to tissue hypoxia. There is also a decrease in the tissue content of ATP and, therefore, a decrease in the availability of energy-rich phosphate compounds for cell function. Reduced cellular phosphorus concentration also stimulates the irreversible deamination of AMP, which depletes intracellular adenosine nucleotide stores and further impairs the cell's ability to generate ATP. Finally, in phosphorus-deficient alkalosis and in dogs with experimental phosphorus deficiency, the resting transmembrane electrical potential difference across muscle cells is abnormally low and may be the cause of the profound weakness experienced by phosphorus-deficient patients (30,57).

An especially important hypophosphatemic syndrome is that seen in seriously ill patients managed for prolonged periods of time with intravenous fluids. Typically, a patient is in an intensive care unit setting, may be postoperative, and has been intubated. The patient cannot be extubated at the expected time or, if extubated, develops progressive weakness and progressive respiratory failure characterized by impairment of respiratory muscle and diaphragm function, hypercarbia, hypoxia, and respiratory acidosis (53–57). Neurologic events may also occur and may include ascending paralysis resembling the Guillain–Barré syndrome, mental confusion, and seizure activity. In these cases, the serum phosphorus concentration usually falls to values less than 1.0 mg/dL. Correction of hypophosphatemia quickly improves the respiratory muscle and diaphragm function and cures the respiratory failure. Neurologic dysfunction, however, improves more slowly (50).

Treatment of Hypophosphatemia

The major question in the evaluation of a patient with hypophosphatemia is whether the low serum phosphorus concentration is indicative of a true phosphorus deficiency syndrome (Table 6). It is reemphasized that less than 0.05% of total body phosphorus is present in the extracellular fluid pool; accordingly, hypophosphatemia does not necessarily denote phosphorus deficiency, since it may represent no more than an intracellular shift. For example, in a previously healthy subject, acute hyperventilation, which induces an acute and transient shift of extracellular fluid phosphorus to the intracellular space, can cause a degree of hypophosphatemia similar to that observed after prolonged nausea and vomiting in a chronic alcoholic patient with alcoholic ketoacidosis. The hypophosphatemia in the previously healthy subject with acute hyperventilation, however, is associated with normal body phosphorus stores and does not require treatment, whereas the same degree of hypophosphatemia in the alcoholic patient most likely represents phosphorus deficiency and requires phosphate replacement therapy.

Since most of the clinical consequences of hypophosphatemia are caused by decreased levels and impaired synthesis of 2,3-DPG in erythrocytes, and of ATP in all cells (including erythrocytes), the measurement of erythrocyte 2,3-DPG and ATP levels would be most helpful in determining whether the decrease in serum phosphorus concentration is associated with a critical decrease in cellular phosphorus. In addition, magnetic resonance spectroscopy can also accurately measure intracellular phosphorus and ATP content. However, until such measurements become routine in the clinical chemistry laboratory or in the radiology suite, the clinician has to resort to less perfect, yet quite adequate, means of assessing the patient with hypophosphatemia.

In most cases of hypophosphatemia, a careful history, physical examination, review of the medications and intravenous fluid therapy, and laboratory data (including arterial pH and blood gases, urinary phosphorus, and urinary creatinine for calculation of fractional excretion of phosphorus) can help establish the cause of the hypophosphatemia and determine whether the patient needs phosphate replacement therapy.

In patients with moderate hypophosphatemia (1.0–2.5 mg/dL), if there is no history of previous renal or gastrointestinal losses, and if there is no evidence of the expected consequences of phosphorus depletion, then there is no need for phosphate replacement. This is especially true if the hypophosphatemia is caused by hyperventilation or nutrient administration, either of which result in a transient shift of phosphorus from extracellular to intracellular sites. In most of these cases, the identification and treatment of the primary cause usually results in restoration of the blood phosphorus concentration to normal. On the other hand, if the hypophosphatemia occurs in patients who are suspected of having previous renal and gastrointestinal phosphorus losses, who have evidence of malnutrition or increased catabolism, and who most importantly, have evidence of the phosphorus depletion syndrome, then careful replacement of the phosphorus deficiency is indicated.

Patients with severe and sustained hypophosphatemia (<1.0 mg/dL) usually have depletion of total body phosphorus stores and may require replacement therapy to normalize plasma phosphorus concentration and tissue 2,3-DPG and ATP levels. An important exception is the common patient with diabetic ketoacidosis whose serum phosphorus is often normal or elevated when first measured, but falls to levels approaching 1.0 mg/dL or less following insulin and fluids. In diabetic ketoacidosis, 2,3-DPG levels are usually lower than normal; furthermore, because of its predictable effects on hemoglobin oxygen affinity, 2,3-DPG was long believed to cause tissue hypoxemia and to play a major role in the pathogenesis of diabetic coma. Phosphate replacement therapy was advocated to enhance recovery of 2,3-DPG levels (61,62). Recent controlled studies, however, have not shown any statistical difference between recovery of erythrocyte 2,3-DPG levels, glucose utilization rates, or the clinical course of recovery from diabetic ketoacidosis in patients who were randomly assigned to conventional treatment alone or combined with phosphate infusions (63,64). Therefore, treatment with insulin and fluids, which corrects the acidosis in diabetic ketoacidosis, results in improvement of the erythrocyte 2,3-DPG levels in spite of the persistent hypophosphatemia (65).

Routine phosphate replacement therapy is therefore not necessary in most patients with diabetic ketoacidosis. It should only be reserved for the occasional patient with severe and persistent hypophosphatemia. As described earlier in this chapter in the discussion dealing with pathogenesis, one should be alert for the typically young, new-onset, type I diabetic who has been developing diabetic ketoacidosis for many days or weeks before he or she is admitted to a hospital. In these cases, the presence of severe hypophosphatemia before treatment has been initiated, despite coexistent metabolic acidosis, indicates a severe phosphorus deficiency that demands treatment.

In most patients with other causes of severe hypophosphatemia, phosphorus replacement may be delayed if the underlying causes, such as phosphorus-binding antacids, alcohol, diuretics, and osmotic diuresis due to uncontrolled diabetes, can be identified and treated and/or discontinued. However, in spite of these measures, if the hypophosphatemia persists, and especially if the patient is symptomatic, then phosphorus therapy should be initiated.

If the patient is able to tolerate oral intake, the safest and most efficient mode of therapy is the administration of skim or low-fat (0.5% fat) milk, which contains approximately 0.9 mg of phosphorus per milliliter. Milk is also a rich source of calcium, potassium, magnesium, and protein, and its use is ideal in malnourished patients. A typical patient with severe hypophosphatemia would require between four and eight cartons of milk (8 oz of milk per carton) per day, because each 8 oz contains approximately 235 mg of elemental phosphorus and because the average patient requires 1000–2000 mg of phosphorus per day to have body stores repleted within 7–10 days.

If the patient is unable to tolerate milk, he or she can be given any of the oral preparations listed in Table 7. The intravenous administration of phosphorus is usually reserved for patients with severe hypophosphatemia who cannot take milk or tablets, or who are overtly symptomatic and have evidence of erythrocyte, platelet, and leukocyte dysfunction; cardiomyopathy; respiratory muscle weakness; or altered mental status as a result of the severe hypophosphatemia (Table 6). Since we do not have adequate means to determine the degree of intracellular phosphorus depletion, we also do not have a satisfactory means to determine the amount of phosphorus that needs to be replaced. An earlier study suggested 2.5–5.0 mg of elemental phosphorus per kilogram of body weight be administered intravenously every 6 h to replete phosphorus in patients with severe hypophosphatemia (66), although the efficacy of this therapy was not

TABLE 7. Commonly available phosphorus-containing preparations

Preparations	Phosphorus	Sodium	Potassium
Oral			
K-Phos neutral tablets (Beach)	250 mg/tab	12 mEq/tab	2 mEq/tab
K-Phos tablets (Beach)	114 mg/tab		3.65 mEq/tab
Neutra-Phos-K capsules (Willen Drug Co.)	250 mg/cap		14 mEq/cap
Neutra-Phos capsules (Willen Drug Co.)	250 mg/cap	7 mEq/cap	7 mEq/cap
Fleet Phospho Soda (C.D. Fleet Co.)	149 mg/mL	6 mEq/mL	
Parenteral			
Hyper-Phos-K (Davies, Rose-Hoyt)	67 mg/mL		3.3 mEq/mL
In-Phos (Davies, Rose-Hoyt)	25 mg/mL	1.6 mEq/mL	0.2 mEq/mL
Sodium phosphate (Abbott)	93 mg/mL	4 mEq/mL	
Potassium phosphate (Abbott)	93 mg/mL		4 mEq/mL

validated. A more recent study administered 9 mM phosphorus in 0.5 N saline intravenously as a continuous infusion over a period of 12 h, which corresponds to approximately 2 mg/kg body weight every 6 h (67). Mean serum phosphorus concentration increased from baseline value of 0.81 mg/dL to 1.27 mg/dL in 12 h, to 1.67 mg/dL in 24 h, 2.07 mg/dL in 36 h, and 2.80 mg/dL in 48 h. Once a serum phosphorus concentration of 2.0–2.5 mg/dL is achieved, it would be most safe to switch to oral replacement therapy.

An important factor that should also be considered in the treatment of patients with hypophosphatemia is that most of these patients may also have low serum magnesium levels. Of note, phosphorus deficiency may result in increased urinary magnesium excretion, and magnesium deficiency may also result in increased urinary phosphorus excretion. Therefore, in selected patients, the hypomagnesemia, if present, may need to be corrected for the successful correction of the hypophosphatemia. In this regard, milk is also a good source for magnesium, since each 8 oz of milk contains 34 mg of this element.

Side Effects and Complications of Treatment of Hypophosphatemia

The major side effects of phosphorus replacement therapy are as follows: diarrhea, especially with oral preparations; hyperphosphatemia; hypocalcemia; hyperkalemia if potassium phosphate salts are employed; metabolic acidosis; and volume expansion, especially with intravenous sodium phosphate preparations.

The diarrhea is a dose-related phenomenon, and it can be generally avoided if phosphorus tablets are given in divided doses and if the total dose is limited to four tablets a day.

The hyperphosphatemia is a direct consequence of excessive phosphorus administration. Since the intracellular phosphorus depletion cannot be correctly estimated, and since the initial serum concentration response to intravenous phosphorus replacement does not indicate the degree of depletion and also does not predict the serum concentration response to further therapy, one has to carefully monitor the serum phosphorus concentration every 12 h during intravenous replacement therapy.

One of the consequences of acute hyperphosphatemia is that it can cause acute hypocalcemia and result in hypotension and cardiac arrest (68). In addition, acute hyperphosphatemia can cause widespread vascular calcification resulting in impairments in pulmonary gas exchange and renal perfusion.

Hyperkalemia may occur in patients with decreased renal function and oliguria, since most of the phosphorus preparations contain potassium. Therefore, serum potassium should be closely monitored during phosphorus administration.

Finally, some of the phosphorus preparations such as oral phosphosoda (pH 4.8), acid sodium phosphate (pH 4.9), intravenous sodium phosphate (pH 5.7), and potassium phosphate (pH 6.6) are acidic and, when administered in large doses, may result in metabolic acidosis.

Hyperphosphatemia

Definition

Hyperphosphatemia is defined as a serum phosphorus concentration exceeding 5 mg/dL in adults, although serum phosphorus concentration of up to 6 mg/dL may be considered physiologic in children and adolescents. Hyperphosphatemia usually indicates total body phosphorus excess; however, it may also occur under circumstances in which total body phosphorus stores are normal, as in situations associated with acute redistribution of phosphorus from intracellular to extracellular fluid.

Causes of Hyperphosphatemia

Hyperphosphatemia can result from (a) reduced renal phosphorus excretion, because of either decreased glomerular filtration rate or increased tubular reabsorption of phosphorus (Table 8), (b) increased gastrointestinal intake and absorption, or intravenous administration of phosphorus (Table 8), and (c) redistribution and/or increased release of intracellular phosphorus (Table 9).

Recently, spurious hyperphosphatemia has been reported in patients with dysglobulinemia (69–71). The pseudohyperphosphatemia results from the interference of monoclonal immunoglobulins with the phosphomo-

TABLE 8. *Causes of hyperphosphatemia: decreased renal excretion, increased tubular reabsorption, and increased gastrointestinal absorption*

Decreased renal excretion of phosphorus
Decrease in glomerular filtration rate
   Chronic renal failure
   Acute renal failure
Increased tubular reabsorption of phosphorus
Hypoparathyroidism
Pseudohypoparathyroidism type I and II
Tumoral calcinosis
Pseudoxanthoma elasticum
Hyperostosis
Hyperthyroidism
Glucocorticoid deficiency
Biphosphonate therapy
Increased gastrointestinal absorption of phosphorus
Ingestion and/or administration of phosphorus laxatives and
   enemas
Pharmacologic therapy with vitamin D metabolites
Clinical disorders associated with increased vitamin D levels

TABLE 9. *Causes of hyperphosphatemia: redistribution and intracellular release*

Redistribution of intracellular phosphorus
Acute respiratory acidosis
Acute metabolic acidosis
Increased release of intracellular phosphorus
Burkitt's lymphoma
Lymphoblastic lymphoma
Acute lymphoblastic leukemia
Metastatic small-cell bronchogenic carcinoma
Metastatic breast adenocarcinoma
Rhabdomyolysis
Thyrotoxicosis
Autoimmune hemolytic anemia

lybdate colorimetric assay for phosphorus determination used in several automated systems. Removal of the immunoglobulins by sulfosalicylic acid precipitation or ultrafiltration results in accurate determination of serum phosphorus concentration.

Renal Causes of Hyperphosphatemia

One of the most common causes of hyperphosphatemia is decreased urinary excretion of phosphorus as a result of reduced glomerular filtration rate associated with chronic or acute renal failure. In chronic and progressive renal failure, phosphorus homeostasis is maintained by a stepwise increase in phosphorus excretion per functioning nephron. As renal insufficiency progresses and the number of functioning nephrons decreases, however, phosphorus homeostasis can no longer be maintained and hyperphosphatemia develops. Hyperphosphatemia is also very common in acute renal failure, especially in acute renal failure resulting from rhabdomyolysis and tumor lysis syndrome.

Increased renal tubular reabsorption of filtered phosphate can also result in hyperphosphatemia. PTH is an important regulator of tubular reabsorption of phosphorus, and the absence of PTH (as in surgical or traumatic hypoparathyroidism) and the tubular resistance to PTH (as in pseudohypoparathyroidism type I and type II) result in hyperphosphatemia due to the increase in the tubular transport maximum for phosphorus. Hyperphosphatemia is also reported with primary or genetic disorders such as (a) the syndrome of familial tumoral calcinosis and (b) pseudoxanthoma elasticum; in the latter disorder there is an increase in the tubular transport maximum for phosphorus (72,73). In tumoral calcinosis and pseudoxanthoma elasticum, abnormal vitamin D metabolism may also play an important pathogenic role, since $1,25(OH)_2D_3$ levels are either normal or increased and can thus result in hyperphosphatemia by causing both increased gastrointestinal absorption and renal tubular reabsorption of phosphorus. Another genetic cause of hyperphosphatemia is hyperostosis (74,75). Hyper-

phosphatemia can also occur in acromegaly, hypothyroidism, and glucocorticoid deficiency after surgical correction of hypercortisolism in patients with Cushing's syndrome (76). Finally, biphosphonates, which are used in the treatment of Paget's disease of bone (77), surgically untreatable hyperparathyroidism, and hypercalcemia of malignancy associated with metastatic bone disease, can also result in hyperphosphatemia, partly due to enhanced renal tubular reabsorption of phosphate.

Gastrointestinal Causes of Hyperphosphatemia

Hyperphosphatemia can result from an increased oral intake of phosphorus tablets or laxatives and vitamin D therapy, which would result in increased intestinal absorption of phosphorus. Another common cause of hyperphosphatemia is sodium phosphate enemas, which can result in very high levels of hyperphosphatemia and subsequent death in individuals with renal insufficiency. A recent study has shown that phosphorus is certainly absorbed by the colon, and therefore that phosphate enemas should be prescribed with great caution—especially in children and in patients with renal insufficiency (78,79).

Pharmacologic Causes of Hyperphosphatemia

Hyperphosphatemia may result from increased intravenous phosphorus administration during the treatment of hypophosphatemia or in patients receiving total parenteral nutrition (TPN) (80).

Hyperphosphatemia Resulting from Redistribution

A common cause of hyperphosphatemia is acute respiratory acidosis, which results in redistribution of phosphorus from intracellular pools to the extracellular fluid. Acute metabolic acidosis is also associated with hyperphosphatemia and may be partially responsible for (a) the hyperphosphatemia seen in patients with diabetic ketoacidosis prior to insulin therapy (29) and (b) the hyperphosphatemia in patients with chronic renal failure (81,82).

Hyperphosphatemia Resulting from Increased Release of Intracellular Phosphorus

Hyperphosphatemia resulting from increased entry into the extracellular fluid is most dramatically seen in patients with acute renal failure associated with the crush syndrome or in the acute tumor lysis syndrome. In the latter, marked hyperphosphatemia, hyperkalemia, and hyperuricemia appear shortly after chemotherapy. It is especially appropriate to follow such treatment for lymphomas, including lymphoblastic lymphoma, Burkitt's lymphoma, and acute lymphoblastic leukemia (83). This syndrome sometimes happens (even in the absence of chemotherapy) in conditions associated with high cell turnover (84); the syndrome has also been reported as a complication of chemotherapy for extensive small-cell bronchogenic carcinoma or for metastatic breast adenocarcinoma, as well as during radiotherapy of metastatic medulloblastoma.

In patients with severe rhabdomyolysis due to trauma or with extensive tissue destruction secondary to infarction or infection, and especially in intestinal necrosis associated with lactic acidosis, hyperphosphatemia of a pronounced degree may serve as an indication for surgical débridement or removal of the affected tissue. Each of these conditions is generally associated with severe volume depletion and renal failure.

Clinical Consequences of Hyperphosphatemia (Table 10)

One of the most striking clinical consequences of hyperphosphatemia is related to the reciprocal fall in the serum calcium concentration, which occurs in all cases of hyperphosphatemia, with the exception of tumoral calcinosis, pseudoxanthoma elasticum, cortical hyperostosis, and thyrotoxicosis, where serum calcium levels are normal because of the associated increase in $1,25(OH)_2D_3$ levels and the increase in gastrointestinal calcium absorption. In all the other cases, hyperphosphatemia produces hypocalcemia by several mechanisms, including decreased synthesis of $1,25(OH)_2D_3$, decreased absorption of calcium from the gastrointestinal tract, and precipitation of calcium. The hypocalcemia can result in impaired myocardial contractility, conduction abnormalities, decreased systemic vascular reactivity, hypotension, and increased neuromuscular excitability, including tetany, seizure activity, and convulsions.

Another serious side effect of hyperphosphatemia is the high incidence of ectopic calcification, which is caused by the precipitation of $Ca-P_i$ in the form of hydroxyapatite crystals. The factors that control $Ca-P_i$ precipitations include the $Ca-P_i$ concentration product, local pH, circulating levels of PTH, and, most importantly, prior cell injury. Thus, if the calcium phosphorus product rises above 60, especially in the presence of an alkaline pH, metastatic calcification is likely. This explains the common occurrence of metastatic calcification in patients with Burnet's (milk alkali) syndrome. High levels of PTH also favor ectopic calcification. The ectopic calcification can occur in virtually every organ system, including the heart, lung, brain, muscle, eye, skin, and the periarticular space of the large joints. Vascular calcification can also occur, resulting in necrosis and gangrene of the upper and lower extremities. Finally, it should be noted that there can be ectopic calcification of the kidney as well, resulting in worsening of renal function, which would only further aggregate the hyperphosphatemia (85).

Treatment of Hyperphosphatemia (Table 11)

The treatment of hyperphosphatemia depends on the cause, whether it is acute or chronic, and whether renal function is intact. The major treatment modalities include inhibition of gastrointestinal absorption and/or enhancement of urinary excretion of phosphorus.

In acute hyperphosphatemic disorders that are mainly caused by rhabdomyolysis, tumor lysis syndrome, and similar conditions that are associated with (a) an increased entrance of phosphorus from intracellular stores to ECF, (b) administration of phosphate enemas and laxatives, or (c) administration of phosphorus-containing intravenous fluids and total parenteral nutrition, if renal function is adequate the goal is to induce phosphaturia.

TABLE 10. *Clinical consequences of severe hyperphosphatemia*

Hypocalcemia
Impaired myocardial contractility
Conduction abnormalities
Decreased systemic vascular tone
Hypotension
Increased neuromuscular excitability

Ectopic calcification
Vascular
Soft tissue
Skeletal muscle
Cardiac muscle
Periarticular space

TABLE 11. *Treatment of hyperphosphatemia*

Acute hyperphosphatemia
Increased renal excretion of phosphorus
  Intravenous volume expansion
  Bicarbonate
  Carbonic anhydrase inhibitors
Shift into intracellular stores
  Glucose-insulin
  Removal from extracellular fluid

Chronic hyperphosphatemia
Dietary phosphorus restriction
Decreased gastrointestinal absorption
  Aluminum salts
    Alternagel
    Amphogel
    Basaljel
    Alu-Caps
    Alu-Tabs
  Magnesium salts
    Magnesium carbonate
    Magnesium hydroxide
  Calcium salts
    Calcium carbonate
    Calcium citrate
    Calcium acetate
  Sucralfate

This can be most optimally achieved by ECF volume expansion with intravenous saline, and also by administration of sodium bicarbonate and acetazolamide, a carbonic anhydrase inhibitor. Each of these modalities reduces tubular reabsorption of filtered phosphorus and results in increased urinary excretion of phosphorus. In the treatment of hyperphosphatemia associated with rhabdomyolysis and tumor lysis syndrome, this form of therapy may also be helpful toward prevention of acute tubular necrosis and hyperkalemia. Allopurinol, a xanthine oxidase inhibitor, is also administered to prevent the hyperuricemia that accompanies the hyperkalemia and hyperphosphatemia associated with the tumor lysis syndrome.

In acute hyperphosphatemic disorders associated with impaired renal function, additional treatment modalities include (a) administration of intravenous insulin and glucose and (b) hemodialysis or peritoneal dialysis. Insulin and glucose administration cause a shift of ECF phosphorus to the intracellular space; however, the effects are only transient. Dialysis is an effective mode of therapy for sustained removal of ECF phosphorus in these conditions. Peritoneal dialysis (PD) may be the preferred mode of dialysis, because frequent exchanges (every 1 or 2 h) utilized in acute peritoneal dialysis allow for the continuous removal of ECF phosphorus. Continuous arteriovenous hemodialysis (CAVHD) may also be quite suitable in the treatment of patients with severe and sustained hyperphosphatemia.

In chronic hyperphosphatemic disorders associated with renal insufficiency, or enhanced gastrointestinal absorption caused by increased vitamin D levels, the goal is to inhibit gastrointestinal absorption of phosphorus. Since dietary phosphorus restriction to the degree that is required to satisfactorily reduce the serum phosphorus concentration is impractical, the major mode of therapy is the use of certain phosphorus-binding salts, including aluminum, magnesium, and calcium salts.

Side Effects and Complications of Treatment of Hyperphosphatemia (Table 12)

Aluminum hydroxide and aluminum carbonate gel and capsules, which are commercially available as Alternagel, Basaljel, Amphogel, and Alu-Tab, have been the traditional form of therapy very effectively used in the control of hyperphosphatemia. The major side effects of the aluminum gels are severe constipation and, in the very compliant patient, hypophosphatemia with phosphate depletion, resulting in osteomalacia (86). In addition, it has clearly become evident that aluminum in these compounds can be absorbed from the gastrointestinal tract, can result in aluminum accumulation in several organs, and can cause chronic anemia, disabling osteomalacia, myopathy, and often fatal encephalopathy (87–92). Therefore, the present-day strategy is to use

TABLE 12. *Complications related to treatment of hyperphosphatemia*

General
Hypophosphatemia
Specific
Aluminum salts
Constipation
Aluminum toxicity
Anemia
Osteomalacia
Encephalopathy
Magnesium salts
Diarrhea
Magnesium toxicity
Neuromuscular
Hypotension
Calcium salts
Calcium toxicity
Ectopic calcification

phosphate-binding salts other than aluminum gels. Magnesium salts are effective phosphate binders (93); however, since magnesium is also absorbed from the gastrointestinal tract and can result in neuromuscular toxicity, its use is limited in patients with chronic renal failure. At the present time the most commonly used phosphate-binding salts are the calcium salts, including calcium carbonate and calcium acetate (94–102). The calcium salts are at least as effective as aluminum gels in binding dietary phosphorus and controlling hyperphosphatemia. They also have the potential advantage that the increase in gastrointestinal calcium absorption may normalize the calcium deficiency that occurs in patients with chronic renal failure. One major side effect, however, is that the increase in gastrointestinal calcium absorption can result in hypercalcemia and can increase the risk to metastatic calcification. Active research is underway to develop and test new nonsoluble and nonabsorbable aluminum compounds and calcium-charged polymers, and ketoacids, which are effective phosphate binders but which potentially lack the side effects associated with aluminum, magnesium, and calcium salts (103–105).

MAGNESIUM DISORDERS

Magnesium is the fourth most abundant cation in extracellular fluid, and in intracellular fluid it is exceeded only by potassium. Like potassium, magnesium is primarily an intracellular ion. A 70-kg person contains about 1750 mEq of magnesium, or 25 mEq/kg; slightly more than 1% of this magnesium is in the extracellular compartment, with the rest in cells (31%) or in bone (67%). In normal adults the serum magnesium is 1.7 ± 0.3 mEq/L (mean ± 2 SD), and 24-h urine magnesium is 10 ± 6 mEq (106). Magnesium levels are customarily reported as either mEq/L or mg/dL. Values reported as mEq/L can be converted to mg/dL simply by multiplying by 1.2.

Approximately 20% of serum magnesium is protein-bound. The important biologic effects of magnesium depend on its capacity to form weak chelates with enzymes and other structures of the cell (e.g., protein, nucleic acids, and phospholipids). The cellular magnesium content of most tissues is 6–9 mM/kg wet weight, and most of this magnesium is localized in membrane structures (e.g., microsomes, mitochondria, and plasma membranes) (107). The much smaller pool of free magnesium in the cell is in an exchanging equilibrium with the bound magnesium in membranes. This buffer system maintains the intracellular free magnesium concentration at about 1 mM during periods of magnesium excess or magnesium depletion. Moreover, this concentration is the optimal magnesium concentration for most intracellular enzyme systems (107). This unbound intracellular magnesium has a critical role in cellular physiology and catalyzes enzymic processes concerned with the transfer, storage, and utilization of energy (108). Phosphatases that hydrolyze and transfer organic phosphate groups are activated by magnesium, as are reactions that involve ATP. Because of the pivotal role of ATP in the metabolism of carbohydrates, fats, nucleic acids, and proteins as well as the many ATP-energy-dependent cellular processes, magnesium deficiency has the potential to impair many critical cellular functions.

The daily requirement for magnesium is estimated to be 18–33 mEq (109). This figure approximates the average dietary magnesium intake in the United States; thus the average U.S. diet could be considered borderline deficient. Meat, green vegetables, grains, and seafoods are the main dietary sources of magnesium.

Magnesium Deficiency States

The predominantly intracellular location of magnesium often makes it difficult to interpret the clinical reports and studies concerned primarily with changes in the relatively small extracellular phase of this ion. The serum levels of magnesium may be high, normal, or low in the presence of cellular depletion (110–114). For example, in untreated diabetic ketoacidosis, initially high serum levels may fall to frankly hypomagnesemic levels with insulin therapy. In this latter condition, serum magnesium movement pre- and post-insulin is similar to that of serum potassium. Determinations of magnesium in red blood cells, bone, and muscle—by direct measurement in biopsy samples, or noninvasively by use of magnetic resonance spectroscopy—give a more accurate assessment of total body magnesium levels, but these determinations have been used primarily as research tools.

In experimental human magnesium deficiency, serum magnesium levels correlate well with progressive magnesium deficiency (115). When complicating factors develop, serum magnesium may be a less useful guide. Since magnesium bound to serum proteins accounts for only 20% of the total, disorders involving a change in serum protein concentration (e.g., nephrotic syndrome and malnutrition) have a much smaller effect on serum magnesium than they are known to have on the more highly bound calcium ion. After measurement of the serum magnesium level, the second step should be a determination of the 24-h urinary magnesium excretion. If both of these tests are normal, it is unlikely that significant magnesium deficiency exists. However, if the serum magnesium is less than 1.0 mEq/L and urinary magnesium excretion is less than 1 mEq/day, this strongly implies a magnesium deficiency state (108). In the research setting, biopsies of muscle and bone have been used to assess total body magnesium. Chronically alcoholic patients, with or without cirrhosis, may have normal serum magnesium, whereas their muscle magnesium is substantially reduced (111,112). Alcoholic patients studied by balance techniques in the period of recovery from magnesium deficiency retain 40–80 mEq of magnesium over a 6- to 7-day period (116,117). To circumvent the need for muscle and bone biopsies, erythrocyte magnesium levels have been measured as an index of total body magnesium; they generally correlate with serum magnesium. There is a correlation between serum and erythrocyte magnesium content in a variety of clinical disorders (114); for any given patient, however, erythrocyte magnesium had a poor predictive value. A more predictive correlation existed between serum magnesium and bone magnesium content. Skeletal muscle magnesium has also been used to estimate total body magnesium, particularly in patients with clinical conditions predisposing to magnesium deficiency (112,113).

Exchangeable magnesium has been used to estimate total body stores and distribution of magnesium (118,119); in normal individuals this accounts for only about 4.5 mEq/kg of the total body magnesium, which is estimated at 25 mEq/kg. Use and interpretation of this tracer is difficult (120). Plasma magnesium concentration falls progressively with aging, apparently independently of underlying diseases or medications ingested (121,122). Whether these lower plasma magnesium values in the elderly necessarily indicate an magnesium-deficient state is unclear since concurrent urinary magnesium excretion data are not available.

In summary, measurements of serum magnesium and urinary magnesium constitute the easiest and clinically most satisfactory way to diagnose magnesium deficiency.

Relationship Between Magnesium Deficiency and Potassium and Calcium Balance

In the body there is a close relationship between the movement of magnesium and potassium. In general, a change in the serum level of one ion causes the other to deviate in the same direction. In one study, six of seven patients made magnesium-deficient developed a fall in serum potassium and an increase in urinary potassium excretion (115). Reinstitution of magnesium into the diet resulted in a prompt and marked positive balance in those patients. In the presence of magnesium deficiency, replacing potassium alone is difficult (112–125). However, in the absence of potassium replacement, magnesium replacement alone is sufficient to correct hypokalemia (115). The link between these ions is further supported by the observations that a deficiency state of either ion produces clinical symptoms with much overlap and that the replacement of one ion without the other often produces symptoms characteristic of deficiency of the ion not replaced (126).

Cellular levels of magnesium and potassium also tend to rise and fall together during periods of magnesium (114,116,127–129) or potassium (114,127,130,131) deficiency. Since dietary magnesium restriction has little effect on renal potassium excretion, the alteration in cellular potassium content during magnesium deficiency must be a consequence of some effect at the tissue level, rather than a defect in renal potassium conservation (132). Although a magnesium-deficient diet in young rats leads to a significant decrease in skeletal muscle potassium concentration and a decrease in the concentration of [³H]ouabain binding sites, there is no evidence that the reduction in [³H]ouabain binding sites (i.e., Na,K-ATPase units) is due, per se, to magnesium deficiency (133). In isolated potassium deficiency, a marked decrease in Na-K- pumps has been shown (134). In muscle cells, in addition to this relationship between cellular potassium and magnesium, there are similar fixed ratios for potassium and phosphorus and for magnesium and phosphorus (127). In alcoholics withdrawing from alcohol, skeletal muscle magnesium deficiency correlates with reduced skeletal muscle phosphorus (116). The precise relationship of the movements of these three ions is not clear, but clinical observations support the possibility of a linkage. In diabetic ketoacidosis, repair of the cellular deficits of magnesium, potassium, and phosphorus requires the simultaneous administration of all three ions (135). And following initial insulin therapy for diabetic acidosis, serum content of all three ions falls simultaneously; this fall presumably results from the movement of these ions from extracellular fluid into cells (136). The failure of cells to take up potassium despite heavy supplementation during periods of magnesium deficiency suggests that cellular magnesium deficiency prevents them from establishing a normal transcellular gradient for potassium. Since the bulk of cellular magnesium is bound to the membrane structures of the cell while free cytosolic magnesium is maintained constant at about 1 mM over wide ranges of extracellular magnesium, magnesium deficiency syndromes primarily affect membrane-bound magnesium, which

exerts important effects on membrane permeability to sodium, potassium, and calcium (107). In turn, it is these resulting ionic changes (e.g., reduced intracellular potassium and elevated intracellular sodium and calcium) that lead to the clinical and metabolic effects of magnesium deficiency. This intriguing formulation explains the apparent key role of magnesium in restoring cellular potassium content.

In humans, hypocalcemia is a prominent manifestation of experimental magnesium deficiency. With replacement of magnesium in the diet, both serum magnesium and serum calcium rise to normal (115). In the dog, too, there is a close relationship between falls in serum magnesium and in serum calcium (137). Many of the early studies in experimental magnesium deficiency utilized the rat. In this species the changes in serum calcium during magnesium depletion depend on dietary calcium intake; a normal or high calcium intake causes hypercalcemia to develop (138), whereas dietary calcium restriction causes serum calcium to fall (139). In humans and most other species, however, the characteristic response to magnesium deficiency is hypocalcemia.

Because neuromuscular symptoms of magnesium deficiency rarely occur in the absence of hypocalcemia, it was once felt that calcium deficiency was the cause of the symptoms. However, there is little evidence, either experimental or clinical, that magnesium deficiency leads to calcium deficiency. Indeed, the reverse may be true. In experimental animals, magnesium depletion is associated with an increased concentration of calcium in soft tissue, bone, and total carcass (138,140,141). Urinary calcium excretion falls rapidly during experimental human magnesium deficiency despite a constant calcium intake (115). Also, the neuromuscular symptoms seen in magnesium deficiency respond poorly, if at all, to calcium replacement alone, and a sustained response is only noted after magnesium replacement. These observations indicate that in magnesium deficiency states the regulatory mechanisms for maintaining serum calcium in the normal range are impaired.

Several theories have been proposed to explain the hypocalcemia of magnesium deficiency: (a) end-organ resistance to PTH; (b) impaired synthesis and/or release of PTH; (c) presence of excess osteoid tissue; and (d) altered equilibrium between calcium in extracellular fluid and in bone. Parathyroid extract had neither a calcemic nor a phosphaturic effect in eight alcoholic patients who were both hypocalcemic and hypomagnesemic, but both defects disappeared following correction of magnesium depletion. This finding suggested end-organ resistance to the effect of PTH (142). In patients with intestinal malabsorption of magnesium, end-organ response to parathyroid extract appears to have a different pattern. Patients with intestinal malabsorption often have radiographic bone changes, bone pain, osteomalacia, and minor, if any, hypocalcemia. However, in a few patients with malabsorption, very low serum calcium with tetany may develop in the absence of radiographic or symptomatic bone disease, suggesting that secondary hyperparathyroidism has failed to mobilize bone or to increase serum calcium (143). The concomitant presence of magnesium deficiency, which blocks the effect of PTH on bone, may explain this paradox; in five of nine patients with hypomagnesemia and hypocalcemia due to intestinal malabsorption, PTH increased phosphaturia but failed to raise serum calcium until magnesium was replenished (144). Thus magnesium deficiency in intestinal malabsorption could be regarded as protective, since secondary hyperparathyroidism failed to produce reabsorption of calcium from bone.

When the clinical observations were investigated in experimental magnesium deficiency in animals, results were mixed. The studies demonstrated normal endorgan responsiveness to PTH (145,146), impaired responsiveness (137), and total lack of responsiveness (147). The explanation for these differences is not known, but factors that must be considered are (a) the species studied and (b) the age of the animal. Magnesium deficiency in growing animals may have a different effect on PTH sensitivity in bone when compared to that in adult animals or in humans. Unfortunately, direct assay of PTH has not given a clear answer to the problem. A low-to-undetectable level of PTH was reported in a patient with isolated intestinal malabsorption of magnesium that responded promptly to magnesium replacement (148). Additional evidence for parathyroid gland failure with primary intestinal malabsorption came from another study which showed that both bone and kidney responded normally to parathyroid extract and that low levels of PTH, serum magnesium and serum calcium all responded to magnesium replacement (149). However, undetectable levels of PTH have not been a universal finding in the hypocalcemia of magnesium deficiency, and frankly high levels are reported (150,151). In general, most patients have either low or inappropriately normal PTH in the face of hypocalcemia (150).

Two clinical studies suggest that the impairment of parathyroid function may not be a failure to synthesize PTH but that it may, instead, be a failure to release PTH in response to the appropriate stimulus. A rapid rise in immunoreactive PTH within minutes of the intravenous administration of magnesium sulfate to magnesium-deficient subjects has been demonstrated (150), suggesting that in some patients impaired release, rather than synthesis of PTH, is the problem. Enhanced de novo synthesis cannot be expected to be so rapid. Besides the impaired release or PTH, there probably was an additional element of end-organ resistance to PTH, since there was a lag in the response of serum calcium to the elevated PTH level.

Clinical variability in the responses of magnesium-deficient patients to parathyroid extract can be summarized as follows: (a) Most cases of primary hypomagnese-

mia have a normal calcemic response to parathyroid extract and (b) unresponsive patients have usually been alcoholics and patients with malabsorption not previously treated with magnesium. The major factor determining the calcemic response to PTH infusion is probably the degree of magnesium deficiency. A normal response to PTH in rats with a serum magnesium of 0.79 mEq/L (146), in contrast to refractoriness to PTH in rats with a serum magnesium of 0.38 mEq/L (152), has been reported. The same appears to hold for the response of severely hypomagnesemic patients to PTH (150). Where end-organ resistance to the action of endogenous or exogenous PTH or extract is shown, the mediator of this action is not clear. Magnesium is required by the enzyme adenylate cyclase for the conversion of ATP to cyclic AMP, a mediator of the peripheral action of PTH. However, the results of measurements of cyclic AMP generation following PTH administration are mixed: Some reports have shown normal generation during the hypocalcemia of magnesium deficiency (149,153), whereas others have shown reduced generation (150). The level of response of this system may also depend on the severity of magnesium depletion (150).

Calcium-deficient bone per se, independent of magnesium deficiency, may be less responsive to PTH. Skeletal tissue from dogs on diets deficient in calcium alone or in vitamin D and calcium showed excess unmineralized osteoid and poor calcemic response to the administration of parathyroid extract (154). This mechanism could be operative in magnesium-deficient states, since magnesium-deficient chicks have been shown to develop increased osteoid tissue (147). However, there is no evidence that such an increase in osteoid tissue is present in the bone of magnesium-deficient humans.

The hypocalcemia of magnesium deficiency may also result from a deficiency in the normal physicochemical exchange of calcium and magnesium between the hydration shell of bone and the blood. Magnesium may substitute for calcium in the hydration of bone (155), but calcium exchange in vitro has been shown to occur to a lesser extent in bone from magnesium-depleted rats (152). Also, the total calcium content of bone has been shown to be greater in magnesium-depleted rats than in normal ones (146). These experimental observations are totally consistent with the clinical observations that hypocalcemic, magnesium-deficient patients have a reduced urinary calcium excretion, normal bone calcium concentration (110,111), positive calcium balance, and normalization of serum calcium following restoration of magnesium stores alone (115).

Causes of Magnesium Deficiency

In clinical situations, magnesium deficiency usually results from one or a combination of the following factors: (a) redistribution of magnesium from the extracel-

TABLE 13. *Causes of magnesium deficiency: gastrointestinal disorders*

Decreased dietary intake
Decreased intestinal absorption
Malabsorption syndromes
Short-bowel syndrome
Bowel and biliary fistulas
Prolonged nasogastric suction
Parenteral hyperalimentation
Prolonged diarrhea
Laxative abuse
Alcoholism
Protein-calorie malnutrition
Pancreatitis

TABLE 14. *Causes of magnesium deficiency: renal disorders*

Primary tubular disorders
Primary renal magnesium wasting
Welt's syndrome
Bartter's syndrome
Renal tubular acidosis
Secondary or acquired tubular disorders
Diuretic phase of acute tubular necrosis
Postobstructive diuresis
Postrenal transplantation
Drug-induced losses
Diuretics
Aminoglycosides
Digoxin
Cisplatin
Cyclosporine
Pentamidine
Hormone-induced losses
Aldosteronism
Hyperthyroidism
Hypoparathyroidism
Hypercalcemia
Volume expansion
Glucose, urea, or mannitol diuresis
Phosphate depletion
Alcohol

lular to the intracellular space (caused by insulin administration, hungry bone syndrome, catecholamine excess states, acute respiratory alkalosis, or acute pancreatitis), (b) decreased gastrointestinal absorption of magnesium (Table 13), or (c) decreased renal tubular reabsorption of magnesium (Table 14).

Gastrointestinal Disorders

Symptomatic magnesium deficiency occurs most often in patients with gastrointestinal disorders (108). Familial hypomagnesemia was first described in 1965 (156). It is primarily a disease of children, with the usual age of onset being 2–4 weeks. The etiology seems to be a specific defect in intestinal absorption of magnesium (157). Renal tubular handling of magnesium is normal, and chronic dietary supplementation with magnesium salts results in normal growth and development (158).

Magnesium depletion frequently accompanies nontropical sprue, short-bowel syndrome, and other disorders associated with steatorrhea. It may occur in the postoperative period in association with prolonged nasogastric suction or following parenteral hyperalimentation with magnesium-deficient fluids. A decreased serum magnesium in 15 of 42 patients with intestinal malabsorption has been reported; four of the 15 patients, each having serum magnesium concentrations of less than 1 mEq/L, had symptoms (159). Steatorrhea, through the formation of magnesium soaps, appears to be the major cause of magnesium loss. In children with protein-calorie malnutrition, electrocardiographic abnormalities and symptoms of neuromuscular irritability were associated with low serum magnesium levels, and magnesium repletion in most cases had a beneficial effect (160,161). In acute pancreatitis the serum magnesium may be decreased; in addition, magnesium measurements on necrotic omentum have demonstrated increased quantities of magnesium presumably resulting from precipitation of insoluble magnesium soaps (162).

Endocrine Disorders

Although hypomagnesemia may occur in both hyperparathyroidism and hypoparathyroidism, it is not known whether PTH affects magnesium directly or secondarily through its effect on calcium. Serum magnesium in hyperparathyroidism is usually normal (163). Thyrotoxicosis is associated with hypomagnesemia and negative magnesium balance (164), but the specific mechanism for this effect is not known.

The role of aldosterone in magnesium homeostasis is unclear. One of the first reported cases of primary hyperaldosteronism was accompanied by hypomagnesemia and tetany (165). The mechanism of the effect of aldosterone on magnesium excretion is probably not direct. Acute mineralocorticoid administration in dogs and in humans had no significant effect on magnesium excretion (166). However, chronic desoxycorticosterone acetate (DOCA) administration in dogs progressively increased magnesium and calcium excretion, an effect that occurred only after development of sodium retention and expansion of the extracellular fluid volume (167).

Plasma magnesium concentration in well-controlled, insulin-dependent diabetic patients is lower than that in normal patients (1.60 ± 0.04 versus 1.80 ± 0.04; 0.02 mEq/L; $p < 0.001$), but skeletal muscle magnesium content in the former group is not different from that in the latter group (168). However, the magnesium content of iliac crest biopsies from insulin-dependent patients is reduced, and bone has been shown to be a better index of total body magnesium stores than has skeletal muscle (169). Hypomagnesemia may be a risk factor for diabetic retinopathy (170), since diabetics with severe retinopathy have a lower mean serum magnesium concentration than do those with normal or only minimal abnormalities. This observation is particularly interesting in view of data relating decreased content of magnesium in coronary arteries to sudden death. In contrast to the mild hypomagnesemia of stable diabetes, patients with diabetic ketoacidosis may show an elevated serum magnesium in a pattern similar to that for potassium, despite the demonstration that there is an actual magnesium deficit. The initially elevated serum magnesium may fall rapidly with insulin and fluid therapy and may produce symptomatic hypomagnesemia as magnesium is driven inside the cell.

Renal Disorders

In the presence of magnesium depletion, a urinary excretion of magnesium exceeding 1 mEq/day indicates renal magnesium wasting. Renal magnesium wasting may be either hereditary (171,172) or acquired (173–178). In either form, the diagnosis is established by the presence of hypomagnesemia with an inappropriately high urinary magnesium excretion. Although not well-studied as a group, patients with congenital renal magnesium wasting seem to share several characteristics, including a propensity for chondrocalcinosis, nephrocalcinosis, histologic renal damage that is interstitial rather than glomerular, and well-maintained glomerular filtration (171). The location in the nephron of the defect that causes magnesium wasting is unknown.

The serum magnesium level in insulin-dependent diabetic children is significantly lower than that in nondiabetic controls, a finding attributable to higher urinary magnesium clearances in the diabetic children (173). Improved diabetic control caused serum magnesium to rise.

Acute and chronic ingestion of alcohol are both associated with increased renal magnesium losses (177–179). Thirty percent of all alcoholics and 86% of patients with delirium tremens have hypomagnesemia during the first 24–48 h after admission to the hospital (180). In the presence of a normal serum magnesium level, marked skeletal muscle depletion of magnesium may exist in alcoholic patients withdrawing from alcohol (111). Tracer studies indicate that exchangeable magnesium is reduced in chronic alcoholics (116,119). Magnesium deficiency in alcoholic patients results from several factors: (a) decreased intake, (b) starvation ketosis, (c) gastrointestinal loss, and (d) increased urinary excretion. A diet in which the primary source of calories is alcohol is severely magnesium-deficient. Starvation with moderately severe ketosis can cause a net negative balance of as much as 10 mEq of magnesium per day (181). Vomitus and diarrhea fluids, particularly in the presence of malabsorption, may be rich in magnesium. Acute ingestion of alcohol causes an increase of urinary magnesium excretion, but chronic exposure to alcohol appears to have no lasting effect on magnesium excretion (177–179). The explana-

tion for this apparent discrepancy between the effects of alcohol on magnesium excretion in normal and magnesium-deficient individuals is unknown. The mechanism of acute, alcohol-induced magnesuria is unknown, but two possibilities are favored: either (i) a direct effect of alcohol on tubular resorption of magnesium or (ii) an increased production of a metabolic intermediate (e.g., lactate) with the potential to bind magnesium when excreted by the kidney (108). The latter theory is supported by the strong correlation between urinary magnesium and lactate excretion following alcohol ingestion (182).

Whether magnesium deficiency is a cause or an effect of the alcohol withdrawal syndrome is unsettled. However, a veterinary problem of considerable economic importance offers several parallels to this syndrome. "Grass staggers" is a syndrome that sometimes develops in cattle, and it is characterized by hypomagnesemia and a variety of neuromuscular disturbances. The syndrome occurs shortly after cattle are allowed to graze in lush pastures in the spring or fall, particularly when the pasture has been heavily fertilized with nitrogen, potassium, or both. Although the mechanism of magnesium deficiency is not known, it may be that the high ammonium content of this spring grass results in the formation of poorly absorbable magnesium-ammonium phosphate in the bowel (183,184). Use of pastures that contain magnesium-rich species of plants (clover, herbs) seems to prevent the problem.

Several observations on patients withdrawing from alcohol have led to the theory that magnesium deficiency is a central factor responsible for the withdrawal syndrome. Following withdrawal of alcohol, serum magnesium rapidly falls, suggesting that magnesium shifts between body pools (116,185). The demonstration that exogenous catecholamines reduce plasma magnesium and the presence of agitation which are so characteristic of the patient withdrawing from alcohol may explain in part the propensity of these patients to hypomagnesemia. Also, hypomagnesemia and respiratory alkalosis developing in the first 48 h after the withdrawal of alcohol are strongly associated with increased susceptibility to seizures (186). Investigators have theorized that hypomagnesemia and the known ability of respiratory alkalosis to trigger seizures may compound during alcohol withdrawal, thereby producing spontaneous seizures (186). However, the relationship of hypomagnesemia and magnesium deficiency to other aspects of the withdrawal syndrome, particularly delirium tremens, is less well defined. Alcoholic patients with delirium tremens and marked hypomagnesemia may be more prone to develop Wernicke–Korsakoff syndrome (186). However, no studies have been able to correlate hypomagnesemia and the onset of delirium tremens. If delirium tremens were due solely to magnesium deficiency, magnesium replacement would be mandatory for recovery. However, patients do survive and recover from delirium tremens without magnesium replacement. Nevertheless, magnesium deficiency in nonalcoholic humans and in experimental animals causes personality changes, neuromuscular irritability, and seizures, and it seems likely that the presence of magnesium deficiency aggravates the alcohol withdrawal syndrome. Therefore, it is justifiable to treat all patients withdrawing from alcohol with oral magnesium and, if particularly ill, with parenteral magnesium salts.

Prolonged treatment (usually longer than 2 weeks) with aminoglycoside antibiotics has been associated with hypomagnesemic tetany (187–191). These patients invariably have hypocalcemia which is refractory to therapy with calcium if the magnesium deficiency is not first corrected. The hypomagnesemia may occur in the absence of other evidence of renal impairment. A recent study found a significant correlation between the total cumulative dose of gentamicin and serum magnesium concentration, as well as between the renal wasting of magnesium and the total cumulative dose of gentamicin administered. Furthermore, gentamicin-induced magnesium depletion is most likely to occur when the drug is given to older patients in large doses over extended periods of time (191).

Cisplatin, a potentially nephrotoxic chemotherapy agent used against epithelial neoplasms, causes hypomagnesemia and renal magnesium wasting in a dose-related manner that appears to be relatively specific for the magnesium ion (192). As occurs with hereditary forms of renal magnesium wasting, renal magnesium wasting resulting from drug toxicity is commonly associated with hypokalemia, kaliuresis, volume depletion, and secondary hyperaldosteronism.

While the loop diuretics (furosemide, bumetanide, and ethacrynic acid) are the most potent magnesuric diuretics, long-term administration of thiazide diuretics also may lead to mild hypomagnesemia. However, the role of thiazide diuretics in causing magnesium depletion has not been universally found (193), and those patients that do become hypomagnesemic (approximately 15% in a large clinical trial) may represent a high-risk subpopulation (194).

Studies with the potassium-sparing diuretics—amiloride, spironolactone, and triamterene—show that they increase skeletal muscle magnesium and potassium content in patients on long-term diuretics for the treatment of congestive heart failure or hypertension (195). However, another study did not show a significant magnesium-sparing effect from spironolactone (196). The magnesium-sparing action of amiloride in the rat appears to be due to a direct renal action, since it reduced fractional excretion of magnesium without affecting systemic blood pressure, glomerular filtration rate, extracellular fluid volume, plasma pH, ultrafilterable magnesium, or plasma aldosterone (197). The effect of

amiloride on the renal handling of magnesium is only approximately 10% of its effect on potassium (198). The mechanism by which potassium-sparing diuretics are magnesium-sparing is unknown, but reduction of the transepithelial potential difference would tend to favor reabsorption of a divalent cation (198).

Renal allograft recipients treated with cyclosporine show a significant reduction in serum magnesium concentration and an increase in total and fractional excretion of magnesium (199). Magnesium supplementation is warranted in such patients. The use of cyclosporine in bone marrow transplantation is also associated with hypomagnesemia (200). A recent study in the rat found that cyclosporine administration caused a fall in serum magnesium concentration, primarily as a result of renal magnesium wasting and possibly as a result of a shift of magnesium to the tissue compartments, with no discernible effect on gastrointestinal handling of magnesium (201).

Recently, intravenous pentamidine, which is used to treat *Pneumocystis carinii* pneumonia (PCP) in acquired immunodeficiency syndrome (AIDS) patients, has also been reported to result in hypomagnesemia (202).

Symptoms of Magnesium Deficiency

To study signs and symptoms of pure magnesium deficiency, several studies in humans have attempted to create and examine the magnesium deficiency state by reducing the dietary intake of magnesium alone (115,120,203–205). However, in only one study was magnesium deficiency of sufficient magnitude to create symptoms (115,205). In this study, seven subjects were evaluated during normal magnesium intake (40 mEq/day), during a depletion period (0.7 mEq/day) that lasted between 1.5 and 8 months, and during an magnesium repletion period. Following removal of magnesium from the diet, urinary magnesium excretion fell within a week to less than 1 mEq/day. Urinary calcium excretion also fell rapidly with magnesium deficiency. Symptoms and clinically detectable evidence of magnesium deficiency occurred in six or seven patients but were not marked or persistent unless they occurred in the presence of hypokalemia and hypocalcemia. Table 15 lists the signs and

TABLE 15. *Signs and symptoms of magnesium depletion*

Signs	Symptoms
Trousseau's sign	Apathy
Chvostek's sign	Weakness
Muscle fasciculations	Anorexia
Tremors	Nausea
Muscular spasticity	Vomiting
Hyporeflexia	
Grand mal seizures	
Cardiac conduction disturbances	
Sudden death	

symptoms seen in this study as well as those noted in other studies. The most common was Trousseau's sign, which occurred in five patients with a variable time of onset. In two patients it was the only sign of magnesium deficiency that developed. The other neuromuscular signs were less frequent. Electromyographic changes consisted of myopathic-like configurations characterized by rapidly firing, high-pitched potentials of short duration occurring on active contraction of muscles. Lethargy and generalized weakness were noted in four subjects and perhaps were the clinical counterpart of electromyographic changes. The behavioral and gastrointestinal signs and symptoms occurred late and tended to herald the onset of neuromuscular changes. When magnesium was added to these patients' diets, all the signs and symptoms attributable to the deficiency reversed. Most of the neuromuscular signs disappeared within hours of the initial repletion dose, but Trousseau's sign was an exception and could be elicited in several patients with decreasing intensity for several days. The neurologic abnormalities described receded within a few hours to a few days of treatment with magnesium. The presence of downbeat nystagmus with magnesium depletion may indicate more extensive neurologic injury, since treatment with magnesium salts in two patients resulted in either no improvement or very slow recovery (206).

In another study involving two normal subjects who were depleted of magnesium for 39 and 49 days, respectively, it was reported that although both patients developed a cumulative negative magnesium balance of approximately 180 mEq (8–10% of body magnesium), neither hypomagnesemia, hypocalcemia, nor symptoms of magnesium deficiency developed (203). Also, muscle magnesium remained normal, leading the authors to conclude that the source of the negative magnesium balance must have been bone. Another study investigated the effect of prolonged fasting on magnesium excretion in obese males (207). More than 20% of total body magnesium was lost in some subjects during the 2-month study period. Most of the magnesium loss occurred via the kidneys. Despite a marked reduction in skeletal muscle magnesium content, serum magnesium remained normal. Unlike experimental isolated magnesium deficiency in which urinary magnesium excretion falls to less than 1 mEq/day, these fasting patients had urinary excretion levels four to five times higher. The etiology of this continued magnesium excretion was postulated to be a consequence of the metabolic acidosis seen in fasting subjects. A prompt reduction in urinary magnesium excretion following the ingestion of glucose was also noted, presumably reflecting a reduction in the production of ketoacids and the movement of magnesium from plasma to the intracellular compartment. Symptoms of magnesium deficiency did not occur in these starving patients. This study offers further proof that serum and urinary magnesium levels are better indicators of magnesium deficiency than is skeletal muscle magnesium concentration.

In a prospective study of 20 patients with severe hypomagnesemia, only 3 patients were noted to have symptoms (tremor and muscle twitching); each of these patients was hypocalcemic (208). None of the 20 had tetany, a positive Trousseau's sign, cardiac arrhythmias, or an abnormal electrocardiogram.

Clinical Consequences of Magnesium Deficiency

Recent reports suggest a relationship between decreased magnesium content of cardiac muscle and coronary arteries and mortality from sudden death ischemic heart disease (SDIHD). The incidence of SDIHD is highest in geographic areas with magnesium-poor soil or soft drinking water (209–211). Also, patients with severe angiographic evidence of coronary artery disease have significantly lower serum magnesium levels than do angiographically normal controls. However, diuretic agents were used significantly more often in the former group, making a cause-and-effect link between magnesium deficiency and coronary artery disease less clear. In the laboratory, in vitro studies indicate that removal of magnesium from the bathing medium enhances the reactivity of several species' vascular tissues toward neurohumoral agents (212). Isolated canine coronary arteries develop increased tension when exposed to a zero-magnesium bath, suggesting that sudden death with hypomagnesemia could result from progressive coronary artery vasoconstriction (213). Conversely, agents known to dilate vascular tissue (prostaglandins and isoproterenol) are less active in the presence of hypomagnesemia (212). In addition, basal tone of isolated vascular tissue depends on the ambient magnesium concentration. The mechanism by which magnesium changes vascular tone may be the altering of membrane permeability to calcium, thus changing the distribution of calcium in smooth muscle cells. Experiments with isolated vascular smooth muscle show that when magnesium is lowered in the extracellular compartment, calcium influx and intracellular content are increased (214). Thus magnesium, acting at the smooth-muscle-cell membrane, functions as a physiologic regulator of calcium entry. The suggestion has been made that alterations in magnesium–calcium exchange in smooth muscle cells may underlie many of the vascular complications seen in diabetes (214).

The demonstrated effects of magnesium on vascular tone may explain (a) the association between hypomagnesemia and hypertension (215) and (b) the effect of an magnesium-deficient diet to further increase arterial blood pressure in the spontaneously hypertensive rat by increasing systemic vascular resistance (216). In addition to the effect of magnesium deficiency on the coronary circulation, magnesium deficiency may also produce further hemodynamic deterioration and ventricular arrhythmias in patients with congestive heart failure (217). Finally, hypomagnesemia can also induce bronchial hyperreactivity and worsen symptoms of asthma and COPD (218).

Diuretic agents—including mercurials, loop diuretics, and thiazides—increase urinary magnesium excretion (219,220). However, loop diuretics appear to be the most potent in this regard. Thus diuretics may be the important link between the reported increase in a variety of cardiac arrhythmias and hypomagnesemia. The arrhythmias are usually, but not invariably, associated with the use of digitalis (221). In experimental animals the uptake of digoxin by myocardial cells is enhanced in the presence of magnesium depletion (222). The mechanism by which hypomagnesemia predisposes to cardiac arrhythmias is unclear, but hypomagnesemia causes a prolongation of the Q–T interval, a change known to predispose to ventricular arrhythmias. Perhaps more important, though, is the potassium depletion known to accompany magnesium depletion. The role of magnesium therapy in treating cardiac arrhythmias is, however, controversial. Intravenous magnesium salts failed to significantly reduce the frequency of extrasystolic beats in a group of patients with plasma or erythrocyte hypomagnesemia (223), indicating that other factors were involved in the origin of the arrhythmia.

Treatment of Magnesium Deficiency

In mild magnesium deficiency, restoration of body stores occurs quickly after ingesting a diet high in magnesium (meat, sea foods, green vegetables, dairy products, and cereals). In more severe magnesium deficiency, parenteral magnesium salts are safe and effective but must be used cautiously in patients with renal insufficiency. Parenteral magnesium is especially useful in patients with symptomatic hypomagnesemia or malabsorption. Initial treatment of the magnesium-deficient state requires 8–12 g of intravenous or intramuscular magnesium sulfate (16–24 mL of 50% $MgSO_4 \cdot 7H_2O$ or 64–96 mEq of Mg^{2+}) in a divided dose over the first 24 h, followed by 4–6 g daily (32–48 mEq) for 3–4 days (224,225). Because of the T_m relationship for magnesium, parenteral magnesium must be given frequently (4- to 6-h intervals), since as much as 50% of each dose will be excreted in the urine despite the presence of total body magnesium depletion. These large doses of $MgSO_4$ are required to ensure retention of 1.0 mEq per kilogram of body weight, the mean retention found in balance studies of magnesium-deficient chronic alcoholics (116). During replacement, serum magnesium and deep tendon reflexes should be monitored closely. A marked depression of deep tendon reflexes indicates a serum magnesium in the range of 4–7 mEq/L, and no further magnesium should be administered. For magnesium deficiency developing in the recovery period of diabetic ketoacidosis, 1 mL (4 mEq) of 50% $MgSO_4$ may be added to each liter of intravenous fluids. In the alcoholic patient with minimal symptoms of withdrawal, oral magnesium is quite effective in restoring the magnesium deficit. Magnesium oxide (MgO) is supplied as 60-mg tablets containing 30 mEq of magnesium per tablet. Several days of four to six tablets per day should suffice to restore the deficit in most patients. Symptomatic renal magnesium wasting may be successfully treated with as little as 80 mg of MgO in four divided doses (171). Most neuromuscular signs of magnesium deficiency disappear within hours of the initial parenteral dose of magnesium, but Trousseau's sign may take up to several days to resolve (115). If the initial dose of magnesium is not followed by repeated doses, serum magnesium may fall and symptoms may recur. This latter finding suggests that the retained magnesium is rapidly taken up by bone or muscle. In patients having simultaneous deficits of magnesium and potassium (most patients), both ions should be replaced, or symptoms of deficiency of the ion not replaced may be produced.

Magnesium Excess

Since magnesium is not routinely measured with other cations, serious hypermagnesemia may go undetected. Therefore, to make a diagnosis of hypermagnesemia, the clinician must maintain a high degree of wariness.

States of magnesium excess usually result from overly vigorous therapeutic doses of magnesium or from conventional doses in the presence of impaired renal function (Table 16). In patients with impaired renal function, injudicious use of antacids containing magnesium may result in excessive and symptomatic levels of magnesium in the blood (226). Five milliliters of Maalox, Gelusil, or Mylanta contains 6.9 mEq of magnesium, whereas 5 mL of the higher-potency preparations of each of these medi-

TABLE 16. *Causes of magnesium excess*

Redistribution
Acidosis
Pheochromocytoma
Increased gastrointestinal absorption
Increased oral intake
Magnesium-containing laxatives
Magnesium-containing antacids
Magnesium-containing enemas
Decreased renal excretion
Extracellular volume depletion
Hypocalcemia
Potassium-sparing diuretics
Lithium
Antidiuretic hormone excess
Glucagon excess
Calcitonin excess

TABLE 17. *Symptoms and signs of magnesium excess*

Symptoms/signs	Serum Mg (mEq/L)
Nausea and vomiting	3–5
Sedation	4–7
Decreased deep tendon reflexes	4–7
Muscle weakness	4–7
Hypotension, bradycardia	5–10
Absent deep tendon reflexes, coma, respiratory paralysis	10–15
Cardiac arrest	>15

cations contains 13.7 mEq of magnesium (227). In addition, magnesium-containing cathartics which are used in the treatment of drug intoxication, including salicylate and theophylline intoxication, may also result in significant hypermagnesemia (228,229).

The only known condition in which there is documented chronic excess of total body magnesium is chronic renal failure (230). It is not known whether this excess magnesium is responsible for any of the complications of uremia, but magnesium is incorporated into the soft-tissue calcifications of uremic patients (231,232).

The symptoms of hypermagnesemia, along with the corresponding serum magnesium levels at which they develop, are listed in Table 17. The therapy of hypermagnesemia is directed first at removal of the source of magnesium and then it is directed at enhancing removal if the serum level of magnesium poses a threat to survival. If vital centers are affected (usually with serum levels of over 7–10 mEq/L), the acute administration of calcium will produce a rapid but short-lived reduction in the serum magnesium and an often dramatic improvement in the patient's clinical condition. High serum levels in the presence of impaired renal function may require either peritoneal dialysis or hemodialysis against a magnesium-free dialysate solution. Since magnesium is easily dialyzed, a rapid and sustained response to this treatment can be expected (226).

ACKNOWLEDGMENTS

The authors would like to thank Ms. Regina E. Citizen for excellent secretarial assistance.

REFERENCES

1. Betro MG, Pain RW. Hypophosphataemia and hyperphosphataemia in a hospital population. *Br Med J* 1972;1:273–6.
2. Juan D, Elrazak MA. Hypophosphatemia in hospitalized patients. *JAMA* 1979;242:163–4.
3. Larson L, Rebel K, Sorbo B. Severe hypophosphatemia—a hospital survey. *Acta Med Scand* 1983;214:221–3.
4. King AL, Sica DA, Miller G, Pierpaoli S. Severe hypophosphatemia in a general hospital population. *South Med J* 1987;80:831–5.
5. Berner YN, Shike M. Consequences of phosphate imbalance. *Annu Rev Nutr* 1988;8:121–48.
6. Editorial Review. Postoperative hypophosphatemia: a multifactorial problem. *Nutr Rev* 1989;47:111–6.
7. Trivedi B, Sanforth WH. Effect of pH on the kinetics of frog muscle phosphofructokinase. *J Biol Chem* 1966;211:4110–4.
8. Mostellar ME, Tutle EP. Effect of alkalosis on plasma and urinary excretion of inorganic phosphate in man. *J Clin Invest* 1964;43:138–51.
9. Hoppe A, Metler M, Berndt TJ, et al. Effect of respiratory alkalosis on renal phosphate excretion. *Am J Physiol* 1982;241(*Renal Fluid Electrolyte Physiol* 12):F471–5.
10. Brautbar N, Leibovici H, Massry SG. On the mechanism of hypophosphatemia during acute hyperventilation: evidence for increased muscle glycolysis. *Miner Electrolyte Metab* 1983;9:45–50.
11. Brady HR, Ryan F, Cunningham J, et al. Hypophosphatemia complicating bronchodilator therapy for acute severe asthma. *Arch Intern Med* 1989;149:2367–8.
12. Laaban JP, Waked M, Laromiguiere M, et al. Hypophosphatemia complicating management of acute severe asthma. *Ann Intern Med* 1990;112:68–9.
13. Laaban JP, Grateau G, Psychoyos I, et al. Hypophosphatemia induced by mechanical ventilation in patients with chronic obstructive pulmonary disease. *Crit Care Med* 1989;17:1115–20.
14. Fiaccadori E, Coffrini E, Ronda N, et al. Hypophosphatemia in course of chronic obstructive pulmonary disease. Prevalence, mechanisms, and relationships with skeletal muscle phosphorus content. *Chest* 1990;97:857–67.
15. Lichtman MA, Miller DR, Cohen J, et al. Reduced red cell glycolysis, 2,3-diphosphoglycerate and adenosine triphosphate concentration, and increased hemoglobin-oxygen affinity caused by hypophosphatemia. *Ann Intern Med* 1971;740:562–8.
16. Travis SF, Sugerman HJ, Ruberg FL, et al. Alterations of red-cell glycolytic intermediates and oxygen transport as a consequence of hypophosphatemia in patients receiving intravenous hyperalimentation. *N Engl J Med* 1971;285:763–8.
17. Silvis SE, DiBartolomeo AG, Aaker HM. Hypophosphatemia and neurological changes secondary to oral caloric intake. A variant of hyperalimentation syndrome. *Am J Gastroenterol* 1980;73:215–22.
18. Weinsier RL, Krumdieck CL. Death resulting from overzealous total parenteral nutrition: the refeeding syndrome revisited. *Am J Clin Nutrition* 1980;34:393–9.
19. Hayek ME, Eisenberg PG. Severe hypophosphatemia following the institution of enteral feedings. *Arch Surg* 1989;124:1325–8.
20. Kalbfleisch JM, Lindeman RD, Ginn HE, et al. Effects of ethanol administration on urinary excretion of magnesium and other electrolytes in alcoholic and normal subjects. *J Clin Invest* 1963;42:1471–5.
21. Stein JH, Smith WO, Ginn HE. Hypophosphatemia in acute alcoholism. *Am J Med Sci* 1966;252:78–83.
22. Blachley JD, Ferguson ER, Carter NW, et al. Chronic alcohol ingestion induces phosphorus deficiency and myopathy in the dog. *Trans Assoc Am Physicians* 1980;93:110–22.
23. Knochel JP. Hypophosphatemia in the alcoholic. *Arch Intern Med* 1980;140:613–5.
24. Ryback RS, Eckardt MJ, Paulter CP. Clinical relationships between serum phosphorus and other blood chemistry values in alcoholics. *Arch Intern Med* 1980;140:673–7.
25. Adler AJ, Gudis S, Berlyne GM. Reduced renal phosphate threshold concentration in alcoholic cirrhosis. *Miner Electrolyte Metab* 1984;10:63–6.
26. De Marchi S, Cecchin E, Grimaldi F. Reduced renal phosphate threshold concentration in chronic alcoholics. One component of a more complex tubule dysfunction? *Miner Electrolyte Metab* 1986;12:147–8.
27. Schafer RM, Teschner M, Heidland A. Alterations of water, electrolyte and acid–base homeostasis in the alcoholic. *Miner Electrolyte Metab* 1987;13:1–6.
28. Urbano-Marquez A, Estruch R, Navarro-Lopez F, et al. The effects of alcoholism on skeletal and cardiac muscle. *N Engl J Med* 1980;15:409–15.
29. Kebler R, McDonald FD, Cadnapaphonchai P. Dynamic changes in serum phosphorus levels in diabetic ketoacidosis. *Am J Med* 1985;79:571–6.

30. Bohannon NJ. Large phosphate shifts with treatment for hyperglycemia. *Arch Intern Med* 1989;149:1423–5.

31. Mezoff AG, Gremse DA, Farrell MK. Hypophosphatemia in the nutritional recovery syndrome. *Am J Dis Child* 1989;143:1111–2.

32. Zamkoff KW, Kirshner JJ. Marked hypophosphatemia associated with acute myelomonocytic leukemia. Indirect evidence of phosphorus uptake by leukemic cells. *Arch Intern Med* 1980;140:1523–4.

33. Matzner Y, Prococimer M, Polliack A, et al. Hypophosphatemia in a patient with lymphoma in leukemic phase. *Arch Intern Med* 1981;141:805–6.

34. Aderka D, Shoenfeld Y, Santo M, et al. Life-threatening hypophosphatemia in a patient with acute myelogenous leukemia. *Acta Haematol* 1980;64:117–9.

35. Lenquist S, Lindell B, Nordstrom H, et al. Hypophosphatemia in severe burns. *Acta Chir Scand* 1979;145:1–6.

36. Moorhead JF, Ahmed KY, Varghese Z, et al. Hypophosphataemic osteomalacia after cadaveric renal transplantation. *Lancet* 1974;20:694–7.

37. Ward HN, Pabico RC, McKenna BA, et al. The renal handling of phosphate by renal transplant patients: correlation with serum parathyroid hormone (SPTH), cyclic 3′,5′-adenosine monophosphate (cAMP) urinary excretion, and allograft function. *Adv Exp Med Biol* 8f1977;81:173–81.

38. Nielsen HE, Christensen MS, Melsen F, et al. Bone disease, hypophosphatemia and hyperparathyroidism after renal transplantation. *Adv Exp Med Biol* 1977;81:603–10.

39. Farrington K, Varghese Z, Newman SP, et al. Dissociation of absorptions of calcium and phosphate after successful cadaveric renal transplantation. *Br Med J* 1979;1:712–4.

40. Nielsen HE, Melsen F, Christiensen MS. Spontaneous fractures following renal transplantation. Clinical and biochemical aspects, bone mineral content and bone morphometry. *Miner Electrolyte Metab* 1979;2:323–30.

41. Walker GS, Peacock M, Marshall DH, et al. Factors influencing the intestinal absorption of calcium and phosphorus following renal transplantation. *Nephron* 1986;26:225–9.

42. Kovarik J, Graf H, Stummvoll HK, et al. Tubular phosphate handling after successful kidney transplantation. *Klin Wochenschr* 1980;58:863–9.

43. Friedman A, Chesney R. Fanconi's syndrome in renal transplantation. *Am J Nephrol* 1981;1:45–7.

44. Rosenbaum RW, Hruska KA, Korkor A, et al. Decreased phosphate reabsorption after renal transplantation: evidence for a mechanism independent of calcium and parathyroid hormone. *Kidney Int* 1981;19:568–78.

45. Lucas PA, Brown RC, Bloodworth L, et al. Vitamin D₃ metabolites in hypercalcemic adults after kidney transplantation. *Proc EDTA* 1983;20:213–9.

46. Bonomini V, Feletti C, Di Felice A, Buscaroli A. Bone remodelling after renal transplantation. *Adv Exp Med Biol* 1984;178:207–16.

47. Sakhaee K, Brinker K, Helderman JH, et al. Disturbances in mineral metabolism after successful renal transplantation. *Miner Electrolyte Metab* 1985;11:167–72.

48. Felsenfeld AJ, Gutman RA, Drezner M, et al. Hypophosphatemia in long-term renal transplant recipients: effects on bone histology and 1,25-dihydroxycholecalciferol. *Miner Electrolyte Metab* 1986;12:333–41.

49. Parfit AM, Kleerekoper M, Cruz C. Reduced phosphate reabsorption unrelated to parathyroid hormone after renal transplantation: implications for the pathogenesis of hyperparathyroidism in chronic renal failure. *Miner Electrolyte Metab* 1986;12:356–62.

50. Knochel JP. Neuromuscular manifestations of electrolyte disorders. *Am J Med* 1982;72:521–35.

51. Venditti FJ, Marotta C, Panezai FR, et al. Hypophosphatemia and cardiac arrhythmias. *Miner Electrolyte Metab* 1987;13:19–25.

52. Davis SV, Olichwier KK, Chakko SC. Reversible depression of myocardial performance in hypophosphatemia. *Am J Med Sci* 1988;295:183–7.

53. Aubier M, Murciano D, Lecocguic Y, et al. Effect of hypophos-

phatemia on diaphragmatic contractility in patients with acute respiratory failure. *N Engl J Med* 1985;313:420–4.

54. Rie MA. Hypophosphatemia and diaphragmatic contractility. *N Engl J Med* 1986;314:519–20.

55. Hasselstrom L, Wimberley PD, Nielsen VG. Hypophosphatemia and acute respiratory failure in a diabetic patient. *Intensive Care Med* 1986;12:429–31.

56. Lewis JF, Hodsman AB, Driedger AA, et al. Hypophosphatemia and respiratory failure: prolonged abnormal energy metabolism demonstrated by nuclear magnetic resonance spectroscopy. *Am J Med* 1987;83:1139–43.

57. Gravelyn TR, Brophy N, Siegert C, et al. Hypophosphatemia-associated respiratory muscle weakness in a general inpatient population. *Am J Med* 1988;84:870–6.

58. Rasmussen A, Segel E, Hessov I, et al. Reduced function of neutrophils during routine postoperative glucose infusion. *Acta Chir Scand* 1988;154:429–33.

59. Rasmussen A, Kimose HH, Segel E, et al. Postoperative and glucose-induced hypophosphatemia in relation to adenosine triphosphate and 2,3-diphosphoglycerate in erythrocytes. *Acta Chir Scand* 1989;155:81–7.

60. Lumlertgul D, Harris DCH, Burke TJ, et al. Detrimental effect of hypophosphatemia on the severity and progression of ischemic acute renal failure. *Miner Electrolyte Metab* 1986;12:204–9.

61. Kanter Y, Gerson JR, Bessman AN. 2,3-Diphosphoglycerate, nucleotide phosphate, and organic and inorganic phosphate levels during the early phases of diabetic ketoacidosis. *Diabetes* 1977;26:429–33.

62. Keller U, Berger W. Prevention of hypophosphatemia by phosphate infusion during treatment of diabetic ketoacidosis and hyperosmolar coma. *Diabetes* 1979;87–95.

63. Wilson HK, Keuer SP, Lea AS, et al. Phosphate therapy in diabetic ketoacidosis. *Arch Intern Med* 1982;142:517–20.

64. Fisher JN, Kitabchi AE. A randomized study of phosphate therapy in the treatment of diabetic ketoacidosis. *J Clin Endocrinol Metab* 1983;57:177–80.

65. Kono N, Kuwajima M, Tarui S. Alteration of glycolyticintermediary metabolism in erythrocytes during diabetic ketoacidosis and its recovery phase. *Diabetes* 1981;30:346–53.

66. Lentz RD, Brown DM, Kjellstrand CM. Treatment of severe hypophosphatemia. *Ann Intern Med* 1978;89:941–4.

67. Vannatta JB, Whang R, Papper S. Efficacy of intravenous phosphorus therapy in the severely hypophosphatemic patient. *Arch Intern Med* 1981;141:885–7.

68. Nemer WF, Teba L, Schiebel F, et al. Cardiac arrest after acute hyperphosphatemia. *South Med J* 1988;8:1068–9.

69. Busse JC, Gelbard MA, Byrnes JJ, et al. Pseudohyperphosphatemia and dysproteinemia. *Arch Intern Med* 1987;147:2045–6.

70. Adler SG, Laidlaw SA, Lubran MM, et al. Hyperglobulinemia may spuriously elevate measured serum inorganic phosphate levels. *Am J Kidney Dis* 1988;11:260–3.

71. Weinberg J, Adler AJ. Spurious hyperphosphatemia in patients with dysglobulinemia. *Miner Electrolyte Metab* 1989;15:185–6.

72. Mallette LE, Mechanick JI. Heritable syndrome of pseudoxanthoma elasticum with abnormal phosphorus and vitamin D metabolism. *Am J Med* 1987;83:1157–62.

73. Weisinger JR, Mogollon A, Lander R, et al. Massive cerebral calcifications associated with increased renal phosphate reabsorption. *Arch Intern Med* 1986;146:473–7.

74. Talab YA, Mallouh A. Hyperostosis with hyperphosphatemia: a case report and review of the literature. *J Pediatr Orthop* 1988;8:338–41.

75. Wilson MP, Lindsley CB, Warady BA, et al. Hyperphosphatemia associated with cortical hyperostosis and tumoral calcinosis. *J Pediatr* 1989;114:1010–3.

76. Takuwa Y, Yamamoto M, Matsumoto T, et al. Hyperphosphatemia after surgical correction of hypercortosolism in patients with Cushing's syndrome. *Miner Electrolyte Metab* 1986;12:119–24.

77. Challa A, Norrwall AA, Bevington A, et al. Cellular phosphate metabolism in patients receiving biophosphonate therapy. *Bone* 1986;7:255–9.

78. Martin RR, Lisehora GR, Braxton M, et al. Fatal poisoning from sodium phosphate enema. *JAMA* 1987;257:2190–2.

79. Wason S, Tiller T, Cunha C. Severe hyperphosphatemia, hypo-

calcemia, acidosis, and shock in a 5-month-old child following the administration of an adult fleet enema. *Ann Emerg Med* 1989;18:696–700.

80. Suzuki NT. Hyperphosphatemia in nondialyzed TPN patients. *J Parenter Enter Nutrition* 1987;11:512.

81. Barsotti G, Lazzeri M, Cristofano C, Cerri M, Lupetti S, Giovannetti S. The role of metabolic acidosis in causing uremic hyperphosphatemia. *Miner Electrolyte Metab* 1986;12:103–6.

82. De Marchi S, Cecchin E. More on the role of metabolic acidosis in causing uremic hyperphosphatemia. *Miner Electrolyte Metab* 1987;13:67–8.

83. Saleh RA, Graham-Pole J, Cumming WA. Severe hyperphosphatemia associated with tumor lysis in a patient with T-cell leukemia. *Pediatr Emerg Care* 1989;5:231–3.

84. Stark ME, Dyer MCD, Coonley CJ. Fatal acute tumor lysis syndrome with metastatic breast carcinoma. *Cancer* 1987;60:762–4.

85. Lumlertgul D, Burke TJ, Gillum DM, Alfrey AC, Harris DC, Hammond WS, Schrier RW. Phosphate depletion arrests progression of chronic renal failure independent of protein intake. *Kidney Int* 1986;29:658–66.

86. Delmez JA, Fallon MD, Harter HR, Hruska KA, Slatopolsky E, Teitelbaum SL. Does strict phosphorus control precipitate renal osteomalacia? *J Clin Endocrinol Metab* 1986;62:747–52.

87. Weberg R, Berstad A. Gastrointestinal absorption of aluminum from single doses of aluminum containing antacids in man. *Eur J Clin Invest* 1986;16:428–32.

88. Slanina P, Frech W, Ekstrom L-G, Loof L, Slorach S, Cedergren A. Dietary citric acid enhances absorption of aluminum in antacids. *Clin Chem* 1986;32:539–41.

89. Froment DPH, Molitoris BA, Buddington B, et al. Site and mechanism of enhanced gastrointestinal absorption of aluminum by citrate. *Kidney Int* 1989;36:978–84.

90. Molitoris BA, Froment DH, Mackenzie TA, et al. Citrate: A major factor in the toxicity of orally administered aluminum compounds. *Kidney Int* 1989;36:949–53.

91. Burnatowska-Hledin MA, Doyle TM, Eadie MJ, Mayor GH. 1,25-Dihydroxyvitamin D_3 increases serum and tissue accumulation of aluminum in rats. *J Lab Clin Med* 1986;108:96–102.

92. Slatopolsky E. The interaction of parathyroid hormone and aluminum in renal osteodystrophy. *Kidney Int* 1987;31:842–54.

93. O'Donovan R, Hammer M, Baldwin D, Moniz C, Parsons V. Substitution of aluminum salts by magnesium salts in control of dialysis hyperphosphatemia. *Lancet* 1986;19:880–3.

94. Slatopolsky E, Weerts C, Lopez-Hilker S, et al. Calcium carbonate as a phosphate binder in patients with chronic renal failure undergoing dialysis. *N Engl J Med* 1986;315:157–62.

95. Salusky IB, Coburn JW, Foley J, Nelson P, Fine RN. Effects of oral calcium carbonate on control of serum phosphorus and changes in plasma aluminum levels after discontinuation of aluminum-containing gels in children receiving dialysis. *J Pediatr* 1986;5:767–70.

96. Alon U, Davidai G, Bentur L, Berant M, Better OS. Oral calcium carbonate as phosphate-binder in patients and children with chronic renal failure. *Miner Electrolyte Metab* 1986;12:320–5.

97. Herez G, Kraut JA, Andress DA, Howard N, Roberts C, Sinaberger JH, Sherrard DJ, Coburn JW. Use of calcium carbonate as a phosphate binder in dialysis patients. *Miner Electrolyte Metab* 1986;12:314–9.

98. Andreoll SP, Dunson JW, Bergstein JM. Calcium carbonate is an effective phosphorus binder in children with chronic renal failure. *Am J Kidney Dis* 1987;3:206–10.

99. Almirall J, Campistol JM, Torras A, Revert L. Calcium carbonate as phosphate binder in dialysis. *Lancet* 1987;10:799–800.

100. Anelli A, Brancaccio D, Damasso R, et al. Substitution of calcium carbonate for aluminum hydroxide in patients on hemodialysis. Effects on acidosis, on parathyroid function, and on calcemia. *Nephron* 1989;52:125–32.

101. Sheikh MS, Maguire JA, Emmett M, et al. Reduction of dietary phosphorus absorption by phosphorus binders. *J Clin Invest* 1989;83:66–73.

102. Mai ML, Emmett M, Sheikh MS, et al. Calcium acetate, an effective phosphorus binder in patients with renal failure. *Kidney Int* 1989;36:690–695.

103. Schnider HW, Kulbe KD, Weber H, Streicher E. *In vitro* and *in vivo* studies with a non-aluminum phosphate-binding compound. *Kidney Int* 1986;29(Suppl 18):S120–3.

104. Larson EA, Ash SR, White JL, Hem SI. Phosphate binding gels: balancing phosphate absorption and aluminum toxicity. *Kidney Int* 1986;29:1131–5.

105. Schaefer K, von Herrath D, Asmus G, et al. The beneficial effect of ketoacids on serum phosphate and parathyroid hormone in patients with chronic uremia. *Clin Nephrol* 1988;30:93–6.

106. Evans RA, Watson L. Urinary excretion of magnesium in man. *Lancet* 1966;1:522–3.

107. Gunther T. Biochemistry and pathobiochemistry of magnesium. *Artery* 1981;9:1967–81.

108. Wacker WEC, Parisi AF. Magnesium metabolism. *N Engl J Med* 1968;278:658–62, 712–7, 772–6.

109. Jones JE, Manalo R, Flink EB. Magnesium requirements in adults. *Am J Clin Nutr* 1967;20:632–5.

110. Lim P, Dong S, Khoo OT. Intracellular magnesium depletion in chronic renal failure. *N Engl J Med* 1969;280:981–4.

111. Lim P, Jacob E. Magnesium status of alcoholic patients. *Metabolism* 1972;21:1045–51.

112. Lim P, Jacob E. Magnesium deficiency in liver cirrhosis. *Q J Med* 1972;163:291–300.

113. Lim P, Jacob E. Tissue magnesium level in chronic diarrhea. *J Lab Clin Med* 1972;80:313–21.

114. Alfrey AC, Miller NL, Butkus D. Evaluation of body magnesium stores. *J Lab Clin Med* 1974;84:153–62.

115. Shils ME. Experimental human magnesium depletion. *Medicine* 1969;48:61–82.

116. Jones JE, Shane SR, Jacobs WH, et al. Magnesium balance studies in chronic alcoholism. *Ann NY Acad Sci* 1969;162:935–46.

117. McCollister RJ, Flink EB, Doe RP. Magnesium balance studies in chronic alcoholism. *J Lab Clin Med* 1960;55:98–104.

118. Lemann J, Piering WF, Lennon EJ. Studies of the acute effects of aldosterone and cortisol on the interrelationship between renal sodium, calcium and magnesium excretion in normal man. *Nephron* 1970;7:117–30.

119. Mendelson JH, Barnes B, Mayman C, et al. The determination of exchangeable magnesium in alcoholic patients. *Metabolism* 1965;14:88–98.

120. Wacker WC. *Magnesium and man.* Cambridge, MA: Harvard University Press, 1980;54.

121. Hollifield JW. Magnesium depletion, diuretics and arrhythmias. *Am J Med* 1987;82(Suppl 3A):30–7.

122. Touitou Y, Godard JP, Ferment O, et al. Prevalence of magnesium and potassium deficiencies in the elderly. *Clin Chem* 1987;33:518–23.

123. Ryan MP, Hingerty D. Effects of magnesium deficiency on restoration of potassium and sodium levels in potassium-depleted muscle. *Ir J Med Sci* 1969;2:137–40.

124. Webb S, Schade DS. Hypomagnesemia as a cause of persistent hypokalemia. *JAMA* 1975;233:23–4.

125. Medalle R, Waterhouse C. A magnesium-deficient patient presenting with hypocalcemia and hyperphosphatemia. *Ann Intern Med* 1973;79:76–9.

126. Flink EB, McCollister RJ, Prasad AS, et al. Evidence for clinical magnesium deficiency. *Ann Intern Med* 1957;47:956–68.

127. Baldwin D, Robinson PK, Zierler KL, et al. Interrelations of magnesium, potassium, phosphorus, and creatinine in skeletal muscle of man. *J Clin Invest* 1952;31:850–8.

128. Whang R, Welt LG. Observations in experimental magnesium depletion. *J Clin Invest* 1963;42:305–13.

129. Grace ND, O'Dell BL. Effect of magnesium deficiency on the distribution of water and cations in the muscle of the guinea pig. *J Nutr* 1970;100:45–50.

130. Alleyne GAO, Millward DJ, Scullard GH. Total body potassium, muscle electrolytes, and glycogen in malnourished children. *J Pediatr* 1970;76:75–81.

131. Duarte C. Magnesium metabolism in potassium-depleted rats. *Am J Physiol* 1978;234:466–71.

132. Carney SL, Wong NLM, Dirks HJ. Effect of magnesium deficiency and excess on renal tubular potassium transport in the rat. *Clin Sci* 1981;60:549–54.

133. Kjeldsen K, Norgaard A. Effect of magnesium depletion on ^{3}H-

ouabain binding site concentration in rat skeletal muscle. *Magnesium* 1987;6:55–60.

134. Norgaard A, Kjeldsen K, Clausen T. Potassium depletion decreases the number of ^{3}H-ouabain binding sites and the active Na-K transport in skeletal muscle. *Nature* 1981;293:739–41.

135. Butler AM. Diabetic coma. *N Engl J Med* 1950;243:648–59.

136. Martin HE, Wertman M. Serum potassium and calcium levels in diabetic acidosis. *J Clin Invest* 1947;26:217–28.

137. Levi J, Massry SG, Coburn JW., et al. Hypocalcemia in magnesium depleted dogs: evidence for reduced responsiveness to parathyroid hormone and relative failure of parathyroid gland function. *Metabolism* 1974;23:323–35.

138. Gitelman HJ, Kukolj S, Welt LG. The influence of parathyroid glands on the hypercalcemia of experimental magnesium depletion in the rat. *J Clin Invest* 1968;47:118–26.

139. MacManus J, Heaton FW. The effect of magnesium deficiency on calcium homeostasis in the rat. *Clin Sci* 1969;36:297–306.

140. Heaton FW, Anderson CK. The mechanism of renal calcification induced by magnesium deficiency in the rat. *Clin Sci* 1965; 28:99–106.

141. Elin RJ, Armstrong WD, Singer L. Body fluid electrolyte composition of chronically magnesium-deficient and control rats. *Am J Physiol* 1971;220:543.

142. Estep H, Shaw WA, Watlington C, et al. Hypocalcemia due to hypomagnesemia and reversible parathyroid hormone unresponsiveness. *J Clin Endocrinol Metab* 1969;29:842–8.

143. Bernstein D, Kleeman CR, Dowling JT. Steatorrhea, functional hypoparathyroidism, and metabolic bone defect. *Arch Intern Med* 1962;109:43–9.

144. Muldowney FP, McKenna TJ, Kyle LH., et al. Pharathormone-like effect of magnesium replenishment in steatorrhea. *N Engl J Med* 1970;282:61–8.

145. Suh SM, Csima A, Fraser D. Pathogenesis of hypocalcemia in magnesium depletion. *J Clin Invest* 1971;50:2668–78.

146. Hahn TJ, Chase LR, Avioli LV. Effect of magnesium depletion on responsiveness of parathyroid hormone in parathyroidectomized rats. *J Clin Invest* 1972;51:886–91.

147. Reddy CR, Coburn JW, Hartenbower DL, et al. Studies on mechanisms of hypocalcemia of magnesium depletion. *J Clin Invest* 1973;52:3000–10.

148. Anast CS, Mohns JM, Kaplan SL, et al. Evidence for parathyroid failure in magnesium deficiency. *Science* 1972;177:606–8.

149. Suh SM, Tashjian AH, Matsuo N, et al. Pathogenesis of hypocalcemia in primary hypomagnesemia: normal end-organ responsiveness to parathyroid hormone, impaired parathyroid gland function. *J Clin Invest* 1973;52:153–60.

150. Rude RK, Oldham SB, Singer FR. Functional hypoparathyroidism and parathyroid hormone end-organ resistance in human magnesium deficiency. *Clin Endocrinol* 1976;5:209–24.

151. Chase LR, Slatopolsky E. Secretion and metabolic efficacy of parathyroid hormone in patients with severe hypomagnesemia. *J Clin Endocrinol Metab* 1974;38:363–71.

152. MacManus J, Heaton FW, Lucas PW. Decreased response to parathyroid hormone in magnesium deficiency. *J Endocrinol* 1971;49:253–8.

153. Anast CS, Winnacker JL, Forte LR, et al. Impaired release of parathyroid hormone in magnesium deficiency. *J Clin Endocrinol Metab* 1976;42:707–17.

154. Jowsey J. Calcium release from the skeleton of rachitic puppies. *J Clin Invest* 1972;51:9–15.

155. Pak CYC, Diller EC. Ionic interaction with bone mineral. V. Effect of magnesium, citrate, fluoride, and sulfate on the solubility, dissolution, and growth of bone mineral. *Calcif Tissue Res* 1969;4:69–77.

156. Paunier L, Radde IC, Kooh SW, et al. Primary hypomagnesemia with secondary hypocalcemia. *J Pediatr* 1965;67:945.

157. Skyberg D, Stromme JH, Nesbakken R, et al. Neonatal hypomagnesemia with selective malabsorption of magnesium. *Scand J Clin Lab Invest* 1968;21:355–63.

158. Stromme JH, Steen-Johnson J, Harnaes K, et al. Familial hypomagnesemia—a follow-up examination of three patients after 9 to 12 years of treatment. *Pediatr Res* 1981;15:1134–9.

159. Booth CC, Babouris N, Hanna S, et al. Incidence of hypomagnesemia in intestinal malabsorption. *Br Med J* 1963;2:141–4.

160. Caddell JL. Studies in protein-calorie malnutrition. I. *N Engl J Med* 1967;276:535–40.

161. Caddell JL. Studies in protein-calorie malnutrition. II. *N Engl J Med* 1967;276:540–5.

162. Edmondson HA, Berne CJ, Homann RE, et al. Calcium, potassium, magnesium, and amylase disturbances in acute pancreatitis. *Am J Med* 1952;12:34–42.

163. Heaton FW, Pyrah LN. Magnesium metabolism in patients with parathyroid disorders. *Clin Sci* 1963;25:475–85.

164. Doe RP, Flink EB, Prasad AS. Magnesium metabolism in hyperthyroidism. *J Lab Clin Med* 1959;54:805.

165. Mader IJ, Iseri LT. Spontaneous hypopotassemia, hypomagnesemia, alkalosis, and tetany due to hypersecretion of corticosterone-like mineralocorticoid. *Am J Med* 1955;19:976–88.

166. Massry SG, Coburn JW, Chapman LW, et al. The acute effect of adrenal steroids on the interrelationship between the renal excretion of sodium, calcium, and magnesium. *J Lab Clin Med* 1967;70:563–70.

167. Massry SG, Coburn JW, Chapman LW, et al. The effect of long-term desoxycorticosterone acetate administration on the renal excretion of calcium and magnesium. *J Lab Clin Med* 1968; 71:212–9.

168. Levin GE, Mather HM, Pilkington TRE. Tissue magnesium status in diabetes mellitus. *Diabetologia* 1981;21:131–4.

169. DeLeeuw I, Verommen J, Abs R. The magnesium content of the trabecular bone in diabetic subjects. *Biomedicine* 1978;29:16–7.

170. McNair P, Christiansen C, Madsbad S, et al. Hypomagnesemia, a risk factor for diabetic retinopathy. *Diabetes* 1978;27:1075–7.

171. Evans RA, Carter JN, George CRP, et al. The congenital "magnesium losing kidney." *Q J Med* 1981;50:395–52.

172. Geven WB, Monnens LA, Willems HE, et al. Renal magnesium wasting in two families with autosomal dominant inheritance. *Kidney Int* 1987;31:1140–4.

173. Fort P, Lifshitz F. Magnesium status in children with insulin-dependent diabetes mellitus. *J Am Coll Nutr* 1986;5:69–78.

174. Schwartz JS, Kempa JS, Vasilomanoloski EC, et al. Viomycin-induced electrolyte abnormalities. *Respiration* 1980;40:284–92.

175. Holmes AM, Hesling CM, Wilson TM. Capreomycin-induced serum electrolyte abnormalities. *Thorax* 1970;25:608–11.

176. Blachley JD, Hill JB. Renal and electrolyte disturbances associated with cisplatin. *Ann Intern Med* 1981;95:628–32.

177. McCollister RJ, Flink EB, Lewis MD. Urinary excretion of magnesium in man following the ingestion of ethanol. *Am J Nutr* 1963;12:415–20.

178. Kalbfleisch JM, Linderman RD, Ginn HE, et al. Effects of ethanol administration on urinary excretion of magnesium and other electrolytes in alcoholic and normal subjects. *J Clin Invest* 1963;42:1471–5.

179. Flink EB. Magnesium deficiency in alcoholism. *Alcoholism* 1986;10:590–4.

180. Sullivan JF, Wolpert PW, Williams R, et al. Serum magnesium in chronic alcoholism. *Ann NY Acad Sci* 1969;162:947–62.

181. Jones JE, Albrink MJ, Davidson PC, et al. Fasting and refeeding of various suboptimal isocaloric diets. Effect on mineral and nitrogen balances in obese patients. *Am J Clin Nutr* 1966;19:320–8.

182. Sullivan JF, Lankford HG, Robertson P. Renal excretion of lactate and magnesium in alcoholism. *Am J Clin Nutr* 1966;18: 231–6.

183. Allen WM, Davies DC. Milk fever, hypomagnesemia, and the "downer cow" syndrome. *Br Vet J* 1981;137:435–41.

184. Dirks JH, Alfrey AC. Normal and abnormal magnesium metabolism. In: Schrier RW, ed. *Renal and electrolyte disorders,* 3rd ed. Boston: Little, Brown & Co., 1986.

185. Mendelson J, Wexler D, Kubyzansky P, et al. Serum magnesium in delirium tremens and alcoholic hallucinosis. *J Nerv Ment Dis* 1959;128:352–7.

186. Victor M. The role of hypomagnesemia and respiratory alkalosis in the genesis of alcoholic withdrawal symptoms. *Ann NY Acad Sci* 1973;215:235–48.

187. Wilkinson R, Lucas GL, Heath A, et al. Hypomagnesemic tetany associated with prolonged treatment with aminoglycosides. *Br Med J* 1986;292:1272–3.

188. Bar RS, Wilson HE, Mazzaferri EL. Hypomagnesemic hypocalcemia secondary to renal magnesium wasting. A possible conse-

quence of high dose gentamicin therapy. *Ann Intern Med* 1975;82:646–9.

189. Zumkley H, Losse H, Spieker C, et al. Effects of drugs on magnesium requirements. *Magnesium* 1987;6:12–7.

190. Chernow B, Bamberger S, Stoiko M, et al. Hypomagnesemia in patients in postoperative intensive care. *Chest* 1989;95:391–7.

191. Kes P, Reiner Z. Symptomatic hypomagnesemia associated with gentamicin therapy. *Magnesium Trace Elem* 1990;9:54–60.

192. Lam M, Adelstein DJ. Hypomagnesemia and renal magnesium wasting in patients treated with cisplatin. *Am J Kidney Dis* 1986;8:164–9.

193. Cohen L, Kitzes R, Schnaider H. The myth of longterm thiazide-induced magnesium deficiency. *Magnesium* 1985;4:176–81.

194. Kuller L, Farrier N, Caggiula A, et al. Relationship of diuretic therapy, and serum magnesium levels among participants in the Multiple Risk Factor Intervention Trial. *Am J Epidemiol* 1985;122:105–9.

195. Kyckner T, Wester PO. Intracellular magnesium loss after diuretic administration. *Drugs* 1984;28(Suppl 1):161–6.

196. Robinson PJ, Morgan DB, Davidson C, et al. Effects of amiloride and spironolactone on plasma magnesium in furosemide-treated patients with cardiac failure. *Br J Clin Pharmacol* 1984;18:268P.

197. Devane J, Ryan MP. Evidence for a magnesium sparing action by amiloride during renal clearance studies in rats. *Br J Pharmacol* 1983;78:891–6.

198. Ryan MP. Magnesium- and potassium-sparing diuretics. *Magnesium* 1986;5:282–92.

199. Barton CH, Vaziri ND, Martin DC, et al. Hypomagnesemia and renal magnesium wasting in renal transplant recipients receiving cyclosporine. *Am J Med* 1987;83:693–9.

200. June CH, Thompson CB, Kennedy MS, et al. Profound hypomagnesemia and renal magnesium wasting associated with the use of cyclosporine for marrow transplantation. *Transplantation* 1985;39:620–4.

201. Barton CH, Vaziri ND, Mina-Araghi S, et al. Effects of cyclosporine on magnesium metabolism in rats. *J Lab Clin Med* 1989;114:232–6.

202. Burnett RJ, Reents, SB. Severe hypomagnesemia induced by pentamidine. *Diagn Imag Clin Med* 1990;24:239–40.

203. Dunn MJ, Walser M. Magnesium depletion in normal man. *Metabolism* 1964;15:884–95.

204. Fitzgerald MG, Fourman P. An experimental study of magnesium deficiency in man. *Clin Sci* 1956;15:635–47.

205. Shils ME. Experimental human magnesium depletion. *Am J Clin Nutr* 1964;15:133–43.

206. Saul RF, Selhorst JB. Downbeat nystagmus with magnesium depletion. *Arch Neurol* 1981;38:650–2.

207. Drenick EJ, Hunt IF, Swendseid ME. Magnesium depletion during prolonged fasting of obese males. *J Clin Endocrinol* 1969;29:1341–8.

208. Kingston ME, Al-Siba'i MB, Skooge WC. Clinical manifestations of hypomagnesemia. *Crit Care Med* 1986;14:950–4.

209. Anderson TW, Leriche WH, MacKay JS. Sudden death and ischemic heart disease. Correlation with hardness of local water supply. *N Engl J Med* 1969;280:805–7.

210. Chipperfield B, Chipperfield JR. Differences in metal content of the heart muscle in death from ischemic heart disease. *Am Heart J* 1978;95:732–7.

211. Manthey J, Stoeppler M, Morgenstern W, et al. Magnesium and trace metals: risk factors for coronary heart disease. *Circulation* 1981;64:722–9.

212. Altura BM, Altura BT. Magnesium ions and contraction of vascular smooth muscle: relationship to some vascular diseases. *Fed Proc* 1981;40:2672–9.

213. Turlapaty PD, Altura BM. Magnesium deficiency produces spasms of coronary arteries: relationship to etiology of sudden death ischemic heart disease. *Science* 1980;208:198–200.

214. Turlapaty PD, Altura BM. Extracellular magnesium ions control calcium exchange and content of vascular smooth muscle. *Eur J Pharmacol* 1978;52:421–3.

215. Sangal AK, Kevwitch M, Rao DS, et al. Hypomagnesemia and hypertension in primary hyperparathyroidism. *South Med J* 1989;82:1116–8.

216. Chrysant SG, Ganousis L, Chrysant C. Hemodynamic and metabolic effects of hypomagnesemia in spontaneously hypertensive rats. *Cardiology.* 1988;75:81–9.

217. Gottlieb SS. Importance of magnesium in congestive heart failure. *Am J Cardiol* 1989;63:39G–42G.

218. Rolla G, Bucca C. Hypomagnesemia and bronchial hyperreactivity. A case report. *Allergy.* 1989;44:519–21.

219. Wacker WEC. The effect of hydrochlorothiazide on magnesium excretion. *J Clin Invest* 1961;40:1086–7.

220. Duarte CG. Effects of ethacrynic acid and furosemide on urinary calcium, phosphate, and magnesium. *Metabolism* 1968;17:867–76.

221. Iseri LT, Freed J, Bures AR. Magnesium deficiency and cardiac disorders. *Am J Med* 1975;58:837–46.

222. Goldman RH, Kleiger RE, Schweizer E, et al. The effect of myocardial ^{3}H-digoxin of magnesium deficiency. *Proc Soc Exp Biol Med* 1971;136:747–9.

223. Pignide L, Hersch R. Efficacy and limits of magnesium therapy in extrasystole. *Magnesium* 1985;4:272–9.

224. Graber TW, Yee AS, Baker FJ. Magnesium: physiology, clinical disorders, and therapy. *Ann Emerg Med* 1981;10:49–57.

225. Oster JR, Epstein M. Management of magnesium depletion. *Am J Nephrol* 1988;8:349–54.

226. Ferdinandus J, Pederson JA, Whatg R. Hypermagnesemia as a cause of refractory hypotension, respiratory depression, and coma. *Arch Intern Med* 1981;141:669–70.

227. Abate MA. Magnesium content of antacids. *Am J Hosp Pharm* 1981;38:1662.

228. Gren J, Woolf A. Hypermagnesemia associated with catharsis in a salicylate-intoxicated patient with anorexia nervosa. *Ann Emerg Med* 1989;18:200–3.

229. Weber CA, Santiago RM. Hypermagnesemia. A potential complication during treatment of theophylline intoxication with oral activated charcoal and magnesium-containing cathartics. *Chest* 1989;95:56–9.

230. Contiguglia SR, Alfrey AC, Miller NL, et al. Total body magnesium excess in chronic renal failure. *Lancet* 1972;1:1300–2.

231. Contiguglia SR, Alfrey AC, Miller NL, et al. Nature of soft tissue calcifications in uremia. *Kidney Int* 1973;4:229–35.

232. LeGeros RZ, Contiguglia SR, Alfrey AC. Pathological calcifications associated with uremia: two types of calcium-phosphate deposits in uremia. *Calcif Tissue Res* 1973;13:173–85.

PART VI

Disorders of Stone Formation

Disorders of Bone and Mineral Metabolism,
edited by Fredric L. Coe and Murray J. Favus,
© 1992 by Raven Press, Ltd. All rights reserved.

CHAPTER 29

Physical–Chemical Processes in Kidney Stone Formation

Charles M. Brown and Daniel L. Purich

One might justifiably assert that urolithiasis is quite unlike other forms of biomineralization in that the healthy condition is characterized by inhibited aggregation and that pathology arises when biomineral deposition and retention occur. For example, in bones and teeth, crystal growth is exquisitely controlled through a sequence of well-defined physiological mechanisms of deposition and resorption, and the disease state represents some interruption or modification of that set of metabolic processes. By contrast, crystallization in the urinary tract seems to happen opportunistically and quite freely, and the disease state arises apparently when unknown processes enable assembly of crystallites into flow-obstructing stones. In principle, such assembly might take place as a consequence of either (a) altered crystal surface properties, (b) changes at the level of the cell surfaces in the urinary tract, or (c) physiological changes that cause retention of crystallites and allow time for processes which, under normal conditions, progress slowly. Any of these scenarios can be exacerbated by uncontrolled biosynthesis of oxalate (primary hyperoxaluria), elevated phosphate (phosphaturia), or excessive dietary intake of oxalate-rich foodstuffs. Nonetheless, stone formation remains an idiopathic disease in most cases. From this perspective, formation and presence of crystallites is a typical renal function directed at concentrating oxalate and phosphate for more effective, irreversible elimination. The abnormal condition results from the agglomeration and further growth of these crystallites. Because crystals are observed quite commonly in most urine, the real mystery may relate to why more people are not stone-formers, and physical chemical investigations promise to provide a means for elucidating some of the processes that contribute to both the prevention and promotion of stone formation. Thus, while the pathophysiology of urolithiasis can be linked in general terms to the insolubility of certain metal ion complexes or metabolites, precise determinations of the driving forces and pathways for stone formation are the goal of physical–chemical studies, with the hope of providing effective clinical intervention.

This chapter presents aspects of the evolving physicochemical picture of urolithiasis. This picture has a stratified appearance, starting with solution and surface phenomena upon which such events as nucleation, crystal growth, and aggregation are based; once these two hierarchies have been described, the processes which lead to the formation of matrix and the large-scale structure of stones can be considered. The goal of developing such a picture is to move gradually from vague descriptions of urolithiasis to increasingly detailed, accurate depictions of what specific ions and molecules are doing at specific times, at particular sites, in response to certain environmental conditions, and so on. Most of our examples deal with oxalate stone formation, but the principles discussed could be applied just as well to other stone-forming substances. In writing this chapter, we have sought to provide more than a review alone by attempting to refine and focus the debate over some physical–chemical issues.

GENERAL OVERVIEW OF CRYSTALLIZATION

Because mechanistic urolithiasis is necessarily rooted in physical chemistry, many readers may wish to refresh their understanding of the physical–chemical underpin-

C. M. Brown and D. L. Purich: Center for the Study of Lithiasis and Pathological Calcification and Department of Biochemistry and Molecular Biology, University of Florida College of Medicine, Gainesville, Florida 32610

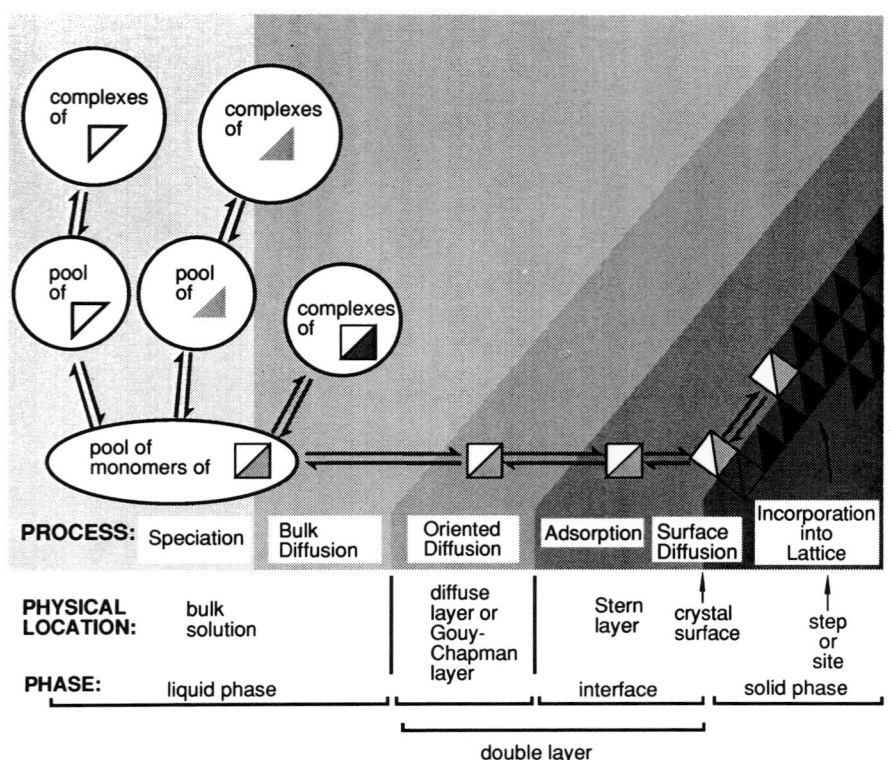

FIG. 1. Schematic representation of various processes that play a role in crystal growth in aqueous solution. The diagram shows the relationship between processes taking place in the bulk solution (speciation and transport), in the interfacial region (adsorption), and on the surface (surface diffusion and incorporation into the lattice).

ning of crystallization processes. Accordingly, we start with a discussion of real electrolyte solutions in which the concentration of a stone-forming substance exceeds its thermodynamically defined solubility. In such a case, the presence of a coexisting crystal surface will lead to crystal growth as depicted schematically in Fig. 1. On the left side of the figure, we see the various stone-forming components in their complexed and uncomplexed forms (shown here as light and dark triangles) that can combine to form a pool of monomers (half-filled squares). The formation of these monomers from pools of uncomplexed precursors can be competitively blocked by the presence of other substances that form complexes with the precursors and thereby deplete the precursor concentration through mass action. The diagram also shows a second phase that helps to explain the nature of oriented diffusion and subsequent adsorption of the monomers. This so-called "double-layer region" is treated as two defined layers: The first is known as the "diffuse layer" or "Gouy–Chapman layer," and the second is called the "Stern layer." This double-layer model allows one to rationalize the forces that monomers experience within the gradient charge field created by the surface in a manner that encourages attractive or repulsive diffusion of the monomer. Furthermore, as the monomer nearly contacts the surface of the crystal, the Stern layer is encountered, and a combination of local electrostatic and chemical forces begins to dominate. Finally, after arriving at the crystal lattice surface, the monomer diffuses in a two-dimensional fashion until it is stabilized

by a favorable lattice interaction leading to net incorporation into the growing crystal surface. Frequently, such sites of incorporation are viewed as discontinuities in the crystal surface such as a step from one lattice layer line to the next. Once formed, crystals can interact with each other and with their environment. Primarily, this interaction will involve some kind of adhesion. Adhesion can occur between crystals directly to form larger structures which may act as the nidus of a stone, or crystals can interact with tissues to form such structures. The role and composition of matrix may be critical to understanding the large-scale structure of stones.

From this perspective, the reader will readily recognize that crystallization is indeed an intriguingly complex process, especially when one considers the solution and surface behavior in the urinary tract or where electrolytes, metabolites, proteins, and even cells can alter the course of the stone-forming processes. To facilitate acquisition of a sufficient working knowledge, we now recursively characterize the events described in the preceding paragraph by retracing the path taken by monomers from solution into the lattice and by providing a glossary of physical–chemical terminology arranged according to the physical phases described in Fig. 1.

Liquid-Phase Behavior

We begin by considering a liquid phase which contains some dissolved substances and is in contact with a particulate solid phase which is partially dissolved; for our purposes, the "liquid phase" is a term synonymous with "aqueous phase," and all processes discussed in this chapter take place in aqueous solutions. The dissolved monomers of the solid phase are formed in equilibrium with their uncomplexed components. Such components may be ions (which are charged atoms or molecules), and ions interact with each other (to reform the monomers) or with other substances to form other complexes. Concentrations of the uncomplexed ions, therefore, depend upon the concentrations of all chemical substances competing for them; the extent of any one complexation reaction is defined by either a solution equilibrium constant (K_a = [complex]/[component x][component y]) or a solubility product constant (K_{sp} = [component A][component B]). Accordingly, if a certain ion undergoes complexation with a number of other substances, then the free or uncomplexed concentration is defined as the total analytical concentration of the ion minus the concentrations of each complexed form of that ion. In other words, the total amount of an ion in solution is divided between its ionic form (uncomplexed form) and its various complexed forms. In some cases, mineral salts are so weakly associated in solution that their ionic forms predominate; such is the case with sodium chloride. We shall use the term "speciation" to designate the ionic and complex species in solution, to account for the equilibria interconnecting such species, and to quantitatively define each of their concentrations. To achieve this, one must explicitly know all of the possible complexation reactions that ions can undergo, and one must have a stability constant (synonymous with "formation constant" or "association constant" in this presentation) to relate the concentration of the complex to the product of the uncomplexed concentrations of its constituent ions. The magnitude of a stability constant is expressed in reciprocal molar units and depends on the temperature and ionic strength of the solution. The reader may recall that ionic strength may be defined as one-half the sum of a series of terms, each corresponding to the concentration of a particular species multiplied by its charge.

So far, we have expressed the number of ions per unit volume by concentration, but physical chemists prefer the concept of "activity" to understand ionic behavior in both dilute and concentrated solution. Indeed, as a solution becomes more concentrated (as the ionic strength increases), ions behave as if there were fewer of them present than would be indicated by their analytical concentrations. Activity of a particular component is related to its concentration by a proportionality constant known as an "activity coefficient." Obviously, this becomes important in fluids such as urine, which can be quite concentrated in terms of a variety of solutes. An extension of this treatment is the use of the "activity product" to represent the mathematical product of the activities of a set of ions.

Most simply, "solubility" is the measure of the amount of a solid that can be held in solution, and this is achieved when a solution remains in contact with the solid for a sufficient period to ensure equilibration (saturation). Usually, solubility is expressed as an activity product which is generally called the "solubility product constant." Perhaps a more useful way of expressing the degree of saturation is provided by the "relative supersaturation," which can be regarded as the activity product of a solid in solution divided by the solubility product constant. This ratio defines how much of a solid is in solution compared to how much should remain dissolved under stable, equilibrium conditions. Relative supersaturation is the driving force for nucleation and crystal growth. It is useful to remember that solutions can be made supersaturated with respect to a particular solid by combining solutions of the constituent ions of the solid, or by lowering the temperature of a saturated solution, or, in the renal context, by urine volume changes. Usually, the temperature dependence of saturation is not very high, so that lowering the temperature is a more gentle means of supersaturating a solution.

Substances in solution are in constant motion as a result of their intrinsic motional energy (i.e., their temperature). If there is a site of chemical activity in a solution (such as a growing crystal), ions in solution must diffuse to this surface through the bulk medium containing an agitated and disordered crowd of other ions and solvent molecules. This process is relatively fast, occurring on the order of centimeters per second for low-molecular-weight ions; nonetheless, such bulk diffusion does introduce a time delay into reactions taking place in solution. In the laboratory, this delay is overcome by stirring. In the urinary tract, flow rates are not high enough to overcome diffusion completely, and transport of reactants to the site of reaction must be taken into account at some point.

Macroscopically, the boundary between the water in a glass container and the surface of the glass itself seems distinct and well-defined. On a microscopic level, however, the boundaries between solids and liquids—referred to as "interfaces"—are usually complicated transition zones where the physical theories that treat liquids or solids alone no longer apply. Physical theories for interfacial behavior are therefore required. This is especially true in the case of crystals in aqueous environments. The surfaces of these crystals often possess characteristic charges ("surface charge") which influence the composition of the solution near the surface. The prevalent approach for describing the electrically influenced zone near a surface is referred to as "double-layer theory." The theory regards the electrically influenced region of the solution as divisible into two parts: a layer near the surface that has a charge excess whose sign is opposite to that of the surface itself (because opposite charges attract) and, outside this layer, a second region of charge opposite to that of the first (and therefore the same charge as the surface), making the whole system electrically neutral. Though this remains a theoretical construct, double-layer theory has proven very useful in the interpretation of interfacial electrical phenomena.

The inner layer of the double-layer theory is usually referred to as the "Stern layer." Ions and molecules in this layer experience a combination of electrostatic and chemical attachment to the surface. The composition of this layer gives rise to many of the distinctive behaviors of particles in solution, especially influencing aggregation. A very important parameter characterizing this layer is the so-called "Debye–Hückel length," which expresses the thickness of this layer and is strongly dependent on the ionic strength of the solution. The "Gouy–Chapman layer" is the outer layer in the double-layer theory, and it is frequently called the "diffuse layer." Ions and molecules in this layer are not bound but are influenced by the electrostatic nature of the Stern layer. Whereas it is meaningful to talk about definite amounts of specific moieties in the Stern layer, the Gouy–Chapman layer is best thought of as possessing only a total charge. "Oriented diffusion" is a term coined for the influence that solutes may experience in different ways by the charge structure of the double-layer region. This influence could amount to a facilitation or obstacle with regard to the participation of certain substances in surface processes.

Certain ions or molecular substances may become attached to surfaces by a mixture of electrostatic and chemical forces. This process is known as "adsorption"; the substances which adhere to the surface are called "adsorbates." Various theories describe the gross features of this phenomenon, and they are usually characterized by an "isotherm," a hyperbolic curve that relates the surface concentration of a substance to the solution concentration. The most well known of these is the Langmuir isotherm. This isotherm is the basis for the Stern theory, though other isotherms could be used as well. To help the reader appreciate the distinction drawn here: An isotherm describes the gross, or macroscopically observed, behavior of adsorbates, whereas the Stern theory is a way of describing adsorption on a molecular level while taking into account the specific properties of the adsorbates and the surfaces. Though many isotherms have been developed based on varying assumptions about how different substances adsorb, the Langmuir has remained the most generally useful because its underlying assumptions of monomolecular coverage and reversible attachment are so widely applicable.

Surface Events

Ions and molecules adsorbed to the surface are not usually rigidly attached and can move across the surface to other points of attraction where they may remain for a time. This is called "surface diffusion." The interface may be pictured as an active region where molecules and ions approach and attach, detach and diffuse, or detach and return to the bulk solution. Some substances may anchor themselves more or less irreversibly to the surface, and this appears to be a particularly important viewpoint for larger biomolecules which may have multiple points of attachment, so-called "polypodal attachment." Such a molecule may release one or two points of attachment, but releasing all points of attachment simultaneously becomes much more unlikely with every additional possible attachment. Naturally, some of the substances from the solution attached to the surface are those of which the solid itself is composed, and the subunits of these substances can interact with the surface in a unique way; because the solid is composed of them, their attachment to the surface is unusually stable. The distinction between incorporated subunits and adsorbed subunits should be kept in mind. Incorporation of these subunits into the solid is "crystal growth." Likewise, subunits of the solid lattice exposed to the interface can occasionally leave and return to solution ("dissolution"). Some lattices may have just the right structure so that other solid lattices can begin to build up on them; when a crystal of one composition gives rise to a crystal of another composition in this way, it is usually called "epitaxy" or "epitaxial growth," but the term "oriented overgrowth" may also be seen.

For a homogeneous solution, supersaturated with respect to solute, crystallization cannot take place in the absence of a higher-order organizational process known as "nucleation." In one sense, "nucleation" refers to any process affording a route for a substance from one physical phase to another, usually in the direction of greater order. Examples are the slow formation of bubbles in carbonated beverages and the condensation of water vapor into droplets. Of greatest interest to this discussion is the sudden appearance of microscopic crystals from supersaturated solutions.

SOLUTION AND SURFACE CHEMISTRY

Some of the physical processes that most directly affect stone formation include ionic speciation, relative supersaturation, and surface adsorption. Over the past decade, the research group headed by the late Birdwell Finlayson developed computational protocols under the general title of EQUIL to deal with these phenomena rigorously. In this regard, we are continuing the effort to make the EQUIL software sufficiently versatile and accessible for scientists focusing on biomineralization. Accordingly, this section emphasizes the utility of EQUIL, and more extended discussions of this software are presented elsewhere.

Speciation

Traditionally, the concentration of substances in urine has been reported in terms of the total mass of substance excreted in a certain urine volume. Patient samples taken to the clinical laboratories were analyzed for a series of important ions and metabolites, such as creatinine and magnesium. Total masses of urinary substances given per unit volume or for 24 hours, including urinary volume itself, allowed detection of certain disease states. When studies of this type were applied to the discrimination between stone-formers and non-stone-formers, much confusion resulted. It was quite natural to ask if stone disease was basically caused by the excretion (in the stone-former's urine) of a preponderance of crystals or urinary stone components, but when this hypothesis failed, the question arose as to how to properly examine the solution properties of urine.

Given the inadequacy of total excretion rates for understanding stone disease, a deeper analysis was required. Such an analysis necessitated some standard framework so that (a) hypotheses could be critically tested, (b) the range of phenomena to be considered could be expanded, and (c) results from various workers could be rationally compared. The tools provided by the physical chemistry of solutions was the obvious set to employ because urine is an aqueous solution, albeit highly concentrated, and the study of the physical chemistry of such solutions is much advanced. Firstly, in considering urine from a physical chemical point of view, we must consider substances in urine on the basis of their molar concentrations. From a theoretical point of view, the activity concept, which represents the effective concentration, is the most important and accurate way of expressing concentrations in solutions; however, molar concentration is what can be determined most easily in the laboratory. Activity can be measured directly through electrochemical means, but the concept of activity is not precisely defined for larger molecules. Secondly, the ideas of ionic concentration and complexation give a new point of view about what a particular substance is doing in solution.

Ions are in a constant state of interaction. Ions in solution are complexed with water molecules (hydration), and to say that a certain ion is uncomplexed really means that it is complexed only with water molecules.

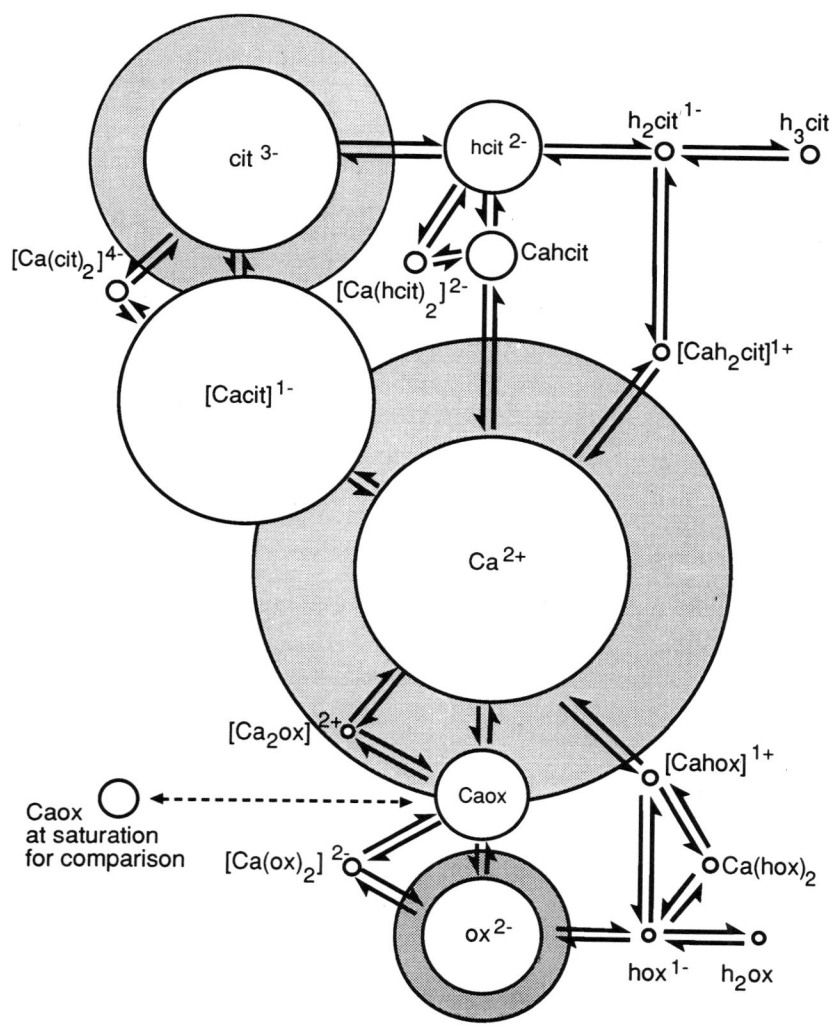

FIG. 2. "Pool diagram" showing all complexes resulting from the interaction of calcium ions, oxalate, and citrate in aqueous solution. The areas of the circles are proportional to the concentrations of the complexes they represent. This steady-state relationship among the various complexes is referred to as the "speciation" of the solution.

Stability constants quantitate the extent to which an ion is complexed with any particular substance in solution, and they allow comparisons of the relative affinity of different complexing agents for a particular chemical substance. For example, calcium ion can form complexes with many substances in urine; the EQUIL program includes stability constants for approximately 25 calcium complexes. Speciation is a chain of interactions in solution which may be best represented graphically as "pool diagrams." These diagrams show the relative concentrations of the various complexes in solution, and the reversible equilibria existing between these pools are shown by the arrows. Figure 2 represents such a diagram constructed with the aid of the EQUIL software, and the size of each circle indicates relative concentration of a particular substance. Very small circles indicate a negligible concentration of complex. Locate the circle labeled "Cacit" on the diagram; the diameter of this circle corresponds to a concentration of approximately 1.4 mM. This circle is linked to two other circles, its components calcium and citrate. The linkage between all the circles through various pathways is a graphical display of the fact that a change in the concentration of any complex or component on the diagram will be transmitted to all other circles on the diagram. For example, if citrate is reduced, the calcium which was bound as calcium citrate complex will be released, and this will increase the available calcium; increased available calcium will, in turn, compete with other cations for phosphate, sulfate, and so on. The net result will be an increased concentration of all other calcium complexes, a reduction of all other cation complexes, and an increase in the uncomplexed cations. Because of the number of complexes in the scheme, the effect of small changes in any one constituent is buffered. The key to the physical success of the scheme is that all the reactions in it are reversible; that is, though the complexes are stable relative to the component activities, if those activities decrease, there is nothing preventing the complexes from breaking down into their components. Irreversible reactions change the way this scheme works; such reactions could be the irreversible binding of a cation or anion, reactions of complexing agents with extremely high affinities, or, as we shall consider in the next section, the precipitation of insoluble salts.

Relative Supersaturation

The free energy in a solution that drives the processes of nucleation and crystal growth is directly related to the relative supersaturation (RS): $\Delta G = -RT \ln (\text{RS})$. The higher the relative supersaturation, the more likely nucleation becomes and the faster crystal growth proceeds.

Underlying RS mechanistically are the processes that lead to dissolution and sustain the equilibrium between solid and liquid phases. Molecules or ions will remain dissolved provided that the conditions are energetically favorable. However, all molecules above a certain threshold solution activity will remain in, or become part of, the solid phase. Molecules are in equilibrium between the solid state and the dissolved state. The extent to which the equilibrium balance favors the dissolved phase indicates the degree of solubility.

Stone salts are highly insoluble, and, once formed through nucleation, the solid phase will grow until the activity of the complex from which the solid phase is formed reaches its equilibrium value. These solid phases are connected to the components in Fig. 2, with which they are in reversible equilibrium. For example, if magnesium were added to a complex solution containing solid calcium oxalate monohydrate (COM), the magnesium would compete with calcium for an increased share of the oxalate; this would reduce the amount of the calcium oxalate complex, and finally a small amount of calcium oxalate solid would dissolve to restore the complex concentration to its equilibrium value. In urine, this picture must be extended to account for the molecular substances that coat crystals and reduce access of the solution to the surface; coated crystals do not redissolve readily.

RS calculations remain the most appropriate characterization of stone risk because there is as yet no detailed mechanistic understanding of the formation of stones from sparingly soluble salts in urine. These calculations are also quite useful because they take into account the impact on each stone salt of all solution components, not just the components of the stone salt itself. We can examine stone risk from both points of view using EQUIL. Figure 3 shows contours of RS for COM [RS(COM)] as a function of both calcium ion and oxalate concentration.

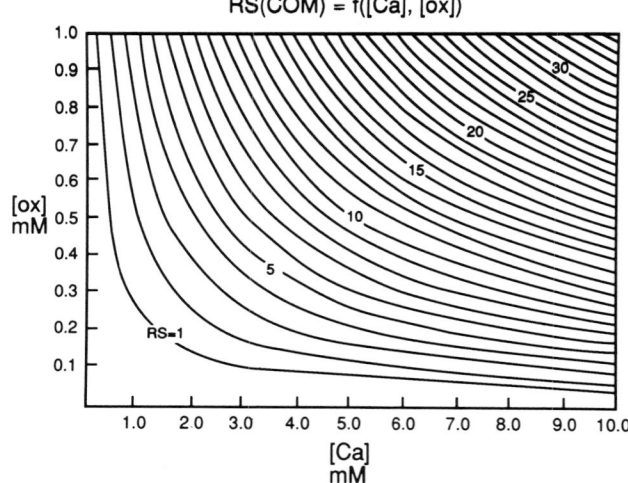

FIG. 3. Graph of RS of typical human urine as a function of calcium ion and oxalate concentrations. The range of concentrations has been chosen to include the physiological range. The symmetry of the diagram reflects the fact that oxalate has roughly 10 times the impact on RS than does calcium ion under these solution conditions.

TABLE 1. *RS(COM) as a function of citrate and magnesium ion concentration[a]*

[Mg], mM	[citrate], mM				
	1	3	5	7	9
1	8.37	7.07	5.93	4.99	4.23
3	7.86	6.83	5.89	5.06	4.36
5	7.39	6.56	5.78	5.07	4.44
7	6.95	6.28	5.63	5.03	4.47
9	6.56	6.01	5.47	4.95	4.46

[a] Values were calculated by EQUIL.

The concentration ranges are not identical but are chosen to include the typical physiological concentration near the center of each axis. The most apparent observation, therefore, is that the calcium ion scale is 10 times the oxalate scale. Given the symmetry of the contours, we could say that oxalate has about 10 times the effect of calcium ion on the RS of this stone salt. The figure also shows that simultaneous changes in both calcium and oxalate have a much more profound impact than does the manipulation of either component by itself. Complexing agents such as magnesium ion or citrate tend to complex oxalate and calcium ion, respectively, thus releasing the counterion; the increase in the counterion mitigates the impact of the complexing agent, and changes in the RS(COM) will be much more modest. This is demonstrated in Table 1, which shows how RS(COM) varies as a function of both magnesium ion and citrate. Table 1 shows that citrate has a stronger effect on RS(COM) than does magnesium because citrate has a higher affinity for calcium ion than does magnesium ion for oxalate. Curiously, at higher citrate concentrations, increases in magnesium ion cause RS(COM) to go through some local maxima rather than to smoothly decrease; increasing magnesium ion compromises the effect of citrate. In this case, the effect is relatively insignificant but does demonstrate the possibility of counterintuitive results.

While beyond the scope of this discussion, Pak's laboratory has developed a stone risk estimator based primarily on the use of EQUIL to calculate RS values.

Adsorption

Assuming the presence of crystal surfaces in the urinary tract, adsorption is the process most actively affecting their nature. Adsorbates alter the chemical, physical, and electrical properties of surfaces; by doing so, they affect crystal growth and aggregation. Whereas one might tend to identify a solid by its bulk composition, it is the surface composition with which the solution interacts. Again, this is a more complex way of understanding the interaction of solids and solutions, but physical chemistry makes theoretical tools for treating this situation available, and EQUIL makes those tools computationally available.

Currently, we are able to treat the surface adsorption of only 13 ions and complexes onto the COM surface using the EQUIL software. Even with this partial information, however, we can begin to develop an understanding of the crystal surface. This can be developed in three stages: (i) the nature of the crystal surface itself (briefly treated above), (ii) the crystal surface in simple solutions, and (iii) some observations concerning the crystal in full urine.

Using COM as our preferred example, the bulk composition of this stone salt will be one calcium ion to one oxalate ion to one water molecule; Deganello and Piro (1) clarified the disposition of these constituents in the crystal lattice. The surface composition depends on how the crystal is sliced, so to speak, and different crystal faces can have different ratios of calcium to oxalate; furthermore, because these ratios need not be strictly one-to-one, the different faces can have different charges. This is seen when certain crystals, when cleaved in air, exhibit static electric charges on the cleaved faces. When such surfaces are immersed in water the situation becomes complicated by the dissolution from the surface of component ions. Each face of the crystal will have a specific surface charge; usually, of course, it is impractical to try to view the charging on such a microscopic level, and the overall charging of the crystal is determined by electrophoretic means. Nonetheless, there is still no consensus regarding the sign of the surface charge on COM crystals in distilled water. From the above explanation, this charge is not a fixed property of COM as are its bulk properties, and we have found that the electrophoretic mobility of calcium oxalate particles can depend on the provenance of a particular sample.

In order to examine the behavior of COM crystals in a solution containing a variety of urinary solutes, we have summarized (see Table 2) double-layer and adsorption results calculated by EQUIL. The basis of these calculations is a hypothetical urine based on average concentrations of urinary components as given in *Documenta Geigy* (2). We use these values because of the completeness of the Geigy tables and because of their wide availability. In this table, the alternation of charge previously described is seen clearly. The surface charge is predicted to be positive owing to the high calcium-to-oxalate ratio in urine; however, the charge in the Stern layer is negative because of the large number of negative charges adsorbed, and the charge in the Gouy–Chapman layer is positive. Note that the most charged layer is the Stern layer. Referring to the lower part of Table 2, we can examine the composition of the Stern layer more thoroughly. Two columns of numbers are given: On the left are the ionic concentrations of the ions or complexes listed; on the right are their charge contributions (in coulombs per square centimeter) to the adsorbed layer

TABLE 2. *Double-layer values for the Geigy urine as calculated by EQUIL; adsorbed species are ranked from largest positive charge contribution to the Stern layer down to the largest negative contribution*

Summary of double-layer calculations
Surface charge = 4.055×10^{-7} coulombs/cm^2
Stern potential = -1.611×10^{-2} V
Stern charge = -1.480×10^{-6} coulombs/cm^2
Gouy charge = 1.074×10^{-6} coulombs/cm^2

Adsorbed species	Moles adsorbed per cm^2	Charge contribution (coulombs/cm^2)
Dicalcium oxalate complex ion	4.439×10^{-6}	2.717×10^{-6}
Calcium ion	1.527×10^{-3}	9.917×10^{-7}
Magnesium ion	9.777×10^{-4}	2.198×10^{-7}
Sodium citrate complex ion	1.335×10^{-10}	-3.820×10^{-18}
Sodium pyrophosphate complex ion	3.181×10^{-7}	-8.215×10^{-16}
Hydrogen pyrophosphate ion	9.716×10^{-6}	-2.509×10^{-14}
Calcium citrate complex ion	1.384×10^{-3}	-6.186×10^{-11}
Pyrophosphate	1.249×10^{-7}	-1.634×10^{-10}
Calcium dioxalate complex ion	9.482×10^{-8}	-1.513×10^{-9}
Oxalate	1.344×10^{-4}	-2.342×10^{-8}
Sulfate	4.292×10^{-2}	-2.061×10^{-7}
Hydrogen phosphate ion	1.651×10^{-2}	-2.779×10^{-7}
Citrate	8.205×10^{-4}	-4.899×10^{-6}

(Stern layer), ranked from largest positive contribution to largest negative contribution. It is obvious that negative adsorbates outweigh positive ones, both in number of species adsorbing and in total charge contribution. Perhaps surprisingly, oxalate makes relatively little of the negative contribution, which is dominated by citrate. Also surprisingly, the majority of the positive charge is contributed by the dicalcium oxalate complex. Finally, we offer a few comments concerning adsorption of macromolecules. In general, the composition of the Stern layer is controlled by the relative concentrations of competitive adsorbates, the number of available surface sites, and the energy of interaction (both chemical and electrostatic) between surface site and adsorbate. The adsorption behavior of macromolecules, which are often polyanionic, differs from that of the small molecules we have considered up to now in that, through polypodal attachment, they can conceivably cover more than one surface site at a time. Adsorption by such molecules may be irreversible, because desorption is dependent on a series of coordinated statistical events (i.e., many attachments must be broken at the same time). Adequate theory to treat such substances in a general way is not yet available when the statistical issues and their kinetic implications are taken into account; the "train–loop–tail" theory de-

veloped by Scheutjens and Fleer (3) is an example of an innovative approach to, and the statistical complexity of, macromolecular adsorption. We conclude by noting the observations of Khan and Hackett (4): After demineralization, stone crystals were found to have been completely enclosed in a thin organic hull.

NUCLEATION

Nucleation is the initial process that allows for (a) transformation from the liquid phase and (b) creation of a new phase organizationally related to the crystal lattice. This process permits solutions that are of high relative supersaturation to crystallize and thereby reach equilibrium with regard to the liquid and solid phases. Nucleation occurs when the local concentration of components that will comprise the solid phase exceeds a threshold level through short-range fluctuations in the bulk solution, and the kinetics of nucleation reflect the frequency and duration of such fluctuations. In Fig. 4, we illustrate five different conditions that arise in the initial absence or presence of crystals as the relative supersaturation is increased on the horizontal axis. In the case where crystals are initially present, only two conditions are seen:

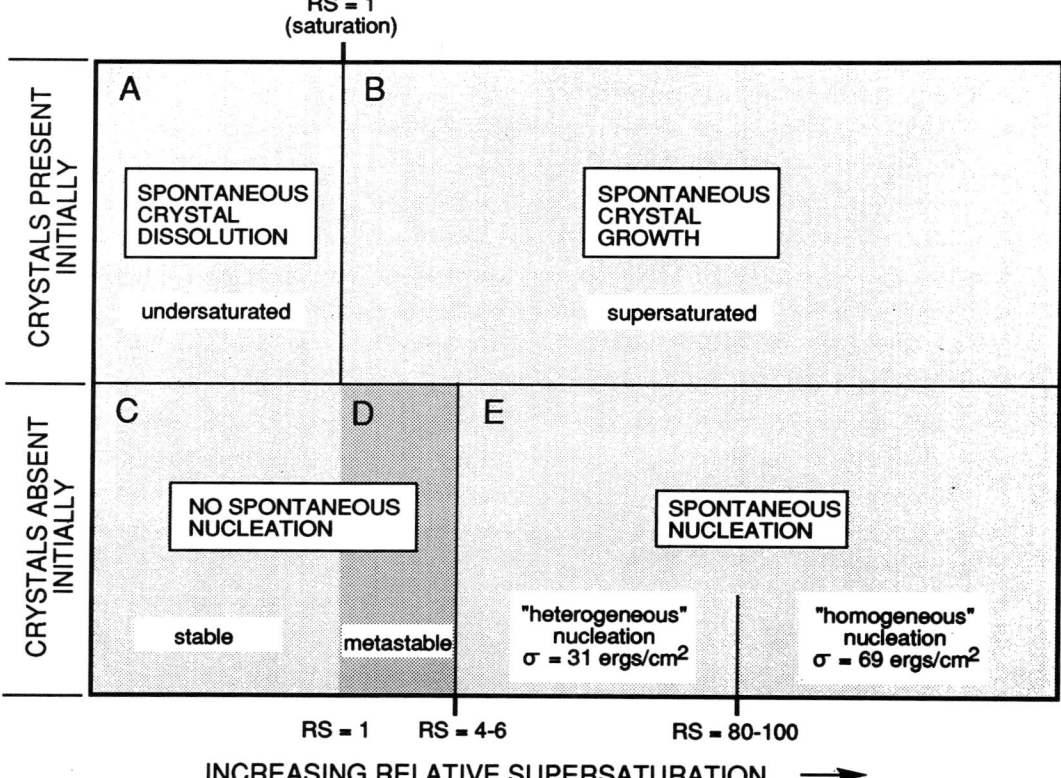

FIG. 4. Diagram showing the free energy regimes of COM behavior in aqueous solution. The horizontal axis is schematic. Region A represents a situation in which crystals are present in an undersaturated solution, and in which they would spontaneously dissolve. Region B represents the addition of COM crystals to a supersaturated solution in which the crystals would undergo spontaneous growth. Addition of crystals could be artificial or the result of nucleation. This area could conceivably be divided into smaller regions representing different growth mechanisms. Regions C and D represent solutions (no crystals present) containing calcium and oxalate which are sufficiently supersaturated to nucleate spontaneously. Note the darker area in which the solution is supersaturated with respect to crystal growth but does not possess sufficient free energy to initiate precipitation. Region E represents solutions (no crystals present) containing calcium and oxalate which are sufficiently supersaturated to nucleate spontaneously. Within this region, two kinds of nucleation have been distinguished according to differences in their apparent interfacial energies and total particle production.

The first, at RS values less than 1, represents the undersaturated phase; the second, where the solution is supersaturated, will undergo spontaneous crystal growth until the relative supersaturation falls to unity. In the case where crystals are absent initially, one can identify so-called "stable" and "metastable" states which do not undergo spontaneous nucleation despite the fact that the metastable condition is somewhat supersaturated. At higher levels of relative supersaturation (here shown as RS 4–6 for COM), one can observe spontaneous nucleation. We should note that this region of spontaneous nucleation can be conceptually divided into two regions based on the magnitude of the liquid–solid interfacial tension (σ): Heterogeneous nucleation, a process that occurs when foreign substances reduce the metastable limit, is characterized by a σ value of approximately 30 erg/cm², whereas homogeneous nucleation is a process

that requires considerably higher relative supersaturation (hence higher σ values) to allow local concentration fluctuations to be the primary route for forming nuclei. To be sure, homogeneous nucleation can occur even at the relative supersaturation values commonly associated with heterogeneous nucleation because free energy reflects a probabilistic distribution indicating a much lower frequency of occurrence as the relative supersaturation value drops. Nonetheless, in the kidney, heterogeneous nucleation is favored both by the presence of many different surfaces and by the unlikelihood of exceeding relative supersaturations of 20–25. Furthermore, Robertson (5) has estimated the crystal particle count in urine of stone-formers to be about 10^4 per milliliter, and Trump et al. (6) showed that cellular debris in the urinary tract can participate in heterogeneous nucleation.

The rate of depleting the supersaturated components through crystal growth depends on the concentration of nuclei. The inhibitory action of various agents reflects a lowering of the nuclei concentration either through inhibition of nuclei formation or through promotion of nuclei dissolution, and promotors of nucleation must act to either increase the rate of nucleation or decrease the loss of nuclei from the solution. Inhibition or promotion of nucleation must be analyzed under conditions where the relative supersaturation remains the same. Thus, we should stress that these definitions do not include mechanisms which could be explained as resulting merely from changes in the relative supersaturation, as would be the case for calcium ion and oxalate complexing agents.

In attempts to quantitatively analyze nucleation, Christiansen and Nielsen (7) have used the induction time, τ, for the precipitation process, where $\tau = gC^n$. C is the square root of the molar ion concentration product of the precipitating salt, and g and n are empirical constants. In this respect, n represents the apparent molecularity for nucleation; for calcium oxalate at 25°C, these investigators obtained values for g and n of 1.03×10^{-7} s and -3.33, respectively. Accordingly, the induction period for concentrated urine is about 3 min, well within the transit time across the kidney. More recently, Brown et al. (8) analyzed nucleation experimentally using the unaided eye or a microscope to detect the first appearance of crystals as a function of initial relative supersaturation (RSI) and mechanical stirring. The data were fitted to the Gibbs–Thomsen nucleation equation, and other computer simulation efforts showed a direct relationship between the measured and calculated turbidity. It is of interest to note that their rate data indicated that both homogeneous and heterogeneous nucleation can take place depending upon the RSI value and are reflected by a change in slope. Indeed, the interfacial energy from the upper limb of similar plots gave values of 69 erg/cm² (9), agreeing well with the published value of 67 erg/cm², whereas the lower limb gave a value of 31.1 erg/cm².

CRYSTAL AND PARTICLE GROWTH

After successful nucleation has occurred, crystal growth ensues until the RS approaches unity. During this course, crystals can remain as single growing units or they can aggregate to form larger particles. In this regard, one should distinguish between crystal size distributions and particle size distributions, the former arising from growth of crystallites in the absence of aggregation and the latter reflecting a summation of individual crystal growth as well as that arising from aggregation. In the context of urinary precipitates, one is particularly interested in conditions that lead to particle diameters of luminal dimensions. In practice, few urinary stones arise

from a single crystal; in this respect, one might consider crystal growth as a more conceptual framework, particularly in light of Finlayson's analysis of free versus fixed urinary stone disease (10). Briefly, he formulated an expression for the diameter of free particles, accounting for the grams of oxalate excreted per day, the number of ducts of Bellini per papilla, the number of papillae per kidney, the density of whewellite, and the transit time through the kidney. He reasoned that if all the oxalate mass issuing through the duct of Bellini over a transit time were incorporated into a single spherical whewellite stone, he could estimate the stone diameter to be 0.0057 cm, as compared to the 0.02-cm diameter of a duct of Bellini. He cited the finding of Robertson (5) that one may expect about 7200 crystals/mL of urine, estimating that about 11 particles per duct would be present over the transit time. This indicated that if all the particles grew at the same rate, the maximal expected particle size would be about 0.0025 cm, a dimension that would allow for ready passage through a duct of roughly 10 times that size. With the elimination of the free particle theory based on crystal growth arguments and with the observation that urinary stones are typically polycrystalline, one must now consider processes that could either (a) fix the stone nidus in the urinary tract or (b) lead rapidly to large particle diameters (i.e., aggregation).

Although the detailed history of any single urinary stone remains elusive, a fully developed stone represents the product of many different chemical and physical interactions. While crystal growth studies remain important in stone research, recent interest has centered on solid-state transformation as a primary lithogenic process. The increasing frequency of observation of calcium oxalate trihydrate in urine has led some to the view that this is a primary precipitating intermediate on the pathway to dihydrate and monohydrate forms of calcium oxalate (11,12). Interestingly, Brown et al. (13) observed that calcium oxalate dihydrate formation was preferred when citrate and magnesium were present while maintaining the RS. Additionally, other factors affecting the transformation of single crystals into a polycrystalline stone are likely to include (a) sites of retention, (b) adsorption of ions and metabolites, including proteins, and (c) aggregation itself.

Aggregation can be regarded as a higher-order process in which particles in aqueous media associate and form extended structures. The charged surfaces on particles can interact to bond them together, forming the larger structures or aggregates. Understanding the composition of the Stern layer is therefore an essential basis to a detailed account of the aggregation behavior of suspended particles. Aggregation is strongly dependent on the hydrodynamic forces in the medium, and it is divided broadly into two categories: (i) orthokinetic aggregation, in the presence of stirring, and (ii) perikinetic aggregation, in the effective absence of stirring. Because flow rates in the urinary tract are usually too small to rise above the orthokinetic minimum, aggregation there is necessarily perikinetic. When particles aggregate so tightly that they merge together, they are said to be "sintered." Aggregation might be effected also by substances that can cross-link surfaces by a sort of gluing phenomenon. Rumpf and Schubert (14) have identified six basic mechanisms by which aggregates are held together; in order of increasing energy, they are electrostatic attraction, van der Waals forces, liquid bridging, capillarity, viscous binder effects, and solid bridging. Because of the zeta potential of particles in urine, the electrostatic forces will be repulsive. Beyond this, relatively little is known about the detailed pathway(s) of aggregation in kidney stone formation.

Finlayson (9) warned that it may be appropriate to be skeptical about the significance of aggregation in stone disease. In treating aggregation in a manner akin to Smoluchowski agglomeration, he concluded that even in the presence of 10^6 particles/mL in crystalluria [a value 100 times that reported by Robertson (5)], the expected aggregation would be so slow that no appreciable aggregation could occur. Whether the Smoluchowski model remains useful in the case of urinary fluid flow past retained particles is a matter open to debate. In particular, Smoluchowski agglomeration takes into account the diffusion coefficient of the particles and treats the system as a diffusion-controlled process following Fick's law. Moreover, in simplest form, Smoluchowski agglomeration does not take into account the zeta potential and surface potential of suspended crystallites, and particle–particle interactions are considered in the absence of any role of RS in driving further annealing and curing of aggregated particles. The latter point might explain the small difference between the density of stones and the density of crystals.

PROSPECTS FOR MECHANISTIC UROLITHIASIS

We have come to appreciate the term "mechanistic urolithiasis" to represent that analytical endeavor to understand the biological, chemical, and physical processes that lead to stone formation. This definition also accommodates the clinical management of stone disease insofar as such management involves efforts to alter the course of stone development, as opposed to removal through surgery. In fact, mechanistic urolithiasis will probably also include extracorporeal shock wave lithotripsy (ESWL) through efforts to understand how the physical chemistry of stone structure affects the efficient absorption of shock wave energy. In this chapter, we have described some of the chemical and physical events that occur in real solutions, emphasizing (where possible) the properties of urine that may influence stone for-

mation. Although much has been accomplished over the last two decades (9,15), there remain many lacunae in our knowledge of the mechanistic issues, and we discuss some likely areas for future clarification.

Efforts to extend solution physical chemistry to account for the properties of urine are clearly warranted. Indeed, we must add additional equilibria to account for the many complexation reactions associated with urinary solutes, and we must reach a greater level of sophistication with regard to defining the activity coefficients and thermodynamic parameters associated with the equilibria that link these solutes. At the same time, it is only fair to acknowledge that EQUIL, sophisticated to the degree that it is, does not provide any account of macromolecular interactions with urinary crystallites. Obviously, retention of stone crystals in the urinary tract implies that such crystals must interact with such cellular components as membranes and excreted proteinaceous substances. In this regard, studies by Khan et al. (16) observed that phospholipids promote stone formation, suggesting that renal cell damage can influence the course of urolithiasis. More recent work by Mandel's group has shown that cultured papillary cells display the capacity to bind COM crystals as a function of crystal number concentration. We should also note that Ryall and Marshall have shown that the Tamm–Horsfall proteins appear to modulate the nucleation and growth of calcium oxalate monohydrate uroliths. In all of these cases, crystallite–metabolite adsorption must be a driving force, but little is known about how biomacromolecules alter the adsorption properties of crystals in the urinary tract. Other related physiological factors that require further elucidation are: the effects of oxalate and calcium ion transport; the effect of the inner and outer phospholipid bilayer components on nucleation; the influence of other macromolecules, including nephrocalcin; changes in urolithogenic capacity during infection; and the nature of stone matrix.

Although we have already described many features of the EQUIL software, the power and scope of EQUIL is complemented, at least in part, by the PSD software. PSD models the kinetic processes of nucleation, crystal growth, aggregation, and breakup (17), relying on EQUIL to define many of the pertinent solution parameters. Using this software, one can simulate the time evolution of the particle size distribution (hence the name PSD) for comparison of theoretical models and experimental data. One application of PSD is illustrated in a recent report by Brown et al. (8), who analyzed nucleation of COM. Turbidimetric and microscopic observations of nucleation lag times were analyzed with PSD to obtain thermodynamic parameters governing the formation of nuclei.

In closing, we feel that we have largely succeeded in our unstated goal of avoiding the presentation of the complicated mathematical expressions that are used to

complicated mathematical expressions that are used to characterize many of these processes. Nonetheless, as pointed out by Finlayson (17), mathematical modeling holds great promise in accounting for the complicated physical chemistry and biology within the urinary tract. He even suggested that urolithiasis should ultimately be analyzed by treating quantitatively all of the domains of consideration relevant to urolithiasis.

REFERENCES

1. Deganello S, Piro O. The crystal structure of calcium oxalate monohydrate (whewellite). *N Jb Miner Mh (Stuttgart)* 1981; 2:81–8.
2. Lentner C, ed. *Geigy scientific tables,* 11th ed. West Caldwell, NJ: Ciba–Geigy, 1981;53–107.
3. Scheutjens JMHM, Fleer GJ. Statistical theory of the adsorption of interacting chain molecules. 2. Train, loop, and tail size distribution. *J Phys Chem* 1980;84:178–90.
4. Khan SR, Hackett RL. Microstructure of decalcified human calcium oxalate urinary stones. *Scan Electron Microsc* 1984;2:935–41.
5. Robertson WG. A method for measuring calcium crystallization. *Clin Chim Acta* 1969;26:105–10.
6. Trump BF, Berezesky IK, Laiho KU, Osornio AR, Mergner WJ, Smith MW. The role of calcium in cell injury. A review. *Scan Electron Microsc* 1980;2:437–62.
7. Christiansen JA, Nielsen AE. On the kinetics of formation of sparingly soluble salts. *Acta Chim Scand* 1951;5:673–4.
8. Brown CM, Purich DL, Finlayson B. Nucleation of calcium oxalate monohydrate: use of turbidity measurements and computer-assisted simulations in characterizing early events in crystal formation. *J Crystal Growth* 1991 in press.
9. Finlayson B. Physiochemical aspects of urolithiasis. *Kidney Int* 1978;13:344–60.
10. Finlayson B. Where and how does urinary stone disease start? An essay on the expectation of free- and fixed-particle urinary stone diseases. In: van Reen R, ed. *Proceedings of the symposium on idiopathic urinary bladder stones. Fogarty International Center Proceedings,* vol. 37. Washington DC: Fogarty-NIH Pub., 1976; 7–31.
11. Hesse A, Berg W, Schneider HJ, Hienzsch E. A contribution to the formal mechanism of calcium oxalate urinary calculi. *Urol Res* 1976;4:157–60.
12. Sheehan ME, Nancollas GH. The kinetics of crystallization of calcium oxalate trihydrate. *J Urol* 1984;132:158–63.
13. Brown P, Ackermann D, Finlayson B. Calcium oxalate dihydrate (weddelite) production. *J Crystal Growth* 1989;98:285–92.
14. Rumpf H, Schubert H. Adhesion forces in agglomeration processes. In: Onoda G, Hench L, eds. *Sciences of ceramic processing before firing.* New York: John Wiley & Sons, 1977; 357–76.
15. Robertson WG, Peacock M. Pathogenesis of urolithiasis. In: Schneider H-J, ed. *Urolithiasis: etiology–diagnosis.* Berlin: Springer-Verlag, 1985;183–84.
16. Khan SR, Hackett RL. In vitro precipitation of calcium oxalate in the presence of whole matrix or lipid components of the urinary stones. *J Urol* 1988;139:418ff.
17. Finlayson B. Comment of the round table discussion on theoretical models related to urolithiasis. In: Schwille PE, Smith LH, Robertson WG, Vahlensieck W, eds. *Urolithiasis and related clinical research.* New York: Plenum, 1985;929–33.

Disorders of Bone and Mineral Metabolism,
edited by Fredric L. Coe and Murray J. Favus,
© 1992 by Raven Press, Ltd. All rights reserved.

CHAPTER 30

Mechanisms of Stone Disruption and Dissolution

James E. Lingeman

Calculi in the urinary system have plagued humankind since the earliest civilizations. Patients with stones suffered not only from the agony associated with calculous disease but also endured the sometimes barbarous attempts—with crude tools and without anesthesia—to have the offending stones removed.

Advances in the treatment of urolithiasis were minimal for many centuries, with efforts focusing primarily on techniques of perineal lithotomy for the treatment of bladder calculi. With the advent of the industrial revolution and the coincident increased occurrence of renal and ureteral calculi, a variety of elegant surgical techniques were developed for the removal of offending calculi. Unfortunately, these operations represented major surgical procedures with their attendant morbidity. Advances in technology for the removal of symptomatic upper urinary tract calculi have accelerated tremendously in the last decade and include the advent of percutaneous nephrostolithotomy (PCNL), ureteroscopic stone removal (URS), and most important, extracorporeal shock wave lithotripsy (ESWL).

MODERN SURGICAL TECHNIQUES: HISTORICAL BACKGROUND

Percutaneous Techniques

Although Hugh Hampton Young passed a pediatric cystoscope into a massively dilated ureter and renal pelvis in a child in 1912, the percutaneous application of endoscopic techniques to the kidney did not begin until

the 1940s. Rupel and Brown from Indianapolis removed a stone in 1941 through a nephrostomy tract which previously had been established surgically, and Trattner in 1948 used a cystoscope to examine the renal collecting system at open renal surgery (1,2).

The placement of a nephrostomy tube percutaneously for the purpose of providing drainage to a grossly hydronephrotic kidney was first reported by Goodwin and associates in 1955 (3). The nephrostomy tube in their patient was placed without the benefit of imaging. However, it was not until 1976 that Fernstrom and Johannson established percutaneous access with the specific intention of removing a renal stone (4). Advances in endoscopes, fluoroscopic imaging equipment, and other instruments, such as ultrasonic lithotripsy probes, allowed urologists and radiologists to refine percutaneous techniques during the late 1970s and early 1980s into well-established methods for the removal of upper urinary tract calculi. The term *endourology* was coined to encompass antegrade and retrograde techniques for the closed manipulation of the urinary tract (5).

Extracorporeal Shock Wave Lithotripsy (ESWL)

The observation that sound waves are focusable has been known for centuries. The ancient Greeks under Dionysios utilized this knowledge to construct vaults which allowed them to overhear the conversations of their imprisoned enemies. In the 18th and 19th centuries, cabinets with echo or sound mirrors were created that were capable of transmitting the ticking of a pocket watch over a distance exceeding 60 ft.

High-energy shock waves have been recognized for many years. Examples of high-energy shock waves include the potentially window-shattering sonic boom created when aircraft pass beyond the speed of sound and the blast effect associated with explosions. Engineers at Dornier Medical Systems in what was then West Ger-

J. E. Lingeman: Methodist Hospital of Indiana, Institute for Kidney Stone Disease, Indianapolis, Indiana 46202

This chapter is dedicated in the memory of Dr. Birdwell Finlayson, a man of rare intellect and insight in the field of urolithiasis. His contributions were many and will be of lasting value.

many, during research on the effects of shock waves on military hardware, demonstrated that shock waves are reflectable and, therefore, focusable. The application of mechanical shock waves to human tissue was discovered when, by chance, a test engineer touched a target body at the very moment of impact of a high-velocity projectile. The engineer felt a sensation similar to an electric shock, although the contact point at the skin showed no damage at all (6). This observation and its potential military application led Dornier to pursue techniques for the generation of a reproducible shock wave.

Beginning in 1969, through the German Ministry of Defense, Dornier began studying the effects of shock waves on tissue. Specifically, the study was to determine if shock waves, generated by projectiles hitting the wall of a tank, would damage the lungs of a tank crew member leaning against the same wall. During this study, Dornier engineers developed techniques to reproduce shock waves and found that shock waves generated in water could pass through living tissue except for the lung without discernible damage, but that brittle materials were destroyed by the shock waves.

At some point, a possible medical application of shock waves became apparent. If the shock wave could safely pass through tissue but fragment brittle materials, perhaps they could be used to break up kidney stones. Subsequently, Dornier engineers found that the lower-energy shock waves appropriate for medical application could be generated by an electrical spark discharge underwater and predictably reproduced.

In 1972, based on preliminary studies performed by Dornier Medical Systems, an agreement was reached with Professor Egbert Schmiedt, Director of the Urologic Clinic at the University of Munich, to proceed with further investigation of the therapeutic potential for this technology (7). The work was supported by the Federal Ministry of Research and Technology in West Germany and the development of the Dornier lithotripter progressed through several prototypes, culminating in the first treatment of a human with ESWL in February 1980. The production and distribution of the Dornier HM3 lithotripter began in late 1983. ESWL was approved by the Federal Drug Administration (FDA) in 1984. Since Dornier's pioneering work, numerous other companies have demonstrated that shock waves capable of stone fragmentation may be generated utilizing electromagnetic induction, microexplosions, focused lasers, and piezoelectric crystals. To date, over 400 lithotripters of all manufacturers have been placed worldwide and well over 1.5 million patients have been treated.

NEW TECHNIQUES FOR KIDNEY STONE REMOVAL

When confronted with the symptomatic urolithiasis patient, the urologist must consider a number of factors —including the short- and long-term goals of therapy, the indications for intervention, and the results of the preoperative evaluation—in order to make a decision regarding the most appropriate form of treatment. In former years, the decision-making process was relatively simple. Approximately 80% of patients could pass their stones spontaneously; the rest had surgery.

Today, since the advent of ESWL and endourologic techniques, the spectrum of options available for the management of patients with symptomatic urolithiasis has increased dramatically. Although these new techniques represent a considerable lessening of morbidity for the patient who previously required an open surgical procedure, the many new techniques now available to the urologist have increased the complexity of judgment involved in choosing the most efficacious approach to a given patient's stone problem. Confusion regarding the relative roles of the various options available is not surprising, as only limited data on new techniques have been published to date. In addition, comparison of experiences with different new techniques from various institutions can be difficult, given the lack of uniformity in procedures, classification of stone burden, and definitions of success. Furthermore, endourologic techniques and ESWL have yet to stand the test of time; only as extensive, long-term follow-up data are collected will it be possible to evaluate comprehensively the risks and the results associated with these exciting techniques.

The current options for the management of symptomatic upper urinary tract urolithiasis are listed in order of decreasing invasiveness in Table 1. The majority of patients presenting with renal colic have small (4 mm or less) ureteral calculi that have a high likelihood of spontaneous passage. Therefore, the conservative or expectant management of ureteral calculi remains a cornerstone of therapy. Surgical procedures such as pyelolithotomy and ureterolithotomy are rarely, if ever, indicated in the present era. Nephrolithotomy (either anatrophic as preferred in the United States, or extended pyelolithotomy combined with multiple radial lithotomies as preferred in Europe) may continue to have a role in the management of extremely complex staghorn calculi. However, currently at the Methodist Hospital of Indiana (MHI), less than 0.5% of patients requiring intervention for upper urinary tract calculi require open surgical procedures.

TABLE 1. *Current options for the management of nephrolithiasis*

Open surgery (nephrolithotomy, pyelolithotomy, ureterolithotomy)
Percutaneous nephrostolithotomy (PCNL)
Ureterorenoscopic stone removal (URS)
Extracorporeal shock wave lithotripsy (ESWL)
Observation

TABLE 2. *Radiographic and clinical features of cystine calculi*

Low radiodensity for the size of the calculus
Large calculi, particularly those associated with multiple peripheral satellite stones
Staghorn calculi
Bilateral stones
Ground-glass appearance of stones
Stones with smooth edges

Because nephrolithotomy is a well-described procedure in the urologic literature and is infrequently indicated, it is not reviewed in detail. Rather, the technical aspects of the newer procedures for kidney stone removal (ESWL, PCNL, and ureterorenoscopy) are presented.

Preoperative Evaluation

The evaluation of patients with urolithiasis in the era of PCNL and ESWL has not changed substantially from the prior era of open stone surgery. Good-quality radiographs and adequate contrast studies are necessary to document the extent of stone material within the upper urinary tract and the function/anatomy of the involved renal unit. Nephrotomography, computed tomography, radionuclide studies, and retrograde contrast studies are occasionally necessary in the evaluation of these patients. Bacteriologic evaluation of the urine is appropriate in all instances.

The composition of any previous stone material passed or removed from the patient is extremely important. If previous stones have contained more than 30% calcium oxalate monohydrate (whewellite) or brushite, fragmentation with ESWL may be expected to be more difficult. If such a stone is of borderline large size, the urologist may be swayed toward a percutaneous procedure rather than ESWL. The presence of cystinuria may be revealed by previous stone analysis. Any patient

TABLE 3. *Radiographic and clinical features suggesting the need for perioperative antibiotics*

Radiographic features suggestive of struvite
  Staghorn calculi
  Laminated calculi
  Low-density calculi

Clinical features suggestive of struvite
  History of previous struvite calculus
  History of recurrent urinary tract infections
  Positive urine culture[a]
  Instrumentation (i.e., ureteral stent, retrograde stone displacement, etc.) at time of ESWL
  Indwelling ureteral stent/catheter
  Nephrostomy tube

[a] Pyuria is commonly present with nephrolithiasis and is therefore not a reliable sign of urinary tract infection.

whose stone or stones have radiographic features compatible with cystine (Table 2) should be screened for cystinuria prior to treatment, as these stones are often not well treated with ESWL.

Many stones may harbor bacteria even though bacteriuria is only intermittently present. This is particularly true in the patient who has been on antibiotics in the recent past. Parenteral antibiotics should be administered preoperatively in any patient where urinary infection is suspected (Table 3). In addition, patients undergoing percutaneous debulking for staghorn calculi (the majority of which are infectious in nature) should receive 24 h of preoperative parenteral antibiotics.

PERCUTANEOUS NEPHROSTOLITHOTOMY

The percutaneous approach to the kidney has advanced to a remarkable degree since the first percutaneous nephrostomy was performed by Goodwin et al. in 1955 (3). That procedure was done without benefit of imaging in a patient with gross hydronephrosis. Today, achieving such goals as satisfactory renal drainage, stone removal, endopyelotomy, and so on, are dependent in large part on the ability to perform precise puncture of the intrarenal collecting system. Knowledge of renal anatomy and of various puncture techniques is essential whether access is achieved by the radiologist or by the urologist. Achievement of the desired goals for the percutaneous procedure requires that the individual performing access be cognizant of the problems at hand and the limitations of percutaneous instrumentation.

The success of percutaneous endourologic procedures is dependent on the following factors. First, the patient needs to have a good understanding of why the procedure is being performed and its inherent risks. Second, the urologist must have patience and persistence. Third, instrumentation must be adequate, including at a minimum both rigid and flexible nephroscopes as well as the capability to perform ultrasonic and electrohydraulic lithotripsy. Fourth, a healthy imagination and a willingness to try new techniques are perhaps the most important aspects of this rapidly evolving field.

Ureteral Catheter

At the MHI, the initial step of PCNL is the cystoscopic placement of an occlusion balloon ureteral catheter, positioned just below the ureteropelvic junction (UPJ) under fluoroscopic guidance. The balloon at the tip of the catheter is inflated until the proximal ureter is occluded. This maneuver is very helpful when performing complicated access procedures, as it allows for the retrograde instillation of contrast material or carbon dioxide and for distention of the collecting system. Additionally, the balloon is inflated during the ultrasonic lithotripsy of large calculi in order to prevent the potentially trouble-some problem of fragment migration into the ureter. If the patient has undergone urinary diversion, the ureteral catheter can almost always be placed by performing endoscopy of the intestinal segment with the flexible nephroscope. Visualization of the upper urinary tract in patients with urinary diversion can also be achieved in many instances by placing a Foley in the intestinal segment and performing a loopogram.

Patient Positioning

Percutaneous procedures are performed with the patient in the prone position with the stone-containing side elevated on a foam pad to approximately 30 degrees. This position aids in ventilation of the patient and tends to bring the posterior calices into a vertical position, which is helpful during puncture of the collecting system. Careful padding of pressure points is essential, and attention should be given to arm position (Fig. 1). The down arm should be placed at the side and the up arm flexed at the elbow and placed on an arm board. The down arm should never be flexed at the shoulder, as this may predispose to brachial plexus injury. Intravenous extension tubing is placed on the occlusion balloon catheter ports and brought out under the sterile drape between the patient's legs to provide easy access for contrast instillation and inflation/deflation of the balloon.

Imaging

Adequate imaging arrangements are necessary for all endourologic procedures. While the majority of trans-urethral procedures and some straightforward percutane-ous procedures can be performed with a fixed fluoro-scopic unit, or even with ultrasound guidance, complicated access problems (such as staghorn calculi, horseshoe kidneys, calyceal diverticula) are best performed with multiplane imaging as provided with a C-arm fluoroscopic unit.

Since PCNL is an invasive, surgical procedure and is usually performed with regional or general anesthesia, the operating room is preferred over the radiology department. Utilizing an image table and a portable C-arm is an efficient and relatively inexpensive imaging arrangement within the budget of most hospitals (Fig. 2). Such an arrangement is preferred at the MHI and is well suited for all endourologic procedures. In addition, the image table doubles as a satisfactory general operating-room table, while the C-arm can provide imaging for other surgical services (general surgery, orthopedics). Most portable C-arms can be combined with a matrix camera to provide hard copy for documentation purposes.

Renal Access

Satisfactory access to the desired portion of the renal collecting system is a prerequisite for successful endourologic procedures. Percutaneous puncture of the kidney is an invasive procedure and thus not without risks and discomfort for the patient. These risks can be minimized by precise puncture technique, fluoroscopic imaging utilizing a C-arm, and by having available all necessary angiographic wires and catheters required to negotiate the intricacies of the intrarenal collecting system and ureter.

Close communication and cooperation between the radiologist (if involved) and the urologist are essential,

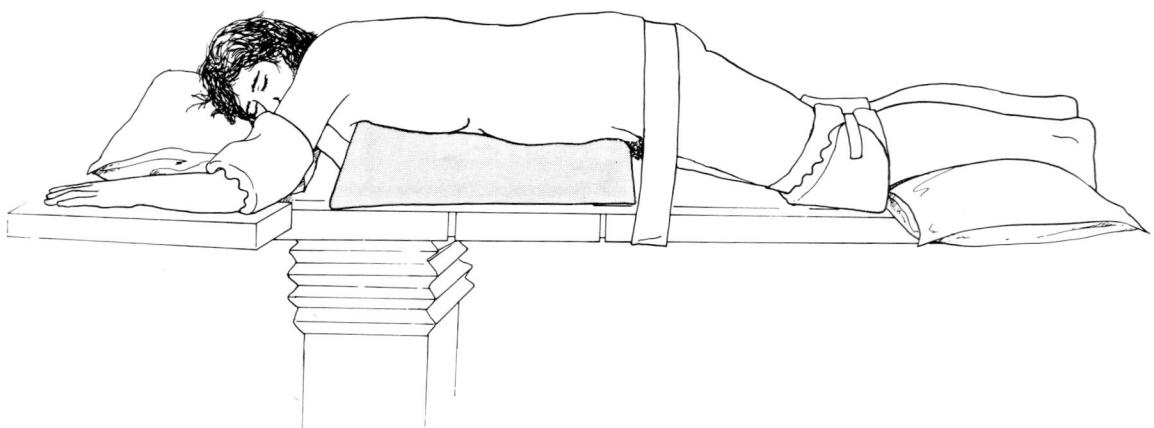

FIG. 1. Patient position for percutaneous procedures. Note that the side to be treated is elevated approximately 30 degrees and that all pressure points are carefully padded. The down arm should be placed at the patient's side and the up arm should be placed in an abducted position. The patient should be placed far enough down on the table so that movement of the C-arm is not impeded by the center post of the table during imaging of the kidney.

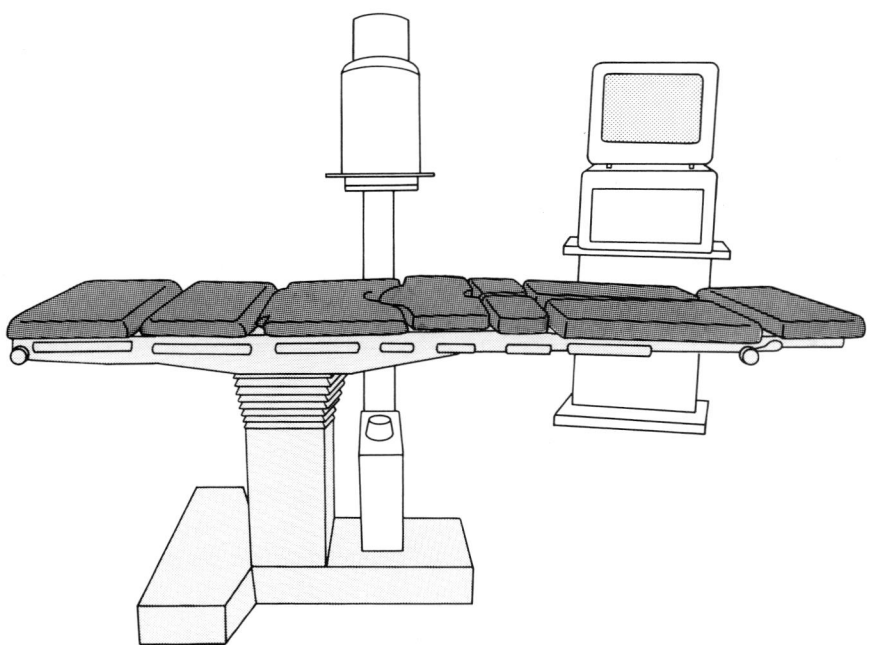

FIG. 2. Portable C-arm and image table in position for percutaneous nephrostolithotomy.

particularly when dealing with specialized access problems such as those encountered with staghorn calculi and calyceal diverticula. Safely achieving a foothold in the renal collecting system is the single most difficult aspect of these procedures. When dealing with staghorn calculi, the collecting system is typically entirely filled with stone material, and caliectasis is usually present. Furthermore, these patients have commonly had previous surgical procedures resulting in perirenal fibrosis, which makes the task of the physician performing access even more difficult.

For the foregoing reasons, it is strongly recommended that the percutaneous procedure be done as a single stage with both the physician performing the access and the urologist utilizing the access working together. This team effort ensures close cooperation and will maximize the chance for a successful outcome. Needle puncture for renal access during PCNL is always performed inside the posterior axillary line, as this approach minimizes the risk of injuring the colon. In general, a lower pole posterior calix is preferred for renal access for the following reasons. First, lower pole access is usually the best location to ensure removal of all stone material from the dependent regions of the kidney. Second, direct puncture into a posterior calix traverses the avascular plane between the anterior and posterior segmental arteries of the kidney, thereby, in theory, reducing chances of damage to the arterial vasculature. Third, the pleural reflection is avoided.

Upper pole access should be considered when treating staghorn calculi with substantial upper pole stone burden or complex lower pole calyceal architecture. Although this approach carries an increased risk of pleural

injury, serious sequela are uncommon (8,9). Renal access through the upper pole more closely parallels the axis of the renal collecting system than does the lower pole approach, because the kidney is oriented in such a way that the upper pole lies closer to the skin than the lower pole (Fig. 3). Also, access to the UPJ and the upper ureter is facilitated by upper pole puncture. Complications of upper pole access are discussed later in this chapter.

Two different renal puncture techniques are possible, utilizing C-arm fluoroscopy. One approach is to adjust the C-arm so that the x-ray beam is parallel to and exactly centered over the needle used for renal puncture. With this technique, the needle appears as a dot directly overlying the calix to be punctured. Thus parallax is eliminated and one may be confident that as the needle is advanced, it will eventually penetrate the desired calix. The C-arm is periodically rotated 90 degrees to allow for the depth of the puncture to be monitored. Although this technique sounds simple, in practice, aligning the C-arm and the puncture needle can be rather tedious. Additionally, the operator's hand lies directly within the x-ray beam.

A second technique, which is essentially a simple triangulation procedure and is preferred at the Methodist Hospital Institute for Kidney Stone Disease, involves the rotation of the C-arm back and forth through 90 degrees as the needle is advanced, placing the x-ray beam alternatively parallel to and perpendicular to the puncture needle. An advantage of this technique is that the C-arm can be positioned by angling the x-ray beam in a direction opposite that of the line of puncture so that the operator's hands need never come close to the x-ray

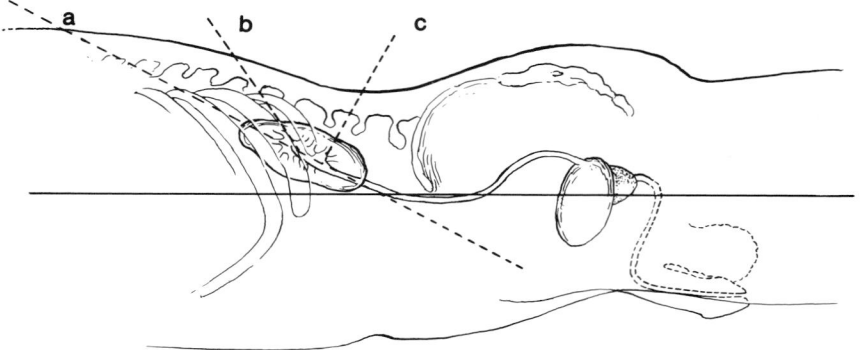

FIG. 3. Angle of entry. Lateral view of abdomen demonstrating (a) renal axis. Because the upper pole of the kidney lies closer to the skin than the lower pole, renal access during PCNL through the upper pole (b) will provide a less acute angle of entry into the collecting system than will access into the lower pole (c).

beam. As the needle is advanced, ventilation of the patient is suspended to minimize renal motion. If supracostal puncture is elected, two caveats should be borne in mind. First, the site of skin puncture should be kept as medial as possible because the lower pole of the kidney tends to be more medial than the lower pole and also to avoid injury to the spleen on the left and to the liver on the right. Second, the needle should always be advanced during expiration to minimize the possibility of pleural injury.

Ideally, following puncture of the desired calix, a J-tipped, Teflon-coated movable core guide wire is negotiated into the renal pelvis and across the UPJ into the distal ureter. However, when dealing with staghorn calculi or calyceal diverticula, it may not be possible to advance the wire out of the calix of puncture. As long as the PCNL is being done as a single-stage procedure, the inability to advance the wire does not present an insurmountable problem. Core is removed from the guide wire and as much wire as possible is coiled into the calix (or diverticulum) of puncture (Fig. 4). The nephrostomy tract is then dilated in the standard fashion, always utilizing a safety wire. When access is achieved in this manner, it is essential that dilating implements and working sheaths not be overadvanced; otherwise, perforation of the medial wall of the calix may occur, resulting in considerable bleeding. As experience and confidence are gained with this approach, considerable time (and radiation exposure to the patient) can be saved by minimizing attempts to negotiate a wire out of an obstructed calix or calyceal diverticulum.

Occasionally, if the tract is extremely long or if fibrosis from previous surgery is present, difficulty may be encountered in passing dilators over the wire into the collecting system. Changing to a stiffer guide wire will often provide sufficient stability for the passage of dilators and balloons. If an extra stiff wire still is inadequate, the 8-Fr. coaxial catheter should be placed down to the point of resistance in the nephrostomy tract and the tract dilated to 14 Fr. with the Amplatz dilators. At this point, if the

dilator is left in place, sufficient stability is provided for the coaxial catheter (or angiographic catheter) to be advanced successfully. If fibrosis from previous surgery is resistant to all attempts at dilation, a small scalpel adapted to a guide wire may be passed to incise the cicatrix (fascial incising needle, Cook Urological).

When dilation of the nephrostomy tract proves impossible or should brisk bleeding occur, the largest possible nephrostomy tube should be placed and the procedure deferred, allowing the nephrostomy tract to mature for a minimum of a week.

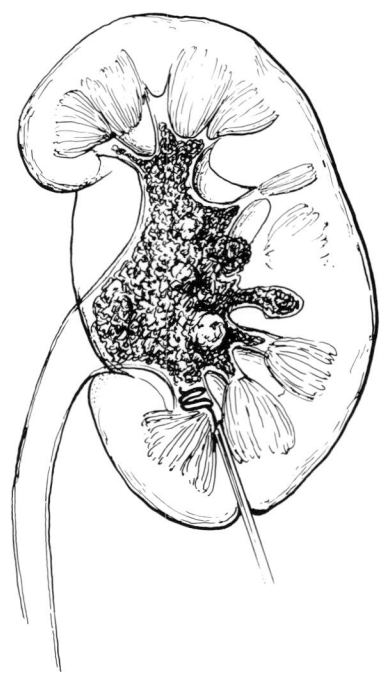

FIG. 4. Staghorn calculus access. Occasionally, a guide wire cannot be negotiated beyond the obstructing infundibular portion of a staghorn calculus. When this situation is encountered, as much wire as possible is coiled into the desired calix, always being sure that the solid core of the wire lies within the collecting system.

Nephroscopy with Closed versus Open Irrigating System

The operating nephroscopes currently available may be utilized with an Amplatz working sheath (open irrigating system) or without such a sheath (closed irrigating system). The advantages and disadvantages of a working sheath are listed in Table 4. A larger nephrostomy tract is required when an Amplatz sheath is used. If an Amplatz sheath is not used, the nephroscope can be passed over a series of telescoping metal dilators which are nondisposable and reusable. However, a closed system is a low-flow, high-pressure system (except during actual lithotripsy, when suction is applied to the ultrasound probe). Absorption of irrigant into the circulation is therefore more likely with a closed system than when using an open system where a flow of irrigant is rapid but intrarenal pressure does not exceed the height of the proximal end of the working sheath above renal collecting system ($\leq$15 cm of water).

The ease and completeness of stone removal are enhanced when vision of the intrarenal collecting system is maximized. Having the capability to switch back and forth from one nephroscope or cystoscope to another facilitates the debulking of large, complicated, and/or multiple calculi. Additionally, the internal diameter of the Amplatz sheath is larger than that of the operating nephroscope, allowing for the grasping or basketing of larger stone fragments.

One drawback to the use of an open sheath is the need to have a system to control the drainage of irrigant. A number of satisfactory draping systems are available. Adherence of the drape is enhanced by spraying the patient's flank with tincture of benzoin.

Several authors have reported the successful extraction of renal calculi with Randall's forceps or Mazzariello-Caprini forceps (modified to allow passage over a guide wire) (10,11). Even when performed under fluoroscopic guidance, this technique is essentially a blind maneuver and as such, preceded the development of current access systems allowing for easy visual inspection of the renal collecting system. The use of such forceps is currently not recommended, as they provide no advantage in the removal of stones that could not be reached and extracted more easily and safely under direct vision using baskets or grasping forceps.

Ultrasonic Lithotripsy

Any stone material larger than 8–9 mm requires fragmentation prior to its removal during PCNL. Ultrasonic lithotripsy through an operating nephroscope (Wolf, Storz, Olympus) (Fig. 5) is preferred in this situation. These instruments allow the stone fragments to be aspirated continuously as they are generated during lithotripsy. High-intensity ultrasound has proven to be an effective mechanism for fragmenting urinary calculi, either percutaneously or transurethrally (12,13). Lithotripsy with ultrasound-based devices relies on the ability of piezoelectric crystals when stimulated by a rapidly alternating electrical current to generate ultrasonic energy at a fixed frequency. The piezoelectric crystal is rigidly coupled to a probe (which may be solid or hollow), causing the probe to oscillate or vibrate thousands of times per second. When the probe is applied directly to calculous material, the resultant mechanical energy causes the probe to act as a mini-jackhammer, fragmenting the stone. Transmission of this mechanical energy requires direct contact between the tip of the probe and the renal calculus. The features of the operating nephroscopes and ultrasonic lithotripsy systems currently available are compared in Table 5.

Efficient ultrasonic lithotripsy requires a proper balance between the inflow of irrigant and the suction applied to the ultrasound probe. Although many manufacturers provide an integrated power and suction foot switch for their ultrasonic instruments, wall suction with intermittent clamping of the suction tubing by an assistant is preferred at the MHI. Generally, suction is applied only when the ultrasonic instrument is on. Suction pressures in the range 60–80 cm of water are sufficient to maintain adequate flow of irrigant during ultrasonic lithotripsy. Suction pressures higher than this will tend to draw air bubbles into the system, impeding vision.

When performing ultrasonic lithotripsy, the stone should first be trapped between the probe and the urothelium. The application of gentle pressure to the stone will enhance fragmentation. The temptation to push too hard should be avoided since calculi can easily be pushed through urothelium, particularly when working in the renal pelvis. When performing ultrasonic lithotripsy of large calculi, especially staghorn calculi, care should be taken to keep the field clear of the innumerable small fragments created by the lithotripsy process, reducing the likelihood that fragments might migrate into inaccessible locations such as peripheral calices or the ureter. The removal of fragments that have migrated into the ureter during ultrasonic lithotripsy can be troublesome

TABLE 4. *Open versus closed systems for percutaneous access*

	Open	Closed
Size of sheath (Fr.)	32–34	24.5–26
Intrarenal pressure of irrigant	Low	High
Potential for irrigant absorption	Low	High
Use of other nephroscopes (i.e., flexible cytoscope)	Easy	Difficult or impossible

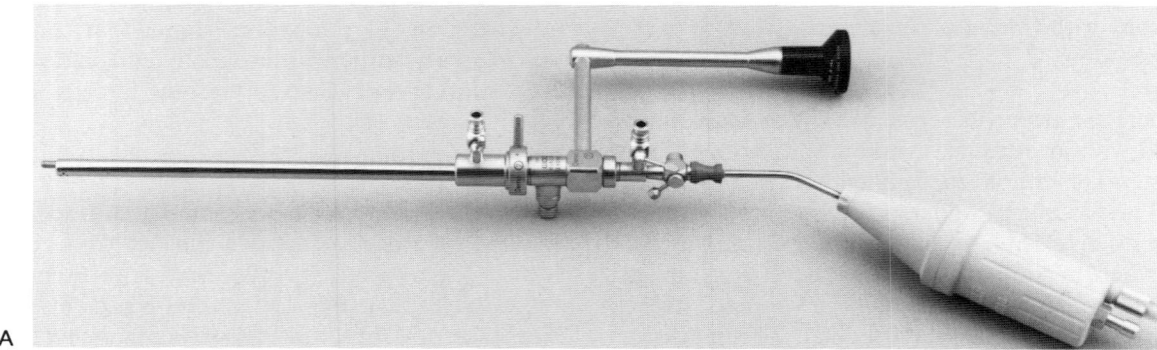

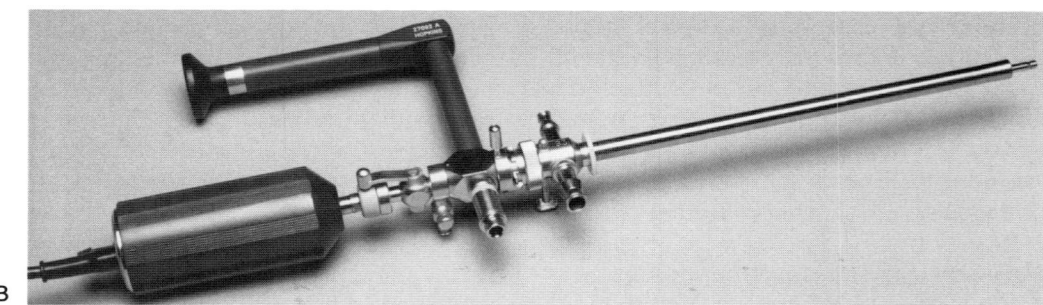

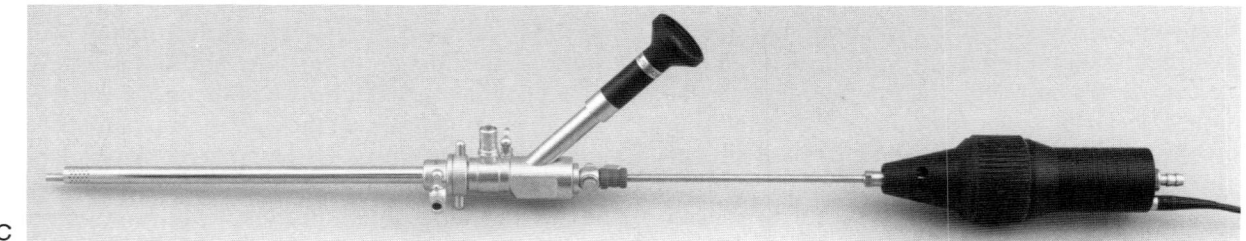

FIG. 5. Operating nephroscopes: (**A**) Wolf; (**B**) Storz; (**C**) Olympus.

and time consuming. This problem is prevented by inflating the previously placed occlusion balloon catheter prior to beginning lithotripsy.

Significant fluid absorption during ultrasonic lithotripsy is unusual with the concomitant use of an Amplatz sheath, because intrarenal pressure from the flow of irrigant is minimized (14). Nonetheless, isotonic irrigation, preferably normal saline, should always be used during ultrasonic lithotripsy. If significant fluid absorption occurs, perforation of the collecting system or extravasation intraabdominally or intrapleurally should be suspected (15). If a lengthy percutaneous procedure is anticipated, the irrigant should be warmed to avoid excessive cooling of the patient.

Electrohydraulic Lithotripsy

Electrohydraulic lithotripsy (EHL) fragments stones with unfocused shock waves generated by an underwater electrical discharge or spark. EHL should be available when performing PCNL, as occasionally stones will be encountered that are difficult to fragment with ultrasound but will yield to EHL. Another advantage of EHL is that the probes are flexible and small, allowing them to be utilized with the flexible nephroscope.

When utilizing EHL, the largest probe that can be accommodated by the nephroscope should be selected.

The lowest power setting sufficient for stone fragmentation should be chosen when performing EHL, for the following reasons. First, because the shock wave produced by EHL is powerful, by using the lowest power setting, trauma to urothelium is minimized, although some mucosal bleeding is common when utilizing EHL. Second, the shock wave is powerful enough to damage the fragile optics of nephroscopes (especially flexible nephroscopes). This risk can also be minimized by keeping the tip of the EHL probe as far away from the telescope as is practical during lithotripsy. Third, the EHL

TABLE 5. *Characteristics of available rigid nephroscopes and ultrasonic lithotrites*

Manufacturer and number	Working length (mm)	Weight (g)	Sheath size (Fr.)	Instrument channel	Optics (angle of view)	Ultrasonic frequency (KHz)	Ultrasonic probe diameter (mm)	Configuration of probe tip
Wolf Sheath 8962.05 Telescope 8962.31	177	232	24.5	12	5-degree rod lens; parallel eyepiece	23–25	2.4 3.5	Smooth Hollow-fixed
Storz Sheath 27093B Telescope 27092 AM	190	259	26	14	0-degree parallel eyepiece	24	3.5 3.5	Oscillating Sawtooth
Olympus Sheath A2465 Telescope A2461	191	277	27	12.6	5-degree angled-offset eyepiece	23	3.4 4.0	Smooth Hollow-fixed

probe is rapidly worn out by the shock waves generated around its tip and its life is prolonged at lower power settings.

Direct contact between the EHL probe and the calculus is neither necessary nor desirable during lithotripsy. It is not the probe but, rather, the shock wave produced that fragments calculi. Multiple probes should be available when performing EHL. The probes must not be overused. Once the insulation has begun to wear away, the probes should be discarded because the shock waves generated are less efficient and pieces of the probe could break off and become lost in the renal collecting system. The smaller-diameter probes (1.9 Fr., 3 Fr., 5 Fr.) are particularly prone to break if overused. Stone fragmentation with EHL (and ultrasound) is enhanced by directing the probe (and shock wave) toward the roughest surface of the calculus. Once the stone has fractured with EHL,

the lithotripsy process often can be more efficiently completed by switching back to ultrasound.

Flexible Nephroscopy

Only the most simple of intrarenal collecting systems can be completely inspected with a rigid nephroscope via a single access site. The complete inspection of the intrarenal collecting system and proximal two-thirds of the ureter requires flexible nephroscopes. The features of flexible nephroscopes currently available are listed in Table 6. The small diameter (16 Fr.) of flexible nephroscopes will allow their passage through most infundibula and the UPJ. The 6-Fr. working port of flexible nephroscopes limits flow of irrigant, particularly when occupied by an instrument (guide wire, catheter, basket, grasping or biopsy forceps). For this reason, irrigant should al-

TABLE 6. *Features of major flexible nephroscopes*

	Olympus CHR-P10	ACMI APN-37	Pentax FCN-15H	Storz Cytoscope/ nephroscope S11275
Field of view (H2O) (deg)	64	60	83	83
Depth of field (mm)	3–50	1–40	3–50	3–50
Focus	Focusable	Focusable	Focusable	Focusable
Distal tip diameter (mm)	4.8	5	4.8	4.8
Working channel (Fr.)	6	5.5	6	6
Deflection (deg)	160/130	180/180	160/130	220/90
Total length (mm)	645	700	640	680
Working length (mm)	330	370	350	400
Angulation lock	Yes	Yes	Yes	No
Immersible	Yes	Yes	Yes	Yes
Outer diameter (Fr.)	14.7	15	14.7	14.4
Irrigation flow control button	No	No	Yes	Yes

ways be pressurized. The results achieved with PCNL of large and/or complex renal calculi will parallel the urologist's skill and persistence in flexible nephroscopy.

Nephrostomy Tubes

A nephrostomy tube is mandatory to tamponade bleeding from renal parenchyma following every primary percutaneous procedures. Clayman has demonstrated experimentally that PCNL without concomitant use of a nephrostomy tube may be associated with sufficient perirenal bleeding to be life threatening (16). Other advantages of the nephrostomy tube are that it provides good drainage following PCNL, minimizing the risk of urosepsis. In addition, if ESWL is anticipated, the tube provides another route for the egress of gravel following lithotripsy. Maintaining access following ESWL allows flexible nephroscopy, which is invaluable in removing residual stone fragments. Contrast material can be instilled through the nephrostomy tube during ESWL to aid in localization of low-density or radiolucent stones, and the tube is also useful for chemolysis. The only disadvantage in utilizing nephrostomy tubes is the possibility of bacteria gaining access to the renal collecting system; however, the risk of bacteriuria is minimized with appropriate antibiotic coverage.

Complications

PCNL, while representing a major advance in urology, is an invasive procedure and, as such, is associated with several recognized complications (Table 7). Given the extremely vascular nature of the organ, bleeding from renal parenchyma occurs to some degree in every PCNL. Bleeding sufficient to require transfusion is the most common major complication of PCNL. Significant blood loss is more likely to occur when treating staghorn calculi as opposed to simple PCNL. Life-threatening renal hemorrhage secondary to traumatic AV fistulas or false aneurysms occurs in about 1 PCNL out of 200 (17). AV fistulas are usually heralded by an abnormal amount of hemorrhage during PCNL and/or intermittent, brisk bleeding through the nephrostomy tube afterward. If an unusual amount of bleeding occurs during or after PCNL, the first maneuver should be to exchange the nephrostomy tube for a Kaye nephrostomy tamponade balloon catheter (Cook Urological). This nephrostomy tube incorporates a low-pressure, 12-mm balloon which may be left inflated for prolonged periods of time to tamponade bleeding from the nephrostomy tract. Bleeding from the nephrostomy tract following PCNL can be a frightening experience, and it is recommended that anyone performing PCNL have a Kaye nephrostomy tube

TABLE 7. *Complications of percutaneous nephrostolithotomy*

	Incidence (Ref)
Hemorrhage	
Requiring transfusion	5% to 12% (35,85)
Arteriovenous fistula or false aneurysm	0.6% (17)
Perforation/extravasation	5.4% to 26% (49,85)
Damage to contiguous organs	
Colon perforation	1% (8,21,22,86)
Pneumo/hydrothorax	
Liver	
Spleen	
Duodenum	
Ureteral obstruction (temporary)	
Ureteral or UPJ stricture	1.7% to 4.9% (21,85)
Water intoxication	0.9% (35,86)
Infection	
Fever	10.9% (35)
Urosepsis	3% (85)

available should the need arise. Once the Kaye nephrostomy tube has been placed, then immediate angiography should be performed to identify possible AV fistulas or false aneurysms. Angiography is both diagnostic and therapeutic as AV fistula and false aneurysms are best managed by embolization (Fig. 6). In the rare event that bleeding cannot be controlled with angiography, partial nephrectomy is usually necessary.

As with traditional open surgical procedures, the possibility of damage to contiguous organs also exists. Injuries to the pleura, liver, spleen, duodenum, and colon have been described (18–22). The absorption of irrigant via the retroperitoneum, celomic, or pleural cavities may be life threatening (15). Pneumothorax is a possibility whenever puncture above the twelfth rib is performed (8). The use of a working sheath will tend to minimize extravasation into the pleural cavity during PCNL as intrarenal pressure is low. Whenever supracostal puncture is performed, a radiograph of the chest should be obtained immediately following the procedure. Should problems occur intraoperatively, the C-arm can be utilized to examine for pneumothorax or hydrothorax. If greater than 10% pneumothorax or hydrothorax occurs, aspiration generally is sufficient, as lung injury is extremely rare (assuming that the puncture has been performed during expiration). Should the pneumothorax recur, a chest tube must be placed. Any time that significant hyponatremia occurs in association with PCNL, loss of irrigant intraabdominally or intrapleurally should be suspected as fluid absorption is rare with an open sheath (low-pressure) irrigating arrangement.

Temperature elevation greater than 38°C is common for 24–48 h following PCNL of struvite calculi. Because the interstices of a calculus provide a privileged sanc-

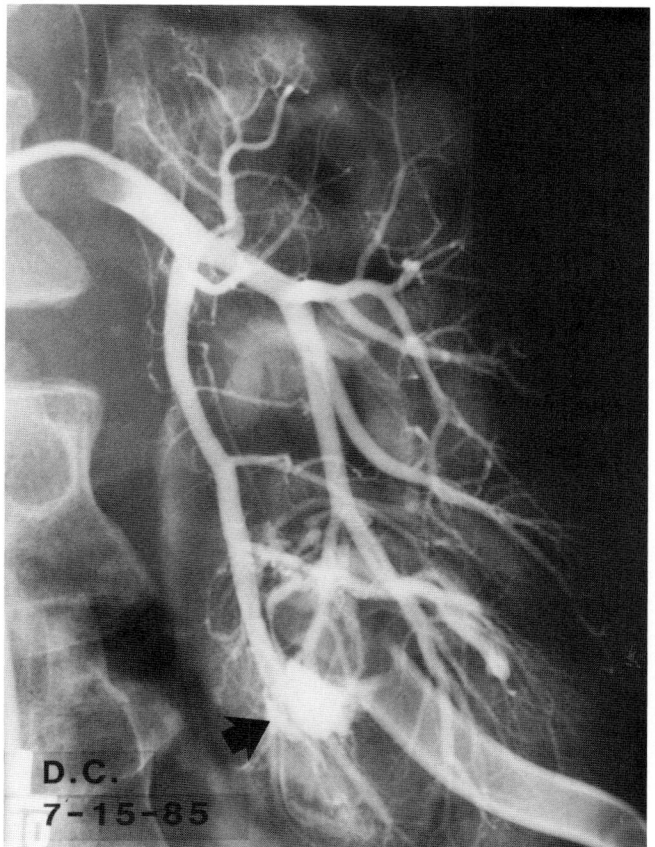
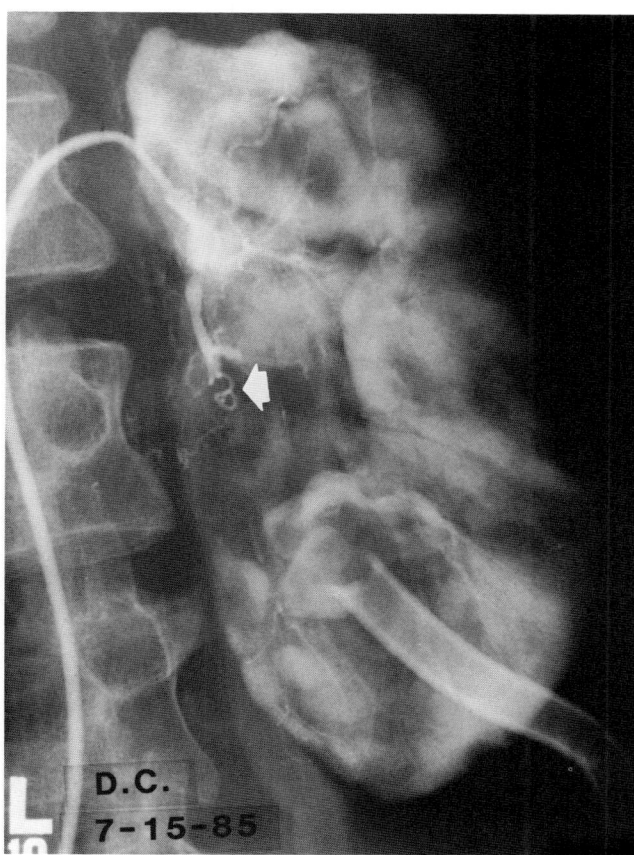

FIG. 6. A: Renal arteriogram demonstrating an arteriovenous fistula (*arrow*) in the lower pole following PCNL. **B:** Same patient following embolization with a coil (*arrow*) of the segmental renal artery feeding the arteriovenous fistula.

tuary for bacteria, urosepsis will rarely occur despite all precautions. Intravenous antibiotic coverage for 24 h prior to PCNL is appropriate to minimize the risk of this potentially devastating complication. Although sepsis is a recognized complication with any approach for the treatment of staghorn calculi, one advantage of PCNL is that it does assure adequate drainage following the procedure.

In summary, PCNL is an elaborate, highly technical procedure requiring advanced angiographic and endoscopic skills. In the era of ESWL, most PCNL procedures will be complex. Therefore, a definite learning curve is to be anticipated for PCNL procedures, even for urologists possessing basic endourologic skills. A considerable investment of time and patience is required if the best results are to be achieved.

URETEROSCOPY

Dilation of the lower ureter for manipulation of calculi as first reported by Young in 1902 has long been a valuable tool to the urologist (23). Ureteral dilatation

with multiple catheters and ureteral balloons was described in detail by Dourmashkin in 1945 with an overall success rate of 81.5% in the treatment of ureteral calculi (24). The use of a pediatric cystoscope for examination of the pelvic ureter in a female as described by Lyon et al. in 1978 began the era of ureteroscopy (25). The development of a long ureteroscope was reported by Perez-Castro and Martinez-Pineiro in 1980, markedly changing the management of ureteral disease, extending transurethral procedures to the renal pelvis (26–28).

The rigid ureteroscope is actually nothing more than a long-narrow cystoscope, and, as such, it is an instrument that requires very little orientation for the experienced endoscopist. However, vision with this instrument is considerably more limited than the cystoscope, and the instrument's small diameter makes it exceedingly fragile. In addition, the ureter is a thin-walled, easily traumatized organ and therefore must be treated with the utmost delicacy. The two cardinal rules of ureteroscopy are patience and avoidance of excessive force. Typically, lack of the former leads to excessive application of the latter and results in trauma to and/or perforation of the ureter.

Anatomic Considerations in Ureteroscopy

The ureter is a retroperitoneal organ varying from 20 to 26 cm in length and is anything but straight, a fact that must constantly be borne in mind by the ureteroscopist. If the course of the ureter is considered in a retrograde fashion, it can be seen to extend from the bladder laterally and posteriorly within the true pelvis. The pelvic portion of the ureter is usually mobile and easily straightened and is capacious enough to accept most ureteroscopes unless there has been previous pelvic surgery or radiation.

As the iliac vessels are approached, the ureter begins to course anteriorly up and out of the true pelvis. The ureter is typically slightly narrowed as it crosses the iliac vessels. These anatomic considerations make this portion of the ureter the most challenging area to negotiate during rigid ureteroscopy. The lumbar ureter typically courses more medially and is the straightest portion of the ureter unless distal obstruction has caused it to be elongated and tortuous. Because the kidney lies cephalad and posterior to the psoas musculature, the course of the ureter at the UPJ is usually slightly posterior. The UPJ nearly always will be of sufficient size to accept the rigid ureteroscope, although renal ptosis may cause considerable angulation at this point.

The ureter is a fragile structure composed of an inner mucosal layer, a thin layer of muscle, and an outer loosely applied fibrous layer (the tunica adventitia). Nerve fibers, lymphatics, and blood vessels course through the tunica adventitia. The marked mobility of the ureter within its tunica adventitia allows it to be converted from its normal serpentine course into a completely straight structure by the ureteroscope. This remarkable mobility and elasticity of the ureter can be affected by surgery, tumors, or radiation, and such factors should be kept in mind when attempting rigid ureteroscopy.

The intramural portion of the ureter deserves special mention as this is the most narrow portion of the ureter (2 mm). The muscularis of the ureter is somewhat attenuated in this most distal aspect of the ureter. However, distention of the ureter at this level rather than being facilitated is greatly restricted by the strength of the detrusor musculature surrounding the intramural ureter, especially in the male patient. Distortion of the intramural ureter and ureteral meatus is commonly encountered due to prostatic enlargement and less commonly to tumors or previous ureteral, bladder, or prostatic surgery.

Indications for Ureteroscopy

The primary advantage of the ureteroscope is that it allows diagnosis and therapeutic maneuvers under direct vision. The potential applications of this technology are

TABLE 8. *Indications for ureteroscopy*

Diagnostic
Radiolucent filling defects
  Tumors
  Radiolucent calculi
  Blood clots
  Sloughed papillae

Obstruction
  Tumors
  Calculi
  Strictures

Unilateral hematuria
  Tumors
  Papillitis
  Arteriovenous malformations

Positive cytology, negative cystoscopy

Therapeutic
Tumor
  Biopsy
  Fulguration and/or resection
  Surveillance

Calculi
  Basketing
  Lithotripsy
    Ultrasonic
    Electrohydraulic
    Laser
  Retrograde displacement (pre-ESWL)

Strictures
  Guide wire/stent placement
  Balloon dilatation
  Direct vision ureterotomy
  Endopyelotomy

Fistula
  Guide wire/stent placement

Foreign body extraction (usually proximally migrated ureteral stents)

listed in Table 8. The vast majority of ureteroscopic procedures are performed for the management of ureteral calculi. However, the ureteroscope may also be an extremely valuable instrument in the detection, biopsy, resection, and follow up of low-grade urothelial neoplasms of the ureter. This process is similar to the endoscopic management of lesions in the bladder. Higher grade/stage ureteral neoplasms are not suitable for primary treatment with the ureteroscope. The adage that a picture is worth a thousand words is certainly applicable to ureteroscopy for the diagnosis of unilateral hemorrhagic lesions of the upper urinary tract.

Imaging and Patient Positioning

The capability of performing fluoroscopic monitoring of ureteroscopy is essential for the safety of the procedure and for achieving the most satisfactory result. Any standard cystoscopic table adapted for fluoroscopy is suitable, although at the MHI the combination of an image table and a portable C-arm as described above is preferred. The portable C-arm may also be utilized with many stationary cystoscopic tables with the buckey pushed out of the way. The advantages of the portable C-arm for ureteroscopic procedures are: It is already available in many operating rooms; current units provide excellent image quality; the x-ray source is below the patient, minimizing radiation scatter to the urologist and other operating room personnel; and current technology allows for hard copy of the fluoroscopic image to be generated for documentation purposes.

The standard lithotomy position is preferred for ureteroscopic procedures. It is often helpful to abduct the contralateral hip as far as it will comfortably allow, enabling the ureteroscopist to align the ureteroscope parallel to the initial pelvic course of the ureter, which aids in the passage of the instrument. If hip abduction is limited and more room is required, it is sometimes possible to flex the hip, raising the leg into an extremely cephalad location, which permits the endoscopist to be positioned underneath the leg.

Examination of the lumbar and UPJ region of the ureter is sometimes facilitated by placing the patient in a steep Trendelenburg position, as this position causes the kidney to migrate in a cephalad direction, straightening the proximal ureter.

Guide Wires

All transurethral procedures should begin with the placement of a safety guide wire into the kidney. Guide wires come with straight or curved tips. Teflon-coated wires facilitate the passage of catheters, stents, and dilators. A guide wire that has a removable central core should be used, allowing the length of the floppy tip to be varied according to the urologist's preference.

The presence of a safety guide wire should be maintained during any manipulation of the ureter (i.e., ureteroscopy, basketry, or grasping forceps). If the urologist prefers to pass the ureteroscope over a wire, a second working wire should be utilized so that the safety wire need not be removed. Should trauma to the ureter occur, drainage can always be established with the safety wire. The presence of the wire has not been found to be a deterrent to the passage of the ureteroscope or to the management of ureteral calculi (i.e., lithotripsy, basketry, etc.).

Ureteral Dilation

Some dilation of the intramural ureter is usually required before a ureteroscope can be passed. Currently, rigid ureteroscopes as small as 7.2 Fr. are available. If it

seems likely that the ureter will accept an instrument of this size, a gentle attempt at passage is often warranted prior to dilation. When performing ureteroscopy on pregnant women, it is unusual for the ureter to require dilation. Ureteral dilation may be accomplished acutely with dilators, bougies, or balloons, or gradually, by leaving an indwelling ureteral stent for 7–10 days. The gradual approach, although requiring two stages, is safer and should always be considered when there are problems dilating the ureter or passing the ureteroscope.

All implements for dilating the ureter should be passed over a guide wire to minimize the chance of perforating the ureter. Usually, dilation of the intramural ureter is all that is required; more proximal dilation is not necessary unless the ureteroscope cannot be passed. When dilating the ureter prior to removal of a stone in the lower ureter, the dilating instrument should be passed to just below the stone and not up next to it, to minimize the chance of ureteral perforation or pushing the stone through the wall of the ureter. Although the incidence of ureteral stricture in humans following dilation and ureteroscopy appears to be low, routine stenting following manipulation of the ureter seems prudent.

Instrumentation

The first rigid ureteroscopes were essentially long pediatric cystoscopes. A 5-Fr. port was available for the passage of flexible instruments. Prior to the development of offset lenses, the telescopic viewing system had to be removed to allow passage of the rigid ultrasound probe when fragmenting ureteral calculi, thus making it a blind procedure. The development of an offset lens system with or without interchangeable sheaths has greatly facilitated ureteroscopic stone procedures, allowing for ultrasonic lithotripsy to be performed under direct vision (Fig. 7).

Flexible ureteroscopes are currently evolving at a rapid rate and are of two basic types: those with passive deflection systems and those with active ones, with the latter being substantially larger in diameter. Vision is considerably more limited with flexible devices and working ports are smaller, limiting instrumentation and irrigation. The advantages of flexible ureteroscopes are their ability to allow for inspection of the ureter (in the small percentage of cases where a rigid instrument cannot be passed) and of the entirety of the intrarenal collecting system. However, the expense of these instruments and their extreme fragility currently limit their practicality for most endoscopists.

Urologists performing ureteroscopy should avail themselves of two basic types of rigid ureteroscopes. In general, the smaller the instrument, the less likely that additional ureteral dilatation will be required and the greater the ease of passage of the instrument. Therefore,

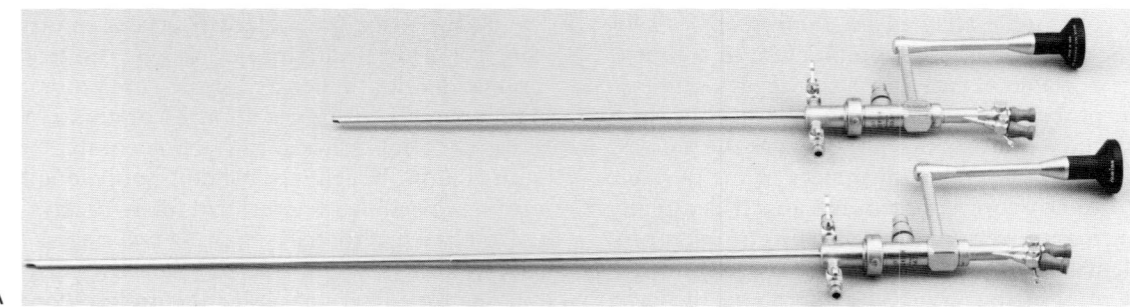

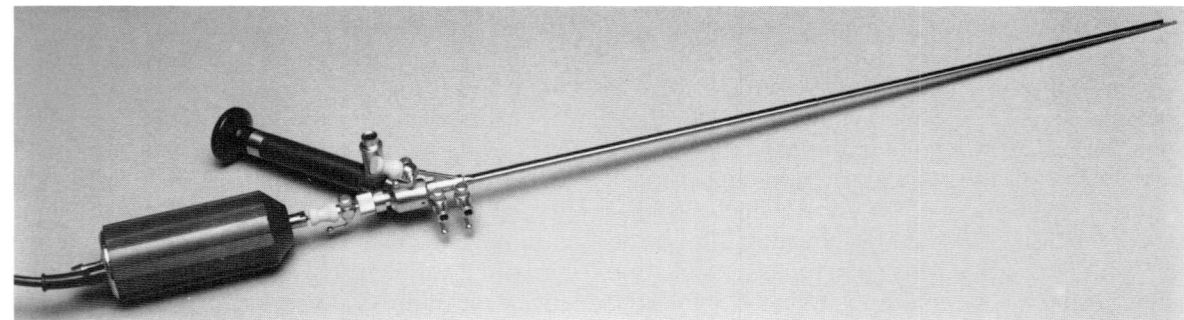

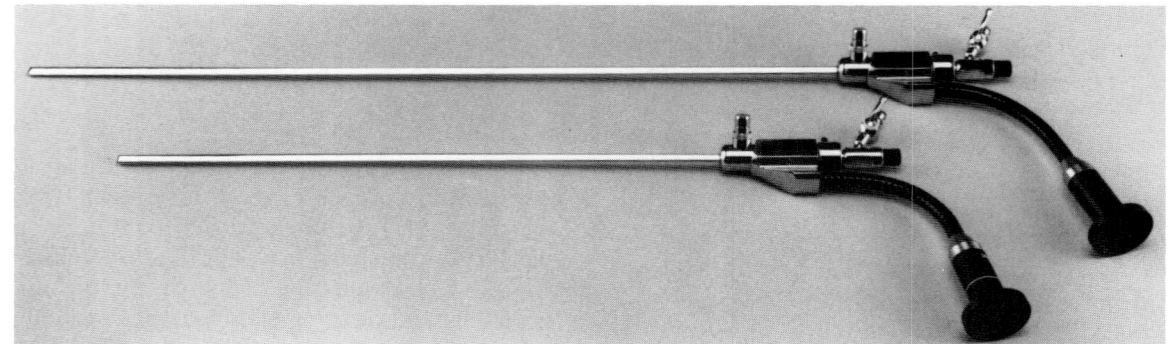

FIG. 7. Ureteroscopes: (**A**) Wolf; (**B**) Storz; (**C**) ACMI.

a small-diameter (7.2 to 9.5 Fr.), direct-vision uretero-scope should be utilized whenever possible. When ultra-sonic lithotripsy is required, an instrument with an offset lens and larger diameter (11 to 12.5 Fr.) (with or without an interchangeable sheath system) is utilized. A variety of baskets and grasping and biopsy forceps are available for use through the rigid ureteroscopes.

Passing the Ureteroscope

The ureteroscope is best passed through the urethra into the bladder under direct vision; otherwise, the small diameter of the instrument may allow it to create a false passage. Ureteroscopy is always initiated with a 0-degree to 5-degree lens. The small field of view can sometimes make location of the ureteral orifice surprisingly difficult (and irritating!). This problem can be avoided by placing the ureteroscope at the bladder neck in the midline and

gradually rotating the instrument laterally toward the desired ureter, searching for the guide wire. Once lo-cated, the guide wire can easily be followed up to the ureteral orifice.

If a ureteroscope is being used with a sharply angu-lated beak, its passage into the ureteral orifice and intra-mural ureter is occasionally facilitated by rotating the instrument 180 degrees and entering the ureter in an upside-down fashion. Once the instrument is in the intra-mural ureter, it may be rotated back to its normal posi-tion. This maneuver minimizes the chance that the lead edge of the instrument may become caught on the ure-teral meatus. With the more snub-nosed instruments, this maneuver is usually not required and it is merely necessary to "dip" the tip of the instrument down as the meatus is entered.

The intramural portion of the ureter is typically trau-matized and hemorrhagic following acute dilation, so vision in this area may be difficult. This is, however, the portion of the ureter, which is the most easily perforated. The instrument should be advanced only when lumen is visible; however, a narrowing of the lumen and/or "gripping" of the instrument by the intramural ureter is occasionally encountered. To ensure safe passage of the instrument through this area, several techniques may be considered. A second wire may be passed up into the renal pelvis and the ureteroscope passed over this wire, guiding the tip of the instrument in the proper direction. Monitoring the direction of passage of the instrument with the fluoroscope is also useful in this circumstance. The use of a 10-cm³ syringe on the bridge of the ureteroscope to augment the flow of irrigant also is useful in clearing away blood and debris as well as distending the lumen in front of the instrument. If considerable resistance to the passage of the instrument is encountered or if the lumen cannot be discerned with sufficient confidence to allow advancement, further dilation of the intramural ureter is required. It is foolhardy to attempt to force the ureteroscope through a lumen that is too small to accept it, as perforation will inevitably occur.

Typically, once the intramural ureter has been traversed, the lumen will open up into the more capacious pelvic ureter. The ureteroscope passes easily through the pelvic ureter unless there has been previous surgery or unless reaction is present due to the presence of a ureteral calculus.

Once the back wall of the true pelvis is reached, the ureter begins to angulate sharply anteriorly. At this point, the urologist should brace the ureteroscope at the urethral meatus while depressing the eyepiece in a posterior direction and attempting to follow the upward course of the ureter (Fig. 8). This maneuver is necessary to minimize bowing of the instrument, which not only reduces the field of vision but subjects the instrument to risk of breakage. The passage of the instrument anteriorly out of the pelvis and over the iliac vessels is the most difficult part of the ureteroscopic procedure and limits the effectiveness of the rigid instrument in the proximal ureter.

During the passage of the ureteroscope over the iliac vessels, the ureteral lumen often is not visible to the endoscopist. However, as long as ureteral mucosa appears to be slipping beneath the beak of the instrument, it is appropriate to continue with gentle and slow passage of the instrument. During this process, the portion of the ureter through which the ureteroscope has already passed often stretches out, whereas the ureter immediately proximal to the instrument tends to telescope. This situation can impede passage of the instrument and may be a prelude to perforation of the ureter. The problem can often be minimized by periodically backing up the ureteroscope to straighten out the proximal portion of the ureter. Frequently, by pausing for a minute or so, any

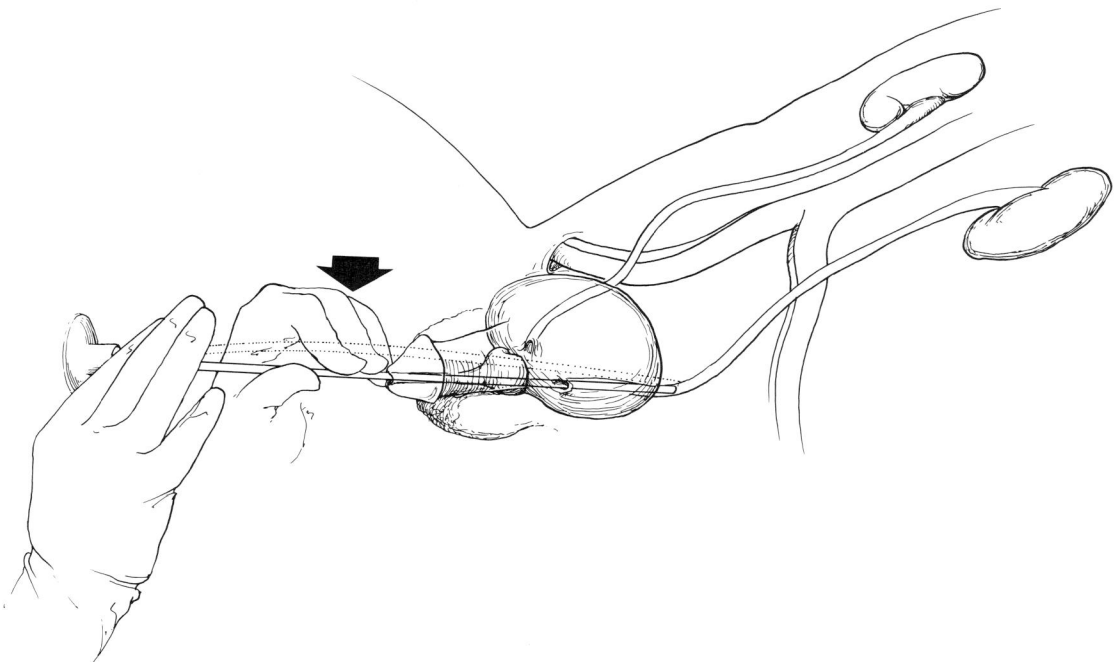

FIG. 8. Supporting the ureteroscope. The middle portion of the ureter lies anterior to the distal ureter. Movement of the instrument in an anterior direction requires downward pressure on the eyepiece of the ureteroscope, often causing it to bow. This can result in loss of visual field and may contribute to damage to the ureteroscope. To prevent this problem, downward pressure should be applied with the urologist's left hand (*arrow*) as close as possible to the urethral meatus.

spasm created by pressure on the ureter from the beak of the ureteroscope will resolve and the instrument can then be advanced more safely. Extreme caution should be exercised when there has been extensive previous surgery in the pelvis (AP resection, radical hysterectomy, etc.), as the ureter may be fixed and easily traumatized by a rigid instrument in this circumstance.

Once the instrument has been passed over the iliac vessels and the lumbar portion of the ureter is reached, the instrument is usually more easily passed. As the instrument passes proximal to the iliac vessels, it is important for the urologist to recall that the lumbar ureter courses more medially so that proper orientation of the ureteroscope can be maintained. Usually, the lumbar ureter is relatively straight and easily traversed with the ureteroscope. However, if the ureter is obstructed, it may become tortuous. Such doubling back of the ureter will give the appearance of folds as the ureteroscope is being advanced. Such a tortuous ureter can often be difficult to traverse without straightening. Passing a guide wire prior to instrumentation helps to straighten the ureter. If tortuosity is still a problem, passage of another wire through the ureteroscope into the renal pelvis may be helpful. Occasionally, passage of a 5-Fr. ureteral catheter through the ureteroscope to allow for decompression of the proximal ureter and renal pelvis will also reduce tortuosity. In a situation where all maneuvers fail, placing a ureteral stent and leaving it for a few days will usually decompress the kidney and thus reduce ureteral length and tortuosity.

Passage of the ureteroscope through the UPJ often requires movement of the tip of the instrument in a posterior direction due to the more posterior location of the kidney and renal pelvis. Usually, however, mobility of the instrument is severely restricted at this point. Often, gentle pressure at the UPJ while waiting for a short period of time will allow the renal pelvis to accommodate itself by peristalsis over the tip of the instrument, and thus just by being patient, the endoscopist will often be able to enter the renal pelvis. Once again, if difficulty is encountered traversing this area, the passage of a catheter or wire through the ureteroscope into the renal pelvis may be useful.

Once the renal pelvis has been entered, passage of the instrument directly into an upper pole calix is usually a comparatively simple maneuver. If a larger instrument with an interchangeable sheath system has been passed, a 70-degree lens may be substituted at this point to allow for inspection of the entire renal pelvis and mid pole calices. Visualization of the lower pole collecting system is usually incomplete with the rigid ureteroscope.

Passage of the ureteroscope is not a procedure for the impatient. Maximizing results and minimizing trauma to the ureter mandate that adequate time be allowed for the performance of the procedure. If the "comfort level" of the urologist is exceeded at any time during the procedure, it is best to terminate the procedure, to place a double-J stent and to bring the patient back at a later time, after allowing the ureter to dilate and/or straighten.

Choice of Irrigant

Significant absorption of fluid may occur during ureteroscopic procedures. Absorption is of particular concern if perforation of the ureter has occurred. Therefore, isotonic fluids (normal saline, 1.5% glycine, 3% sorbitol) should be used at all times. The flow of irrigant through the tiny channels of the ureteroscope is often limited, especially when instruments are being used through the working port. This problem sometimes requires that the pressure of the irrigant be raised to 60 cm or even 90 cm of water. Routinely, however, this additional pressure is not necessary and in a situation where the flow of irrigant is inadequate, it is probably safer to use the previously described syringe method and leave the bags of irrigant at a lower level (i.e., 30 cm).

Techniques for Stone Removal

When approaching a calculus ureteroscopically, some care must be taken to prevent proximal stone migration if access to ESWL is not readily available. Typically, proximal stone migration is more likely to occur if the ureter above the stone is grossly dilated or if the stone is at or above the level of other iliac vessels. It is unusual for stones in the pelvic ureter to migrate out of reach during passage of the ureteroscope. When attempting to remove a stone ureteroscopically, irrigation should be minimized as the stone is approached. Sometimes the reverse Trendelenburg position may be helpful in minimizing the risk of proximal migration, as this position will compensate for the more posterior location of the upper ureter and kidney relative to the mid-ureter. If contrast studies suggest a nonimpacted stone or a very dilated ureter proximal to the stone, a 3 Fr. balloon catheter may be passed beyond the calculus and then inflated to prevent the stone from moving.

Once the stone has been visualized, an attempt should be made to engage it in a basket as soon as possible. If the diameter of the stone is not greater than that of the ureter, it is preferable to remove the stone under direct vision with the basket. The ureter is observed carefully as the ureteroscope is withdrawn to ensure that binding of the stone does not occur. If movement of the stone relative to the ureter ceases (typically, at the iliac vessels or ureterovesical junction), excessive traction should not be applied, as there is a significant chance of ureteral disruption. In this circumstance the stone is carried back proximally and placed in a portion of the ureter where it can be easily viewed, and then it is fragmented with ultrasound, electrohydraulic, or laser lithotripsy. One significant advantage of the ureteroscope over blind basketry is the opportunity to minimize trauma to the ureter by having visual control of the basket, the ureter, and the stone at all times.

Occasionally, a situation is encountered where the stone is impacted and difficulty is encountered in passing a basket beyond the stone. In this circumstance the stone should be fragmented with lithotripsy and, as soon as a lumen is identified, a basket should be passed. Another option is to negotiate a wire beyond the stone under direct vision (which is almost always possible). A 4.5-Fr. Cook stone basket sheath can then be passed over the wire and the wire exchanged for a stone basket.

At the Methodist Hospital Institute for Kidney Stone Disease, several methods of fragmentation are available and a stone has yet to be encountered that could not be fragmented utilizing one of the following techniques. Our general preference is to use a pulsed-dye laser (Candela Corporation) which allows the use of a small ureteroscope. The Candela laser utilizes a coumarin dye circulated through the laser head. As the coumarin green dye is exposed to the flashlamp in the laser head, pulses of green light 1 μs in duration with a wavelength of 504 nm are emitted. The laser energy is delivered through a quartz fiber 250–320 μm in diameter. The combination of a short pulse duration and the small diameter of the fiber produces high power density at the fiber tip, resulting in the generation of tiny shock waves but with minimal heat production. Pulse energies of 30–80 mJ appear to be sufficient to fragment most calculi, but even when the fiber touches the ureteral wall, no visible epithelial injury occurs, because the wavelength of the laser chosen (504 nm) provides maximum absorption of the light energy by the stone but minimum absorption by hemoglobin and tissue. As the pulses are emitted from the fiber tip, the light is efficiently absorbed by the stone surface, resulting in plasma formation and subsequently an acoustic shock wave. The shock wave then fragments the stone in a mechanism identical to that utilized with electrohydraulic lithotripsy and ESWL. The utility of the laser is limited by its extremely high purchase price ($250,000).

If a laser is not available, a 1.9 Fr. or 3-Fr. electrohydraulic probe is another device that can be utilized through the smaller instruments. If ultrasonic lithotripsy is elected, with the current availability of an offset lens system, fragmentation should be done under direct vision at all times. Removing the telescope and blindly attempting to fragment a calculus with the ultrasonic probe is not advisable, as blind fragmentation is associated with a significantly higher risk of ureteral perforation. One of the advantages of ultrasonic lithotripsy is that fragments are aspirated through the probe while they are being created, whereas with electrohydraulic or laser lithotripsy, extraction of fragments is often necessary. A solid wire ultrasonic device is manufactured by

Storz (TUUL). This instrument is significantly more powerful than the hollow ultrasound probes and is capable of fragmenting a calculus with either side-to-side or to-and-fro vibration of the wire. A continuous flow irrigation system does not exist with this device, but the sheath required for using this instrument is slightly smaller (10.5 Fr.) than that required for hollow ultrasound probes. These procedures are tedious and time consuming, and the urologist should never risk ureteral avulsion by giving too strong a tug on a large fragment in the hope that it might pop through a narrowed segment of the ureter. Small fragments (<2 mm) will pass without difficulty following lithotripsy and need not be completely eliminated at the time of the ureteroscopic procedure, especially since they can be difficult to basket. Compulsion in their complete removal is required only if there has been significant perforation of the ureter and there is concern about losing them into the periureteral space.

Following ureteroscopic stone removal, a ureterogram should be performed by injecting contrast material through the ureteroscope to check for possible perforations of the ureter. This ureterogram is necessary to determine the length of postoperative ureteral stenting. In most instances following removal of ureteroscope, a double-J ureteral stent is placed. Stenting allows the performance of ureteroscopic procedures on an outpatient basis or with an extremely short hospitalization. Another alternative is to utilize an open-ended ureteral catheter for 24–48 h. However, this approach causes significant discomfort because of the required indwelling Foley catheter and does not obviate ureteral colic following catheter removal in approximately 10% of patients.

Ureteral Stents

Ureteral stenting has become a common adjunct to endourologic procedures. The indications for the use of ureteral stents are listed in Table 9. The placement of ureteral stents should always be preceded by the passage of a guide wire and by the confirmation fluoroscopically

TABLE 9. *Indications for internal (double-J) ureteral stents*

Following acute ureteral dilation/ureteroscopy

Ureteral perforation

Ureteral fistula

Ureteral dilation
 In conjunction with ESWL of renal calculi > 2 cm
  in diameter
 To facilitate ureterorenoscopy
 For the treatment of ureteral strictures

Relief of obstruction

Following ureteral surgery (i.e., pyeloplasty,
 ureteroneocystostomy)

To hold calculi in the kidney following retrograde ureteral
 stone displacement in anticipation of ESWL

of its satisfactory position within the renal pelvis and/or upper pole calix. Accurate stent placement is aided by opacification of the collecting system. The length of the ureter is then measured from the radiograph or with a ureteral catheter. It is important that the stent not be too long, as extra length may increase vesical irritability. Removal of a double-J stent is facilitated by attaching a suture to it prior to placement.

Management of Complications

The most common complication of ureteroscopy is ureteral perforation. Perforation with guide wires or catheter is common and usually heals within 48 hours. Perforation with the ureteroscope, stone baskets, or dilating implements are more serious but usually will heal if adequate drainage is provided by a ureteral stent. When a significant perforation of the ureter has occurred, demonstration of integrity of the ureter with a contrast study should be performed prior to removal of the stent.

Ureteral strictures appear to be uncommon following ureteral manipulation, although long-term follow up has yet to be reported extensively. One important predisposing factor to stricture formation at the ureterovesical junction is concomitant percutaneous drainage. If the ureter has been traumatized and/or dilated acutely, it may rapidly stricture closed if no urine is passing through it. Therefore, the use of a ureteral stent is mandatory in these situations.

Endourologic procedures by their nature are clean rather than sterile procedures, and appropriate preoperative antibiotic coverage should be utilized. The urine should be sterile at the time of ureteroscopy. If pyonephrosis is encountered, drainage should be established and ureteroscopy should be delayed until the infection has resolved; otherwise, urosepsis may be precipitated.

Vesicoureteral reflux is an uncommon sequela of ureteral dilation and has never been of long-term significance at the MHI.

Whenever ureteral perforation has occurred, the possibility of fluid extravasation/absorption should be considered. The patient's abdomen should be carefully inspected periodically during the procedure. If significant perforation has occurred, a stent should be placed, the procedure abandoned, and the ureter allowed to heal before proceeding further. If fluid absorption is suspected, the administration of diuretics is usually appropriate. Adverse sequela are unlikely if isotonic irrigant has been utilized. In the absence of ureteral perforation, clinically significant fluid absorption is exceedingly rare.

EXTRACORPOREAL SHOCK WAVE LITHOTRIPSY

Extracorporeal shock wave lithotripsy (ESWL) is currently the preferred mode of therapy for the majority of symptomatic upper urinary tract calculi. The rapid acceptance and distribution of this treatment modality reflects the remarkable design achievement of Dornier Medical Systems and the department of urology at the University of Munich, resulting in the HM3 lithotripter. The Dornier HM3 lithotripter is fast, reliable, and easy to use, and it achieves stone fragmentation in a high percentage of cases. Because of the success of the Dornier device and the large potential market for lithotripsy, numerous other design concepts have been and are being developed by manufacturers around the world. ESWL is therefore a technology that is still in rapid evolution.

Shock waves capable of fragmenting calculi may be produced by underwater electrical discharges, piezoceramic crystals, electromagnetic induction, and even microexplosions. Immersion in a water bath, while the theoretic ideal for shock wave coupling, is not essential for stone fragmentation, and many lithotripters currently utilize water bags for shock wave coupling. Ultrasound for stone localization has been incorporated into a number of lithotripters in lieu of x-rays. All of the aforementioned variables have some impact on the ease of stone fragmentation, stone visualization, and the cost of lithotripsy. It is not the purpose of this chapter to review in detail the technical features of currently available lithotripter. However, there are a number of treatment principles common to lithotripsy that will be of use to urologists no matter which lithotripter is being utilized.

Theoretical Aspects of ESWL

A shock wave is a pressure wave characterized by a rapid rise in pressure and a gradual decay (Fig. 9). Although both shock waves and ultrasound waves are subject to the physical laws of acoustics, they differ fundamentally in that ultrasound represents a sinusoidal pressure wave with a positive and negative component that is typically created at a fixed frequency, whereas shock waves are a positive pressure wave associated with a small negative pressure or reflective (tensile) component. Additionally, shock waves, when generated, span a spectrum of frequencies. It is believed that the lower-frequency pressure waves created by an underwater spark discharge (as with the Dornier devices) pass from water into and through body tissue with less attenuation than the higher-frequency pressure waves associated with ultrasound, allowing sufficient pressure to be delivered to a calculus to achieve stone fragmentation. The most common system for the generation of shock waves for lithotripsy involves the discharge of an electrical spark underwater. The spark vaporizes the water near the electrodes so rapidly that a cavitation bubble is generated. The expanding cavitation bubble creates a spherical hydrodynamic pressure wave (shock wave). A second, much less powerful shock wave is released a few milliseconds later as the bubble collapses.

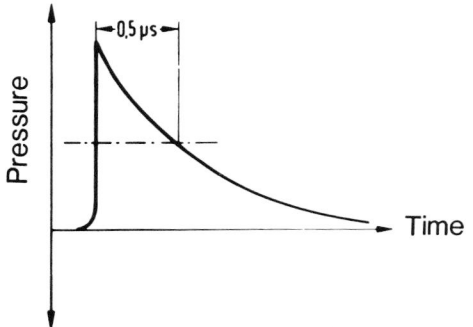

FIG. 9. The pressure/time relationships of a hydrodynamic shock wave.

All ESWL units utilize focused shock waves so that the targeted stone may be subjected to high pressures while maintaining much lower pressures in the tissues surrounding the stone. The underwater spark-generated shock waves are focused by releasing the pressure wave at the first focal point of an ellipsoidal reflector. The shock wave propagates spherically, strikes the wall of the ellipsoid, and is reconcentrated at the second focal point of the ellipsoid. Shock waves may also be focused with an acoustic lens as is utilized in the Siemens Lithostar and the Storz Pulsolith. Piezoelectric-generated shock waves differ in that they do not rely on reflection for focusing; rather, they are aligned in spherical fashion with each individual unit being targeted to the same point. This system allows for much sharper (i.e., smaller) focal zoners of high pressure than with the ellipsoidal reflectors or acoustic lens focusing systems.

The shock wave utilized for ESWL must be generated in a medium with an acoustical impedance similar to that of body tissue. Therefore, all lithotripters generate their shock wave in water. Many systems utilize degasified water as the presence of microscopically dissolved air in water will attenuate the shock wave slightly. Coupling of the shock wave to the body is ideally accomplished by placing the patient's flank in a water bath as is utilized by the Dornier HM3 device. Alternatively, a membrane capable of transmitting the shock wave may be interposed between the water and the skin, allowing for a water bag to be substituted for a water bath. Although some reflection of the shock wave energy may be expected with water bag arrangements, numerous lithotripters capable of generating sufficient pressures for stone fragmentation have been devised utilizing this system. The features of various lithotripters currently being manufactured are listed in Table 10.

A shock wave generated underwater will pass through the tissues between the skin and the kidney stone with only slight attenuation because of the relatively similar acoustical impedence of bodily tissue vis-à-vis water. However, when the shock wave passes from a zone of high acoustical impedance (water or tissue density) to a zone of much lower acoustical impedance (kidney stone), the pressure wave is reflected, transmitting com-

pressive forces to the calculous material. Kidney stones are inhomogeneous structures, resulting in multiple reflections of the shock wave as it passes through the stone. The variation in the acoustical density presented by a calculus is potentiated as the stone develops fracture planes and begins to crumble. As the shock wave leaves the stone and passes back into a medium of lower acoustical density, energy is once again reflected. In this circumstance, however, the forces created are tensile or reflective in nature as opposed to the compressive forces generated as the pressure wave entered the stone. The tensile forces generated as the shock wave leaves the stone are probably of a lower order of magnitude than the compressive forces, as the shock wave probably has been significantly attenuated during its passage through the calculous material. However, tensile forces may still be an important mechanism in stone fragmentation, as renal calculi are more sensitive to tensile stresses than compression stresses by a factor of 7 (29).

The process of stone fragmentation accelerates as the stone begins to fragment and multiple fracture planes present innumerable differences in acoustical impedence to the passing shock wave. Fragmentation of calculi during ESWL appears to begin peripherally and then proceeds to the center of the stone. As the periphery of the stone disintegrates, the efficiency of stone disintegration is enhanced if there is sufficient room for the particles created by lithotripsy to disperse, minimizing the buffering effect of these particles, which may protect unfragmented stone material at the core of the stone. This buffering effect may explain why impacted stones in the ureter and renal infundibula are more resistant to fragmentation during ESWL, as there is no room available for particles to separate from the central stone mass as they are created.

Principles of Therapy

Patient Positioning

A hydraulically controlled, immersible gantry is required for treatment in the water bath of the Dornier HM3. Although manufacturers' guidelines limit treatment to individuals under 6 ft 6 in. tall (198 cm) and with weights of no more than 300 lb (135 kg), experience at the MHI suggests that there is sufficient variability in body habitus that occasionally patients exceeding these parameters are treatable. A good general rule is that any patient with unusual body habitus or who is near the limits of the aforementioned parameters should first be simulated in the lithotripter prior to initiation of anesthesia to determine if satisfactory positioning is feasible.

The flank of the kidney to be treated should be rotated down toward the ellipsoid. The closer the stone to be treated lies to the spine, the greater the degree of rotation required to allow the stone to be visible on both fluoroscopic units of the HM3 or HM4 devices (Fig. 10). When the stone is located in the upper ureter, rotation of the

TABLE 10. *Lithotripters*

Lithotripter	Shock wave generation	Focusing	Coupling	Locating	Clinical use since
Dornier					
HM3	Underwater electrode	Semiellipsoid 15 cm/17 cm	Complete water bath	2 under patient x-ray tables	1980/1986
HM3 modified	Underwater electrode	Semiellipsoid 17 cm	Complete water bath	2 under patient x-ray tables	1980/1986
HM4	Underwater electrode (40 nf)	Semiellipsoid 17 cm	Water cushion	2 under patient x-ray tables	1986
MPL 9000	Underwater electrode (60 nf)	Semiellipsoid 21 cm	Water cushion	1 lateral ultrasonic + 1 coaxial ultrasonic	1987
MFL 5000	Underwater electrode (40 nf)	Semiellipsoid 17 cm	Water cushion	1 rotating under patient tube	1988
Technomed					
Sonolith 3000	Underwater electrode (50,000 shocks per electrode set)	Semiellipsoid 20.5 cm	Partial water bath	1 lateral ultrasonic + 1 coaxial ultrasonic	1985
Siemens					
Lithostar	Electromagnetic element	Acoustic lens aperture 12 cm	Water cushion	2 over patient x-ray tubes	1986
Wolf					
Piezolith 2300	3000 piezoelectric elements	Spherical alignment aperture 30 cm	Partial water bath	2 coaxial ultrasonic scanners	1987
EDAP					
LT01	300 piezoelectric elements	Spherical alignment aperture 54 cm	Water cushion	1 coaxial ultrasonic scanner	1986
Yachiyoda					
Extracorporeal microexplosion	Lead azide pellet	Semiellipsoid	Complete water bath	1 rotating C-arm/x-ray	1986
Medstone					
1050	Underwater electrode	Semiellipsoid	Water cushion	1 rotating over patient x-ray	1987
Northgate					
SD-3	Underwater electrode	Semiellipsoid	Water cushion	Coaxial ultrasound	1987
Direx					
Tripter X7	Underwater electrode	Semiellipsoid	Water cushion	Portable C-arm	1987

patient must be further exaggerated. Calculi between L_5 and the pelvic brim cannot be successfully treated through the bony pelvis, but may be approached successfully with the patient in the prone position (30).

While treatment in the prone position is possible with the Dornier HM3 lithotripter, ESWL in the prone position is more easily accomplished with the Dornier MFL 5000 lithotripter as well as most other second-generation

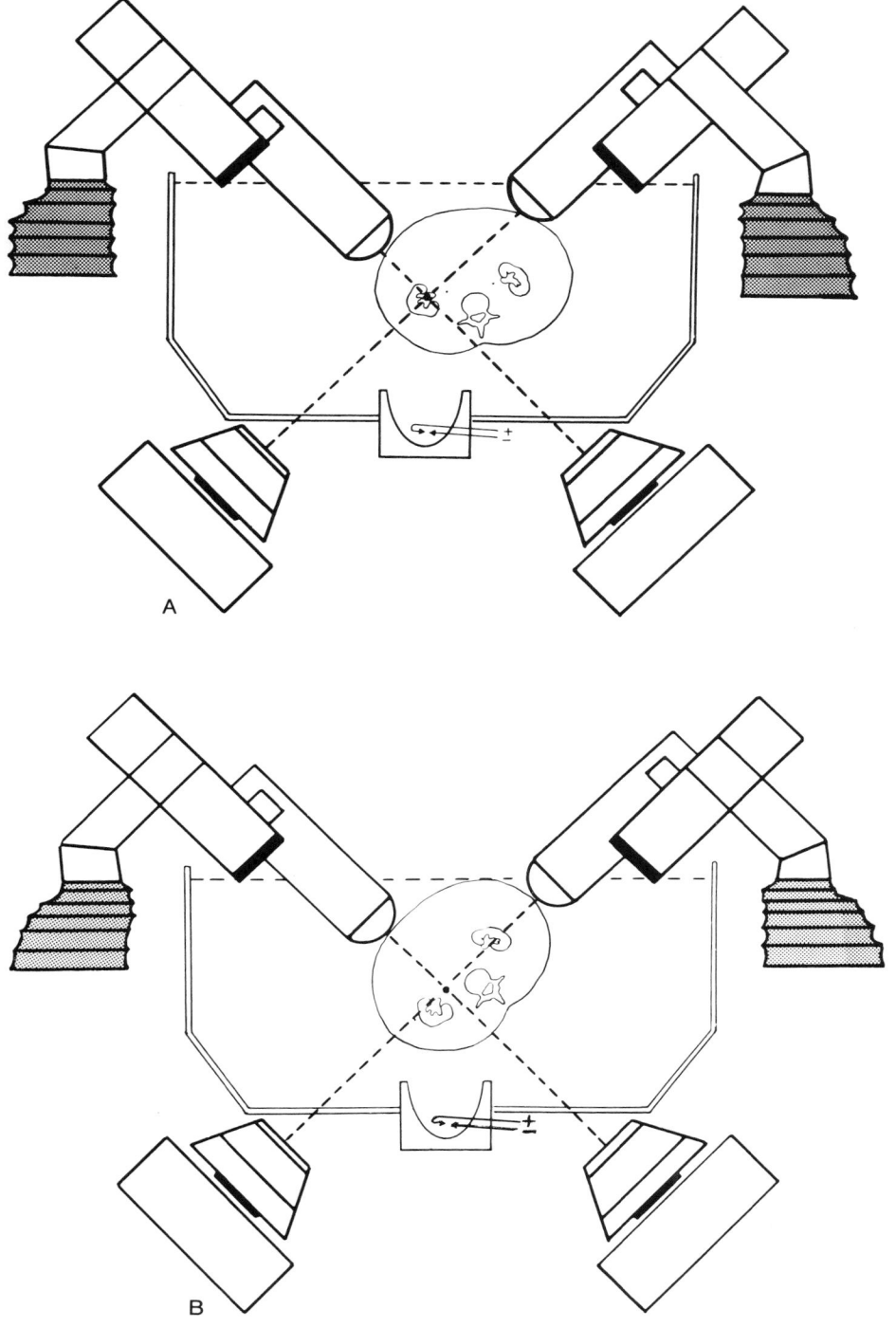

FIG. 10. Patient positioning during ESWL. Patient positioning during ESWL is influenced by the proximity of the stone to be treated to the spine. The closer the stone is to the spine, the greater the degree of rotation required to allow satisfactory imaging of the stone in both fluoroscopic monitors. Insufficient rotation will result in the stone being projected behind the spine, obscuring vision. **A:** The stone to be treated is in the renal pelvis, and minimal rotation of the patient is required. **B:** The stone is in the ureter, and more rotation of the patient in the gantry is required for satisfactory imaging.

lithotripters. The indications for prone ESWL are listed in Table 11.

Solitary Stones

As a general rule, ESWL should be initiated at the point to the stone nearest to UPJ, ensuring that the stone material likely to enter ureter first is sufficiently fragmented. Treatment should then proceed toward the periphery of the kidney. If the stone material is deemed likely to be easily treatable in a single session of ESWL, rationing of the number of shock waves given to any particular region of the stone during therapy is not required. If the stone is large but a single treatment is still a possibility, the shock wave energy should be distributed evenly over the stone mass, saving approximately 10% of

TABLE 11. *Indications for prone ESWL*

Ectopic pelvic kidney
Horseshoe kidney (especially inferior and medial calices)
Transplant kidney
Severe kyphoscoliosis
Mid-ureteral and distal calculi

the total number of shock waves to be delivered for treatment of the regions of the stone that are judged to have fragmented least well during therapy. If fragmentation seems uniform, this final "bolus" of shock waves may be delivered to the portion of the stone fragments nearest to the UPJ, minimizing the possibility of a large lead fragment retarding passage of the rest of the stone fragments.

The assessment of fragmentation is easiest when treating renal pelvic calculi since stone fragments will commonly disperse into the renal pelvis or calices during lithotripsy. The assessment of fragmentation during ESWL of calyceal or ureteral stones is more difficult because fragments have little room to disperse during treatment. To ensure adequate pulverization, it is prudent to empirically administer a larger number of shock waves to calyceal or ureteral stones than for comparable renal pelvic stones. However, the routine administration of a maximum number of shock waves with each ESWL session is to be discouraged.

Multiple Stones

When treating patients with multiple calculi, ESWL should be initiated with the stone lying in the most dependent area of the renal collecting system and then should progress in a cephalad direction, as this will prevent accumulation of stone fragments around an untreated calculus in a dependent location. The presence of such particles will absorb some of the shock wave energy, retarding the efficiency of ESWL.

Impacted Stones

The treatment of impacted calculi, whether they are calyceal or ureteral in location, is more difficult. Many investigators suggest that these stones are resistant to fragmentation because of the absence of a fluid interface around the stone (31,32). The degree of impaction (and difficulty in fragmentation) is related directly to the amount of obstruction associated with the stone. Larger numbers of shock waves and higher pressures (22–26 kV with the Dornier HM3 device) are necessary to achieve fragmentation in these cases. Ten to 20% of impacted calculi will not be fragmentable with ESWL (33).

Treatment of Substantial Stone Burden

Most of the problems associated with ESWL occur when treating renal units containing stones larger than 2 cm in diameter or multiple stones, and relate to difficul-

ties in the passage of gravel. If kidneys with calculi greater than 2 cm in aggregate diameter are treated with ESWL, the pretreatment placement of an indwelling ureteral stent will significantly reduce the incidence of ureteral colic, ureteral obstruction, and *steinstrasse* (34). Ureteral stents facilitate the expulsion of fragments following ESWL by dilating the intramural ureter and inducing ureteral atony. Although some ureters may undergo the aforementioned changes within 48 h to stent placement, at the MHI stents are left at least 7–10 days to maximize ureteral dilation. Smaller stone fragments will commonly pass around the stents. The placement of a ureteral stent may be accomplished under the same anesthesia planned for ESWL, and a suture attached to the stent will facilitate its removal at a later date.

The routine use of ureteral stents in conjunction with ESWL is not required. The great majority of renal calculi are small, and the likelihood of significant problems associated with the passage of gravel for the treatment of calculi less than 2 cm in diameter is low enough that the morbidity and expense of the stent in this circumstance cannot be justified (35–37). However, ureteral stenting is indicated when treating calculi less than 2 cm in diameter in the presence of a solitary kidney.

The routine treatment with ESWL monotherapy of calculi larger than 3 cm in diameter or staghorn calculus is not recommended because complications rise rapidly in this category of patients, while the possibility of achieving a stone-free result is low (35). These calculi are more appropriately pursued with percutaneous nephrostolithotomy. If ESWL is attempted, an indwelling ureteral stent is mandatory, and multiple sessions of ESWL probably will be required.

Low-Density/Radiolucent Calculi

Upper urinary tract calculi vary widely in their radiodensity. The treatment of calculi which are of low radiodensity or which are radiolucent is greatly facilitated by the placement of a ureteral catheter at the time of ESWL. The ureteral catheter quickly allows the operator to locate the kidney, reducing x-ray exposure to the patient, and if the stone is not easily identified on fluoroscopy, contrast material can be injected through the ureteral catheter and the appropriate area of the renal collecting system treated. Although ultrasound has been touted as an important advantage in the treatment of radiolucent calculi, such stones are easily treated with fluoroscopy using ureteral catheters and contrast material.

The treatment of cystine calculi greater than 2 cm with ESWL is generally not recommended for several reasons. First, these calculi are sometimes dissolvable with an adequate regimen of systemic chemolysis, and chemolysis should be the initial approach when symptoms permit. Second, cystine stones are resistant to fragmentation with ESWL. Higher voltage and a larger number of shock waves are required, even for the treatment of calculi less than 2 cm in diameter (38). Third, cystinuria is frequently associated with staghorn calculi or large, multiple, and/or bilateral calculi. Kidneys with such stone burden are inappropriate for ESWL monotherapy and are best approached percutaneously if intervention is required. Fourth, the relatively radiolucent character of these stones makes assessment of fragmentation difficult during ESWL.

Bilateral Simultaneous ESWL

Renal calculi commonly are present bilaterally, and if the contralateral renal unit contains calculi 5 mm or greater in diameter, bilateral simultaneous ESWL should be considered.

Shock Wave Dosage

The amount of shock wave energy that may safely be applied to a kidney with any ESWL device is presently unknown. ESWL produces changes in the kidney similar to that of renal trauma, consisting primarily of intraparenchymal and perirenal hemorrhage and edema. Since the efficiency of ESWL declines as fragments accumulate during treatment, the routine administration of greater than 2000 shock waves in a single session should be avoided when treating with an unmodified Dornier HM3 device. While the optimal interval between sessions of ESWL is not established, at the MHI, a minimum of 48 h between ESWL treatments is preferred to allow fragments created with the initial ESWL session to disperse and/or pass. It is hoped that experimental and clinical parameters will soon be developed that define treatment parameters for the safe performance of ESWL.

Complications of ESWL

Although ESWL is well tolerated by most patients, complications can occur (Table 12). Most of the problems associated with ESWL are related to the passage (or nonpassage) of gravel following lithotripsy. Approximately one-third of patients will have significant colic following ESWL with the Dornier HM3 lithotripter (39,40). The likelihood of pain following ESWL is di-

TABLE 12. Complications of ESWL

Complications related to stone fragments
Colic
Steinstrasse
Incomplete fragmentation
Acute complications of shock waves
Skin bruising
Perinephric hematoma
Pancreatitis (rare)
Urosepsis

rectly related to the amount of stone material treated in the kidney and the resulting gravel that must be expelled by the ureter (39,40). The accumulation of stone particles in the ureter (usually distally) is termed *steinstrasse* (street of stone) and is a common occurrence following ESWL. Most *steinstrasse* are short and pass with minimal symptoms to the patient; however, in approximately 7% of patients treated during the U.S. trials of the Dornier HM3 lithotripter, symptomatic *steinstrasse* required intervention of some sort. The likelihood of developing a *steinstrasse* requiring intervention is directly related to the stone burden and the occurrence of *steinstrasse* can be reduced with the judicious use of indwelling ureteral stents placed prior to ESWL of kidney containing moderate or large stone burden (34,35).

The management of symptomatic *steinstrasse* varies depending on whether they are classified as simple or complex *steinstrasse*. Simple *steinstrasse* are defined as columns of gravel less than 5 cm in length in a patient who has no signs of urosepsis. Complicated *steinstrasse* are columns of gravel greater than 5 cm in length or in patients exhibiting signs of urosepsis. Simple *steinstrasse* have a limited number of stone particles present in the ureter and can usually be efficiently and safely removed with ureteroscopy and/or stone basketing. The manipulation of *steinstrasse* transurethrally should not be attempted unless a safety guide wire can first be passed beyond the offending stone material. If a guide wire cannot be passed, the risk of ureteral perforation during manipulation is greatly increased and may result in extravasation of stone particles in or around the ureter. Following transurethral removal of *steinstrasse,* an indwelling ureteral stent should be placed for 7–10 days.

Another alternative for the management of symptomatic *steinstrasse* is in situ ESWL to the portion of the ureter where fragments are lodged. Miller and colleagues have reported that a successful outcome may be expected in 90% of patients so treated (41).

Patients presenting with complicated *steinstrasse* (representing a large volume of stone material in the ureter or signs of urosepsis) should not be managed transurethrally. The large number of stone particles in the ureter is extremely difficult to remove with the ureteroscope and the chance of ureteral perforation/injury rises significantly. Additionally, transurethral manipulation is hazardous and usually contraindicated in patients with signs of urosepsis. Complicated *steinstrasse* are better managed with the placement of a percutaneous nephrostomy for drainage of the affected renal unit. Renal colic is relieved and urosepsis will usually resolve promptly with adequate drainage and appropriate antibiotics. The ureter will continue to peristalse, and the *steinstrasse* will almost always pass spontaneously even in the absence of urine flow.

Lithotripters that deliver lower pressure into smaller focal points appear to be associated with a reduced incidence of renal colic, believed to be due to the production of smaller fragments during the lithotripsy process (42,43). Although complications related to the passage of stone fragments appear to be reduced, higher numbers of shock waves and multiple ESWL sessions also result from this treatment philosophy.

The most dramatic acute effect of shock waves on the kidney is clinically apparent perirenal hemorrhage, which has been noted following 0.66% of treatments with the Dornier HM3 device (44). Perirenal hemorrhage is always manifested by pain in the flank, usually sufficient to require parenteral narcotics. At the MHI any patient experiencing severe flank pain or a hemoglobin decrease of greater than 2 gm % 24 h following ESWL is examined with renal ultrasound to check for the possibility of a perinephric hematoma. Bleeding sufficient to cause hypotension, albeit rare, is possible. The risk of perirenal bleeding appears to be increased if the patient has a history of hypertension or is hypertensive at the time of lithotripsy (44). Chaussy has suggested that the administration of salicylate-type components may be a factor in the occurrence of this complication, and when possible, discontinuation of such medications two weeks prior to ESWL is advisable if possible (7). The management of clinically apparent perinephric bleeding following ESWL is generally conservative. Hematomas following ESWL generally resolve in 3–6 months but in a number of instances may persist for a year or more following their occurrence. The long-term sequela of perinephric hematomas is unknown at this time.

Because urinary calculi are commonly associated with bacteriuria, urosepsis is an ever-present danger no matter what form of therapy is applied. Temperature elevation is uncommon following ESWL, occurring in less than 2% of cases. Gram-negative septicemia with shock occurred in 0.2% of cases treated at the MHI during FDA trials of the lithotripter (39). Urosepsis, when it occurs, usually implies the concomitant presence of obstruction and constitutes a urologic emergency. This complication can be minimized by the judicious use of ureteral stents, and the administration of parenteral antibiotics whenever lithotripsy is performed on calculi with an associated history of urinary tract infection.

In summary, ESWL, while representing a significant reduction in morbidity for patients, does require attention to innumerable technical details to assure satisfactory treatment. Adequate imaging is a prerequisite for successful lithotripsy. The results achieved with ESWL will be maximized and the complications minimized with the realization that lithotripsy is not for all calculi, particularly large and complex stones. The judicious use of ureteral stents will reduce ureteral morbidity following lithotripsy. Although acute complications of ESWL are infrequent, awareness of the potential adverse effects of shock waves is essential to the treating urologist, particularly when treating patients on an outpatient basis.

CONCLUSIONS

The fields of endourology and ESWL are in their infancy, and not surprisingly, techniques and equipment continue to evolve rapidly. The techniques presented above are not intended to be all inclusive; rather, they represent approaches which have become preferred at the Methodist Hospital Institute for Kidney Stone Disease and are designed to allow for the broadest application to upper urinary tract calculi. Instrumentation continues to be further miniaturized and new technology continues to be developed at a bewildering rate. However, the vast majority of symptomatic, upper urinary tract calculi can be managed effectively with the basic instrumentation and techniques described.

INDICATIONS FOR EXTRACORPOREAL SHOCK WAVE LITHOTRIPSY, PERCUTANEOUS NEPHROSTOLITHOTOMY, AND URETEROSCOPY

Physicians should realize that symptomatic urolithiasis represents a tremendous spectrum of disease. An understanding of the factors involved in each urolithiasis case is particularly important today, given the expanded indications for intervention with new, less invasive procedures. Conditions in years past that might not have justified major surgery now may be deemed appropriate for less invasive procedures. Many factors are involved in a given patient's stone problem. These include the size and number of stones, their location in the kidney or ureter, the presence or absence of obstruction, dilatation and/or infection, function of the renal unit, and composition of the stone. The success of an individual patient's treatment is dependent on the careful consideration of these various factors, and it is becoming increasingly evident that no single technique is appropriate for all types of calculi. Extracorporeal shock wave lithotripsy (ESWL) open surgery, percutaneous nephrostolithotomy (PCNL), ureteroscopy (URS), and other endourologic techniques have their relative advantages and disadvantages in the management of urolithiasis. In the remainder of this chapter we present the rationale utilized at the Methodist Hospital Institute for Kidney Stone Disease for treating the stone patient with the procedure that is most likely to achieve the goals of therapy with the lowest risk of side effects and complications. In general, the least invasive procedure (ESWL) is preferred when possible, but it is important to realize that ESWL may not always be associated with the lowest morbidity or the best result.

Goals of Therapy

When treating a patient with urolithiasis, the goals of therapy must be established prior to making a decision as

TABLE 13. *Short-term goals of therapy*

Eliminating the symptomatic calculus

Achieving a stone-free state

Eradicating stone-related bacteriuria

Choosing the procedure
  with the lowest morbidity
  that is least invasive
  that is least costly
  that provides for the lowest likelihood of residual fragments

to which procedure would be preferred. For example, is the goal of treatment to remove the symptomatic stone, or is it to achieve a completely stone-free state? These goals are not necessarily synonymous.

The previous concept of success versus failure must be expanded when determining both the goals of therapy and the results of treatment. Procedures performed on urolithiasis patients may be deemed successful without rendering the patient entirely stone-free. As in the era of open stone surgery, small asymptomatic fragments may remain in the upper urinary tract following treatment with ESWL, percutaneous nephrostolithotomy, or ureteroscopy. If these fragments are small enough (≤4 mm) to allow a high likelihood of spontaneous passage and are not associated with recalcitrant bacteriuria, further therapy is rarely required and the treatment may be considered a short-term success. However, when dealing with struvite or infected stones, the risks of recurrence is substantial unless the patient is rendered entirely stone-free (45). It would seem, therefore, inappropriate to consider patients with retained struvite particles following therapy a success of treatment, even when the fragments are few in number and small in size.

The patient with urolithiasis should be educated to the need for both short-term and long-term goals of therapy. Short-term goals of therapy are listed in Table 13. Most of the long-term goals in the management of the urolithiasis patient relate to the future prevention of crystal growth and thus stone recurrence. This goal requires attention to the metabolic factors associated with urolithiasis.

Nonstaghorn Renal Calculi

PCNL has been demonstrated to be applicable to the removal of a wide variety of upper urinary tract calculi (10,20,46), and presently virtually any stone can be removed by this method. ESWL also appears to be applicable to the great majority of upper urinary tract calculi (38,47), making these two new techniques of great significance to the recurrent stone former who has multiple previous surgical procedures and who is at risk for increased morbidity and loss of renal parenchyma with further open surgery (48). Given the success of ESWL and PCNL, it seems safe to state that presently most

open surgical procedures for the removal of renal calculi (i.e., nephrolithotomy, pyelolithotomy) will be relegated to historic status. That these new techniques are here to stay is unquestioned. What remains controversial, however, is their relative roles.

In this section we review the results and morbidity of 110 patients undergoing PCNL and 982 patients having ESWL at MHI. The PCNLs were performed primarily as a single-stage procedure, as described previously. All ESWL treatments were performed on the Dornier HM3 lithotripter. In these 982 patients, 1020 kidneys were treated and a total of 1146 ESWL treatments were applied.

The two procedures were compared with respect to treatment parameters such as the number of procedures per case, duration of the procedure, and blood loss. Morbidity as measured by postoperative temperature elevation, pain medication usage, postoperative stay, complications, and adjunctive procedures required was also contrasted. The results of therapy were stratified by the size, number, and location of stone material treated. No patients with staghorn calculi are included in this comparative analysis.

The procedures were considered successful if the patient was either stone-free or had only clinically insignificant residual fragments (CIRF) following treatment. CIRF were defined as asymptomatic fragments ≤ 4 mm, not composed of struvite, and associated with sterile urine.

Results

The groups were generally quite similar, and the distribution of stone size and stone location is listed in Table 14. There was a higher percentage of calculi greater than 3 cm in the PCNL group, suggesting that these larger stones tend not to do as well when treated with ESWL monotherapy.

TABLE 14. *Distribution of stone size and stone location*

	PCNL	ESWL
Location		
Pelvis	50 (45%)	462 (46%)
Calix	27 (25%)	377 (37%)
Upper	4	87
Mid	4	64
Lower	19	226
Ureter	33 (30%)	169 (17%)
Upper	19	132
Mid	11	36
Lower	3	1
Size (cm)		
<1	38 (35%)	394 (38%)
1–2	47 (43%)	494 (48%)
2–3	9 (8%)	123 (12%)
>3	16 (14%)	13 (1%)

TABLE 15. *Comparisons of treatment morbidity*

Morbidity measure	PCNL	ESWL
Blood loss		
Pretreatment Hgb	13.7	14.6
Post-treatment Hgb	12.2	14.1[a]
Blood transfusion required	5.5%	0.2%
Maximum temperature (°C)		
≥39	12 (11%)	4 (0.5%)
38	37 (34%)	111 (15%)
<38	60 (55%)	635 (85%)
Maximum pain medication		
None	10 (9%)	586 (51%)
Oral	15 (14%)	191 (17%)
IM narcotic	85 (77%)	369 (32%)
Postoperative stay	5.9	3.0[b]

[a] p < 0.05 (PCNL versus ESWL).
[b] p < 0.001 (PCNL versus ESWL).

Of 1030 renal units treated with ESWL, a single treatment was sufficient in 927 (90%), while 93 (9%) kidneys required two treatments and 10 (1%) kidneys required three or more treatments. This pattern was remarkably similar to the 110 kidneys treated with PCNL, as 100 (91%) of these cases required only a single session, whereas two treatments were required in seven (6%) kidneys and three or more in three (3%) kidneys. Morbidity for the entire groups, as measured by total blood loss, maximum temperature elevation, length of postoperative stay, and pain medication required is listed in Table 15. Even when stratified by stone size, no category of ESWL patients needed more pain medication than comparable PCNL patients. However, the likelihood of experiencing pain following ESWL has been documented to increase with increasing stone size (40). Cystoscopy with stone basketing, ureteroscopy, or percutaneous nephrostomy for drainage was occasionally necessary following ESWL or PCNL to remove or assist in the passage of stone fragments created by the treatment process. The need for these adjunctive procedures is listed in Table 16, which also lists the open surgical procedures required following PCNL or ESWL. Complications necessitating surgery included a UPJ stricture after percutaneous removal of a long-standing impacted proximal ureteral stone, and a large perirenal hematoma that was explored because computed tomography erroneously suggested splenic bleeding. As shown in Table 17, nonsurgical complications were not common but were more frequent with PCNL than ESWL. The average time for PCNL, including access, was 155 min versus 37 min for ESWL ($p \leq .0001$). The length of postoperative stay was directly correlated with the size of stone treated (Fig. 11) but was significantly less ($p \leq .0001$) for ESWL than PCNL in all categories. The overall results of treatment are listed in Table 18 and indicate that when a variety of stone cases are treated, PCNL is significantly more effective in rendering kidneys free of stone material than ESWL ($p \leq .001$). The number of cases requiring further therapy (i.e., either multiple treatments or ancillary procedures) did not differ significantly between ESWL and PCNL when the stones were located in the renal pelvis or calix. The two procedures had comparable success rates (stone-free plus CIRF) when treating solitary stones in the renal pelvis or calix.

As stone size and number (i.e., total stone burden) increased, so did the need for retreatment with both procedures (Fig. 12 and Table 19). However, the need for ancillary procedures such as cystoscopy and stone manipulation, ureteroscopy, or percutaneous nephrostomy to aid in the elimination of gravel following treatment was

TABLE 16. *Other procedures required*

	PCNL	ESWL
Adjunctive procedures		
Cystoscopy/stone manipulation preoperative	0	46 (4%)
Cystoscopy/stone manipulation postoperative	2 (1.8%)	68 (6.9%)
Nephrostomy tube	NA	13 (1.3%)
PCNL	NA	
Total procedures	2 (1.8%)	139 (13.5%)[a]
Open surgery		
Ureterolithotomy	2 (1.8%)	2 (0.2%)[b]
Pyelolithotomy with pyeloplasty	0	1 (0.1%)[b]
Pyeloplasty	1 (0.9%)	0
Nephrectomy	0	1 (0.1%)[c]
Exploration/perirenal hematoma	0	1 (0.1%)
Total kidneys treated	110	1030

[a] p < .01 (PCNL versus ESWL).
[b] One ureterolithotomy done at another institution.
[c] Done at another institution.

TABLE 17. *Nonsurgical complications*

	PCNL	ESWL
Fever > 39°C	12 (10.9%)	4 (0.4%)
Pulmonary	0	2 (0.2%)
Cardiovascular problems		
MI	0	2 (0.2%)
CVA	0	3 (0.3%)
Pancreatitis	0	1 (0.1%)
Bleeding		
Transfusion	6 (5.5%)	2 (0.2%)
Perirenal hematoma	0	5 (0.5%)
Post-nephrostomy tube bleeding	1 (0.9%)	0
Water intoxication	1 (0.9%)	0
Ileus	0	1 (0.1%)
Perforation	6 (5.5%)	0
Machine malfunction	0	7 (0.7%)
Total kidneys treated	110	1030

directly related to stone burden with ESWL but not following PCNL (Fig. 13). If the need for any further procedures (including retreatments, stone manipulation, percutaneous nephrostomy, etc.) is examined (Fig. 14), it can be seen that for stones of diameter 2 cm or greater, significantly more procedures are necessary to complete therapy if ESWL is performed as the initial treatment rather than PCNL.

Less than half of patients whose largest stone was greater than 2 cm in diameter became free of stone material following treatment with ESWL (Fig. 15). However, increasing stone size did not reduce the effectiveness of PCNL, demonstrating the ability of this technique to remove substantial amounts of stone material from the kidney. Additionally, patients with multiple calculi treated with ESWL fared significantly less well than their PCNL counterparts (Table 19). Seventy-five percent of such patients treated by PCNL became free of all stone material, whereas only 51% achieved the same result with ESWL ($p \leq .05$).

Although there can be little doubt that extracorporeal shock wave lithotripsy and percutaneous nephrostolithotomy represent significant improvements in the management of symptomatic upper urinary tract calculi, the data above, generated at the MHI, emphasize that these procedures have their relative advantages and disadvantages. Both treatment modalities are applicable to a wide variety of upper urinary tract calculi, with about 10% of cases being expected to require more than one treatment. The occasional need for a secondary procedure is a general rule applicable to all endourologic and lithotripsy procedures. The need for secondary procedures for the PCNL cases in this series was comparable to previous reports (10,49,50).

ESWL is the procedure of choice for most stones less than 2 cm in diameter because the morbidity as measured by blood loss, pain, fever, and postoperative stay was significantly less than with PCNL (Table 15). However, further procedures (retreatments plus ancillary procedures) after the initial procedure were required signifi-

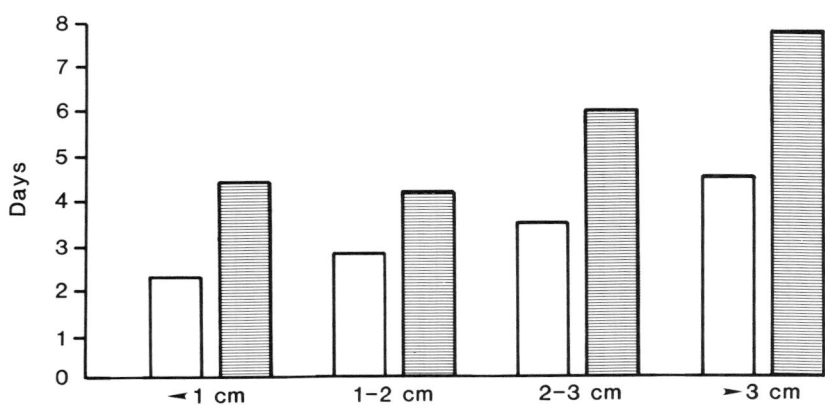

FIG. 11. ESWL (*clear bar*) versus PCNL (*gray*). Postoperative stay in days, by stone size.

TABLE 18. *Comparisons of treatment outcomes*

	PCNL	ESWL
Success[a]	108 (98%)	545 (96%)
Stone-free	100 (91%)	407 (72%)[b]
Clinically insignificant residual fragments	8 (7%)	138 (24%)[b]
Open stone surgery/failure	2 (2%)	24 (4%)
Total patients with 3-month follow-up	110	569

[a] Stone-free and clinically insignificant residual fragments.
[b] $p < .001$ (PCNL versus ESWL).

cantly more often with ESWL. The success of the two methods (if defined as stone-free plus clinically insignificant residual fragments) was comparable for the two groups, although PCNL patients were more likely to be stone-free (Fig. 16). This finding may be important in that the fate of residual fragments remaining in the upper urinary tract (predominantly in dependent calices) is unclear and understandably controversial. Long-term follow-up of such cases is only now becoming available. Analysis of patients followed for at least 2 years at the Institute for Kidney Stone Disease suggests that the recurrence rate for kidneys rendered stone free by ESWL is approximately 9% annually, a rate that compares favorably with recurrence rates following other stone removal procedures. However, if fragments remained in the upper urinary tract following "successful" ESWL, the recurrence rate rose to 22% annually (51). If this finding is substantiated, the success of ESWL for the approximately 25% of patients with residual fragments following treatment may need to be reevaluated.

Some stones less than 2 cm in diameter should still be considered for PCNL. (The indications for PCNL versus ESWL are reviewed in Table 20.) These include cystine stones greater than 1 cm in diameter (if multiple) because cystine is not easily fragmented with ESWL (38). Symptomatic cystine stones smaller than this are uncommon. In addition, some stones residing in dependent calices may be better candidates for PCNL. If the calix is dilated, the likelihood of residual fragments following ESWL is high (51). Thus if rendering the patient entirely stone free is a high priority (such as for struvite), PCNL should be performed instead of ESWL.

Calculi contained in most calyceal diverticula are less than 2 cm in diameter, but the reported results of ESWL in this situation suggest that less than 20% of these patients can be rendered stone-free with this technique (52,53). This is not surprising given the extremely narrow communication of the diverticulum with the renal collecting system (usually ≤2 mm) and the virtual lack of urine circulation through these nonsecretory diverticula. Although percutaneous access may be complex in these cases, they can be treated successfully with PCNL in a high percentage of cases (53).

For stones between 2.1 and 3 cm in diameter, the reduction in hospital stay and pain following ESWL are offset by the more frequent need for retreatment and the increased need for ancillary procedures to assist in the passage of fragments. In addition, although 83% of ESWL patients in this category were considered to have had a successful result, only 39% were actually rendered stone-free compared to 90% of PCNL-treated patients. The placement of indwelling ureteral stents in association with ESWL treatment can significantly reduce ureteral morbidity when treating stones in this category.

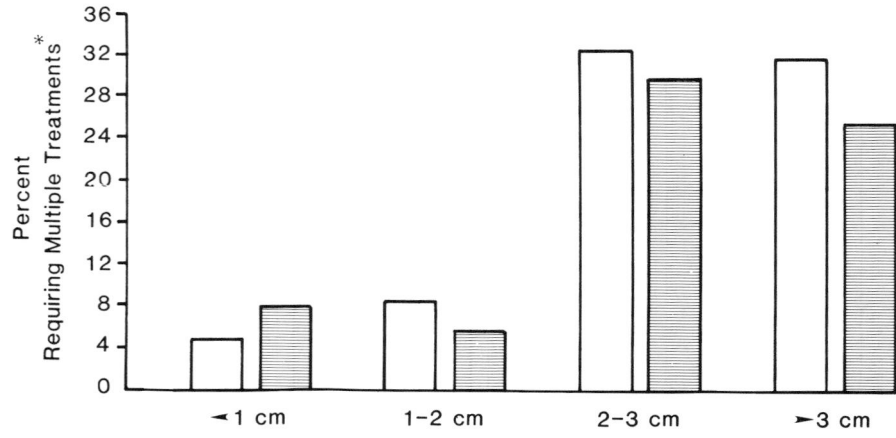

FIG. 12. ESWL (*clear bar*) versus PCNL (*gray*). Frequency of multiple treatments, by stone size. *Multiple treatments equals repeat ESWL or repeat PCNL.

TABLE 19. *Treatment results stratified by number of stones*

	Single stone		Multiple stones	
	PCNL	ESWL	PCNL	ESWL
At time of hospitalization				
Multiple treatments	5 (7%)	53 (8%)	7 (22%)	54 (16%)
Ancillary procedures[a]	2 (3%)	70[b] (10%)	0 (0%)	69[c] (20%)
Mean postoperative stay	4.5	2.6	4.9	3.0
Total patients	76	684	32	340
At time of 3-month follow-up				
Success	75 (98%)	371 (98%)	31 (97%)	17 (92%)
Stone-free	71 (93%)	311[b] (82%)	24 (75%)	96[b] (51%)
Clinically insignificant residual fragments	4 (5%)	60[b] (16%)	7 (22%)	78[b] (41%)
Treatment failures or significant fragments	1 (1%)	8 (2%)	1 (3%)	16 (8%)
Total patients	76	379	32	190

[a] Cystoscopy/stone manipulation pre- or post-ESWL, percutaneous nephrostomy, or nephrostolith-otomy required following treatment.
[b] $p < .05$ (PCNL versus ESWL).
[c] $p < .01$ (PCNL versus ESWL).

Ureteral stents are not without their own expense and morbidity (36,37), however, and they have not been demonstrated to improve the stone-free rate in a series reported by Libby (34). If all stones larger than 2 cm in diameter are compared, the differences between PCNL and ESWL are further exaggerated (Fig. 15). Further procedures are necessary twice as often with ESWL, suggesting that morbidity with this noninvasive technique is not actually less than that for PCNL. In addition, the success rates—especially the stone-free rates—are significantly less for these larger stones (staghorn calculi excluded from this analysis). There appears to be a critical mass of gravel that may be produced by ESWL that exceeds the ability of the renal collecting system to effectively eliminate it. Although a number of ways exist for determining stone burden, the data above suggest that 2.0 cm appears to be near the maximum size for the routine application of ESWL monotherapy.

While ESWL may be utilized for stones larger than 2 cm, other factors, such as stone composition, location, and the need to render the patient stone-free, must be carefully considered prior to recommending this approach. Because of the frequent need for further procedures (repeat ESWL, placement of double-J stents, etc.), the cost of this approach also exceeds that of PCNL (54). Therefore, the investment in resources can be substantial relative to the expectation of a stone-free result.

As indicated earlier, few stones larger than 3 cm in diameter can be treated successfully with ESWL alone. This includes most staghorn calculi. Of 13 nonstaghorn stones greater than 3 cm treated with ESWL monotherapy, 77% required further treatment, only 29% were rendered stone free, and 57% had to be considered treatment failures. For these reasons, large stones (and especially staghorn calculi) are best approached initially percutaneously. ESWL may then be used to treat small remaining fragments which are not easily accessed percutaneously. The experience at the Institute for Kidney Stone Disease suggests that a stone-free status approaching 100% for large *nonstaghorn* calculi may be achieved with combined PCNL and ESWL.

Chaussy et al. (55) reported in 1984 a stone-free rate of

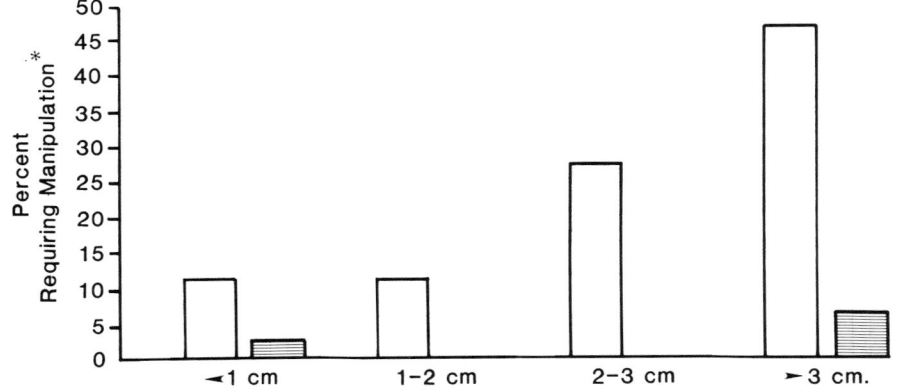

FIG. 13. ESWL (*clear bar*) versus PCNL (*gray*). Frequency of post-treatment manipulation, by stone size. *Manipulation equals cystoscopy, stone basketing, ureteroscopy, or insertion of ureteral stent.

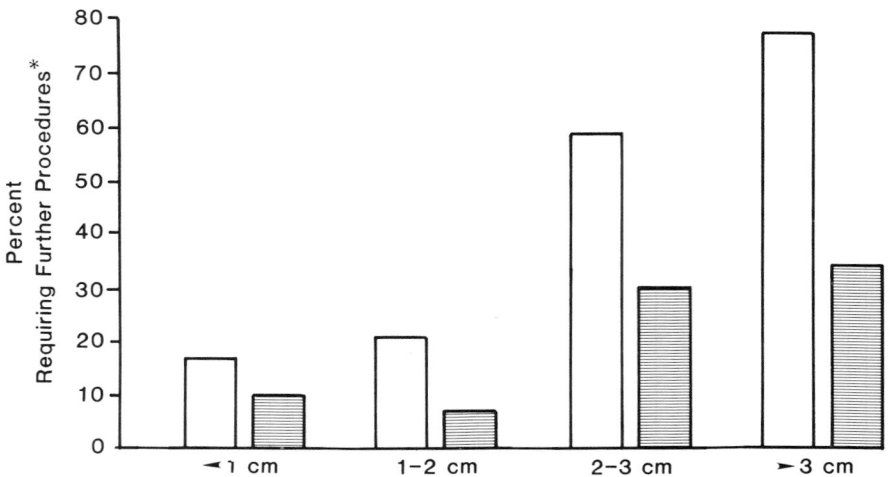

FIG. 14. ESWL (*clear bar*) versus PCNL (*gray*). Frequency of further procedures by stone size. *Further procedures: post-treatment manipulations plus retreatments.

90% following ESWL, a number substantially higher than that observed at the MHI and other series (39,56,57). The patients treated in Munich during early trials of the Dornier lithotripter were not stratified by stone size or number, but Chaussy and Schmiedt (55) did state: "We initially treated only stones approximately the size of a cherry." Of the patients with solitary renal pelvic stones less than 2 cm in diameter treated with ESWL at the MHI, 91.3% were found to be free of all stone material at 3 months (39), a result that is remarkably similar to Chaussy's. This extremely high stone-free rate contrasts sharply with the 67% stone-free rate reported by the United States Study Group of ESWL (40) and demonstrates that interpretation of the results of ESWL therapy is impossible without stratification of cases by stone burden, location, and composition.

The results presented above document that the morbidity of ESWL is lowest overall, but morbidity as well as costs rise significantly in patients with substantial stone burden. Such cases, which represent a minority of urolithiasis patients, are better served with PCNL. While the current trend toward the aggressive use of indwelling ureteral stents at many ESWL centers may reduce the incidence of post-ESWL manipulation for obstructive ureteral gravel (so-called *steinstrasse*), stents are not likely to reduce the rate of retreatment or the ultimate likelihood of achieving stone-free status. The extremely low morbidity of ESWL may lead to a tendency to overutilize this remarkable new technology and should be resisted.

Staghorn Renal Calculi

Staghorn calculi, which have been defined traditionally as renal pelvic stones with extension into at least two calyceal groups, have always represented an extremely challenging problem for urologists. The majority of these stones are composed of struvite (57) and, as such, are

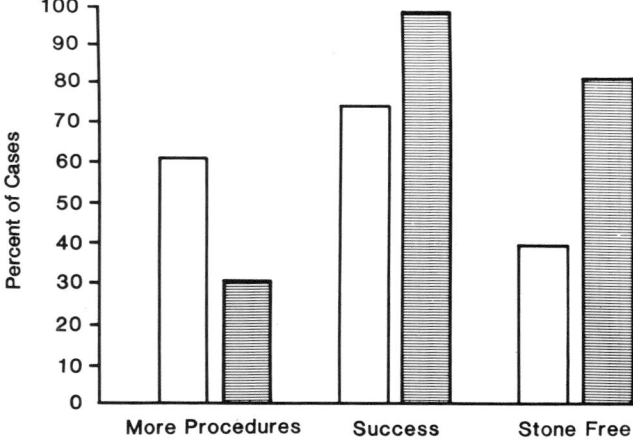

FIG. 15. ESWL (*clear bar*) versus PCNL (*gray*). The need for further procedures, success, and stone-free rates for renal calculi greater than 2 cm in diameter.

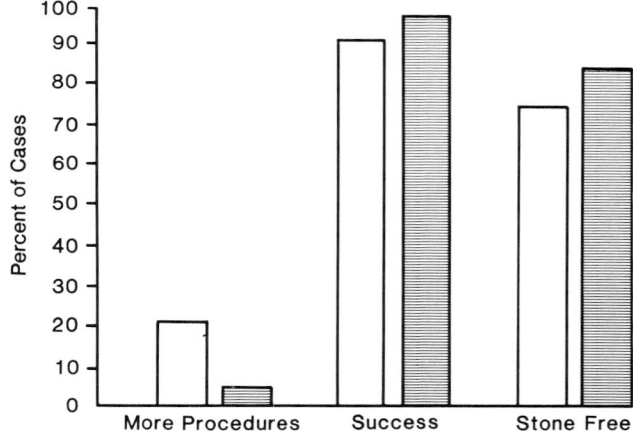

FIG. 16. ESWL (*clear bar*) versus PCNL (*gray*). The need for further procedures, success, and stone-free rates for calculi less than 2 cm in diameter.

TABLE 20. *Indications PCNL versus ESWL*

Calculi ≤ 2 cm: ESWL unless:
  Cystine
  Calyceal diverticula   } PCNL
  Struvite in dilated dependent calix

Calculi ≥ 2.1 cm and ≤3 cm:
  ESWL and double-J stent for suspected calcium oxalate
    dihydrate (low-density) stones
  PCNL for brushite, suspected calcium oxalate
    monohydrate (radiodense), struvite,[a] cystine,
    stones associated with chronic bacteriuria

Calculi ≥ 3.1 cm: PCNL (followed by ESWL if needed)

[a] Can do ESWL with stent if renal collecting system nondilated.

present in these patients and need to be identified and treated appropriately. Segura et al. found contributory metabolic abnormalities in 62% of 75 patients with struvite calculi treated at the Mayo Clinic (61). There is nothing more frustrating to both patient and urologist than to have achieved complete stone removal and then be confronted with a metabolic stone that has recurred in absence of urinary infection.

Second, anatomical abnormalities contributing to stasis within the urinary tract must be addressed. Some obstructive lesions, such as strictures, may be treated endourologically in conjunction with stone removal, while others justify open surgical repair at the time of nephrolithotomy (i.e., infundibuloplasty for infundibular stenosis) (62).

Third, the procedure or combination of procedures most likely to render the patient free of stone material with the lowest morbidity needs to be selected. In the past, most staghorn calculi required nephrolithotomy. Anatrophic nephrolithotomy as popularized by Boyce and colleagues has been performed most commonly in the United States, while multiple radial nephrotomies in combination with pyelolithotomy have been the preferred procedures in Europe (57,62–65). Although these procedures (when combined with intraoperative radiographs) usually render the kidneys free of all stone material, they are associated with substantial morbidity. The hospital stay is often lengthy, even in the absence of renacidin irrigation (63), and hemorrhage necessitating transfusion occurs in the majority of cases (66). Atelectasis, pneumothorax, wound infection, and delayed hemorrhage have been reported with nephrolithotomy (67). The introduction of ESWL provided a new therapy potentially applicable to staghorn calculi (47,68,69). The noninvasive nature of this new technology was very appealing, and initial reports from West Germany suggested that the treatment of staghorn calculi was feasible. However, as experience was gained with ESWL monotherapy, some difficulties became apparent (70). As detailed above, the morbidity of ESWL is clearly dependent on the burden of stone fragments presented to the ureter following treatment (35,39,40). Thus, when ESWL monotherapy is utilized for large nonstaghorn calculi, the patient can anticipate a prolonged treatment process associated with multiple procedures, repeated anesthesias, considerable expense, and a low likelihood of achieving the desired goal of therapy—a stone-free state.

For nonstaghorn calculi, the stone-free rates with PCNL (in contrast to ESWL) are relatively independent of stone burden (Fig. 17). Although the removal of staghorn calculi with multiple dendritic branches is an extremely challenging endourological procedure, multiple authors have demonstrated the feasibility of this approach (10,46,70). However, multiple procedures (and often multiple nephrostomy tracts) are commonly required, and the residual stone rate often remains signifi-

associated with chronic urea-splitting bacteriuria. For many years, some urologists believed that patients with staghorn calculi, particularly those with minimal symptoms, should be treated conservatively, that is, without surgery. But Rous and Turner (58) in 1977 showed that 30% of the patients who did not have surgery died of renal failure or sepsis. Blandy and Singh (59) reported a mortality rate of 28% in patients treated conservatively, with pyonephrosis having developed in most cases.

Struvite stones required special care in their treatment, because of their tendency to grow back from residual fragments. Growth of residual stone material following open surgical procedures may be expected in as many as 30% of cases (45). New stone formation has occurred in 85% of patients undergoing incomplete percutaneous removal of struvite calculi (60). This recurrence rate is in marked contrast to the recurrence rate of only 10% in similar patients who have been rendered completely stone-free by percutaneous nephrostolithotomy (60). Thus it is clear that retained struvite stone material is a significant risk factor for recurring infection, continued ureolysis, and future stone growth. Even when rendered entirely stone-free, many patients with struvite calculi and infection-induced urolithiasis (such as those with neurogenic bladders or urinary diversions) or difficult-to-control metabolic stone disease (i.e., cystinuria, intestinal hyperoxaluria) are at high risk for the development of recurrent stones. Over the years, considerable morbidity has been associated with the repetitive open surgical procedures necessitated in such high-risk patients (48). With the recent development of less invasive modalities for kidney stone removal (percutaneous nephrostolithotomy and ESWL), new approaches for the management of these difficult problems are now available.

Pretreatment Consideration

The ideal management of these challenging cases is threefold. First, metabolic abnormalities are commonly

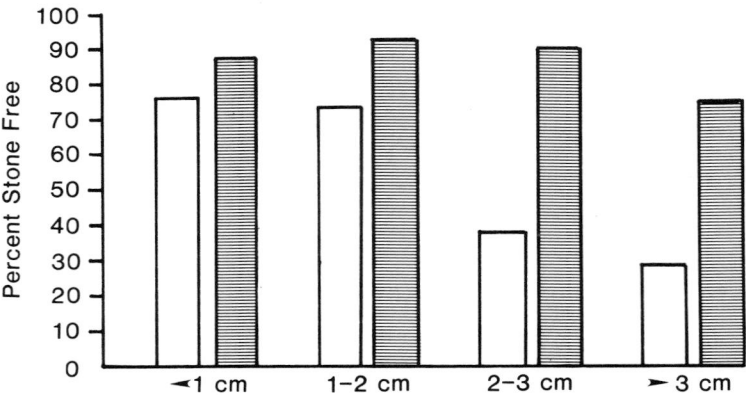

FIG. 17. ESWL (*clear bar*) versus PCNL (*gray*). Stone-free rates by stone size.

cant when these staghorn calculi are treated by percutaneous means alone (20,71).

When combined for the treatment of staghorn calculi, ESWL and PCNL have many complementary features. By adding ESWL to PCNL, all areas of the kidney can be accessed for stone extraction and/or disintegration, thereby minimizing the number of percutaneous punctures required. Investigation of the feasibility of a combined approach as opposed to ESWL alone was begun at MHI in 1984. Between July 1984 and June 1987, 313 kidneys containing staghorn calculi were treated with either ESWL monotherapy or initial percutaneous debulking followed by ESWL, as needed. Adequate follow-up was available on 296 patients (Table 21).

Classification of Staghorn Calculi

The traditional classification of partial versus complete staghorn calculi is inadequate to describe stones which vary greatly in size and complexity. In addition to stone volume, renal anatomy (dilatation), renal function, and stone composition are all important factors to be considered when treating staghorn calculi.

At the MHI, partial staghorn calculi were defined as renal pelvic calculi extending into at least two calyceal groups, while complete staghorn calculi were defined as renal pelvic calculi extending into all major calyceal groups and filling at least 80% of the collecting system. The calculi were then further stratified based on the degree of dilatation of the renal collecting system (Fig. 18). Kidneys containing staghorn calculi with no dilatation of the renal collecting system were placed in group I, those with mild dilatation in group II, those with moder-

ate dilatation in group III, and kidneys with gross dilatation of the renal collecting system were placed in group IV.

When stratified by renal anatomy (dilatation), the number of procedures required per case showed no significant difference between ESWL monotherapy and combination therapy (Fig. 19). Note that no kidneys containing staghorn calculi with gross dilatation of the collecting system were treated initially with ESWL monotherapy due to concern that while fragmentation may occur, stone material, rather than being discharged, would tend to settle in the dependent areas of such systems. If the two treatment approaches are contrasted by the stone volume treated (Fig. 20), once again there is not a significant difference between the number of procedures required. However, ESWL monotherapy of staghorn calculi tends to be a drawn-out process at times. Twenty percent of patients with staghorn calculi treated with ESWL monotherapy required more than one hospitalization to complete treatment versus only 2% of patients treated with combined therapy.

Although postoperative stay (stratified by anatomy) (Fig. 21) was slightly less for ESWL monotherapy, this difference was accounted for primarily by the fact that all struvite staghorn calculi treated with combined therapy (67% of staghorn cases) received 48 h of prophylactic renacidin irrigation following demonstration of stone-free status by endoscopy and nephrotomography. When postoperative stay was stratified by stone volume (Fig. 22), complete staghorn calculi treated with ESWL monotherapy actually had longer hospital stays than did their combination therapy counterparts.

Complications were more frequent in the ESWL monotherapy group than their combination therapy counterparts (55% versus 34%), although serious complications such as bleeding were more common with the latter approach. Ureteral obstruction was by far the most common complication in the ESWL monotherapy patients (33% of cases). The frequency of ureteral obstruction following ESWL has been lowered recently with the more aggressive use of indwelling ureteral stents.

TABLE 21. *Distribution of staghorn calculi*

	ESWL monotherapy	Combined PCNL/ESWL	Total
Partial staghorn	60	87	147
Complete staghorn	13	136	149
Total	73	223	296

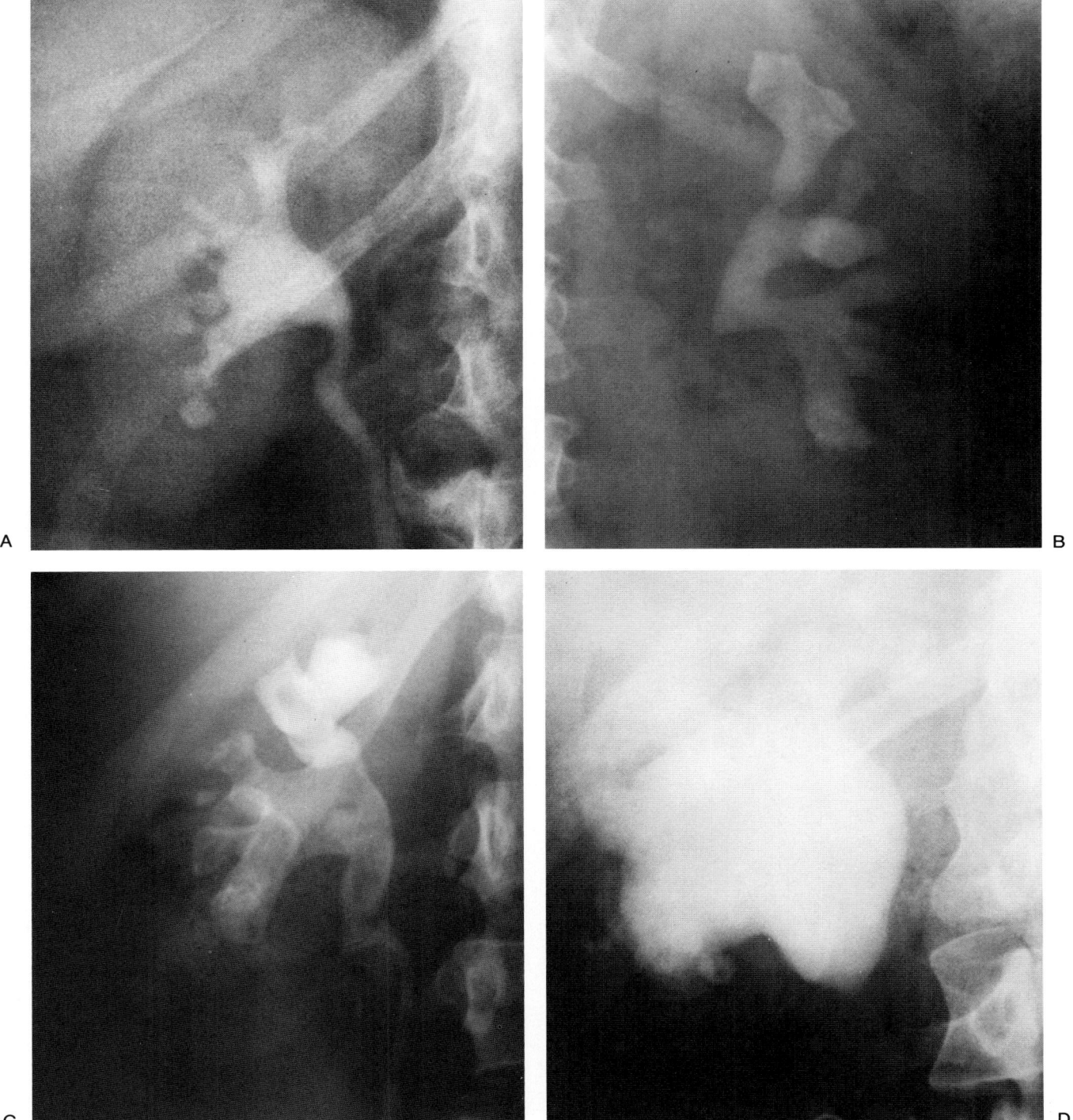

FIG. 18. Staghorn calculi. Degree of renal collecting system dilation. **A:** Group I, no dilatation. **B:** Group II, mild dilatation. **C:** Group III, moderate dilatation. **D:** Group IV, gross dilatation.

Although ESWL correctly has been associated in the minds of both urologists and patients with extremely low morbidity for the majority of stone cases, the data presented above reveal that ESWL monotherapy of staghorn calculi presents a far different picture. Morbidity (as measured by the number of procedures required, the length of postoperative stay, and complications) is not greater when percutaneous debulking is the initial procedure followed by ESWL (if required). Clearly, considerable effort is required in the management of these com-

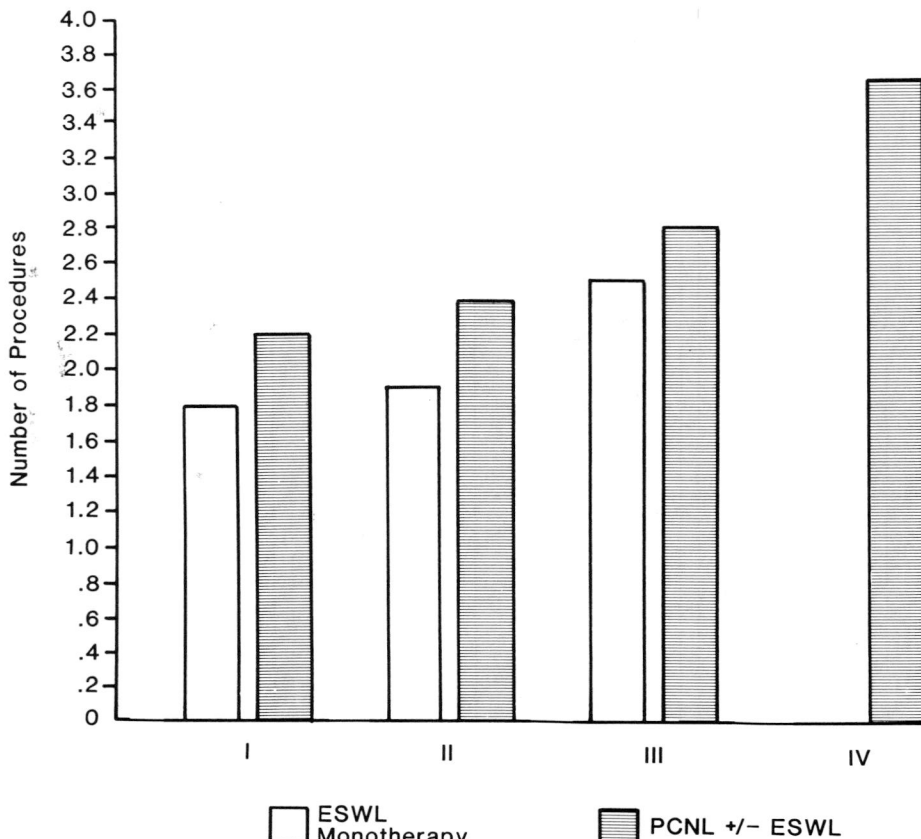

FIG. 19. Staghorn calculi. Number of procedures stratified by renal anatomy.

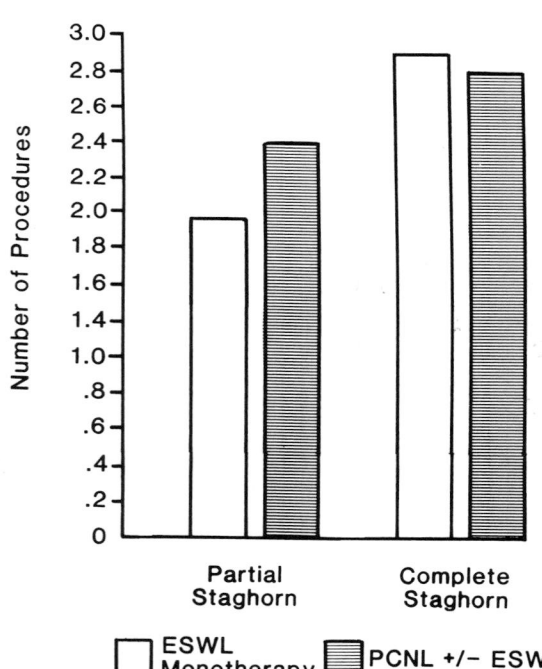

FIG. 20. Staghorn calculi. Number of procedures stratified by stone volume.

plex cases no matter what approach is utilized, making the result expected the most important factor to be considered in selecting the preferred procedure.

Combination therapy achieved stone-free rates superior to ESWL monotherapy for the treatment of partial staghorn calculi no matter what the degree of dilatation of the renal collecting system (Fig. 23). Overall, only 67% of kidneys with partial staghorn calculi treated with ESWL monotherapy became stone free, compared to 92% of similar stones treated with combination therapy ($p = .0002$). ESWL monotherapy produced the best results for partial staghorn calculi when utilized in otherwise normal renal collecting systems (group I), with 84% of such kidneys becoming free of all stone material. The differences between ESWL monotherapy and combined therapy are even greater when complete staghorn calculi are considered (Fig. 24). Less than one-third of complete staghorn calculi treated with ESWL monotherapy became free of all stone material, whereas 91% of similar cases treated with combined therapy were rendered stone-free ($p < .0001$).

The management of complete staghorn calculi in grossly dilated renal units is difficult no matter what approach is elected. Although only 61% of such kidneys

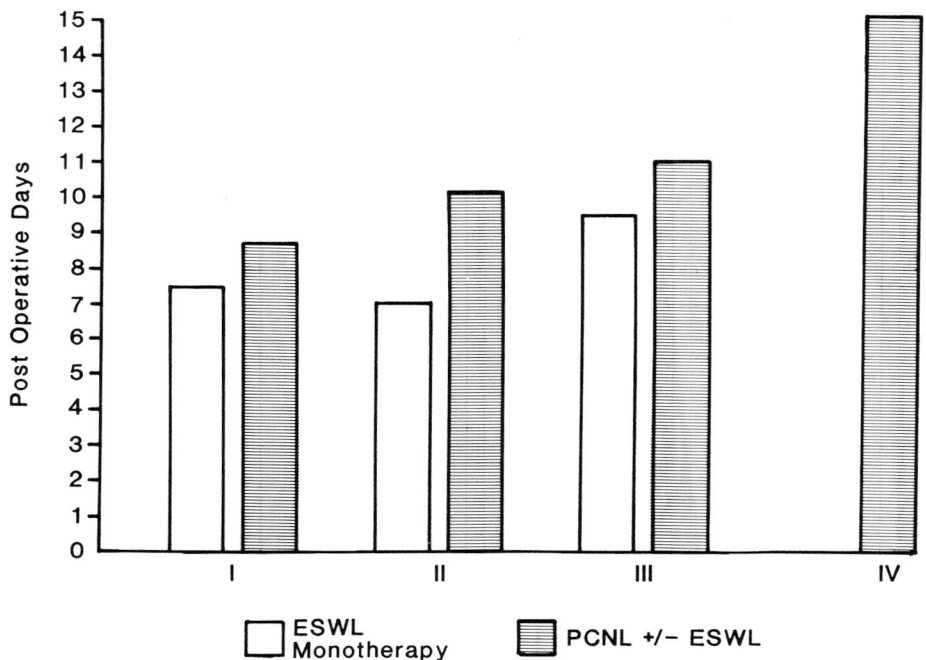

FIG. 21. Staghorn calculi. Length of postoperative stay stratified by renal anatomy.

could be rendered stone-free with combined therapy, it is doubtful that open surgery could achieve any better results. Although the stone-free rates reported with anatrophic nephrolithotomy are in the range 80–90%, previous surgical series have not stratified their cases in a manner

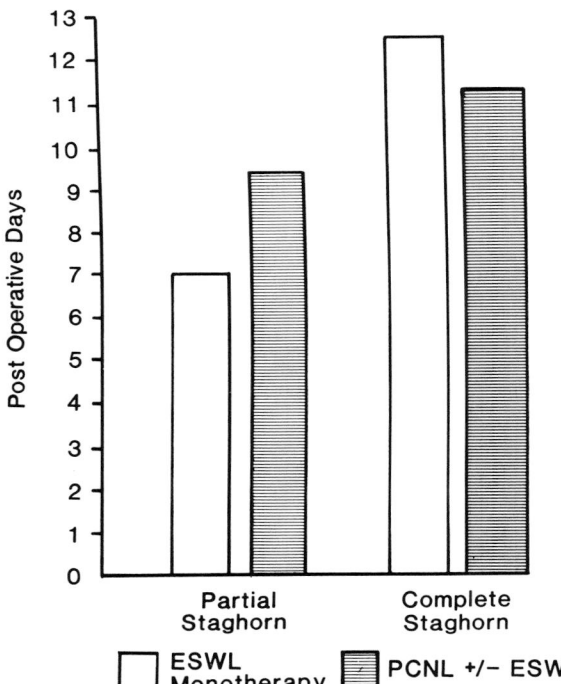

FIG. 22. Staghorn calculi. Length of postoperative stay stratified by stone volume.

such as in this series. The hospital stay and the requirement for multiple procedures (and access) are greatest in patients with grossly dilated collecting systems, and therefore nephrolithotomy might appropriately be considered as a treatment alternative for this special category of cases.

Stone composition is also an important consideration in the management of staghorn calculi (Fig. 25). Struvite is usually easily fragmented with ESWL, but because of the previously described problems with the massive stone burden and difficulties in complete passage of the gravel, only 63% of stones of this type could be rendered stone-free with ESWL monotherapy versus 92% when combined therapy was utilized ($p \leq 0.0001$). Calcium stones were also more successfully treated with combined therapy than with ESWL monotherapy. Cystine staghorn calculi should not be treated with ESWL, as this type of stone material is resistant to fragmentation. Fortunately, it is amenable to the percutaneous approach with 95% of calculi so treated becoming stone-free. Uric acid staghorn calculi should not be treated with ESWL monotherapy for several reasons. First, these are usually very hard stones and difficult to fragment. Second, adequate fragmentation during ESWL is difficult to assess because the stone material is radiolucent. Third, to follow the radiolucent fragments after ESWL, contrast studies are required.

More than 95% of staghorn calculi may be treated with the combined approach of PCNL and ESWL. However, patients who are marginal candidates for ESWL (i.e., those with renal ectopia, kyphoscoliosis, or extreme obesity) should be simulated in the lithotripter before a

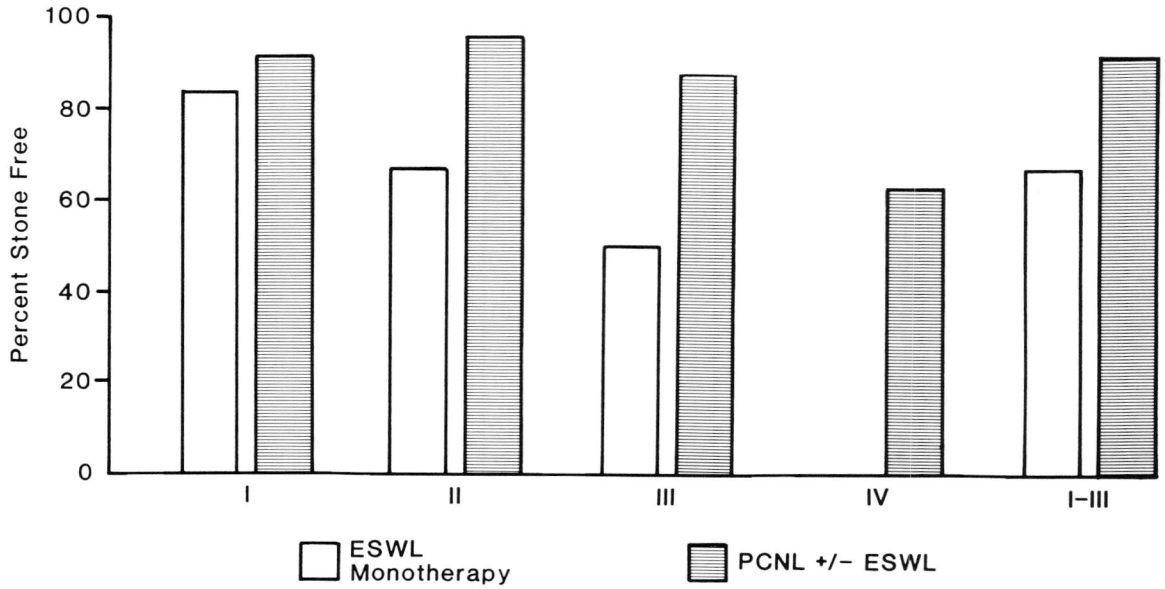

FIG. 23. Stone-free rates for partial staghorn calculi stratified by renal anatomy.

decision is made about the type of approach to be used. Patients who are not candidates for ESWL must have a good chance of being rendered stone free by nephrostolithotomy alone; otherwise, PCNL should not be attempted. In such cases (Fig. 26), open surgery is a better choice. Patients with extremely complex intrarenal architecture (a judgment depending, at least in part, on the operator's endourological skills) or with true infundibular stenosis (which is rare) may be better served by anatrophic nephrolithotomy (62).

Flexible nephroscopy is always performed at the time

the nephrostomy tube is removed, even when no stones are noted on nephrotomography (performed in all cases); otherwise, minute fragments may be missed and may act as a nidus for continued infection and/or further stone formation.

In summary, the results of combination therapy for complete and partial staghorn calculi are superior to ESWL monotherapy in virtually every category examined. Furthermore, the morbidity of combined therapy is not substantially greater than ESWL monotherapy. For these reasons it is the preference at the MHI to treat

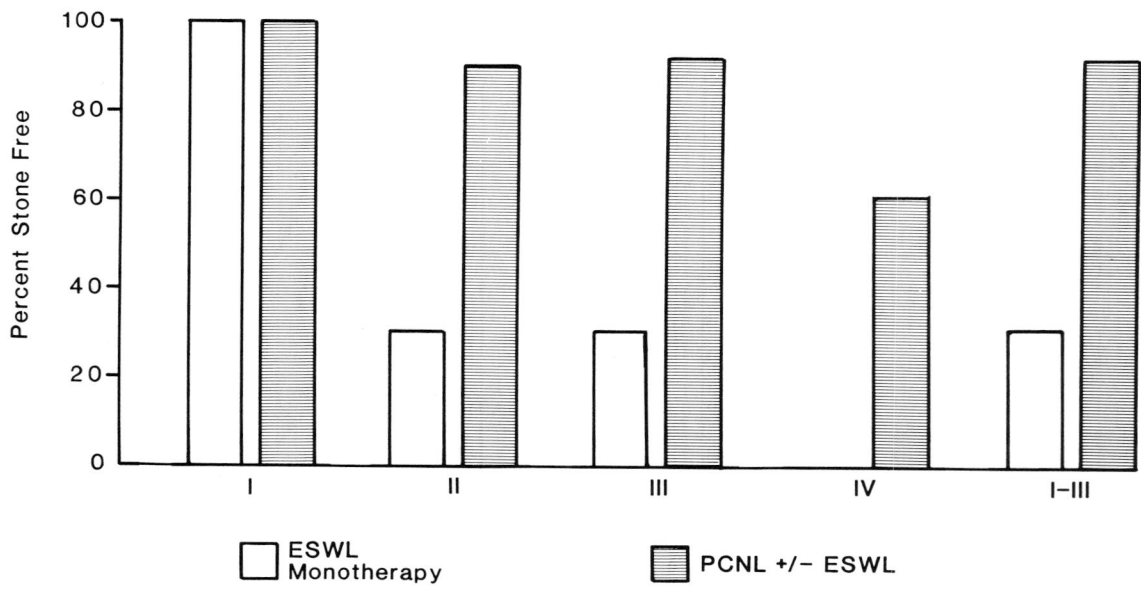

FIG. 24. Stone-free rates for complete staghorn calculi stratified by renal anatomy.

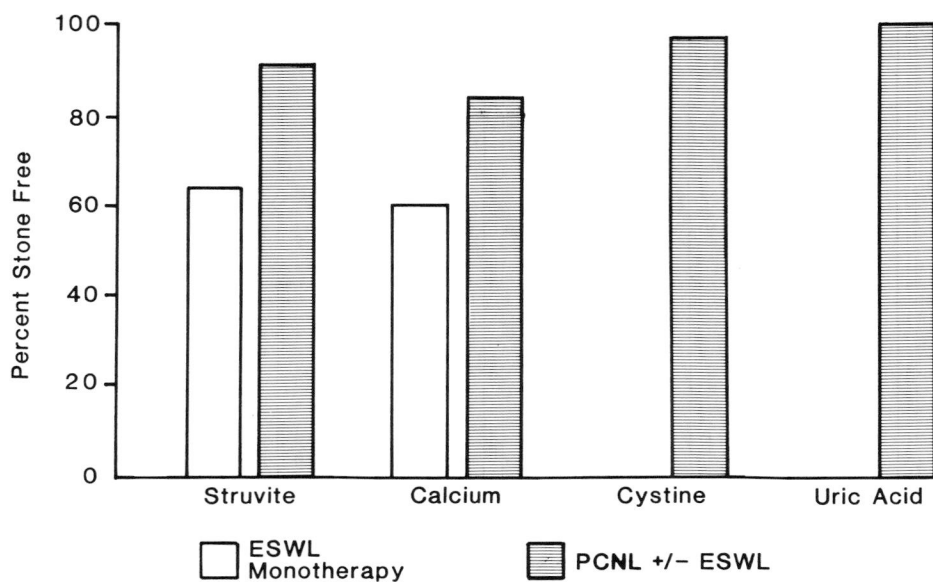

FIG. 25. Staghorn calculi. Stone-free rates stratified by stone composition (groups I–III).

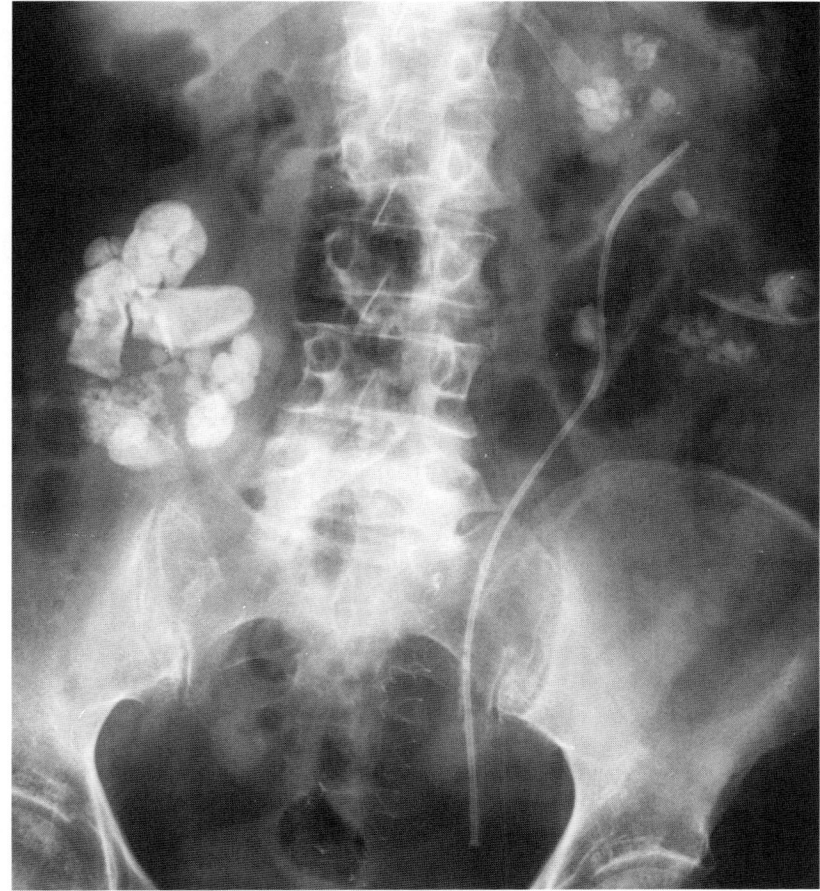

FIG. 26. The staghorn calculus in the right kidney of this 71-year-old woman was associated with such complex calyceal architecture that adequate percutaneous access would be difficult to achieve. Additionally, the lower half of the kidney lay below the pelvic brim, rendering ESWL less effective. Therefore, anatrophic nephrolithotomy was recommended. The broken ureteral stent and multiple stones in the left kidney were removed with PCNL.

all staghorn calculi with combined therapy with the possible exception of low-volume partial staghorn calculi in nondilated collecting systems.

The management of staghorn calculi with a combined approach is technically demanding. A definite learning curve for these complex cases will be evident, even for those facile in endourological techniques.

Ureteral Calculi

A rational approach to the management of ureteral calculi requires an assessment of the efficacy, morbidity, and costs associated with the various treatment options listed in Table 22. The efficacy, morbidity, and costs of the various treatment options available for ureteral calculi will vary depending on the location of the stone.

Prior to the advent of ESWL, PCNL, and URS, when ureterolithotomy was commonly performed, the ureter was divided into thirds, reflecting the various surgical approaches required. The upper ureter extended from the ureteropelvic junction to the upper edge of the sacrum and calculi lodged in this segment of the ureter required a conventional flank incision or a Foley muscle-splitting incision (72,73). The middle portion of the ureter extended from the upper margin of the sacrum to the pelvic brim, encompassing the physiologic narrowing of the ureter as it crosses the iliac vessels. Surgically, the ureter was best approached, for stone removal at this level with a high Gibson incision (74). The lower or pelvic portion of the ureter extended from the pelvic brim (inferior margin of the sacrum) to the ureteral orifice and was generally approached with a modified Gibson or vertical midline incision.

With the shift away from ureterolithotomy at the MHI, the division of the ureter into thirds has been abandoned in lieu of a system dividing the ureter into two sections at the pelvic brim, because it has become apparent that the point where the ureter courses out of the true pelvis across the pelvic brim, and over the iliac vessels provides a significant impediment to the utilization of the rigid ureteroscope. Stones distal to this point are approached much more easily with the ureteroscope. Therefore, the current approach to ureteral stones at the MHI divides the ureter into proximal and distal sections at this point. The proposed management of ureteral calculi that follows will therefore be divided into the management of proximal ureteral calculi (stones above the

pelvic brim) and distal ureteral calculi (stones below the pelvic brim).

Indications for Intervention

The indications for intervention in the management of ureteral calculi clearly have been altered by the increased efficacy and lowered morbidity of PCNL, ESWL, and URS, compared to surgery and blind basketry. With the current array of technologies available, the size of the ureteral calculus is less important than the symptoms it produces. In general, any patient with sufficient symptoms to justify hospital admission should be considered a candidate for stone removal with one of the new techniques. Fortunately, the majority of ureteral calculi are small (≤ 4 mm) and will pass spontaneously with a minimum of discomfort and inconvenience for most patients (75). Patients who have proximal ureteral calculi less than 5 mm in diameter and who have mild enough symptoms to be managed on an outpatient basis with oral pain medication may be followed expectantly. However, calculi 5 mm or larger in diameter presenting in the proximal ureter have a 50% chance at best of spontaneous passage (75,76); therefore, intervention should be considered, as the risks of treatment are extremely low and the results of treatment are excellent (33,77). Another rationale for early intervention for such stones presenting in the proximal ureter is that the longer a stone is present in the ureter without movement, the more impacted it becomes and the more difficult to treat with any technique.

Stones 6 mm or smaller in diameter presenting in the distal ureter can be managed expectantly, assuming that the patient's symptoms are minimal. However, distal stones 7 mm or larger in diameter have a poor rate of spontaneous expulsion; therefore, they should be considered for immediate treatment (75,76).

Urosepsis continues to remain an absolute indication for intervention. Proximal drainage via percutaneous nephrostomy is preferred as the initial procedure at the MHI for two reasons. First, this drainage allows for resolution of urosepsis, reducing the risk of subsequent treatments. Second, the ureteral calculus occasionally will pass during treatment of the patient's infection, obviating the need for further intervention.

Proximal Ureteral Calculi

The treatment of proximal ureteral calculi with ESWL was initially reported by Chaussy and Schmiedt (47) to be highly effective with a 95% stone-free rate for calculi treated in situ in the ureter without prior manipulation. Most of these stones had been lodged in the ureter for fewer than 6 weeks at the time of treatment. However, initial experience at the MHI with 169 ureteral stones treated in similar fashion demonstrated some difficulty

TABLE 22. *Treatment options for ureteral calculi in order of decreasing invasiveness*

Ureterolithotomy
Percutaneous nephrostolithotomy (PCNL)
Ureteroscopy (URS)
Extracorporeal shock wave lithotripsy (ESWL)
Spontaneous passage

with fragmentation as 28% of patients required multiple treatments and/or ancillary procedures (39). In addition, the results of treatment as judged 3 months after ESWL of ureteral stones in situ were not always unsatisfactory, as only 80% of patients became stone-free (33). Other investigators also reported inconsistent fragmentation, particularly with stones impacted in the ureter (30). Although the exact explanation for this observation is unknown, some evidence supports the need for fluid interface between the calculus and the wall of the ureter, providing an expansion chamber during stone fragmentation with ESWL (31). Dissatisfaction with in situ ESWL at the MHI led to a reevaluation of the approach to upper ureteral calculi and to an evaluation of other techniques for the treatment of these stones. Those techniques included manipulation of calculi into the kidney before ESWL and passage of catheters beyond the calculi at the time of ESWL.

Essentially, four options are currently available utilizing ESWL for the treatment of ureteral calculi. The stone may be treated with ESWL in situ without manipulation (group I); the stone may be bypassed with an open-ended ureteral catheter or double-J stent and then treated in situ (group II); the stone may be pushed back into the kidney without concomitant stent placement prior to ESWL (group III); or the stone may be manipulated successfully into the kidney at some time preceding ESWL, with placement of a double-J stent to prevent distal migration of the stone prior to treatment.

The treatments for 724 proximal ureteral calculi at the MHI were reviewed. Only solitary ureteral stones were selected for analysis in order to remove the influence of additional stone burden, leaving a total of 471 treatments in 465 patients.

All patients had pretreatment contrast imaging of the affected renal unit. A KUB and renal ultrasound image were obtained within 24 h of treatment to assess the degree of stone fragmentation and renal obstruction. If these radiographs revealed that the patient was either stone-free or possessing stone debris 2 mm or smaller in greatest diameter, the disintegration was considered successful. All patients had a KUB 3 months following treatment. Fragments remaining in the kidney that were asymptomatic, less than or equal to 4 mm in diameter, and not associated with urinary tract infections were considered clinically insignificant residual fragments

(CIRF). Any fragments remaining in the ureter were considered significant, regardless of size.

The treatment data for patients with solitary ureteral calculi are listed in Table 23. The average stone size varied only 0.07 cm between groups. More shock waves (1347 versus 1017; $p \leq .0001$) were required when calculi were treated in situ in the ureter (groups I and II) compared to calculi treated in the kidney (groups II and IV). Calculi treated in the ureter also required significantly greater application of power (3.06×10^7 versus 2.34×10^7; $p \leq .0001$). Despite this more vigorous treatment, complete disintegration occurred in only 82.9% of the stones treated in situ compared to 94.7% of those treated in the kidney ($p \leq .0001$).

Repeat ESWL treatments, percutaneous nephrostomy, cystoscopy with stone manipulation, and percutaneous nephrostolithotomy were necessary more frequently when the calculus was treated within the ureter (Fig. 27). The retreatment period included the time immediately following treatment through the 3-month evaluation.

Three-month follow-up studies were obtained after 316 treatments, representing 67% of all patients with solitary ureteral stones. For groups III and IV, in which the stone was manipulated successfully preceding ESWL, the success rate (stone-free or CIRF) was significantly higher (99% versus 88.9%; $p \leq 0.001$) than when the stone was treated in situ (groups I and II) (Fig. 28). The stone-free rate for calculi that were repositioned into the kidney successfully prior to ESWL was 90.4% compared to 82.4% for calculi treated in situ, a difference close to statistical significance ($p = .06$). Interestingly, all 56 patients in group IV were stone-free at 3-month follow up, suggesting that ureteral stents may have enhanced stone passage in this group. Complications were uncommon and consisted primarily of ureteral perforations in 15 patients (8 in group II; 7 in group III), perirenal bleeding in four (1 in group II; 2 in group III; 1 in group IV), urosepsis in five (2 in group I; 1 in group II; 2 in group III), and urinary retention in one, pancreatitis in one, and pneumonia in one (all group III). No complication required an open operation, and ureterolithotomy was not necessary in any patient in this series.

Patients who underwent ESWL in situ without prior manipulation or placement of a stent (group I) were examined for possible factors that might have influenced

TABLE 23. *Treatment data*

Group	Treatments	Average stone size (cm)	Average no. of shocks	Average maximum kV	Power ($\times 10^7$)[a]	Complete disintegration
I	123	0.93	1205.3	21.9	2.67	87 (78.2%)
II	47	0.97	1587.1	23.7	3.78	41 (89.1%)
III	245	1.00	1014.2	22.9	2.34	230 (95.9%)
IV	56	0.93	1034.7	22.8	2.37	56 (100%)

[a] Power = no. of shock waves × kV (40).

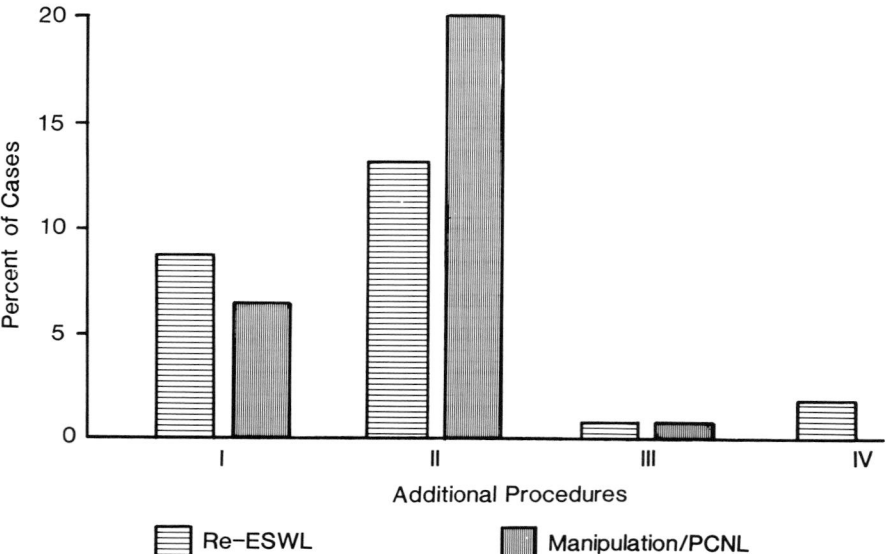

FIG. 27. The need for repeat ESWL or manipulation/PCNL following treatment for proximal ureteral calculi, by group.

the success of their treatment. No correlation was found between successful treatment and previous surgery on the treated side or prior passage of stones from that system. In addition, there was no correlation with body habitus, with sex of the patient, with stone composition, with stone location (left versus right or upper versus mid-ureter), or with the presence of renal malformations. Increasing stone burden has been shown to be inversely related to successful ESWL of renal calculi (33), but stone burden did not seem to be a factor in this series of ureteral calculi. The need for a fluid interface around ureteral calculi was supported by the observation that patients whose stones were associated with minimal obstruction fared better than those with a higher degree of

obstruction (Table 24). Despite the improved results for ESWL in situ when minimal or no obstruction was present, the results still did not approach that achieved when the stone has been repositioned successfully into the kidney prior to ESWL.

Although at the MHI it is recommended that double-J ureteral stents are used to secure manipulated calculi from the kidney in anticipation of ESWL at a later date, the routine use of such stents (when ureteral calculi are successfully dislodged into the kidney immediately before ESWL) is not justified. A number of ESWL units routinely place double-J ureteral stents in this situation but such patients (group III) have extremely low morbidity and infrequently need repeat ESWL or manipulative

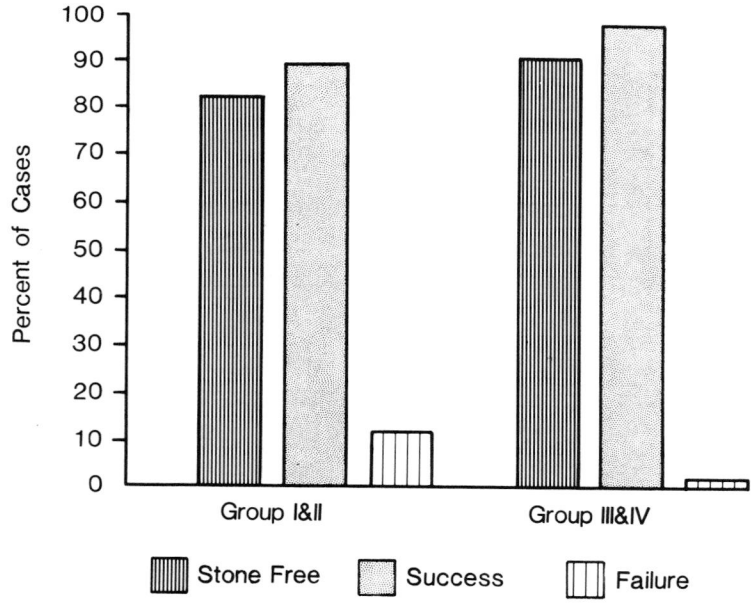

FIG. 28. Stone-free rates, success rates, and failure rates following ESWL treatment of proximal ureteral calculi. Groups I and II represent in situ treatments; groups III and IV represent treatment following successful repositioning of the ureteral calculus into the kidney.

TABLE 24. *ESWL in situ for proximal ureteral calculi: treatment results stratified by degree of obstruction[a]*

Pretreatment obstruction	No. of treatments	Additional therapy	Treatment with 3-month follow-up	3-Month treatment success[a]
None to mild	51	7 (13.7%)	35	33 (94.3%)
Moderate to severe	72	12 (16.7%)	42	34 (81.0%)

[a] $p < .001$.

procedures after treatment (Fig. 27). Since double-J stents are not without expense and morbidity (36), they should not be used following successful dislodgement unless the ureter has been perforated at the time of manipulation or unless ESWL must be delayed. However, a double-J stent should be considered for ESWL treatments in patients with a solitary kidney, in cases of known ureteral stricture, and in patients who have substantial stone burden to be treated within the kidney.

Experience at the MHI demonstrates that 86.5% of all proximal ureteral calculi can be successfully manipulated into the kidney preceding ESWL, utilizing the techniques previously described (33). Since a successful outcome after treatment may be anticipated in 99% of cases (206 of 208 patients—groups III and IV from Fig. 28) in which the ureteral stone was displaced into the kidney, retrograde stone manipulation is attempted at the MHI for all proximal ureteral calculi prior to ESWL. Such results are significantly better than those reported for ureteroscopy when used for similar stones (28,77,78). In addition, the invasiveness and morbidity of retrograde stone manipulation followed by ESWL is low compared to ureteroscopy. The rate of perforation and other trauma to the ureter is lower with retrograde manipulation alone, since dilation of ureterovesical junction and insertion of a rigid instrument into the ureter are not required. Also, ureteral avulsion is avoided. The patient's hospital stay is extremely short, and ureteral catheter drainage and/or placement of a stent are required only infrequently. Actually, ESWL in situ without manipulation achieves results comparable to the best results that have been reported for ureteroscopy (78).

The success rate for the removal of ureteral calculi percutaneously is better than for ureteroscopy of ureteral stones, with reported success rates between 88 and 94% (19,20,35). However, the morbidity of percutaneous stone extraction has been demonstrated to be significantly greater than that associated with ESWL (35). Currently, with access to ESWL being widespread, attempted retrograde stone displacement followed by ESWL is the treatment of choice for symptomatic proximal ureteral calculi.

A nomogram for the management of proximal ureteral calculi with ESWL is presented in Fig. 29. Even if the stone cannot be dislodged, it is almost always possible to pass a catheter or stent successfully beyond the stone. At the MHI, only 2.7% of 334 consecutive proximal ureteral calculi could not be displaced or bypassed with a catheter (33). If the stone cannot be dislodged and a stent is placed, ESWL in situ should be attempted since the patient already is anesthetized, and a successful outcome can be anticipated in approximately 75% of cases. If the stone does not fragment, the patient is discharged and the stent is left indwelling for 2 weeks, allowing the reaction and edema around the calculus to resolve and permitting the ureter to dilate. The stent is then removed, and stone dislodgement is again attempted. In most instances the stone easily can be dislodged and pushed back into the kidney, and ESWL can then be performed. Since ESWL in situ previously has been attempted unsuccessfully, another session of in situ treatment is unlikely to prove successful if the stone is still impacted in the ureter. In this situation (fortunately an uncommon occurrence), ureteroscopy is the least invasive alternative available. The ureteroscopic procedure will be facilitated by the ureteral dilation induced from the previously placed ureteral stent. If the stone cannot be reached with the ureteroscope, PCNL is indicated.

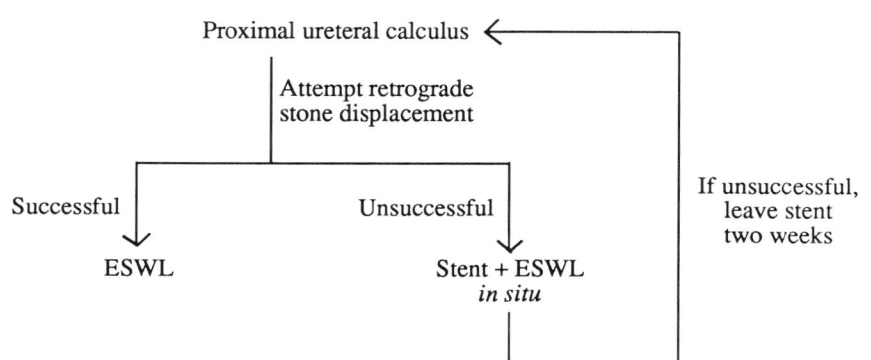

FIG. 29. Nomogram for the management of proximal ureteral calculi.

Only after all of these procedures have been attempted unsuccessfully should ureterolithotomy be considered.

Distal Ureteral Calculi

The rigid ureteroscope is ideally suited for the removal of calculi lodged in the ureter below the pelvic brim. Even when BPH or fixation of the ureter are present, it is often possible to pass a small ureteroscope far enough into the pelvic ureter to accomplish stone removal. At the MHI, the use of ureteroscopy has allowed successful removal of ureteral calculi in 98% of such calculi (79). The smaller ureteroscopes can often be negotiated through the intramural portion of the ureter with minimal or no ureteral dilation. The safety of transurethral manipulation of ureteral calculi is enhanced when the procedure can be performed under endoscopic control. For this reason the ureteroscope is used at the MHI in virtually every instance when approaching distal ureteral calculi.

Currently at the MHI, ureteroscopy is preferred over ESWL for distal ureteral calculi for the following reasons. First, the results of ureteroscopy for distal ureteral calculi are superior to those reported for ESWL (Table 25). Second, at the MHI the cost of ureteroscopy is significantly less than for ESWL (80). Third, although ESWL is a noninvasive procedure, multiple treatments are more commonly required for the treatment of distal ureteral calculi than when ureteroscopy is utilized, and the morbidity of ureteroscopy is very low, frequently allowing its performance on an outpatient basis.

The complications of ureteroscopy consist primarily of ureteral perforations and are reviewed earlier. Two patients undergoing ureteroscopy who suffered complete strictures at the ureteral orifice deserve special mention, however. In both instances, following failure to retrieve the stone, nephrostomy drainage without a stent was used to relieve obstruction, leaving the traumatized distal ureter without urine flow. In both cases, further intervention was necessary to reestablish ureteral continuity. Therefore, if the intramural ureter has been acutely dilated in the presence of proximal urinary diversion, a stent must be left in the ureter until urinary drainage is reestablished.

Distal ureteral calculi can be removed via percutaneous nephrostolithotomy in the rare instance when ureterorenoscopy and ESWL fail. Ureterolithotomy has been relegated to an almost historic status. It is an extraordinarily rare stone that cannot be removed by one of the aforementioned techniques with lower morbidity than might be anticipated with ureterolithotomy.

The Future

The current rationale at the MHI for the management of patients with ureteral calculi is influenced by the fact that ESWL (utilizing the unmodified Dornier HM3) and ureteroscopy require regional or general anesthesia. Such anesthesia requirements tend to favor treatment options that minimize the need for multiple treatments, such as combining retrograde stone displacement with ESWL. Although retrograde ureteral stone displacement, when combined with ESWL clearly reduces the need for subsequent treatment, invasiveness is increased, as is the risk, albeit slight, of ureteral perforation. As lithotripters are developed that allow ESWL under local or no anesthesia, the inconvenience and expense of ESWL treatments may be reduced. It is conceivable that for some patients the benefits of minimal or no anesthesia and of no instrumentation may outweigh the drawbacks of multiple sessions of ESWL. The balance of the equation between completely noninvasive therapy (ESWL in situ) and slightly invasive therapy (stone displacement plus ESWL) will depend on several factors. First, the efficiency of fragmentation of ureteral stones in situ by new lithotripters will be crucial. As demonstrated in the data above, higher pressures appear to be necessary to fragment some ureteral calculi. The ability of new lithotripters to allow lithotripsy with little or no anesthesia is at least partially dependent on treatment at lower pressures. In addition, the incorporation of larger ellipsoids/reflectors into most of the new lithotripters results in the shock wave intensity being less concentrated at the point of entry into the body. Although this concept also facilitates anesthesia-free treatments, this feature may be a disadvantage when treating upper ureteral calculi because the close proximity of these stones to the spine may result in a higher percentage of the shock wave en-

TABLE 25. *Results of ureteroscopy and ESWL for distal ureteral calculi (%)*

Reference	Success	Multiple treatments	Complications
Ureteroscopy			
Lingeman et al., 1990 (79)	98	2	8
Smith and Lyon, 1988 (78)	99	2	1
ESWL			
Miller and Hautmann, 1987 (41)	94	16	0
Jenkins, 1987 (30)	83	22	8
Becht et al., 1988 (87)	95	18	5

ergy being absorbed by bone. Ureteral calculi associated with minimal or no obstruction may be amenable to anesthesia-free ESWL with acceptable retreatment rates, whereas the more difficult-to-fragment, impacted calculi may have unacceptably high retreatment rates. In these cases it may remain appropriate to perform pre-ESWL displacement of the stone into the kidney despite attendant anesthetic requirements (79).

The role of ureteroscopy in the management of lower ureteral stones could also be diminished by anesthesia-free ESWL. ESWL of stones or *steinstrasse* in the lower ureter is feasible (41). Although the success rate for ESWL in situ of approximately 80% with a single session is less than that achievable with ureteroscopy, the noninvasive nature of anesthesia-free ESWL in situ may be sufficiently appealing to justify acceptance of a high retreatment rate (30).

CONCLUSIONS

The field of endourology is in its infancy, and not surprisingly, techniques and equipment continue to evolve rapidly. The techniques presented are not intended to be all inclusive; rather, they represent approaches that have been preferred at the Methodist Hospital Institute for Kidney Stone Disease and are designed to allow for the broadest application to upper urinary tract calculi, strictures, stenting, and neoplasms. Instrumentation continues to be further miniaturized and new technology (i.e., the pulsed-dye laser) continues to be developed at a bewildering rate. However, the vast majority of endourologic problems can be effectively managed with the basic instrumentation and techniques described above.

Traditional indications for open surgical procedures (pyelolithotomy, nephrolithotomy, ureterolithotomy, etc.) in the patient with urolithiasis have been significantly diminished by the advent of new techniques for kidney stone removal. Almost all upper urinary tract calculi previously requiring such procedures may now be approached with ESWL, percutaneous nephrostolithotomy, or combinations thereof. Exceptions include: first, staghorn calculi with exceedingly complex intrarenal anatomy or with true infundibular stenosis; second, patients whose physical characteristics, such as excessive obesity or severe kyphoscoliosis, might preclude positioning in a lithotripter or would prevent satisfactory percutaneous access; and third, those stone-bearing kidneys in which another indication for surgical intervention exists (i.e., UPJ obstruction).

The traditional indications (pain, infection, or obstruction) for intervention in the patient with urolithiasis have not been changed by the advent of new stone technology. However, as has been the case whenever a new, less invasive procedure has been introduced into medical practice, patients with symptoms too mild to warrant the

TABLE 26. *Indications for treatment of asymptomatic renal calculi*

Calculus affecting work status (i.e., airline pilot)
When treating a symptomatic stone with ESWL in the contralateral kidney
Multiple calyceal stones in a patient with repetitive disabling episodes of renal colic
Solitary kidney

morbidity associated with a major surgical procedure can be and should be considered for treatment with procedures associated with greatly lessened morbidity.

The potential application of ESWL to kidney stones previously thought to be nonsurgical has raised concerns about overutilization (82). The substitution of ESWL and PCNL in patients who would otherwise have been candidates for surgical procedures (as presented above) is clearly appropriate. In addition, there may exist a population of patients who previously did not have sufficient symptoms to justify the potential risks and morbidity of an open surgical procedure but appropriately may be considered for procedures with greatly lowered morbidity, lowered costs, and shorter convalescence (80,83). Many patients with calyceal stones fit into this category (84).

The application of ESWL and endourology to asymptomatic upper urinary tract calculi remains controversial. Huebner et al. documented in 1984 that almost half of "asymptomatic" calyceal renal calculi will eventually become symptomatic within two years (81). Therefore, intervention in this category of patient may be justified. Given the large potential pool of patients in this category, the impact on health care expenditures would probably be substantial; therefore, further study will be required before the routine treatment of asymptomatic calculi can be recommended. However, there are certain instances where asymptomatic stones can be and should be considered for treatment (Table 26).

The results achieved with ESWL and PCNL at the MHI provide a rational basis for choosing the most effective procedure with the lowest morbidity for the patient with upper urinary tract calculi. ESWL is the preferred method of treatment for the majority of symptomatic upper urinary tract calculi (since most of these stones are small), but ESWL centers must be prepared to provide suitable PCNL support; otherwise, the best possible results will not be achieved. Although the urologist's new armamentarium has resulted in decreased morbidity, the complexity of judgment required to treat the current urolithiasis patient has, if anything, increased.

REFERENCES

1. Rupel E, Brown R. Nephroscopy with removal of stone following nephrostomy for obstructive calculus anuria. *J Urol* 1941;46:177.

2. Trattner HR. Instrumental visualization of the renal pelvis and its communications: proposal of a new method: preliminary report. *J Urol* 1948;60:817.

3. Goodwin WE, Casey WC, Woolf W. Percutaneous trocar (needle) nephrostomy in hydronephrosis. *JAMA* 1955;157:891.

4. Fernstrom I, Johannson B. Percutaneous pyelolithotomy: a new extraction technique. *Scand J Urol Nephrol* 1976;10:257.

5. Smith AD. Foreword. *Urol Clin North Am* 1982;9:1.

6. Hepp W. *Survey of the development of shock wave lithotripsy,* Dornier Medizintechnik GmbH, September 1984.

7. Chaussy CG, ed. *Extracorporeal shock wave lithotripsy: technical concept, experimental research, and clinical application.* Basel: S. Karger, 1986.

8. Young AT, Hunter DW, Castaneda-Zuniga WR, et al. Percutaneous extraction of urinary calculi: use of the intercostal approach. *Radiology* 1985;154:633.

9. Forsyth MJ, Fuchs EF. The supracostal approach for percutaneous nephrostolithotomy. *J Urol* 1987;137:197.

10. Clayman RV, Surya A, Miller RP, et al. Percutaneous nephrolithotomy: an approach to branched and staghorn renal calculi. *JAMA* 1983;250:73.

11. Smith AD, Castaneda-Zuniga WR. Techniques for removal of kidney stones intact. In: Smith AD, Castaneda-Zuniga WR, Bronson JC, eds. *Endourology: principles and practice.* New York, Georg Thieme, 1986.

12. Alken P, Hutschenreiter G, Gunther R, et al. Percutaneous stone manipulation. *J Urol* 1981;125:463.

13. Segura JW, Patterson DE, LeRoy AJ, et al. Percutaneous removal of kidney stones: preliminary report. *Mayo Clin Proc* 1982;57:615.

14. Kahnoski RJ, Lingeman JE, Coury TA, et al. Combined percutaneous and extracorporeal shock wave lithotripsy for staghorn calculi: an alternative to anatrophic nephrolithotomy. *J Urol* 1986; 135:679.

15. Schultz PE, Hanna PM, Wein AJ, et al. Percutaneous ultrasonic lithotripsy choice of irrigant. *J Urol* 1983;130:858.

16. Clayman RV, Elbers J, Palmer JO, et al. Experimental extensive balloon dilatation of the distal ureter: immediate and long-term effects. *J Endourol* 1987;1:19.

17. Patterson DE, Segura JW, LeRoy AJ, et al. The etiology and treatment of delayed bleeding following percutaneous lithotripsy. *J Urol* 1985;133:447.

18. Brannen GE, Bush WH, Correa RJ, et al. Kidney stone removal: percutaneous v surgical lithotomy. *J Urol* 1985;133:6.

19. Reddy PK, Hulbert JC, Lange PH, et al. Percutaneous removal of renal and ureteral calculi: experience with 400 cases. *J Urol* 1985;134:662.

20. Segura JW, Patterson DE, LeRoy AJ, et al. Percutaneous removal of kidney stones: review of 1,000 cases. *J Urol* 1985;134:1077.

21. Lee WJ, Smith AD, Cubelli V, et al. Complications of percutaneous nephrostolithotomy. *AJR* 1987;148:177.

22. Winfield HN, Clayman RV. Complications of percutaneous removal of renal and ureteral calculi. *World urology update series,* vol 2, lesson 37, part I, 1985.

23. Young HH. Treatment of calculus of the lower ureter in the male. *Am Med* 1902;4:209.

24. Dourmashkin RL. Cystoscopic treatment of stones in the ureter with special reference to large calculi: based on a study of 1,550 cases. *J Urol* 1945;54:245.

25. Lyon ES, Kyker JS, Schoenberg JW. Transurethral ureteroscopy in woman: a ready addition to the urologic armamentarium. *J Urol* 1978;119:35.

26. Perez-Castro EE, Martinez-Pineiro JA. La ureterorrenoscopia transuretral: un actual proceder urologico. *Arch Esp Urol* 1980;33:445.

27. Huffman JL, Bagley DH, Lyon ES. Treatment of distal ureteral calculi using rigid ureteroscope. *Urology* 1982;20:574.

28. Lyon ES, Huffman JL, Bagley DH. Ureteroscopy and ureteral pyeloscopy. *Urology* 1984;23:29 (special issue).

29. Kaneko H, Watanabe H, Takahasi T, et al. Studies on the application of microexplosion to medicine and biopsy. IV. Strength of wet and dry urinary calculi. *Napon Hinyokika Gakkai Zasshi* 1979;70:61.

30. Jenkins AD. ESWL of ureteral stones below the pelvic brim. *Probl Urol* 1987;1:641.

31. Mueller SC, Wilbert D, Thueroff JW, et al. Extracorporeal shock wave lithotripsy of ureteral stones: clinical experience and experimental findings. *J Urol* 1986;135:831.

32. Rassweiler J, Hath U, Bub P, et al. Extracorporeal shock wave lithotripsy (ESWL) for distal ureteral calculi. *Endourology* 1986;1:15.

33. Lingeman JE, Shirrell WL, Newman DM, et al. Management of upper ureteral calculi with extracorporeal shock wave lithotripsy. *J Urol* 1987;138:720.

34. Libby JM, Meacham RB, Griffith DP. Role of silicon ureteral stents in extracorporeal shock wave lithotripsy of large renal calculi. *J Urol* 1988;139:15.

35. Lingeman JE, Coury TA, Newman DM, et al. Comparison of results and morbidity of percutaneous nephrostolithotomy and extracorporeal shock wave lithotripsy. *J Urol* 1987;138:485.

36. Pollard SG, McFarlane R. Symptoms arising from double-J ureteral stents. *J Urol* 1988;139:37.

37. Pryor JL, Jenkins AD. Use of double-J stents in extracorporeal shock wave lithotripsy. *J Urol* 1990;143:475.

38. Hockley NM, Lingeman JE, Hutchinson CL. Relative efficacy of extracorporeal shock wave lithotripsy and percutaneous nephrostolithotomy in the management of cystine calculi. *J Endourol* 1989;3:273.

39. Lingeman JE, Newman DM, Mertz JHO, et al. Extracorporeal shock wave lithotripsy: The Methodist Hospital of Indiana experience. *J Urol* 1986;135:1134.

40. Drach GW, Dretler SP, Fair WR. Report of the United States cooperative study of ESWL. *J Urol* 1986;135:1127.

41. Miller K, Hautmann R. Treatment of distal ureteral calculi with ESWL: experience with more than 100 consecutive cases. *World J Urol* 1987;5:259.

42. Vallancien C, Aviles J, Munoz R, et al. Piezoelectric extracorporeal lithotripsy by ultrashort waves with EDAP LT01 device. *J Urol* 1988;139:689.

43. Marberger M, Turk C, Steinkogler I. Painless piezoelectric extracorporeal lithotripsy. *J Urol* 1988;139:695.

44. Knapp PM, Kulb TB, Lingeman JE, et al. Extracorporeal shock wave lithotripsy induced perirenal hematomas. *J Urol* 1988;139:700.

45. Griffith DP. Infection induced stones. In: Coe FL, ed. *Nephrolithiasis: pathogenesis and treatment.* Chicago: Year Book Medical Publishers, 1978.

46. Elder JS, Gibbons RP, Bush WH. Ultrasonic lithotripsy of a large staghorn calculi. *Urology* 1984;131:1152.

47. Chaussy CG, Schmiedt E. Extracorporeal shock wave lithotripsy (ESWL) for kidney stones: an alternative to surgery? *Urol Radiol* 1984;6:80.

48. Finlayson B. Renal lithiasis in review. *Urol Clin North Am* 1974;1:181.

49. Preminger GM, Clayman RV, Hardeman SW, et al. Percutaneous nephrostolithotomy v open surgery for renal calculi. *JAMA* 1985;254:1054.

50. Clayman RV, Surya V, Miller RP, et al. Percutaneous nephrolithotomy: extraction of renal and ureteral calculi from 100 patients. *J Urol* 1984;131:868.

51. Newman DM, Scott JW, Lingeman JE. Two-year follow up of patients treated with extracorporeal shock wave lithotripsy. *J Endocrinol* 1988;2:163.

52. Psihramis KE, Dretler SP. Extracorporeal shock wave lithotripsy of calyceal diverticula calculi. *J Urol* 1987;138:707.

53. Jones JA, Lingeman JE, Steidle CP. The roles of ESWL and PCNL in the management of pyelocalyceal diverticula. *J Urol* [In press].

54. Mosbaugh PG, Newman DM, Lingeman JE, et al. Cost comparisons of the options currently available in the treatment of upper urinary tract stone disease. In: *Report of the American Urologic Association ad hoc committee to study the safety and efficacy of current technology of percutaneous and noninvasive lithotripsy.* Baltimore, May 16, 1985.

55. Chaussy C, Schuller J, Schmiedt E, et al. Extracorporeal shock wave lithotripsy (ESWL) for treatment of urolithiasis. *Urology* 1984;23:59.

56. Riehle R, Fair WR, Vaughan ED. Extracorporeal shock wave lithotripsy for upper urinary tract calculi. *JAMA* 1986;255:2043.

57. Boyce WH. Surgery of urinary calculi in perspective. *Urol Clin North Am* 1983;10:585.

58. Rous SN, Turner WR. Retrospective study of 95 patients with staghorn calculus disease. *J Urol* 1977;118:902.
59. Blandy JP, Singh M. The case for a more aggressive approach to staghorn stones. *J Urol* 1976;115:505.
60. Patterson DE, Segura JW, LeRoy AJ. Long-term follow up of patients treated by percutaneous ultrasonic lithotripsy for struvite staghorn calculi. *J Endourol* 1987;1:177.
61. Segura JW, Erickson SB, Wilson et al. Infected renal lithiasis: results of long-term surgical and medical management. In: Smith LH, Robertson WG, Finlayson B, eds. *Urolithiasis: clinical and basic research.* New York: Plenum Press, 1981.
62. Assimos DG, Boyce WH, Harrison LH, et al. The role of open stone surgery since extracorporeal shock wave lithotripsy. *J Urol* 1989;142:263.
63. Boyce WH, Elkins IB. Reconstructive renal surgery following anatrophic nephrolithotomy: follow up of 100 consecutive cases. *J Urol* 1974;111:307.
64. Wickham JEA, Coe N, Ward JP. One hundred cases of nephrolithotomy under hypothermia. *J Urol* 1974;112:702.
65. Harrison LH, Assimos DG. Anatrophic nephrolithotomy. In: Harrison LH, Kandel LB, eds. *Techniques in urologic stone surgery.* Mount Kisco, NY: Futura Publishing Co., 1986.
66. Stubbs AJ, Resnick MI, Boyce WH. Anatrophic nephrolithotomy in the solitary kidney. *J Urol* 1978;119:457.
67. Boyce WH. Nephrolithotomy. In: Glenn JF, ed. *Urologic surgery,* 3rd ed. Philadelphia: JB Lippincott, 1983.
68. Chaussy C, Schmiedt E, Jocham D, et al. First clinical experience with extracorporeally induced destruction of kidney stones by shock waves. *J Urol* 1982;127:417.
69. Chaussy C, Schmiedt E. Shock wave treatment for stones in the upper urinary tract. *Urol Clin North Am* 1983;10:743.
70. Winfield HN, Clayman RV, Chaussy CG, et al. Monotherapy of staghorn renal calculi: comparative study between percutaneous nephrolithotomy and extracorporeal shock wave lithotripsy. *J Urol* 1988;139:895.
71. Segura JW, Patterson DE, LeRoy AJ, et al. Percutaneous removal of staghorn calculi: review of 86 cases. *J Urol* 1985;133:182A(abstr).
72. Foley FEB. Management of ureteral stone. *JAMA* 1935;104:13.
73. Hughes J. Ureterolithotomy. In: Glenn JF, ed. *Urologic surgery,* 3rd ed. Philadelphia: JB Lippincott, 1983.
74. Koontz WW, Klein FA, Smith MJV. Surgery of the ureter. In: Walsh PC, Gittes RB, Perlmutter AD, et al., eds. *Campbell's urology,* 5th ed. Philadelphia: WB Saunders, 1986.
75. Ueno A, Kawamura T, Ogawa A, et al. Relation of spontaneous passage of ureteral calculi to size. *Urology* 1977;10:544.
76. Carstensen HE, Hansen TS. Stones in the ureter. *Acta Chir Scand Suppl* 1973;433:66.
77. Lingeman JE, Sonda LP, Kahnoski RJ, et al. Ureteral stone management: emerging concepts. *J Urol* 1986;135:1172.
78. Smith FL, Lyon E. Eleven years of ureteroscopy: the University of Chicago experience. *J Urol* 1988;139:474A (abstr).
79. Lingeman JE, Saint R, Newman DM, et al. Management of ureteral calculi: current and future concepts. *J Urol* 1990; 143:247A(abstr).
80. Lingeman JE, Saywell RM, Woods JR, et al. Cost analysis of extracorporeal shock wave lithotripsy relative to other surgical and nonsurgical treatment alternatives for urolithiasis. *Med Care* 1986;24:1151.
81. Huebner W, Haschek H, Schramek P. Der Kelchstein: Verlaufskontrolle bei 63 patienten ueber 1-21 jahre. *Verh Detsch Ges Urol* 36 Tagung, 1984;3:6.
82. Mulley AG. Shock wave lithotripsy: assessing a slam-bang technology (editorial). *N Engl J Med* 1986;314:845.
83. Lingeman JE, Woods JR, Toth PD, et al. The role of lithotripsy and its side effects. *J Urol* 1989;141:793.
84. Coury TA, Sonda LP, Lingeman JE, et al. Treatment of painful calyceal stones. *Urology* 1988;32:119.
85. Lingeman JE, Smith LH, Woods JR, et al. Staghorn calculi. In: *Urinary calculi: ESWL, endourology, and medical therapy.* Philadelphia: Lea & Febiger, 1989;chap 3.2:163.
86. Vallancien G, Capdeville R, Viellon B, et al. Colonic perforation during percutaneous nephrostomy. *J Urol* 1985;134:1185.
87. Becht E, Moll V, Neisius D, et al. Treatment of prevesical ureteral calculi by extracorporeal shock wave lithotripsy. *J Urol* 1988;139:916.

CHAPTER 31

Primary Hyperparathyroidism as a Cause of Calcium Nephrolithiasis

Aaron Halabe and Roger A. L. Sutton

HISTORICAL ASPECTS

The early history of the discovery of the parathyroid glands and of their role in the regulation of the plasma calcium concentration has been reviewed by several authors (1,2). Owen published the first description of the glands in the Indian rhinocerus in 1862, and named them the parathyroids (3). Salvesen (4) is credited with establishing the relationship of the parathyroid glands to calcium metabolism in 1923. Collip (5) produced a clean, potent parathyroid extract in 1925 with which Albright and Ellsworth in 1929 (6) demonstrated the hypercalcemic and hypophosphatemic effects. Von Recklinghausen (7) had recognized osteitis fibrosis cystica generalisata in 1891. Askanazy in 1903 (8) noted the association of bone disease with a tumor in the neck, initially identified as of thyroid origin, but later suggested to be parathyroid (9), and Erdheim (10) erroneously concluded in 1907 that the parathyroid lesion was a secondary, compensatory response to bone disease. The first parathyroidectomy for hyperparathyroidism with osteosis fibrosa cystica was performed by Mandl in Vienna in 1926 (11), after he had first unsuccessfully tried parathyroid extract followed by autologous parathyroid transplants as treatment. Albright and associates (12) recognized in 1929 that hypercalcemia was a consistent feature of primary hyperparathyroidism (PHP).

Barr and Bulger in 1930 (13) were probably first to recognize an association of nephrolithiasis with primary hyperparathyroidism, although Mandl had noted that his patient's urine caked the walls of the glass container,

and earlier patients had been described with bone disease and renal calculi (1,14).

The group at the Massachusetts General Hospital, including Aub, Bauer, and Albright, soon recognized that hyperparathyroidism with severe osteitis fibrosa cystica represented the end stage of chemical events predictable from the action of parathyroid hormone, and by 1937 had recognized that primary hyperparathyroidism might present either with renal stones or with bone disease. Albright and colleagues discovered many cases of primary hyperparathyroidism among patients with renal stones at the Massachusetts General Hospital at a time when the disease was generally thought to be rare (15).

INCIDENCE OF RENAL CALCULI IN PRIMARY HYPERPARATHYROIDISM

The incidence of renal stones among patients with diagnosed primary hyperparathyroidism has progressively decreased since the condition was first recognized. Albright and Reifenstein reported an incidence of 80% of renal calculi among their patients (16). They also appreciated that many patients had neither bone nor stone disease. Broadus (17) summarized the results of nine studies published between 1961 and 1979 reporting an incidence of stones in patients with primary hyperparathyroidism between 39 and 78%, with an average of 55%. More recently, as the diagnosis of primary hyperparathyroidism has become more frequent in consequence of the more widespread determination of the serum calcium concentration, the incidence of bone and stone disease has fallen sharply to less than 10% of diagnosed cases (18,19). At the same time, primary hyperparathyroidism is now being discovered in as many as 25 per 100,000 population per year, or in older women, the group at greatest risk, as many as 188 per 100,000 per year (18).

A. Halabe: Metabolic Unit, Belinson Medical Center, Petach-Tikua, Israel.

R. A. L. Sutton: Department of Medicine, Vancouver General Hospital, Vancouver, British Columbia, Canada, V5Z 4E3.

While the incidence of stones among diagnosed cases of primary hyperparathyroidism has decreased, the incidence of primary hyperparathyroidism among patients with renal calculi has remained in the range 2–13% between 1960 and 1988 (17,20–22). Although the incidence of primary hyperparathyroidism among patients with renal calculi is therefore relatively low, this remains an important diagnosis to make among these patients, since further stone formation can frequently be prevented by appropriate treatment of primary hyperparathyroidism.

CLINICAL PICTURE

Calcium nephrolithiasis associated with primary hyperparathyroidism is generally clinically indistinguishable from other varieties of calcium nephrolithiasis. Occasional patients may have other clinical manifestations of primary hyperparathyroidism, such as peptic ulcer, symptoms of hypercalcemia, pancreatitis, and so on, but more commonly these patients have no clinical manifestations other than renal calculi. The renal stones may be unilateral or bilateral, single or multiple, and may cause pain, infection, or hematuria. In addition to stones within the collecting system, primary hyperparathyroidism may cause nephrocalcinosis. Although nephrocalcinosis and renal calculi may occur together, several authors have pointed out that nephrocalcinosis is more commonly seen in patients with renal impairment and osteitis fibrosa than in patients with simple nephrolithiasis (23).

Medullary sponge kidney (MSK) may coexist with renal calculi and hyperparathyroidism (24–27). The nature of the association between hyperparathyroidism and MSK is not clear. Only limited data are available on the incidence of primary hyperparathyroidism in MSK. Maschio et al. (27) reported 7 cases of MSK among 28 with surgically proven primary hyperparathyroidism. Parks et al. (28) studied 799 stone patients (175 females, 624 males) in whom 33 females and 73 males had MSK. From the total of 106 MSK patients, two (<2%) had primary hyperparathyroidism, and both were women. The authors did not find a higher frequency of primary hyperparathyroidism among their patients with MSK than in other calcium stone formers. These data are similar to those reported previously by the same authors (21).

The calculi in primary hyperparathyroidism consist of calcium salts of phosphate and/or oxalate (29). Several authors have reported that there is a higher incidence of calcium phosphate relative to calcium oxalate in primary hyperparathyroidism than in idiopathic calcium stones (30,31). However, the majority of stones, even in primary hyperparathyroidism, consist of calcium oxalate (21). As in other calcium stone formers, the urinary tract of patients with primary hyperparathyroidism may become secondarily infected with urea-splitting organisms, and as a result they may form mixed stones consisting largely of struvite.

The biochemical hallmark of the stone patient with primary hyperparathyroidism is hypercalcemia, which is commonly mild but may be moderate or severe. Although there are other causes of hypercalcemia associated with renal calculi, such as sarcoidosis or vitamin D intoxication, primary hyperparathyroidism is overwhelmingly the commonest cause. The hypercalcemia is most often relatively mild, and may be intermittent, and hence it is recommended that patients with calcium stones have the serum calcium determined carefully (preferably fasting and without venous stasis) on at least two occasions. Where the total serum calcium level is borderline, it may be helpful, in addition, to obtain an ionized calcium determination, which may on occasion clearly identify a patient as having true hypercalcemia (32,33). Problems in the diagnosis of primary hyperparathyroidism are considered further in a later section.

CLINICAL PRESENTATION OF PRIMARY HYPERPARATHYROIDISM

The clinical presentation of primary hyperparathyroidism can be quite varied, and several hypotheses have been proposed to account for these different clinical presentations. Albright, recognizing that the condition may be present with or without bone disease, proposed that bone disease might be more likely to develop in patients with an inadequate calcium intake that might predispose them to a negative overall calcium balance (16). Patients with nephrolithiasis commonly have an elevated urinary calcium excretion but are usually in normal overall calcium balance, the hypercalciuria being offset by enhanced net intestinal calcium absorption. Dent and colleagues (34), following up on Albright's hypothesis of different calcium intakes, surveyed the dietary calcium intakes of their patients and found no differences between patients with and without bone disease. Dent proposed that the parathyroid glands might produce two hormones, one causing hypercalcemia and the other acting on the bone and engendering nephrocalcinosis and azotemia. It is now known, however, that all of the actions of parathyroid hormone are produced by the 1 to 84 polypeptide hormone. Lloyd (35) undertook a retrospective analysis of 138 cases of primary hyperparathyroidism collected by Dent. Lloyd found that there were two groups of cases, those with large tumors, more marked hypercalcemia, less hypercalciuria, less stone disease, and more bone disease. The second group had smaller tumors, less marked hypercalcemia, more marked hypercalciuria, more stone disease, and very little osteitis fibrosa cystica. This analysis suggested that the tumors associated with bone disease tended to be more rapidly growing, larger, and more aggressive, while those associated with stone disease were smaller, less active, and more indolent.

Peacock (36) studied intestinal calcium absorption in 111 patients with primary hyperparathyroidism, including 63 patients with renal stone disease. The patients with stone disease showed, as a group, a striking hyperabsorption of calcium, whereas the patients without renal stone disease had a significantly lower calcium absorption. Urinary calcium excretion correlated positively with intestinal calcium absorption. Peacock concluded that the action of parathyroid hormone (PTH) on the gut (perhaps through vitamin D metabolism) resulted in intestinal calcium hyperabsorption in the patients with stone disease, who showed minimal changes in bone resorption, while patients without stone disease who did not hyperabsorb calcium tended to develop bone disease with increased bone resorption and osteopenia. Peacock suggested that the latter patients represent a failure of PTH to act on the gut, probably through its action on vitamin D metabolism.

A recent study from Paris by Patron et al. (37) has confirmed and extended the observations of Peacock. These authors studied 102 patients with primary hyperparathyroidism, including 33 with recurrent stones, 60 with nonspecific symptoms, and 9 with overt bone disease. They determined PTH, 25-hydroxyvitamin D [25(OH)D], and 1,25-dihydroxyvitamin D (calcitriol) levels as well as urinary nephrogenous cyclic AMP levels, and the calciuric response to an oral calcium load. The key results are summarized in Table 1. The three groups of patients did not differ significantly with respect to serum total calcium concentration. The patients with bone disease had significantly higher PTH levels, higher nephrogenous cyclic AMP excretions, lower glomerular filtration rates, lower 25(OH)D levels, and lower calci-

triol levels, as well as diminished calciuric responses to the oral calcium load in comparison with the other groups. By contrast, the patients with renal calculi were characterized by a greater calciuric response to the oral calcium load, normal 25(OH)D levels, higher calcitriol levels, higher glomerular filtration rates, and a lower mean age than the non-stone-forming groups.

These data appear to have finally clarified the reasons for the different clinical presentations of primary hyperparathyroidism. The presentation with renal calculi appears to be associated with increased intestinal calcium absorption, a consequence of elevated calcitriol levels. Those patients who achieve higher calcitriol levels tend to be younger and to have better renal function (higher glomerular filtration rates) as well as a more plentiful supply of the substrate, 25(OH)D. Of particular interest, in this group of patients from Paris, 4 of the 9 patients with bone disease were immigrants from North Africa with low estimated vitamin D intakes who stayed at home and avoided sunlight. Patron et al. note that PTH levels were higher in the patients with bone disease, and they make the interesting suggestion that the lower calcitriol levels in this group would not exert a tonic suppression of PTH release to the same extent as in the stone patients with higher calcitriol levels.

More recently, Patron et al. (38) have reported that the intravenous administration of calcitriol resulted in a marked suppression of the PTH level in a patient with primary hyperparathyroidism and osteitis fibrosa cystica, not attributable to changes in plasma calcium levels, providing direct evidence in support of the hypothesis that lower calcitriol levels may engender more severe hypersecretion of PTH. In this discussion, bone disease refers to patients with overt, radiologically apparent osteitis fibrosa cystica. Using the more sensitive techniques of bone densitometry and bone biopsy, Silverberg et al. (39) found that over 80% of 52 patients without radiological osteitis fibrosa cystica had a cortical width below the

TABLE 1. *Characteristics of patients with different clinical presentations of primary hyperparathyroidism*[a]

Groups of patients	25(OH)D (nmol/L)	NcAMP (nmol/dL GF)	iPTH (pg/mL)	Serum phosphorus (mmol/L)	1,25(OH)$_2$D$_3$ (pmol/L)	Calciuric response to oral load of 1 g calcium (μmol/dL GF)	Fasting calciuria (μmol/dL GF)
I. Renal stone (n = 33)	44	4.2***	110	0.73***	222***	7.04***	4.81***
p value (I vs. II)	<.05	NS	NS	NS	<.001	<.001	NS
II. Nonspecific symptoms (n = 60)	28	4.2***	119	0.76***	157*	4.00	5.03***
p value (II vs. III)	<.05	<.001	<.001	<.01	<.01	<.05	NS
III. Bone disease (n = 9)	8.5**	12.0***	328	0.60***	83	0.77*	7.04***
p value (III vs. I)	<.001	<.001	<.001	<.05	<.001	<.001	NS
Normal subjects (n = 40)	33	1.28	<76	1.06 (n = 18)	101	3.8	1.75 (n = 18)

Source: Patron et al. (38).

[a] Values are means (SD omitted). Significance of the differences between values for a group and values for the normal subjects; * = $p < .05$; ** = $p < .01$, *** = $p < .001$. NS, not significant.

mean, while over 80% had a cancellous bone volume above the mean. Radial (cortical) density averaged 79% of the expected value. Thus these techniques are able to demonstrate skeletal abnormalities in many of the patients in the category "without bone disease."

PATHOGENESIS OF STONES

Hypercalciuria

Hypercalciuria, which characterizes the group of patients with primary hyperparathyroidism who present with renal stones, has been assumed to be a major risk factor in the pathogenesis of the stones. The characteristic combination, however, of mild (often minimal) hypercalcemia with marked hypercalciuria has caused considerable interest, particularly in view of the direct effect of PTH to enhance renal tubular calcium reabsorption (40–42). Broadus (17) reviewed the conflicting data on urinary calcium excretion in primary hyperparathyroidism with renal calculi. He noted that in early studies, patients were frequently studied on a restricted dietary calcium intake, and under these circumstances patients with primary hyperparathyroidism frequently did not have striking hypercalciuria. By contrast, the use of a high-normal calcium intake brings out more clearly features related to increased intestinal calcium absorption (43,44). The latter studies employed a calcium load test in which, following an oral load containing 1000 mg of elemental calcium, the calcemic response, the calciuric response, and the degree of parathyroid supressibility as assessed by reduction in nephrogenous cyclic AMP were examined.

In 50 patients with primary hyperparathyroidism a highly significant positive correlation was seen between the calciuric response and the baseline serum calcitriol level; also, the 24-h urine calcium excretion was strongly correlated with serum calcitriol levels. The patients were subdivided into those who showed an abnormal calciuric response to the calcium tolerance test [greater than 0.20 mg of calcium per 100 mL of glomerular filtration (GF)] or a normal response (less than 0.20 mg of calcium per 100 mL of GF). The patients with the abnormal calciuric response exhibited higher calcitriol levels and a higher incidence of stones as well as a higher 24-h urinary calcium excretion. Fasting calcium excretion was not different between the two groups. In this study the reason for the higher calcitriol levels in the hypercalciuric group was not clear. PTH, glomerular filtration rate (GFR), age, and 25(OH)D levels were not different between the two groups. With respect to parathyroid suppression, patients with abnormal hypercalciuria showed a greater calcemic response and a greater suppression of nephrogenous cyclic AMP (cAMP). A suppression of nephrogenous cAMP was also seen on increasing the dietary calcium intake from 400 to 1000

mg/day, indicating that parathyroid responsiveness is likely to be of physiological importance in primary hyperparathyroidism. In summary, the studies of Broadus indicated that patients with renal calculi are characterized by increased intestinal absorption of calcium, a greater calcemic response, greater parathyroid suppression, and therefore greater urinary calcium excretion than patients without calculi. These data of Broadus are somewhat in conflict with the data of Pak et al. (45) in which patients with primary hyperparathyroidism were divided into those with and without renal calculi, and no difference in mean serum calcitriol levels was found.

In the studies of Patron et al. (37) discussed above, calcitriol levels were higher in patients with calculi than in those with osteitis fibrosa cystica, and this appeared to be related to better renal function and higher 25(OH)D levels. The determinants of calcitriol levels in primary hyperparathyroidism have been examined in other studies. Hulter et al. (46) gave intravenous PTH continuously to normal human subjects, sufficient to induce moderate hypercalcemia and hypophosphatemia, and observed a decrease in plasma calcitriol levels. In experiments in dogs, these authors showed that a similar reduction in plasma calcitriol concentration was not seen if the hypercalcemia was prevented during PTH infusion by simultaneous EGTA infusion. In the latter animals PTH resulted in a sustained increase in the plasma calcitriol concentration. These data suggested that hypercalcemia can prevent and even reverse the elevated calcitriol level associated with chronic hypersecretion of PTH.

It is of interest to note that patients with primary hyperparathyroidism and renal calculi typically have only minimally elevated plasma calcium levels, which would therefore have little action to attenuate the rise in calcitriol levels produced by increased PTH secretion. Lo Cascio et al. (47) administered 25(OH)D 50 μg daily for a month to normal volunteers and to patients with primary hyperparathyroidism. In the normal subjects calcitriol levels did not increase, whereas in the patients with primary hyperparathyroidism a sharp increase in calcitriol occurred, and 25(OH)D and calcitriol levels were significantly positively correlated. Thus, as concluded by Patron et al. (37), in patients with primary hyperparathyroidism, unlike normal subjects, calcitriol levels are dependent on the supply of the precursor 25(OH)D.

Although the observations above help to explain the occurrence of hypercalciuric hyperparathyroidism with minimal hypercalcemia, occasional patients are actually normocalcemic. Gardin and Paillard (48) examined a group of patients with primary hyperparathyroidism and found that the degree of hypercalcemia was not correlated with either PTH or nephrogenous cyclic AMP levels. Examination of the relationship between urinary calcium excretion and serum calcium level, however, showed that tubular reabsorption of calcium was increased in the hypercalcemic patients but was normal or subnormal in the patients with normal serum calcium levels. These data suggest that the main determinant of the plasma calcium value in primary hyperparathyroidism is the tubular reabsorption of calcium. Since differences in PTH levels did not account for the differences in tubular calcium reabsorption, these authors suggested that undetermined factors must interfere with the tubular action of PTH in normocalcemic patients. After correction of hyperparathyroidism, fasting hypercalciuria and intestinal calcium absorption return to normal, indicating that these patients were not suffering from preexisting "renal hypercalciuria" (49). Data from experiments in the hamster (50), a species that shows unusual sensitivity to the hypocalciuric effect of PTH, showed that under certain circumstances calcitriol appears to antagonize the effect of PTH on renal tubular calcium reabsorption. These data are difficult to reconcile with those of Yamamoto et al. showing that repletion of vitamin D–depleted rats with vitamin D enhanced tubular calcium reabsorption (51). It is possible, however, that exogenous calcitriol, or supraphysiological levels, might interact in some manner with PTH to promote hypercalciuria.

Insulin and growth hormone may lead to hypercalciuria by enhancing intestinal calcium absorption (52,53). Insulin also has a direct calciuric action (54). Patients with primary hyperparathyroidism and urolithiasis may have abnormal glucose metabolism and hyperinsulinemia (55–57) due to sustained endogenous insulin resistance (58). Although these hormonal abnormalities are not known to cause renal stones, it is possible that they might contribute to the hypercalciuria in primary hyperparathyroidism.

Although hypercalciuria is not a direct effect of PTH, as discussed above, it is commonly observed in primary hyperparathyroidism. Several constituents of a normal diet may enhance the risk of stone formation. Urinary calcium excretion is induced by a diet rich in proteins (59,60). An increase in urinary uric acid excretion (61) and a decrease in urinary pH (62), both potential contributors to stone formation, also result from increased protein intake. A calciuric response to carbohydrate ingestion has also been reported by Lemann et al. (63) and Tschope et al. (64). Increased salt intake increases calcium excretion even in normal people (65). Muldowney et al. (66) showed that a decrease in sodium excretion from 177 mEq/day to 73 mEq/day was associated with a significant decrease in calcium excretion from 384 mEq/day to 278 mg/day. Although the studies above indicate that dietary factors may contribute to the production of hypercalciuria, it is not certain whether stone formation in primary hyperparathyroidism may be influenced by these dietary factors.

Factors Other Than Hypercalciuria

In addition to hypercalciuria, several other factors have been suggested as being contributory to calcium stone formation in primary hyperparathyroidism. These include the presence of renal tubular acidosis, hyperuricosuria, changes in urine pH, and changes in quantities of various inhibitors or promoters of stone formation.

With respect to renal tubular acidosis, a mild hyperchloremic metabolic acidosis has been noted in patients with primary hyperparathyroidism and has been attributed to the inhibition of proximal bicarbonate reabsorption by PTH (67,68). However, this mechanism could only account for a proximal renal tubular acidosis, which, unlike distal renal tubular acidosis, is usually not associated with renal calculi or nephrocalcinosis (69). Furthermore, the degree of hyperchloremic metabolic acidosis is mild and variable in primary hyperparathyroidism. The issue of whether chronic PTH hypersecretion does lead to metabolic acidosis has been addressed in a number of studies. Hulter and Peterson (70) showed only a mild transient renal acidosis followed by sustained mild alkalosis associated with increased hydrogen ion excretion. Bichara et al. (71) recently confirmed in the rat that PTH caused an increase in net acid excretion, with enhanced reabsorption of bicarbonate in Henle's loop counterbalancing the inhibition in the proximal tubule. Thus renal tubular acidosis appears to be an unlikely cause of the stone forming tendency in primary hyperparathyroidism. A major factor in renal tubular acidosis leading to calcium stone formation is hypocitraturia. Although Smith et al. (72) reported a reduction in urinary citrate in patients with primary hyperparathyroidism and active stone disease in contrast to patients without stone disease, other investigators have not noted an abnormal citrate excretion in primary hyperparathyroidism.

Although hyperuricosuria is an important risk factor in the formation of calcium oxalate stones, there is no convincing evidence that urinary uric acid excretion is elevated in patients with primary hyperparathyroidism. Ljunghall and Akerstrom (73) have reported a positive correlation between 24-h uric acid excretion and serum calcium in primary hyperparathyroidism, which disappeared after parathyroidectomy. Broulik et al. (74) examined urate clearance in 25 hyperparathyroid patients and control subjects. This study showed that hyperparathyroid patients have a lower urate clearance than healthy controls. From these studies we can conclude that hyperuricosuria is not an important risk factor for stone formation in primary hyperparathyroidism.

With respect to other inhibitors and promoters of stone formation, Pak and Holt (75) studied the nucleation and growth of brushite and calcium oxalate in urinary stone formers and found an increased activity product ratio of brushite and calcium oxalate in the urine of patients with primary hyperparathyroidism compared with that of normal subjects, attributable to the hypercalciuria. The formation product ratio for brushite and calcium oxalate was lower in synthetic solutions (devoid of inhibitors of nucleation) than in primary hyperparathyroidism and in other stone formers, suggesting the possibility of the presence of promoters of nucleation. In addition, crystal growth of brushite and calcium oxalate was significantly enhanced in primary hyperparathyroidism but not in idiopathic stone formers, suggesting the possibility of a promoter of crystal growth in primary hyperparathyroidism.

Koide et al. (76) have recently compared the effect of normal urine and urine from patients with primary hyperparathyroidism and renal calculi in promoting calcium oxalate crystal growth and aggregation. Whereas normal urine did not differ from distilled water in terms of the resulting crystals, urine from primary hyperparathyroid patients resulted in the formation of crystals of a larger size distribution which, on microscopic examination, proved to be mainly due to crystal aggregation. These data suggest that the urine of patients with primary hyperparathyroidism contains either a promoter of crystal aggregation or a blocker of the inhibitors of aggregation present in normal healthy urine.

Another factor in primary hyperparathyroidism that may render the normal inhibitors less effective than usual may be the recently demonstrated effect of hypercalciuria to influence the urinary inhibitory activity against calcium oxalate precipitation. Zerwekh et al. (77) gave calcium supplements of 600 mg/day to 11 patients with nephrolithiasis and demonstrated a significant fall in the urinary inhibitory activity against calcium oxalate precipitation, as indicated by a decline in the formation product ratio. In subsequent in vitro studies the influence of calcium on the activities of citrate, chondroitin sulfate, and naturally occurring macromolecular inhibitors was examined. The authors concluded that hypercalciuria can attenuate the inhibitory activities of citrate and chondroitin sulfate against calcium oxalate precipitation, while at the same time accentuating the inhibitory activity of the naturally occurring macromolecular inhibitors. The final outcome will depend on which inhibitors exert a dominant role in a particular patient.

PROBLEMS OF DIAGNOSIS OF PRIMARY HYPERPARATHYROIDISM WITH STONES

In patients presenting with renal stones consisting of calcium oxalate and/or calcium phosphate, the recognition of underlying primary hyperparathyroidism usually hinges on the demonstration of hypercalcemia. With the general availability of precise methods for determination of total serum calcium, and with appropriate allowance

for variations in serum albumin or serum protein concentrations, the diagnosis of hypercalcemia is generally straightforward. Although there are numerous causes of hypercalcemia, primary hyperparathyroidism is by far the most common cause among patients with renal calculi, particularly in patients in whom the hypercalcemia has been known to be present for a long time. In this regard old records may be helpful. Serum phosphate levels are of limited importance but tend to be lower in patients with hypercalcemia mediated either by PTH or by the PTH-like peptide produced by solid tumors than in vitamin D–mediated hypercalcemia or in milk-alkali syndrome or hematologic malignancies. Determination of 24-h urinary calcium is of little diagnostic value in the patient with renal calculi and primary hyperparathyroidism. However, it is important in the asymptomatic hypercalcemic patient in whom familial hypocalciuric hypercalcemia is a consideration.

Difficulties with the identification of primary hyperparathyroidism among stone formers relate largely to patients with normocalcemia or intermittent hypercalcemia. Among these patients the main differential diagnosis is idiopathic hypercalciuria. Henneman et al. explored the necks of many of their early patients to determine that they did not have primary hyperparathyroidism (78).

Although the existence of normocalcemic primary hyperparathyroidism has been disputed (79), many authors have agreed that it can occur (48,80–82). Hypercalcemia may be masked by vitamin D deficiency or magnesium deficiency, but such patients usually do not present with renal calculi. As discussed above, it is typical of patients with primary hyperparathyroidism and renal calculi that the hypercalcemia is mild and it may be intermittent. It is rarely persistently absent. Broadus (17) suggests that the diagnosis should be considered in patients demonstrating a mean total serum calcium greater than 10.0 mg/dL (2.5 mM) on three determinations performed under fasting conditions with minimal venous stasis.

Although the hypercalcemia may be intermittent, evidence of parathyroid overactivity in the form of elevated PTH or urinary cAMP levels is persistent. Abnormal parathyroid suppressibility can also be demonstrated (83) and calcitriol levels may be elevated. Attempts to develop provocative tests using thiazide or vitamin D have been relatively unsuccessful. None of these tests has proved to be reliable.

Use of the serum ionized calcium provides a further refinement in the diagnosis of hypercalcemia (32,33). Recent improvements in ionized calcium electrodes have made the method simpler and more widely available.

Parathyroid hormone assays have been available for a number of years, and originally antisera directed against the carboxyterminal end of the PTH molecule proved to be the most useful in clinical practice (84). Subsequently,

N-terminal assays were developed and refined and appeared to give somewhat improved results. More recently, immunoradiometric (IRMA) assays against intact PTH have become commercially available and appear to represent a further improvement in diagnosing borderline primary hyperparathyroidism (85).

The measurement of urinary cAMP (82,86) provided useful information at a time when PTH assays were less well developed, but at the present time they have a limited role in the diagnosis of primary hyperparathyroidism. Suppression tests add useful information to static measurements: for example, the oral calcium tolerance test as used by Broadus et al. With this test (43,83) patients with primary hyperparathyroidism exhibit abnormal hypercalcemia following the calcium load, together with abnormal (decreased) suppression of nephrogenous cyclic AMP (and presumably also PTH).

SURGICAL TREATMENT

First Exploration

The definitive treatment for primary hyperparathyroidism is surgery. Active stone disease is one of the specific indications for surgery. Surgery should be undertaken by an experienced parathyroid surgeon who will usually attempt to identify all four glands even if the enlarged parathyroid has been localized preoperatively by one of the new noninvasive methods. With an experienced surgeon and pathologist, a success rate as high as 95% has been reported for a first parathyroid operation (87). However, Lafferty and Hubay (88), Sivula and Ronni-Sivula (89), and Palmér et al. (90–92) have recently reported higher rates of persistent or recurrent hypercalcemia (5.4, 8.9, and 13%, respectively) after parathyroidectomy. Failure to locate the abnormal gland has been reported at around 3%, whereas recurrent hyperparathyroidism (i.e., hypercalcemia developing after at least 1 year of normocalcemia following surgery) was observed in 4.4%.

Although the diagnosis of primary hyperparathyroidism is established prior to surgery, the pathology of the parathyroid disorder (whether adenoma, hyperplasia, or carcinoma) is generally made only during surgery. In identifying hyperfunctioning parathyroid tissue, some pathologists advocate the use of fat stains because intracellular fat is absent or markedly decreased in 90% of adenomatous and hyperplastic parathyroid glands.

Preoperative imaging to localize hyperfunctioning parathyroid tissue is not essential in a patient undergoing an initial exploration. The role of noninvasive techniques such as ultrasound examination of the neck (93,94) or double-tracer subtraction scanning (95) under these circumstances is controversial (96). Successful localization using these methods may result in a shorten-

ing of the operation time and therefore in reduced morbidity. In addition, intrathyroid adenomas that might otherwise be overlooked may also be localized (97).

The operative strategy is to identify four or more parathyroid gland(s). Paloyan et al. (98) initially removed only the adenoma but then changed to the removal of $3\frac{1}{2}$ glands because of the high rate of recurrence of hyperparathyroidism. In 1973 the policy was modified again, leaving half of each of two normal glands in the neck at surgery. In 292 patients in whom this approach was used during the period 1965–1981, 97.6% were cured by the first operation and only 1% had long-term hypoparathyroidism. A reasonable alternative approach in patients with adenoma is to remove the enlarged gland and biopsy one of the apparently normal gland(s) (99) while preserving the remaining normal glands in the neck. There is still controversy about the best surgical management of a parathyroid adenoma. Although those advocating the conservative approach of removing an adenoma and inspecting the remaining parathyroid glands point to a very low rate of postoperative hypocalcemia (100,101), these studies involve a short follow-up of less than 1 year, which may lead to underestimation not only of permanent hypoparathyroidism but also of recurrent hypercalcemia.

In patients with hyperplasia of all four glands, some surgeons recommend the removal of $3\frac{1}{2}$ glands, leaving the equivalent of one normal and well-vascularized gland (40 mg), while others advocate total parathyroidectomy with autotransplantation of multiple 1-mm³ parathyroid fragments into the patient's forearm muscle. Patients who are known to have multiple endocrine neoplasia, in which parathyroid hyperplasia is the usual finding, should have a total parathyroidectomy with autotransplantation, or if autotransplantation is not available, excision of $3\frac{3}{4}$ glands. In cases where more extensive dissections and biopsies are undertaken, there is an increased risk of short- and long-term damage to the residual parathyroids and also to the recurrent laryngeal nerves. Transplantation of adenomatous tissue is not recommended because of the tendency of this tissue to grow and to present problems with recurrent hypercalcemia.

The complications of parathyroid surgery from five studies in the literature are presented in Table 2. Studies of Lafferty and Hubay (88), Sivula and Ronni-Sivula (89), and Palmér et al. (91,92) with a 5.3- to 7.7-year mean follow-up interval found higher rates of postsurgical complications (17.7, 18.7, and 19.2%) than in the other groups. In these studies there is a difference in the rate of hypoparathyroidism (8.8% versus 3.8 and 1.2%, respectively) coupled with a rate of persistent (1.0% versus 3.7 and 5.4%) and recurrent hypercalcemia (4.4% versus 5.2 and 7.6%, respectively), due to the difference in the surgical techniques. While Lafferty and Hubay biopsied all identified normal glands, Sivula and Ronni-Sivula (89) attempted to visualize all glands at surgery,

TABLE 2. *Complications of parathyroid surgery*

	Satava et al. (148) 1975	Russell and Edis (93) 1982	Sivula and Ronni-Sivula (89) 1985	Palmér et al. (90–92) 1986–87	Lafferty and Hubay (88) 1989
No. operated on[a]	327	500	334	441	100
No. seen at final follow-up[b]			289	312	68
Mean follow-up, y	1	1	5.3	7.7	4.3
Mortality (%)[c]	0	0.2	0.9	0.7	0
Negative exploration (%)	6	3.4		4.3	3
Persistent hypercalcemia (%)	5	4.4	5.4	3.7	1
Recurrent hypercalcemia (%)			7.6	5.2	4.4
Vocal cord paralysis (%)					
Transient	2.4	2.7	2.1		2
Persistent	0.3	0.2	1.5		0[d]
Permanent Hypoparathyroidism (%)	1	2	1.2	3.8	8.8
Total morbidity (%)	14.7	12.9	18.7	17.7	19.2

Source: Lafferty and Hubay (88).

[a] The number of patients operated on was used in the calculation of percentages for mortality, negative exploration, persistent hypercalcemia, and transient vocal cord paralysis.

[b] The final follow-up number was used in calculating the percentages of recurrent hypercalcemia, permanent vocal cord paralysis, and permanent hypoparathyroidism.

[c] Mortality refers to patients operated on who died within 2 months of neck exploration.

[d] Occasional hoarseness occurred in 4.4%.

but rarely confirmed them by biopsy. A higher rate of permanent hypoparathyroidism, and a lower rate of persistent or recurrent hypercalcemia, may result from the practice of biopsying normal parathyroid glands in patients with parathyroid adenoma. Nevertheless, it is justified, because second explorations also carry a higher morbidity: for example, hypoparathyroidism in 41%, transient vocal paralysis in 5%, permanent vocal paralysis in 1% and death in 2% (88). Lafferty and Hubay (88) conclude that medical follow-up is a reasonable alternative to surgery in the mild, asymptomatic, compliant patient over 50 years of age.

Reexploration

In patients in whom previous parathyroid exploration was unsuccessful, there are advantages in locating, or at least lateralizing, the abnormal gland prior to subsequent surgery. One approach is to measure PTH levels in blood sampled from the thyroid veins (102,103). Using this method, the abnormal parathyroid tissue has been identified in 75–90% of cases. Arteriography increased the success of localization but is associated with significant morbidity since the injection of contrast material can cause transient ischemia of the cervical spinal cord. Levy et al. (104) identified six out of seven tumors by using digital subtraction angiography. By this method the contrast material is administered into the superior vena cava via an antecubital vein catheter. Ultrasonography (94) and mediastinal computerized tomography (105,106) are promising noninvasive techniques whose

precision is dependent on the resolution of available equipment. Intraoperative urinary cyclic AMP determination has been used as a guide to the success of parathyroid surgery (107). Among the 20 patients reported by Spiegel et al., cAMP/GFR fell in 18 who were cured and failed to fall in the 2 who remained hypercalcemic after surgery. In patients who have had previous parathyroid surgery, such intraoperative proof of successful surgery may be helpful.

Patients in whom the risk of mortality or morbidity from parathyroid surgery is high may benefit from ultrasound-guided percutaneous ethanol ablation of the parathyroid adenoma (108,109). An alternative approach is the arterial embolisation or dye infarction of the parathyroid gland as reported by Goohoed et al. (110).

Effect on Biochemical Parameters

Successful parathyroidectomy results in a rapid fall in the serum calcium concentration, accompanied by a significant decrease in urinary calcium excretion (111). Coe and Parks also reported a reduction in urinary oxalate excretion and in the urinary calcium oxalate concentration product ratio following surgery (79). A fall in concentration product ratio for oxalate was also observed by Pak (112), who in addition noted a rise in the formation product ratio for calcium oxalate and brushite, indicating that the urine became less saturated with respect to these salts, resulting in a decreased risk of new stone formation.

Stone Recurrence after Parathyroidectomy

The likelihood of development of renal calculi cannot be predicted from the urinary calcium level. In fact, 30% of hyperparathyroid patients with or without renal calculi are normocalciuric (21,113). The reported incidence of active renal stone formation, defined as the passage, operative removal, or roentgenographic evidence of enlargement or the appearance of new calculi within 1 year following parathyroid surgery has varied between several studies. The prospective study of Purnell et al. (114) reported an incidence of stone formation of less than 11%.

McGeown (115) studied 68 hyperparathyroid patients with renal stones. In 59 patients hyperparathyroidism was confirmed on exploration of the neck, and in the other 9 the parathyroid glands appeared normal at operation, but biochemical and clinical remission occurred and persisted for 2–5 years. Fifty-six of the 59 patients who underwent parathyroidectomy were kept under observation for a 1- to 5-year period. In this study the duration of the disease was measured from the year in which the first stone was diagnosed, either by x-rays or by the passage of a stone, to the time of operation. In the preoperative period, 99 stones were formed during 401 patient-years, whereas in the postoperative period only 8 stones were formed in 158 patient-years. From this study it was concluded that the rate of stone formation is reduced after parathyroidectomy.

Parks et al. (21) studied 48 patients with primary hyperparathyroidism and renal stones. Parathyroidectomy abolished the hypercalciuria in all patients and eliminated the kidney stone problem in 90–95%. The results of this study are similar to those of Siminovitch et al. (116), who followed 448 patients undergoing parathyroidectomy for presumed hyperparathyroidism. Of these patients 184 had associated renal calculi, in 72 of whom (16%) stone disease was metabolically active. Out of 72, 48 had adenomas, 18 had hyperplasia, and 6 had normal glands. None of the adenoma patients has had recurrent calculi, whereas calculi continued to form in 45% of the patients with hyperplastic glands and in 50% of those with normal glands.

Recently, Deaconson et al. (117) reported changes in the rates of new stone formation in 71 patients with primary hyperparathyroidism followed for 1–15 years (mean, 5 years) after surgery. The study included patients with stones, hypercalcemia, and inappropriately elevated PTH concentrations. All these values returned to normal in 69 of 71 patients after parathyroidectomy. Only 4 patients have passed renal stones since undergoing surgery, and the rate of stone formation per patient per year is 0.02 in contrast to 0.36 prior to surgery. Two of the four patients with recurrent stone events also had hypercalcemia and evidence of persistent or recurrent hyperparathyroidism.

Ronni-Sivula and Sivula (118) followed 289 patients who underwent parathyroidectomy over a period of 5 years. Out of 99 patients, 87 had single adenoma and 12 had multiglandular disease. Renal stones were the presenting symptom in 99 patients (57% of the men and 27% of the women). In this study, stones did not recur in 88 patients (89%). Six of the 87 adenoma patients and 4 of the 12 with multiglandular disease had recurrent renal stones during the follow-up period. Lafferty and Hubay (88) followed 100 cases, of whom 18% had stones over a 5-year period. The majority of studies, therefore, have shown a marked decrease in recurrent stone formation following parathyroidectomy in patients in whom adenoma is the cause of hyperparathyroidism. Posen et al. (119), however, observed a 50% chance of further stone formation or the passage of preexisting stones among 77 patients followed up for 7.8 years after parathyroidectomy. By contrast, patients without a previous history of renal calculi were unlikely to form stones even if they remain hypercalcemic and hypercalciuric.

Recurrent stone formation may also occur despite the cure of the clinical hyperparathyroidism in cases in which hypercalciuria of the so-called renal or absorptive type persists. Urinary calcium excretion should therefore be determined following parathyroidectomy in patients with a history of renal stones.

Natural History

The study reported by Scholz and Purnell (120) included 107 patients with mild asymptomatic primary hyperparathyroidism followed for a mean period of 10 years, of whom 22% underwent parathyroid exploration, 48% showed no progression, and 30% died from other causes. Only 6% developed new renal calculi during follow-up. Posen et al. (119) reported a similar incidence of 5% of new renal calculi among 90 patients followed for a mean period of 5.2 years.

Surgery for Normocalcemic Hyperparathyroidism

Parathyroidectomy should be undertaken only with extreme caution in patients with renal stones and normocalcemia since it may not prevent recurrent stone formation in such cases. Normocalcemic hyperparathyroidism is defined as a normal serum calcium concentration associated with surgical evidence of parathyroid disease. Kristofferson et al. (121) reported a retrospective study of 82 so-called normocalcemic patients subjected to parathyroidectomy with a median postoperative follow-up of 96 months. Of the 19 patients with severe stone formation, 12 were apparently cured by parathyroidectomy. These cured patients were found at operation to have parathyroid adenoma or hyperplasia, or even normal glands. Although these patients were reported as normocalcemic, 50% of them had episodic hypercalcemia. The results of this study are difficult to interpret since the definition of normocalcemia appears to differ from that of other investigators.

Siminovitch et al. (122) studied 21 patients with renal calculi and normocalcemia who underwent parathyroidectomy. Five patients had serum calcium levels from 10.7 to 11 mg/dL. Of the 21, 1 had an adenoma, 9 had hyperplasia, and 11 had normal glands. Of the 19 patients followed, 6 (32%) did not form stones, while 8 (42%) had recurrent stones. In 5 of these patients the glands were reported to be hyperplastic, while in 3, the glands were normal.

Persistence of Hypercalciuria After Parathyroidectomy

A varying incidence of hypercalciuria has been observed following parathyroidectomy. Fabris et al. (123) reported an incidence of 30%, whereas Siminovitch et al. (122) reported that of the 5–10% of patients with primary hyperparathyroidism who continued to form stones after surgery, 90% had some form of hypercalciuria.

There are several hypothetical explanations for persistent hypercalciuria after successful parathyroidectomy:

1. So-called renal hypercalciuria may have antedated, and actually caused the development of, the autonomous hyperparathyroidism. In such cases renal hypercalciuria may be expected to persist following parathyroidectomy (49). An example of this mechanism is described by Maschio et al. (124), who reported a patient with bilateral recurrent calcium nephrolithiasis, hypercalciuria, and hypercalcemia, and in whom a parathyroid adenoma was removed. The patient remained hypercalciuric despite the cure of hyperparathyroidism and on repeat surgical exploration a diffuse adenomatous parathyroid gland and another gland with pure hyperplasia were excised. The patient again remained normocalcemic and hypercalciuric despite a low-calcium diet. The patient was treated with hydrochlorothiazide 50 mg/day, leading to normalization of urinary calcium excretion. This patient could have had hyperplasia of the parathyroid glands throughout, or on the other hand, a primary renal leak of calcium may have caused a continuous stimulation of the parathyroid glands, resulting initially in hyperplasia and later in the development of an autonomous adenoma.

2. Hypercalciuria may be secondary to renal tubular damage caused by sustained hypercalcemia or hypercalciuria in patients with primary hyperparathyroidism.

3. Absorptive hypercalciuria and primary hyperparathyroidism, both of which are common disorders, may coincidentally both be present so that after parathyroidectomy "absorptive" hypercalciuria persists. Breslau and Pak (125) recently reported five hyperparathyroid patients who had persistent hypercalciuria of the absorp-

tive type following surgery. Four of these five patients developed a new kidney stone. Postoperatively, the patients showed increased 24-h urinary calcium excretion, enhanced response to an oral calcium load, and persistent elevation in fractional intestinal ^{47}Ca absorption and calcitriol levels despite normalization of serum calcium and PTH levels. In this study no explanation was given for the persistent elevated calcitriol levels. This study suggests that both diseases may coexist. Whether the hypercalciuria is mediated by calcitriol or by other factors needs to be clarified (126).

MEDICAL TREATMENT

There is no specific treatment other than surgery which has been proved to reduce the risk of stone recurrence in patients with primary hyperparathyroidism. However, in those patients in whom surgery is contraindicated, has been refused, or has failed, various forms of medical treatment may be considered.

Calcium Intake

In many patients with primary hyperparathyroidism and renal calculi there is hyperabsorption of calcium from the gut due to increased calcitriol levels. Calcium-restricted diets used to be recommended for such patients. Insogna et al. (127) reported that patients who received a 1000-mg calcium diet have lower PTH and calcitriol levels than patients on a 400-mg calcium diet. It therefore appears that a low-calcium diet might have negative consequences, such as further stimulation of PTH secretion, greater mobilization of calcium from bone, and a more negative calcium balance. Dietary calcium restriction may therefore not be advisable in these patients. Avoidance of a high-calcium intake, however, appears prudent, together with strict avoidance of calcium supplements and vitamin D supplements, which would be expected to increase the risk of stone formation.

Protein Intake

Excessive ingestion of foods rich in animal proteins should probably be avoided in patients with primary hyperparathyroidism and renal stones, since it tends to lower urinary pH and citrate, and increase urinary uric acid as well as urinary calcium, potentially increasing the risk of stone formation in these patients.

Sodium Intake

The role of dietary sodium in primary hyperparathyroidism and kidney stones has not been examined in detail. However, a high sodium intake may contribute to calcium stone formation by enhancing the renal excretion of calcium and producing sodium urate-induced crystallization of calcium salts (128). To overcome these problems, moderate sodium restriction (100 mEq/day) may be helpful in these patients.

Fluid Intake

A high fluid intake is the only nutritional modification that is universally agreed to be useful in all forms of nephrolithiasis (129). Although a high fluid intake per se does not prevent stone formation in patients with primary hyperparathyroidism, patients should be advised to increase their daily water intake and avoid volume depletion which may lead to a further increase in the serum calcium level. An increase in urine flow rate reduces the concentration of insoluble urinary constituents and decreases the risk of stone formation. A high fluid intake has been reported to increase renal oxalate excretion (130), but this has not been confirmed by other investigators.

Drug Therapy

The acute administration of furosemide or ethacrynic acid together with saline infusion will lower serum calcium, by enhancing urinary calcium excretion due to inhibition of calcium reabsorption in the ascending limb of Henle's loop (131–133). Both drugs are frequently used in the treatment of severe hypercalcemia. However, they have no place in the chronic treatment of renal stones and hyperparathyroidism since an increase in the urinary calcium excretion could increase the risk of stone formation, and in any case the hypocalcemic effect may not be sustained with chronic administration of these drugs. Thiazide diuretics are commonly used for the prevention of idiopathic calcium stones (134). These diuretics enhance calcium reabsorption in the distal tubule and may also stimulate proximal tubular reabsorption of calcium secondary to extracellular volume depletion. Thiazide diuretics should be avoided, however, in patients with stones and primary hyperparathyroidism, since they may exacerbate the hypercalcemia (135).

A theoretically attractive approach to the nonsurgical treatment of hyperparathyroidism would be by inhibiting PTH secretion. The initial encouraging reports of beneficial effects of cimetidine (136) and beta-adrenergic blockers (137,138) in primary hyperparathyroidism have not been confirmed (139,140).

Calcitriol may decrease PTH secretion both in the normal parathyroid (141,142) and in patients with primary hyperparathyroidism, osteitis fibrosa, and vitamin D deficiency (38). However, calcitriol is clearly contraindicated in patients with primary hyperparathyroidism

and renal stones, in whom baseline calcitriol levels tend to be elevated.

Another approach in the treatment of primary hyperparathyroidism would be to inhibit the peripheral action of PTH on bone. Phosphate administered orally or intravenously decreases the serum calcium by causing a shift of calcium out of the extracellular fluid into bone, and also by inhibiting the effect of PTH on bone resorption. Phosphate treatment can reduce the frequency of idiopathic calcium oxalate stones, probably via several mechanisms, including complexing calcium in the intestinal lumen, decreasing calcitriol synthesis, and enhancing the excretion of pyrophosphate, an inhibitor of calcium phosphate and oxalate crystal formation. The disadvantages of this treatment may include metastatic calcification, acute renal failure, and a further increase in PTH levels.

Broadus et al. (143) studied 10 patients (8 women and 2 men, mean age 53 years) with primary hyperparathyroidism and high calcitriol levels prior to and following 1 year of oral phosphate therapy. Six of the ten patients had a history of one or more renal stone events. An increase in PTH levels was accompanied by an increase in urinary cAMP and phosphorus excretion, with no change in creatinine clearance. In this study, no patient experienced a stone event, formed new stone material, or showed growth of preexisting stones. Although phosphate treatment reduces calcitriol levels and decreases calcium hyperabsorption, its effectiveness in the prevention of recurrent stone formation requires further clinical studies, and phosphate is not currently recommended for primary hyperparathyroidism with renal calculi.

The incidence of hyperparathyroidism is high in postmenopausal women (18,144). Treatment with estrogens was first reported in 1972 (146). In a recent study, 10 of 14 postmenopausal women with primary hyperparathyroidism showed a reduction in serum calcium during estrogen therapy (147). Basal 24-h urinary calcium and hydroxyproline excretion as well as serum alkaline phosphatase were also reduced, indicating reduced bone turnover. Although the urinary calcium/creatinine ratio decreased during estrogen therapy, no data on stone formation rate were presented in these studies. Similar results have been reported by Gallagher and Nordin (145) and by Selby and Peacock (147). In conclusion, therefore, there is no proven medical therapy for the prevention of stones in persisting primary hyperparathyroidism, and hence parathyroid surgery is generally the treatment of choice.

REFERENCES

1. Fourman P, Royer P. *Calcium metabolism and the bone.* Oxford: Blackwell Scientific, 1968;chap 3.
2. Kleeman, CR, Salehmoghaddam S, Hercz G. Primary hyperpara-

thyroidism (PHP) revisited. In: Massry SG, Olmer M, Ritz E, eds. *Phosphate and mineral homeostasis,* vol 208. New York: Plenum Press, 1986;17–45.

3. Cave AJE. Richard Owen and the discovery of the parathyroid glands. In Underwood EA, ed. *Science, medicine and history,* vol ii. Oxford: Oxford University Press, 1953;217–22.
4. Salvesen HA. Studies on the physiology of the parathyroids. *Acta Med Scand* 1923;6:1–160.
5. Collip JB. The extraction of a parathyroid hormone which will prevent or control parathyroid tetany and which regulates the level of blood calcium. *J Biol Chem* 1925;63:395–438.
6. Albright F, Ellsworth R. Studies on the physiology of the parathyroid glands. I. Calcium and phosphorus studies on a case of idiopathic hypoparathyroidism. *J Clin Invest* 1929;7:183–201.
7. von Recklinghausen FD. Die fibrose oder deformirende osteitis die osteomalacie und die osteoplastische carcinose in ihren gegenseitigen Beziehungen In: *Festschrift Rudolph Virchow zu seinem 71 Geburtstage.* Berlin: G Reiner, 1891;1–89, Pl 1–5.
8. Askanazy M. Ueber osteitis deformans ohne osteides Gewebe. *Arb Pathol Anat Bakteriol Tuebingen* 1904;4:398–422.
9. Askanazy M. Uber ein Adenom der Glandula Parathyroidea. *Verh Dtsch Ges Pathol* 1906;10:85.
10. Erdheim J. Uber Epithelkorperbefunde bei Osteomalacie SB. *Akad Wiss Wien Math Naturwiss Kl* 1907;116:311–70.
11. Mandl F. Therapeutischer Versuch bei einem Falle von Ostitis fibrosa generalisata mittels Extirpation eines Epithelkorperchentumors. *Zbl Chir* 1926;53:260–4.
12. Albright F, Bauer W, Ropes M, Aub JC. Studies of calcium and phosphorus metabolism. IV. The effect of parathyroid hormone. *J Clin Invest* 1929;7:139–81.
13. Barr DP, Bulger HA. The clinical syndrome of hyperparathyroidism. *Am J Med Sci* 1930;179:471–3.
14. Davies-Colley N. Bones and kidneys from a case of osteomalacia in a girl aged 13. *Trans Pathol Soc Lond* 1884;35:285–97.
15. Albright F, Sulkowitch HW, Bloomberg E. Further experience in the diagnosis of hyperparathyroidism, including a discussion of cases with a minimal degree of hyperparathyroidism. *Am J Med Sci* 1937;193:800–12.
16. Albright F, Reifenstein EC. *The parathyroid glands and metabolic bone disease.* Baltimore: Williams & Wilkins, 1948;393.
17. Broadus A. Nephrolithiasis in primary hyperparathyroidism. In: Coe F, Brenner B, Stein J, eds. *Nephrolithiasis.* New York: Churchill Livingston, 1980.
18. Heath HW III, Hodgson SF, Kennedy MA. Primary hyperparathyroidism: incidence, morbidity and potential economic impact on the community. *N Engl J Med* 1980;302:189–93.
19. Mundy GR, Cove DH, Fisken R. Primary hyperparathyroidism: changes in the pattern of clinical presentation. *Lancet* 1980;1:1317–20.
20. Fetter TR, McCuskey BM. Hyperparathyroidism and urolithiasis. *J Urol* 1960;84:213–8.
21. Parks J, Coe F, Favus M. Hyperparathyroidism in nephrolithiasis. *Arch Intern Med* 1980;140:1479–81.
22. Fuss M, Pepersack T, Corvilain J, et al. Infrequency of primary hyperparathyroidism in renal stone formers. *Br J Urol* 1988;62:4–6.
23. Dent, CE. Some problems of hyperparathyroidism. *Br Med J* 1962;ii:1419–25, 1495–1500.
24. Rao DS, Frame B, Block MA, et al. Primary hyperparathyroidism: a cause of hypercalciuria and renal stones in patients with medullary sponge kidney. *JAMA* 1977;237:1353–5.
25. Gremillion DH, Kee JW, McIntosh DA. Hyperparathyroidism and medullary sponge kidney: a chance relationship? *JAMA* 1977;237:799–800.
26. Hellman DE, Kartchner M, Komar N, et al. Hyperaldosteronism, hyperparathyroidism, medullary sponge kidneys, and hypertension. *JAMA* 1980;244:1351–3.
27. Maschio G, Tessitore N, D'Angelo A, et al. Medullary sponge kidney and hyperparathyroidism: a puzzling association. *Am J Nephrol* 1982;2:77–84.
28. Parks JH, Coe FL, Strauss AL. Calcium nephrolithiasis and medullary sponge kidney in women. *N Engl J Med* 1982;306:1088–91.

29. Hellstrom J. Experience from one hundred and five cases of hyperparathyroidism. *Acta Chir Scand* 1957;113:501–5.
30. Hodgkinson A, Peacock M, Nicholson M. Quantitative analysis of calcium-containing urinary calculi. In: Hodgkinson A, Nordin BEC, eds. *Renal stone research symposium.* London: J&A Churchill, 1969.
31. Gault, MH, Robertson WG, Senciall D. The oxalate: phosphate ratio in urinary tract calculi by infrared revised analysis. *Clin Chim Acta* 1987;166:103–5.
32. Muldowney FP, Freaney R, McMullin JP, et al. Serum ionized calcium and parathyroid hormone in renal stone disease. *Q J Med* 1976;45:75–86.
33. Yendt ER, Gagne RJA. Detection of primary hyperparathyroidism, with special reference to its occurrence in hypercalciuric females with normal or borderline serum calcium. *Can Med Assoc J* 1968;98:331–6.
34. Dent CE, Hartland BV, Hicks J, Sykes ED. Calcium intake in patients with primary hyperparathyroidism. *Lancet* 1961;2:336–8.
35. Lloyd HM. Primary hyperparathyroidism; an analysis of the role of the parathyroid tumor. *Medicine* 1968;47:53–71.
36. Peacock M. Renal stone disease and bone disease in primary hyperparathyroidism and their relationship to the action of parathyroid hormone on calcium absorption. In: *Calcium regulating hormones, proceedings of the fifth parathyroid conference,* Amsterdam: Exerpta Medica, 1975;78.
37. Patron P, Gardin JP, Paillard M. Renal mass and reserve of vitamin D: determinants in primary hyperparathyroidism. *Kidney Int* 1987;31:1174–80.
38. Patron P, Gardin JP, Borensztein P, Prigent A, Paillard M. Marked direct suppression of primary hyperparathyroidism with osteitis fibrosis cystica by intravenous administration of 1,25 dihydroxy coli-calciferol, *Miner Electrolyte Metab* 1989;15(6):321–5.
39. Silverberg SJ, Shane E, de la Cruz L, et al. Skeletal disease in primary hyperparathyroidism. *J Bone Miner Res* 1989;4:283–291.
40. Talmage RV, Kraintz FW. Progressive changes in renal phosphate and calcium excretion in rats following parathyroidectomy or parathyroid administration. *Proc Soc Exp Biol (NY)* 1954;87:263–7.
41. Widrow SH, Levinsky NG. The effect of parathyroid extract on renal tubular calcium reabsorption in the dog. *J Clin Invest* 1962;41:2151–9.
42. Shareghi GT, Agus ZS. Magnesium transport in the cortical thick ascending limb of Henle's loop of the rabbit. *J Clin Invest* 1982;69:759–69.
43. Broadus AE, Domingues M, Bartter FC. Pathophysiological studies in idiopathic hypercalciuria; use of an oral calcium tolerance test to characterize distinctive hypercalciuric subgroups. *J Clin Endocrinol Metab* 1978;47:751–60.
44. Broadus EE, Their SO. Metabolic basis of renal stone disease. *N Engl J Med* 1979;300:839–45.
45. Pak CYC, Nicar MJ, Peterson R, Zerwekh JE, Snider W. A lack of unique pathophysiologic backgrounds for nephrolithiasis of primary hyperparathyroidism. *J Clin Endocrinol Metab* 1981;53:536–42.
46. Hulter HN, Halloran BP, Toto RD, Peterson JC. Long-term control of plasma calcitriol concentration in dogs and humans. *J Clin Invest* 1985;76(2):695–702.
47. Lo Cascio V, Adami S, Galvanini G, Ferrari M, Cominacini L, Tartarotti D. Substrate–product relation of 1-hydroxylase activity in primary hyperparathyroidism. *N Engl J Med* 1985;313:1123–5.
48. Gardin JP, Paillard M. Normo-calcemic primary hyperparathyroidism: resistence to PTH effect on tubular reabsorption of calcium. *Miner Electrolyte Metab* 1984;10:301–308.
49. Bordier P, Ryckewart A, Gueris J, Rasmussen H. On the pathogenesis of so-called idiopathic hypercalciuria. *Am J Med* 1977;363:398–409.
50. Burnatowska MA, Harris CA, Sutton RAL, Seely JF. The effects of vitamin D on renal handling of calcium, magnesium and phosphate in the hamster. *Kidney Int* 1985;27:864–70.

51. Yamamoto M, Kawanobe Y, Takahashi H, Shimazawa E, Kimura S, Ogata E. Vitamin D deficiency and renal calcium transport in the rat. *J Clin Invest* 1984;74:507–13.
52. Rümenapf G, Issa S, Schwille PO. The influence of progressive hyperinsulinemia on duodenal calcium absorption in the rat. *Metabolism* 1987;36:60–5.
53. Beck JC, McGarry EE, Dyrenfurth D. Metabolic effects of human and monkey growth in man. *Science* 1957;125:884–6.
54. DeFronzo RA, Cooke CR, Andres R, Faloona GR, Davis PJ. The effect of insulin on renal handling of sodium, potassium, calcium and phosphate in man. *J Clin Invest* 1975;55:845–55.
55. Schwille PO, Scholz D, Hagemann G, Sigel A. Metabolic and glucose load studies in uric acid, oxalate, and hyperparathyroid stone formers. *Adv Exp Biol Med* 1974;41B:485–91.
56. Rao PN, Gordon C, Davies D, Blacklock NJ. Are stone formers maladapted to refined carbohydrates? *Br J Urol* 1982;54:575–7.
57. Scholz D, Schwille PO, Sigel A. Response of gastrointestinal hormones and intestinal calcium absorption during an oral carbohydrate meal. In: Smith LH, Robertson WG, Finlayson B, eds. *Urolithiasis: basic and clinical research.* New York: Plenum Press, 1981;795–800.
58. Prager H, Kovarik J, Schernthaner G, Woloszczuk W, Willvonseder R. Peripheral insulin resistance in primary hyperparathyroidism. *Metab Clin Exp* 1983;32:800–5.
59. Robertson WG, Peacock M. Review of risk factors in calcium urolithiasis. *World J Urol* 1983;1:114–8.
60. Linkswiler HM, Zemel MB, Hegsted M, Schuette S. Protein-induced hypercalciuria. *Fed Proc* 1981;40:2429–33.
61. Coe FL, Favus MJ. Disorders of stone formation. In: Brenner BM, Rector F, eds. *The kidney,* 3rd ed. Philadelphia: WB Saunders, 1986;1403–42.
62. Lutz J. Calcium balance and acid–base status of women as affected by increased protein intake and by sodium bicarbonate ingestion. *Am J Clin Nutr* 1984;39:281–8.
63. Lemann J, Piering WF, Lennon EJ. Possible role of carbonate-induced calciuria in calcium oxalate kidney-stone formation. *N Engl J Med* 1969;280:232–7.
64. Tschope W, Ritz E, Schellenberg B. Plasma phosphate and urinary calcium in recurrent stone formers: effects of age, blood pressure and diet. *Miner Electrolyte Metab* 1980;4:237–45.
65. McCarron DA, Rankin LI, Bennett WM, et al. Urinary calcium excretion at extremes of sodium intake in normal man. *Am J Nephrol* 1981;1:84–90.
66. Muldowney FP, Freaney R, Moloney MF. Importance of dietary sodium in the hypercalciuria syndrome. *Kidney Int* 1982;22:292–6.
67. Muldowney FP, Carroll DV, Donohoe JF, Freaney R. Correction of renal bicarbonate wastage by parathyroidectomy. *Q J Med* 1971;40:487–98.
68. Bank N, Aynedjian HC. A micropuncture study of the effect of parathyroid hormone on renal bicarbonate reabsorption. *J Clin Invest* 1976;58:336–44.
69. Brenner RJ, Spring DB, Sebastian A, et al. Incidence of radiographic evident bone disease, nephrocalcinosis, and nephrolithiasis in various types of renal tubular acidosis. *N Engl J Med* 1982;307:217–21.
70. Hulter HN, Peterson JC. Acid–base homeostasis during chronic PTH excess in humans. *Kidney Int* 1985;28:187–92.
71. Bichara M, Mercier O, Paillard M, Leviel F. Effects of parathyroid hormone on urinary acidification. *Am J Physiol* 1986;251:F444–53.
72. Smith LH, Vandenberg CJ, Wilson DM, Scholz DA, Purnell DC. Urolithiasis in primary hyperparathyroidism. *Proceedings of the American Society of Nephrology,* 1977;9A.
73. Ljungall S, Akerstrom G. Urate metabolism in primary hyperparathyroidism. *Urol Int* 1982;37:73–8.
74. Broulik PD, Stepán JJ, Pacovsky V. Primary hyperparathyroidism and hyperuricaemia are associated but not correlated with indicators of bone turnover. *Clin Chim Acta* 1987;170:195–200.
75. Pak CYC, Holt K. Nucleation and growth of brushite and calcium oxalate in urine of stone formers. *Metabolism* 1976;25:665.
76. Koide T, Yoshioka T, Oka T, Sonoda T. Promotive effect of urines from patients with primary hyperparathyroidism on calcium oxalate crystal aggregation. In: Walker V, Sutton RAL, Cameron EC, Pak CYC, Robertson WG, eds. *Urolithiasis.* New York: Plenum Press, 1989;109–11.
77. Zerwekh JE, Hwang TIS, Poindexter J, Hill K, Wendell G, Pak CYC. Modulation by calcium of the inhibitor activity of naturally occurring urinary inhibitors. *Kidney Int* 1988;33:1005–8.
78. Henneman PH, Benedict PH, Forbes AP, Dudley HR. Idiopathic hypercalciuria. *N Engl J Med* 1958;259:802–7.
79. Coe FL, Parks JH, eds. *Nephrolithiasis: pathogenesis and treatment,* 2nd ed. Chicago: Year Book Medical Publishers, 1988.
80. Johnson RD, Conn JW. Hyperparathyroidism with a prolonged period of normocalcemia. *JAMA* 1969;210:2063–6.
81. Yendt ER, Gagne RJA. Detection of primary hyperparathyroidism, with special reference to its occurrence in hypercalciuric females with "normal" or borderline serum calcium. *Can Med Assoc J* 1968;98:331–6.
82. Wills MR, Pak CYC, Hammond WG, et al. Normocalcemic primary hyperparathyroidism. *Am J Med* 1969;47:384–91.
83. Broadus AE, Horst RL, Littledike ET, Mahaffey JE, Rasmussen H. Primary hyperparathyroidism with intermittent hypercalcemia: serial observations and simple diagnosis by means of an oral calcium tolerance test. *Clin Endocrinol* 1980;12:225–35.
84. Arnaud CD, Goldsmith RS, Bordier PJ, Sizemore GW, Larsen JA, Gilkinson J. Influence of immunoheterogeneity of circulating parathyroid hormone on results of radioimmunoassays of serum in man. *J Clin Invest* 1974;56:785–93.
85. Hackeng WHL, Lips P, Netelenbos JC, Lips CJM. Clinical implications of estimation of intact parathyroid hormone (PTH) versus total immunoreactive PTH in normal subjects and hyperparathyroid patients. *J Clin Endocrinol Metab* 1986;63:447–53.
86. Chase LR, Aurbach GD. Renal adenyl cyclase: anatomically separate sites for parathyroid hormone and vasopressin. *Science* 1968;159:545–6.
87. Clark OH, Way LW, Hunt TK. Recurrent hyperparathyroidism. *Ann Surg* 1976;184:391–402.
88. Lafferty FW, Hubay CA. Primary hyperparathyroidism: a review of the long-term surgical and nonsurgical morbidities as a basis for a rational approach to treatment. *Arch Intern Med* 1989;149:780–96.
89. Sivula A, Ronni-Sivula H. Observations on 334 patients operated on for primary hyperparathyroidism. *Ann Chir Gynaecol* 1985;74:66–73.
90. Rudberg C, Akerström G, Palmér M, et al. Late results of operation for primary hyperparathyroidism in 441 patients. *Surgery* 1986;99:643–51.
91. Palmér M, Adami HO, Bergström R, et al. Mortality after surgery for primary hyperparathyroidism: a followup of 441 patients operated on from 1956 to 1979. *Surgery* 1987;102:1–7.
92. Palmér M, Ljunghall S, Akerström G, et al. Patients with primary hyperparathyroidism operated on over a 24 year period: temporal trends of clinical and laboratory findings. *J Chronic Dis* 1987;40:121–30.
93. Russell CF, Edis AJ. Surgery for primary hyperparathyroidism: experience with 500 consecutive cases and evaluation of the role of surgery in the asymptomatic patient. *Br J Surg* 1982;69:244–7.
94. Brewer WH, Walsh JW, Newsome HH Jr. Impact of sonography on surgery for primary hyperparathyroidism. *Am J Surg* 1983;145:270–2.
95. Ferlin G, Borsato N, Camerani M, Conte N, Zotti D. New perspectives in localising enlarged parathyroids by technetium–thallium subtraction scan. *J Nucl Med* 1983;24:438–41.
96. Winzelberg GG. Parathyroid imaging. *Ann Intern Med* 1987;107:64–70.
97. Mallette LE. Review: primary hyperparathyroidism, an update: incidence, etiology, diagnosis, and treatment. *Am J Med Sci* 1987;293:239–49.
98. Paloyan E, Lawrence AM, Oalopa R, Shah KH, Ernst K, Hofmann C. Subtotal parathyroidectomy for primary hyperparathyroidism: long term results in 292 patients. *Arch Surg* 1983;118:425–30.
99. Aetiology and treatment of primary hyperparathyroidism (editorial). *Lancet* 1983;1:1367–8.
100. Edis AJ, Beahrs OH, van Heerden JA, et al. "Conservative" ver-

sus "liberal" approach to parathyroid neck exploration. *Surgery* 1977;82:466–73.

101. Kaplan EL, Bartlett S, Sugimoto J, et al. Relation of postoperative hypocalcemia to operative techniques: deleterious effect of excessive use of parathyroid biopsy. *Surgery* 1982;92:827–34.

102. Eisenberg H, Pallotta J, Sherwood LM. Selective arteriography, venography and venous hormone assay in diagnosis and localization of parathyroid lesions. *Am J Med* 1974;56:810–20.

103. Bilezikian JP, Doppman JL, Powell D, et al. Preoperative localization of abnormal parathyroid tissue: cumulative experience with venous sampling and arteriography. *Am J Med* 1973;55:505–14.

104. Levy JM, Hessel SJ, Dippe SE, McFarland JO. Digital subtraction angiography for localization of parathyroid lesions. *Ann Intern Med* 1982;97:710–2.

105. Doppman JF. CT localization of cervical parathyroid glands. *J Comput Assist Tomogr* 1982;6:519.

106. Whitley NO, Bohlman M, Connor TB, McCrea ES, Mason GR, Whitley JE. Computed tomography for localization of parathyroid adenomas. *J Comput Assist Tomogr* 1981;5:812.

107. Spiegel AM, Eastman ST, Attie MF, et al. Intraoperative measurements of urinary cyclic AMP to guide surgery for primary hyperparathyroidism. *New Engl J Med* 1980;303:1457–60.

108. Charboneau JW, Hay ID, van Heerden JA. Persistent primary hyperparathyroidism: successful ultrasound-guided percutaneous ethanol ablation of an occult adenoma. *Mayo Clin Proc* 1988;63:913–7.

109. Müller-Gärtner HW, Beil FU, Schneider C, Ringe JD, Greten H. Percutaneous transthyroidal instillation treatment of parathyroid adenoma with ethanol in primary hyperparathyroidism. *Dtsch Med Wochenschr* 1987;112:1459–61.

110. Goolhoed GW, Krudy AG, Doppmann JL. Long term follow-up of patients with hyperparathyroidism treated by transcatheter staining with contrast agent. *Surgery* 1983;94:849–62.

111. Hodgkinson A. Biochemical aspects of primary hyperparathyroidism: analysis of 50 cases. *Clin Sci* 1963;25:231–42.

112. Pak, CYC. Effect of parathyroidectomy on crystallization of calcium salts in urine of patients with primary hyperparathyroidism. *Invest Urol* 1979;17:146–8.

113. Kyle LH, Beisel WR, Emary JJ. Evaluation of relative value of diagnostic tests in hyperparathyroidism. *Ann Intern Med* 1962;57:957–62.

114. Purnell DC, Smith LH, Scholz DA, Elveback LR, Arnaud CD. Primary hyperparathyroidism: a prospective clinical study. *Am J Med* 1971;50:670–8.

115. McGeown, MG. Effect of parathyroidectomy on the incidence of renal calculi. *Lancet* 1961;1:586–7.

116. Siminovitch JMP, Caldwell BE Jr, Straffon RA. Renal lithiasis and hyperparathyroidism: diagnosis, management and prognosis. *J Urol* 1981;126:720–2.

117. Deaconson TF, Wilson SD, Lemann J Jr. The effect of parathyroidectomy on the recurrence of nephrolithiasis. *Surgery* 1987;102:910–3.

118. Ronni-Sivula H, Sivula A. Long-term effect of surgical treatment on the symptoms of primary hyperparathyroidism. *Ann Clin Research* 1985;17:141–7.

119. Posen S, Clifton-Bligh P, Reeve TS, et al. Is parathyroidectomy of benefit in primary hyperparathyroidism? *Q J Med* 1985;54:241–51.

120. Scholz DA, Purnell DC. Asymptomatic primary hyperparathyroidism: ten year prospective study. *Mayo Clin Proc* 1981;56:473–8.

121. Kristoffersson A, Boquist L, Holmlund D, Järhult J. Long-term effects of surgery for normocalcaemic hyperparathyroidism. *Acta Chir Scand* 1987;153:331–6.

122. Siminovitch JMP, James RE, Esselstyne CB Jr, Straffon RA, Banowsky LH. The effect of parathyroidectomy in patients with normocalcemic calcium stones. *J Urol* 1980;123:335–7.

123. Fabris A, Ortalda V, D'Angelo A, Giannini S, Maschio G. Biochemical and clinical studies after parathyroidectomy in primary hyperparathyroidism. In: Walker V, Sutton RAL, Cameron EC, Pak CYC, Robertson WG, eds. *Urolithiasis.* New York: Plenum Press, 1989;637–40.

124. Maschio G, Vecchioni R, Tessitore N. Recurrence of autonomous hyperparathyroidism in calcium nephrolithiasis. *Am J Med* 1980;69:607–9.

125. Breslau NA, Pak YC. Combined primary hyperparathyroidism and absorptive hypercalciuria: clinical implications. In: Walker V, Sutton RAL, Cameron EC, Pak CYC, Robertson WG, eds. *Urolithiasis.* New York: Plenum Press, 1989;627–30.

126. Hino M, Yamamoto I, Shigeno C, et al. Evidence that factors other than 1,25 dihydroxyvitamin D may play a role in augmenting intestinal calcium absorption in patients with primary hyperparathyroidism. *Calcif Tissue Int* 1986;38:193–6.

127. Insogna KL, Mitnick ME, Stewart AF, et al. Sensitivity of parathyroid hormone-1,25 dihydroxyvitamin D axis to variations in calcium intake in patients with primary hyperparathyroidism. *N Engl J Med* 1985;313:1126–30.

128. Pak CYC. *Renal stone disease: pathogenesis, prevention and treatment.* Hingham, Mass: Martinus Nijhoff, 1987.

129. Pak CYC, Sakhaee K, Crowther C, Brinkley L. Evidence justifying a high fluid intake in treatment of nephrolithiasis. *Ann Intern Med* 1981;93:36–9.

130. Zarembski PM, Hodgkinson A. Some factors influencing the urinary excretion of oxalic acid in man. *Clin Chim Acta* 1969;25:1–10.

131. Imai M. Effect of bumetanide and furosemide on the thick ascending limb of Henle's loop of rabbits and rats perfused in vitro. *Eur J Pharmacol* 1977;41:409–16.

132. Burg M, Green N. Effect of ethacrynic acid on the thick ascending limb of Henle's loop. *Kidney Int* 1973;4:301.

133. Duarte CG. Effects of ethacrynic acid and furosemide on urinary calcium, phosphate, and magnesium. *Metabolism* 1968;17:867–76.

134. Yendt ER, Gagne RJA, Cohanim M. The effects of thiazides in idiopathic hypercalciuria. *Trans Am Clin Climatol Assoc* 1975;77:96.

135. Duarte CG, Winnacker KL, Becker KL, Pace A. Thiazide-induced hypercalcemia. *N Engl J Med* 1971;284:828–30.

136. Sherwood JK, Ackroyd FW, Garcia M. Effect of cimetidine on circulating parathyroid hormone in primary hyperparathyroidism. *Lancet* 1980;1:616–20.

137. Caro JF, Castro JH, Glennon JA. Effect of long-term propranolol administration on parathyroid hormone and calcium concentration in primary hyperparathyroidism. *Ann Intern Med* 1979;91:740–1.

138. Heath H. Biogenic amines and the secretion of parathyroid hormone and calcitonin. *Endocrine Rev* 1980;1:319–38.

139. Palmer FJ, Sawyers TM, Wierzbinski SJ. Cimetidine and hyperparathyroidism. *N Engl J Med* 1980;302:692.

140. Heath H. Cimetidine and hyperparathyroidism. *Lancet* 1980;1:980.

141. Chan YL, McKay C, Dye E, Slatopolsky E. The effects of 1,25 dihydrocholecalciferol on parathyroid hormone secretion by monolayer cultures of bovine parathyroid cells. *Calcif Tissue Int* 1986;38:27–32.

142. Cantley LK, Russell J, Lettieri D, Sherwood LM. 1,25-dihydroxy vitamin D_3 suppresses parathyroid hormone secretion from bovine parathyroid cells in tissue culture. *Endocrinology* 1985;117:2114–9.

143. Broadus AE, Magee JS, Mallette LE, et al. A detailed evaluation of oral phosphate therapy in selected patients with primary hyperparathyroidism. *J Clin Endocrinol Metab* 1983;56:953.

144. Boonstra CE, Jackson CE. Hyperparathyroidism detected by routine serum calcium analysis: prevalence in a clinic population. *Ann Intern Med* 1963;63:468–74.

145. Gallagher JC, Nordin BEC. Treatment with estrogens of primary hyperparathyroidism in post-menopausal women. *Lancet* 1972;1:503–7.

146. Marcus R, Madvig P, Crim M, Pont A, Kosek J. Conjugated estrogens in the treatment of post menopausal women with hyperparathyroidism. *Ann Intern Med* 1984;100:633–40.

147. Selby PL, Peacock M. Ethinyl estradiol and norethindrone in the treatment of primary hyperparathyroidism in post-menopausal women. *N Engl J Med* 1986;314:1481–6.

148. Satava RM, Beahrs OH, Scholz DA. Success rate of cervical exploration for hyperparathyroidism. *Arch Surg* 1975;110:625–7.

Disorders of Bone and Mineral Metabolism,
edited by Fredric L. Coe and Murray J. Favus,
© 1992 by Raven Press, Ltd. All rights reserved.

CHAPTER 32

Pathogenesis of Idiopathic Hypercalciuria and Nephrolithiasis

Jacob Lemann, Jr.

Approximately 80% of all kidney stones are composed of calcium oxalate and/or apatite (1,2). The average prevailing urinary Ca concentration, as determined by the daily rate of Ca excretion relative to the excretion of water, is thus one of the factors that determines the crystallization of calcium oxalate and calcium phosphate in the urine and the growth of such crystals. Figure 1 (3) illustrates the relative supersaturation (RSR) with respect to calcium oxalate of a solution having a composition similar to normal urine as a function of daily urine volume in relation to a range of daily rates of Ca excretion. The urine (solution) is increasingly supersaturated with respect to calcium oxalate as daily rates of Ca excretion increase and as daily urine volumes decrease, especially at urine volumes < 1.5 L/day, because both increasing daily urine Ca excretion rates and decreasing urine volumes increase the average prevailing urine Ca concentration.

This chapter summarizes current knowledge regarding the occurrence, mechanisms, and treatment of hypercalciuria among patients with Ca-containing kidney stones in relation to urinary Ca excretion rates in healthy individuals and the factors known to affect those rates. Quantitative data are, with some exceptions, presented in molar units: 1 mmol Ca = 40 mg Ca and 1 mmol Ca = 2 mEq Ca.

Following the development of chemical methods to measure Ca in biological samples more than 50 years ago, Flocks (4,5) observed that patients with Ca-containing kidney stones often exhibit hypercalciuria. As shown in Table 1, he found that Ca-stone formers exhibited higher rates of urinary Ca excretion than did healthy subjects regardless of whether those groups ate diets providing little or large amounts of Ca. Subsequently, Al-

bright (6) and Henneman (7) and their associates distinguished a group of Ca-stone formers, predominantly men, who exhibited hypercalciuria without hypercalcemia, hypophosphatemia, and normal skeletal radiographs. These patients did not give a history of vitamin D use or excessive consumption of Ca, as in Ca-containing antacids. They had no clinical evidence of diseases that may be accompanied by hypercalciuria including sarcoidosis, hyperthyroidism, Cushing's syndrome, cancer, rapid bone loss (Paget's disease or other circumstances accompanied by accelerated bone turnover together with immobilization), or renal tubular acidosis. Their serum total Ca concentrations were persistently normal and their net rates of intestinal Ca absorption, as assessed by metabolic balances, were increased. In addition, negative surgical exploration of the neck in seven patients provided evidence that they did not have hyperparathyroidism. Albright and Henneman (6,7) introduced the term *idiopathic hypercalciuria* (IH) to describe these patients. Subsequent and continuing studies have suggested that IH reflects a group of disorders, remaining to be precisely defined, which ultimately are expressed by hypercalciuria and Ca-nephrolithiasis.

THE QUANTITATIVE DEFINITION AND PREVALENCE OF HYPERCALCIURIA

Healthy adults, who are no longer growing and who are not yet exhibiting the gradual losses of body components that occur with senescence, are in Ca balance (e.g., Ca intake − Ca excretion = approximately zero). There is effective homeostatic integration of both internal and external Ca transport including bone resorption and bone formation as well as net intestinal Ca absorption and urinary Ca excretion; bone structure is normal. Thus, urinary Ca excretion in the steady-state in health must predominantly reflect the net rate of dietary Ca

J. Lemann, Jr.: Nephrology Division, Medical College of Wisconsin, Froedfert Memorial Lutheran Hospital, 9200 West Wisconsin Avenue, Milwaukee, Wisconsin 53226.

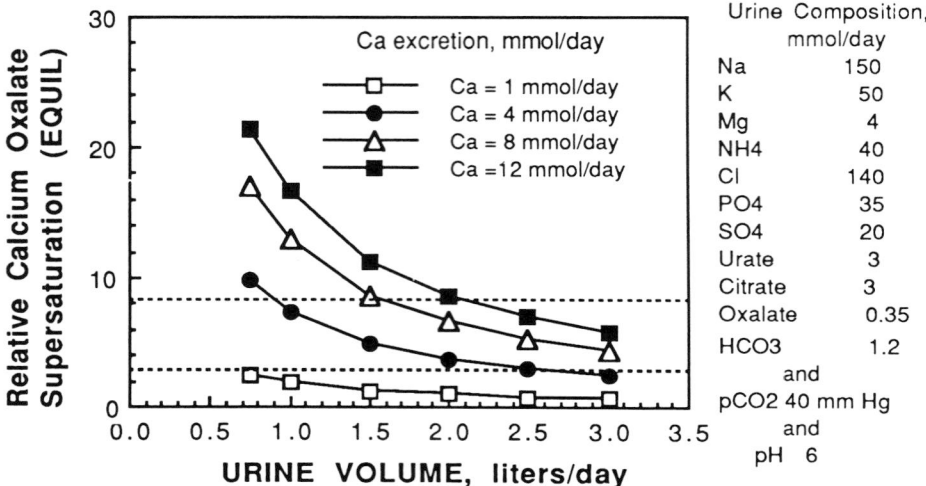

FIG. 1. Relative supersaturation (RSR) with respect to calcium oxalate of a solution having a mineral content comparable to normal urine (Na 150, K 50, Mg 5, NH_4 40, Cl 140, PO_4 35, urate 3, SO_4 20, HCO_3 1.2, citrate 3, and oxalate 0.35 mmol/day; pH 6.0) as a function of daily urine volume for a family of rates of Ca excretion ranging from 1 to 12 mmol/day. Estimated using EQUIL (3).

entry into the extracellular fluid (ECF) across the intestine; there is no net entry of Ca from bone, the site of >99% or more of body stores of Ca, if rates of bone formation and of bone resorption are equal. Based on the ranges for urinary Ca excretion in a large number of healthy men and women eating their customary self-selected diets, Hodgkinson and Pyrah (8) proposed that urinary Ca excretion rates > 7.50 mmol/day (300 mg/day) in men or >6.25 mmol/day (250 mg/day) in women can serve to define hypercalciuria. Another widely accepted definition for subjects eating *ad libitum* is the urinary excretion of >0.1 mmol Ca/kg body weight/day (>4 mg/kg/day), regardless of sex or age (8,9). Figure 2 shows the average relationships between daily urinary Ca excretion and dietary Ca intake from several studies of healthy adults fed constant diets of known composition (10–15). Among healthy adults eating diets providing normal amounts of Ca—10 to 25 mmol/day (400 to 1000 mg/day)—urinary Ca averages about 4 mmol/day (160 mg/day) and, on average, does not exceed 7.5 mmol/day (mean + 2 SD) even when dietary Ca intake is as high as 40 mmol/day (2000 mg/day). Moreover, the relative increase in urinary Ca as diet Ca intake increases (slope) averages only about 8%.

By contrast, among patients with IH urinary Ca excretion is, on average, twofold higher across a similar range of dietary Ca intakes. Thus, the increase in urinary Ca as dietary Ca intake is increased (slope) among patients with IH averages about 20%, a value approximately twice that observed among healthy subjects and that reflects the more efficient intestinal Ca absorption present in IH. Note also in Fig. 2 that even at the lowest dietary Ca intakes, patients with IH excrete greater than normal quantities of Ca into their urine suggesting that they are poised to withdraw skeletal Ca-stores at a greater than normal rate.

Using these definitions of hypercalciuria approximately 2–5% (20–50 per thousand) of healthy adults exhibit hypercalciuria (8). On the other hand the incidence of nephrolithiasis, about 80% being Ca-stones, is about 2 or 3% (20–30 per thousand) in the population (16) and at most about 50% of the Ca-stone formers exhibit hypercalciuria (10–15 per thousand). Therefore, some healthy individuals must exhibit hypercalciuria but do not form kidney stones. Moreover, hypercalciuria may be present among patients with hyperparathyroidism, with glucocorticoid excess (Cushing's syndrome), with various neoplasms, and with sarcocoid or other granulomatous dis-

TABLE 1. Urinary Ca excretion in normal adults and Ca-stone formers

Group	Number of subjects	Urinary Ca excretion (mmol/day)	
		Diet Ca 7.5 mmol/day	Diet Ca 62.5 mmol/day
Healthy adults	11	2.5–3.75	6.25–7.5
Ca-stone formers	23	6.25–15	11.25–18

Source: adapted from Refs. 4 and 5.

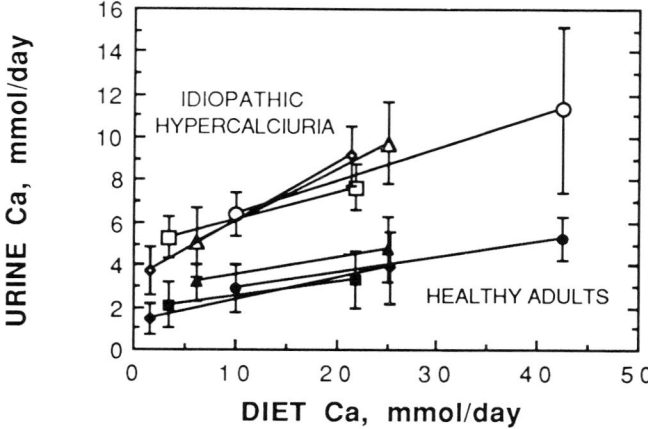

FIG. 2. Mean daily urine Ca excretion in relation to dietary Ca intake for groups of healthy adults (*solid symbols*) and groups of patients with IH (*open symbols*). Adapted from Refs. 10–15.

eases without the formation of kidney stones. These considerations thus indicate that other factors including limited water intake or accelerated water losses in sweat or diarrheal stools with low urine flow rates, increased urinary oxalate concentrations, low urinary citrate excretion rates, and abnormalities of normal urinary inhibitors of calcium oxalate crystal growth such as nephrocalcin, etc. must be equally or even more important than hypercalciuria in the pathogenesis of kidney stones. Nevertheless, as reviewed subsequently, measures that reduce urinary Ca excretion among patients with IH prevent or reduce stone recurrence rates thus emphasizing the clinical relevance of hypercalciuria to the formation of kidney stones.

OVERVIEW OF THE MECHANISMS FOR HYPERCALCIURIA

The ultimate source of the additional Ca excreted into the urine of patients with IH could, theoretically, be only the diet as a consequence of more efficient intestinal Ca absorption or the skeleton that contains 99% or more of body Ca stores or from both sources. Thus, overall mechanisms that could account for hypercalciuria include: (i)

a primary increase of intestinal Ca absorption or activation of factors stimulation intestinal Ca absorption with excretion of the Ca into the urine, (ii) increased net bone resorption, (iii) a primary defect in renal tubular reabsorption of Ca filtered across the glomeruli with a physiologic compensatory increase of intestinal Ca absorption (and net bone resorption), or (iv) a more generalized acceleration of Ca transport affecting all of these processes. Early views of the pathogenesis of IH considered that hypercalciuria could be the result of either primary augmentation of intestinal Ca absorption or a renal Ca-leak (impaired renal tubular reabsorption of filtered Ca). In subsequent pioneering studies summarized in Table 2 (12,17,18), Pak and associates divided patients with hypercalciuria into three major categories: (i) absorptive hypercalciuria defined by a fall in daily and fasting urinary Ca excretion rates to the range observed in healthy subjects in response to the ingestion of diets low in Ca or the additional administration of sodium cellulose phosphate to bind dietary Ca within the lumen of the gut and minimize Ca absorption; (ii) renal hypercalciuria defined by fasting hypercalciuria, a trend toward hypocalcemia and consequent secondary hyperparathyroidism; and, separately, (iii) resorptive hypercalciuria, typified by primary hyperparathyroidism, and characterized by fasting hypercalciuria and evidence of accelerated bone turnover or reduced bone mass. More recently, Coe and Favus (19) have reviewed all of the published metabolic balance studies that have been observed in patients with IH fed diets providing constant and accurately known quantities of Ca in comparison to comparable studies in healthy adults. These data are summarized in Fig. 3, daily urinary Ca excretion rates are plotted in relation to average daily net intestinal absorption rates (dietary Ca intake minus fecal Ca excretion) for each subject. The diagonal dashed lines in Fig. 3 indicate equivalent rates of net intestinal Ca absorption and urinary Ca excretion, the zero balance line. In comparison to healthy subjects, the patients with IH exhibited increased rates of intestinal Ca absorption and even greater rates of urinary Ca excretion so that the majority of the patients with IH, although not all, were in negative Ca balance, most of the data points lying above and to the left of the zero balance line. All of the data points for the patients with IH were above the 95% confidence band for the observations in

TABLE 2. *Absorptive and renal hypercalciuria*

	Normals	Absorptive hypercalciuria	Renal hypercalciuria
Serum Ca, mg/dL	9.8	9.8	9.5
Serum P, mg/dL	3.8	3.9	3.7
Fasting Urine Ca/Cr, mg/mg	0.057	0.078	0.17
Serum iPTH, mg Eq/ml	0.42	0.28	1.25
Fasting Urine cAMP/Cr, mmol/g	4.02	3.22	6.17

Source: adapted from Refs. 12, 17, 18.

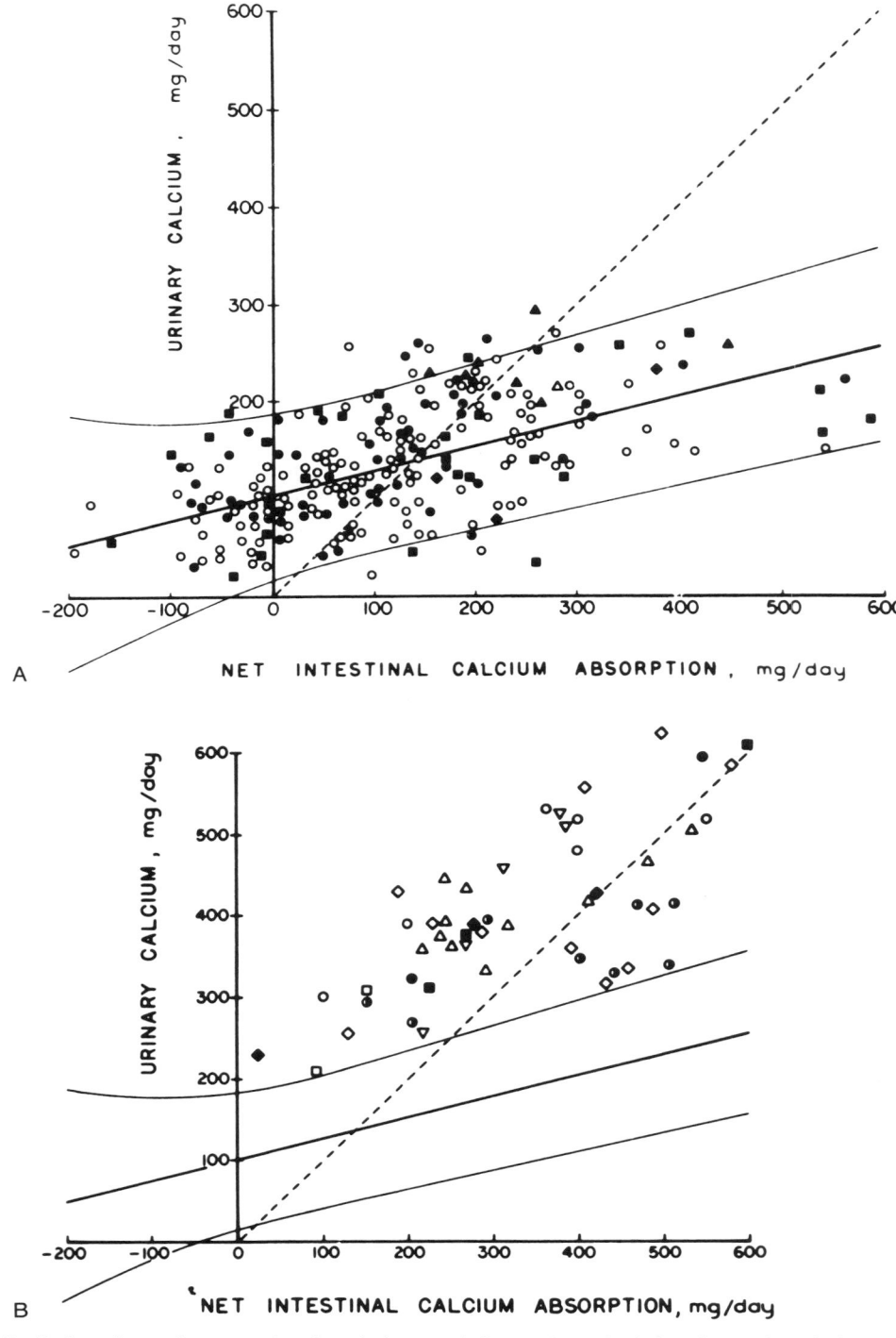

FIG. 3. Daily urinary Ca excretion in relation to daily net intestinal Ca absorption during metabolic balance studies in healthy adults (**A**) and in patients with IH (**B**). The dashed lines indicate equivalent rates of urinary Ca excretion and net intestinal Ca absorption, the zero balance line. The solid lines indicate the 95% confidence band about the mean regression relationship observed in health. Reproduced with permission from Coe and Favus (19).

healthy subjects. These observations demonstrate that while intestinal Ca absorption is increased among patients with IH, greater rates of urinary Ca excretion must reflect a subtle renal Ca leak in many patients perhaps reflecting a more generalized acceleration of Ca transport that can, potentially, cause negative Ca balances.

INTESTINAL Ca ABSORPTION IN HEALTH AND IH

As previously illustrated in Fig. 3, patients with IH exhibit increased rates of intestinal Ca absorption. The quantity of Ca that is absorbed by the intestine is determined by the availability of Ca in the diet and the capacity of the intestine to absorb Ca. In general, intestinal Ca absorption represents the sum of two transport processes, saturable transcellular absorption that is physiologically regulated and non-saturable paracellular absorption that is dependent on the Ca concentration within the lumen, in turn largely determined by the quantity of Ca in the diet.

While occasional patients with IH give a history of excessive intake of Ca-rich foods, especially milk, cheese, and ice cream, or a history of using antacids containing $CaCO_3$, the vast majority do not, thus implying enhanced intestinal absorption of Ca in IH is not the consequence of higher concentrations of Ca in the gut lumen and greater rates of non-saturable paracellular transport. Further support for this view is provided by the data in Fig. 4 that compares average daily rates of net intestinal Ca absorption observed during balance studies of patients with IH to those in healthy subjects (11,13,20–36) when both groups were eating diets providing comparable and normal quantities of Ca, 23.6–25 mmol (=944–1000 mg) Ca/day. Net intestinal Ca absorption in IH was almost twice that observed in health. Data from these and other balance studies, as well as studies assessing absorption of isotopic Ca, also confirming enhanced in-

testinal Ca absorption in IH are summarized in Table 3 (37). Collectively, these data thus indicate that intestinal Ca absorption is most likely increased in IH because of greater active transcellular Ca transport. Furthermore, direct support for this view are observations that isotopic Ca uptake into intestinal mucosa obtained by biopsy from patients with IH is increased when compared to normal subjects (38).

Currently, the hormonal metabolite of the vitamin D endocrine system, $1,25(OH)_2D$ (calcitriol), is the only documented physiological stimulus that can act to augment intestinal Ca absorption (39). Figure 5 summarizes measurements of intestinal Ca absorption in health and disease (18,40–42), expressed as a percent to minimize differences due to variations in Ca administered (intake) and using several methods, in relation to simultaneously measured serum $1,25(OH)_2D$ concentrations. Ca absorption is exquisitely sensitive to prevailing serum $1,25(OH)_2D$ levels increasing by about 0.2%/pmol $1,25(OH)_2D/L$ or about 0.5%/pg $1,25(OH)_2D/mL$. The observations are, on the average, independent of the method used to assess Ca absorption since the slopes of the lines are similar. When assays for serum $1,25(OH)_2D$ concentrations first became available, Pak and his associates (18) were the first to demonstrate that serum $1,25(OH)_2D$ concentrations are higher than normal among some patients with IH, especially those considered to have a renal Ca leak. As summarized in Table 4 (18,43–47a), a number of subsequent studies, although not all, have confirmed that serum $1,25(OH)_2D$ concentrations are higher among patients with IH averaging about 146 pmol/L (61 pg/mL) as compared to an average of about 94 pmol/L (39 pg/mL) among normal subjects, thus suggesting that activation of $1,25(OH)_2D$ synthesis could account for the increase in intestinal Ca absorption. Moreover, as summarized in Fig. 6, $1,25(OH)_2D_3$ production rates among patients with IH, as measured by the equilibrium infusion of ^3H-

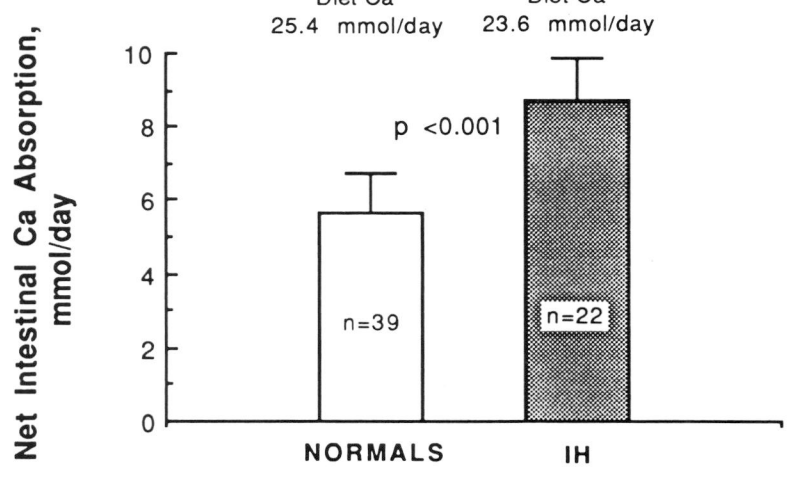

FIG. 4. Net intestinal Ca absorption during metabolic balance studies among healthy adults and among patients with IH fed constant diets providing comparable normal quantities of Ca. Adapted from data in Refs. 11, 13, 20–36.

TABLE 3. *Intestinal Ca absorption in normal adults and in idiopathic hypercalciuria patients*

Method	Normal subjects			Idiopathic hypercalciurics			p
	Number of subjects	Net Ca absorption (mmol/day)	Percent Ca absorption	Number of subjects	Net Ca absorption (mmol/day)	Percent Ca absorption	
Metabolic balance (diet intake minus fecal excretion)	62	4.35 ± 3.12[a]	19 ± 12	31	9.12 ± 2.82	39 ± 11	<0.001
Isotopic Ca absorption (oral ^{47}Ca, +i.v. ^{45}Ca)	27		28 ± 8	22		48 ± 11	<0.001
Fecal recovery of oral ^{47}Ca							
400-mg diet	6		50 ± 8	9		73 ± 7	<0.001
1,700-mg diet	6		31 ± 5	9		51 ± 6	<0.001

Source: adapted from Lemann (37).
[a] Variance shown as ±SD.

labeled-1,25(OH)$_2$D$_3$, have been shown to be increased without a decrease in the metabolic clearance of 1,25(OH)$_2$D$_3$ (48).

Possible mechanisms accounting for activation of 1,25(OH)$_2$D$_3$ synthesis in some IH patients remain incompletely understood. In health, most 1,25(OH)$_2$D is presumed to be produced in the kidneys (39) by a proximal tubular mitochondrial 25(OH)D$_3$-1α-hydroxylase, a heme-containing cytochrome P450 enzyme that has not yet been isolated and characterized. Some physiological studies suggest that there may be two distinct enzyme activities in the renal tubule (49). Synthesis of 1,25(OH)$_2$D is known to be stimulated by parathyroid hormone (PTH), by hypophosphatemia or dietary PO$_4$

deprivation, and by hypocalcemia either directly or indirectly via the effect of hypocalcemia to enhance PTH secretion (39). A few patients with IH and fasting hypercalciuria, as evidence of a renal Ca-leak, in association with elevated serum PTH levels or increased rates of urinary excretion of cAMP or nephrogenous cAMP (excreted minus filtered cAMP) as evidence of the action of PTH on the kidneys have been reported (12). However, as summarized in Table 5, most studies of patients with IH have demonstrated that neither serum PTH levels nor urinary cAMP excretion rates are high among patients with IH. Thus, PTH-mediated activation of 1,25(OH)$_2$D is unlikely among a significant number of patients with IH unless there is enhanced sensitivity of

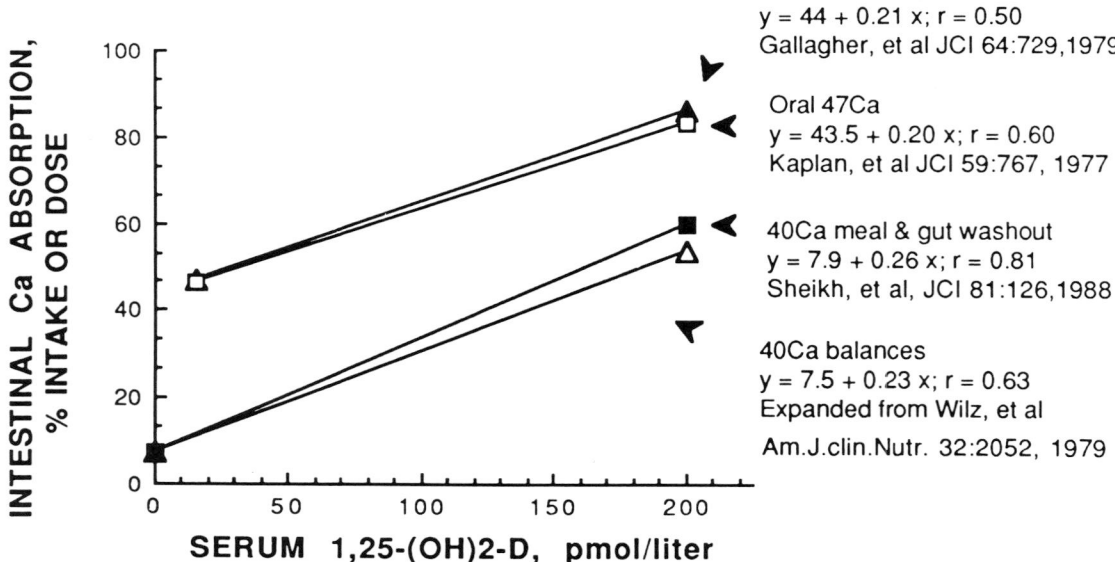

Oral 47Ca + iv 45Ca
y = 44 + 0.21 x; r = 0.50
Gallagher, et al JCI 64:729,1979

Oral 47Ca
y = 43.5 + 0.20 x; r = 0.60
Kaplan, et al JCI 59:767, 1977

40Ca meal & gut washout
y = 7.9 + 0.26 x; r = 0.81
Sheikh, et al, JCI 81:126,1988

40Ca balances
y = 7.5 + 0.23 x; r = 0.63
Expanded from Wilz, et al
Am.J.clin.Nutr. 32:2052, 1979

FIG. 5. Intestinal Ca absorption, expressed as percent intake or percent of dose of isotopic calcium, in relation to prevailing serum 1,25(OH)$_2$D concentrations, using four methods. From data in Refs. 12, 38–41.

TABLE 4. *Serum 1,25(OH)₂D concentrations in normal subjects and idiopathic hypercalciuria (IH) patients*

Reference	Normal	IH	p
18	82 ± 22[b] (11)[a]	115 ± 29 (24)	<0.001
43	82 ± 17 (17)	130 ± 46 (15)	<0.001
44	87 ± 29 (48)	150 ± 74 (26)	<0.001
45	82 ± 17 (9)	99 ± 14 (24)	NS
46, 46a	106 ± 26 (56)	185 ± 30 (50)	<0.001
47	82 ± 17 (15)	117 ± 43 (21)	<0.001
47a	120 ± 38 (12)	166 ± 30 (32)	<0.001

[a] Numbers in parentheses indicate number of subjects.
[b] Variances shown as ±SD.

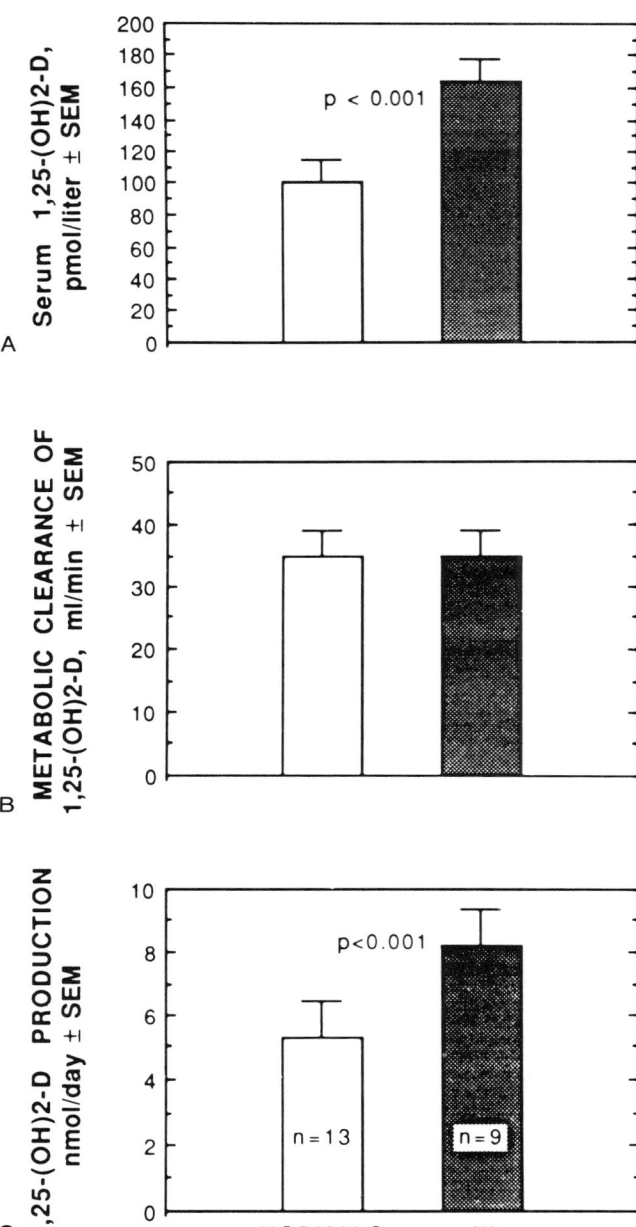

FIG. 6. Mean serum 1,25(OH)₂D concentrations (**A**), 1,25(OH)₂D₃ metabolic clearances (**B**) and 1,25(OH)₂D₃ production rates (**C**) in health and in IH. Adapted from Insogna et al. (48).

the proximal tubule to normal serum PTH levels via some as yet unknown mechanism. Albright and associates (6,7) observed mild hypophosphatemia when they originally defined IH and subsequent studies, summarized in Table 6, and also provided evidence that many, although again not all, patients with IH have mildly low serum PO_4 concentrations. Moreover, as shown in Fig. 7, patients with IH appear to exhibit delayed achievement of maximal renal PO_4-conservation in response to the ingestion of a synthetic low PO_4-diet and elevated fasting saliva/serum PO_4-concentration ratios suggesting the possibility of a subtle and more generalized PO_4 "leak" (50). Dietary PO_4-deprivation in healthy adults (51–53) and in children with mild chronic renal failure (54) has been shown to increase serum 1,25(OH)₂D concentrations. In animals, dietary PO_4-deprivation increases synthesis of 1,25(OH)₂D in the kidney (55), an effect that is independent of PTH (56) but abolished by hypophysectomy (57). The augmentation of renal 1,25(OH)₂D synthesis in hypophysectomized animals in response to PO_4-deprivation is restored by growth hormone (GH) and by somatomedin C (SM-C; IGF-1) (58,59). Moreover, other maneuvers that reduce serum SM-C levels in animals such as dietary protein restriction (4% of diet) or induction of experimental diabetes also blunt the effect of dietary PO_4-deprivation to activate renal 1,25(OH)₂D synthesis (60). Thus, the effect of hypophosphatemia to increase 1,25(OH)₂D synthesis appears to be permissively dependent on normal pituitary function and normal availability of SM-C. There is no clinical evidence for GH excess in IH and SM-C levels have not been reported. More direct evidence for a potential role for hypophosphatemia in activating vitamin D metabolism in humans is provided by the report of a family with afflicted members demonstrating hereditary hypophosphatemia of varying degree, accompanied by

elevated serum 1,25(OH)₂D levels and hypercalciuria among those with mild hypophosphatemia and, additionally, osteomalacia among those with severe hypophosphatemia (61). Thus, subtle hypophosphatemia may play a role to activate vitamin D metabolism among at least a subset of patients with IH. Rare patients with IH exhibit an overt renal Ca leak, mild hypocalcemia, and secondary hyperparathyroidism resulting in increased serum 1,25(OH)₂D concentrations (12). However, most patients with IH have normal serum Ca con-

TABLE 5. *Serum PTH concentrations and urinary excretion of cAMP or nephrogenous cAMP in normal subjects and idiopathic hypercalciuria (IH) patients*

Serum PTH reference	Units	Normal	IH	p
12	μg Eq/mL	0.42 ± 0.29 (20)	0.28 ± 0.24 (22)	NS
43	pg/mL	357 ± 78 (17)	238 ± 55 (15)	<0.001
44	μL Eq/mL	6.5 ± 3.6 (48)	6.3 ± 2.1 (26)	NS
49a	μL Eq/mL	60 (upper normal limit)	111 ± 68 (27)	<0.001
Urine cAMP				
45	nmol/mg creatinine	4.3 ± 0.9 (9)	2.8 ± 1.6 (13)	<0.05
Nephrogenous cAMP				
49b	nmol/100 ml GFR	1.4 ± 2.2 (25)	1.3 ± 4.0 (50)	NS

centrations so that hypocalcemia alone or with elevations in PTH seldom appears to account for activation of the vitamin D endocrine system.

The increased intestinal absorption of Ca that is regularly observed among patients with IH may also be independent of $1,25(OH)_2D$ or the result of other factors that affect the ways by which $1,25(OH)_2D$ interacts with its specific intestinal cytosolic receptor to initiate transcription and translation of Ca-binding protein (CaBP) and, speculatively, other factors that ultimately result in enhanced lumen to blood translocation of Ca. As shown in Fig. 8, Pak and associates (18) observed that among patients with IH and absorptive hypercalciuria, intestinal absorption of ^{47}Ca was increased out of proportion to prevailing serum $1,25(OH)_2D$ concentrations, in comparison to the relationship observed among normal subjects, together with stone-formers with a renal Ca leak or without hypercalciuria and patients with hyperparathyroidism, thus suggesting $1,25(OH)_2D$-independent Ca absorption. Subsequent balance studies, shown in Fig. 9 (62), have also shown that net intestinal Ca absorption among patients with IH (expressed as a percent of di-

etary Ca intake to take account of small differences in dietary Ca intake between subjects) is also increased out of proportion to the relationship between percent Ca absorption and serum $1,25(OH)_2D$ concentrations observed in healthy subjects (Fig. 9A and B). However, when similar data for healthy subjects given $1,25(OH)_2D_3$ to experimentally increase serum $1,25(OH)_2D$ concentrations were additionally considered, the slope of percent Ca absorption in relation to serum $1,25(OH)_2D$ concentrations was observed to double and the data for the patients with IH fell within the 95% confidence band for this new relationship (Fig. 9C and D). $1,25(OH)_2D$ is now known to up-regulate the apparent numbers of its own receptor in the intestine of rats (63) and in the parathyroids of humans (64). Such increased expression of the receptor in the intestine would be expected to enhance intestinal Ca absorption. Thus it seems reasonable to consider that the effects of $1,25(OH)_2D$ may be amplified in IH by such up-regulation of the receptor or by other factors that influence the receptor when serum $1,25(OH)_2D$ levels are normal (Fig. 8) or by $1,25(OH)_2D$ itself when $1,25(OH)_2D$ concentrations are only mildly elevated (Fig. 9). Direct measurements of apparent or actual $1,25(OH)_2D$-receptor numbers are needed to directly evaluate this possible mechanism. Other studies have also provided evidence that the augmentation of intestinal Ca absorption in IH may be independent of $1,25(OH)_2D$. The patterns of intestinal Ca and Mg absorption along the perfused small intestine have been reported to differ from those seen among normal subjects given $1,25(OH)_2D_3$ (65,66). In addition, among a group of rats inbred to exhibit hypercalciuria, intestinal Ca absorption was found to be increased despite normal or reduced serum $1,25(OH)_2D$ concentrations (67). Further studies are clearly needed to explore the regulation of intestinal Ca transport in IH in an effort to clarify the role of $1,25(OH)_2D$ and to precisely identify vitamin D-independent mechanisms.

TABLE 6. *Serum phosphate concentrations in normal subjects and idiopathic hypercalciuria (IH) patients*

Reference	Normal	IH	p
6	1.1	0.90	not available
45	1.10 ± 0.19[a] (9)[b]	1.04 ± 0.19	NS
43	1.19 ± 0.10 (17)	0.94 ± 0.19 (15)	<0.001
44	1.25 ± 0.19 (48)	1.10 ± 0.18 (26)	<0.001
18	1.20 ± 0.23	1.19 ± 0.16	NS
47a	1.05 ± 0.41 (12)	0.88 ± 0.20 (32)	NS

[a] Variations shown as ±SD.
[b] Number in parentheses indicate number of subjects.

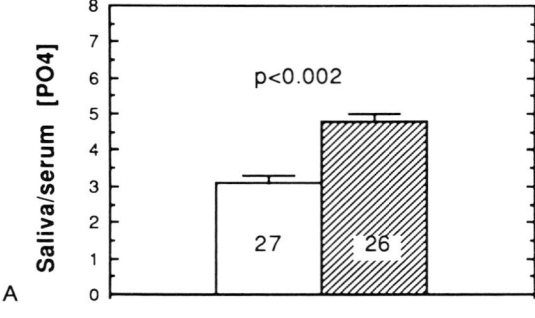

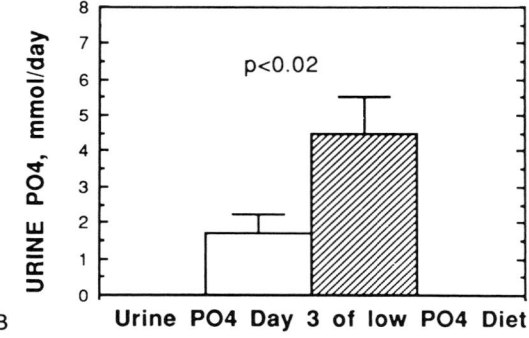

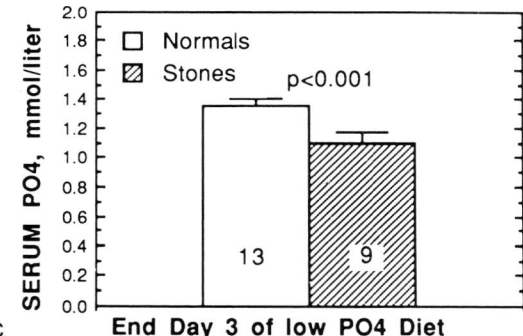

FIG. 7. Fasting saliva/serum concentration ratios (**A**) and daily urine PO_4 excretion and fasting serum PO_4 concentrations on the third day of dietary PO_4^- deprivation (**B and C**) in health and in IH. Adapted from Lemann et al. (50).

REGULATION OF URINARY Ca EXCRETION IN HEALTH AND IH

Increased urinary Ca excretion may be the consequence of increases in glomerular filtration of Ca, usually due to hypercalcemia and/or inhibition of net renal tubular Ca reabsorption. The major factors currently known to increase or decrease urinary Ca excretion are listed in Table 7 (68).

The initial process in the urinary excretion of Ca is the glomerular filtration of Ca. Glomerular filtration of Ca is determined by the plasma concentration of ultrafilterable Ca, normally averaging 60% of plasma total Ca con-

centration, and by the glomerular filtration rate. Thus, hypercalciuria in IH could be the consequence of either an increase in plasma ultrafilterable Ca concentrations or of increased GFR or both. Neither, however appear to be present. As shown in Table 8 (69,70), renal clearance studies have documented higher rates of fractional excretion of Ca filtered across the glomeruli among patients with IH as compared to healthy subjects. Moreover, as illustrated in Fig. 10, across comparable ranges among healthy subjects and patients with IH for GFR, for serum ultrafilterable Ca concentrations, and for rates of glomerular filtration of Ca, patients with IH exhibit greater than normal urinary Ca excretion rates (expanded from Ref. 71). Observations, such as these suggest that the greater rates of Ca excretion in IH at any given rate of filtration of Ca are the consequence of reduced net renal tubular reabsorption of filtered Ca.

Parathyroid hormone (PTH) is known to augment distal renal tubular reabsorption of filtered Ca (72). Thus, it would be anticipated that at any given rate of filtration of Ca, a lower than normal rate of PTH secretion, resulting in lower prevailing plasma PTH concentrations or, theoretically, impaired responsiveness of the renal tubule to PTH, would reduce net renal tubular Ca reabsorption and enhance urinary Ca excretion. As previously shown in Table 4, some studies, although not all, have shown that serum immunoreactive PTH concentrations, generally employing assays that use antibodies recognizing primarily COOH-terminal sequences of the molecule, may be in the lower part of the normal range in some patients with IH. Additional studies using current immunoassays specific for intact PTH (73) are needed to clarify whether subtle reductions in PTH contribute to the apparent inhibition of net renal tubular Ca reabsorption in IH, as might be expected if serum $1,25(OH)_2$ concentrations were raised because of the known effects of $1,25(OH)_2$ to inhibit transcription and secretion of PTH (74) or in relation to hypophosphatemia since dietary PO_4-deprivation is accompanied by a fall in serum PTH levels (75). Moreover, several studies of patients with IH have shown that some (12,76) may exhibit increased serum immunoreactive PTH concentrations suggesting that either impaired responsiveness of the renal tubule at the PTH-sensitive sites of Ca reabsorption or defective Ca reabsorption at other sites ("renal Ca-leak") may result in a trend toward hypocalcemia and compensatory secondary hyperparathyroidism (12).

Increasing NaCl intake, either in the diet or by intravenous saline, is well known to inhibit net renal tubular Ca reabsorption and to increase urinary Ca excretion. Some data illustrating this effect among healthy adults and patients with IH are illustrated in Fig. 11 (77–80). On the average, among healthy adults, urinary Ca excretion increases by about 0.6 mmol/day for every 100 mmol/day increase in urinary Na excretion (77–79). The studies of

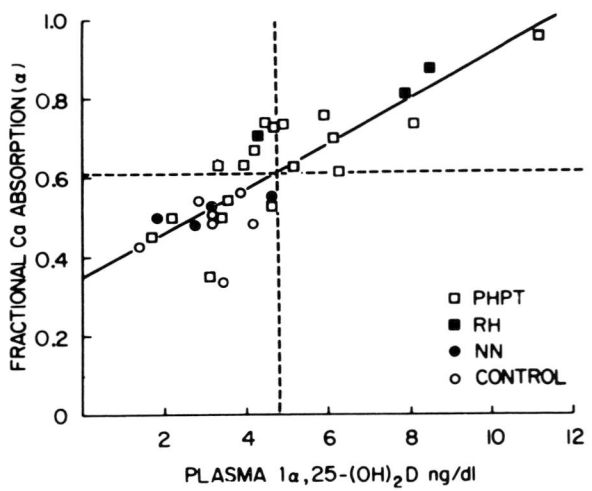
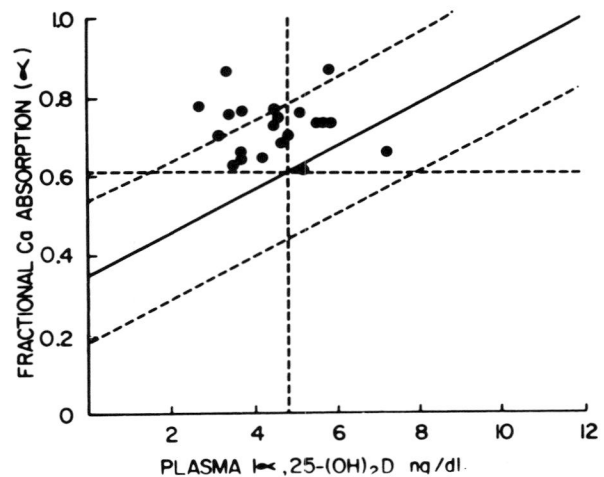

FIG. 8. Percent intestinal absorption of ^{47}Ca in relation to prevailing serum 1,25(OH)$_2$D concentrations in normal subjects (control, ○), normocalciuric nephrolithiaisis (NN, ●), nephrolithiais with a renal Ca leak (RH, ■), and primary hyperparathyroidism (PHPT, □) (**A**), and for patients with absorptive hypercalciuria superimposed on the 95% confidence band for the relationship in the other subjects (**B**). Reproduced with permission from Kaplan et al. (18).

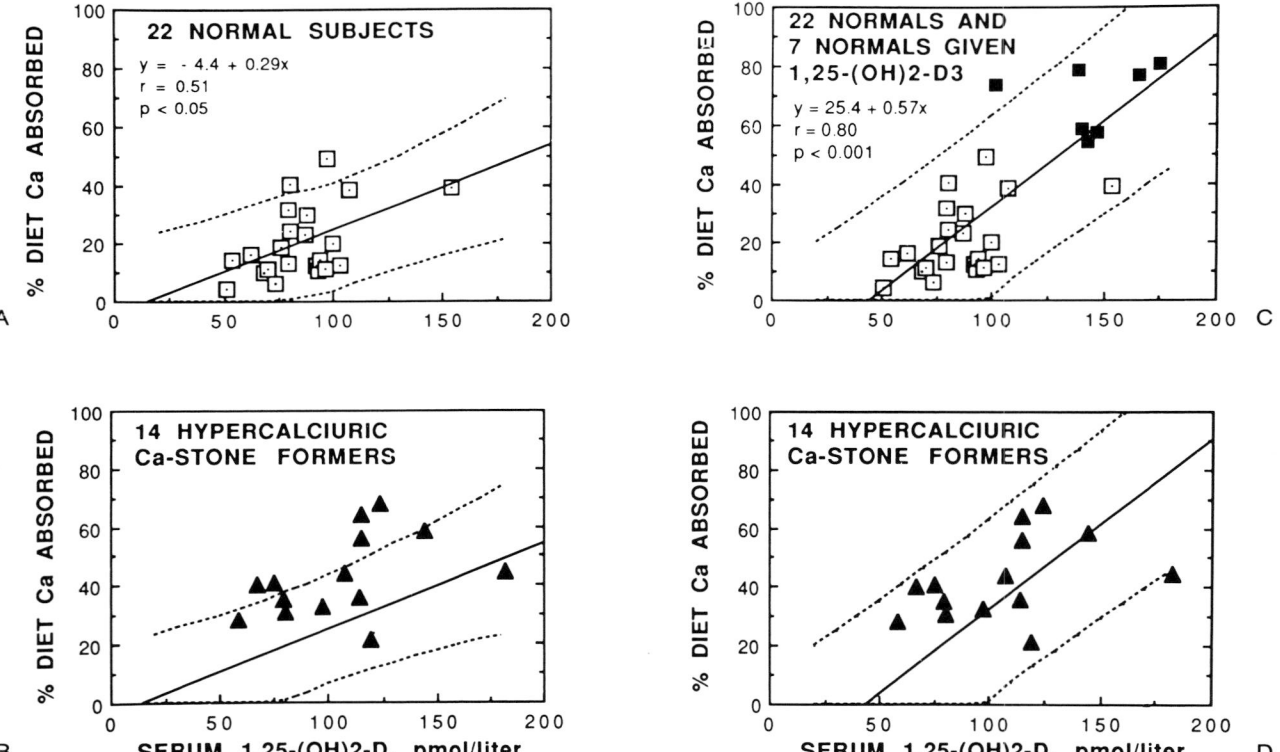

FIG. 9. Percent intestinal Ca absorption measured during balance studies in relation to prevailing serum 1,25(OH)$_2$D concentrations among healthy adults (**A**), patients with IH superimposed on the mean relationship and 95% confidence band for the relationship in normals (**B**), together with the same relationship among normals and normals also given 1,25(OH)$_2$D$_3$ (**C**), and the data for patients with IH superimposed on this second 95% confidence band (**D**). Adapted from Lemann and Gray (62).

TABLE 7. *Factors increasing or decreasing urinary Ca excretion*

FACTORS INCREASING URINARY CA EXCRETION
Increased filtered Ca
Dietary Ca intake
Hypercalcemia

Reduced tubular Ca reabsorption
Reduced PTH
NaCl intake (volume expansion)
Protein intake
Glucose, sucrose, ethanol
Potassium restriction
Phosphate restriction
Magnesium
Furosemide, bumetanide, ethacrynic acid

FACTORS DECREASING URINARY CA EXCRETION
Reduced filtered Ca
Hypocalcemia
Low GFR

Increased tubular Ca reabsorption
Increased PTH
Base ingestion (HCO_3^-)
Potassium
Thiazides, chlorthalidone, indapamide, amiloride

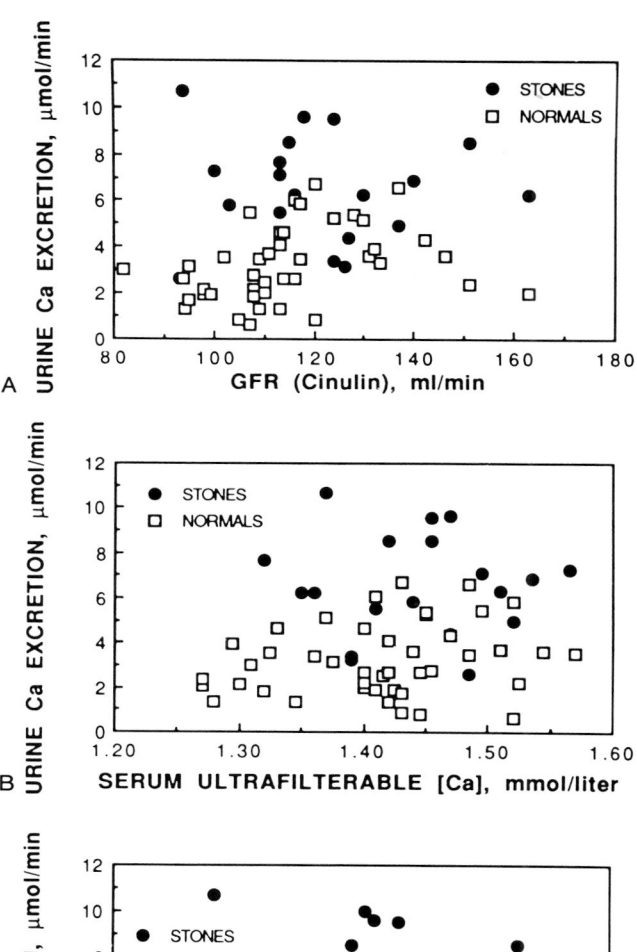

FIG. 10. Urinary Ca excretion rates in healthy adults and patients with IH observed during renal clearance studies during water diuresis after overnight fasting in relation to glomerular filtration rates (**A**), serum ultrafilterable Ca concentrations (**B**) and estimated rates of glomerular filtration of Ca (**C**). Expanded from Lemann et al. (71).

patients with IH eating controlled, but not constant, diets at home show that urinary Ca excretion is higher than among normal subjects in relation to simultaneous rates of Na excretion (Fig. 11) but that restriction of dietary NaCl intake may be accompanied by a decrease in urinary Ca excretion even into the normal range among some patients (80). Thus, excessive salt intake may contribute to hypercalciuria among some patients with IH. However, hypercalciuria persists among patients with IH even when they are fed fixed diets containing 100 mmol NaCl/day (12). Moreover, as shown in Fig. 12, across comparable ranges of urinary Na excretion, measured either in 24-hour urines or during renal clearance studies, urinary Ca excretion is higher among patients with IH than among healthy subjects (71,81). Therefore, it is unlikely that a persistently higher salt intake is responsible for the hypercalciuria among the majority of patients with IH, although increased dietary NaCl intake and the consequent increase in urinary Na excretion could aggravate hypercalciuria.

TABLE 8. *Urinary Ca excretion as percent glomerular filtration of Ca in normal subjects and idiopathic hypercalciuria (IH) patients*

Reference	Normal	IH	p
69	0.94% (7)	2.14% (14)	<0.001
70	1.27% (5)	4.25% (9)	<0.01

Number in parentheses indicates number of subjects.

Increasing dietary protein intake augments urinary Ca excretion. As shown in Fig. 13 (82–85), urinary Ca excretion increased by about 0.04 mmol/day for each increase of 1 g/day protein intake (about 1.5 mg Ca/g protein) when dietary protein intake was varied among healthy men and women. The effect of increased protein intake to augment Ca excretion may be mediated by several mechanisms. The oxidation of amino acid sulfur to inorganic sulfate augments acid production (86). Acido-

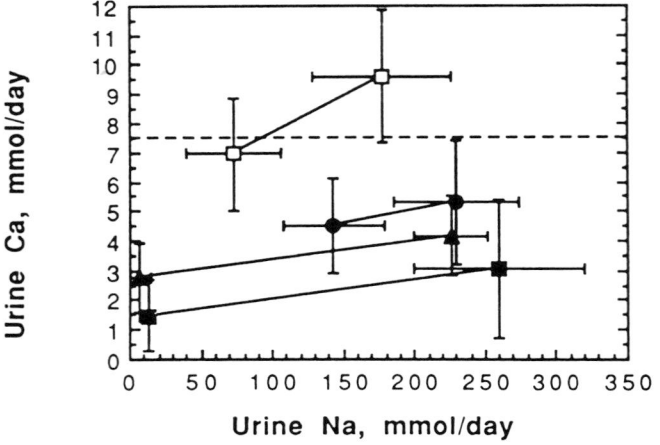

FIG. 11. Mean daily urinary Ca excretion in relation to mean daily urinary Na excretion for groups of normal subjects (*solid symbols*) and for a group of patients with IH (*open symbols*) eating diets providing varying amounts of NaCl. Vertical and horizontal error bars indicate ±SD. Adapted from Refs. 77–80.

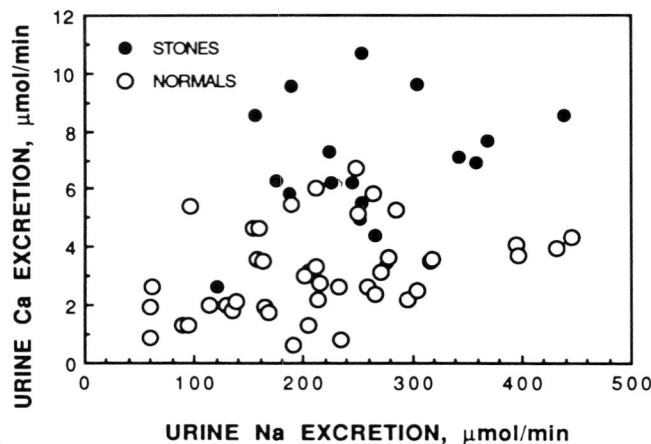

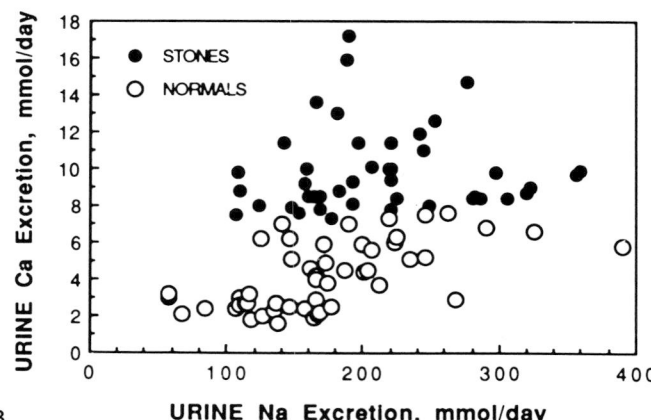

FIG. 12. Urinary Ca excretion in relation to urinary Na excretion among patients with IH (*solid symbols*) and normal subjects (*open symbols*) observed during renal clearance studies during water diuresis (**A**) and in 24-hour urine collections (**B**). Expanded from Refs. 71 and 81.

sis, produced experimentally by the administration of ammonium chloride, is accompanied by inhibition of renal tubular Ca reabsorption (87) as well as by increased rates of net bone resorption (88,89) without a change in rates of intestinal Ca absorption (90). In addition, the divalent anion sulfate is not readily reabsorbed by the renal tubules and when present in tubular fluid in increased concentration, sulfate can complex Ca and augment urinary Ca excretion; urinary Ca excretion is increased to a greater extent by the infusion of Na_2SO_4 than by the infusion of Na at a similar rate as NaCl (91). When dietary protein is increased and urinary Ca excretion rises, Ca excretion can be reduced by the additional administration of $NaHCO_3$ (85) despite continuing the higher protein intake and the persistence of increased rates of sulfate excretion into the urine. Thus, the mild systemic acidosis accompanying higher protein intakes may be of most significance in mediating the effect of protein to augment urinary Ca excretion. Epidemiological data implicate a role for dietary protein in the incidence of kidney stones. The incidence of stones among various nations throughout the world has been found to be correlated to protein intake, especially animal protein (92) but whether this relationship is mediated by the calciuric effect of protein is not known. However, as shown in Fig. 14 (71) urinary Ca excretion is higher among Ca-stone formers than among healthy subjects despite comparable ranges of urinary sulfate excretion, as a reflection of protein intake. Moreover, urinary Ca excretion is higher among stone formers than among normal subjects in relation to comparable rates of net acid excretion (93). While excessively high rates of dietary protein intake may cause hypercalciuria in some patients or further increase urinary Ca excretion in others, these data

suggest high protein intakes are unlikely to be a primary cause of hypercalciuria or the inhibition of renal tubular Ca reabsorption in IH.

The ingestion of glucose, as well as other rapidly metabolizable nutrients such as sucrose, protein, and ethanol, are known to be accompanied by transient calciuria and by magnesuria (94), probably related to an effect of insulin (95). Among patients with IH, the administration of glucose or sucrose causes an exaggerated transient increase in urinary Ca, but not Mg, excretion (71). The mechanism for this observation has not been clarified. It seems reasonable to suspect that higher rates of Ca excretion following meals rich in purified carbohydrates, by transiently increasing urinary Ca concentrations, could increase the relative supersaturation of the urine with respect to Ca-oxalate and favor Ca-oxalate crystalluria or stone growth. However, there has been no direct confirmation of such events. Moreover, the administration of glucose is accompanied by acidification of

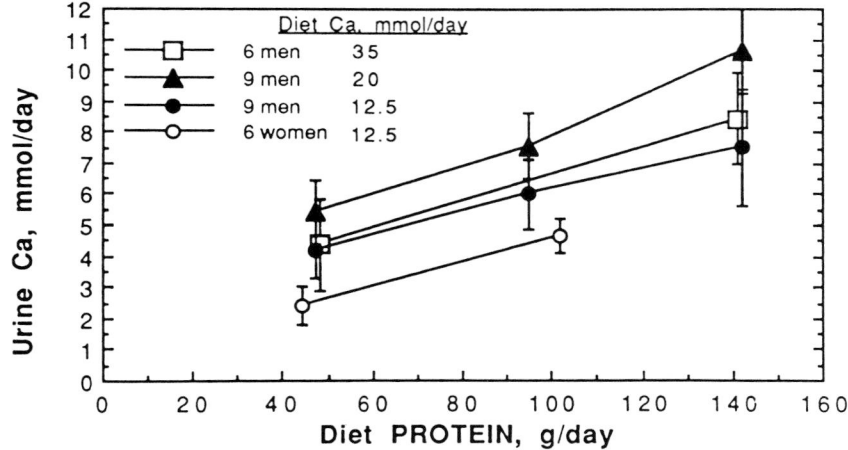

FIG. 13. Urinary Ca excretion in relation to dietary protein intake among men and women fed varying amounts of Ca during metabolic balance studies. Adapted from Refs. 82–85.

the urine (71,96) that would cause relatively more urinary phosphate to be present as $H_2PO_4^-$ rather than HPO_4^{2-}, thus lessening the risk for crystallization of brushite, $CaHPO_4 \cdot 2\ H_2O$.

Recent studies in healthy adults have demonstrated that dietary potassium deprivation is accompanied by increased urinary Ca excretion, regardless of whether K is removed from the diet with Cl^- or with HCO_3^- (79). In addition, the administration of KCl was found to prevent the increase in urinary Ca excretion that accompanies the administration of NaCl while the administration of $KHCO_3$ reduced urinary Ca excretion, whereas the administration of equivalent amounts of $NaHCO_3$ did not change urinary Ca excretion (79,97). The quantitative relationship between the changes in urinary Ca excretion and the changes in urinary K excretion observed in these studies is summarized in Fig. 15: Δ Urine Ca, mmol/day = 0.29 − 0.0147 Δ Urine K, mmol/day; an increase in urinary K of 20 mmol/day thus reducing urinary Ca by about 0.3 mmol Ca/day (12 mg/day). The

mechanisms responsible for the effects of K administration to decrease and K deprivation to increase urinary Ca excretion are not definitively known but may include: (i) ECF-volume contraction related to the long known saliuretic effects of the administration of K-salts and ECF-volume expansion accompanying renal Na and Cl retention during K deprivation, and (ii) the effect of K administration to increase distal renal tubular PO_4 reabsorption (98) and slightly raise serum PO_4 concentrations, thus reducing serum $1,25(OH)_2D$ levels (79,99). No data exist, however, to indicate that patients with IH habitually eat diets low in K that could contribute to hypercalciuria. In fact, as shown in Fig. 16, urinary Ca excretion rates among patients with IH are higher than those observed in healthy subjects across comparable ranges of urinary K excretion (71,81). Thus, reductions in dietary K intake, like increased dietary intake of NaCl, protein and purified carbohydrate, may worsen hypercalciuria but does not account for IH.

Dietary PO_4-deprivation is known to be accompanied

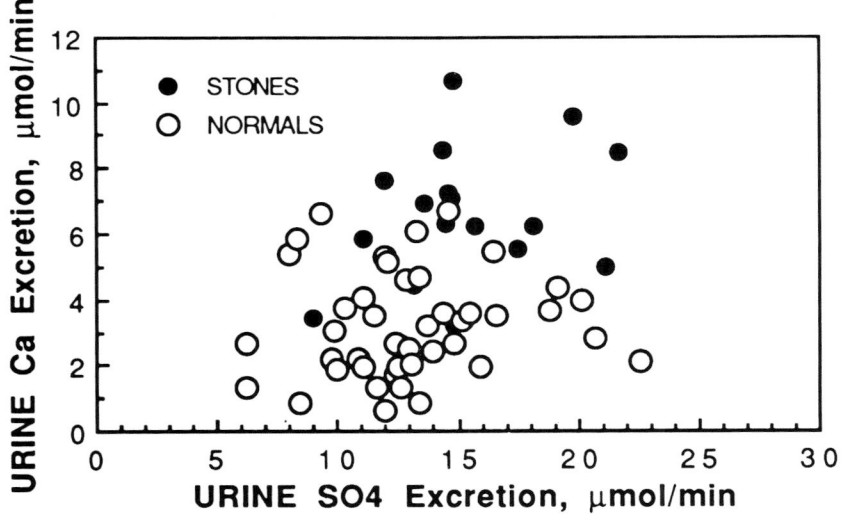

FIG. 14. Urinary Ca excretion in relation to urinary SO_4 excretion as a reflection of protein intake among patients with IH (*solid symbols*) and normal subjects (*open symbols*) observed during renal clearance studies during water diuresis. Expanded from Lemann et al. (71).

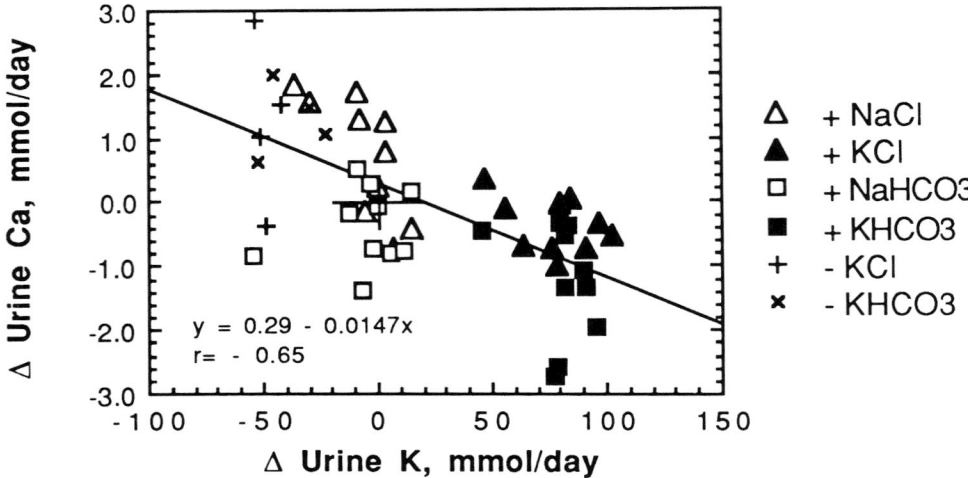

FIG. 15. The changes (△) in daily urinary Ca excretion in relation to the changes in daily urinary K excretion observed on the fourth day of dietary K-deprivation or the on going administration of NaCl, KCl, NaHCO₃, or KHCO₃. Reproduced with permission from Lemann et al. (79).

by increased rates of urinary Ca excretion (75), probably reflecting the previously described effect of even subtle hypophosphatemia to activate the vitamin D endocrine system and thereby enhance intestinal Ca absorption when Ca is available in the diet or enhance net bone resorption when dietary Ca intake is very low (100,101). There are no data to support the view that habitually reduced levels of dietary PO_4 intake contribute to hypercalciuria in IH. Once again, as shown in Fig. 17, urinary Ca excretion rates among patients with IH are higher than among healthy adults, across comparable rates of urinary PO_4 excretion. The defect in regulation of serum PO_4 concentration causing hypophosphatemia that appears to be present in a subset of patients with IH thus appears to reflect a subtle defect in tubular PO_4-reabsorption, at an undefined tubular site.

Bicarbonate is known to enhance renal tubular Ca reabsorption both in the proximal tubule (102) and in the distal tubule (103). Experimental NH_4Cl acidosis, with reductions in serum HCO_3 concentrations, is accompanied by increased rates of daily urinary Ca excretion and of fasting urinary Ca excretion, the latter reflecting net bone resorption (89). Moreover, the hyperchloremic metabolic acidosis caused by defective final acidification of the urine in classic distal renal tubular acidosis may also be accompanied by increased rates of urinary Ca excretion (19). Although subtle defects in urinary acidification have been described among some patients with IH (104), most patients exhibit normal serum HCO_3 concentrations and appear to acidify their urine normally.

IH may be familial (105) and a hereditary defect in renal tubular transport may account for hypercalciuria. Pharmacological studies have provided evidence for defective proximal renal tubular Ca reabsorption in IH

(106). The enzyme, Ca-Mg-ATPase is present in the distal tubule (107) and could participate in the processes leading to Ca reabsorption. A similar, if not the same enzyme, is present in red blood cells. Recent studies have demonstrated that the activity of RBC Ca-Mg-ATPase is increased among patients with IH (108). Furthermore, that same report demonstrated that in family studies there was a significant correlation between Ca-Mg-ATPase activity in children and the mean of the enzyme activities in their parents as well as a significant correlation between urinary Ca excretion rates in the children and the mean Ca excretion rates in their parents. These observations have provided initial clues as to possible genetically determined enzymatic defects in Ca transport in IH and confirmation of these data and additional studies are needed.

THE SKELETON IN IDIOPATHIC HYPERCALCIURIA

The skeleton cannot be the source of a significant proportion of the additional Ca excreted into the urine of patients with IH since hypercalciuria may persist for many years and, if urinary Ca excretion was increased from a normal mean value of about 4 mmol/day (160 mg/day) to 10 mmol/day (400 mg)/day, the increment in urinary Ca above normal of 6 mmol/day (240 mg/day) would result in the loss of about 9% per year of the approximately 25,000 mmol of Ca contained in the skeleton of an adult of average size. Such rates of Ca loss could not be sustained without the development of overt bone disease, which patients with IH do not exhibit. Thus, the bulk of the extra Ca appearing in the urine of patients with IH must reflect more efficient intestinal Ca

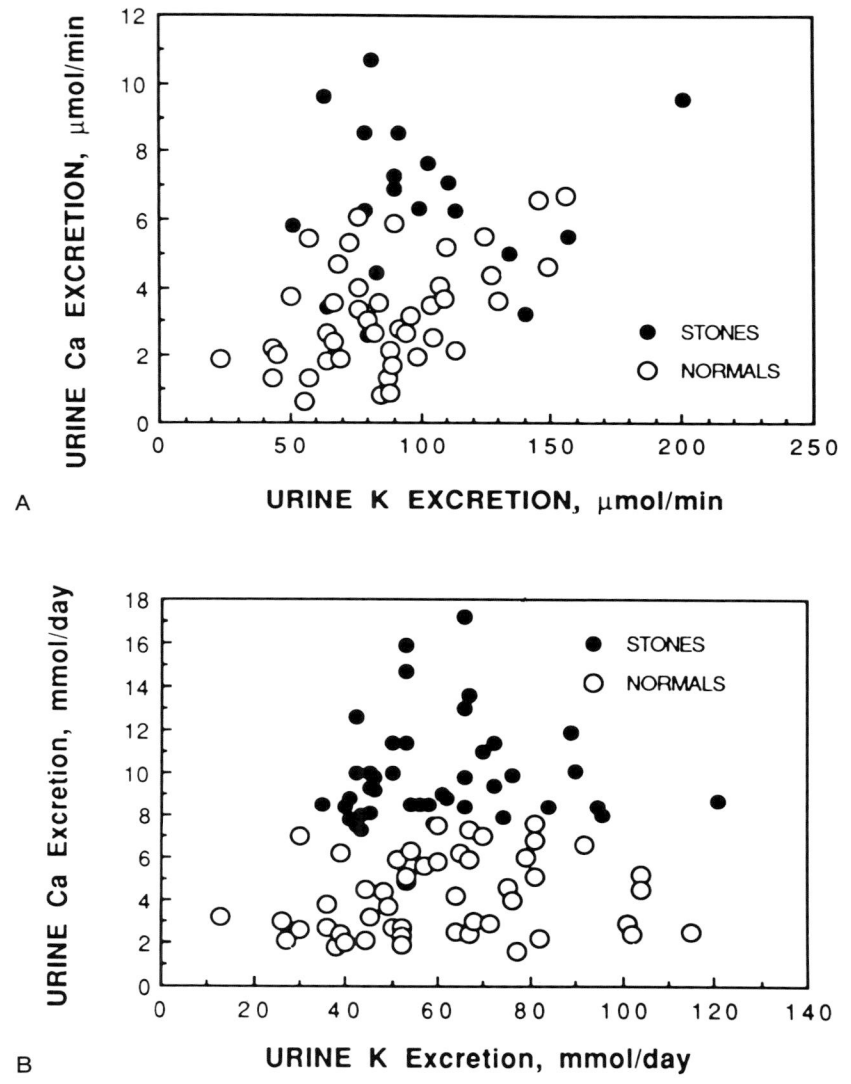

FIG. 16. Urinary Ca excretion in relation to urinary K excretion among patients with IH (●) and normal subjects (○) observed during renal clearance studies during water diuresis (**A**) and in 24-hour urine collections (**B**). Expanded from Refs. 71 and 81.

absorption. Nonetheless, a series of studies have provided evidence for the participation of the skeleton in IH. Studies of the turnover of injected radiocalcium, summarized in Table 9 (29), have demonstrated that patients with IH, in comparison to normals, exhibit enlarged pools of exchangeable Ca and increased rates of both bone formation and bone resorption, implying accelerated bone remodeling. The acute intravenous administration of Ca to patients with IH results in rapid distribution of most of the administered Ca to sites outside of the plasma (and ECF) volume (109), reflecting more efficient "buffering" of the Ca load, presumably in bone. In response to the ingestion of diets providing only 0.05 mmol Ca/kg body weight/day (2 mg/kg/day), patients with IH were unable to reduce their urinary Ca

excretion rates to levels as low as did normal subjects eating similar diets, the patients with IH exhibiting a spectrum of individually higher rates of urinary Ca excretion, the additional Ca, in part, having been derived from bone (45). Some patients with IH have been observed to exhibit reduced bone density as measured by photon absorptiometry in the forearm as compared to age- and sex-matched normal subjects (37,110,111). Similarly, in vivo neutron activation assessment of bone mineral content in the trunk and upper thighs has demonstrated lower than normal values among patients with IH with such estimates of body Ca content being found to be lower as fasting rates of urinary Ca excretion increased (112). Increased rates of urinary hydroxyproline excretion, an index of bone resorption, have been ob-

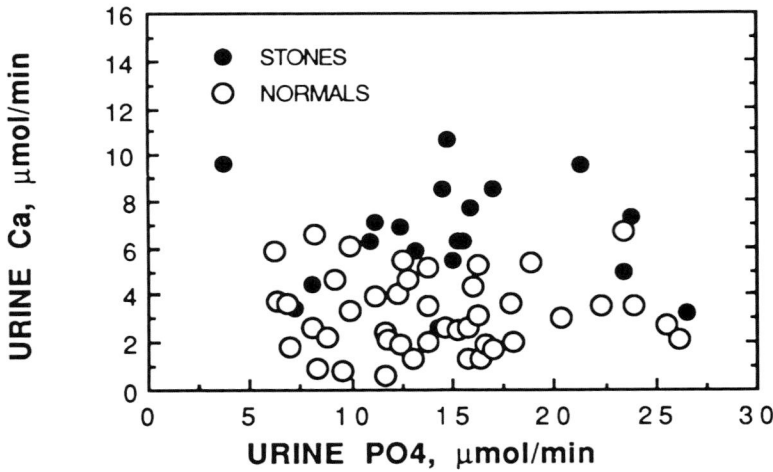

FIG. 17. Urinary Ca excretion in relation to urinary PO4 excretion among patients with IH (●) and normal subjects (○) observed during renal clearance studies during water diuresis. Expanded from Lemann et al. (71).

served in IH (113). Several histomorphometric analyses of bone biopsies in IH have also been reported but a uniform pattern of disordered bone structure and turnover has not been recognized. Increased osteoclastic resorptive surfaces with or without increased osteoid or increased osteoid and reduced trabecular bone formation, either suggesting net bone resorption, have been observed (76,114). Another study described a prolonged mineralization lag time and prolonged bone formation period with increased extension of eroded surfaces, without evidence of hyperparathroid changes, that were interpreted to be best explained by hypophosphatemia and a slight mineralization defect (115). Collectively, all of these observations support the view that bone participates in the overall acceleration of Ca transport that occurs in IH. Speculatively, similar defects in Ca transport may be present in gut, kidney, and bone in IH or alternatively, a primary transport defect in one organ may initiate compensatory physiological responses that affect the others.

A SUMMARY OF POSSIBLE MECHANISMS FOR IH

Based on the foregoing, IH currently appears to represent a spectrum of disorders and the possible mechanisms are summarized in the diagram shown in Fig. 18. Beginning in the kidney, hypercalciuria may first of all reflect a defect in renal tubular reabsorption of filtered Ca that results in mild hypocalcemia, activation of PTH secretion, stimulation of renal $1,25(OH)_2D_3$ synthesis, and consequent enhanced intestinal Ca absorption when Ca is available in the diet and potentially enhanced bone resorption when dietary Ca intake is limited. Alternatively, IH may reflect a primary defect in renal tubular phosphate reabsorption resulting in mild hypophosphatemia, activation of vitamin D metabolism and again enhanced intestinal Ca absorption. Other factors

could, speculatively, directly activate the synthesis of $1,25(OH)_2D$ in the kidney leading to enhanced intestinal Ca absorption and hypercalciuria. Moreover, the effects of $1,25(OH)_2D$ activation by any of these mechanisms could be further increased by the direct effect of $1,25(OH)_2D$ to up-regulate expression of its own receptor or, alternatively, by other factors, not yet clarified that similarly act to up-regulate the receptor for $1,25(OH)_2D$ or the subsequent events that are involved in activating intestinal Ca transport. The underlying defect in IH could also reflect an increase in vitamin D-independent intestinal Ca absorption. While there is no current evidence to support such a view, it is also conceivable that a primary acceleration of bone turnover, independent of PTH, could result in compensatory signals activating intestinal Ca transport and resulting in hypercalciuria. Finally, a more generalized defect in the cellular mechanisms for Ca transport, as indicated by the recent documentation of genetically determined activation of Ca-Mg-ATPase (108), may be the underlying process.

TABLE 9. ^{47}Ca kinetics in normal subjects and idiopathic hypercalciuria (IH) patients

	Normal (3)	IH (9)	p
Exchangeable Ca pool, g	3.8	5.6	<0.001
Ca turnover rate, g/day	0.8	1.2	<0.001
Bone formation rate, g/day	0.54	0.79	<0.025
Bone resorption rate, g/day	0.42	0.77	<0.001
Urinary Ca, mg/day	140	404	<0.005
Endogenous fecal Ca, mg/day	127	99	NS
True intestinal Ca absorption as a percent of Ca intake	38	61	<0.01

Source: adapted from Liberman et al. (29)
Number in parentheses indicate number of subjects.

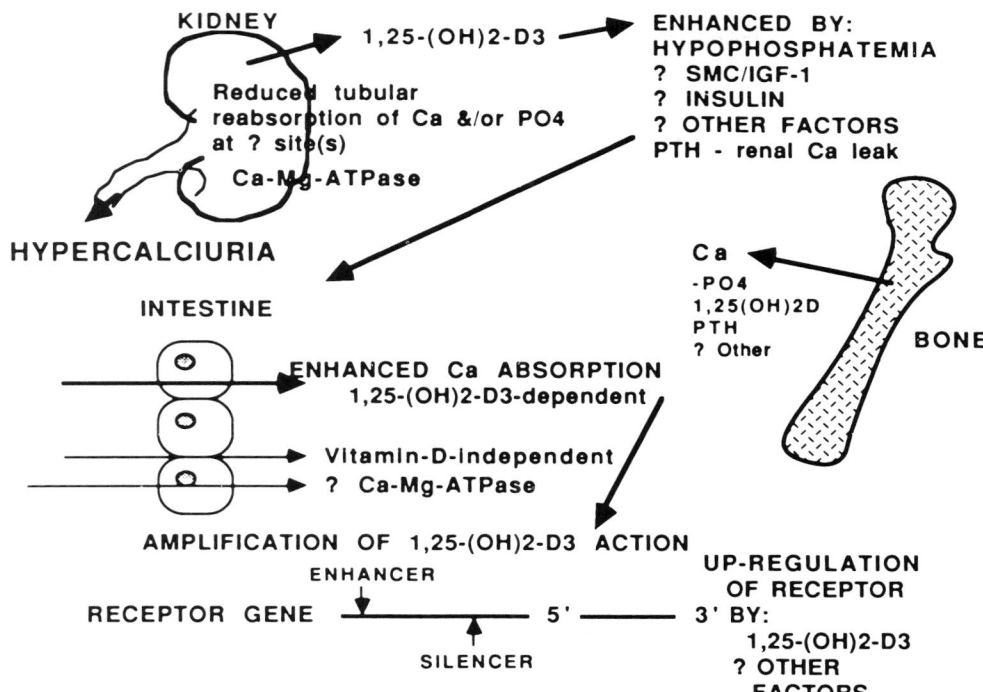

FIG. 18. An overview of possible mechanisms for IH (see text).

TREATMENT

If, in an individual patient, the precise underlying mechanism for IH were understood, the selection of treatment would optimally be directed toward correction of the underlying abnormality for Ca transport. In the instance of patients found to have renal hypercalciuria (renal Ca leak), treatment with thiazide diuretics, long known to augment renal tubular calcium reabsorption (116), has been shown to reduce urinary Ca excretion, correct secondary hyperparathyroidism that had accompanied hypercalciuria, and also reduce intestinal Ca absorption (47). However, for many patients the precise underlying mechanism for hypercalciuria is not readily apparent. Moreover, other individual patient characteristics require consideration, including the severity of stone disease as reflected by the number and frequency of previous stone episodes, the need for urological procedures, including lithotripsy, and the presence of residual stones. In addition, the age of the patient, and the simplicity and cost of treatment that determines long term compliance also require consideration.

All new patients having formed Ca-containing kidney stones require evaluation for IH. Initial efforts should be directed towards excluding the presence of other diseases known to be associated with hypercalciuria, especially primary hyperparathyroidism, sarcoidosis or other gran-ulomatous diseases, and Cushing's syndrome. Nephrolithiasis appears to be very rare among patients with hypercalciuria in association with neoplasia or hyperthyroidism. In addition to measurement of 24-hour urinary Ca excretion, including measurement of urinary creatinine excretion to assure the accuracy of the collection in relation to the patient's age, sex, and weight, urinary excretion rates of sodium, as a reflection of salt intake, of urea nitrogen as a reflection of protein intake, of potassium, of oxalate, and of citrate should be measured. Obviously, a history of excessive intake of calcium rich foods, the abuse of calcium containing antacids, or the abuse of antacids containing aluminum hydroxide which can result in hypophosphatemia, hypercalciuria, and stones (117) should be sought. The urine volume should also be noted.

For a young patient who has spontaneously passed a single stone and who has only mild hypercalciuria, for example 8 mmol/day (320 mg/day), it might be quite reasonable to recommend only general nutritional advice including restriction in the dietary intake of dairy products to only one serving per day of either milk, cheese, or ice cream, an increase in water intake to maintain a urine volume above 1.5–2.0 L/day (preferably using water), a reduction in dietary salt intake, limitation of animal protein intake to one serving per day (118), sufficient calories being consumed as fruits, vegetables,

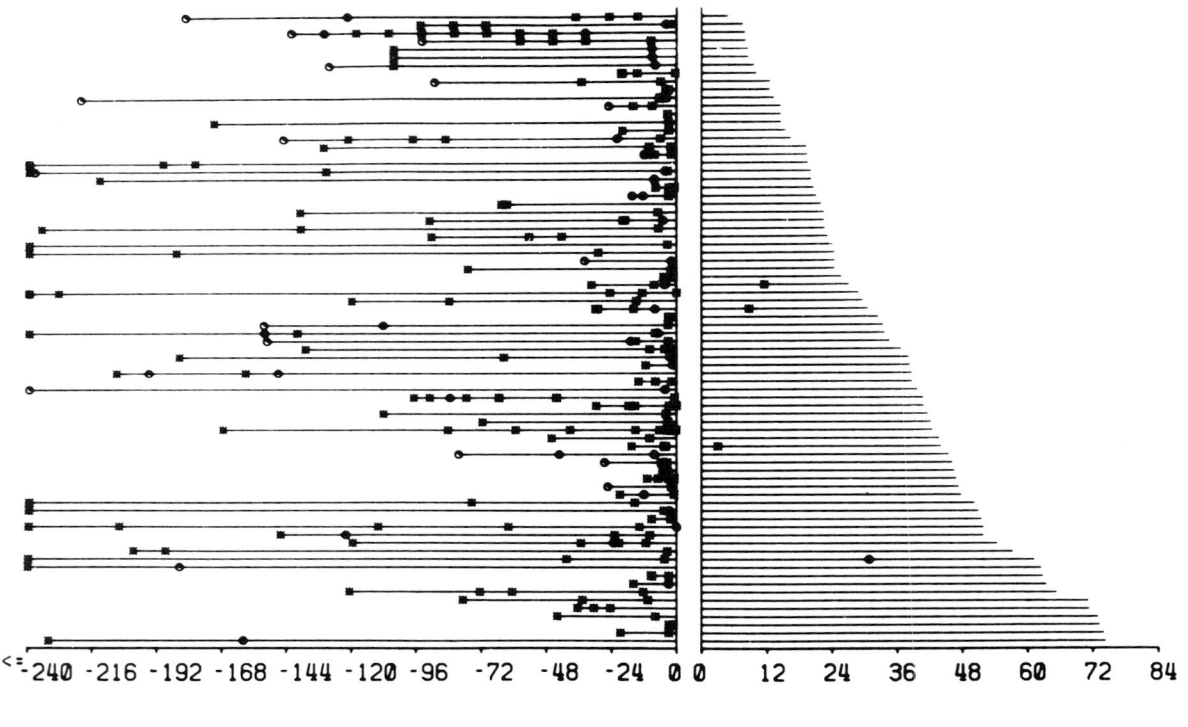

MONTHS BEFORE TREATMENT   MONTHS AFTER TREATMENT

FIG. 19. Effect of thiazide diuretics on stone recurrence in IH. Each horizontal line indicates one patient and the symbols along the line indicate the time of stone episodes, before treatment on the left and during treatment on the right. Reproduced with permission from Coe et al. (121).

and cereals that would assure a relatively greater intake of potassium and actual or potential base. Such efforts, if successful, would avoid the need and expense of ongoing treatment of asymptomatic patients who frequently find it difficult to comply. There have, however, been no long term studies of such a therapeutic approach and it can only be undertaken bearing in mind that stone formers in general have an approximate 80% risk of forming another stone within five years of the first and virtually all stone formers will have a second stone if followed for 20 years or more (119,120).

Patients with IH who have had more than a single stone or who have required urological extraction or lithotripsy, should receive additional treatment. The thiazide diuretics, chlorthalidone, indapamide, and amiloride have all been shown to be anticalciuric. The thiazide diuretics have long been known to reduce urinary Ca excretion by about 50% among treated patients with IH (116). In addition, as illustrated in Fig. 19 and in Table 10, thiazide diuretics effectively reduce the frequency of recurrent stones (9,116). The thiazides act by augmenting distal renal tubular Ca reabsorption. In addition, metabolic balance studies before and after ongoing treatment of IH with chlorthalidone have demonstrated that chlorthalidone causes Ca and PO_4 balances to become

more positive (121). Similarly, the administration of hydrochlorothiazide to healthy men was also accompanied by more positive calcium and phosphate balances as well as a reduction in urinary hydroxyproline excretion, reflecting an inhibition of bone resorption (122). Long term treatment of patients with hypertension with thiazide diuretics is accompanied by a slight but significant increase in bone density (123). There has been concern that chronic thiazide therapy could lead to ectopic calcification, because in several studies, increased rates of intestinal Ca absorption among patients with hypercalciuria were not reduced during thiazide treatment although urinary Ca excretion rates were reduced (47). Thus far, there appear to have been no reports of ectopic calcification in patients with IH who have received thiazide therapy for many years although that remains a theoretical possibility. It should be noted that many hypertensives have received thiazides as part of their treatment for many years without apparent reports of ectopic calcification and, since thiazide therapy reduces urinary Ca excretion even in normal subjects (122), the resulting potential for calcium retention must, over the long term, be offset by some degree of calcium deposition in bone as well as eventually a reduction in net intestinal Ca absorption.

TABLE 10. *Effect of thiazide treatment to reduce stone recurrence in idiopathic hypercalciuria*

Reference	9		116	
Number of patients	78		67	
	Before	Thiazide Rx	Before	Thiazide Rx
Patient-years of observation	811	229	686	136
Number of recurrent stones	256	5	241	8
Predicted number of new stones without treatment		73		48
Percent reduction in recurrence (observed/predicted)		93%		83%

Currently, treatment might best be initiated by chlorthalidone or indapamide because of their longer duration of action that requires that patients take treatment only once daily rather than using hydrochlorothiazide which would have to be taken twice a day. The relative expense and convenience requires consideration for individual patients. Mild hypokalemia regularly accompanies the administration of the anticalciuric diuretics but is seldom sufficiently severe to demand supplementary K administration. If K supplements are required, they are best administered as K-citrate or effervescent mixtures of K-citrate-acetate-bicarbonate. Such alkaline K salts increase urinary citrate excretion thus enhancing complexation of urinary Ca and limiting Ca-oxalate precipitation. Urinary citrate excretion may be reduced in IH (124) and K-citrate administration has been shown to provide additional therapeutic benefit to reduce stone recurrence when thiazide diuretics alone have not drastically reduced stone recurrence (125).

Among patients with IH considered to have absorptive hypercalciuria, efforts to directly limit gastrointestinal Ca absorption by the administration of sodium cellulose phosphate to bind Ca within the lumen of the gut and prevent its absorption have been used with effective reduction in urinary Ca excretion (126). However, the administration of cellulose phosphate was accompanied by an increase in urinary oxalate excretion that offset the effect of the fall in urinary Ca excretion to reduce the relative degree of saturation of the urine with respect to calcium oxalate (126–128). For this reason and because cellulose phosphate must be taken with each meal to be maximally effective, there has not been widespread use of this agent in the treatment of IH.

With respect to the treatment of IH with anticalciuric diuretics, further studies are needed to determine whether treatment needs to be continued indefinitely or whether after some, as yet undetermined period, treatment can be discontinued without a significant risk of stone recurrence. If IH is most often determined by a constitutional genetic and irreversible defect, then treatment would likely best be continued indefinitely.

REFERENCES

1. Prien EL, Frondel C. Studies in urolithiasis. I. Composition of urinary calculi. *J Urol* 1947;57:949.
2. Mandel NS, Mandel GS. Urinary tract stone disease in the United States veteran population: II. Geographical variation in composition. *J Urol* 1989;142:1516.
3. Finlayson B. Calcium stones: some physical and clinical aspects. In: David DS, ed. *Calcium metabolism in renal failure and nephrolithiasis.* New York: John Wiley, 1977;337.
4. Flocks RH. Calcium and phosphorus excretion in the urine of patients with renal or ureteral calculi. *JAMA* 1939;113:1466.
5. Flocks RH. Calcium urolithiasis: the role of calcium metabolism in the pathogenesis and treatment of calcium urolithiaisis. *J Urol* 1940;43:214.
6. Albright F, Henneman P, Benedict PH, Forbes AP. Idiopathic hypercalciuria. A preliminary report. *Proc R Soc Med Lond [Biol]* 1953;46:1077.
7. Henneman PH, Benedict PH, Forbes AP, Dudley HR. Idiopathic hypercalciuria. *N Engl J Med* 1958;259:802.
8. Hodgkinson A, Pyrah LN. The urinary excretion of calcium and inorganic phosphate in 344 patients with calcium stone of renal origin. *Br J Surg* 1958;48:10.
9. Coe FL. Treated and untreated recurrent calcium nephrolithiasis in patients with idiopathic hypercalciuria, hyperuricosuria, or no metabolic disorder. *Ann Intern Med* 1977;87:404.
10. Litin RB, Diessner GR, Keating FR. Urinary excretion of calcium in patients with renal lithiasis. *J Urol* 1961;86:17.
11. Edwards NA, Hodgkinson A. Metabolic studies in patients with idiopathic hypercalciuria. *Clin Sci* 1965;29:237.
12. Pak CYC, Ohata M, Lawrence EC, Snyder W. The hypercalciurias: causes, parathyroid functions, and diagnostic criteria. *J Clin Invest* 1974;54:387.
13. Marshall RW, Cochran M, Hodgkinson A. Relationships between calcium and oxalic acid intake in the diet and their excretion in the urine of normal and stone forming subjects. *Clin Sci* 1972;49:91.
14. Adams ND, Gray RW, Lemann J Jr. The effects of CaCO$_3$ loading and of dietary calcium deprivation on plasma 1,25(OH)$_2$D concentrations in healthy adults. *J Clin Endocrinol Metab* 1979;48:1008.
15. Lemann J Jr, Lennon EJ. The limits of renal calcium conservation in patients with idiopathic hypercalciuria. *J Clin Invest* 1973;52:51a.
16. Coe FL, Parks JH. *Nephrolithiasis: pathogenesis and treatment,* 2nd ed. Chicago: Year Book Medical, 1988.
17. Pak CYC. A simple test for the diagnosis of absorptive, resorptive and renal hypercalciurias. *N Engl J Med* 1975;292:497.
18. Kaplan RA, Haussler MR, Deftos LJ, Bone H, Pak CYC. The role of 1α-25-dihydroxyvitamin D in the mediation of intestinal hyperabsorption of calcium in primary hyperparathyroidism and absorptive hypercalciuria. *J Clin Invest* 1977;59:756.
19. Coe FL, Favus MJ. Nephrolithiasis. In: Brenner BM, Rector FC

Jr, eds. *The kidney,* 4th ed. Philadelphia: WB Saunders, 1991;1742.

20. Bogert LJ, McKittrick EJ. Studies in inorganic metabolism. 1. Interrelationships between calcium and magnesium metabolism. *J Biol Chem* 1922;54:363.

21. Breiter H, Mills R, Dwight J, McKey B, Armstrong W, Outhouse J. The utilization of the calcium of milk by adults. *J Nutr* 1941;21:351.

22. Chu HI, Liu SH, Hsu HC, Chao JC, Cheu SH. Calcium, phosphorus, nitrogen and magnesium metabolism in normal young Chinese adults. *Chin Med J Engl* 1941;59:1.

23. Davis RH, Morgan DB, Rivlin RS. The excretion of calcium in the urine and its relation to calcium intake, sex and age. *Clin Sci* 1970;39:1.

24. Dent CE, Harper CM, Parfitt AM. The effect of cellulose phosphate on calcium metabolism in patients with hypercalciuria. *Clin Sci* 1964;27:417.

25. Heaney RP, Skillman TG. Secretion and excretion of calcium by the human gastrointestinal tract. *J Lab Clin Med* 1964;64:29.

26. Heaton FW, Hodgkinson A, Rose GA. Observations on the relation between calcium and magnesium metabolism in man. *Clin Sci* 1964;27:31.

27. Hunscher HA, Donelson E, Erickson BN, Macy IG. Results of the ingestion of cod liver oil and yeast on calcium and phosphorus metabolism in women. *J Nutr* 1934;8:341.

28. Jackson WPU, Doncaster C. A consideration of the hypercalciuria in sarcoidosis, idiopathic hypercalciuria, and that produced by vitamin D. A new suggestion regarding calcium metabolism. *J Clin Endocrinol Metab* 1959;19:658.

29. Liberman UA, Sperling O, Atsmon A, Frank M, Modan M, de Vries A. Metabolic and calcium kinetic studies in idiopathic hypercalciuria. *J Clin Invest* 1968;47:2580.

30. Nordin BEC, Smith DA, Shimmins J, Oxby C. The effect of dietary calcium on the absorption and retention of radiostrontium. *Clin Sci* 1967;32:39.

31. Parfitt AM, Higgins BA, Nassim JR, Collins JA, Hilb A. Metabolic studies in patients with hypercalciuria. *Clin Sci* 1964;27:463.

32. Phang JM, Kales AN, Hahn TJ. Effect of divided calcium intake on urinary calcium excretion. *Lancet* 1968;2:84.

33. Schwartz E, Chokas WV, Panariello VA. Metabolic balance studies of high calcium intake in osteoporosis. *Am J Med* 1964;36:233.

34. Spencer H, Scheck J, Lewin I, Samachson J. Comparative absorption of calcium from calcium gluconate and calcium lactate in man. *J Nutr* 1966;89:283.

35. Steggerda FR, Mitchell HH. The calcium requirement of adult man and the utilization of the calcium in milk and in calcium gluconate. *J Nutr* 1939;17:253.

36. Wiley FH, Wiley LL, Waller DS. The effect of the ingestion of sodium, potassium and ammonium chlorides and sodium bicarbonate on the metabolism of inorganic salts and water. *J Biol Chem* 1933;101:73.

37. Lemann J Jr. Idiopathic hypercalciuria. In: Coe FL, ed. *Nephrolithiasis.* In: Brenner BM, Stein JH, eds. *Contemporary issues in nephrology,* vol 5. New York: Churchill Livingstone 1980;86.

38. Duncombe VM, Watts RWE, Peters TJ. Studies on intestinal calcium absorption in patients with idiopathic hypercalciuria. *Q J Med* 1984;209:69.

39. Norman AW. The vitamin D endocrine system. *Physiologist* 1985;28:219.

40. Gallagher JC, Riggs BL, Eisman J, Hamstra A. Intestinal calcium absorption and serum vitamin D metabolites in normal subjects and osteoporotic patients. *J Clin Invest* 1979;64:729.

41. Sheikh MS, Ramirez A, Emmett M, et al. Role of vitamin D-dependent and vitamin D-dependent mechanisms in absorption of food calcium. *J Clin Invest* 1988;81:126.

42. Wilz DR, Gray RW, Dominguez JH, Lemann J, Jr. Plasma 1,25(OH)$_2$-vitamin D concentrations and net intestinal calcium, phosphate and magnesium absorption in humans. *Am J Clin Nutr* 1979;32:2052.

43. Shen FH, Baylink DJ, Nielson RL, Sherrard DJ, Ivey JL, Haussler MR. Increased serum 1,25-dihydroxyvitamin D in the idiopathic hypercalciuria. *J Lab Clin Med* 1977;90:955.

44. Gray RW, Wilz DR, Caldas AE, Lemann J Jr. The importance of phosphate in regulating plasma 1,25(OH)$_2$-vitamin D levels in humans: studies in healthy subjects, in calcium-stone formers and in patients with primary hyperparathyroidism. *J Clin Endocrinol Metab* 1977;45:299.

45. Coe FL, Favus MJ, Crockett T, Strauss LM. Effects of low-calcium diet on urine calcium excretion, parathyroid function and serum 1,25(OH)$_2$D$_3$ levels in patients with idiopathic hypercalciuria and in normal subjects. *Am J Med* 1982;72:25.

46. Broadus AE, Dominguez M, Barter FC. Pathophysiological studies in idiopathic hypercalciuria; use of an oral calcium tolerance test to characterize distinctive hypercalciuric subgroups. *J Clin Endocrinol Metab* 1978;47:751.

46a. Broadus AE, Magee JS, Mallette LE, et al. A detailed evaluation of oral phosphate therapy in selected patients with primary hyperparathyroidism. *J Clin Endocrinol Metab* 1983;56:953.

47. Zerwekj JE, Pak CYC. Selective effects of thiazide therapy on serum 1α-25-hydroxyvitamin D and intestinal calcium absorption in renal and absorptive hypercalciurias. *Metabolism* 1980;29:13.

47a. Bataille P, Bouillon R, Fournier A, Renaud H, Gueris J, Idrissi A. Increased plasma concentrations of total and free 1,25(OH)$_2$D$_3$ in calcium stone formers with idiopathic hypercalciuria. *Contrib Nephrol* 1987;58:137–142.

48. Insogna KL, Broadus AE, Dreyer BE, Ellison AF, Gertner JM. Elevated production rate of 1,25-dihydroxyvitamin D in patients with absorptive hypercalciuria. *J Clin Endocrinol Metab* 1985;61:490.

49. Kawashima H, Torikai S, Kurokawa K. Calcitonin selectivity stimulates 25-hydroxyvitamin D$_3$-1α-hydroxylase in the proximal straight tubule of the rat kidney. *Nature* 1981;291:327.

49a. Coe FL, Canterbury JM, Firpo JJ, Reiss E. Evidence for secondary hyperparathyroidism in idiopathic hypercalciuria. *J Clin Invest* 1973;52:134.

49b. Broadus AE, Insogna KL, Lang R, et al. A consideration of the hormonal basis and phosphate leak hypothesis of absorptive hypercalciuria. *J Clin Endocrinol Metab* 1984;58:161.

50. Lemann J Jr, Dominguez JH, Gray RW. The effects of dietary phosphate deprivation in men and women: similarities and differences. In: Avioli L, Bordier P, Fleisch H, et al., eds. *Phosphate metabolism and bone.* Paris: Amour Montague, 1986;387.

51. Lufkin EG, Kumar R, Heath H III. Hyperphosphatemic tumoral calcinosis: effects of phosphate depletion on vitamin D metabolism, and of acute hypocalcemia on parathyroid hormone secretion and action. *J Clin Endocrinol Metab* 1983;56:1319.

52. Insogna KL, Broadus AE, Gertner JM. Impaired phosphorus conservation and 1,25-dihydroxyvitamin D generation during phosphorus deprivation in familial hypophosphatemic rickets. *J Clin Invest* 1983;71:1562.

53. Maierhofer WJ, Gray RW, Lemann J Jr. Phosphate deprivation increases serum 1,25-(OH)$_2$-vitamin D concentrations in healthy men. *Kidney Int* 1984;25:571.

54. Portale AA, Halloran BP, Murphy MM, Morris RC Jr. Oral intake of phosphorus can determine the serum concentration of 1,25-dihydroxyvitamin D by determining its production rate in humans. *J Clin Invest* 1986;77:7.

55. Gray RW, Napoli JL. Dietary phosphate deprivation increases 1,25-dihydroxyvitamin D$_3$ synthesis in rat kidney in vitro. *J Biol Chem* 1983;258:1152.

56. Hughs MR, Haussler MR, Wergedal J, Baylink DJ. Regulation of serum 1,25(OH)$_2$D by calcium and phosphate in the rat. *Science* 1975;190:578.

57. Gray RW. The control of plasma 1,25(OH)$_2$-vitamin D concentrations by calcium and phosphorus in the rat: effects of hypophysectomy. *Calcif Tissue Int* 1982;33:485.

58. Gray RW, Garthwaite TL, Phillips LS. Growth hormone and triiodothyronine permit an increase in plasma 1,25(OH)$_2$D concentrations in response to dietary phosphate deprivation in hypophysectomized rats. *Calcif Tissue Int* 1983;35:100.

59. Halloran BP, Spencer EM. Dietary phosphorus and 1,25-dihydroxyvitamin D metabolism: influence and insulin-like growth factor I. *Endocrinology* 1988;123:1225.

60. Gray RW. Evidence that somatomedins mediate the effect of hypophosphatemia to increase serum 1,25-dihydroxyvitamin D$_3$ levels in rats. *Endocrinology* 1987;121:504.

61. Tieder M, Modai D, Shaked U, et al. "Idiopathic" hypercalciuria and hereditary hypophosphatemic rickets. *N Engl J Med* 1987;316:125.

62. Lemann J Jr, Gray RW. 1,25(OH)$_2$D$_3$ in humans: regulation in health and role in urolithiasis. In: Walker VR, Sutton RAL, Cameron EC, et al., eds. *Urolithiasis.* New York: Plenum Press, 1989; 603.

63. Favus MJ, Mangelsdorf DJ, Tembe V, Coe BJ, Haussler MR. Evidence for in vivo up-regulation of the intestinal vitamin D receptor during dietary calcium restriction in the rat. *J Clin Invest* 1988;82:218.

64. Korkor AB. Reduced binding of ^{3}H-1,25-dihydroxyvitamin D$_3$ in the parathyroid glands of patients with renal failure. *N Engl J Med* 1987;316:1573.

65. Brannan PG, Vergne-Marini P, Pak CYC, Hull AR, Fordtran JS. Magnesium absorption in the human small intestine. Results in normal subjects, patients with chronic renal disease and patients with idiopathic hypercalciuria. *J Clin Invest* 1976;57:1412.

66. Brannan PG, Morawski S, Pak CYC, Fordtran JS. Selective jejunal hyperabsorption of calcium in absorptive hypercalciuria. *Am J Med* 1979;66:425.

67. Bushinsky DA, Krieger NS, Geisser DI, Grossman EB, Coe FL. Effects of pH on bone calcium and proton fluxes in vitro. *Am J Physiol* 1983;245.

68. Suki WN, Rouse D. Renal transport of calcium, magnesium and phosphorus. In: Brenner BM, Rector FC Jr, eds. *The kidney,* 4th ed. Philadelphia: WB Saunders, 1991;380.

69. Edwards NA, Hodgkinson A. Studies of renal function in patients with idiopathic hypercalciuria. *Clin Sci* 1965;29:327.

70. Peacock M, Nordin BEC. Tubular reabsorption of calcium in normal and hypercalciuric subjects. *J Clin Pathol* 1968;2:355.

71. Lemann J Jr, Piering WF, Lennon EJ. Possible role of carbohydrate-induced calciuria in calcium oxalate kidney-stone formation. *N Engl J Med* 1969;280:232.

72. Widrow SH, Levinsky NG. The effect of parathyroid extract on renal tubular Ca reabsorption in the dog. *J Clin Invest* 1962;41:2151.

73. Nussbaum SR, Zahtsfnik RJ, Lavigne JR, et al. Highly sensitive two-site immunoradiometric assay of parathyroid and its clinical utility in evaluating patients with hypercalcemia. *Clin Chem* 1987;33:1364.

74. Silver J, Russell J, Sherwood LM. Regulation of vitamin D metabolites of messenger ribonucleic acid for preproparathyroid hormone in isolated bovine parathyroid cells. *Proc Natl Acad Sci USA* 1985;82:4270.

75. Dominguez JH, Gray RW, Lemann J Jr. Dietary phosphate deprivation in woman and men: effects on mineral and acid balances, parathyroid hormone and the metabolism of 25-OH-vitamin D. *J Clin Endocrinol Metab* 1976;43:1056.

76. Bordier P, Ryckewart A, Gueris J, Rasmussen H. On the pathogenesis of so-called idiopathic hypercalciuria. *Am J Med* 1977;63:398.

77. Breslau NE, McGuire JL, Zerwekh JE, Pak CYC. The role of dietary sodium on renal excretion and intestinal absorption of calcium and on vitamin D metabolism. *J Clin Endocrinol Metab* 1982;55:369.

78. McCarron DA, Rankin LI, Bennett WM, Krutzik S, McClung MR, Luft FC. Urinary calcium excretion at extremes of sodium intake in normal man. *Am J Nephrol* 1981;1:84.

79. Lemann J Jr, Pleuss JA, Gray RW, Hoffmann RG. Potassium administration reduces and potassium deprivation increases urinary calcium excretion in healthy adults. *Kidney Int* 1991; in press.

80. Muldowney FP, Freaney R, Moloney MF. Importance of dietary sodium in the hypercalciuria syndrome. *Kidney Int* 1972;22:292.

81. Lemann J Jr, Worcester EA, Gray RW. Hypercalciuria and stones. (Finlayson colloquium on urolithiasis) *Am J Kidney Dis* 1991;17:386.

82. Johnson NE, Alcantara EN, Linkswiler HM. Effect of level of protein intake on urinary and fecal calcium and calcium retention of young adult males. *J Nutr* 1970;100:1425.

83. Walker RM, Linkswiler HM. Calcium retention in the adult human male as affected by protein intake. *J Nutr* 1972;102:1297.

84. Anand CR, Linkswiler HM. Effect of protein intake on calcium balance of young men given 500 mg calcium daily. *J Nutr* 1974;104:695.

85. Lutz J. Calcium balance and acid-base status of women as affected by increased protein intake and by sodium bicarbonate ingestion. *Am J Clin Nutr* 1984;39:281.

86. Lemann J Jr, Relman AS. The relation of sulfur metabolism to acid-base balance and electrolyte excretion: the effects of DL-methionine in normal man. *J Clin Invest* 1959;38:2215.

87. Lemann J Jr, Litzow JR, Lennon EJ. Studies of the mechanism by which chronic metabolic acidosis augments urinary calcium excretion in man. *J Clin Invest* 1967;46:1318.

88. Lemann J Jr, Litzow JR, Lennon EJ. The effects of chronic acid loads in normal man: further evidence for the participation of bone mineral in the defense against chronic metabolic acidosis. *J Clin Invest* 1966;45:1608.

89. Lemann J Jr, Gray RW, Maierhofer WJ, Cheung HS. The importance of renal net acid excretion as a determinant of fasting urinary calcium excretion. *Kidney Int* 1986;29:743.

90. Lemann J Jr, Adams ND, Gray RW. Urinary calcium excretion in human beings. *N Engl J Med* 1979;301:535.

91. Walser M. Calcium clearance as a function of sodium clearance in the dog. *Am J Physiol* 1961;200:1099.

92. Robertson WG, Peacock M, Heyburn PJ, et al. Epidemiological risk factors in calcium stone disease. *Scand J Urol Nephrol* 1980;53:15.

93. Lemann J Jr. Urinary calcium excretion and net acid excretion: effects of dietary protein, carbohydrate and calories. In: Schwille PO, Smith LH, Robertson WG, et al., eds. *Urolithiasis and related clinical research.* New York: Plenum, 1985;53.

94. Lindemann RD, Adler S, Yiengst MJ, et al. Influence of various nutrients on urinary divalent cation excretion. *J Lab Clin Med* 1967;70:236.

95. DeFronzo RA, Cooke CR, Andres R, et al. The effect of insulin on renal handling of sodium, potassium, calcium and phosphate in man. *J Clin Invest* 1975;55:845.

96. Lennon EJ, Lemann J Jr, Piering WF, Larson LS. The effect of glucose on urinary action excretion during chronic extracellular volume expansion in normal man. *J Clin Invest* 1974;53:1424.

97. Lemann J Jr, Gray RW, Pleuss JA. Potassium bicarbonate, but not sodium bicarbonate, reduces urinary calcium excretion and improves calcium balance in healthy men. *Kidney Int* 1989; 35:688.

98. Jaeger P, Bonjour JP, Karlmark B, et al., Influence of acute potassium loading on renal phosphate transport in the rat kidney. *Am J Physiol* 1983;245:F601.

99. Sebastian A, Hernandez RE, Portale AA, Colman J, Tatsuno J, Morris RC Jr. Dietary potassium influences kidney maintenance of serum phosphorus concentration. *Kidney Int* 1990;37:1341.

100. Maierhofer WJ, Gray RW, Cheung HS, Lemann J Jr. Bone resorption stimulated by elevated serum 1,25(OH)$_2$D concentrations in healthy men. *Kidney Int* 1983;24:555.

101. Maierhofer WJ, Gray RW, Lemann J Jr. Dietary calcium and serum 1,25(OH)$_2$-vitamin D concentrations in healthy men. *Kidney Int* 1984;25:571.

102. Bomsztyk K, Calalb MB. Bicarbonate absorption stimulates active calcium reabsorption in the rat proximal tubule. *J Clin Invest* 1988;81:1455.

103. Sutton RAL, Wong NLM, Dirks JH. Effects of metabolic acidosis and alkalosis on sodium and calcium transport in the dog kidney. *Kidney Int* 1979;15:520.

104. Backman U, Danielson BG, Johansson S, Ljunghall S, Wilkstrom B. Incidence and clinical importance of renal tubular defects in recurrent renal stone formers. *Nephron* 1980;25:96.

104a. Nutahara K, Higashihara E, Ishiii Y, Niijima T. Renal hypercalciuria and acidification defect in kidney stone patients. *J Urol* 1989;141:813.

104b. Tessitore N, Ortalda V, Fabris A, et al. Renal acidification defects in patients with recurrent calcium nephrolithiasis. *Nephron* 1985;41:325.

105. Coe FL, Parks JH, Moore ES. Familial idiopathic hypercalciuria. *N Engl J Med* 1979;300:337.

106. Sutton RAL, Walker VR. Responses to hydrochlorothiazide and acetazolamide in patients with calcium stones. Evidence suggesting a defect in renal tubular function. *N Engl J Med* 1980;302:709.

107. Borke JL, Minami J, Verma A, et al. Monoclonal antibodies to human erythrocyte membrane Ca^{++}-Mg^{++}-adenosine triphosphatase pump recognize an epitope in the basolateral membrane of human kidney distal tubule cells. *J Clin Invest* 1987;80:1225.

108. Bianchi G, Vezzoli G, Cusi D, et al. Abnormal red-cell calcium pump in patients with idiopathic hypercalciuria. *N Engl J Med* 1988;319:897.

109. Nunziata V, Giannattasio R, di Giovanni G, Corrado MF, Galletti F, Mancini M. Altered kinetics of an intravenous calcium load in idiopathic hypercalciuria. *Metabolism* 1989;38:826.

110. Lawoyin S, Sismilich S, Browne R, Pak CYC. Bone mineral content in patients with calcium urolithiasis. *Metabolism* 1979;28:1250.

111. Alhava EM, Juuti M, Karjalainen P. Bone mineral density in patients with urolithiasis. *Scand J Urol Nephrol* 1976;10:154.

112. Barkin J, Wilson DR, Manuel A, Bayley A, Murray T, Harrison J. Bone mineral content in idiopathic calcium nephrolithiasis. *Miner Electrolyte Metab* 1985;11:19.

113. Sutton RAL, Walker VR. Bone resorption and hypercalciuria in calcium stoneformers. *Metabolism* 1989;35:485.

114. Malluche HH, Tschoepe W, Ritz E, Meyer-Sabellek W, Massry SG. Abnormal bone histology in idiopathic hypercalciuria. *J Clin Endocrinol Metab* 1980;50:654.

115. Steiniche T, Mosekilde L, Christensen MS, Melsen F. A histomorphometric determination of iliac bone remodeling in patients with recurrent renal stone formation and idiopathic hypercalciuria. *APMIS* 1989;97:309.

116. Yendt ER, Cohanim M. Prevention of calcium stones with thiazides. *Kidney Int* 1978;13:397.

117. Cooke N, Teitelbaum S, Avioli L. Antacid-induced osteomalacia and nephrolithiasis. *Arch Intern Med* 1978;138:1007.

118. Kontessis P, Jones S, Dodds R, et al. Renal, metabolic and hormonal responses to ingestion of animal and vegetable proteins. *Kidney Int* 1990;38:136.

119. Williams RE. Long term survey of 530 patients with upper urinary tract stones. *Br J Urol* 1963;35:416.

120. Blacklock NJ. The pattern of urolithiasis in the Royal Navy. In: Hodgkinson A, Nordin BEC, eds. *Proceedings in renal stone research symposium.* London: JA Churchill, 1969;33.

121. Coe FL, Parks JH, Bushinsky DA, Langman CB, Favus MJ. Chlorthalidone promotes mineral retention in patients with idiopathic hypercalciuria. *Kidney Int* 1988;33:1140.

122. Lemann J Jr, Gray RW, Maierhofer WJ, Cheung HS. Hydrochlorothiazide inhibits bone resorption in men despite experimentally elevated serum 1,25-dihydroxyvitamin D concentrations. *Kidney Int* 1985;28:951.

123. Wasnich RD, Benfante RJ, Yano K, Heilbrun L, Vogel JM. Thiazide effect on the mineral content of bone. *N Engl J Med* 1983;309:344.

124. Nicar MJ, Skurla C, Sakhaee K, Pak CYC. Low urinary citrate excretion in nephrolithiasis. *Urology* 1983;21:8.

125. Pak CYC, Peterson R, Sakhaee K, Fuller C, Preminger G, Reisch J. Correction of hypocitraturia and prevention of stone formation by combined thiazide and potassium citrate therapy in thiazide-unresponsive hypercalciuric nephrolithiasis. *Am J Med* 1985;79:284.

126. Hayasaki Y, Kaplan RA, Pak CYC. Effect of sodium cellulose phosphate therapy on crystallization of calcium oxalate in urine. *Metabolism* 1975;24:1273.

127. Hautmann R, Hering FJ, Lutzeyer W. Calcium oxalate stone disease: effects and side effects of cellulose phosphate and succinate in long-term treatment of absorptive hypercalciuria and hyperoxaluria. *J Urol* 1978;120:712.

128. Backman U, Danielson BG, Johansson G, et al. Treatment of recurrent calcium stone formation with cellulose phosphate. *J Urol* 1980;123:9.

CHAPTER 33

Hyperoxaluric States

Lynwood H. Smith

Oxalate and its calcium oxalate salt are of importance in most biological systems (1). Oxalate is a major source of energy for bacteria that contain oxalate degrading enzymes (2). Digestion and production of oxalate occur in fungi (3,4). In plants oxalate appears to be important in maintaining calcium homeostasis (5). If a tree finds itself in an environment too rich in calcium, it cannot move to a more favorable environment. Oxalate can be produced in the leaves and bark to precipitate excess calcium as calcium oxalate, which is stored as crystalline deposits within vacuoles of cells allowing the maintenance of normal calcium balance within the plant. Periodically the leaves and bark are shed representing a pattern of excretion that allows the tree to be rid of the excess calcium. Other roles for oxalate in plants may be present but are less well defined. In animals oxalate appears less welcome and is a potential source of pathological processes. Oxalate is produced as a waste product of normal endogenous metabolism. The problems that occur are not due to this endogenous production of oxalate but instead seem to be on a dietary basis. In the spring ruminant animals who are allowed in fresh pastures with plants that are rich in oxalate may develop acute oxalosis (6,7). These animals normally can eat oxalate rich plants without problems due to the presence of oxalate degrading bacteria in their stomachs. During the winter months these animals have been on a diet with a low oxalate content. Because of the lack of this nutrient, these bacteria disappear from the intestinal tract. In the spring when oxalate is reintroduced into the diet, the intestine and stomach are recolonized. Once this is accomplished, the animal has no problem with a diet rich in oxalate. Examples of acute oxalosis and death in big cats when exposed to precursors of oxalate have been noted (8,9). Domestic dogs whose diet is more and more like that of man in industrialized countries have been noted to form calcium oxalate urinary calculi with increasing frequency (10). In the past their stones were usually calcium phosphate and magnesium ammonium phosphate, so this may represent a significant change.

In humans the formation of urinary calculi within the urinary tract is the third most common affliction of this organ system (11). At least 5% to 15% of the population in industrialized countries that reach age 70 will have had at least one episode with a urinary stone (12–14). The principal crystal contained in 70% to 80% of these stones is calcium oxalate as the monohydrate and dihydrate phases (15–17). There is a subset of these patients who have hyperoxaluria associated with the formation of their stones within the urinary tract (18–21). Mild hyperoxaluria is present in from 15% to 50% of the patients with the syndrome of idiopathic calcium oxalate urolithiasis. More severe hyperoxaluria most often is secondary to intestinal malabsorption from primary intestinal disease, bowel resection, or small bowel bypass for obesity. A small group of patients with hyperoxaluria will have an inborn error of metabolism causing an overproduction of oxalate. In the severe hyperoxaluric states, the potential for rapid stone formation, nephrocalcinosis, renal insufficiency, and generalized oxalosis with early death exists (22).

This chapter reviews oxalate as it relates to humans in health and in disease states, normal metabolism and transport of oxalate, calcium oxalate crystal formation, diet and oxalate, and the measurement of oxalate in biological fluids. A detailed review of the clinical disorders that may be associated with hyperoxaluria will also be presented.

PRODUCTION AND METABOLISM

The major metabolic pathways involved in the production of oxalate are outlined in Fig. 1. Detailed reviews of

L. H. Smith: Department of Medicine, Mayo Medical School, Rochester, Minnesota 55905.

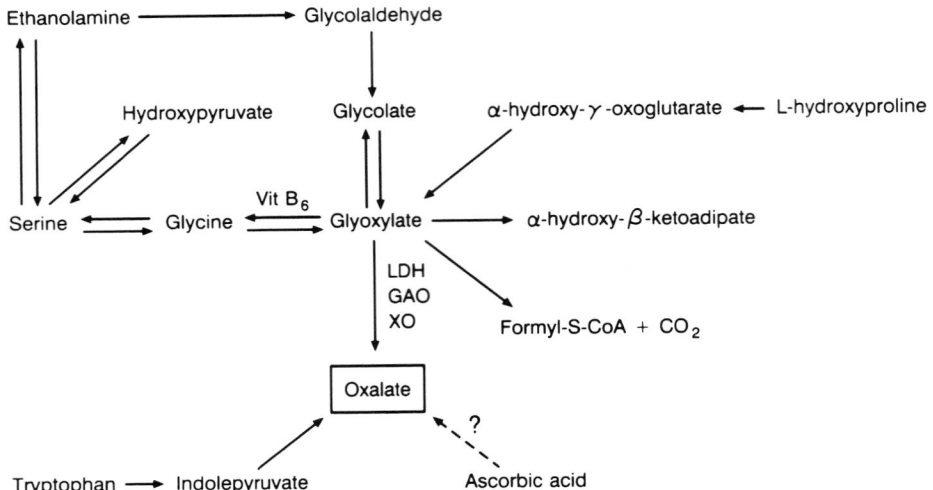

FIG. 1. Metabolic pathways of oxalate production (see text).

the metabolism of oxalate are available in the literature (1,5,22). In health, 10–15% of the oxalate excreted in the urine is derived from the diet with the remainder coming from the endogenous production of oxalate (23). It has been thought that the major precursors of oxalate are glycine and ascorbic acid with each contributing about 40% of the oxalate normally present in urine. Hydroxyproline, tryptophan, and perhaps other compounds have been thought to contribute no more than 5% of the oxalate present in urine. In humans, the pathway that leads to the production of oxalate from ascorbic acid is not defined. Radioisotope studies have suggested that oxalate is derived from C-1 and C-2 of ascorbic acid (24–26). Outlined in Fig. 2 is a theoretical pathway of ascorbic acid metabolism that could lead to the production of oxalate. Recent studies have challenged the older data in regard to the relative contribution of ascorbic acid to the urinary excretion of oxalate (27,28). As will be discussed subsequently, ascorbic acid can be converted to oxalate when it is present in the urine during the period of collection and during the procedures of chemical analysis. Clearly, the role of ascorbic acid in the endogenous production of oxalate in humans needs to be readdressed using currently available techniques that avoid these potential problems during collection and analysis.

Glyoxylate is another major precursor of oxalate that is involved in a number of metabolic routes (1,5,22). Glycolate and glycine are precursors and products of glyoxylate metabolism. Glycolate oxidase (GAO) and lactate dehydrogenase (LDH) are the two major enzymes involved in the oxidative conversion of glyoxylate to oxalate (1,22,29,30). Also, the conversion of glycolate to glyoxylate can be catalyzed by glycolate oxidase which is located in the peroxisome. Lactate dehydrogenase is located in the cytosol suggesting a two-compartment model including peroxisome and cytosol for the normal synthesis of oxalate (31). Although xanthine oxidase also has been suggested as having a role in the conversion of glyoxylate to oxalate, its contribution to this reaction appears to be minimal at best (32). In some animals, there would appear to be a second pathway involved in the production of oxalate with the direct conversion of glycolate to oxalate bypassing glyoxylate (33). This conversion is catalyzed by the enzyme glycolic acid dehydrogenase. To date this alternate pathway has not been demonstrated in humans.

Xylitol, a five-carbon sugar alcohol, is an intermediate in the glucuronate-xylulose pathway in humans, animals, and plants (34–37). Its use in parenteral nutrition was suggested because of its desirable characteristics

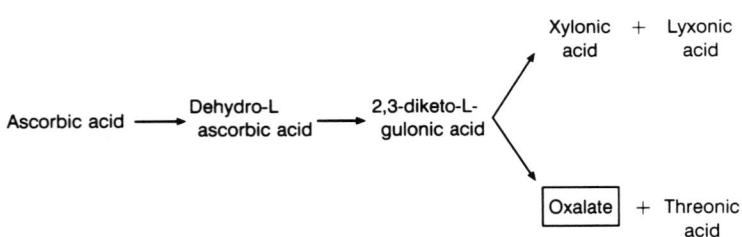

FIG. 2. Theoretical pathway of ascorbic acid metabolism.

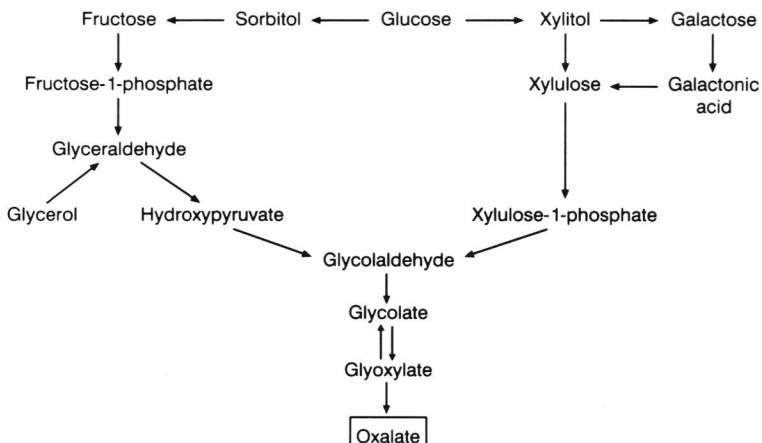

FIG. 3. Additional metabolic pathways of oxalate production (see text).

(38). These include entry into cells independent of insulin, efficient utilization without serious hyperglycemia, less stimulation of insulin secretion than glucose, and decreased irritation to veins when compared to glucose in hyperosmolar solution. Its use became available in Australia in 1969. This was followed by a series of deaths that were attributed to the xylitol infusions. Similar observations were noted in Germany, Japan, and Denmark. Patients who were given xylitol as parenteral infusions developed renal, liver, and cerebral dysfunction with metabolic acidosis and tissue oxalosis involving the brain, kidney, and heart. At the time the precipitation of calcium oxalate was not predicted since there was no known metabolic pathway that would explain the production of oxalate from xylitol. Subsequent studies have defined specific pathways from sugars and sugar alcohols through glycoaldehyde to oxalate (Fig. 3) (28). It has been thought that these metabolic pathways are a minor contributor to oxalate production in healthy humans. When sugars and sugar alcohols are given in excess, these pathways become important with increased endogenous production of oxalate. That these metabolic pathways may have a more subtle role in the mild hyperoxaluria of some patients with idiopathic calcium oxalate urolithiasis has been suggested, but further study is needed to establish a relationship (28).

Up to this point, oxalate has been considered a waste product of normal metabolism. It has been considered an unfortunate choice as a waste product because of its tendency to precipitate as calcium oxalate causing pathologic disorders of crystal deposition. Recent observations summarized in detail by Hamilton suggest that oxalate may be of critical importance to animal metabolism (39). Oxalate inhibits several important familiar enzymes including lactate dehydrogenase, glycolate oxidase, pyruvate kinase, pyruvate carboxylase, and malic enzyme. This inhibition by oxalate of lactate dehydrogenase and glycolate oxidase would prevent an excess build up of oxalate catalyzed by these enzymes. Oxalate inhibi-

tion of the other three enzymes will have an effect on gluconeogenesis, glycolysis, and NADPH formation. Hamilton suggests another possible role for oxalate in the mitochondria (39). The potential activity product of calcium oxalate within the mitochondria may exceed the solubility product for calcium oxalate. If so, then calcium oxalate may precipitate within the mitochondria forming crystalline spherulites like those formed with calcium phosphate (40,41). If this occurs, then the concentration of oxalate could regulate the mitochondrial calcium concentration and influence metabolism within the mitochondria. Although these observations are incomplete at this time, it is clear that the role of oxalate in many metabolic pathways in humans needs to be reexamined with a broader approach to these studies.

A little known observation in regard to the deposition of calcium oxalate crystals has been described in normal thyroid tissue (42,43). In pathological states of thyroid these crystals decrease in number or disappear. Their role (if any) in the health and metabolism of the thyroid remains to be defined.

OXALATE TRANSPORT

Renal Clearance

Clearance of oxalate by the kidney has been studied in a variety of species using labeled ^{14}C-oxalate. Cattell et al. examined the clearance of ^{14}C-oxalate in dogs and compared it with a clearance of inulin, creatinine, and paraaminohippuric acid (PAH) (44). Glomerular filtration and tubular secretion were involved in oxalate excretion. There also was evidence for passive tubular reabsorption. Tubular secretion was inhibited by caronamide, probenecid, and PAH. They felt that from their studies, tubular excretion of oxalate was localized to the proximal tubule.

Using free-flow micropuncture technique, Weinman et al. demonstrated that oxalate was secreted early in the proximal convoluted tubule by the observation that the fractional excretion of ^{14}C-oxalate was 120% of the filtered load (45). Reabsorption occurred later in the proximal segment when only 85% of the intratubular microinjection of ^{14}C-oxalate could be recovered. Collections made further down the proximal segment showed complete recovery of the ^{14}C-oxalate suggesting additional secretion. Subsequent microperfusion studies by Knight et al. examined the transepithelial secretory flux of ^{14}C-oxalate (46). Increases in the concentration of oxalate in the capillary solution resulted in progressively higher rates of oxalate secretion into the lumen up to a concentration of 4.3 mM. Further increase in capillary concentration of oxalate showed a tendency toward a plateau in oxalate excretion. The addition of sodium, cyanide, indanyloxyacetic acid, parachloromercuribenzoate, furosemide, and paraaminohippurate lowered the secretory flux of oxalate. Probenecid inhibited oxalate secretion when the oxalate concentration and capillary solution was between 1.1 and 4.3 mM. At higher capillary concentrations of oxalate, it had no effect on oxalate secretion. It was suggested that oxalate secretion in the proximal tubule of the rat was an active carrier mediated process. When put together with previous studies, it was felt that there may be more than one oxalate secretory system present in the rat proximal tubules. Clearance studies in humans using ^{14}C-oxalate have consistently shown net tubular secretion of oxalate with a fractional excretion ranging from 1.54 to 2.15 (47–49). In two recent studies where plasma oxalate was measured without radioisotope, the fractional excretion of oxalate ranged from 0.86 to 1.12 with a majority of the normal subjects from the two studies being less than 1 (50,51). These data in a small group of normal subjects from two laboratories using different methods to measure plasma oxalate suggest that the majority of the normal subjects had net tubular reabsorption of oxalate. Additional studies examining this question in normal subjects are needed.

Renal Transport

Recent studies have examined the transcellular transport of oxalate through specific membranes. The first set of studies examined the apical membrane using a membrane vesicle preparation from rabbits (52). An apical transporter was identified exchanging oxalate for chloride and formate. Sulfate and bicarbonate did not affect oxalate exchange. This apical transport of oxalate was inhibited by the anion transport inhibitor 4,4'-diisothiocyanato-stilbene-2-2'-disulfonic acid (DIDS). Additional studies have examined the basolateral membrane using a membrane vesicle preparation (53). Here oxalate was exchanged for bicarbonate and sulfate. Sodium did not affect the transport of oxalate, and the uptake was inhibited by DIDS, furosemide, and bumetanide.

Gastrointestinal Transport

The oxalate concentration within the intestinal contents is dependent upon dietary oxalate in healthy subjects. In the presence of gastrointestinal disease with bacterial overgrowth, oxalate content can be altered as will be discussed later. The oxalate content of a normal diet is normally between 80 and 120 mg of oxalate per day. Much of this is bound by dietary calcium and subsequently excreted with the feces. On a normal diet no more than 20% of the ingested oxalate is available for absorption. Oxalate can be absorbed throughout the intestinal tract although it would appear that the majority of the absorption is from the distal ileum and colon. This may, in part, be related to calcium absorption. As the calcium concentration in the intestinal contents decreases, more oxalate is available as the oxalate ion. In health, oxalate absorption from the intestinal tract is by an active transport mechanism being inhibited by the anion transport inhibitor 4-acetamido-4'-isothiocyanato-stilbene-2-2'-disulfonic acid (SITS) (54,55). Studies using ileal membrane vesicles from the rabbit showed that oxalate could exchange with hydroxal and chloride ions (56). This transport system appeared to be localized to the brush border membrane and was not present in basolateral membrane vesicles. The transport of oxalate was diminished by several anion transport inhibitors including DIDS, SITS, probenecid, furosemide, and bumetanide. Oxalate transport also can occur by passive diffusion through the tight junctions, but this appears to more important in disease state and will be reviewed in the discussion of enteric hyperoxaluria (57).

CALCIUM OXALATE CRYSTAL FORMATION

A detailed discussion of calcium oxalate crystal formation is presented in Chapter 29. In a discussion of hyperoxaluric states, it is important to emphasize some aspects of the formation of calcium oxalate crystals. Illustrated in Fig. 4 are examples of calcium oxalate crystals as they appear in urine. A third crystal phase, calcium oxalate trihydrate, may occur transiently at the time of initial precipitation, but it has not been recognized as a consistent part of calcium oxalate stones formed within the urinary tract (16,17,58,59). Calcium oxalate monohydrate (whewellite) is the most stable phase and the one most often found in urinary stones. In vitro, this is the crystalline phase that precipitates from aqueous solutions of calcium and oxalate. Calcium oxalate dihydrate (weddellite) is extremely difficult to grow in the laboratory, yet when calcium oxalate precipitates in normal urine, it is as the dihydrate phase (60–62). The predominant calcium oxalate phase in patients with idiopathic calcium oxalate urolithiasis is dihydrate. Inhibitors of calcium oxalate crystal formation that occur

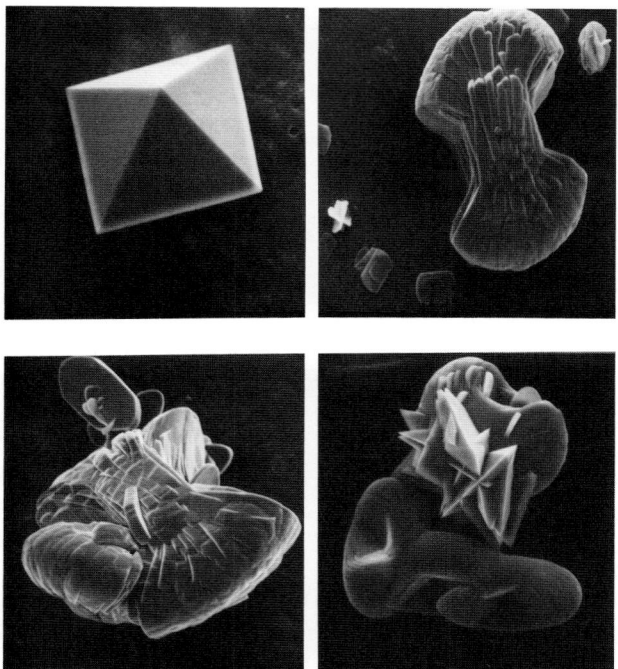

FIG. 4. Examples of calcium oxalate crystalluria present in freshly voided urine obtained from patients with hyperoxaluria. Observations are made with scanning electron microscopy. **Upper left:** Calcium oxalate dihydrate (weddellite). **Upper right:** Calcium oxalate monohydrate (whewellite). **Lower left:** Crystal aggregate of calcium oxalate monohydrate. **Lower right:** Crystal aggregate containing both crystal phases.

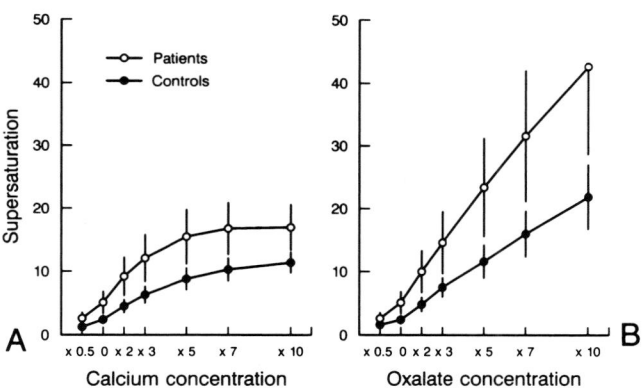

FIG. 5. The effect of changing calcium concentration (**A**) or oxalate concentration (**B**) on supersaturation of calcium oxalate using EQUIL2 (141).

normally in urine stabilize the dihydrate phase (63). When significant hyperoxaluria is present with massive crystalluria, the predominant crystal phase becomes calcium oxalate monohydrate (62). It has been suggested that this change in the crystal phase may occur because of the large amount of crystal formation going on in the urine. When crystals are formed, natural inhibitors are absorbed to the crystal surface affectively removing them from urine. With their removal, the dihydrate phase can no longer be stabilized, and calcium oxalate monohydrate is formed. Supporting this hypothesis is the fact that total inhibition for calcium oxalate crystal formation is reduced in patients with primary hyperoxaluria who have massive calcium oxalate monohydrate crystal formation (64). When the crystal formation is stopped or greatly decreased with treatment, the amount of inhibition of calcium oxalate crystal formation returns to normal and the predominant crystal becomes calcium oxalate dihydrate. A second element in the consideration of crystal formation and hyperoxaluria relates to the free ion activity of calcium and oxalate. The stoichiometric relationship between calcium and oxalate in the crystal is 1:1. At that ratio, the largest crystalline mass is produced. In urine from normal subjects the ratio between calcium and oxalate is approximately 5:1. As

one moves away from the 1:1 ratio in either direction, the effects on supersaturation and crystalline mass decrease. Following these observations, one would anticipate that even small increases in the free ion activity of oxalate would have a much greater effect than increases in calcium ion activity in urine (20,65). As can be seen in Fig. 5, increasing oxalate concentration affects the supersaturation of calcium oxalate much more than increasing calcium concentration.

DIET AND OXALATE

It is important to review some general considerations about the role of diet in the urinary excretion of oxalate. As stated earlier, 10% to 15% of the oxalate excreted in the urine comes from the diet in normal subjects. As will be reviewed subsequently, this percentage can increase significantly when there are disturbances of intestinal absorption. Data available to dietitians in regard to the oxalate content of specific foods is marginal at best. Most published methods for the measurement of oxalate in foods involve homogenization of the food followed by cold or hot extraction of the homogenate with hydrochloric acid, extraction with diethyl ether, precipitation with calcium, and estimation with potassium permanganate (1). Some methods omit ether extraction, and some have determined both the water soluble and the acid soluble (total) oxalate fractions. There are many problems with these methods. The data available at this time lacks the preciseness one usually expects with food analysis. The problem is complicated further by the fact that the oxalate content of many foods, particularly plants, vary with age (66). This variation is not only in terms of total oxalate content but also the form of oxalate that is present (67,68). Oxalate may be present in a soluble or an insoluble form with the former being absorbed better from the intestinal tract. Also, the calcium and magnesium content of the food may influence oxalate bioavailability. To date, newer techniques available for the measurement of oxalate have not been applied to food analysis. All of these factors make it extremely difficult for dietitians to measure the dietary intake of oxalate and instruct patients in diets that are accurate in terms of oxalate content. There is a real need for the analysis of foods in terms of oxalate content and bioavailability using current analytical techniques.

Outlined in Table 1 are some dietary factors that affect the urinary excretion of oxalate. In considering these, it is important to remember that elements of the diet can serve as precursors to oxalate being metabolized through the metabolic pathways outlined in Figs. 1 to 3. These include certain amino acids, sugars and sugar alcohols, protein, and ascorbic acid (1,5,22,28,69). Also present in the diet are elements that can decrease urinary oxalate. Calcium and dietary fiber bind oxalate in the colon and limit its absorption (70–75). Calcium is especially important when one considers the intestinal absorption of oxalate. Outlined in Fig. 6 are situations where calcium can influence the bioavailability of oxalate and its intestinal absorption. If the diet is low in calcium with normal oxalate, oxalate absorption will increase with an increase in urinary oxalate. Early studies by Zarembski and Hodgkinson examine the relationship between urinary oxalate and the dietary intake of calcium (70). They noted a significant increase in the urinary excretion of oxalate when subjects were given a low calcium diet. This increase was magnified when oral EDTA was added to the low calcium diet. If calcium absorption is increased in the small bowel due either to increased 1,25-dihydroxyvitamin D or increased passive absorption, the calcium content of the intestine will decrease and the bioavailability of oxalate will increase (76–80). Finally, if calcium is complexed with such things as fatty acids or calcium binders, oxalate bioavailability is increased (81–84). Pyridoxine deficiency will increase the urinary excretion of oxalate. Pyridoxine is a co-enzyme in the conversion of glyoxylate to glycine (see Fig. 1), and when there is a deficiency of pyridoxine, there will be an increased endogenous production of oxalate with subsequent hyperoxaluria (85–87). As will be discussed subsequently, pyridoxine has been suggested as having a role

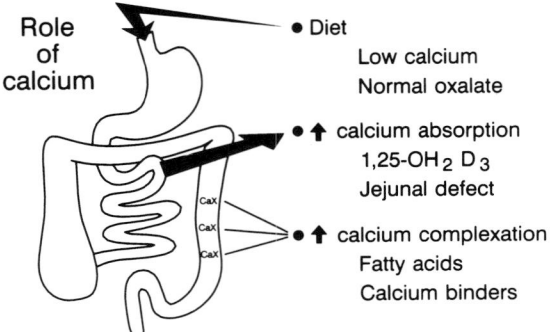

FIG. 6. Intestinal absorption of oxalate.

in the treatment of mild hyperoxaluria in patients with idiopathic calcium oxalate urolithiasis.

MEASUREMENT OF OXALATE

A primary problem in the study of oxalate is its measurement when present in biological solutions (88–90). Even today, all of the factors present in urine and plasma that can modify the analytical results when measuring oxalate are not defined. Although oxalate would seem to be a very simple compound, one which would be easy to measure, this has not been the case. Since Archer et al. published a method to measure oxalate in 1957, there have been published at least 86 different methods to measure oxalate in biological fluids (67). Many of the titles for these papers use descriptive terms such as "simple," "rapid," and "precise." Only recently have any of these descriptive terms applied to the analysis of oxalate in biological fluids.

Wandzilak and Williams recently summarized the many techniques that have been suggested over the years to measure oxalate in urine, plasma, amniotic fluid, cerebrospinal fluid, tissue, bone, feces, and food (90). Today, enzymatic, ion chromotographic, gas chromotographic, and bioluminescent methods provide accurate measurement of oxalate in biological samples if these samples are collected and handled correctly in the laboratory (91–97).

Ascorbic acid presents a particularly difficult problem in the analysis of oxalate and can alter the final results (89,90,98,99). When ascorbic acid is present, it can be metabolized to oxalate by a nonenzymatic chemical reaction. The rate of this reaction increases as pH increases. This can be a particular problem in urine where a significant amount of ascorbate may be present particularly in patients taking vitamin C supplementation. If the urine is collected at the voided pH and allowed to stand at room temperature until the 24-hour urine collection is completed, ascorbic acid can be converted to oxalate causing an apparent hyperoxaluria. This artifact can be

TABLE 1. *Dietary factors affecting urinary oxalate excretion*

Increased excretion
  Oxalate
  Protein
  Some amino acids
  Sugars and sugar alcohols
  Ascorbic acid

Decreased excretion
  Calcium
  Dietary fiber
  Pyridoxine

prevented if hydrochloric acid is added to the collection container prior to the collection so that the urine pH is at 2.0 or below. Refrigeration during the collection is also helpful. If one pays attention to these details and analyzes the sample promptly on completion of the collection, then the risk of conversion is eliminated.

With the new microtechniques for the analysis of oxalate in both urine and plasma, opportunities are now present to study oxalate transport in health and in disease states.

Increased glycolate excretion in the urine of patients with calcium oxalate stones has been used as an indicator of increased endogenous production of oxalate (1,5,18,22). Methodologies to measure glycolate have included isotope dilution, chemical, colorimetric, chromotographic, and enzymatic techniques (100). Problems exist with each of these procedures. The chemical and colorimetric methods are nonspecific, and the chromotographic and HPLC methods require complex isolation and derivitization steps. Enzyme methods have been widely used but also have several problems. Glycolate and lactate are isolated together from urine during a charcoal absorption step. This requires a second separate assay for lactate with subsequent subtraction to correct for the glycolate values. Automation has not been possible, and the enzymatic preparation is not stable. Recently, a method using automated ion chromotography has been described (100). This appears to avoid many of the problems with the other assays.

CLINICAL DISORDERS COMPLICATED BY HYPEROXALURIA

Enteric Hyperoxaluria

The formation of stones within the urinary tract by patients who have underlying gastrointestinal disorders with malabsorption has been well recognized (18). Gelzayd and his associates reviewed the case histories on 885 patients with inflammatory bowel disease noting the occurrence of nephrolithiasis in 64 (7.2%) (101). Previous surgery of the gastrointestinal tract had been performed in 179 (20%) of the patients. Of these, 29 (16%) subsequently developed urinary calculi. The frequency of the formation of calculi within the urinary tract in these patients with gastrointestinal disorders was much greater than the overall estimated prevalence of urinary calculi in the United States. Of special interest in this study was the fact that 46 (72%) of the patients had stones that contained calcium salts and were radiopaque.

The association of calcium oxalate urolithiasis and hyperoxaluria in patients who have had small bowel resection was noted in 1970 (102). Following this initial observation, a series of studies confirming the association were reported (103–106). These studies have provided

an increased understanding of this complication in terms of etiology and potential approaches to treatment. Any cause of intestinal malabsorption can produce enteric hyperoxaluria if at least a portion of the colon is intact. Clinical disorders of the gastrointestinal tract that have been associated with the development of enteric hyperoxaluria are listed in Table 2.

The presence of enteric hyperoxaluria and recurrent calcium oxalate urolithiasis has been especially common in patients who have had small bowel bypass for obesity at least in part due to the massive steatorrhea that these patients often have (107–109). In this setting the prevalence of stone formation has ranged from 17% to 32%.

The formation of stones within the urinary tract of these patients may be due to multiple factors (18). Clearly, the hyperoxaluria that occurs is a major stress factor in the stone formation. Other abnormalities secondary to the intestinal malabsorption can promote the formation of urinary calculi. For the purpose of this chapter, hyperoxaluria will be considered first followed by a discussion of the other nonspecific abnormalities due to malabsorption that promote stone formation.

The hyperoxaluria in this syndrome is due to increased oxalate absorption from the intestinal tract, principally the colon (110,111). As Fig. 7 illustrates three factors influence the hyperoxaluria. Dietary oxalate is critical. To date, there is no evidence supporting increased endogenous production of oxalate in these patients so that the increased urinary excretion of oxalate must come from the oxalate that is absorbed from the gastrointestinal tract. A special situation in these patients may influence intestinal oxalate. If bacterial overgrowth has occurred with colonization of the proximal intestine, two situations theoretically may exist influencing intestinal oxalate. The first situation could decrease oxalate concentration. If the flora overgrowing the upper intestinal tract included anaerobic oxalate degrading bacteria such as *Oxalobacter formigenes,* at least some of the dietary oxalate could be metabolized by the oxalate degrading enzymes of these bacteria (2,6,112,113). A second situation with bacterial overgrowth would have the

TABLE 2. *Gastrointestinal disorders associated with enteric hyperoxaluria*

Primary diseases
    Regional enteritis
    Nontropical sprue
    Blind loop syndrome
    Bacterial overgrowth syndrome
    Chronic pancreatitis
    Biliary tract disease

Postsurgical causes
    Small bowel resection
    Pancreatectomy
    Small bowel bypass for obesity

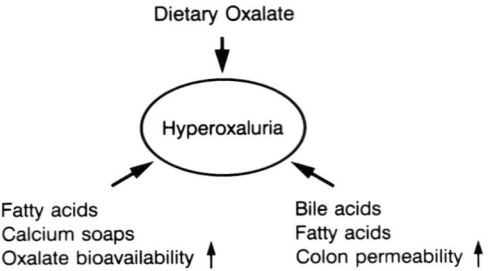

FIG. 7. Factors influencing oxalate absorption.

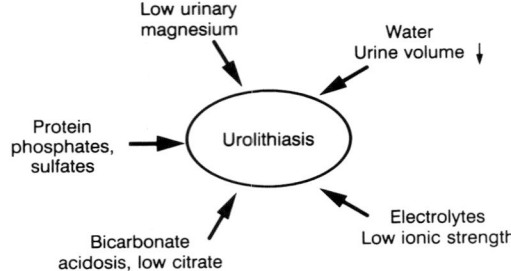

FIG. 8. Nonspecific abnormalities favoring urolithiasis.

opposite effect (114). In this situation, precursors of oxalate in the diet such as proteins, amino acids, sugar and sugar alcohol, and vitamin C could be metabolized by the intestinal bacterial flora to oxalate increasing the oxalate content of the intestinal tract. Although theoretically possible, the regular occurrence of either of these situations remains to be established.

A second abnormality contributing to the hyperoxaluria is fatty acid malabsorption with steatorrhea (115–118). Two factors may influence oxalate absorption in this situation. First, calcium within the intestinal contents is bound to the fatty acids forming calcium soaps. This effectively reduces the calcium concentration that is available to complex oxalate and limits its absorption. As a result, oxalate bioavailability increases. Fatty acids also increase the permeability of the colon to organic compounds like oxalate (57). The third factor, bile acid malabsorption, also increases colon permeability to oxalate (57,118). The changes in colon permeability appear to relate to passive transport of oxalate through channels such as the tight junctions, and more of these channels may become available. Size and charge selectivity is not altered, and the active membrane transport of oxalate does not appear to be a primary factor in the increased oxalate absorption. Another factor that may influence oxalate absorption by the colon is the pH of the colonic contents (119). Acidification, perhaps from bacterial overgrowth, can increase the absorption of oxalate.

Another nonspecific group of abnormalities secondary to intestinal malabsorption favor the formation of calculi within the urinary tract (18). These disturbances that can alter dramatically the physicochemical balance in urine are often overlooked or not sought in the workup of patients with enteric hyperoxaluria. Yet these abnormalities may be primary in the patient's stone formation. Unless they are identified and corrected, treatment failure is likely. Figure 8 outlines the major nonspecific abnormalities that favor the formation of urinary calculi. Malabsorption with diarrhea causes increased water loss in the stool with a decrease in urine volume. This can be a major problem when bile acid diarrhea is present. The decreased urine volume due to reduced water absorption from the intestinal tract causes increased concentration of urinary solute (mg/L) such as

calcium or oxalate without changes in excretion rates (mg/24 hr). The loss of univalent ions such as sodium, potassium, and chloride in the stool may occur causing a decrease in the urinary excretion of these ions. Since monovalent ions are the principal contributor to the ionic strength of the urine, it is decreased reducing the solubility of ions such as calcium and oxalate (120). Magnesium absorption often is reduced with malabsorption causing a decrease in the urinary excretion of magnesium (18,121,122). Magnesium is an important complexor of oxalate. When its concentration is reduced in urine, there is an increase in the portion of oxalate present as the free ion. Bicarbonate loss commonly occurs with malabsorption, and a mild compensated metabolic acidosis can develop. With this, the urinary excretion of citrate often is too low to measure (18,123,124). Additional factors already discussed that may influence citrate excretion and intracellular metabolic acidosis are the malabsorption of potassium and magnesium (125). A deficiency of either can create or aggravate an intracellular metabolic acidosis and the hypocitric aciduria. Citrate is an important complexor of calcium (120,126). In urine it also acts as an inhibitor of calcium apatite and calcium oxalate crystal formation (127,128). These patients may have protein malabsorption with an associated reduction in the absorption of phosphate and sulfate from the diet. This can cause a reduction in the urinary excretion of phosphate and sulfate. Depending upon the pH of the urine, these anions are important in the complexation of calcium (120). A reduction in their concentration increases the free calcium ion activity. With the reduction in phosphate excretion, the urinary excretion of pyrophosphate also is reduced (129). Pyrophosphate is a surface inhibitor of calcium apatite and calcium oxalate crystal formation (127,128).

Because of the changes with malabsorption, another etiologic factor may play a role in the stone formation in some of these patients. The uric acid excretion rate is normal in most patients with enteric hyperoxaluria. This uric acid must be excreted into urine of low volume which typically is very acidic, an ideal situation for the precipitation of uric acid (130–133). With the changes previously discussed promoting the supersaturation of the urine in terms of calcium oxalate, this is an ideal

TABLE 3. *Hyperoxaluric states*

Mole/mole creatinine[a]	Normal subjects n = 16	Enteric hyperoxaluria n = 15	Primary hyperoxaluria n = 12
Calcium	0.32 ± 0.03	0.33 ± 0.05	0.34 ± 0.06
Oxalate[b]	0.03 ± 0.003	0.11 ± 0.01	0.22 ± 0.05
Magnesium[c]	0.5 ± 0.03	0.2 ± 0.04	0.6 ± 0.05
Citrate[c]	0.3 ± 0.03	0.08 ± 0.02	0.3 ± 0.08
Phosphate[c]	2.7 ± 0.2	2.0 ± 0.1	3.1 ± 0.3
Sulfate[c]	1.4 ± 0.1	0.8 ± 0.1	1.4 ± 0.2
Potassium[c]	7.0 ± 0.5	4.0 ± 0.6	7.9 ± 0.7
Supersaturation CaC_2O_4[b]	2.45 ± 0.6	11.23 ± 1.4	7.61 ± 0.8

[a] Mean ± SE.
[b] Each group differs from each other.
[c] Enteric hyperoxaluria differs from other groups.

setting for the heterogeneous nucleation of calcium oxalate by uric acid (134–139). An alternate hypothesis with the co-precipitation of calcium oxalate by uric acid in this setting has been suggested (140).

To emphasize the importance of the multiple factors involved in the precipitation of calcium oxalate in the formation of urinary calculi in these patients, data from normal subjects (n = 16) and patients with enteric hyperoxaluria (n = 15) and primary hyperoxaluria (n = 12) are presented (Table 3). These subjects were studied in a metabolic research center for a 60-hour period on their normal diet and fluid intake. None of the patients were on specific treatment at the time of the study. Two 24-hour urine collections were made during the period, and the data from the analysis of these urine collections were averaged in each subject. By measuring pH and the major ion species including sodium, potassium, chloride, calcium, magnesium, citrate, sulfate, phosphate, oxalate, ammonia, and bicarbonate, it was possible to estimate ionic strength, free ion activity, activity product, and supersaturation for the major urinary crystal systems. To make these estimates, an iterative computer

program previously described (EQUIL2) was utilized (141). The urinary concentration of calcium was not different in the three groups. Oxalate concentration was elevated in the patients with enteric hyperoxaluria, but it was much greater in the patients with primary hyperoxaluria (0.11 versus 0.22 mol/mol of creatinine). Magnesium, citrate, phosphate, pyrophosphate, sulfate, and potassium were decreased significantly in the urine of the patients with enteric hyperoxaluria. Because of these changes and their effect on ionic strength and complexation, the calcium oxalate supersaturation was greater in the patients with enteric hyperoxaluria than in the patients with primary hyperoxaluria. This emphasizes the need in these patients to look beyond excretion rates and solute concentration to the more subtle elements of supersaturation including pH, ionic strength, and complexation (120). Examples of the extensive calcium oxalate stone formation that can occur in patients with intestinal malabsorption and enteric hyperoxaluria are presented in Figs. 9 and 10.

A number of specific treatment programs have been developed for these patients to reduce hyperoxaluria and

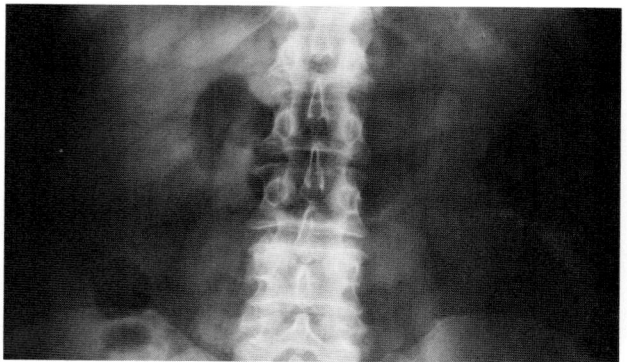 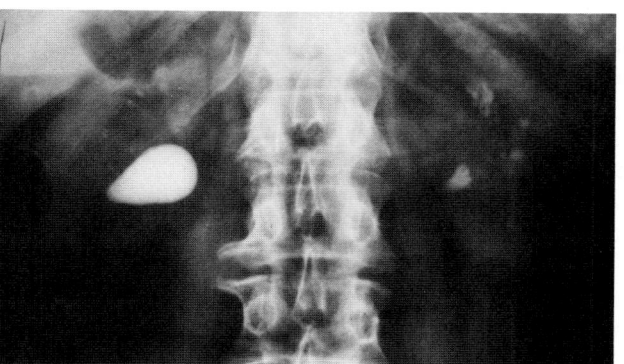

FIG. 9. A: A 64-year-old woman with enteric hyperoxaluria. Flat plate of abdomen prior to partial resection of small bowel. **B:** KUB roentgenogram 3 years later showing huge calcium oxalate stone in the right renal pelvis, a smaller calcium oxalate stone in the left renal pelvis, and multiple caliceal stones bilaterally.

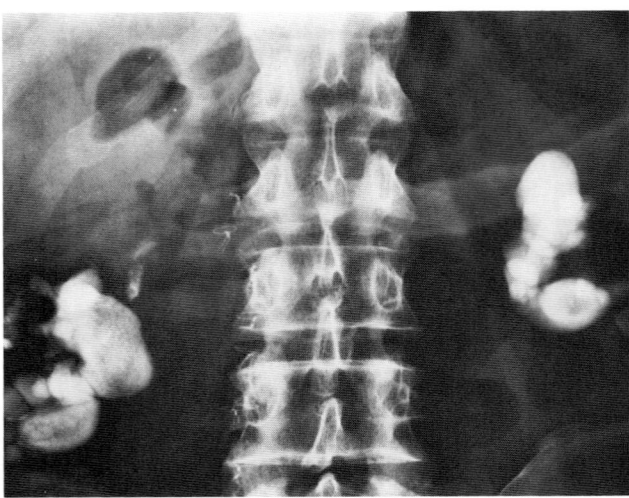

FIG. 10. KUB roentgenogram from a 63-year-old man with enteric hyperoxaluria showing a large collection of calcium oxalate stones in both kidneys that formed within one year following partial resection of the small bowel for regional enteritis.

control or prevent stone formation within their urinary tract (18,75,142,143). Reported response to these treatment programs has been variable. For instance, oxalate excretion may be decreased to normal, but stone formation continues to occur in some patients. In part, this may be due to the lack of consideration of the specific disturbances present in the individual patient responsible for their stone formation. One cannot emphasize enough the need to evaluate these patients carefully and identify all of the abnormalities present in their urine created by the intestinal malabsorption. At the time of the initial evaluation, one should identify all of the specific abnormalities that are present promoting the stone formation. A treatment program should be applied in stages beginning with an attempt to eliminate the hyperoxaluria. As with all patients who form urinary calculi, fluid intake should be maximized. In these patients with malabsorption, drinking small amounts (4–6 ounces) of fluid frequently may be better tolerated in terms of the malabsorption with more effective absorption of the fluid. Avoiding or taking a minimal amount of fluid at mealtime also can help to avoid overloading the absorptive surfaces of the intestine. Dietary oxalate should be reduced to an absolute minimum. During the evaluation stool fat should be quantitated, and if there is significant steatorrhea, a diet reduced in fat (±50 g fat diet) should be used along with the oxalate restriction. Patients will often accept this diet since it will greatly reduce the volume and number of stools. When they cheat with their diet taking in excess fat, their diarrhea will promptly return reminding them of the importance of the diet. Calcium supplementation up to 1 g/day can help to decrease the bioavailability of intestinal oxalate. This is best sup-

plied by calcium carbonate which also will provide much needed alkali to the patient. If bile acid malabsorption is a contributing factor to the diarrhea, cholestyramine given as 4 g three to four times daily will bind the bile acids and reduce their effect on diarrhea and colon permeability.

Table 4 outlines the treatment approaches to patients with enteric hyperoxaluria.

The first stage of treatment is directed toward correcting the hyperoxaluria with increased fluid intake and diet to restrict oxalate and fat. If stone formation continues then corrections of other abnormalities caused by the malabsorption should be considered. Of these, the easiest to treat is hypocitric aciduria. Alkali replacement as potassium citrate or a mixture of sodium and potassium citrate is usually adequate. Absorption seems to be better when this is given in liquid form to provide 30 mEq of base three to four times daily. If there has been a significant potassium wasting with potassium depletion, using the potassium salt of citrate is advisable. Citrate excretion should return to normal with adequate replacement therapy. If there is a significant magnesium depletion, this will not occur until magnesium stores are replaced. Magnesium replacement represents a second approach to treatment of nonspecific abnormalities. This is used when there is evidence of magnesium depletion. Unfortunately, replacement must be given by intramuscular injection as magnesium sulfate, 1 g weekly. If the deficiency is severe, daily injections may be needed until body stores are replaced. A new approach to the hyperoxaluria has been suggested by several groups (75,76). This involves the use of specific anion complexors that will bind oxalate within the intestine and prevent its absorption. Unfortunately, these compounds are nonspecific anion complexors so that other important anions such as phosphate and sulfate may be bound preventing their absorption. Safety and clinical response to the use of these compounds remains to be established.

TABLE 4. *Treatment approaches in enteric hyperoxaluria*

All patients
    Maximum fluid intake
    Low oxalate diet

Treatment for specific abnormalities
    Steatorrhea with fatty acid malabsorption
        Low fat diet
        Calcium supplement
    Bile acid malabsorption
        Cholestyramine
    Metabolic acidosis with hypocitric aciduria
        Alkali replacement
        Potassium replacement
        Magnesium replacement, if needed
    Magnesium deficiency
        Magnesium replacement
    Combinations

Small bowel bypass for obesity may create a special set of circumstances in patients with enteric hyperoxaluria (107–109). Many of these patients have profound steatorrhea with marked abnormalities in their urine secondary to the malabsorption. By nature, they have been unwilling to diet and may not do well with the dietary restriction of oxalate and fat. A subset of these patients will develop marked hyperoxaluria (>150 mg/24 hr), progressive stone formation, nephrocalcinosis, renal insufficiency, and increasing plasma oxalate (144–147). These patients must be convinced that their bypass should be taken down even though it has effectively controlled their weight problems. If this is not done, they will progress to renal failure and systemic oxalosis. In these patients, if the treatment approaches outlined above are unsuccessful, the bypass should be taken down before it is too late and significant renal insufficiency develops.

IDIOPATHIC CALCIUM OXALATE UROLITHIASIS

Most patients who form calcium oxalate calculi within the urinary tract have a heterogeneous syndrome termed by some idiopathic calcium oxalate urolithiasis (148). A variety of abnormalities promoting their calcium oxalate stone formation have been identified in these patients (149–152). In the past, the presence of hypercalciuria secondary to several abnormalities received the greatest attention by workers in the field. Other abnormalities included hyperuricosuria, hyperoxaluria, hypocitruria, and reduced inhibitors of crystal formation. These specific abnormalities are not mutually exclusive commonly occurring together to varying degrees in individual patients with idiopathic calcium oxalate urolithiasis (153). In trying to make some sense of all of this, Robertson et al. offered an alternative approach to the classification of these patients that has been helpful in developing treatment programs to prevent further stone formation (149). They examined urine composition in a group of patients with idiopathic calcium oxalate urolithiasis and recurrent stone formation. From this, they were able to identify a group of specific risk factors in the urine of the patients that correlated with the activity of their stone formation. These included low urine volume, hyperoxaluria, low urinary inhibitors of crystal formation, hyperuricosuria, hypercalciuria, and high urine pH. Low urine volume had the best correlation with hyperoxaluria closely behind. It is the purpose of this chapter to review current knowledge in regard to identified and theoretical causes of the hyperoxaluria and to emphasize the importance of mild increases in the urinary excretion of oxalate. As discussed earlier, these mild increases will have a much greater effect on calcium oxalate supersaturation and crystal mass than increases in urine calcium.

Mild hyperoxaluria (0.5–1.15 mmol/24 hr) has been reported to occur in from 15% to 50% of the patients with idiopathic calcium oxalate urolithiasis (154). Possible causes of the hyperoxaluria in these patients are outlined in Table 5. Of the causes listed, it is quite clear that diet and intestinal absorption has a well-established role in the development of this abnormality (71). It is important to emphasize again the several aspects of diet in addition to oxalate intake that can influence the urinary excretion of oxalate. As discussed earlier, oxalate precursors can increase, and oxalate binders can decrease the total oxalate excretion.

The role of diet and its composition in causing the mild hyperoxaluria in patients with this syndrome seems to be well established. The early work by Zarembski and Hodgkinson previously cited clearly established the relationship between calcium and oxalate in the diet (70). Hesse et al. reported that 52.7% of males and 18.8% of females had mild hyperoxaluria on a free diet (155). After one week of a standard diet in a metabolic research center, the occurrence of hyperoxaluria decreased to 18.9% in the males and 6.3% in the females. The standard diet included 100 g of protein, 250 g of carbohydrate, 90 g of fat, 1 g of calcium, 100 mg of oxalate, and 2.41 liters of fluid. Robertson and Peacock examined two groups of stone formers including those with a single stone and those who had recurrent stone formation (65). Their results were compared with a group of normal subjects. The patients were studied initially when they were seen in the urology clinics with a problem related to a specific stone. A 24-hour urine was collected for oxalate at that time. They were studied again six to eight weeks later in a stone clinic when the 24-hour urine collection for oxalate was repeated. Two percent of normal subjects had mild hyperoxaluria defined as greater than 0.46 mmol/day. At the time of the initial study, 27% of the single stone formers and 43% of the recurrent stone formers had hyperoxaluria. At the time of restudy in the stone clinic, this had decreased to 13% of the single stone formers and 23% of the recurrent stone formers. It was thought that this decrease reflected modification in diet following the initial visit. A recent study from our stone clinic analyzed the diet in 96 patients with idiopathic calcium oxalate urolithiasis (154). Calcium intake in this

TABLE 5. *Possible causes of hyperoxaluria in idiopathic calcium oxalate urolithiasis*

Increased calcium absorption
    Calcium restricted diet
    Calcium hyperabsorption
    Calcium binders

Transport defects
    Membrane
    Kidney

Endogenous metabolism

group was 7.4 ± 4.8 mg/kg/24 hr. This compares with 14.6 ± 7.3 mg/kg/24 hr in normal subjects ($P < 0.001$). Fifty-three of the patients had metabolically active stone formation. In them, the diet was not different from the total group of patients. It is typical in patients that have formed calcium oxalate stones that they are told to avoid calcium containing foods especially dairy products. If oxalate intake is not restricted, then the expected benefit from reducing urine calcium is quickly overcome by an increase in urine oxalate.

Calcium hyperabsorption is a primary or secondary defect that is present in the patients with idiopathic calcium oxalate urolithiasis who have hypercalciuria. Two primary abnormalities have been described. The first relates to an increase in 1,25-dihydroxyvitamin D in some of the patients with absorptive hypercalciuria (76,156,157). A second abnormality involves a selective hyperabsorption of calcium unrelated to magnesium absorption in the jejunum (78). This appears to be independent of 1,25-dihydroxyvitamin D. A third defect is secondary to a renal leak of phosphate in a subset of these patients (158). The hypophosphatemia that occurs stimulates the production of 1,25-dihydroxyvitamin D and increased calcium absorption in a secondary fashion. In the patients who have hypercalciuria with renal leak, the problem is thought to begin in the kidney with calcium loss (159). This stimulates the release of parathyroid hormone and the production of 1,25-dihydroxyvitamin D resulting in increased absorption of calcium from the intestine. Each of these abnormalities effectively decreased the calcium concentration within the intestinal contents increasing the bioavailability of oxalate and promoting its increased intestinal absorption. To illustrate the relationship between calcium hyperabsorption and hyperoxaluria, it may be helpful to review several studies that examined this question. Bataille et al. examined the effect of low calcium diet given for five days to control subjects and patients with idiopathic calcium oxalate urolithiasis (160). The patients were divided into four groups including those with normocalciuria, absorptive hypercalciuria type 1, absorptive hypercalciuria type 2, and renal hypercalciuria. This classification followed the screening procedure of Pak et al. (161). Oxalate excretion increased in all groups including the control subjects. The greatest increase was in those patients with the greatest hyperabsorption of calcium (absorptive hypercalciuria type 1). The authors suggested that the increased absorption of calcium decreased calcium availability within the intestinal tract causing decreased complexation of oxalate with increased bioavailability of oxalate for absorption. In our own study of 96 patients with idiopathic calcium oxalate urolithiasis, we were able to demonstrate increased oxalate excretion in the group of patients who had increased intestinal absorption of calcium as demonstrated by their urine calcium/diet calcium ratio while on their normal diet (154).

Finally, substances within the intestine that bind cal-

cium increase the bioavailability of oxalate and its absorption. The role of fatty acids in the syndrome of enteric hyperoxaluria was reviewed in detail in the previous section. Another example of a calcium binder is cellulose phosphate which has been used in some patients with type 1 absorptive hypercalciuria (162). If there is not a restriction of dietary oxalate when this treatment program is used, urine oxalate will increase significantly overcoming the benefit of reducing hypercalciuria.

Perhaps one of the best examples in nature of the role of dietary factors in hyperoxaluria and the formation of calcium oxalate stones is present in Saudi Arabia where oxalate excretion in the urine in normal Saudi males is almost twice that in the western industrialized countries (163,164). The diet in Saudi Arabia when compared with the English diet shows significant differences. Calcium intake is approximately one-half of the calcium intake in England while oxalate is 2.5 times greater than the English diet. Animal protein is also increased. If one adds calcium to the diet, oxalate decreases toward normal. As one would predict, the prevalence of calcium oxalate stones is very high in Saudi Arabia with approximately 20% of the males having had a symptomatic episode with kidney stones by the age of 70.

A second possible cause of hyperoxaluria in these patients has been suggested by several studies examining the transport of oxalate. Baggio et al. examined the uptake of oxalate by the red blood cell membrane in a subset of patients with idiopathic calcium oxalate urolithiasis (165). Of 98 patients studied, 78 had red blood cell membrane uptake of oxalate that was above the upper limit of normal. An additional study in five pairs of brothers with one member of each pair having an abnormality in oxalate flux suggested that there was increased intestinal absorption of oxalate in the subjects that had abnormal flux. ^{14}C-oxalate excretion in the urine from a test meal was increased during collections at two hours and four hours following the meal. These increases were significantly different from the brothers with normal flux suggesting an abnormality in intestinal absorption. Further studies were done in 33 of the patients with abnormal oxalate flux. Oral hydrochlorothiazide, amiloride, or both restored to normal or nearly normal the oxalate flux.

Preliminary studies by two independent groups using different methodology to measure oxalate noted a significant increase in the fractional excretion of oxalate in patients with idiopathic calcium oxalate urolithiasis (50,51). Plasma oxalate was lower than the plasma oxalate in normal subjects, and the fractional excretion of oxalate was significantly higher than the fractional excretion in normal subjects. These preliminary observations would be compatible with a possible membrane transport abnormality within the kidneys of these patients with idiopathic calcium oxalate urolithiasis. Studies to confirm and expand these observations are needed.

Another possible cause of hyperoxaluria in patients

with idiopathic calcium oxalate urolithiasis relates to reports suggesting increased endogenous production of oxalate (166). Mild hyperoxaluria was noted in a subset of these patients with idiopathic calcium oxalate urolithiasis. Glycolate excretion was also increased, a situation that could occur if there was increased endogenous production of oxalate. Pyridoxine given in therapeutic range reduced to normal oxalate and glycolate excretion in some of these patients. Response was variable with some showing no effect. In others the response occurred only after a period of treatment. Still others apparently responded immediately. A major problem with these studies related to the fact that the diet was not controlled. Yendt and Cohanim also have observed mild hyperoxaluria and hyperglycolic aciduria in their patients with idiopathic calcium oxalate urolithiasis (167). In their studies, they could find no correlation between these two abnormalities. In a subset of the patients, pyridoxine had no effect when given orally. The increased urinary excretion of glycolate correlated in a positive fashion with the protein content of the diet and the urinary excretion of uric acid. It was their feeling that the increased excretion of glycolate was on a dietary basis. The possibility that there could be a subset of patients with idiopathic calcium oxalate urolithiasis that have a mild or incomplete form of primary hyperoxaluria remains. As we learn more about the genetic defects that are present in patients with primary hyperoxaluria, answers to whether or not this possibility exists should be available.

Approaches to treatment of patients with idiopathic calcium oxalate urolithiasis and mild hyperoxaluria are outlined in Table 6. As with any patient who forms stones, the foundation of therapy is adequate fluid intake. Ideally, these patients should take in a glass (8 ounces) of fluid approximately hourly while awake and again at night one time if up to void. Half of this should be as water. The other half can be of their choosing. The goal of fluid intake is a daily urine volume of at least 2.5 liters in men and at least 2.0 liters in women. To accomplish this goal, one must take the time to explain to the patient what is expected in terms of fluid intake and what is achieved in terms of diluting solute.

As has been emphasized, diet can be a very important factor in the mild hyperoxaluria that occurs in these patients. Not only must attention be paid to the oxalate content of the diet, but also one needs to consider calcium and potential precursors to oxalate such as protein, amino acids, sugars and sugar alcohols, and ascorbic acid. The goal of the dietary history would be to identify specific excesses or deficiencies in these dietary elements and provide a diet that eliminates identified abnormalities. Depending upon the clinical history and the amount of inadequacy with fluid intake and diet, a decision is made in regard to management at this point. If there is room for improvement, it is advisable to manage the patient conservatively with fluid and diet for a period of observation assessing the metabolic activity of his or her stone formation. Once this program is shown to be inadequate, then specific medication should be added.

Orthophosphate given as the neutral salt to provide 1.5 to 2.0 g of elemental phosphorus in three or four divided doses has been effective in preventing stone formation in not only these patients but also patients with primary hyperoxaluria discussed in the next section (168–173). Its use was first described by Howard et al. when they noted that oral orthophosphate would convert "evil" (mineralizing) urine of the stone former to "good" (nonmineralizing) urine of the non-stone former (174). Orthophosphate is not a simple program for the patient, and it is associated with side effects. The cathartic action of orthophosphate is the most common side effect usually occurring at the initiation of treatment. Often this subsides without further difficulty. In 13 of 172 patients with idiopathic calcium oxalate urolithiasis treated with orthophosphate, diarrhea was severe enough to interfere with therapy (171). Patients who have underlying gastrointestinal disorders, including irritable bowel, do not tolerate orthophosphate well. Old stones present when orthophosphate treatment is initiated may pass. This is not unique with orthophosphate and may occur with any effective treatment program. In a long-term study of patients treated with orthophosphate, 40% of the patients lost stone mass, and in 43% this occurred without symptoms. Only 10% of the patients required surgical intervention to manage the symptomatic stones. Orthophosphate must be limited if there is reduced renal function. It is contraindicated if the glomerular filtration rate is less than 30 mL/min and must be used cautiously when the glomerular filtration rate is between 30 and 50 mL/min. In these patients, serum creatinine, calcium, and phosphorus must be carefully monitored. Orthophosphate is also contraindicated in patients who have obstruction and/or infection playing a role in the stone formation. In these situations, the mechanism of stone formation is different and orthophosphate may actually promote stone growth. The mechanisms by which orthophosphate prevents stone formation will be reviewed in the subsequent section.

Potassium citrate also may be effective in these patients particularly if the urinary excretion of citrate is low (175). This is given to provide 20 to 30 mEq of base and potassium twice daily. Potassium citrate has some of the beneficial effects that occur with orthophosphate includ-

TABLE 6. *Treatment approaches in idiopathic calcium oxalate urolithiasis with mild hyperoxaluria*

Fluid intake
Diet modification
Orthophosphate
Potassium citrate
Magnesium
Pyridoxine

ing the increased complexation of calcium secondary to the increased concentration of citrate and the increased pH which makes both the citrate and phosphate a more effective complexor. Citrate also acts as an inhibitor of the crystal formation of calcium salts, and in that role its increased concentration is beneficial. A systematic long-term treatment trial of potassium citrate in patients with idiopathic calcium oxalate urolithiasis and hyperoxaluria has not been done.

Other forms of possible treatment have included magnesium and pyridoxine (176–178). Magnesium is an important complexor of oxalate so that an increased urinary excretion of magnesium will decrease the free ion activity of oxalate. One treatment trial in patients with idiopathic calcium oxalate urolithiasis suggested control of stone formation with magnesium hydroxide (179). Oxalate excretion was not reported in these patients, so it was not possible to know whether or not mild hyperoxaluria was present in the patients that responded to treatment. The use of pyridoxine in patients with mild hyperoxaluria has already been discussed. Unfortunately, the studies that have been reported did not control diet so that it was not possible to know what role the pyridoxine had in those patients who reduced their oxalate excretion with treatment.

PRIMARY HYPEROXALURIA

Primary hyperoxaluria is the most malignant of the conditions complicated by the formation of urinary calculi if left without treatment (18,22). In 1964 Hockaday et al. summarized 64 cases of primary hyperoxaluria from the world's literature (180). In 40 patients by the age of 4 symptoms or signs of the disease were present, 28 had died of their disease by the age of 20, and only 2

lived beyond the age of 40. Examples of the type of stone formation that may occur in these patients are shown in Fig. 11. The natural progression of the disease in the untreated patient is to move from stone formation to nephrocalcinosis to renal insufficiency and systemic oxalosis. The deposition of calcium oxalate outside of the kidney (oxalosis) occurs first in bone marrow and blood vessels. Bone deposition of calcium oxalate with replacement of the calcium apatite bone crystal is common in the latter stages of the disease. An example of the extent of oxalosis is shown in Fig. 12.

Two enzymatic defects in patients with primary hyperoxaluria have been described. Type 1 glycolic aciduria is due to a deficiency of alanine:glyoxylate aminotransferase in the peroxisomal membrane of liver cells (181–184). This defect is outlined in Fig. 13. In these patients, the urinary excretion of oxalate and glycolate is increased. It is thought that the majority of patients with primary hyperoxaluria have this enzyme defect. Recent studies have suggested that several abnormalities may be present (185–188). In addition to an absolute deficiency of alanine:glyoxylate aminotransferase, there would appear to be a subset of patients in whom there is a trafficking defect. In this situation, alanine:glyoxylate aminotransferase is located in the mitochondria instead of the peroxisome where it cannot function to convert glyoxylate to glycine. Absolute amounts of alanine:glyoxylate aminotransferase are normal within the liver, but the enzyme is located in an organelle where it appears to have no beneficial effect.

Type 2 L-glyceric aciduria is due to a deficiency of D-glyceric dehydrogenase which can be demonstrated in peripheral blood leukocytes from patients with this disorder (189). Urinary excretion of oxalate and L-glycerate is increased while glycolate is normal. A recent study by Mistry et al. identified a deficiency of glyoxylate reductase in addition to D-glyceric dehydrogenase in a patient

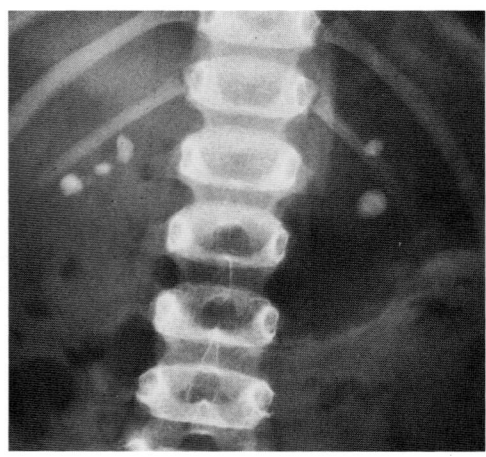
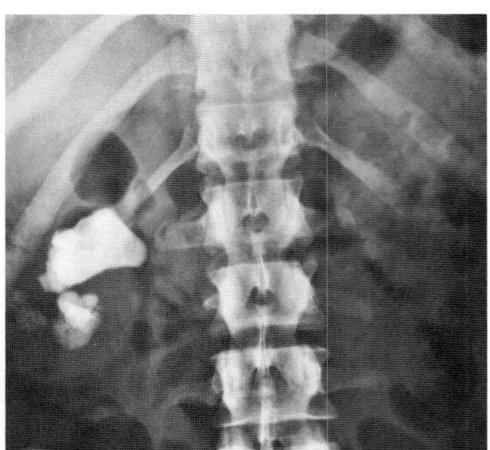

FIG. 11. **A:** KUB roentgenogram showing 5 large calcium oxalate stones in a $2\frac{1}{2}$-year-old girl with primary hyperoxaluria, type 1. **B:** KUB roentgenogram showing the large amount of calcium oxalate stone formation in the solitary kidney of a 20-year-old man with primary hyperoxaluria, type 1.

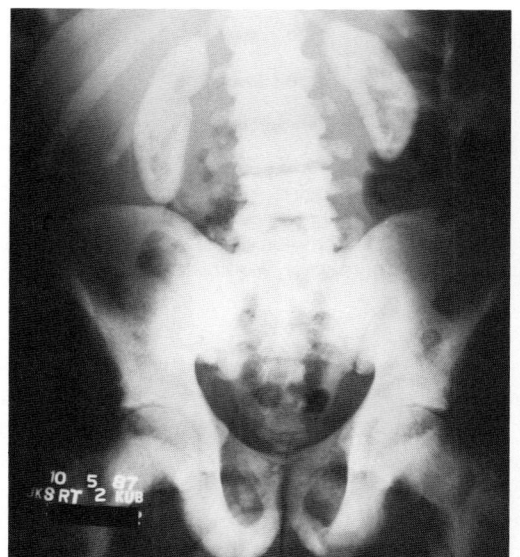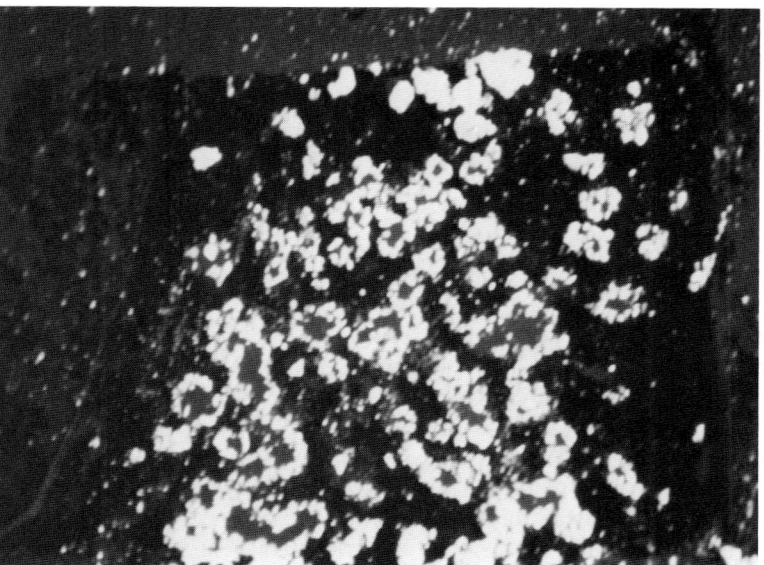

A   B

FIG. 12. A: A 29-year-old man with primary hyperoxaluria—type 1, renal failure, and massive oxalosis after 7 years of anuria and dialysis. KUB roentgenogram showing extensive nephrocalcinosis and dense bones compatible with calcium oxalate deposition in the bones. **B:** Bone biopsy showing extensive calcium oxalate crystal deposition with polarized light. X-ray defraction of the bone showed no hydroxy-apatite—only calcium oxalate.

with type 2 primary hyperoxaluria (190). This second enzyme abnormality may explain, at least in part, the hyperoxaluria that occurs in these patients. Glyoxylate reductase is important in the reduction of glyoxylate to glycolate in the cell cytoplasm. With the glyoxylate reductase deficiency, glyoxylate accumulates and is oxidized to oxalate by lactic dehydrogenase. Both disorders cause the increased endogenous production of oxalate, hyperoxaluria, urolithiasis, nephrocalcinosis, and renal insufficiency. The inheritance patterns of these enzyme disorders appear to be autosomal recessive. As more is learned about the specific abnormalities, it may be that there will be present some recognizable biochemical abnormalities in the heterozygote which currently is not the case.

Medical treatment of patients with primary hyperoxaluria has involved three specific approaches. It is im-

portant to emphasize that these approaches to medical treatment must be started before significant renal insufficiency has occurred. This emphasizes the need for early diagnosis and treatment in these patients. The first treatment program involves the use of pyridoxine (191–195). Pyridoxine is a co-enzyme in the conversion of glyoxylate to glycine (see Fig. 1). A subgroup of patients with type 1 primary hyperoxaluria will respond to therapeutic doses of pyridoxine reducing their urinary excretion of oxalate to normal or near normal. As many as 30% of the patients with type 1 primary hyperoxaluria will respond when pyridoxine is given as 200 mg per day. A few patients have been reported to need as much as 1 g per day although there is a risk of significant side effects with a continued dose at this level. Even though a patient may get only a partial response, any reduction of the urinary excretion of oxalate in this condition is beneficial, and

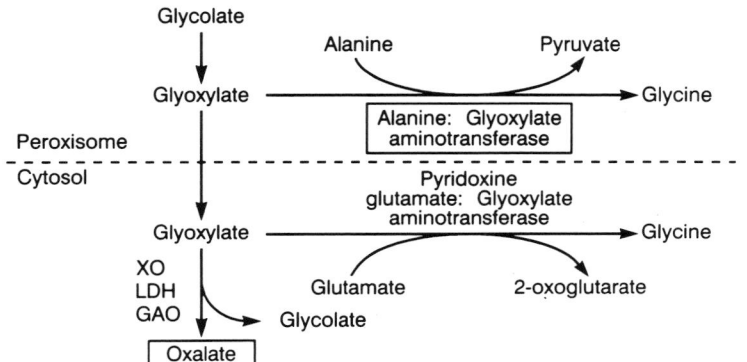

FIG. 13. Glyoxylate metabolism within the peroxisome and the cytosol alanine:glyoxylate aminotransferase deficiency increases cytosolic glyoxylate and causes increased production of oxalate.

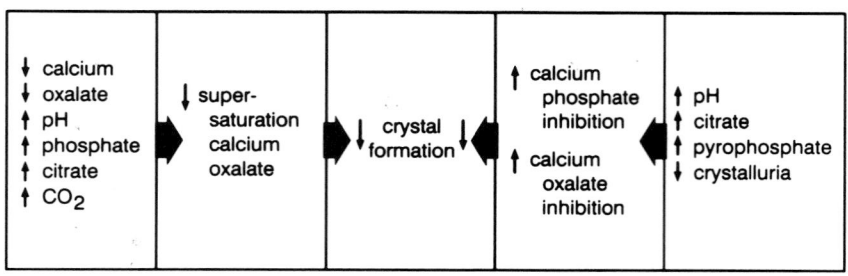

FIG. 14. The mechanisms of orthophosphate and pyridoxine treatment in patients with primary hyperoxaluria (see text).

the pyridoxine should be included as part of the treatment program. Patients with type 2 primary hyperoxaluria would not be expected to respond to pyridoxine treatment.

Magnesium supplements as magnesium oxide (450 mg/day) or magnesium hydroxide (210 mg/day) have been reported to prevent stone formation in 8 of 12 patients with primary hyperoxaluria treated for up to 11 years (196–198). Magnesium forms a soluble complex with oxalate in urine reducing free ion activity and decreasing the supersaturation of calcium oxalate.

Oral orthophosphate as its neutral salt was first used by Frederick et al. in two patients with primary hyperoxaluria (199). Later, it was suggested that pyridoxine should be combined with orthophosphate to obtain the potential added benefits of both treatment programs (192). The combination of orthophosphate and pyridoxine has been reported to prevent stone formation and renal insufficiency in 12 of 13 patients with type 1 primary hyperoxaluria over a mean treatment period of 15 years (200). The mechanism by which orthophosphate and pyridoxine alter the physical chemistry of urine is shown in Fig. 14. Calcium and oxalate are decreased while pH, phosphate, citrate, and CO_2 are increased in urine. This means that excretion rate of solute decreases while complexation increases causing a decrease in the supersaturation of calcium oxalate. Changes that occur in terms of inhibition of crystal formation include an increase in citrate and pyrophosphate with an increase in pH. The increase in pH makes both of these surface inhibitors more effective preventors of calcium oxalate crystal formation. Crystalluria decreases significantly preventing the removal of inhibitors of calcium oxalate crystal formation which would normally be absorbed to the crystal surface. This restores the concentration of these important inhibitors to normal further preventing crystal formation. With supersaturation down and inhibitors up, stone formation is prevented. In adults, the dosage of elemental phosphorus is usually 2 g as the neutral salt in four divided doses. In children up to 30 mg/kg may be used. The complications and contraindications have been discussed in the previous section.

Treatment becomes especially difficult in patients with primary hyperoxaluria when renal failure develops. Current forms of dialysis are not able to remove oxalate at a rate equal to or greater than endogenous oxalate production (201–203). As a result there is gradual accumulation of oxalate within the body and the development of significant oxalosis. Renal transplantation has been effective in a small group of patients who have developed renal failure with primary oxaluria (204–206). This should be done prior to the development of significant oxalosis since body stores of oxalate will be mobilized after successful renal transplantation putting the new kidney at significant risk for calcium oxalate precipitation. With a successful renal transplant, it is critical that the patient be placed on medical treatment as described above to prevent recurrence of the complications. Watts et al. have reported combined liver/kidney transplantation in selected patients who have renal insufficiency and are pyridoxine resistant (207–211). When successful, the enzymatic defect is corrected and the urinary excretion of glycolate and oxalate is restored to normal. To date, this approach has been used in a limited number of patients. A recent report summarized the results in nine patients from three centers. Four of the nine patients are alive and doing well 36 to 50 months post-transplant (212). Of the patients that died, all five had severe oxalosis and four of the five had been on dialysis for five to nine years prior to the transplantation. The patients who are doing well had only short-term dialysis before transplantation and three of the four had no evidence of systemic oxalosis. It is clear from this review that patients who have developed extensive oxalosis have not done well and that if this combined transplant is to be used, it should be done before the development of extensive oxalosis. The question of whether or not renal transplant should be done first before the more involved combined transplant is not resolved.

REFERENCES

1. Hodgkinson A. *Oxalic acid in biology and medicine.* New York: Academic Press, 1977.
2. Allison MJ, Dawson KA, Mayberry WR, Foss JG. Oxalobacter formigenes gen. nov., sp. nov.: oxalate-degrading anaerobes that inhabit the gastrointestinal tract. *Arch Microbiol* 1985;141:1–7.
3. Foster JW. *Chemical activities of fungi.* New York: Academic Press, 1949;326–50.
4. Martin SM. Formation of carboxylic acids by molds. In: Ruhland W., ed. *Encyclopedia of plant physiology,* vol 12, part 2. Berlin: Springer, 1960;605–39.

5. Franceschi VR, Horner HT Jr. Calcium oxalate crystals in plants. *The Botanical Review* 1980;46:361–427.
6. Allison MJ, Reddy CA. Adaptations of gastrointestinal bacteria in response to changes in dietary oxalate and nitrate. In: Klug MJ, Reddy CA, eds. *Current perspectives in microbial ecology.* Washington, D.C.: American Society for Microbiology, 1984;248–56.
7. Argenzio RA, Liacos JA, Allison MJ. Intestinal oxalate-degrading bacteria reduce oxalate absorption and toxicity in guinea pigs. *J Nutr* 1988;118:787–92.
8. Atkins CE, Johnson RK. Clinical toxicities of cats. *Vet Clin North Am* 1975;5:623–52.
9. Silberman MS, Blue J, Mahaffey E. Antifreeze (ethylene glycol) poisoning in a captive cheetah (*Acinonyx jubatus*) population. *Proc Am Assoc Zoo Vets* 1977;121–2.
10. Osborne CA, Poffenbarger EM, Klausner JS, Johnston SD, Griffith DP. Etiopathogenesis, clinical manifestations, and management of canine calcium oxalate urolithiasis. *Vet Clin North Am Small Anim Pract* 1986;16:133–71.
11. Hiatt RA, Friedman GD. The frequency of kidney and urinary tract diseases in a defined population. *Kidney Int* 1982;22:63–8.
12. Johnson CM, Wilson DM, O'Fallon WM, Malek RS, Kurland LT. Renal stone epidemiology: a 25-year study in Rochester, Minnesota. *Kidney Int* 1979;16:624–31.
13. Shuster J, Finlayson B, Scheaffer R, Sierakowski R, Zoltek J, Dzegede S. Water hardness and urinary stone disease. *J Urol* 1982;128:422–5.
14. Hiatt RA, Dales LG, Friedman GD, Hunkeler EM. Frequency of urolithiasis in a prepaid medical care program. *Am J Epidemiol* 1982;115:255–65.
15. Prien EL, Frondel C. Studies in urolithiasis. I. The composition of urinary calculi. *J Urol* 1947;57:949–94.
16. Prien EL. Crystallographic analysis of urinary calculi: a 23-year survey study. *J Urol* 1963;89:917–24.
17. Herring LC. Observations on the analysis of ten thousand urinary calculi. *J Urol* 1962;88(4):545–62.
18. Smith LH. Enteric hyperoxaluria and other hyperoxaluric states. In: Coe FL, Brenner BM, Stein JH, eds. *Contemporary issues in nephrology,* vol 5. New York: Churchill Livingstone, 1980;136–64.
19. Williams HE. Oxalic acid and the hyperoxaluric syndromes. *Kidney Int* 1978;13:410–7.
20. Larsson L, Tiselius H-G. Hyperoxaluria. *Miner Electrolyte Metab* 1987;13:242–50.
21. Williams HE, Wandzilak TR. Oxalate synthesis, transport and the hyperoxaluric syndromes. *J Urol* 1989;141:742–7.
22. Williams HE, Smith LH Jr. Primary hyperoxaluria. In: Stanbury JB, Wyngaarden JB, Fredrickson DS, eds. *The metabolic basis of inherited disease,* 4th ed. New York: McGraw-Hill, 1978;182–204.
23. Wyngaarden JB, Elder TD. Primary hyperoxaluria and oxalosis. In: Standbury JB, Wyngaarden JB, Fredrickson DS, eds. *The metabolic basis of inherited disease,* 2nd ed. New York: McGraw-Hill, 1966;189–212.
24. Banay M, Dimant E. On the metabolism of L-ascorbic acid in the scorbutic guinea pig. *Biochim Biophys Acta* 1962;59:313–9.
25. Baker EM, Saari JC, Tolbert BM. Ascorbic acid metabolism in man. *Am J Clin Nutr* 1966;19:371–8.
26. Hornig D. Metabolism of ascorbic acid. *World Rev Nutr Diet* 1975;23:225–58.
27. Schmidt KH, Oberritter H, Hagmaier V, Hornig DH, Rutishauser G. Studies on the metabolic conversions of ascorbate with special regard to oxalate urolithiasis. In: Ryall RL, Brockis JG, Marshall VR, Finlayson B, eds. *Urinary stone.* Edinburgh: Churchill Livingstone, 1984:295–9.
28. Conyers RAJ, Bais R, Rofe AM. The relations of clinical catastrophes, endogenous oxalate production, and urolithiasis. *Clin Chem* 1990;36:1717–30.
29. Smith LH, Bauer RL, Williams HE. Oxalate and glycolate synthesis by hemic cells. *J Lab Clin Med* 1971;78:245–54.
30. Gibbs DA, Watts RWE. The identification of the enzymes that catalyze the oxidation of glyoxylate to oxalate in the 100,000 g. supernatant fraction of human hyperoxaluric and control liver and heart tissue. *Clin Sci* 1973;44:227–41.
31. Danpure CJ. Recent advances in the understanding, diagnosis

32. and treatment of primary hyperoxaluria type 1. *J Inherited Metab Dis* 1989;12:210–24.
32. Gibbs DA, Watts RWE. An investigation of the possible role of xanthine oxidase in the oxidation of glyoxylate to oxalate. *Clin Sci* 1966;31:285–97.
33. Liao LL, Richardson KE. The metabolism of oxalate precursors in isolated perfused rat liver. *Arch Biochem Biophys* 1972;153:438–48.
34. Rofe AM, Thomas DW, Edwards RG, Edwards JB. [^{14}C]oxalate synthesis from [U-^{14}C]xylitol: in vivo and in vitro studies. *Biochem Med* 1977;28:440–51.
35. James HM, Bais R, Edwards JB, Rofe AM, Conyers RAJ. Models for the metabolic production of oxalate from xylitol in humans: a role for fructokinase and aldolase. *Aust J Exp Biol Med Sci* 1982;60:117–22.
36. Hauschidt S, Brand K. [^{14}C]oxalate formation from [U-^{14}C]-glucose and [U-^{14}C]xylitol in rat liver homogenate. *Biochem Med* 1979;21:55–61.
37. Dills WL, Barngrover DA, Covey TR. Metabolism of 1-^{3}H-D-xylitol and 5-^{3}H-D-xylitol in isolated rat hepatocytes. *Int J Vitam Nutr Res* 1985;(Suppl 28):59–64.
38. Georgieff M, Moldawer LL, Bistrian BR, Blackburn GL. Xylitol, an energy source for intravenous nutrition after trauma (review). *J Parenter Enter Nutr* 1985;9:199–209.
39. Hamilton GA. Peroxisomal oxidases and suggestions for the mechanism of action of insulin and other hormones. *Adv Enzymol* 1985;57:86–178.
40. Lehninger AL. Mitochondria and calcium ion transport. *Biochem J* 1970;119:129–38.
41. Meyer JL, McCall JT, Smith LH. Inhibition of calcium phosphate crystallization by nucleoside phosphates. *Calcif Tissue Res* 1974;15:287–93.
42. Reid JD, Choi C-H, Oldroyd NO. Calcium oxalate crystals in the thyroid. Their identification, prevalence, origin, and possible significance. *Am J Clin Pathol* 1987;87:443–54.
43. MacMahon HE, Lee HY, Rivelis CF. Birefringent crystals in human thyroid. *Acta Endocrinol* 1968;58:172–6.
44. Cattell WR, Spencer AG, Taylor GW, Watts RWE. The mechanism of the renal excretion of oxalate in the dog. *Clin Sci* 1962;22:43–52.
45. Weinman EJ, Frankfurt SJ, Ince A, et al. Renal tubular transport of organic acids. Studies with oxalate and para-aminohippurate in the rat. *J Clin Invest* 1978;61:801–6.
46. Knight TF, Sansom SC, Senekjian HO, Weinman EJ. Oxalate secretion in the rat proximal tubule. *Am J Physiol* 1981;240:F295–8.
47. Hodgkinson A, Wilkinson R. Plasma oxalate concentration and renal excretion of oxalate in man. *Clin Sci Mol Med* 1974;46:61–73.
48. Osswald H, Hautmann R. Renal elimination kinetics and plasma half-life of oxalate in man. *Urol Int* 1979;440–50.
49. Williams HE, Johnson GA, Smith LH. The renal clearance of oxalate in normal subjects and patients with primary hyperoxaluria. *Clin Sci* 1971;41:213–8.
50. Wilson DM, Smith LH, Erickson SB, Torres VE, Liedtke RR. Renal oxalate handling in normal subjects and patients with idiopathic renal lithiasis: primary and secondary hyperoxaluria. In: Walker VR, Sutton RAL, Cameron ECB, Pak CYC, Robertson WG, eds. *Urolithiasis.* New York: Plenum Press, 1989, 453–5.
51. Schwille PO, Manoharan M, Rümenapf G, Wölfel G, Berens H. Oxalate measurement in the picomol range by ion chromatography: values in fasting plasma and urine of controls and patients with idiopathic calcium urolithiasis. *J Clin Chem Clin Biochem* 1989;27:87–96.
52. Karniski LP, Aronson PS. Anion exchange pathways for Cl-transport in rabbit renal microvillus membranes. *Am J Physiol* 1987;253:F513–21.
53. Kuo S, Aronson PS. Oxalate transport via the sulfate/HCO$_3$ exchanges in rabbit renal basolateral membrane vesicles. *J Biol Chem* 1988;263:9710–7.
54. Freel RW, Hatch M, Earnest DL, Goldner AM. Oxalate transport across the isolated rat colon. A re-examination. *Biochim Biophys Acta* 1980;600:838–43.
55. Hatch M, Freel RW, Goldner AM, Earnest DL. Oxalate and chlo-

ride absorption by the rabbit colon: sensitivity to metabolic and anion transport inhibitors. *Gut* 1984;25:232–7.

56. Knickelbein RG, Aronson PS, Dobbins JW. Oxalate transport by anion exchange across rabbit ileal brush border. *J Clin Invest* 1986;77:170–5.

57. Kathpalia SC, Favus MJ, Coe FL. Evidence for size and charge permselectivity of rat ascending colon. Effects of ricinoleate and bile salts on oxalic acid and neutral sugar transport. *J Clin Invest* 1984;74:805–11.

58. Tomazic B, Nancollas GH. The kinetics of dissolution of calcium oxalate hydrates. *J Crystal Growth* 1979;6:355–61.

59. Heijnen W, Jellinghaus W, Klee WE. Calcium oxalate trihydrate in urinary calculi. *Urol Res* 1985;13:281–3.

60. Robertson WG. A method for measuring calcium crystalluria. *Clin Chim Acta* 1969;26:105–10.

61. Dyer R, Nordin BEC. Urinary crystals and their relation to stone formation. *Nature* 1967;215:751–2.

62. Werness PG, Bergert JH, Smith LH. Crystalluria. *J Crystal Growth* 1981;53:166–81.

63. Martin X, Smith LH, Werness PG. Calcium oxalate dihydrate formation in urine. *Kidney Int* 1984;25:948–52.

64. Smith LH. Application of physical, chemical and metabolic factors to the management of urolithiasis. In: Fleisch H, Robertson WG, Smith LH, Vahlensieck W, eds. *Urolithiasis research.* New York: Plenum Press, 1976;199–211.

65. Robertson WG, Peacock M. The cause of idiopathic calcium stone disease: hypercalciuria or hyperoxaluria? *Nephron* 1980; 26:105–10.

66. Snigh PP, Saxena SN. Effect of maturity on the oxalate and cation contents of six leafy vegetables. *Indian J Nutr Dietetics* 1972;9:269–76.

67. Archer HE, Dormer AE, Scowen EF, Watts RWE. Studies on the urinary excretion of oxalate by normal subjects. *Clin Sci* 1957;16:405–11.

68. Brinkley LJ, Gregory J, Pak CYC. A further study of oxalate bioavailability in foods. *J Urol* 1990;144:94–6.

69. Goldfarb S. Dietary factors in the pathogenesis and prophylaxis of calcium nephrolithiasis. *Kidney Int* 1988;34:544–55.

70. Zarembski ZM, Hodgkinson A. Some factors influencing the urinary excretion of oxalic acid in man. *Clin Chim Acta* 1969;25:1–10.

71. Marshall RW, Cochran M, Hodgkinson A. Relationships between calcium and oxalic acid intake in the diet and their excretion in the urine of normal and renal-stone-forming subjects. *Clin Sci* 1972;43:91–9.

72. Hodgkinson A. Evidence of increased oxalate absorption in patients with calcium-containing renal stones. *Clin Sci* 1978; 54:291–4.

73. Pinto B, Bernshtam J. Diethylaminoethanol-cellulose in the treatment of absorptive hyperoxaluria. *J Urol* 1978;119:630–2.

74. Bannwart C, Hagmaier V, Simonet C, Rutishauser G, Seiler H. Reduction of exogenous oxalate in urine of rats by binding with aluminium-oxyhydrate (Andursil) and an anion-exchanger (Colestid) in the intestinal tract. *Urol Res* 1982;10:209–11.

75. Lindsjö M, Fellström B, Ljunghall S, Wikström B, Danielson BG. Treatment of enteric hyperoxaluria with calcium-containing organic marine hydrocolloid. *Lancet* 1989;2:701–4.

76. Kaplan RA, Haussler MR, Deftos LH, Bone H, Pak CYC. The role of $1\alpha,25$-dihydroxyvitamin D in the mediation of intestinal hyperabsorption of calcium in primary hyperparathyroidism and absorptive hypercalciuria. *J Clin Invest* 1977;59:756–60.

77. Lemann J Jr, Piering WF, Lennon EJ. Possible role of carbohydrate-induced calciuria in calcium oxalate kidney-stone formation. *N Engl J Med* 1969;280:232–7.

78. Brannan PG, Morawski S, Pak CYC, Fordtran JS. Selective jejunal hyperabsorption of calcium in absorptive hypercalciuria. *Am J Med* 1979;66:425–8.

79. Caldas AE, Gray RW, Lemann J Jr. The simultaneous measurement of vitamin D metabolites in plasma: studies in healthy adults and in patients with calcium nephrolithiasis. *J Lab Clin Med* 1978;91:840–9.

80. Coe FL, Favus MJ, Crockett T, et al. Effects of low-calcium diet on urine calcium excretion, parathyroid function and serum $1,25(OH)_2D_3$ levels in patients with idiopathic hypercalciuria and in normal subjects. *Am J Med* 1982;72:25–32.

81. Earnest DL, Johnson G, Williams HE, Admirand WH. Hyperoxaluria in patients with ileal resection: an abnormality in dietary oxalate absorption. *Gastroenterology* 1974;66(6):1114–22.

82. Dobbins JW, Binder HJ. Effect of bile salts and fatty acids on the colonic absorption of oxalate. *Gastroenterology* 1976;70:1096–100.

83. Blacklock NJ, Macleod MA. The effect of cellulose phosphate on intestinal absorption and urinary excretion of calcium. Some experience in its use in the treatment of calcium stone formation. *Br J Urol* 1974;46:385–92.

84. Pak CYC, Delea CS, Bartter FC. Successful treatment of recurrent nephrolithiasis (calcium stones) with cellulose phosphate. *N Engl J Med* 1974;290:175–80.

85. Gershoff SN, Faragalla FF, Nelson DA, Andrus SB. Vitamin B_6 deficiency and oxalate nephrocalcinosis in the cat. *Am J Med* 1959;27:72–80.

86. Faber SR, Feitler WW, Bleiler RE, Ohlson MA, Hodges RE. The effects of an induced pyridoxine and pantothenic acid deficiency on excretions of oxalic and xanthurenic acid in the urine. *Am J Clin Nutr* 1963;12:406–12.

87. Mayer GG, Chase T, Farvar B, et al. Metabolic studies on the formation of calcium oxalate stones with special emphasis on vitamin B_6 and uric acid metabolism. *Bull N Y Acad Med* 1968;44:28–44.

88. Hodgkinson A. Determination of oxalic acid in biological material. *Clin Chem* 1970;16:547–57.

89. Robertson WG, Rutherford A. Aspects of the analysis of oxalate in urine—a review. *Scand J Urol Nephrol* 1980;53:85–95.

90. Wandzilak TR, Williams HE. The hyperoxaluria syndromes. In: Smith LH, ed. *Endocrinology and metabolism clinics of North America.* Philadelphia: WB Saunders, 1990:19:851–67.

91. Chalmers AH, Cowley DM. Urinary oxalate by rate analysis compared with gas chromatographic and centrifugal analyzer methods. *Clin Chem* 1984;30:1891–2.

92. Kasidas GP, Rose GA. Continuous-flow assay for urinary oxalate using immobilised oxalate oxidase. *Ann Clin Biochem* 1985;22:412–9.

93. Parkinson IS, Kealey T, Laker MF. The determination of plasma oxalate concentrations using an enzyme/bioluminescent assay. *Clin Chim Acta* 1985;152:335–45.

94. Kasidas GP, Rose GA. Measurement of plasma oxalate in healthy subjects and in patients with chronic renal failure using immobilised oxalate oxidase. *Clin Chim Acta* 1986;154:49–58.

95. McWhinney BC, Cowley DM, Chalmers AH. Simplified column liquid chromatographic method for measuring urinary oxalate. *J Chromatography* 1986;383:137–41.

96. Classen A, Hesse A. Enzymatic and ion chromatographic measurement of urinary oxalate. *Contrib Nephrol* 1987;58:85–8.

97. Schwille PO, Manoharan M, Rümenapf G, Wölfel G, Berens H. Oxalate measurement in the picomol range by ion chromatography: values in fasting plasma and urine of controls and patients with idiopathic calcium urolithiasis. *J Clin Chem Clin Biochem* 1989;27:87–96.

98. Fituri N, Allawi N, Bentley M, Costello J. Urinary and plasma oxalate during ingestion of pure ascorbic acid: a re-evaluation. *Eur Urol* 1983;9:312–5.

99. Chalmers AH, Cowley DM, McWhinney BC. Stability of ascorbate in urine: relevance to analyses for ascorbate and oxalate. *Clin Chem* 1985;31:1703–5.

100. Wandzilak TR, Hagen LE, Hughes H, Sutton RAL, Smith LH, Williams HE. Quantitation of glycolate in urine by ion-chromatography. *Kidney Int* 1991;39:765–70.

101. Gelzayd EA, Breuer RI, Kirsner JB. Nephrolithiasis in inflammatory bowel disease. *Am J Digest Dis* 1968;13:1027–34.

102. Smith LH, McCall JT, Hofmann AF, Thomas PJ. Secondary hyperoxaluria in patients with ileal resection and oxalate nephrolithiasis. *Clin Res* 1970;18:541.

103. Admirand WH, Earnest DL, Williams HE. Hyperoxaluria and bowel disease. *Trans Assoc Am Physicians* 1971;84:307–12.

104. Dowling RH, Rose GA, Sutor DJ. Hyperoxaluria and renal calculi in ileal disease. *Lancet* 1971;1:1103–6.

105. Smith LH, Fromm H, Hofmann AF. Acquired hyperoxaluria, nephrolithiasis, and intestinal disease: description of a syndrome. *N Engl J Med* 1972;286:1371–5.

106. Stauffer JQ, Humphreys MH, Weir GJ. Acquired hyperoxaluria in patients with regional enteritis after ileal resection: role of dietary oxalate. *Ann Intern Med* 1973;79:383–91.

107. O'Leary JP, Thomas WC Jr, Woodward ER. Urinary tract stone after small bowel bypass for morbid obesity. *Am J Surg* 1974;127(2):142–7.

108. Dickstein SS, Frame B. Urinary tract calculi after intestinal shunt operations for the treatment of obesity. *Surg Gynecol Obstet* 1973;136:257–60.

109. Gregory JG, Starkloff EB, Miyai K, Schoenberg HW. Urologic complications of ileal bypass operation for morbid obesity. *J Urol* 1975;113:521–4.

110. Dobbins JW, Binder HJ. Importance of the colon in enteric hyperoxaluria. *N Engl J Med* 1977;296(6):298–301.

111. Saunders DR, Sillery J, McDonald GB. Regional differences in oxalate absorption by rat intestine: evidence for excessive absorption by the colon in steatorrhoea. *Gut* 1975;16:543–8.

112. Daniel SL, Hartman PA, Allison MJ. Intestinal colonization of laboratory rats with Oxalobacter formigenes. *Appl Environ Microbiol* 1987;53:2767–70.

113. Argenzio RA, Liacos JA, Allison MJ. Intestinal oxalate-degrading bacteria reduce oxalate absorption and toxicity in guinea pigs. *J Nutr* 1988;118:787–92.

114. Hofmann AF, Laker MF, Dharmsathaphorn K, Sherr HP, Lorenzo D. Complex pathogenesis of hyperoxaluria after jejunoileal bypass surgery. Oxalogenic substances in diet contribute to urinary oxalate. *Gastroenterology* 1983;84:293–300.

115. Earnest DL, Johnson G, Williams HE, Admirand WH. Hyperoxaluria in patients with ileal resection: an abnormality in dietary oxalate absorption. *Gastroenterology* 1974;66(6):1114–22.

116. Andersson H, Jagenburg R. Fat-reduced diet in the treatment of hyperoxaluria in patients with ileopathy. *Gut* 1974;15:360–6.

117. McDonald GB, Earnest DL, Admirand WH. Hyperoxaluria correlates with steatorrhea in patients with celiac sprue. *Gastroenterology* 1975;68:A-92/949.

118. Dobbins JW, Binder HJ. Effect of bile salts and fatty acids on the colonic absorption of oxalate. *Gastroenterology* 1976;70:1096–100.

119. Diamond KL, Fox CC, Barch DH. Role of cecal pH in intestinal oxalate absorption in the rat. *J Lab Clin Med* 1988;112:352–6.

120. Smith LH. Pathogenesis of renal stones. *Miner Electrolyte Metab* 1987;13:214–9.

121. Oliver J, MacDowell M, Whang R, Welt LG. The renal lesions of electrolyte imbalance. *J Exp Med* 1966;124:263–77.

122. Wacker WEC, Vallee BL. Magnesium metabolism (concluded). *N Engl J Med* 1958;259:475–82.

123. Elliot JS, Soles WP. Excretion of calcium and citric acid in patients with small bowel disease. *J Urol* 1974;111:810–2.

124. Rudman D, Dedonis JL, Fountain MT, et al. Hypocitraturia in patients with gastrointestinal malabsorption. *N Engl J Med* 1980;303(12):657–61.

125. MacIntyre I, Davidsson D. The production of secondary potassium depletion, sodium retention, nephrocalcinosis and hypercalcaemia by magnesium deficiency. *Biochem J* 1958;70:456–62.

126. Meyer JL, Selinger AH. Effect of citrate on calcium phosphate phase transitions. *Miner Electrolyte Metab* 1980;3:207–16.

127. Fleisch H. Inhibitors and promoters of stone formation. *Kidney Int* 1978;13:361–71.

128. Meyer JL, Smith LH. Growth of calcium oxalate crystals. II. Inhibition by natural urinary crystal growth inhibitors. *Invest Urol* 1975;13:36–9.

129. Fleisch H, Bisaz S, Care AD. Effect of orthophosphate on urinary pyrophosphate excretion and the prevention of urolithiasis. *Lancet* 1964;1:1065–7.

130. Atsmon A, Frank M, Lazebnik J, Kochwa S, de Vries A. Uric acid stones: a study of 58 patients. *J Urol* 1960;84(1):167–76.

131. Gutman AB, Yü TF. Uric acid nephrolithiasis. *Am J Med* 1968;45:756–79.

132. Bennett RC, Jepson RP. Uric acid stone formation following ileostomy. *Aust N Z J Surg* 1966;36(2):153–8.

133. Reisner GS, Wilansky DL, Schneiderman C. Uric acid lithiasis in the ileostomy patient. *Br J Urol* 1973;45:340–3.

134. Coe FL, Raisen L. Allopurinol treatment of uric-acid disorders in calcium-stone formers. *Lancet* 1973;1:129–31.

135. Coe FL, Kavalach AG. Hypercalciuria and hyperuricosuria in patients with calcium nephrolithiasis. *N Engl J Med* 1974;291(25):1344–50.

136. Pak CYC, Waters O, Arnold L, Holt K, Cox C, Barilla D. Mechanism for calcium urolithiasis among patients with hyperuricosuria. *J Clin Invest* 1977;59:426–31.

137. Sarig S. The hyperuricosuric calcium oxalate stone former. *Miner Electrolyte Metab* 1987;13:251–6.

138. Meyer JL, Bergert JH, Smith LH. The epitaxially induced crystal growth of calcium oxalate by crystalline uric acid. *Invest Urol* 1976;14:115–9.

139. Meyer JL. Nucleation kinetics in the calcium oxalate–sodium urate monohydrate system. *Invest Urol* 1981;19:197–201.

140. Ryall RL, Grover PK, Marshall VR. Urate and calcium stones—picking up a drop of mercury with one's fingers? *Am J Kidney Dis* 1991;17:426–30.

141. Werness PG, Brown CM, Smith LH, Finlayson B. EQUIL2: a BASIC computer program for the calculation of urinary saturation. *J Urol* 1985;134:1242–4.

142. Williams HE. Oxalic acid and the hyperoxaluric syndromes. *Kidney Int* 1978;13:410–7.

143. Gregory JG. Hyperoxaluria and stone disease in the gastrointestinal bypass patient. *Urol Clin North Am* 1981;8(2):331–51.

144. Cryer PE, Garber AJ, Hoffsten P, Lucas B, Wise L. Renal failure after small intestinal bypass for obesity. *Arch Intern Med* 1975;135:1610–2.

145. Miller MJ, Frame B, Parfitt AM. Nephrocalcinosis in intestinal bypass patients. *Arch Intern Med* 1977;137:1743–4.

146. Drenick EJ, Stanley TM, Border WA, et al. Renal damage with intestinal bypass. *Ann Intern Med* 1978;89:594–9.

147. Gelbart DR, Brewer LL, Fajardo LF, Weinstein AB. Oxalosis and chronic renal failure after intestinal bypass. *Arch Intern Med* 1977;137:239–43.

148. Lingeman JE, Smith LH, Woods JR, Newman DM. *Urinary calculi: ESWL, endourology, and medical therapy.* Philadelphia: Lea & Febiger, 1989:92–104.

149. Robertson WG, Peacock M, Heyburn PJ, Marshall DH, Clark PB. Risk factors in calcium stone disease of the urinary tract. *Br J Urol* 1978;50:449–54.

150. Pak CYC, Britton F, Peterson R, et al. Ambulatory evaluation of nephrolithiasis. Classification, clinical presentation and diagnostic criteria. *Am J Med* 1980;69:19–30.

151. Coe FL. Treated and untreated recurrent calcium nephrolithiasis in patients with idiopathic hypercalciuria, hyperuricosuria, or no metabolic disorder. *Ann Intern Med* 1977;87:404–10.

152. Smith LH. Idiopathic calcium oxalate urolithiasis. In: Smith LH, ed. *Endocrinology and metabolism clinics of North America.* Philadelphia, WB Saunders, 1990;937–48.

153. Smith LH, Werness PG, Erickson SB, Phillips SF. Postprandial response to a normal diet in patients with idiopathic calcium urolithiasis. In: Ryall RL, Brockis JG, Marshall VR, Finlayson B, eds. *Urinary stone.* New York: Churchill Livingstone, 1984;47–56.

154. Smith LH. Diet and hyperoxaluria in the syndrome of idiopathic calcium oxalate urolithiasis. *Am J Kidney Dis* 1991;17:370–5.

155. Hesse A, Strenge A, Vahlensieck W. Oxalic acid excretion of calcium oxalate stone formers and of healthy persons. In: Ryall R, Brockis JG, Marshall V, Finlayson B, eds. *Urinary stone.* New York: Churchill Livingstone, 1984;57–62.

156. Broadus AE, Insogna KL, Lang R, Ellison AF, Dreyer BE. Evidence for disordered control of 1,25-dihydroxyvitamin D production in absorptive hypercalciuria. *N Engl J Med* 1984;311:73–80.

157. Erickson SB, Cooper K, Broadus AE, et al. Oxalate absorption and postprandial urine supersaturation in an experimental human model of absorptive hypercalciuria. *Clin Sci* 1984;67:131–8.

158. Pak CYC. Physiological basis for absorptive and renal hypercalciurias. *Am J Physiol* 1979;237:F415–23.

159. Coe FL, Canterbury JM, Firpo JJ, Reiss E. Evidence for second-

ary hyperparathyroidism in idiopathic hypercalciuria. *J Clin Invest* 1973;52:134–42.

160. Bataille P, Charransol G, Gregoire I, et al. Effect of calcium restriction on renal excretion of oxalate and the probability of stones in the various pathophysiological groups with calcium stones. *J Urol* 1983;130:218–23.

161. Pak CYC, Kaplan R, Bone H, Townsend J, Waters O. A simple test for the diagnosis of absorptive, resorptive and renal hypercalciurias. *N Engl J Med* 1975;292(10):497–500.

162. Pak CYC. Sodium cellulose phosphate: mechanism of action and effect on mineral metabolism. *J Clin Pharmacol* 1973;13:15–27.

163. Robertson WG, Nisa M, Husain I, et al. The importance of diet in the etiology of primary calcium and uric acid stone formation: the Arabian experience. In: Walker VR, Sutton RAL, Cameron ECB, Pak CYC, Robertson WG, eds. *Urolithiasis.* New York: Plenum Press, 1989;735–9.

164. Robertson WG, Qunibi W, Husain I, et al. The calculation of stone risk in the urine of middle eastern men and western expatriates living in Saudi Arabia. In: Walker VR, Sutton RAL, Cameron ECB, Pak CYC, Robertson WG, eds. *Urolithiasis.* New York: Plenum Press, 1989;669–71.

165. Baggio B, Gambaro G, Marchini F, et al. An inheritable anomaly of red-cell oxalate transport in "primary" calcium nephrolithiasis correctable with diuretics. *N Engl J Med* 1986;314:599–604.

166. Harrison AR, Kasidas GP, Rose GA. Hyperoxaluria and recurrent stone formation apparently cured by short courses of pyridoxine. *Br Med J* 1981;282:2097–8.

167. Yendt ER, Cohanim M. Hyperoxaluria in idiopathic oxalate nephrolithiasis. In: Leklem JE, Reynolds RD, eds. *Clinical and physiological applications of vitamin B-6.* New York: Alan R. Liss, 1988;229–44.

168. Thomas WC Jr. Effectiveness and mode of action of orthophosphates in patients with calcareous renal calculi. *Trans Am Clin Climatol Assoc* 1971;83:113–24.

169. Bernstein DS, Newton R. The effect of oral sodium phosphate on the formation of renal calculi and on idiopathic hypercalciuria. *Lancet* 1966;2:1105–7.

170. Fleisch H, Bisaz S, Care AD. Effect of orthophosphate on urinary pyrophosphate excretion and the prevention of urolithiasis. *Lancet* 1964;1:1065–7.

171. Smith LH, Thomas WC Jr, Arnaud CD. Orthophosphate therapy in calcium renal lithiasis. In: Cifuentes Delatte L, Rapado A, Hodgkinson A, eds. *Urinary calculi: recent advances in aetiology, stone structure and treatment.* Basel: Karger, 1973;188–97.

172. Thomas WC Jr. Use of phosphates in patients with calcareous renal calculi. *Kidney Int* 1978;13:390–6.

173. Sarig S, Garti N, Azoury R, Perlberg S, Wax Y. Follow-up of drug therapy efficacy to prevent recurrence of calcium oxalate kidney stone formation. *J Urol* 1983;129:1258–61.

174. Howard JE, Thomas WC Jr, Mukai T, Johnston RA Jr, Pascoe BJ. The calcification of cartilage by urine, and a suggestion for therapy in patients with certain kinds of calculi. *Trans Assoc Am Physicians* 1962;75:301–5.

175. Pak CYC. Citrate and renal calculi. *Miner Electrolyte Metab* 1987;13:257–66.

176. Melnick I, Landes RR, Hoffman AA, Burch JF. Magnesium therapy for recurring calcium oxalate urinary calculi. *J Urol* 1971;105:119–22.

177. Gershoff SN, Prien EL. Effect of daily MgO and vitamin B$_6$ administration to patients with recurring calcium oxalate kidney stones. *Am J Clin Nutr* 1967;20:393–9.

178. Prien EL Sr, Gershoff SF. Magnesium oxide-pyridoxine therapy for recurrent calcium oxalate calculi. *J Urol* 1974;112:509–12.

179. Johansson G, Backman U, Danielson BG, Fellström B, Ljunghall S, Wikström B. Biochemical and clinical effects of the prophylactic treatment of renal calcium stones with magnesium hydroxide. *J Urol* 1980;124:770–4.

180. Hockaday TDR, Clayton JE, Frederick EW, Smith LH Jr. Primary hyperoxaluria. *Medicine* 1964;43:315–45.

181. Danpure CJ, Jennings PR. Peroxisomal alanine:glyoxylate aminotransferase deficiency in primary hyperoxaluria type I. *FEBS Lett* 1986;201:20–4.

182. Danpure CJ, Jennings PR, Watts RWE. Enzymological diagnosis of primary hyperoxaluria type 1 by measurement of hepatic alanine:glyoxylate aminotransferase activity. *Lancet* 1987;1:289–91.

183. Danpure CJ, Jennings PR. Further studies on the activity and subcellular distribution of alanine:glyoxylate aminotransferase in the livers of patients with primary hyperoxaluria type 1. *Clin Sci* 1988;75:315–22.

184. Cooper PJ, Danpure CJ, Wise PJ, Guttridge KM. Immunocytochemical localization of human hepatic alanine:glyoxylate aminotransferase in control subjects and patients with primary hyperoxaluria type 1. *J Histochem Cytochem* 1988;36:1285–94.

185. Danpure CJ, Jennings PR. Enzymatic heterogeneity in primary hyperoxaluria type 1 (hepatic peroxisomal alanine: glyoxylate aminotransferase deficiency). *J Inherited Metab Dis* 1988;11:205–7.

186. Danpure CJ, Cooper PJ, Wise PJ, Jennings PR. An enzyme trafficking defect in two patients with primary hyperoxaluria type I:peroxisomal alanine/glyoxylate aminotransferase rerouted to mitochondria. *J Cell Biol* 1989;108:1345–52.

187. Purdue PE, Takada Y, Danpure CJ. Identification of mutations associated with peroxisome-to-mitochondrion mistargeting of alanine/glyoxylate aminotransferase in primary hyperoxaluria type 1. *J Cell Biol* 1990;111:2341–51.

188. Danpure CJ. Molecular and clinical heterogeneity in primary hyperoxaluria type 1. *Am J Kidney Dis* 1991;17:366–9.

189. Williams HE, Smith LH Jr. L-Glyceric aciduria. A new genetic variant of primary hyperoxaluria. *N Engl J Med* 1968;278:233–9.

190. Mistry J, Danpure CJ, Chalmers RA. Hepatic D-glycerate dehydrogenase and glyoxylate reductase deficiency in primary hyperoxaluria type 2. *Biochem Soc Trans* 1988;16:626–7.

191. Gibbs DA, Watts RWE. The action of pyridoxine in primary hyperoxaluria. *Clin Sci* 1970;38:277–86.

192. Smith LH Jr, Williams HE. Treatment of primary hyperoxaluria. *Mod Treat* 1967;4:522–30.

193. Alinei P, Guignard J-P, Jaeger P. Pyridoxine treatment of type I hyperoxaluria. *N Engl J Med* 1984;311:798–9.

194. Yendt ER, Cohanim M. Response to a physiologic dose of pyridoxine in type I primary hyperoxaluria. *N Engl J Med* 1985;312:953–7.

195. Watts RWE, Veall N, Purkiss P, Mansell MA, Haywood EF. The effect of pyridoxine on oxalate dynamics in three cases of primary hyperoxaluria (with glycolic aciduria). *Clin Sci* 1985;69:87–90.

196. Silver L, Brendler H. Use of magnesium oxide in management of familial hyperoxaluria. *J Urol* 1971;106:274–9.

197. Dent CE, Stamp TCB. Treatment of primary hyperoxaluria. *Arch Dis Child* 1970;45:735–45.

198. Watts RWE, Chalmers RA, Gibbs DA, Lawson AM, Purkiss P, Spellacy E. Studies on some possible biochemical treatments of primary hyperoxaluria. *Q J Med* 1979;48:259–72.

199. Frederick EW, Rabkin MT, Richie RH Jr, Smith LH Jr. Studies on primary hyperoxaluria. I. In vivo demonstration of a defect in glyoxylate metabolism. *N Engl J Med* 1963;269(16):821–9.

200. Smith LH. Hyperoxaluria. In: Walker VR, Sutton RAL, Cameron ECB, Pak CYC, Robertson WG, eds. *Urolithiasis.* New York: Plenum Press, 1989;405–9.

201. Watts RWE, Veall N, Purkiss P. Oxalate dynamics and removal rates during haemodialysis and peritoneal dialysis in patients with primary hyperoxaluria and severe renal failure. *Clin Sci* 1984;66:591–7.

202. Ramsay AG, Reed RG. Oxalate removal by hemodialysis in end-stage renal disease. *Am J Kidney Dis* 1984;4:123–7.

203. Morgan SH, Purkiss P, Watts RWE, Mansell MA. Oxalate dynamics in chronic renal failure. Comparison with normal subjects and patients with primary hyperoxaluria. *Nephron* 1987;46:253–7.

204. Whelchel JD, Alison DV, Luke RG, Curtis J, Diethelm AG. Successful renal transplantation in hyperoxaluria. A report of two cases. *Transplantation* 1983;35:161–4.

205. Binswanger U, Keusch G, Frei D, Bammatter F, Müller U, Largiadèr F. Kidney transplantation in primary hyperoxaluria of adult patients. *Transplant Proc* 1986;18:14–5.

206. McCarthy JT, Perkins JD, Wilson DM, Wiesner RH, Smith LH. Management of renal failure in patients with type 1 primary hy-

peroxaluria. In: Vahlensieck W, Gasser G, Hesse A, Schoeneich G, eds. *Urolithiasis.* The Netherlands: Excerpta Medica, 1990; 164–6.

207. Watts RWE, Calne RY, Williams R, et al. Primary hyperoxaluria (type I): attempted treatment by combined hepatic and renal transplantation. *Q J Med* 1985;57:697–703.

208. Watts RWE, Rolles K, Morgan SH, et al. Successful treatment of primary hyperoxaluria type 1 by combined hepatic and renal transplantation. *Lancet* 1987;2:474–5.

209. Smith LH, Perkins J, Wilson D, McCarthy J, Wiesner R. Biochemical correction of type I primary hyperoxaluria with combined liver-kidney transplant. *Kidney Int* 1988;33(1):209.

210. Morgan SH, Watts RWE, Calne RY, et al. Primary hyperoxaluria type 1—combined hepatic and renal transplantation in 4 patients —a rational approach to management. *Eur J Clin Invest* 1988;18:A28.

211. McDonald JC, Landreneau MD, Rohr MS, DeVault GA Jr. Reversal by liver transplantation of the complications of primary hyperoxaluria as well as the metabolic defect. *N Engl J Med* 1989;321:1100–3.

212. Watts RWE, Morgan SH, Danpure CJ, et al. Combined hepatic and renal transplantation in primary hyperoxaluria type 1: clinical report of nine cases. *Am J Med* 1991;90:179–88.

Disorders of Bone and Mineral Metabolism,
edited by Fredric L. Coe and Murray J. Favus,
© 1992 by Raven Press, Ltd. All rights reserved.

CHAPTER 34

Calcium Nephrolithiasis and Renal Tubular Acidosis

Vardaman M. Buckalew, Jr.

Renal tubular acidosis (RTA) is a syndrome in which metabolic acidosis results from a specific defect or defects in renal tubular function. The earliest reported cases had nephrocalcinosis and/or nephrolithiasis, an important association that has been amply confirmed by the literature, as research on RTA has expanded (1). It can be argued that nephrolithiasis represents the most important complication of the most common type of RTA in adults (1,2). Although RTA is not a common cause of kidney stones, the unique relationship between the disorders of renal tubular function and the pathophysiology of stone formation in RTA justify a separate discussion.

RENAL ACID EXCRETION AND THE PATHOPHYSIOLOGY OF RENAL TUBULAR ACIDOSIS

Renal acid excretion can be conveniently divided into two processes according to physiologic function. The reabsorption of filtered bicarbonate, which takes place primarily in the proximal tubule, preserves acid-base balance by preventing the excretion of bicarbonate from the plasma stores. Generation of new bicarbonate, which occurs in both the proximal and distal tubules, is needed to buffer fixed acid produced from the metabolism of dietary protein and carbohydrate.

Bicarbonate Reabsorption

Approximately 2500 mEq of bicarbonate is filtered per day, about 85% of which is reabsorbed in the proxi-

mal tubule and the remainder in the early distal tubule (3). Hydrogen-ion secretion by the luminal membrane of the tubular epithelium converts the filtered bicarbonate to CO_2 and water, both of which are readily reabsorbed. The secretion of hydrogen ions derived from carbonic acid results in the production of bicarbonate ions which are transported across the basolateral membrane into the blood. The net result is that filtered bicarbonate is reabsorbed, although the bicarbonate ions that are filtered are not those that are reabsorbed.

The set point (or "renal threshhold") for bicarbonate reabsorption is normally about 25 mEq/L of glomerular filtrate (3,4). This means that the renal tubules reabsorb sufficient filtered bicarbonate to maintain the bicarbonate concentration in the filtrate (or by implication, in plasma) at approximately 25 mEq/L. The operation of this system can be illustrated by the following example. Suppose that a person weighing 70 kg with a normal plasma bicarbonate concentration of 25 mEq/L is given a 100-mEq bolus of sodium bicarbonate intravenously. This would cause a rapid rise in the plasma bicarbonate (and in the glomerular filtrate) concentration to approximately 32 mEq/L (100 mEq distributed in 20% of the body weight). However, the renal tubules would reabsorb only that amount of bicarbonate necessary to maintain a filtrate concentration of 25 mEq/L. Thus the 100-mEq bolus of bicarbonate would be rapidly excreted, returning the plasma bicarbonate to baseline.

It should be appreciated that this system does not operate in the reverse direction. That is, reduction in the plasma bicarbonate concentration below 25 mEq/L by the ingestion of acid (e.g., ammonium chloride) cannot be compensated by a change in bicarbonate reabsorption. It can only be corrected by production of new bicarbonate, a process to be described below.

It should also be pointed out that the set point for

V. M. Buckalew, Jr.: Department of Medicine, Bowman Gray School of Medicine, Wake Forest University, Winston-Salem, North Carolina 27103

bicarbonate reabsorption is not fixed. It is inversely proportional to plasma volume and directly proportional to plasma PCO_2 (4). For example, plasma volume contraction such as occurs in many metabolic alkaloses increases the set point and maintains the elevated plasma bicarbonate (4). Similarly, the increased set point accompanying respiratory acidosis is an essential feature of the renal compensation for that acid-base disturbance (4).

Fixed Acid Production

Biochemical reactions that generate energy from food may produce or consume hydrogen ions. Western cultures prefer a diet that generates more hydrogen ions than are actually consumed and has therefore an *acid ash*. The generation of so-called *fixed acid* (as distinguished from CO_2, which is *volatile acid*) is usually discussed in terms of a paradigm that employs the concept of cation–anion balance and electroneutrality (5,6). According to one version of this scheme, reactions in which anions are produced from neutral compounds, or neutral compounds are produced from cations, will generate hydrogen ions in order to maintain electroneutrality (5). Conversely, hydrogen ions are consumed (bicarbonate is generated) to preserve electroneutrality when anions are converted to neutral compounds or neutral compounds

are converted to cations (5). We refer to hydrogen ions and bicarbonate generated by these reactions as *excess* because they are generated in the presence of normal oxidation/reduction potentials and a steady state of energy balance and cause acidosis or alkalosis if not buffered or excreted by normal processes described below. The term *excess* is used, therefore, in much the same sense as Huckabee used it in referring to "excess lactic acid" (7).

Biochemical Reactions

The electroneutrality paradigm, which emphasizes net effects of metabolic pathways, provides no insight into the actual biochemical reactions that produce excess hydrogen ions and excess bicarbonate. The most important of these reactions are summarized in Table 1. The most fundamental reaction that generates hydrogen ions is ATP hydrolysis. ATP may be hydrolyzed to ADP and 1 hydrogen ion or to AMP and 2 hydrogen ions. ATP can be regenerated directly from ADP by oxidative phosphorylation in a reaction consuming 1 hydrogen ion. The reaction in which ATP is hydrolyzed directly to AMP is essentially irreversible because two high-energy phosphate bonds are destroyed (8). However, since 1 AMP and 1 ATP can be converted to 2 ADP in a reaction catalyzed by adenylate kinase (8), ATP can essen-

TABLE 1. *Major reactions generating excess hydrogen ion and bicarbonate[a]*

A. Excess Hydrogen Ions
1. Hydrolysis of ATP
   $ATP^{4-} + H_2O \rightleftharpoons ADP^{3-} + Pi^{2-} + H^+$
   $ATP^{4-} + H_2O \rightarrow AMP^{2-} + 2Pi^{2-} + 2H^+$
2. Formation of carbamoyl phosphate
   $CO_2 + NH_4^+ + 2ATP^{4-} + H_2O \rightarrow$ carbamoyl phosphate$^{2-} + 2ADP^{3-} + Pi^{2-} + 3H^+$
3. Conversion of ornithine to citrulline
   ornithine$^+$ + carbamoyl phosphate$^{2-} \rightarrow$ citrulline + $Pi^{2-} + H^+$
4. Ornithine oxidation
   ornithine$^+ + O_2 \rightarrow$ glutamate$^-$ + urea + $NH_4^+ + H^+$
5. Hydrolysis of urocanate
   urocanate + THF^{2-} + $2H_2O$ + $H^+ \rightarrow$ formimino-THF^{2-} + glutamate$^-$ + $2H^+$
6. Oxidation of homogentisate
   homogentisate$^-$ + $O_2 \rightarrow$ 4-maleylacetoacetate^{2-} + H^+
7. Hydrolysis of 4-fumarylacetoacetate
   4-fumarylacetoacetate^{2-} + $H_2O \rightarrow$ fumarate^{2-} + acetoacetate$^-$ + H^+
8. Carboxylation of propionyl-CoA
   propionyl CoA + HCO$_3^-$ + $ATP^{4-} \rightarrow$ methylmalonyl CoA$^-$ + AMP^{2-} + $2Pi^{2-}$ + $2H^+$
9. Carboxylation of pyruvate
   pyruvate$^-$ + CO_2 + ATP^{4-} + $H_2O \rightarrow$ oxaloacetate^{2-} + ADP^{3-} + Pi^{2-} + $2H^+$
10. Renal excretion of organic anion

B. Excess Bicarbonate
1. Oxidation of NADH
   $NADH + H^+ + \frac{1}{2}O_2 \rightleftharpoons NAD^+ + H_2O$
2. Regeneration of ATP
   $ADP^{3-} + Pi^{2-} + H^+ \rightleftharpoons ATP^{4-} + H_2O$
   $AMP^{2-} + 2Pi^{2-} + 2H^+ \rightarrow ATP^{4-} + 2H_2O$[b]

Source: Adapted from Ref. 8.
[a] Pi, orthophosphate; THF, tetrahydrofolate.
[b] This reaction as written here is the net of two reactions (see the text).

tially be regenerated from AMP in a two-step process consuming 2 hydrogen ions (Table 1). In a steady state of energy metabolism, the ATP/ADP ratio would be kept constant by the regeneration of ATP from ADP or AMP. Therefore, the hydrolysis of ATP under most circumstances generates no excess hydrogen ion and has no effect on acid-base balance in the steady state. Also, hydrogen ions consumed in regenerating ATP from ADP or AMP are, in most cases, hydrogen ions that have been generated by the hydrolysis of ATP. Therefore, the conversion of ADP or AMP to ATP will usually not produce excess bicarbonate. The exceptions to this general rule are of interest and will be discussed subsequently.

The formation of carbamoyl phosphate from CO_2 and ammonium (NH_4^+), 2 ATP, and H_2O generates 3 H^+ (8), two of which would be utilized in regenerating 2 ATP. Therefore, the reaction generates a net of 1 excess H^+. Another reaction that generates 1 excess H^+ is the conversion of ornithine to citrulline (8). This reaction does not involve ATP hydrolysis. The carboxylation of propionyl CoA to methylmalonyl CoA utilizes bicarbonate instead of CO_2 (8) and therefore generates 1 excess hydrogen ion. (The 2 hydrogen ions generated by the hydrolysis of ATP to AMP would be consumed in regenerating the ATP.) The conversion of two amino acids, ornithine and urocanate, to glutamate results in the production of 1 excess hydrogen ion (8). The conversion of homogentisate to 4-maleylacetoacetate produces 1 hydrogen ion, as does the conversion of 4-fumarylacetoacetate to fumarate and acetoacetate (8). Finally, carboxylation of pyruvate to oxaloacetate yields a net of 1 excess hydrogen ion because the other hydrogen ion generated by the reaction is consumed by regeneration of 1 ATP from ADP (8).

The other process listed in Table 1 that results in excess hydrogen ion production is the excretion of organic anion in the urine. Most organic anions, such as citrate, lactate, and pyruvate, are metabolized by the citric acid cycle, a series of reactions that result in consumption of hydrogen ion (see below). Therefore, the excretion of these organic anions is the same as though base were excreted (9).

The two most important reactions that consume hydrogen ion are the oxidation of the electron carrier NADH to NAD^+ and the conversion of ADP and AMP to ATP (Table 1). These two reactions are coupled in the process of oxidative phosphorylation. The oxidation of 1 NADH yields about 3 ATP; the number of molecules of orthophosphate Pi incorporated into ADP per atom of oxygen consumed (the P:O ratio) is, therefore, 3 (8). Thus oxidation of one NADH yields 3 ATP and 4 bicarbonate. As noted above, the hydrogen ion consumed (bicarbonate generated) in converting ADP to ATP and NADH to NAD^+ is for the most part hydrogen ion, which has been generated by ATP hydrolysis and reduction of NAD^+ and produces no net effect on acid-base

TABLE 2. *Biochemical "sites" of excess hydrogen ion and bicarbonate generation*

Reaction	Site
Excess Hydrogen Ions	
1. Hydrolysis of ATP to ADP	Glycolysis
2. Formation of carbamoyl phosphate	Urea cycle
3. Conversion of ornithine to citrulline	Urea cycle
4. Ornithine oxidation	Degradation of arginine, proline
5. Hydrolysis of urocanate	Histidine degradation
6. Oxidation of homogentisate	Degradation of phenylalanine, tyrosine
7. Oxidation of 4-fumarylacetoacetate	Degradation of phenylalanine, tyrosine
8. Carboxylation of propionyl-CoA	Oxidation of methionine, isoleucine; fatty acid oxidation (odd-numbered)
9. Carboxylation of pyruvate	Gluconeogenesis
Excess Bicarbonate	
1. Oxidation of NADH	Oxidative phosphorylation
2. Conversion of ADP and AMP to ATP	Oxidative phosphorylation

balance. The biochemical "sites" of the reactions that produce excess hydrogen and bicarbonate ions are shown in Table 2 and include glycolysis, the urea cycle, the degradation of amino acids and fatty acids, gluconeogenesis, and oxidative phosphorylation.

Glycolysis

Glucose is converted to 2 pyruvate in a reaction that consumes 2 Pi, 2 ADP, and 2 NAD^+, yielding 2 ATP, 2 NADH, 2 H_2O, and 2 H^+ in addition to the 2 pyruvate (8). Regeneration of the 2 NAD^+ utilized from the 2 NADH will consume the 2 hydrogen ions. Hydrolysis of the 2 ATP generated by glycolysis to ADP produces 2 excess hydrogen ions. The net effect, therefore, of converting glucose to 2 pyruvate would be the generation of 2 excess hydrogen ions, assuming constancy of the NAD^+/NADH and ATP/ADP ratios. This stoichiometry is consistent with electroneutrality wherein one neutral molecule (glucose) is converted to two anions (2 pyruvate).

Citric Acid Cycle

The net reaction of the citric acid cycle is as follows: 1 acetyl-CoA, 3 NAD^+, 1 FAD, 1 GDP, 1 Pi, and 2 H_2O are converted to 1 CoA, 3 NADH, 1 $FADH_2$, 1 GTP, 2

H^+, and 2 CO_2 (8). Regeneration of 3 NAD^+ from NADH consumes 3 hydrogen ions, one more than is produced by the cycle. (The regeneration of 3 NAD^+ from NADH would also convert 9 ADP to ATP, generating 9 bicarbonate. However, as already noted, the hydrogen ion consumed by ATP generation replaces ATP consumed and hydrogen ion generated in other biochemical pathways.)

Although the generation of GTP from GDP by the citric acid cycle does not utilize a hydrogen ion, reconversion of GTP to GDP occurs by a reaction between GTP and ADP, catalyzed by nucleoside diphosphokinase, which generates 1 ATP (8). Hydrolysis of the ATP produced in this reaction to ADP would be required to maintain the ATP/ADP ratio constant, generating a hydrogen ion. Therefore, the net effect of one turn of the citric acid cycle beginning with acetyl-CoA is zero, assuming constancy of the NAD^+/NADH, ATP/ADP, and GTP/GDP ratios. This stoichiometry is consistent with electroneutrality, wherein acetyl-CoA is converted to CoA and a neutral compound (CO_2).

Finally, the fact that one turn of the citric acid cycle will utilize 1 acetyl-CoA must be considered. If the acetyl-CoA/CoA ratio is held constant by the conversion of pyruvate to acetyl-CoA, 1 additional NAD^+ will be utilized, regeneration of which generates 1 excess bicarbonate. As a result, the net effect of one turn of the citric acid cycle beginning with pyruvate is the generation of 1 excess bicarbonate. This stoichiometry is consistent with electroneutrality wherein one anion (pyruvate) is converted to a neutral compound (CO_2).

Gluconeogenesis

The net reaction for gluconeogenesis beginning with pyruvate is as follows: 2 pyruvate, 4 ATP, 2 GTP, 2 NADH, and 6 H_2O are converted to 1 glucose, 4 ADP, 2 GDP, 6 Pi, 2 NAD^+, and 2 H^+ (8). Regeneration of the 2 NADH from NAD^+ generates 2 additional hydrogen ions, while regeneration of 4 ATP and 2 GTP consumes 6 hydrogen ions. Thus the net effect of converting 2 pyruvate to 1 glucose is the production of 2 excess bicarbonate. This stoichiometry is consistent with the conversion of two anions (2 pyruvate) to a neutral compound (glucose).

Gluconeogenesis from oxaloacetate yields a different result. The net reaction is as follows: 2 oxaloacetate, 2 ATP, 2 GTP, 2 NADH, 2 H^+, and 4 H_2O are converted to 1 glucose, 2 ADP, 2 GDP, 4 Pi, and 2 NAD^+ (8). Regeneration of 2 ATP and 2 GTP generates 4 excess bicarbonate. Regeneration of 2 NADH from 2 NAD^+ would replace the 2 H^+ utilized. Therefore, the net reaction generates 4 excess bicarbonate. This stoichiometry is consistent with the conversion of four anions (2 oxaloacetate) to a neutral compound (glucose). Therefore, metabolism of 1 oxaloacetate via gluconeogenesis gener-

ates 2 bicarbonate. Oxaloacetate could also be metabolized by the citric acid cycle, in which case only one excess bicarbonate would be generated. This difference in stoichiometry is important in considering the role of ammonia excretion by the kidney in maintaining acid-base balance, as will be discussed subsequently.

Urea Cycle

The net reaction of the urea cycle is as follows: 1 CO_2, 1 NH_4^+, 3 ATP, 3 H_2O, and 1 aspartate are converted to 1 urea, 2 ADP, 2 Pi, 1 AMP, 1 fumarate, and 6 hydrogen ions (8). Three hydrogen ions are produced by the formation of carbamoyl phosphate from NH_4^+, CO_2, and 2 ATP (Table 1). One hydrogen ion is produced by the conversion of ornithine to citrulline (Table 1), and two others are produced by hydrolysis of 1 ATP to AMP in the reaction converting citrulline and aspartate to argininosuccinate. Two of the 6 hydrogen ions generated by the net reaction would be consumed in regenerating 2 ATP from 2 ADP, and 2 would be consumed by regenerating 1 ATP from 1 AMP. Thus one turn of the urea cycle would produce a net of 2 excess hydrogen ions. This stoichiometry is consistent with electroneutrality wherein one cation (NH_4^+) is converted to a neutral compound (urea) and one anion (aspartate) is converted to two anions (fumarate), and with the net reaction, as is sometimes written, in which 2 bicarbonate are consumed (6).

There is one further consideration that influences the net effect of the urea cycle on acid-base balance. If the fumarate generated by the urea cycle enters the citric acid cycle, 1 additional excess bicarbonate would be generated. In that case, one turn of the urea cycle generates a net of 1 excess hydrogen ion. However, if fumarate is diverted to gluconeogenesis by way of oxaloacetate, 2 bicarbonate will be generated and one turn of the urea cycle will have no effect on acid-base balance.

Fatty Acid Oxidation

Fatty acids are oxidized by a stepwise removal of 2 carbons per reaction cycle, the first step of which is the coversion of the fatty acid, 1 CoA, 1 ATP, and 1 H_2O to 1 acyl-CoA, 1 AMP, 2 Pi, and 2 H^+ (8). The acyl-CoA is shortened by two carbons in a reaction that utilizes 1 FAD, 1 NAD^+, 1 CoA, and 1 H_2O, yielding 1 shortened acyl-CoA, 1 acetyl-CoA, 1 $FADH_2$, 1 NADH, and 1 H^+ (8). The net reaction of one cycle, therefore, generates 3 hydrogen ions, 2 of which are utilized in regenerating 1 ATP from AMP and 1 in regenerating NAD^+ from NADH. Utilization of the acetyl-CoA generated by each reaction cycle by the citric acid cycle would not generate or consume hydrogen ion. Therefore, the net effect of fatty acid oxidation on acid-base balance is zero.

Metabolism of Foodstuffs

Having outlined these fundamental reactions, we are now in a position to examine the effect of metabolism of the basic foodstuffs glucose, protein, and fatty acid on acid-base balance.

Glucose

Dietary glucose is metabolized first to pyruvate by glycolysis and then to CO_2 by the citric acid cycle. As noted above, the conversion of 1 glucose to 2 pyruvate generates 2 excess hydrogen ions, and the conversion of 2 pyruvate to CO_2 by two turns of the citric acid cycle generates 2 excess bicarbonate. Thus the metabolism of 1 glucose to 6 CO_2 by glycolysis and the citric acid cycle has no net effect on acid-base balance. This stoichiometry is compatible with the conversion of a neutral compound (glucose) to a neutral compound (CO_2).

Amino Acids

The pathways by which amino acids are oxidized vary with the individual amino acids. The common denominator is the removal of amino groups that enter the urea cycle as NH_4^+ and the formation of carbon skeletons that can enter the citric acid cycle or the pathway for gluconeogenesis. Thus the effect of amino acid oxidation on acid-base balance is determined in part by the relationship between the acidifying effect of the urea cycle and the alkalinizing effect of the citric acid cycle and the pathway for gluconeogenesis. As noted, one turn of the urea cycle generates zero or 1 excess hydrogen ion, one turn of the citric acid cycle generates 1 excess bicarbonate, and gluconeogenesis generates 1 or 2 bicarbonate (-1 or -2 hydrogen ions), depending on the precursor (1 pyruvate or 1 oxaloacetate).

Five amino acids (glycine, alanine, serine, cysteine, and threonine) are converted to pyruvate and NH_4^+ by reactions that do not generate excess hydrogen ions or bicarbonate (8). If pyruvate formed by this pathway is metabolized by the citric acid cycle and NH_4^+ by the urea cycle, there would be no effect on acid-base balance or the generation of 1 excess bicarbonate (zero to 1 hydrogen ion generated by the urea cycle minus 1 from the citric acid cycle). Leucine and isoleucine are converted to NH_4^+ and acetyl-CoA (8), causing the same net effect on acid-base balance as those amino acids converted to pyruvate.

Degradation of amino acids such as arginine, histidine, and proline involve several intermediate steps that generate 1 NH_4^+, 1 glutamate, and 1 excess hydrogen ion (8). The pathway by which arginine (and proline) is converted to glutamate involves the oxidation of ornithine, a reaction that produces 1 excess hydrogen ion (Table 1). The conversion of histidine to glutamate involves a reaction between urocanate and tetrahydrofolate (THF) which also produces 1 excess hydrogen ion (Table 1). The final common pathway in the degradation of these amino acids is the deamination of glutamate to form α-ketoglutarate (8). Thus degradation of these amino acids produces 1 hydrogen ion, 2 NH_4^+, and 1 α-ketoglutarate. If α-ketoglutarate enters the citric acid cycle, the degradation of these amino acids would generate zero to 2 excess hydrogen ions (1 from reactions generating glutamate, zero to 2 from two turns of the urea cycle, minus 1 from the citric acid cycle). Alternatively, if the α-ketoglutarate were diverted to gluconeogenesis, degradation of these amino acids would generate +1 to -1 excess hydrogen ions. Glutamine is another amino acid that donates two NH_4^+ groups to the urea cycle (Fig. 1). Most glutamine is formed in the liver from glutamate and is transferred to the kidney, where it plays a special role in regulating acid-base balance, as will be discussed subsequently.

Intermediate steps in the degradation of phenylalanine, tyrosine, methionine, and isoleucine also involve reactions that produce excess hydrogen ions (8) (Tables 1 and 2). The first step in the degradation of phenylalanine is its conversion to tyrosine in a reaction that consumes 1 NADH and 1 hydrogen ion. Assuming a constant $NAD^+/NADH$ ratio, this step has no effect on acid-base balance. Tyrosine is metabolized to fumarate, acetoacetate, NH_4^+, and CO_2 by a series of four reactions, two of which produce excess hydrogen ions (Tables 1 and 2). The net effect of phenylalanine and tyrosine degradation is, therefore, the generation of zero to 2 excess hydrogen ions (zero to 1 from the urea cycle, 2 from the intermediate reactions, minus 1 to 2 from the metabolism of fumarate).

Methionine and isoleucine deamination occurs by a reaction resulting in the formation of propionyl-CoA (8). The latter is converted to succinyl-CoA in a reaction that utilizes 1 bicarbonate ion and involves the hydrolysis of 1 ATP molecule to AMP and 2 hydrogen ions (8) (Table 1). ATP regeneration from AMP consumes the 2 hydrogen ions; the net reaction, therefore, generates 1 excess hydrogen ion. The entry of NH_4^+ in the urea cycle generates zero to 1 additional excess hydrogen ion, whereas succinyl-CoA metabolism by the citric acid cycle generates 1 excess bicarbonate. The net effect of methionine and isoleucine degradation by this pathway, therefore, is the production of zero to 1 excess hydrogen ion. If succinyl-CoA were metabolized to glucose by way of oxaloacetate, 2 excess bicarbonate would be generated and the net effect of methionine and isoleucine degradation would be zero to 1 excess bicarbonate.

Fatty Acids

The oxidation of fatty acids contributes no excess hydrogen ions or bicarbonate as discussed above.

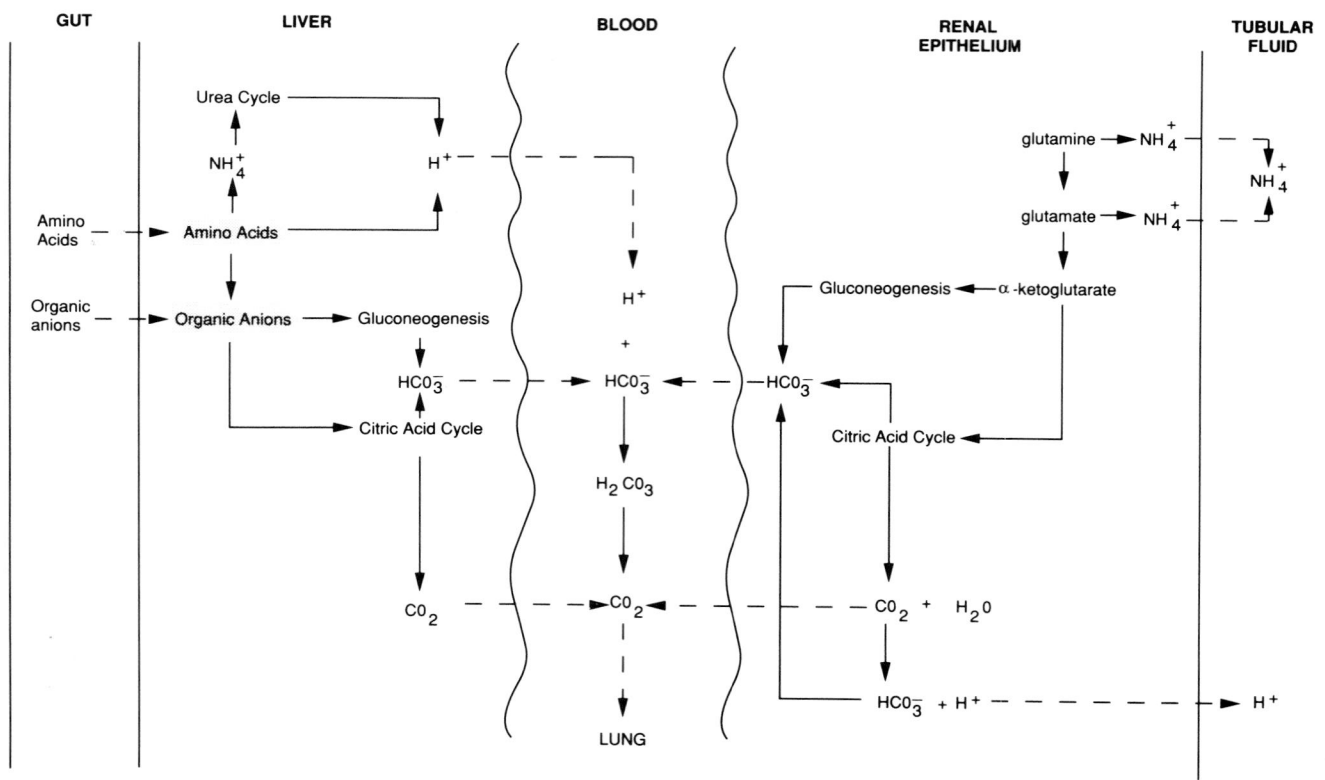

FIG. 1. Role of liver, kidney, and lungs in regulating acid-base balance. Degradation of dietary amino acids generates an excess of hydrogen ions which convert blood bicarbonate to CO_2 and the latter is exhaled by the lungs. "New bicarbonate" needed to maintain balance is generated by oxidative phosphorylation linked to the citric acid cycle and gluconeogenesis in liver and kidney, and by renal hydrogen-ion secretion. The kidney, in addition, excretes a potential source of hydrogen ions (NH_4^+). Arrows with solid lines indicate biochemical pathways, those with dashed lines indicate direction of net transport of indicated chemical species across biological membranes. See the text for a full discussion of the figure.

Organic Anions

The diet of Western societies contains a small amount of organic anion, which represents absorbable alkali (10). The actual amount of alkali absorbed from the diet can be estimated by subtracting the anion gap of food from that of feces (all the "noncombustible" ions must be measured, including calcium, magnesium, and phosphorus) (10). Presumably, these organic anions absorbed from the diet are metabolized to CO_2 by the citric acid cycle, generating one bicarbonate for each organic anion that enters the cycle.

Summary

The foodstuffs that affect acid-base balance are amino acids and organic anions. Metabolism of some of the former generates hydrogen ions, while metabolism of the latter generates bicarbonate. The diet of Western civilizations generates a net excess of hydrogen ions because the amount of hydrogen ion forming amino acids in the diet as protein exceeds the amount of bicarbonate forming amino acids and organic anions. The net excess hydrogen ion production from the diet is approximately 1 mEq/kg body weight per day (5).

Renal Regulation of Acid-Base Balance

Metabolism of Fixed Acid

Excess hydrogen ions generated from metabolism of foodstuffs are termed *fixed acid* to distinguish them from the *volatile acid* generated by CO_2 production. The quantity of volatile acid present in body fluids is, of course, regulated within tightly controlled limits by alveolar ventilation. The quantity of fixed acid present in body fluids during steady-state conditions is reflected by the plasma bicarbonate concentration, as illustrated in Fig. 1. Excess hydrogen ions generated from amino acid degradation and from the urea cycle do, in fact, represent strong acids that require buffering. Hydrogen ions from this source are, therefore, buffered by bicarbonate in a reaction that is irreversible because the resulting CO_2 is excreted by the lungs. (The reader should realize that plasma contains buffers other than bicarbonate which participate in the buffering of strong acid. The process described is the net effect.) The bicarbonate thus consumed is replaced by the generation of "new bicarbonate" from the metabolism of organic anions by the citric acid cycle and gluconeogenesis in both the kidney and liver. In the kidney, the major organic anion from which new bicarbonate is generated is α-ketoglutarate. In the liver, new bicarbonate is generated from organic anions derived from the diet and from amino acid degradation. The generation of new bicarbonate by the kidney is dependent on NH_4^+ and hydrogen ion excretion in the urine.

Renal Hydrogen Ion and Ammonia Excretion

It has been clearly understood for many years that the generation of new bicarbonate by the kidney depends on the secretion of hydrogen ions from distal tubular cells to tubular lumen and the generation of ammonia by tubular cells (11). Lately, however, the understanding of the mechanism by which these tubular processes are related to bicarbonate generation has undergone some revision (12). The old scheme can be summarized as follows: New bicarbonate is generated when hydrogen ions produced from carbonic acid in tubular cells are secreted into the tubular lumen and excreted in the urine, leaving an equal amount of new bicarbonate ions for transport to the blood. Secreted hydrogen ion is buffered by and is, therefore, dependent on the tubular fluid concentration of monohydrogen phosphate, creatinine, and ammonia (NH_3). Phosphate and creatinine concentrations are, of course, determined by glomerular filtration and tubular reabsorption. Tubular fluid NH_3 concentration is determined by nonionic diffusion of the gas generated in tubular cells from glutamine, and "trapping" in the lumen by conversion of NH_3 to ammonium (NH_4^+). Net hydrogen ion secretion (and hence new bicarbonate generation) is, therefore, the sum of urinary titratable acid (the amount of hydrogen ion excreted as dihydrogen phosphate and acidified creatinine) and NH_4^+, minus the urinary excretion of real or potential base (bicarbonate and/or organic acids). Quantitatively, NH_4^+ excretion accounts for more than 75% of net acid excretion (11).

The new formulation involves a different understanding of the products of glutamine metabolism; that is, deamination of glutamine produces NH_4^+ and α-ketoglutarate, not free NH_3 (Fig. 1). This creates a problem for the older scheme. If NH_4^+ is the major product of glutamine metabolism, its transport to the tubular lumen and excretion in the urine would not result in net removal of hydrogen ions. However, the stoichiometric relationship between NH_4^+ excretion and net new bicarbonate generation on which the old scheme was based might be preserved in the following way: Glutamine is hydrolyzed to glutamate and NH_4^+; the glutamate is then converted to α-ketoglutarate, yielding a second NH_4^+. If α-ketoglutarate is metabolized by the citric acid cycle, 1 molecule of new bicarbonate would be produced. If the 2 NH_4^+ produced from glutamine were excreted in the urine, and the α-ketoglutarate were metabolized by the citric acid cycle, new bicarbonate generation would be only one-half the amount of NH_4^+ excreted. On the other hand, if the α-ketoglutarate were metabolized by way of acetoacetate to glucose, generating 2 new bicarbonate, the amount of NH_4^+ excreted would equal the amount of new bicarbonate generated.

This new formulation implies that the main effect of renal ammonia excretion is to prevent its transfer to the liver, where it would enter the urea cycle. If any NH_4^+ generated from glutamate were not excreted in the urine, the same stoichiometric considerations outlined above would obtain. If NH_4^+ not excreted were transported to the liver for conversion to urea, 1 or 2 hydrogen ions would be produced for every NH_4^+ that entered the cycle. These would be balanced by an equal amount of bicarbonate if α-ketoglutarate were metabolized to glucose by gluconeogenesis or to CO_2 by the citric acid cycle.

Since the major portion of NH_4^+ addition to the tubular fluid occurs in the proximal tubule, it follows that the major site of new bicarbonate generation is probably the proximal tubule (13,14). The implications of this new scheme for current concepts of the pathophysiology of RTA are discussed below.

Classification of RTA

RTA can be classified into two pathophysiologic types based on the distinction between bicarbonate reabsorption and generation (Table 3).

Decreased Bicarbonate Reabsorption

Impairment of bicarbonate reabsorption in the proximal tubule (lowered set point) causes bicarbonate losses in the urine of sufficient magnitude to cause metabolic acidosis (3,5). The pathophysiology of the acidosis in type II RTA is divided into two phases: generation and maintenance. During the generation phase, which is not usually observed clinically, the plasma bicarbonate concentration falls from a normal value to some lower value that varies depending on the severity of the defect. During the maintenance phase, the plasma bicarbonate concentration is maintained in a steady state at this lower value.

TABLE 3. *Pathophysiology of RTA variants*

Tubular abnormality	RTA type
1. Decreased bicarbonate reabsorption	Type II (proximal)
2. Decreased bicarbonate generation	Type I (classic; distal); type IV

The distal tubule mechanism of hydrogen-ion secretion is intact; however, it cannot function properly during the generation phase of the acidosis because the distal tubule is flooded by bicarbonate from the proximal tubule, preventing development of a sufficient hydrogen-ion gradient. During the maintenance phase of the acidosis, however, all of the filtered bicarbonate is reabsorbed proximally, allowing the distal mechanisms to maintain plasma bicarbonate in a steady state at a lower than normal level.

This type of tubular acidosis may have been the first to be reported (15). However, differentiation between this condition and the type of tubular acidosis caused by decreased bicarbonate generation did not occur until after the latter was recognized, hence the designation type II RTA. Other names attached to this syndrome, which derive from its pathophysiology, are *proximal* and *bicarbonate wasting*.

Type II RTA, which may occur rarely in a pure form, is seen most commonly as a component of Fanconi syndrome in children with a variety of inherited metabolic disorders (16,17), or in adults with a variety of conditions listed in Table 5. Type II RTA may occasionally be associated with nephrolithiasis, as will be discussed subsequently.

Decreased Bicarbonate Generation

There are two types of RTA associated with abnormalities in bicarbonate generation (Table 1). Although both are associated with defects in distal tubular function, the term *distal RTA* is usually reserved for the condition known as type I or *classic RTA*. As noted, type I RTA (RTA-1) was not the first to be described, but was the first in which the pathophysiology was correctly characterized, hence the term "classic." Hypercalciuria, nephrolithiasis, and nephrocalcinosis were prominent features of the earliest described cases (18,19) and are important contributors to the morbidity resulting from this condition (20,21). Accordingly, RTA-1 is discussed extensively in this chapter.

The other distal disorder is referred to as type IV or hyperkalemic RTA. The most recently described form of tubular acidosis (3), it is typically caused by hypoaldosteronism and is always accompanied by hyperkalemia (3,16,22). Acidosis is due primarily to impairment of ammonia generation secondary to hyperkalemia (22). Although these individuals have a complex defect in hydrogen-ion secretion (22), its role in the pathophysiology of the acidosis is unclear. Since pure type IV RTA is not associated with nephrolithiasis or any other disorder of mineral metabolism, it will not be considered extensively here. Nephrolithiasis may occur, however, in patients with mixed type I and IV RTA. The reader is referred to several recent reviews for a comprehensive discussion of type IV RTA (16,22).

TYPE I RENAL TUBULAR ACIDOSIS

Etiology and Nosology

RTA-1 is associated with eight major clinical manifestations that occur with varying frequency (Table 4). Four of these, hypercalciuria, nephrolithiasis, nephrocalcinosis, and osteomalacia, fall in the category of disorders of bone and mineral metabolism. The syndrome of RTA-1 has multiple etiologies, occurs in a bewildering variety of settings (Table 5) (23), and many classification schemes have been proposed. Our approach to classification, outlined in Table 5, essentially divides etiology into two categories: hereditary (primary or secondary) and acquired (secondary or idiopathic) (2). Hereditary RTA-1 may occur as a primary disorder, or secondary to any one of several hereditary metabolic diseases (Table 5). Primary hereditary RTA-1 is usually an autosomal dominant condition, although two recessive forms have been reported, one associated with nerve deafness (24,25), and one with deficient erythrocyte carbonic anhydrase B (26,27). The most common form of secondary hereditary RTA-1 appears to be that associated with hereditary, idiopathic hypercalciuria, which is also an autosomal dominant condition (2,20).

RTA-1 may be acquired from a variety of nonhereditary conditions that damage the distal tubule. The most common "cause" of RTA in this category is a group of autoimmune disorders such as Sjogren's syndrome and systemic lupus erythematosus (2). Other causes of acquired RTA are drugs such as amphotericin, lithium, and analgesics, toxins such as heavy metals and myeloma proteins, and conditions such as obstructive uropathy and medullary sponge kidney.

Under idiopathic, acquired RTA-1 we include all cases that do not have an obvious familial association or any obvious cause of distal tubule damage (2). It seems likely that some cases of apparent idiopathic RTA-1 are in reality hereditary forms (2). It should be noted that one could classify all cases of RTA-1 due to hereditary metabolic causes under the category of "secondary" (2). In that case, RTA-1 would be classified into three categories: primary (meaning primary hereditary), secondary,

TABLE 4. *Major clinical manifestations of Type I RTA*

1. Not associated with abnormal mineral metabolism
   a. Metabolic acidosis
   b. Hyperexcretion of monovalent cation (Na, K)
   c. Growth retardation
   d. Renal insufficiency
2. Abnormal mineral metabolism
   a. Hypercalciuria
   b. Nephrolithiasis
   c. Nephrocalcinosis
   d. Osteomalacia

TABLE 5. *Classification of renal tubular acidosis*

Site: Proximal Tubule		Site: Distal Tubule, ctd.	
Hereditary RTA Type II	*Acquired RTA Type II*	*Hereditary RTA Type I, ctd.*	*Acquired RTA Type I, ctd.*
Familial	Drugs	Ehlers-Danlos	Primary hyperparathyroidism
Transient (infants)	Acetazolamide	syndrome	with nephrocalcinosis
	Mafenide acetate	Fabry's disease	Galactorrhea with
	Sulfanilamide	Hereditary	hyperprolactinemia
	Chronic active hepatitis	eliptocytosis	Idiopathic hypercalciuria
	Associated with tetralogy of	Medullary sponge	Hypomagnesemia
	Fallot	kidney	Hypergammaglobulinemic states
Fanconi's Syndrome	Fanconi's syndrome	Polycystic kidney	Idiopathic
Familial	Drugs	disease	Hyperglobulinemic purpura
Cystinosis	Outdated tetracycline	Wilson's disease	Cryoglobulinemia
Wilson disease	Methyl-5-chrome	Associated with nerve	Sjogren's syndrome
Galactosemia	6-Mercaptopurine	deafness	SLE
Hereditary fructose	Cephalothin	Associated with	Sarcoidosis
intolerance	Gentamicin	deficient carbonic	Hodgkin's disease
Lowes syndrome	Heavy metals: Pb, Cd, Hz, V	anhydrase	Tuberculosis
Tyrosinemia, type 1	Secondary		Takayusu's arteritis
Pyruvate carboxylase	hyperparathyroidism		Chronic active hepatitis
deficiency	Immunologic disorders		Thyroiditis
	Multiple myeloma		Starvation and malnutrition
	Monoclonal gammopathy		Hepatic cirrhosis
	Systemic lupus		Primary biliary cirrhosis
	Sjogren's syndrome		Acute tubular necrosis
	Renal transplantation		Pyelonephritis
	Amyloidosis		Renal transplantation
	Burkitt's lymphoma		Obstructive uropathy
	Interstitial nephritis		Drugs
	Balkan nephropathy		Lithium
	Nephrotic syndrome		Amphotericin B
	Osteopetrosis		Toluene
	Paroxysmal nocturnal		Analgesic nephropathy
	hemoglobinuria	*Hereditary RTA Combined Types I and IV*	*Acquired RTA Combined Types I and IV*
Site: Distal Tubule		SS hemoglobinopathy	Secondary
Hereditary RTA Type I	*Acquired RTA Type I*	SC hemoglobinopathy	Chronic renal parenchymal
Primary	Idiopathic		disease
Secondary	Metabolic disorders		Obstructive uropathy
Hypercalciuria	Hyperthyroidism with		Medullary sponge kidney
Hereditary fructose	nephrocalcinosis		Drugs
intolerance	Hypothyroidism		Amiloride
			Triamterene

Source: Reprinted with permission from *Current Nephrology*, vol 6, HC Gonick, ed., copyright 1983 by John Wiley & Sons, Inc.

and sporadic (meaning nonhereditary with no obvious cause) (28).

Regardless of the scheme one uses, the difficulty in correctly classifying an isolated case of RTA-1 can be illustrated by a person with hypercalciuria and a family history of kidney stones and RTA. The question arises as to whether this person has primary RTA-1 or RTA-1 secondary to hereditary hypercalciuria. The only way this distinction can be made is to show that all members of the family with RTA-1 have hypercalciuria and that some family members without RTA-1 have hypercalciuria (2). This may be difficult when cases occur in individuals from small families. In isolated cases of RTA-1 with no family history of kidney stones or RTA-1, the patient should be investigated, for an autoimmune dis-

ease since the RTA-1 may become manifest before the classic signs and symptoms of the autoimmune disease become manifest (29).

Pathophysiology of Clinical Manifestations Other Than Disorders of Bone and Mineral Metabolism

Hyperchloremic Metabolic Acidosis

Acidosis in RTA-1 results from a defect in the ability of the distal tubule to lower urine pH appropriately (3,16). This defect could be due to an abnormality in the hydrogen pump itself or to an abnormality in generation of the electrical gradient that promotes hydrogen-ion secretion in the distal tubule (Table 6) (3,5,16,30). The

TABLE 6. *Postulated transport defects in Type I RTA*

1. Decreased hydrogen-ion secretion
   a. Pump defect
   b. Decreased electrical gradient
2. Increased back leak
   a. Hydrogen ion
   b. Carbonic acid

defect could also be caused by increased back-leak of hydrogen ion or of carbonic acid due to increased permeability of the distal tubule (Table 6) (3,5,16,30). The type of defect may be cause specific. For example, lithium may cause a defect in generation of the electrical gradient (30), amphotericin may cause increased permeability of the distal tubule to hydrogen ion (28), and toluene may reduce proton conductance (31). Thus heterogeneity almost certainly exists among patients, depending on the etiology and pathogenesis of their particular form of RTA-1 and possibly on the particular segment of the distal nephron that is damaged (5,32). It should be noted, however, that no differences in the clinical manifestations of RTA-1 have ever been attributed to any possible difference in the mechanism of the distal tubular defect.

Most of the speculation about the mechanism of the defect in urine acidification in RTA-1 is based on theoretical considerations derived from direct observations in patients, from experimental models, and from in vitro experiments performed on transporting epithelia (9,30). Perhaps the most important observation in patients was the demonstration that urine PCO_2 did not rise normally when urine pH was raised by bicarbonate administration (33). The interpretation of this phenomenon is based on the generally accepted notion of the origin of the CO_2 dissolved in urine. It has been known for some time that PCO_2 of alkaline urine is higher than that of plasma (34). This was explained by postulating that hydrogen-ion secretion by the distal tubule into the bicarbonate-rich urine results in the formation of carbonic acid, which dissociates into CO_2 and water, to a large extent, in the urinary bladder rather than in the distal tubule lumen. The "delayed dehydration" of carbonic acid, therefore, results in a urine PCO_2 value higher than that of plasma (34). Although other interpretations are possible, it seems reasonable to postulate that failure to raise urine PCO_2 normally during bicarbonate administration results from a defect in hydrogen-ion secretion in the distal tubule (5). Since most patients with RTA-1 cannot raise urine PCO_2 normally when urine pH is high (5), it seems likely that most patients have a defect in the hydrogen-ion pump.

The consequences of a defect in distal hydrogen-ion secretion are predictable from the concepts developed earlier in this chapter. Bicarbonate generation is impaired because of decreased titration of those urinary buffers that depend on a pH below 6.0 (phosphate and

creatinine) and an inability to trap ammonia in the tubular lumen. Since NH_4^+ accounts for most of new bicarbonate generated, the defect in NH_4^+ excretion is by far the most important in the pathogenesis of metabolic acidosis in RTA-1. As will be discussed below, the impairment of NH_4^+ excretion in RTA-1 is only partly due to the characteristic defect in hydrogen-ion secretion.

In discussing the defect in ammonia excretion in RTA-1, some consideration must be given to the implications of the new concepts regarding ammonia metabolism discussed earlier. Although this new scheme localizes the new bicarbonate generated from ammonia metabolism to the proximal rather than the distal tubule, the net generation of new bicarbonate from ammonia metabolism remains a function of urinary NH_4^+ excretion. In the old scheme, urine NH_4^+ was derived from deamination of glutamine in the distal tubule cells. In the new scheme, NH_4^+ added to the proximal tubular fluid is then carried by the Na, K, Cl cotransporter as a substitute for K from the lumen of the thick ascending limb to the cell, where it becomes NH_3 and H^+ (11,13). (The H^+ may be secreted back into the lumen of the ascending limb, where it effects the reabsorption of any bicarbonate that has escaped reabsorption in the proximal tubule.) The NH_3 so generated then diffuses across the medullary interstitium and into the distal tubular lumen, where it is converted again to NH_4^+ by hydrogen ions secreted by distal tubular cells (i.e., ammonia trapping). Thus a defect in distal hydrogen secretion results in a defect in NH_4^+ trapping (and therefore to a defect in bicarbonate generation) in both schemes.

However, the defect in NH_4^+ excretion actually observed in RTA-1 is not due simply to reduced NH_4^+ trapping. Reduced NH_4^+ excretion in RTA-1 may also be due to decreased NH_4^+ production, an insight gained from studies of the *forme frust* of RTA-1, usually referred to as "incomplete" RTA (IRTA).

Patients with IRTA have a defect in lowering urinary pH, but they do not have acidosis (1,11). Two differences observed between patients with complete and incomplete RTA help elucidate the pathophysiology of acidosis in RTA-1. First, minimum urinary pH is lower in IRTA; that is, patients with IRTA have milder defects than those with acidotic RTA (2,35). Second, the glomerular filtration rate (GFR) is higher in IRTA than in RTA (2,11). In a recently published series from our institution, we found that acidosis did not occur in RTA patients with creatinine clearances greater than 80 mL/min (2). Third, most patients with IRTA have normal net acid excretion (i.e., they do not have impaired renal bicarbonate generation, at least under normal circumstances) (2). It should also be noted that reduced citrate excretion reduces the need for bicarbonate generation since urine organic acid represents a loss of base to the organism (9). Therefore, the reduced citrate excretion observed in many cases of IRTA contributes to the ability of these patients to avoid the development of metabolic acidosis. However, low urine citrate may be found in both acidotic and incomplete RTA (2).

These observations are compatible with Wrong and Davies's suggestion that the kidneys in patients with IRTA excrete ammonia in sufficient amounts to avoid systemic acidosis despite the defect in lowering urine pH (11). In the absence of renal parenchymal damage, urine ammonia excretion becomes a higher percentage of total acid excretion, compensating for the impairment in titration of phosphate and creatinine induced by mild defects in urine acidification. This may be possible because the pK of ammonia of 9.2 is much higher than that for the other two buffers. It is well known that renal parenchymal damage of any type impairs renal ammonia generation (11), a phenomenon that holds true in RTA-1 (11). Thus patients with RTA-1 develop acidosis when they have sufficient generalized renal failure to impair ammonia generation, when they have a defect in lowering urine pH sufficiently severe to decrease ammonia excretion, or when they have a combination of these two that cumulatively interferes sufficiently with ammonia excretion. There is no reason to think that patients with IRTA have an occult systemic acidosis. This is an important issue in the pathophysiology of hypocitraturia and nephrolithiasis in RTA and is discussed later.

When acidosis occurs in RTA-1 it is typically the type with a normal anion gap (hyperchloremic). The anion gap is normal because acidosis develops before renal failure has progressed to the point where decreased glomerular filtration causes undetermined anion retention. Hyperchloremia is the inexorable consequence of the law of electroneutrality and the fall in plasma bicarbonate concentration in the absence of a rise in undetermined anion; however, the mechanism by which the rise in plasma chloride concentration occurs has not been fully elucidated (1). It could be due to an increase in the amount of chloride in ECF, to a decrease of ECF volume, or to a combination of the two. If the rise were due to chloride retention, the amount of chloride retained would equal the bicarbonate deficit assuming that the volume of distribution of bicarbonate and chloride were the same. However, bicarbonate is distributed in approximately 40% of total body weight, while chloride is contained almost exclusively in the ECF, or approximately 20% of body weight. Therefore, the rise in plasma chloride concentration could equal the bicarbonate fall if the amount of chloride retained were approximately half the bicarbonate deficit. For the same reason, a pure contraction in ECF volume would have unequal effects on the concentrations of chloride and bicarbonate. A decrement in ECF volume would cause a rise in chloride concentration by the same percentage as the fall in ECF volume. However, a rise in plasma bicarbonate concentration due to ECF volume contraction would tend to increase ECF pH, causing a shift of bicarbonate into in-

tracellular fluid (or, more accurately, a shift in hydrogen ions from intracellular to extracellular fluid). Thus a decrement in ECF volume would have a larger effect on plasma chloride concentration than on plasma bicarbonate concentration.

The relative effect of changes in chloride balance and ECF volume on plasma chloride concentration has not been well studied in RTA-1. Sketchy reports of studies in two patients (36,37) are relevant to these questions. When alkali therapy was withdrawn with the patients on severe sodium and chloride restriction, plasma bicarbonate concentration fell with no rise in chloride concentration. Although not reported, this result implies that the plasma sodium concentration also fell if the anion gap did not change. As might be expected, when these studies were repeated with the subjects on normal dietary sodium chloride, plasma chloride concentration rose by an increment equal to the decrement in bicarbonate concentration. No studies were performed on urinary chloride excretion or chloride balance, but the results suggest that the rise in chloride concentration was due to a positive chloride balance. It should be noted that achievement of a positive chloride balance in patients with RTA-1 could be facilitated by their low urine ammonia concentration. Since urine chloride concentration is a direct function of the sum of urine cation concentrations (38), a decrease in ammonia concentration in the absence of an increase in urine sodium or potassium concentration would decrease the urine chloride concentration (38). It should also be noted that patients with RTA-1 who develop advanced renal failure develop increased anion gap and normal chloride concentration, as do all other patients with severe, generalized renal failure (20).

Hyperexcretion of Monovalent Cation

Potassium

Hypokalemia due to renal potassium wasting occurs in RTA-1 with a frequency that has not been determined. In our series recently published, we noted hypokalemia in only 28% of 58 cases (2). The mechanism of potassium wasting is probably multifactorial and is not completely understood. Earliest speculations attempted to link the wasting of potassium with the defect in hydrogen-ion secretion (19,39) and were based on the hypothesis that sodium–hydrogen exchange in the distal tubule is reciprocally related to sodium–potassium exchange (40) and the observation that correction of acidosis in RTA-1 resulted in correction of the potassium wasting (39).

There are now several reasons for rejecting the hypothesis. If potassium wasting were linked to the defect in urine acidification, potassium wasting would occur in every case. While subclinical degrees might occur in all cases, potassium wasting of sufficient magnitude to cause clinical hypokalemia probably occurs in a minority of cases (see above). Furthermore, current concepts of the control of potassium secretion by the distal tubule are not compatible with the reciprocal relationship with hydrogen-ion secretion originally postulated (41).

Acidosis itself might increase potassium excretion by increasing sodium and water delivery to the distal tubule (41). Additionally, increased excretion of sodium and water might cause volume depletion and increased activity of the renin–angiotensin–aldosterone system (39,42). Again, there are several reasons to reject this speculation. The most important comes from the only careful study of the issue wherein correction of acidosis in RTA-1 was found to ameliorate but did not completely correct potassium wasting (42). Furthermore, in this same study, although correction of acidosis reduced aldosterone secretion, it remained inappropriately high for the serum potassium concentration (42). Finally, potassium wasting has been reported in several patients with the incomplete form of RTA-1 in which acidosis is not present (43).

The question as to why hyperaldosteronism might persist despite correction of acidosis and volume depletion remains open. One possible explanation for this phenomenon was suggested by the finding in one patient where indomethacin reduced plasma renin activity to normal and ameliorated, but did not correct, potassium wasting (44). This observation suggests that at least in some cases, increased activity of the renin–angiotensin–aldosterone system and potassium wasting might be due to increased prostaglandin secretion. The increased prostaglandin secretion might be secondary to potassium depletion, resulting from a primary defect in tubular potassium reabsorption as has been postulated in Bartter syndrome (45,46).

Sodium

Overt sodium wasting with severe volume depletion is rare in RTA-1, although the exact prevalence is not known. Occult defects in conservation of sodium that become apparent only when sodium intake is restricted may be more common (47). The mechanism of sodium wasting when it occurs is not known. It is not due to the acidosis (47), nor can it be linked to the defect in hydrogen-ion secretion, although both defects could be due to the same underlying mechanism. It may be more common in children. Because of its rarity in RTA-1, the problem has received little attention.

Growth Retardation

Children with RTA-1 commonly manifest growth retardation. This is a problem that children with both types I and II share, probably because it is due entirely to the acidosis. In a classic study, McSherry and Morris showed that earlier studies in which correction of acidosis did not correct abnormal growth were due to inadequate treatment of the acidosis (48). Interestingly, their study showed that very large doses of bicarbonate were needed to correct the acidosis completely because bicarbonate administration induced bicarbonate wasting in some children with RTA-1 (48). This phenomenon apparently occurs almost exclusively in children.*

Renal Insufficiency

As originally pointed out by Wrong and Davies (11), renal insufficiency is common in RTA-1 (2). It should be noted, however, that there is probably a marked difference in the prevalence of renal insufficiency between adults and young children. In our series, all 12 infants with RTA-1 had normal BUN and serum creatinine, whereas 17 of 44 older children and adults (39%) had renal insufficiency, as indicated by an elevated serum creatinine concentration (2). As we have pointed out in the forgoing discussion, generalized renal failure is an important feature in the pathophysiology of metabolic acidosis in these patients.

The mechanism of renal failure when it occurs is not understood. Earlier studies indicated that interstitial nephritis secondary to medullary calcification and recurrent pyelonephritis was common in RTA-1 (51–53). All these factors in combination may play a role in causing renal failure since, in our series, creatinine clearance tended to be lower in patients with a history of urinary tract infection, in patients with staghorn calculi, and in those with nephrocalcinosis (2). When each of these factors was considered alone, however, no significant effect on GFR was observed (2).

It is reasonable to assume that patients with RTA-1 secondary to an autoimmune disorder such as SLE or Sjogren's syndrome have CRF secondary to autoimmune interstitial nephritis. In these cases, in contrast to those with most other etiologies, CRF and the defect in tubular hydrogen ion secretion are due to the same disorder. Interestingly, CRF in RTA-1 is rarely progressive. In this author's experience, only two cases have resulted in dialysis dependent end-stage renal disease. In one of those type I diabetes mellitus was also present.

Diagnosis

Presentation

Patients with RTA-1 may present with one or more of the major clinical manifestations outlined in Table 4. Children having sporadic RTA-1 most often present with acidosis and growth retardation in the general setting of failure to thrive (2). The presentation in adults is

---

* The phenomenon of bicarbonate wasting in infants treated with bicarbonate is probably the explanation for the condition originally described as type III RTA (49,50).

more variable. It may be due to signs and symptoms of an underlying cause of RTA-1 such as SLE. However, nephrolithiasis is probably the most common condition for which adults with RTA-1 seek medical attention (2). Acidosis is usually mild and is detected most often incidentally. Muscle weakness or polyuria caused by potassium depletion may be the presenting abnormality (54,55). Occasionally, potassium depletion may be sufficiently severe to cause periodic paralysis (55). This phenomenon may be more common in individuals of Oriental extraction with Sjogren's syndrome (55). Osteomalacia is rarely seen and if present, is found in patients with long-standing RTA since childhood.

It should be noted that patients suspected of having RTA-1 because of the typical plasma electrolyte pattern of high chloride, low bicarbonate, and low potassium concentrations and an alkaline urine pH could have chronic respiratory alkalosis. The author has seen more than one patient referred with this constellation of abnormalities for a workup for RTA in which chronic respiratory alkalosis due to anxiety has been the correct diagnosis. In some cases, therefore, unless the diagnosis is obvious, arterial blood gases should be obtained.

Urine Acidification

Diagnosis of RTA-1 usually involves demonstrating the typical defect in urine acidification discussed in the forgoing section. This can be done either by detecting an inappropriately elevated urine pH in patients with spontaneous hyperchloremic acidosis or by performing one of the standard tests of urine acidification.

Urine pH and Ammonia in Patients with Hyperchloremic Acidosis

It is generally agreed that urine pH in response to ammonium chloride induced metabolic acidosis in normal subjects should fall below 5.5 (1). Accordingly, if urine pH is not below 5.5 in patients with spontaneous hyperchloremic acidosis, a diagnosis of RTA-1 is justified (some exceptions will be noted below). Some have argued that the diagnosis cannot be made unless a "fixed" defect is demonstrated by showing that urine pH does not go below 5.5 despite the superimposition of severe metabolic acidosis upon mild metabolic acidosis (15). We have argued that the defect in RTA-1 is not fixed and that patients with mild metabolic acidosis and urine pH above 5.5 have RTA-1 even if their urine pH falls below 5.5 when more severe acidosis is superimposed by ammonium chloride administration (2).

An additional controversy has recently been raised by the "Canadian school," who have proposed a "pathophysiologic" (as opposed to "clinical") classification of RTA based on the serum potassium concentration and three physiologically determined parameters: the amount of urinary ammonia and the urine pH during metabolic acidosis (either spontaneous or induced by ammonium chloride), and the urine PCO_2 during bicarbonate administration (the latter test is described below) (5,56). Introduction of this new approach to the diagnosis of distal tubular acidosis is based on the contention that since urine pH is affected by the amount of urinary ammonia (57), errors in diagnosis may occur if urine pH is relied on as the sole criterion (56).

Although it is true that reliance on urine pH alone may lead to some errors, the issue should be put into perspective by considering the type of errors that may occur. These are most easily appreciated by comparing the criteria used by the two schemes for diagnosing the various types of distal RTA as summarized in Table 7. Analysis of the differences between the criteria reveals very little difference between the two schemes and indicates, in fact, that the new scheme is more cumbersome than the old. In the old scheme, RTA-1 is diagnosed when urine pH is above 5.5 in the presence of metabolic acidosis. In the new scheme, the same criteria are used; the only difference is that the new scheme differentiates between the pump defect and the back-leak defect, a distinction without any clinical significance except as to possible etiology (see above). Type IV RTA is diagnosed in the old scheme by the combination of hyperkalemia and a urine pH less than 5.5 during metabolic acidosis. Exactly the same criteria are used by the new scheme. The same criteria are used by both schemes to diagnose the combination of type I + type IV: patients with metabolic acidosis, hyperkalemia, and urine pH greater than 5.5.

There are two situations in which the old scheme may lead to an error that would be avoided by the new scheme. The first error would involve patients with metabolic acidosis, hypokalemia, and urine pH less than 5.5. If this syndrome were due to an unlikely situation in which renal medullary disease caused an ammonia defect and renal potassium wasting with an intact distal hydrogen-ion pump, it would be incorrectly diagnosed by the old scheme as the untreated, maintenance phase of type II RTA. Therefore, to diagnose these rare cases correctly it is necessary to estimate urine ammonia by measuring the urine anion gap (see below).

Reliance on urine pH during metabolic acidosis and the serum potassium concentration as the sole criteria for diagnosing the various types of distal RTA may lead to one other diagnostic error. Patients with severe, chronic diarrhea may have metabolic acidosis, hypokalemia, and a urine pH greater than 5.5 [the latter being due to high urine ammonia (5,38)], leading to a diagnosis of RTA-1. These patients can be identified and correctly diagnosed by the history unless they engage in surreptitious laxative abuse. In that case, measurement of the urine anion gap would be necessary (38). To avoid missing the rare individual with diarrhea and RTA-1 concomitantly, determination of the urine PCO_2 during bi-

TABLE 7. *Two proposed classifications of distal RTA*

Old scheme		New scheme	
Nomenclature	Criteria	Nomenclature	Criteria
Type I	Urine pH > 5.5[a]	Primary pump failure	Urine pH > 5.5[a] plus Urine PCO_2 < 70[b]
		Backleak of H^+	Urine pH > 5.5[a] plus Urine PCO_2 > 70[b]
Type IV	Urine pH < 5.5[a] plus Hyperkalemia	Ammonia defect with hyperkalemia	Urine pH < 5.5[a] plus Hyperkalemia
Types I and IV	Urine pH > 5.5[a] plus Hyperkalemia	Voltage defect	Urine pH > 5.5[a] plus Hyperkalemia
None corresponding	—	Ammonia defect with hypokalemia	Urine pH < 5.5[a] plus Urine PCO_2 > 70[b] plus Low urine NH_4^+

[a] Urine pH during metabolic acidosis.
[b] Urine PCO_2 during bicarbonate loading.

carbonate loading would be necessary. It is unlikely, however, that making this fine distinction would have any important clinical significance.

Urine Acidification Tests

Two types of tests of urine acidification have been proposed. Determination of urine pH following the administration of ammonium chloride measures the ability of the distal tubule to generate a hydrogen-ion gradient (11). The measurement of urine PCO_2 during the administration of a bicarbonate load reflects the ability of the distal tubule to secrete hydrogen ion from cell to tubular lumen in the absence of a hydrogen-ion gradient as discussed earlier in this chapter. One or both of these tests are indicated in patients suspected of having RTA-1 who either do not have spontaneous acidosis (they may have IRTA) or in whom very mild or borderline acidosis is indicated on arterial blood gas determination.

Ammonium chloride testing has been the "gold standard" for more than 30 years (11). In the long test, 100 mg/kg is administered in divided doses for 3 days, with a 24-h urine being collected on the third day (58). More easily performed is the short test in which the same dose is administered over a 1-h period and urine is collected hourly for several hours after the load. In either test, urine pH should fall below 5.5 (11,58). No measurements other than urine pH are absolutely required during these tests. However, it is usually recommended that arterial blood gasses be obtained before and following ammonium chloride to determine the degree of metabolic acidosis that is induced and to make certain that

the patient has ingested adequate amounts of ammonium chloride (15).

Measurement of urine PCO_2 during bicarbonate loading is a relatively new test that is still evolving. It is based on the concept of delayed dehydration of carbonic acid. Hydrogen-ion secretion by the distal tubule in the presence of bicarbonate results in the formation of carbonic acid that dissociates into CO_2 and water. Because of the time lag between the formation of carbonic acid and its dehydration, a significant portion of the latter takes place in the late distal tubule and bladder urine (34). Under these circumstances, bladder urine PCO_2 becomes an index of distal tubule and collecting duct hydrogen-ion secretion (59). Not surprisingly, urine PCO_2 is a function of urine bicarbonate concentration, and defects in hydrogen-ion secretion can be detected reliably only at urine bicarbonate concentrations in excess of about 80 mEq/L (5,31). Attainment of this very high value requires administration of large amounts of bicarbonate and cannot be achieved in all patients (31).

Several protocols have been described in the literature. A bicarbonate load of 500 mEq can be given intravenously during metabolic acidosis (31,60). Alternatively, an oral load of 0.5–2.0 mEq/kg can be given to subjects whose plasma bicarbonate concentration has been normalized (5). During bicarbonate administration, urine is collected until its pH has reached a high enough value to ensure that urine bicarbonate is greater than 80 mEq/L, or somewhere between 7.4 (5) and 7.8 (31,60). Under these conditions, normal individuals should have urine PCO_2 greater than 70 mmHg or more than 30 mmHg greater than arterial blood (5,31,60). However, it may be necessary to relate urine PCO_2 to urine bicarbonate concentration to detect mild defects (5,61,62).

Determination of urine PCO_2 can substitute for the ammonium chloride loading test. As already noted, a theoretical advantage for the urine PCO_2 test has been claimed for differentiating the various types of RTA. Although we do not accept the scope of this claim, it is interesting to note that several patients have been reported with IRTA in which the ammonium chloride loading test was normal, but the bicarbonate loading test was abnormal (63). This suggests that the bicarbonate loading test can detect mild defects not detectable by the ammonium chloride loading test. Further studies are needed to confirm the validity of this interpretation and its possible clinical significance.

Urine Anion Gap

The concept of an anion gap in urine is the same as that for plasma. The difference is that when one calculates the urine anion gap using those ions usually measured in urine, sodium, potassium, and chloride, the value is negative (i.e., measured anions are greater than measured cations) because the largest unmeasured ion in urine is NH_4^+, a cation (38). It has recently been pointed out that the urine anion gap is a reasonably good index of urine ammonia concentration and a useful diagnostic tool in evaluating patients with hyperchloremic acidosis (5,38,56). Thus in patients with RTA-1 and hyperchlor-

emic acidosis, the urine anion gap is positive and the urine pH is above 5.5. The urine anion gap is most useful in differentiating between patients with acidotic RTA-1 and those with hyperchloremic acidosis due to gastrointestinal loss of bicarbonate. The latter may be mistakenly diagnosed as RTA-1 since the patients may have a defect in urine acidification because of a combination low urine sodium secondary to ECF volume contraction, and high urine NH_4^+ concentration. However, they can be differentiated from RTA-1 and other types of distal RTA by their normal urine anion gap (5,38,56).

Summary

We suggest the following approach to the diagnosis of RTA in patients with a history of nephrolithiasis (Fig. 2). If the serum electrolyte concentration shows hyperchloremia, a simultaneous arterial blood gas, urine pH, and urine anion gap should be determined. If hyperchloremic acidosis is present with an arterial pH less than 7.33, a urine pH greater than 5.5, and a positive anion gap, a diagnosis of RTA-1 is indicated and no further studies are necessary. (Further studies to define the mechanism of stone formation are indicated, however, as will be discussed subsequently.) If hyperchloremic acidosis is present with a negative urine anion gap, a history of diarrhea or surreptitious cathartic ingestion should be sought. If urine pH less than 5.5 and a negative anion gap is found in a patient with normal or low serum potas-

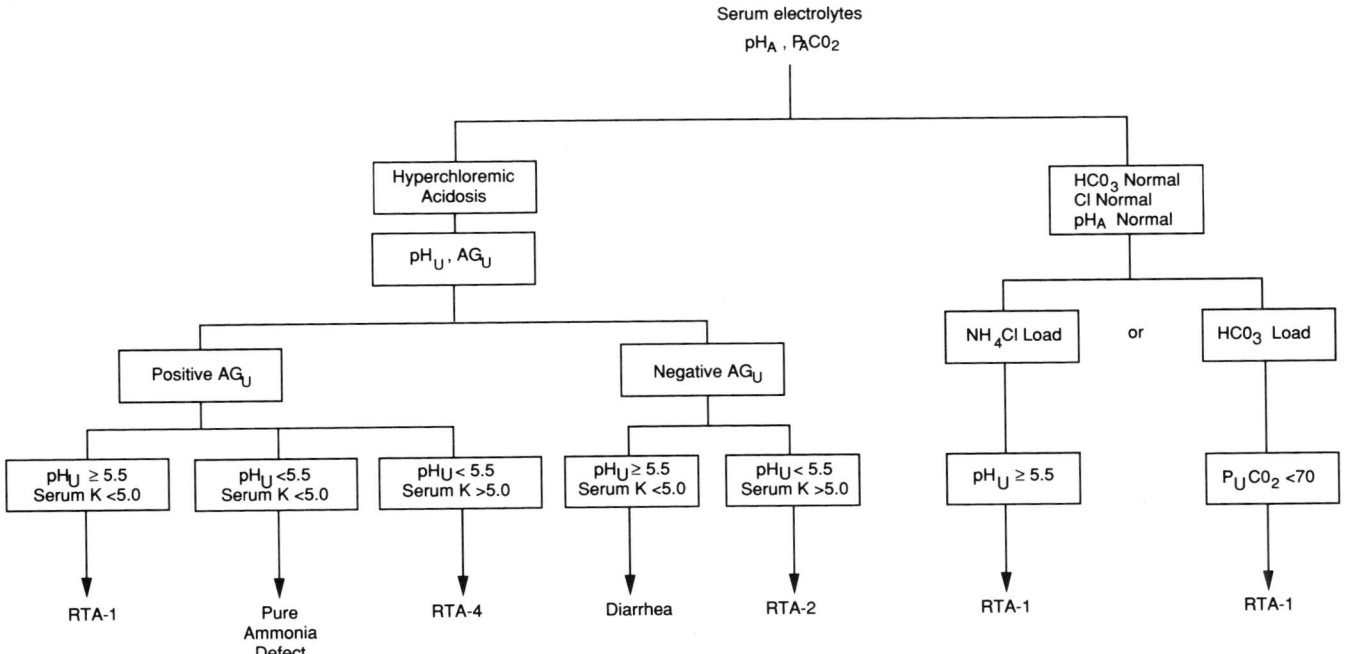

FIG. 2. Algorithm for the diagnosis of various types of RTA and conditions that mimic RTA. Patients with spontaneous hyperchloremic acidosis can be correctly identified by determination of urine pH (pH_u) and urine anion gap (AG_u). Patients without hyperchloremic acidosis who might have incomplete RTA can be diagnosed by either an ammonium chloride loading test or a bicarbonate loading test. See the text for description of these tests.

sium, a diagnosis of RTA-2 is indicated. If a mild hyperchloremic acidosis with a pH between 7.33 and 7.35 is present or if acidosis is not found, an ammonium chloride loading study or determination of urine PCO_2 during bicarbonate loading should be performed, either of which can accurately diagnose RTA-1.

Nephrolithiasis in Type I RTA

Clinical Features

Incidence and Prevalence

The prevalence of RTA in the population of patients with nephrolithiasis has been reported to vary between 0.3 and 8% (64–70). The incidence of nephrolithiasis in the population of patients with RTA-1 is not known. The prevalence of nephrolithiasis in known cases of RTA-1 is rarely reported. In one series reported from San Francisco, it was 7% in 29 adults, while no cases were observed in children (71). In another series from the Mayo Clinic, the prevalence was 48% in 48 adults (54). In our series from North Carolina the overall prevalence of 59% was the highest reported to date (2). When 14 infants under 2 years of age were excluded, the prevalence was 77%. These high values undoubtedly reflect the fact that our institution is a referral center for patients with complicated stone disease.

Nephrolithiasis may occur as a complication in any patient with RTA-1 regardless of etiology or associated condition (2), and in both the acidotic and nonacidotic (incomplete) forms (2,11,29,43). Nephrolithiasis is particularly prevalent in the hereditary form of RTA-1 (2,20).

Stone Number

Three series have reported the number of stones in patients with RTA-1 (2,72,73). In two of these the number has not been remarkable (72,73). In our series, by contrast, the average number of stone-forming events was 51 ± 14 per patient (2). Our patients, therefore, resemble two anecdotal cases of type I with prodigious stone formation (66,74), and the group of 71 patients with accelerated stone formation reported by Coe et al. (75). Apparently, none of the patients in the series of Coe et al. had RTA-1.

Stone Type

Composition of stones is not often reported in patients with RTA-1. Theoretical considerations would predict, and several small series have reported only or predominantly calcium phosphate stones in these patients (61,72,73,76). However, there are two anecdotal reports of cases with mixed calcium phosphate and calcium oxalate stones (43,74). More recently, we have reported the largest series to date in which 30 stones from 26 patients were analyzed with somewhat surprising results (2). Only 4 were pure calcium phosphate, while 6 were pure calcium oxalate, 7 were struvite, and 13 were mixtures of calcium oxalate, phosphate, carbonate, and struvite. Thus the distribution of stone types in RTA-1 appears not to be radically different from that found in the entire population of calcium stone formers (77). The possible reasons for this will be examined.

Nephrocalcinosis

Many patients with RTA-1 have nephrocalcinosis, some of whom may not have nephrolithiasis. The overall prevalence is approximately 55% in hereditary RTA-1 (20) and may be approximately the same in the nonhereditary cases (71). It is interesting to note that Brenner et al. found that 73% of adults (age 18 years or greater) but only 29% of children had nephrocalcinosis (71). In our series, only 2 of 16 (6%) patients with RTA-1 less than age 18 had nephrocalcinosis, whereas 23 of 44 (52%) patients 18 years or greater had nephrocalcinosis (2). These observations suggest that nephrocalcinosis may be a function of the duration of the disease process (71), a possibility we discuss in more detail subsequently.

Pathophysiology

Nephrolithiasis and nephrocalcinosis in RTA-1 are promoted by a unique combination of risk factors that are not observed in other stone-forming states. These are hypercalciuria, low urine citrate concentration, and elevated urine pH. In addition, hyperuricosuria has recently been reported in some patients with RTA-1 and nephrolithiasis (2). In this section we review the pathophysiology of hypocitraturia and hypercalciuria. The mechanism of the elevated urine pH has been discussed earlier in this chapter.

Hypocitraturia

Decreased excretion of citrate, originally described by Fourman and Robinson in 1953 (78) and subsequently confirmed by numerous investigators (e.g., 79–82), is probably the most commonly occurring risk factor for stone formation in RTA-1. It appears to be present in most, but not all, cases of RTA-1 with nephrolithiasis (2,21).

Citrate, an organic anion formed by the Krebs cycle, undergoes glomerular filtration and reabsorption by the proximal tubules (83,84). Although some evidence suggests that tubular secretion of citrate can occur (85,86), this mechanism probably does not contribute significantly to urine citrate under most circumstances. The most important aspect of renal citrate handling for this discussion is the fact that citrate excretion is decreased by systemic acidosis and increased by alkalosis (83,87–

89). Recent studies have suggested several mechanisms that may account for this effect.

Tubular reabsorption of citrate occurs via a sodium-dependent synporter located on the brush border membrane which has high structural specificity for Krebs cycle intermediates (90–92). Several mechanisms have been identified by which changes in systemic acid base balance might alter citrate transport by this synporter. Most speculation has centered on the well-established fact that alkalosis increases and acidosis decreases renal tubular cell citrate content (93,94). This effect is probably due to the fact that alkalosis reduces citrate transport into mitochondria by inhibiting the mitochondrial tricarboxylate carrier, or that alkalosis reduces mitochondrial citrate uptake by inhibiting mitochondrial citrate oxidation (94,95). In either case the conclusion is that tubular reabsorption of citrate is inhibited by alkalosis and stimulated by acidosis because of the effects of acidosis and alkalosis on the tubular lumen to cell concentration gradient of citrate.

More recently, a different mechanism has been proposed to explain these observations. It has been shown that citrate uptake by brush border membrane vesicles (BBMV) increases with decreasing pH, an effect that may be due to changes in the concentration of the various ionic species of citrate (96–98). A similar effect of pH may explain observations in the isolated, perfused proximal tubule. Brennan et al. found that decreasing peritubular pH increased citrate reabsorption, an effect that could be abolished by preventing secondary alterations in luminal pH (99). These studies suggest that lowered intraluminal pH stimulates tubular citrate reabsorption by increasing the luminal concentration of the divalent form of citrate. This suggestion is compatible with the known pK_a values of citrate (2.91, 4.34, and 5.62) and the fact that divalent citrate appears to be the predominant form transported by the luminal synporter (96).

As a result of these various mechanisms, citrate excretion is exquisitely sensitive to changes in systemic acid-base balance and/or urine pH. For example, citrate excretion can be reduced by the mild acidification stimulus provided by a high-protein diet and increased by a low-protein diet (100). Potassium depletion, which also reduces citrate excretion, may do so by decreasing intracellular pH (87,101,102).

An effect of glomerular filtration rate on citrate excretion is possible, whereby decreased filtered load of citrate could reduce citrate excretion if fractional reabsorption remained constant. This effect may account in part for the fact that renal failure of whatever cause is associated with low citrate excretion (103–106).

These considerations have relevance to the question of why patients with RTA-1 have hypocitraturia. It may be that some patients have low citrate because of the combination of low GFR, acidosis, and/or potassium deple-

tion (21). However, a number of cases of IRTA have been reported with hypocitraturia who had neither hypokalemia nor low GFR (21). We have analyzed two reported series of IRTA with hypocitraturia for the presence or absence of known causes of hypocitraturia (2,21,107). In the series from Winston-Salem (2,21), 15 of 16 patients had at least one of the conditions known to cause hypocitraturia, whereas in the series from Dallas (107), only one of nine patients had one of these conditions. Despite this difference in incidence of known causes of hypocitraturia, citrate excretion was reduced to about 30% of normal in both groups (21). This similarity in the magnitude of reduction in citrate excretion suggests that acidosis, low GFR, and hypokalemia may not contribute substantially to the hypocitraturia of RTA-1. These observations are compatible with the suggestion that hypocitraturia in RTA-1 is due to a primary defect of proximal tubule function (1,2,16). Some have speculated that hypocitraturia and the defect in hydrogen ion secretion in RTA-1 is due to the same underlying cause (11,16). However, no direct evidence to support this speculation has been reported.

It has been suggested that hypocitraturia in IRTA may be due to the presence of an occult, intracellular acidosis (108), based on the observation that very large doses of bicarbonate are needed to correct the metabolic acidosis in some children with RTA-1 (48,109) and to increase urine citrate to normal in some patients with RTA (110,111). We think it unlikely that these observations indicate a generalized intracellular acidosis in patients without extracellular acidosis for the following reasons. First, the large amounts of bicarbonate required to correct acidosis in children with RTA-1 has been shown to be due to renal bicarbonate wasting (48). Second, most patients with IRTA in our experience do not require large doses of bicarbonate to normalize citrate excretion. Third, as noted, most patients with IRTA have normal net acid excretion despite a defect in lowering urine pH. There is no proposed mechanism by which individuals with normal blood bicarbonate, normal blood pH, and normal net acid excretion could generate or maintain a generalized intracellular acidosis. As we have noted, intracellular acidosis may be the cause of hypocitraturia associated with potassium depletion (92–94). However, potassium depletion severe enough to cause hypocitraturia should be associated with hypokalemia. Although some patients with IRTA and hypocitraturia have hypokalemia, many do not (21) and there is no reason to believe that patients with IRTA with a normal serum potassium concentration have an occult potassium depletion.

It is possible that an intracellular acidosis confined to the proximal tubule cells might explain decreased citrate excretion. If so, this would probably be due to some primary abnormality in proximal cell function which would not be predicted from any current understanding of the pathophysiology of RTA-1. In this regard it is interesting to note the suggestion that urine citrate excretion is an indirect index of proximal tubule cell pH (94) and the recent proposal that isolated proximal RTA (RTA-2) is due to a relative alkaline pH of proximal tubular cells (112). It could be that patients with IRTA have an abnormality of proximal tubule function opposite to that found in patients with isolated RTA-2.

Hypocitraturia of uncertain cause has also been found in patients with nephrolithiasis (104,105,113,114), some of whom have idiopathic hypercalciuria (IH) (115) (see Chs. 32 and 35). Hypocitraturia in the general stone-forming population has been attributed to renal failure (104,105) and to the acidifying effect of a high-protein diet (100,113). However, there have been few studies of citrate excretion in the general stone-forming population aimed at elucidating the mechanism of hypocitraturia and the possibility remains that, at least in some patients, the mechanism may be the same as that in RTA-1. As noted, when several characteristics of two reported series of patients with RTA-1 and hypocitraturia are compared with two reported series of patients with idiopathic hypocitraturic calcium oxalate nephrolithiasis, the most striking difference is the more severe degree of hypocitraturia in IRTA (21). Patients with IRTA excreted approximately 30% of the normal amount of citrate, whereas those with idiopathic nephrolithiasis excreted approximately 75% of the normal amount (21). It is possible that this marked difference in magnitude of abnormal citrate excretion indicates that hypocitraturia is due to a different mechanism in the two conditions. Alternatively, it could be that the two conditions share a similar mechanism with the more severe defect expressed in patients with RTA-1. This possibility is discussed more fully in a subsequent section of this chapter.

Clearly, the explanation for reduced citrate excretion in RTA and IH and for the difference in magnitude of the defect between the two conditions remains to be elucidated. Whatever the explanation may be, the large difference in excretion of citrate probably accounts for the fact that patients with IRTA form stones at more than a 10-fold faster rate than those with idiopathic hypocitraturic calcium oxalate nephrolithiasis (21).

Hypercalciuria

It was originally proposed that hypercalciuria in RTA-1 was due to some consequence of metabolic acidosis (18,19). It is now clear that this mechanism applies only to some patients with RTA-1. In others, hypercalciuria precedes the development of RTA and, in fact, is probably responsible for the development of RTA.

The concept that hypercalciuria is a consequence of the acidosis in RTA-1 is based on two lines of evidence. It has been shown that alkali therapy in some patients with the acidotic form of RTA-1 reduces calcium excretion (25,48,116). In addition, experimental metabolic acidosis induced by ammonium chloride loading increases renal calcium excretion by inhibiting tubular calcium reabsorption and by titrating bone calcium salts (117–119). However, it is clear that not all patients with acidotic RTA-1 have hypercalciuria. The reported prevalence of hypercalciuria in RTA has varied from 3 to 36% (28,119–121). In our series, hypercalciuria was present in 7 of 8 cases of hereditary RTA and 5 of 18 sporadic cases (2). It was found in none of 18 cases of secondary RTA. This kind of distribution is not supportive of the notion that hypercalciuria is caused by metabolic acidosis. Furthermore, some patients with the nonacidotic, *forme fruste* of RTA may have hypercalciuria (1,2,20). Although it is possible that the lack of hypercalciuria in some acidotic patients may be due to the presence of renal failure (2,20,43), the presence of hypercalciuria in the absence of acidosis clearly requires another explanation.

The explanation for the latter phenomenon was suggested by studies of a large family with hereditary RTA-1. Four cases of RTA were found in three successive generations, three of whom had IRTA (20). All four had hypercalciuria, nephrocalcinosis, and recurrent nephrolithiasis. In addition, 15 family members had hypercalciuria, none of whom had RTA and only two of whom had nephrocalcinosis or nephrolithiasis. Thus most of the individuals affected had asymptomatic hypercalciuria, which would not have been detected otherwise. These studies led to the hypothesis outlined in Fig. 3, which suggests that RTA may be due to distal tubule damage resulting from longstanding, hereditary hypercalciuria. One large family showing a similar pathophysiology has been reported in detail since the original one (122), and four small families observed in our series have recently been reported in brief (2). In addition, one other large family with similar findings has been investigated but not yet reported (O. Wrong, personal communication).

The suggestion that hypercalciuria in these families is hereditary is supported by recent evidence indicating that idiopathic hypercalciuria is familial in most cases (123,124) (see Chapter 32). Thus hereditary RTA with hypercalciuria is, in many cases, probably a variant of familial idiopathic hypercalciuria (20). If this hypothesis is correct, the fact that a majority of families with hypercalciuria do not develop nephrocalcinosis and RTA-1 represents an interesting puzzle.

The existence of this pathophysiology for hypercalciuria also raises an interesting nosologic dilemma. In one sense, RTA in patients with familial hypercalciuria is secondary to the hypercalciuria and they should be classified as having secondary RTA. However, since this type of RTA usually occurs in families and is probably a variant of a genetic condition, it can be classified as a hereditary form of RTA, as we have suggested (20).

Thus hypercalciuria in RTA-1 appears to have two causes: metabolic acidosis and a heredo-familial disorder of uncertain nature. For purposes of genetic counseling it may be important to determine which of the two causes is operative. In individuals with incomplete RTA and hypercalciuria, the genetic disorder is probably present. In individuals with metabolic acidosis, the response of urine calcium excretion to alkali therapy may be informative, although somewhat difficult to interpret. It would be expected that alkali therapy would reduce calcium excretion in any person with metabolic acidosis (117–119). In fact, alkali therapy in the form of potassium citrate may reduce calcium excretion in individuals without metabolic acidosis (125,126), including those with incomplete RTA (127). Presumably, this is due to the effect of intraluminal pH on renal tubular calcium reabsorption (126). Interestingly, the hypocalciuric effect is not observed with alkali in the form of sodium salts (128), possibly because the tendency for sodium salts to reduce tubular calcium reabsorption cancels out the effect of the alkali to increase tubular calcium reabsorption (128). Accordingly, acidotic patients with RTA-1 may respond to alkali with a reduction in calcium excretion. In that case, determination that a heredo-familial disorder was present would require study of family members.

Hyperuricosuria

Hyperuricosuria is a well-recognized risk factor for stone development in the non-RTA stone-forming population (see Chapter 35). We have recently reported increased uric acid excretion in 8 of 31 (23%) RTA patients with nephrolithiasis (2). This is a prevalence similar to that found in the general population of patients with stones (129). Curiously, the patients with hyperuricosuria had fewer stones than those without it (2).

Lithogenesis

The physiochemical basis for calcium stone formation is detailed in Chs. 29, 31–33, 35. Therefore, we discuss this topic in relation to RTA only briefly. As noted, stone formation in patients with RTA-1 is promoted by three factors found in some patients without RTA-1: hypocitraturia, hypercalciuria, and hyperuricosuria. In addition, patients with RTA-1 have increased urine pH. It is not known whether other abnormalities such as decreased excretion of protein inhibitors of crystal growth occur in RTA-1.

The relative importance of these lithogenic factors in RTA-1 is not known. Elevated urine pH increases activity product of the calcium phosphate salts and the activity product ratio for brushite, octocalcium phosphate, and hydroxyapatite (130,131). Therefore, since calcium phosphate stones are rare in idiopathic stone formers, their formation in patients with RTA-1 is undoubtedly due primarily to increased urine pH. However, as noted, patients with RTA-1 do not form calcium phosphate stones exclusively (2). Citrate reduces urinary saturation of calcium phosphate and calcium oxalate (132) and inhibits the spontaneous nucleation of calcium phosphate (133), which might secondarily reduce nucleation of calcium oxalate since the former may promote heterogenous nucleation of the latter (131). Trace metal citric acid complexes may inhibit calcium phosphate and calcium oxalate crystal growth (134,135). In addition, citrate has recently been shown to have a major inhibitory effect on calcium oxalate crystal agglomeration (136). Therefore, since many patients with RTA-1 have increased activity product for calcium oxalate as well as calcium phosphate (107,130), it seems likely that hypocitraturia plays a major role in promoting calcium oxalate stone formation. This hypothesis is also supported by the effect of alkali therapy to reduce stone formation in hypocitraturic RTA-1 despite the fact that it also increases urine pH (see below).

The prevalence of the risk factors that increase the risk of nephrolithiasis is not known with certainty. As we noted earlier, hypercalciuria has been reported in from 3 to 36% of cases (28,119–121) and was 32% in our recent series of 34 cases (2). Hypocitraturia is probably present in most cases. However, several patients have been reported with hypercalciuria without hypocitraturia (21,137). No patients have been reported with nephrolithiasis who did not have either hypercalciuria or hypocitraturia, although that circumstance remains a possibility.

There are some interesting similarities between stone formation in the general population of calcium stone formers and those with RTA-1. As noted, the two populations share three of the same risk factors: hypercalciuria, hypocitraturia, and hyperuricosuria. Furthermore, the prevalence of the common risk factors in patients with idiopathic hypocitraturia and calcium nephrolithiasis and patients with RTA-1 with hypocitraturia are similar, as shown in Table 8. The major difference between the two groups appears to be the number of stones formed in the patients with RTA-1. This could be due to the fact that citrate excretion on average is much lower in RTA-1 than in idiopathic hypocitraturia (21).

These similarities suggest some underlying connection between the pathophysiology of nephrolithiasis in RTA-1 and in some patients with idiopathic nephrolithiasis. Furthermore, it is possible that there is some underlying connection between the presence of risk factors for stone formation and the pathophysiology of RTA-1. One such connection has already been recognized. That is, some cases of RTA-1 are caused by idiopathic hypercalciuria (20). Since the latter is a hereditary disorder (123,124), it seems likely that many kindred with hereditary RTA-1 actually have hereditary idiopathic hypercalciuria. As discussed earlier (Fig. 3), it is postulated that hypercal-

TABLE 8. *Idiopathic hypocitraturic calcium-oxalate nephrolithiasis versus hypocitraturic RTA-1*

	Idiopathic		RTA-1	
	Pak and Fuller	Kok and Associates	Caruana and Buckalew	Preminger and Nicar and Associates
Number of cases	37	7	16	9
Urine citrate				
(% low normal)	70	80 ± 7	34 ± 8	29
Hypercalciuria (%)	18 (49)	0	6 (37.5)	? (<100)[a]
Hyperuricosuria (%)	2 (17)	0	5/14 (36)	0
Stone rate				
(no./yr; 3 yr)	136 ± 245	—	52 ± 14	13.1 ± 26.6

Source: Reprinted with permission from Ref. 21.
[a] Mean calcium excretion ± standard deviation 238 ± 73 mg/dL (intake 400 mg/dL).

ciuria causes a defect in acidification either because of prolonged exposure of the lumenal membrane of the distal tubule to high relative saturation ratios of calcium salts or because of tissue damage produced by the development of recurrent nephrolithiasis and/or overt nephrocalcinosis.

It is possible that hypocitraturia may also lead to distal tubule damage and the development of RTA-1 by an analogous mechanism (21). Similar to hypercalciuria, hypocitraturia can lead to increased relative saturation ratios of calcium salts and recurrent nephrolithiasis and/or nephrocalcinosis. Although there is no direct evidence for the hypothesis that hypocitraturia can cause a distal defect in acidification, there is one piece of indirect evidence. If idiopathic hypocitraturia were the primary hereditary defect in families with RTA-1 and hypocitraturia, there should be some cases in which hypocitraturia occurs in the absence of a defect in urine acidification. Thus it is interesting to note that in the family reported by Norman et al. (111), a 5-year-old female with profound hypocitraturia but without a defect in acidification was reported.

These considerations led us to suggest the following hypothesis (21). Both hypercalciuria and hypocitraturia are primary defects determined by independent genetic mechanisms which may occur alone or in combination. When either one occurs alone, it may lead to the appear-

ance of three basic phenotypes. For example, hypocitraturia may occur as idiopathic hypocitraturia, as idiopathic hypocitraturia with nephrolithiasis, or as idiopathic hypocitraturic RTA-1. Similarly, idiopathic hypercalciuria may occur as idiopathic hypercalciuria with or without hematuria (138), as idiopathic hypercalciuria with nephrolithiasis, or as RTA-1 with hypercalciuria. In some cases, idiopathic hypocitraturia and hypercalciuria may occur in the same person. In that case, three additional phenotypes would be found, which would be combinations of the three basic phenotypes caused by the primary defect alone. Thus two genetically determined primary abnormalities could result in the appearance of nine phenotypes.

This hypothesis extends the one proposed previously (20) to account for the appearance of several phenotypes in families with RTA-1 and hypercalciuria. It can be tested by more extensive studies of families in which RTA-1 occurs with hypocitraturia without hypercalciuria and by studies of the families of individuals with idiopathic hypercalciuria and hypocitraturia.

Treatment

The treatment of stones in RTA-1, as in any other stone-forming condition, involves modification of the risk factors that lead to stone formation. Except for the

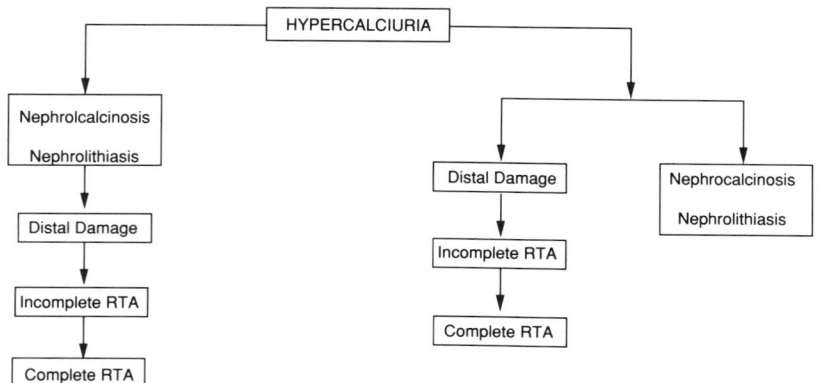

FIG. 3. Proposed pathophysiology of type I RTA in patients with hereditary hypercalciuria. In one group of families (*left*), hypercalciuria appears to cause a defect in distal hydrogen secretion by causing nephrocalcinosis and nephrolithiasis. In another group of families (*right*), hypercalciuria appears to cause distal tubular damage and a defect in hydrogen ion secretion directly and may also cause nephrocalcinosis and nephrolithiasis. (Reprinted from Ref. 1, p. 365, by courtesy of Marcel Dekker, Inc.)

tendency for an inappropriately alkaline urine, the stone-promoting risk factors vary in different individuals with RTA. Yet elevated urine pH is the one risk factor about which nothing can be done. Therefore, therapy for stones in patients with RTA-1 is similar to therapy in the general stone-forming population. Those patients with hypercalciuria without hypocitraturia should be treated with measures to reduce calcium excretion. Those patients with hypocitraturia without hypercalciuria should be treated with measures that increase urine citrate excretion. Patients with both hypercalciuria and hypocitraturia may require measures to reduce both risk factors. This potentially complex situation is simplified by the fortuitous fact that certain forms of alkali therapy can both reduce calcium excretion and increase urine citrate excretion.

Alkali

Alkali has been used to treat metabolic acidosis in RTA-1 since the condition was first described (18). The observation that alkali reduced calcium excretion in these cases led to the suggestion that hypercalciuria in RTA-1 was caused by metabolic acidosis (48), a point we discussed earlier in this chapter. Although alkali was first shown to have beneficial effects on nephrocalcinosis and nephrolithiasis in acidotic RTA-1 in 1957 (74), its regular use to reduce stone formation in complete and incomplete RTA is a relatively recent development.

After some initial confusion (73,79,80,82,140), it was shown unequivocally in 1963 that alkali could increase renal citrate excretion in RTA-1 with hypocitraturia (110). As a result, the suggestion was made that alkali would be an appropriate treatment for nephrolithiasis and nephrocalcinosis in incomplete RTA (139). However, there was a reluctance to treat patients with hypocitraturic incomplete RTA-1 and nephrolithiasis with alkali because it was feared that the increase in urine pH might increase stone formation by increasing the saturation indices for calcium phosphate (130,131). Nevertheless, the first few cases were treated with alkali in the early 1960s without deterioration. If anything, there was improvement (139). These observations have led to more recent studies which have confirmed this impression (21).

Sodium bicarbonate was the alkalinizing agent used initially. However, recent studies have pointed out the advantages of potassium citrate (107,115,133,141–145). Both salts are equally effective in increasing urine citrate excretion. However, citrate, but not bicarbonate salts, can be formulated into wax matrix tablets, which produces a more prolonged, sustained effect. The use of potassium rather than sodium as the cation is based on the fact that potassium citrate causes a reduction in calcium excretion in IRTA, whereas sodium bicarbonate does not (107,128). The mechanism for this difference is not

entirely clear but may be explained by the effect of sodium on renal calcium excretion. Alkali administration should reduce calcium excretion because of the effect of increased intratubular pH to increase tubular calcium reabsorption. Conversely, sodium salts, including bicarbonate, might tend to decrease tubular calcium reabsorption by increasing extracellular fluid volume. This volume expansion effect would not occur with a potassium salt. Thus the opposing effects of sodium bicarbonate may result in no change in renal calcium excretion.

The effects of potassium citrate on nine patients with IRTA and nephrolithiasis have recently been reported (107). The relative saturation ratio for calcium oxalate was reduced from 5.73 ± 2.08 to 3.14 ± 1.23 with no effect on the RSR for brushite or sodium urate. Citrate excretion increased from 221 ± 163 to 494 ± 304 mg/day and calcium excretion decreased from 238 ± 73 to 164 ± 61 mg/day. Urine pH increased from 6.47 ± 0.28 to 7.05 ± 0.16. Stone formation rate decreased dramatically from 13.1 ± 26.6 to 1.15 ± 2.23 per year. These studies show clearly that the increase in urine pH does not increase lithogenesis in hypocitraturia RTA-1. Rather, the increase in citrate concentration and the decrease in calcium excretion bring about a beneficial decrease in RSR for calcium oxalate. It should be noted that the decrease in lithogenic potential occurs only for calcium oxalate. Thus citrate therapy might not be expected to decrease the number of phosphate stones as dramatically as calcium oxalate stones. The fact that citrate therapy did reduce stones dramatically underscores the fact, noted earlier in this chapter, that most stones in RTA-1 are calcium oxalate or mixed calcium oxalate/phosphate, not pure calcium phosphate as had been suggested earlier.

Other Therapies

These considerations would suggest that potassium citrate might be beneficial in all patients with RTA-1 and nephrolithiasis. However, as we discussed, some patients with RTA-1 have hypercalciuria without hypocitraturia. This is most likely to occur in families in which RTA-1 is secondary to idiopathic hypercalciuria. In those cases, the same measures used to treat idiopathic hypercalciuria, discussed fully in Chapter 32, might be beneficial. We have reported one such patient in whom a thiazide diuretic reduced renal calcium excretion. In another such case (unreported), thiazide diuretic therapy eliminated stone formation. Other therapies such as orthophosphate and cellulose phosphate might be useful in these patients.

Mild hyperparathyroidism of uncertain cause has been reported in RTA-1 (146). One case with refractory nephrolithiasis and hyperparathyroidism has been reported in which subtotal parathyroidectomy caused reduction in the number of stones formed (76).

Genetic Considerations

The familial occurrence of RTA-1 has therapeutic implications. It is common to obtain a family history of stones in patients with nephrolithiasis (see Chs. 31–33). A history of stones in other family members raises the possibility that the family has a hereditary form of RTA. If this possibility proves to be true, and if the family has the hypercalciuric type of hereditary RTA, it is likely that some family members have asymptomatic hypercalciuria. If the family has RTA with hypocitraturia, it is possible that some family members have asymptomatic hypocitraturia. If the hypothesis that long-standing hypercalciuria or hypocitraturia leads to the development of nephrocalcinosis and distal tubule damage is correct (Fig. 3), it is possible that this complication could be prevented by early treatment of the hypercalciuria and/or the hypocitraturia. These considerations would be particularly relevant and important with regard to children.

Based on these considerations, we recommend that patients with nephrolithiasis and hypercalciuria or hypocitraturia and a positive family history for nephrolithiasis should be investigated to determine whether they have RTA-1. If they do, first-degree relatives should be investigated for hypercalciuria or hypocitraturia regardless of whether they have a history of stones or not. Any individuals found to have hypercalciuria should be counseled to avoid a high-calcium diet and to consume an adequate fluid intake. Any individuals found to have hypocitraturia should be treated with potassium citrate to normalize citrate excretion.

TYPE II RENAL TUBULAR ACIDOSIS

Etiology and Nosology

Type II RTA is a much rarer condition than RTA-1. It may occur as an isolated condition, sometimes in families (147). More commonly, type II RTA is observed as one component of Fanconi syndrome (FS), a diffuse disorder of proximal tubular function including decreased reabsorption of bicarbonate (16,17). FS is the result of a variety of disorders that are listed in Table 5.

Pathophysiology of Metabolic Acidosis

As noted earlier, the metabolic acidosis of type II RTA results from decreased reabsorption of bicarbonate by the proximal tubule. The generation of metabolic acidosis in this condition can be simulated and has been studied carefully in three situations: in patients with hereditary fructose intolerance on a low-fructose diet who are infused with fructose (148), in patients whose acidosis has been corrected with bicarbonate loading in whom the bicarbonate is discontinued (3,16,49,50), and in dogs and rats given maleic acid (16).

The pathogenesis of the acidosis includes a transient generation phase and a steady-state maintenance phase. The generation phase occurs as the plasma bicarbonate falls from a normal value to its steady-state reduced value. The actual value of the plasma bicarbonate during the maintenance phase is a manifestation of the "set point" or renal threshold for bicarbonate reabsorption, and varies among individuals with the condition. For most patients, the value is in the range 15–16 mEq/L (16,49,50). During generation of the acidosis, urine pH is abnormally alkaline (i.e., above 5.5). During the maintenance phase, however, urine pH is less than 5.5 and urine ammonia is not reduced since distal acid excretion mechanisms are intact (16).

Metabolic acidosis accounts for growth retardation in children with type II RTA (48). Other clinical manifestations associated with type II RTA and FS, except for those related to mineral metabolism, will not be discussed here.

Hypercalciuria, Nephrolithiasis, and Nephrocalcinosis

Hypercalciuria is not a common feature of type II RTA with FS except in cases of Wilson's disease (WD) (16). Because of this apparent unique feature of WD, it will be discussed separately later in this chapter. There are a few reported cases of FS with hypercalciuria, with or without nephrolithiasis and nephrocalcinosis who did not have WD (16,149–153). Most of these cases have had concomitant bone disease and one was found to have a high-normal plasma concentration of 1,25-dihydroxy vitamin D_3 (153). Although not well studied, it appears that hypercalciuria when it does occur in FS is corrected or markedly reduced by correction of the acidosis and healing of the bone disease (151). Urine citrate excretion, when measured, has been normal in FS despite the presence of metabolic acidosis and hypokalemia (154,155). This may be due to decreased tubular reabsorption of citrate secondary to the diffuse abnormality in proximal tubular transport (155). It is possible that in contrast to RTA-1, normal urine citrate may prevent to some extent the development of nephrolithiasis and nephrocalcinosis when hypercalciuria is also present (154).

As we have already noted, it is not clear why all patients with type II RTA do not have hypercalciuria. Considerable evidence suggests that renal tubular calcium reabsorption is pH sensitive such that metabolic acidosis should inhibit tubular calcium reabsorption (118,156). Therefore, any metabolic acidosis should be accompanied by hypercalciuria. Two explanations have been offered to explain this apparent anomaly. It has been shown in dogs that increased bicarbonate delivery to the distal tubule causes increased distal calcium reabsorption (125). Therefore, during the generation phase of type II RTA, bicarbonate flooding of the distal tubule could prevent the developing acidosis from causing hypercalciuria. However, during the maintenance phase of the acidosis, proximal bicarbonate is complete, so that there is no increase in distal bicarbonate delivery (see above). This mechanism does not explain, therefore, the lack of hypercalciuria in the steady state.

Another possible explanation is based on the concept of acid balance. It has been shown that net hydrogen ion production from the metabolism of acid producing foods and the excretion of organic anions (Tables 1 and 2) exactly equals the excretion of acid by the kidney (117). Accordingly, normal individuals are in "acid balance." Patients with the acidosis of chronic renal failure are in positive acid balance. That is, they produce more hydrogen ions than are excreted (117). It has been postulated that the retained hydrogen ions are buffered by calcium carbonate in bone, resulting in titration of bone and an increased calcium excretion by the kidney (117). It is implied from the pathophysiology of type II RTA discussed earlier that patients with steady-state acidosis would have an intact ability to generate new bicarbonate and would therefore be able to maintain acid balance normally. In that case, bone mineral would not be titrated preventing the development of hypercalciuria. This explanation, like the foregoing one, does not explain why the acidosis itself does not decrease tubular calcium reabsorption.

Type II RTA in Patients with Nephrolithiasis

Renal bicarbonate wasting (type II RTA) has been reported to occur with varying frequency in several series of patients with nephrolithiasis (157–159). In the study of Backman et al., 34 of 310 stone formers (11%) were said to have an "incomplete" form of type II RTA (157). This diagnosis was based on the fact that during acid loading, urine pH as a function of plasma bicarbonate concentration was shifted to the left of normals with urine pH of less than 5.0 eventually being obtained at plasma bicarbonate concentrations less than 15 mEq/L. This finding was interpreted by these investigators as indicating the presence of a proximal leak of bicarbonate insufficient to cause metabolic acidosis, but sufficient to prevent the full expression of normal distal acidifying capacity, hence "incomplete" type II RTA.

Using bicarbonate loading studies, these investigators also found 3 patients (1%) with classic type II RTA (metabolic acidosis plus a reduced renal tubular maximum for bicarbonate reabsorption). In addition, they found 4 other patients (1%) who excreted 15% or more of the filtered load of bicarbonate during bicarbonate loading, none of whom had metabolic acidosis.

There are several problems with the interpretation of these studies by Backman et al. In the first place, the concept of an "incomplete" form of type II RTA is not in accord with current concepts of the pathophysiology of metabolic acidosis in that condition as discussed earlier. Accordingly, a decrease in the tubular maximum for proximal bicarbonate reabsorption should always produce a metabolic acidosis with a urine pH of less than 5.5 in the maintenance phase. Second, the shift in the urine pH versus bicarbonate curve observed by these investigators is consistent with a defect in acidification mechanisms intrinsic to the distal tubule (i.e., RTA-1) (1). Thus patients with RTA-1 may lower urine pH to less than 5.5 if the plasma bicarbonate concentration is low enough (1). According to this argument, most of the patients that Backman et al. labeled as incomplete type II RTA would be diagnosed as having incomplete RTA-1, some of whom have bicarbonate wasting during bicarbonate loading.

Another problem with the report by Backman et al. is the four patients who excreted more than 15% of the filtered load of bicarbonate yet did not have metabolic acidosis. According to current concepts, all patients with a defect in bicarbonate reabsorption of that magnitude should have metabolic acidosis (16).

Tessitore et al. (158) reported a study in 28 adults with recurrent calcium nephrolithiasis, 19 of whom had "renal hypercalciuria." The latter designation was based on an elevated fasting urinary calcium. Eight of 28 stone formers (26%), all of whom had hypercalciuria, had a reduced tubular maximum for bicarbonate associated with a decreased plasma bicarbonate concentration indicating the presence of type II RTA. This study suggests a very high prevalence of type II RTA in renal hypercalciuria which has not been reported by other investigators.

Jaeger et al. found that 13 of 37 (35%) stone formers had an increased fractional excretion of bicarbonate during loading with alkali salts of calcium (159). Calcium salts were used rather than sodium salts to prevent the stimulation of PTH secretion by a fall in serum-ionized calcium which itself might interfere with proximal bicarbonate reabsorption (16). These investigators also showed a number of other defects in tubular function in many of the stone formers, including increased fractional excretion of glucose, insulin, phosphate, and enzymes such as lysozyme and γ-glutamyltransferase (159). Of interest was the fact that these abnormalities of tubular function were not confined to any type of condition, but appeared to be distributed among all the diagnostic groups, which included primary hyperparathyroidism, medullary sponge kidney, hyperuricemia, cystinuria, struvite stone disease, idiopathic hypercalciuria, and normocalciuric idiopathic urolithiasis. Their interpretation of this observation was that the abnormalities in tubular function were secondary to the stone disease, an idea supported by the fact that the defects were related to the presence of large stones in the pelvocalyceal system. Although this interpretation is reasonable based on their findings, the issue as to the type, incidence, and cause of renal tubular defects in stone-forming populations raised by these and other studies (160) has not been finally settled.

WILSON'S DISEASE

Wilson's disease (WD) is a rare, autosomal recessive disorder in which excess copper accumulates in various tissues. The condition affects the kidneys (Table 9), but the exact prevalence of renal involvement is not known. Of importance for this discussion is the fact that some patients have hypercalciuria, nephrolithiasis, and both types I and II RTA. In this section we discuss the relationships among these complications.

Hypercalciuria

Hypercalciuria was first reported in Wilson's disease in 1950 (161). The first series of cases was reported from the Mayo Clinic in 1959, showing that 4 of 5 patients with Wilson's disease had hypercalciuria (162). Most other reports of hypercalciuria have been isolated, single cases (163–169).

The cause of hypercalciuria in WD is not known. It has been suggested that hypercalciuria in WD is a component of FS (168). However, hypercalciuria is not always present in FS and when present is usually accompanied by metabolic acidosis, as we have already noted. In WD, most reported cases with hypercalciuria do not have acidosis. Playoust and Dale reported an interesting case in 1961 in which hypercalciuria developed fully 3 years after the diagnosis of WD was first made (163). The only evidence of renal involvement at the time hypercalciuria was first noted was aminoaciduria and a renal biopsy was normal. Cortisone administration reduced renal calcium excretion without affecting intestinal calcium absorp-

tion. These investigators suggested that hypercalciuria was due to a skeletal disorder, perhaps secondary to copper deposits in bone (163).

Renal Tubular Acidosis

An abnormally alkaline urine in WD was first reported in 1957, but no investigation into its cause was performed (170). In 1968, two series were published almost simultaneously showing that a defect in lowering urine pH (i.e., RTA-1) was common in WD (165,171). In the report by Walshe (171), the defect in acidification was found to be reversible by long-term penicillamine therapy, showing that the defect in tubular function was due to copper deposits, not to penicillamine. The first report of type II RTA in WD was in 1974 (166). In that report, only 2 of 13 patients had type II RTA, whereas 9 of 13 had type I. Thus although WD is often cited as a cause of type II RTA, RTA-1 is actually more common in these patients. There appears to be no correlation between the presence of RTA and hypercalciuria since many of the reported cases of RTA do not have hypercalciuria (165,167).

Nephrolithiasis

In 1959, Litin et al. reported one case of WD with bilateral nephrocalcinosis and one with a stone in one kidney (162). One of 12 patients reported by Fulop et al. in 1968 had nephrocalcinosis (165). In a series published in 1974 from the Mayo Clinic 2 of 13 patients had nephrolithiasis (166). In a larger series from the same clinic in 1979, 7 of 45 patients had nephrolithiasis (167). It is not clear whether the two cases reported in 1974 are included in the 1979 publication.

With so few cases reported, it is not surprising that the pathophysiology of nephrolithiasis in WD is unclear. The best information is contained in the report of seven cases from the Mayo Clinic (167). Three of the seven had hypercalciuria. Only five were studied by ammonium chloride loading, four of which had RTA-1. Tubular maximum for bicarbonate reabsorption was determined in four stone formers, one of which had RTA-2. It was not clear from the paper whether the one patient with RTA-2 also had RTA-1. It was also not clear whether the patients with RTA were the ones who also had hypercalciuria. Stones from two patients were composed mainly of calcium phosphate and some calcium carbonate.

These studies suggest that nephrolithiasis in WD is a consequence of RTA-1 and hypercalciuria. This impression is supported by the other reported cases, most of which had either RTA-1, hypercalciuria, or both. There is only one documented case of nephrolithiasis in a patient with WD who had isolated RTA-2 (169). That patient had hypercalciuria, which appeared to be due to the

TABLE 9. Renal abnormalities in Wilson's disease

1. Hematuria
2. Proximal tubular dysfunction
   a. Proteinuria (low molecular weight)
   b. Aminoaciduria
   c. Fanconi syndrome
      i. Phosphaturia
      ii. Uricosuria
      iii. Bicarbonaturia (type II RTA)
3. Distal tubular dysfunction
   a. Acidification defect (type I RTA)
   b. Concentrating defect (nephrogenic DI)
4. Hypercalciuria
5. Nephrolithiasis and nephrocalcinosis
6. Renal failure
   a. Acute (secondary hemolytic anemia)
   b. Chronic
7. Complications of penicillamine

acidosis, since it was largely corrected by alkali treatment.

REFERENCES

1. Buckalew VM Jr, Caruana RJ. The pathophysiology of distal (type 1) renal tubular acidosis. In: Gonick HC, Buckalew VM Jr, eds. *Renal tubular disorders: pathophysiology, diagnosis, and management.* New York: Marcel Dekker, 1985;357–86.
2. Caruana RJ, Buckalew VM Jr. The syndrome of distal (type 1) renal tubular acidosis: clinical and laboratory findings in 58 cases. *Medicine* 1988;67:84–99.
3. Morris RC Jr. Renal tubular acidosis: mechanisms, classification and implications. *N Engl J Med* 1969;281:1405–13.
4. Batlle DC, Kurtzman NA. Renal regulation of acid-base homeostasis: integrated response. In: Seldin DW, Giebish G, eds. *The kidney: physiology and pathophysiology.* New York: Raven Press, 1985;539–1565.
5. Halperin ML, Goldstein MB, Stinebaugh BJ, Richardson RMA. Renal tubular acidosis. In: Maxwell MH, Kleeman CR, Narins RG, eds. *Clinical disorders of fluid and electrolyte metabolism.* New York: McGraw-Hill, 1987;675–89.
6. Walser M. Roles of urea production, ammonium excretion, and amino acid oxidation in acid-base balance. *Am J Physiol* 1986;250:F181–8.
7. Huckabee WE. Relationship of pyruvate and lactate during anaerobic metabolism. I. Effects of infusion of pyruvate or glucose and of hyperventilation. *J Clin Invest* 1958;37:244–54.
8. Stryer L. *Biochemistry,* 3rd ed. New York: WH Freeman, 1988.
9. Brown JC, Packer RK, Knepper MA. Role of organic anions in renal response to dietary acid and base loads. *Am J Physiol* 1989;257:F170–6.
10. Lennon EJ, Lemann J Jr, Litzow JR. The effects of diet and stool composition on the net external acid balance of normal subjects. *J Clin Invest* 1966;45:1601–7.
11. Wrong O, Davies HEF. The excretion of acid in renal disease. *Q J Med* 1959;28:259–313.
12. Halperin ML, Goldstein MB, Stinebaugh BJ, Jungas RL. Biochemistry and physiology of ammonium excretion. In: Seldin DW, Giebisch G, eds. *The kidney: physiology and pathophysiology.* New York: Raven Press, 1985;1471–90.
13. Halperin ML. How much "new" bicarbonate is formed in the distal nephron in the process of net acid excretion? *Kidney Int* 1989;35:1277–81.
14. Knepper MA, Burg MB. Renal acid-base transport. In: Schrier RW, Gottschalk CW, eds. *Diseases of the kidney.* Boston: Little, Brown: 1988;211–39.
15. Edelmann CM Jr. Isolated proximal (type 2) renal tubular acidosis. In: Gonick HC, Buckalew VM Jr, eds. *Renal tubular disorders: pathophysiology, diagnosis, and management.* New York: Marcel Dekker, 1985;261–79.
16. Morris RC Jr, Sebastian A. Renal tubular acidosis and Fanconi syndrome. In: Stanbury JB, Wyngaarden JB, Frederickson DS, Goldstein JL, Brown MS, eds. *The metabolic basis of inherited disease,* 5th ed. New York: McGraw-Hill, 1983;1808–43.
17. Brewer ED. The Fanconi syndrome: clinical disorders. In: Gonick HC, Buckalew VM Jr, eds. *Renal tubular disorders: pathophysiology, diagnosis, and management,* New York: Marcel Dekker, 1985;475–544.
18. Albright F, Consolazio WV, Coombs FS, Sulkowitch HW, Talbott JH. Metabolic studies and therapy in a case of nephrocalcinosis with rickets and dwarfism. *Bull Johns Hopkins Hosp* 1940;66:7–33.
19. Albright F, Reifenstein EC Jr. *The parathyroid glands and metabolic bone disease: selected studies.* Baltimore: Williams & Wilkins, 1948.
20. Buckalew VM Jr, Purvis ML, Shulman MG, Herndon CN, Rudman D. Hereditary renal tubular acidosis: report of a 64 member kindred with variable clinical expression including idiopathic hypercalciuria. *Medicine* 1974;53:229–54.
21. Buckalew VM Jr. Nephrolithiasis in renal tubular acidosis. *J Urol* 1989;141:731–7.
22. Sebastian A, Schambelan M, Hulter HN, et al. Hyperkalemic renal tubular acidosis. In: Gonick HC, Buckalew VM Jr, eds. *Renal tubular disorders: pathophysiology, diagnosis, and management,* New York: Marcel Dekker, 1985;307–56.
23. Caruana RJ, Buckalew VM Jr, Lorentz WB. Renal tubular disorders. In: Gonick HC, ed. *Current nephrology,* vol 6. New York: John Wiley & Sons, 1983;51–73.
24. Nance WE, Sweeney A. Evidence for autosomal recessive inheritance of the syndrome of renal tubular acidosis with deafness. *Birth Defects* 1971;7:70–2.
25. Bentur L, Alon U, Mandel H, Pery M, Berant M. Familial distal renal tubular acidosis with neurosensory deafness: early nephrocalcinosis. *Am J Nephrol* 1989;9:470–4.
26. Shapira E, Ben-Yoseph Y, Eyal FG, Russell A. Enzymatically inactive red cell carbonic anhydrase B in a family with renal tubular acidosis. *J Clin Invest* 1974;53:59–63.
27. Sly WS, Whyte MP, Sundaram V, et al. Carbonic anhydrase II deficiency in 12 families with the autosomal recessive syndrome of osteopetrosis with renal tubular acidosis and cerebral calcification. *N Engl J Med* 1985;313:139–45.
28. Wrong OM, Feest TG. The natural history of distal renal tubular acidosis. *Contrib Nephrol* 1980;21:137–44.
29. Caruana RJ, Barish CF, Buckalew VM Jr. Complete distal renal tubular acidosis in systemic lupus: clinical and laboratory findings. *Am J Kidney Dis* 1985;6:59–63.
30. Batlle DC, Kurtzman NA. The defect in distal (type 1) renal tubular acidosis. In: Gonick HC, Buckalew VM Jr, eds. *Renal tubular disorders: pathophysiology, diagnosis, and management,* New York: Marcel Dekker, 1985;281–305.
31. Batlle DC, Sabatini S, Kurtzman NA. On the mechanism of toluene-induced renal tubular acidosis. *Nephron* 1988;49:210–8.
32. Berry CA, Warnock DG. Acidification in the in vitro perfused tubule. *Kidney Int* 1982;22:507–18.
33. Halperin ML, Goldstein MB, Haig A, Johnson MD, Stinebaugh BJ. Studies on the pathogenesis of type I (distal) renal tubular acidosis as revealed by the urinary PCO2 tensions. *J Clin Invest* 1974;53:669–77.
34. Berliner RW. Carbon dioxide tension of alkaline urine. In: Seldin DW, Giebisch G, eds. *The kidney: physiology and pathophysiology.* New York: Raven Press, 1985;1527–37.
35. Tannen RL, Falls WF Jr, Brackett NC Jr. Incomplete renal tubular acidosis: Some clinical and physiological features. *Nephron* 1975;15:111–23.
36. Seldin DW, Rector FC, Portwood R, Carter N. Pathogenesis of hyperchloremic acidosis in renal tubular acidosis. In: *Proceedings of the 1st international congress of nephrology,* Geneva, 1961;725.
37. Seldin DW, Wilson JD. Renal tubular acidosis. In: Stanbury JB, Wyngaarden JB, Fredrickson DS, eds. *The metabolic basis of inherited disease,* 2nd ed. New York: McGraw-Hill, 1966;1230.
38. Batlle DC, Hizon M, Cohen E, Gutterman C, Gupta R. The use of the urinary anion gap in the diagnosis of hyperchloremic metabolic acidosis. *N Engl J Med* 1988;318:594–9.
39. Gill JR Jr, Bell NH, Bartter FC. Impaired conservation of sodium and potassium in renal tubular acidosis and its correction by buffer anions. *Clin Sci* 1967;33:577–92.
40. Berliner RW. Renal mechanisms for potassium excretion. *Harvey Lect* 1960;55:141–71.
41. Wright FS, Giebisch G. Regulation of potassium excretion. In: Seldin DW, Giebisch G, eds. *The kidney: physiology and pathophysiology.* New York: Raven Press, 1985;1223–49.
42. Sebastian A, McSherry E, Morris RC Jr. Renal potassium wasting in renal tubular acidosis (RTA): its occurrence in types 1 and 2 RTA despite sustained correction of systemic acidosis. *J Clin Invest* 1971;50:667–78.
43. Buckalew VM Jr, McCurdy DK, Ludwig GD, Chaykin LB, Elkinton JR. Incomplete renal tubular acidosis: physiologic studies in three patients with a defect in lowering urine pH. *Am J Med* 1968;45:32–42.
44. Caruana RJ, Buckalew VM Jr. Improvement of hypercalciuria, potassium wasting and hyperreninemia in incomplete distal renal tubular acidosis by indomethacin. *Nephron* 1979;24:232–5.
45. Buckalew VM Jr, Lorentz WB Jr, Fraser DS. Renal tubular disorders. In: Gonick HC, ed. *Current nephrology.* Boston: Houghton-Mifflin, 1980;39–75.

46. Ferris TF. Prostaglandins, potassium, and Bartter's syndrome. *J Lab Clin Med* 1978;92:663–8.

47. Sebastian A, McSherry E, Morris RC Jr. Impaired renal conservation of sodium and chloride during sustained correction of systemic acidosis in patients with type 1, classic renal tubular acidosis. *J Clin Invest* 1976;58:454–69.

48. McSherry E, Morris RC Jr. Attainment and maintenance of normal stature with alkali therapy in infants and children with classic renal tubular acidosis. *J Clin Invest* 1978;61:509–27.

49. McSherry E, Sebastian A, Morris RC Jr. Renal tubular acidosis in infants: the several kinds, including bicarbonate-wasting, classic renal tubular acidosis. *J Clin Invest* 1972;51:499–514.

50. Sebastian A, Morris RC Jr. Renal tubular acidosis. *Clin Nephrol* 1977;7:216–30.

51. Milne MD. Renal tubular dysfunction. In: Straus MB, Welt LG, eds. *Diseases of the kidney,* 2nd ed. Boston: Little, Brown, 1971;1071–138.

52. Chan JCM. Acid-base, calcium, potassium and aldosterone metabolism in renal tubular acidosis. *Nephron* 1979;23:152–8.

53. Feest TG, Lockwood CM, Morley AR, Uff JS. Renal histology and immunopathology in distal renal tubular acidosis. *Clin Nephrol* 1978;10:187–90.

54. Harrington TM, Bunch TW, Van den Berg, CJ. Renal tubular acidosis: a new look at treatment of musculoskeletal and renal disease. *Mayo Clin Proc* 1983;58:354–60.

55. Pun KK, Wong CK, Tsui EYL, Tam SCF, Kung AWC, Wang CCL. Hypokalemic periodic paralysis due to the Sjogren syndrome in Chinese patients. *Ann Intern Med* 1989;110:405–6.

56. Goldstein MB. Insights derived from the urine in acid–base disturbances. *AKF Nephrol Lett* 1989;6:19–25.

57. Madison LL, Seldin DW. Ammonia excretion and renal enzymatic adaptation in human subjects, as disclosed by administration of precursor amino acids. *J Clin Invest* 1958;37:1615–27.

58. Elkinton JR, Huth EJ, Webster GD Jr, McCance RA. The renal excretion of hydrogen ion in renal tubular acidosis. I. Quantitative assessment of the response to ammonium chloride as an acid load. *Am J Med* 1960;29:554–75.

59. DuBose TD Jr, Caflisch CR. Validation of the difference in urine and blood carbon dioxide tension during bicarbonate loading as an index of distal nephron acidification in experimental models of distal renal tubular acidosis. *J Clin Invest* 1985;75:1116–23.

60. Batlle DC, Gaviria M, Grupp M, Arruda JAL, Wynn J, Kurtzman NA. Distal nephron function in patients receiving chronic lithium therapy. *Kidney Int* 1982;21:477–85.

61. Gougoux A, Vinay P, Lemieux G, et al. Studies on the mechanism whereby acidemia stimulates collecting duct hydrogen ion secretion in vivo. *Kidney Int* 1981;20:643–8.

62. Stinebaugh BJ, Schloeder FX, Tam SC, Goldstein MB, Halperin ML. Pathogenesis of distal renal tubular acidosis. *Kidney Int* 1981;19:1–5.

63. Batlle D, Grupp M, Gaviria M, Kurtzman NA. Distal renal tubular acidosis with intact capacity to lower urinary pH. *Am J Med* 1982;72:751–8.

64. Melick RA, Henneman PH. Clinical and laboratory studies of 207 consecutive patients in a kidney stone clinic. *N Engl J Med* 1958;259:307–14.

65. Coe FL, Kavalach AG. Hypercalciuria and hyperuricosuria in patients with calcium nephrolithiasis. *N Engl J Med* 1974; 291:1344–50.

66. Cintron-Nadal E, Lespier LE, Roman-Miranda A, Martinez-Maldonado M. Renal acidifying ability in subjects with recurrent stone formation. *J Urol* 1977;118:704–6.

67. Drach GW, Perin R, Jacobs S. Outpatient evaluation of patients with calcium urolithiasis. *J Urol* 1979;121:564–7.

68. Backman U, Danielson BG, Johansson G, Ljunghall S, Wilstrom B. Incidence and clinical importance of renal tubular defects in recurrent renal stone formers. *Nephron* 1980;25:96–101.

69. Coe FL, ed. *Nephrolithiasis: pathogenesis and treatment.* Chicago: Year Book Medical Publishers, 1978.

70. Rapado A, Mancha A, Castrillo JM, Traba ML, Santos M, Cifuentes Delatte L. Etiological classification of renal lithiasis: a study based on 1936 patients. In: Fleisch H, Robertson WG, Smith LH, Vahlensieck W, eds. *Urolithiasis research.* New York: Plenum Press, 1976;495–8.

71. Brenner RJ, Spring DB, Sebastian A, et al. Incidence of radiographically evident bone disease, nephrocalcinosis and nephrolithiasis in various types of renal tubular acidosis. *N Engl J Med* 1982;307:217–21.

72. Cochran M, Peacock M, Smith DA, Nordin BEC. Renal tubular acidosis of pyelonephritis with renal stone disease. *Br Med J* 1968;2:721–9.

73. Coe FL, Parks JH. Stone disease in hereditary distal renal tubular acidosis. *Ann Intern Med* 1980;93:60–1.

74. Wilansky DL, Schneiderman C. Renal tubular acidosis with recurrent nephrolithiasis and nephrocalcinosis. *N Engl J Med* 1957;257:399–403.

75. Coe FL, Parks JH, Strauss AL. Accelerated calcium nephrolithiasis. *JAMA* 1980;244:809–10.

76. Lee DBN, Drinkard JP, Gonick HC, Coulson WF, Cracchiolo A III. Pathogenesis of renal calculi in distal renal tubular acidosis. *Clin Orthop* 1976;121:234–42.

77. Prien EL, Prien EL Jr. Composition and structure of urinary stone. *Am J Med* 1968;45:654–72.

78. Fourman P, Robinson JR. Diminished urinary excretion of citrate during deficiencies of potassium in man. *Lancet* 1953; 2:656–7.

79. Harrison HE, Chisolm JJ Jr, Harrison HC. Congenital renal tubular acidosis. *AMA J Dis Child* 1958;96:588–90.

80. Dedmon RE, Wrong O. The excretion of organic anion in renal tubular acidosis with particular reference to citrate. *Clin Sci* 1962;22:19–32.

81. Hodgkinson A. Citric acid excretion in normal adults and in patients with renal calculus. *Clin Sci* 1962;23:203–12.

82. Nordin BEC, Smith DA. Citric acid excretion in renal stone disease and in renal tubular acidosis. *Br J Urol* 1963;35:438–44.

83. Grollman AP, Harrison HC, Harrison HE. The renal excretion of citrate. *J Clin Invest* 1961;40:1290–6.

84. Brennan TS, Klahr S, Hamm LL. Citrate transport in rabbit nephron. *Am J Physiol* 1986;251:F683–9.

85. Runeberg L, Lotspeich WD. Krebs cycle acid excretion with isotopic split renal function techniques. *Am J Physiol* 1966;211:467–75.

86. Cohen RD, Prout RES. Studies on the renal transport of citrate using ^{14}C-citrate. *Clin Sci* 1965;28:487–97.

87. Crawford MA, Milne MD, Scribner BH. The effects of changes in acid–base balance on urinary citrate in the rat. *J Physiol (Lond)* 1959;149:413–23.

88. Evans BM, MacIntyre I, MacPherson CR, Milne MD. Alkalosis in sodium and potassium depletion (with especial reference to organic acid excretion). *Clin Sci* 1957;16:53–65.

89. Jenkins AD, Dousa TP, Smith LH. Transport of citrate across renal brush border membrane: effects of dietary acid and alkali loading. *Am J Physiol* 1985;249:F590–5.

90. Kippen I, Hirayama B, Klinenberg JR, Wright EM. Transport of tricarboxylic acid cycle intermediates by membrane vesicles from renal brush border. *Proc Natl Acad Sci USA* 1979;76:3397–400.

91. Wright SH, Kippen I, Klinenberg JR, Wright EM. Specificity of the transport system for tricarboxylic acid cycle intermediates in renal brush borders. *J Membr Biol* 1980;57:73–82.

92. Wright SH, Wunz TM. Succinate and citrate transport in renal basolateral and brush-border membranes. *Am J Physiol* 1987;253:F432–9.

93. Adler S, Anderson B, Zemotel L. Metabolic acid-base effects on tissue citrate content and metabolism in the rat. *Am J Physiol* 1971;220:986–92.

94. Simpson DP. Citrate excretion: a window on renal metabolism. *Am J Physiol* 1983;244:F223–34.

95. Simpson DP. Regulation of renal citrate metabolism by bicarbonate ion and pH: observations in tissue slices and mitochondria. *J Clin Invest* 1967;46:225–38.

96. Barac-Nieto, M. Effect of pH, calcium, and succinate on sodium citrate cotransport in renal microvilli. *Am J Physiol* 1984; 247:F282–90.

97. Jorgenson KE, Kragh-Hansen U, Roigaard-Peterson H, Sheikh MI. Citrate uptake by basolateral and luminal membrane vesicles from rabbit kidney cortex. *Am J Physiol* 1983;244:F686–95.

98. Wright SH, Kippen I, Wright EM. Effect of pH on the transport

of Krebs cycle intermediates in renal brush border membranes. *Biochim Biophys Acta* 1982;684:287–90.

99. Brennan S, Herring-Smith K, Hamm LL. Effect of pH on citrate reabsorption in the proximal convoluted tubule. *Am J Physiol* 1988;255:F301–6.

100. Goldfarb S. Dietary factors in the pathogenesis and prophylaxis of calcium nephrolithiasis. *Kidney Int* 1988;34:544–55.

101. Cooke RE, Segar WE, Cheek DB, Coville FE, Darrow DC. The extrarenal correction of alkalosis associated with potassium deficiency. *J Clin Invest* 1952;31:798–805.

102. Adler S, Zett B, Anderson B. The effect of acute potassium depletion on muscle cell pH in vitro. *Kidney Int* 1972;2:159–63.

103. Hodgkinson A. Citric acid excretion in normal adults and in patients with renal calculus. *Clin Sci* 1962;23:203–12.

104. Hodgkinson A. The relation between citric acid and calcium metabolism with particular reference to primary hyperparathyroidism and idiopathic hypercalciuria. *Clin Sci* 1963;24:167–78.

105. Conway NS, Maitland AIL, Rennie JB. Urinary citrate excretion in patients with renal calculi. *Br J Urol* 1949;21:30–8.

106. Breslau NA, Brinkley L, Hill KD, Pak CYC. Relationship of animal protein-rich diet to kidney stone formation and calcium metabolism. *J Clin Endocrinol Metab* 1988;66:140–6.

107. Preminger GM, Sakhaee K, Skurla C, Pak CYC. Prevention of recurrent calcium stone formation with potassium citrate therapy in patients with distal renal tubular acidosis. *J Urol* 1985;134:20–3.

108. Discussion. National Institute of Health concensus development conference on prevention and treatment of kidney stones. *J Urol* 1989;141:748–9.

109. McSherry E. Renal tubular acidosis in childhood. *Kidney Int* 1981;20:799–809.

110. Morrissey JF, Ochoa M Jr, Lotspeich WD, Waterhouse C. Citrate excretion in renal tubular acidosis. *Ann Intern Med* 1963;58:159–66.

111. Norman ME, Feldman NI, Cohn RM, Roth KS, McCurdy DK. Urinary citrate excretion in the diagnosis of distal renal tubular acidosis. *J Pediatr* 1978;92:394–400.

112. Halperin ML, Kamel KS, Ethier JH, Magner PO. What is the underlying defect in patients with isolated, proximal renal tubular acidosis? *Am J Nephrol* 1989;9:265–8.

113. Hosking DH, Wilson JWL, Liedtke RR, Smith LH, Wilson DM. Urinary citrate excretion in normal persons and patients with idiopathic calcium urolithiasis. *J Lab Clin Med* 1985;106:682–9.

114. Schwille PO, Scholz D, Paulus M, Engelhardt W, Sigel A. Citrate in daily and fasting urine: results of controls, patients with recurrent idiopathic calcium urolithiasis, and primary hyperparathyroidism. *Invest Urol* 1979;16:457–62.

115. Pak CYC, Fuller C. Idiopathic hypocitraturic calcium-oxalate nephrolithiasis successfully treated with potassium citrate. *Ann Intern Med* 1986;104:33–7.

116. Nash MA, Torrado AD, Greifer I, Spitzer A, Edelmann CM Jr. Renal tubular acidosis in infants and children. *J Pediatr* 1972;80:738–48.

117. Goodman AD, Lemann J Jr, Lennon EJ, Relman AS. Production, excretion and net balance of fixed acid in patients with renal acidosis. *J Clin Invest* 1965;44:495–506.

118. Lemann J Jr, Lennon EJ, Goodman AD, Litzow JR, Relman AS. The net balance of acid in subjects given large loads of acid or alkali. *J Clin Invest* 1965;44:507–17.

119. Lemann J Jr, Litzow JR, Lennon EJ. The effects of chronic acid loads in normal man: further evidence for the participation of bone mineral in the defense against chronic metabolic acidosis. *J Clin Invest* 1966;45:1608–14.

120. Perez GO, Oster JR, Vaamonde CA. Incomplete syndrome of renal tubular acidosis induced by lithium carbonate. *J Lab Clin Med* 1975;86:386–94.

121. Robertson WG, Peacock M. Calcium oxalate crystalluria and inhibitors of crystallization in recurrent renal stone-formers. *Clin Sci* 1972;43:499–506.

122. Hamed IA, Czerwinski AW, Coats B, Kaufman C, Altmiller DH. Familial absorptive hypercalciuria and renal tubular acidosis. *Am J Med* 1979;67:385–91.

123. Bianchi G, Vezzoli G, Cusi D, et al. Abnormal red-cell calcium

pump in patients with idiopathic hypercalciuria. *N Engl J Med* 1988;319:897–901.

124. Coe FL, Parks JH, Moore ES. Familial idiopathic hypercalciuria. *N Engl J Med* 1979;300:337–40.

125. Sutton RAL, Wong NLM, Dirks JH. Effects of metabolic acidosis and alkalosis on sodium and calcium transport in the dog kidney. *Kidney Int* 1979;15:520–33.

126. Peraino RA, Suki WN. Urine HCO_3^- augments renal CA^{2+} absorption independent of systemic acid-base changes. *Am J Physiol* 1980;238:F394–8.

127. Preminger GM, Sakhaee K, Skurla C, Pak CYC. Prevention of recurrent calcium stone formation with potassium citrate therapy in patients with distal renal tubular acidosis. *J Urol* 1985;134:20–3.

128. Sakhaee K, Nicar M, Hill K, Pak CYC. Contrasting effects of potassium citrate and sodium citrate therapies on urinary chemistries and crystallization of stone-forming salts. *Kidney Int* 1983;24:348–52.

129. Coe FL. Hyperuricosuric calcium oxalate nephrolithiasis. *Kidney Int* 1978;13:418–26.

130. Robertson WG, Peacock M, Nordin BEC. Activity products in stone-forming and non-stone-forming urine. *Clin Sci* 1968;34:579–94.

131. Pak CYC, Hayashi Y, Arnold LH. Heterogeneous nucleation with urate, calcium phosphate and calcium oxalate. *Proc Soc Exp Biol Med* 1976;153:83–7.

132. Hastings AB, McLean FC, Eichelberger L, Hall JL, Da Costa E. The ionization of calcium, magnesium, and strontium citrates. *J Biol Chem* 1934;107:351–70.

133. Pak CYC. Citrate and renal calculi. *Miner Electrolyte Metab* 1987;13:257–66.

134. Meyer JL, Thomas WC Jr. Trace metal–citric acid complexes as inhibitors of calcification and crystal growth. II. Effects of Fe(III), Cr(III) and Al(III) complexes on calcium oxalate crystal growth. *J Urol* 1982;128:1376–8.

135. Meyer JL, Thomas WC Jr. Trace metal–citric acid complexes as inhibitors of calcification and crystal growth. I. Effects of Fe(III), Cr(III) and Al(III) complexes on calcium phosphate crystal growth. *J Urol* 1982;128:1372–5.

136. Kok DJ, Papapoulos SE, Bijvoet OLM. Excessive crystal agglomeration with low citrate excretion in recurrent stone-formers. *Lancet* 1986;1:1056–8.

137. Gyory AZ, Edwards KDG. Renal tubular acidosis: a family with an autosomal dominant genetic defect in renal hydrogen ion transport, with proximal tubular and collecting duct dysfunction and increased metabolism of citrate and ammonia. *Am J Med* 1968;45:43–62.

138. Stapleton FB, Roy S III, Noe HN, Jerkins G. Hypercalciuria in children with hematuria. *N Engl J Med* 1984;310:1345–8.

139. Elkinton JR, McCurdy DK, Buckalew VM Jr. Hydrogen ion and the kidney. In: Black DAK, ed. *Renal disease*, 2nd ed. Philadelphia: FA Davis, 1967;110–35.

140. Brodwall EK, Westlie L, Myhre E. The renal excretion and tubular reabsorption of citric acid in renal tubular acidosis. *Acta Med Scand* 1972;192:137–9.

141. Nicar MJ, Skurla C, Sakhaee K, Pak CYC. Low urinary citrate excretion in nephrolithiasis. *Urology* 1983;21:8–14.

142. Pak CYC, Peterson R, Sakhaee K, Fuller C, Preminger G, Reisch J. Correction of hypocitraturia and prevention of stone formation by combined thiazide and potassium citrate therapy in thiazide-unresponsive hypercalciuric nephrolithiasis. *Am J Med* 1985;79:284–8.

143. Nicar MJ, Peterson R, Pak CYC. Use of potassium citrate as potassium supplement during thiazide therapy of calcium nephrolithiasis. *J Urol* 1984;131:430–3.

144. Pak CYC, Fuller C, Sakhaee K, Preminger GM, Britton F. Long-term treatment of calcium nephrolithiasis with potassium citrate. *J Urol* 1985;134:11–9.

145. Nicar MJ, Hsu MC, Fetner C. Urinary response to oral potassium citrate therapy for urolithiasis in a private practice setting. *Clin Ther* 1986;8:219–25.

146. Coe FL, Firpo JJ Jr. Evidence for mild reversible hyperparathyroidism in distal renal tubular acidosis. *Arch Intern Med* 1975;135:1485–9.

147. Brenes LG, Brenes JN, Hernandez MM. Familial proximal renal tubular acidosis: a distinct clinical entity. *Am J Med* 1977;63:244–52.
148. Morris RC Jr. An experimental renal acidification defect in patients with hereditary fructose intolerance. II. Its distinction from classic renal tubular acidosis; its resemblance to the renal acidification defect associated with the Fanconi syndrome of children with cystinosis. *J Clin Invest* 1968;47:1648–63.
149. Soriano JR, Houston IB, Boichis H, Edelmann CM Jr. Calcium and phosphorus metabolism in the Fanconi syndrome. *J Clin Endocrinol Metab* 1968;28:1555–63.
150. Sirota JH, Hamerman D. Renal function studies in an adult subject with the Fanconi syndrome. *Am J Med* 1954;16:138–52.
151. Wilson DR, Yendt ER. Treatment of the adult Fanconi syndrome with oral phosphate supplements and alkali: reports of two cases associated with nephrolithiasis. *Am J Med* 1963;35:487–511.
152. Smith R, Lindenbaum RH, Walton RJ. Hypophosphataemic osteomalacia and Fanconi syndrome of adult onset with dominant inheritance: possible relationship with diabetes mellitus. *Q J Med* 1976;45:387–400.
153. Wen S, Friedman AL, Oberley TD. Two case studies from a family with primary Fanconi syndrome. *Am J Kidney Dis* 1989;13:240–6.
154. Milne MD, Stanbury SW, Thomson AE. Observations on the Fanconi syndrome and renal hyperchloraemic acidosis in the adult. *Q J Med* 1952;21:61–82.
155. De Toni E Jr, Nordio S. The relationship between calcium-phosphorus metabolism, the "Krebs cycle" and steroid metabolism. *Arch Dis Child* 1959;34:371–82.
156. Lemann J Jr, Litzow JR, Lennon EJ. Studies of the mechanism by which chronic metabolic acidosis augments urinary calcium excretion in man. *J Clin Invest* 1967;46:1318–28.
157. Backman U, Danielson BG, Johansson G, Ljunghall S, Wikstrom B. Incidence and clinical importance of renal tubular defects in recurrent renal stone formers. *Nephron* 1980;25:96–101.
158. Tessitore N, Ortalda V, Fabris A, et al. Renal acidification defects in patients with recurrent calcium nephrolithiasis. *Nephron* 1985;41:325–32.
159. Jaeger P, Portmann L, Ginalski JM, Jacquet AF, Temler E, Burckhardt P. Tubulopathy in nephrolithiasis: consequence rather than cause. *Kidney Int* 1986;29:563–71.
160. Sutton RAL, Walker VR. Responses to hydrochlorothiazide and acetazolamide in patients with calcium stones: evidence suggesting a defect in renal tubular function. *N Engl J Med* 1980;302:709–13.
161. Cooper AM, Eckhardt RD, Faloon WW, Davidson CS. Investigation of the aminoaciduria in Wilson's disease (hepatolenticular degeneration): demonstration of a defect in renal function. *J Clin Invest* 1950;29:265–78.
162. Litin RB, Randall RV, Goldstein NP, Power MH, Diessner GR. Hypercalciuria in hepatolenticular degeneration (Wilson's disease). *Am J Med Sci* 1959;238:614–20.
163. Playoust MR, Dale NE. Metabolic balance studies in a patient with Wilson's disease and hypercalcuria. *Metabolism* 1961;10:304–14.
164. Reynolds ES, Tannen RL, Tyler HR. The renal lesion in Wilson's disease. *Am J Med* 1966;40:518–27.
165. Fulop M, Sternlieb I, Scheinberg IH. Defective urinary acidification in Wilson's disease. *Ann Intern Med* 1968;68:770–7.
166. Wilson DM, Goldstein NP. Bicarbonate excretion in Wilson's disease (hepatolenticular degeneration). *Mayo Clin Proc* 1974;49:394–400.
167. Wiebers DO, Wilson DM, McLeod RA, Goldstein NP. Renal stones in Wilson's disease. *Am J Med* 1979;67:249–54.
168. Carpenter TO, Carnes DL Jr, Anast CS. Hypoparathyroidism in Wilson's disease. *N Engl J Med* 1983;309:873–7.
169. Morgan HG, Stewart WK, Lowe KG, Stowers JM, Johnstone JH. Wilson's disease and the Fanconi syndrome. *Q J Med* 1962;31:361–84.
170. Bearn AG. Wilson's disease: an inborn error of metabolism with multiple manifestations. *Am J Med* 1957;22:747–57.
171. Walshe JM. Effect of penicillamine on failure of renal acidification in Wilson's disease. *Lancet* 1968;1:775–8.

Disorders of Bone and Mineral Metabolism,
edited by Fredric L. Coe and Murray J. Favus,
© 1992 by Raven Press, Ltd. All rights reserved.

CHAPTER 35

Inhibitors and Promoters of Calcium Oxalate Crystallization

Their Relationship to the Pathogenesis and Treatment of Nephrolithiasis

Fredric L. Coe, Joan H. Parks, and Yashushi Nakagawa

Certainly, clinicians will recognize few features of this subject that interest them, but measurement of certain inhibitors has become a part of what we do for our patients. Citrate, for example, and one promoter, uric acid, are recognized as putative causes of calcium oxalate stones, high levels of urine uric acid and low levels of urine citrate are treated, lately, as ways of preventing stones. In writing this review, we encountered an earlier one (1) and commend it as a valuable contribution.

NATURE OF THE PROBLEM

As they conserve water, kidneys concentrate whatever solutes remain in the tubule lumen, such as calcium, and anions like oxalate and phosphate with which calcium forms insoluble salts, so water conservation creates calcium oxalate and calcium phosphate salt supersaturations. Supersaturation (described in Chapter 00), means salts exist in solution above their solubility and so are able to change phase and become solids given proper provocation, either in the form of seed nuclei or unrelated solid phases such as cell debris or protein precipitates, which can act as surface to promote crystallization. It is not mainly diet, but rather the design of the kidney that gives rise to calcium oxalate and calcium phosphate

supersaturations, which are therefore not easily eliminated and do not arise mainly because of culture or habit.

Blood calcium ion levels approximate 1.2 mM and tubule calcium reabsorption never rises above 99% (see Chapter 1); so at least 1% of filtered calcium load reaches the urine, or about 50–100 mg daily, and usual urine levels exceed this number, ranging from 100 to 200 mg (2). Oxalate excretion involves filtration and tubule secretion (3,4) (which are the only ways to remove this toxic material from the body), and create urine levels of oxalate ranging from 20 to 40 mg daily (2), enough to cause 2- to 10-fold supersaturations (5). Phosphate in urine approximates 500–1000 mg daily (see Chapters 1 and 3), enough to cause supersaturations with respect to brushite and apatite. A low-calcium diet cannot lower urine calcium enough to abolish supersaturations, and in stone formers, idiopathic hypercalciuria occurs frequently (see Chapter 32), raises urine calcium much above normal levels, and may predispose to bone disease if dietary calcium is lowered greatly (6). Low-oxalate diet cannot reduce urine oxalate below usual normal values, which mainly reflect endogenous oxalate production. Low-phosphate diet raises urine calcium excretion (see Chapter 1) and could not be considered a reasonable treatment. Given these restrictions, supersaturations of urine seem a part of human life not easily prevented, nearly universal, and more marked in stone formers than in normals.

F. L. Coe, J. H. Parks, and Y. Nakagawa: Departments of Medicine and Physiology, University of Chicago, Pritzker School of Medicine, Chicago, Illinois 60637.

INHIBITORS

Semantics partly governs one's view of the word "inhibitors," which could include molecules that form soluble salts with calcium or oxalate and reduce calcium oxalate supersaturation or factors (such as ionic strength) that reduce ion activities and also reduce supersaturations. We prefer to limit the term to molecules that raise the supersaturation needed to initiate nucleation, that inhibit secondary nucleations, or that reduce the growth rate and the rate of aggregation of crystal nuclei. We know of two proteins, as well as three other types of naturally occurring molecules in urine, that possess some or all of these properties. In addition, many papers have documented the general role of urine, and of urine macromolecules of undefined character, as inhibitors.

Undefined Inhibitors

Urine

Calcium Phosphate

Urine at 2.2% added to an inorganic salt system increased the supersaturation needed to initiate the formation of calcium phosphate crystals, measured as the formation product or ion product at the point of first detectable nucleation, from 53 to 105 mg% (7), and almost all of the activity was removed by passing urine through a Dowex anion-exchange column. Inorganic pyrophosphate was identified in urine, and by plotting formation product against measured pyrophosphate concentration, about one-half to one-fourth of the increase that urine produced could be ascribed to the pyrophosphate it contained, leaving a considerable amount unexplained.

The importance of pyrophosphate was explored in a later paper using an ingenious technique not often exploited (8). Urines were brought to a constant supersaturation by equilibration with a brushite (calcium hydrogen phosphate) column, then seeded with apatite crystals in increasing solid-to-liquid ratios, stirred, and incubated for 24 h at 37°C, and the calcium phosphate product at the end was expressed as a fraction of that at the start. When at equilibrium with brushite, urine is supersaturated with respect to apatite, so all urines started out supersaturated to an equal degree. As crystals were added, inhibitors coated their surfaces, so they could not induce crystallization, but as the amount of apatite crystals increased, their surface gradually exceeded the coating capacity of the available inhibitors, and ions were lost from solution during the 24 hours of incubation. The amount (expressed in milligrams) of apatite needed to achieve a 50% reduction of the calcium phosphate product served as the index of inhibitor capacity, and it varied smoothly with the percent of urine in the incuba-

tion. Citrate, magnesium, and pyrophosphate together accounted for about 20% or less of the effects of urine; citrate was probably the most important of the three, and magnesium was almost negligible in effect. One wonders if this technique later was applied using calcium oxalate crystals, as we have not found such papers.

In an in vitro study, Robertson (9) showed that inorganic pyrophosphate and diphosphonates (carbon analogues of pyrophosphate that are stable and not degraded by pyrophosphatases) both inhibit the precipitation of calcium phosphates from solution, and the diphosphonate inhibited growth of apatite crystals in a metastably supersaturated calcium phosphate solution. In addition, this study shows efficient heterogeneous nucleation of calcium phosphates by calcium oxalate crystals.

Calcium Oxalate

Urine also increases the formation product for calcium oxalate. By adding both ions, slowly, to urine, Dent and Sutor (10) observed less crystallization in urine of normals than in that of hypercalciuric but non-stone-forming patients, and the most crystallizations occurred in urine of patients with stones. Using a different method [i.e., by adding diluted urine to an acetate buffer (pH 6) containing calcium (3 mM) and oxalate (0.3 mM) and determining the amounts of calcium crystallized, as judged by retention by a 0.45-μm filter], Rose (11) found marked inhibition by urine (at 0.5–15% by volume) added to the system.

Using oxalate addition or calcium chloride addition, Pak and Holt (12) found an elevated formation product ratio (the ratio of the formation product to the ion product at equilibrium) in urine from normals versus urine from stone-forming patients, and the urine from stone formers also was more supersaturated; both facts led to the satisfying conclusion that in stone patients, high supersaturation coexisted with reduced nucleation inhibitors. Ryall et al. (13), 10 years later, found the same results, but they ascribed the lower formation product of stone-former urine to higher urine volume—in other words, to dilution of inhibitors. Pak and Holt (12) had shown no differences whatsoever between the urine volume of patients and that of normals, so the failure of Ryall et al. (13) to confirm their work seems difficult to understand. Elsewhere, Pak and Galosy (14) combined supersaturation and formation product ratio to create a discriminant function that successfully separated stone formers from normals, as the earlier paper predicts must happen. These investigators also showed that treatments moved this index toward normal, by reducing supersaturation and increasing the formation product ratio.

A rather unusual measurement of whole urine effects, partly dissected in terms of citrate interactions, used light scattering as an estimate of particle size. Urine from four patients placed in a fluorometer scattered light after calcium and oxalate were added to achieve concentrations of 1.30 mM each in addition to concentrations already in the urine (in other words, sufficient to raise the ion concentration product above the threshold of metastability), because the additions caused calcium oxalate spontaneous precipitations (15). The greater the particle density, the greater the light scattering, so that light scattering measured particle density. In addition, crystals were imaged optically. Citrate reduced the amounts and average size of particles at added concentrations of 2–3 mM in three of four urines, but it was ineffective in the fourth. Pyrophosphate and magnesium seemed mainly ineffective. The method used urine nearly unaltered, except for its calcium oxalate product and selected additions, though the measurements seem a bit indirect, and the reasons for great variability among patients are unclear.

Another paper (16), using the same methods, found a citrate effect on crystal development measured by light scattering and optical visualization in urine from 13 of 21 stone formers, who seemed to differ from those not responding to citrate in being less hypercalciuric. This conclusion seems unconvincing to us, since no multivariate discriminant analysis was used, and the original data do not show a dramatic difference among urine measurements.

In other experiments, in which optical measurements of crystal number and size alone were made (17), calcium oxalate crystallization was promoted by calcium phosphate or uric acid seed additions. Citrate, magnesium, and pyrophosphate reduced amounts and sizes of crystals produced with and without added seeds, but chondroitin sulfate inhibited only effects of seed addition.

Using a less supersaturated calcium oxalate solution, produced in vitro and artificially, rather than in whole urine [calcium (1 mM) and oxalate (0.2 mM), pH 6, seeded with 20 μg/mL of calcium oxalate seed crystals], Robertson and Peacock (18) showed that undisturbed seed crystals increased their average size by a mixture of particle growth and aggregation, that urine at 5% by volume reduced the particle size, and that urine from patients who formed stones reduced particle size less than did urine from normal people who did not form stones.

Meyer and Smith (19) used a similar system [calcium and oxalate (both 0.4 mM), pH 6.7, seeded with calcium oxalate monohydrate crystals, 625 μg/mL], in which growth of crystals was assayed by rate of disappearance of calcium, measured by atomic absorption spectrophotometry in medium filtered through a 0.22-μm filter. The rate at which calcium disappeared varied as the square of the difference between the calcium concentration in the solution and the concentration at thermodynamic equilibrium, the point at which the crystals in the solution no longer grew nor shrank. Using this fact, an integrated rate law was derived from which they ex-

tracted a simple growth rate parameter. Inorganic pyrophosphate and human urine progressively reduced the growth rate parameter with increasing concentration, and did so in a manner consistent with the assumptions of the Langmuir-type isotherm, from whose slope an apparent dissociation constant for the inhibitors could be derived. Inorganic pyrophosphate inhibited growth rate by 50% at 16 μM concentration, urine achieved this same reduction at a dilution factor of 62-fold, at which dilution the concentration of pyrophosphate could account for less than 2% of the total inhibition found. Citrate inhibited crystal growth, even after allowing for effects on supersaturation from ion pairing, a 30% reduction occurred at about 0.5 mM citrate concentration, which is below the levels in urine of normal women (2). This study, perhaps more clearly than any before its time, documented that unknown inhibitors comprised almost all of the inhibition power of urine when diluted and studied in a seeded crystal growth system, at very modest supersaturation, and with respect to growth inhibition in particular.

Using the same system they used earlier [calcium (1 mM) and oxalate (0.2 mM), pH 6, seeded with calcium oxalate monohydrate seeds, (presumably 20 μg/mL)] and assaying combined growth and aggregation of the seeds by particle size increase measured by Coulter counter, Robertson et al. (20) found that 1% by volume of urine from eight patients with calcium oxalate stones inhibited particle size increase to a lesser extent than did urine from eight normal members of the hospital staff, though with considerable overlap. Furthermore, the urines from the stone-forming patients were more supersaturated with respect to calcium oxalate, also with considerable overlap; but when supersaturation and inhibitory power were plotted against one another, the control- and patient-derived points separated cleanly along the diagonal of a discriminant function (Fig. 1). One might say that this paper marked the climax of a decade of work, showing the clinical importance of reduced inhibition in stone-former urine, a lack of correlation between supersaturation and inhibition evident in the figure, and a reason to try to measure inhibitors in patients, isolate them, and find out what they might be made of. An editorial praised the work, cautiously.

Yet another demonstration of urine as crystal growth inhibitor used a constant composition technique (21), in which consumption of calcium by growth of seed crystals in modestly supersaturated calcium oxalate solution (supersaturation 1.3) led to automatic replacement of calcium and oxalate by parallel pumps, so pump rate could index ligand consumption and supersaturation could remain constant. At 1 to 3%, whole urine inhibited ligand consumption strongly.

In a short report, Robertson et al. (22) showed that the main inhibitors in human urine with molecular weights above 10 kD (as determined by ultrafiltration) could be

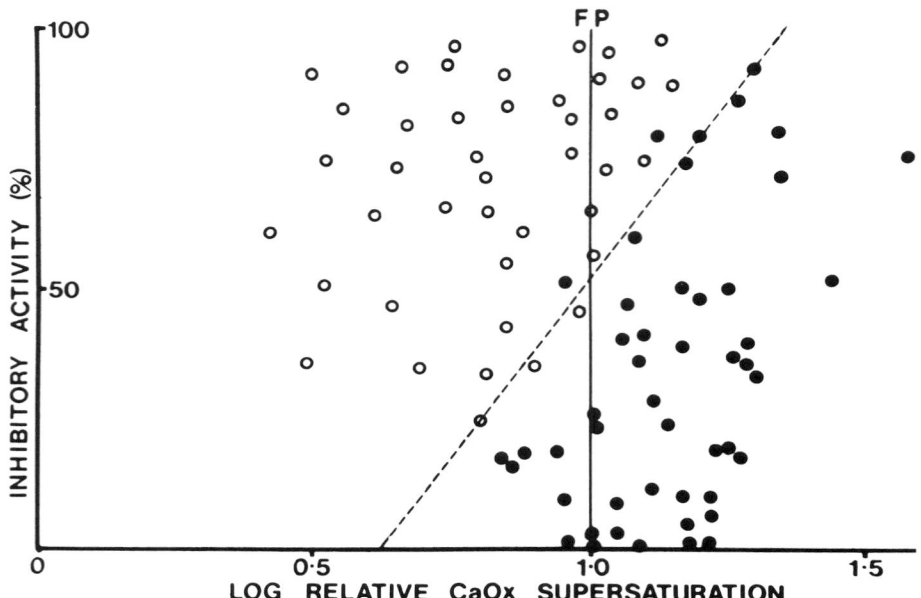

FIG. 1. Scattergram of inhibitory activity plotted against log of relative calcium oxalate (CaOx) supersaturation in the urine samples of the patients with recurrent stone formation (●) and the controls (○). The full line represents the formation product (FP) of calcium oxalate, and the dashed line represents the calculated discriminant function. [From Robertson et al. (20).]

precipitated using cetylpyridinium chloride and, after precipitation, showed infrared features of carboxyl, hydroxyl, and sulfate groups, supporting the notion that the inhibitory material could be made up of acid mucopolysaccharides (AMPS). Degree of inhibition varied smoothly with measured concentration of AMPS, adding further support. In addition, sodium hydrogen urate seed crystals seemed to interact with AMPS, as more urate diminished inhibition and removal of urate increased inhibition. They proposed that increased urine urate could raise risk of stones, possibly by forming some colloidal association with AMPS, which could then do less well in inhibition. This brief paper seems to be the first of a group of reports concerned with mucopolysaccharides as urine calcification inhibitors. The urate interactions repeat earlier work (23) showing linkages between uric acid excess and calcium oxalate stone disease, reviewed later in this chapter.

With the same system as that of Robertson et al. (20), but using as an assay for aggregation the flow rate through a 20-μm-pore-diameter filter, which rate falls as pores plug with aggregates of such a size, Felix et al. (24) found a marked inhibition of particle size increase by urine at 1% and 5%. They also found: (a) that Tamm–Horsfall glycoprotein (THP), which they called "uromucoid," had no effects on particle size increase; (b) inhibitors in the urine could be removed by ultrafiltration and could be adsorbed on an anion-exchange column from which they eluted in progressive steps with increasing NaCl concentration; and (c) that eluted inhibitors migrated during Sephadex G-75 column chromatography in several apparent molecular-weight peaks between 14 and 200 kD. At the high dilutions involved, inorganic pyrophosphate could have played no role (in Felix et al.'s opinion), though in undiluted urines the pyrophosphate

concentration would have been high enough to have contributed importantly.

We (25) used the Meyer–Smith assay modified to use [^{14}C]oxalate disappearance as an estimate of crystal growth to measure inhibition by urine from normal people and from patients with calcium oxalate stone disease, and we also measured urine calcium oxalate supersaturation with the concentration product method of Pak and Galosy (14). Like Robertson et al. (22), we observed the following: (a) Supersaturation and inhibition are independent of one another, (b) there are higher supersaturations and lower inhibitions in urine from patients with stones than in urine from normal people, and (c) low inhibition predicted stone-forming very accurately, but the use of a multivariate discriminant function added nothing to the separation of normals from stone formers. Patients with hypercalciuria had lower inhibitor levels than did those with hyperuricosuria, suggesting some interactions between urine calcium and inhibition.

Finally, one must mention work using an altogether different kind of technique, known as "mixed suspension mixed product removal" (MSMPR), in which calcium and oxalate solutions enter a mixing chamber, with the calcium at 30 mM, the oxalate at 1.50 mM, or at a calcium-to-oxalate ratio of 20 to 1 and an extreme supersaturation that causes immediate nucleation (26). In such a system, the entry streams keep creating nuclei, but in the mixing chamber the stirred crystal mass keeps the solution at a lower level of supersaturation, as crystals take up ions from the solution in proportion to their mass, surface, growth rate constant, and degree of initial supersaturation. The particles that leave are analyzed for size distribution, from which one can estimate growth and nucleation rates. Compared to salt solutions, urine from patients and normals reduced the total mass of crystals, the growth rate of crystals, and the mean particle size of crystals but increased nucleation rate. Compared to urine from normal people, urine from patients with stones reduced growth rate, increased nucleation rate, and resulted in smaller crystals, results exactly opposite to what one would expect from all other experiments. The best explanation is that stone-forming urine promotes nucleation, raising the number of nuclei and using up a higher proportion of the supersaturation in new nuclei, leaving fewer nuclei for growth. Other methods do not include such extreme supersaturations or nucleation rates as seen here, and isolate growth, or aggregation and growth, from nucleation, so they can respond to growth inhibition directly.

On reading over these papers from what we could call the first era of research on inhibitors, much of the work still seems important, not so much in defining the inhibitors but in showing the robust nature of the inhibition effect—especially the rather consistent failure of urine from stone formers to inhibit as well as normal urine, despite the use of many types of assays. One problem involves the use of highly diluted urine, a situation which always emphasizes the role of high-affinity inhibitors (inhibitors that bind to crystals at low concentration and with a high avidity) and diminishes the role of inhibitors with lower affinities that could be very important in undiluted urine, such as citrate and inorganic pyrophosphate. Another concern is the confusion of aggregation and growth in all assays that measured particle size, because they used metastably supersaturated buffers that supported growth and the extremely different picture one gets of urine effects when one works at very high supersaturations, where nucleation predominates, compared to systems of low supersaturations containing preformed crystal seeds. Inhibitors of only aggregation could seem inactive when growth and aggregation are combined by measurements of particle size, since both growth and aggregation would increase particle size. Finally, one must separate the problems of calcium oxalate and calcium phosphate inhibition. The former seems mainly due to molecules other than pyrophosphate or citrate, although undiluted urine does contain such high concentrations of both that they could play a significant role, and the latter could be in significant measure due to pyrophosphate and citrate, especially in undiluted urine.

Defined Inhibitors

Macromolecules

Because passage of urine through anion-exchange columns removed most of the high-affinity inhibitors, and most activity could be removed using cetylpyridinium chloride precipitation, Ito and Coe (27) assessed the inhibitory potential of candidate urine anions, including RNA, gastric pepsin, and synthetic poly-L-aspartic and

glutamic acid, all of which inhibited growth of seed crystals in a system very similar to that of Meyer and Smith (19), except for use of [^{14}C]oxalate disappearance instead of calcium disappearance from filtrates of medium and use of 1 mM calcium and 0.2 mM oxalate instead of equimolar concentrations. Treating urine with pronase (a protein-digesting enzyme) immobilized on beads, but not with RNAase immobilized on beads, reduced inhibition significantly, suggesting that the inhibitor was partly a protein. Subsequent purification of inhibiting material on diethylaminoethyl (DEAE)-cellulose followed by G50 Sephadex eluted an inhibitory fraction comprised mainly of a protein whose amino acid composition departed from general urine proteins in having a preponderance of aspartic and glutamic acids over lysine and arginine. For example, the ratio of Asp + Glu to Lys + Arg was 2.74 in dialyzed urine, but it reached 9.1 in the most purified inhibitor fractions, achieved by rechromatographing active material on gel exclusion columns (Fig. 2). At that time, the role of RNA seemed unclear, as RNA migrated with the protein, but preparative electrophoresis separated them, and inhibition eluted much before the RNA. The purest product from electrophoresis and subsequent gel filtration inhibited crystal growth by about 50% at about 3 mg/L. Given our current knowl-

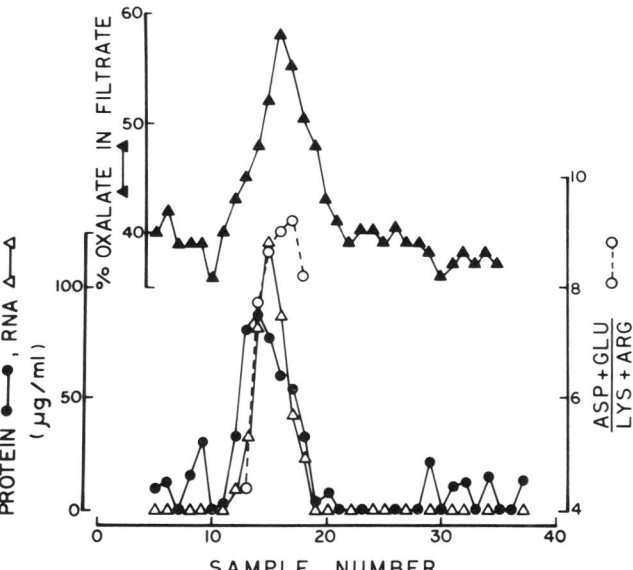

FIG. 2. Rechromatography of second peak. Tubes 13 through 17 from Fig. 3 of Ref. 27 were pooled, reduced to 2 mL in volume, reapplied to same G-50 column, and eluted in 0.05 M Tris buffer, pH 7.3, NaCl 0.15 M; 0.2 mL of each sample was assayed. No void volume peak was present. Inhibition eluted in an irregular peak at same position observed in previous experiment. Amino acid compositions of tubes 12–18 were determined. Ratio of diacidic to dibasic amino acid rose steeply to about 9 in tubes 15 through 17, which were also the most actively inhibiting samples. [From Ito and Coe (27).]

edge (not then available to us) that the main urine inhibitor has a monomeric molecular weight of about 14 kD, the approximate affinity of our purified material then would have been about 0.1 μM.

If urine is evaporated to high osmolalities of 1450 mOsm/kg, crystals of calcium oxalate form, and if pH is kept at 6.8 or higher, calcium phosphate crystals form at lower osmolalities of 1250 mOsm/kg (28). Passing urine through an ultrafilter of 12-kD cutoff reduced the size of the crystal deposits, and addition of uromucoids, which here means all proteins precipitated by high NaCl concentrations and includes THP, increased crystal yield and the size of deposits. This study arose from a line of research begun long before the modern age, which held that urine proteins promote crystallization.

Somewhat later, we (29) improved our procedure for isolating inhibitors from human urine by using batch DEAE-cellulose extraction followed by linear elution of inhibitor from a column of DEAE-cellulose and subsequent Biogel P 100 chromatography. The inhibitor was clearly the same one found by Ito and Coe (27), but additional measurements confirmed it to be a glycoprotein that also contained gamma-carboxyglutamic acid (Gla).

Long after this work (and after the work described below on specific molecules), the urine inhibitor isolated by ion-exchange chromatography and gel filtration (much like our own procedure) was studied along with chondroitin sulfate and citrate for its effects on the calcium oxalate formation product in vitro, in relation to the effects of calcium ion on the elevation of formation product (30). As calcium ion level increased from 0.25 to 6 mM, citrate lost its effects, chondroitin sulfate as well, but the urine macromolecules increased in effect; the latter was an unexpected finding. By 2 mM calcium, chondroitin sulfate barely raised the calcium oxalate formation product (in $M^2 \times 10^{-8}$) from 1.81 ± 0.09 to 2.11 ± 0.11, whereas macromolecules gave 2.73 ± 0.20, and by 4 mM the corresponding values were 1.97 ± 0.10 versus 2.80 ± 0.22.

Here, in an arbitrary way, we draw a line to end a phase of exposition, even though the actual research that follows merges into the papers we have just reviewed. During the decade from 1980 to now, most attention turned to characterizing particular molecules, to clarifying the role (or lack of role) of AMPS, and studying the effects of molecules already well-characterized, like THP. In leaving the work, we recognize how dangerous the leap to highly diluted urines was, how it distorted the question, to focus not so much on what molecules might actually inhibit most in the kidney but on molecules that could inhibit even at low concentrations—in other words, on molecules with a high affinity for the crystals of interest. The results have led to much understanding of high-affinity inhibitors, and one hopes their eventual cloning and sequencing will clarify their exact roles in the nephron. We also recognize that methods and obser-vations tend to be forgotten, and we hope that our review may prompt some to use the methods that were used 10 or 20 years ago.

Nephrocalcin

This section derives mainly from our own laboratory, which has been alone, thus far, in the work. Naturally, we expect subsequent editions of this book will contain materials about nephrocalcin from other investigators. At this time, no one has determined the primary sequence of the protein, so what we mean by the term "nephrocalcin" requires special clarification. Whereas prior sections concern both calcium phosphate and calcium oxalate crystallizations, this concerns only calcium oxalate [actually only calcium oxalate monohydrate crystals (COM), since no others have been tested to date]. In addition, we consider virtually only growth rate inhibition at high dilutions, not because this is the only interesting property but because of technical resources and time, with the main objective being to purify and characterize a molecular inhibitor and not to explore all facets of the inhibition process.

What We Mean by Nephrocalcin

From urine or other sources, we can extract an acidic glycoprotein containing a predominance of acidic versus basic amino acids (containing Gla, as well, in most instances), having a minimum molecular weight of 14 kD but aggregating to higher-molecular-weight forms that can be disaggregated to the monomer by ethylenedi-aminetetraacetic acid (EDTA) incubation, and possessing an ability to inhibit the growth of calcium oxalate monohydrate (COM) seed nuclei at concentrations in the range of 0.1 μM, or—to put another way—an affinity for the COM crystal of 0.1–0.5 μM as judged by inhibition assays. Furthermore, nephrocalcin (NC) creates very stable films at the air–water interface, with high collapse pressures, an unusual characteristic. Finally, the NC elutes from DEAE-cellulose in specific ranges of ionic strength. For some years, we have had antibodies available that add a level of identification, though, of course, in the absence of a sequence, the gold standard remains a cluster of biochemical and biophysical characteristics. The name, "nephrocalcin" incidentally, was not used at first, so several interim names or phrases appear among our papers.

Cell Culture

The first fully successful purification of NC was not from urine but was, instead, from medium conditioned by a renal cell line that belonged to a commercial concern (Collaborative Research, Waltham, Massachusetts) gracious enough to give us large amounts of the crude eluate from ion exchange (31). As an assay, we used the

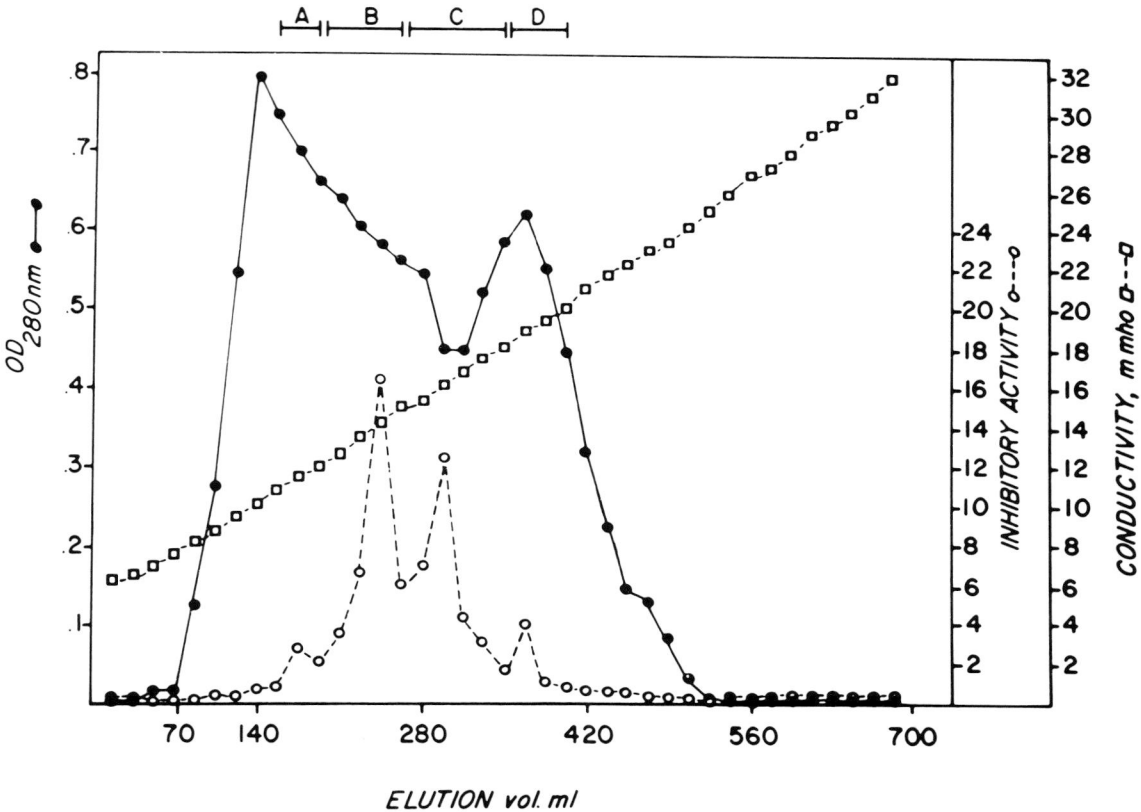

FIG. 3. Isolation of inhibitor from human kidney tissue culture medium using DEAE-cellulose chromatography (2 × 15 cm). Elution was carried out using a linear NaCl gradient from 0.05 to 0.5 M in 0.05 M Tris-HCl, pH 7.3 (600 mL of each solution). The fractions (3 mg/tube) were collected in test tubes containing one drop of 1% NaN$_3$ aqueous solution. Protein was monitored by absorption at 280 nm, and salt concentration was determined using a Radiometer conductivity meter. [From Nakagawa et al. (31).]

modified Meyer–Smith system (27), from which we extracted the second-order kinetic growth rate constant. The value of the constant at different concentrations of inhibiting protein was plotted against the concentration in the Langmuir-type isotherm plot, in which the term $k_0/(k_0 - k_{exp})$ varies linearly with $1/I$, where I is the pro-

tein inhibitor concentration and where "exp" represents the k value with inhibitors present.

From DEAE-cellulose, inhibiting proteins eluted in four different ionic strength regions (Fig. 3). The large peak, B, chromatographed on Sephacryl S200, gave a main peak and several smaller peaks, indicating multiple

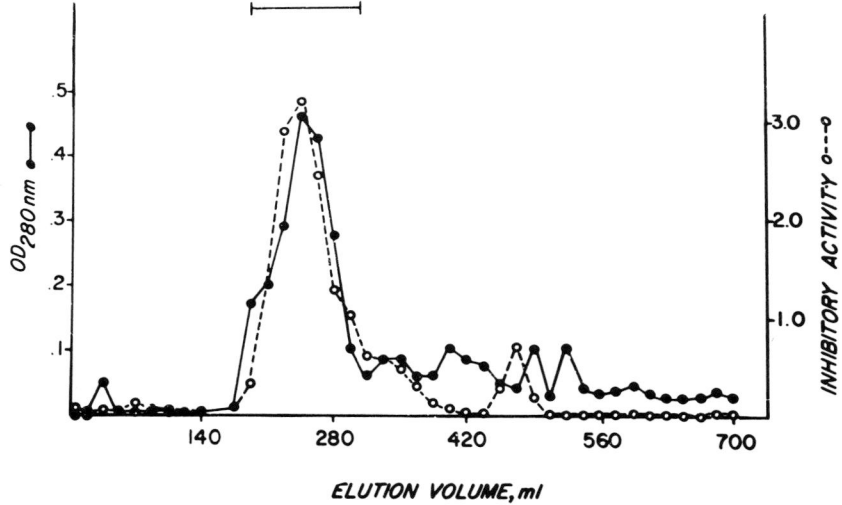

FIG. 4. Rechromatography of the main inhibitory peak from the previous step (Fig 2). Using Sephacryl S-200 (4 × 113 cm) with the same buffer system, protein was monitored at 280 nm. [From Nakagawa et al. (31).]

molecular-weight forms, and when the predominant peak was rechromatographed, protein and inhibitor elutions matched well (Fig. 4) in a main peak, but a minor peak reappeared, all consistent with disaggregation of a polymerized molecule. The main peak treated with EDTA migrated at the position of the minor peak seen before EDTA treatment, confirming this idea (Fig. 5). The purification attained was 82-fold in 0.4% of the initial protein, with a total yield of 22.5 mg from 5178 mg of crude protein starting material. The purified material showed an amino acid composition (Table 1) and carbohydrate composition (Table 2) like that of the material Ito and Coe (27) found. Gla was not found. The protein seemed to have a calculated minimum amino acid content of 73 residues, with a protein molecular weight of 8194 daltons; by ultracentrifugation of the molecular weight was found to be 13.3 kD. Using an air–water film interfacial balance technique, the molecular weight was found to be 13.9 kD. The ultraviolet (UV) absorption spectrum (Fig. 6) showed very weak absorption at 280

nm because of very few aromatic amino acid residues (Table 1).

The Langmuir-type isotherm plot (Fig. 7) showed linearity, and from the slope the affinity was found to be 0.019 μM. The linear fit supports a mechanism of protein adsorption governed by a single dissociation constant, with coated sites not growing and all growth from uncoated sites. To test this assumed mechanism further, crystals were electrophoresed in an electrical field, and their mobility was determined as a function of the protein concentration with which they were preincubated (Fig. 8). With progressive increase in the incubation protein concentration, growth rate fell and the mobility changed direction—from movement toward the anode (like a crystal with net positive charge) to movement toward the cathode.

This study laid the foundation for much of what came after, in showing the molecular weight, anion-exchange column heterogeneity, self-aggregation characteristics, crystal adsorption, and compositional characteristics.

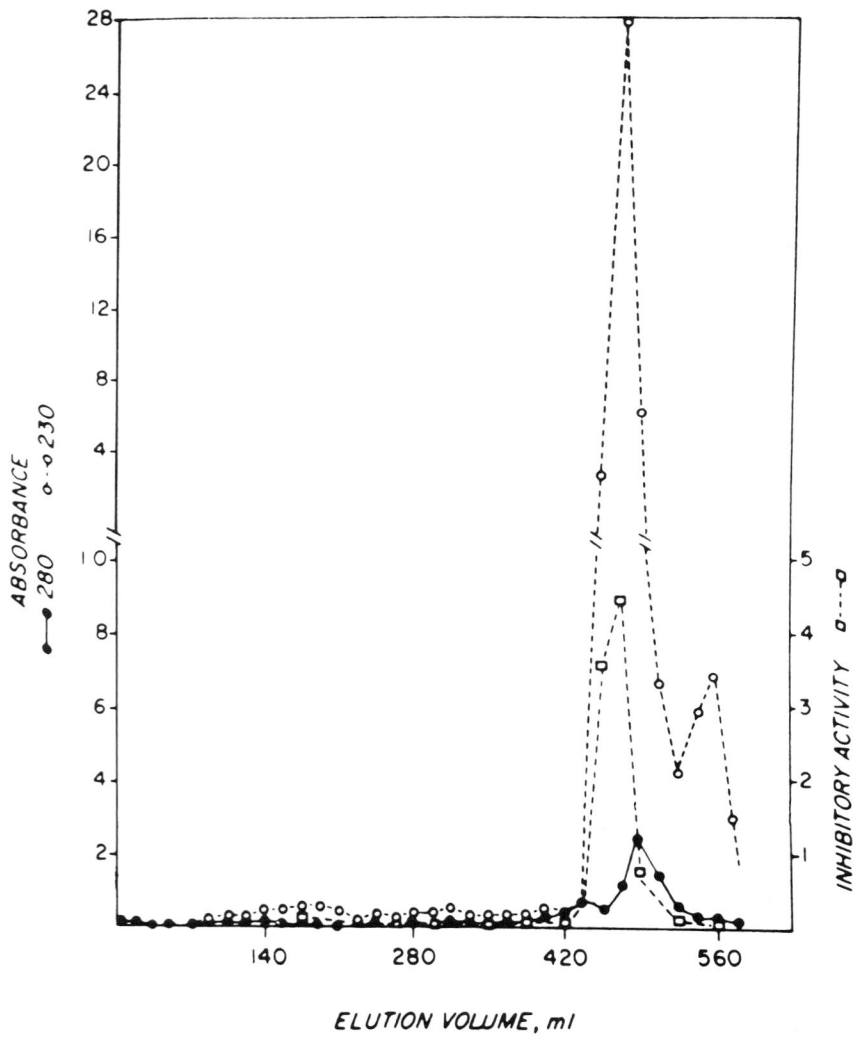

FIG. 5. Column chromatography of the EDTA-treated inhibitor. The purified inhibitor was incubated with EDTA, and then it was chromatographed on a column of Sephacryl S-200 (4 × 113 cm). The elution buffer was the same one as used previously. [From Nakagawa et al. (31).]

TABLE 1. *Amino acid composition of calcium oxalate crystal growth inhibitor isolated from human kidney tissue culture medium*

Amino acid	Number of residues/ $M_r = 1.33 \times 10^3$	Nearest integer
Lysine	3.0	3
Histidine	2.2	2
Arginine	2.4	2
Aspernine	15.1	15
Threonine	4.6	5
Serine	6.7	7
Glutamic acid	9.7	10
Proline	4.3	4
Glycine	5.3	5
Alanine	2.7	3
Valine	5.3	5
Methionine	1.4	1
Isoleucine	1.3	1
Leucine	4.1	4
Tyrosine	1.4 (1.2[a])	1
Phenylalanine	1.8	2
Cysteine	1.6	2
Tryptophan	0 (0.8[a])	1

Source: After Nakagawa et al. (31).
[a] These values were determined spectrophotometrically.

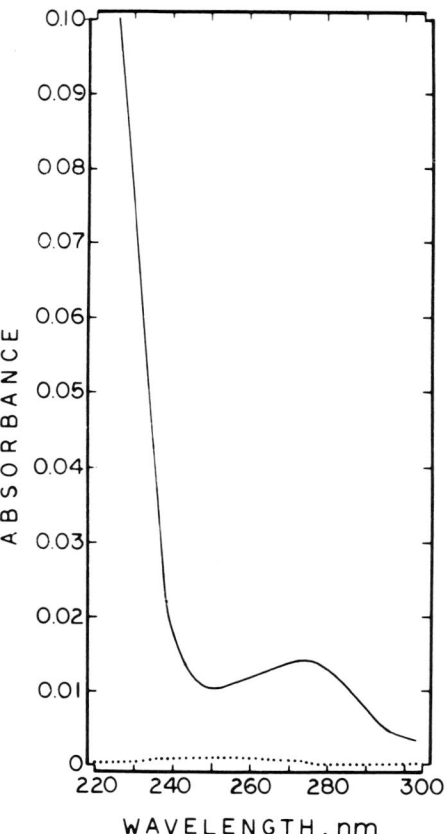

FIG. 6. UV absorption spectrum of the isolated inhibitor. The inhibitor was dissolved in 0.01 M Tris-HCl (pH 7.2) to give 0.19 mg/mL, and the spectrum of the resultant solution was scanned between 220 and 300 nm using a Cary 15 spectrophotometer with 0.01 scale expansion (*solid line*). Background absorption of the buffer solution was also recorded (*dotted line*). [From Nakagawa et al. (31).]

The protein seems designed to masquerade as a carbohydrate polymer, as it does not absorb light well at 280 nm, reacts little with the Lowry technique, and stains poorly with Coomasie blue, usual traits of proteins. We guessed, then, that the AMPS of Robertson et al. (22) contained nephrocalcin.

Human Urine

We isolated a very similar inhibitor from human urine using the same methods, but we incorporated an additional step to remove an obvious brown stain by incubating the DEAE-cellulose eluates with 50% formamide and passing the mixture over a BioGel P-10 column that separated the protein from the chromogen (32). Sedimentation equilibrium centrifugation (Fig. 9) gave a molecular weight of 14 kD. As with cell culture inhibitor, multiple

TABLE 2. *Carbohydrate composition of the isolated inhibitor*

	Weight %	Number of residues	Nearest integer
Fucose	1.9	1.7	2
Galactose	11.3	9.3	9
Glucose	3.2	2.6	3
N-Acetylneuraminic acid	17.0	7.8	8
Glucosamine[a]		0.3	3
Galactosamine[a]		0.8	1

Source: After Nakagawa et al. (31).
[a] The results were obtained from amino acid analysis.

molecular-weight fractions eluted from DEAE-cellulose, but they could be disaggregated to a single 14-kD monomer (Fig. 10). The purified product following EDTA disaggregation showed a single band on gel electrophoresis (Fig. 11) and exhibited amino acid and carbohydrate compositions very similar to those of the cell culture material (Tables 1 and 2), and it also contained Gla. Inhibition followed the Langmuir-type isotherm (Fig. 12), with an affinity of 0.5 μM. At the air–water interface, the protein formed a very strong film (Fig. 13), with a collapse pressure of 41.5 dyne/cm; the molecular weight of this protein was found to be 16 kD.

This paper (32) created the main comparison between cell culture and urine inhibitor, and it also showed their similarities; moreover, it demonstrated that almost all of the inhibition produced by diluted urine was accounted for by the protein we isolated, which was a very pure protein as judged by polyacrylamide gel electrophoresis (PAGE) and high-performance liquid chromatography (HPLC). The lack of Gla in the cell culture material vs

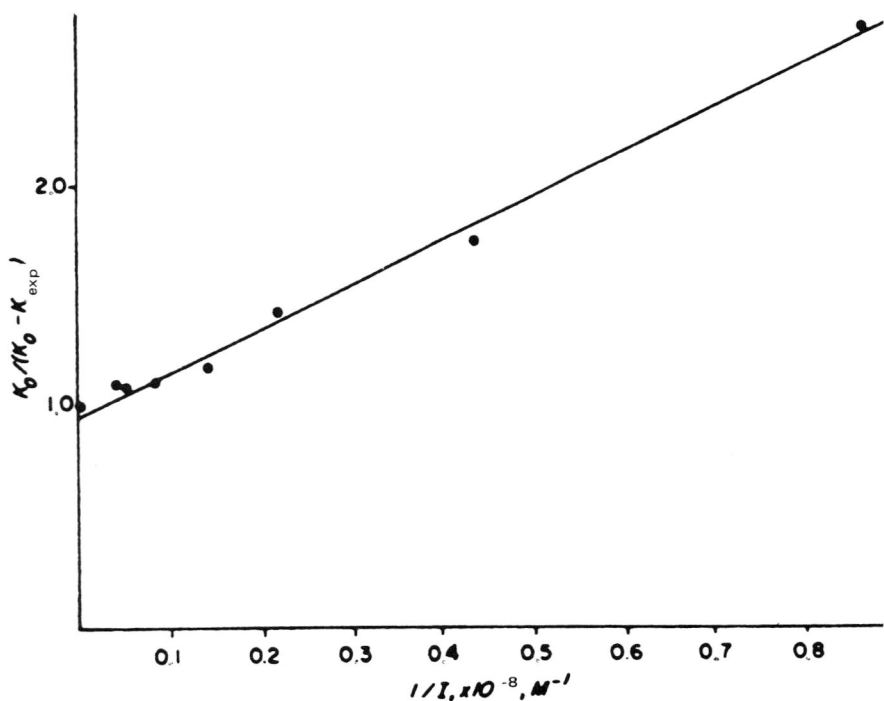

FIG. 7. Langmuir-type adsorption isotherm plot showing the effect of kidney tissue culture inhibitor on the rate of calcium oxalate monohydrate crystal growth. Values of k_0 and k_{exp} represent the rate constants in the absence and presence of inhibitor, respectively. The line drawn represents a linear regression fit to the data ($r = 0.996$). [From Nakagawa et al. (31).]

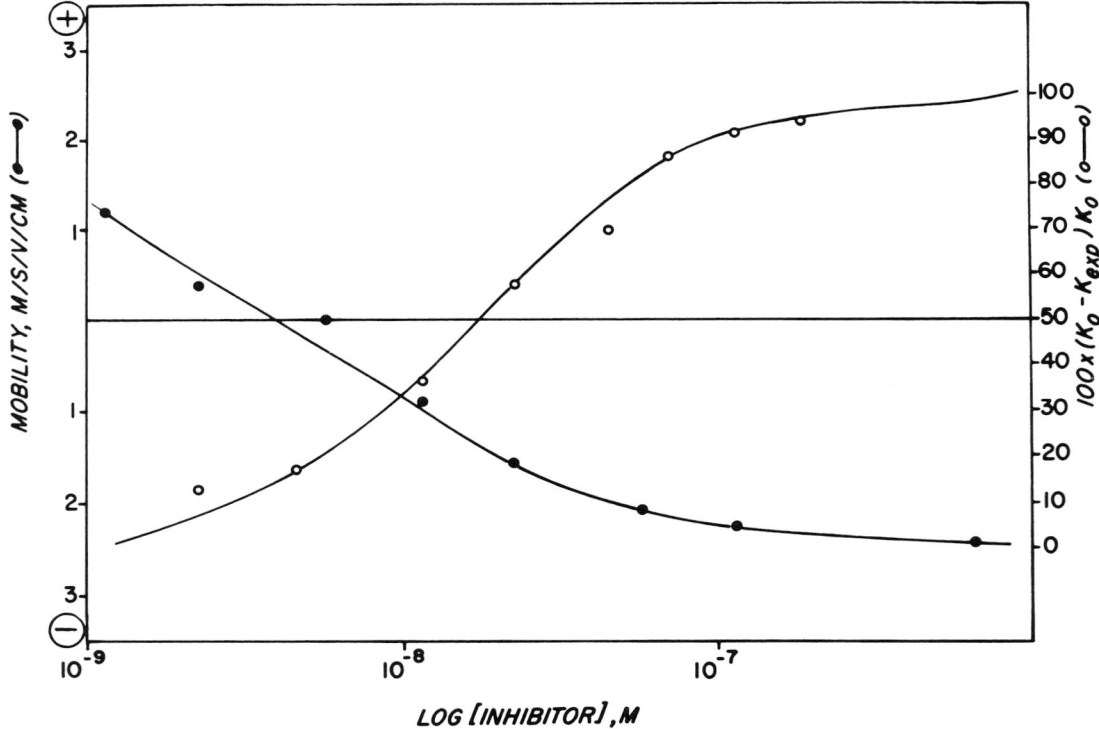

FIG. 8. The effect of kidney tissue culture inhibitor on the electrophoretic mobility of calcium oxalate monohydrate. Mobility measurements were made at 37°C (pH 5.7), using a commercially available Zeta-meter. The extent of inhibition, $(k_0 - k_{exp})/k_0$, as a function of inhibitor concentration, is also shown to emphasize the correlation between mobility changes and extent of inhibition. [From Nakagawa et al. (31).]

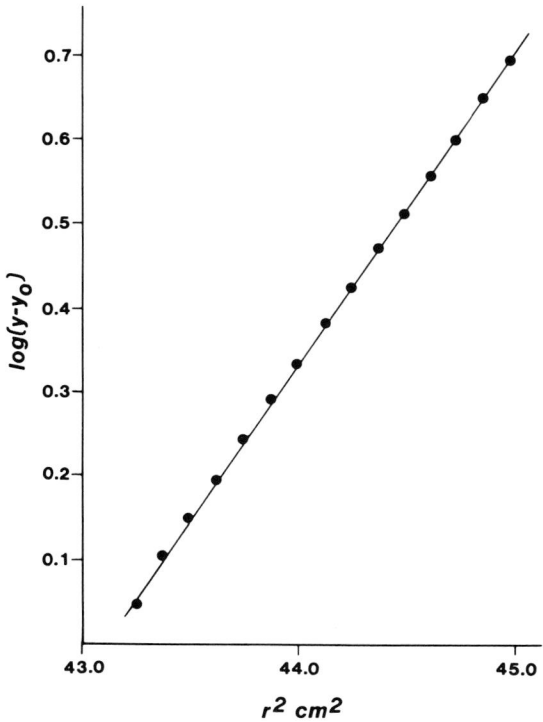

FIG. 9. Sedimentation equilibrium centrifugation of human urinary inhibitor. Protein concentration was 0.3 mg/mL in 0.05 M Tris-HCl plus 0.1 M NaCl (pH 7.3). The running conditions were at 20°C and 30,000 rpm for 48 h. The optical densities were recorded by a photoelectric scanner. [From Nakagawa et al. (32).]

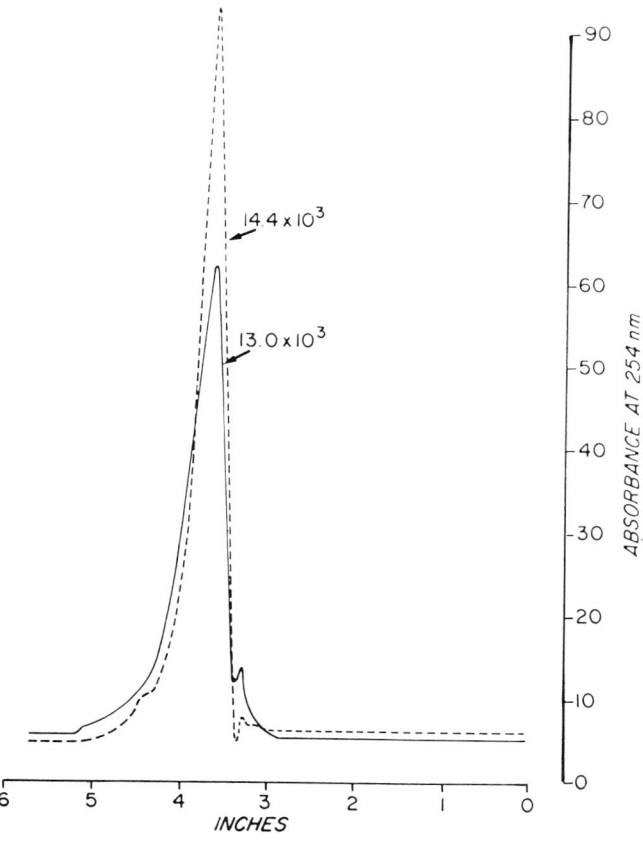

FIG. 10. Elution of the inhibitor from a Toyo–Soda column using high-performance liquid chromatography (HPLC). The chromatogram was developed by the use of 0.05 M Tris-HCl (pH 7.5) containing 0.1 M NaCl and 0.02% NaN_3. High-molecular-weight inhibitors were incubated with 0.01 M EDTA (pH 8.5) for 4 days at 4°C. The solid line indicates the small-molecular-weight inhibitor (1.3×10^4); the dashed line indicates the high-molecular-weight inhibitor (2.7×10^4), whose fraction was injected on the HPLC column after 4 days of incubation with a solution containing EDTA. Chart speed, 8 inches/hr. [From Nakagawa et al. (32).]

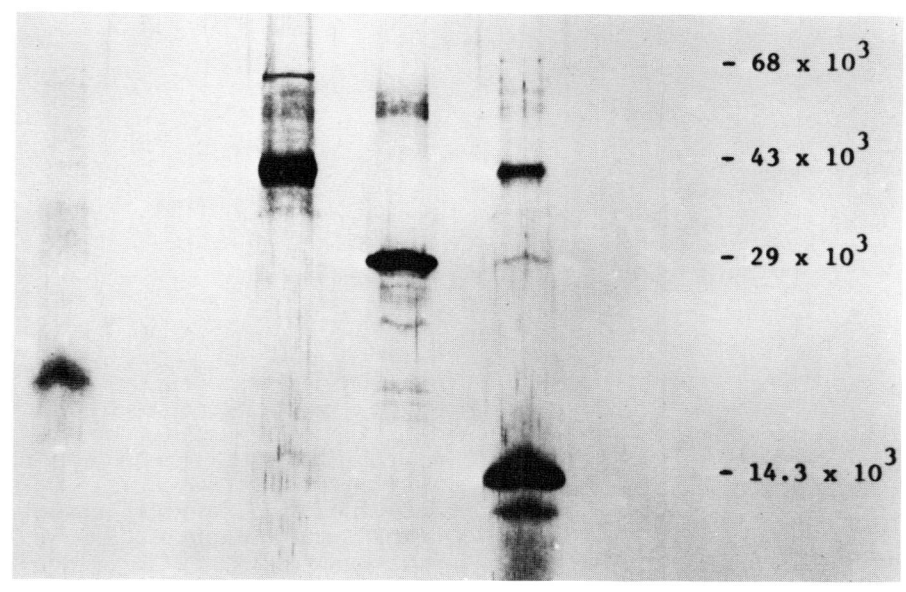

FIG. 11. Sodium dodecyl sulfate–polyacrylamide gel electrophoresis (SDS–PAGE). The SDS–polyacrylamide gel electrophoretogram (0.8-mm thickness) was stained by silver nitrate, and then it was dried with a gel slab dryer (BioRad). Lane 1, purified human urinary inhibitor, 5.1 μg ($M_r = 6.8 \times 10^4$); lane 2, ovalbumin ($M_r = 4.3 \times 10^4$); lane 3, carbonic anhydrase ($M_r = 2.9 \times 10^4$); lane 4, lysozyme (egg white, $M_r = 1.43 \times 10^4$). [From Nakagawa et al. (32).]

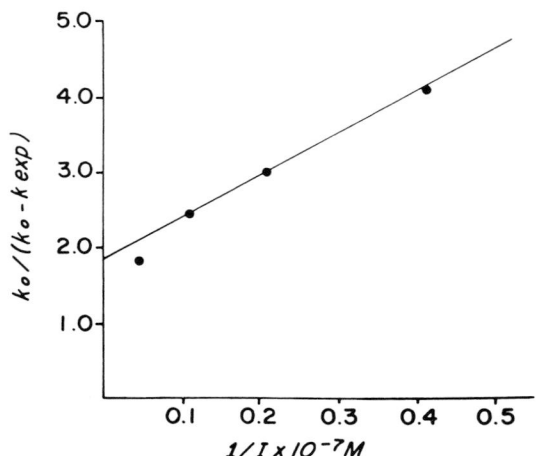

FIG. 12. Langmuir-type adsorption plot for inhibition of calcium oxalate monohydrate crystal growth by human urinary inhibitor. Values of k_0 and k_{exp} represent the rate constants in the absence and presence of inhibitor, respectively. [From Nakagawa et al. (32).]

material in urine seemed to be due to the lack of vitamin K supplementation of the culture, since Gla depends upon a vitamin-K-dependent enzyme.

Rat Kidney and Urine

Using the same methods, we (33) isolated inhibitors from rat kidney tissue and rat urine, then showed that they contained Gla, were indistinguishable in their amino acid compositions, and, on chromatography, behaved like each other and like human urine and cell culture materials. Traits that we observed in human urine and cell culture inhibitor we found here: (a) self-aggregation disruptions using EDTA and not EGTA, (b) a monomer of 14 kD, (c) multiple elution peaks from DEAE-cellulose, and (d) properties very likely to cause confusion between the glycoprotein and a carbohydrate polymer. Carbohydrate composition of urine and tissue materials differed, which we ascribed to probable enzyme effects in urine to remove some carbohydrate. Affinities towards the COM crystal judged from isotherm plots were 0.087 and 0.14 μM for tissue and urine materials. We did this work because we reasoned that kidney could produce the inhibitor (because a renal cell culture produced it), and we found so much inhibitor in kidney tissue that we believed the kidney could indeed produce it, although secretion and filtration from blood could not be ruled out. We also wondered if species other than

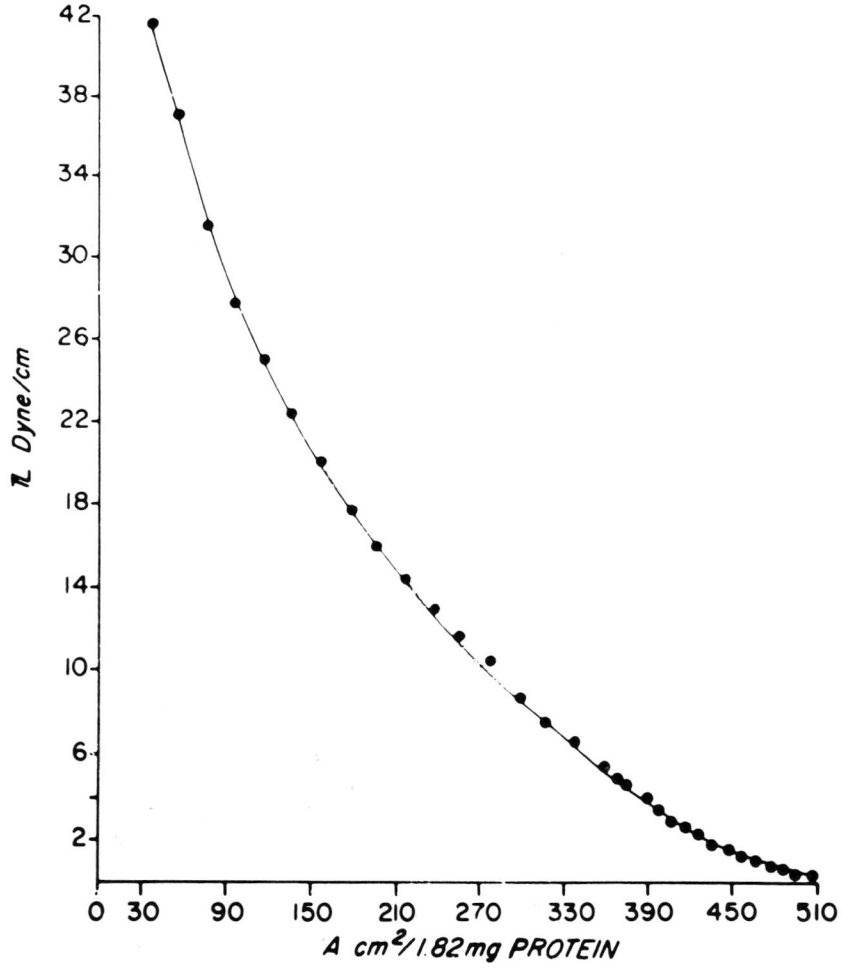

FIG. 13. Surface pressure curve of monolayer of the urinary inhibitor at the air–water interface. The inhibitor solution was dissolved in 0.01 M Tris-HCl plus 0.1 M NaCl (pH 7.4), and the monolayer was compressed and expanded reversibly between 700 and 200 cm² at a rate of 2.2 cm²/s. [From Nakagawa et al. (32).]

humans produced an inhibitor of this special character —in other words, if we were working with a biologically conserved material.

Stone-Former Urine

Naturally, the main reason to study the inhibitors was stone disease. If stone disease occurs because of abnormal inhibitors, then urine from stone formers must contain abnormal inhibitors. By prediction, the stone-former inhibitor should have a low affinity for the COM crystal or should have some other trait that would reduce its ability to inhibit. In Ref. 33, we coined the abbreviation 'GCI' to stand in place of the cumbersome description "urine protein crystal growth inhibitor" and its variants. Later on, we regretted this choice, for its rather ugly appearance, and dropped it for another and a better name.

From urine of men and women, with and without stones, we (34) isolated GCI using the methods already used for rat cell culture, rat urine, and rat tissue. Men and women differed not at all, so the 4 groups were collapsed into 2, normals and stone formers. In both, the fractions of GCI that eluted in each of the four DEAE-cellulose ion-exchange chromatography fractions (which we have always labeled A to D, for want of a better system) were not different (Fig. 14).

The proteins all followed the Langmuir-type isotherms, but they differed in affinity: The C and D materials from patients had very high values, which means low affinities for the COM crystal (Fig. 15). At the air–water interface, normal urine GCI created the usual stable films—except for the D fraction, the one that elutes at the highest ionic strength and whose films col-

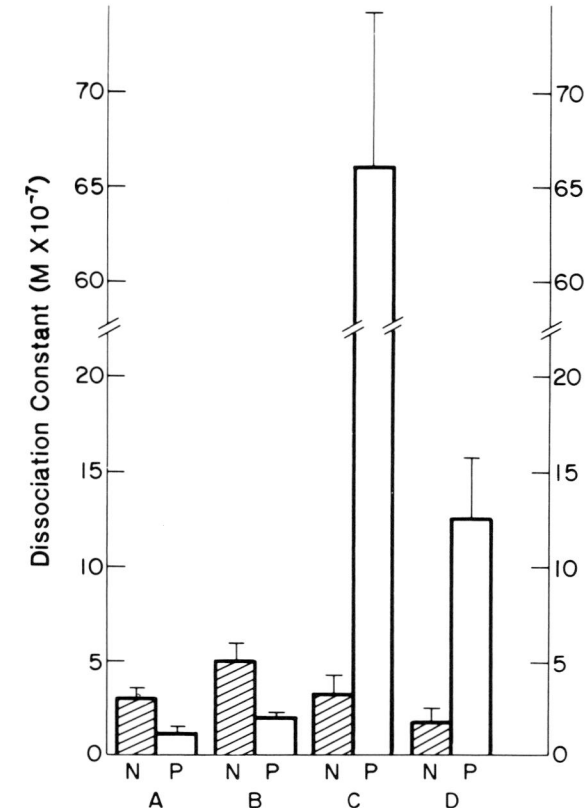

FIG. 15. Langmuir adsorption coefficients. Values are means ± SEM for normals (N) and patients (P) for the A–D fractions depicted in Fig. 14. The ordinate shows the slopes of Langmuir-type isotherm regressions depicted in Fig. 3A–D in Ref. 34. Patients and normals differed, $p < 0.01$ for A and B; and $p < 0.001$ for C and D. (Note changed scale indicated by broken ordinate line.) [From Nakagawa et al. (34).]

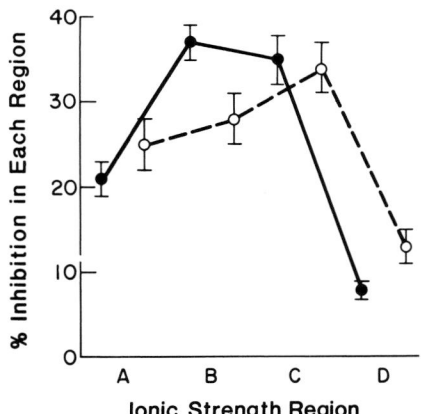

FIG. 14. Distribution of A–D GCI molecules in patients (○) and normal subjects (●). Values are means ± SEM. A through D refer to the ionic strength at which inhibitory molecules elute from DEAE-cellulose. The ordinate shows the percentage of total calcium oxalate crystal growth inhibition within each of the four fractions. Normal percentage B exceeds patients ($p < 0.01$); patient percentage D exceeds normals ($p < 0.01$). [From Nakagawa et al. (34).]

lapsed at relatively low pressures. The normal GCI from fractions A to C contained Gla, but the D fraction contained none. Stone-former GCI from all four fractions formed weak films and contained no Gla.

We interpreted this study to mean that Gla confers upon the molecule some critical properties that endow it with strong film-forming abilities, most likely well-defined and separated hydrophilic regions (which keep the protein on the water surface) and hydrophobic regions (which prevent the protein from dissolving in the water). Because Gla binds calcium, as does GCI, we think that the Gla could form calcium-centered bridges within the molecule to stabilize its tertiary structure in such a way that hydrophobic and hydrophilic regions remain separate and well-defined.

Clearly, the absence of Gla does not lower the affinity of the protein for crystals, as the affinity of patient GCI fractions A and B equaled that of normal GCI A and B though the patient material contained no Gla, and normal D fraction affinity equaled the affinities of normal A to C material but contained no Gla. We reason that inhibitor from patients must have two defects, one concerning the Gla and another concerning its ability to bind to the crystals and inhibit growth.

One might ask, "what importance can film-forming properties have in defense against stone formation?" We can offer only a speculative answer. If an inhibitor, such as poly-L-aspartic acid, binds to COM crystals, being symmetrical it offers to solution ions the same charge spacing it offers to the crystal surface, so calcium ions in solution can bind to the protein and can build up on the protein coating a new layer of COM crystals. As an instance of such overgrowth, mineral substrates can induce crystallization of four different proteins (35). GCI, being amphiphilic, must offer the crystal surface its charged regions, and could present the ions in solution its hydrophobic regions, which should offer only sparse charged sites for their attachment.

Sites of Renal Production

Because kidney tissue offered a rich source of inhibitor, kidney suggested itself as a likely site of synthesis, and Lopez et al. (36) studied this question using an antibody localization protocol. Nakagawa et al. (37) prepared GCI from a single normal male, disaggregated a portion using EDTA, and left the remainder aggregated. THP was purified conventionally, except for a final gel filtration step at pH 7.2 in 4 M urea, and lyophilized. Rabbits were immunized with monomeric and aggregated GCI, and IgG purified from serum after sevenfold titers had been attained. Some IgG was affinity-purified using immobilized monomeric GCI. The antibody to monomeric GCI stained thick ascending limbs of Henle's loop (TAHL) in a pattern identical to that of staining with antibodies to THP. Antibody to aggregated GCI also stained proximal tubules along with Bowman's capsule and Bowman's space, but with progressive dilution it stained TAHL alone.

As a routine interpretation of this experiment, GCI could have been THP or contaminated with THP, but immunodiffusion studies showed that after EDTA treatment, THP produced two bands against the anti-THP antibody and one band against the anti-GCI antibody; the latter band ran continuously with the band that antibody created against GCI itself (Fig. 16). In a multiple comparison immunodiffusion (Fig. 17), the anti-GCI antibody produced a single band continuous with one of two bands produced by the anti-THP antibody. On sodium dodecyl sulfate–polyacrylamide gel electrophoresis (SDS–PAGE) gel, THP migrated at the expected 84-kD region, but after EDTA treatment it showed an additional band at 14 kD, not different from the 14-kD band produced by monomeric GCI (Fig. 18). Protein blotting of a nitrocellulose transfer from the gel showed staining of the 14-kD GCI band and of the 14- and 84-kD bands of the EDTA-treated THP. The best interpretation is that THP adsorbed and was contaminated with GCI and that even though no obvious 84-kD band could be found, the monomeric GCI was contaminated with enough THP to create anti-THP determinants in the anti-GCI antibody.

The value of the work, despite evident flaws, was to highlight the possible interactions between THP and GCI so that GCI can—perhaps—adsorb or attach to THP and remain attached despite 4 M urea treatment yet dissociate with EDTA treatment. It also pointed to TAHL as a possible site of GCI production. Unfortunately, the two proteins could not, then, be completely separated, and the properties of THP as a crystal growth inhibitor were unexplored except for some provisional and unpublished work.

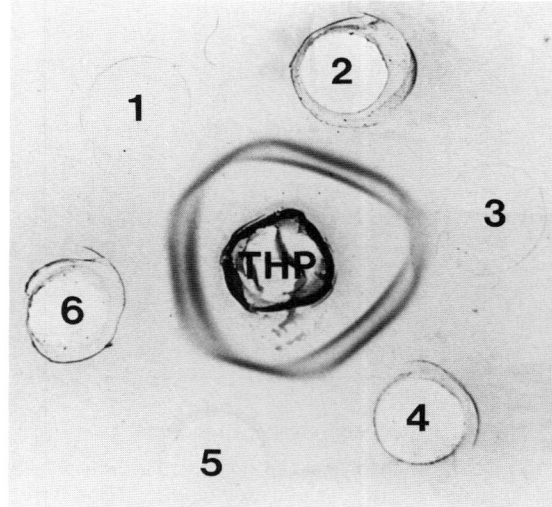

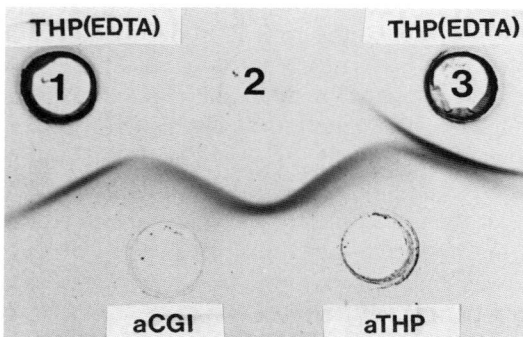

FIG. 16. Immunodiffusion of anti-CGI and anti-THP against monomeric CGI and THP treated with EDTA. Note that anti-CGI reacts with THP in spite of EDTA treatment of THP (site 1); this is identical to the reaction with CGI. In addition, anti-THP reacts with another determinant of THP (site 3), not identified on CGI (site 2). [From Lopez et al. (36).]

FIG. 17. Immunodiffusion of anti-THP (sites 2, 4, and 6) at 1:4 dilution and anti-CGI (sites 1, 3, and 5) at dilutions of 1:1 (site 1), 1:4 (site 3), and 1:16 (site 5) against THP (treated with EDTA). Note the single determinant identified by aCGI and two determinants of anti-THP. [From Lopez et al. (36).]

SILVER STAIN

WESTERN STAIN
aff aCGI, Biotin-GaRG,
Streptavidin-peroxidase

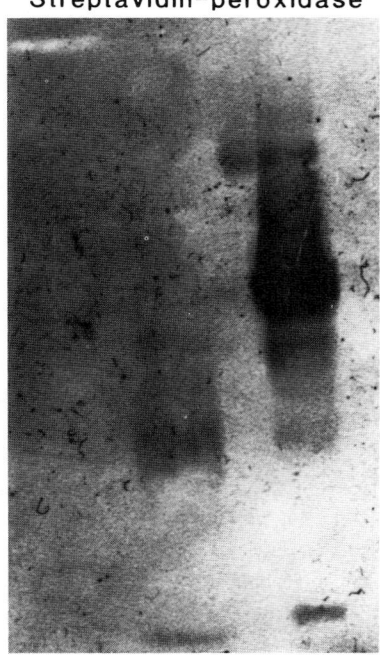

94K —
67K —
40K —
20K —
14.4K —

STD
1

CGI
2

THP(EDTA)
3

STD
4

CGI
5

6 THP

FIG. 18. SDS–PAGE in the presence of 0.05 *M* EDTA. Silver stained (lanes 1, 2, and 3) and Western blot (lanes 4, 5, and 6) with AFaCGI. [From Lopez et al. (36).]

Kidney Stone Nephrocalcin

Because of the urine findings, we sought to confirm Gla deficiency of inhibitors from stone formers and chose to elute inhibitor from calcium oxalate stones themselves, reasoning such material was of certain provenance. Early on in Ref. 37 we introduced the term "nephrocalcin," which came from the idea that the kidney is a likely source of origin and that the inhibitor is calcium-associated. Bone Gla protein carries the name "osteocalcin," which served as the template for the word "nephrocalcin"; hereafter we will use the latter term, with the reservation that to this date the primary sequence remains undiscovered. We abandoned the GCI abbreviation gladly, as we found it ugly and cumbersome in use.

Reference 37 also introduced a refined growth assay using calcium and oxalate (each 1 m*M*) in a stirred quartz cuvette kept at 37°C, monitored at 214-nm wavelength. Seed crystals grow in such a medium rather rapidly, since the supersaturation is high, and disappearance of optical density (OD) at 214 nm follows oxalate disappearance exactly, since calcium chloride has virtually no absorbance at that wavelength. The continuous record-

ing of oxalate disappearance provides hundreds of points for fitting the kinetic rate law, so the growth rate constant can be calculated with great precision using online computer data processing.

The main findings paralleled those of urine nephrocalcin (NC). Stone NC formed weak air–water interfacial films and altogether lacked Gla. The affinity of all four DEAE-cellulose NC fractions towards the COM crystal fell in the range of 0.02–0.2 μM, like normal NC, perhaps because stones would predictably adsorb the highest-affinity inhibitors from urine. This illustrated the complete dissociation between Gla content and affinity and showed the close correspondence between Gla content and film-forming capacity.

Studies of Crystal Adsorption

The work by Lopez et al. (36) provoked us to raise new antisera, and especially to sort out the effects of THP and NC. The antiserum was raised using cell-culture-derived NC (to avoid THP cross-reactivity altogether) and was named "tN1" (38). THP was purified from normal urine using the same methods as for the Lopez et al. (36) paper, and a monoclonal antibody to THP was obtained as a gift. Using the antibody, we could track the adsorption of NC to COM crystals (Fig. 19) and could show progressive inhibition of crystal growth in parallel with protein adsorption. Furthermore, the dissociation constant for adsorption and the slope of the Langmuir-type isotherm derived from parallel inhibition studies on the same batches of crystals showed almost identical values. THP could not be shown to adsorb to the COM crystals as judged using the monoclonal antibody to THP at a protein concentration in the incubation medium of 0.5 μM, and it did not inhibit growth of COM crystals. Albumin binds to COM crystals, but it did not slow their growth at even 3 μM concentration.

What did this study add to our knowledge? We already knew from electrophoretic studies that NC binds to COM crystals, and that binding and inhibition progress in parallel, so why redo the work indirectly with antibodies? Our reason was to dissociate THP and albumin (both plentiful in urine) from NC by using NC from cell culture that had no THP. Such NC inhibited COM crystal growth, and THP could not; the antibody could not have been, unbeknownst to us, tracking the adsorption of contaminating THP in the NC preparation—in this study at least. From the work, we could be sure that whatever the relationship between THP and NC, THP was not the inhibitor in which we were interested.

The Reason for Multiple DEAE Elution Peaks of NC

A puzzling characteristic of NC always was the multiple elution peaks from DEAE-cellulose, which peaks we have called A to D, and which differ in Gla and film stability. Using ^{31}P-NMR (39), NC purified from bovine kidneys showed a major peak (Fig. 20) characteristic of phosphoserine, at +1.75 ppm; treatment with alkaline phosphatase, which cleaves phosphate from phosphoserine, deleted this peak and drastically altered the elution of the NC from DEAE-cellulose. The latter is shown by comparing the elution of the unaltered NC (Fig. 21) (which gave a large C region peak) to the elution of the C peak after alkaline phosphatase treatment, whereupon the NC eluted entirely in the lowest ionic strength region (Fig. 22). Alkaline phosphatase reduced the phosphate content of the C material from 1338 μg/mg protein to 614 μg/mg protein, and it deteriorated the K_d from 0.218 μM to 2.3 μM, a 10-fold change.

Presumably, NC carries many phosphoserine residues, which confer an important part of its inhibitory ability and which account for much of the DEAE-cellulose elution heterogeneity. In addition, NC contains other forms of phosphate, given the residual phosphate after enzyme treatment. This means that post-translational processing plays a role crucial to production of

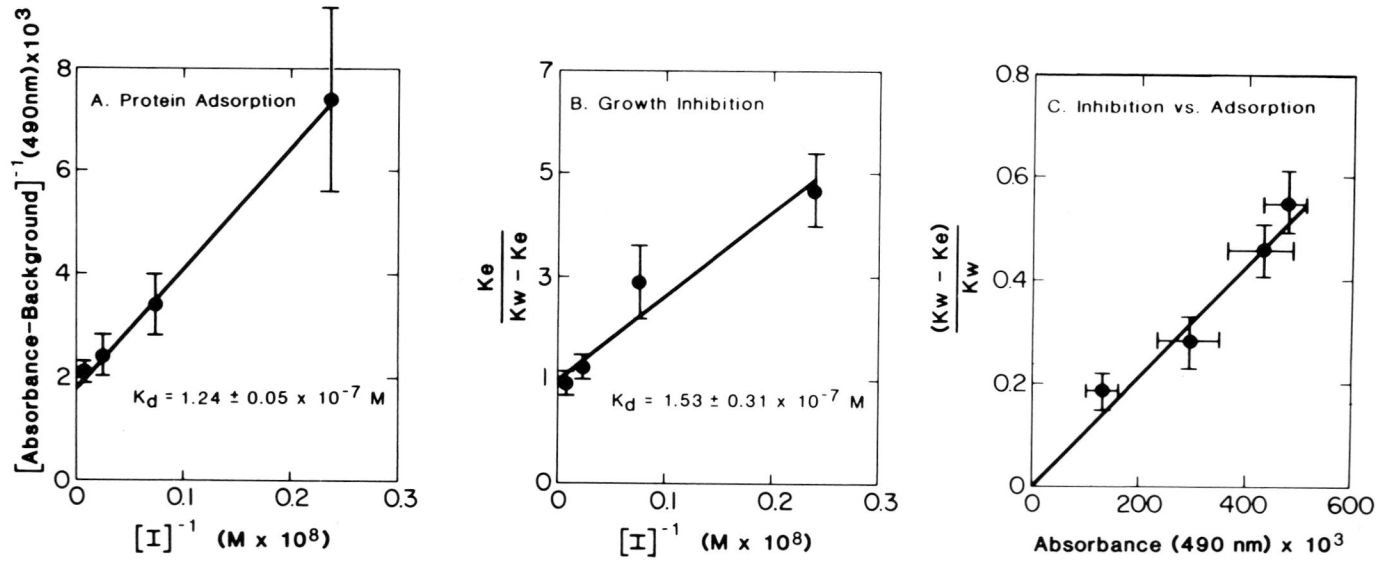

FIG. 19. **A:** Adsorption of NC to calcium oxalate crystals measured using serum from single rabbit (tN1) (*ordinate*) versus NC concentration (*abscissa*) in incubation medium. Crystals of calcium oxalate monohydrate were incubated with NC for 2 h, and then they were probed using tN1; after washing, tN1 was probed using peroxidase-labeled goat anti-rabbit immunoglobulin (IgG). Values ± SEM do not depart from the linear relationship predicted by simple mass action for a double-reciprocal plot. Slope of regression is 2.32 ± 0.053, intercept is 1.85; dissociation constant, calculated from ratio of slope to intercept, is 1.24 ± 0.028 × 10^{-7} M. The regression is significant (F = 1865, p < 0.001). **B:** Reduction of growth of same crystals by NC followed a Langmuir-type isotherm with dissociation constant of 1.53 ± 0.3 × 10^{-7} M. Regression was significant (F = 24, p < 0.105). **C:** Relationship between reduction of calcium oxalate crystal growth (*ordinate*) and adsorption of NC to calcium oxalate crystals (*abscissa*). Incubations and measurements are the same as in **A** and **B**. Fall in growth rate constant (k_e) compared to control growth rate (k_w) did not depart from linear dependence on protein absorption. [From Worcester et al. (38).]

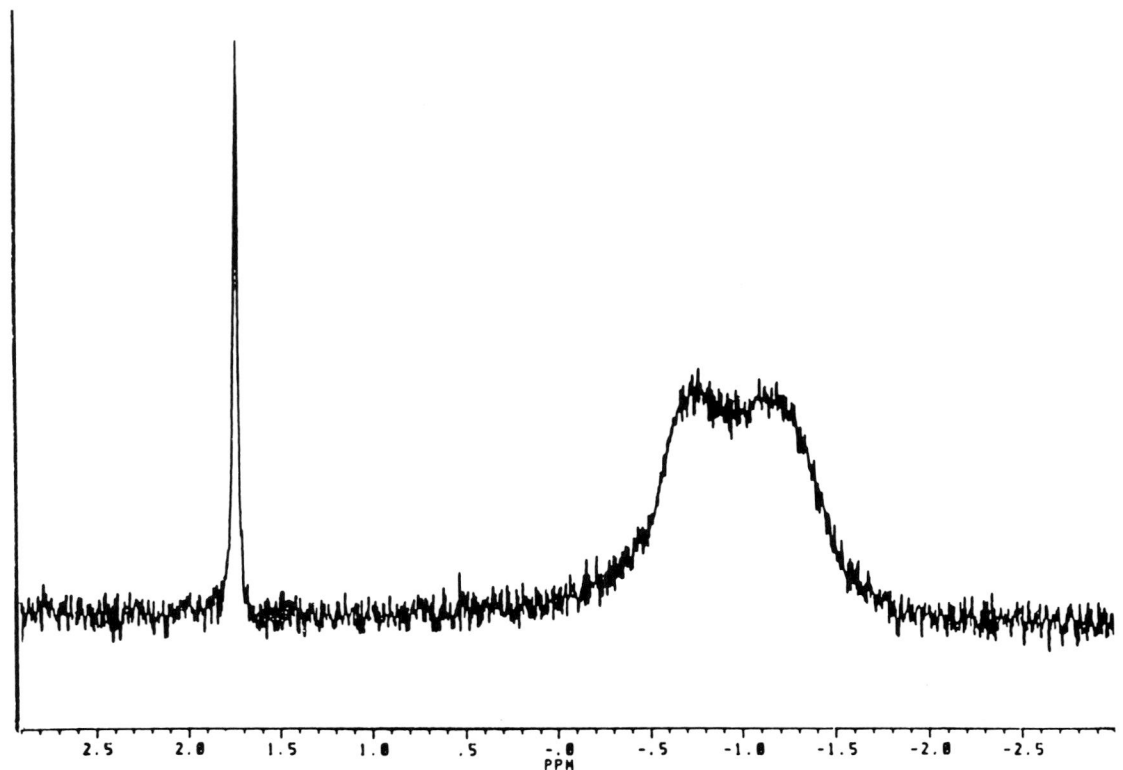

FIG. 20. NMR spectrum of NC fraction C. Reprinted by permission of the publisher from: Elucidation of multiple forms of nephrocalcin by 31P-NMR spectrometer by Y. Nakagawa, T. Otsuki, and F. L. Coe, *FEBS Lett* 250:187–90. Copyright 1989 by Elsevier Science Publishing Co. Inc.

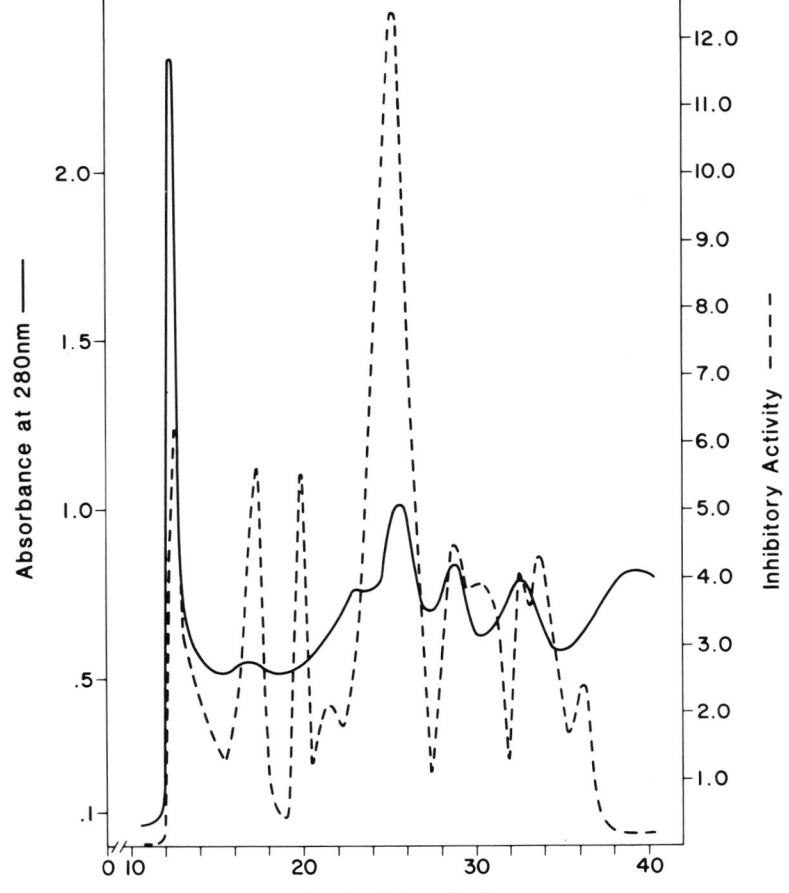

FIG. 21. Elution profile of NC from DEAE-cellulose column. Bovine kidney homogenate was prepared by a manner similar to that described previously, and four fractions of NC were separated by DEAE-cellulose column chromatography (2 × 15 cm) using a linear NaCl gradient from 0.1 *M* to 0.5 *M* in 0.05 *M* Tris-HCl (pH 7.3). Reprinted by permission of the publisher from: Elucidation of multiple forms of nephrocalcin by 31P-NMR spectrometer by Y. Nakagawa, T. Otsuki, and F. L. Coe, *FEBS Lett* 250:187–90. Copyright 1989 by Elsevier Science Publishing Co. Inc.

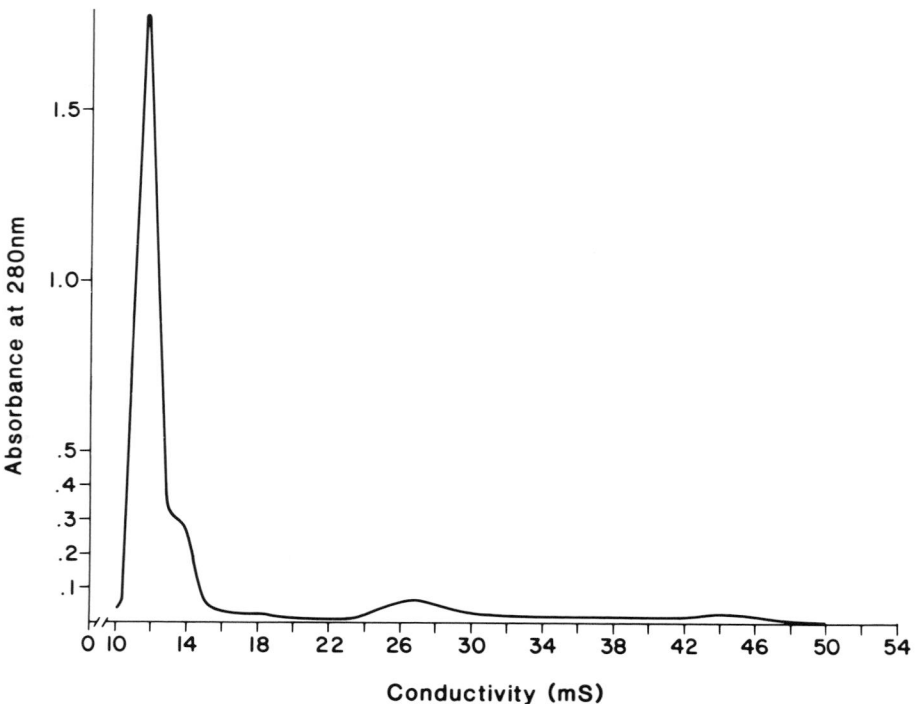

FIG. 22. Elution pattern of dephosphorylated NC fraction C. Fraction was dephosphorylated by alkaline phosphatase and was chromatographed under conditions identical to those described in Fig. 21. Reprinted by permission of the publisher from: Elucidation of multiple forms of nephrocalcin by 31P-NMR spectrometer by Y. Nakagawa, T. Otsuki, and F. L. Coe, FEBS Lett 250:187–90. Copyright 1989 by Elsevier Science Publishing Co. Inc.

finished and effective NC inhibitor, leaving many mechanisms for production of abnormal inhibitors besides simple alterations of primary structure.

Proximal Tubule Origin of NC

Given the Lopez et al. (36) work, we would have preferred to culture TAHL cells, since they probably produce NC. However, we cultured proximal tubule cells using primary cultures grown to confluence, and we were still able to produce calcitriol from vitamin D substrate; as a result, we found strong evidence for NC pro-

duction (40). The proximal tubules are isolated from mouse kidneys, purified as tubule fragments on a density gradient, and then plated out on culture dishes. The cells grow out from the tubule fragments and form a confluent monolayer. For our antibody, we used one prepared against human urinary NC, since we thought that proximal tubules could not produce THP. This antibody, EW1, could recognize THP.

The medium conditioned by the cells contained COM crystal growth inhibitor, which eluted from DEAE-cellulose in the usual way as urine NC (Fig. 23). The EW1 antibody stained all cells in the cultures (Fig. 24), as

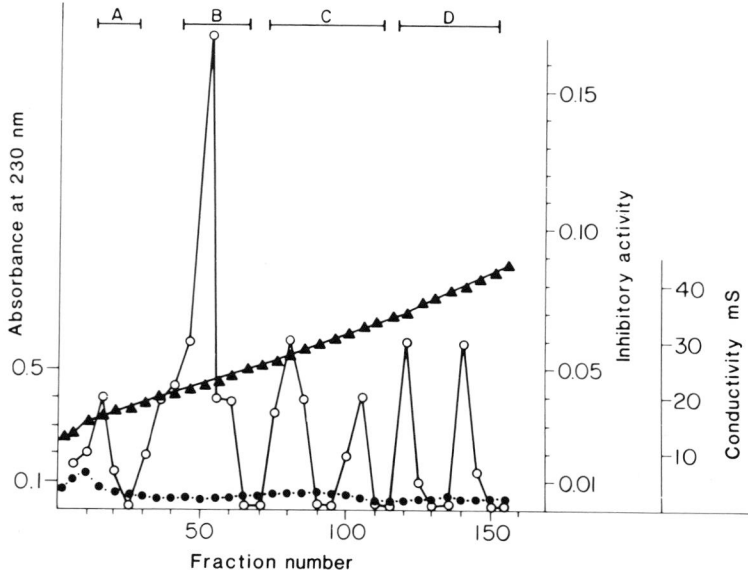

FIG. 23. Elution profile of NC from DEAE-cellulose column. Supernatant of proximal tubule cell culture was subjected to a DEAE-cellulose column with a linear NaCl gradient, from 0.1 M to 0.4 M, for purification of NC. ●, absorbance at 230 nm; ○, inhibitory activity; ▲, conductivity of each fraction (A, B, C, and D, respectively). [From Sirivongs et al. (40).]

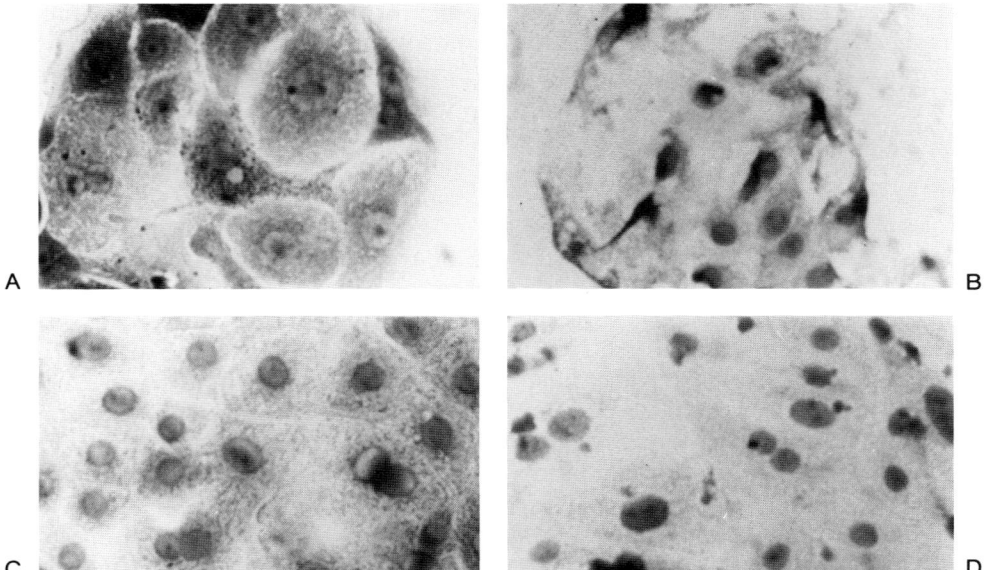

FIG. 24. Immunoperoxidase staining of F4 cell cultured proximal tubule cells. Immunoperoxidase reaction stains cells incubated with EW1 (**A** and **C**), but it does not stain cells incubated with nonimmune serum (**B** and **D**). Dark cytoplasmic pigment is in all cells. Original magnification ×400. [From Sirivongs et al. (40).]

opposed to no staining with nonimmune serum, and by enzyme-linked immunosorbent assay (ELISA), EW1 cross-reacted with all four DEAE-cellulose fractions (Fig. 25). Amino acid compositions of the four fractions showed the characteristic pattern of low basic and aromatic amino acids and high acidic amino acids, along with 1.7 residues/mole of Gla in fraction A. All four fractions inhibited COM crystals strongly, with K_d values ranging from 0.05 to 0.1 μM. The use of primary cell culture supports the notion that the in vitro results mimic in vivo conditions, whereas a cell line could have lost so many characteristics of its original progenitor that it expresses proteins never expressed in the natural set-

ting. That our cells could produce calcitriol added a strong evidence of differentiation.

Where Things Stand

As we write this chapter and review the published data, we feel reasonably certain that NC is a protein of renal origin, probably not one that already has been described, and probably one that depends for its function on post-translational modifications. Given less-than-perfect rigor, one could confuse NC with a carbohydrate polymer, since it reacts poorly with standard protein reagents, absorbs light weakly at 280 nm, and on gels stains

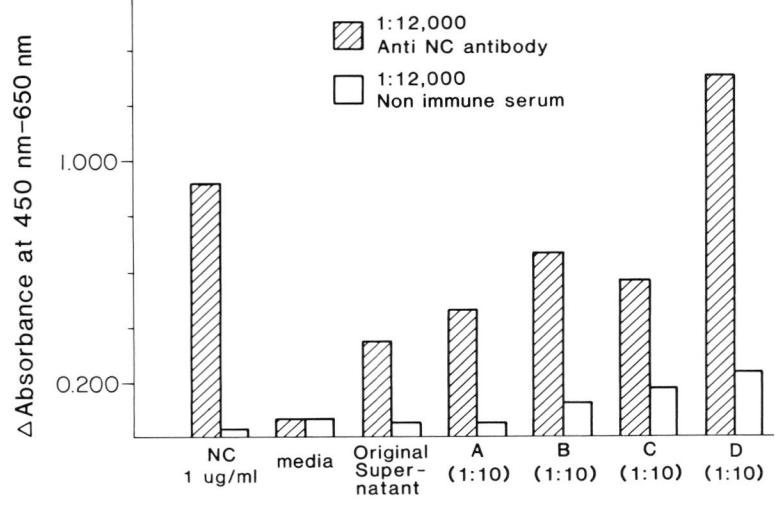

FIG. 25. Direct ELISA of NC fractions from DEAE-cellulose column. An original supernatant and 1:10 dilution of all four fractions (A–D) from DEAE-cellulose chromatography were tested using EW1. All four show cross-reactivity. [From Sirivongs et al. (40).]

poorly with usual protein stains. Being acidic, rather acid-resistant, and a glycoprotein, NC could get into many types of AMPS and glycosaminoglycan preparations, but it is not in any way related to such molecules, since it contains no glucuronic acid. Certainly, it inhibits COM crystal growth very strongly, and at high dilutions. In native urine, at high concentrations, it will also inhibit, although its role relative to other inhibitors of low affinity but high molar concentration remains unclear. The Gla deficiency and low affinity of stone-former NC and NC from human calcium oxalate stones suggests that NC defects play a role in the disease.

One should mention parallel papers to ours describing urine inhibitor products that may be very related to NC. Using ultrafiltration and gel exclusion chromatography, Kitamura et al. (41) extracted COM growth inhibitors containing protein and very little uronic acid or glycosaminoglycans, and they found that stone-formers excreted less inhibiting materials; their procedure should have included some NC. Stone matrix protein, either hydrolyzed (42) or extracted and hydrolyzed (43), showed high values for aspartic and glutamic acids, as in NC; THP surely comprised part of the matrix as well. Urinary matrix calculi from hemodialysis patients (44) also showed high aspartic and glutamic acid contents. Lian et al. (45) found gamma-carboxyglutamic acid residues in stone matrix protein also rich in aspartic and glutamic acids.

Tamm–Horsfall Glycoprotein (THP)

Very copious in urine (about 50–100 mg excreted daily), THP has always attracted attention in this field as a promoter, inhibitor, or suspect bystander in the crystallization process. Perhaps its best established property is formation of urinary casts (46). Attempts to implicate THP in tubulointerstitial renal disease have yielded mixed results (47). Present evidence favors its role as an inhibitor of aggregation, but much depends upon how aggregation is measured, whether or not growth and aggregation can be separated in the assay, and whether the THP used has been separated from other proteins, including NC.

Unlike NC, THP has been sequenced (48). The protein contains 48 cysteine residues that can support up to 24 disulfide bonds, through which this protein may self-aggregate into a gel (49), presumably a normal pathway in formation of urinary casts. Originally, THP was isolated as an inhibitor of viral hemagglutination (50); later on, THP was found to be uromodulin, an inhibitor of interleukin production (48).

Promotion of Crystal Formation

If urine is evaporated to increase its concentration of salts, crystals form, which are said to be mainly calcium oxalate at pH 5.3 (51). The amount of crystal, judged by microscopic counting or by amount of radioactive oxalate incorporated into precipitate, was higher in whole urine than in urine passed through an ultrafiltration cell to remove high-molecular-weight materials. Adding back THP purified by NaCl precipitation, but not using subsequent column chromatography, increased the numbers of crystals. Albumin had no such effect.

A problem with this kind of research is the nature of the concentrating step, which concentrates sodium and potassium chloride (as well as urea, nonspecifically) to reach a predetermined osmolality (1250 mOsm/kg in this case) and a low urine pH. Low pH and high ionic strength cause THP to self-aggregate strongly, into a fibrous material (52); using flow viscometry (53), rotating cylinder viscometry (54–56), or light scattering (57), aggregation occurs to a very large extent when NaCl concentrations exceed 200 mM and pH falls below 5.5, especially when calcium ion concentration rises to as high as 1 μM. In evaporated undialyzed urine such as used here, concentrations of NaCl (not given) in the final evaporate should have been more than twice normal values (usually 100–200 mM), and calcium concentrations should have been up to 5 or even 10 mM. The state of THP under such circumstances should have been a fibrous mass.

Inhibition of Crystal Growth and Nucleation

In another kind of experiment, THP did not promote calcium oxalate crystallization (58). THP was isolated from urine of six normals and nine stone-forming patients by NaCl precipitation, and it was lyophilized for later use. To 1 mM CaCl$_2$ (pH 6.5) and 136 mM NaCl, oxalate can be added in steps to find the concentration sufficient to initiate CaOx precipitation, as judged by clouding and confirmed by solution ion depletion—in other words, the formation product. The ratio of the calcium oxalate ion activity product at that point (determined by graphical interpolation of plots of concentration product vs ion depletion) to the activity product measured at thermodynamic equilibrium in the same system, called the "formation product ratio" (FPR), rose from 8 in the basic system to 10 when THP concentration was 100 mg/L, about the highest level expected in normal urine. Second-order growth rate constants of seed crystals in the Meyer–Smith metastable growth medium (59) fell by 50% (a significant amount) with THP addition.

This experiment used conditions in which THP should have remained in solution relatively disaggregated, since pH was high and NaCl concentration was moderate. However, the THP was purified with no gel filtration step, so the product could have contained other glycoproteins, even NC. Certainly, the conflict between the two papers we just reviewed cannot be resolved, since the methods have almost nothing in common.

Effects on Growth and Aggregation

Robertson and Scurr (60) used the MSMPR technique (calcium 6 mM, oxalate 0.6 mM in final mixed solution, 12 mM calcium and 1.2 mM oxalate in the feed solutions, pH 5.8, ionic strength 0.33), in which particle size distribution from the mixing chamber is used to give estimates of nucleation and growth rate and aggregation (agglomeration); the latter is obtained from the difference between the number of particles between 2.5 and 51.2 μm (predicted from the steady-state crystal distribution equation) and the observed numbers from a given set of experimental conditions. RNA inhibited nucleation and growth and aggregation, for example, so the system could respond to polyanions at concentrations in the range of 0.1 μM, but THP polymerized and formed particles, and the particles could not be distinguished from crystal particles, so THP could not be studied. Presumably, the same occurred in the Rose and Sulaiman (51) experiment, since urine was evaporated.

Later (61) the same authors used their system at lower ionic strength of 0.161 (pH 6.0) and found that THP could inhibit aggregation at concentrations between 0.05 and 1 μM, but they found that THP self-aggregated above that concentration. They could see masses of crystals and aggregated THP under the microscope. Inhibition of aggregation correlated with change in the zeta potential, the apparent surface charge on COM crystals whose rate and direction of migration are studied in an electrical field. These results echo an earlier presentation of much the same data by these authors (62).

Elsewhere (63), they explored the zeta potential effects of THP with other coating polyanions, asking whether THP could influence binding of other materials and thereby reduce their ability to prevent aggregation. In other words, because zeta potential and aggregation inhibition moved in parallel, zeta potential was taken as a marker for materials that could inhibit aggregation, and effects of zeta potential were taken as markers for effects on aggregation inhibitors—a dangerously long chain of inferences. THP, as well as fresh urine, interfered with binding of such materials as RNA to COM crystals, as evidenced by reduced effects of RNA on zeta potential. Whether or not RNA, for example, can reduce the ability of THP to inhibit COM crystal aggregation remains unknown.

Inhibition of Aggregation Under Zero Growth Conditions

Hess et al. (64) used an aggregation measurement uncomplicated by crystal growth. COM crystals in an equilibrium calcium oxalate solution aggregate when stirred slowly, and their rate of fall can be monitored in a cuvette with continuous recording at 620 nm. The slope of the OD decline after stirring has ceased, and particles fall at limiting velocities that vary inversely with their radii, gives an index of the mean of those radii.

Whole urine inhibited aggregation, as measured by particle radius (Fig. 26), and even extreme dilution did not lower the inhibition below 30%. Urine proteins also inhibited aggregation (Fig. 27); THP was the greatest inhibitor, followed by NC. Stone-former urine NC and kidney stone NC inhibited much less well than did normal NC. Albumin and beta-2 microglobulin also inhibited, but at concentrations above those expected in normal urine. Citrate did no inhibiting at all. THP and NC both altered zeta potential, but THP did it to a greater extent than did NC, though both inhibited aggregation equally in the ranges of concentration used (Fig. 28). Thus, zeta potential and aggregation inhibition did not move in parallel in this case.

Clinical Studies

Finally, one should note attempts at clinical distinctions such as low or high THP excretion in stone disease.

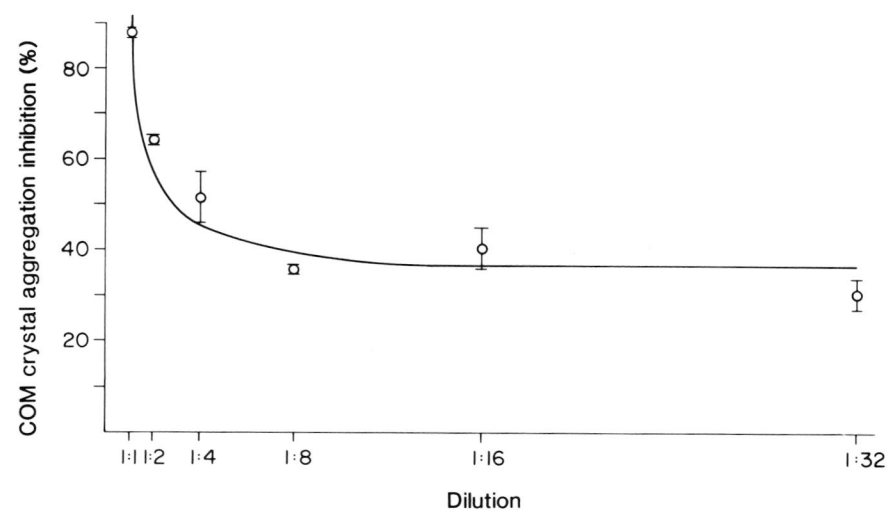

FIG. 26. COM crystal aggregation inhibition by dialyzed human urine. Urine, dialyzed against a 10 mM Tris-HCl buffer (pH 7.2) containing 90 mM NaCl, inhibited COM crystal aggregation as judged by T_s, in a concentration-dependent manner. [From Hess et al. (64).]

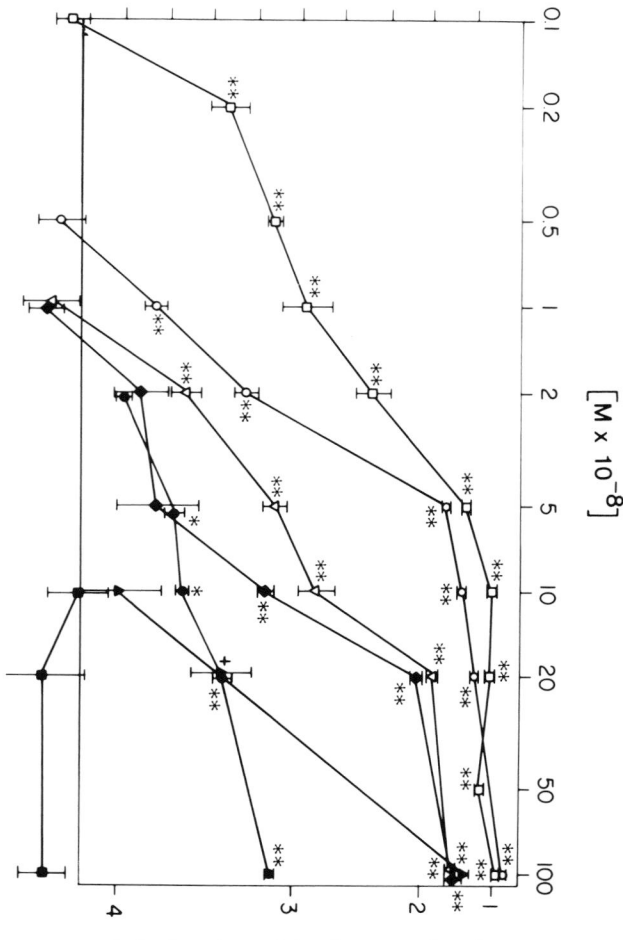

Calculated particle diameter (μm)

FIG. 27. Effects of inhibitors on COM crystal aggregation. Inhibition of COM crystal aggregation (*y*-axis, *left*) by THP (□), normal urine NC (○), albumin (▽), B2-MG (◆), stone-former urine NC (●), NC from stones (▲), and citrate (■) increased as their concentrations increased (*x*-axis). All values are means ± SEM. The plus sign (+) indicates that the value differs from control value ($p < 0.05$); *$p < 0.01$; **$p < 0.001$. Citrate is also without effect at $1 \times 10^{-3} M$ (not shown). Particle diameters (*y*-axis, *right*) are calculated. [From Hess et al. (64).]

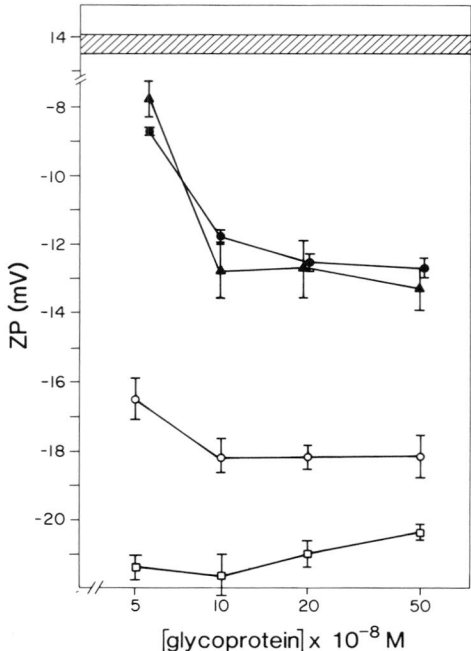

[glycoprotein] x 10^{-8} M

FIG. 28. Surface charge (zeta potential) of COM crystals. Zeta potential (*y*-axis) of crystals incubated with THP (□), normal urine NC (○), stone-former urine NC (●), and stone NC (▲) became negative when compared to control (hatched region, above broken *y*-axis). Above $10^{-7} M$, increasing concentration did not increase negativity of potential. [From Hess et al. (64).]

Using an antibody method, Bichler et al. (65) found that normals excreted 50 mg and that calcium oxalate stone formers excreted 65 mg ($p > 0.5$). Among uric acid stone-formers, however, THP excretion was low (40 mg, $p < 0.05$ versus normal), perhaps because of an acid urine pH. Among six people with renal tubular acidosis (RTA) and staghorn calculi, THP excretion was very low, (17 mg, $p < 0.05$ versus normal), certainly not because of low urine pH but perhaps due to renal damage.

An Overview

Whatever Nature intended THP to do, the protein interacts very strongly with COM crystals, and what it does to the crystals probably depends upon its own state, ag-

gregated or not, and whether the crystals are growing or not. Evaporating urine probably aggregates THP, makes it into particles, and exaggerates the size of crystal deposits. In dilute systems that support COM growth and aggregation, separating the two could be a problem, and if THP inhibits only aggregation but not growth, as we believe (38), growth could enlarge particles and give the illusion that THP was not a good inhibitor of aggregation. In the Scurr papers, an intrinsic source of confusion could be growth mimicking aggregation. Furthermore, the THP must be free of NC, and we attempt to separate them using a gel filtration step after NaCl precipitation. If NC contaminates THP preparations, COM growth inhibition may be found, as in the paper by Kitamura and Pak (58).

THP clearly adsorbs to COM crystals, and our own failure to document adsorption using antibodies (38) illustrates inherent weaknesses of such methods in crystal work, perhaps related to our using a monoclonal antibody for tracking THP. That zeta potential and aggregation inhibition correlate well using some polyanions, and not well when NC and THP are compared, suggests that zeta potential and aggregation are related to each other through other shared features, not through a direct linkage.

When urine is concentrated and of high ionic strength, THP aggregates, forming fibers and eventually urinary casts. The protein self-aggregation removes the protein from solution and presumably interferes with its binding to COM crystals and inhibits the aggregation of the COM crystals. Possibly, THP fibers could themselves promote crystallizations, either by acting as a surface for heterogeneous nucleation or by matting together small crystal nuclei into a protein crystal mass, whose size could become large enough to occlude tubule lumens. Furthermore, aggregated THP can provoke neutrophil degranulation (50) and release of leukotrienes, so possibly such aggregates could create localized foci of inflammation in tubules if epithelial surfaces were disrupted by, for example, crystal-induced cell injury.

Factors that could influence this phenomenon include the contribution of urea versus NaCl to the final osmolality, since high ionic strength promotes THP self-aggregation but urea does not, and this balance depends upon sodium and protein intakes. The inherent tendency for THP to self-aggregate certainly may be a major factor, since THP from diabetics seems to self-aggregate more readily than does normal THP (66); THP from some stone formers could possibly do the same. Finally, small proteins in urine, such as Bence Jones proteins, promote THP self-aggregation and also reduce the efficiency of TAHL NaCl reabsorption, thereby increasing lumen NaCl concentration (in principle). Therefore, these proteins could influence the effects of THP on crystals (67). Relationships to nephrolithiasis seem tenuous.

Other Examples of Inhibition Outside of Kidney and Urine

Fish Antifreeze Proteins

Nature has expressed herself most clearly about crystal inhibitors in fashioning, for fish that live in freezing cold waters, proteins for their blood that prevent the formation of ice, itself a well-studied crystal that is very destructive in blood and in cells (68). At least four kinds of antifreeze proteins exist. One is a glycoprotein, made up of a repeating three-amino-acid sequence (alanine, alanine, threonine) repeated from 4 to 40 times, with a disaccharide on the threonine. The other three are diverse, and they are also different from the glycoprotein. One is an alanine-rich α-helical protein found in flounders. Another is a cystine-rich protein found in sea ravens. The third, found in eel pouts, seems heterogeneous, existing in up to 12 variants, all sharing considerable amino acid sequence. Of great interest, despite the wide variety of structures, the proteins all exhibit similar actions on ice crystals, abridging their growth along one plane. The α-helical antifreeze protein is amphiphilic, and it appears to adsorb to ice on its charged areas. It also presents the solution with its hydrophobic side, which impedes ice overgrowth. Furthermore, glycopeptide from one arctic fish (69) inhibits melting of ice crystals.

To us, the extreme importance of fish antifreeze proteins is their ability to lower the freezing point of blood for fish that live in cold water. Thus, one can be quite sure that at least once in evolution Nature has created proteins specialized as crystallization inhibitors. One cannot as yet be so sure for urine proteins, which may indeed inhibit crystallization but which could also have some other primary purpose in the biology of the animal, since the inhibition of renal crystallization has not yet been elevated to as clear a biological importance as prevention of freezing of blood in cold water fish.

Saliva

Salivary glands produce an acidic peptide called "statherin" (70); it contains 43 amino acids, is rich in tyrosine and glutamic acid, and is able to block the nucleation and growth of calcium phosphate crystals that tend to form in saliva, given its alkaline pH. Using the sequence (70), a cDNA clone was isolated (71) and was used to map the chromosomal locale of statherin.

Pancreatic Stones

From human stones, a 15-kD protein has been isolated and sequenced that can form helical protein threads and that inhibits calcium carbonate crystallization (72). The protein is not rich in aspartic and glutamic acids, contains six cystines, and contains considerable tyrosine and tryptophan, and thus it differs greatly from NC.

Gallstones

Human bile is supersaturated with respect to cholesterol, which can crystallize into stones (73). Bile proteins contain an inhibitor of cholesterol nucleation (74). Acting on a reasonable hypothesis, apolipoprotein A-I and A-II, which occur in bile, were tested and found to be efficient inhibitors of cholesterol crystallization (75). From human gallstones, Shimizu et al. (76) isolated a low-molecular-weight, highly acidic protein that inhibits calcium carbonate crystallization and that seems different from the pancreatic protein, though it shares with NC an excess of glutamic and aspartic residues, low lysine and arginine. The protein contained no Gla, but neither does human kidney stone NC.

Citrate

By serving as a calcium ligand, forming a soluble salt with calcium and thereby reducing the availability of calcium for reaction with oxalate and phosphate, citrate "inhibits" stone disease, a topic explored in the chapter on supersaturation (Chapter 29). Here we consider interactions of citrate with crystal growth, aggregation, and nucleation, direct inhibitions of the transition from solution to solid-phase structure.

Citrate Effects on Urine Crystallization

We already noted (19) that citrate at 0.5 mM reduces the second-order COM crystal growth rate constant by one-third (measured in a seeded metastable crystal growth system), even after correction for ligand formation. Using the apatite seed addition method devised by Bisaz, Bisaz et al. (8) found that citrate, at concentrations between 0.5 and 2 mM, inhibits apatite crystallization after allowing for ligand binding, although these studies show no effects of urine ultrafiltration, so macromolecules seem to play no role. Using Robertson's continuous crystallizer method, Robertson and Scurr (60) found that citrate promoted nucleation and reduced crystal growth for COM, but only in proportion to its reduction of supersaturation by calcium binding. Urine citrate concentrations are approximately 2.53 and 1.83 mM in normal women and men, respectively (2), and are approximately 1.79 and 1.35 mM among women and men with stones. Thus, citrate must be presumed to contribute to the COM crystal growth inhibition of whole urine, and because its concentration is lower in stone formers, citrate could contribute to stone formation when low.

Using an assay that measures agglomeration and crystal growth at the same time, Kok et al. (77) found that 1:5 diluted urines from stone formers inhibited calcium oxalate monohydrate crystal growth and agglomeration to a lesser degree than did normal urine, and they also found that inhibition of aggregation varied as a regular function of urine citrate concentration. In this assay, COM seeds are added to a supersaturated calcium oxalate solution ($0.14 \ \mu M^2$), their growth is measured by uptake of ^{45}Ca into the seeds, and the effects of agglomeration are measured as a depression of growth rate from that expected using a mathematical model of the growth process. These same investigators presented data (78) showing that citrate inhibits COM crystal aggregation. We (64), however, found just the opposite–that under conditions of equilibrium, when growth does not occur, aggregation of crystals is unaffected by citrate. We must presume that the discrepancy reflects the presence or absence of growth in the two experiments.

Among seven normal people and four elderly male patients with recurrent calcium oxalate stones, magnesium citrate and magnesium oxide (given four times daily) each raised urine citrate, from 521 mg to 663 mg and 619 mg, respectively; the concentration of the citrate preparation was higher than that of the oxide, and both were above control levels (79). Neither treatment altered supersaturation or formation product for calcium oxalate or brushite. In a substudy involving these medications given with meals to four normals and three of the four patients, the magnesium citrate reduced calcium oxalate supersaturation below control levels, and it raised the calcium oxalate formation product above control; thus the subset of subjects, or the use of the treatments with meals, or both, seems to affect outcome.

A crucial subgroup of patients who may most particularly need citrate consists of those with RTA (see Chapter 34), either complete (i.e., with metabolic acidosis) or incomplete (i.e., unable to lower urine pH normally but without metabolic acidosis). RTA patients form calcium phosphate stones because of elevated urine pH, have low urine citrate because acid excretion (even when sufficient to prevent overt metabolic acidosis) is less than normal, and fail to lower urine pH below 5.5 after an ammonium chloride challenge. Among six such patients (four men and two women), Preminger et al. (80) found that sodium or potassium citrate raised urine citrate (from 312 to above 500 mg daily, and to an equal extent), but potassium citrate lowered urine calcium (from 214 to 178 mg daily) whereas sodium citrate did not. Thus potassium citrate lowered supersaturation with respect to calcium oxalate. Of interest, calcium phosphate supersaturation for brushite did not fall with either agent, because urine pH rose, furthermore, supersaturations actually rose with sodium citrate. One must suppose that potassium citrate could reduce the calcium oxalate component of stones in RTA.

Urine Citrate Levels

The issue of urine citrate in stone disease, particularly the frequency, gender differences, and reasons for low urine citrate in stone-forming people, expected for a putative cause of stones, seems less than settled to us. If citrate inhibits nucleation, growth, and aggregation apart from its effects on supersaturation, as much evidence suggests, and since citrate also can reduce supersaturation, urine citrate could protect against stones while low citrate could promote stones. Is citrate really reduced in urine of stone-formers?

We (2) found a great difference between the sexes: Normal women have high urine citrate, stone-forming women have lower urine citrate; normal men have urine citrate levels similar to those of stone-forming women, and men with stones have the same daily citrate excretions as normal men but exhibit relative polyuria (Fig. 29). As a result, normal women seem to make up a class of their own (see the upper left-hand corner of the graph), with all the rest being less protected, suggesting, perhaps, a reason why four of every five stone-formers are men.

Hosking et al. (81) found nothing the same as our results. Men and women alike excreted similar amounts of citrate, which increased with age. Among women aged 39 or less, patients and normals excreted like amounts, and for men the amounts were alike for age 49 or less. Citrate excretion rose with age in normals of both sex but did not rise among patients, accounting for the age-

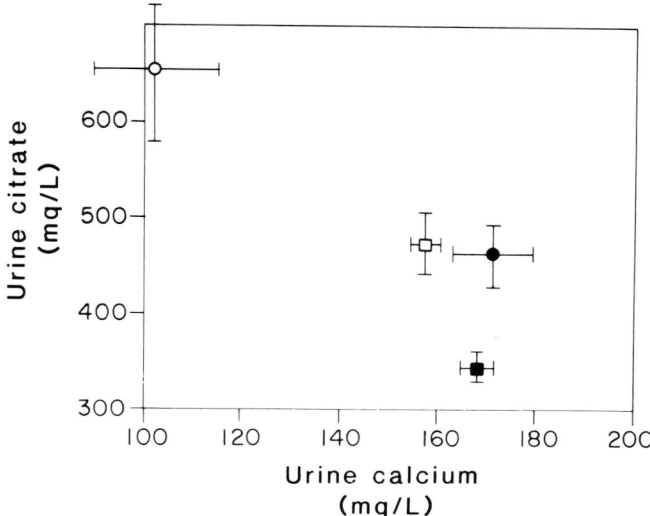

FIG. 29. Urine citrate versus calcium concentration (±SEM) in women (○, □) and men (●, ■) with (□, ■) and without (○, ●) calcium oxalate nephrolithiasis. [From Parks and Coe (2).]

hypercalciuria and those without hypercalciuria were analyzed separately, urine calcium was found to be higher in the former than in the latter. Allowing for what seems to be a confused presentation, low urine citrate among stone-formers could be documented.

Nikkila et al. (83) studied 14 women and 22 men normals, who had urine citrate/creatinine ratios of 0.21 ± 0.03 versus 0.15 ± 0.02, respectively. The ratio for males was clearly lower, than the ratio for females. The ratio for female stone-formers was 0.13 ± 0.03, clearly like the ratio for normal men. Finally, the ratio for stone-forming men was 0.08 ± 0.01, which was the lowest of all. These data match ours. For female normals versus stone-formers, the difference of 0.08 was statistically insignificant ($p > 0.01$); however, the difference for men, 0.07, was statistically significant ($p < 0.01$), probably because so many more men were studied. It is unclear as to why we found higher urine citrate excretion among women than among men without a need to correct for urine creatinine or body weight.

Minisola et al. (84) found citrate excretions (mM/ mM) of urine creatinine of 0.43 ± 0.13 and 0.23 ± 0.08 in normal women and men, respectively, a clear excess in women. Women with stones excreted 0.28 ± 0.17, whereas men with stones excreted 0.16 ± 0.09; these results exactly like ours.

What do we conclude at this time? Three of five studies agree in the gender difference, though not in the need to correct for body size or muscle mass. The others found lower citrate concentrations among stone-formers but found no gender difference. If we summarize the three comparable studies, all presented in the same units (Table 3), the following results stand out: (a) higher urine citrate concentrations in females than in males and (b) a remarkable similarity between normal male and stone-former female citrate concentrations.

Citrate as Treatment

One can find two indices of treatment: (i) reduced stone rate and (ii) improvement in urine chemistries related to stone formation, such as supersaturation. Of the two, the former convinces more completely. In the future, it would be most desirable to perform a placebo-controlled trial.

Pak and Fuller (85) treated 37 patients (6 women, 31 men) who formed calcium-oxalate-containing stones. Of

related deficiencies of the patients. Groups are small because of the many subdivisions, and the only significant differences were between men patients and normals aged 50–59 years and between women patients and normals aged 40–49 years and aged 50–59, with patients' citrate excretion always lower.

Considering the fact that we both chose subjects from among routine populations, it is hard to determine why we should disagree regarding a stable measurement. As for hypocitraturia, we (2) found it as a trait of women stone-formers, whereas Hosking et al. (81) found it to be age-related and among both sexes. No one doubts that metabolic acidosis reduces urine citrate, and low urine values were reported by Hosking et al. (81) among patients with RTA or bowel disease. We and Hosking et al. excluded such patients from the general comparison between patients and normals.

Conte et al. (82) found lower urine citrate concentrations among patients (300 mg/L) than among normals (517 mg/L) but did not describe a sex difference and did not give separate values for men and women, so we could analyze them. Like ourselves, they plotted urine citrate versus calcium, and found, as we did not, a correlation, perhaps because both are related somehow to size effects not properly analyzed. Also, when patients with

TABLE 3. *Summary of urine citrate excretions*[a]

Study	Normal men	Normal women	Men patients	Women patients
Parks and Coe (2)	0.29 ± 0.028	0.58 ± 0.056	0.27 ± 0.011	0.46 ± 0.029
Minisola et al. (84)	0.23 ± 0.021	0.43 ± 0.027	0.16 ± 0.019	0.28 ± 0.038
Nikkila et al. (83)	0.15 ± 0.02	0.21 ± 0.03	0.08 ± 0.01	0.13 ± 0.03

[a] Values are urine citrate/urine creatinine in 24-h collections, ± SEM.

these, 25 took potassium citrate alone and of the 25, 15 had low urine citrate as the sole detected abnormality. Urine citrate (mg/24 h) rose from control of 223 ± 92 to between 475 and 578 during the six follow-up periods over 2 years of treatment, and urine pH also rose. Urine volume rose and urine calcium oxalate supersaturation fell, mainly because of the increase in volume. Only three of the patients formed a new stone during treatment. This was so impressive a reduction that we reprint the figure for your inspection (Fig. 30).

Among 13 hypercalciuric patients with recurrent stones, who continued to form stones despite thiazide treatment that lowered urine calcium excretion rate, Pak et al. (86) found that potassium citrate, when added, reduced the stone formation rate in 10 during 1–2 years of follow-up, even though the citrate did not lower urine calcium further; moreover, the thiazide therapy had not lowered urine citrate below control (i.e., pretreatment) levels, which were, for the group, very low (250 ± 86 mg daily) and which rose to between 473 and 557 mg daily during treatment with added citrate. Urine pH also rose.

In a review, Pak (87) mentions (a) a 91% improvement in stone rate and 67% remission rate among nine patients with RTA, who ought to respond to citrate, and (b)

an 88% improvement in stone rate and 67% remission rate among nine patients with chronic diarrheal syndrome, who also would be expected to have low urine citrate and pH from intestinal bicarbonate losses. As certainly expected, citrate virtually cured uric acid stones among 17 patients, but almost any alkali therapy should do as well. To date, we have found no other stone trials.

In principle, oral citrate should reduce calcium absorption, if given with meals, since the citrate could bind to calcium and prevent its efficient transport by enterocytes. Eight normal men (88) absorbed much more calcium given alone than with citrate, as judged from measurement of blood radioactivity from radioactive calcium given orally as a marker with 5 mM of $CaCl_2$. This technique measures unidirectional calcium uptake by intestine. In another study, of 28 stone formers (9 women), and 28 normal subjects (14 women) (89), citrate enhanced absorption of oral calcium carbonate over a 6-h interval, as judged by urine calcium excretion, and it did so for normals and stone formers alike.

The absolute contradiction between these two studies may be due to technique, since the first includes a more direct measure of intestinal calcium absorption. Should citrate reduce renal tubule calcium reabsorption, for ex-

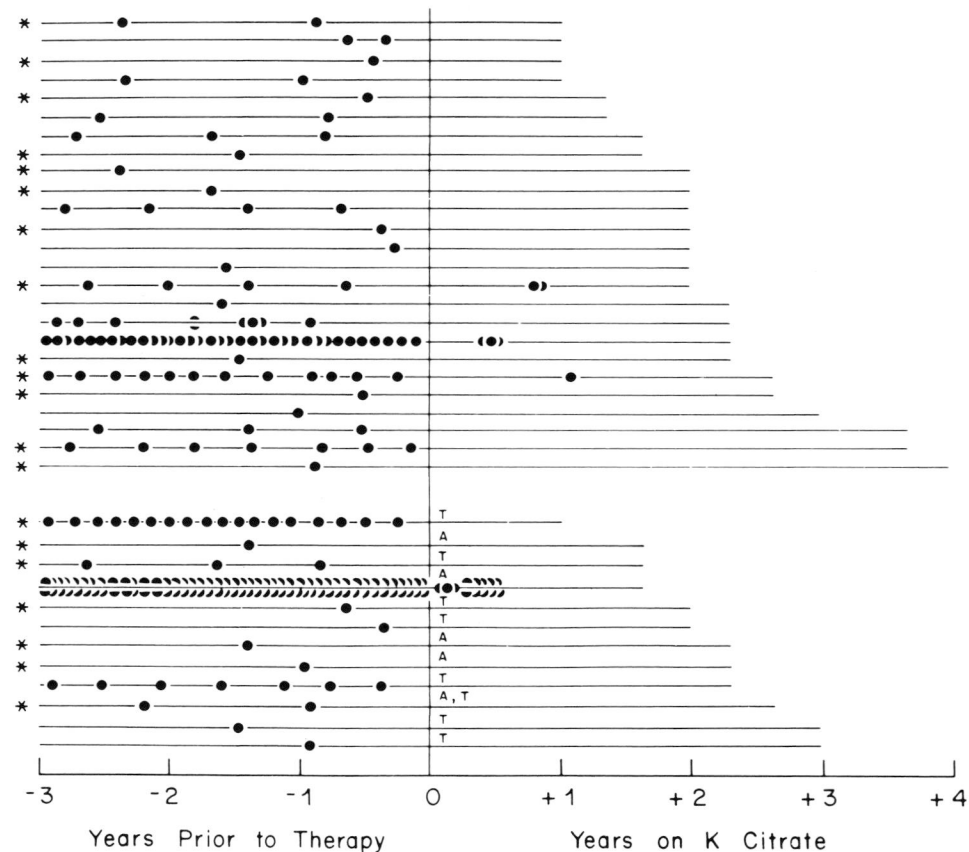

FIG. 30. Effect of thiazide treatment and thiazide–potassium-citrate treatment on new stone formation. Each line represents the study in separate patients. Each point indicates new stone formation. Thiazide–potassium-citrate treatment was begun immediately after thiazide treatment. [From Pak and Fuller (85).]

ample, urine calcium could rise with no increase of intestinal calcium absorption. In that regard, citrate infusion increases urine calcium of thyroparathyroidectomized rats given replacement parathyroid hormone (90), even though the filtered load of calcium falls, which is sure evidence that citrate can reduce tubule calcium reabsorption, all things being equal. Whether this occurs in people with intact parathyroid glands seems uncertain.

We were interested in Cowley et al.'s paper (89) for a reason other than the effect of citrate: These investigators found urine calcium excretions above oral calcium intake in 12 of 20 hypercalciuric stone formers ingesting 150 mg of calcium daily, as well as in only one of eight normals concurrently studied—an exact echo of our results (not otherwise duplicated to our knowledge), published years before (6) and (rather surprisingly) not quoted by these authors.

We would have assumed citrate to be an innocuous compound, given its natural occurrence in blood and urine, but Nature occasionally surprises us. Aluminum, a potential toxin in normals and surely very undesirable in the bodies of patients with chronic renal failure, may be absorbed at higher-than-normal rates after oral citrate treatment (91). In rats, aluminum citrate penetrated into mucosa of everted gut sacs from duodenum to a greater extent than did aluminum lactate, and evidence pointed to opening of mucosal tight junctions by the citrate salt. Because citrate could increase aluminum uptake as well as uptake of other metals (such as lead) (91,92), its use in stone-formers may require some additional studies on amounts absorbed. In particular, one should avoid aluminum antacids while taking citrate for stone disease, and patients with reduced renal function should perhaps avoid citrate.

Magnesium

This ion can affect COM crystal growth, as measured by change in particle number using Coulter-counter methods with a modestly supersaturated calcium oxalate solution, such that $2 \mu M/mL$ of Mg caused a 50% reduction (93). Inhibition followed Langmuir-type isotherm plots, with an affinity of about 1.07 mM. Furthermore, magnesium forms a soluble complex with oxalate, reducing calcium oxalate supersaturation. Low urine magnesium is not a feature of stone-formers (94). Using high supersaturations giving spontaneous crystallizations, Sutor (95) could find no effects of magnesium additions, illustrating the effects of techniques on results. Magnesium treatment has never been studied well.

Pyrophosphate, Glycosaminoglycans (GAGs), Acid Mucopolysaccharides (AMPs), RNA, Unknown Materials

Here, at the end of a wearisome encounter with molecules that can affect crystals, we return to this collection.

Some of them are important, some are minor actors in a large drama, and others are simply mistakes along the way.

Pyrophosphate

Pyrophosphate certainly deserves continued attention, because it is in urine at concentrations that affect both calcium oxalate and calcium phosphate crystallizations. An interesting survey (96) presents urine pyrophosphate levels in young and old men and women with and without stones, which we summarize for clarity (Table 4). Given the general range of $20–40 \mu M$ pyrophosphate excreted daily, and that pyrophosphate inhibits COM seed crystal growth by about 50% at $16 \mu M$ concentration, urine pyrophosphate levels seem sufficient to inhibit crystal growth, and this effect surely can matter in whole urine even though as urine is diluted, inhibition persists long after the pyrophosphate concentration has fallen below the level needed for inhibition. In other words, whole urine inhibitions must involve pyrophosphate, and low urine pyrophosphate certainly could matter in whole urine, even though molecules such as NC can inhibit despite a much greater dilution of urine because of a higher affinity. Of interest to us, the range of urine pyrophosphate excretions is very great within such groups as normal men and women or corresponding stone-forming patients, and thus some patients excrete 10% of the amounts excreted by others. Such differences could be very important for an inhibitor.

Inorganic pyrophosphate itself consists of a chain of phosphates linked through oxygen molecules, which can be degraded rapidly by urine (97) or serum pyrophosphatases. Diphosphonates replace the phosphate–oxygen skeleton with a phosphate–carbon skeleton, preserving the side-chain oxygen groups; moreover, they mimic the inhibition of pyrophosphates while offering the advantage of great stability. Ethane-1-hydroxy-1,1-diphosphonate (EHDP) increases the FPR and reduces COM crystal growth rate in vitro (98); it also protects rats against calcium oxalate or calcium phosphate stones when given ethylene glycol (an agent causing hyperoxaluria) or excess vitamin D, but it does not protect them against spontaneous struvite stones. EHDP given to three stone-forming patients reduced the average size of urine crystals and the ability of urine to inhibit COM

TABLE 4. *Urine inorganic pyrophosphate (PP$_i$) excretions*[a]

Age (years)	MN	MSF	WN	WSM
20–40	40	36	30	14
>40	55	33	20	27

Source: Adapted from Schwille et al. (96).
[a] Values are median micromoles PP$_i$ excreted per 24 h; MN and MSF, men normals and men stone formers, WN and WSF, women normals and women stone formers.

crystal growth (99), but it also increased urine oxalate levels, so supersaturations increased.

Subsequent studies showed that EHDP, like all other diphosphonates, inhibited much more efficiently at pH 6.0 and above than at pH 5, by a 100-fold order of magnitude (100), and that a dose sufficient to affect urine reliably toward greater inhibition would probably raise risk of EHDP effects on bone mineralization. Bone et al. (101) treated 12 patients with EHDP for up to 30 months, and found rather poor effects on stone formation, since five of the 12 showed no reduction; several patients showed marginal evidence of osteomalacia. Of interest, controlled-release EHDP implants seem to reduce calcifications on heart valve implants (102).

Oral orthophosphate increases urine pyrophosphate excretion (103), and oral phosphate in 11 patients with stones reduced calcium oxalate supersaturation, but it increased the FPR in only some patients and often increased COM crystal growth rate. We (104) have summarized phosphate trials, which have generally been disappointing.

GAGs, AMPs, RNA

GAGs, AMPS, RNA, and related molecules can inhibit calcium oxalate crystal growth and nucleation, are in urine, and have been offered as important factors in the normal inhibition process. We (27) found inhibition of calcium oxalate crystal growth by RNA, synthetic polyadenylates, and gastric pepsin (an acidic urine protein) at micromolar concentration of the pepsin or the constituent nucleotide of the polymers, which means that the polymers were at about 0.01 μM of intact chain. Scurr et al. (62) precipitated urine constituents with Alcian blue, a process that produces a mixture of AMPS, and measured their amounts and their inhibitory activities using a batch crystallizer of the mixed suspension type. Stone formers excreted less Alcian blue precipitable material and smaller quantities of GAGs, THP, and RNA. In the crystallizer, RNA inhibited aggregation (as measured simultaneously with crystal growth), as did heparin, chondroitin sulfate, and pyrophosphate; similar findings were reported by Robertson et al. (105) 10 years earlier.

Cetylpyridinium chloride precipitation (22) removes much of urine inhibitors with high affinities, and the inhibitors can be recovered in the precipitate along with AMPS, hinting at a link between the molecule type and the main urine inhibitor, but NC will also precipitate into such a mixture, as we have already mentioned.

A recent paper (106) used better methods than past workers have used, and it explored the excretion rates of GAGs in urine of normals and stone formers. Urine was dialyzed and vacuum-dried, aliquots were electrophoresed on agarose, and GAG migration regions were stained with toluidine blue for quantification. Cetyl-pyridinium bromide precipitates were similarly electrophoresed and GAGs were quantified; BioGel P4 gel chromatography of urine was used with uronic acid measurements for quantification. The methods gave different values for GAG excretion, but the investigators chose one of these methods, namely, agarose gel electrophoresis after dialysis; this method produced lower-than-normal GAGs in urine of stone formers. One can feel intrigued by such findings as these (namely, low levels of an inhibitor in stone-former urine) and may come to believe that GAGs must play some role, somehow, in protection against crystallization and, when deficient, permit stones to form; but only more evidence, and of a different kind, could ever convince us of the aforementioned. We observed that some urine macromolecules delay the transition of calcium oxalate dihydrate to COM (107); furthermore, transition delay can be done using intact urine, and thus it could help elucidate the role of various materials.

Overview

Somehow, the polyanions in urine remain suspected but unconvicted as inhibitors, very likely to play a role if for no reason other than their abilities to interact with crystals, but we lack clear evidence that specific urine GAGs or AMPS, or urine RNA fragments, when purified completely, actually do contribute to COM crystal growth or aggregation inhibition to any important extent when compared with NC and THP. One could say as much about THP and NC, but with greater difficulty, because THP in very pure form surely inhibits aggregation and also because NC products nowadays are very pure and inhibit both growth and aggregation, and both inhibit to such an extent that in whole urine their effects must be very strong. NC, unlike THP, does not seem to inactivate itself through protein self-aggregation, and thus NC may emerge as the main inhibitor of both processes. Our prejudices naturally favor proteins with which we have worked.

PROMOTORS

As we said about inhibitors, this word rouses uncertainties that we wish to eliminate by a careful focusing. Crystal nuclei form by coalescence of solution ions into molecular aggregates that structure themselves into organized lattice structures, and the coalescence usually occurs on preformed discontinuities such as bubbles (in vitro), container irregularities, or any solid phase in solution; thus "heterogeneous" nucleation predominates strongly, and homogeneous nucleation (pure coalescence of solution ions without any preformed solid phase) is considered a great rarity.

In vivo, cell surfaces, cell debris, protein aggregates, and other crystals probably serve as heterogeneous nuclei for COM, and such surfaces "promote" COM formation because any preformed surface lowers the supersaturation required to achieve de novo nucleation, so at a given supersaturation, nuclei may form on a given surface but may not form in its absence. We use the term "promoter" to describe substances in urine or kidney on which COM can form, either because the surface is particularly suitable as a template or simply because the surface happens to be present in the tubule lumen and urine. Reduced formation products seem to be the surest evidence of promotion.

Uric Acid

Our focus on uric acid comes entirely from empirical evidence and not from theory, and we presume that further research will identify other materials that serve a similar purpose. We discuss apatite for reasons that are partly theoretical, to stimulate others in their investigations.

Clinical Evidence

Association of Uric Acid and Calcium Oxalate Stones

Before our work, uric acid and calcium stones seemed to commingle. Yu (108) reported that 23% of 2038 gout patients formed stones, 17% of which contained calcium oxalate, alone or with uric acid, the rest being pure uric acid. This gives a frequency of 4% for calcium oxalate stone-forming, much above usual estimates for populations, which usually lie below 1%. Also, 17% of the stones contained calcium oxalate, but urine abnormalities in the gout patients consisted of acid urine pH and higher-than-normal levels of undissociated urine uric acid and total urine uric acid. In secondary gout, resulting from myeloproliferative diseases, almost all stones were uric acid, raising the interesting idea that perhaps low urine pH affects calcium oxalate formation in primary gout, because secondary gout patients would tend to lack the peculiarly low urine pH levels of primary gout patients.

In quite another kind of work, Lonsdale (109) pointed out the strong geometrical correspondence between uric acid, uric acid dihydrate, and calcium oxalate mono- and dihydrate crystals, as well as between apatite and calcium oxalate monohydrate crystals, and suggested that oriented overgrowths of one on a surface of the other could easily occur. We accept as commonplace that apatite occurs in most calcium oxalate stones, and we have noted elsewhere (110) that uric acid occurred in stones of 109 of 821 calcium oxalate stone formers, or 13%.

We (111) found a shift of frequency distribution of urine uric acid excretion rates between normals and stone-forming patients, so that 34% of the male patients excreted above 800 mg of uric acid versus 12% of normal

males, a 22% surplus, and for females, the corresponding values were 14% versus 0%.

Fellstrom et al. (112) reported no differences in uric acid excretions, but, in fact, about 13% of their male patients excreted above 800 mg of uric acid versus 6% of normal men, a doubling. Given the diet basis for hyperuricosuria, and the fact that the studies were performed in two different countries, this correspondence seems very important, and it also highlights that the hyperuricosuria always involves a thickening of the high value tail of a skewed distribution, which is not well detected by comparisons of mean values.

Hodgkinson (113) studied 132 male stone formers and found that 17% excreted uric acid at levels above the range for his normal male population, not far from our 22% surplus. He concluded that his work failed to confirm ours, for reasons we cannot understand, but he indicated that he found high urine uric acid levels in stone-former patients as a result of diet.

Overall, we found similar observations in all three studies (ours and the other two) but found differences in the interpretation of data. In one case a long tail of high values in patients versus normals was neglected, and in another case the tail was explicitly recognized and matched one that we found; however, the dietary origin of the hyperuricosuria is taken to mean that the finding is not intrinsic to the biology of the patients but to their diets. We found the same, and we believe that high-protein diets (i.e., high in purine) increase urine uric acid, and that stone formers, especially males, seem more prone than normals to select such diets.

Schwille et al. (114) studied fasting urine uric acid levels in stone formers and controls of both sex, and they found a significant excess among male stone formers under age 40. When men and women were pooled, the difference held for those under age 40. Serum urate levels and filtered loads of urate were not different, so increased fractional urate excretion was the cause of the fasting hyperuricosuria. Of interest, fasting urine pH was higher among the stone formers, urine phosphate levels were lower than those of normals, and the patients had lower serum phosphorus levels.

Allopurinol Treatment of Calcium Oxalate Stones

The original 21 patients given allopurinol as sole therapy for calcium oxalate stones seemed to be candidates for such a treatment simply because of hyperuricosuria and no other discernible defect, and one of us prescribed the drug in the hope of doing some good (23). The data simply showed (a) 73 new stones during 183 patient-years before treatment and (b) one new stone during 39 patient-years of treatment. Naturally, being an open trial, all types of bias could have weighted the dice (the desire of a young man to publish, for example, high fluid intake by patients impressed by the advice of a young

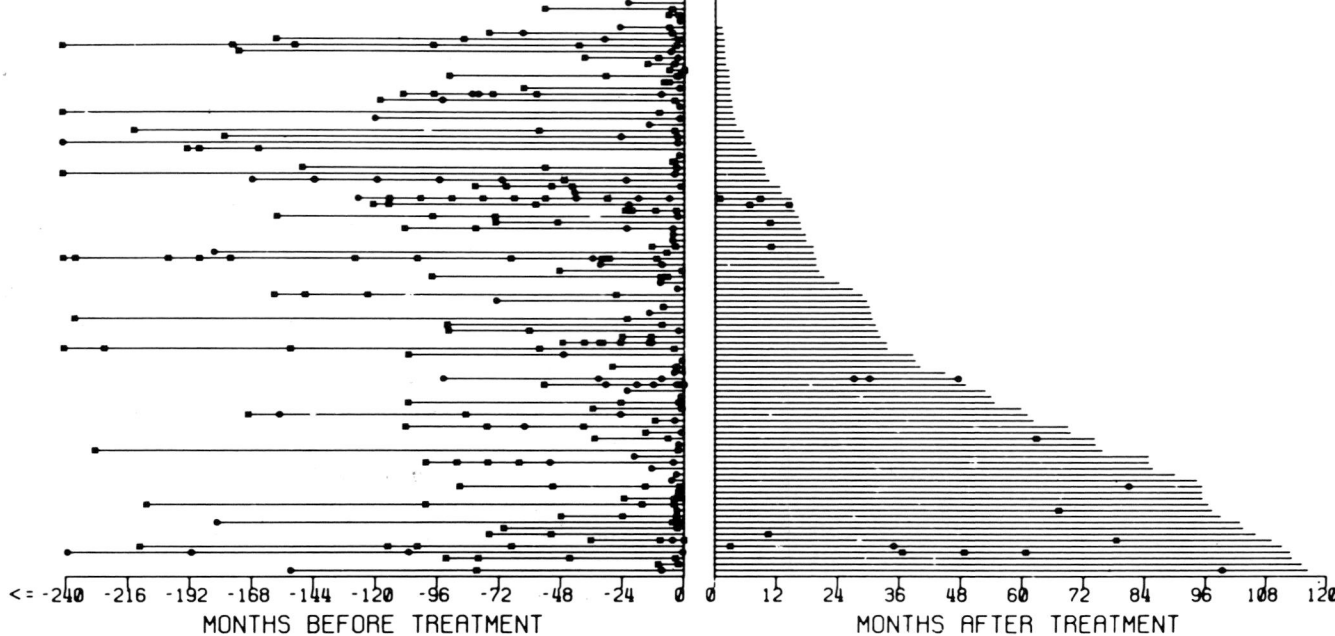

FIG. 31. Calcium stone formation before and during treatment of hyperuricosuria with allopurinol. Each patient is shown as a horizontal line; new stones are represented as closed symbols, and multiple stones in clusters are represented as open symbols. [From Coe (117).]

clinician), but even so, only one stone attracted attention, and should have.

Later on, as more people received the treatment, 32 patients who had formed 90 new stones during 258 patient-years before treatment formed only four new stones during 68 patient-years of treatment (115). Time went on, and by 1977 48 patients who had formed 152 stones during 408 patient-years before treatment formed only eight stones during 186 patient-years of follow-up (116). The discrepancy between the numbers of stones predicted and observed struck us as extraordinary, even

allowing for all types of bias. In 1983, a review paper included our last summary of the data (117) (Fig. 31), by which time 91 patients had been observed. We would have gone on counting forever, but others (118) did a double-blind prospective placebo trial (Fig. 32) which proved that bias did not cause our results, leaving allopurinol as the main factor.

In this study, pretreatment stone events were calculated as we calculate them, as the number of stones passed or appearing on radiographs not present on a prior radiograph. During treatment, we always count the

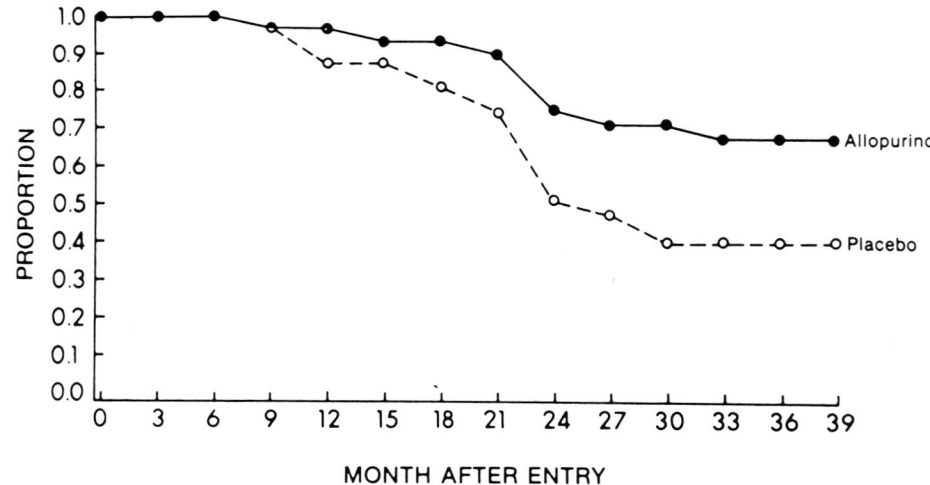

FIG. 32. Life-table plot showing proportion of patients without calculous events during treatment with allopurinol or placebo. [From Ettinger et al. (118).]

same way, but Ettinger includes as "calculus events" the enlargement of preformed stones. Enlargement accounted for 44% of the treatment failures in allopurinol-treated patients, which included nine of the original 29 patients, or 31%. Of the nine, four failures were from enlargement, and five patients (17%) actually formed a new stone—similar to our own data. Among placebo recipients, 39% failed by showing enlargement, leaving 61% of the 18 failures (or 11 of the original 31 placebo patients, a total of 35%) as failures from new stones.

We argue that enlargement offers a poor index of allopurinol effects, since stone growth must reflect the uptake of calcium and oxalate from urine onto preformed calcium oxalate crystals, a process no one would expect allopurinol to alter, whereas formation of new stones is precisely the event one would hope allopurinol would reduce. For this reason, and though we present the original data, we believe the correct interpretation of the study is that the drug reduced new stone formation from 31% to 17% over a period of 3 years.

Allopurinol itself, as well as its main metabolites oxypurinol and allopurinol riboside, could have produced these effects by complexations that affect supersaturation, or by altering kinetics of COM crystal growth. The two metabolites (119) do not adsorb to COM crystals (as judged by solution depletion or alteration of COM crystal zeta potential), nor do they alter kinetics of seed crystal growth, nor the particle number nor size distribution produced by spontaneous COM crystallization, and the same negative results were found by the same investigators using the same methods for allopurinol itself (120).

A report by Tiselius et al. (121) describes giving allopurinol at random to 99 patients in an open, prospective study; not surprisingly, these investigators found a poor result, namely, that recurrence was high after 5 years of treatment. Their results neither conflict with, challenge, nor elaborate upon those of any other study, since allopurinol has no intrinsic anti-stone actions apart from those on uric acid, which were not particularly abnormal in most patients they treated. Fellstrom et al. (122) treated 32 patients (five with idiopathic hypercalciuria, eight with hyperuricosuria, six with both IH and hyperuricosuria, and 13 with no defect) with allopurinol for an average of 2 years. Among the eight patients with hyperuricosuria alone, six remained free of stones (a 75% remission), as opposed to about 20–50% remission in the rest. Groups were too small to permit any conclusions. This paper quotes an early Ettinger paper showing an allopurinol effect, but it draws the conclusion that the drug either was ineffective or had a contradictory effect.

Another paper in the random treatment category, by Marangella et al. (123), described the effects of allopurinol (for an average of 17 months) given to 38 patients (11 with no disorder, five with idiopathic hypercalciuria, nine with hyperuricosuria, six with hyperoxaluria and seven with both idiopathic hypercalciuria, and hyperuri-

cosuria. Allopurinol produced a 33% reduction in total stone or gravel passage events, a result that was no different from that of 38 similar patients given no drug. The near-uselessness of studies of this type (i.e., very short treatment period, illogical use of drugs, no separation of new stones from passage of old stones) is sufficient reason for rendering them unpublishable.

Smith et al. (124) observed high serum uric acid levels in calcium stone formers, and treated such patients with allopurinol, observing an excellent response in a double-blind, placebo-type trial. Urine data were not originally presented. Later, Smith (125) reported that if only the presence or absence of new stones was the criterion for success, then 60% of allopurinol-treated subjects and less than 10% of placebo subjects met the criterion—a very strong effect.

One should mention complications of allopurinol, along with alternatives not yet proven but rational. Oxypurinol, the main metabolite of allopurinol, can crystallize into stones when the drug is given at high dosage (126,127). Hepatotoxicity is well known (128,129). Stevens–Johnson syndrome can occur. Since high urine uric acid arises mainly from diet, lowering of protein food intake can be as effective as allopurinol, though change of habit may be difficult and irregularly maintained. Of interest, low-protein diets, in the range of 19 g daily, may reduce oxypurinol clearance, thereby increasing its blood levels and increasing the possible risks of side reactions (130).

In retrospect, nothing about the problem of allopurinol as treatment seems confusing, except the manner of presentation in some papers. Our prospective work, of ample duration and involving many well-characterized patients, showed a strong effect that was confirmed in the only placebo trial using similar patients and in another placebo trial using less well selected patients; the rest of our work involves mixtures of patients, usually divided into unusably small groups from which no conclusions should have been sought. Danielson et al. (131) came to this same conclusion in a review, namely, that allopurinol seemed surely effective.

Because allopurinol and its metabolites are inert with respect to COM crystallization itself, it must either (a) affect calcium oxalate stone disease through altering urine calcium, oxalate, pH, or some other level related to COM crystallization or (b) act through its main effect, to lower urine uric acid. We tested the former hypothesis many times and found a negative result, which we never published. Ettinger et al. (118) showed a lack of effect of allopurinol on urine calcium.

Citrate Treatment

Pak and Peterson (132) treated 19 hyperuricosuric calcium oxalate stone formers with potassium citrate; three of them also took thiazide. The rate of new stone formation fell from 1.55 to 0.38 stones/patient-year (during a mean of 2.35 treatment-years), and new stones formed in only three patients. The citrate lowered urine calcium oxalate supersaturation (as expected) as well as dihydrogen urate supersaturation, but it did not lower monosodium urate supersaturation. However, in vitro, citrate greatly inhibited heterogeneous nucleation of calcium oxalate by seeds of monosodium hydrogen urate, even at a fixed calcium oxalate supersaturation, supporting a mechanism for citrate treatment effects.

Studies of Mechanism

Naturally, an observation unsupported by theory exasperates clinical investigators and their basic science col-

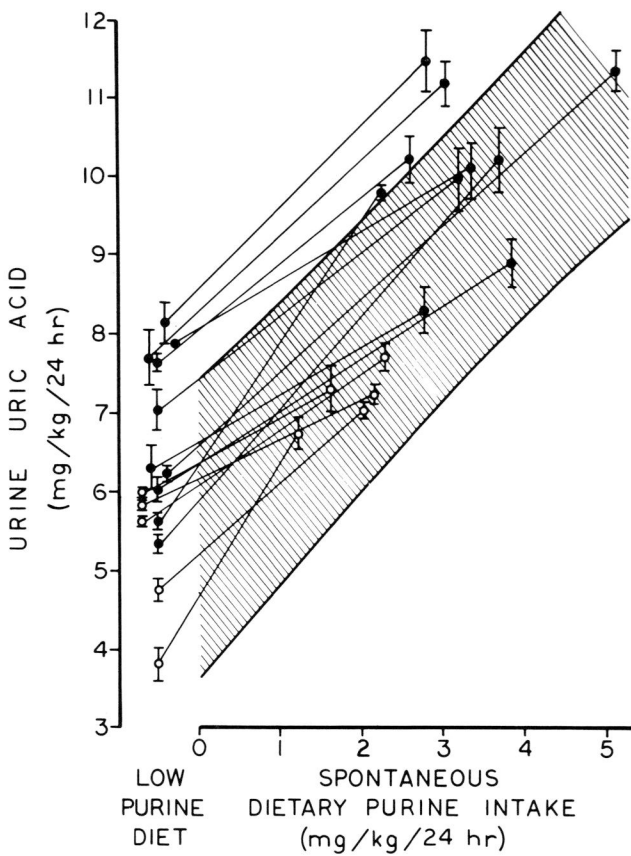

FIG. 33. Relation between urine urate excretion and purine intake in patients and normal subjects on ambient and low-purine diets. Each point on the right panel compares mean (±1 SEM) urate excretion by a patient (●) or normal subjects derived from three 24-h samples (○) to average spontaneous purine intake on the 3 days during and before each urine collection. Hatched area shows the confidence band derived from five normal subjects. The band was computed so that the probability would be less than 5% that the mean of three values from the normal population would fall outside the band. Urate excretion by three patients was excessive in terms of purine intake. Mean (±1 SEM) urate excretion during low purine intake is shown on the left panel. The four patients with values considerably above those of normal subjects suggested urate overproduction; five were clearly normal, and one was borderline. [From Coe and Kavalach (115).]

leagues, reminiscent of the story about bumble bees that should not, given the state of knowledge of aerodynamics in 1950, have been able to fly, and many investigators have busied themselves trying to explain how allopurinol could have worked, since the drug alone has no apparent effect on calcium crystallizations. In other words, since the effect of the drug must be through lowering of urine uric acid, uric acid and its salts must somehow promote calcium crystallizations, but no one can be exactly sure how. Present work mostly amplifies and contends with Lonsdale's idea of uric acid as a substrate for calcium oxalate crystallizations, or it follows the theory that uric acid salts can adsorb inhibitors. Naturally, the contentiousness of the investigators exceeds the importance of their work in almost all cases, as one would expect in such a narrow corner of science.

Cause of Hyperuricosuria

It seems that the only uncontroversial issue is the cause of hyperuricosuria, which we find to be due almost always to dietary excess of purine. When diet purine varied from very low to normal, urine uric acid varied also (Fig. 33), in a way most compatible with purine excess (115). It seemed that the source of extra purine was simply substitution (Fig. 34) of meat, fish, and poultry for breads grains and starches (133). Others came to conclusion that renal tubule urate handling is normal in hyperuricosuric calcium stone formers (134).

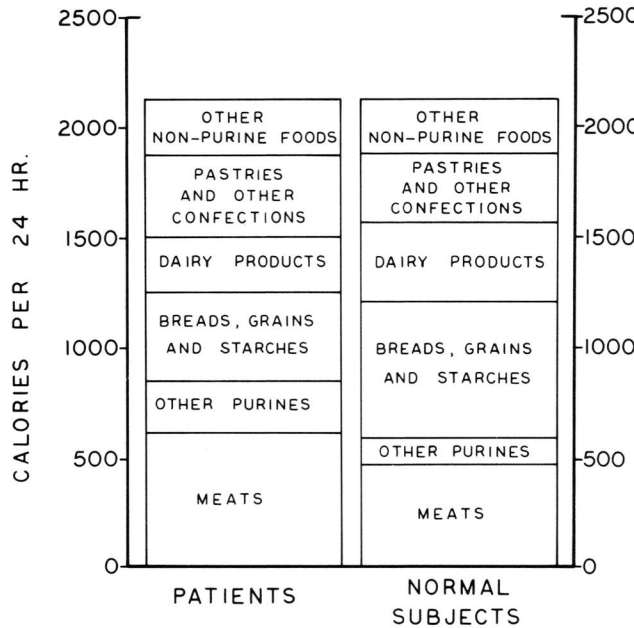

FIG. 34. Diets of patients and normal subjects. Calories consumed in each of six broad food categories are similar for the two groups except for meats and other high-purine foods and for breads, grains, and starches, which differ markedly. [From Coe et al. (133).]

The Main Urate Phase Involved

Pak et al. (135) worked out the solubility of sodium monohydrogen urate in human urine, and they showed that urine with modestly high sodium concentration and total urate concentration could reach supersaturation with the salt, so that the salt could crystallize. Potassium and ammonium salts of monohydrogen urate, also supersaturated in human urine, could not promote calcium oxalate crystallization. This paper did not include screening for supersaturations in urine from a group of stone formers.

We studied urine supersaturations in patients with hyperuricosuric calcium urolithiasis, asking with which phase of uric acid or salt the urine seemed most supersaturated (136). Possible phases included undissociated uric acid itself—in other words, dihydrogen urate, sodium monohydrogen urate, or another salt such as potassium or ammonium urate. We found that dihydrogen urate supersaturation in patient urine exceeded normal, whereas sodium hydrogen urate supersaturation did not, mainly because urine pH was lower among hyperuricosuric patients than among normals or patients with idiopathic hypercalciuria (Table 5).

In contrast, Pak et al. (137) found no difference in pH between seemingly comparable patients with hyperuricosuria and others with hypercalciuria, though his urine pH value for the hypercalciuric patients matched ours, at

about 6.0. This difference surprises us, since both laboratories have always tended to find similar results; our patient groups seem well-matched otherwise, and high-purine diets should lower urine pH because of the acid-loading effects of the meat. Because of the higher pH, sodium hydrogen urate predominated in supersaturation.

We attempted to glean some additional insights from patients who formed mixed stones (i.e., stones consisting of calcium oxalate and uric acid) (110,138). Of 821 calcium oxalate stone formers, 109 produced such mixed stones (110), and their urine pH values were below those of the other calcium stone formers (Table 6). Urine supersaturations with calcium oxalate and dihydrogen urate were higher in mixed stone formers (Fig. 35) than in calcium oxalate or uric acid stone formers. In a way, this paper showed very similar data for mixed stone formers (whose stones actually contained measurable amounts of uric acid and calcium oxalate together) and for patients with hyperuricosuric calcium oxalate stones (whose stones themselves did not contain measurable amounts of uric acid). On the other hand, the two types of patients could differ in their supersaturations, given the conflict between ourselves and Pak; thus the matter remains unsettled.

Harvey and Pak (139) published a case that was rather supportive of our ideas. The patient had gout, and he passed six calcium oxalate dihydrate stones over a period

TABLE 5. *Summary of urinary uric acid saturation measurements*[a]

24-Hour urine values	Metabolic group				
	Normal ($n = 20$)	IH ($n = 24$)	HU ($n = 12$)	Both ($n = 14$)	Neither ($n = 17$)
Number of samples:	24	69	36	42	51
Total uric acid (mg/L):	503 ± 32	421 ± 23	575 ± 28	616 ± 27^g	462 ± 32
Urine volume (mL):	1268 ± 65	$1717 \pm 133^{h,i}$	1501 ± 79^f	1397 ± 70	1387 ± 90
Urine pH:	6.22	5.92	5.62^g	5.74^g	5.67^h
Undissociated uric acid[b] (mg/L):	57 ± 8^j	84 ± 11	155 ± 21^h	150 ± 16^i	128 ± 18^g
CPR, monosodium urate:	2.8 ± 0.3^e	2.2 ± 0.2	2.7 ± 0.2	3.1 ± 0.2	2.2 ± 0.2
Initial [Na] $\times$ [urate][c] ($M^2 \times 10^{-5}$):	37 ± 4	27 ± 3	35 ± 4	42 ± 3^j	29 ± 3
Final [Na] $\times$ [urate][d] ($M^2 \times 10^{-5}$):	13.2 ± 0.7	11.0 ± 0.5	12.0 ± 0.6	12.9 ± 0.5	13.2 ± 1.0
Sodium concentration (mEq/L):	131 ± 8^j	118 ± 7	130 ± 7	149 ± 7^k	132 ± 7^j

Source: After Coe et al. (136).

[a] All values, except for the numbers of samples and the numbers of people in each metabolic group (in parentheses), are the means $\pm$ SEM. Abbreviations used are: IH, idiopathic hypercalciuria; HU, hyperuricosuria; CPR, concentration product ratio; [Na], sodium concentration (mEq/L); [urate], urate concentration (mmol/L).

[b] The mean equilibrium value, determined in 26 urine samples of pH below 5.6, after 48 h of incubation with crystals of uric acid, was 90.5 mg/L.

[c] Before incubation with crystals of sodium hydrogen urate.

[d] After 48 h of incubation with crystals of sodium hydrogen urate.

[e] Based upon the study of the 16 of the 20 normal subjects who had CPR measurements.

[f] $p < 0.05$, compared with control.

[g] $p < 0.02$, compared with control.

[h] $p < 0.01$, compared with control.

[i] $p < 0.001$, compared with control.

[j] $p < 0.05$, men versus women.

[k] $p < 0.02$, men versus women.

TABLE 6. *Selected laboratory characteristics*

Characteristics	Type of calcium (n = 821)	Stones mixed (n = 109)	Uric acid (n = 22)
Serum creatinine (mg/dL)	0.98 ± 0.01	1.02 ± 0.02[c]	1.06 ± 0.05
Serum uric acid (mg/dL)	5.70 ± 0.04	6.38 ± 0.14	5.96 ± 0.33
Serum calcium (mg/dL)	9.48 ± 0.01	9.55 ± 0.43	9.35 ± 0.06[b]
Serum phosphorus (mg/dL)	3.17 ± 0.48	3.23 ± 0.62	3.25 ± 0.08
Urine volume (L)	1.59 ± 0.06	1.53 ± 0.05	1.51 ± 0.12
Urine calcium (mg/24 h)	231 ± 4	216 ± 10	175 ± 25[d]
Urine calcium (mg/kg/24 h)	3.06 ± 0.05	2.62 ± 0.12[e]	2.12 ± 0.28[e]
Urine uric acid (g/24 h)	700 ± 40	665 ± 20	669 ± 40
Urine pH	6.0 ± 0.4	5.7 ± 0.4[e]	5.5 ± 0.4[e]
Urine oxalate (mg/24 h)	39 ± 16	38 ± 1	36 ± 3

Source: After Millman et al. (110).
[a] All values are mean ± SEM.
[b] Value differs from mixed, $p < 0.05$.
[c] Value differs from calcium, $p < 0.05$.
[d] Value differs from calcium, $p < 0.01$.
[e] Value differs from calcium, $p < 0.001$.

of 2 years. Urine chemistries were normal except for low urine pH (5.31 and 5.35) and low urine citrate. Alkali and allopurinol treatment seemed successful until the patient developed hypercalcemic sarcoidosis, with subsequent hypercalciuria and recurrent stones.

Tiselius and Larsson (140) studied diurnal variation of urine urate, not 24-h averages, and found a correlation

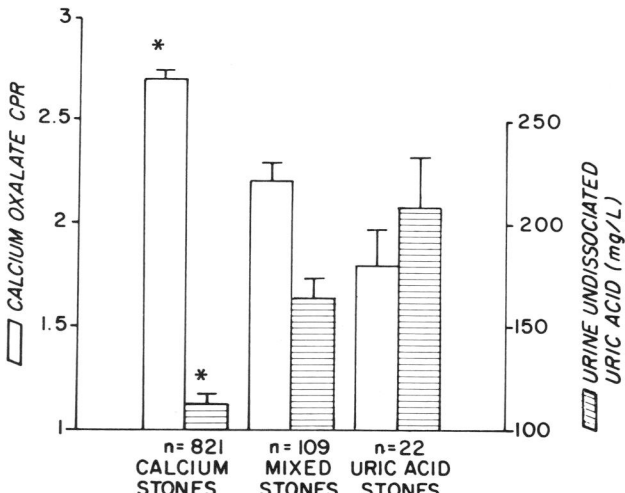

FIG. 35. Calcium oxalate and undissociated uric acid supersaturation in stone-forming patients. Values for concentration product ratio (CPR) (*unhatched bars*) of above 1 indicate supersaturation. The solubility of undissociated uric acid (*hatched bars*) in urine is 96 mg/L, so supersaturations can be calculated by dividing the concentrations by 96. The figure presents all available measurement in patients with calcium oxalate, mixed calcium oxalate and uric acid, and pure uric acid stones. For CPR, there were values from 431, 56, and 9 patients for calcium oxalate, mixed calcium oxalate and uric acid, and pure uric acid stone formers, respectively; corresponding numbers of patients providing undissociated uric acid values were 821, 109, and 22. All values are means ± SEM. Asterisk indicates that the value differs from mixed and uric acid stones ($p < 0.001$). [From Millman et al.]

(during the morning hours) between the highest concentrations of total urate species in urine and the lowest urine pH values, so that dihydrogen urate would have been the phase most prone to crystallize. Sodium hydrogen urate supersaturations always remained below the metastable limit. In other words, peaks of supersaturation for uric acid seemed the rule, so that this phase could be prone to bursts of crystallization, especially during the morning hours.

The Theory of Heterogeneous Nucleation

The structural similarities pointed out by Lonsdale (109) served as a stimulus for Pak and Arnold (141) and our group (142) to assay the ability of sodium urate and dihydrogen urate to promote ion depletion from a modestly supersaturated calcium oxalate solution, and we both found urate to be very effective, and that dihydrogen urate was almost ineffective for about an hour, but after that it was effective. Inorganic pyrophosphate inhibited the urate nucleation.

Five years later, Koutsoukos et al. (143) used a constant composition system metastably supersaturated with respect to calcium oxalate monohydrate, and found an immediate induction by uric acid or sodium hydrogen urate seeds of solution ion depletion. They also found the rate of ion consumption to be higher with uric acid seeds, in accordance with their better match with calcium oxalate monohydrate crystals (Fig. 36).

In the same volume of the same journal, Burns and Finlayson (144) studied the same question. However, they used as their assay the particle size distribution in a mixed suspension system, in which calcium oxalate crystals were created by very high supersaturation (1 μM^2); uric acid and urate seeds had no effects on the crystals produced, but at less extreme supersaturations (of about one-third that level) the urate seeds promoted calcium oxalate crystallization. They found the results unimpres-

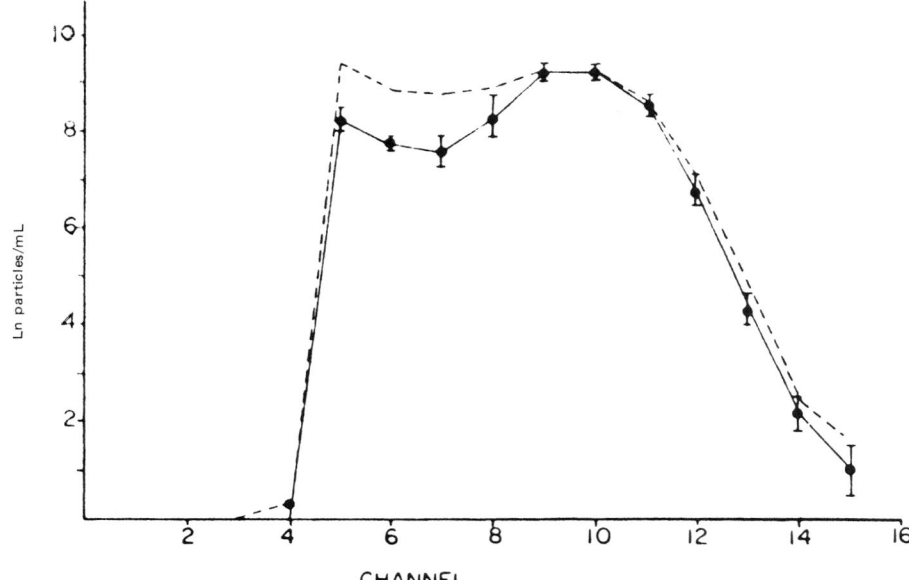

FIG. 36. Calcium oxalate precipitation with added sodium hydrogen urate (NaHUr) seed crystals (*solid line*), standard curve (*dashed line*). Ln total particles = 10.69 ± 0.44. Error bars represent the SEM. [From Burns and Finlayson (144).]

sive and ascribed the urate nucleation to "nonspecific" effects, even though Koutsoukos et al. (143) showed electron photomicrographs of calcium oxalate monohydrate overgrowths on uric acid and urate seeds suggestive of oriented, epitaxial, overgrowths, as one would expect from the matching of the lattice dimensions of the crystals. The methods differ greatly in supersaturation, so that calcium oxalate will not crystallize in the Koutsoukos system without some added seed but will crystallize in the Burns system, so the Burns model may apply only to urines greatly supersaturated with calcium oxalate.

Tiselius (145) found no effects of uric acid or sodium hydrogen urate seeds on calcium oxalate crystallization in metastably supersaturated solutions of calcium oxalate (0.2 μM^2), whose concentration was very similar to that used by Koutsoukos et al. (143), so these two experiments, both concerned with seed effects on solution ion depletion, disagree. One suspects that this complete disagreement is best explained by the type of seed crystals used and by the available seed surface, but details of seed preparation are not given by Tiselius (145). In metastably supersaturated urine, he found that both seeds accelerated calcium oxalate crystallization. This acceleration could have reflected reduction of urine inhibitors, as proposed in the alternative theory of urate action presented below.

Hallson et al. (146) lowered urine urate using bead-immobilized uricase, or they raised urine urate by adding some uricase, then they evaporated water off the urine to raise supersaturation and provoke crystallization, asking whether the uric acid or urate level was important. They determined the number of crystals formed or the amount of radioactive oxalate incorporated into crystals, and neither of these changed when urine urate

changed, so they believed that urine urate was without effect. This left them with the difficulty of explaining how allopurinol prevents stones, which they ascribed to its ability to lower urine oxalate. Allopurinol does not lower urine oxalate.

We believe that their experiments lacked basic elements of good design. To use uricase, urine pH was raised to 8.2 by adding NaOH, so crystals formed, presumably calcium phosphates and sodium hydrogen urates. These solids were removed by centrifugation, then they were added back after passing the urine through glass coils of the immobilized uricase, when pH had been lowered back to 5.3 with HCl. Sodium oxalate was added to raise final urine oxalate by 0.22 mM/L above the original concentration. Water was then evaporated to raise osmolality to 1050 mOsm/kg.

This osmolality would have been made up of the original urine constituents along with the added Na and Cl from the base and acid treatments, which was very different from urine, where salts are reabsorbed with water and urea makes up a major portion of the osmolality. The ionic strength (not measured) must have been raised greatly, and the entire ionic composition of the material must have been distorted from the original. The reason for the experiment was to mimic in vivo conditions, which cleaner and simpler models cannot achieve, but to us this montage of nearly arbitrary compositions does not mimic the interior of the kidney at all.

Deganello and Chou (147) studied human stones containing calcium oxalate and uric acid, looking for evidence that one phase controlled the growth of the other. In general, the two phases grew coaxially along one of their axes, a fact predicted from their similar dimensions, but the orientations of crystals in the stones seemed to be influenced by the organic matrix (presumably THP, NC, and other materials), so all they could be sure of was that the matrix played a major template role in the complex stone milieu. In an earlier paper, Deganello and Coe (148) showed oriented overgrowths of calcium oxalate on a substrate of uric acid. This result proved the possibility of epitaxial overgrowth, but apparently in the complicated conditions of actual stone formation, epitaxy occurs too rarely for detection in stones, and stone protein matrices alter crystal interactions greatly.

Sarig (149) performed a fascinating experiment in which she duplicated past results demonstrating that uric acid is a poor promoter of calcium oxalate crystallization and that sodium hydrogen urate is better. She also revealed new information: Uric acid seeds are best when given at a concentration of 5 ppm of glutamic acid (5 mg/L, or 30 μM) added to the incubation mixture (Fig. 37). Her explanation was that glutamic acid could bind to uric acid seeds and could provide a charged site for calcium attraction, making it an efficient promoter. Urine does contain glutamic acid (at levels above 30 μM), so uric acid crystals in urine have access to this amino acid.

One should always come to some conclusion, and ours is that the uric acid and calcium oxalate monohydrate crystals certainly can interact to promote crystallizations, firstly because they have matching lattice parameters so that formal epitaxy can occur, but mainly because experiments by Pak, our group, and others have shown that one can seed a solution containing ions of the other and promote crystallization. The Sarig experiment stands out from most others, since it offers a fruitful area of experimental work concerning effects of adsorbed small molecules on crystal seeds. To our knowledge, this work has not been repeated. The real system that creates stones in kidneys seems greatly complicated, so crystal interactions can be only one of many factors, even though we must state this disclaimer, we generally disdain complexity as an excuse for still coping with many possibilities despite years of research. We hope that new work will limit the present range of alternatives.

Reduced Inhibition by Urates or Uric Acid

An alternative, or perhaps supplement, to the crystal interaction idea posits crystals of urate adsorbing urine inhibitors whereby urine loses a protective element and

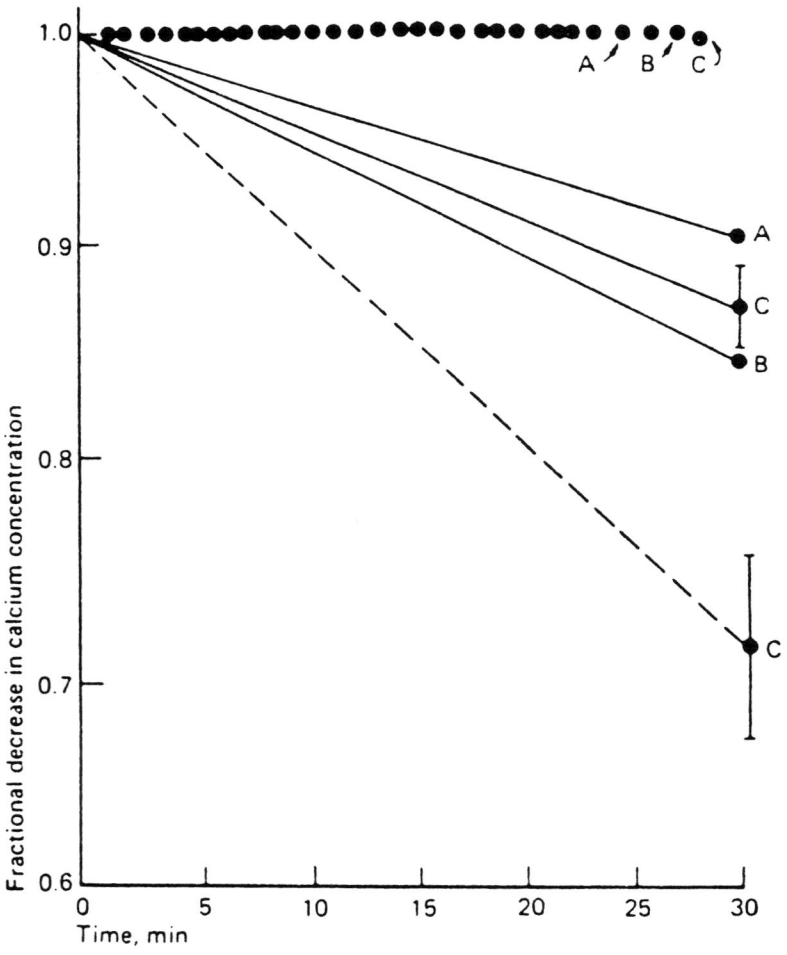

FIG. 37. Decrease in calcium concentration caused by seeds of uric acid species in supersaturated calcium oxalate solutions from which precipitation did not occur spontaneously during the time of measurement. The data are from the study of Pak and Arnold (A), the study of Coe et al. (B), and the study of Sarig et al. (C). Dotted line represents seeds of uric acid; solid lines represent seeds of sodium urate; dashed line represents seeds of uric acid with the admixture of 5 ppm glutamic acid. [From Sarig (149).]

calcium oxalate crystals can form and grow—a kind of distracting of the watchdog. Such a theory has natural appeal, since (a) uric acid is plentiful in urine, (b) large amounts of its crystals could form in a short time, and (c) therefore much of the THP or NC, or other inhibitors, could be removed.

We have already mentioned the observation of Tisselius (145) that, in vitro, urate seeds affected no aspect of calcium oxalate crystallization but did promote calcium oxalate crystallization from highly supersaturated urine. In other studies, urine from patients given allopurinol, when added in great dilution to a seeded crystal growth system, inhibited COM crystal growth to a greater extent than did urine from the same subjects before the treatment (150)—more evidence for reduced inhibitor content. Oxypurinol had no effects on the inhibition level, as Finlayson had found. These kinds of observations favor adsorption or other inactivation of inhibitors by urates, reduced with allopurinol presumably because the drug reduces urate concentrations.

Pak et al. (151) varied urine uric acid from high to low using high or low levels of purine or allopurinol, and found that as the sodium hydrogen urate supersaturation fell, the calcium oxalate formation product ratio rose, and vice versa (Fig. 38)—strong evidence that this salt promoted calcium oxalate crystallization. Passing urine supersaturated with respect with sodium hydrogen urate through 0.22-μm filters did not alter the urate concentration, arguing against crystal formation, but membrane ultrafiltration did reduce the urate concentration (this reduction was greatest when supersaturation was highest), raising the notion of (a) urate bound to proteins

or (b) formation of a urate colloid, by which these investigators must have meant molecular aggregates of very small size. This paper could be classified either in the "distracted watchdog" category or in the "crystal interaction" category, since one could envision either mechanism causing what was observed. We place it in the "distracted watchdog" category, since the authors clearly favored the distraction hypothesis.

Perhaps the progenitor of the "distracted watchdog" studies, performed by Robertson et al. (22), showed that urine calcium oxalate monohydrate inhibition could be correlated with urine AMPS concentration (as discussed earlier in the chapter) and that calcium oxalate stone-former urine [whose urine total urate levels exceeded (by 200%) those of calcium oxalate/calcium phosphate stone-former urine, inhibited COM growth and aggregation about half as well, given its measured content of AMPS. In other words, the natural excess of urate seemed to be associated with lower effectiveness of the AMPS in inhibition. Even if one discounts the AMPS themselves as major inhibitors, as we do, the low inhibition of the urine with high urate levels stands out. This paper spawned a school of similar papers, all concerned with interactions between particular—and often not surely naturally occurring—inhibitors and urate crystals.

Heparin adsorbed onto powders of sodium acid urate (152), and calcium ion promoted the adsorption. In vitro, chondroitin sulfate and heparin increased the COM formation product (as one would expect for an inhibitor), and increases in monosodium hydrogen urate concentration lowered the formation product ratio back down (as one would expect if the inhibitors were being adsorbed) (153). In another paper, uric acid inactivated heparin less efficiently than did sodium hydrogen urate, and potassium or ammonium acid urate were ineffective (137).

Fellstrom et al. (154) harvested non-ultrafilterable macromolecules (10-kD filter) from human urine; and they found that these macromolecules inhibited the second-order growth rate constant of COM seeds in a metastable, calcium (3–4 mM) oxalate (0.22 mM) solution, and that preincubation of the ultrafilter retentate with uric acid or sodium hydrogen urate seeds reduced inhibition only 10% and 18%, respectively, whereas COM crystals removed almost all of the inhibition. If the macromolecules were preincubated in metastably supersaturated calcium oxalate solutions, the uric acid crystals removed 55% of inhibition while the sodium hydrogen urate removed 75%. This paper argues that adsorption of inhibitors can occur and that calcium promotes adsorption, as prior investigations (151) suggested.

After using a 50-kD filter to prepare macromolecules from normal human urine, Zerwekh et al. (155) used the preparation to raise the formation product ratio for calcium oxalate. They then showed that sodium hydrogen

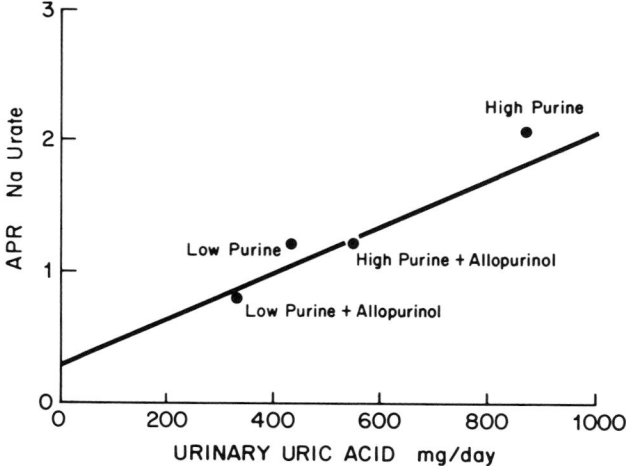

FIG. 38. The relationship between the urinary activity product ratio of monosodium urate and uric acid. The diagonal line represents the regression line obtained from the mean of each 3-day study period from each of nine patients ($r = 0.50$, $p < 0.01$). The four points indicate mean values for the whole group of patients during four study periods. [From Pak et al. (151).]

urate crystals and uric acid crystals could reverse the formation product back down, compatible with adsorption of inhibitors, and that for uric acid crystals to match the effects of sodium hydrogen urate crystals in adsorption, twice the crystal surface was required. Furthermore, the macromolecules lowered the growth rate constant for COM seeds in a metastable growth system (0.44 mM calcium and oxalate); and the two crystals offset the molecules, and they did so equally when uric acid surface surpassed sodium hydrogen urate surface by twofold.

Almost exactly opposed to Zerwekh et al. (155) and to Fellstrom et al. (154), Ryall et al. (156) preincubated urine samples with monosodium urate crystals, found the upper limit of metastability, found the crystal growth rate and the amount of crystals formed unchanged, and ascribed the difference to using intact urine instead of urine fractions subject to prior dilutions. In another paper, published the same year, Ryall et al. (157) studied (a) crystal growth measured by an increase in particle diameter and (b) aggregation as percent decrease in crystal number using a Coulter-counter method. They found that inhibition of crystal growth by heparin, but not by chondroitin sulfate, could be reduced by preincubation with sodium hydrogen urate seeds, and that crystal aggregation inhibition by both was reduced by such preincubation. A 1% addition of urine reduced growth and aggregation rates, and urate preincubation with the urine exerted little effect upon either inhibition.

No resolution of these contradictory studies is readily apparent, but most plausible is the simple notion that urine contains many possible inhibitors, and those that act at high dilutions and that have high affinities for the calcium oxalate crystal may also have modest concentrations and adsorb well to urate crystals, whereas low-affinity inhibitors may act on calcium oxalate crystals in undiluted urine and not adsorb well to urate crystals. This theme reminds us of the earliest papers on inhibitors—that is, those published before the present emphasis upon purification of high-affinity inhibitors, which remain uncharacterized.

Even so, Pak showed the effects of increased urate, and of decreasing urate with diet or drugs using intact urine and measuring upper limits of metastability and crystal growth in intact urine, whereas Ryall reported the opposite in papers which seem reasonable technically. These discrepancies may not be a result of quantitative differences but may, instead, be a result of technical peculiarities that affect outcomes and that could be resolved by repeating one another's experiments exactly.

Elsewhere, Grover et al. (158), from the Ryall group, redid the Hallson et al. (146) experiment by removing uric acid from urine using uricase immobilized on tubing, but they studied the urine differently—for metastable limits, volume of crystal formed in 90 min, and crystal aggregation using particle counting—and found no effects of lowering urate levels on any of the three mea-

sured indices. Samples of urine had their THP removed, because the protein forms aggregates that interfere with particle counting.

Unlike the previous paper, this one seems without merit. The average total urate concentration of the urine was 470 mg/L (a very low value), and pH and sodium concentrations were not given. Assuming a pH of 6 and common sodium concentrations of 150 mEq/L, supersaturations with uric acid and sodium hydrogen urate would be absent and modest, respectively, and would lower urate concentrations via an elaborate enzyme system, without any effect. It is important that the investigators use urine from patients with hyperuricosuria or that they induce hyperuricosuria, otherwise the test is of no validity at all; without supersaturation, inhibitor adsorption and heterogeneous nucleation both disappear and cannot be made to disappear to a greater extent by removing urate.

An Attempt at an Overview

One might say that the state of this field remains unsettled, mainly because the methods all seem different, and in a few cases, similar methods give contradictory results. We need a few experiments with internal controls, in which methods giving contradictory results can be repeated in one laboratory, side by side, so that the reasons for the contradictions can be determined. For example, the Burns versus Koutsoukos papers and the Pak versus Ryall papers seem absolutely contradictory, yet they used methods not so very different from one another. Sarig (149) offered a crucial idea, namely, that intrinsically inert urine molecules such as glutamic acid can activate a seed crystal of uric acid experiment; this hypothesis needs further testing.

Apatite

An interesting observation by Meyer et al. (159) shows that apatite seeds cause solution ion depletion from a metastably supersaturated calcium oxalate solution (Fig. 39) with virtually no time delay, and scanning electron micrographs show calcium oxalate crystals on surfaces of the apatite seeds. The converse experiment—seeds of calcium oxalate in a metastably supersaturated calcium phosphate system—causes no ion depletion, and this is ascribed to the fact that the initial phase of calcium phosphate is not apatite but rather a precursor of different structure.

We (160) have shown that tubule fluid in the thin segment of Henle's loop is supersaturated with respect to brushite, an early calcium phosphate phase, and that solutions modeled after tubule fluid using low, normal, or highest values reported from micropuncture experiments can create apatite crystals in vitro (Table 7). Furthermore, urine is supersaturated with respect to bru-

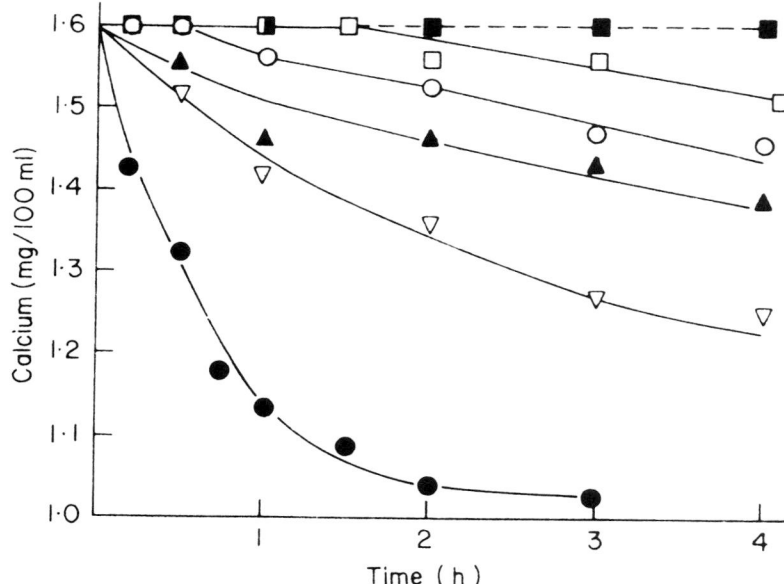

FIG. 39. Effect of surface area of seed on growth of calcium oxalate crystals at $S = 2.1$. Seed added: ■, none; □, hydroxyapatite, 3.7 cm²/mL; ○, hydroxyapatite, 7.7 cm²/mL; ▲, hydroxyapatite, 11.5 cm²/mL; ▽, hydroxyapatite, 19.3 cm²/mL; ●, calcium oxalate monohydrate (0.8 cm²/mL). [From Meyer et al. (159).]

shite (161), so brushite phases could easily form and can convert to apatite. Stone-former urine is more supersaturated than normal urine with respect to brushite (12).

We suspect that the reason for the very common occurrence of apatite in renal stones could be spontaneous thin-segment supersaturation, and we also suspect that apatite crystals may exist normally in the kidney. This work adds the possibility that such crystals could promote calcium oxalate crystallization, especially because high collecting-duct pH or hypercalciuria raises the likelihood that apatite could survive into the late nephron and also because collecting-duct calcium oxalate supersaturations are raised by hypercalciuria.

Cell Interactions

Here, at the very end of the chapter, we introduce some ideas concerning crystal interactions with cells. These share the conjecture that crystals can injure cells, stick to cells, enter cells, and promote cell growth, and that cell effects may lead to local disturbances inside the

nephrons that either obstruct their lumens, allow crystals to penetrate into the interstitium, or at least lodge so they can grow at leisure into stones.

Dulbecco and Elkington (162) noticed what they thought was growth stimulation of resting cultured fibroblasts by calcium ion, which turned out to be due to calcium phosphate crystallization (163); thus, it was determined that cell proliferation depends upon numbers of particles. Polystyrene beads, barium sulfate crystals, and kaolin particles all stimulated growth similarly. Rubin and Sanui (164) confirmed that calcium stimulation depends upon phosphate ion and upon formation of particulates.

In cultured synovial fibroblasts, crystalline calcium oxalate monohydrate and sodium hydrogen urate crystals stimulated collagenase production (165) and prostaglandin release, whereas poorly crystallized calcium oxalates stimulated these to a much smaller extent. Hemolytic ability of the two crystals that most provoked fibroblasts was very modest, showing that hemolytic potential tracks cell stimulation poorly.

Calcium oxalate and sodium hydrogen urate crystals can activate granulocytes to produce superoxide (166), to aggregate, and to attach to endothelium, and the effect seemed to be due to activation of complement. The authors considered these effects to be possible causes of the vasculitis of acute oxalosis.

Most pertinent to our concerns, sodium hydrogen urate crystals seem to adhere to cultured renal cells (MDCK line) and enter the cells (167), and at this site, the cells pile up on one another to form multicellular layers of crystal-laden cells. The affected cells release intracellular enzymes, suggesting cell injury, but they remain seemingly viable. The cells release prostaglandins. Diamond crystals, particulate but of different structure,

TABLE 7. *Summary of in vitro experiments*

Material	1	2	3	4	5
Calcium	N	N	N	N	N
Phosphorus	N	L	H	L	N
Sodium	N	N	N	L	L
Brushite	−	−	++++	−	−
Hydroxyapatite	+++	−	++	−	++
Calcite	+	LM	−	LM	++

+, X-ray crystallography; number of plus signs indicates quantity; N, normal; L, low; H, high; LM, seen by light microscopy.

elicit no responses. Uric acid crystals seem to cause the same effects as the sodium hydrogen urate. The authors believe that gouty nephropathies could arise, in part, from the mechanisms they observed in vitro, and we wonder if crystals do this in kidney tubules as part of renal stone formation.

Mandel et al. (168) found that putative inhibitors of crystallizations, such as EHDP, AMPS, GAGs, and RNA, could reduce hemolysis from calcium oxalate crystal interactions with red blood cells; all of these substances have about the same degree of effect. The same materials enhanced hemolysis from apatite crystals, and they had virtually no effect on brushite hemolysis. One possibility is that they interact at different places on these crystals. A natural conjecture is that calcium oxalate, brushite, uric acid, sodium hydrogen urate, and apatite crystals all may be able to provoke local cell injuries and proliferations, and that the so-called inhibitors may act most beneficially by inhibiting cell effects. We have taken this nice idea most seriously.

ACKNOWLEDGMENT

This work was supported by Grant AM 33949.

REFERENCES

1. Fleisch H. Inhibitors and promotors of stone formation. *Kidney Int* 1978;13:361–71.
2. Parks JH, Coe FL. A urinary calcium-citrate index for the evaluation of nephrolithiasis. *Kidney Int* 1986;30:85–90.
3. Senekjian HO, Weinman EJ. Oxalate transport by proximal tubule of the rabbit kidney. *Am J Physiol* 1982;243:F271–5.
4. Knight TF, Sansom SC, Senekjian HO, Weinman EJ. Oxalate secretion in the rat proximal tubule. *Am J Physiol* 1981; 240:F295–8.
5. Weber DV, Coe FL, Parks JH, Dunn MS, Tembe V. Urinary saturation measurements in calcium nephrolithiasis. *Ann Intern Med* 1979;90:180–4.
6. Coe FL, Favus MJ, Crockett T, et al. Effects of low-calcium diet on urine calcium excretion, parathyroid function and serum 1,25(OH)$_2$D$_3$ levels in patients with idiopathic hypercalciuria and in normal subjects. *Am J Med* 1982;72:25–32.
7. Fleisch H, Bisaz S. Isolation from urine of pyrophosphate, a calcification inhibitor. *Am J Physiol* 1962;203:671–5.
8. Bisaz S, Felix R, Neuman WF, Fleisch H. Quantitative determination of inhibitors of calcium phosphate precipitation in whole urine. *Miner Electrolyte Metab* 1978;1:74–83.
9. Robertson WG. Factors affecting the precipitation of calcium phosphate in vitro. *Calcif Tissue Res* 1973;11:311–22.
10. Dent CE, Sutor DJ. Presence or absence of inhibitor of calcium-oxalate crystal growth in urine of normals and of stone-formers. *Lancet* 1971;1:776–8.
11. Rose MB. The inhibitory effect of urine on calcium oxalate precipitation. *Invest Urol* 1975;12:428–33.
12. Pak CYC, Holt K. Nucleation and growth of brushite and calcium oxalate in urine of stone formers. *Metabolism* 1976; 25:665–73.
13. Ryall RL, Hibberd CM, Mazzachi BC, Marshall VR. Inhibitory activity of whole urine: a comparison of urines from stone formers and healthy subjects. *Clin Chim Acta* 1986;154:59–67.
14. Pak CY, Galosy RA. Propensity for spontaneous nucleation of calcium oxalate: quantitative assessment by urinary FPR–APR discriminant score. *Am J Med* 1980;69:681–9.
15. Grases F, Genestar C, March P, Conte A. Variations in the activity of urinary inhibitors in calcium oxalate urolithiasis. *Br J Urol* 1988;62:515–20.
16. Grases F, Genestar C, Conte A, March P, Costa-Bauza A. Inhibitory effect of pyrophosphate, citrate, magnesium and chondroitan sulfate in calcium oxalate urolithiasis. *Br J Urol* 1989;64: 235–7.
17. Grases F, Gil JJ, Conte A. Urolithiasis inhibitors and calculus nucleation. *Urol Res* 1989;17:163–6.
18. Robertson WG, Peacock M. Calcium oxalate crystalluria and inhibitors of crystallization in recurrent renal stone formers. *Clin Sci* 1972;43:499–506.
19. Meyer JL, Smith LH. Growth of calcium oxalate crystals. II. Inhibition by natural urinary crystal growth inhibitors. *Invest Urol* 1975;13:36–9.
20. Robertson WG, Peacock M, Marshall RW, Marshall DH, Nordin BEC. Saturation–inhibition index as a measure of the risk of calcium oxalate stone formation in the urinary tract. *N Engl J Med* 1976;294:249–52.
21. Lanzalaco AC, Sheehan ME, White DJ, Nancollas GH. The mineralization inhibitory potential of urines: a constant composition approach. *J Urol* 1982;128:845–9.
22. Robertson WG, Knowles F, Peacock M. Urinary acid mucopolysaccharide inhibitors of calcium oxalate crystallisation. In: Fleisch H, Robertson WG, Smith LH, Vahlensieck W, eds. *Urolithiasis research.* London: Plenum, 1976;331–40.
23. Coe FL, Raisen L. Allopurinol treatment of uric-acid disorders in calcium-stone formers. *Lancet* 1973;1:129–31.
24. Felix R, Monod A, Broge L, Hansen NM, Fleisch H. Aggregation of calcium oxalate crystals: effect of urine and various inhibitors. *Urol Res* 1977;5:21–8.
25. Coe FL, Margolis HC, Deutsch LH, Strauss AL. Urinary macromolecular crystal growth inhibitors in calcium urolithiasis. *Miner Electrolyte Metab* 1980;3:268–75.
26. Drach GW, Thorson S, Randolph A. Effects of urinary organic macromolecules on crystallization of calcium oxalate: enhancement of nucleation. *J Urol* 1980;123:519–23.
27. Ito H, Coe FL. Acidic peptide and polyribonucleotide crystal growth inhibitors in human urine. *Am J Physiol* 1977;233:F455–63.
28. Hallson PC, Rose GA. Uromucoids and urinary stone formation. *Lancet* 1979;1:1000–1.
29. Nakagawa Y, Kaiser ET, Coe FL. Isolation and characterization of calcium oxalate crystal growth inhibitors from human urine. *Biochem Biophys Res Commun* 1978;84:1038–44.
30. Zerwekh JE, Hwang TI, Poindexter J, Hill K, Wendell G, Pak CY. Modulation by calcium of the inhibitor activity of naturally occurring urinary inhibitors. *Kidney Int* 1988;33:1005–8.
31. Nakagawa Y, Margolis HC, Yokoyama S, Kezdy FJ, Kaiser ET, Coe FL. Purification and characterization of a calcium oxalate monohydrate crystal growth inhibitor from human kidney tissue culture medium. *J Biol Chem* 1981;256:3936–44.
32. Nakagawa Y, Abram V, Kezdy FJ, Kaiser ET, Coe FL. Purification and characterization of the principal inhibitor of calcium oxalate monohydrate crystal growth in human urine. *J Biol Chem* 1983;258:12594–600.
33. Nakagawa Y, Abram V, Coe FL. Isolation of calcium oxalate crystal growth inhibitor from rat kidney and urine. *Am J Physiol* 1984;247:F765–72.
34. Nakagawa Y, Abram V, Parks JH, Lau HS, Kawooya JK, Coe FL. Urine glycoprotein crystal growth inhibitors. Evidence for a molecular abnormality in calcium oxalate nephrolithiasis. *J Clin Invest* 1985;76:1455–62.
35. McPherson A, Shlichta P. Heterogeneous and epitaxial nucleation of protein crystals on mineral surfaces. *Science* 1988; 238:385–6.
36. Lopez M, Nakagawa Y, Coe FL, Tsai C, Michael AF, Scheinman JI. Immunochemistry of urinary calcium oxalate crystal growth inhibitor (CGI). *Kidney Int* 1986;29:829–33.
37. Nakagawa Y, Ahmed M, Hall SL, Deganello S, Coe FL. Isolation from human calcium oxalate renal stones of nephrocalcin, a glycoprotein inhibitor of calcium oxalate crystal growth. Evidence that nephrocalcin from patients with calcium oxalate nephroli-

thiasis is deficient in gamma-carboxyglutamic acid. *J Clin Invest* 1987;79:1782–7.

38. Worcester EM, Nakagawa Y, Wabner CL, Kumar S, Coe FL. Crystal adsorption and growth slowing by nephrocalcin, albumin, and Tamm–Horsfall protein. *Am J Physiol* 1988;255:F1197–205.

39. Nakagawa Y, Otsuki T, Coe FL. Elucidation of multiple forms of nephrocalcin by ^{31}P-NMR spectrometer. *FEBS Lett* 1989; 250:187–90.

40. Sirivongs D, Nakagawa Y, Vishny WK, Favus MJ, Coe FL. Evidence that mouse renal proximal tubule cells produce nephrocalcin. *Am J Physiol* 1989;257:F390–8.

41. Kitamura T, Zerwekh JE, Pak CY. Partial biochemical and physicochemical characterization of organic macromolecules in urine from patients with renal stones and control subjects. *Kidney Int* 1982;21:379–86.

42. Warpehoski MA, Buscemi PJ, Osborn DC, Finlayson B, Goldberg EP. Distribution of organic matrix in calcium oxalate renal calculi. *Calcif Tissue Int* 1981;33:211–2.

43. Spector AR, Gray A, Prien EL Jr. Kidney stone matrix; differences in acidic protein composition. *Invest Urol* 1976;13:387–9.

44. Bommer J, Ritz E, Tschope W, Waldherr R, Gebhardt M. Urinary matrix calculi consisting of microfibrillar protein in patients on maintenance hemodialysis. *Kidney Int* 1979;16:722–8.

45. Lian JB, Prien EL Jr, Glimcher MJ, Gallop PM. The presence of protein-bound gamma-carboxyglutamic acid in calcium-containing renal calculi. *J Clin Invest* 1977;59:1151–7.

46. Hoyer JR, Seiler MW. Pathophysiology of Tamm–Horsfall protein. *Kidney Int* 1979;16:279–89.

47. Chambers R, Groufsky A, Hunt JS, Lynn KL, McGiven AR. Relationship of abnormal Tamm–Horsfall glycoprotein localization to renal morphology and function. *Clin Nephrol* 1986;26:21–6.

48. Pennica D, Kohr WJ, Kuang WJ, et al. Identification of human uromodulin as the Tamm–Horsfall urinary glycoprotein. *Science* 1987;236:83–8.

49. Hamlin LM, Fish WW. Physical properties of Tamm–Horsfall glycoprotein and its glycopolypeptide. *Int J Pept Protein Res* 1977;10:270–6.

50. Horton JK, Davies M, Topley N, Thomas D, Williams JD. Activation of the inflammatory response of neutrophils by Tamm–Horsfall protein. *Kidney Int* 1990;37:717–26.

51. Rose GA, Sulaiman S. Tamm–Horsfall mucoproteins promote calcium oxalate crystal formation in urine: quantitative studies. *J Urol* 1982;127:177–9.

52. Wiggins RC. Uromucoid (Tamm–Horsfall glycoprotein) forms different polymeric arrangements on a filter surface under different physicochemical conditions. *Clin Chim Acta* 1987;162:329–40.

53. Curtain CC. The viscometric behavior of a mucoprotein isolated from human urine. *Aust J Exp Biol Med Sci* 1953;31:255–66.

54. Stevenson FK, Cleave AJ, Kent PW. The effect of ions on the viscometric and ultracentrifugal behavior of Tamm–Horsfall glycoprotein. *Biochim Biophys Acta* 1971;236:59–66.

55. Stevenson FK. The viscosity of Tamm–Horsfall mucoprotein. *Biochim Biophys Acta* 1968;160:296–8.

56. Stevenson FK. The viscosity of Tamm–Horsfall mucoprotein and its relation to cystic fibrosis. *Clin Chim Acta* 1969;23:441–7.

57. McQueen EG, Engel GB. Factors determining the aggregation of urinary proteins. *J Clin Pathol* 1966;19:392–6.

58. Kitamura T, Pak CY. Tamm and Horsfall glycoprotein does not promote spontaneous precipitation and crystal growth of calcium oxalate in vitro. *J Urol* 1982;127:1024–6.

59. Meyer JL, Smith LH. Growth of calcium oxalate crystals. I. A model for urinary stone growth. *Invest Urol* 1975;13:31–5.

60. Robertson WG, Scurr DS. Modifiers of calcium oxalate crystallization found in urine. I. Studies with a continuous crystallizer using an artificial urine. *J Urol* 1986;135:1322–6.

61. Scurr DS, Robertson WG. Modifiers of calcium oxalate crystallization found in urine. II. Studies on their mode of action in an artificial urine. *J Urol* 1986;136:128–31.

62. Scurr DS, Latif AB, Sergeant V, Robertson WG. Polyanionic inhibitors of calcium oxalate crystal agglomeration in urine. *Proc Eur Dial Transplant Assoc* 1983;20:440–4.

63. Scurr DS, Robertson WG. Modifiers of calcium oxalate crystallization found in urine. III. Studies on the role of Tamm–Horsfall mucoprotein and of ionic strength. *J Urol* 1986;136:505–7.

64. Hess B, Nakagawa Y, Coe FL. Inhibition of calcium oxalate monohydrate crystal aggregation by urine proteins. *Am J Physiol* 1989;257:F99–106.

65. Bichler KH, Kirchner C, Ideler V. Uromucoid excretion of normal individuals and stone formers. *Br J Urol* 1976;47:733–8.

66. Rambausek M, Dulawa J, Jann K, Ritz E. Tamm Horsfall glycoprotein in diabetes mellitus: abnormal chemical composition and colloid stability. *Eur J Clin Invest* 1988;18:237–42.

67. Sanders PW, Booker BB, Bishop JB, Cheung HC. Mechanisms of intranephronal proteinaceous cast formation by low molecular weight proteins. *J Clin Invest* 1990;85:570–6.

68. Davies PL, Hew CL. Biochemistry of fish antifreeze proteins. *FASEB J* 1990;4:2460–8.

69. Knight CA, DeVries AL. Melting inhibition and superheating of ice by an antifreeze glycopeptide. *Science* 1989;245:505–7.

70. Schlesinger DH, Hay DL. Complete covalent structure of statherin, a tyrosine-rich acidic peptide which inhibits calcium phosphate precipitation from human parotid saliva. *J Biol Chem* 1977;252:1689–95.

71. Sabatini LM, Carlock LR, Johnson GW, Azen EA. cDNA cloning and chromosomal localization (4q11–13) of a gene for statherin, a regulator of calcium in saliva. *Am J Hum Genet* 1987;41:1048–60.

72. De Caro AM, Bonicel JJ, Rouimi P, De Caro JD, Sarles H, Rovery M. Complete amino acid sequence of an immunoreactive form of human pancreatic stone protein isolated from pancreatic juice. *Eur J Biochem* 1987;168:201–7.

73. Holan KR, Holzbach RT, Hermann RE, Cooperman AM, Claffey WJ. Nucleation time: a key factor in the pathogenesis of cholesterol gallstone disease. *Gastroenterology* 1979;77:611–7.

74. Holzbach RT, Kibe A, Thiel E, Howell JH, Marsh M, Hermann RE. Biliary proteins: unique inhibitors of cholesterol crystal nucleation in human gallbladder bile. *J Clin Invest* 1984;73:35–45.

75. Kibe A, Holzbach RT, LaRusso NF, Mao SJT. Inhibition of cholesterol crystal formation by apolipoproteins in supersaturated model bile. *Science* 1984;225:514–6.

76. Shimizu S, Sabsay B, Veis A, Ostrow JD, Rege RV, Dawes LG. Isolation of an acidic protein from cholesterol gallstones, which inhibits the precipitation of calcium carbonate in vitro. *J Clin Invest* 1989;84:1990–6.

77. Kok DJ, Papapoulos SE, Bijvoet OLM. Crystal agglomeration is a major element in calcium oxalate urinary stone formation. *Kidney Int* 1990;37:51–6.

78. Kok DJ, Papapoulos SE, Blomen LJ, Bijvoet OL. Modulation of calcium oxalate monohydrate crystallization kinetics in vitro. *Kidney Int* 1988;34:346–50.

79. Lindberg J, Harvey J, Pak CYC. Effect of magnesium citrate and magnesium oxide on the crystallization of calcium salts in urine: changes produced by food–magnesium interaction. *J Urol* 1990;143:248–51.

80. Preminger GM, Sakhaee K, Pak CY. Alkali action on the urinary crystallization of calcium salts: contrasting responses to sodium citrate and potassium citrate. *J Urol* 1988;139:240–2.

81. Hosking DH, Wilson JWL, Liedtke RR, Smith LH, Wilson DM. Urinary citrate excretion in normal persons and patients with idiopathic calcium urolithiasis. *J Lab Clin Med* 1985;106:682–9.

82. Conte A, Roca P, Gianotti M, Grases F. On the relation between citrate and calcium in normal and stone former subjects. *Int Urol Nephrol* 1989;21:369–73.

83. Nikkila M, Koivula T, Jokela H. Urinary citrate excretion in patients with urolithiasis and normal subjects. *Eur Urol* 1989;16:382–5.

84. Minisola S, Rossi W, Pacitti MT, et al. Studies on citrate metabolism in normal subjects and kidney stone patients. *Miner Electrolyte Metab* 1989;15:303–8.

85. Pak CY, Fuller C. Idiopathic hypocitraturic calcium-oxalate nephrolithiasis successfully treated with potassium citrate. *Ann Intern Med* 1986;104:33–7.

86. Pak CYC, Peterson R, Sakhaee K, Fuller C, Preminger GM, Reisch J. Correction of hypocitraturia and prevention of stone formation by combined thiazide and potassium citrate therapy in

thiazide-unresponsive hypercalciuric nephrolithiasis. *Am J Med* 1985;79:284–8.

87. Pak CYC. Citrate and renal calculi. *Miner Electrolyte Metab* 1987;13:257–66.

88. Rumenapf G, Schwille PO. The influence of oral alkali citrate on intestinal calcium absorption in healthy man. *Clin Sci* 1987;73:117–21.

89. Cowley DM, McWhinney BC, Brown JM, Chalmers AH. Effect of citrate on the urinary excretion of calcium and oxalate: relevance to calcium oxalate nephrolithiasis. *Clin Chem* 1989; 35:23–8.

90. Borensztein P, Patron P, Bichara M, Gardin J, Paillard M. Effects of citrate on urinary calcium excretion. *Miner Electrolyte Metab* 1989;15:353–8.

91. Froment DH, Molitoris BA, Buddington B, Miller N, Alfrey AC. Site and mechanism of enhanced gastrointestinal absorption of aluminum by citrate. *Kidney Int* 1989;36:978–84.

92. Molitoris BA, Froment DH, MacKenzie TA, Huffer WH, Alfrey AC. Citrate: a major factor in the toxicity of orally administered aluminum compounds. *Kidney Int* 1989;36:949–53.

93. Desmars JF, Tawashi R. Dissolution and growth of calcium oxalate monohydrate. I. Effect of magnesium and pH. *Biochim Biophys Acta* 1973;313:256–67.

94. Welshman SG, McGeown MG. The relationship of the urinary cations, calcium, magnesium, sodium and potassium, in patients with renal calculi. *Br J Urol* 1975;47:237–42.

95. Sutor DJ. Growth studies of calcium oxalate in the presence of various ions and compounds. *Br J Urol* 1969;41:171–8.

96. Schwille PO, Rumenapf G, Wolfel G, Kohler R. Urinary pyrophosphate in patients with recurrent urolithiasis and in healthy controls: a reevaluation. *J Urol* 1988;140:239–45.

97. Wakid NW, Kutayli F, Buri H. Inorganic pyrophosphatase in human urine. *Clin Chim Acta* 1970;30:527–9.

98. Pak CY, Ohata M, Holt K. Effect of diphosphonate on crystallization of calcium oxalate in vitro. *Kidney Int* 1975;7:154–60.

99. Robertson WG, Peacock M, Marshall VR, Knowles F. The effect of ethane-1-hydroxy-1,1-diphosphonate (EHDP) on calcium oxalate crystalluria in recurrent renal stone-formers. *Clin Sci Mol Med* 1974;47:13–22.

100. Meyer JL, Lee KE, Bergert JH. The inhibition of calcium oxalate crystal growth by multidentate organic phosphonates; effect of pH. *Calcif Tissue Res* 1977;28:83–6.

101. Bone HG III, Zerwekh JE, Britton F, Pak CYC. Treatment of calcium urolithiasis with diphosphonate: efficacy and hazards. *J Urol* 1979;121:568–71.

102. Levy RJ, Wolfrum J, Schoen FJ, Hawley MA, Lund SA, Langer R. Inhibition of calcification of bioprosthetic heart valves by local controlled release diphosphonate. *Science* 1985;228:190–2.

103. Russell RGG, Bisaz S, Fleisch H. The influence of orthophosphate on the renal handling of inorganic pyrophosphate in man and dog. *Clin Sci Mol Med* 1976;51:435–43.

104. Coe FL, Parks JH. Idiopathic stone formers. In: *Nephrolithiasis: pathogenesis and treatment.* Chicago: Year Book Medical Publishers, 1988;232–49.

105. Robertson WG, Peacock M, Nordin BEC. Inhibitors of the growth and aggregation of calcium oxalate crystals in vitro. *Clin Chim Acta* 1973;43:31–7.

106. Michelacci YM, Glashan RQ, Schor N. Urinary excretion of glycosaminoglycans in normal and stone forming subjects. *Kidney Int* 1989;36:1022–8.

107. Martin X, Smith LH, Werness PG. Calcium oxalate dihydrate formation in urine. *Kidney Int* 1984;25:948–52.

108. Yu T. Urolithiasis in hyperuricemia and gout. *J Urol* 1981;126:424–30.

109. Lonsdale K. Epitaxy as a growth factor in urinary calculi and gallstones. *Nature* 1968;217:56–8.

110. Millman S, Strauss AL, Parks JH, Coe FL. Pathogenesis and clinical course of mixed calcium oxalate and uric acid nephrolithiasis. *Kidney Int* 1982;22:366–70.

111. Coe FL. Hyperuricosuric calcium oxalate nephrolithiasis. *Kidney Int* 1978;13:418–26.

112. Fellstrom B, Backman U, Danielson BG, Johansson G, Ljunghall S, Wikstrom B. Urinary excretion of urate in renal calcium stone

113. Hodgkinson A. Uric acid disorders in patients with calcium stones. *Br J Urol* 1976;48:1–5.

114. Schwille P, Samberger N, Wach B. Fasting uric acid and phosphate in urine and plasma of renal calcium-stone formers. *Nephron* 1976;16:116–25.

115. Coe FL, Kavalach AG. Hypercalciuria and hyperuricosuria in patients with calcium nephrolithiasis. *N Engl J Med* 1974; 291:1344–50.

116. Coe FL. Treated and untreated recurrent calcium nephrolithiasis in patients with idiopathic hypercalciuria, hyperuricosuria, or no metabolic disorder. *Ann Intern Med* 1977;87:404–10.

117. Coe FL. Uric acid and calcium oxalate nephrolithiasis. *Kidney Int* 1983;24:392–403.

118. Ettinger B, Tang A, Citron JT, Livermore B, Williams T. Randomized trial of allopurinol in the prevention of calcium oxalate calculi. *N Engl J Med* 1986;315:1386–9.

119. Finlayson B, Burns J, Smith A, Du Bois L. Effect of oxipurinol and allopurinol riboside on whewellite crystallization: in vitro and in vivo observations. *Invest Urol* 1979;17:227–9.

120. Finlayson B, Reid F. The effect of allopurinol on calcium oxalate (whewellite) precipitation. *Invest Urol* 1978;15:489–91.

121. Tiselius HG, Larsson L, Hellgren E. Clinical results of allopurinol treatment in prevention of calcium oxalate stone formation. *J Urol* 1986;136:50–3.

122. Fellstrom B, Backman U, Danielson BG, et al. Allopurinol treatment of renal calcium stone disease. *Br J Urol* 1985;57:375–9.

123. Marangella M, Tricerri A, Sonego S, et al. Critical evaluation of various forms of therapy for idiopathic calcium stone disease. *Proc Eur Dial Transplant Assoc* 1983;20:434–9.

124. Smith MJ, Hunt LD, King JS Jr, Boyce WH. Uricemia and urolithiasis. *J Urol* 1969;101:637–42.

125. Smith MJV. Placebo versus allopurinol for renal calculi. *J Urol* 1977;117:690–2.

126. Stote RM, Smith LH, Dubb JW, Moyer TP, Alexander F, Roth JLA. Oxypurinol nephrolithiasis in regional enteritis secondary to allopurinol therapy. *Ann Intern Med* 1980;92:384–5.

127. Landgrebe AR, Nyhan WL, Coleman M. Urinary-tract stones resulting from the excretion of oxypurinol. *N Engl J Med* 1975;292:626–7.

128. Al-Kawas FH, Seeff LB, Berendson RA, Zimmerman HJ, Ishak KG. Allopurinol hepatotoxicity: report of two cases and review of the literature. *Ann Intern Med* 1981;95:588–90.

129. Swank LA, Chejfec G, Nemchausky BA. Allopurinol-induced granulomatous hepatitis with cholangitis and a sarcoid-like reaction. *Arch Intern Med* 1978;138:997–9.

130. Berlinger WG, Park GD, Spector R. The effect of dietary protein on the clearance of allopurinol and oxypurinol. *N Engl J Med* 1985;313:771–6.

131. Danielson BG, Pak CY, Smith LH, Vahlensieck W, Robertson WG. Treatment of Idiopathic calcium stone disease. *Calcif Tissue Int* 1983;35:715–9.

132. Pak CY, Peterson R. Successful treatment of hyperuricosuric calcium oxalate nephrolithiasis with potassium citrate. *Arch Intern Med* 1986;146:863–7.

133. Coe FL, Moran E, Kavalich AG. The contribution of dietary purine over-consumption to hyperpuricosuria in calcium oxalate stone formers. *J Chronic Dis* 1976;29:793–800.

134. Fellstrom B, Backman U, Danielson BG, Johansson G, Ljunghall S, Wikstrom B. Renal handling of urate in patients with calcium stone disease. *Nephron* 1982;31:31–6.

135. Pak CYC, Waters O, Arnold L, Holt K, Cox C, Barilla DE. Mechanism for calcium urolithiasis among patients with hyperuricosuria. *J Clin Invest* 1977;59:426–31.

136. Coe FL, Strauss AL, Tembe V, Le Dun S. Uric acid saturation in calcium nephrolithiasis. *Kidney Int* 1980;17:662–8.

137. Pak CYC, Holt K, Britton F, Peterson R, Crowther C, Ward D. Assessment of pathogenetic roles of uric acid, monopotassium urate, monoammonium urate and monosodium urate in hyperuricosuria calcium oxalate nephrolithiasis. *Miner Electrolyte Metab* 1980;4:130–6.

138. Coe FL. Calcium-uric acid nephrolithiasis. *Arch Intern Med* 1978;138:1090–3.

139. Harvey JA, Pak CY. Gouty diathesis and sarcoidosis in patient with recurrent calcium nephrolithiasis. *J Urol* 1988;139:1287–9.

140. Tiselius HG, Larsson L. Urinary excretion of urate in patients with calcium oxalate stone disease. *Urol Res* 1983;11:279–83.

141. Pak CY, Arnold LH. Heterogeneous nucleation of calcium oxalate by seeds of monosodium urate. *Proc Soc Exp Biol Med* 1975;149:930–2.

142. Coe FL, Lawton RL, Goldstein RB, Tembe V. Sodium urate accelerates precipitation of calcium oxalate in vitro. *Proc Soc Exp Biol Med* 1975;149:926–9.

143. Koutsoukos PG, Lam Erwin CY, Nancollas GH. Epitaxial considerations in urinary stone formation. I. The urate–oxalate–phosphate system. *Invest Urol* 1980;18:178–84.

144. Burns JR, Finlayson B. The effect of seed crystals on calcium oxalate nucleation. *Invest Urol* 1980;18:133–6.

145. Tiselius HG. Effects of sodium urate and uric acid crystals on the crystallization of calcium oxalate. *Urol Res* 1984;12:11–5.

146. Hallson PC, Rose GA, Sulaiman S. Urate does not influence the formation of calcium oxalate crystals in whole human urine at pH 5.3. *Clin Sci* 1982;62:421–5.

147. Deganello S, Chou C. The uric acid–whewellite association in human kidney stones. *Scan Electron Microsc* 1984;927–33.

148. Deganello S, Coe F. Epitaxy between uric acid and whewellite: experimental verification. *N Jb Miner Mh* 1983;6:270–6.

149. Sarig S. The hyperuricosuric calcium oxalate stone former. *Miner Electrolyte Metab* 1987;13:251–6.

150. Tiselius HG. Inhibition of calcium oxalate crystal growth in urine during treatment with allopurinol. *Br J Urol* 1980;52:189–92.

151. Pak CY, Barilla DE, Holt K, Brinkley L, Tolentino R, Zerwekh JE. Effect of oral purine load and allopurinol on the crystallization of calcium salts in urine of patients with hyperuricosuric calcium urolithiasis. *Am J Med* 1978;65:593–9.

152. Finlayson B, DuBois L. Adsorption of heparin on sodium acid urate. *Clin Chim Acta* 1978;84:203–6.

153. Pak CY, Holt K, Zerwekh JE. Attenuation by monosodium urate of the inhibitory effect of glycosaminoglycans on calcium oxalate nucleation. *Invest Urol* 1979;17:138–40.

154. Fellstrom B, Backman U, Danielson BG, Holmgren K, Ljunghall S, Wikstrom B. Inhibitory activity of human urine on calcium oxalate crystal growth: effects of sodium urate and uric acid. *Clin Sci* 1982;62:509–14.

155. Zerwekh JE, Holt K, Pak CY. Natural urinary macromolecular inhibitors: attenuation of inhibitory activity by urate salts. *Kidney Int* 1983;23:838–41.

156. Ryall RL, Hibberd CM, Marshall VR. The effect of crystalline monosodium urate on the crystallisation of calcium oxalate in whole human urine. *Urol Res* 1986;14:63–5.

157. Ryall RL, Harnett RM, Marshall VR. The effect of monosodium urate on the capacity of urine, chondroitin sulphate and heparin to inhibit calcium oxalate crystal growth and aggregation. *J Urol* 1986;135:174–7.

158. Grover PK, Ryall RL, Potezny N, Marshall VR. The effect of decreasing the concentration of urinary urate on the crystallization of calcium oxalate in undiluted human urine. *J Urol* 1990;143:1057–61.

159. Meyer JL, Bergert JH, Smith LH. Epitaxial relationships in urolithiasis: the calcium oxalate monohydrate–hydroxyapatite system. *Clin Sci Mol Med* 1975;49:369–74.

160. Deganello S, Asplin J, Coe FL. Evidence that tubule fluid in the thin segment of the loop of Henle normally is supersaturated and forms a poorly crystallized hydroxyapatite that can initiate renal stones. *Kidney Int* 1990;37:472–72.

161. Pak CYC, Hayashi Y, Finlayson B, Chu S. Estimation of the state of supersaturation of brushite and calcium oxalate in urine: a comparison of three methods. *J Lab Clin Med* 1977;89:891–909.

162. Dulbecco R, Elkington J. Induction of growth in resting fibroblastic cell cultures by Ca++. *Proc Natl Acad Sci USA* 1975;72:1584–8.

163. Barnes DW, Colowick SP. Stimulation of sugar uptake and thymidine incorporation in mouse 3T3 cells by calcium phosphate and other extracellular particles. *Proc Natl Acad Sci USA* 1977;74:5593–7.

164. Rubin H, Sanui H. Complexes of inorganic pyrophosphate, orthophosphate, and calcium as stimulants of 3T3 cell multiplication. *Proc Natl Acad Sci USA* 1977;74:5026–30.

165. Hasselbacher P. Stimulation of synovial fibroblasts by calcium oxalate and monosodium urate monohydrate. A mechanism of connective tissue degradation in oxalosis and gout. *J Lab Clin Med* 1982;100:977–85.

166. Boogaerts MA, Hammerschmidt DE, Roelant C, Verwilghen RL, Jacob HS. Mechanisms of vascular damage in gout and oxalosis: crystal induced, granulocyte mediated, endothelial injury. *Thromb Haemost* 1983;50:576–80.

167. Emmerson BT, Cross M, Osborne JM, Axelsen RA. Reaction of MDCK cells to crystals of monosodium urate monohydrate and uric acid. *Kidney Int* 1990;37:36–43.

168. Mandel NS, Mandel GS, Hasegawa AT. The effect of some urinary stone inhibitors on membrane interaction potentials of stone crystals. *J Urol* 1987;138:557–62.

Disorders of Bone and Mineral Metabolism,
edited by Fredric L. Coe and Murray J. Favus,
© 1992 by Raven Press, Ltd. All rights reserved.

CHAPTER 36

Noncalcium Nephrolithiasis

Malachy J. Gleeson, Kyoichi Kobashi, and Donald P. Griffith

Noncalcium nephrolithiasis encompasses a heterogeneous group of urinary calculi of varying compositions and widely differing causative factors. This chapter is divided into four sections that deal with urate calculi, cystine calculi, struvite calculi, and a miscellaneous group of less common calculi. Calculi of different compositions are discussed individually with regard to their pathophysiology, diagnosis, and treatment.

URATE RENAL CALCULI

Urate calculi may form as ammonium acid urate or uric acid stones. Ammonium acid urate calculi account for about 0.2% of lithiasis in industrial countries compared to as high as 69% of lithiasis in developing countries such as Turkey and Pakistan (1–3). Ammonium acid urate calculi can be separated into type I and type II according to their morphology (2). Type I stones are composed of large, yellowish crystals with a needle-like configuration which are often mixed with magnesium ammonium phosphate crystals. These calculi are thought to arise if urealytic infections occur in urine that is already oversaturated with uric acid. Similar stones occur secondary to urinary tract infections in dalmatian dogs because of a congenital deficiency in tubular reabsorption of uric acid. Type II ammonium acid urate stones are composed of small crystals that are organized into spheruliths. They occur in sterile urine in association with calcium oxalate monohydrate crystals. This type of stone is particularly common in children in endemic areas (developing countries) and is caused by dietary deficiencies in calories, phosphorus, proteins, and vitamin A. Children's diets in underdeveloped countries are commonly deficient in milk and rich in cereals. The organic phosphate esters (phytic acid) present in cereals are poorly absorbed in the human intestine in the presence of protein and vitamin A deficiencies because of the relative deficiency in phytase that is required for hydrolysis. The subsequent hypophosphatemia results in an increased endogenous ammonia production that reacts with free H^+ ions in urine to form ammonium ions. A purine-rich diet (pinto beans) in conjunction with a low fluid intake (carbonated soda) was postulated to be the cause of ammonium acid urate urolithiasis in three Navajo Indian children in New Mexico (4). The chemical dissolution of ammonium urate calculi has not been described in vivo. As the urinary pH decreases, ammonium urate solubility increases but uric acid precipitation may occur (5). In alkaline urine, ammonium urate crystals are stabilized. The treatment must therefore consist of calculus removal and the prevention of further stone formation with an adequate diet and the administration of allopurinol.

Uric acid is an end product of purine metabolism which plays a fundamental role in nucleic acid production (Fig. 1). Three forms of renal disease are attributable to excess uric acid or urate deposition: acute uric acid nephropathy, chronic urate nephropathy, and uric acid nephrolithiasis (6). Uric acid nephrolithiasis accounts for about 10% of renal calculi (7,8).

Pathophysiology

The daily input and output of uric acid is shown in Fig. 2 (14,15). In the kidney uric acid is handled in four different ways (Fig. 3) (16). About 5% of uric acid is bound to plasma proteins and the rest is freely filtered at the glomerulus. Approximately 99% of this filtrate is reabsorbed in the proximal tubule; 50% is then secreted and most of this is reabsorbed at the postsecretory reabsorption sites to leave only 10% excreted in the urine

M. J. Gleeson and D. P. Griffith: Scott Department of Urology, Baylor College of Medicine, Houston, Texas 77030

K. Kobashi: Department of Biochemistry, Toyama Medical and Pharmaceutical University, Toyama-Shi, Japan

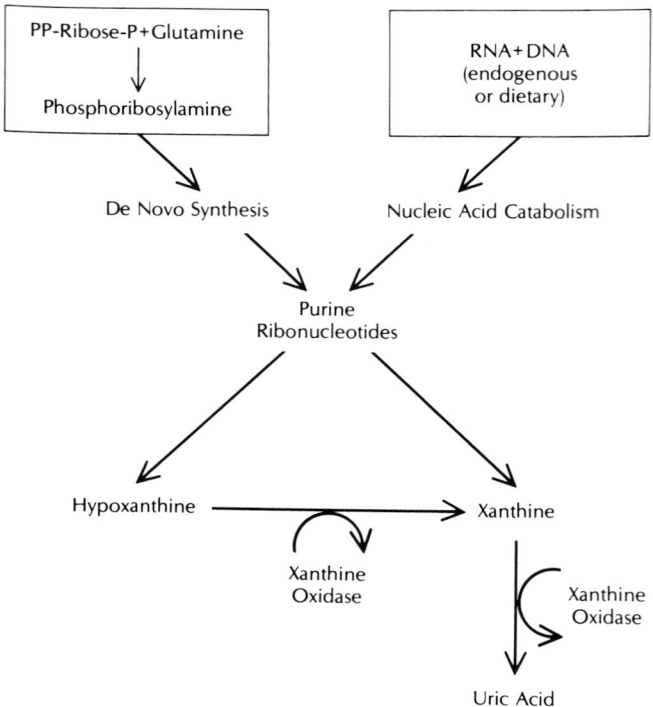

FIG. 1. Purine metabolism.

(16,17). Approximately half of the daily pool turns over daily.

Uric acid has a dissociation constant (pK_a) of 5.46 so that at urinary pH values below 6, most of the uric acid is in the undissociated form, which is unsoluble in acid urine (7). At acid pH levels, urine is supersaturated with uric acid so that crystalluria is relatively common. As urinary pH rises, uric acid dissociates to give the relatively soluble urate ion so that at a pH of 6.5, urine is undersaturated with regard to uric acid and preexisting crystals dissolve (Fig. 4) (7).

The fundamental predisposing factor leading to uric acid urolithiasis is low urinary pH, although low urinary volume and hyperuricosuria also play a role (18,19). A

uric acid crystallization inhibitor has also been reported, but its structure and significance are as yet unknown (20,21).

It has been reported that urinary pH in uric acid stone formers is lower than in those with mixed renal calculi, but this is not a consistent finding (19,22). However, low urinary pH may result secondary to extrarenal bicarbonate loss because of diarrhea, ileostomy drainage, or chronic renal failure. The normal diet supplies about 50 mEq of acid daily, which may be reduced by a high vegetable intake or increased by a high animal protein and fat intake (see Chapter 34). The diurnal variation in urinary pH (Fig. 5) is attributed to the diet, as the early part of digestion causes a loss of stomach acid and results in alkaline urine, whereas these changes are reversed later when the food passes through the small intestine. However, the overall urinary pH is dependent on the total protein, fat, and vegetable content of the diet (7). A familial form of uric acid stone formation has also been reported and may be due to a hereditary defect in urinary acidification (7).

Low urinary volumes result in a raised concentration of uric acid, relative hyperuricosuria, and increased urinary acidity. Common causes of oliguria are low fluid intake, inflammatory bowel disease, ileostomies, colostomies, and warm climates (23,24). The majority of patients with idiopathic uric acid calculi are accounted for by some combination of the known risk factors. The causes of hyperuricosuria are outlined in Table 1. Of those with secondary uric acid stones, gout is probably the commonest associated disease, with stone formation resulting from hyperuricosuria and abnormally low urinary pH in some patients. Gout, which is characterized by hyperuricemia, has three clinical phases: acute gouty arthritis, a period of interval gout, and chronic tophaceous gout. Uric acid nephrolithiasis may occur during any of these phases or may rarely be the presenting sign (9). Although Sydenham associated gout with nephrolithiasis in 1683, this was not confirmed until Scheele isolated uric acid from calculi in 1776 and Wollaston isolated it from tophi of patients with gout in 1797

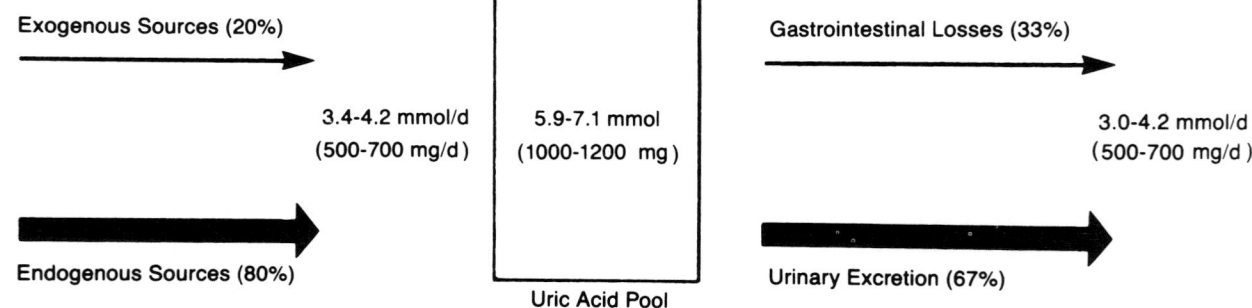

FIG. 2. Daily uric acid balance in human beings. (Reproduced with permission from D. Dykman, E. E. Simon, and L. V. Aviole, *Arch Intern Med* 1987;147:1341–1345; copyright 1987, American Medical Association.)

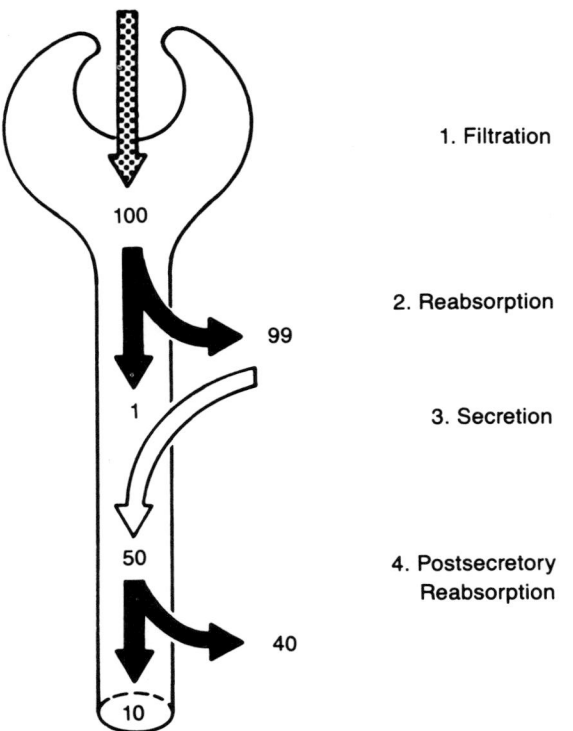

1. Filtration

2. Reabsorption

3. Secretion

4. Postsecretory Reabsorption

FIG. 3. Renal handling of uric acid. (Reproduced with permission from D. Dykman, E. E. Simon, and L. V. Aviole, *Arch Intern Med* 1987;147:1341–1345; copyright 1987, American Medical Association.)

order that leads to increased PRPP production. PRPP is both a substrate and an activator of the first enzyme committed to de novo synthesis of purines (Fig. 1). This enzyme abnormality usually appears before 10 years of age with nephrolithiasis and arthritis appearing later.

Glucose-6-phosphatase deficiency (type I glycogen storage disease) is an autosomal recessive disorder that usually presents with arthritis in the teens and tophaceous gout and nephropathy in adulthood. The mechanisms of the hyperuricemia are (a) decreased feedback inhibition of de novo purine synthesis, (b) increased PRPP production with resultant increased de novo purine synthesis, and (c) hyperlactacidemia which decreases renal clearance of uric acid.

Lesch-Nyhan syndrome (hypoxanthine guanine phosphoribosyltransferase deficiency) (HGPRT) is an X-linked recessive disorder in males characterized by gout, hyperuricosuria, uric acid calculi, spasticity, choreoathetosis, mental retardation, and self-mutilation. A partial deficiency of the enzyme may also occur with less severe neurological symptoms. The enzyme deficiency results in increased substrate and decreased feedback inhibition of de novo purine synthesis. All enzyme defects are rare but should be considered in children with gout so that early management and genetic counseling can be undertaken (9).

Australia is an example of a country that has a high animal protein intake with resultant high dietary purine intake which, together with a warm climate, combine to give a high prevalence of uric acid stones (25,26).

Myeloproliferative disorders such as polycythemia rubra vera, secondary polycythemia, myeloid metaplasia, and multiple myeloma have increased nucleic acid turnover with resultant enhanced uric acid production. Hyperuricemia and hyperuricosuria are especially common

(10–12). Over 20% of patients with primary gout and 40% of patients with secondary gout will develop uric acid nephrolithiasis (13).

Phosphoribosyl pyrophosphate (PRPP) synthetase overactivity is a heterogeneous X-linked dominant dis-

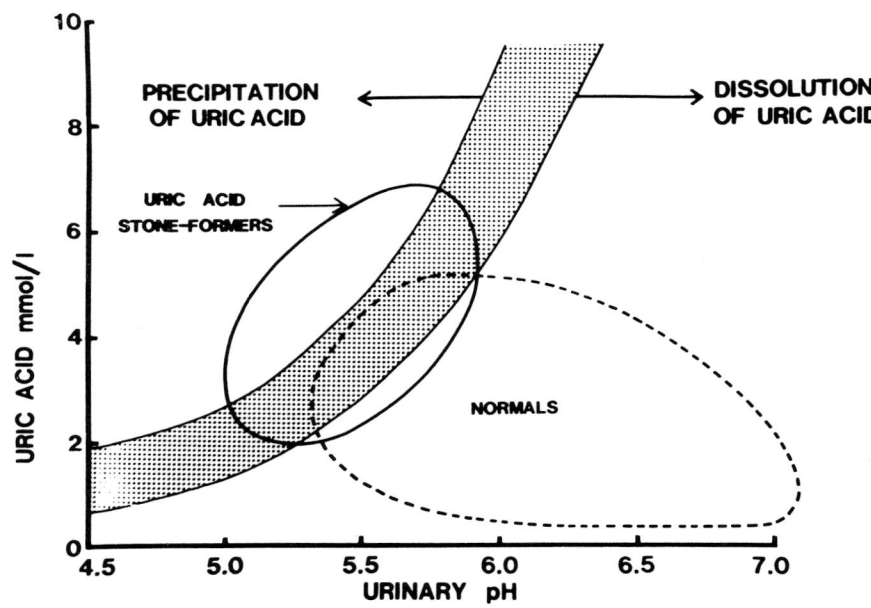

FIG. 4. Saturation curve of uric acid with regard to urinary pH. (Reproduced with permission from Ref. 7.)

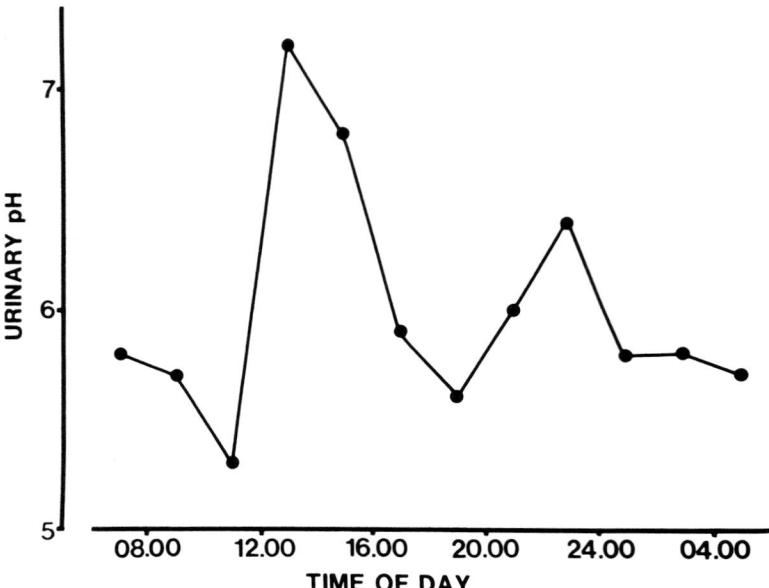

FIG. 5. Normal diurnal urinary pH variation. (Reproduced with permission from Ref. 7.)

in patients with leukemias and lymphomas after the initiation of treatment due to the large amount of tissue breakdown (26). For this reason, prophylactic allopurinol is usually prescribed concurrent with cytotoxic chemotherapy (27).

Drugs that alter uric acid metabolism are outlined in Table 2. Hyperuricemia and hyperuricosuria alone do not invariably result in urolithiasis. With regard to renal transplant recipients, there have been five case reports of uric acid calculus formation secondary to cyclosporin A immunosuppression (28). Hyperuricemia occurs in 56% of cyclosporin-treated patients and results in gout in 12% of these cases (29). The causative mechanism has been attributed to a renal tubular abnormality in the presence of a low urinary pH (28,30).

Presentation

The clinical presentation of uric acid calculi is similar to other types of urolithiasis. Calculi are more common in men than women, with the peak prevalence after 50 years of age (31). Most patients present with renal colic and hematuria. The presence of a low urinary pH should suggest the diagnosis to the clinician. Investigation with

TABLE 1. *Causes of hyperuricosuria*

Primary gout
Enzymatic defects
   Phosphoribosyl pyrophosphate (PRPP) synthetase
     overactivity
   Glucose-6-phosphatase deficiency
   Lesch-Nyhan syndrome
Increased purine intake
Myeloproliferative disorders
Uricosuric drugs

standard radiographs will not demonstrate calculi, as uric acid stones are radiolucent. However, they may be demonstrated using ultrasonography or computed tomography (without contrast). Typically, retrieved calculi are friable and have smooth surfaces. They are composed of a mixture of anhydrous and dihydrate uric acid crystals (1,32).

Treatment

The treatment of uric acid urolithiasis rests with (1) increasing urinary volume, (2) decreasing uricosuria by decreasing dietary purine intake or by allopurinol medication, (3) increasing urinary pH, and (4) operative intervention.

Increasing Urinary Volume

A urinary output of 2.5–3 L/day will decrease urinary uric acid concentration and therefore increase its solubility (18). To attain this urine volume, a variable intake is required, depending on individual patient factors such as degree of perspiration and fluid loss in the feces.

Decreased Dietary Purine Intake

Reduction of animal protein intake (e.g., red meat, fish, and fowl) reduces uricosuria and can be monitored by checking uricosuric levels (25). Severe dietary restrictions are infrequently warranted, as only 20% of uric acid intake is derived from dietary sources (Fig. 2).

Allopurinol Therapy

Allopurinol reduces uric acid synthesis by inhibiting xanthine oxidase and has resulted in xanthine stone for-

TABLE 2. *Drugs that alter uric acid metabolism*

Hyperuricemic Drugs	Hypouricemic Drugs Cont.
INCREASE URATE PRODUCTION	Chlorprothixene
4-Amino-5-imidazolecarboxamide riboside	Cinchophen
B$_{12}$ (acute administration)	Citrate
Cytotoxic drugs	Dicumarol
Ethanol	Diflumidone
2-Ethylamino-1,3,4-thiadiazole	Diuretics (acutely, before extracellular volume contraction)
Fructose	Estrogens
Nicotinic acid	Ethyl biscoumacetate
Pancreatic extract	Ethyl *p*-chlorophenoxyisobutyric acid
	Glycerol guaiacolate
DECREASE URATE EXCRETION	Glycine
Cyclosporin A	Glycopyrrolate
Diuretics	Halofenate
Acetazolamide	Iodopyracet
Amiloride	Iopanoic acid
Chlorthalidone	Meglumine iodipamide
Furosemide	*p*-Nitrophenylbutazone
Organomercurials	Orotic acid
Thiazides	Phenolsulfonphthalein
Triamterene	Phenylbutazone
Ethambutol	Phenylindandione
Ethanol	Probenecid
Laxative abuse (alkalosis)	Salicylates (>15 mg/dL, high dose)
Levodopa	Sodium diatrizoate
Methoxyflurane	Sulfaethylthiadiazole
Nicotinic acid	Sulfinpyrazone
Pyrazinamide	Tetracyclines (outdated ones)
Salicylates (5–10 mg/dL, low dose)	X-ray contrast agents
	Zoxazolamine
Hypouricemic Drugs	
	DECREASE URATE EXCRETION
INCREASE URATE EXCRETION	Allopurinol
Acetohexamide	Azauridine
Benzbromarone and benziodarone	Orotic acid
Calcium ipodate	Oxypurinol

mation in a few cases (33–35). The standard dose is 300 mg/day. It may cause side effects, such as a skin rash in less than 1% of patients (18). However, severe toxic side effects have been reported, primarily in patients with diminished renal function. The toxic reaction includes rash, pyrexia, deteriorating renal function, eosinophilia, leukocytosis, hepatitis, and possibly death (36). It has been postulated that the toxic reaction is secondary to high levels of oxypurinol, which is the major end product of allopurinol metabolism and is excreted primarily in the urine. Therefore, smaller than normal doses are advised in patients with renal failure. It has been recommended that allopurinol therapy should be initiated prior to urine alkalinization if the patient's initial urinary pH is not low and if the patient has clinical gout (37).

Urinary Alkalinization

Alkalinization of urine is the most important component of therapy. The ideal objective is to maintain a urinary pH of 6.4–6.7. Further alkalinization increases the risk of calcium phosphate (brushite) crystallization on the surface of existing uric acid stones (37). Sodium bicarbonate has been used as an alkalinizer, but it increases the risk of hypertension, congestive heart failure, and possibly the calculogenesis of calcium calculi (22,38). The mechanism of calculogenesis is that the increased sodium load causes increased urinary saturation of sodium urate, which induces crystallization of calcium oxalate (39). Calcium phosphate lithiasis is a result of increased urinary pH, which causes phosphate dissociation and raises calcium phosphate saturation (40).

Sodium citrate has the same systemic and alkalinizing effects as sodium bicarbonate. Alkali therapy generally reduces calciuria, but the sodium load increases calciuria and/or the increased saturation of monosodium urate coupled with offsetting effects on calciuria, but this is not the case with this drug, as it probably results in little net effect on the calculogenesis of calcium stones (38).

Potassium citrate also alkalinizes urine and reduces calciuria (22). The absence of a sodium load maintains urinary undersaturation with regard to monosodium urate. Urinary citrate excretion increases, which inhibits calcium phosphate and calcium oxalate crystallization. Potassium citrate may have a more prolonged effect than other potassium alkalis because of the delay in conversion of citrate to alkali (22). The usual daily dose of potassium citrate is 60 mEq/day in four divided doses; the dose may be tailored by monitoring urinary pH with pH-sensitive dipsticks and alteration of the dose accordingly (18).

Operative Intervention

Operative intervention is indicated in the case of severe renal colic or an obstructing stone. In the patient with renal colic, the site of the calculus will be determined with an intravenous urogram. In many cases the retrograde passage of a ureteric catheter or indwelling ureteral stent will relieve symptoms and allow an adequate time to effect peroral pharmacologic chemolysis. An obstructing calculus may be treated similarly or by insertion of a percutaneous nephrostomy tube. Tube drainage relieves symptoms, improves renal function, and provides time to treat the patient medically, with irrigation chemolysis, peroral chemolysis, or with extracorporeal shock wave lithotripsy (ESWL). Should irrigation be contemplated, the patient must receive antibiotic prophylaxis and a renal pelvic pressure of ≤30 cm of water be maintained. Agents used include sodium bicarbonate, tris(hydroxymethyl)aminomethane (THAM) and THAM-E (with added electrolytes) (41–44). THAM and THAM-E have been demonstrated to dissolve calculi faster than sodium bicarbonate in vitro, but the higher pH has the potential disadvantage of inducing calcium phosphate crystallization (43). ESWL is also effective. Because of the radiolucent nature of uric acid stones, contrast introduction via ureteral catheters is necessary to visualize the calculi using lithotriptors with fluoroscopic localization systems. In vitro studies have shown that uric acid calculi, together with calcium oxalate dihydrate calculi, are in fact the easiest renal calculi to fragment with shock waves (45).

CYSTINE CALCULI

Cystinuria is a cellular disorder of amino acid transport affecting the brush border of the epithelial cells of the proximal renal tubules and the gastrointestinal tract. It is inherited as an autosomal recessive trait, resulting in defective transport of cystine, lysine, arginine, and ornithine. The mutant gene has not yet been mapped to a specific chromosomal locus. Cystinuria's sole clinical manifestation is in the development of urolithiasis. Lysine, arginine, and ornithine are freely soluble in urine and do not cause calculi or precipitate on the cystine nidus (46).

History

1810 Wollaston analyzed two bladder stones, which he called "cystic oxide" (47).

1824 Stromeyer noted hexagonal platelike crystals in the urine of patients with cystinuria (48).

1833 Berzelius renamed stone composition "cystine" (49).

1902 Friedman defined the chemical structure of cystine (50).

Pathophysiology

In 1908, Garrod described cystinuria as an inborn error of metabolism and it was considered as such for the next 40 years (51). In 1947, Yeh et al. demonstrated lysinuria and argininuria in patients with cystinuria (52). Stein demonstrated associated ornithinuria 4 years later (53). Dent et al. showed that cystine and the dibasic amino acids had structural similarities. They also showed that their plasma levels were normal or low and postulated that a single cellular transport mechanism located in the membrane of the renal tubule, which was shared by all these amino acids, was defective or absent in cystinuria (54,55). Two transport mechanisms for cystine have been demonstrated in the rat (56,57). One has a high affinity for cystine, which is shared with the dibasic amino acids, and the other has a low affinity for cystine, which is unshared.

In cystinuric patients cystine clearance in the kidney may exceed creatinine clearance, which is interpreted as evidence of a concurrent renal tubular secretion of cystine (58). Cystinurics also have a defect in the single absorption transport mechanism of cystine and dibasic amino acids from the intestine which has been confirmed by in vitro studies on jejunal biopsies (59). In normal individuals, the upper limits for cystine excretion in urine is about 18 mg/g creatinine or less than 100 mg/day (60).

Harris et al. classified cystinurics into heterozygotes, incompletely recessive heterozygotes, and homozygotes (61). Heterozygotes are completely recessive and have normal amino acid excretion. Incompletely recessive heterozygotes excrete between 150 and 300 mg of cystine per 24 h but usually do not form calculi. Homozygotes excrete greater than 400 mg of cystine per day and are at high risk of stone formation. More than 50% of asymptomatic homozygotes will develop renal calculi (62). More recently, both homozygotes and heterozygotes have been further subclassified into types I, II, and III on the basis of their intestinal mucosal transport patterns, but this has limited clinical application (46,63). Infants under 6 months of age have immature tubular function, which may result in excess cystine excretion in heterozygotes, so that they may be incorrectly classified as homozygotes and counseled and treated accordingly (64).

Presentation

The overall prevalence is about 1 in 7000 (65). In England it is 1 in 2000, in Australia 1 in 4000, in the United

States 1 in 15,000, and in Sweden 1 in 100,000. The disease occurs equally in both sexes, although males are more severely affected and have a higher mortality rate. This has been postulated to be related to their greater likelihood of developing urethral obstruction (1). The disease is predominant in whites, but there are occasional reports in blacks and Asians (66,67).

Cystine calculi account for 1% of all uroliths (68). Radiographically, they have a homogeneous or "ground-glass," faintly opaque appearance. The disulfide bond of cystine renders stones radiopaque, although less dense than calcium stones. Macroscopically, the stones are yellow-brown in color. As with all renal calculi, the most common presentation is with renal colic. The calculi tend to be multiple or staghorns. Stone recurrence is common. The peak of clinical expression is in the second and third decades, although cases may present in the first year of life to the ninth decade (69).

Cystinuria has been associated with hyperuricemia, hemophilia, retinitis pigmentosa, muscular dystrophy, muscular hypotonia, hereditary pancreatitis, and mental retardation (69). However, in vitro studies have demonstrated different transport systems in the brain compared to the kidney and the intestine, which make it unlikely that cystinuric patients are at risk because of transport abnormalities in the central nervous system (41). Cystinuria may also occur as an isolated aminoaciduria with hypocalcemic tetany.

The relationship of cystine solubility to urinary pH was clearly demonstrated by Dent and Senior (Fig. 6) (80). Cystine has a maximum insolubility at pH 3.8. The change in solubility is slight with pH increases up to 7.0, but at a pH of 7.5 solubility has increased 50% and at a pH of 9 has increased 1400%.

Diagnosis

The diagnosis should be entertained in all patients with renal calculi, but especially in those with recurrent calculi. Microscopic examination of urinary sediment, preferably the first morning specimen, often shows typical hexagonal cystine crystals, which are diagnostic. However, although their presence is pathognomonic of the condition, they may only be present in 26% of patients (70).

The cyanide–nitroprusside colorimetric test is the most widely applied chemical screening procedure. The lower limit of sensitivity of the reaction is 75–125 mg/g creatinine, which will result in detection of all homozygotes (71). False positive reactions may occur due to sulfur-containing drugs, ampicillin, or N-acetylcysteine and has been reported in Fanconi's syndrome (72). The other most commonly used screening and detection techniques in use are thin-layer amino acid chromatography, colorimetric estimations of cystine and lysine, and ion-exchange amino acid chromatography. Of these four techniques, thin-layer chromatography has been re-

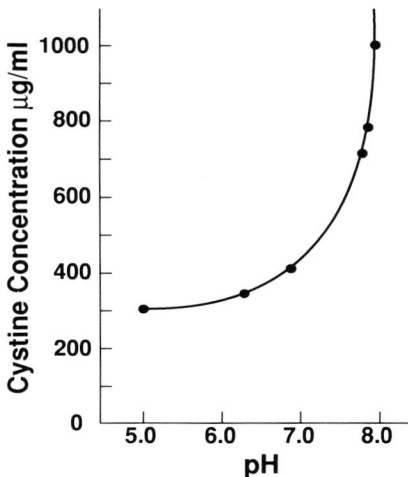

FIG. 6. Solubility of cystine in relation to urinary pH. (From Ref. 80; reproduced with permission from Churchill Livingstone, Edinburgh.)

ported to be the most sensitive and colorimetric estimations the least sensitive (63).

Treatment

The treatment of cystinuria is designed to reduce cystine excretion and increase its solubility in urine. Medical therapy may be classified as:

1. Dietary restriction aimed at reducing cystine production and excretion.
2. Efforts to increase cystine solubility.
3. Efforts to convert cystine to a more soluble compound.

Surgical therapy may be classified as:

1. Attempts to dissolve cystine calculi by irrigation.
2. Removal of calculi by open surgery, percutaneous endoscopy, or shock wave lithotripsy.
3. Renal transplantation to replace kidneys destroyed by cystinuria.

Dietary Therapy

Cystine production arises from the essential amino acid methionine, which is abundant in animal proteins such as milk, eggs, cheese, and fish. Restriction of these may lower cystinuria and decrease urinary acidity (72). However, to be effective, dietary methionine must be reduced to 1 g/day, which corresponds to 0.5 mg of animal protein per kilogram per day (73). The effectiveness of methionine restriction has, however, not been reported to reduce cystinuria uniformly (62,74,75). Vegetarian diets are generally considered unpalatable and protein restriction is undesirable in the growing child. In the event of restriction of animal protein, protein supplements may be given in the form of peanut butter.

In renal and intestinal brush border membranes, basic amino acid transport is partially Na^+ dependent (76). In the kidney, cystine transport is completely dependent on sodium, oxygen, and pH (77). Although the exact mechanism is unknown, the excretion of cystine and related dibasic amino acids is a function of sodium intake down to levels of about 50 mmol/day (3 g of salt) (78). Although long-term studies are lacking, restriction of dietary sodium appears to be a simple, yet effective new means of reducing cystinuria. In patients with a high sodium intake (300 mmol/day) glutamine has an anticystinuric effect via an unknown mechanism that ceases at a sodium intake of 150 mmol/day (79).

Alteration of Cystine Solubility

The solubility of cystine in urine is roughly 250–300 mg/L. Supersaturation of urine with cystine can thus be prevented by a urine output of 2 ml/min (62). To achieve this, an intake of 600 ml every 4 h throughout the day and night is required. An adequate diuresis is demonstrated by maintaining the urinary specific gravity at 1.010 or less (72). This regimen, although effective, is generally poorly tolerated by patients, although Dent et al. demonstrated that patients started on this treatment at the time of initial presentation generally had better compliance than those who initially began alternative treatments. Adherence to a constant diuresis has been shown to result in stone dissolution in addition to the prevention of new stone formation (62).

Urine alkalinization to a pH of about 7.5 is recommended with sodium bicarbonate (13.5–22.7 g/day), sodium citrate, or potassium citrate (80–135 ml/day) in equally divided daily doses. Urinary pH must be monitored and maintained below 8 to avoid precipitation of calcium salts (81). Patient tolerance to large doses of alkali may be limited by abdominal pain, bloating, or diarrhea. Alkalinization has also been reported using acetazolamide (Diamox). This inhibits carbonic anhydrase, which normally accelerates urine acidification. Alkaline urine results because bicarbonate ion excretion is increased. The recommended dosage is 250 mg of acetazolamide and 1 g of sodium bicarbonate three times per day (82).

Cystine Conversion to a More Soluble Compound

In the event of continuing crystalluria after treatment with hydration and alkalinization, the use of a thiol may be indicated to convert cystine to a more soluble compound. In 1954, Tabachnick et al. noted that penicillamine (β,β-dimethylcysteine), one of the degradation products of penicillin, reacted with cystine to form a mixed disulfide, penicillamine cysteine (83). The mechanisms are facilitated by an alkaline medium and are outlined on Fig. 7. Penicillamine can also undergo a disulfide interchange to form a mixed disulfide. Penicil-

lamine cysteine is 50 times more soluble than cystine (84). Its clinical use in 1963 demonstrated a reduction in cystinuria and in stone size (85). Cystinuria can usually be reduced to 200 mg/g creatinine by 1–2 g of D-penicillamine hydrochloride in four divided doses. Only the D isomer should be used clinically, as the L isomer is toxic and has an antipyridoxine (vitamin B_6) effect (86). Twenty-five milligrams of vitamin B_6 twice daily is recommended as supplementation for patients taking D-penicillamine. D-Penicillamine can safely be prescribed in childhood and in doses up to 1 g/day in pregnancy (87,88). Doses of 2 g/day in pregnancy may cause connective tissue dysplasia in the fetus (89). Side effects of D-penicillamine therapy may occur in up to 84% of patients and require cessation of therapy in up to 69% (90). Reported side effects are listed in Table 3. Side effects should initially be treated by dose reduction or cessation in conjunction with steroids and antihistamines. In many cases patients can then be desensitized by restarting treatment at low dosage with slowly increasing increments until the full dose is reached. N-Acetyl-D-penicillamine, a related compound, is also effective in disulfide formation and is reported to have fewer side effects (91).

α-Mercaptopropianylglycine (α-MPG) is a mercaptan with a 30% higher dissolution rate for cystine compared to penicillamine in vitro (92). About a quarter of the orally taken dose of α-MPG appears in the urine to participate in a thiol–disulfide exchange with cystine as penicillamine does (93). Side effects are listed in Table 3. These are less common than with D-penicillamine (75% versus 84%) and are also less likely to result in cessation of therapy (90). α-MPG has no teratogenic effect and recommended dosage is 100–1000 mg/day (94). The effectiveness of D-penicillamine or α-MPG therapy should be monitored regularly with an effective quantitative screen such as the cyanide-nitroprusside test.

Captopril is an antihypertensive agent that has been used with good effect in two patients for 2 and 6 months, respectively (277). The mechanism of action is partly related to the formation of captopril–cysteine disulfide, which is 200 times more soluble than cystine. Urinary cystine excretion was decreased by 70 and 93% in the two patients studied to date. Chlordiazepoxide has also been found to decrease cystine crystalluria, but as yet the mechanism is unknown (95).

Irrigant Dissolution

The first report of irrigant dissolution of a renal cystine calculus was by Crowell in 1924. He successfully dissolved a cystine calculus by oral alkalinization with sodium bicarbonate in conjunction with renal pelvic irrigation of mercurochrome and saline through a ureteric catheter. Mercurochrome is alkaline as well as being an antiseptic (96).

Dissolution of cystine calculi by irrigation through a percutaneous nephrostomy tube was initially described

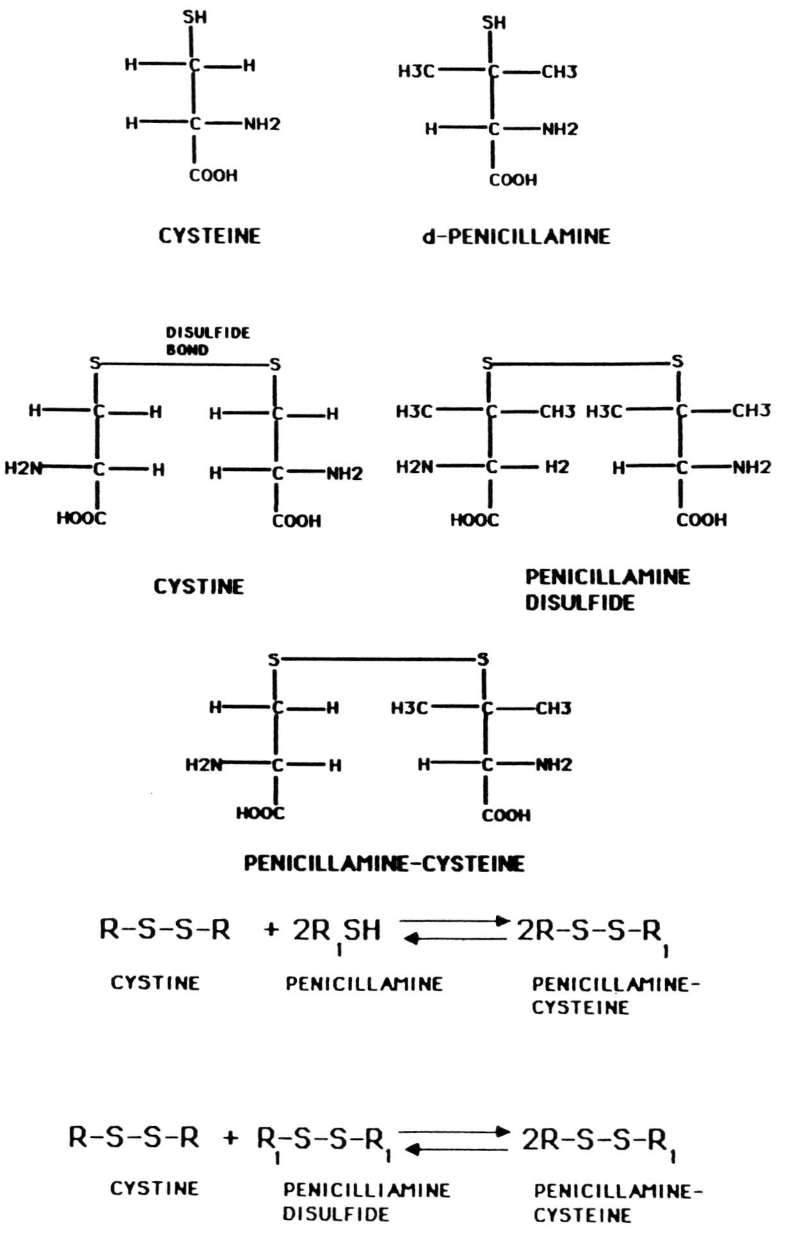

FIG. 7. Mechanism of action of penicillamine.

by Smith et al. in 1979 (97). The two most commonly used irrigant solutions are N-acetylcysteine (Mucomyst) and tromethamine-E (THAM-E), but sodium bicarbonate and D-penicillamine have also been used (98). Like penicillamine, *N-acetylcysteine* forms soluble disulfide complexes with cystine when applied as an alkaline solution together with sodium hydroxide (pH 9.0). Acetylcysteine in its natural state, however, has a pH of 2.0 (99). A 2% solution is now generally recommended for use. Although irrigation in rats causes an acute inflammatory response at 3 days, this is healed almost completely at 4 weeks (100). THAM-E is an organic amine buffer of pH 10.2. Its use is based on the increased solubility of cystine in a highly alkaline medium. Stone dissolu-

tion has been reported after periods of irrigation of 5 to 37 days (72). To date, comparative in vitro dissolution studies have shown that N-acetylcysteine is more effective than THAM-E (99,100).

Lithotomy, PCNL, and ESWL

Prior to the present era of percutaneous nephrolithotomy (PCNL) and extracorporeal shock wave lithotripsy (ESWL) treatment for renal calculi, open surgical lithotomy was required for obstructing calculi and those causing intractable pain. The recently introduced term of *stone fragility* has confirmed the relative resistance of cystine stones to fragmentation, which has made their treatment with ESWL inadvisable (45). Together with

TABLE 3. *Side effects of D-penicillamine and α-MPG*

Side effects	
Gastrointestinal:	Nausea, emesis, diarrhea, anorexia, abdominal pain, flatus
Taste and smell:	Impairment
Dermatological:	Rash, pruritis, urticaria, pemphigus, pharyngitis, oral ulcers, elastosis perforans serpiginosa
Hypersensitivity:	Laryngeal edema, dyspnea, fever, arthralgia, myalgia, lymphadenopathy
Hematological:	Increased bleeding, anemia, leukopenia, eosinophilia
Hepatic:	Abnormal liver function tests
Renal:	Proteinuria, nephrosis, foul-smelling urine
Others:	Vaginitis, impotence, headache, chest pain, cough

calcium oxalate monohydrate calculi, cystine calculi have been shown to be the most difficult to fragment with shock waves. PCNL is the preferable form of surgical intervention, which allows direct access to the calculi, which may be fragmented using electrohydraulic or ultrasonic probes (101). In many cases ultrasound is unable to erode the calculi and may in fact result in "plugging" of the probe with minute fragments. PCNL debulking of large calculi also allows ready access to the renal collecting system to facilitate irrigant chemolysis of small residual stones.

Transplantation

Occasionally, cystinuria may result in chronic renal failure. As the hyperexcretion transport defect is in the renal tubules, a donor kidney from a noncystinuric patient should not result in calculus formation. To date, normal amino acid excretion has been reported over 3 years after such a case was treated by renal transplantation (102).

STRUVITE CALCULI

Archaeological studies have shown that urolithiasis has affected humans for thousands of years. Excavations at El Amrah, Egypt, by G. Elliot Smith in 1901 discovered one case of vesical calculi and two cases of renal calculi which dated to 4800 B.C. (103). In 1905, Shattock reported that an Egyptian renal calculus dated 4200 B.C. was composed of calcium carbonate, calcium phosphate, and calcium oxalate (104). A struvite and calcium oxalate renal calculus has been found in a late bronze age burial mound in Hungary (105). In 387 B.C. Hippocrates documented renal calculi associated with putrefaction and loin abscess (107). In 1817, Marcet noted the association of putrefaction, ammoniacal urine, alkalinity, and the production of phosphate calculi (107).

In 1901, Brown proposed the theory that the splitting of urea by bacteria resulted in ammoniacal urine, alkalinity, and stone formation (111). Urine cultures in his six patients revealed *Proteus vulgaris* and staphylococci. *P. vulgaris* was also grown from the center of one calculus. In all cases stone analysis showed "phosphates and carbonates of calcium and magnesium." Hagar and Ma-

gath suggested in 1925 that a bacterial protein called urease was responsible for the hydrolysis of urea (112). In the following year Sumner reported that he had isolated a new protein from the jack bean, *Canavalia ensiformis* (113). This enzyme (urease) hydrolyzed urea and was in the form of colorless octahedra crystals. He was later awarded the Nobel prize for this work in isolating the first known enzyme. In the early part of the nineteenth century, the mineral $MgNH_4PO_4 \cdot 6H_2O$ was identified in bat guano by Ulex, a Swedish geologist. He named it "struvite" in honor of his mentor, Baron H. C. G. von Struve, a Russian diplomat and naturalist (1772–1851) (106). Struvite calculi are composed of magnesium ammonium phosphate ($MgNH_4PO_4 \cdot 6H_2O$) and carbonate apatite [$Ca_{10}(PO_4)_6 \cdot CO_3$]. Throughout the world literature, struvite calculi have also been referred to as "infection," "infection-induced," "urease," "phosphatic," and "triple-phosphate" stones. The term *triple-phosphate* arises from early chemical analyses of stones wherein three cations (Ca^{2+}, Mg^{2+}, and NH_4^+) were found in association with one anion (PO_4^{3-}) (107). Although progress has been made in understanding the underlying pathogenesis of these stones, treatment is frustrating because of persistent urinary tract infections and high stone recurrence rates.

Stoichiometry

Crystallization occurs when the solubility products of the component solutes are exceeded. Human urine is replete with calcium, phosphate, magnesium, and urea. Only in the presence of accelerated ureolysis are urine alkalinity and the concentrations of ammonia, bicarbonate, and carbonate sufficient for crystallization of struvite and carbonate apatite. Struvite will not crystallize if the urine pH is less than 7.19 or if urine alkalinity is not also associated with ammoniuria (108,109). Urease-producing bacteria cause hydrolysis of urea:

$$NH_2-CO-NH_2 + H_2O \xrightarrow{urease} 2NH_3 + CO_2$$

Further hydrolysis converts ammonia to ammonium:

$$NH_3 + H_2O \rightleftharpoons NH_4^+ + OH^-$$

The carbonate found in carbonate apatite crystals arises from further hydrolysis:

$$CO_2 + H_2O \rightleftharpoons H_2CO_3 \rightleftharpoons H^+ + HCO_3^- \rightleftharpoons 2H^+ + CO_3^{2-}$$

$$pK(NH_3) = 9.03 \qquad pK(HCO_3^-) = 6.33$$

$$pK(CO_3^{2-}) = 10.1$$

The biochemical changes occurring during a 2-h period following the addition of urease to normal human urine are shown in Fig. 8 (110). The factor determining the relative proportions of struvite and carbonate apatite in infection stones is uncertain, but it may be due to differing solute concentrations and differing rates of crystallization for either salt with varying urinary pH. The cause-and-effect relationship between urea-splitting bacteria and infection stones is now well recognized.

Bacteriology

Urinary infection with urease-synthesizing organisms is an essential prerequisite for infection stone formation. The most widely used method of identifying urease-producing bacteria was described by Christensen in 1946 (114). This technique identifies color changes in urea agar which are caused by the pH change as urea is hydrolyzed. Recently, the *spot test* has been developed for a more rapid detection of bacterial urease activity (115). Most commonly encountered urease-producing bacteria are gram-negative organisms, as shown in Table 4. Silverman and Stamey reported that 87% of their 46 infection-induced calculi were caused by *Proteus mirabilis* infections (116). This varies considerably from reports in the first half of this century when staphylococcal species were the commonest causative organisms (117). Recently, ureaplasma urealyticum has been cited as a causative organism, the detection of which requires specialized culturing techniques (118). Its calculogenic activity has also been demonstrated in vitro (119).

Glycosaminoglycans (GAGs) are highly charged macromolecules that are present in normal urine (see Chapter 35). Normal bladder mucosa is covered by a layer of GAGs which acts as a defense against bacterial adherence and infection (120). Using the rabbit model, Parsons et al. showed that ammonium interfered with the GAGs layer and thus increased the ability of bacteria to adhere to the bladder mucosal surface. The mecha-

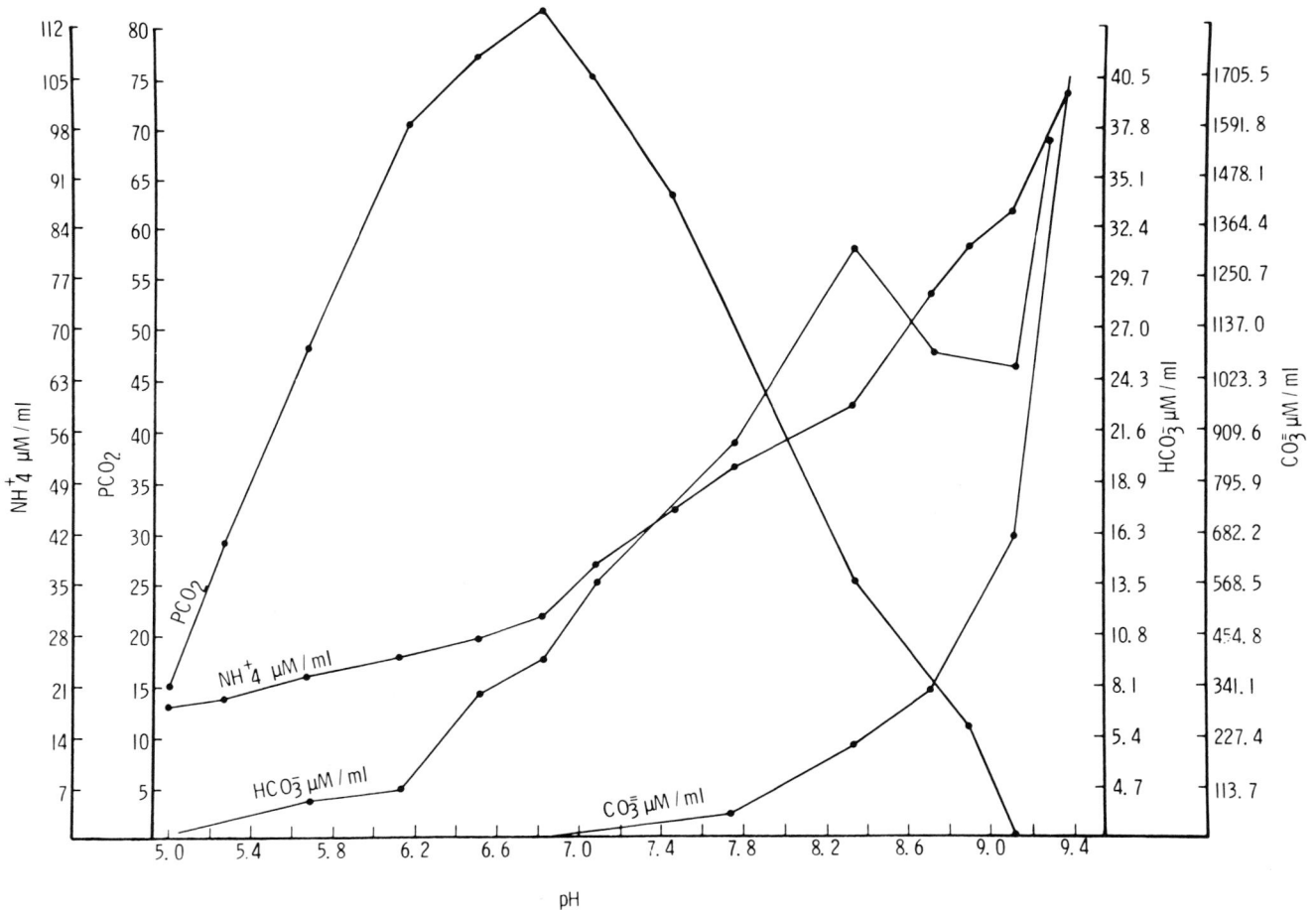

FIG. 8. Biochemical changes occurring during a 2-h period following the addition of urease to normal human urine (Reproduced with permission from Ref. 110.)

TABLE 4. *Organisms that may produce urease*

Organisms	Usually (>90% of isolates)	Occasionally (5–30% of isolates)
BACTERIA		
Gram-negative	*Proteus rettgeri*	*Klebsiella pneumoniae*
	P. vulgaris	*K. oxytoca*
	P. mirabilis	*Serratia marcescens*
	P. morganii	*Haemophilus parainfluenzae*
	Providencia stuartii	*Bordetella bronchiseptica*
	H. influenzae	*Aeromonas hydrophila*
	B. pertussis	*Pseudomonas aeruginosa*
	Bacterioides corrodens	*Pasteurella* spp.
	Yersinia enterocolitica	
	Brucella spp.	
	Flavobacterium spp.	
Gram-positive	*Staphylococcus aureus*	*S. epidermidis*
	Micrococcus varions	*Bacillus* spp.
	Corynebacterium ulcerans	*C. murium*
	C. renale	*C. equi*
	C. ovis	*Peptococcus asaccharolyticus*
	C. hofmanii	*Clostridium tetani*
		Mycobacterium rhodochrous group
MYCOPLASMA	*T-strain mycoplasma*	
	Ureaplasma urealyticum	
YEASTS	*Cryptococcus*	
	Rhodotorula	
	Sporobolmyces	
	Candida humicola	
	Trichosporon cutaneum	

nism of action is thought to be that ammonium combines with the sulfate group of the GAGs and thus impairs its hydrophilic activity (121). Recently, it has been shown that the removal of the GAGs layer from rat bladders increases the adherence of struvite and calcium phosphate crystals five to six times compared to that of intact rat bladders (122).

These studies seem to confirm Griffith's theory of intrarenal struvite calculogenesis (Fig. 9) (107). He proposed that the end products of ureolysis in urinary tract infections damaged the urothelial GAGs layer and facilitated bacterial adherence with resultant encrustation. However, the exact role of matrix in the pathogenesis of infection stones is unclear. Boyce et al. showed that the bulk of matrix was made up by a low-molecular-weight mucoprotein which they called matrix substance A (123). Matrix stones are characterized by the presence of poorly mineralized, gelatinous, organic stone material in kidneys with advanced parenchymal damage. Nickel et al. have studied the ultrastructure of infection stones and have demonstrated bacteria growing as microcolonies within an organic matrix (124). The organic matrix or glycocalyx may result from capsules that are inherent in the bacterial cell walls. Some of the normally soluble urinary macromolecules (polysaccharides and microproteins) may also be "salted out" in microenvironments adjacent to the organisms wherein ureolysis increases osmolality. Bacterial organic material (glycocalyx) has also been described in relation to infected pros-

theses, such as cardiac pacemakers, peritoneal dialysis catheters, and hip joints. This insoluble organic matrix action may protect bacteria from destruction by antimicrobials.

Thus a source of some of the matrix may be the bacteria themselves. Khan et al. have also demonstrated that urinary macromolecules are absorbed onto crystal surfaces, which may explain a further passive mechanism of matrix formation (125).

Clinical Manifestations

Struvite calculi account for between 7 and 31% of all renal tract calculi in the Western world (126). Although calcium oxalate calculi have been reported to be the commonest type in the United States, Sarmina et al. have recently reported that struvite–carbonate apatite calculi were the most common type in black patients in Ohio (127).

Females are more commonly affected than males, in a ratio of 2:1, presumably because of their increased susceptibility to urinary tract infections (128). Comarr et al. have reported that 8% of spinal cord injury patients will develop infection stones (129). The incidence is highest in complete and upper motor neuron lesions (130). Infection stones are prone to occur in patients with neurogenic bladders, urinary diversions, indwelling Foley catheters, and lower-tract voiding dysfunction with abnormal cystometry (131). Correcting the cystometric ab-

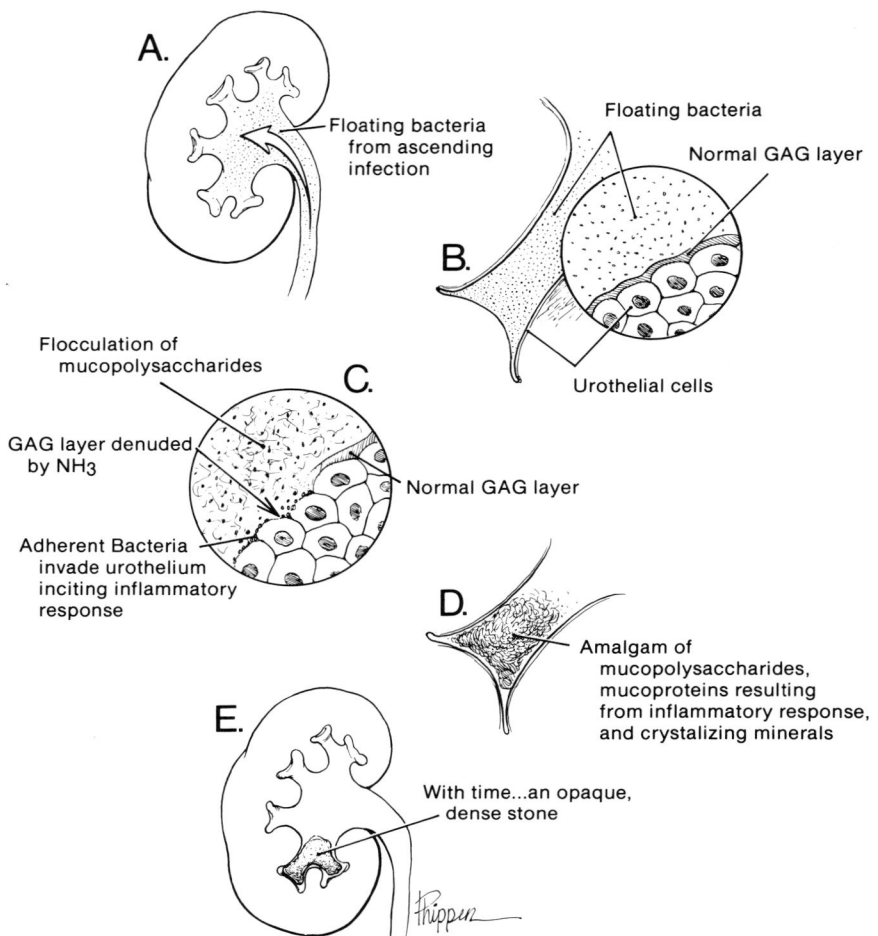

FIG. 9. Glycosaminoglycans and struvite calculogenesis. **A:** Renal infection originates from bacteriuria introduced into the lower urinary tract and ascending to the kidney. **B:** A glycosaminoglycan (GAG) layer normally protects urothelium from bacterial adherence. **C:** End products of urealysis damage urothelial GAG layer and thereby facilitate (1) bacterial adherence to cells and (2) tissue invasion by bacteria. Urealysis-induced hyperosmolality probably contributes to flocculation of organic compounds. Tissue inflammation brought on by local irritation (mostly ammonia) and bacterial invasion increased the quantity of these organic compounds. **D:** Matrix concretions composed of poorly soluble organic compounds, struvite and carbonate apatite crystals, inflammatory cells, and bacteria form rapidly into immature stone. **E:** With time, the immature stone becomes progressively mineralized due to continued urealysis by bacteria trapped within the concretion, and the concretion matures into a dense, hard stone. (From Ref. 107; reproduced with permission from S. Karger AG, Basel.)

normalities should eliminate the risk of calculus formation. The correlation between vesicoureteral reflux and the formation of staghorn calculi remains controversial (132,133).

The clinical presentation is variable but may include pyrexia, loin pain, dysuria, frequency, and hematuria. Acute pyelonephritis and hydronephrosis may progress to form acute pyonephrosis and renal or perirenal abscesses. Occasionally, xanthogranulomatous pyelonephritis may occur, which is characterized by replacement of renal parenchyma with granulomatous tissue containing macrophages. Up to 25% of cases may be completely asymptomatic and detected during investigations for unrelated problems (134). Radiographically, infection stones are usually branched and may grow rapidly to form a cast of the renal collecting system, the so-called staghorn calculus. Approximately 75% of staghorn calculi are composed of struvite–carbonate apatite–matrix, with the remaining 25% being composed of calcium oxalate, calcium phosphate, or cystine. Most infection stones are radiopaque, but poorly mineralized matrix stones are faintly radiopaque or radiolucent. Most infection stones are renal in site but occasionally

may be found in the bladder, especially in patients with long-term indwelling catheters. Ureteric calculi composed of struvite–carbonate apatite are rare.

In patients with dual pathology such as renal calculi and chronic prostatitis, it may be helpful to try to localize the site of infection accurately by taking consecutive selective ureteral urine samples (135). In the era of open surgical therapy, culture of pelvic urine aspirate and stone washings both before and after crushing were useful to get bacterial documentation to aid treatment (136).

Treatment

Nonoperative management of staghorn calculi was reported in 1976 to result in a 28% mortality during 20 years of follow-up with all survivors having persistent pain and urinary tract infections (137). Vargas and associates later confirmed the rarity of the "silent staghorn calculus" with only 1 (4.5%) of 22 staghorns managed nonsurgically remaining asymptomatic and 17 (77%) resulting in significant complications, 2 of which resulted in death after a follow-up period of 1–6 years (138). Treatment rests with surgical ablation of all stone material, followed by the various medical options to eliminate or retard urinary infection.

Open Surgical Procedures

Surgical removal has been the cornerstone of treatment for infection stones. The first successful nephrectomy for stone disease was performed by Gustav Simon in 1871 (106). Attempted stone removal from pyonephritic kidneys in 1872 and 1874 both resulted in patient deaths. In 1879, Heinecke performed the first successful pyelolithotomy, which was followed in the following year by a successful nephrolithotomy performed by Morris (107,139). The open operative alternatives include nephrectomy, partial nephrectomy, pyelolithotomy, extended pyelolithotomy (Gil-Vernet) (140), dismembered pyelolithotomy (Ohshima et al.) (141), anatrophic nephrolithotomy (Smith and Boyce) (142), radial nephrolithotomy (Wickham et al.) (143), and bench surgery with autotransplantation (Turini et al.) (144). These techniques may be used in conjunction with operative nephroscopy, coagulum pyelolithotomy, and hypothermia, and either regional or systemic inosine to minimize ischemic renal damage. In Great Britain in 1976, intravenous, intraarterial, or intraperitoneal administration of inosine was shown to preserve renal function for up to 1 h of warm ischemia, enabling safer transparenchymal surgery (145). Inosine use has not been approved by the U.S. Food and Drug Administration. Controversy still exists as to which procedures cause the least parenchymal damage. Fitzpatrick et al. studied renal function and morphology in dogs 48 h after surgery using creatinine, inulin, and PAH clearance (146). They found no functional or parenchymal loss after the extended sinus approach (Gil-Vernet), 30% functional loss and significant parenchymal loss with the anatrophic intersegmental approach, and 50% functional loss with considerable parenchymal loss after bivalving the kidney. The following year Stage and Lewis reported no difference in postoperative functional loss between pyelolithotomy and anatrophic nephrolithotomy in patients who had differential quantitative renal scans using [^{99}Tc]diethylene triaminepentaacetic acid (DTPA) or [^{131}I]hippuran (147). All procedures may im-

prove renal function by relieving intrarenal obstruction. The overall residual stone rate after open surgery is approximately 15%, with a 30% stone recurrence rate over 6 years and a 40% risk of recurrent urinary tract infection (148).

Percutaneous Nephrolithotomy Monotherapy

Percutaneous nephrostolithotomy (PCNL) was described in 1976 by Fernstrom and Johannson (149). Initially, only small calculi were removed percutaneously, but with the aid of electrohydraulic and ultrasonic lithotripsy, the procedure has been extended to include staghorn calculi (150,151). PCNL has been used to treat staghorn calculi with stone-free results in 60–90% of kidneys (Table 5). Adams et al. defined staghorns as calculi conforming to the branched configuration of two or more calices but did not refer to stone burden (152). With an average hospitalization time of 18 days, they rendered 7 of 11 kidneys (63%) stone-free with PCNL monotherapy. Kerlan et al. reported 90% (18 of 20 kidneys) stone-free with calculi which "filled the caliceal collecting structures and renal pelvis" (150).

Using a staghorn definition as a branched calculus > 5 cm in greatest diameter, Young et al. rendered 68% of their 25 kidneys stone-free (153). Sixteen of these calculi were <8 cm and 9 were ≥8 cm in longest dimension. Snyder and Smith, using a more standard staghorn definition of a calculus that filled the renal pelvis and at least two major calices, rendered 64 of 75 kidneys (85%) stone-free with PCNL and had an average hospitalization time of 13.3 days (154). This series was updated more recently by Lee et al. and reported a similar stone-free rate (85%) at time of discharge on 124 kidneys treated (155). After 6 months of follow-up, spontaneous passage of residual calculi < 5 mm increased the stone-free rate to 92%.

Eisenberger et al. reported their updated series on 151 partial or complete staghorn calculi in 1987 (156). All calculi filled the renal pelvis and at least two branched calices, and the mean follow-up was 18 months. The stone-free rate at the time of discharge was 69% on 42 kidneys treated with PCNL monotherapy, and this increased to 77% on follow-up with a 4% stone recurrence rate. However, long-term results were based on only 89 kidneys (59%) of their total series with adequate follow-

TABLE 5. *Staghorn calculi treated with percutaneous nephrolithotomy monotherapy*

Author	Kidneys	Treatments per kidney	Stone-free at 3 months (%)
Adams et al. (152)	11	2.2	63
Kerlan et al. (150)	20	1.8	90
Young et al. (153)	25	2.9	68
Snyder and Smith (154)	75	1.24	85
Lee et al. (155)	124	1.3	85
Eisenberger et al. (156)	42	1.3	69
Gleeson et al. (157)	30	1.43	60

up. Our own experience has resulted in 18 out of 30 kidneys (60%) being stone-free 3 months postoperatively (157).

Experimental studies in dogs have shown PCNL does not cause any loss of renal function, but these studies referred to a single percutaneous tract rather than multiple tracts as are commonly required for removal of staghorn calculi (158). Comparative studies of PCNL and anatrophic nephrolithotomy show PCNL to be less expensive, and to result in a smaller need for blood transfusion, a shorter hospital stay, and a more rapid return to work (154,159,160).

Extracorporeal Shock Wave Lithotripsy Monotherapy

Extracorporeal shock-wave lithotripsy (ESWL) was introduced clinically in 1980 (161). Its use initially was for small pelvic calculi, but considerable success has resulted in its application to calculi in all parts of the collecting system (162–164). ESWL monotherapy has generally resulted in stone-free results ranging from 30 to 66% (Table 6). Eisenberger et al. treated 26 partial and 5 complete staghorns with ESWL monotherapy (156). While only 6 (19%) were stone-free at the time of discharge, 8 of 16 kidneys (50%) followed for 18 months became stone-free. Rocco et al. reported that 53 of 84 kidneys (63%) were rendered stone-free with the added use of in situ irrigation in 20 cases (165).

A large series of 140 partial staghorns (mean burden = 30 ± 10 mm) and 34 complete staghorns (mean burden = 62 ± 16 mm) treated by Wirth and Frohmuller had a 54% stone-free rate at 3 months which increased to 61% at 1 year (166). However, the results were based on a follow-up rate of 65%. Although the total number of procedures per kidney was not reported, 29% of partial staghorns and 48% of complete staghorns required more than one treatment.

Harada et al. rendered 9 of 19 complete staghorn calculi (45%) and 15 of 28 partial staghorns (54%) stone-free, resulting in an overall stone-free rate of 51% (167).

Pode et al. have recently reported a 44% stone-free rate with 41 complete staghorn calculi (168). Complete staghorns were defined as filling the renal pelvis and at least two calices.

As part of a multicenter prospective randomized study comparing ESWL monotherapy to PCNL-ESWL combination therapy, Sohn et al. have reported that 20 of 33 patients were treated with ESWL monotherapy and only 6 of these (30%) have become stone-free (169). This compares with 7 of 13 staghorns (54%) rendered stone-free in the combination PCNL-ESWL group.

In our department, 12 of 18 kidneys (66%) have been rendered stone-free with a mean number of treatments of 1.4 per kidney (157). Our criteria for this treatment selection included calculi, which were less radiopaque than the adjacent ribs and absence of obstruction or calycectasis on the preoperative intravenous urogram.

PCNL/ESWL Combination Treatment

The large stone burden of staghorn calculi has resulted in many reports advocating combination PCNL and ESWL, with ESWL being used to treat residual stones after primary removal with PCNL (156,170,171). Combination PCNL-ESWL has reportedly resulted in stone-free rates between 23 and 92% (Table 7). Although only 23% of 78 staghorns treated with combination PCNL-ESWL by Eisenberger et al. were stone-free at the time of discharge, this increased to 60% after 18 months (156).

Kahnoski et al. treated 52 staghorn calculi of which 36 had combination PCNL-ESWL therapy (172). Their stone-free outcome for combination therapy was 85% with a mean hospital stay of 12.6 days. A recent update on this series from Indianapolis has reported that 92% of kidneys with partial staghorns and 91% with complete staghorns become stone-free following three-stage procedures consisting of (a) PCNL, (b) ESWL, and (c) flexible PCNL with lavage of residual debris (173).

A particularly low stone-free rate with struvite staghorns from the Mayo Clinic was attributed to a less aggressive effort at initial PCNL; these authors now favor an aggressive PCNL approach to staghorns (174). The

TABLE 6. *Staghorn calculi treated with extracorporeal shock wave lithotripsy monotherapy*

Author	Kidneys	Stone-free at 3 months (%)
Eisenberger et al. (156)	31	50[a]
Rocco et al. (165)	84	63[b]
Wirth and Frohmuller (166)	174	54
Harada et al. (167)	47	51
Sohn et al. (169)	20	30
Pode et al. (168)	41	44
Gleeson et al. (157)	18	66

[a] Stone-free rate after 18 months.
[b] Rocco EXL catheter used in 20 cases.

TABLE 7. *Staghorn calculi treated with combination percutaneous nephrolithotomy and extracorporeal shock wave lithotripsy*

Author	Kidneys	Stone-free at 3 months (%)
Eisenberger et al. (156)	78	60
Kahnoski et al. (172)	36	85[a]
Segura et al. (174)	16	23[b]
Lingeman (173)	313	91–92
Schulze et al. (171)	87[c]	58
Gleeson et al. (157)	22	55

[a] Includes cases treated with ESWL and PCNL monotherapy.
[b] 6 months follow-up.
[c] 77 calculi were partial or complete staghorns.

"sandwich" technique of multiple procedures in a relatively short period was introduced by Streem and is now being used with good effect in Indianapolis (173,175). However, Schulze et al. treated 77 partial and complete staghorns with combination therapy and had only a 58% stone-free rate at 3 months despite a mean hospital stay of 19 days (171). Our treatment outcome with 12 of 22 kidneys (55%) being stone-free is similar with a much shorter hospital stay of 10.3 days (157).

Urinary Acidification

Alkaline urine, which occurs in patients with urease-producing urinary tract infections, is necessary for urine to become supersaturated with struvite and carbonate apatite. Urinary acidification should therefore be of benefit to increase the solubility of struvite and carbonate apatite. Ascorbic acid has generally been unsuccessful in acidifying urine, although Murphy et al. have reported acidification with the concomitant use of antimicrobial therapy in the presence of urease-producing bacteria (176–178). Vermeulen et al. used ammonium chloride to acidify urine in rats and thus promoted stone dissolution and prevented stone formation (179). This work was successfully applied to the ranch mink industry, which was previously plagued by deaths secondary to struvite urolithiasis (180). Although short-term acidification has been achieved in humans with ammonium chloride, no long-term studies have been reported (181). It has been shown that ammonium chloride results in increased ammonia excretion after 6 days, thus counteracting earlier acidification (182).

In 1978, Froeling used ammonium nitrate (NH_4NO_3) to acidify urine in humans, but no long-term studies were performed (183). In 1987, Pizzarelli and Peacock reported their experience with urinary acidification with ammonium sulfate [$(NH_4)_2SO_4$] (184). All patients were treated for a minimum of 2 years. Acidic urine and persistent reduction in the relative saturation of calcium phosphate and stone formation rate were reported. They also noted that metabolic acidosis did not occur in the presence of normal renal function. This is of vital importance as urinary calcium and phosphate excretion increase during acute or chronic metabolic acidosis (185,186). Coe et al. have, however, shown that hypercalciuria can be prevented in chronic metabolic acidosis by a low-sodium diet (187).

Lavage Chemolysis

In 1938, Hellstrom reported his experience with lavage chemolysis for struvite calculi (117). He used varying combinations of urinary antiseptics and acidifying agents. Albright et al. reported their in vitro and in vivo experience with acidic solutions in 1939 (188). They selected citric acid as the most likely effective substance. The resulting equation demonstrates the reaction that occurs:

$$3Ca^{2+} + 2Cit^{2-} \rightarrow Ca_3Cit_2 \rightarrow Ca^{2+} + 2(CaCit)^-$$

The addition of citrate ions to a solution containing calcium ions results in a two-thirds reduction of free calcium ions. The tertiary citrate (Ca_3Cit_2) is produced only in an alkaline pH. At acidic pH levels, primary [$Ca(H_2Cit)_2$] and secondary (CaHCit) citrates are formed, and as these are weakly dissociated, there is a similar reduction in free calcium ions.

Albright noted that solutions with a pH of 4.0 caused little tissue irritation. In vitro dissolution of calcium phosphate/calcium carbonate calculi were achieved with a sodium citrate–citric acid mixture of 154 mm/L (isotonic) at a pH of 4.0. In vivo experiments were performed in four patients, but successful dissolution occurred only in one patient who had multiple bladder calculi.

In 1943, Suby and Albright reported the development of Solution G and their experience with its use (189). Original research with citric acid caused marked irritation of rabbit bladder mucosa. This was reduced by the addition of magnesium ions and was thus applied clinically. Solution G was used in six patients and in all cases resulted in partial or complete dissolution of calculi. The irrigant was introduced via nephrostomy tubes in four patients and via ureteral catheters in two patients.

Mulvaney later reported in vitro dissolution of struvite calculi with a similar solution (10% hemiacidrin) (190). He also dissolved one patient's renal pelvic calculi by irrigation with 7% hemiacidrin through a nephrostomy tube. The main differences between Suby's solution G and 10% hemiacidrin are that Suby's G contains the carbonic acid in the sodium salt rather than as the calcium salt and hemiacidrin contains additional magnesium salt and D-gluconic acid (Table 8). Both are equally effective in dissolving calculi in vitro (135). The theoretical mode of action is that a calcium ion in the stone is exchanged for a magnesium ion to form the equivalent magnesium salt, which is soluble in the gluconocitrate solution (136). The U.S. Food and Drug Administration later banned renal pelvic irrigation with renacidin (10%

TABLE 8. *Comparison of Suby's solution G and 10% hemiacidrin (renacidin)*

	Suby's G	10% Hemiacidrin
pH	~4.0	3.9
Citric acid	32.25 g hydrous	28.2 g
Magnesium oxide	3.84 g anhydrous	0
Sodium carbonate	4.37 g anhydrous	0
Calcium carbonate	0	1 g
D-Gluconic acid	0	5 g
Magnesium hydrocarbonate	0	14.5 g
Magnesium acid citrate	0	2.5 g
H_2O	1000 mL	1000 mL

hemiacidrin) after four deaths were reported (135). Nemoy and Stamey emphasized that the deaths may have been the result of urosepsis rather than the irrigant solution used (136). They outlined the precautions necessary when using irrigant chemolysis, which include (1) maintenance of sterile urine, (2) unobstructed inflow and outflow, (3) intrapelvic pressure maintenance < 30 cm H_2O, (4) absence of extravasation, and (5) careful monitoring of magnesemia. Hypermagnesemia is more likely to occur in patients with compromised renal function (191). Using the aforementioned irrigation precautions, Nemoy and Stamey successfully dissolved renal calculi in eight patients (136). There have also been reports of successful staghorn stone dissolution through percutaneous nephrostomy tubes and ileal conduit urinary diversions (192,193). Recently, outpatient irrigation with 10% hemiacidrin has been advocated under carefully controlled conditions (194). Palmer et al. treated 13 patients in this way with stone dissolution in 78% and a 17% rehospitalization requirement. Chemolytic irrigation may decrease the incidence of stone recurrences (116). Silverman and Stamey irrigated 46 kidneys after open surgery and dissolved calculi in 10 out of 11 kidneys with residual stones. After a mean follow-up of 7 years, the only stone recurrence that occurred was in the kidney with a residual calculus post irrigation.

Dietary Supplementation

In the 1930s, hypovitaminosis A was implicated as a cause of struvite calculogenesis, but dietary supplementation is of doubtful value (195–197).

Substrate Depletion

In 1945, Shorr proposed the theoretical advantages of using estrogens and aluminum hydroxide gels in patients with struvite calculi (198). Citric acid was known to enhance calcium solubility, but when administered orally it was thought to be mostly metabolized with little excreted in the urine. The use of estrogens were suggested as they increase urinary citric acid and decrease calciuria. The mechanism of action of aluminum hydroxide gel is that it binds with phosphate in the gastrointestinal tract to form insoluble aluminum phosphate. Thus less phosphate absorption occurs and urinary phosphate is decreased. It was hoped that this combination coupled with a low-phosphorus diet would provide protection against calcium phosphate precipitation, even in alkaline urine. Five years later, Shorr and Carter reported their experience with low-calcium, low-phosphorus diets together with aluminum gels in 22 patients (199). Patients were treated for 2–7 years. Basic aluminum carbonate gel (Basaljel) was found to be effective in reducing urinary phosphorus excretion. This combination treatment enhanced stone dissolution in 23% of stones and prevented stone growth in a further 67%. Lavengood and Marshall have reported their experience using the Shorr regimen (200). They recorded dramatic urinary phosphorus reductions in their patients who were taking 40 cm^3 of basic aluminum gel (Basaljel) after meals and at bedtime, 3 L of fluid, and a daily diet containing less than 1300 mg of phosphorus. Stone recurrence occurred in 9.8% of infected patients on the regimen for 3.5 years compared to 30% of infected patients not on the regimen. Recurrences in uninfected patients were 0% in patients on the regimen compared to 22% of those not on the regimen. Dietary compliance was difficult and many patients developed constipation. The use of aluminum hydroxide must be monitored carefully, as it may cause anorexia, malaise, lethargy, bone pain, and hypercalciuria (201).

Antimicrobial Agents

The aim of antimicrobial therapy is to sterilize the urine and thus render it undersaturated with respect to struvite. In vitro and in vivo studies have shown that struvite calculi may partially dissolve in the presence of sterile urine (202,203). The long-term treatment with suppressive agents such as sulfa, methenamine, and nitrofurantoin has generally resulted in poor suppression of infection. Methenamine is particularly unsuitable, as rapid passage through the upper renal tracts does not allow time for the conversion of methenamine to formaldehyde (204,205). Long-term culture-specific antimicrobials may reduce the magnitude of the urinary infection even if sterility does not result. A reduction of the colony count from 10^7–10^5 ml^{-1} reduces the urease production by 99% (107). In many cases sterile urine will not be achieved because bacteria are situated within the interstices of the stones and are thus not exposed to the antimicrobial therapy (136). The majority of urease-producing infections are caused by *Proteus mirabilis*. Over 90% of these are sensitive to penicillin or ampicillin at a concentration of 20 μg/mL urine (206). Standard doses of oral penicillin (500 mg every 6 h) or ampicillin (250 mg every 6 h) will produce urinary levels of 150 to 300 μg/mL of urine, respectively (202). Feit and Fair maintained sterile urine in 16 of their 20 patients with long-term oral penicillin.

Tetracyclines are of similar value in patients with *Pseudomonas* or *Ureaplasma urealyticum* urinary tract infections (118,207). *U. urealyticum* lacks a rigid cell wall and does not synthesize folic acid. It is therefore resistant to antimicrobials, which act by interfering with cell wall formation or folic acid synthesis, such as penicillins, cephalosporins, and sulfonamides (118). Recently, fluorquinolones such as ciprofloxacin and norfloxacin have been reported to offer improved coverage against *Pseudomonas,* but they are more expensive than tetracyclines (208,209). Griffith et al. maintained sterile urine in nine patients with struvite calculi, who were treated with long-term culture-specific antibiotics, including ampicillin, cephalosporin, nalidixic acid, nitro-

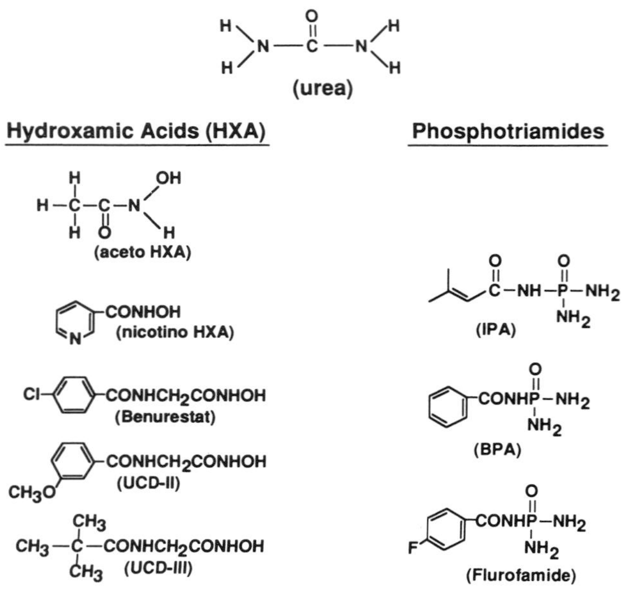

FIG. 10. Molecular structure of urea and examples of urease inhibitors.

furantoin, penicillin, sulfisoxazole-trimethoprim, and tetracycline (203). Five patients had significant stone dissolution, three had no change in stone size, and one had considerable stone growth requiring surgery. They also treated 17 patients (25 stone-containing kidneys) with recalcitrant urinary tract infections with intermittent or continuous antibiotics for up to 4 years. Stone growth occurred in 21 kidneys, slight stone dissolution occurred in two kidneys, and no change occurred in two kidneys. The long-term use of antibiotics, while possibly preventing stone growth and recurrence, will subject the patient to the risk of developing resistant organisms and the alteration of native bacterial flora. Long-term, low-dose, culture-specific antimicrobials are probably the best suppression if surgery is contraindicated or if stone clearance is not complete following surgery. The realistic expectation of such therapy is to inhibit stone growth rather than cause stone dissolution.

Preoperative and perioperative antibiotics are vital to prevent urosepsis and to sterilize the renal parenchyma and urine during open surgery, percutaneous nephrolithotomy, extracorporeal shock wave lithotripsy, and lavage chemolysis.

Methylene Blue

In the 1950s methylene blue was theorized to inhibit struvite stone growth and cause stone dissolution by the exchange of ions of dye for ions of crystal (210–212). The questionable benefits of cationic dye therapy has resulted in its infrequent use.

Urease Inhibitors

In 1962, Kobashi et al. noted that hydroxamic acids had a similar molecular structure to urea (Fig. 10) and caused specific inhibition of urease at a concentration of 10^{-6} M (213). The site of urease inhibition is the R-CONHOH group, which characterizes the hydroxamate family (214). Aromatic hydroxamic acids inhibit urease competitively, whereas fatty acyl hydroxamic acids inhibit it noncompetitively. Heptylo- and caprylohydroxamic acids (fatty acyl derivatives) have the greatest urease inhibitory power. Recently, phosphotriamide derivatives have been reported to cause greater inhibition of urease of plant and bacterial origin at a concentration of 10^{-8} M (215,216). Table 9 outlines the concentration of hydroxamic acids and phosphotriamides, which cause a 50% inhibition (I_{50}) of urease activity from various sources.

The ideal urease inhibitor should have three properties for in vivo usage. First, the drug must inhibit urease activity in viable bacterial cells, as more than 90% of the urease is distributed within bacterial cells (217). All urease inhibitors listed in Fig. 10 have this property. Hydroxamic acid and phosphotriamide derivatives also have weak antimicrobial activity but cannot be expected to reduce the viable urinary cell number in vivo (216,218). However, two phosphotriamide derivatives; N-benzoylphosphotriamide (BPA) and fluorofamide have been shown to be bacteriocidal toward U. urealyticum at a concentration of 10^{-5} M (219,220).

The second necessary property is that the drug must be easily metabolized and have a high renal clearance. Acetohydroxamic acid (AHA) is rapidly absorbed from the gastrointestinal tract when administered orally and reaches peak plasma levels after about 1 h (221). The two major metabolites in humans are acetamide and carbon dioxide. Carbon dioxide is eliminated in the breath and accounts for 20–45% of the administered dose. Acetamide is excreted in the urine and accounts for 9–14% of

TABLE 9. I_{50} urease values of hydroxamic acid and phosphotriamides

Urease origin	Hydroxamic acid (µM)		Phosphotriamides (nM)	
	Caprylo-	Nicotino-	N-Benzoyl-	N-Isopentenoyl-
Jack bean	0.84	2.9	6.5	4.9
Proteus mirabilis	4.1	41	7.9	7.8
Morganella morganii	6.0	14	270	190
Klebsiella pneumoniae	6.6	7.6	6.1	5.8
Ureaplasma urealyticum	2.2	2.7	7.0	2.0

the dose administered. The remaining dose (19–48%) is excreted as intact AHA in the urine. AHA metabolism in the rat is different, as acetamide is the major metabolite (222). There is a positive linear relationship between AHA half-life and creatinine clearance in humans. The half-life is 3.5–10 h in normal subjects, 9–13 h in patients with cirrhosis, and 15.3–23.7 h in patients with diminished renal function (223,224). The effectiveness of AHA depends on its concentration in the urine. At the recommended dose of 250 mg every 8 h, urinary concentrations of 15–30 mg/dL are usually achieved in patients with normal renal function (225). When the serum creatinine exceeds 2 mg/dL, full therapeutic concentrations of AHA are unachievable. The inhibitory power of AHA is moderate ($I_{50} = 1 \times 10^{-5}$ M) compared to that of caprylo- and nicotinohydroxamic acid ($I_{50} = 8.4 \times 10^{-7}$ M and 2.9×10^{-6} M, respectively). However, only 0.3 and 0.5% of these compounds are excreted in the urine when taken orally (226). These hydroxamic acids have been developed for the inhibition of intestinal urease activity as a therapeutic agent in patients with hyperammonemia or hepatic coma (227,228). Attempts to develop new potent inhibitors have resulted in the development of m-methoxyhippurohydroxamic acid (UCD-II) and 2,2'-dimethylpropionylglycinohydroxamic acid (UCD-III) in Japan (229,230). In rats, 15 and 11%, respectively, are excreted in the urine within 6 h of oral administration. In human urine, 50% inhibition (I_{50}) of Proteus mirabilis urease activity is demonstrated at concentrations of 13 and 45 μM, respectively. The inhibitory effects on struvite stone formation in rats with typical hydroxamic acid derivatives are outlined in Table 10. These data were obtained separately from different research groups and may not be comparable. However, urinary alkalinization and stone formation were inhibited in all cases.

The incidence and severity of pyelonephritis in the treated groups were also much lower than those in the control, although they had no effect on bacterial cell number in urine. These advantageous effects were attributable to decreased ammonia production. The effective-

ness of combining urease inhibitors and antibiotics has resulted in the suggestion that antibiotics such as cephalexin enhance the inhibitory action of urease inhibitors on intracellular urease by damaging bacterial cell wall synthesis, while urease inhibitors potentiate the antibacterial activity of the antibiotics by reducing the pH elevation in the urine (232,235). In rats, 20–30% of orally administered phosphotriamide derivatives are excreted intact in the urine within 4 h (236).

The third necessary property of effective urease inhibitors is that their long-term administration be safe. The greatest clinical experience worldwide is with AHA. Although it is noncarcinogenic, it has been shown to be teratogenic when administered to female beagle dogs (236). Pups born to bitches receiving AHA had significantly lower birthweights, higher perinatal mortality, and congenital cardiac and coccygeal anomalies. Hernias also occurred more frequently. Table 11 outlines the results of three double-blind, placebo-controlled clinical trials of AHA in patients with infection induced renal calculi. In each study treatment with 250–1000 mg of AHA daily was compared with a mannitol placebo. Concurrent antimicrobial agents were given in the Cornell study and were given intermittently in the VA and Baylor studies. Sterile urine was not achieved in any patient group. Similar symptomatic side effects occurred in all three trials. In the Cornell study these included deep venous thrombosis, tremulousness, and intolerable headache. In the VA cooperative study they included palpitations, edema, nausea, vomiting, diarrhea, headache, tremulousness, loss of taste, hallucinations, rash, alopecia, abdominal pain, anemia, hematocrit decrease, and reticulocyte increase. In the Baylor study 22% of patients withdrew because of similar side effects. All side effects reversed upon cessation of AHA and no attributable deaths were recorded (239). Propionohydroxamic acid (PHA) has been used less extensively in patients but has been associated with few side effects (240). Biosuppressin (hydroxycarbamide), an antineoplastic agent, has been shown to decrease urinary ammonia and pH in in vitro studies (241). Its use for this purpose has not been applied clinically because of its leukopenic action.

The search for an ideal urease inhibitor continues. The ideal qualities are (1) specific urease inhibition, (2) antibacterial action, and (3) potentiation of antimicrobial drugs. It should also achieve high urinary concentrations, which are nontoxic, nonteratogenic, and nonmutagenic (242). In conclusion, although the epidemiology and pathogenesis of infection stones are well documented, effective curative treatment remains problematic.

Nonoperative treatment leads to progressive renal damage, so treatment rests with attempted surgical clearance of the stones followed by elimination of urinary tract infections. Although the long-term effects of PCNL and ESWL are not well documented, combination

TABLE 10. *Effect of hydroxamic acids on struvite calculi formation in rats*

	Dose (mg/kg)	Weight of stone (mg)	
		Untreated	Drug-treated
Aceto HXA (231)	100	52	8.0
NicotinoHXA (226)	100	18.8	3.9
Benurestat (232)	100	30.1	13.6
UCD-II (233)	100	29.0	18.3
UCD-III (234)	Drinking water[a]	35.8	11.5
UCD-III + cephalexin (235)	100 + 5	74	38

[a] Saturated solution in drinking water.

TABLE 11. *Double-blind, placebo-controlled clinical trials of acetohydroxamic acid in patients with infection calculi[a]*

	Cornell (237)	VA (238)	Baylor (239)
Patients	37	210	94
Patient population	N + SCI	SCI	N + SCI
STONE GROWTH OR RECURRENCE			
Placebo (%)	58 (19 months)	60 (12 months)	46 (18 months)
		60 (24 months)	
AHA (%)	22 (16 months)	33 (12 months)	17 (18 months)
		42 (24 months)	
Side effects (%)	45	68	22

Source: Cornell University College of Medicine (237), Baylor College of Medicine (239), and the Veterans Administration (VA) Cooperative Study Group (238).
[a] N, normal; SCI, spinal cord injury.

PCNL-ESWL appears to offer the patient a less morbid surgical alternative than standard open surgery. Adjunctive medical therapy such as culture-specific antibiotics, urease inhibitors, and urine acidification are worthwhile to reduce the morbidity associated with persistent urinary tract infections and further stone recurrence.

RARE CALCULI

This section of the chapter deals with calculi composed of crystallized drugs, dihydroxyadenine lithiasis, and xanthine calculi.

Urolithiasis Secondary to Drug Crystalluria

In 1936, the effectiveness of sulfanilamide against hemolytic streptococcal infections dramatically altered the management of bacterial disease (243). The most commonly used sulfonamides were N'-heterocyclic derivatives of sulfanilamide such as sulfadiazine (2-sulfanilamidopyrimidine), sulfamerazine (2-sulfanilamido-4-methylpyrimidine), and sulfamethazine (2-sulfanilamido-4-6-dimethylpyrimidine). When sulfapyrimidines are absorbed into the bloodstream, a percentage of them undergo acetylation of their primary amino groups in the liver. It is these acetyl derivatives that crystallize in the urine, especially if the urine volume and pH are low. The percentage of acetylated sulfapyrimidines in the urine ranges from 25 to 50% (244). The crystals originally form in the convoluted tubules and may pass into the calices, where their affinity for one another causes aggregation (245). The propensity for crystalluria is further compounded by the fact that these are short-acting sulfonamides which are excreted in the urine within 4 h of oral administration, so very large doses are necessary to maintain effective blood levels (246). In the 1940s, efforts to decrease crystalluria by using mixtures of three sulfonamides were partially effective (247). The theoretical basis for this was that sulfonamides dissolve independently in urine. Although equally effective sulfonamides with greater urinary solubility were introduced in 1951, occasional reports of sulfonamide urolithiasis are still published (246,248,249). Before making a diagnosis of sulfonamide crystalluria, it is vital to confirm that the urine sample temperature is 37°C because crystal formation is induced by cooling (250). When sulfonamides are used clinically, precautionary measures that should be taken include (a) the use of sulfonamide mixtures, (b) avoiding sulfonamides that are largely excreted as their acetylated derivatives, (c) alkalinization of the urine, and (d) maintaining high urinary output (243).

Tiramterene is a pteridine that has been used as a diuretic for more than 20 years (251,252). When taken orally it is rapidly absorbed and metabolized to parahydroxytriamterene and parahydroxytriamterene sulfate (253). The half-life is 1.5–2.5 h and the drug and its metabolites are excreted in bile and urine (251). The urinary excretion of the metabolites is three times that of the parent drug. In 1979, Ettinger et al. reported the first case of a triamterene renal calculus, which encouraged them to investigate the incidence more thoroughly (252). Of 50,000 calculi studied, they found 181 renal calculi (0.4%) which were partially or totally composed of triamterene and its metabolites (254). Calculi also contained calcium oxalate monohydrate or uric acid. Pure triamterene calculi are mustard- or gold-colored with a smooth outer surface and concentric lamellae which are visible on crushing (254). They may appear as radiolucent filling defects on intravenous urography, which can be identified correctly as calculi using computed tomography. Their attenuation value is 132 Hounsfield units (255). Treatment rests with stone removal and discontinuation of the drug.

Silica stones are very rare in humans and occur only in patients taking antacids (256). In 1941, Page et al. demonstrated increased urinary silica excretion after the administration of magnesium trisilicate (257). Occasional case reports of silica urolithiasis have been reported from Europe and the United States (256,259,260). After oral administration, the breakdown products in the digestive tract include various silica acids which are soluble and are absorbed (7). These are gradually excreted in urine and may precipitate as a gel composed of silicon dioxide (7,258). Calculi may also be partially composed of calcium salts (260). Radiologically, the calculi are faintly opaque and may be demonstrated as filling defects on an intravenous urogram. Stone analysis can be performed using x-ray crystallography after heating to 1000°C to convert the silica to tridymite. Stone recurrence can be prevented by discontinuing the drug. Even rarer cases of drug crystal-induced calculi include mefenamic acid, which is the major component of many analgesics such as ponstan, and ioxaglic acid, which is the active ingredient of many radiological contrast media (248).

2,8-Dihydroxyadenine Calculi

2,8-Dihydroxyadenine (DHA) lithiasis has only been described since 1974, probably because stone analysis mistook 2,8-DHA as uric acid (261). Dihydroxyadeninuria is transmitted by an autosomal recessive gene that controls the production of the enzyme adenine phosphoribosyl transferase (APRT). Gene coding for APRT is located on the long arm of chromosome 16 (261). APRT catalyzes the synthesis of adenosine monophosphate from the purine adenine (Fig. 11). In the absence of APRT, the only alternative route for adenine metabolism involves oxidation to its hydroxylated metabolites, 8-hydroxyadenine and 2,8-dihydroxyadenine (262). 2,8-DHA is only sparingly soluble in urine over the pH range 5–7.4, so it tends to crystallize and form calculi (263). The only clinical manifestations of APRT deficiency are crystalluria and urolithiasis.

Heterozygosity for the trait has been reported to be 1 per 100 people, whereas the incidence of homozygotes is about 1 per 50,000 people (261). Heterozygotes are normally asymptomatic, with APRT levels about 25% of the normal mean. However, 39 of these patients have formed calculi in Japan (276). The large number of cases reported from Japan has been attributed to the widespread distribution of a unique mutant gene (APRT*J) (276). At least 30 homozygotes worldwide have been reported to have developed urolithiasis (261,262,264). Of these the majority have been male children. The diagnosis should be considered in all male children who present with radiolucent calculi. Homozygotes can be identified by the presence of adenine in the urine (265). Heterozygotes can be detected by measuring the erythrocyte APRT activity (266). DHA crystals appear as spheres bearing maltese crosses when viewed under the microscope with polarized light (263). The calculi are pale gray in color and are rough and friable (261,263).

Treatment rests with stone removal endoscopically, percutaneously, or with extracorporeal shock wave lithotripsy. Urinary alkalinization has been shown to be of no use; thus a radiolucent calculus that does not dissolve with alkalinization may be composed of 2,8-DHA rather than the more commonly found uric acid (261,262).

Preventative measures against stone recurrence include maintaining a high fluid intake and a low purine diet and use of allopurinol, which inhibits xanthine oxidase (261,262). Allopurinol therapy is beneficial because adenine is more soluble in urine than its derivatives (263). This rare disease may not present until the fourth or fifth decades and can cause chronic renal failure requiring dialysis (261,262).

Xanthine Lithiasis

Xanthine calculi account for less than 0.04% of calculi analyzed (267,268). Urolithiasis occurs secondary to increased urinary xanthine excretion in only two conditions. The first of these is hereditary xanthinuria, which is transmitted by an autosomal recessive gene. This condition was described initially in 1954 and is characterized by a deficiency of xanthine oxidase activity (269). This leads to an increase in blood and urinary xanthine and hypoxanthine with a corresponding fall in plasma and urinary uric acid (Fig. 11) (270). Fifty to 80% of the purine load is excreted as xanthine, with the remainder

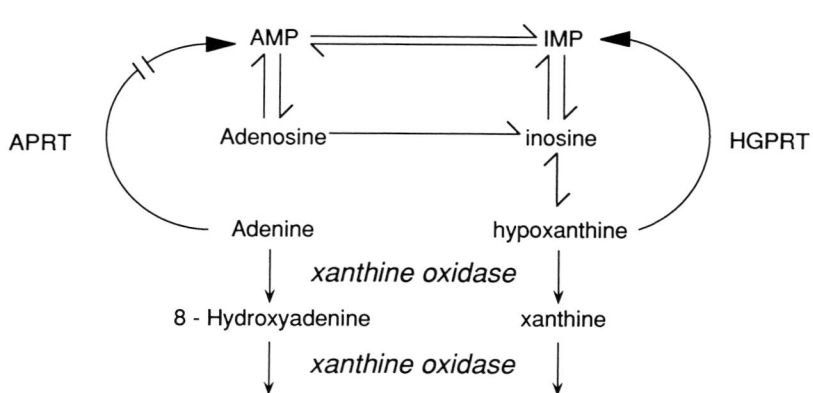

FIG. 11. Pathway of purine degradation and salvage metabolism demonstrating production of 2,8-dihydroxyadenine. APRT, adenine phosphoribosyltransferase; AMP, adenosine monophosphate; IMP, inosine monophosphate; HGPRT, hypoxanthine guanine phosphoribosyltransferase.

being excreted as hypoxanthine (271). The reasons that xanthine is the major product excreted are that the residual xanthine oxidase is able to oxidize some hypoxanthine to xanthine, and hypoxanthine is a substrate for the salvage enzyme hypoxanthine guanine phosphoribosyltransferase (HGPRT), which converts hypoxanthine to guanine (263,272). The diagnosis should be considered in all children with radiolucent calculi, although some cases may not present until adult life. The presence of low serum and very low urinary uric acid are suggestive of the condition (271). Xanthine calculi are usually smooth, friable, and brown in color. Paper chromatography, differential spectrophotometry, and x-ray crystallography confirm the calculus composition (263). The recommended treatment is removal of all calculi and the initiation of preventative measures. These should include maintenance of a high urinary output (3–4 L) and consumption of a low-purine diet. The benefits of urinary alkalinization are controversial (263,271). Allopurinol treatment is of benefit because it blocks the residual xanthine oxidase activity, which reverses the urinary xanthine/hypoxanthine ratio (263). Hypoxanthine is more soluble than xanthine, so the overall degree of oxypurine supersaturation is decreased.

Urolithiasis may also arise in patients with hyperuricemia who are taking allopurinol. To date there have been a small number of such cases reported in patients with Lesch-Nyhan syndrome and leukemia (273–275).

REFERENCES

1. Lansdale K, Mason P. Uric acid, uric acid dihydrate and urates in urinary calculi, ancient and modern. *Science* 1966;152:1511–2.
2. Klohn M, Bolle JF, Reverdin NP, Susini A, Baud CA, Graber P. Ammonium urate urinary stones. *Urol Res* 1986;14:315–8.
3. Shahjehan S, Ataur Rahman M. Studies on the etiology of urolithiasis in Karachi. *Am J Clin Nutr* 1971;24:32–7.
4. Borden TA, Dean WM. Ammonium acid urate stones in Navajo indian children. *Urology* 1979;14:9–12.
5. Bowyer RC, McCulloch RK, Brockis JG, Ryan GD. Factors affecting the solubility of ammonium hydrogen urate. *Clin Chim Acta* 1979;95:17–22.
6. Maierhofer WJ. Renal disease from excess uric acid. *Postgrad Med* 82(4):1987;123–9.
7. Robertson WG, Peacock M. Pathogenesis of urolithiasis. In: Schneider H-J, ed. *Urolithiasis: etiology diagnosis,* vol 17(1). Berlin: Springer-Verlag, 1985;251–334.
8. Gutman AB, Yu T-F. Uric acid nephrolithiasis. *Am J Med* 1968;45:756–79.
9. German DC, Holmes EW. Gout and hyperuricemia: diagnosis and management. *Hosp Prac* 1986;21:119–32.
10. Synderham T. Cited by Robertson WG, Peacock M. Pathogenesis of urolithiasis. In: Schneider H-J, ed. *Urolithiasis: etiology diagnosis,* vol 17(1). Berlin: Springer-Verlag, 1985;251–334.
11. Scheele KW. Examen chemicum calculi urinarii. *Opuscula* 1776;2:73–90.
12. Wollaston WH. On gouty and urinary concretions. *Philos Trans R Soc Lond* 1797;87:386–400.
13. Yu TF, Gutman AB. Uric acid nephrolithiasis in gout: predisposing factors. *Ann Intern Med* 1967;67:1133–48.
14. Chonko AM, Grantham JJ. Disorders of urate metabolism and excretion. In: Brenner BM, Rector FC Jr, eds. *The kidney.* Philadelphia: WB Saunders, 1981;1023–55.
15. Weinman EJ, Knight TF. Uric acid and the kidney. In: Suki WN, Eknoyan G, eds. *The kidney in systemic disease.* New York: John Wiley & Sons, 1981;285–306.
16. Steele TH. Urate secretion in man: the pyrazinamide suppression test. *Ann Intern Med* 1973;79:734–7.
17. Postlethwaite AE, Gutman RA, Kelley WN. Salicyclate-mediated increase in urate removal during haemodialysis: evidence for urate binding to protein in vivo. *Metabolism* 1974;23:771–7.
18. Preminger GH. Pharmacologic treatment of uric acid calculi. *Urol Clin North Am* 1987;14(2):335–8.
19. Coe FL. Uric acid and calcium oxalate nephrolithiasis. *Kidney Int* 1983;24:392–403.
20. Sperling O, DeVries A, Kedem O. Studies on the etiology of uric acid lithiasis. IV. Urinary non-dialyzable substances in idiopathic uric acid lithiasis. *J Urol* 1965;94:286–92.
21. Porter P. Colloidal properties of urates in relation to calculus formation. *Res Vet Sci* 1966;7:128–37.
22. Pak CYC, Sakhaee K, Fuller C. Successful management of uric acid nephrolithiasis with potassium citrate. *Kidney Int* 1986;30:422–8.
23. Clarke AM, McKenzie RG. Ileostomy and the risk of urinary uric stones. *Lancet* 1969;2:395–7.
24. Gigax JH, Leach JR. Uric acid calculi associated with ileostomy for ulcerative colitis. *J Urol* 1971;105:797–9.
25. Bateson EM. Renal tract calculi and climate. *Med J Aust* 1973;2:111–3.
26. Lavan JN, Neale FC, Posen S. Urinary calculi: clinical, biochemical and radiological studies in 619 patients. *Med J Aust* 1971;2:1049–61.
27. Curtis JR. Drug-induced renal disease. *Drugs* 1979;18:377–91.
28. Dieckmann K-P, Schwarz A, Klan R, Offermann G. Uric acid calculus complicating renal transplantation. *Clin Transplant* 1988;2:211–3.
29. West C, Carpenter BJ, Hakala TR. The incidence of gout in renal transplant recipients. *Am J Kidney Dis* 1987;10:369–72.
30. Tiller DJ, Hall BM, Horvath JS, Duggin GG, Thompson JF, Sheil AGR. Gout and hyperuricaemia in patients on cyclosporin and diuretics. *Lancet* 1985;1:453.
31. Peacock M, Robertson WG. The biochemical aetiology of renal lithiasis. In: Wickham JEA, ed. *Urinary calculous disease.* Edinburgh: Churchill Livingstone, 1979;69–95.
32. Hesse A, Schneider H-J, Berg W, Hienzsch E. Uric acid dihydrate as urinary calculus component. *Invest Urol* 1975;12:405–9.
33. Dykman D, Simon EE, Avioli LV. Hyperuricemia and uric acid nephropathy. *Arch Intern Med* 1987;147:1341–5.
34. Coe FL, Strauss AL, Tembe V, Dun S-L. Uric acid saturation in calcium nephrolithiasis. *Kidney Int* 1980;17:662–8.
35. Greene ML, Fujimoto WY, Seegmiller JE. Urinary xanthine stones: a rare complication of allopurinol therapy. *N Engl J Med* 1969;280(8):426–7.
36. Hande KR, Noone RM, Stone WJ. Severe allopurinol toxicity. *Am J Med* 1984;76:47–56.
37. Rose GA. Other metabolic causes of stones. In: Rose GA, ed. *Urinary stones: clinical and laboratory aspects.* Baltimore: University Park Press, 1982;233–55.
38. Parfitt AM. Acetazolamide and sodium bicarbonate induced nephrocalcinosis and nephrolithiasis. *Arch Intern Med* 1969;124:736–40.
39. Pak CYC, Waters O, Arnold L, Holt K, Cox C, Barilla D. Mechanism of calcium urolithiasis among patients with hyperuricosuria: supersaturation of urine with respect to monosodium urate. *J Clin Invest* 1977;59:426–41.
40. Pak CYC, Diller EC, Smith GW, Howes ES. Renal stones or calcium phosphate: physicochemical basis for their formation. *Proc Soc Biol Med* 1969;130:753–7.
41. Freiha FS, Hemady K. Dissolution of uric acid stones: alternative to surgery. *Urology* 1976;8:334–5.
42. Gordon MR, Carrion HM, Politano VA. Dissolution of uric acid calculi with THAM irrigation. *Urology* 1978;12:393–7.
43. Sadi MV, Saltzman N, Feria G, Gittes RF. Experimental observations on dissolution of uric acid calculi. *J Urol* 1985;134:575–9.
44. Ebisuno S, Fukatani T, Yoshida M, Kumeda K, Ohkawa T. Percutaneous dissolution of uric acid calculi with THAM irrigation. *Urol Radiol* 1987;9:146–8.

45. Dretler SP. Stone fragility: a new therapeutic distinction. *J Urol* 1988;139:1124–6.
46. Segal S, Thier SO. Cystinuria. In: Stanbury JB, Wyngaarden JB, Fredrickson DS, Goldstein JL, Brown MS, eds. *The metabolic basis of inherited disease,* 5th ed. New York: McGraw Hill, 1983;1774–91.
47. Wollaston WH. On cystic oxide: a new species of urinary calculus. *Philos Trans R Soc Lond* 1810;100:223–30.
48. Noehden GH. Scientific notices: chemistry, cystic oxide, communicated in a letter from Dr. Noehden to Mr. Children. *Ann Philos* 1824;7:146.
49. Berzelius JJ. Calculus urinaries. *Traite Chem* 1833;7:424.
50. Friedman E. Der Kreislauf des Schwefels in der organischen Natur. *Ergeb Physiol* 1902;1:15.
51. Garrod AE. Inborn errors of metabolism. *Lancet* 1908;2 (lecture I, p. 1–7, lecture II, p. 73–9, lecture III, p. 142–8, lecture IV, p. 214–20).
52. Yeh HL, Frankl W, Dunn MS, Parker P, Hugher B, Gyorgy P. The urinary excretion of amino acids by a cystinuric subject. *Am J Med Sci* 1947;214:507.
53. Stein WH. Excretion of amino acids in cystinuria. *Proc Soc Exp Biol Med* 1951;78:705.
54. Dent CE, Rose GA. Amino acid metabolism in cystinuria. *Q J Med* 1951;20:205–20.
55. Dent CE, Senior B, Walshe JM. The pathogenesis of cystinuria. II. Polarographic studies of the metabolism of sulphur-containing amino acids. *J Clin Invest* 1954;33:1216–26.
56. Foreman JW, Hwang SM, Segal S. Transport interactions of cystine and dibasic amino acids in isolated rat renal tubules. *Metabolism* 1980;29:53.
57. Segal S, McNamara PD, Pepe LM. Transport interaction of cystine and dibasic amino acids in renal brush border vesicles. *Science* 1977;197:169.
58. Frimpter GW, Horwith M, Furth E, Fellows RE, Thompson DD. Inulin and endogenous amino acid renal clearances in cystinuria: evidence of tubular secretion. *J Clin Invest* 1962;41:281.
59. Milne MD, Asatoor AM, Edwards KDG, Loughridge LW. The intestinal absorption defect in cystinuria. *Gut* 1961;2:323–37.
60. Crawhall JC, Watts RWE. Cystinuria. *Am J Med* 1968;45:736–55.
61. Harris H, Mittwoch U, Robson EB, et al. Phenotypes and genotypes in cystinuria. *Ann Hum Genet* 1955;20:57–91.
62. Dent CE, Friedman M, Green H, Watson LCA. Treatment of cystinuria. *Br Med J* 1965;1:403–8.
63. Gingliani R, Ferrari I, Greene LJ. An evaluation of four methods for the detection of heterozygous cystinuria. *Clin Chim Acta* 1987;164:227–33.
64. Scriver CR. Cystinuria. *N Engl J Med* 1986;315(18):1155–7.
65. Levy HL. Genetic screening. In: Harris H, Hirschorn K, eds. *Advances in human genetics,* vol 4. New York: Plenum Press, 1973;1.
66. Fleming WH, Avery GB, Morgan RL, et al. Gastrointestinal malabsorption associated with cystinuria: report of a case in a negro. *Pediatrics* 1963;32:358–70.
67. Pruzanski W. Cystinuria: report of 56 cases. *Urol Int* 1965;20:154–62.
68. Schneider HJ. Epidemiology of urolithiasis. In: Schneider HJ, ed. *Urolithiasis: etiology diagnosis,* vol 17(1). Berlin: Springer-Verlag, 1985;146.
69. Thier SO. Cystinuria. In: Wyngaarden JB, Smith LH, eds. *Cecil textbook of medicine,* vol 1. Philadelphia: WB Saunders, 1985;611.
70. Dahlberg PJ, VanDenberg CJ, Kurtz SB, et al. Clinical features and management of cystinuria. *Mayo Clin Proc* 1977;52:533–41.
71. Hambraeus L. Comparative studies of the value of two cyanide-nitroprusside methods in the diagnosis of cystinuria. *Scand J Lab Clin Invest* 1963;15:657.
72. Pahira JJ. Management of the patient with cystinuria. *Urol Clin North Am* 1987;14(2):339–46.
73. Smith DR, Kolb FO, Harper HA. The management of cystinuria and cystine stone disease. *J Urol* 1959;81:61–9.
74. Zinneman HH, Jones JE. Dietary methionine and its influence on cystine excretion on cystinuric patients. *Metabolism* 1966;15:915–21.
75. Kolb FO, Earll JM, Harris HA. Disappearance of cystinuria in a patient treated with prolonged low methionine diet. *Metabolism,* 1967;16:378.
76. White MF. The transport of cationic amino acids across the plasma membrane of mammalian cells. *Biochem Biophys Acta* 1985;822:355–74.
77. Segal S, Crawhall JC. Characteristics of cystine and cysteine transport in rat kidney cortex slices. *Proc Natl Acad Sci USA* 1968;59:231–4.
78. Editorial. Cystinuria is reduced by low-sodium diets. *Nutr Rev* 1987;45(3):79–82.
79. Jaeger P, Portmann L, Saunders A, Rosenberg LE, Thier SO. Anticystinuric effects of glutamine and of dietary sodium restriction. *N Engl J Med* 1986;315(18):1120–3.
80. Dent CE, Senior B. Studies in the treatment of cystinuria. *Br J Urol* 1955;27:317.
81. Smith LH. Medical evaluation of urolithiasis: etiologic aspects and diagnostic evaluation. *Urol Clin North Am* 1974;1:241–60.
82. Freed SZ. The alternating use of an alkalizing salt and acetazolamide in the management of cystine and uric acid stones. *J Urol* 1975;113:96–9.
83. Tabachnick N, Eisen HN, Levine B. New mixed sulfide: penicillamine cysteine. *Nature* 1954;174:701–2.
84. Lotz M, Potts JT Jr, Holland JM, et al. D-Penicillamine therapy in cystinuria. *J Urol* 1966;95:257–63.
85. Crawhall JC, Scowen EF, Watts RWE. Effect of penicillamine on cystinuria. *Br Med J* 1963;1:585.
86. Kuchinaskas EJ, Horuath A, DuVigneaud V. An anti-vitamin B$_6$ action of L-penicillamine. *Arch Biochem* 1957;68:69–75.
87. Watts RW. Problems of inborn errors of metabolism and urinary stone disease. In: Brockis JG, Findlayson B, eds. *Urinary calculus.* Littleton, Mass: PSG Publishing, 1981.
88. Crawhall JC, Scowen EF, Thompson CJ, et al. Dissolution of cystine stones during D-penicillamine treatment of a pregnant patient with cystinuria. *Br Med J* 1967;2:216–8.
89. Mjoluerod OK, Dommerud SA, Rasmussen K, et al. Congenital connective tissue defect probably due to D-penicillamine treatment in pregnancy. *Lancet* 1971;1:673–5.
90. Pak CYC, Fuller C, Sakhaee K, Zerwekh JE, Adams BV. Management of cystine nephrolithiasis with α-mercaptopropionylglycine. *J Urol* 1986;136:1003–8.
91. Stokes GS, Potts JT, Lotz M, Bartter F. A new agent in the treatment of cystinuria: N-acetyl-D-penicillamine. *Br Med J* 1968;1:284.
92. Kallistratos G, Malorny G. Experimentelle Untersuchungen zur Frage der chemisohen Auflösung von Cystinsteinen. *Arzneimittelforschung* 1972;22:1434.
93. Toshioka N, Mita I, Chiba T. *Proceedings of the international symposium on thiola.* Osaka, Japan: Santen Pharmaceutical Co., 1970;1.
94. King JS Jr. Treatment of cystinuria with α-mercaptopropionylglycine: a preliminary report with some notes on column chromatography of mercaptans. *Soc Exp Biol Med* 1968;129:927–32.
95. Fariss BL, Kolb FO. Preliminary communications: factors involved in crystal formation in cystinuria. *JAMA* 1968;205:138.
96. Crowell AJ. Cystin nephrolithiasis: report of case with roentgenographic demonstration of disintegration of stone by alkalinization. *Surg Gynecol Obstet* 1924;38:87–91.
97. Smith A, Lange P, Miller R, et al. Dissolution of cystine calculi by irrigation with acetylcysteine through percutaneous nephrostomy. *Urology* 1979;13:422–3.
98. Stark H, Savir A. Dissolution of cystine calculi by pelviocaliceal irrigation with D-penicillamine. *J Urol* 1980;124:895.
99. Saltzman N, Gittes RF. Chemolysis of cystine calculi. *J Urol* 1986;136:846–9.
100. Burns JR, Hamrick LC Jr. In vitro dissolution of cystine urinary calculi. *J Urol* 1986;136:850–2.
101. Kandel LB, Harrison LH. ESWL, percutaneous nephrostolithotomy, and medical management of uric acid and cystine calculi. In: McCullough DL, Paulson DF, eds. *Problems in urology, calculous disease,* vol 1(4). Philadelphia: JB Lippincott, 1987;668–81.
102. Kelly S, Nolan DP. Letter to the editor. *JAMA* 1980;243:1897.

103. Wershub LP. *Urology: from antiquity to the 20th century.* St Louis, MO: Warren H Green, 1970;35–6.
104. Shattock SG. A prehistoric or predynostic Egyptian calculus. *Trans Pathol Soc Lond* 1905;61:275–90.
105. Schneider HJ. Epidemiology of urolithiasis. In: Schneider HJ, ed. *Urolithiasis: etiology diagnosis.* Berlin: Springer-Verlag, 1985;137–84.
106. Dana ES. *Descriptive minerology.* New York: John Wiley & Sons, 1920;806.
107. Griffith DP, Osborne CA. Infection (urease) stones. *Miner Electrolyte Metab* 1987;13:278–85.
108. Elliot JS, Sharp RF, Lewis L. The solubility of struvite in urine. *J Urol* 1959;81:366–8.
109. Pitts RF. Production and excretion of ammonia in relation to acid-base regulation. In: Orloff J, Berlinger RW, eds. *Renal physiology.* Washington, DC: American Physiological Society, 1973;455.
110. Griffith DP. Struvite stones. *Kidney Int* 1978;13:372–82.
111. Brown TR. On the relation between the variety of microorganisms and the composition of stone in calculous pyelonephritis. *JAMA* 1901;36:1395–7.
112. Hagar, BH, Magath TB. The etiology of encrusted cystitis with alkaline urine. *JAMA* 1925;85:1352–5.
113. Sumner JB. The isolation and crystallization of the enzyme urease. *J Biol Chem* 1926;69:435–41.
114. Christensen WB. Urea decomposition as a means of differentiating *Proteus* and *Paracolon* cultures from each other and from *Salmonella* and *Shigella* types. *J Bacteriol* 1946;52:461–6.
115. Qadri SMG, Zubairi S, Hawley HP, Ramirez EG. Simple spot test for rapid detection of urease activity. *J Clin Microbiol* 1984;20:1198–9.
116. Silverman DE, Stamey TA. Management of infection stones: the Stanford experience. *Medicine* 1983;62:44–51.
117. Hellstrom J. The significance of staphylococci in the development and treatment of renal and ureteric stones. *Br J Urol* 1938;10:348–78.
118. Hedelin H, Brorson JE, Grenabo L, Pettersson S. Ureaplasma urealyticum and upper urinary tract stones. *Br J Urol* 1984;56(3):244–9.
119. Takebe S, Numata A, Kobashi K. Stone formation by ureaplasma urealyticum in human urine and its prevention by urease inhibitors. *J Clin Microbiol* 1984;20:869–73.
120. Parsons CL, Greenspan C, Moore SW, Mulholland SG. Role of surface mucin in primary antibacterial defense of bladder. *Urology* 1977;9:48–52.
121. Parsons CL, Stauffer C, Mulholland SG, Griffith DP. The effect of ammonium on bacterial adherence to bladder transitional epithelium. *J Urol* 1984;132:365–6.
122. Grenabo L, Hedelin H, Pettersson S. Adherence of urease-induced crystals to rat bladder epithelium. *Urol Res* 1988;16:49–52.
123. Boyce WH, King JS Jr, Fielden ML. Total nondialyzable solids (TNDS) in human urine. XIII. Immunological detection of a component peculiar to renal calculous matrix and to urine of calculous patients. *J Clin Invest* 1962;41:1180–9.
124. Nickel JC, Eintage J, Costerton JW. Ultrastructural microbial ecology of infection-induced urinary stones. *J Urol* 1985;133:622–7.
125. Khan SR, Finlayson B, Hackett RL. Stone matrix as proteins absorbed on crystal surfaces; a microscopic study. *Scanning Electron Microsc* 1983;1:379–81.
126. Peacock M, Robertson WC. The biochemical aetiology of renal lithiasis. In: Wickham JEA, ed. *Urinary calculous disease.* Edinburgh: Churchill Livingstone, 1979;69–95.
127. Sarmina I, Spirnak JP, Resnick MI. Urinary lithiasis in the black population: an epidemiological study and review of the literature. *J Urol* 1987;138:14–7.
128. Resnick MI. Evaluation and management of infection stones. *Urol Clin North Am* 1981;8(2):265–76.
129. Comarr AE, Kawaichi GK, Bors E. Renal calculosis in patients with traumatic cord lesions. *J Urol* 1962;85(5):647–56.
130. Bors E. Neurogenic bladder. *Urol Surv* 1957;7(3):177–250.
131. Koff SA, Lapides J. Altered bladder function in staghorn calculus disease. *J Urol* 1977;117:577–80.

132. Amar AD, Hutch JA, Katz I. Coexistence of urinary calculi and vesicoureteral reflux. *JAMA* 1968;206:2312–3.
133. Lue TF, Macchia RJ, Pastore L, Waterhouse K. Vesicoureteral reflux and staghorn calculi. *J Urol* 1982;127:247–8.
134. Rous SN, Turner RW. Retrospective study of 95 patients with staghorn calculus disease. *J Urol* 1977;118:902–4.
135. Shortliffe LMD, Spigelmann SL. Infection stones: evaluation and management. *Urol Clin North Am* 1986;13:717–26.
136. Nemoy NJ, Stamey TA. Surgical, bacteriological, and biochemical management of "infection stones." *JAMA* 1971;215:1470–6.
137. Blandy JP, Singh M. The case for a more aggressive approach to staghorn stones. *J Urol* 1976;115:505–6.
138. Vargas AD, Bragin SD, Mendez R. Staghorn calculus: its clinical presentation, complications and management. *J Urol* 1982;127:860–2.
139. Murphy LJT. *The history of urology.* Springfield, Ill: Charles C Thomas, 1972;191–271.
140. Gil-Vernet J. New concepts in removing renal calculi. *Urol Int* 1965;20:255–88.
141. Ohshima S, Ono Y, Mitsuya H. Dismembered pyelolithotomy: new procedure for removal of renal calculi. *Urology* 1981;17:22–5.
142. Smith MJV, Boyce WH. Anatrophic nephrotomy and plastic calyhaphy. *J Urol* 1968;119:521–7.
143. Wickham JEA, Coe N, Ward JP. One hundred cases of nephrolithotomy under hypothermia. *J Urol* 1974;112:702–5.
144. Turini D, Nicita G, Fiorelli C, Masini GC, Gazzarrini O. Staghorn renal stones: value of bench surgery and autotransplantation. *J Urol* 1977;118:905–1.
145. Fernando AR, Armstrong DMG, Griffiths JR, et al. Enhanced preservation of the ischemic kidney with inosine. *Lancet* 1976;1:555–7.
146. Fitzpatrick JM, Sleight MW, Braack A, Marberger M, Wickham JEA. Intrarenal access: effects on renal function and morphology. *Br J Urol* 1980;52:409–14.
147. Stage KH, Lewis S. Pre- and postoperative evaluation of renal function in patients with staghorn calculi utilizing quantitative renal scanning. *Urology* 1981;17:29–32.
148. Griffith DP, Gibson JR, Clinton CW, Musher DM. Acetohydroxamic acid: clinical studies of a urease inhibitor in patients with staghorn renal calculi. *J Urol* 1978;119:9–15.
149. Fernstrom I, Johannson B. Percutaneous pyelolithotomy: a new extraction technique. *Scand J Urol Nephrol* 1976;10:257–9.
150. Kerlan RK, Kahn RK, Laberge JM, Pogany AC, Ring EJ. Percutaneous removal of renal staghorn calculi. *AJR* 1985;145:797–801.
151. Clayman RV, Surya V, Miller RP, Castaneda-Zuniga WR, Amplatz K, Lange PH. Percutaneous nephrolithotomy: an approach to branched and staghorn renal calculi. *JAMA* 1983;250:73–5.
152. Adams GW, Oke EJ, Dunnick NR, Carson CC. Percutaneous lithotripsy of staghorn calculi. *AJR* 1985;145:803–7.
153. Young AT, Hulbert JC, Cardella JF, et al. Percutaneous nephrolithotomy: application to staghorn calculi. *AJR* 1985;145:1265–9.
154. Snyder JA, Smith AD. Staghorn calculi: percutaneous extraction versus anatrophic nephrolithotomy. *J Urol* 1986;136:351–4.
155. Lee WJ, Smith AD, Cubelli V, Vernace FM. Percutaneous nephrolithotomy: analysis of 500 consecutive cases. *Urol Radiol* 1986;8:61–6.
156. Eisenberger F, Rassweiler J, Bub P, Kallert B, Miller K. Differentiated approach to staghorn calculi using extracorporeal shock-wave lithotripsy and percutaneous nephrolithotomy: an analysis of 151 consecutive cases. *World J Urol* 1987;5:248–54.
157. Gleeson MJ, Lerner S, Griffith DP. Treatment of staghorn calculi with extracorporeal shock-wave lithotripsy and percutaneous nephrolithotomy. *Urology.* [In press].
158. Webb DR, Fitzpatrick JM. Percutaneous nephrolithotripsy: a functional and morphological study. *J Urol* 1985;134:587–91.
159. Charig CR, Webb DR, Payne SR, Wickham JEA. Comparison of treatment of renal calculi by open surgery, percutaneous nephrolithotomy and extracorporeal shock-wave lithotripsy. *Br Med J* 1986;292:879–82.
160. Lingeman JE, Saywell RM Jr, Woods JR, Newman DM. Cost analysis of extracorporeal shock-wave lithotripsy relative to other

surgical and nonsurgical treatment alternatives for urolithiasis. *Med Care* 1986;24:1151–60.

161. Chaussy C, Brendel W, Schmiedt E. Extracorporally induced destruction of kidney stones by shock waves. *Lancet* 1980; 2:1265–8.

162. Gleeson MJ, Shabsigh R, Griffith DP. Outcome of ESWL in patients with multiple renal calculi based on stone burden and location. *J Endourol* 1988;2:145–9.

163. Miller K, Hautmann R. Treatment of distal ureteral calculi with ESWL: experience with more than 100 consecutive cases. *World J Urol* 1987;5:259–61.

164. Salvini A, Faustini S, Pizzi P, Quadraccia A. Treatment of urinary bladder stone by ESWL. Presented at *4th Symposium on shock-wave lithotripsy: state-of-the-art,* Indianapolis, Ind. (Mar 5–6, 1988).

165. Rocco F, Larcher P, Caimi D, Decobelli O, Musci R, Meroni T. Treatment of renal staghorn calculi with ESWL monotherapy using the Rocco EXL catheter. Presented at *4th Symposium on shock-wave lithotripsy: state-of-the-art,* Indianapolis, Ind. (Mar 5–6, 1988).

166. Wirth MP, Frohmuller HGW. Results of primary treatment of staghorn calculi with extracorporeal shock-wave lithotripsy. Presented at *4th Symposium on shock-wave lithotripsy: state-of-the-art,* Indianapolis, Ind. (Mar 5–6, 1988).

167. Harada M, Okuda Y, Maeda H, et al. ESWL treatment of staghorn calculi and large stones. Presented at *4th Symposium on shock-wave lithotripsy: state-of-the-art,* Indianapolis, Ind. (Mar 5–6, 1988).

168. Pode D, Verstandig A, Shapiro A, Katz G, Caine M. Treatment of complete staghorn calculi by extracorporeal shock-wave lithotripsy monotherapy with special reference to internal stenting. *J Urol* 1988;140:260–5.

169. Sohn M, Deutz FJ, Rohrmann D, Fischer N, Rubben H. Anesthesia-free ESWL monotherapy with double J stents versus PCNL/ESWL combined approach in staghorn disease: a prospective randomized study. Presented at *4th Symposium on shock-wave lithotripsy: state-of-the-art,* Indianapolis, Ind. (Mar 5–6, 1988).

170. Gilhuis R, Carpentier PJ. Treatment of staghorn calculus by percutaneous lithotripsy followed by ESWL. *J Urol* 1987;137:279A.

171. Schulze H, Hertle L, Graff J, Funke PJ, Senge T. Combined treatment of branched calculi by percutaneous nephrolithotomy and extracorporeal shock-wave lithotripsy. *J Urol* 1986;135:1138–41.

172. Kahnoski RJ, Lingeman JE, Coury TA, Steele RE, Mosbaugh PG. Combined percutaneous and extracorporeal shock-wave lithotripsy for staghorn calculi: an alternative to anatrophic nephrolithotomy. *J Urol* 1986;135:679–81.

173. Lingeman JE. Results of 313 staghorn treatments. Presented at the *4th Symposium on shock-wave lithotripsy: state-of-the-art,* Indianapolis, Ind. (Mar 5–6, 1988).

174. Segura JW, Patterson DE, LeRoy AJ. Combined percutaneous ultrasonic lithotripsy and extracorporeal shock-wave lithotripsy for struvite staghorn calculi. *World J Urol* 1987;5:245–7.

175. Streem SB, Zelch MG, Risius B, Geisinger MA. Planned endourologic "sandwich" therapy for extensive staghorn calculi. *J Urol* 1987;137:705A.

176. McLeod DC, Nabata MC. Inefficiency of ascorbic acid as a urinary acidifier. *N Engl J Med* 1977;296(24):1413.

177. Hetey SK, Kleinberg ML, Parker WC, Johnson EW. Effect of ascorbic acid on urine PH in patients with injured spinal cords. *Am J Hosp Pharm* 1980;37:235–7.

178. Murphy FJ, Zehman S, Mau W. Ascorbic acid as a urinary acidifying agent. 2. Its adjunctive role in chronic urinary infection. *J Urol* 1965;94:300–3.

179. Vermeulen CW, Ragins HD, Grove WJ, Goetz R. Experimental urolithiasis. III. Prevention and dissolution of calculi by alteration of urinary pH. *J Urol* 1951;66:1–5.

180. Nielsen IM. Urolithiasis in mink: pathology, bacteriology and experimental production. *J Urol* 1956;75:602–14.

181. Cintron-Nadad E, Lespier LE, Roman-Mircuda A, Martinez-Maldonado M. Renal acidifying ability in subjects with recurrent stone formation. *J Urol* 1977;118:704–6.

182. Rector FC Jr, Seldin DW, Copenhaver JH. The mechanism of ammonia excretion during ammonium chloride acidosis. *J Clin Invest* 1955;34:20–6.

183. Froeling PGAM. Akute zuurbelastingen. In: *De Zuuruitscheiding bis de Behandeling von Mensen met Nierstenen.* 1978;93–106.

184. Pizzarelli F, Peacock M. Effect of chronic administration of ammonium sulfate on phosphatic stone recurrence. *Nephron* 1987;46:247–52.

185. Leman J Jr, Litzow JR, Lennon EJ. Studies of the mechanism by which chronic metabolic acidosis augments urinary calcium excretion in man. *J Clin Invest* 1967;46:1318–28.

186. Mahnensmith R, Thier SO, Cooke CR, Broadus A, DeFronzo RA. Effect of acute metabolic acidemia on renal electrolyte transport in man. *Metabolism* 1979;28:831–42.

187. Coe FL, Firpo JJ, Hollandsworth DL, Segil L, Canterbury JM, Reiss E. Effect of acute and chronic metabolic acidosis on serum immunoreactive parathyroid hormone in man. *Kidney Int* 1975;8:262–73.

188. Albright F, Sulkowitch HW, Chute R. Nonsurgical aspects of the kidney stone problem. *JAMA* 1939;113:2049–53.

189. Suby HI, Albright F. Dissolution of phosphatic urinary calculi by the retrograde introduction of a citrate solution containing magnesium. *N Engl J Med* 1943;228:81–91.

190. Mulvaney WP. A new solvent for certain urinary calculi: a preliminary report. *J Urol* 1959;82:546–8.

191. Cato AR, Tulloch AGS. Hypermagnesemia in a uremic patient during renal pelvis irrigation with renacidin. *J Urol* 1974; 111:313–4.

192. Brock WA, Nachtseim DA, Parsons CL. Hemiacidrin irrigation of renal pelvic calculi in patients with ileal conduit urinary diversion. *J Urol* 1980;123:345–7.

193. Dretler SP, Pfister RC, Newhouse JH. Renal stone dissolution via percutaneous nephrostomy. *N Engl J Med* 1979;300:341–3.

194. Palmer JM, Bishai MB, Mallon DS. Outpatient irrigation of the renal collecting system with 10 per cent hemiacidrin: cumulative experience of 365 days in 13 patients. *J Urol* 1987;138:262–5.

195. Higgins CC. Urinary lithiasis: experimental production and solution with clinical application and end results. *J Urol* 1936; 36:168–77.

196. McCarrison R. Causation of stone in India. *Br Med J* 1931;1:1009–15.

197. Racic J. Calculus of bladder in Dalmatia. *Urol Cutaneous Rev* 1935;39:158–63.

198. Shorr E. The possible usefulness of estrogens and aluminum hydroxide gels in the management of renal stone. *J Urol* 1945; 53:507–20.

199. Shorr E, Carter AC. Aluminum gels in the management of renal phosphatic calculi. *JAMA* 1950;144(18):1549–56.

200. Lavengood RW Jr, Marshall VF. The prevention of renal phosphatic calculi in the presence of infection by the Shorr regimen. *J Urol* 1972;108:368–71.

201. Lotz M, Zisman E, Bartter FC. Evidence for a phosphorus depletion syndrome in man. *N Engl J Med* 1968;278(8):409–15.

202. Stamey TA, ed. *Infection stones in urinary infections.* Baltimore: Williams & Wilkins, 1972;213.

203. Griffith DP, Moskowitz PA, Carlton CE Jr. Adjunctive chemotherapy of infection-induced staghorn calculi. *J Urol* 1979; 121:711–5.

204. Hamilton-Miller JMT, Brumfitt W. Methenamine and its salts as urinary tract antiseptics: variables affecting the antibacterial activity of formaldehyde, mandelic acid and hippuric acid in vitro. *Invest Urol* 1977;14:287–91.

205. Heathcote RSA. Hexamine as a urinary antiseptic. I. Its rate of hydrolysis at different hydrogen ion concentrations. II. Its antiseptic power against various bacteria in urine. *Br J Urol* 1935;7:9–32.

206. Feit RM, Fair WR. The treatment of infection stones with penicillin. *J Urol* 1979;122:592–4.

207. Musher D, Minuth J, Thorsteinsson SB, Holmes T. Effectiveness of achievable urinary concentrations of tetracyclines against "tetracycline-resistant" pathogenic bacteria. *J Infect Dis* 1975; 131(suppl):40–4.

208. Cox CE, McCabe RE, Grad C. Oral norfloxacin versus parenteral treatment of nosocomial urinary tract infections. *Am J Med* 1987;82(suppl 6B):59–64.

209. Scully BE, Neu HC, Parry MF, Mandell W. Oral ciprofloxacin

therapy of infections due to *Pseudomonas aeruginosa*. *Lancet* 1986;1:819–22.

210. Boyce WH, McKinney WM, Long TT, Drach GW. Oral administration of methylene blue to patients with renal calculi. *J Urol* 1967;97:783–9.

211. Sobel AE, Burger M. Calcification: investigation of role of chondroitin sulfate in calcifying mechanism. *Proc Soc Exp Biol Med* 1954;87:7–13.

212. Van't Riet B, McKinney WM, Brandt EA, Currey AE, Taylor DM. Dye effects on inhibition and dissolution of urinary calculi. *Invest Urol* 1964;1:446–56.

213. Kobashi K, Hase J, Uehara K. Specific inhibition of urease by hydroxamic acid. *Biochim Biophys Acta* 1962;65:380–3.

214. Kobashi K, Kumaki K, Hase J. Effect of acyl residues of hydroxamic acids on urease inhibition. *Biochim Biophys Acta* 1971; 227:429–41.

215. Dixon NE, Cassola C, Watters JJ, Blakeley RL, Zerner B. Inhibition of Jack bean urease (EC 3.5.1.5) by acetohydroxamic acid and by phosphoramide: an equivalent weight for urease. *J Am Chem Soc* 1975;97:4130–1.

216. Kobashi K, Takebe S, Numata A. Specific inhibition of urease by N-acylphosphoric triamide. *J Biochem* 1985;98:1681–8.

217. Takeuchi H, Yoshida O, Takebe S, Kobashi K, Hase J. Urease activity in infected urine: relation of stone formation. *Acta Urol Jpn* 1977;23:647–51 (in Japanese).

218. Hase J, Kobashi K, Kawaguchi N, Sakamoto K. Antimicrobial activity of hydroxamic acids. *Chem Pharm Bull* 1971;19:363–8.

219. Takebe S, Numata A, Kobashi K. Stone formation by *Ureaplasma urealyticum* in human urine and its prevention by urease inhibitors. *J Clin Microbiol* 1984;20:869–73.

220. Kenny GE. Inhibition of the growth of *Ureaplasma urealyticum* by a new urease inhibitor, flurofamide. *Yale J Biol Med* 1983;56:717–22.

221. Putcha L, Griffith DP, Feldman S. Pharmacokinetics of acetohydroxamic acid in patients with staghorn renal calculi. *Eur J Clin Pharmacol* 1985;28:439–45.

222. Putcha L, Griffith DP, Feldman S. Disposition of ^{14}C-acetohydroxamic acid and ^{14}C-acetamide in the rat. *Drug Metab Dispos* 1984;12:438–43.

223. Feldman S, Putcha L, Griffith DP. Pharmacokinetics of acetohydroxamic acid: preliminary investigations. *Invest Urol* 1978; 15:498–501.

224. Summerskill WHJ, Thorsell F, Feinberg HJ, Aldrete JS. Effects of urease inhibition in hyperammonemia: clinical and experimental studies with acetohydroxamic acid. *Gastroenterology* 1967; 54:20–6.

225. Griffith DP, Khonsari F, Skurnick JH, James KE, Osborne C. Experimental and clinical trials of lithostat (acetohydroxamic acid—AHA). In: Martelli A, Buli P, Marchesini B, eds. *Inhibitors of crystallization in renal lithiasis and their clinical application.* Acta Med 1988;229–35.

226. Takeuchi H, Yoshida O, Kobashi K, Takebe S, Hase J. Prevention of infected urinary stones by urease inhibitor. II. Urinary excretion of hydroxamic acids and prevention of infected bladder stones in rats. *Acta Urol Jpn* 1977;23:113–8 (in Japanese).

227. Fishbein WM, Carbone PD, Hochertein HD. Acetohydroxamate; bacterial urease inhibitor with therapeutic potential in hyperammonemia states. *Nature* 1965;208:46–8.

228. Summerskill WH, Thorsell F, Feinberg JH, Aldrete JS. Effects of urease inhibition in hyperammonemia; clinical and experimental studies with acetohydroxamic acid. *Gastroenterology* 1967; 54:20–6.

229. Kobashi K, Munakata K, Takebe S, Hase J. Therapy for urolithiasis by hydroxamic acids. II. Urease inhibitory potency and urinary excretion rate of hippurohydroxamic acid derivatives. *J Pharm Dyn* 1980;3:444–50.

230. Munakata K, Kobashi K, Takebe S, Hase J. Therapy for urolithiasis by hydroxamic acids. III. Urease inhibitory potency and urinary excretion rate of N-acylglycinohydroxamic acids. *J Pharm Dyn* 1980;3:451–6.

231. Griffith DP, Musher DM. Urease; principal cause of infection stones. In: Fleisch H, Robertson WG, Smith LH, Vanlensieck W, eds. *Urolithiasis Research.* New York: Plenum Press, 1976; 451–4.

232. Anderson JA. Benurestat, a urease inhibitor for the therapy of infected ureolysis. *Invest Urol* 1975;12:381–6.

233. Takeuchi H, Kobashi K, Yoshida O. Prevention of infected urinary stones in rats by urease inhibitor, a new hydroxamic acid derivative. *Invest Urol* 1980;18:102–5.

234. Kobashi K, Munakata K, Takebe S, Hase J, Takeuchi H, Yoshida O. Therapy for urolithiasis by urease inhibitor, hydroxamic acid. In: Kehl H, et al., eds. *Chemistry and hydroxamic acids.* Basel, S Karger, 1982;104–10.

235. Takeuchi H, Okuda Y, Kobashi K, Yoshida O. Treatment of infected urinary stones in rats by a new hydroxamic acid "N-(pivaroyl)glycinohydroxamic acid." *Urol Res* 1982;10:217–9.

236. Bailie NC, Osborne CA, Leininger JR, et al. Teratogenic effect of acetohydroxamic acid in clinically normal beagles. *Am J Vet Res* 1986;471(12):2604–11.

237. Williams JJ, Rodman JS, Peterson CM. A randomized double-blind study of acetohydroxamic acid in struvite nephrolithiasis. *N Engl J Med* 1984;311:760–4.

238. Griffith DP, Khonsari F, Skurnick JH, James KE. VA Cooperative Study Group. A randomized trial of acetohydroxamic acid for the treatment and prevention of infection induced urinary stones in spinal cord injury patients. *J Urol* 1988;140:318–24.

239. Griffith DP, Lee H, Lonunet R, Deman R, Earle N. Double-blind clinical trial of Lithostat (acetohydroxamic acid) in the palliative treatment of infection-induced urinary stones. [Unpublished report].

240. Martelli A, Buli P, Spatafora S. Clinical experience with low dosage of propionohydroxamic acid (PHA) in infected renal stones. *Urology* 1986;28(5):373–5.

241. Javor A, Frang D, Nagy Z. Applicability of Biosuppressin as a urease-inhibitor. *Int Urol Nephrol* 1984;16(3):191–4.

242. Rosenstein I. Therapeutic applications of urease inhibitors. *J Antimicrob Chemother* 1982;10:159–61.

243. Flippin HF. Sulfonamide concretions and calculi. In: Butt AJ, ed. *Etiologic factors in renal lithiasis.* Springfield, Ill: Charles C Thomas, 1956;151–61.

244. Clark JK, Murphy FD, Flippin HF. Absorption, excretion, and distribution of sulfamethazine in man. *J Lab Clin Med* 1943;28:1828–34.

245. Prien EL. Mechanism of renal complications in sulfonamide therapy. *N Engl J Med* 1945;232:63–8.

246. Dorfman LE, Smith JP. Sulfonamide crystalluria: a forgotten disease. *J Urol* 1970;104:482–3.

247. Flippin HF, Reinhold JG. An evaluation of sulfonamide mixtures and various adjuvants for control of sulfonamide crystalluria. *Ann Intern Med* 1946;25:433–43.

248. Asper R, Schmucki O. Critical aspects of urine and stone analysis: appearance of iatrogenic urinary calculi. *Urol Int* 1986;41:334–42.

249. Siegel WH. Unusual complication of therapy with sulfamethoxazole-trimethoprim. *J Urol* 1977;117:397.

250. Alfthan OS, Liewendahl K. Investigation of sulfonamide crystalluria in man. *Scand J Urol Nephrol* 1976;6:44–6.

251. Pruitt AW, Winkel JS, Dayton PG. Variations in the fate of triamterene. *Clin Pharmacol Ther* 1977;21(5):610–9.

252. Ettinger B, Weil E, Mandel NS, Darling S. Triamterene-induced nephrolithiasis. *Ann Intern Med* 1979;91(5):745.

253. Hollander JB. Triamterene bladder calculus. *Urology* 1987; 30:154–5.

254. Ettinger B, Oldroyd NO, Sorgel F. Triamterene nephrolithiasis. *JAMA* 1980;244(21):2443–5.

255. Guevara A, Springmann KE, Drach GW, Hillman BJ. Triamterene stones and computerized axial tomography. *Urology* 1986;27(2):104–6.

256. Lagergren C. Development of silica calculi after oral administration of magnesium trisilicate. *J Urol* 1962;87:994–6.

257. Page RC, Heffner RR, Frey A. Urinary excretion of silica in humans following oral administration of magnesium trisilicate. *Am J Dig Dis* 1941;8:13–5.

258. Levison DA, Crocker PA, Banim S, Wallace DM. Silica stones in urinary bladder. *Lancet* 1982;1:704–5.

259. Hammartsen G, Helldorf I, Magnasson W, Rieton T. Dubbelsidiga njurstenor av hiselyra efter bruk av silikathaltigt antacidum. *Sven Lahort* 1953;50:1242.

260. Joekes AM, Rose GA, Sutor J. Multiple renal silica calculi. *Br Med J* 1973;1:146–7.
261. Simmonds HA. 2,8-Dihydroxyadenine lithiasis. *Clin Chim Acta* 1986;160:103–8.
262. Manzak MJ, Frensilli FJ, Miller HC. 2,8-Dihydroxyadenine urolithiasis: report of an adult case in the United States. *J Urol* 1987;137:312–4.
263. Rose GA. Inborn errors of metabolism. In: Rose GA, ed. *Urinary stones: clinical and laboratory aspects.* Baltimore: University Park Press, 1982;215–32.
264. Nobori T, Yamanaka H, Kamatani N, Nishioka K, Mikanagi K. The prevalence of metabolic disorders in Japan (abstr). *Pediatr Res* 1985;19:767.
265. Simmonds HA, Barratt TM, Webster DR, et al. Spectrum of 2,8-dihydroxyadenine urolithiasis in complete APRT deficiency. *Adv Exp Med Biol* 1980;122A:337.
266. Nishida Y, Hirano S, Miyamoto T. A mutant adenine phosphoribosyltransferase in 2,8-dihydroxyadenine urolithiasis. *Arch Intern Med* 1986;146:2068–70.
267. Herring LC. Observations on the analysis of ten thousand urinary calculi. *J Urol* 1962;88:545–62.
268. Hesse A, Schneider H-J. Results of the standardization and centralization of stone analysis in the German Democratic Republic. In: Fleisch H, Robertson WG, Smith LH, Vahlensieck W, eds. *Urolithiasis research.* New York: Plenum Press, 1976;295–8.
269. Dent CE, Philpot GR. Xanthinuria an inborn error (or deviation) of metabolism. *Lancet* 1954;1:182–5.
270. Watts RWE. Xanthinuria and xanthine stone formation. In: Williams DI, Chisholm GD, eds. *Scientific foundations of urology,* vol 1. London: Heinemann, 1976;310–5.
271. Lutzeyer W, Hering F. Drug therapy of urinary calculi and prevention of recurrence. In: Schneider H-J, ed. *Urolithiasis: therapy-prevention.* London: Springer-Verlag, 1986;53.
272. Ayvazian JH, Skupp S. The study of purine utilization and excretion in a xanthinuric man. *J Clin Invest* 1965;44:1248–60.
273. Potter JL, Silvidi AA. Xanthine lithiasis, nephrocalcinosis, and renal failure in a leukemia patient treated with allopurinol. *Clin Chem* 1987;33(12):2314–6.
274. Brock WA, Golden J, Kaplan GW. Xanthine calculi in the Lesch-Nyhan syndrome. *J Urol* 1983;130:157–9.
275. Greene ML, Fujimoto WY, Seegmiller JE. Urinary xanthine stones: a rare complication of allopurinol therapy. *N Engl J Med* 1969;280(8):426–7.
276. Kamatani N, Sonoda T, Nishioka K. Distribution of patients with 2,8-dihydroxyadenine urolithiasis and adenine phosphoribosyltransferase deficiency in Japan. *J Urol* 1988;140:1470–2.
277. Sloand JA, Izzo JL Jr. Captopril reduces urinary cystine excretion in cystinuria. *Arch Intern Med* 1987;147:1409–12.

PART VII

Disorders of Bone

Disorders of Bone and Mineral Metabolism,
edited by Fredric L. Coe and Murray J. Favus,
© 1992 by Raven Press, Ltd. All rights reserved.

CHAPTER 37

Primary Osteoporosis

Robert Lindsay and Felicia Cosman

DEFINITION

The term *osteoporosis* refers to a group of conditions in which the mass and structure of the skeleton are altered in such a way that increases the risk of fracture. Primary osteoporosis refers to the occurrence of the condition among the aging population where a secondary predisposing condition cannot be found. Thus the primary condition includes both postmenopausal osteoporosis and osteoporosis of aging, the commonest forms of the disorder, as well as a few rare forms. Osteoporosis is a generic term used to define the reduction in mass and increased porosity of the skeleton that alters fracture risk. It is often not used until patients present with fracture, the term osteopenia being used for the preclinical state. However, this semantic distinction serves little purpose, may cause considerable confusion, and the diagnostic term for the skeletal problem should be osteoporosis, whether fracture has occurred or not.

INTRODUCTION

Osteoporosis is a common condition among the aging female population (1). In a referral clinic, more than 90% of the cases of primary osteoporosis can be expected among women over the age of 50 years. Recent data have highlighted the importance of loss of ovarian function as the principal predisposing factor that leads to bone loss and hence increased risk of fracture in this group (2). As the population ages, osteoporosis among postmenopausal women will continue to be the major clinical expression of the disorder seen by clinicians.

R. Lindsay: Department of Internal Medicine, Columbia University, College of Physicians and Surgeons, New York, New York 10032; and Regional Bone Center, Helen Hayes Hospital, West Haverstraw, New York 10993.

F. Cosman: Department of Internal Medicine, Columbia University, College of Physicians and Surgeons, New York, New York 10032; and Regional Bone Center, Helen Hayes Hospital, West Haverstraw, New York 10993.

The problem of osteoporosis is not unique to the twentieth century. Several descriptions exist of osteoporotic changes in the skeletons of individuals living in prehistoric times (3–7). Comments from Hippocrates, Paulus Aeginata (~600 AD) and others have noted conditions of the elderly that appear to be reasonable descriptions of osteoporosis (7). Studies by Armelagos and Perzigian (3,5,6) showed age-related changes in the skeletons of individuals from ancient Nubia and among North American Indians apparently starting at an age prior to menopause (8) which occurred between age 50 and 55 years even in those times (4). Osteoporotic changes were more common among Nubian women than men (4), however, much as is true in most societies today.

Throughout history, a variety of descriptions of osteoporosis can be found. The most classic is that of Sir Astley Cooper who described the bones of old age as "thin in their shell and spongy in their texture" and also pointed out the likelihood of hip fracture after modest trauma (9). In general these clinical descriptions describe the effects of the changes that can now be observed in the skeleton as age increases, that is bone mass declines with age and the reduction is more marked among women than men. The increased prevalence of osteoporosis noted in the latter half of the twentieth century is thought to result at least in part from the increased life expectancy from birth that has been so marked in this century. Therefore, the increased numbers of patients with osteoporotic fracture reflect the greater number of individuals surviving to old age, but also possibly reflect the great reduction in infant mortality that resulted in survival of more frail children, who might be expected to have prejudiced skeletons as they age, for a variety of reasons, at least some of which will be environmental rather than genetic.

Osteoporosis must be distinguished from other metabolic bone disorders, and is often a diagnosis by exclusion. In some populations the distinction between osteo-

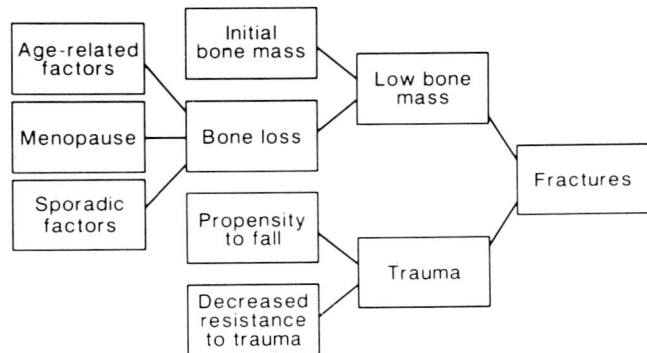

FIG. 1. Model of risk factors for osteoporotic bone loss and fractures. From Melton (10), with permission.

porosis and osteomalacia is a frequent problem and one that can only be resolved by the examination of bone biopsy material after tetracycline labeling. Not infrequently this is the case in the very elderly, especially the institutionalized elderly, who are particularly at risk of hip fracture.

Postmenopausal osteoporosis expresses itself clinically as fracture. The most common fractures are those of the spine (vertebral crush fractures), femoral neck, and distal radius (Colles' fractures), although fracture of any bone can occur (10–13). Data gathered over the past 20 years or so, since non-invasive techniques to measure bone mass have become available, have demonstrated that there is a prolonged period of asymptomatic bone loss that precedes fracture. The risk of fracture is proportional to the amount of bone present per unit volume of the skeleton and mass gives bone 80% or more of its strength (14). However, as bone tissue is lost, there are other skeletal alterations such as changes in architecture, aging of the tissue itself, and accumulation of microdamage that add to fracture risk. The combination of these changes creates a skeleton that is liable to collapse on modest or minimal injury. In most circumstances, however, there must be some traumatic skeletal injury to cause the fracture. Thus the likelihood of fracture and clinical expression of osteoporosis depends on both skeletal status (mass, architecture, and bone age) as well as the frequency of falls or other traumatic events (Fig. 1). The latter events are least frequently evident for vertebral crush fractures which often appear to occur spontaneously or with such minimal injury that the precipitating event is often not identifiable. Hip fracture, on the other hand, most commonly follows trauma, usually a fall from a standing height.

EPIDEMIOLOGY

The incidence of fractures in the population is greatest in the young and very old (10–13). Fractures that are considered to be osteoporotic are those that occur most

commonly among the older population. In all *adult* populations studied thus far, overall fracture frequency generally increases with age, although the increment varies significantly among skeletal sites and among populations. Generally in the United States, those fractures that increase with age are also more frequent among women, and result from minimal trauma. In addition to the classic fractures of vertebral bodies (crush fracture), distal radius (Colles' fracture), and proximal femur, fractures of the pelvis and proximal humerus must be included, and data suggest that other limb fractures follow a similar pattern (Fig. 2). The most classic clinical description of osteoporosis is that of Fuller Albright, who in describing the fracture syndromes, differentiated the condition from other metabolic bone disorders, and noted the high frequency of oophorectomy among his patients (15,16).

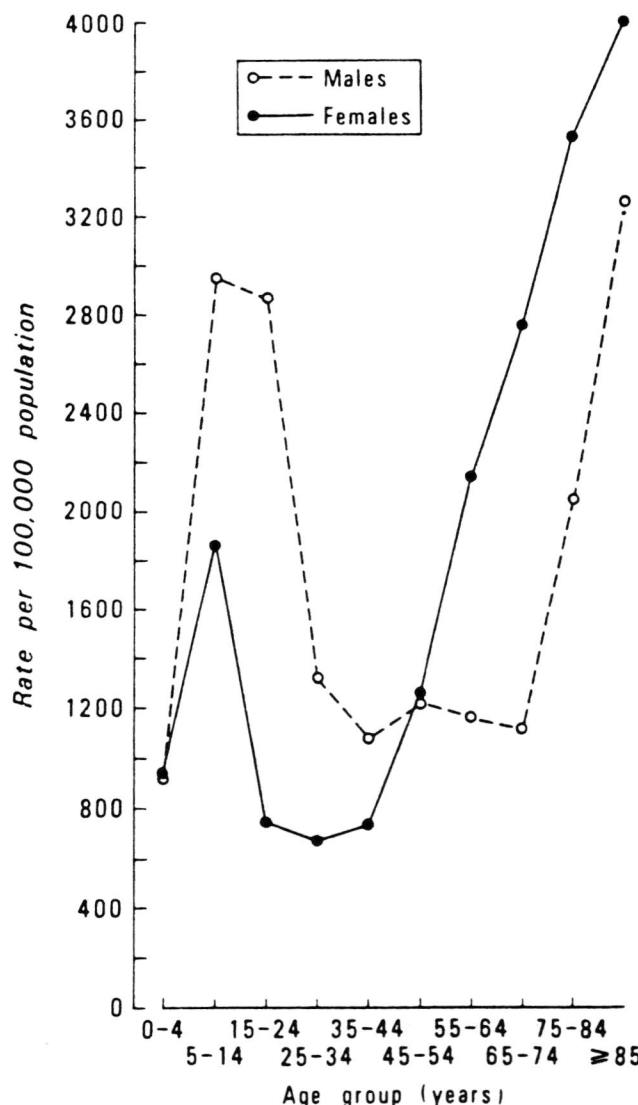

FIG. 2. Age- and sex-specific incidence of all limb fractures among the residents of Rochester, Minnesota, 1969–1971. From Garraway et al. (11), with permission.

Much of our present day understanding of the disorder is based on these skillful clinical observations of Albright, made before the availability of non-invasive techniques for bone mass quantitation.

Osteoporosis is now recognized as a major public health problem in many countries, particularly in the United States and northern Europe, with significant health care costs (Table 1). At present, at least 1.5 million osteoporotic fractures occur each year in the United States (12,13). Vertebral crush fractures are probably most common, although reliable epidemiological data about the prevalence and incidence of these fractures are difficult to find. It is estimated that more than 0.5 million such fractures occur annually in the United States, with a female to male ratio of at least 10 to 1. Hip fracture represents the most serious medical complication of osteoporosis and the one for which there is the most epidemiological data. About 300,000 fractures of the hip occur each year in the United States, mostly in individuals over the age of 70 years (10–13). At age 50 the average woman has a lifetime risk of 15% for hip fracture, and one in three of the very old will have had a hip fracture (12). Fractures of the hip are about 2–3 times as common in women as in men, although about 80% of these fractures occur in women since more women live to an older age. The current annual incidence of hip fracture in the United States is about 1 per 10,000 person years at age 40 increasing to >300 per 10,000 person years at age 85 (10) and incidence doubles with each 5 year increment after age 50.

It is common clinical experience that patients with one type of age-related fracture are more likely to suffer another. Patients presenting with hip fractures are several times more likely to have had one or more vertebral fractures, and twice as likely to have had a Colles' fracture (10,17). However, most individuals who suffer an osteoporotic fracture are, in fact, unlikely to have another osteoporotic fracture, and it is impossible to predict for any individual patient the outcome of the disorder when she presents for the first time. This heterogeneity in clinical expression of the disorder presents a major problem in the design of good clinical studies of the established disorder.

Hip Fracture

The incidence of hip fracture (Fig. 3) varies across populations, with the highest rates reported for the northern European countries and for the United States (10–13). The lowest incidence is in the Bantu although curiously they do not have markedly increased bone mass at least as measured by morphometry (18). Part of the marked variability in fracture frequency among populations may be related to inaccurate recording of fracture data, but the general conclusion from world data is that people who live in latitudes further from the equator appear to have a higher incidence of hip fracture. Further data are required to validate this. However, if it is indeed true it may, at least in part, be related to a proposed pathogenetic role for subtle alterations in the metabolism of vitamin D in osteoporosis of aging. Latitude changes may not be evident within countries, and the relationship could be spurious (Fig. 4) (760). An alternative explanation might be that fractures are related to industrialization, since there is some relationship between gross national product and fracture occurrence. Hip fracture rates are generally higher among whites than non-whites,

TABLE 1. Annual cost of fractures in the United States

DIRECT COSTS		
Hospital inpatient services	4,467,440,000	1,136,030,000
Outpatient and emergency room institutional services	88,410,000	2,530,000
Outpatient diagnostic and therapeutic services	3,200,400,000	24,650,000
Patient inpatient services	1,570,340,000	739,310,000
Physician office, outpatient, and emergency room services	356,850,000	10,220,000
Other practitioner services	211,990,000	82,450,000
Drugs	120,020,000	3,440,000
Nursing home services	4,534,520,000	4,001,930,000
Prepayments and administration	654,750,000	27,030,000
Non-health sector goods and services	2,182,500,000	900,080,000
Total direct costs	17,387,220,000	7,170,670,000
INDIRECT COSTS		
Lost earnings (wage earners)	425,960,000	9,240,000
Lost earnings (homemakers)	330,870,000	83,400,000
Total indirect costs	756,830,000	92,640,000
Total costs	18,144,050,000	7,263,340,000

From Holbrook et al. (13), with permission.

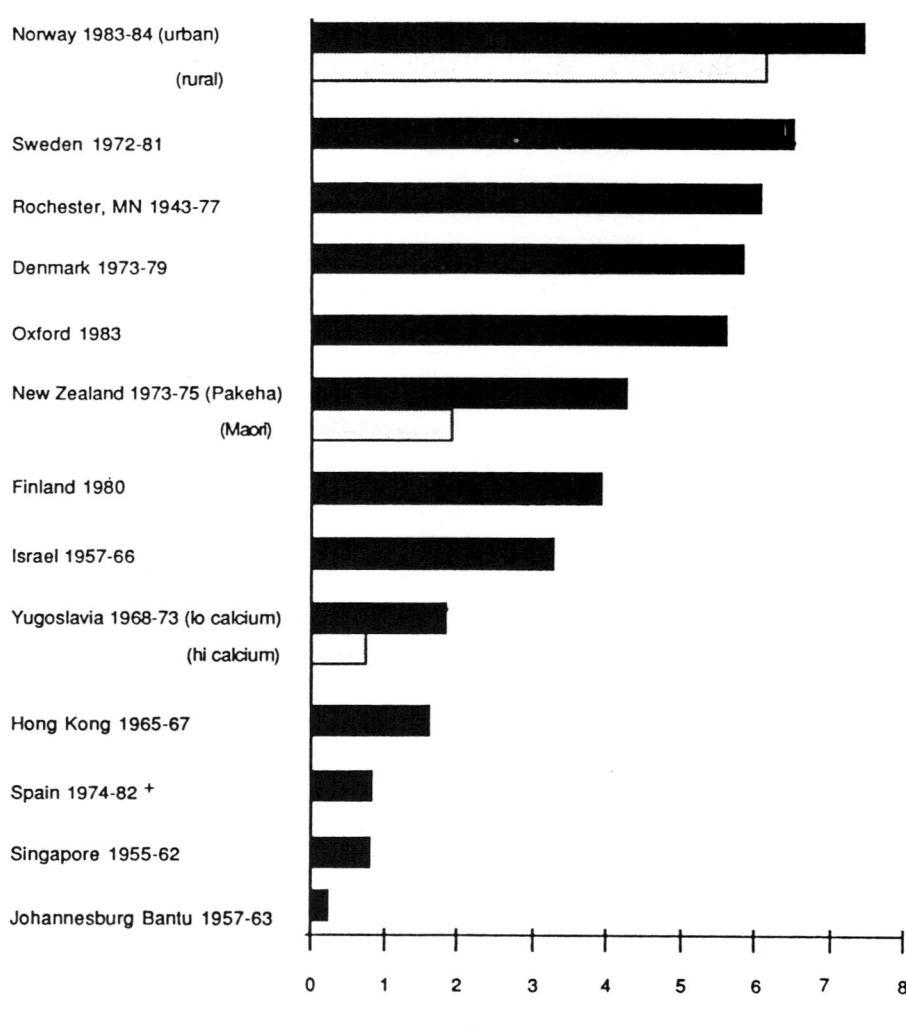

Norway 1983-84 (urban)

(rural)

Sweden 1972-81

Rochester, MN 1943-77

Denmark 1973-79

Oxford 1983

New Zealand 1973-75 (Pakeha)

(Maori)

Finland 1980

Israel 1957-66

Yugoslavia 1968-73 (lo calcium)

(hi calcium)

Hong Kong 1965-67

Spain 1974-82 +

Singapore 1955-62

Johannesburg Bantu 1957-63

Rate (per 1,000)

0 1 2 3 4 5 6 7 8

FIG. 3. Age-adjusted annual incidence of hip fractures in women over 50 years of age. +Trochanteric fractures only. *Standardized to the US population in 1986. Adapted from Melton (10), with permission.

and in almost all areas, greater among females than males (Fig. 5). The sex ratio appears to be between 2 and 3 to 1 in most studies, although among a few groups, such as the Bantu (18), and the Malay and Chinese in Singapore (19), fracture rates appear to be proportionately higher among males; in the Maori race male fracture frequency is equal to the female rate (20). Data from northern Europe have convincingly demonstrated an increase in the age-specific incidence of hip fracture (21–24), over the past several decades. Similar data have been suggested for Canada (25) and the United States (26), although in one study of fractures in Minnesota no recent secular changes in hip fracture were seen (27,28). In general, however, most studies agree that there has been an increase in the absolute number of hip fractures over time (Fig. 6). The question is whether all of that increase can be explained by an increase in the population at risk, an increase in the true prevalence of osteoporosis in the elderly, or changes in other factors such as the risk of

falls. In our data at least 50–60% of the increment in hip fracture occurrence between 1970 and 1980 could be explained by the population change (26). The remainder may represent a real increase in the age-specific occurrence of hip fracture or an increase in readmission for complications of fracture (such as secondary admission for joint replacement after initial internal fixation), since such admissions cannot easily be traced in our discharge data. Even if there is no increase in age-independent hip fracture occurrence, however, it is clear that hip fracture is currently a major public health problem that will increase over the next 50 years or so as the elderly population increases. We expect the number of hip fractures to increase from about 300,000 per year to 500,000 in the early part of next century. The acute care costs will increase from about $7 billion in 1985 dollars to $16 billion as fractures near the half million mark (29), somewhere in the early part of the next century.

In addition to the dollar cost, hip fracture extracts a

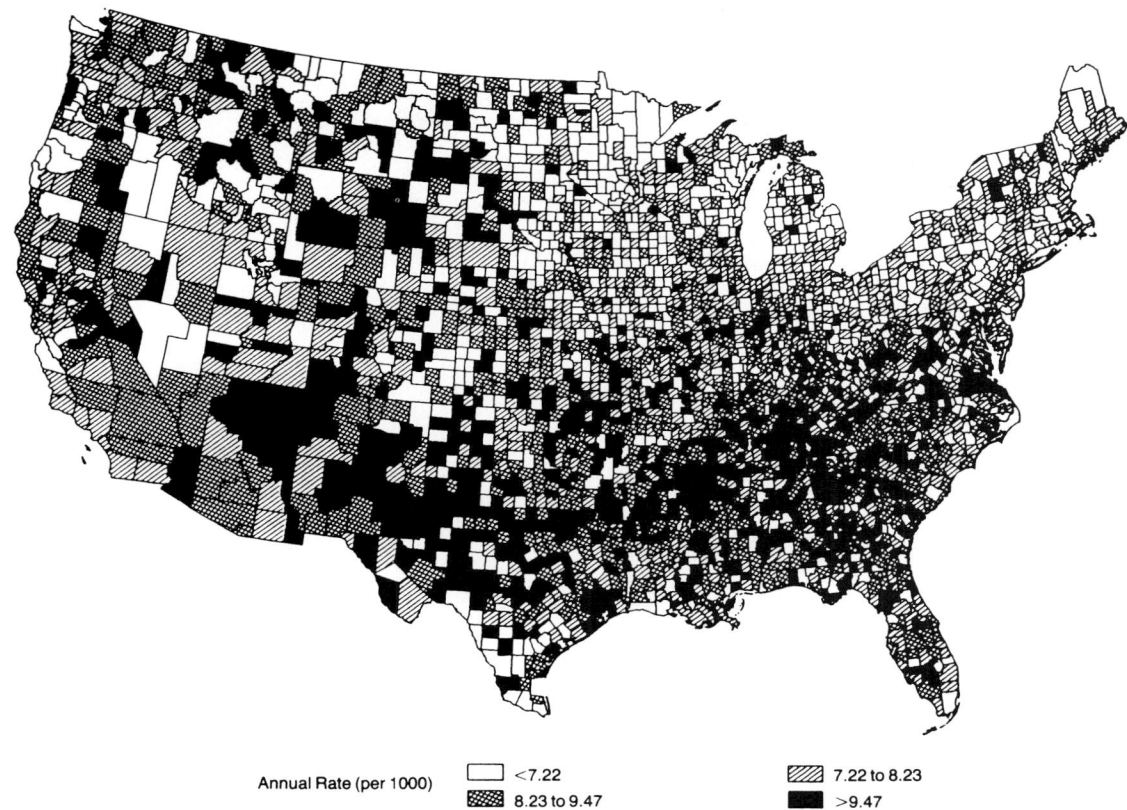

Annual Rate (per 1000) □ <7.22   ▨ 7.22 to 8.23
                        ▦ 8.23 to 9.47   ■ >9.47

FIG. 4. Age-adjusted annual incidence of hip fracture among white women aged 65 years and older by county of residence, 1984 through 1987. From Jacobsen et al. (760), with permission.

human cost from those who suffer the problem. Within the first year after hip fracture there is a death rate of 5–20% in excess of that expected in control populations of a similar age (30) (Fig. 7). Approximately one half of patients who were able to ambulate independently prior to the fracture cannot walk independently after the event, and one third become totally dependent. The recent enactment of prospective payment schedules in the United States denies rehabilitation for hip fracture, and appears to have significantly worsened the outcome (31).

Falls and Osteoporotic Hip Fracture

The majority of fractures of the hip, both intertrochanteric and femoral neck, require some degree of trauma (10–13). From most patients a history of a fall from a standing height can be elicited, although occasionally it appears as though the fracture precedes the fall. The incidence of falls increases with increasing age (Fig. 8) (32–34) and falls appear to be commoner among older women at least to age 75 years (35). After age 70

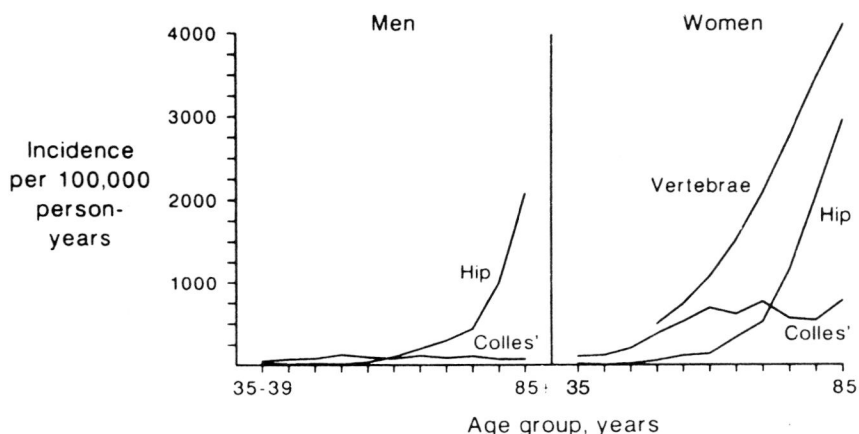

FIG. 5. Incidence of osteoporotic fractures as a function of age in men (*left*) and women (*right*). Adapted from Melton (10), with permission.

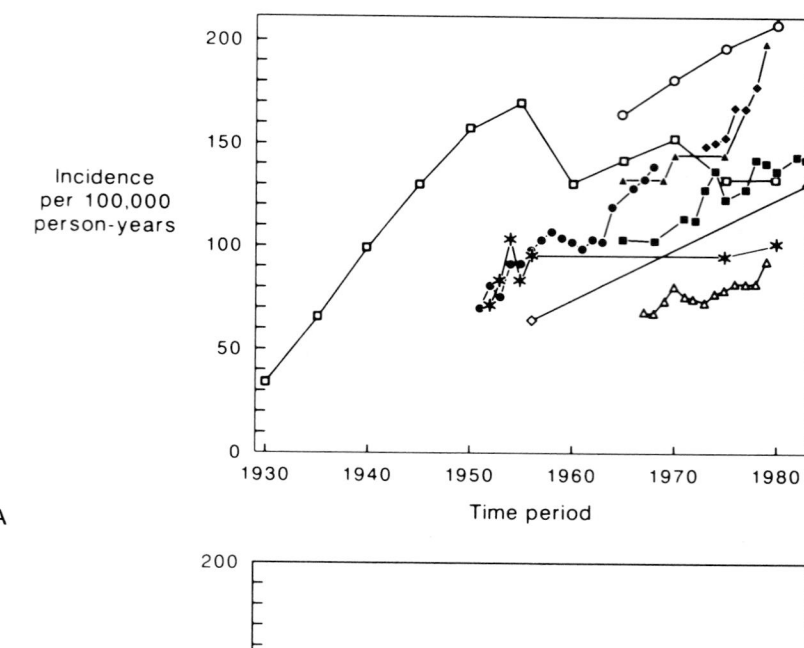

A

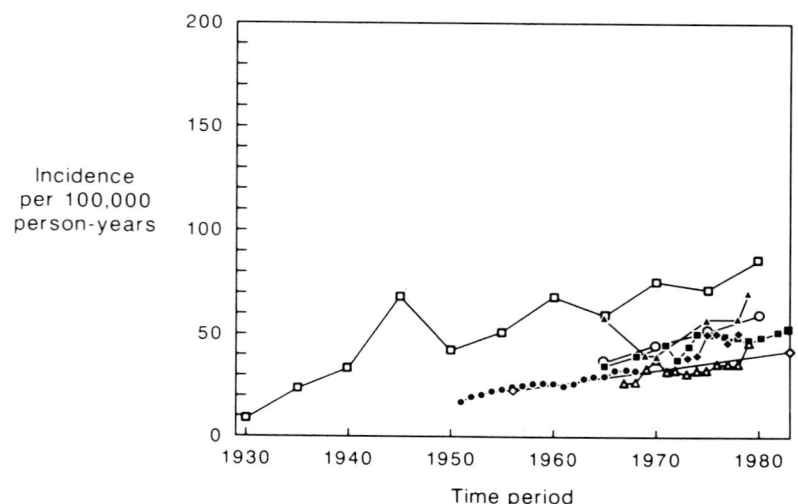

B

FIG. 6. Incidence of hip fractures as reported from various studies of women (**A**) and men (**B**). From Melton (10), with permission.

years falls occur among one person in four, and individuals who fall once have a much higher chance of falling again (36). Falls are commoner among the infirm and very elderly, groups especially at risk of hip fracture (34) and the number of falls increases per person per year with age and infirmity. It has been estimated that only 6% of falls result in fractures (33) and only 1% result in hip fracture (34). The reasons for this have been inadequately evaluated in prospective studies but probably are multifactorial. Most falls generate sufficient force even to fracture a normal hip if the hip suffers the direct impact, a rare occurrence (37). However as gait slows with age, and as balance deteriorates, the likelihood of a direct fall upon the hip increases. In addition, loss of protective reflex contraction of the gluteal muscles pulling the hip into the joint, and declining fat which could act as a cushion, may both contribute. Finally, increased use of alcohol, tranquilizing medicines (38), and confusion among the elderly (39) also contribute to increased risk of injury (33). Intrinsic and extrinsic factors that alter the risk of falling are shown in Tables 2A and 2B.

Since most hip fractures occur after a fall, the energy from the fall must be focused through the neck of the femur and not absorbed by other tissues or diverted away from this site. The fall must satisfy several criteria, therefore, before resulting in fracture. First, the patient must land on, or in the region of, the hip itself. This seems most likely to happen at slow gait speeds, or senile gait (41) which may result from neurological impairment. Syncope also produces falls more likely to impact upon the hip (34). Second, protective responses must fail. This includes using hands and arms for protection and is dependent on strength and reaction time. Next, local shock absorption must be reduced because of reduced fat or muscle mass (42). Finally, the strength of the bone must be insufficient to withstand the energy transmitted from the fall. Bone strength is related principally to mass (43) but also can be changed if quality, age, and trabecular geometry are altered (44). All of these factors change with age but to varying degrees. Models that describe the changes that occur in hip fracture frequency with age may help in understanding the relative

SURVIVAL, PER CENT

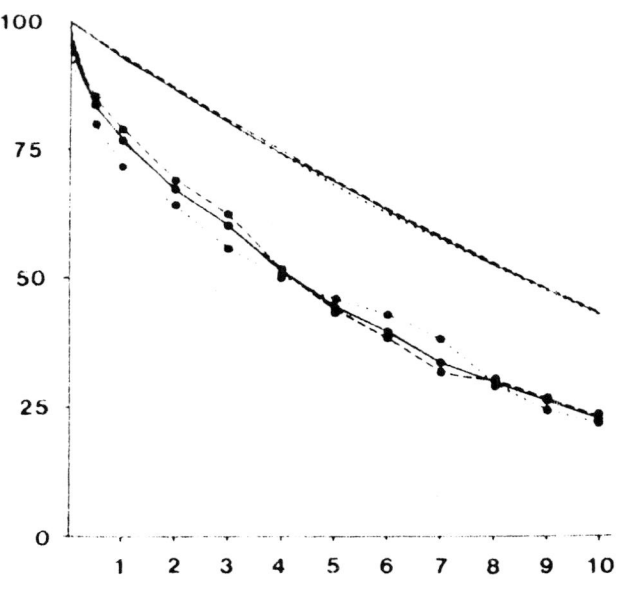

FIG. 7. Survival of all 288 patients, 207 women and 81 men, after hip fracture. Survival of the age-matched population is shown: all (---), females (– – –), and males (· · ·) as well as survival of the fracture patients: all (● — ●) females (● --- ●), and males ● · · ·●). From Elmerson et al. (767), with permission.

TABLE 2A. *Intrinsic factors altering risk of falling, among the elderly*

LONG-TERM
Neurologic disease
Parkinson's disease
Hemiparesis
Alzheimer type dementia
Cognitive Disorders
Vision
Hearing
Vestibular function
Proprioception
Musculoskeletal disorders
Muscle weakness
Slow gait (senile gait)
Medications
Sedatives, tranquilizers
Hypotensive agents
Diuretics
Anticonvulsants
Alcohol
SHORT TERM
Acute illness (or acute exacerbation of chronic illness)
Postural hypotension
Medications

proportion of fracture risk that can be ascribed to each of the changing variables (45). However, although the importance of the intrinsic skeletal changes has been questioned (46), it would appear as though low bone mass is a necessary but not sufficient cause of fracture. The data suggest a 58% fall in bone mass in the hip of women from age 20 to 90 years [30% in men (47)] without compensa-

tion, as happens at some other long bone sites, by increased width (48). Since the decline in bone mineral leads to a decline in bone strength (49–51), it is not surprising that there is a gradient of risk for hip fracture as bone mass declines (52). Mean bone density begins to fall below the point at which fracture risk begins at about

TABLE 2B. *Extrinsic factors altering risk of falling, among the elderly*

Lighting
Glare
Excessive shadows
Floors
Rug
Trailing cords
Small objects (litter)
Waxed surfaces
Stairs
Lighting
Rails
Contrasting steps
Adequate repair
Kitchen
Cupboards within reach, etc.
Bathroom
Grab bars, showers, toilets, baths
Non-skid floor on shower
Shower chair
Footwear
Form-fitting shoes
Non-skid
Outdoors
Ice, snow
Terrain uneven
Tools, etc.
Lighting

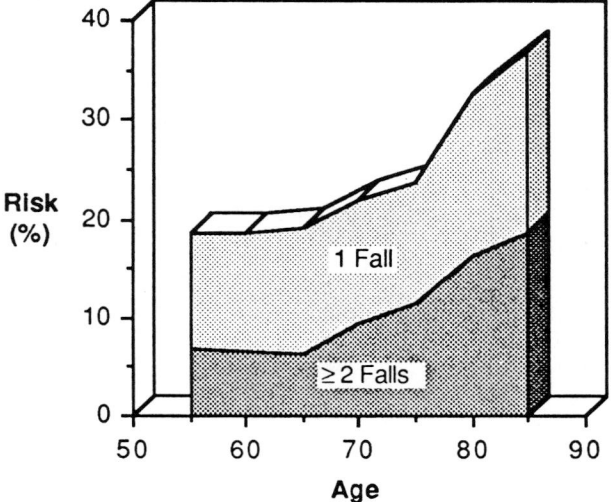

FIG. 8. Annual risk of falling, among older women. From Cummings and Nevitt (34), with permission.

age 65 years, and by age 90 years, most women will be in the "at risk" range, awaiting the sequence of events noted above.

Vertebral Fracture

Despite the morbidity and mortality of hip fracture, vertebral crush fractures are equally feared by postmenopausal women. Although these fractures are never a direct cause of mortality, their visibility among the aging female population, because of the deformity that they produce, induces this concern. Vertebral fractures are thought to be mostly asymptomatic (1,17,54) but nonetheless can result in significant acute back pain, requiring rest and adequate analgesia. Rarely are patients admitted to a hospital and thus good epidemiological data are difficult to obtain. The prevalence of vertebral fractures estimated from radiographs suggests their occurrence among a high proportion of the aging population (55). Prevalence rates vary from 15–75% for the population 70 years or older (53–55,57). Part of this variability is caused by the lack of agreement about the definition of a vertebral fracture. Complete vertebral collapse (Fig. 9) is easy to diagnose, but whether minor degrees of anterior wedging commonly seen in elderly individuals should be classified as osteoporotic fractures is not at all clear. Such changes, mostly asymptomatic, might occur gradually, produced by modeling of vertebral shape in response to increased stress and pressure at the anterior ends of vertebral bodies by virtue of gravitational forces. The erect posture and natural dorsal kyphosis might, in some individuals, be sufficient to produce changes in vertebral configuration of this type.

From cross-sectional data, it has been estimated that more than 500,000 women will have a first vertebral fracture each year (53) equivalent to an incidence rate of almost 20/1000 person years. The prevalence of vertebral fracture increases as vertebral bone mass declines exceeding 40% at bone mass levels of less than 0.6 g/cm² (1,58,59). Fracture of any bone is generally assumed to require a degree of trauma sufficient to overcome the ability of the bone to withstand the load, and declines in bone strength, therefore, are associated with reductions in the degree of trauma required for fracture. For osteoporotic vertebral fracture, a history of trauma is rarely obtained (54,60). Normal daily activities load the spine significantly. For example, during standing in the erect position, the compressive load on each vertebral body is equal to the body weight plus that exerted by ligament and muscle tension required to maintain the erect posture (61). In addition, during simple postural changes such as bending, the force exerted on the lumbar spine can be greater than body weight (62), and lifting a load in the forward bending position can exert a force many times greater than the load itself (63). The protection

against these forces is afforded by the intervertebral disc and by compression of the vertebral bodies themselves (48). Declining bone mass with age causes declining strength (64) principally due to loss of trabecular bone (65). Although the decline in strength is somewhat greater than the decline in density alone. Because the forces generated are sufficient to fracture the weakened bone, fracture risk closely follows bone mineral density (48).

Colles' Fractures

Fractures of the distal radius, of the most part consisting of those of the Colles' type, represent the third most common of the osteoporotic fractures (1,12). As with other fractures of this type, the incidence of Colles' fracture increases after the menopause. However, unlike other fractures, there is no continuous increase with age (17), and incidence plateaus after age 60 years (Fig. 5). Many hypotheses have been formulated to account for this difference between Colles' fractures and other osteoporotic fractures. Perhaps the current likely hypothesis suggests that the phenomenon is created by the changing

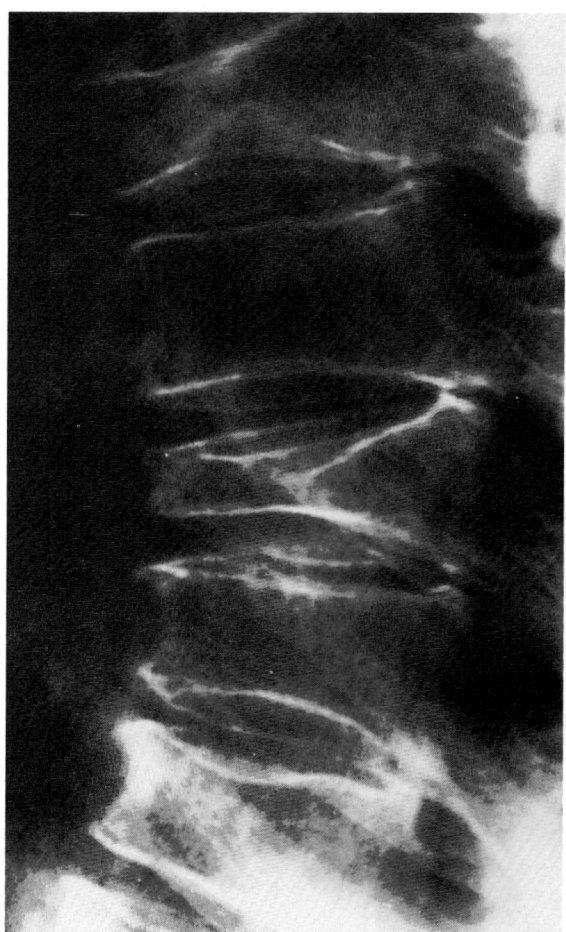

FIG. 9. Multiple vertebral deformities in a patient with osteoporosis.

gait pattern of the elderly. As gait slows, falls are less likely to occur upon the outstretched hand and more likely to involve a direct trauma to the hip (66). This remains to be confirmed. Colles' fractures do tend to be seasonal, occurring more frequently during winter, especially in the northerly and therefore icy climates (10).

Approximately 150,000–200,000 Colles' fractures occur each year in the United States. These fractures result, population wide, in only modest morbidity and no mortality, although they account for some considerable costs to the health care system. Some data suggest similar secular changes in Colles' fracture (67) although as for vertebral fracture, the data are limited.

Other Fractures

Although those are the commonest osteoporotic fractures, fractures of other bones can and do occur as primary osteoporosis is a generalized disorder of the skeleton. Most frequent are fractures of the pelvis, proximal humerus, and tibial table. Eighty-three percent and 64% of proximal humerus and pelvic fractures, respectively, occur in persons over the age of 35 years (10), while 74% and 69%, respectively, occur among women (10,68). Other age-related fractures include the ankle and distal femur (69,70).

PATHOPHYSIOLOGY

The development of non-invasive techniques to measure bone mass has enabled us to follow changes in skeletal mass that occur with age. It is now clear that bone mass in young adulthood is somewhat greater in men than in women and that difference becomes more

marked after the menopausal period (71–74). Bone mass also tends to be somewhat higher (by about 5% or so) among black women, who have about one half of the risk of white women for hip fracture (75,76). Measurements of bone mass in patients with fractures have consistently shown that this population overlaps the normal age-matched population, leading to questions about the importance of bone mass in the pathogenesis of the fracture (77–82). However, the prevalence of vertebral fracture and the incidence of hip fracture are inversely related to bone mass at the fracture site (1,10) (Fig. 10), and thus low bone mass can be used as a marker for the disorder.

Control of Peak Bone Mass

The amount of bone that is present in the skeleton at any point in life is the algebraic sum of skeletal mass accumulated during growth and consolidation (peak skeletal mass) and the subsequent alterations that take place as bone is continually remodeled throughout life. Both peak bone mass and the subsequent rate and duration of bone loss are important in determining whether skeletal status at any point in life will be sufficiently impaired to result in fracture.

Peak bone mass appears to be principally controlled by genetic factors (83–86). In studies of monovular and binovular twins, the concordance between mass measurements is greater in the monovular twins (85). Discordance increases with age after early adult life (83,86). Preliminary data suggest that peak bone mass may be modified during growth and perhaps also in the early adult years. During growth the skeleton must increase from a size of 100 gm to almost 900 gm, an increase that requires the net retention of some 150 mg per day. While

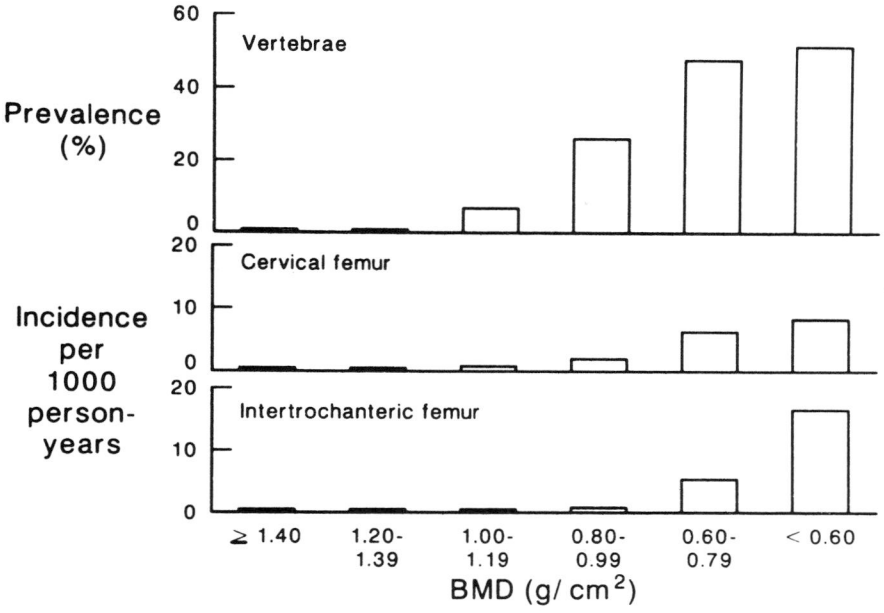

FIG. 10. Estimated prevalence of vertebral fractures by lumbar spine bone mineral density (BMD) and estimated incidence of cervical and intertrochanteric hip fractures by cervical and intertrochanteric BMD, respectively, among Rochester, Minnesota women ≥ 35 years of age. From Riggs and Melton (1), with permission.

there are only modest data on calcium homeostasis during childhood, if we assume that absorption and utilization efficiency are at least as good as during adult life, this would require an intake of at least 1000 mg per day. Nutritional calcium requirement would increase at the time of the prepubertal growth spurt to at least 1500 mg, a figure significantly greater than that achieved by many, if not all, teenagers (87). Thus, it is perhaps not surprising that preliminary data suggest that increasing calcium intake at this stage in life will positively affect peak bone mass (88). The evidence that in turn there will be a reduction in the frequency of fractures among the elderly comes from a study by Matkovic and co-workers who demonstrated a reduced age-related increment in fracture of the proximal femur with a comparatively small increase in peak bone mass thought to have been effected by a higher lifetime calcium intake (Fig. 11) (89). This study is, however, not entirely free from other confounding factors that might have positively influenced bone mass in the village noted to have a high (~980 mg/day) calcium intake. The various important factors that influence skeletal mass throughout life are demonstrated in Table 3.

It has been suggested that there is a period during early adult life when bone mass continues to increase although linear growth has ceased. The amount of bone accrual during this period, often called consolidation, is potentially modifiable, although consolidation may be a phe-

TABLE 3. *Proposed risk factors for osteoporosis*

Genetic
  Race
  Sex
  Familial prevalence
Nutritional
  Low calcium intake
  High alcohol
  High caffeine
  High sodium
  High animal protein
Lifestyle
  Cigarette use
  Low physical activity
Endocrine
  Menopausal age (oophorectomy)
  Obesity

nomenon that occurs mostly in cortical bone through periosteal apposition of new bone (90–92). Our cross-sectional data (93) suggest that in women of average age 30 years, there is a 5% advantage in bone mass if calcium intake can be maintained above 1000 mg per day and a similar increase in mass if activity levels exceed 400 kcal per day (the equivalent of a 4 mile walk). If both calcium intake and exercise level are high the total mass that can be accrued by the skeleton may be as much as 15% over that achieved when calcium intake and activity are low (i.e., normal) particularly in the vertebral bodies where activity seems to have a greater impact than nutrition.

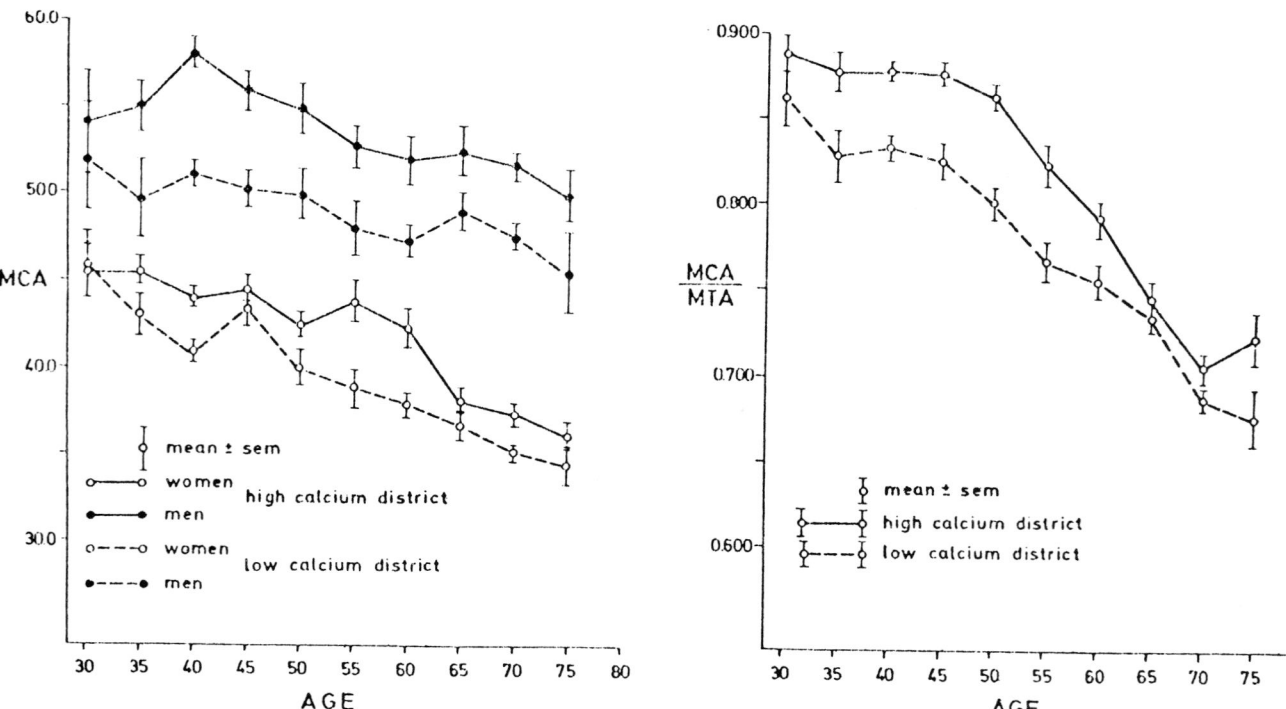

FIG. 11 A and B. **A:** Metacarpal cortical area (MCA) in women and men in both districts in relation to age. **B:** Metacarpal cortical/total area ratio (MCA/MTA) in women in both districts in relation to age. From Matkovic et al. (89), with permission.

While these data are only preliminary and clearly require confirmation with prospective data, there is abundant evidence that weight-bearing exercise is associated with increased peak bone mass (94–96).

Low bone mass in adults has been reported in a variety of situations. It has been suggested that Anglo-Saxon women have lower bone mass than women of Hispanic origin (97), and that Chinese and Japanese, whether American or Asian born have lower bone mass than caucasian Americans (97A). Low peak bone mass has also been found among American Eskimos (98,99). In this group, the reduced bone mass may be compatible with smaller body size (98), decreased calcium intake, or the high acid protein diet. High circulating levels of $1,25(OH)_2D$ with concomitantly low $24,25(OH)_2D$ have been recorded in the Eskimo population and may be due to low calcium intake (100). As we have noted, peak bone mass tends to be somewhat higher among the black female population (75,76,101–104), although the difference may in part be accounted for by differences in fat distribution between the races (75,76,103,104). Low peak bone mass is also associated with Turner's syndrome, Klinefelter's syndrome, and other chromosome abnormalities, β-thalassemia, and pseudo-pseudohypoparathyroidism (105–111). Recent studies suggest that bone mass may be lower among daughters of women presenting with osteoporosis (112,113), perhaps suggesting that there is some familial tendency to develop the disorder, as is suggested from clinical practice, where a family history of osteoporotic fracture is commonly obtained from patients presenting with their first osteoporotic fracture.

Peak bone mass can also be reduced by alterations in ovarian function and several studies have demonstrated reduced bone mass in women with amenorrhea from a variety of causes (Fig. 12) (114–124). Thus, both hypothalamic amenorrhea of exercise and the reduced ovarian function found in hyperprolactinemia result in low bone mass (124). Two groups have reported an increase in vertebral bone mass after previously amenorrheic runners have resumed ovarian activity (125,126) usually by reducing the training program with an accompanying increase in weight. Amenorrhea occurs also in anorexia nervosa and results in low bone mass (127) and we have seen severe osteonecrosis of the hip in a young adult ballet dancer with anorexia nervosa (128).

The Role of the Menopause

From around the end of the fourth decade of life there is a gradual, continuous loss of bone mass, particularly among women, that continues until late in life. This appears to be a universal process that has been found in all populations studied thus far (1). The capability of measuring bone mass using non-invasive techniques has

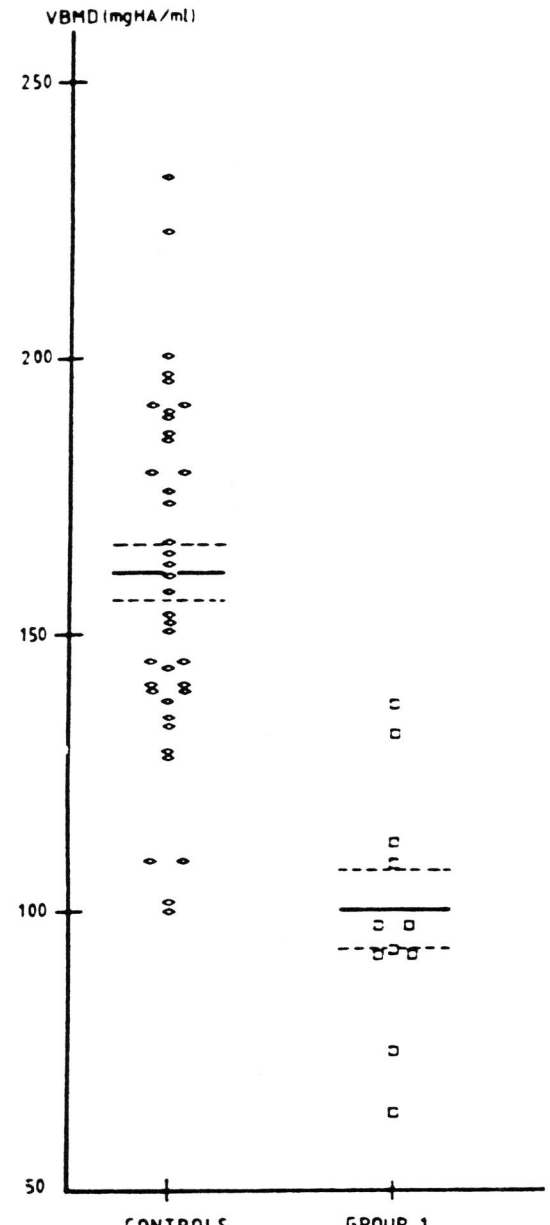

FIG. 12. Vertebral bone mineral density (VBMD) assessed by quantitative CT in 39 healthy controls and 22 women with primary ovarian failure. Controls are represented as lozenges, patients without estrogen replacement (group 1) as squares. Horizontal lines represent mean ± standard error of the mean values in each group.

proven to be a powerful tool in examining this essentially asymptomatic process. Our early studies of this phenomenon demonstrated that the important factor in determining the rate of bone loss appeared not to be age, but loss of ovarian function (129). Within just 2–3 years of surgery, women who had bilateral oophorectomy had significantly less bone than women of the same age who still had adequate ovarian function after hysterectomy alone (Fig. 13). More recent studies have confirmed

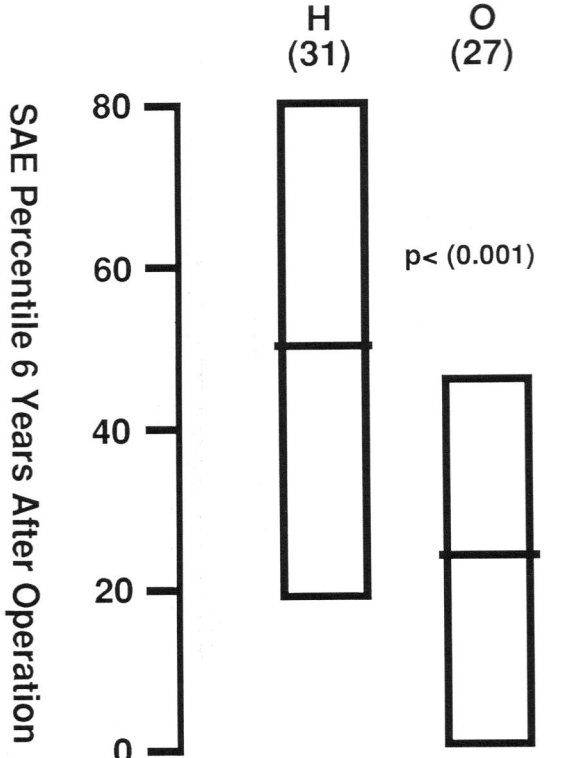

FIG. 13. Bone mass in ovariectomized individuals three years after surgical procedure. Bone mass is measured by radiographic absorptiometry (SAE percentile) and ovariectomized (O) women are compared with hysterectomized (H) women who still have ongoing ovarian function. From Aitken et al. (129), with permission.

these findings and demonstrated that the cancellous bone of vertebral bodies appears to be particularly sensitive to declining sex hormone production, with bone loss beginning earlier and being most rapid at that site (130). In one elegant study designed to differentiate the effects of age from those of ovarian failure, mean bone mass at three skeletal sites was examined in women aged 50 and 70 years (131). Both groups had suffered ovarian failure 20 years previously, the former having had bilateral oophorectomy at the average age of 30 while the latter had gone through a normal menopause at the expected average age of 50. The decrement in bone mass from the mean young normal figure was similar in both groups when measured in the spine, hip, or radius, suggesting that indeed the time spent without ovarian function, 20 years for both groups, was more important than chronological age.

Recent data have suggested that there is significant loss of bone among premenopausal women (47). The rate of loss is less than among women immediately after the menopause, and appears to be associated with declining ovarian activity. In prospective data reductions in circulating estradiol below mean values of 110 pg/mL and 40 pg/mL are associated with bone loss in the mid-

shaft and distal radius, respectively (130). Among postmenopausal or oophorectomized women we demonstrated that the rate of loss is dependent on the remaining endogenous estrogen supply (Fig. 14) (132), data that have been confirmed by others (Fig. 15) (389). In these circumstances when the range of estradiol values is relatively restricted, the relationship between rate of loss and estradiol, is perhaps not unexpectedly, relatively weak. Moreover, single measurements of estrogen levels among postmenopausal women do not adequately represent the ongoing level of estrogen supply, and thus are not by themselves insufficiently predictive of rate of bone loss to be useful clinically.

Using the calcium balance technique coupled with kinetic studies using calcium isotopes, Heaney, in an elegant series of studies, demonstrated clearly that the efficiency of intestinal calcium absorption declines across menopause. He also showed an increase in urinary calcium loss, revealing an overall reduced efficiency in the use of dietary calcium (87,133–135). The data indicate that these changes in external calcium balance are accompanied by an increased transfer of calcium into and out of bone. It is possible to deduce what might be the primary event from analysis of the probable physiologic consequences (Fig. 16). For example, if the primary defect is increased loss of calcium from the kidney, producing a "calcium drain," this would be expected to improve the efficiency of calcium absorption across the intestine as well as to increase mobilization of calcium from bone. Using this deductive process, one is left with the conclusion that the increased calcium transport into and out of the skeleton must be the primary change that occurs after estrogen deficiency. Recent evidence that bone is a target tissue for estrogens supports this concept. Putative receptors for estrogens have been demonstrated

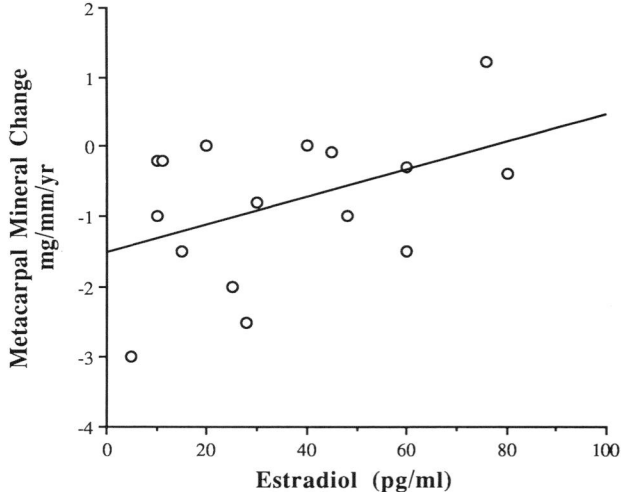

FIG. 14. The relationship of change in skeletal mass to circulating estradiol levels. From Lindsay et al. (132), with permission.

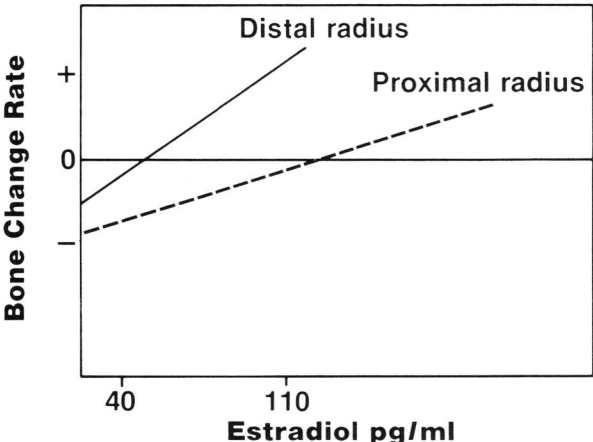

FIG. 15. The changes in bone mass and circulating estradiol levels in perimenopausal women. After Slemenda et al. (389).

in cells of the osteoblast lineage (136,137), and physiological responses to bone cells in vitro have been found in response to application of 17 β-estradiol in doses equivalent to those found in premenopausal cycling women (137,139–142).

The loss of bone mass that occurs after the reduction in ovarian function is relatively rapid and in excess of the decline in skeletal muscle mass that occurs with age (143,769) (Fig. 17). Immediately following cessation of overt evidence of ovarian activity the rate of bone loss may be as rapid as 5% per year or more in trabecular bone and 1–2% per year in cortical bone (129,144–152), the rates being somewhat greater with quantitative computed tomography (QCT) than by dual photon absorptiometry (DPA). Cross-sectional data suggest that bone loss follows an exponential function, gradually slowing to a basal rate in most individuals that continues into very old age (51,52), although this requires confirmation by longitudinal data. It is still not clear if patients likely to develop osteoporosis continue to lose bone at a more rapid rate for a longer time period

(153). It is also not clear whether or not other of the so-called risk factors can influence either the rate or the duration of accelerated bone loss after menopause. The evidence tends to suggest that loss of ovarian steroids is an overwhelming offence to the skeleton, that cannot be overcome by the lifestyle and nutritional factors that are normally thought of as important in the development of osteoporosis.

As we have noted previously, other situations in which there is reduction in the circulating concentrations of ovarian hormones, are also associated with low bone mass, including, for example, amenorrhea induced by exercise (114–121), anorexia nervosa, or hyperprolactinemia (122–124), and Turner's syndrome (105–107). It is logical to expect that, if the stimulus to increased bone remodeling is indeed loss of sex steroids, then similar alterations in skeletal metabolism would be expected, irrespective of the cause of ovarian insufficiency or the age of onset. Osteoporosis occurs commonly in association with Turner's syndrome and can be associated with severe vertebral collapse, hip fracture, and protrusion acetabulae (105,106,154). Cortical thickness appears to be reduced even before puberty, suggesting that the reduction in bone mass might be part of the genetic syndrome as well as secondary to estrogen deficiency (107). It is also possible that these patients are relatively sex hormone deficient during childhood and that this accounts for the early evidence of skeletal changes. Skeletal maturation is delayed in Turner's syndrome and that may itself account for the reduced mineral content in young adults with the disorder. Iliac crest biopsy from patients with Turner's syndrome suggests increased skeletal remodeling, and increased alkaline phosphatase levels have been reported (154). Elite female athletes, especially runners, have a high incidence of hypothalamic amenorrhea, with consequent circulating estradiol levels in the postmenopausal range (155). Several studies have now demonstrated significant reduction in skeletal mineral in these athletes when compared to normally men-

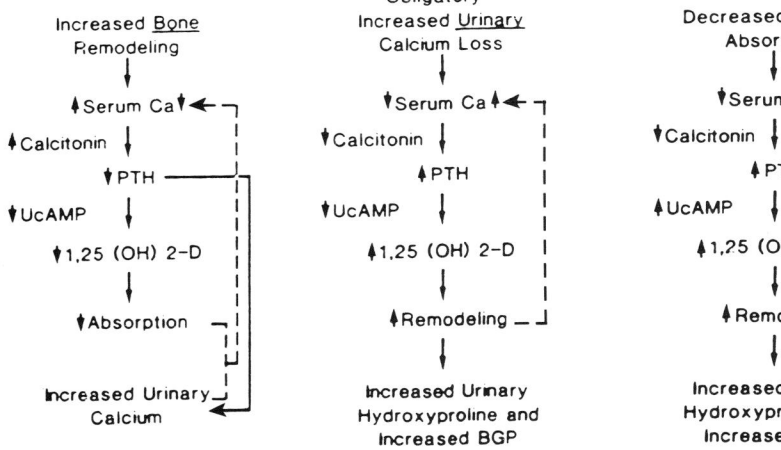

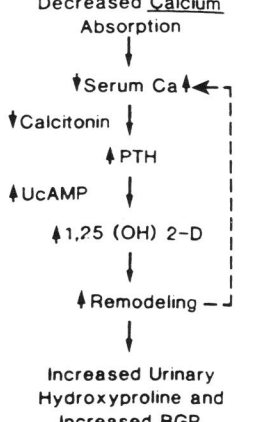

FIG. 16. Postulated impairments in hormonal control of calcium metabolism which might occur after menopause and account for the observed changes in mineral and skeletal homeostasis. From Avioli and Lindsay (404), with permission.

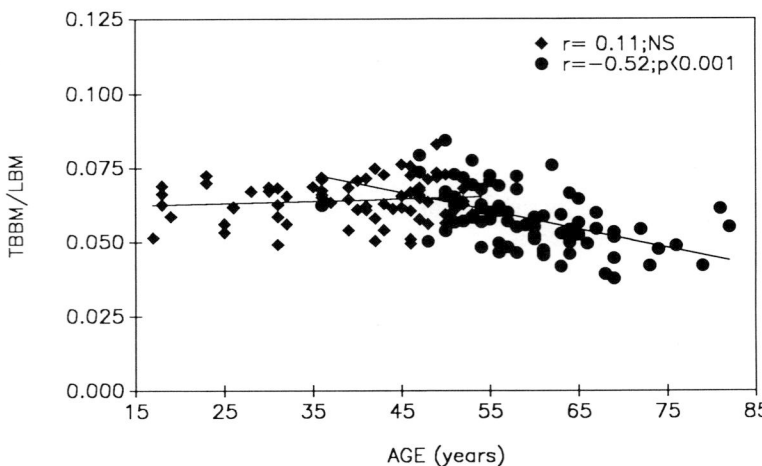

FIG. 17. Changes in the proportion of lean body mass occupied by the skeleton (TBBM/LBM) in pre- (♦) and postmenopausal (●) women with age. From Lindsay and Cosman (769).

struating women exercising to a similar extent (Fig. 12), or even sedentary controls (114–121). The majority of the data are cross-sectional, however, and do not exclude the possibility that those who are of lightest frame (and lowest bone mass) are the very athletes most predisposed to amenorrhea. The more recent demonstration that the return of menses is associated with small but significant increases in bone mass tends, however, to support the argument that it is loss of ovarian function that is the determinant. Loss of bone mass resulting from a prolonged period of amenorrhea may not be completely regained (155), especially once individual remodeling units have been completed (v.i.) Hyperprolactinemia when associated with amenorrhea is also accompanied by reductions in bone mass (122–124). The mere presence of high circulating levels of prolactin alone, in the presence of normal ovarian function, does not appear to influence skeletal mass (124). Anorexia nervosa and bulimia are also associated with reduced bone mass (127), although the situation is confounded by the primary eating disorder. It should be noted that athletic amenorrhea is also often associated with nutritional aberrations that may negatively affect the skeleton. These aberrations are not characteristically seen in hyperprolactinemic amenorrhea, however. Periods of menstrual disturbance (both oligomenorrhea and amenorrhea) are, therefore, risk factors for low bone mass prior to overt menopause. In contrast, the use of estrogen containing oral contraceptives tends to be associated with a small but significant increase in bone mass in some (156) but not all studies (158,159).

Bone Remodeling and Bone Loss

The quantum concept of bone remodeling is described in detail in Chapter 15 of this volume. It is important to consider bone loss in terms of the remodeling cycle since this is the major cellular process by which bone is resorbed and replaced in the adult (Fig. 18). The changes that occur with age and estrogen deficiency can be accounted for in terms of perturbations of the remodeling cycle (161–163).

In the young adult, it is proposed that in each remodeling unit, the amount of newly synthesized bone is equal to the quantity of bone resorbed by each team of osteoclasts. As age progresses, localized imbalances appear within each remodeling cycle, such that the amount of bone resorbed is now greater than the quantity with which it is replaced, particularly on the endosteal surface of cortical bone and in cancellous bone (162,163). These changes could result from an increase in resorption depth, a decrease in the volume of new bone formed, or a combination of both. Once this local imbalance has been created at the level of the bone remodeling unit, the overall or total body rate of bone loss is controlled principally by the frequency with which new remodeling cycles are activated (164). The evidence available, to date, tends to

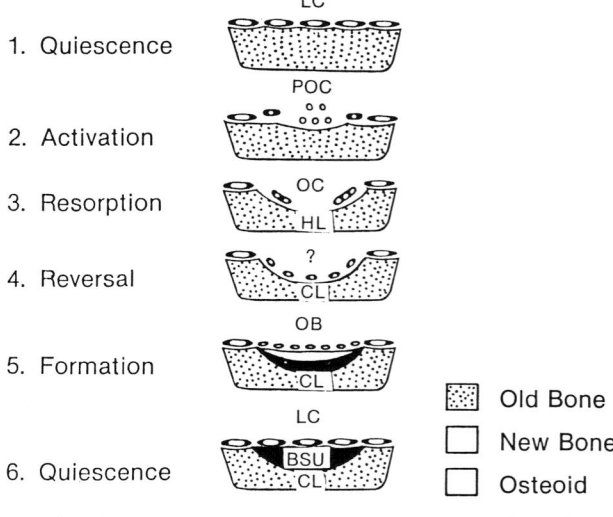

FIG. 18. Normal bone remodeling. From Parfitt (160).

suggest that estrogen deficiency increases both the activation frequency and the local imbalance between resorption and formation (161,164,165), confirming the data obtained by kinetic studies of calcium homeostasis at menopause (133–135).

Biopsy data on normal pre- and postmenopausal women are available (166–169) but the data are too limited for us to be dogmatic about the exact cellular changes that occur across the menopause. Increased activation frequency by itself given remodeling imbalance could result in the loss of complete trabecular elements, the specific pathologic lesion within cancellous bone (161). However, the rapidity of postmenopausal bone loss suggests that further factors must be at work. Two possibilities exist. The first is the noted decline in wall thickness in aging individuals (166,169,170) and presumably therefore a decline in the work performed by teams of osteoblasts. Adjusted appositional rate declines with age (166,171) implying slower work rate for osteoblast teams. However, recent data confirm that trabecular thickness does not decline with age in postmenopausal women (166,172,173). Alteration in wall thickness cannot be responsible for the decline in trabecular number, without evidence of global thinning of trabeculae. Thus, the decline in wall thickness in this scenario can only increase the amount of unremodeled bone (174) which might by itself decrease the mechanical strength (175). The second hypothesis proposes increased avidity of osteoclasts, the so-called "killer osteoclasts" (161). This phenomenon has not been observed directly in humans, but reconstruction of the complete remodeling sequence suggests that it might occur (165). Our observations of trabecular structures in the scanning electron microscope support the view that such a phenomenon might be responsible for perforation of trabecular plates, conversion of these to rods, and finally loss of the rods (176). In this situation, one could speculate that the loss of stress on the disconnected trabecula creates a form of localized disuse osteoporosis in which complete elimination of the trabecula rapidly occurs (Fig. 19). A somewhat similar phenomenon has been observed in a primate model of osteoporosis (161). Bone loss would, therefore, be driven principally by increased activation frequency following estrogen deprivation and thereby increased likelihood of trabecular penetration on a random basis. This process would then be exacerbated by the local "disuse" phenomenon, accounting for the phenomenon of loss of trabecular structures without global thinning of trabeculae seen in female fracture patients (173).

An understanding of skeletal remodeling status is important in the decision about therapy for osteoporotic patients. The status of the skeleton may well be considerably different when the patient presents after fracture, than in the immediate postmenopausal stage. In the latter there may be increased activation of remodeling, with

perhaps evidence for increased osteoclast activity. Antiresorptive agents, or agents which reduce activation frequency, such as estrogen (164) will prevent further loss of bone mass. However, in patients with established disease, there is a more marked variability of all histologic findings. In younger patients, usually presenting with vertebral fractures, there is a predominant deficit in cancellous bone (177). In these patients, marked variability in turnover status of the remaining cancellous bone has also been reported based on histological appearances (178). In this study, 31% of patients with vertebral osteoporosis had increased eroded surfaces and abnormally extended osteoid surface, and the authors considered these patients to have increased remodeling rates. These findings have been confirmed by others (179,180). However, these findings are not specific for true increased remodeling based on increased activation frequency. In the original study (178) 21% of patients were found to have increased activation rates, while 25% had prolonged formation periods (resulting from a reduction in the rate of synthesis of new osteoid presumably due to impaired function of osteoblast teams). In the majority of these patients, no histological abnormalities of remodeling could be demonstrated and others have found only a few patients with true increased turnover (181,182). In general, reduced activation frequency, and inefficient osteoblast teams are the dominant findings. The latter contributes to a decline in trabecular thickness and relates closely to overall bone loss in osteoporosis (172). In addition, the slower rate of turnover tends to increase the age of the residual bone (173) which must be a determinant of fatigue failure (175).

In addition, the correlations seen in normal individuals between biochemical indices of bone remodeling and histological parameters demonstrate the increase in coupled remodeling after menopause (174). Among patients with osteoporosis, these correlations are lost, and there is an increase in the amount of eroded surface, but no increase in osteoclast number (175,176) suggesting a delay in the onset of bone formation after completion of resorption. Estimation of resorption rate (which is done indirectly from formation rate) is thus reduced, and especially so in trabecular bone (185). Thus the generalization is true that patients with clinical fracture syndromes have evidence of low, or low-normal turnover on biopsy, but with significant heterogeneity in the population.

The specific mechanisms controlling the rate of bone loss among postmenopausal women are not clear. In general bone mass is lost at a rate that is greater than the loss of lean body mass, and it is presumed that this excess loss is estrogen dependent. As noted earlier, the recent demonstration of estrogen receptors within the skeleton provided the first evidence of a direct effect of sex steroids on bone cells (136,137). Data from in vitro studies have subsequently demonstrated physiological responses of these cells to appropriate concentrations of 17-β-estra-

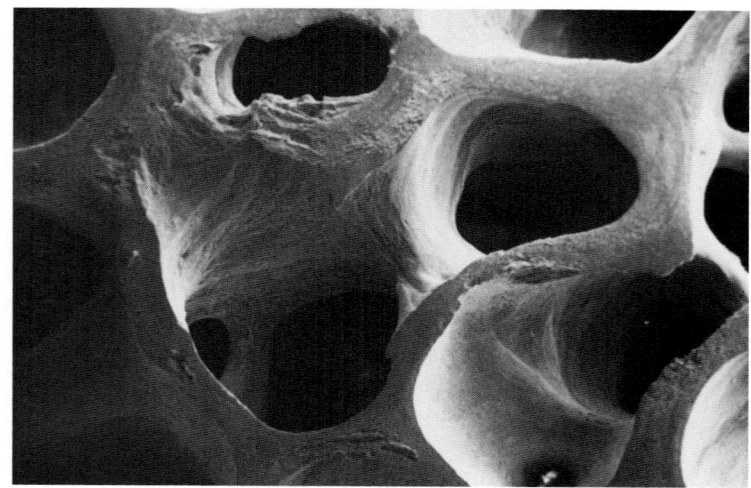

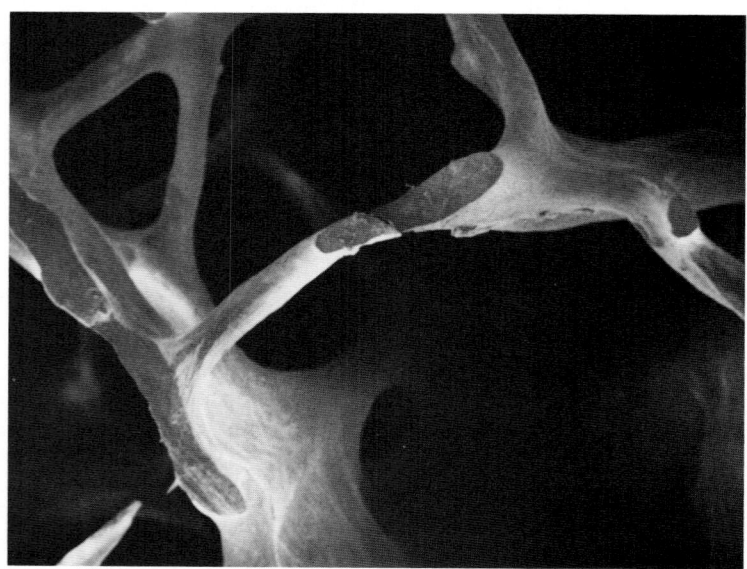

FIG. 19. Scanning electron micrographs of normal and osteoporotic cancellous bone. Normal cancellous bone has trabecular plates interconnecting with small regular marrow spaces (**A**). As bone is lost the trabeculae are penetrated, become rod-like and eventually are completely resorbed (**B**). All stages of this process can be observed. From Dempster et al. (176).

diol (138–142). Estrogen stimulates the production of a variety of growth factors including TGF-β, IGF-1, and IGF-2 (141,142). In addition factors that are known stimulants of bone resorption have been found to be increased in situations of estrogen deprivation (184,185). In particular, monocyte production of interleukin-1 appears to be increased in osteoporotic women and in women after menopause (184,186) and is suppressed by estrogen therapy (186) although not all the data agree (187). In addition prostaglandin E, a potent stimulator of bone resorption (188) is increased after oophorectomy in rats (185). Thus several potential mechanisms exist within bone to account for the changes in bone remodeling that occur across the menopause.

Some considerable time prior to the discovery of mechanisms of estrogen action within bone, Heaney proposed that estrogens decreased the sensitivity of the skeleton to PTH (189). Indeed this may well be the net effect since

PTH and prostaglandins act synergistically within the skeleton, as do PTH and interleukin-1 (190).

Other mechanisms for the interaction between estrogen deficiency and bone loss have been proposed and are not excluded by the presence of receptors within the skeleton. Some studies have shown that estrogens can stimulate circulating levels of calcitonin in postmenopausal women (191–193), although again there are disagreements (194). Calcitonin is a potent inhibitor of osteoclast function (195) and estrogen can also be shown in vitro to stimulate release of calcitonin from medullary cells (196). It is tempting to speculate that the increased loss of bone that occurs with estrogen deficiency may in part be related to a decline in calcitonin production which some studies do find after menopause or in osteoporosis (197–201). Parathyroid hormone secretion also appears to be under control of estrogen, at least in vitro (202,203) but not in vivo (204,205) although this has not been tested rigorously as yet. In hyperparathyroidism estrogen treatment does not cause an increase in circulating PTH (206,207). The relevance of the in vitro data is therefore in question. Other potential mechanisms for estrogen action on the skeleton include alterations in growth hormone and insulin-like growth factors. Growth hormone levels in response to stimuli are modified by menopause and estrogen (208), and as noted above estrogens are stimulants for production of insulin-like growth factors in bone (141,142) and potential exists, as yet unexamined, for a role for this axis in the pathogenesis of postmenopausal bone loss (209).

Other Factors Influencing Bone Loss

Riggs and Melton have proposed a metabolic defect that might provide a mechanism for bone loss occurring in both sexes with advancing age (Fig. 20) (210). In this hypothesis, it is proposed that the primary event is a reduced capacity of the kidney to synthesis and secrete the active metabolite of vitamin D, 1,25(OH)$_2$D, in response to appropriate stimuli. This is presumably caused by an age-related decline in the 1α-hydroxylase activity. In an attempt to maintain adequate circulating concentrations of 1,25(OH)$_2$D for physiological functions, it is further proposed that there must be increases in PTH secretion to compensate for the flagging hydroxylase. The increments in PTH, it is argued, would cause increases in bone remodeling and loss of skeletal tissue.

The concept has some attractive features. Serum 1,25(OH)$_2$D levels have been reported in some (211,212), but not all (213,214) studies to decline with age. When renal function is maintained there may be little decline in circulating 1,25(OH)$_2$D with age at least until the age of 65 years (215). Further, PTH immunoreactivity increases with age (215–219), and bioactivity seems to behave similarly (219). In a proportion of patients with osteoporosis PTH levels may be increased (216).

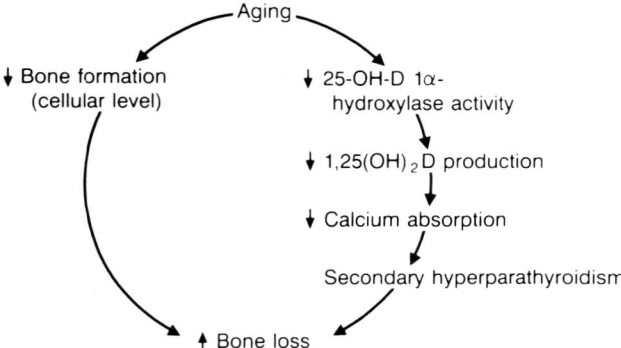

FIG. 20. Type II osteoporosis, "senile." From Riggs and Melton (1), with permission.

Testing the responsivity of the 1-α hydroxylase has produced somewhat conflicting results. In general the response of the enzyme to stimulation by infusion of PTH declines with age, but without clear evidence of a more marked reduction in response in patients with osteoporosis (212,220). It is also not entirely clear if modifications in the PTH-vitamin D relationships can be produced by estrogen or estrogen withdrawal (221–223). Suppression of 1-α-hydroxylase activity, following administration of phosphate occurs more readily in osteoporotic women than in age-matched controls (224), and it was suggested recently that exaggeration of the PTH increase following phosphate loading was a mechanism by which this suppressibility of the renal enzyme could be overcome in normal aging women (225), something that seems unlikely on basic physiological principles. Thus the precise etiological role of abnormalities in the PTH-vitamin D system, which almost certainly do occur with age in at least some individuals, in the phenomenon of aging bone loss still remain undecided.

Calcium

It is not surprising that skeletal status is equated with calcium nutrition, since 99% of the calcium in the body is stored within the skeleton. The issue remains, however, controversial (226–228) and perhaps no other issue in this field is so polarized. It is clear, and probably not disputed by anyone, that calcium deficiency at the low extreme of intake causes bone loss and osteoporosis. There are considerable animal data that indicate that a low calcium diet results in loss of bone mass in adult cats and dogs, growing rats, and in monkeys (229–234). Although the histology of the bone is similar, the relevance of this disorder to the human syndrome of osteoporosis is not decided.

Since maintenance of serum calcium is of vital importance, it is simple economics that when intake is less than output the difference has to come from body stores. The dilemma lies in identification of the state of deficiency for any individual. Average calcium intake in the United States was estimated during the 1970s to be around 500 mg with around 25% of individuals consuming less than 300 mg (Fig. 21) (235). The estimated intake averaged across a large number of studies suggests that to achieve calcium balance a range of 830–1700 mg with a mean of 1040 mg would be required (236,237). Thus average intake is less than requirement for the majority of individuals and requirement is more than the Recommended Daily Allowance (RDA) of 800 mg and even slightly greater than the United States Recommended Dietary Allowance (U.S. RDA) of 1000 mg.

Considerable epidemiological data have been accumulated seeking to evaluate the relationship between cal-

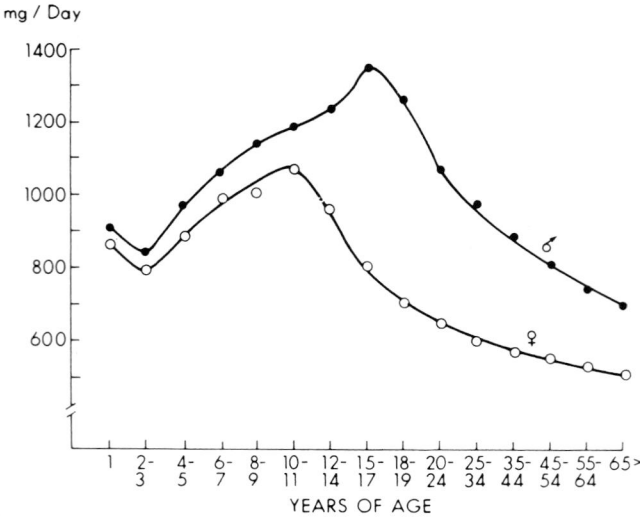

FIG. 21. Mean calcium intakes of men and women in the United States National Health Survey from 1971 to 1974. From ref. 235.

cium intake and bone health with mixed results. Garn was unable to detect any influence of current calcium intake on bone mass in young or elderly subjects (238), and the same author found similar rates of bone loss in different countries despite a broad range of calcium intakes (239). However, these data are confounded by racial differences, and in another evaluation of prevalence of osteoporosis in Finland where calcium intake is greater than 1200 mg/day the prevalence of osteoporotic fractures was the lowest of the 12 countries studied (237). Within country, studies are equally conflicting. Swiss investigators could find no relationship between skeletal status and calcium intake (240), while in the United States a weak but positive relationship was found between calcium intake and bone mass in the Ten-State Nutrition Survey (241). The most famous of the epidemiological data are those of Matkovic and co-workers (Fig. 11) who were able to demonstrate increased bone mass in young adults from a village in Yugoslavia with high calcium intake (~940 mg) in comparison to a village with low calcium intake (~450 mg). The difference, already present at age 30 years persisted into old age and although age-related bone loss occurred in both populations, the higher intake group had a reduced prevalence of hip fracture (89). It is possible that the effects of increased calcium intake are most evident during growth when the demands of the skeleton are much greater than in adult life. This would be particularly true during the growth spurt at puberty, when increased calcium intake might influence peak skeletal mass (88,93,242).

Calcium absorption declines with age, in addition to the decline across the menopause noted above (211,243,244). In part this may be related to the decline in supply of 1,25(OH)$_2$D also noted above, but also may be related to increased resistance of the intestine to the

action of 1,25(OH)$_2$D (245). At this time, calcium intake also declines (237), in part perhaps due to the increased incidence of lactose intolerance among the elderly and the avoidance of dairy products (246,247). However, even in this age group some data support the concept that a high calcium intake may reduce the subsequent risk of fractures. In one study in the United States a reduction in fracture risk was demonstrated among elderly men with the highest calcium intake (248), although another British study could not find an effect (249).

Studies of calcium intervention have produced equally varied results. For the most part these have been undertaken in perimenopausal or immediately postmenopausal women in whom data indicate that the rate of bone loss is independent of calcium intake (250,251). In view of the dominant effect of estrogen lack on bone loss, not unexpectedly the consensus of these studies in postmenopausal women is that there are in general modest effects (if any) on the rate of cortical bone loss but no effect on cancellous bone loss (252–258).

Several reasons exist as to why there are conflicting data about calcium. First, it seems unlikely that calcium is completely irrelevant. It is more likely that investigators have been searching for an effect that will occur only in a segment of the population that they are examining. If not all women being studied are calcium deficient, then any effect observed in those who are will be diluted by the lack of effect in those who are not. The relationship between calcium and osteoporosis can be considered to be similar to the relationship between iron and anemia. Deficiency of the mineral causes the disorder; but not all types of the disorder are caused by mineral deficiency. Thus treatment of all anemias with iron would lead to variable results dependent on the proportion of patients included who had true iron deficiency as the cause of their anemia. This is the case with all trials of calcium conducted thus far. The problem is created because unlike the situation with iron there is no readily available test for calcium deficiency. Calcium absorption is highly variable (Fig. 22; 259) and cannot be tested clinically in most centers. This wide variability leads to vastly different requirements for calcium among individuals (Fig. 23; 259) with, of necessity, significant and variable numbers of calcium-replete individuals included in studies.

In an attempt to overcome these problems with conflicting data the 1984 Consensus Development Conference sponsored by the National Institutes of Health (260) recommended a calcium intake of 1000 mg/day for premenopausal women increasing to 1500 mg/day for estrogen-deficient women. In 1987 the recommendations were modified somewhat to indicate 1500 mg/day only for those considered at high risk of osteoporosis. These intakes are generally safe, can be achieved by dietary modification in most individuals, and if not a modest calcium supplement will suffice.

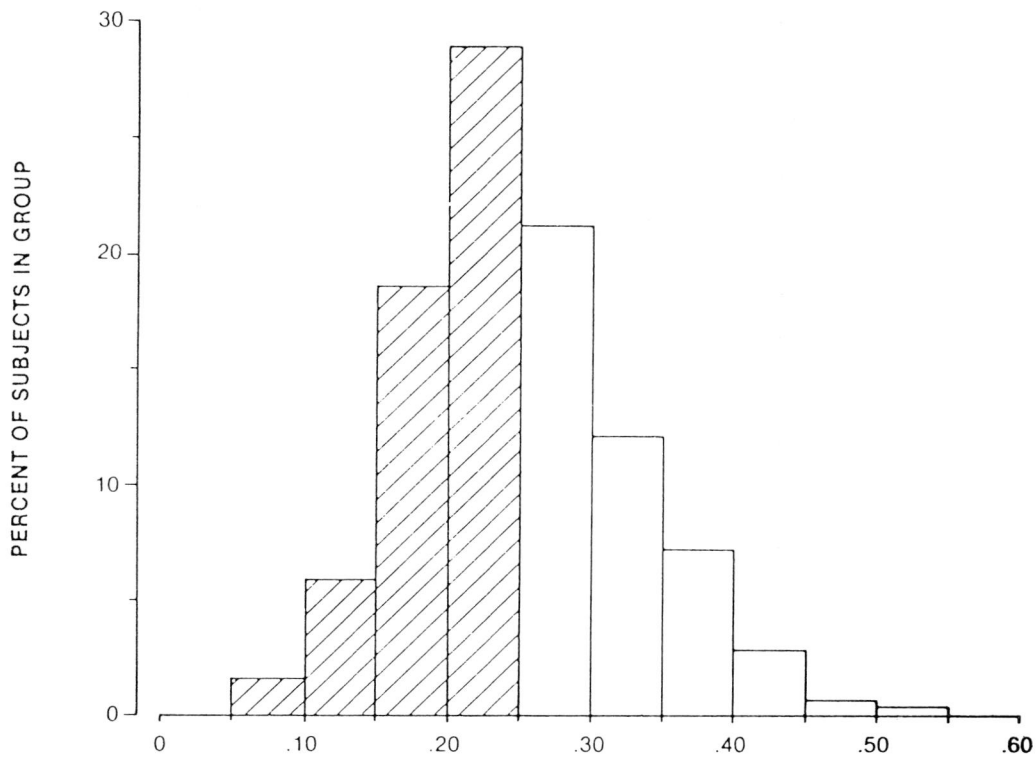

FIG. 22. Fractional calcium absorption in perimenopausal women corrected to an intake of 800 mg/day. From ref 259.

Other Dietary Factors

For the most part other dietary factors are likely to modify risk of osteoporosis by interacting or interfering with calcium utilization (261). In general it goes almost

without saying that good nutrition is as important for skeletal integrity as for any other organ system. Wide deviations such as protein malnutrition, and starvation including anorexia nervosa have marked detrimental effects on bone (127,262–266). The importance of dietary

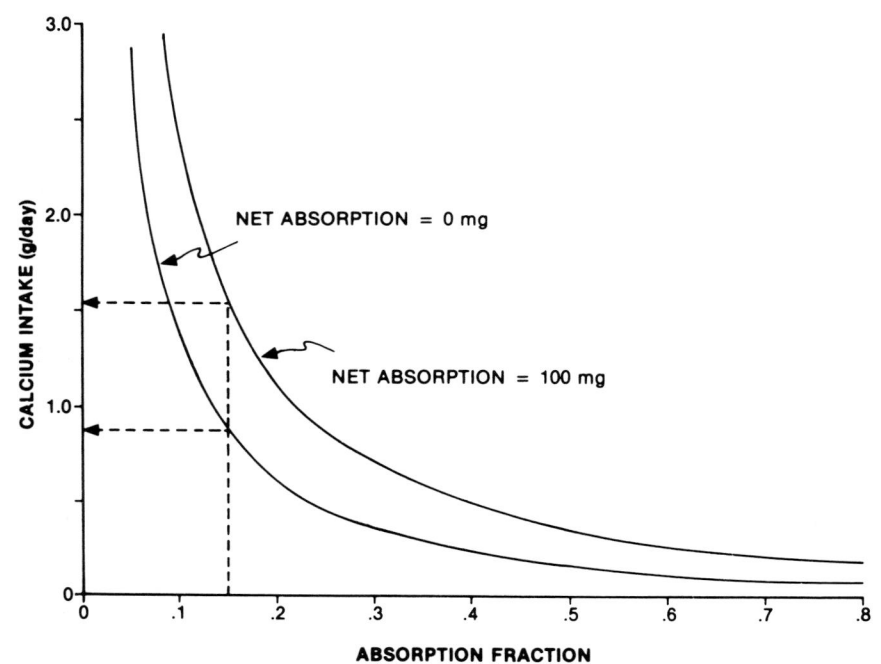

FIG. 23. Calcium intake required to produce specified net absorption at different absorptive efficiencies. From ref. 259.

variation within normal practice is more difficult to document. An excessive intake of protein, particularly animal protein which provides an acid load has received some recent popularity. Administration of protein or amino acid mixtures with high sulfate contents to normal adults causes calciuria (237,267–271). There are, however, no studies linking fracture and protein intake within the normal ranges of intake, although a high protein intake is one possible explanation of the relatively high rates of cortical bone loss found among Eskimos (272).

Phosphate administration causes secondary hyperparathyroidism (224,272), but the effect is short-lived and phosphorus intake does not seem to influence skeletal homeostasis within normal ranges of intake although the use of phosphorus-containing antacids at low calcium intakes may be deleterious (237,273). There is also the possibility among the elderly that with modest nutritional intakes phosphate deficiency might occur, particularly if calcium intake is maintained at a relatively high level. Since low serum phosphate stimulates bone resorption (274) this might exacerbate other causes of bone loss among the elderly. Excess caffeine intake may have some detrimental effect on calcium balance (267,275), but again within normal ranges of intake long-term effects on bone have not been studied. Osteoporotic individuals do have relatively high intakes of caffeine (275). In rats caffeine does not influence skeletal remodeling at ranges of intake similar to those found among adults (768).

Perhaps of more importance is the role of alcohol. The abuse of alcohol clearly increases the risk of osteoporosis for both sexes (276–279). In severely affected alcoholics, the loss of protein intake contributes to the specific toxic effects of ethanol (279–281) which can depress osteoblast function and reduce bone formation (281). Sodium has marked effects on urine calcium which are complex, but in general increasing sodium intake increases calcium excretion (282,283) and increases $1,25(OH)_2D$ production (284). The fasting excretion of sodium increases in estrogen deficiency along with the increased urinary calcium (285). Effects of sodium on bone mass and fracture have not been studied. Similarly the effects of other minor nutrients and trace metals which have been only reported in observational studies remain unknown. These include zinc (286,287), vitamin B_{12} and folate (286), boron (288), silicon (289), and vitamin C (290). Fluoride deserves special mention in view of its disputed role in treatment. In two studies that have examined the effects of high intakes from natural sources divergent results have been reported (291,292). It is therefore not clear if fluoride supplementation in drinking water can affect skeletal health in a positive fashion. Excess fluoride ingestion causes fluorosis, a painful condition associated with extra-osseous calcification and brittle bones (293).

Physical Activity

Mechanical activity is clearly an important stimulus to the skeleton. It has been known for some time that disuse, immobilization, or denervation paralysis resulted in bone loss (294–308). Somewhat similar loss of skeletal tissue was observed during prolonged spaceflight (309–313), although the magnitude was significantly less and loss was most evident in the os calcis. However, the deficit was not completely recouped upon return to earth (314). The effects of complete bed rest, on the other hand, can be extremely severe and rapid. A loss of 0.9% per week has been documented by dual photon absorptiometry (306), with even greater rates of loss recorded among immobilized adolescent girls with scoliosis (315). In most circumstances the loss is self-limiting when about 30% of skeletal mass has been lost (300,316).

In contrast, prolonged excessive physical activity is associated with increased bone mass (317–323). In these mostly cross-sectional evaluations athletes competing in a wide variety of sports can be found to have significantly greater bone mass in the commonly used limbs than either controls or in the limbs not required for that particular sport. The response generally appears to be related to the magnitude of the stress. Ex vivo data suggest that the dose response for the effects of physical stress on bone formation is steep at low levels of stress but may be much flatter at higher stress magnitudes or rates (324–327). Since load bearing is one function of the skeleton, it is perhaps not surprising that the skeleton can adapt to increases in functional load bearing by increasing its capacity (327). Thus while generally genetic factors must establish the general shape and size of the skeleton, if external stresses are applied in addition, it is reasonable to expect the skeleton of the young individual at least to respond by increasing in mass. Thus relationships between indicators of activity and bone mass can be found in young individuals (93,328–332). Among premenopausal women these relationships are critically dependent on maintenance of normal ovarian function (114–121).

Prospective data are important to allow determination of that portion of the increment in peak skeletal mass related primarily to the activity. In other words, do heavy-boned individuals self select exercise? In one recent prospective study of weight-lifting among premenopausal women an increment of only 0.81% in spinal mineral was achieved after one year (333). This in itself would be insufficient to significantly improve peak skeletal mass unless maintained over a long period. Moreover that study demonstrated the greatest drawback to the use of activity since there was a 49% dropout rate in the exercise group over the year despite inducements, this being a typical figure of most exercise programs (334).

More studies have been conducted among postmenopausal women or in men to determine if intervention with exercise can reduce the rate of bone loss (335–344). The results of these have been mixed at best, although there do appear to be some small effects that occur only in the specific regions of the skeleton involved in the activity. Confounding factors in some studies undoubtedly have been the seasonal changes in calcium homeostasis and bone mass seen in localities with specific seasons (345–347). It appears on balance that some beneficial effects can be achieved and exercise should be encouraged for its general effects on health.

The mechanism of the effects of activity on the skeleton are obscure. Since the response of the skeleton is to the strain which is applied, it appears likely that a local mechanism is involved. It is plausible that stress applied to a skeletal site produces a local electrical signal, in particular, streaming potentials (348), which could create alkaline conditions at the cathode in favor of new bone formation (349). It has also been suggested that release of prostaglandins locally may mediate the stress effect (350–351). The exercise effects on IGF production (329,352) and the effects on vitamin D metabolism (353) are other possible more general mediators of the exercise effects on the skeleton.

CLINICAL CHARACTERISTICS

Occasionally the patient presents to the physician after a fracture, often a vertebral crush fracture (Fig. 9). The symptoms may include sudden onset of severe lancing back pain that is worse on movement and relieved by rest. The pain may be sufficiently severe to cause breathlessness, pallor, nausea and vomiting, which exacerbate the problem as does coughing or sneezing. In the acute phase, tenderness may be elicited over the affected vertebrae. The pain often radiates laterally following a dermatomal distribution, and is accompanied in many patients with severe spasms of the paraspinal muscles. Clinical examination confirms the locality of the pain and the fracture. There is loss of lumbar lordosis if the lower thoracic or the lumbar vertebrae are involved. The patient is uncomfortable in most positions and is stiff, with difficulty in getting to sitting posture. Mild to moderate kyphosis may be observed especially if the patient has had previous fractures. This acute pain gradually subsides within 2–6 weeks.

In contrast to this acute picture, the majority (~80% or more) of vertebral crush fractures cause no pain and are discovered incidentally on routine radiographs, often of the chest. The reasons why pain is a prominent accompaniment of these fractures in some individuals and not in others is not clear. Many patients are referred for evaluation after a radiograph reveals the deformities. Others seek medical care when they or a relative becomes concerned about loss of height or kyphosis, both outcomes of multiple vertebral fractures. Increasingly,

however, physicians are seeing asymptomatic patients, prior to vertebral fracture, seeking advice about their risk of contracting the disorder. Commonly, these are young or middle-aged women, some of whom have a family history of the disorder. Others may have read about the disorder in the popular press, while many are perimenopausal women who wish to make a decision about the necessity for preventive therapy. Rarely do we see patients after a fracture of the distal radius referred for assessment of osteoporosis. The reasons for this are not clear. Patients who are seen after surgical intervention for hip fracture are often at a late stage in the disorder, are significantly older than other groups, and have different requirements for evaluation and therapy.

The acute pain from vertebral crush fracture lasts from several days to 2–6 weeks and may initially require bed rest, analgesics, and antispasmodics. We prefer to mobilize patients as early as possible, and the use of a spinal support or water environment (therapeutic pool) is often helpful. After about 10–14 days, pain may be completely gone or the patient left with modest or moderate back pain. As soon as is feasible, the patient should be weaned from narcotic analgesia, antispasmodics, and the spinal support. At this stage the use of alternative modalities for pain relief, including transcutaneous nerve stimulation (TENS), hot packs, and ultrasound are often helpful. Calcitonin therapy may also have a therapeutic role in pain relief (vi).

Spinal osteoporosis not presenting as an acute fracture is often accompanied with a chronic dull low back ache, elicited by history. The pain may be throbbing in nature and is often difficult to localize accurately. It may radiate laterally and mimic the pain of nerve root compression, although in osteoporosis it is probably referred periosteal pain. It is difficult to explain why some patients have pain as a prominent feature of their disorder while others have no pain despite similar skeletal status. In part, this may be explained by chronically aching muscles extended abnormally around the kyphotic deformity. Thoracic kyphosis changes the center of gravity, partially compensated for by increased lumbar lordosis. Both of these may be related to muscular and ligamental strain which produces back pain.

Physical examination should include measurements of height, weight, and arm span (which is a rough estimate of original height in young adult life). Complete examination of the back should be performed to evaluate the degree of spinal deformity, and other overt lesions. The examination should be performed in good light with the patient undressed, and standing erect. The examiner should determine symmetry, locate and palpate the spinous processes and paraspinal muscles to evaluate both deformity and pain. Mobility of the spine should be tested in all six directions (flexion, extension, bending to left and right and rotation to both sides). Neurological examination should also be performed, including position sense, and the cremasteric and bulbocavernosus reflexes. Gait should be evaluated by asking the patient to walk at a normal pace across the room and back. A general systemic examination should also be performed. Height loss can be demonstrated by measuring pubis to crown and pubis to heal. The latter remains one half of the arm span while the former is reduced.

Progressive vertebral fractures lead to downward angulation of the ribs. Eventually the 12th rib comes to rest on the iliac crest as the gap between the ribs and the ilium gradually narrows. Patients may complain of pain or discomfort as the ribs rub across the crest during breathing or motion. The reduction in lumbar height reduces the size of the abdominal cavity and abdominal protrusion, distension, constipation, and eructation become common symptoms. Prominent horizontal skin creases can be seen across the abdomen. In severely affected patients pseudospondylolisthetic abnormalities with a forward pelvic tilt, hamstring contractures, hip joint flexion, and pronated feet are characteristic. The gait is shuffling, unsteady and slow, and chronic low back pain is a major problem.

DIFFERENTIAL DIAGNOSIS

As osteoporosis usually presents with back pain, deformity, or asymptomatic fractures the differential diagnosis is that of these presenting symptoms. Kyphosis, the usual deformity, is usually of gradual onset, occurring later in life. Younger individuals present often with more rapidly developing kyphosis that must be distinguished from juvenile kyphosis or Scheuermann's syndrome, which may also predispose to osteoporosis. In both cases pain may or may not be a feature. Kyphosis may also be congenital, occur after trauma or radiation, or in inflammatory disease of the spine (e.g., ankylosing spondylitis). Other disorders that may present with kyphosis include osteomalacia, tumors, osteogenesis imperfecta, skeletal dysplasias, and collagen disorders (Marie-Strümpell disease).

Multiple vertebral fractures can present without pain, but pain when present can mimic spinal conditions other than osteoporosis. Osteomalacia is commonly associated with more severe longstanding pain than osteoporosis, and there is often marked bony tenderness. Malignancies, including multiple myeloma, can be difficult to distinguish especially in their early stages. All other causes of chronic low back pain must be excluded by history, physical examination, or radiological evaluation. Occasionally patients with persistent low back pain without an obvious etiology may be labeled as osteoporotic on the basis of radiological "thinning" of the bone. However, the presence of pain secondary to osteoporosis in the absence of vertebral fractures is questionable. More often in the absence of fracture, back pain is associated with other causes such as osteoarthritis, degenerative disc disease, spondylolisthesis, or enthesopathy.

When the differential diagnosis is in doubt or osteomalacia is considered a possibility, a bone biopsy, usually at the ilial site following tetracycline labeling, should be performed. Quantitative histomorphometric evaluation of nondecalcified sections should be performed (see Chapter 21).

In addition to these non-osteoporotic disorders it is important to determine the presence of conditions that may cause secondary osteoporosis or exacerbate the primary condition. Information on history and physical examination should seek to elicit symptoms and signs of Cushing's syndrome, intestinal malabsorption, renal stone disease, renal dysfunction, thyrotoxicosis, liver disease, major surgery particularly gastrointestinal, rheumatoid arthritis, and alcohol and cigarette consumption. A complete drug history should be obtained including specifically the use of diuretics, thyroid replacement, steroids, anticonvulsants, and vitamin supplements.

Dietary evaluation should be performed to obtain an estimate of calcium intake, and in addition to be used as a base for dietary advice in discussing treatment options. In practice we use dietary evaluation also as a base upon which to broaden the discussion to those other disorders of aging, particularly cardiovascular disease, which are affected by nutrition.

LABORATORY INVESTIGATION

In general laboratory tests are used to assist in the differential diagnosis, since most results in patients with postmenopausal osteoporosis are within the normal range. Baseline investigations include automated biochemistry and hematology, and 24 h urinary calcium and creatinine. In most individuals, particularly the elderly, we also routinely evaluate thyroid function and perform protein electrophoresis in serum and urine. Cortisol is only measured when there is a clinical reason to suspect Cushing's syndrome, and estrogen levels are not measured in postmenopausal patients since the commercial assays are generally not sensitive enough to evaluate circulating estradiol levels of less than 20–40 pg/mL. In a few patients assessment of vitamin D status (serum 25-hydroxyvitamin D) is of value to rule out coexisting vitamin D deficiency prior to considering a bone biopsy. Parathyroid hormone levels may also be useful to rule out hyperparathyroidism, but must be interpreted along with serum calcium (preferably ionized calcium). PTH increases with age and occasionally elevations occur associated with low-renin hypertension (354), patients on corticosteroid therapy (355), and in familial hypocalciuric hypercalcemia (356).

Elevations in alkaline phosphatase occur in a variety of metabolic bone diseases, including Paget's disease, hyperparathyroidism, renal osteodystrophy, osteomalacia, hypercortisolism, and healing fractures. The increase in serum alkaline phosphatase after a fracture can be found only after 7–10 days (357). Other causes of elevated alkaline phosphatase include most liver diseases, hyperthyroidism, polymyalgia rheumatica, pulmonary embolism, thyroiditis, heart failure, osteomyelitis, malignancies, and a plethora of drugs. The measurement of bone specific alkaline phosphatase may help exclude most of these latter conditions.

New biochemical markers of bone remodeling are now being evaluated clinically and may prove of use in determining skeletal status (358). Tartrate-resistant acid phosphatase, that portion of the acid phosphatase in circulation derived from bone, specifically the osteoclast population, is a marker for increased bone resorption for which good assays have been developed and are now being evaluated clinically (359,360). Urinary deoxypyridinoline has recently been shown to be an index of collagen breakdown, specific for bone (361) which may also prove useful as an indicator of increased bone breakdown. Serum bone-gla-protein (osteocalcin, BGP) is thought to be an indicator of bone formation (358,359) and correlates with histologically-derived bone formation rate in mixed patient populations (362,363). The use of these and other biochemical markers of remodeling currently remains investigational.

RADIOLOGICAL EVALUATION

The radiological assessment of patients with postmenopausal osteoporosis relies on the presence of fractures that have occurred as a consequence of relatively trivial trauma (364–366). In addition there may be subjective evidence of reduced bone mass, or general demineralization on spinal radiographs. These latter changes are often misleading in the absence of direct quantification of bone mass because the radiographic appearance of the vertebral bodies can be influenced markedly by technique. More reliable radiographic assessment can be obtained by searching for characteristic morphological changes affecting the vertebrae (366). Early changes include loss of horizontal trabeculae, creating a more prominent appearance of the remaining vertical trabeculae, vertebral biconcavity, and anterior vertebral wedging (Fig. 9) (367,368). Schmorl's nodes (invaginations of the disc into the vertebral body) are often seen also, but are not pathognomonic for osteoporosis as is commonly stated (366,369). Insufficiency fractures, often thought to be pathognomonic for osteomalacia can also be seen in osteoporosis. Complete crush fractures with reductions in both anterior and posterior vertebral height are readily seen on plain radiographs. Insufficiency fractures occur in other bones also, and in older patients femoral neck fractures are the hallmark of advanced loss of bone. Attempts have also been made to quantify bone mass in the hip using routine radiographs, the best known technique being that of Singh (372,373) who advocates using the gradual disappearance of the trabecular pattern of the neck as an index of severity. The index is a poor predictor of fracture, however, and does not correlate

well with bone mass in the hip (374). The use of a noninvasive technique for bone mass measurement [quantitative computed tomography (QCT), dual x-ray or photon absorptiometry (DXA or DPA)] allows some assessment of the severity of the problem (375).

ASSESSMENT OF THE ASYMPTOMATIC WOMAN

Increasingly we are finding that women are requesting evaluation of their risk for osteoporosis. These women are often pre- or perimenopausal. Since osteoporosis is more easily prevented than treated, it would be useful to determine those most at risk and to target that segment of the population for intervention. Unfortunately, at present there is no satisfactory method by which the physician can reliably predict, using clinical means alone, those who will fracture in later life. It is common to use a list of so-called risk factors for evaluation of these patients (Table 4). However, there is no evidence that these factors can predict bone mass either at the time of examination or in the future, nor is there evidence that they can be used to predict fracture. However, since the risk factor list for osteoporosis has many items that are commonly associated with general poor health, we feel that their assessment is of some value in each patient. When uncovered in the individual patient we will initiate our discussion of disease prevention around reduction or elimination of these factors.

There is a close relationship between the strength of a bone and its mass, which explains some 80% or more of the variance in strength when tested in vitro (65). Most cross-sectional studies, as we have noted, demonstrate that bone mass at the site of fracture is somewhat lower than average for age and sex, although usually with considerable overlapping with values in normal individuals (376,377). Indeed, since factors other than bone mass (such as risk of falling) influence the likelihood of fracture it is not surprising that overlap exists. This overlap has led some investigators to the conclusion that bone mass measurements are of little value in hip fracture. This view is unlikely to be correct since hip fracture is related to absolute bone mass and not relative bone mass. Overlap in risk factors among patients and controls is common in all studies of this type. This is especially true of the relationship between cholesterol and myocardial infarction and diastolic blood pressure and stroke (378,379). These risk factors are not diagnostic but define those at higher risk for the clinical event. Those with the highest levels (or lowest for bone mass) will still have a finite risk of experiencing the clinical event (heart attack, stroke, or fracture). Bone mass is, therefore, not used to diagnose a fracture, but recent data suggest that judicious use of bone mass can predict the risk of fracture (379).

Hui and co-workers in a study of 500 individuals followed for 15 years demonstrated that the rate of all non-

TABLE 4. *Factors commonly associated with the female osteoporotic syndromes*

Genetic	*Medical disorders (contd.)*
White or Asiatic ethnicity	Occult osteogenesis imperfecta
Positive family history	Mastocytosis
Small body frame (less than 127 lb)	Rheumatoid arthritis
Lifestyle	"Transient" osteoporosis
Smoking	Prolonged parenteral nutrition
Inactivity	Prolactinoma
Nulliparity	Endometriosis
Exessive exercise (producing amenorrhea)	Partial hysterectomy[a]
Early natural menopause	Tubal ligations[a]
Late menarche	Hemolytic anemia
Nutritional factors	Ankylosing spondylitis
Milk intolerance	*Drugs*
Lifelong low dietary calcium intake	Thyroid replacement therapy
Vegetarian dieting	Glucocorticoid drugs
Excessive alcohol intake	Anticoagulants
Consistently high protein intake	Chronic lithium therapy
Medical disorders	Chemotherapy
Anorexia nervosa	GnRH agonist or antagonist therapy
Acromegaly	Anticonvulsant drugs
Thyrotoxicosis	Extended tetracycline use[b]
Parathyroid overactivity	Diuretics producing calciuria[b]
Cushing's syndrome	Phenothiazine derivatives[b]
Type I diabetes	Cyclosporine A[b]
Alterations in gastrointestinal and hepatobiliary function	

[a] Potential decrease in ovarian function due to vascular insufficiency.
[b] Not yet associated with decreased bone mass although identified as either toxic to bone in animals or inducing calciuria and/or calcium malabsorption in humans.

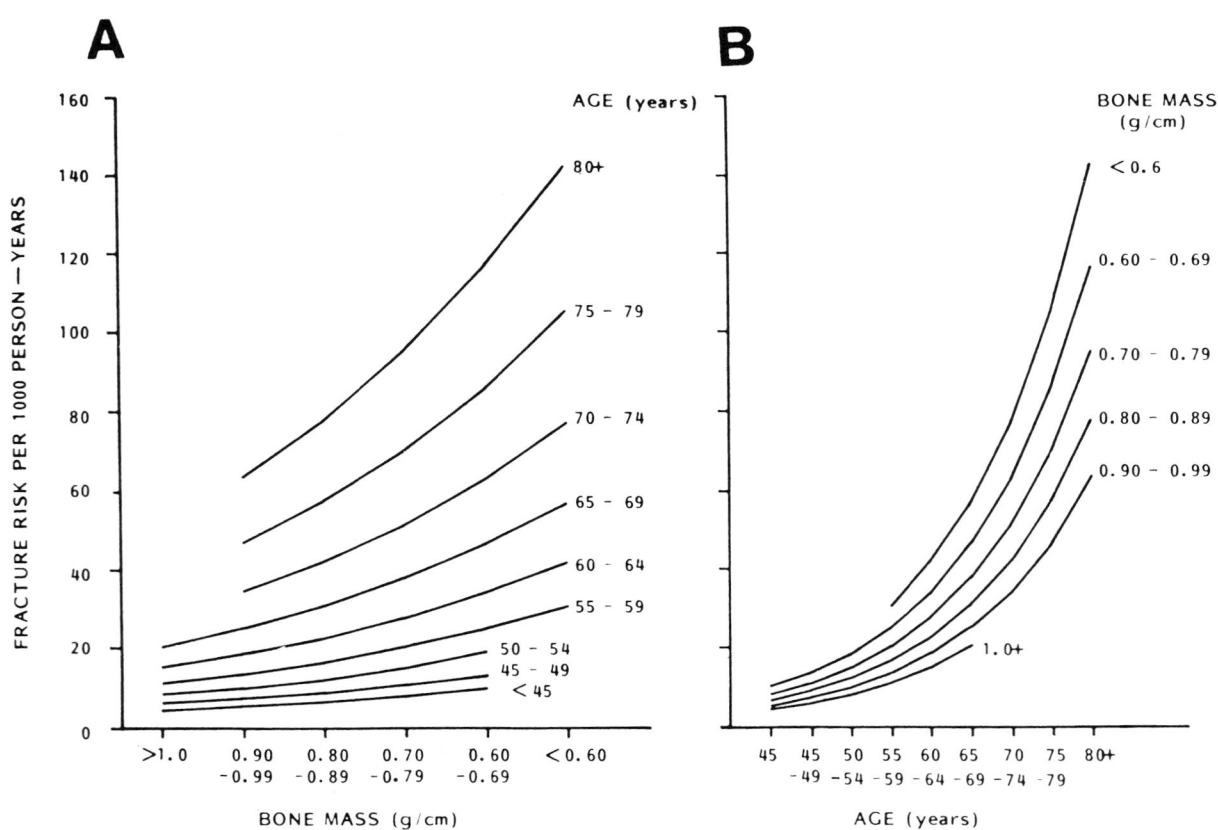

FIG. 24. Estimated incidence of fracture as a function of age and bone mass (**A** and **B**). From ref. 380.

spinal fractures increased with decreasing bone mass, and with increasing age (Fig. 24). These two factors had independent effects on fracture risk (380), although the effects of bone mass were stronger than the effects of age, for fractures other than hip fracture. For women starting around the age of 60 years the relative risk of fracture increases by 1.3 for every standard deviation decrease in bone mass (381) (for ischemic heart disease the risk increases by 1.25 for each SD increase in cholesterol). Thus, bone mass is at least as useful in predicting fracture as cholesterol is in predicting cardiovascular disease. The increase in relative risk may be even greater for younger individuals. Those non-mass factors that influence fracture risk include age itself as well as age-associated factors such as frailty, falling risk, and qualitative changes in skeletal architecture.

At least three studies have demonstrated that baseline bone mass measurements can be used to predict the risk of fracture (380–383). Bone mass measurements made at non-fracture sites predicted fracture risk and performed just as well as measurements made at fracture sites (vertebrae) (Fig. 25). As discussed in another chapter of this volume bone mass can be measured safely, accurately, and precisely using currently available techniques (Chapter 20). It is a common clinical belief that risk factors can be used as a surrogate for bone mass. As discussed earlier, however, at present no adequate study has validated a technique by which individual risk

factors or groups of risk factors can be used to estimate bone mass with reasonable precision (384,385). In some, but not all studies, statistically significant relationships between combinations of factors (e.g., height, weight, age, and serum estrogen) can be demonstrated (386–390). Mostly such studies involve ranges greater than those seen clinically, and the combined risk factors account for less than 50% of the variance in bone mass, making their clinical application limited. Since bone mass predicts fracture we use bone mass as a guide to therapeutic decision making in asymptomatic patients (391). Not all patients require bone mass measurement, and it should only be used clinically when a therapeutic decision will be based on the result (14).

The issue of whether more widespread use should be made of bone mass measurements among the perimenopausal population is at present in question. As yet there is no prospective evidence upon which to base a decision about screening, its costs and its likely impact. It can be suggested that by treating women with the lowest bone mass measurements lifetime risk for the population would fall from 10% to 8% (a risk reduction of 20%) if the use of preventive therapy (estrogen) increased from 15% to 19% (14). In another study it was suggested that the incidence of all osteoporotic fracture would be reduced by 33% if the women with the lowest 47% of bone mass were treated (392). Numerous position papers and editorial articles describe different opinions (391–402). In

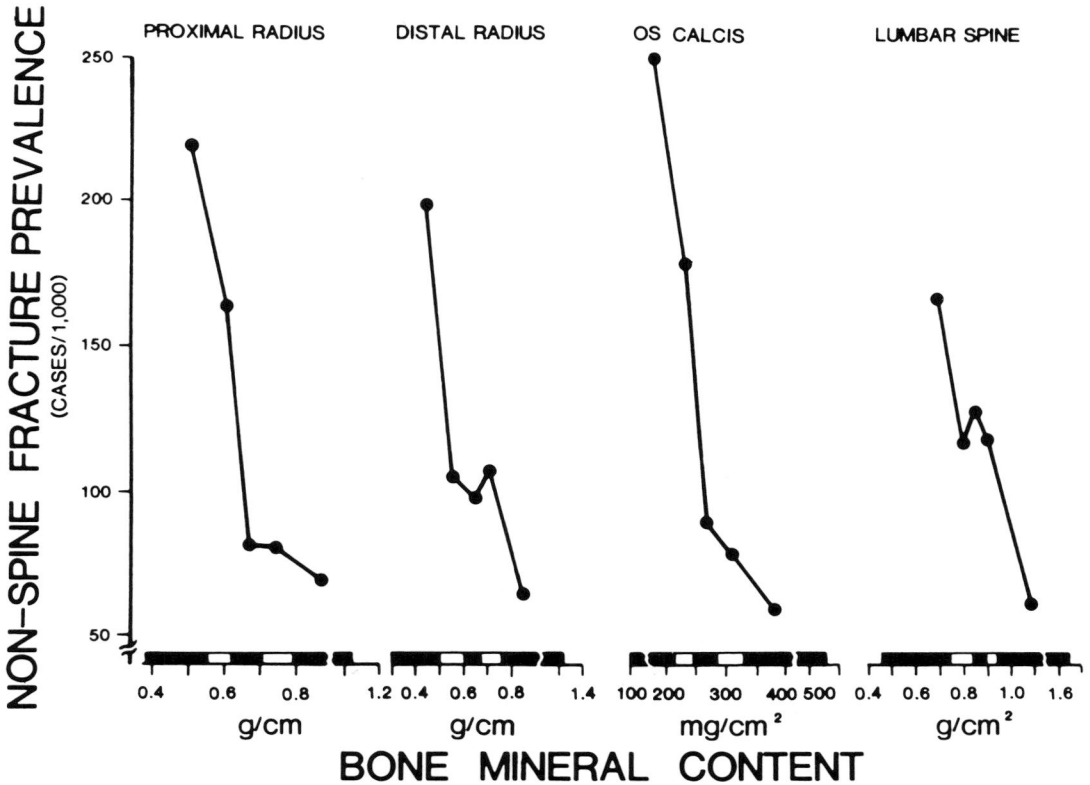

FIG. 25. Unadjusted nonspine fracture prevalence rates by quintile of bone mineral content at four skeletal sites. All fractures preceded bone mineral content measurements. From ref. 383.

clinical practice, however, the position of the Scientific Advisory Committee of the National Osteoporosis Foundation appears to be most rational (14). Bone mass measurements should be performed in estrogen-deficient women to diagnose significantly low bone mass in order to make decisions about hormone replacement therapy. Thus the measurements are indicated when the physician will make use of them in patient management. In addition bone mass measurement is a useful tool to determine the severity of the disorder in patients presenting with their first osteoporotic fracture. There is the potential with the new techniques involving dual energy x-ray to follow individual patients and assess their response to therapy, but this remains an indication for the future (14).

PREVENTION AND TREATMENT

Several options now exist for therapeutic intervention for both prevention and treatment of established osteoporosis (403,404). Since the agents used and the practical approach to the patients have many similarities in the two circumstances both prevention and treatment will be discussed in this section. As for other disorders with multiple etiological factors, reduction or elimination of risk factors is the initial approach to the patient (404). However, in this disorder the absence of an easily measured marker of the success of such maneuvers (for example cholesterol or blood pressure) coupled with the somewhat disappointing outcomes achieved in clinical trials of life style modification have resulted in a general feeling that pharmaceutical intervention is warranted especially if the individual can be demonstrated to be at increased risk.

Calcium

The evidence that calcium deficiency is likely to be a risk factor for bone loss and osteoporosis has already been reviewed (87–89,92,93,226–261). The problem that the physician faces when dealing with individual patients is that even the evaluation of calcium intake does not allow determination of the calcium balance status of that individual. Absorption efficiency for calcium at the recommended dietary allowance can vary from less than 10% to almost 60% (Figs. 22 and 23) (259) for the average woman around menopausal age. Thus, other factors being equal, wide variations in intake are likely to be required to obtain calcium balance. Indeed there are almost no data that answer the question of whether increasing calcium intake can maintain calcium balance over long periods of time although it clearly does so in the short term (405–409). In addition there is convincing evidence that the absorption efficiency for calcium declines with age (243–245,260). Unfortunately no acceptable test of calcium absorption efficiency is generally

available to the clinician, nor is there a test of calcium status, as for example ferritin is for iron status. Clearly some individuals can adapt to chronically low calcium intake but not all will be able to do so.

Some time ago the data assembled by Heaney led to the conclusion that the recommendations for calcium intake were set too low in the United States (410). The current RDA for adults over the age of 25 years remains at 800 mg/day, although it has recently been increased for younger individuals to 1200 mg/day. In 1984 a Consensus Development Conference sponsored by the National Institutes of Health recommended intakes of 1000 mg/day for estrogen-replete women and 1500 mg/day for women who were estrogen deficient (260). This recommendation was modified slightly in 1987 (411) with the recommendation that women at particular risk of osteoporosis increase their intakes to 1500 mg with all other adults (with the exception of pregnancy and lactation) maintaining intakes of 1000 mg. These recommendations are somewhat of a compromise among the factors of achievability, compliance, efficacy, and safety.

Such intakes are achievable, either with dietary modification or with modest supplementation. In the clinical setting this is most commonly achieved by supplementation since dietary modification usually involves increases in dairy produce which many find intolerable. There are no controlled data that have evaluated the effect of increasing calcium intake above 1000 mg/day on bone mass in a randomized controlled clinical trial, *in which only individuals who might be thought to be calcium deficient are included.* Thus it is not surprising perhaps that the results of the studies completed thus far are somewhat mixed (236,237,252–258,412–419). Tables 5 and 6 illustrate the results of most of the studies of calcium supplementation in the literature. These can be summarized by the generalization that there appears in many to be some reduction in the rate of cortical bone loss, but little effect on cancellous bone. In part this may be because many studies (Table 5) have included women in the immediate postmenopausal period when bone loss is clearly dependent on the reduction of estrogen that occurs at this time (252–255,257,412). In addition accurate assessment of intake over the long time periods required for such studies is problematic as is the problem of absorption. It is not surprising, therefore, that calcium supplementation can be found to have only modest effects. Almost no well controlled data address the issue of whether higher intakes of calcium would be more effective. There are few well controlled studies of older women or women with established primary osteoporosis (258,409,415–418,418a). Again the results are variable (Table 6), and generally more negative than positive. Two recent studies in which calcium was the control arm for investigation of another therapeutic modality did suggest some effect (418,420), although we were not able to distinguish a significant effect of calcium in our study of estrogen (465).

TABLE 5. *The effects of calcium supplementation on bone loss in post-menopausal women*

	Subject numbers (age range)	Supplemental calcium dose	Duration of study (years)	Measurement technique	Site measured	Significant difference from control	Slowed rate of bone loss in calcium treated group
banese et al. 1975	12 (78–86)	750	2–3	Radiographic Densitometry	Phalanx	Yes	Yes
orsman et al. 1977	89 (33–65)	800	<2.5	Radiogrammetry SPA	Metacarpacal Distal radius Distal ulna	No No Yes	Yes Yes Yes
ecker et al. 1977	60 (55–65)	1040	2	SPA Radiogrammetry	Distal radius Metacarpal	No Yes	Yes Yes
nith et al. 1981	80 (65–95)	750	3	SPA	Distal radius	Yes	Yes
las et al. 1984	103 (<55)	500	2	SPA	Distal radius	No	No
ecker et al. 1984	22 (45–70)	800 (as milk)	2	SPA	Distal radius	No	Yes
tinger et al. 1987	73 (43–59)	1000	2	QCT SPA Radiogrammetry	Lumbar vertebrae Distal radius Metacarpal	No No No	No No No
s et al. 1987	43 (45–54)	2000	2	SPA	Distal forearm Proximal forearm Lumbar vertebrae Total body calcium	No Yes No Yes	No Yes No Yes
ordin and Polley 1987	348 (?–75)	1000 (Sandocal)	0.75	SPA	Distal radius	Yes	Yes
nith et al. 1987	169 (35–65)	1500	4	SPA	Proximal radius Ulnar Humerus midshaft	No Yes Yes	Yes Yes Yes

SPA; single photon absorptiometry; QCT, quantitative computed tomography.

Three studies have evaluated fracture rate in women with osteoporosis on calcium supplementation (407, 421,422). Only one is of appropriate design. Nevertheless all three suggest that there is a reduction in fracture rate. The fracture reduction may be as much as 50% from that occurring without treatment, although the suboptimal study designs make conclusions difficult. The most recent well controlled study specifically tests the hypothesis that calcium supplementation will reduce fracture recurrence. In addition, two observational studies have evaluated the relationship between hip fracture occurrence and calcium intake (248,249), with one study appearing to demonstrate a positive effect, while the other was essentially negative.

As stated, the levels of calcium intake recommended currently can be considered somewhat of a compromise. Such intakes are almost certainly safe and thus it would be expected that they can be recommended on a public health basis. It can also be deduced from Heaney's data that such intakes would be sufficient to ensure that the majority of individuals would not be in significant calcium deficit (133–135). Arguments have been made against this case (226,227). However, in the absence of data it seems reasonable to recommend this compromise position for all patients with osteoporotic fracture and for those at risk of the disorder. A rough estimation of current calcium intake can be obtained by assessment of dairy produce consumption which provides more than 80% of available calcium in most diets. Intakes can then be adjusted to the required level by modifying dairy produce or by advising a supplement. For most individuals no more than 500–1000 mg/day need be obtained by supplementation.

Increasing calcium intakes using foodstuffs as the source of supply is preferable to tablets, because calcium tablets in the United States are regulated not as drugs but as food supplements, and are not subject to the same rigorous quality control as is required for drug formulations. Many calcium supplements are so poorly formulated that they disintegrate in an acid environment in vitro (423) and therefore the calcium is not available for absorption. In addition, achlorhydria, not uncommon among the elderly, may interfere with the release of calcium from calcium carbonate (424). Calcium absorption from foods ranges from 21–26% including milk, cheese, yogurt, and green vegetables with the exception of spin-

TABLE 6. *Summary of controlled studies on the effect of calcium supplementation on bone loss in post-menopausal women with osteoporosis*

	Subject numbers (age range)	Supplemental calcium dose	Duration of study (years)	Measurement technique	Site measured	Significant difference from control	Slowed rate of bone loss in calcium treated group
Shapiro et al. 1975	10 (36–80)	2400	1–2	SPA	Proximal radius	No	No
Smith et al. 1975	94 (50–80)	1140/1200	1.5–4.5	Radiographic densitometry and radiogrammetry	Metacarpal	No	No
Lamke et al. 1978	40	1000	1	Radiographic spectrophotometry	Femoral neck Femoral shaft	No No	Yes
Nordin et al. 1980	95 (55–72)	1200	Variable	Radiogrammetry	Metacarpal	No	Yes
Ott et al. 1987	71 (unknown)	1000	2	Neutron activation analysis DPA SPA	Total body calcium Lumbar spine Radius		Yes
Riggs et al. 1987	200 (uknown)	1500	4	DPA	Lumbar spine Femoral neck		Yes

SPA, single photon absorptiometry; DPA, dual photon absorptiometry.

ach whose absorbability is only 5% (425,426), and in general, meals improve calcium absorption even from supplements in patients (424). A divided dose schedule results in a greater supply of calcium because of the relationship between dose and absorption efficiency. However, in general, compliance with medication declines as dosing frequency increases. We prefer therefore to provide calcium as one tablet with meals, the equivalent of three times per day. With currently available carbonate preparations, this yields from 600 to 1800 mg elemental calcium, although any available salt can be used provided adequate elemental calcium intake can be achieved.

Physical Activity

The evidence that physical activity is important in the maintenance of skeletal status has also been reviewed. It is clear that disuse results in osteoporosis and that excessive activity can result in hypertrophy. However, within the confines of normal activity it is not entirely clear whether or not increments easily achievable by the general population can result in significant effects on bone mass. In part this may be because of the difficulty in devising and conducting an adequately controlled clini-

cal trial in this area. In general, however, since exercise has multiple beneficial effects on health it seems appropriate to recommend increasing activity for both those at risk of osteoporosis and also those with the clinical disorder. In addition, even if exercise does not alter the rate of bone loss, it may decrease the risk of severe injury after a fall by improving shock absorption through increased muscle mass or decreasing forces acting on a weakened skeleton. The exercise prescription required is not clear. Therefore in our clinical practice for prevention we adhere to the recommendations of the American Heart Association for cardiovascular health. All who are participating in activity for the first time should undergo a physical examination including, if thought necessary, a stress test. Activity programs should be fun and we find that competitive sports are most likely to lead to reasonable patient compliance. The person who has not exercised until the age of 50 is hardly likely to persist in a program of activity undertaken spontaneously by themselves.

For patients with established fracture syndromes the recommendations are more difficult since they rely on the physical status of the individual. For the patient with Colles' fracture as the presenting complaint the guidelines can generally be similar to those used for prevention, in addition to any physical therapy required to reha- bilitate the fractured arm. For those with one or more crush fractures we recommend swimming or water exer- cises in a therapeutic pool particularly if back pain is a problem. Patients can be gradually weaned onto land mobility as the pain decreases. Thereafter activity is on a case by case basis avoiding exercises that produce flexion of the dorsal spine or sudden rotational movements. With time, many patients become very active and inter- ested in their progress. The effects of such incremental programs on bone mass has not been documented. In- deed there is a theoretical possibility that activity in the erect posture in a patient with kyphosis will increase the kyphosis because of excessive modeling at the anterior edges of the vertebral bodies. Patients with marked ky- phosis occasionally report lethargy and exercise intoler- ance that may be related to restriction of lung movement caused by the change in body configuration.

Falls

Among the elderly falls constitute a major problem. Falls increase with age and more so among women than men at least up to the age of 70 years (Fig. 8) (33– 35,40,428–432). Only about 5–6% of falls result in frac- ture and only 1% result in hip fracture (428). The events leading up to falls in the elderly are only gradually being understood as investigation into the pathophysiology of falls has only recently been initiated. Unfortunately many of the factors that lead to increased falling are diffi- cult to correct, including dementia, balance and gait dysfunction, diminished reflexes and strength (33,35,39, 429–435). Others are more amenable to intervention in- cluding household hazards such as loose rugs, trailing electrical cords, poor lighting, stairs without guards, showers without grab bars, etc. (430,436–438). In these instances we find it useful to ask for a home visit from a health professional, usually an occupational therapist, to remedy as many obstacles or hazards as possible. Some medical problems may be amenable to intervention also, including failing eyesight, over-medication, alcohol abuse, etc. (38,430,439–442). Improvements in strength and muscle function can be achieved even in the elderly by regular participation in an activity program. Group programs by experienced physical therapists contribute greatly to patient management. The outcomes expected are less related to skeletal status than to muscle function. Clinical scales have been generated to evaluate the el- derly for risk of falling (38,429,437,444–446). These can be useful in the practice setting, allowing the nurse to evaluate these issues for individual patients and triage patients so that the most important problems can be handled efficiently. This is worth doing in any prac- tice setting that deals with a large population of elderly since falling is a common reason for seeking nursing

home entry and is feared greatly by those diagnosed with osteoporosis.

Estrogen

Since estrogen deficiency is the major cause of bone loss among women, it is not surprising that estrogen re- placement is the main intervention that is of proven effi- cacy in the prevention of osteoporosis. Albright (15,16,447) originally suggested that estrogen would be effective in treatment of osteoporosis. However, it was not until the introduction of non-invasive measure- ments of bone mass that controlled clinical studies could be carried out to determine the efficacy of estrogen in prevention of the disorder in asymptomatic individuals. In our original observations we determined (Fig. 26) that intervention with estrogen reduced the rate of bone loss among oophorectomized women (448–450). Since those observations a large body of data has accumulated con- firming that in estrogen-deficient women estrogen inter- vention is capable of reducing the rate of bone loss signifi- cantly (451–480). Indeed several of these studies indicate that there is virtually no bone loss at any skeletal site over

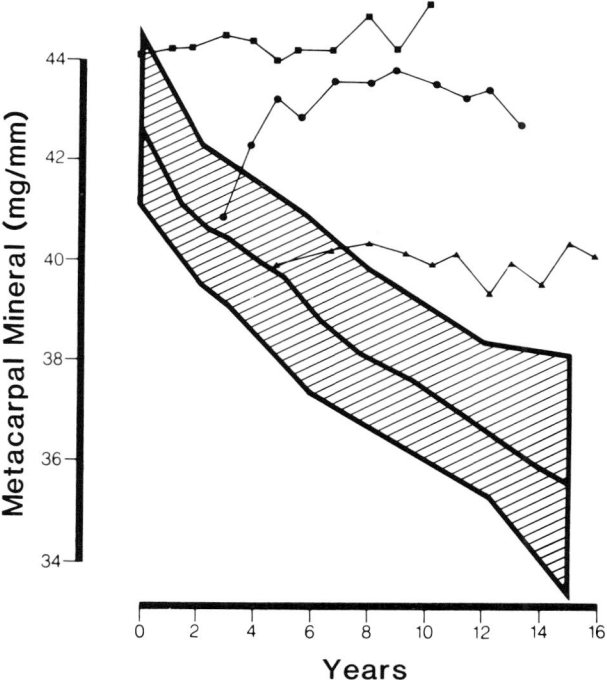

FIG. 26. Long-term prevention of bone loss by estrogen. The hatched areas represent the placebo using (mean ± SD) a prospective controlled study in oophorectomized women. The 3 lines show the mean values only for 3 estrogen treated groups; treatment initiated at the time of oophorectomy (■ — ■), 3 years after (● — ●), or 6 years after oophorec- tomy (▲ — ▲). Bone loss is prevented in all 3 situations. How- ever, the earlier treatment is begun, the better the outcome, in terms of bone mass after 10 years of therapy. From ref. 769.

a two year period. Our data in women followed for ten years suggest that estrogen intervention almost eliminates bone loss at the major sites of osteoporotic fracture (Fig. 27) (482,758). Longitudinal data demonstrated that estrogen eliminated bone loss in cortical bone estimated by single photon absorptiometry (448,450). In the same patients estrogen intervention resulted in a 24% increase in vertebral bone mass (Fig. 27) and a 12% increase in femoral neck bone mass over the placebo-treated patients during ten years of treatment (480). Examination of lateral radiographs confirmed that estrogen had prevented vertebral abnormality. Vertebral deformations including wedging and reduction in central vertebral height were significantly more common among the placebo-treated patients than among those treated with estrogen suggesting that continuation of treatment would result in prevention of vertebral fracture. Calculations based on these data suggest a reduction of almost 80% in vertebral fracture rate with the use of long-term estrogen (Table 7). Cross-sectional data in which radiographs from a Health Maintenance Organization were evaluated also indicated a dramatic reduction in the prevalence of vertebral fractures with estrogen exposure of one year or more (Fig. 28) (454).

The skeleton is extremely sensitive to exogenous estrogen, as might be predicted from the studies in which rate of bone loss was examined as a function of endogenous estrogen. Bone loss is inhibited by endogenous estrogen when circulating concentrations are in the early to mid-follicular range for a premenopausal women. Doses of exogenous estrogen which produce similar blood levels therefore, and perhaps not surprisingly, reduce bone loss. The minimum effective dose for conjugated equine estrogen (Premarin) the most commonly used estrogen in the United States, is 0.625 mg/day (Fig. 29) (458). The skeletal effects of estrogen are independent of the route of administration. There is now evidence that percutaneous (157,466), and transdermal (565) estrogen significantly reduce bone loss.

There is now considerable epidemiological data indicating that estrogen exposure is associated with a decline in the risk of hip fracture (Table 8) (456,481,483–487). The data indicate for the most part a risk reduction of about 50% although there is a considerable variation, in part due to the wide definitions accepted for estrogen use and duration of use. In general it appears as though the earlier that estrogen therapy is introduced the greater the magnitude of risk reduction, a finding that fits with the concept of a postmenopausal acceleration of bone loss and its prevention by estrogen intervention, specifically agreeing with our cross-sectional data. The most recent of these studies from Sweden suggests that for women whose estrogen replacement is not initiated until after age 60 years, there is no evidence for protection against

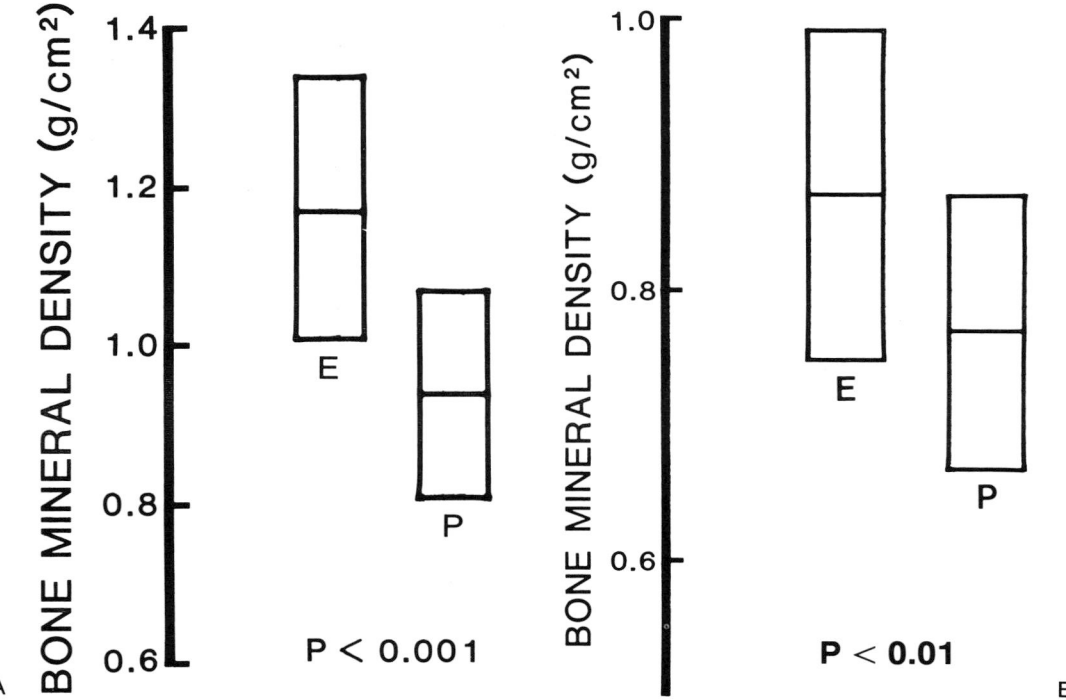

FIG. 27. The effect of ten years of treatment with estrogen on bone mass in the axial skeleton. **A:** Measurements of the lumbar spine. **B:** Measurements of the femoral neck, both using dual photon absorptiometry. E, estrogen; and P, placebo. From Lindsay et al. (758).

TABLE 7. *Radiographic changes following estrogen or placebo treatment for 10 years*

Treatment	Spine score[a]	Percentage positive scores	Crush fractures
Estrogen	0.35	27.6	1
Placebo	1.65	66	5
	$p < 0.01$	$p < 0.01$	

[a] Spine Score was obtained by reviewing all vertebrae from T1 to L5 and scoring 1 for wedge and 2 for "crush" fractures.

hip fracture (489). However, in prospective studies in which bone mass has been measured as the end point, there is clear evidence that bone loss is inhibited at least up to age 70 years (461,465,467). The reason for the discrepancy between the epidemiological data and the bone mass data is not clear. It is possible that the reduction in mass and change in architecture in the immediate postmenopausal period sufficiently weakened the femoral neck such that decreasing further bone loss would be to no avail. Subsequent fracture risk would therefore be more dependent on falls rather than any subsequent reduction in mass. To confound the story some epidemiological studies suggest that the maximum estrogen effect on hip fracture is seen in women currently on estrogen in the age range for hip fracture risk, that is over 70 years (483). One explanation for this finding has nothing to do with the estrogen effects on bone mass. A study only presented in preliminary format thus far, suggests that estrogen intervention in this age group increases the capacity for central neurologic processing of information (488). This improved processing could reduce the risk of injury by reducing falls or improving the protection from injury with more rapid reflex response such that the faller would be able to reach out and perhaps hold onto something to prevent serious injury. We must await further information on this important issue.

Estrogen intervention has other effects which should not be surprising since estrogens are potent hormones that have multiple target organs in premenopausal women.

Estrogens also appear to reduce the risk of ischemic heart disease among postmenopausal women (Table 9) (489–511). General conclusions that can be drawn from the mass of epidemiological data imply that estrogen intervention will reduce the risk of cardiovascular disease and mortality by as much as 50%. Again the greatest benefits appear to accrue to those who initiate therapy early and continue on treatment until old age. The maximum benefit is realized by those currently on treatment. The mechanism of the cardioprotective effect is not entirely clear. Estrogens reduce total serum cholesterol and LDL and increase HDL, all considered to be favorable changes for reduction of cardiovascular risk (492,512). However, in animal models estrogen administration in conjunction with potent progestogens also appear to effectively reduce coronary vascular occlusion despite the absence of lipid changes of a positive nature (513). Estrogen receptors occur in many areas of the vascular system including the coronary vessels, and estrogens appear to be vasodilators, possibly directly influencing arterial function. This is an area of intensive investigation at present. Estrogen also appear to reduce the risk of cerebrovascular accidents in postmenopausal women and are associated with reduced overall mortality at least up to the age of 79 years (514).

Estrogens when given continuously over long periods of time increase the risk of endometrial malignancy (Table 10) (516–532). The increase in risk is dependent on dose and duration of use. The increment is 2–10 times, increasing endometrial carcinoma from an incidence of 1 per 1000 to 2–10 per 1000 in the postmenopausal population. This increase in risk does not cease with termination of estrogen use (527,528). The addition of a proges-

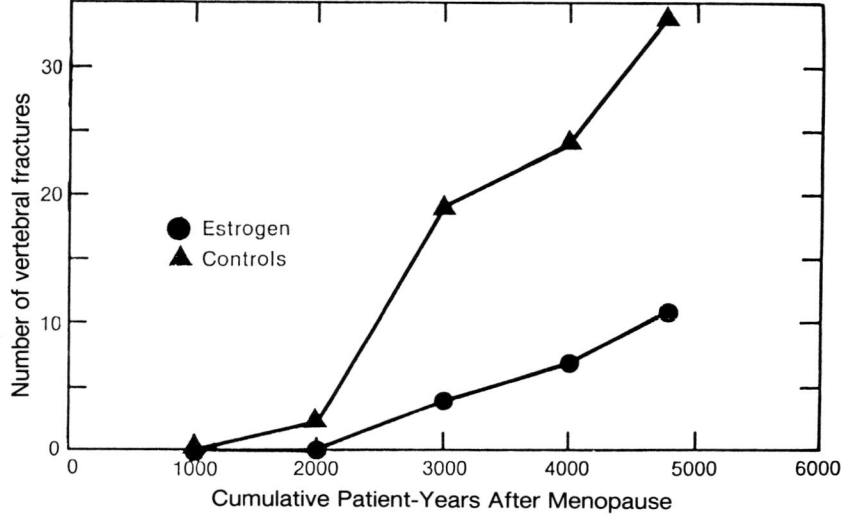

FIG. 28. Prevalence of radiologic vertebral abnormalities in postmenopausal women as a function of estrogen use. From ref. 454, with permission.

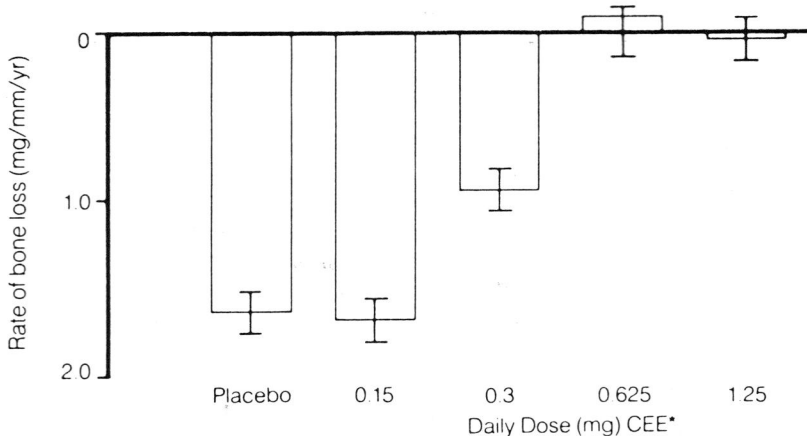

FIG. 29. The effects of various doses of conjugated equine estrogen on bone loss. Allocation to treatment program was done randomly using placebo and 0.15, 0.30, 0.625, and 1.25 mg doses of conjugated estrogens. Rate of loss was calculated for each individual patient over a two-year period. From ref. 458.

togen to the regimen protects from endometrial hyperplasia and reduces the risk of endometrial malignancy to baseline (533,534). This effect of progestins is the sole reason, with our present state of knowledge, for the addition of a progestin to the regimen for postmenopausal women.

A more disturbing feature of long-term estrogen replacement therapy is the potential of an increase in the risk of breast cancer (Fig. 30). Here the data are mixed with some authors finding protective effect, others no effect, but most a small increase in risk usually not clearly evident until after at least ten years of use (535–554). The increment in risk appears to be of the order of 5–20% after prolonged use. Progestogens do not appear to protect the breast tissue in the way that they protect the endometrium (535,536), although some authors disagree (539,540). Other perhaps less well documented effects of estrogens include improvement in psychiatric symptoms (555), neurologic functioning (488), skin (556), the genitourinary symptoms associated with atrophy (557), and sexuality (558,559). Estrogens increase the risk of gall stones by a factor of two (560). Postmenopausal estrogen use does not appear to be associated with an increase in blood pressure (561,562) or a deterioration in glucose control (563).

Estrogen Prescription

Because estrogens influence so many tissues, the reasons for estrogen prescription for the postmenopausal woman vary considerably. In this section the use of estrogen for osteoporosis prevention and treatment will be considered without reference to other reasons for estrogen use. Typically the patients seen in our clinic are perimenopausal, usually asymptomatic women, women referred after their first osteoporotic fracture, or older women late in the progression of their disorder. Guidance about estrogen use has many similarities among all three groups. After a complete history and physical examination, we obtain a bone mass measurement to evaluate accurately the status of the skeleton. For the younger women, if bone mass is above average we recommend no estrogen intervention. For bone mass below average, especially if accompanied by other risk factors, we recommend estrogen intervention. Before supplying the prescription all patients must have an adequate breast examination and mammography. Estrogens can be given by mouth, across the skin, or per vagina. For skeletal protection, the first two routes of administration are preferred. Usually patients choose the oral route and we prescribe conjugated equine estrogen (Premarin) 0.625

TABLE 8. *Studies indicating a reduction in fractures with estrogen use*

Author	Journal	Year	Fracture	Relative risk
Hutchinson	Lancet	1979	H, C	0.17[a]
Johnson	Am J Public Health	1981	H	0.67[a]
Kreiger	Am J Epidemiol	1982	H	0.5[a]
Paganini-Hill	Ann Intern Med	1981	H	0.42[a]
Weiss	N Engl J Med	1980	H, C	0.46[a]
Williams	Obstet Gynecol	1982	H, C	variable
Kiel	N Engl J Med	1987	H	0.65[a]
Ettinger	Ann Intern Med	1985	All	—
Lindsay	Lancet	1980	V	—
Naessen	Ann Intern Med	1990	H	0.79[a]

[a] $p < 0.05$.
H, Hip; C, Colles'; and V, vertebral.

TABLE 9. *Observational and experimental studies of*

Observational studies: population controlled

First author	N	Follow-up (years)	Endpoints	Risk estimate
MacMahon	1,891	12.0	ASHD death	.30[a]
Burch	737	13.3	CHD deaths	.43[a]
Hunt	4,544	5.6	CVD deaths	.51[a]

Observational studies: case control

First author	Cases/ controls	Types of controls/ recency of use	Endpoints	Risk estimate
Talbot	64	Com/C	Sudden death	.34
Sullivan	744	H/C	>70% Stenosis	.44[a]
Rosenberg	336	H/C	Non-fatal MI	.47
Adam	76	Com/C	Non-fatal MI	.79
Szklo	36	H/P	Non-fatal MI	.83
Rosenberg	105	H/C	Non-fatal MI	1.05
La Vecchia	116	H/C	Non-fatal MI	1.62

Observational studies: prospective

First author	N	Percentage users	Follow-up	Endpoints	Risk estimate
Lafferty	124	49%	8.6	MI	0.16[a]
Stampfer	32,317	53%	4.0	All CVD	0.30[a]
Hammond	610	49%	5.0	All CVD	0.33[a]
Bush	2,270	26%	8.5	CVD Death	0.34[a]
Potocki	198	47%	10.0	CHD	0.47
Henderson	8,807	56%	4.5	MI	0.54[a]
Wilson	1,234	24%	7	All CVD	1.21

Experimental studies: clinical trials

First author	N	Follow-up time	Regimen	Endpoints	Risk estimate
Nachtigall	84 matched pairs	10 years	Premarin 2.5 mg/day plus Provera 10 mg/day 7 days/month	MI[a]	0.33

[a] $p < 0.05$; Com, community; H, hospital; C, current; P, past; MI, myocardial infarction; ASHD, atherosclerotic heart disease; CVD, cardiovascular disease; and CHD, coronary heart disease.

mg/day or its equivalent. This has been shown to be the minimum effective dose for prevention of bone loss (Fig. 29) (458,564). For transdermal administration preliminary data indicate that 50 mcg 17 β-estradiol by "patch" changed twice weekly (Estraderm) will reduce loss of

TABLE 10. *Dose relationship of estrogen and endometrial cancer*

Study author	Relative risk, by dose	
	0.625 mg	1.25 mg
Spengler et al.	2.0	4.0
Stavraky et al.	1.9	3.1
	2.9	6.4
Weiss et al.	8.8	7.6
Antunes et al.	3.5	7.1
McDonald et al.	1.4	7.2
Mack	5.0	9.4

bone at all skeletal sites (565). Estrogens are given continuously, and for those with an intact uterus a progestogen is added on an intermittent basis. We use the calender month, asking patients to begin their progestin on the first of each calender month and continue for 12–14 days. Withdrawal bleeding usually occurs between the 11th and 21st day. We generally use medroxyprogesterone acetate in daily doses of 5–10 mg, but norethindrone (1–5 mg) or norgestrel (750 mcg) are alternatives. Newer progestogens are becoming available with better profiles in terms of their effects on the lipid metabolism. We do not add a progestogen if the patient has had a hysterectomy. For those who do not wish the inconvenience of recurrent vaginal bleeding, combination therapy (Premarin 0.625 mg with medroxyprogesterone acetate 2.5 mg) given continuously is an option. About 60% of patients will not bleed on this regimen, but the remainder

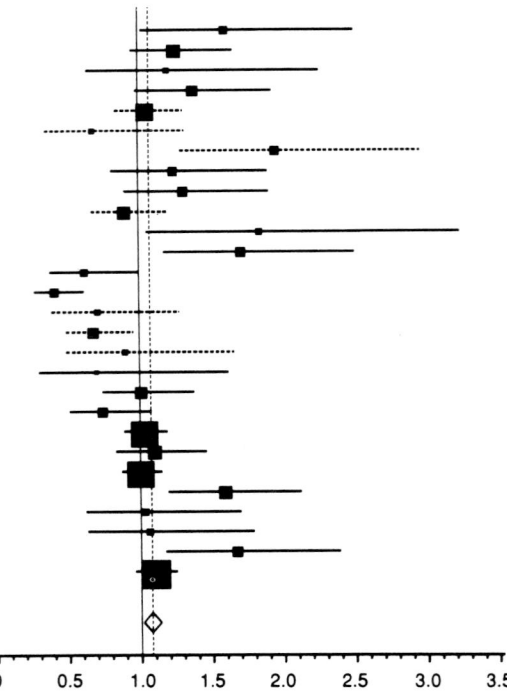

FIG. 30. Relative risks of breast cancer associated with menopausal estrogen therapy that have been reported in the literature in the past 15 years. Risks are relative to women who did not take estrogens. The black squares mark the estimated relative risk for each study. The area of each square is proportional to the information contributed by its study. The horizontal lines indicate 95% confidence intervals for these relative risks. Dashed horizontal lines indicate studies that used hospital controls. The diamond indicates the combined relative risk estimate and 95% confidence interval from all studies. This latter confidence interval is calculated under the assumption that all of the studies are estimating the same relative risk. However, the variability in reported breast cancer risks indicates either that different therapies have been used in the different studies or that factors other than replacement estrogen therapy have had effects on breast cancer risks.

will have intermittent bleeding that may be considerably inconvenient for the first six months. No long-term safety data are available with this regimen.

As the complications are likely to be gynecological we generally ask each patient to review the program with her gynecologist, but general internists can also manage the problems should they arise. Bleeding when unexpected requires investigation as for any postmenopausal woman, but we no longer recommend regular endometrial sampling on less than a 3-year regimen. Annual mammography is a must, as it should be for all women of this age.

The duration of therapy required to obtain reduction in fracture risk is probably 5 years or longer (486). However, we review the benefits and risks of the treatment program with each patient on an annual basis. Most, after the first year, prefer to remain on treatment.

For older patient populations, at present we are looking at long-term, perhaps lifetime treatment. Some data indicate that for the older asymptomatic woman (>60 years) there is little protection against fracture (487), but for the woman who already has an atraumatic fracture, symptomatic improvement and protection against further loss of bone are commonly seen (Fig. 31). As age increases, because of the multiple organs affected by estrogens, we tend to use alternative therapeutic modalities more frequently. The final choice always belongs to the patient, and in practice estrogens are used at least as commonly as all other approaches in almost all classes of patient.

Calcitonin

Alternatives to estrogen are now available for primary osteoporosis. Salmon calcitonin administered subcutaneously is approved in the United States for treatment of patients with established osteoporosis, although experience in the United States is somewhat limited (566,567). Calcitonin in controlled studies produces essentially the same effects as estrogen (566–580). There is preservation of bone mass with doses of salmon calcitonin of 50–100 units daily or on alternate days (Fig. 32). A clear dose response relationship has been described over this limited range (562). Recently one study divided patients biochemically into those with "high" versus "low" turnover and demonstrated a more pronounced therapeutic effect in those with increased skeletal remodeling (Fig. 33) (580). The effects of calcitonin on bone mass may not be the only reason to use calcitonin immediately following fractures such as vertebral fracture whose main symptom is pain. Several reports including controlled experiments in animals indicate that calcitonin in certain circumstances is an effective analgesic agent (Fig. 34) (581–589). Thus immediately following vertebral fracture if pain is a major symptom, calcitonin may speed the recovery of the patient, reducing the requirement for narcotic analgesia, and perhaps shortening the period of bed rest required. The main disadvantage to the use of calcitonin in the United States at present is the necessity for parenteral administration. Recent studies in which preparations of calcitonin have been administered in an intranasal spray have demonstrated that the drug effectively reduces bone loss by this route (Fig. 35) (576–577). Calcitonin is relatively devoid of serious side effects. Flushing, nausea, and abdominal fullness are the most frequent. These are usually transient, and if problematic the dose should be reduced. Initiation of treatment at a low dose, gradually increasing the dose every two to three days until the therapeutic dose is reached is the most effective method of reducing the likelihood of side effects. In addition, since calcitonin is a potent inhibitor of gastric acid secretion, it should be administered sev-

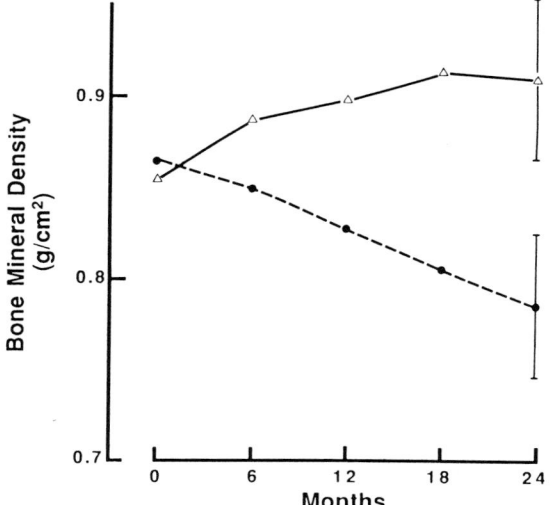

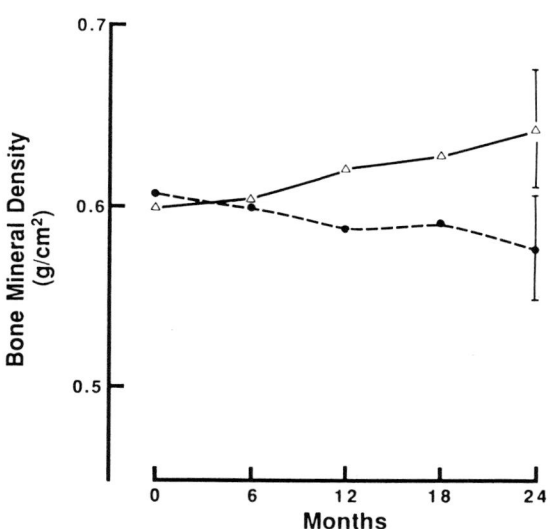

FIG. 31. Mean changes in bone mineral density of the lumbar spine (**A**) and the femoral neck (**B**) during 2 years of therapy with estrogen and calcium (△ — △) or calcium (● – – ●). At the end of 2 years, the mean bone mineral density of the lumbar spine was significantly greater in the calcium and estrogen-treated group than at the initiation of the study ($p < 0.01$) and than the final mean for the calcium-treated group ($p < 0.01$). From ref. 465.

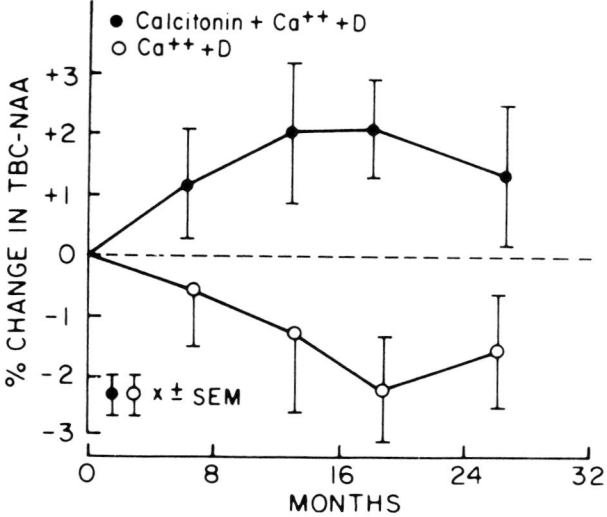

FIG. 32. Effect of synthetic salmon calcitonin (100 units per day), calcium, and vitamin D on total body calcium measured by neutron activation analysis (TBC-NAA) in 24 osteoporotic women (●- - -●). Twenty-one control osteoporotic women (○- - -○) received only 400 units of vitamin D and 1200 mg of calcium as calcium carbonate during the study. Iliac crest bone biopsies revealed a significantly greater percent total bone in calcitonin-treated patients compared to control patients after 2 years of treatment. From ref. 572.

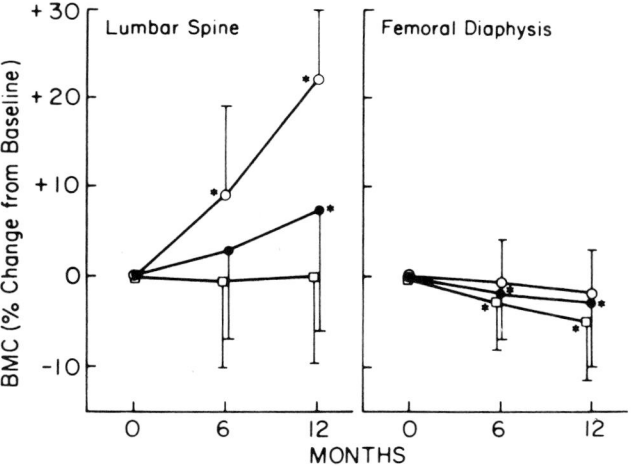

FIG. 33. Percent changes in BMC of the lumbar spine (left) and femoral diaphysis (right), in relation to bone turnover, in a group of postmenopausal osteoporotic women treated with subcutaneous salmon calcitonin for 1 yr, (○) high turnover osteoporosis (n = 17); (□) normal turnover osteoporosis (n = 36); (●) pooled groups (n = 53). Data are mean ± SD. *P < 0.01 vs. time 0 (one-sample t-test for mean + 0; t-test for paired data on the actual BMC values gave the same result. From ref. 580, with permission.

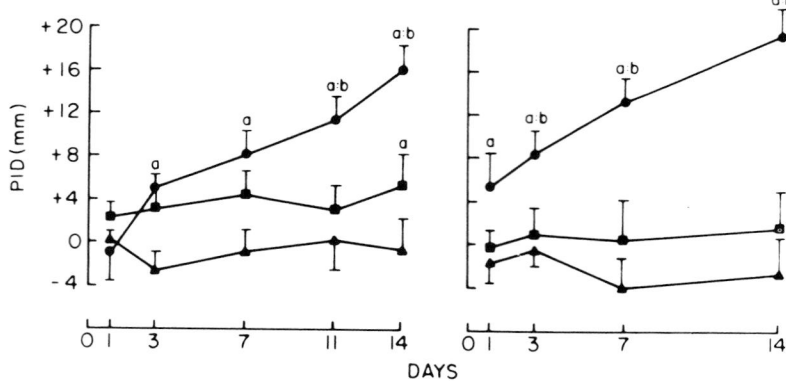

FIG. 34. Time-course of Pain Intensity Difference (PID) (mean ± SEM) in patients with malignancy and bone pain as scored by patients (left panel) and physician (right panel) during treatment with placebo (▲- - -▲), human calcitonin (■- - -■), and salmon calcitonin (●- - -●), "a" = statistically significant versus placebo; "b" = statistically significant versus human calcitonin. Salmon calcitonin was more effective in reducing bone pain than either human calcitonin or placebo. From ref. 571.

eral hours after food (590). We generally administer calcitonin in the evening prior to the patient retiring to minimize the side effects. An antiemetic may be given one-half hour beforehand if nausea is a problem, but is rarely required for longer than a few weeks of therapy.

Calcitonin in the United States is used primarily in the treatment of established osteoporosis. It is our practice to initiate therapy at a relatively low dose (25 IU s.c.) given at night, increasing to 100 IU or maximum tolerated dose by 25 IU increments every 3–4 days. The side effects of flushing and nausea tend to diminish with time, although are generally not a major problem on this regimen. We maintain treatment for 3 months and then reduce to 50–100 IU on alternate days continuing at this dose level for as long as can be tolerated. Most patients easily learn to inject themselves, but this can be a major problem for the elderly. At present no established short-term method for determination of calcitonin response is available in osteoporosis. It is possible that restricting the use of calcitonin to patients with high turnover states will allow the use of newer biochemical markers of bone resorption such as deoxypyridinoline to determine the optimum dose for individual patients. Patients can be followed with serial bone mass measurements if a high precision technique is available. The appearance of antibodies commonly seen in treatment of Paget's disease are to be expected in this situation also but are probably not clinically significant (591). The appearance of resistance, often noted in the treatment of Paget's disease, unrelated to the appearance of antibodies (592) has not

been reported in osteoporosis. The plateau seen in bone mass studies can be explained by the expected effect of an antiresorptive agent which reduces bone turnover and should not be interpreted as resistance.

Bisphosphonates

The effects of bisphosphonates in both prevention of bone loss and in the treatment of osteoporosis have recently been tested in several studies (593–605,608). For the first generation compound etidronate, the only bisphosphonate currently marketed in the United States, the net effects are somewhat similar to those observed with the other antiresorptive agents, calcitonin and estrogen. Bisphosphonates are potent inhibitors of osteoclast action, characterized by two C—P bonds forming a basic P—C—P structure that allows the synthesis of many different forms by the addition of side chains or phosphate esters. The activity of the compounds in inhibiting bone resorption varies greatly, and etidronate is one of the weaker compounds in this regard. The precise mechanism for osteoclast inhibition is still in doubt, but may be a toxic effect since the osteoclast may be exposed to high concentrations of compounds which cannot be metabolized and which can cause lysosomal enzyme inhibition, and reduction in lactic acid and prostaglandin synthesis (602).

Bisphosphonates have generally been used in situations of high bone turnover, in Paget's disease or hypercalcemia of malignancy (606,607,611). Their antiresorp-

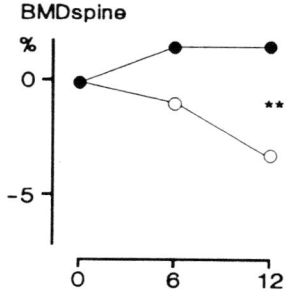

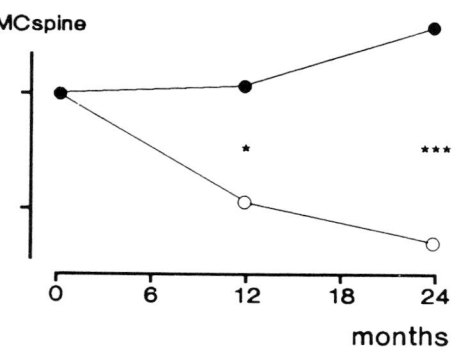

FIG. 35. Effects of intranasal salmon calcitonin on bone loss at the lumbar spine. Early postmenopausal women (○——○) lost bone whereas the nasal spray prevented bone loss (●——●) when given at a dose of 50 units, 5 days a week (A) [From Reginster et al. (576)] and 100 units daily (B) [From Overgaard et al. (759)].

tive activity, oral route of administration, and low systemic toxicity makes them attractive candidates for use in osteoporosis. Several different approaches to their use have been evaluated in the data available thus far. Continuous therapy (601,602) resulted in decline in both resorption and accretion with only a modest effect on calcium balance. The dose of etidronate (20 mg/kg/day) used in that study has since been shown to cause a mineralization defect, a phenomenon associated with few other bisphosphonates (602,605). Lower doses (5 mg/kg) were ineffective in reducing the negative calcium balance in the bed rest model (609), and did not affect loss of calcaneal bone. However, a 3-month course of etidronate did reduce skeletal metabolism measured biochemically immediately following oophorectomy (Figs. 36 and 37) (599). The most recent studies of etidronate evaluated bone mass and fracture recurrence with short intermittent pulses repeated at intervals of approximately 3 months (594,600). The daily dose was 400 mg, approximately 5 mg/kg. Small increments in bone mass occurred during each study compatible with an antiresorptive effect even at this small dose of the drug. In both studies reductions in vertebral fracture recurrence were seen. The use of etidronate in this fashion is important if the data are confirmed in long-term studies. The potentially long half-life of bisphosphonates in the skeleton and their inhibition of metabolism in osteoclasts raises the possibility that prolonged use in osteoporosis will increase the age of the remaining skeletal tissue and increase its potential for fracture. Dogs treated with high doses of bisphosphonate over long periods suffered spontaneous fractures (610) but no such problems have been observed in Paget's patients treated long term with bisphosphonates (606,611). In etidronate-treated patients with Paget's disease fractures do continue, but at a lower rate than might be expected and may be more related to the mineralization defect seen with this compound.

In the absence of long-term data, etidronate remains at present an investigational drug for osteoporosis. However, its safety in the short term makes it an option for treatment which might potentially receive approval in the near future. When used in the fashion described in the most recent publications, etidronate is given by mouth 400 mg/day for a two-week period. To improve compliance we use the beginning of every fourth calender month to begin treatment. The drug must be given on an empty stomach to maximize its absorption and food as well as nutritional supplements should not be consumed for two hours before or after the dose. During the drug-free period (of 3 or 3.5 months) calcium intake should be maintained at 1500 mg/day. Patients should probably be followed with high precision bone mass measurements where these are available.

Calcitriol

The use of the parent compound cholecalciferol (vitamin D_3) in osteoporosis has been widespread for some years often coupled with calcium and sodium fluoride. This in part followed the demonstration of relative malabsorption of calcium in elderly osteoporotic patients (245). Efficacy of vitamin D used in this fashion has never been demonstrated and indeed may be harmful, at least in doses of 50,000 units once or twice per week. These regimens should be discouraged and their use discontinued.

Recently with the availability of the active metabolite of vitamin D, 1,25-dihydroxyvitamin D (calcitriol), several studies have examined its use in patients with established osteoporosis (612–630). The results of these studies are somewhat variable. Calcitriol appears to reduce bone loss and in two studies reduced fracture frequency (612–630). However, other studies have not found significant effects (616,620,625,626,627). In part this may be related to the dose or to the severity of the patients included in the studies. In Japan the results are more encouraging, perhaps suggesting that osteoporosis may have a somewhat different etiology with perhaps a higher incidence of patients with calcium deficiency or calcium malabsorption (618,619,622,623).

Calcitriol is not approved for use in osteoporosis in the United States. The major drawbacks to its general use are the difficulty in clinically detecting individuals with calcium malabsorption, referred to in the preceding text, and the narrow therapeutic window for the drug. Significant hypercalciuria and hypercalcemia can occur during its use at doses within the proposed therapeutic range (613), especially if calcium intake is not controlled. It is possible that the effects of calcitriol are mediated directly on the skeleton, since calcitriol is a potent stimulator of bone resorption in culture (631,632) and stimulates the synthesis of osteocalcin (633) and osteopontin (634). Alternatively it has been proposed that the effects of calcitriol are mediated by correction of abnormal lymphocyte subsets found in some Japanese patients with primary osteoporosis (635). Calcitriol is a potent regulator of cell function and controls cell differentiation (636). Its use in osteoporosis remains investigational at this time. It is possible that other metabolites of vitamin D may prove to be of therapeutic value in osteoporotic patients.

Anabolic Agents

Although the dominant hormonal change that predisposes to osteoporosis is the loss of estrogen from ovarian sources, there is also an age-related decline in androgen production (637). Reductions in the weak androgens androstanedione and dehydroepiandrosterone with age and with osteoporosis or bone density have been reported (637–640). Consequently anabolic agents, essentially modified androgens, have been evaluated in patients with osteoporosis. The results seem somewhat

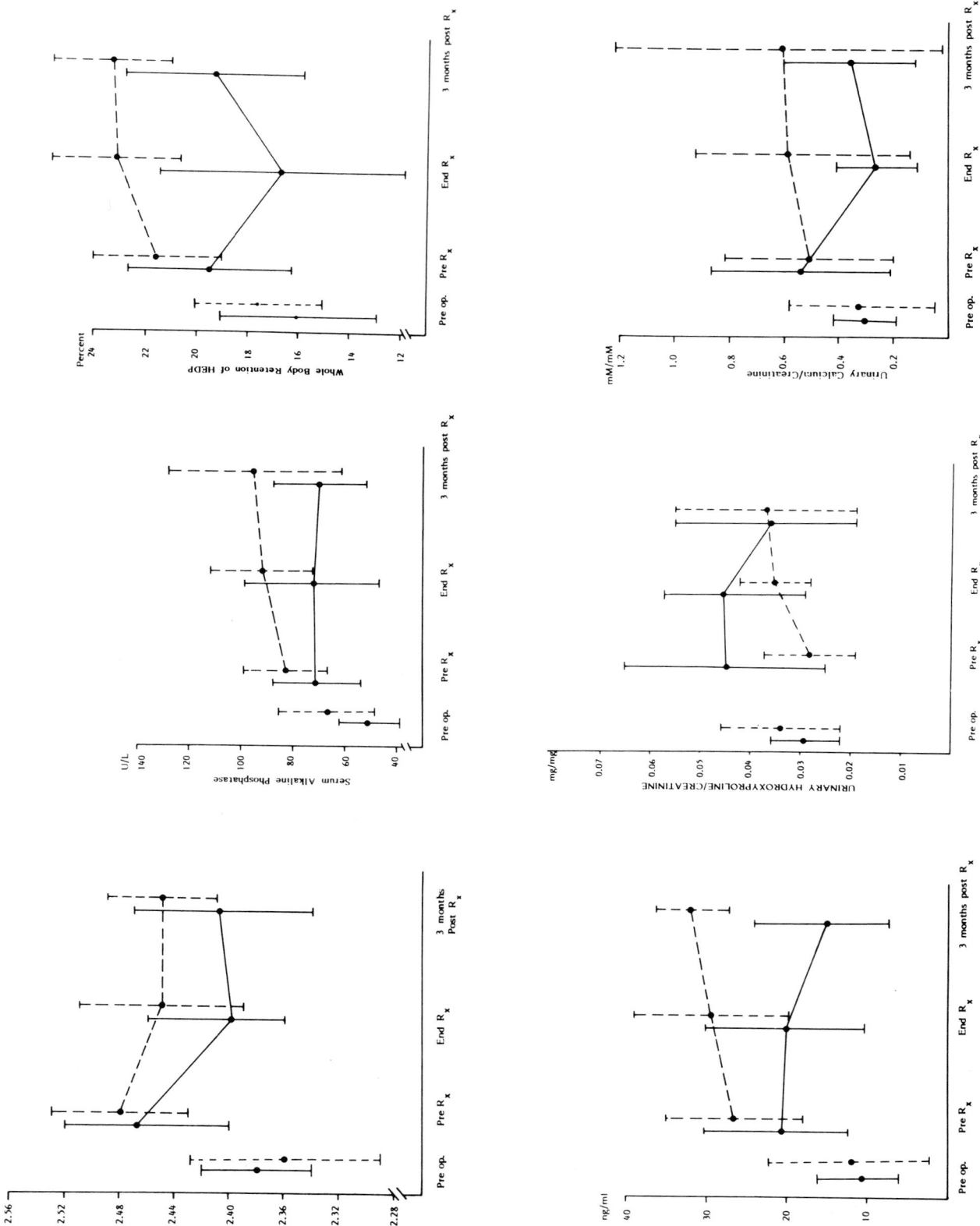

FIG. 36. The changes in biochemical determinants of bone turnover in serum and urine before oophorectomy, after oophorectomy, during treatment with etidronate (400 mg/day) or a placebo for three months, and after treatment. From Smith et al. (599).

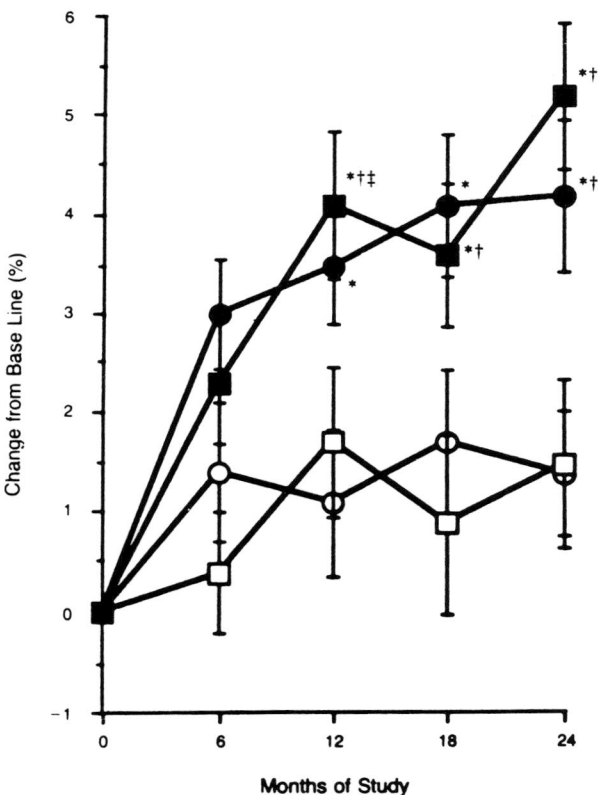

FIG. 37. Mean (±SE) changes in bone mineral density of the spine (as measured by dual photon absorptiometry) in group 1 (placebo and placebo; open circles), group 2 (phosphate and placebo; open squares), group 3 (placebo and etidronate; solid circles), and group 4 (phosphate and etidronate; solid squares). The asterisk indicates a significant change from baseline ($p < 0.017$); the dagger, a significant change as compared with group 1 ($p < 0.01$); and the double dagger, a significant difference as compared with group 2 ($p < 0.01$). From ref. 600, with permission.

similar, in terms of their effects on bone mass, to those that are seen with the use of estrogens (Fig. 38) (641–647). No dramatic increases in bone mass have been reported, and the most that can be expected is reduction in rate of bone loss. Moreover, this may occur in part because of changes in soft tissue, namely the reduction in fat and increased lean body mass interacting with the measurement of bone mass to exaggerate the effect of the drug (648). In vitro, anabolic agents stimulate osteoblasts, (649) and in vivo have been shown to increase serum osteocalcin (650). The relationship between these effects and the observed effects on the skeleton remains obscure.

Anabolic agents remain investigational in the treatment of osteoporosis and while they may have a role, it is likely to be small. Androgenic drugs are poorly tolerated, and their negative effects on lipid metabolism render them riskier to use particularly in younger individuals (648,651). Their role may be in treatment of the frail elderly individual with osteoporotic fractures where their anabolic effects on muscle may be more important than their effects on the skeleton (648).

Fluoride

For many years sodium fluoride has been used in the treatment of osteoporosis. Fluoride is the only available agent that stimulates new bone formation and increases bone mass. Dietary intake of fluoride is usually less than 0.5 mg per day (653), unless water fluoridation is practiced, which increases intake by about 1 mg. Intakes of 1–2 mg are sufficient to reduce dental caries in children, but probably are insufficient to affect the skeleton. Skele-

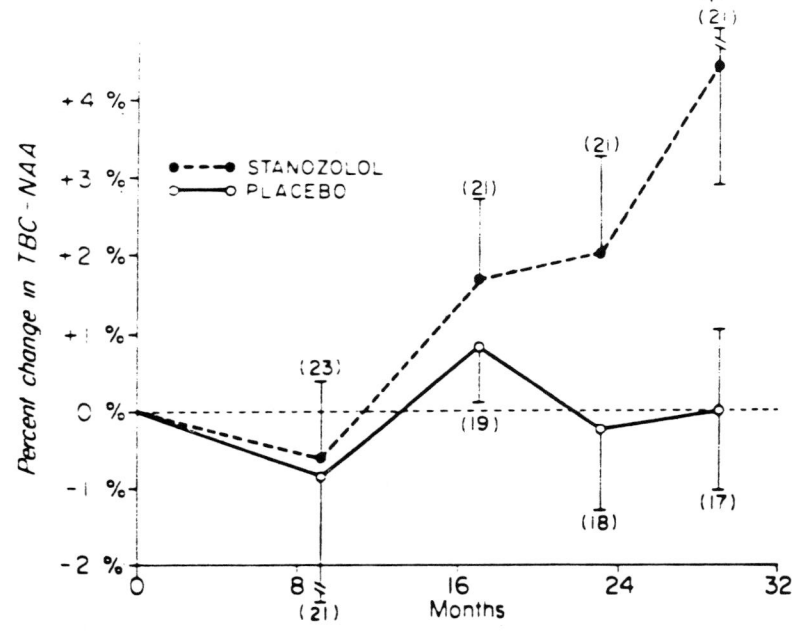

FIG. 38. Percentage of change in TBC (grams) as a function of treatment time in treated and control patients, mean ± SEM (n). *, significantly different from baseline, $p < 0.01$; ², change from baseline between treated and control groups significantly different, $p = 0.03$. From ref. 641, with permission.

tal content of fluoride is proportional to intake over a wide range (653) and about 50% of ingested fluoride is deposited in the skeleton. High fluoride intakes result in fluorosis, a painful crippling disorder associated with dense bones, extraosseous calcification around joints and in ligaments, and bony outgrowths which can produce neurologic deficits (654,655). Asymptomatic osteosclerosis, the precursor of fluorosis, is seen commonly in areas of high fluoride intake (656), where the incidence and prevalence of osteoporosis is notably low (657). This phenomenon led to the use of fluoride in the treatment of osteoporosis initially in 1961 (658). Since then a considerable number of studies have been completed with variable and conflicting results (420,421, 658–693,761).

In most studies fluoride increases bone density of the axial skeleton including the iliac crest in a variable percentage of the patients treated (Fig. 39). The proportion responding appears to depend on dose but is usually about 60%. There is either no change in peripheral bone or a decline in bone mass. Results depend on the use of calcium supplementation which reduces the amount of unmineralized osteoid produced in response to fluoride by an unknown mechanism and prevents the increase in bone resorption that follows treatment, perhaps by reducing PTH secretion. The optimum dose of sodium fluoride appears to be around 50 mg per day, accompanied by sufficient calcium to bring intake up to at least 1500 mg per day. The addition of vitamin D is not necessary except in replacement dose (100 to a maximum of 800 IU/day) for older individuals who may be deficient (693). In studies using regimens similar to this the results appear more convincing with marked increments in vertebral mineral, and cancellous bone volume of the iliac crest (665,669,670,676,678,679,685,687,691–693). Fluoride, however, still remains a controversial treatment in part, at least, because of the high incidence of side effects, including gastrointestinal irritation and a painful syndrome in the periarticular bone in the lower limbs, with an overall occurrence of 30–50%, dependent on dose (693). The gastrointestinal side effects can be reduced using a slow-release preparation (694). However, the painful limb syndrome remains a problem for some patients. The exact cause of this syndrome is still unknown. Pain is associated with positive radionuclide bone scans, and it has been suggested that these are insufficiency fractures that may in some individuals become complete (695,762–764). Further concerns have been raised about the quality of new bone that is formed in response to fluoride (693,765). There is increased osteoid, which is not entirely prevented by the administration of calcium (696) and the architecture may be abnormal (697).

Recently two controlled studies examined the effects of sodium fluoride in doses of 75 mg per day (90 and 60 mg on alternate days (420,692). Increments in spinal

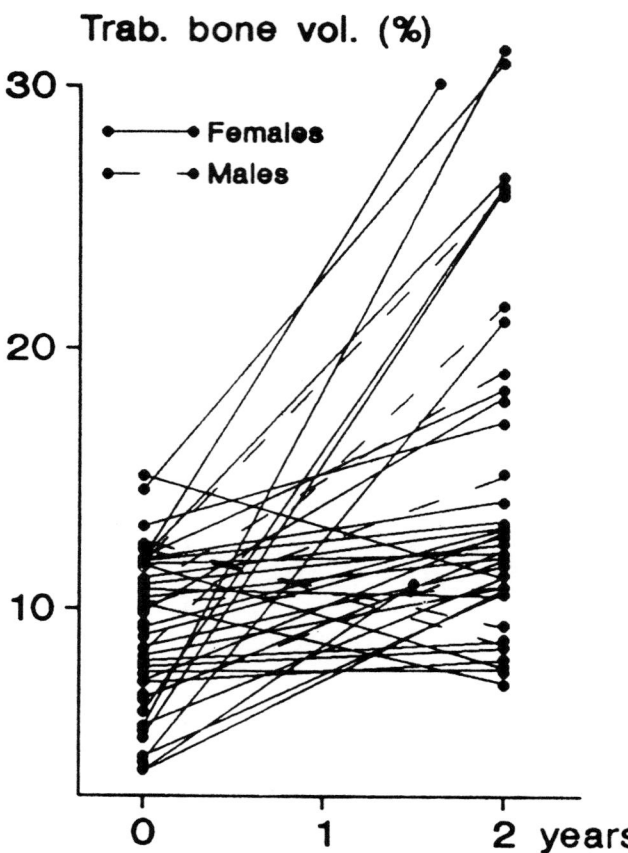

FIG. 39. Measurement of trabecular bone volume in 46 patients before and two years after continuous treatment with sodium fluoride (50 mg daily), vitamin D, and calcium. There was a significant increase in bone matrix volume in the majority of patients, but in one-third of patients no anabolic effect was observed. From Briancon and Meunier, (669).

mineral were seen as expected but no decline in vertebral fracture frequency was observed (Fig. 40). A disturbing feature of one study was an increase in peripheral fractures, in particular hip fractures. There were only 3 hip fractures in the placebo group compared with 7 in the fluoride treated group (Table 11). The possibility that fluoride increases the risk of hip fracture has been noted previously (698–700), but is controversial (701). In one other randomized controlled study a small reduction in new vertebral fractures was observed (691) with a small but insignificant increase in hip fracture risk. At present, therefore, fluoride cannot be recommended for use in osteoporosis, and must remain an investigational drug, at least in the United States. It is possible that other doses or preparations of fluoride, such as monofluorophosphate, may be more effective and safer but also may be associated with greater toxicity (766). We must also learn more about the precise cellular mechanism of the effects of fluoride. The ion stimulates bone cell growth and influences enzymatic activity in osteoblasts (702–704,761).

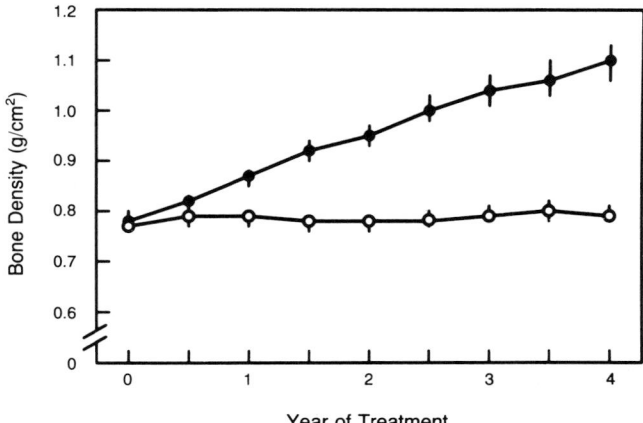

FIG. 40. Mean (±SE) bone density of the lumbar spine in the fluoride group (●——●) and the placebo group (○——○). From ref. 420.

Other Investigational Regimens

The amino-terminal fragment of human parathyroid hormone has received recent attention although Selye first demonstrated the anabolic effects of parathyroid hormone on the skeleton many years ago (705). Several reports suggest increased bone mass with the use of small doses of (1–34)hPTH given subcutaneously to animals (706–714) and in humans (715–723). The results, although uncontrolled for the most part are impressive with dramatic increments in bone mass. The effects appear to require stimulation of 1-α-hydroxylase and increased circulating levels of 1,25(OH)$_2$D (718). How-

ever, the disturbance of skeletal architecture that characterizes osteoporosis may not be correctable and more detailed investigation of this and any other method of increasing bone mass is clearly required.

Frost originally suggested that the bone remodeling cycle could be manipulated to therapeutic advantage (Fig. 41) (652,724). The technique known by its acronym ADFR (for Activate, Depress, Free, Repeat) argues that if a synchronous population of bone remodeling units could be stimulated then the entire active population of osteoclasts could be suppressed (e.g., by calcitonin or a bisphosphonate). At the end of the osteoclast resorption period the suppressing agent is removed and osteoblasts are allowed to form new bone. The cycle is then repeated. The concept requires that the inhibited osteoclasts resorb less bone than normal and that the osteoblast population synthesize (and mineralize) its normal quota of osteoid. This would have the net effect of creating a positive balance at each remodeling site and as each cycle of treatment is completed bone mass would increase, presumably continually until treatment is discontinued. Several attempts at this schedule have been made in patients with osteoporosis (600,725–730,734). Usually phosphate has been used to stimulate endogenous PTH secretion as the activator of remodeling and etidronate used to depress osteoclast function. The results are essentially the same as those obtained using intermittent etidronate alone, or continuous calcitonin or estrogen. In fact in one study in which the ADFR regimen was evaluated in a random design using estrogen as the control, the ADFR protocol was less effective than estrogen (460). In all instances, except one (725) calcium or other agents were given during the free period, and it

TABLE 11. *Non-vertebral fractures during the study in the women with osteoporosis in the fluoride and placebo groups[a]*

Site	Incomplete fractures		Complete fractures		Total fractures	
	Fluoride	Placebo	Fluoride	Placebo	Fluoride	Placebo
Radius (Colles' fracture)	0 (0)	0 (0)	1 (1)	4 (4)	1 (1)	4 (4)
Humerus	0 (0)	0 (0)	5 (6)	1 (1)	5 (6)	1 (1)
Rib	1 (1)	0 (0)	10 (13)	8 (8)	11 (14)	8 (8)
Pelvis	3 (4)	0 (0)	3 (3)	1 (1)	6 (7)	1 (1)
Proximal femur	4 (5)	1 (1)	7 (8)	3 (3)	11 (13)	4 (4)
Tibia	10 (11)	0 (0)	2 (2)	0 (0)	12 (13)	0 (0)
Metatarsus or calcaneus	7 (10)	1 (1)	2 (2)	2 (2)	9 (12)	3 (3)
Other[b]	1 (1)	0 (0)	5 (5)	3 (3)	6 (6)	3 (3)
All sites	7 (10)	1 (1)	2 (2)	2 (2)	9 (12)	3 (3)
Relative risk (95% confidence interval)[c]	16.8 (3.9–71.7)		1.9 (1.1–3.4)		3.2 (1.8–5.6)	

[a] No. of patients (no. of fractures).

[b] Other fractures involved the clavicle (two), the shaft or distal femur (two), and the small bones of the wrist or foot (two) in the fluoride group and the ulna, fibula, and hand in the placebo group.

[c] The fluoride group had 310 person-years of follow-up and the placebo group had 325 person-years of follow-up. Patients were evaluated every six months for non-vertebral fractures.

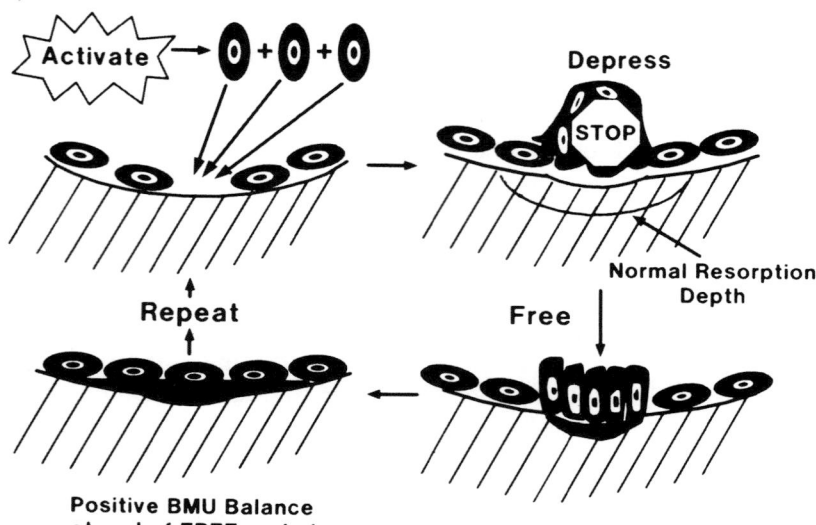

FIG. 41. The "ADFR" approach to increasing bone mass. This currently remains a hypothetical therapy under investigation (A, activation of a large synchronous population of remodeling cycles (vitamin D, parathyroid hormone); D, depression of bone resorption (calcitonin, diphosphonates or estrogen); F, free running bone formation; R, repeat: in theory, osteoclasts will dig smaller holes and osteoblasts will overfill them, giving a positive bone balance).

is possible that the suppressing effects of these agents on activation is one reason for the lack of success of the ADFR schedule. In fact several possibilities exist for the apparent failure of the regimens proposed thus far, including failure to demonstrate activation, the lack of knowledge about osteoclast behavior and the unknown response of the osteoblast population to the reduced size of resorption cavities. Indeed as has been pointed out, the activation burst followed by synchronous resorption might result in an insult to the skeleton and with a temporary reduction in skeletal mass. This might be significant for patients with already prejudiced skeletons such that an increased fracture risk, albeit temporary, might result (730). The use of ADFR regimens cannot be recommended for clinical use at present.

Other intermittent and cyclical strategies not following the strict ADFR protocol have been proposed (731–733), but none has any clear advantage over continuous estrogen or calcitonin or intermittent etidronate.

Growth Hormone

Since bone turnover and bone mass are increased in acromegaly, it is not surprising that growth hormone has been considered for therapeutic use in osteoporosis (735–737). Growth hormone increases bone mass in dogs, and is an activator of skeletal remodeling in humans (738,739). The addition of growth hormone to calcitonin, however, resulted in no significant alteration in skeletal response (733,740,741). More recently growth hormone itself has been used in elderly individuals with a small positive increment in bone mass (742). However, the changes in body composition with increased muscle mass make this a potential future therapy for the frail elderly with osteoporosis.

CONCLUSIONS

Primary osteoporosis occurs in women as a consequence of ovarian failure. In addition, age-related alterations in calcium homeostasis and bone remodeling contribute to loss of bone mass with age in both sexes. Superimposed upon these relentless and universal age-related changes, a wide variety of insults to the skeleton, some of which can themselves result in clinical osteoporosis (e.g., corticosteroid use), can occur. The prevalence and incidence of osteoporotic fractures are increasing, at least in part related to the increase in the numbers of elderly, but there may also be an age-independent increment in risk that has been documented in several countries. Early introduction of estrogen replacement therapy, or more correctly hormone replacement therapy, since progestins are required also if the uterus is intact, reduces bone loss and the subsequent risk of fracture. Patients treated in this fashion have a reduced risk of cardiovascular disease, but after long-term therapy there may be a small (5–20%) increase in the risk of breast cancer. Bone mass measurements can be used to determine those at greatest risk of osteoporotic fracture and therefore target them for intervention. Estrogen/progestin therapy can also be used to treat the established disorder once the patient has presented with fracture. Alternatives to estrogen include calcitonin and the bisphosphonates, both more often used in treatment of the clinical fracture syndrome rather than in prevention, although they might be expected to be more useful as preventive agents. Fluoride, the one available agent that increases axial bone mass does not appear to significantly reduce vertebral fractures, and may actually increase the risk for peripheral fractures, and therefore needs further study. Other therapeutic regimens have been proposed and are currently under investigation. It seems likely that specific approaches to increase skeletal mass will be developed in the near future. Whether any such approach will be successful in eliminating the risk of atraumatic fracture once osteoporosis has occurred, depends on its ability to correct the architectural and other qualitative factors that increase fracture risk in the osteoporotic patient. It may be that osteoporosis will remain a condition more amenable to prevention than treatment.

REFERENCES

1. Riggs BL, Melton LJ III. Involutional osteoporosis. *N Engl J Med* 1986;314:1676–86.
2. Lindsay R. Sex steroids in the pathogenesis and prevention of osteoporosis. In: Riggs BL, Melton LJ III, eds. *Osteoporosis: etiology, diagnosis, and management.* New York: Raven Press, 1988;233–58.
3. Armelagos GJ. Disease in ancient Nubia. Changes in disease patterns from 350 B.C. to A.D. 1400 demonstrate the interaction of biology and culture. *Science* 1969;163:255–9.
4. Amundsen DW, Diers CJ. The age of menopause in classical Greece and Rome. *Hum Biol* 1970;42:79–86.
5. Perzigian AJ. Osteoporotic bone loss in two prehistoric Indian populations. *Am J Phys Anthropol* 1973;39:87–96.
6. Perzigian AJ. The antiquity of age-associated bone demineralization in man. *J Am Geriatr Soc* 1973;21:100–5.
7. Little K. *Bone behavior.* London: Academic Press, 1973;301–2.
8. Bartley MH, Arnold JS. Sex differences in human skeletal involution. *Nature* 1967;214:908–9.
9. Cooper APA. *Treatise on dislocations and on fractures of the joints,* 4th ed. London: Langmen, HWST Recs Ome and Browne, 1824.
10. Melton LJ III. Epidemiology of fractures. In: *Osteoporosis: etiology, diagnosis, and management.* Riggs BL, Melton LJ III, eds. New York: Raven Press, 1988;133–54.
11. Garraway WM, Stauffer RN, Kurland LT, O'Fallon WM. Limb fractures in a defined community. 1. Frequency and distribution. *Mayo Clinic Proc* 1979;54:701–7.
12. Cummings SR, Kelsey JL, Nevitt MC, O'Dowd KJ. Epidemiology of osteoporosis and osteoporotic fractures. *Epidemiol Rev* 1985;7:178–208.
13. Holbrook TL, Grazier K, Kelsey JL, et al. The frequency of occurrence, impact, and cost of musculoskeletal conditions in the United States. Chicago: American Academy of Orthopedic Surgeons, 1984;163–6.
14. Johnston CC Jr, Melton LJ III, Lindsay R, Eddy DM. Clinical indications for bone mass measurements. *J Bone Miner Res* 1989;4(Suppl):2.
15. Albright F, Bloomberg F, Smith PH. Postmenopausal osteoporosis. *Trans Assoc Amer Phys* 1940;55:298–305.
16. Albright F, Reifenstein EC Jr. Metabolic bone disease: osteoporosis. In: Albright F, Reifenstein EC, eds. *The parathyroid glands and metabolic bone disease.* Baltimore: Williams & Wilkins, 1948;145–204.
17. Melton LJ III, Riggs BL. Epidemiology of age-related fractures. In: Avioli LV, ed. *The osteoporotic syndrome.* New York: Grune & Stratton, 1983;45–72.
18. Solomon L. Osteoporosis and fracture of the femoral neck in the South African Bantu. *J Bone Joint Surg* 1968;50B:2–13.
19. Wong PCN. Femoral neck fractures among the major racial groups in Singapore. Incidence patterns compared with non-Asian communities. *Singapore Med J* 1964;5:150–7.
20. Stott S, Gray DH. The incidence of femoral neck fractures in New Zealand. *N Z Med J* 1980;91:6–9.
21. Hedlund R, Aulbom A, Lindgren U. Hip fracture incidence in Stockholm 1972–1981. *Acta Orthop Scand* 1985;57:30–4.
22. Elabdien BSZ, Olerud S, Karlstrom G, Smedley B. Rising incidence of hip fracture in Uppsala 1965–1980. *Acta Orthop Scand* 1984;55:284–9.
23. Finsen V, Benun P. Changing incidence of hip fractures in rural and urban areas of central Norway. *Clin Orthop* 1987;218:104–10.
24. Felch JA, Liebekk A, Slumbaard W. Epidemiology of hip fractures in Norway. *Acta Orthop Scand* 1985;56:12–6.
25. Martin AD, Silverthorn KG, Houston CS. Age-specific increase in hip fractures in Canada. In: Christiansen C, Johansen JS, Riis BJ, eds. *Osteoporosis.* Copenhagen: Osteopres, 1987;111–2.
26. Lindsay R, Dempster DW, Clemens T, Herrington B, Wilt S. Incidence, cost and risk factors of fracture of the proximal femur in the USA. In: Christiansen C, Johansen JS, Riis BJ, eds. *Osteoporosis.* Copenhagen: Osteopres, 1984;311–6.
27. Melton LJ III, O'Fallon WM, Riggs BL. Secular trends in the incidence of hip fracture. *Calcif Tissue Int* 1987;41:57–64.
28. Melton LJ III, Ilstrup DM, Riggs BL, Beckenbaugh RD. Fifty year trend in hip fracture incidence. *Clin Orthop* 1982; 162:144–9.
29. Cummings SR, Rudin SM, Black D. The future of hip fracture in the United States: numbers, costs and potential effects of postmenopausal estrogen. *Clin Orthop Rel Res* 1990;252:163–6.
30. Cummings SR. Osteoporotic fractures: the magnitude of the problem. In: *Osteoporosis 1987,* vol 2. Christiansen C, Johansen JS, Riis BJ, eds. Osteopres: Copenhagen, 1987;1193–6.
31. Fitzgerald JF, Moore PS, Dittus RS. The care of elderly patients with hip fractures. *N Engl J Med* 1988;319:1392–7.
32. Baker SP, Harvey AH. Fall injuries in the elderly. Symposium on falls and the elderly. Biological and Behavioral Aspects. *Clin Geriatr Med* 1985;1:501–8.
33. Gryfe CI, Amies A, Ashley MJ. A longitudinal study of falls in the elderly population: incidence and morbidity. *Age Aging* 1977;6:201–10.
34. Cummings SR, Nevitt MC. Epidemiology of hip fractures and falls. In: Kleerekoper M, Krane S, eds. *Clinical disorders of bone and mineral metabolism.* New York: Mary Ann Liebert, 1989;231–6.
35. Campbell AJ, Remken J, Allan BC, Martinez GS. Falls in old age: a study of frequency and related clinical factors. *Age and Aging* 1981;10:264–70.
36. Prudham D, Evans JG. Factors associated with falls in the elderly: a community study. *Age and Aging* 1981;10:141–6.
37. Frankel VH, Pugh JW. Biomechanics of the hip. In: Frankel VH, ed. *Basic biomechanics of the skeletal system.* Philadelphia: Lea and Febiger, 1980;115–51.
38. Ray WA, Griffin MR, Schaffner W, et al. Psychotropic use and the risk of hip fracture. *N Engl J Med* 1987;316:404–6.
39. Buchner DM, Larson EB. Falls and fractures in patients with Alzheimer type dementia. *J Am* 1987;257:1492–5.
40. Tinetti ME, Speechley M. Prevention of falls among the elderly. *N Engl J Med* 1989;320:1055–9.
41. Koller WC, Glatt SL, Fox JH. Senile gait: a distinct clinical entity. *Clin Geriatr Med* 1985;1:661–9.
42. Melton LJ III, Riggs BL. Risk factors for injury after a fall. *Clin Geriatr Med* 1985;1:1–15.
43. Mastens M, Van Audekarcke R, Delport P, Demeester P, Mulier JC. The mechanical characteristics of cancellous bone at the upper femoral region. *J Biomech* 1983;16:971–83.
44. Parfitt AM. Trabecular architecture in the pathogenesis and prevention of fracture. *Am J Med* 1987;82:68–71.
45. Horsman A, Burkenshow L. Stochastic models of femoral bone loss and hip fracture risk. In: Kleerekoper M, Krane SM, eds. *Clinical disorders of bone and mineral metabolism.* New York: Mary Ann Liebert, 1989;253–60.
46. Cummings SR. Are patients with hip fractures more osteoporotic? Review of the evidence. *Am J Med* 1985;78:487–94.
47. Riggs BL, Wahner HW, Seeman E, et al. Changes in bone mineral density of the proximal femur and spine with aging. Differences between the postmenopausal and senile osteoporosis syndromes. *J Clin Invest* 1982;70:716–23.
48. Melton LJ III, Chao EYS, Lane J. Biomechanical aspects of fracture. In: Riggs BL, Melton LJ III, eds. *Osteoporosis: etiology,*

diagnosis, and management. New York: Raven Press, 1988;111–31.

49. Vose GP, Mack PB. Roentgenologic assessment of femoral neck density as related to fracturing. *Amer J Roentgenol* 1963;89:1296–301.

50. Leichter I, Margulies JY, Weinreb A, et al. The relationship between bone density, mineral content, and mechanical strength in the femoral neck. *Clin Orthop* 1982;163:272–81.

51. Frankel VH, Pugh JW. Biomechanics of the hip. In: Tranzo RG, ed. *Surgery of the hip joint.* New York: Springer-Verlag, 1984;115–31.

52. Melton LJ III, Wahner HW, Richelson LS, O'Fallon WM, Riggs BL. Osteoporosis and the risk for hip fracture. *Am J Epidemiol* 1986;124:254–61.

53. Melton LJ III, Kan SH, Frye MA, Wahner HW, O'Fallon WM, Riggs BL. Epidemiology of vertebral fractures in women. *Am J Epidemiol* 1989;129:1000–11.

54. Gershon-Cohen J, Rechtman AM, Schroeser H, et al. Asymptomatic fractures in osteoporotic spines of the aged. *JAMA* 1953;153:625–7.

55. Jensen GF, Christiansen C, Boesen J, et al. Epidemiology of postmenopausal spinal and long bone fractures. *Clin Orthop* 1982;166:75–81.

56. Hodkinson HM. The pattern of vertebral collapse in elderly women with osteoporosis. *J Clin Exp Geront* 1989;11:21–7.

57. Marshall DH, Horsman A, Simpson M. Fractures in elderly women: prevalence of wrist, spine and femur fractures and their concurrence. In: Christiansen C, Arnaud CD, Nordin BEC, eds. *Osteoporosis.* Denmark: Aalborg Stiftsborgtrykkerri 1984;361–363.

58. Ross PD, Wasnich RD, Vogel JM. Detection of prefracture spinal osteoporosis using bone mineral absorptiometry. *J Bone Miner Res* 1988;3:1–11.

59. Odvina CV, Wergedal JE, Libanati CR, et al. Relationship between trabecular vertebral bone density and fractures: a quantitative definition of spinal osteoporosis. *Metabolism* 1988;37:221–8.

60. Frost HM. Clinical management of the symptomatic patient. *Orthop Clin North Am* 1981;12:671–81.

61. Lindhe M. Biomechanics of the lumbar spine. In: Frankel VH, Nordin M, eds. *Basic biomechanics of the skeletal system.* Philadelphia: Lea and Ferbiger, 1980;255–90.

62. Schultz AB, Andersson GBJ, Haderspeck K, et al. Analysis and measurement of lumbar trunk loads in tasks involving bends and twists. *J Biomech* 1982;15:669–75.

63. Perey O. Fracture of the vertebral end-plate in the lumbar spine: an experimental biomechanical investigation. *Acta Orthop Scand* 1957;25(Suppl):3–101.

64. Bartley MH, Arnold JS, Haslam RK, et al. The relationship of bone strength and bone quantity in health disease and aging. *J Gerontol* 1966;21:517–21.

65. Hansson T, Roos B, Nachemson A. The bone mineral content and ultimate compressive strength of lumbar vertebrae. *Spine* 1980;5:46–54.

66. Evans JG. Epidemiology of proximal femur fractures. *Rec Adv Ger Med* 1982;2:201–14.

67. Bengner V, Jonnell O. Increasing incidence of forearm fractures: a comparison of epidemiologic patterns 25 years apart. *Acta Orthop Scand* 1985;56:158–60.

68. Melton LJ, Sampson JM, Morrey BF, Ilstrup DM. Epidemiologic features of pelvic fractures. *Clin Orthop* 1981;155:43–7.

69. Buhr AJ, Cook AM. Fracture patterns. *Lancet* 1959;i:531–6.

70. Hedlund R, Lindgren U. Epidemiology of diaphyseal femoral fractures. *Acta Orthop Scand* 1987;57:423–7.

71. Robin GC, Steinberg R, Leichter I, Menczel J, Makin M. A comparison of noninvasive methods in the diagnosis of osteoporosis. In: Ed Menzel J, Robin GC, Makin M, Steinberg RJ, eds. *Osteoporosis.* Chichester, England: John Wiley, 1982;71–9.

72. Arnold JS, Bartley MH, Tout SA, Jenkins DP. Skeletal changes in aging and disease. *Clin Orthop* 1966;49:17–38.

73. Lindhol O, Lindgren AGH. Grading of osteoporosis in autopsy specimens. *Acta Orthop Scand* 1960;32:85–7.

74. Smith DA, Anderson JB, Shimmins J, Speirs CF, Barnett E. Changes in metacarpal mineral content and density in normal male and female subjects with age. *Clin Radiol* 1969;20:23–31.

75. Liel Y, Edwards J, Shary J, Spiar KM, Gordon L, Bell NH. The effects of race and body habitus on bone mineral density of the radius, hip and spine in premenopausal women. *J Clin Endocrinol Metab* 1988;66:1247–50.

76. Luckey MM, Meier DE, Mandeli JP, DeCasta MC, Hubbard ML, Goldsmith SJ. Radial and vertebral bone mineral density in white and black women: evidence for racial differences in premenopausal bone homeostasis. *J Clin Endocrinol Metab* 1989;69:762–70.

77. Gallagher JC, Golgar D, Mahoney P, McGill J. Measurement of spine density in normal and osteoporotic subjects using computed tomography. Relationship of spine density to fracture threshold and fracture index. *J Comput Assist Tomogr* 1985;9:634–5.

78. Mack LA, Hanson JA, Kilcoyne RF, Ott SM, Gallagher JC, Chesnut CH. Correlation between fracture index and bone density by CT and dual photon absorptiometry. *J Comput Assist Tomagr* 1985;9:635–6.

79. Powell MR, Kolb FO, Genant HK, Cann CE, Stebler BG. Comparison of dual photon absorptiometry and quantitative computed tomography of the lumbar spine in the same subjects. In: *Clinical disorders of bone and mineral metabolism.* Frame B, Potts JT, eds. Amsterdam: Excerpta Medica, 1983;58–61.

80. Mazess RB, Borden H, Ettinger M, Schulz E. Bone density of the radius, spine and proximal femur in osteoporosis. *J Bone Miner Res* 1987;3:13–18.

81. Firooznia H, Golumbia C, Rafii M, Schwartz MS, Allerman ER. Quantitative computed tomography assessment of spinal trabecular bone. II. In Osteoporotic women with and without vertebral fractures. *J Comput Assist Tomogra* 1984;8:99–103.

82. Harma M, Karjalainen P, Hoikka V, Alhova E. Bone density in women with spinal and hip fractures. *Acta Orthop Scand* 1985;56:380–5.

83. Maller M, Horsman A, Harvald B, Hauge M, Henningsen K, Nordin BEC. Metacarpal morphometry in monozygotic and dizygotic elderly twins. *Calcif Tissue Res* 1978;25:197–201.

84. Pocock NA, Eisman JA, Hopper JL, Yeates MG, Sambrook PN, Ebers S. Genetic determinants of bone mass in adults. *J Clin Invest* 1987;80:706–10.

85. Smith DM, Nance WE, Kang KW, et al. Genetic factors in determining bone mass. *J Clin Invest* 1973;52:2800.

86. Dequeker J, Nijs J, Verstraeten A, Geusens P, Gevers G. Genetic determinants of bone mineral content at the spine and radius: a twin study. *Bone* 1987;8:207–9.

87. Heaney RP. Nutritional factors in bone health. In: Riggs BL, Melton LJ III, eds. *Osteoporosis: etiology, diagnosis, and management.* New York: Raven Press, 1988;359–72.

88. Matkovic V, Tominac C, Fontana D, Chesnut C. Influence of calcium on peak bone mass: a 24-month follow-up. *J Bone Min Res* 1988;3(suppl. 1):S85.

89. Matkovic V, Kostial K, Simonovic I, Brizina R, Brodarec A, Nordin BEC. Bone status and fracture rates in two regions of Yugoslavia. *Am J Clin Nutr* 1979;32:540.

90. Doyle FH. Age-related bone changes in women. A quantitative x-ray study of the distal third of the ulna in normal subjects. In: Whedon GD, Cameron JR, eds. *Progress in methods of bone mineral measurement.* Washington, DC: U.S. Department of Health Education and Welfare, 1968.

91. Frost HM. The skeletal intermediary organization. A synthesis. In: Peck WA, ed. *Bone and mineral research,* vol 3. Amsterdam: Elsevier, 1988;49–107.

92. Kleerekoper M, Talia L, Parfitt AM. Nutritional, endocrine and demographic aspects of osteoporosis. *Orthop Clin North Am* 1981;12:547–56.

93. Kanders B, Dempster DW, Lindsay R. Interaction of calcium, nutrition, and physical activity on bone mass in young women. *J Bone Miner Res* 1988;3:145–9.

94. Nilsson BE, Westlin NE. Bone density in athletes. *Clin Orthop* 1971;77:179.

95. Dalen N, Olsson KE. Bone mineral content and physical activity. *Acta Orthop Scand* 1974;45:170.

96. Aloia JF, Cohn SH, Babu T, et al. Skeletal mass and body composition in marathon runners. *Metabolism* 1978;27:1793.
97. Smith RW Jr, Rizek J. Epidemiologic studies of osteoporosis in women of Puerto Rico and Southeastern Michigan with special reference to age, race, national origin, and to other related or associated findings. *Clin Orthop* 1966;45:31–48.
97a. Proceedings of the First Asian Symposium on Osteoporosis. Edited by Chesnut CH III. Hong Kong: Excerpta Medica, 1988.
98. Mazess RB, Mather W. Bone mineral content of North American Eskimos. *Am J Clin Nutr* 1974;27:916–25.
99. Thompson DD, Posner AS, Loughlin WS, Blumenthal NC. Comparison of bone apatite in osteoporotic and normal Eskimos. *Calcif Tissue Int* 1983;35:392–3.
100. Mazess RB, Borden HS, Christiansen C, et al. Bone mineral and vitamin D in Aleutian Islanders. *Amer J Clin Nutr* 1985;42:143–6.
101. Solomon L. Bone density in aging Caucasian and African populations. *Lancet* 1979;3:1326–9.
102. Bloom RA, Pogrund H. Humeral cortical thickness in female Bantu: its relationship to the incidence of femoral neck fracture. *Skeletal Radiol* 1982;8:590–602.
103. Cohn SH, Abesamis C, Yasamara S, Aloia JF, Zanai I, Ellis KJ. Comparative skeletal mass and radial bone mineral content in black and white women. *Metabolism* 1977;26:171–8.
104. Trotter M. Densities of bones of white and Negro skeletons. *J Bone Joint Surg* 1960;42A:50–8.
105. Beals RK. Orthopedic aspects of the XO Turner's syndrome. *Clin Orthop* 1973;97:19–30.
106. Engel E, Forbes AP. Cytogenetic and clinical findings in 48 patients with congenitally defective or absent ovaries. *Medicine (Baltimore)* 1965;44:135–64.
107. Barr DG. Bone deficiency in Turner's syndrome measured by metacarpal dimensions. *Arch Dis Child,* 1974;49:821–2.
108. Garn SM, Pozranski AK. Transient and irreversible bone losses. In: Barzel US, ed. *Osteoporosis.* New York: Grune & Stratton, 1970;114–23.
109. Smith DAS, Walker MS. Changes in plasma steroids and bone density in Klinefelter's syndrome. *Calcified Tissue Research* 1977;22(suppl.):225–228.
110. de Vernejoul MC, Girot G, Gueris J, et al. Calcium phosphate metabolism and bone disease in patients with homozygous thalessemia. *J Clin Endocrinol Metab* 1982;54:276–81.
111. Avioli LV. Hyperparathyroidism, hypoparathyroidism, pseudohypoparathyroidism, and pseudopseudohypoparathyroidism. In: Goldensohn ES, Appel SH, eds. *Scientific approaches to clinical neurology,* vol 2. Philadelphia: Lea and Febiger, 1977;1871–83.
112. Seeman E, Hopper JL, Bach LA, et al. Reduced bone mass in daughters of women with osteoporosis. *N Engl J Med* 1989;320:554–8.
113. Evans R, Marel GM, Lancaster EK, et al. Bone mass is low in relatives of osteoporotic patients. *Ann Intern Med* 1988;1:870–3.
114. Lindberg JS, Fears WB, Hunt MM. Exercise induced amenorrhea and bone density. *Ann Intern Med* 1984;101:647–9.
115. Linnel SL, Stager MM, Blue PW. Bone mineral content and menstrual regularity in female runners. *Med Sci Sports Exerc* 1989;16:343–8.
116. Marcus R, Cann C, Madvig D. Menstrual function and bone mass in elite women distance runners. *Ann Intern Med* 1985;102:158–63.
117. Klibanski A, Neer RM, Beitins IZ, Ridgway C, Zervas NT, MacArthur J. Decreased bone density in hyperprolactinemic women. *N Engl J Med* 1980;303:1511–4.
118. Sanborn CF, Martin BJ, Wagner WW. Is athletic amenorrhea specific to runners. *Am J Obstet Gynecol* 1982;143:859–61.
119. Cann CE, Martin MC, Genant HK. Decreased spinal mineral content in amenorrheic women. *JAMA* 1984;251:626–9.
120. Drinkwater BL, Nilson KL, Chesnut CH III. Bone mineral content of amenorrheic and eumenorrheic athletes. *N Engl J Med* 1984;311:277–81.
121. Gonzalez ER. Premature bone loss found in some nonmenstruating sportswomen. *JAMA* 1982;248:513–4.
122. Schlechte JA, Sherman B, Martin R. Bone density in amenorrheic women with and without hyperprolactinemia. *J Clin Endocrinol Metab* 1983;56:1120–3.
123. Koppelman MCS, Kurtz DW, Morrish KA, et al. Vertebral body bone mineral in hyperprolactinemic women. *J Clin Endocrinol Metab* 1984;59:1050–3.
124. Nystrome E, Leman J, Lundberg PA, et al. Bone mineral content in normally menstruating women with hyperprolactinemia. *Horm Res* 1988;29:214–7.
125. Drinkwater BL, Nilson K, Ott S, Chesnut CH III. Bone mineral density after resumption of menses in amenorrheic women. *JAMA* 1986;256:380–2.
126. Lindberg JS, Powell MR, Hunt MM, Ducey DE, Wado CE. Increased vertebral bone mineral in response to reduced exercise in amenorrheic women. *West J Med* 1987;146:39–42.
127. Rigotti NA, Nussbaum SR, et al. Osteoporosis in women with anorexia nervosa. *N Engl J Med* 1984;311:1601–6.
128. Warren MF, Shane E, Lee MJ, et al. Osteonecrosis of the hip associated with anorexia nervosa in a 20 year old ballet dancer. *Clin Orthop* 1989;251:171–6.
129. Aitken JM, Hart DM, Anderson JB, Lindsay R, Smith DA. Osteoporosis after oophorectomy for non-malignant disease. *Br Med J* 1973;i:325–8.
130. Johnston CC, Hui SL, Witt RM, Appledorn R, Baker RS, Longcope C. Early menopausal changes in bone mass and sex steroids. *J Clin Endocrinol Metab* 1984;61:905–11.
131. Richelson LS, Wahner HW, Melton LJ, Riggs BL. Relative contributions of aging and estrogen deficiency to postmenopausal bone loss. *N Engl J Med* 1984;311:1273–5.
132. Lindsay R, Coutts JRT, Sweeney A, Hart DM. Endogenous oestrogen and bone loss following oophorectomy. *Calcif Tissue Res* 1977;22:213–6.
133. Heaney RP, Recker RR, Saville PD. Calcium balance and calcium requirements in middle-aged women. *Am J Clin Nutr* 1977;30:1603–11.
134. Heaney RP, Recker RR, Saville PD. Menopausal changes in calcium balance performance. *J Lab Clin Med* 1978;92:953–63.
135. Heaney RP, Recker RR, Saville PD. Menopausal changes in bone remodeling. *J Lab Clin Med* 1978;92:964–70.
136. Eriksen EF, Colvard DS, Berg NJ, et al. Evidence of estrogen receptors in normal human osteoblast-like cells. *Science* 1988;241:84–6.
137. Komm BS, Terpening CM, Benz DJ, et al. Estrogen binding receptor MRNA and biological response in osteoblast-like osteosarcoma cells. *Science* 1988;241:81–4.
138. Ernst M, Schmid C, Fraesch ER. Enhanced osteoblast proliferation and collage gene expression by estradiol. *Proc Natl Acad Sci USA* 1988;85:2307–10.
139. Fukuyama S, Tashjian AH Jr. Direct modulation by estradiol of the response of human bone cells Sa S-2 to human parathyroid hormone PTH and PTH-related protein. *Endocrinology* 1989;124:397–401.
140. Gray TK, Flynn TC, Gray KM, Nabell LM. 1987. 17β-estradiol acts directly on the clonal osteoblast cell line UMR1006. *Proc Natl Acad Sci USA* 1987;84:6267–71.
141. Gray TK, Mohan S, Linkhard TA, Baylink D. Estradiol stimulates *in vitro* the secretion of insulin-like growth factors by the clonal osteoblastic cell line UMR106. *Biochem Biophys Res Commun* 1989;158:407–12.
142. Ernst M, Heath JK, Rodan GA. Estradiol effects on proliferation, messenger ribonucleic acid for collagen and infusion-like growth factor-1, and parathyroid hormone-stimulated adenylate cyclase activity in osteoblastic cells from calvariae and long bones. *Endocrinology* 1989;125:825–33.
143. Cohn SH, Aloia JF, Vaswani AN, Yuen K, Yasumura S, Ellis KJ. Women at risk for developing osteoporosis: determination by total body neutron activation analysis and photon absorptiometry. *Calcif Tissue Int* 1986;38:9–15.
144. Ettinger B, Genant HK, Cann CE. Menopausal bone loss can be prevented by low dose estrogen with calcium supplements. *J Comput Assist Tomogr* 1985;633–4.
145. Genant HK, Cann CE, Ettinger B, Gordan GS. Quantitative computed tomography of vertebral spongiosa: a sensitive method

for detecting early bone loss after oophorectomy. *Ann Intern Med* 1982;97:699–705.

146. Riis B, Thomsen K, Christiansen C. Does calcium supplementation prevent postmenopausal bone loss? *N Engl J Med* 1987;316:173–7.

147. Genant HK, Block JE, Steiger P, Glower CC, Ettinger B, Harris ST. Appropriate use of bone densitometry. *Radiology* 1989; 170:817–22.

148. Stepan JJ, Pospichal J, Presl J, et al. Bone loss and biochemical indices of bone remodeling in surgically induced postmenopausal women. *Bone* 1987;8:279–84.

149. Geusens P, Dequeker J, Verstraeten A, Nijs J. Age-sex- and menopause-related changes of vertebral and peripheral bone: population study using dual and single photon absorptiometry and radiogrammetry. J Nucl Med 1986;27:1540–9.

150. Nilas L, Christiansen C. Bone mass and its relationship to age and the menopause. *J Clin Endocrinol Metab* 1987;65:697–702.

151. Riis BJ, Christiansen C. Measurement of spinal or peripheral bone mass to estimate early postmenopausal bone loss. *Am J Med* 1988;84:646–53.

152. Meema HE, Meema S. Postmenopausal osteoporosis: simple screening method for diagnosis before structural failure. *Radiology* 1987;164:405–10.

153. Christiansen C, Riis BJ, Rodbro P. Prediction of rapid bone loss in postmenopausal women. *Lancet* 1987;i:1105–8.

154. Brown DM, Jowsey J, Bradford DS, Brincat T. Osteoporosis in ovarian dysgenesis. *J Pediatr* 1974;84:816–20.

155. Drinkwater BL. 1989. Preserving strong bones: the young adult female. In: Kleerekoper M, Krane SM. eds. *Clinical disorders of bone and mineral metabolism.* New York; Mary Ann Liebert, 1989;173–8.

156. Lindsay R, Tohme J, Kanders B. The effect of oral contraceptive use on vertebral bone mass in pre- and postmenopausal women. *Contraception* 1986;34:333–49.

157. Savvas M, Studd JWW, Fogelman I. Skeletal effects of oral oestrogen compared with subcutaneous oestrogen and testosterone in postmenopausal women. *Br Med J* 1988;297:331–3.

158. Lloyd T, Buchanan JR, Ursino GR, Myers C, Woodward G, Halbert DR. Long term oral contraceptive use does not affect trabecular bone density. *Am J Obstet Gynecol* 1989;160:402–4.

159. Sowers MFR, Shapiro B, Gilbrath MA, Jannausch M. Health and hormonal characteristics of premenopausal women with lower bone mass. *Osteoporosis* 1990.

160. Hreschehyshyn MM, Hopkins A, Zylstra S, Anbar M. Associations of parity, breast feeding and birth control pills with lumbar spine and femoral neck bone densities. *Am J Obstet Gynecol* 1988;159:318–22.

161. Parfitt AM. Bone remodeling: relationship to the amount and structure of bone, and the pathogenesis and prevention of fractures. In: Riggs BL, Melton LJ III. eds. *Osteoporosis: etiology, diagnosis, and management.* New York; Raven Press, 1988;45–93.

162. Parfitt AM. Bone remodeling in the pathogenesis of osteoporosis. *Medical Times* 1981;109:80–92.

163. Parfitt AM. Age-related structural changes in trabecular and cortical bone: cellular mechanism and biochemical consequences. A. Differences between rapid and slow bone loss. B. Localized bone gain. *Calcif Tissue Int* 1984;36(Suppl):S123–8.

164. Steiniche T, Hasling C, Charles P, Eriksen EF, Mosekilde L, Melsen F. A randomized study on the effects of estrogen/gestagen or high dose oral calcium on trabecular bone remodeling in postmenopausal osteoporosis. *Bone* 1989;10:313–321.

165. Eriksen EF, Melsen F, Mosekilde L. Reconstruction of the resorptive site in iliac trabecular bone: a kinetic model for bone resorption in 20 normal individuals. *Metab Bone Dis Rel Res* 1984;5:235–42.

166. Recker RR, Kimmel DB, Parfitt AM, Davies KM, Keshowarz N, Hinders S. Static and tetracycline-based bone histomorphometric data from 34 normal postmenopausal females. *J Bone Miner Res* 1988;3:133–44.

167. Vedi S, Compston JE, Webb A, Tighe JR. Histomorphometric analysis of bone biopsies from the iliac crest of normal British subjects. *Metab Bone Dis Rel Res* 1982;4:231–6.

168. Vedi S, Compston JE, Webb A, Tighe JR. Histomorphometric

analysis of dynamic parameters of trabecular bone formation in the iliac crest of normal British subjects. *Metab Bone Dis Rel Res* 1983;5:69–74.

169. Melsen F, Mosekilde L. Tetracycline double-labeling of iliac trabecular bone in 41 normal adults. *Calcif Tissue Res* 1978;26:99–102.

170. Lips P, Coupron P, Meunier PJ. Mean wall thickness of trabecular bone packets in the human iliac crest: changes with age. *Calcif Tissue Res* 1978;26:13–7.

171. Parfitt AM. 1989. Surface specific bone remodeling in health and disease. In: Kleerekoper M, Krane SM. eds. *Clinical disorders of bone and mineral metabolism.* New York: Mary Ann Liebert, 1989;7–14.

172. Parfitt AM, Mathews CHE, Villaneuva AR, Kleerekoper M, Frame B, Rao DS. Relationships between surface, volume, and thickness of iliac trabecular bone in aging and in osteoporosis. *J Clin Invest* 1983;72:1396–409.

173. Kleerekoper M, Villaneuva AR, Stanciu J, Rao DS, Parfitt AM. The role of three dimensional trabecular microstructure in the pathogenesis of vertebral compression fractures. *Calcif Tissue Int* 1985;37:594–7.

174. Courpron P, Lepine P, Arlot M, Lips P, Meunier PJ. Mechanisms underlying the reduction with age of the mean wall thickness of trabecular basic structure unit (BSU) in human iliac bone. In: Jee WSS, Parfitt AM, eds. *Bone histomorphometry,* vol III. Paris: Armour Montagu, 1981;323–30.

175. Uhthoff HK, ed. *Current concepts of bone fragility.* Ottowa: University Ottowa Press, 1986.

176. Dempster DW, Shane E, Horbert W, Lindsay R. A simple method for correlative light and scanning electron microscopy of human iliac crest bone biopsies: qualitative and quantitative observations in normal and osteoporotic subjects. *J Bone Miner Res* 1986;1:15–21.

177. Johnston CC, Norton J, Khari MRA, et al. Heterogeneity of fracture syndromes in postmenopausal women. *J Clin Endocrinol Metab* 1985;61:551–6.

178. Meunier PH, Sellami S, Briancon D, Edouard C. Histological heterogeneity of apparently idiopathic osteoporosis. In: DeLuca HF, Frost H, Jee WSS, Johnston CC, Parfitt AM, eds. *Osteoporosis: recent advances in pathogenesis and treatment.* Baltimore: University Park Press, 1981;293–301.

179. Teitelbaum SL, Bergfeld MA, Avioli LV, Whyte MP. Failure of routine biochemical studies to predict the histological heterogeneity of untreated postmenopausal osteoporosis. In: DeLuca HF, Frost H, Jee WSS, Johnston CC, Parfitt AM., eds. *Osteoporosis: recent advances in pathogenesis and treatment.* Baltimore: University Park Press, 1981;303–9.

180. Whyte MP, Bergfeld MA, Murphy WA, Avioli LV, Teitelbaum SL. Postmenopausal osteoporosis: a heterogenous disorder as assessed by histomorphometric analysis of iliac crest bone from untreated patients. *Am J Med* 1982;72:193–201.

181. Parfitt AM, Kleerekoper M. Diagnostic value of bone histomorphometry and comparison of histologic measurements and biochemical indices of bone remodeling. In: Christiansen C, Arnaud CD, Nordin BEC, eds. *Osteoporosis.* Denmark: Aalborg Stiftsbogtrykkeri, 1984;119–20.

182. Dempster DW (personal communication).

183. Arlot M, Edouard C, Meunier PJ, Neer RM, Reeve J. Impaired osteoblast function in osteoporosis: comparison between calcium balance and dynamic histomorphometry. *Br Med J* 1984; 289:517–20.

184. Pacifici R, Rifas L, Teitelbaum S, et al. Spontaneous release of interleukin-1 from human blood monocytes reflects bone formation in idiopathic osteoporosis. *Proc Natl Acad Sci USA* 1987;84:4616–20.

185. Feyen JHM, Raisz LG. Prostaglandin production by calvariae from sham operated and oophorectomized rats: effects of 17 beta-estradiol in vivo. *Endocrinology* 1987;121:819–21.

186. Pacifici R, Rifas L, Vered I, et al. Interleukin-1 secretion from human blood monocytes in normal and osteoporotic women: effect of menopause and estrogen/progesterone treatment. *J Bone Miner Res* 1988;3A:541.

187. Stock JL, Coderre JA, McDonald B, Rosenwasser LJ. Effects of estrogen in vivo and in vitro on spontaneous interleukin-1 release

by monocytes from postmenopausal women. *J Clin Endocrinol Metab* 1989;68:364–8.

188. Raisz LG. Local and systemic factors in the pathogenesis of osteoporosis. *N Engl J Med* 1988;318:818–28.

189. Heaney RP. A unified concept of osteoporosis. *Am J Med* 1965;39:377–80.

190. Dewhurst FE, Ago JM, Peros UT, Stashenko P. Synergism between parathyroid hormone and interleukin-1 in stimulating bone resorption in organ culture. *J Bone Miner Res* 1987;2:127–34.

191. Stevenson JC, Abeyasekera G, Hillyard CJ. Regulation of calcium-regulating hormones by exogenous sex steroids in early postmenopause. *Eur J Clin Invest* 1983;13:481–7.

192. Stevenson JC, White MC, Joplin GF, MacIntyre I. Osteoporosis and calcitonin deficiency. *Br Med J* 1982;285:1010–1.

193. Reginster JY, Derasy R, Albert A, et al. Relationship between whole plasma calcitonin levels, calcitonin, secretory capacity and plasma levels of estrone in healthy women and postmenopausal osteoporosis. *J Clin Invest* 1989;83:1073–7.

194. Tiegs RD, Body JJ, Wahner HW, Barta J, Riggs BL, Heath HH III. Calcitonin secretion in postmenopausal osteoporosis. *N Engl J Med* 1985;312:1097–100.

195. Friedman J, Raisz LG. Thyrocalcitonin: inhibitor of bone resorption in tissue culture. *Science* 1965;150:1465–6.

196. Greenberg C, Kirkreja SC, Bowser EN, Hargis GK, Henderson WT, Williams GA. Effects of estradiol and progesterone on calcitonin secretion. *Endocrinology* 1990;118:2594–8.

197. Milhaud G, Benezech-Lefevre M, Mowkhtar MS. Deficient calcitonin response to calcium stimulation in postmenopausal osteoporosis. *Lancet* 1978;i:475–8.

198. Catherwood B, Onishi T, Deftos LJ. Effect of estrogens and phosphorus depletion on plasma calcitonin in the rat. *Calcif Tissue Int* 1983;35:502–7.

199. Love F, Galli M, Franci M, Mertorelli MT. Calcitonin levels in normal subjects according to age and sex. *Biomed Pharmacother* 1984;38:261–3.

200. Chesnut CH III, Baylink DT, Sisom K, Nelp WP, Roos BA. Basal plasma immunoreactive calcitonin in postmenopausal osteoporosis. *Metabolism* 1980;29:559–62.

201. Taggart H, Chesnut CH III, Ivey JL, Baylink DJ, Sisom K, Huber MB, Ross BA. Deficient calcitonin response to calcium stimulation in postmenopausal osteoporosis. *Lancet* 1982;i:475–8.

202. Duarte B, Hargis GK, Kukreja SC. Effects of estradiol and progesterone on parathyroid hormone secretion from human parathyroid tissue. *J Clin Endocrinol Metab* 1988;66:584–7.

203. Greenberg C, Kukreja SC, Bowser EN, Hargis GK, Henderson WJ, Williams GA. Parathyroid hormone secretion: effect of estradiol and progesterone. *Metabolism* 1987;36:151–4.

204. Stock JL, Coiderre JA, Malette LE. Effects of a short course of estrogen on mineral metabolism in postmenopausal women. *J Clin Endocrinol Metab* 1985;61:595–600.

205. Selby PL, Peacock M, Barkworth SA, Brown WB, Taylor GA. Early effects of ethinyloestradiol and norethisterone treatment in postmenopausal women on bone resorption and calcium regulating hormones. *Clin Sci* 1985;69:265–71.

206. Marcus R, Madvig P, Crim M, Pont A, Kosek J. Conjugated equine estrogens in the treatment of postmenopausal women with hyperparathyroidism. *Ann Intern Med* 1984;100:633–40.

207. Horowitz M, Wishert J, Need AG, Morris H, Philcox J, Nordin BEC. Treatment of postmenopausal hyperparathyroidism with norethindrone. *Arch Intern Med* 1987;147:681–5.

208. Frantz AG, Rabkin MT. Effects of estrogen and sex difference on secretion of human growth hormone. *J Clin Endocrinol Metab* 1965;25:1470–80.

209. Duursma SA, Bislsma LWJ, Van Passen HC, Clootweg MC. Oestrogens and bone metabolism: a hypothesis. *Maturitas* 1986;8:1–6.

210. Riggs BL, Melton LJ III, Wahner HW. Heterogeneity of involutional osteoporosis: evidence for two distinct osteoporotic syndromes. In: Frame B, Potts JT Jr, eds. *Clinical disorders of bone and mineral metabolism.* Amsterdam Excerpta Medica: 1983, 337–41.

211. Gallagher JC, Riggs BL, Eisman JA, Hamstra A, Arnaud SB, DeLuca HF. Intestinal calcium absorption and serum vitamin D

212. Tsai K, Heath HH III, Kumar R, Riggs BL. Impaired vitamin D metabolism with aging in women: possible role in pathogenesis of senile osteoporosis. *J Clin Invest* 1984;73:1668–72.

213. Clemens TL, Zhou XY, Myles M. Serum vitamin D_2 and vitamin D_3 metabolite concentrations and absorption of vitamin D_2 in elderly subjects. *J Clin Endocrinol Metab* 1986;63:656.

214. Halloran BP, Portale AA, Lonergan ET, Morris EC. Production and metabolic clearance of 1,25-dihydroxyvitamin D in men: effect of advancing age. *J Clin Endocrinol Metab* 1989;70:318–23.

215. Epstein S, Bryce G, Hinman JW, et al. The influence of age on bone mineral regulating hormones. *Bone* 1986;7:421–5.

216. Gallagher JC, Riggs BL, Jerpbak M, Arnaud CD. The effect of age on serum immunoreactive parathyroid hormone in normal and osteoporotic women. *J Lab Clin Med* 1990;95:373–85.

217. Sokoll LJ, Morrow FD, Quirbach DM, Dawson-Hughes B. Intact parathyrin in postmenopausal women. *Clin Chem* 1988;34:407–410.

218. Wiske PS, Epstein S, Bell NH, Queener SF, Edmundson J, Johnston CC. Increases in immunoreactive parathyroid hormone with age. *N Engl J Med* 1979;300:1419–21.

219. Forero MS, Klein RF, Nissenson RA, et al. Effect of age on circulating immunoreactive and bioactive parathyroid hormone levels in women. *J Bone Miner Res* 1987;2:363–6.

220. Slovik DM, Adams JS, Neer RM, Holick MF, Potts JT Jr. Deficient production of 1,25-dihydroxyvitamin D in elderly osteoporotic patients. *N Engl J Med* 1981;305:372–4.

221. Cosman F, Shen V, Herrington BS, Seibel M, Ratcliffe A, Lindsay R. Mechanism of estrogen action in osteoporosis treatment as assessed by human (1-34) PTH infusion. In: Christiansen C, Overgaard K, eds. *Osteoporosis III.* Denmark: Osteopres, 1990;976–978.

222. Cheema C, Grant BF, Marcus R. Effects of estrogen on circulating "free" and total 1,25-dihydroxyvitamin D and on the parathyroid-vitamin D axis in postmenopausal women. *J Clin Invest* 1989;83:537–42.

223. Civitelli R, Agnudei D, Nardi P, Zacchei F, Avioli LV, Gennari C. Effects of one-year treatment with estrogens on bone mass, intestinal calcium absorption, and 25-hydroxyvitamin D-1α-hydroxylase reserve in postmenopausal osteoporosis. *Calcif Tissue Int* 1988;42:77–86.

224. Clemens TL, Silverberg S, Dempster DW, et al. Oral phosphate depresses serum 1,25-dihydroxyvitamin D concentrations in osteoporotic patients. In: *Vitamin D: chemical, biochemical and clinical update,* New York: Walter de Gruyter. 1985;1010–1.

225. Silverberg SJ, Shane E, de la Cruz L, et al. Abnormalities in parathyroid hormone secretion and 1,25-dihydroxyvitamin D_3 formation in women with osteoporosis. *N Engl J Med* 1989;320:277–81.

226. Kanis JA, Passmore R. Calcium supplementation of the diet. II. *Br Med J* 1989;298:205–8.

227. Kanis JA, Passmore R. Calcium supplementation of the diet. I. *Br Med J* 1989;298:137–40.

228. Nordin BEC, Heaney RP. Calcium supplementation of the diet justified by present evidence. *Br Med J* 1990;300:1056–60.

229. Bauer W, Aub JC, Albright F. Studies of calcium and phosphorus metabolism: a study of the bone trabeculae as a readily available reserve supply of calcium. *J Exp Med* 1929;49:145–61.

230. Jaffe HL, Bodansky A, Chandler JP. Ammonium chloride decalcification as modified by calcium intake: the relation between generalized osteoporosis and osteitic fibrosa. *J Exp Med* 1932;56:823–4.

231. Nordin BE. Osteomalacia, osteoporosis, and calcium deficiency. *Clin Orthop* 1960;17:235–58.

232. Bell GH, Cuthbertson DP, Orr J. Strength and size of bone in relation to calcium intake. *J Physiol* 1941;100:299–317.

233. Jowsey J, Gershon-Cohen J. Effect of dietary calcium levels of production and reversal of experimental osteoporosis in cats. *Proc Soc Exp Biol Med* 1964;116:437–441.

234. Griffiths HJ, Hunt RD, Zimmerman RE, Finehay H, Cutters J. The role of calcium and fluoride in osteoporosis in rhesus monkeys. *Radiology* 1975;10:263–8.

235. Abraham S, Carrol MD, Dresser CM, Johnson CL. Dietary in-

take findings, U.S., 1971–1974, National Center for Health Statistics, HEW publication No. 77:1647.

236. Irwin MI, Kienholz EW. A consensus of research on calcium requirements. *J Nutr* 1973;7:1019–95.

237. Heaney RP, Gallagher JC, Johnson CC, et al. Calcium nutrition and bone health in the elderly. *Am J Clin Nutr* 1982;36:986–1013.

238. Garn SM. *The earlier gain and the later loss of cortical bone in nutritional perspective.* Springfield, IL: Charles C Thomas, 1970.

239. Garn SM, Rolmann CG, Wagner B, Davila GH, Ascoli W. Population similarities in the onset and rate of adult endosteal bone loss. *Clin Orthop* 1969;65:51–60.

240. Donath A, Indermuhle P, Band R. Influence of the national calcium and fluoride supply and of a calcium supplementation on bone mineral content of a healthy population in Switzerland. *Proceedings of the International Conference on bone mineral measurement.* DHEW publ. no. (NIH) 75–633, 1975;267A.

241. Garn SM, Solomon MA, Friedl J. Calcium intake and bone quality in the elderly. *Ecol Food Nutr* 1981;10:131–3.

242. Miller J, Johnston CC Jr. Relationship of dietary calcium and bone mass in twin children. *J Bone Min Res* 1990;5(suppl):804.

243. Alevizaki CC, Ikkos DJ, Singhelakis P. Progressive decrease of true intestinal calcium absorption with age in normal man. *J Nucl Med* 1973;14:760–2.

244. Bullamore JR, Wilkinson R, Gallagher JC, Nordin BEC. Effect of age on calcium absorption. *Lancet* 1970;2:535–7.

245. Frances RM, Peacock M, Taylor GA, Stoner JH, Nordin BEC. Calcium malabsorption in elderly women with vertebral fracture: evidence for resistance to the action of vitamin D metabolites on the bowel. *Clin Sci* 1984;66:103–7.

246. Birge SJ, Keulmann HT, Cuatrecasas P, Whedon GD. Osteoporosis, intestinal lactase deficiency and low dietary calcium intake. *N Engl J Med* 1967;276:445–8.

247. Newcomer AD, Hodgson SF, McGill DB, Thomas PJ. Lactase deficiency: prevalence of osteoporosis. *Ann Intern Med* 1978;89:218–20.

248. Holbrook TL, Barrett-Connor E, Wingrau DL. Dietary calcium and risk of hip fracture: 14-year prospective study. *Lancet* 1988;ii:1046–9.

249. Cooper C, Barker DJP, Morris J, Briggs RST. Osteoporosis, falls and age in fractures of the proximal femur. *Br Med J* 1987;295:13–5.

250. Riggs BL, Wahner HW, Melton LJ, Richelson LS, Judd HL, O'Fallon WM. Dietary calcium intake and rates of bone loss in women. *J Clin Invest* 1987;80:979–82.

251. Stevenson JC, Whitehead MI, Padwick M, et al. Dietary intake of calcium and postmenopausal bone loss. *Br Med J* 1988;297:15–7.

252. Horsman A, Gallagher JC, Simpson M, Nordin BEC. Prospective trial of estrogen and calcium in postmenopausal women. *Br Med J* 1977;2:789–92.

253. Recker RR, Saville PD, Heaney RP. The effect of estrogens and calcium carbonate on bone loss in postmenopausal women. *Ann Intern Med* 1977;87:649–55.

254. Ettinger B, Genant HK, Cann CE. Postmenopausal bone loss is prevented by treatment with low-dosage estrogen with calcium. *Ann Intern Med* 1987;106:40–5.

255. Riis B, Thomsen K, Christiansen C. Does calcium supplementation prevent postmenopausal bone loss? A double-blind, controlled clinical study. *N Engl J Med* 1987;316:173–7.

256. Smith EL, Reddan W, Smith PE. Physical activity and calcium modalities for bone mineral increase in elderly women. *Med Sci Sports Exerc* 1981;13:60–4.

257. Nilas L, Christiansen C, Rodbro P. Calcium supplementation and postmenopausal bone loss. *Br Med J* 1984;289:1103–6.

258. Smith DA, Anderson JJB, Aitken JM, Shimmons J. The effects of calcium supplementation of the diet on bone mass in women. In: Kuhleracordt F, Krase HP, eds. *Calcium metabolism, bone and metabolic bone diseases.* Berlin: Springer Verlag, 1975;278–82.

259. Heaney RP, Recker RR. Distribution of calcium absorption in middle-aged women. *Am J Clin Nutr* 1986;43:229–305.

260. Consensus Development Conference on Osteoporosis. *J AMA* 1984;252:799–800.

261. Parfitt AM. Dietary risk factors for age-related bone loss and fractures. *Lancet* 1983;ii:1181–4.

262. Adams, Berridge FR. Effects of kwashiorkor on cortical and trabecular bone. *Arch Dis Child* 1969;44:705–9.

263. Garn SM, Guzman MA, Wagner B. Subperiosteal gain and endosteal loss in protein-calorie malnutrition. *Am J Phys Anthropol* 1969;30:153–5.

264. Parsons V, Szmukler G, Brown SJ, Vajpei V, Darby A. Fracturing osteoporosis in young women with anorexia nervosa. *Calcif Tissue Int* 1983;35:A2.

265. Garn SM, Kangas J. Protein intake, bone mass and bone loss. In: DeLuca HF, Frost H, Jee WSS, Johnston CC, Parfitt AM, eds. *Osteoporosis: recent advances in pathogenesis and treatment.* Baltimore: University Park Press, 1981;257–63.

266. Garnell J, Garnell ES, Merdell RJ, Barnard DL. Urinary calcium excretion during ketoacidosis of prolonged total starvation. *Metabolism* 1970;19:502–8.

267. Heaney RP, Recker RR. Effects of nitrogen phosphorus and caffeine on calcium balance in women. *J Lab Clin Med* 1982;99:46–55.

268. Linkswiler HM, Zemel MB, Jegsted M, Schiette S. Protein-induced hypercalciuria. *Fed Proc* 1981;40:2429–33.

269. Trilok G, Draper HH. Sources of protein-induced endogenous acid production and excretion by human adults. *Calcif Tissue Int* 1989;44:335–338.

270. Yuen DE, Draper HH. Effect of dietary protein on calcium metabolism in man. *Nutr Abst Rev Clin Nutr* 1984;54:447–59.

271. Anand CR, Linkswiler HM. Effect of protein intake on calcium balance of young men 500 mg calcium daily. *J Nutr* 1974;104:695–700.

272. Reiss E, Cantebury JM, Kaplan L. The role of phosphate in the secretion of parathyroid hormone in men. *J Clin Invest* 1970;49:2146–9.

273. Spencer H, Kramer L, Osis D, Norris C. Effect of phosphorus on the absorption of calcium and on the calcium balance in men. *J Nutr* 1978;108:447–57.

274. Raisz LG. Bone resorption in tissue culture. Factors influencing the response to parathyroid hormone. *J Clin Invest* 1965;44:103–16.

275. Kiel DP, Felson DT, Hannan MT, et al. Caffeine and the risk of hip fracture: the framingham study. *Am J Epidemiol* 1990;32:675–684.

276. Feitelberg S, Epstein S, Ismail F, D'Amanda C. Deranged bone mineral metabolism in chronic alcoholism. *Metabolism* 1987;36:326–32.

277. Spencer H, Rubio N, Rubio E, Indreika M, Seitam A. Chronic alcoholism: frequently overlooked cause of osteoporosis in men. *Am. J. Med.* 1986;80:393–7.

278. Diamond T, Stiel D, Posen S. Osteoporosis in hemochromatosis: iron excess, gonadal deficiency, or other factors. *Ann Intern Med* 1989;110:430–6.

279. Nilsson BE, Westlin NE. Changes in bone mass in alcoholics. *Clin Orthop Rel Res* 1973;90:229–32.

280. Baran DT, Teitelbaum SL, Bergfeld MA, Parker G, Cruvant EM, Avioli LV. Effect of alcohol ingestion on bone and mineral metabolism in rats. *Am J Physiol* 1980;238:E507–10.

281. Farley JR, Fitzsimmons R, Taylor AK, Jarch UM, Lau KHW. Direct effects of ethanol on bone resorption and formation in vitro. *Arch Biochem Biophys* 1985;237:305–14.

282. Robertson WG. Urinary excretion. In: Nordin BEC, ed. *Calcium phosphate and magnesium metabolism.* Great Britain: Churchill-Livingstone, 1976;113–61.

283. Goulding A. Effects of dietary NaCl supplements on parathyroid function, bone turnover, and bone composition in rats taking restricted amounts of calcium. *Miner Electrolyte Metab* 1980;4:203.

284. Breslaw NA, McGuire JL, Zerwekh JE, Pak CYC. The role of dietary sodium on renal excretion and intestinal absorption of calcium and on vitamin D metabolism. *J Clin Endocrinol Metab* 1982;55:369–73.

285. Goulding A. Fasting urinary sodium/creatinine in relation to calcium/creatinine and hydroxyproline/creatinine in a general population of women. *N Z Med J* 1981;93:294–7.

286. Freudenheim JL, Johnson NE, Smith EL. Relationships between usual nutrient intake and bone-mineral content of women 35–65 years of age: longitudinal and cross-sectional analysis. *Am J Clin Nutr* 1986;44:863–76.

287. Calhoun NR, Smith JC, Becker KL. The role of zinc in bone metabolism. *Clin Orthop* 1974;103:212–34.

288. Nielsen FH, Hunter CD, Mullen LM, Hunt JR. Effect of dietary boron on mineral, estrogen, and testosterone metabolism in postmenopausal women. *FASEB J* 1987;1:394–7.

289. Carlisle EM. Silicon as an essential element. *Fed Proc* 1974;33:1558–66.

290. Lynch SR, Berelowitz I, Seftel HC, et al. Osteoporosis in Johannesburg Bantu males. Its relationship to siderosis and ascorbic acid deficiency. *Am J Clin Nutr* 1967;20:799–807.

291. Bernstein DS, Sadowsky N, Hegsted DM, et al. Prevalence of osteoporosis in high and low-fluoride areas in North Dakota. *JAMA* 1966;198:499–504.

292. Affram PA, Hornberg J, Nilsson BEC. The influence of a high-fluoride content in drinking water on the bone mineral mass in man. *Acta Orthop Scand* 1969;40:137–40.

293. Riggs BL. Treatment of osteoporosis with sodium fluoride: an appraisal. *J Bone Miner Res* 1984;2:266–393.

294. Albright F, Burnett CH, Cope O, Parson W. Acute atrophy of bone (osteoporosis) simulating hyperparathyroidism. *J Clin Endocrinol Metab* 1941;1:711–6.

295. Whedon GD, Shen E. Metabolic studies in paralytic acute anterior poliomyelitis. II. Alterations in calcium phosphorus metabolism. *J Clin Invest* 1957;36:966–81.

296. Issekutz B, Blizzard JJ, Burkhead NC, Rodahl K. Effect of prolonged bed rest on urinary calcium output. *J Appl Physiol* 1966;21:1013–20.

297. Geiser M, Trueta J. Muscle action, bone rarefaction bone formation. *J Bone Joint Surg* 1958;40B:282–311.

298. Howard JE, Parson W, Bigman RS. Studies on patients convalescent from fracture. 3. The urinary excretion of calcium phosphorus. *Bull Johns Hopkins Hosp* 1945;77:291–313.

299. Deitrick JE, Whedon GD, Sherr E. Effects of immobilization upon various metabolic physiologic functions of normal men. *Am J Med* 1948;47:3–36.

300. Minaire P, Meunier PJ, Edouard C, Bernard J, Courpron P, Bournet J. Quantitative histological data on disuse osteoporosis. Comparison with biological data. *Calcif Tissue Res* 1974;17:57–63.

301. Nilsson BE. Post-traumatic osteopenia. A quantitative study of the bone mineral mass of the femur following fracture of the tibia in man using Americium-241 as a photon source. *Acta Orthop Scand* 1966;91:1–55.

302. Westlin NE. Loss of bone after Colles' fracture. *Clin Orthop Rel Res* 1974;20:194–9.

303. Mazess RB, Wheadon GD. Immobilization and bone. *Calcif Tissue Int* 1983;35:265–267.

304. Biering-Sorensen F, Bohr HH, Schaadt OP. Longitudinal study of bone mineral content in the lumbar spine, the forearm lower extremities after spinal cord injury. *Eur J Clin Invest* 1990;20:330–335.

305. Uhthoff HK, Jowarski ZF. Bone loss in response to long-term immobilization. *J Bone Joint Surg* 1978;60B:420–9.

306. Krolner B, Toft B. Vertebral bone loss: an unheeded side effect of therapeutic bed rest. *Clin Sci* 1983;64:537–40.

307. Biering-Sorensen F, Bohr H, Schaadt O. Bone mineral content of the lumbar spine and lower extremities years after spinal cord lesion. *Paraplegia* 1988;26:293–301.

308. Young DR, Niklowitz WJ, Brown RJ, Jee WSS. Immobilization-associated osteoporosis in primates. *Bone* 1986;7:109–17.

309. Whedon GD, Lutwak L, Reid J, et al. Mineral nitrogen metabolic studies on skylab orbital space flights. *Trans Assoc Am Phys* 1974;87:95–110.

310. Smith MC, Rambout PC, Vogel JM, Whittle M. Bone mineral measurement in experiment M078 in biomedical records from Skylab. *NASA Publication* 1977;183–190.

311. Rambaut PC, Goode AW. Skeletal changes during space flight. *Lancet* 1985;2:1050–2.

312. Mack PB, LaChance PA, Vose GP, Vogt FB. Bone demineralization of foot and hand of Gemini-Titan IV, V, VII astronauts during orbital flight. *Am J Roentgenol* 1967;100:503–11.

313. Vogel JM. Bone mineral changes in the Apollo astronauts. In: Mazess RB, ed. *Proceedings of the International Conference on bone mineral measurements*. Bethesda: U.S.-DHEW, 1973;352–61.

314. Tilton FE, Degioanni JJC, Schneider vs. Long-term follow-up of Skylab bone dimineralization. *Aviat Space Environ Med* 1980;51:1209–13.

315. Hansson TH, Roos BO, Nachemson A. Development of osteopenia in the fourth lumbar vertebra during prolonged bed rest after operation for scoliosis. *Acta Orthop Scand* 1975;46:621–30.

316. Heaney RP. Radiocalcium metabolism in disuse osteoporosis in man. *Am J Med* 1962;33:188–200.

317. Jones HH, Priest JD, Hayes WC, Tichenar CC, Nagel DA. Humeral hypertrophy in response to exercise. *J Bone Joint Surg* 1977;59A:204–8.

318. Nilsson BE, Westlin NE. Bone density in athletes. *Clin Orthop* 1971;77:179–82.

319. Huddleston AL, Rockwell D, Kulund DN, Harrison RB. Bone mass in lifetime tennis athletes. *JAMA* 1980;244:1107–9.

320. Aloia JF, Cohn SH, Babu T, Abesamis C, Kalice N, Ellis K. Skeletal mass body composition in marathon runners. *Metabolism* 1978;27:104–7.

321. Dalen N, Olsson KE. Bone mineral content physical activity. *Acta Orthop Scand* 1974;45:170–4.

322. Lane NE, Bloch DA, Jones HH, Marshall WH Jr, Wood PD, Fries JF. Long-distance running, bone density osteoarthritis. *JAMA* 1986;255:1147–51.

323. Montoye HJ, Smith EL, Ferdon DF, Hawley ET. Bone mineral in senior tennis players. *Sc J Sports Sci* 1980;2:26–32.

324. Rubin CT, Lanyon LE. Regulation of bone formation by applied dynamic loads. *J Bone Joint Surg* 1984;66A:767–81.

325. Lanyon LE. Bone loading—the functional determinant of bone architecture and a physiological contributor to the prevention of osteoporosis. In: Smith R, ed. *Osteoporosis*. London: Royal College of Physicians, 63–78.

326. Rubin CT, Lanyon LE. Regulation of bone mass by mechanical strain magnitude. *Calcif Tissue Int* 1985;37:411–7.

327. Lanyon LE. Bone loading-the functional determinant of bone architecture a physiological contributer to the prevention of osteoporosis. In: Smith R, ed. *Osteoporosis 1990*. London: Royal College of Physicians, 1990;63–78.

328. Buchanan J, Myers C, Lloyd T, Leuenberger P, Demers L. Determinants of peak trabecular bone density in women: the role of androgens, estrogens exercise. *J Bone Miner Res* 1988;3:673–84.

329. Davee AM, Rosen CJ, Adler RA. Exercise patterns and trabecular bone density in college women. *J Bone Miner Res* 1990;5:245–50.

330. Snow-Herter C, Bouxsein M, Lewis B, Cherette S, Weinstein P, Marcus R. Muscle strength as a predictor of bone mineral density in young women. *J Bone Miner Res* 1990;5:589–95.

331. Pocock NA, Eisman JA, Gwinn T, et al. Muscle strength, physical fitness but not age predict femoral neck bone mass. *J Bone Miner Res* 1989;4:441–8.

332. Pocock NA, Eisman J, Yeates MG, Sambrook PN, Eberi S. Physical fitness is a major determinant of femoral neck lumbar spine bone mineral density. *J Clin Invest* 1986;78:618–21.

333. Gleeson PB, Protas E, LeBlanc A, Schneider VS, Evans HJ. Effects of weight lifting on bone mineral density in premenopausal women. *J Bone Miner Res* 1990;5:153–8.

334. Oldbridge NB. Compliance with intervention rehabilitation exercise programs: a review. *Prev Med* 1982;2:56–70.

335. Aloia JF, Cohn SH, Ostini J, Cane R, Ellis K. Prevention of involutional bone loss by exercise. *Ann Intern Med* 1978;89:356–8.

336. Krolner B, Toft B, Nielson SP, Tondevold I. Physical exercise as prophylaxis against involutional vertebral bone loss: a controlled trial. *Clin Sci* 1983;64:541–6.

337. Sler RB, Cauley JA, Hom DL, Sashin D, Kriska AM. The effects of walking on the cross-sectional dimensions of the radius in postmenopausal women. *Calcif Tissue Int* 1987;41:65–69.

338. Simkin A, Ayalen J, Leichter I. Increased trabecular bone density due to bone-loading exercises in postmenopausal osteoporotic women. *Calcif Tissue Int* 1987;40:59–63.

339. White MK, Martin RB, Yeates RA, Bulcher RL, Radin EL. The effects of exercise on the bones of postmenopausal women. *Int Orthop* 1990;7:209–14.

340. Smith EL, Reddan W, Smith PE. Physical activity calcium modalities for bone mineral increase in aged women. *Med Sci Sports Exerc* 1981;13:60–4.

341. Smith EL, Gilligan C, McAdam M, Ensign CP, Smith PE. Deterring bone loss by exercise intervention in premenopausal postmenopausal women. *Calcif Tissue Int* 1989;44:312–21.
342. Rundgren A, Aniansson A, Ljungberg P, Wetterquist H. *Arch Gerontol Geriatr* 1984;3:243–8.
343. Chow RK, Harrison JE, Sturtridge U, et al. *Clin Invest Med* 1987;10:59–63.
344. Dalsky GP, Stocke KS, Ehsani AA, et al. Weight bearing exercise training and lumbar bone mineral content in postmenopausal women. *Arch Intern Med* 1988;108:824–8.
345. Aitken JM, Gordon S, Anderson JB, et al. Seasonal variations in calcium phosphorus homeostasis in man. In: Frame B, Parfitt AM, Duncan H, eds. *Clinical aspects of metabolic bone disease.* Amsterdam: Excerpta Medica, 1973;80–3.
346. Aitken JM, Anderson JB, Horton PW. Seasonal variations in bone mineral content after the menopause. *Nature* 1973;241:59–60.
347. Bergstralh EJ, Sinaki M, Offord KP, Wahner HW, Melton LJ III. Effect of season on physical activity score, back extension muscle strength lumbar bone density. *J Bone Miner Res* 1990;5:371–7.
348. Eriksson C. Streaming potentials other water-dependent effects in mineralized tissues. *Ann N Y Acad Sci* 1974;238:321–38.
349. Patt GH. The influence of pH on growth of bone in tissue culture. *Proc Soc Exp Biol Med* 1948;68:288–93.
350. Bindema I, Somjen D, Shimshani Z, Harell A. Role of prostaglandins in bone remodeling induced by physical forces. In: Menczel J, Robin GC, Makin M, Steinberg R, eds. *Osteoporosis.* Chichester: John Wiley, 1982;192–9.
351. Pead MJ, Lanyon LE. Indomethacin modulation of load-related stimulation of new bone formation in vivo. *Calcif Tissue Int* 1989;45:34–40.
352. Nelson ME, Merideth CN, Dawson-Hughes B, Evans WJ. Hormone and bone mineral status in endurance trained and sedentary postmenopausal women. *J Clin Endocrinol Metab* 1988;66:927–33.
353. Bell NH, Godsen RN, Henry DP, Shary J, Epstein S. The effects of muscle-building exercise on vitamin D mineral metabolism. *J Bone Miner Res* 1988;3:369–73.
354. Resnick LM, Miller FB, Laragh JH. Calcium regulating hormones in essential hypertension. Relation to plasma renin activity and sodium metabolism. *Ann Intern Med* 1986;105:649–54.
355. Gennari C, Imbimbo B, Montagnani M, Bernini M, Nardi P, Avioli LV. Effects of prednisone and deflazacort on mineral metabolism and parathyroid hormone activity in humans. *Calcif Tissue Int* 1984;36:245–52.
356. Marx SJ, Stock JL, Altie MF. Familial hypocalciuric-hypercalcemia: recognition among patients referred after unsuccessful parathyroid exploration. *Ann Intern Med* 1980;92:351–6.
357. Nilsson BE, Westlin NE. Plasma concentrations of alkaline phosphatase, phosphorus and calcium following femoral neck fracture. *Acta Orthop Scand* 1972;43:564–7.
358. Epstein S. Serum and urinary markers of bone remodeling: assessment of bone turnover. *Endocr Rev* 1988;9:437–49.
359. Delmas PD. Biochemical markers of bone turnover in osteoporosis. In: Riggs BL, Melton LJ III, eds. *Osteoporosis: etiology, diagnosis, and management.* New York: Raven Press, 1990;297–316.
360. de la Piedra C, Torres R, Rapado A, et al. Serum tartrate resistant acid phosphatase and bone mineral content in postmenopausal osteoporosis. *Calcif Tissue Int* 1989;34:58–60.
361. Black D, Quherson C, Robins SP. Excretion of pyridinium crosslinks of collagen in ovariectomized rats as urinary markers for increased bone resorption. *Calcif Tissue Int* 1989;44:343–7.
362. Brown JP, Delmas PD, Malaval L, Edouard C, Chapuy MC, Meunier PJ. Serum bone gla-protein: a specific marker for bone formation in postmenopausal osteoporosis. *Lancet* 1990;i:1091–3.
363. Lindsay R, Mellish R, Cosman F, Dempster DW. Biochemical markers for bone remodeling. In: Nordin BEC, ed. *Osteoporosis: contributions to modern management.* London: Parthenon, 1990;47–56.
364. Grech P, Martin TJ, Barrington NA, Ell PJ. *Diagnosis of metabolic bone disease.* London: Chapman and Hall, 1985.
365. Siegelman SS. The radiology of osteoporosis. In: Barzel U, ed. *Osteoporosis.* New York: Grune & Stratton, 1970;68–79.
366. Genant HK. The radiology of osteoporosis. In: Riggs BL, Melton

367. Gordan GS, Vaughn C. *Clinical management of the osteoporoses,* Acton: Publishing Sciences Group, 1976.
368. Saville PD. Observations on 80 women with osteoporotic spine fractures. In: Barzel U, ed. *Osteoporosis.* New York: Grune & Stratton, 1970;38–46.
369. McKenna MJ, Kleerekoper M, Ellis BI, et al. Atypical insufficiency fractures confused with looser zones of osteomalacia. *Bone* 1987;8:71–8.
370. Barnett E, Nordin BEC. The radiological diagnosis of osteoporosis: a new approach. *Clin Radiol* 1960;ii:166–74.
371. Kleerekoper M, Parfitt AM, Ellis BI. Measurement of vertebral fracture rates in osteoporosis. In: Christiansen C, Arnaud CD, Nordin BEC, et al., eds. *Osteoporosis.* Denmark: Aalborg Stiftsbogtrykkeri, 1984;103–9.
372. Singh M, Nagrath AR, Meini PS. Changes in trabecular pattern of the upper end of the femur as an index of osteoporosis. *J Bone Joint Surg* 1970;52A:457–67.
373. Singh M, Riggs BL, Beebout JW, Jowsey J. Femoral trabecular-pattern index for evaluation of spinal osteoporosis. *Arch Intern Med* 1972;77:63–7.
374. Bohr H, Schaadt O. Bone mineral content of femoral bone and the lumbar spine measured in women with fracture of the femoral neck, by dual photon absorptiometry. *Clin Orthop* 1983;179:240–5.
375. Cohn SH. Non-invasive measurements of bone mass and their clinical application. Boca Raton, FL: CRC Press, 1981.
376. Genant HK, Ettinger B, Harris ST, Block JE, Steiger P. Quantitative computed tomography in assessment of osteoporosis. In: Riggs BL, Melton LJ III, eds. *Osteoporosis: etiology, diagnosis, and management.* New York: Raven Press, 1988;221–49.
377. Mazess RB, Wahner HM. Nuclear medicine in densitometry. In: Riggs BL, Melton LJ III, eds. *Osteoporosis: etiology, diagnosis, and management.* New York: Raven Press, 1988;251–95.
378. Rose G. Sick individuals and sick populations. *Int J Epidemiol* 1985;14:32–8.
379. Melton LJ, Eddy DM, Johnston CC. Screening for osteoporosis. *Arch Intern Med* 1990;112:516–28.
380. Hui SL, Slemenda CW, Johnston CC. Age and bone mass as predictors of fracture in a prospective study. *J Clin Invest* 1988;81:1804–9.
381. Hui SL, Slemenda CW, Johnston CC Jr. Baseline measurement of bone mass predicts fracture in white women. *Ann Intern Med* 1989;111:355–61.
382. Gardsell P, Johnell O, Nilsson BE. Predicting fractures in women by using forearm bone densitometry. *Calcif Tissue Int* 1989;44:235–42.
383. Wasnich RD, Ross PD, MacLean CJ, Davis JW, Vogel JM. A prospective study of bone mass measurements and spine fracture incidence. In: Christiansen C, Johansen JS, Riis BJ, eds. *Osteoporosis.* Denmark: Osteopres, 1987;377–378.
384. Heidrich F, Thompson RS. Osteoporosis prevention: strategies applicable for general population groups. *J Fam Pract* 1987;25:33–9.
385. Davis MR. Screening for postmenopausal osteoporosis. *Am J Obstet Gynecol* 1987;156:1–5.
386. Sowers KP, Wallace RD, Lemke JM. Correlates of mid-radius bone density among postmenopausal women: a community study. *Am J Clin Nutr* 1985;41:1045–1053.
387. Jones KP, Revnikar VA, Tutchinsky D, Schiff I. Comparison of bone density in amennorheic women due to athletics, weight loss and premature menopause. *Am J Obstet Gynecol* 1987;66:5–7.
388. Evers SE, Orchard JW, Haddad RG. Bone density in postmenopausal North American Indians and Caucasian females. *Hum Biol* 1985;57:719–26.
389. Slemenda CW, Hui SL, Johnston CC, Longcope C. Prediction of bone mass and rate of loss: clinical versus laboratory data. *J Bone Miner Res* 1987;2:A206.
390. Yano K, Wasnich RD, Vogel JM, Heilbrun LK. Bone mineral measurements among middle-aged and elderly Japanese residents in Hawaii. *Am J Epidemiol* 1984;119:751–64.
391. Tohme J, Lindsay R. Bone mineral screening for osteoporosis (letter). *N Engl J Med* 1987;317:315.
392. Ross PD, Wasnich RD, MacLean CJ, Hagina R, Vogel JM. A

model for estimating the potential costs and savings of osteoporosis prevention strategies. *Bone* 1988;9:337–47.

393. Health and Public Policy Committee, American College of Physicians. Radiologic methods to evaluate bone mineral content. *Ann Intern Med* 1984;100:908–11.

394. Health and Public Policy Committee, American College of Physicians. Bone mineral densitometry. *Ann Intern Med* 1987;107:932–6.

395. Cummings SR, Black D. Should perimenopausal women be screened for osteoporosis. *Ann Intern Med* 1986;104:817–23.

396. Hall FM, Davis MA, Baran DT. Bone mineral screening for osteoporosis. *N Engl J Med* 1987;316:212–4.

397. Melton LJ III, Eddy DM, Johnston CC Jr. Screening for osteoporosis. *Ann Intern Med* 1990;11:516–528.

398. Ott SM. Should women get screening bone mass measurements. *Ann Intern Med* 1986;104:874–6.

399. Fogelman I. The case for routine bone mass measurements. *Nucl Med Commun.* 1988;9:541–3.

400. Hall FM. Bone mineral screening for osteoporosis. *Am J Radiol* 1987;149:120–122.

401. Wasnich RD. Screening for osteoporosis. In: Genant HK, ed. *Osteoporosis Update 1987.* Berkeley: University of California Press, 1987;123–7.

402. Raisz LG, Lorenzo JA, Smith JA. Bone mineral screening for osteoporosis (letter). *N Engl J Med* 1987;317:315.

403. Lindsay R. Pathogenesis, prevention, and treatment of osteoporosis. In: Stevenson JC, ed. *New techniques in metabolic bone disease.* London: Wright, 1990;221–31.

404. Avioli LV, Lindsay R. The female osteoporotic syndrome. In: Krane S, Avioli LV, eds. *Metabolic bone disease.* 1990;397–451.

405. Harrison M, Fraser M, Mullan B. Calcium metabolism in osteoporosis. Acute and long-term responses to increased calcium intake. *Lancet* 1961;i:1015–9.

406. Whedon GD. Effects of high calcium intakes on bones, blood and soft tissue: relationship of calcium intake to balance in osteoporosis. *Fed Proc* 18:1112–8.

407. Nordin BEC, Horsman A, Crilly RG, Marshall D, Simpson M. Treatment of spinal osteoporosis in postmenopausal women. *Br Med J* 1980;i:451–4.

408. Rose GA. A study of the treatment of osteoporosis with fluoride therapy and high calcium intake. *Proc R Soc Lond* [*Biol*] 1965;38:436–40.

409. Thalassinos NC, Gutteridge DH, Joplin GF, Fraser TR. Calcium balance in osteoporotic patients on long-term oral calcium therapy with or without sex hormones. *Clin Sci* 1982;221–6.

410. Heaney RP. Nutritional factors in bone health in elderly subjects: methodological and contextual problems. *Am J Clin Nutr* 1989;50:1182–9.

411. National Osteoporosis Foundation report to the National Academy of Sciences. National objectives for disease prevention and health promotion for the year 2000, 1988.

412. Albanese AA, Edelson AH, Lareze EK, Woodhull ML, Wein EH. Problems of bone health in elderly. *N Y State J Med* 1975;75:326–36.

413. Nordin BEC, Polley KJ. Metabolic consequences of the menopause. *Calcif Tissue Int* 1987;41(Suppl 1):1–59.

414. Smith EL, Smith PE, Gilligan C, Sempos CT. Calcium supplement reduces bone loss in middle-aged women over four years. *J Bone Miner Res* 1987;2(Suppl 2):220.

415. Shapiro JR, Moore WT, Jorgensen H, et al. Osteoporosis, evaluation of diagnosis and therapy. *Ann Intern Med* 1975;135:563–7.

416. Lamke R, Sjoborg HE, Sylinen M. Bone mineral content in women with Colles' fracture: effect of calcium supplementation. *Acta Orthop Scand* 1978;49:143–6.

417. Nordin BEC, Horsman A, Crilly RG, Marshall DM, Simpson M. Treatment of spinal osteoporosis in postmenopausal women. *Br Med J* 1980;280:451–4.

418. Ott SM, Chesnut CH III. Calcitriol treatment in patients with postmenopausal osteoporosis. In: Christiansen C, Johansen C, Riis BJ, eds. *Osteoporosis 1987.* Copenhagen: Osteopres, 1987;844–9.

419. Polley JK, Nordin BEC, Baghurst PA, Walker CJ, Chatterton BE. Effect of calcium supplementation on forearm bone mineral content in postmenopausal women: a prospective sequential controlled trial. *J Nutr* 1987;117:1929–35.

420. Riggs BL, Hodgson SF, O'Fallon WM, et al. Effect of fluoride treatment on the fracture rate in postmenopausal women with osteoporosis. *N Engl J Med* 1990;322:802–9.

421. Riggs BL, Seeman E, Hodgson SF, Taves DR, O'Fallon WM. Effect of the fluoride/calcium regimen on vertebral fracture occurrence in postmenopausal osteoporosis. *N Engl J Med* 1982;306:446–50.

422. Dawson-Hughes B, Dallas GE, Krall GE, et al. A controlled trial of the effect of calcium supplementation on bone density in postmenopausal women. *N Engl J Med* 1990;323:878–883.

423. Carr CJ, Shangrow R. Nutritional and pharmaceutical aspects of calcium supplementation. *Am J Pharmacol* 1987;NS27:49–57.

424. Recker RR. Calcium absorption and achlorhydria. *N Engl J Med* 1985;333:70–4.

425. Recker RR, Bammi A, Barger-Lux J, Heaney RP. Calcium absorbability from milk products, or imitation milk and calcium carbonate. *Am J Clin Nutr* 1988;47:93–5.

426. Heaney RP, Weaver CM, Recker RR. Absorbability of calcium from spinach. *Am J Clin Nutr* 1988;47:707–9.

427. Heaney RP. Calcium supplements: practical considerations. *Osteoporosis International* 1990;1:65–71.

428. Gibson MJ. The prevention of falls in later life. A report of the Kellogg International Work Group on the prevention of falls in the elderly. *Dan Med Bull* 1987;34(Suppl 4):1–24.

429. Tideiksaar R. Geriatric falls: assessing the cause, preventing recurrence. *Geriatrics* 1989;44:57–64.

430. Tinetti ME, Speechley M, Ginter SF. Risk factors for falls among elderly persons living in the community. *N Engl J Med* 1988;319:1701:1707.

431. Evans JG. Falls and fractures. *Age Aging* 1988;17:361. In: Christiansen C, Overgaard K, eds. Copenhagen: Osteopres, 1990; 1009–1011.

432. Wild D, Nayak USL, Isaacs B. Characteristics of old people who fall at home. *J Clin Exp Gerontol* 1980;2:271–87.

433. Nickens H. Intrinsic factors in falling among the elderly. *Arch Intern Med* 1985;145:1089–93.

434. Overstall PW, Exton-Smith PN, Imms FJ, Johnson AL. Falls in the elderly related to postural imbalance. *Br Med J* 1977;1:261–4.

435. Rubenstein LZ, Robbins AS, Schulman BL, Rosado J, Osterwell D, Josephson KR. Falls and instability in the elderly. *J Am Geriatr Soc* 1988;36:266–78.

436. Waller JA. Falls among the elderly-human environmental factors. *Accid Anal Prev* 1978;10:21–3.

437. Tideiksaar R. Preventing falls: home hazard checklists to help older patients protect themselves. *Geriatrics* 1986;41:26–8.

438. United States Consumer Product Safety Commission (USCPC). Home safety checklist for older consumers. Washington, DC:USCPC, 1986.

439. Kornzweig AL. Visual loss in the elderly. *Hosp Pract* 1977;12:51–9.

440. Tobis JS, Reinsch S, Swanson JM, Byrd M, Scharf T. Visual perception dominance of falls among community-dwelling adults. *J Am Geriatr Soc* 1985;33:330–3.

441. Lipsitz LA. Syncope in the elderly. *Ann Intern Med* 1983;99:92–105.

442. Cahalan D, Cisin IH, Crosby HM. American drinking practices: a national study of drinking behavior and attitudes. New Brunswick, NJ, Rutgers Center of Alcohol Studies, 1969.

443. Tinetti ME. Performance-oriented assessment of mobility problems in elderly patients. *J Amer Geriatr Soc* 1986;34:119–26.

444. Tinetti ME, Ginter SF. Identifying mobility dysfunctions in elderly patients: standard neuromuscular examination or direct assessment. *JAMA* 1988;259:1190–3.

445. Melton LJ, Riggs BL. Risk factors for injury after a fall. *Clin Geriatr Med* 1985;525:539.

446. Tinetti ME, Williams TF, Mayewski R. Fall risk index for elderly patients based on number of chronic disabilities. *Am J Med* 1986;80:429–34.

447. Albright F. The effect of hormones on osteogenesis in man. *Recent Prog Horm Res* 1947;1:293–353.

448. Lindsay R, Aitken JM, Anderson JB, Hart DM, MacDonald EB, Clark AC. Long-term prevention of postmenopausal osteoporosis by oestrogen. *Lancet* 1976;i:1038–41.

449. Lindsay R, Hart DM, Purdie P, Ferguson MM, Clark AC, Kraszewski A. Comparative effects of oestrogen and a progestogen on

bone loss in postmenopausal women. *Clin Sci Mol Med* 1978;54:193–5.

450. Lindsay R, Hart DM, Forrest C, Baird C. Prevention of spinal osteoporosis in oophorectomized women. *Lancet* 1980; ii:1151–4.

451. Christiansen C, Rodbro P. Does postmenopausal bone loss respond to estrogen replacement therapy independent of bone loss rate. *Calcif Tissue Int* 1983;35:720–2.

452. Christiansen C, Christiansen MS, McNair P. Prevention of early postmenopausal bone loss: conducted 2 years study in 315 normal females. *Eur J Clin Invest* 1980;10:273–9.

453. Davis ME, Lanzl LH, Cox AB. Detection, prevention and retardation of postmenopausal osteoporosis. *Obstet Gynecol* 1970;36:187–98.

454. Ettinger B, Genant HK, Cann CE. Long-term estrogen therapy prevents bone loss and fracture. *Ann Intern Med* 1985;102:319–24.

455. Gallagher JC, Riggs BL, DeLuca HF. Effect of estrogen on calcium absorption and serum vitamin D metabolites in postmenopausal osteoporosis. *J Clin Endocrinol Metab* 1980;51:1359–64.

456. Gordan GS, Picchi J, Roof BS. Antifracture efficacy of long-term estrogens for osteoporosis. *Trans Assoc Am Physicians* 1973;86:326–32.

457. Horsman A, Gallagher JC, Simpson M, Nordin BEC. Prospective trial of estrogen and calcium in postmenopausal women. *Br Med J* 1977;2:789–92.

458. Lindsay R, Hart DM, Clark DM. The minimum effective dose of estrogen for prevention of postmenopausal bone loss. *Obstet Gynecol* 1984;63:759–63.

459. Nachtigall LE, Nachtigall RH, Nachtigall RD. Estrogen replacement therapy I: a 10-year prospective study in the relationship to osteoporosis. *Obstet Gynecol* 1979;53:277.

460. Pacifici R, McMurtry C, Vered I, et al. Coherence therapy does not prevent axial bone loss in osteoporotic women. A preliminary comparative study. *J Clin Endocrinol Metab* 1989;66:747–53.

461. Quigley MET, Martin BL, Burnier AM, Brooks P. Estrogen therapy arrests bone loss in elderly women. *J Obstet Gynecol* 1987;156:1516–23.

462. Recker RR, Saville PD, Heaney RP. The effect of estrogens and calcium carbonate on bone loss in postmenopausal women. *Ann Intern Med* 1977;87:649–55.

463. Riggs BL, Jowsey J, Kelly PJ, Jones JD, Maher FT. Effect of sex hormones on bone in primary osteoporosis. *J Clin Invest* 1969;48:1065–72.

464. Meema S, Bunker ML, Meema HE. Preventive effect of estrogen on postmenopausal bone loss. *Arch Intern Med* 1975;135:1436–40.

465. Lindsay R, Tohme J. Estrogen treatment of patients with established osteoporosis. *Obstet Gynecol* 1990;76:1–6.

466. Riis B, Thomsen K, Strom V, Christiansen C. The effect of percutaneous estradiol natural progesterone on postmenopausal bone loss. *Am J Obstet Gynecol* 1987;156:61–5.

467. Jensen GF, Christiansen C, Transbol I. Treatment of postmenopausal osteoporosis: a controlled therapeutic trial comparing oestrogen/gestagen, 1,25-dihydroxyvitamin D₃ calcium. *Clin Endocrinol* 1982;16:515–24.

468. Caniggia A, Delling G, Nuti R, Vattimo A. Clinical, biochemical and histological results of a double blind trial with 1,25-dihydroxyvitamin D₃, estradiol and placebo in postmenopausal osteoporosis. *Acta Vitaminol Enzymol* 1984;6:117–28.

469. Aitken JM, Hart DM, Anderson JB, Lindsay R, Smith DA. Osteoporosis after oophorectomy for non-malignant disease. *Br Med J* 1973;i:325–8.

470. Christiansen C, Rodbro P. Does oestriol add to the beneficial effect of combined hormonal prophylaxis against postmenopausal osteoporosis? *Br J Gynecol* 1984;91:489–93.

471. Christiansen C, Christiansen MS, Rodbro P, Hagen C, Transbol I. Effect of 1,25-dihydroxyvitamin D₃ by itself of combined with hormone treatment in preventing postmenopausal osteoporosis. *Eur J Clin Invest* 1981;11:305–9.

472. Ettinger B, Genant HK, Cann CE. Postmenopausal bone loss is prevented by treatment with low-dosage estrogen with calcium. *Ann Intern Med* 1987;106:40–5.

473. Finn-Jensen M, Christiansen C, Transbol I. Fracture frequency and bone prevention in postmenopausal women treated with estrogen. *Obstet Gynecol* 1982;60:493–6.

474. Genant HK, Cann C, Ettinger B, Gordan G. Quantitative computed tomography of vertebral spongiosa: a sensitive method for detecting early bone loss after oophorectomy. *Ann Intern Med* 1982;97:699–705.

475. Gotfredsen A, Nilas L, Riis BJ, Thomsen K, Christiansen C. Bone changes occurring spontaneously and caused by oestrogen in early postmenopausal women: a local or generalized phenomenon? *Br Med J* 1986;292:1098–100.

476. Horsman A, James M, Francis R. The effect of estrogen dose on postmenopausal bone loss. *N Engl J Med* 1983;309:1405–7.

477. Lafferty FN, Helmuth DO. Postmenopausal estrogen replacement: the prevention of osteoporosis and systemic effects. *Maturitas* 1985;7:147–59.

478. Linde J, Friis T, Ostergaard E. Oestrogens and postmenopausal bone loss. *Calcif Tissue Res* 1976;21:478–83.

479. Munk-Jensen N, Pors Nielsen S, Obel EB, Eriksen PB. Reversal of postmenopausal vertebral bone loss by oestrogen and progestogen: a double blind placebo controlled study. *Br Med J* 1988;296:1150–2.

480. Al-Azzawi F, Hart DM, Lindsay R. Long-term effect of oestrogen replacement therapy on bone mass as measured by dual photon absorptiometry. *Br Med J* 1987;294:1261–2.

481. Hutchinson TA, Polansky JM, Feinstein AR. Postmenopausal oestrogens protect against fracture of hip and distal radius. *Lancet* 1979;ii482. Johnson RE, Specht EE. The risk of hip fracture in postmenopausal females with and without estrogen drug exposure. *Am J Public Health* 1981;71:138–44.

481a. Riggs BL, Hodgson SF, Muhs J, Wahner HW. Fluoride treatment of osteoporosis: clinical and bone densitometric responses. In: Christiansen C, Overgaard K, eds. Copenhagen: Osteopres, 1987;817–823.

482. Al-Azzawi F, Hart DM, Lindsay R. Long term effect of oestrogen replacement therapy on bone mass as measured by dual photon absorptiometry. *Br Med J* 1987;294:1261–1262.

483. Kiel DP, Felson DT, Anderson JJ, et al. Hip fracture and the use of estrogens in postmenopausal women: the Framingham Study. *N Engl J Med* 1987;317:1169–74.

484. Kreiger N, Kelsey JL, Holford TR. An epidemiological study of hip fracture in postmenopausal women. *Am J Epidemiol* 1982;116:141–8.

485. Paganini-Hill A, Ross RK, Gerkins VR, Henderson BE, Arthur M, Mack TM. Menopausal estrogen therapy and hip fractures. *Ann Intern Med* 1981;95:28–31.

486. Weiss NS, Ure CL, Ballard JH. Decreased risk of fractures of the hip and lower forearm with postmenopausal use of oestrogen. *N Engl J Med* 1980;303:1195–8.

487. Naessen T, Persson I, Adami HO, Bergstrom R, Bergkvist L. Hormone replacement therapy and the risk for first hip fracture. *Ann Intern Med* 1990;113:95–103.

488. Birge S, Price S, McGee S, et al. The role of estrogen in the prevention of hip fracture in women over age 69. In: Christiansen C, Overgaard K, eds. *Osteoporosis, II ed.* Denmark: Osteopres, 1990;1196–1197.

489. Adam S, Williams V, Vessey MP. Cardiovascular disease and hormone replacement treatment: a pilot case-control study. *Br Med J* 1981;282:1277–8.

490. Bain C, Willet W, Hennekins CH. Use of postmenopausal hormones an risk of myocardial infarction. *Circulation* 1981; 64:42–6.

491. Barrett-Connor E, Brown, Turner, Austin, Criqui MH. Heart disease risk factors and hormone use in postmenopausal women. *JAMA* 1979;241:2167–9.

492. Bradley DD, Wingerd J, Petitti DB, Krauss RM, Ramcharan S. Serum high-density lipoprotein cholesterol in women using oral contraceptives, estrogens, and progestins. *N Engl J Med* 1978;299:17–20.

493. Burch JC, Byrd BF, Vaughn WK. The effects of long-term estrogen on hysterectomized women. *Am J Obstet Gynecol* 1974;118:778–82.

494. Bush TL, Barrett-Connor E. Non-contraceptive estrogen use and cardiovascular disease. *Epidemiol Rev* 1985;7:80–104.

495. Bush TL, Barrett-Connor E, Cowan LD, et al. Cardiovascular mortality and noncontraceptive use of estrogen in women: results from the lipid research clinics program follow-up study. *Circulation* 1987;75:1102–9.

496. Criqui MH, Suarez L, Barrett-Connor E, et al. Postmenopausal

estrogen use and mortality, results from a prospective study in a defined, homogenous community. *Am J Epidemiol* 1988;128:606–14.

497. Hammond CB, Jelovser R, Lee KL. Effects of long-term estrogen replacement therapy. II. Neoplasia. *Am J Obstet Gynecol* 1979;133:537–47.

498. Henderson BE, Pike, Ross RK, Mack TM, Lobo R. Reevaluating the role of progestin therapy after the menopause. *Fertil Steril* 1988;49:9S–15.

499. Henderson BE, Ross RK, Paganini-Hill A, Mack TM. Estrogen use and cardiovascular disease. *J Reprod Med* 1985;30:814–20.

500. Jick H, Dinan B, Rothman KJ. Oral contraceptives estrogens and myocardial infarction. *JAMA* 1978;239:1403–6.

501. Nachtigall LE, Nachtigall RH, Nachtigall RD. Estrogen replacement therapy II: a prospective study in the relationship to carcinoma and cardiovascular and metabolic problems. *Obstet Gynecol* 1979;54(1):74–9.

502. Petitti DB, Perlman JA, Sidney S. Postmenopausal estrogen use and heart disease. *N Engl J Med* 1986;315:131–2.

503. Petitti D, Winegerd J, Pellegrin F, Ramcharan S. Risk of vascular disease in women: smoking, oral contraceptives, noncontraceptive estrogens and other factors. *JAMA* 1979;242:1150–6.

504. Pfeffer RI, Whipple GH, Kurosuki TT, Chapman JM. Coronary risk and estrogen use in postmenopausal women. *Am J Epidemiol* 1978;107:479–97.

505. Rosenberg L, Armstrong B, Jick H. Myocardial infarction and estrogen therapy in postmenopausal women. *N Engl J Med* 1976;294:1256–9.

506. Rosenberg L, Slone D, Shapiro S, et al. Noncontraceptive estrogens and myocardial infarction in young women. *J Am A* 1980;244:339–42.

507. Ross RK, Paganini-Hill A, Mack TM, et al. Menopausal oestrogen therapy and protection from death from ischemic heart disease. *Lancet* 1981;i:858–60.

508. Stampfer MJ, Willett WC, Colditz GA, et al. A prospective study of postmenopausal estrogen therapy and coronary heart disease. *N Engl J Med* 1985;313:1044–9.

509. Szklo M, Tonascia J, Gordis L. Estrogen use and myocardial infarction risk: a case control study. *Prev Med* 1984;13:510–6.

510. Gordon T, Kannel WB, Hjortland MC, et al. Menopause and coronary heart disease: the Framingham study. *Ann Intern Med* 1978;89:157–61.

511. Wilson PWF, Garrison RJ, Castelli WP, et al. Postmenopausal estrogen use, cigarette smoking, and cardiovascular morbidity in women over 50: the Framingham study. *N Engl J Med* 1985;313:1038–43.

512. Bush TL, Miller VT. Effects of pharmacologic agents used during the menopause: impact on lipids and lipoproteins. In: Mishell DR Jr, ed. *Menopause: physiology and pharmacology.* Chicago: Year Book Medical 1987;187–208.

513. Adams MR, Clarkson TB, Kloritnik DR, Nash HA. Contraceptive steroids and coronary-artery disease in cynomolagous macaques. *Fertil Steril* 1987;47:1010–8.

514. Paganini-Hill A, Ross RK, Henderson BE. Postmenopausal oestrogen treatment and stroke: a prospective study. *Br Med J* 1988;297:519–22.

515. Bush TL, Cowan LD, Barrett-Connor E, et al. Estrogen uses and all cause mortality. *JAMA* 1983;249:903–6.

516. Antunes CMF, Stolley PD, Rosenshein NB, et al. Endometrial cancer and estrogen use. Report of a large case-control study. *N Engl J Med* 1979;300:9–13.

517. Gray LA, Cristopherson WM, Hoover RN. Estrogens and endometrial cancer. *Obstet Gynecol* 1977;49:385–9.

518. Hoogerland DL, Buchler DA, Crowley JJ, Carr WF. Estrogen use—risk of endometrial carcinoma. *Gynecol Oncol* 1978;6:451–8.

519. Hulka BS. Effects of exogenous estrogen on postmenopausal women: the epidemiologic evidence. *Obstet Gynecol Surv* 1980;35:389–411.

520. Hulka BS, Folwer WC, Kaufman DG, et al. Estrogen and endometrial cancer: cases and two control groups from North Carolina. *Am J Obstet Gynecol* 1980;137:92–105.

521. Hulka BS, Kaufman DG, Fowler WC. Predominance of early endometrial cancers after long-term estrogen use. *JAMA* 1980;244:2419–22.

522. Jelovsek FR, Hammond CB, Woodard BH, et al. Risk of exoge-

523. Kelsey JL, LiVolsi VA, Holford TR, et al. A case-control study of cancer of the endometrium. *Am J Epidemiol* 1982;116:333–42.

524. LaVecchia C, Franceschi S, Gallus G, et al. Oestrogens and obesity as risk factors for endometrial cancer in Italy. *Int J Epidemiol* 1982;11:120–6.

525. Mack TM, Pike MC, Henderson BE, et al. Estrogens and endometrial cancer in a retirement community. *N Engl J Med* 1976;294:1262–7.

526. McDonald TW, Annegers JF, O'Fallon WM, et al. Exogenous estrogens and endometrial carcinoma: case-control and incidence study. *Am J Obstet Gynecol* 1977;127:572–80.

527. Shapiro S, Kaufman DW, Slone D, et al. Recent and past use of conjugated estrogens in relations to adenocarcinoma of the endometrium. *N Engl J Med* 1980;303:485–9.

528. Shapiro S, Kelly JP, Rosenberg L, et al. Risk of localized and widespread endometrial cancer in relation to recent and discontinued use of conjugated estrogens. *N Engl J Med* 1985;313:969–72.

529. Smith DC, Prentice R, Thompson DJ, et al. Association of exogenous estrogens and endometrial cancer. *N Engl J Med* 1975;293:1164–7.

530. Spengler RF, Clarke EA, Woolever CA, et al. Exogenous estrogens and endometrial cancer: a case control study and assessment of potential biases. *Am J Epidemiol* 1981;114:497–506.

531. Weiss NS, Szekely DR, English DR, et al. Endometrial cancer in relation to patterns of menopausal estrogen use. *JAMA* 1979;242:261–4.

532. Ziel HK, Finkle WD. Increased risk of endometrial carcinoma among users of conjugated estrogens. *N Engl J Med* 1975;293:1167–70.

533. Lane G, King R, Whitehead M. The effect of oestrogens and progestogens on endometrial biochemistry. In: Studd SWW, Whitehead MI, eds. *The Menopause.* Oxford: Blackwell, 1988;213–26.

534. Persson I, Adami HO, Bergkvist L, et al. Risk of endometrial cancer after treatment with oestrogens alone or in conjunction with progestogens: results of a prospective study. *Br Med J* 1988;298:147–51.

535. Barrett-Connor E. Postmenopausal estrogen replacement and breast cancer. *N Engl J Med* 1989;321:319–20.

536. Bergkvist L, Adami HO, Persson I, Hoover R, Schairer C. The risk of breast cancer after estrogen and estrogen-progestogen replacement therapy. *N Engl J Med* 1989;321:293–7.

537. Brinton LA, Hoover RN, Szklo M, et al. Menopausal estrogen use and risk of breast cancer. *Cancer* 1981;47:2517–22.

538. Brinton LA, Hoover RN, Fraumeni JF Jr. Menopausal oestrogens and breast cancer risk: an expanded case-control study. *Br J Cancer* 1986;54:825–32.

539. Gambrell D. The menopause: benefits and risks of estrogen-progestogen replacement therapy. *Fertil Steril* 1982;37:457–74.

540. Gambrell D, Maier RC, Sanders BI. Decreased incidence of breast cancer in postmenopausal estrogen-progestogen users. *Obstet Gynecol* 1983;62:435–43.

541. Hiatt RA, Bawol R, Friedman GD, et al. Exogenous estrogens and breast cancer after oophorectomy. *Cancer* 1984;54:139–44.

542. Hoover R, Glass A, Fingle WD, et al. Conjugated estrogens and breast cancer risk in women. *J Natl Cancer Inst* 1981;67:815–20.

543. Hoover R, Gray L, Cole P, et al. Menopausal estrogens and breast cancer. *N Engl J Med* 1976;295:401–5.

544. Hulka BS, Chambless LE, Deubner DC, et al. Breast cancer and estrogen replacement therapy. *Am J Obstet Gynecol* 1982;143:638–44.

545. Jick H, Walker AM, Watkins RN, et al. Replacement estrogens and breast cancer. *Am J Epidemiol* 1980;112:586–94.

546. Kaufman DW, Miller DR, Rosenberg L, et al. Noncontraceptive estrogen use and risk of breast cancer. *J AM A* 1984;252:63–7.

547. Kelsey JL, Fischer DB, Holford JR, et al. Exogenous estrogens and other factors in the epidemiology of breast cancer. *J Natl Cancer Inst* 1981;67:327–33.

548. LaVeccia C, Decarli A, Parazzini F, et al. Noncontraceptive oestrogens and the risk of breast cancer in women. *Int J Cancer* 1986;38:853–8.

549. McDonald JA, Weiss NS, Daling JR, et al. Menopausal estrogen

use and the risk of breast cancer. *Breast Cancer Res Treat* 1986;7:193–9.

550. Nomura AMY, Kolonel LN, Hirohata T, et al. The association of replacement estrogens with breast cancer. *Int Cancer* 1986;37:49–53.

551. Ross RK, Paganini-Hill A, Gerkins VR, et al. A case-control study of menopausal estrogen therapy and breast cancer. *JAMA* 1980;243:1635–9.

552. Sherman B, Wallace R, Bean J. Estrogen use and breast cancer interaction with body mass. *Cancer* 1983;51:1531–7.

553. Thomas DB, Persing JP, Hutchinson WB. Exogenous estrogens and other risk factors for breast cancer in women with benign breast diseases. *J Natl Cancer Institute* 1982;69:1017–25.

554. Wingo PA, Layde PM, Lee NC, et al. The risk of breast cancer in postmenopausal women who have used estrogen replacement therapy. *JAMA* 1987;257:209–15.

555. Dennerstein L. Psychiatric aspects of the climacteric. In: Studd JWW, Whitehead MI, eds, *The menopause*. Oxford: Blackwell, 1988;43–54.

556. Brincat M, Moniz CF, Studd JWW, et al. The long-term effects of menopause and of administration of sex hormones on skin collagen and skin thickness. *Br J Obstet Gynecol* 1985;92:256–9.

557. Versl E, Cardozo LD. Oestrogens and lower urinary tract function. In: JWW Studd, MI Whitehead, eds, *The menopause*. Oxford: Blackwell, 1988;76–84.

558. Sarrel PM, Whitehead MI. Sex and the menopause: defining the issues. *Maturitas* 1985;7:217–25.

559. Bachmann GA, Leiblum SR, Kenmann E, Colburn DW, Swartzman L, Sheldon R. Sexual expression and its determinants in the postmenopausal women. *Maturitas* 1984;6:19–29.

560. Boston Collaborative Drug Surveillance Program. Surgically confirmed gall bladder disease, venous thromboembolism and breast tumors in relation to postmenopausal estrogen therapy. *N Engl J Med* 1974;290:15–9.

561. Hart DM, Lindsay R. Vascular complications of long term estrogen. *Front Horm Res* 1978;5:174–94.

562. Wren BG, Routledge AD. The effect of type and dose of oestrogen on the blood pressure of postmenopausal women. *Maturitas* 1983;5:134–42.

563. Thom MH, Chokrovarti S, Oram DH, Studd JW. Effect of hormone replacement therapy on glucose tolerance in postmenopausal women. *Br J Obstet Gynecol* 1977;84:776–84.

564. Geola FL, Frumar AM, Tataryn IV, et al. Biological effects of various doses of conjugated equine estrogens in postmenopausal women. *J Clin Endocrinol Metab* 1980;51:620–625.

565. Stevenson JC, Cust MP, Gangar KF, et al. Effects of transdermal versus oral hormone replacement therapy on bone density in spine and proximal femur in postmenopausal women. *Lancet* 1990;336(8710):265–9.

566. Fatourechi V, Heath HH III. Salmon calcitonin in the treatment of postmenopausal osteoporosis. *Ann Intern Med* 1987; 107:923–5.

567. McDermott MT, Hidd GS. The role of calcitonin in the development and treatment of osteoporosis. *Endocr Rev* 1987;8:377–90.

568. Gonzalez D, Ghiringhelli G, Mautalen C. Acute antiosteoclastic effect of salmon calcitonin in osteoporotic women. *Calcif Tissue Int* 1986;38:71–5.

569. Caniggia A, Gennari C, Bencini M, et al. Calcium metabolism and ^{47}calcium kinetics before and after long term thyrocalcitonin treatment in senile osteoporosis. *Clin Sci* 1970;38:397–407.

570. Maresca V. Human calcitonin in the management of osteoporosis: a multicentre study. *J Intern Med Res* 1985;13:311–6.

571. Gennari C, Chierichetti SM, Bigazzi S, et al. Comparative effects on bone mineral content of calcium and calcium plus salmon calcitonin given in two different regimens in postmenopausal osteoporosis. *Curr Ther Res* 1985;38:455–64.

572. Gruber HE, Ivey JL, Baylink DJ, et al. Long-term calcitonin therapy in postmenopausal osteoporosis. *Metabolism* 1984;33:295–303.

573. Mazzouli GF, Passeri M, Gennari C, et al. Effects of salmon calcitonin in postmenopausal osteoporosis: a controlled double-blind clinical study. *Calcif Tissue Int* 1986;38:3–8.

574. Wallach S, Cohn SH, Ellis KJ, et al. Effect of salmon calcitonin on skeletal mass in osteoporosis. *Curr Ther Res* 1977;22:556–72.

575. Polatti F, Montrasio MG, Caprotti M, et al. Bone mineral con-

tent after oophorectomy: effects of salmon calcitonin and oral calcium. *Miner Metab Res* 1984;5:159–63.

576. Reginster JY, Denis D, Albert A, et al. 1-Year controlled randomized trial of prevention of early postmenopausal bone loss by intranasal calcitonin. *Lancet* 1987;ii:1481–3.

577. Christiansen C. Intranasal calcitonin for prevention and treatment of osteoporosis. *Ann Chir Gyn* 1988;77:229–34.

578. MacIntyre I, Stevenson JC, Whitehead MI, et al. Calcitonon for prevention of postmenopausal bone loss. *Lancet* 1988;i:900–2.

579. Gennari C, Avioli LV. Calcitonin therapy in osteoporosis. In: Avioli LV, ed. *The osteoporotic syndrome*. New York: Grune & Stratton, 1987;121–43.

580. Civitelli R, Gonnelli S, Zacchei F, et. al. Bone turnover in postmenopausal osteoporosis. *J Clin Invest* 1988;82:1268–1274.

581. Schiraldi GF, Soresi E, Locicero S, Harari S, Scoccia S. Salmon calcitonin in cancer pain: comparison between two different treatment schedules. *Int J Clin Pharmacol Ther Toxicol* 1987; 25:229–232.

582. Fiore CE, Castorina F, Malatino LS, Tamburino C. Antalgic activity of calcitonin: effectiveness of the epidural and subarachnoid routes in man. *Int J Clin Pharmacol Res* 1983;3:257–60.

583. Gennari C, et al. Effects of calcitonin treatment on bone pain and bone turnover in Paget's disease of bone. *Miner Metab Res It* 1981;2:109–13.

584. Gennari C, et al. Dolore osseo, endorfine e calctinonine. In: Gennari C, Segre G, eds. *The effects of calcitonin in man. Proceedings of the First International Workshop*. Masson, ed. 1983;213–22.

585. Welzel D. Analgesic potential of salmon calcitonin in postoperative pain. In: Gennari C, Segre G, eds. *The effects of calcitonin in man. Proceedings of the First International Workshop*. Masson, 1983;223–32.

586. Bates RFL, et al. The interaction of naloxone and calcitonin in the production of analgesia in the mouse. *Br J Pharmacol* 1981;74:279.

587. Szanto J, Sandor P. Preliminary observations on the analgesic effect of salmon calcitonin in osteolytic metastases. *Clin Trials J* 1983;20:266–74.

588. Hindley AC, Hill EB, Leyland MJ, Wiles AE. A double-blind controlled trial of salmon calcitonin in pain due to malignancy. *Cancer Chemother Pharmacol* 1982;9:71–4.

589. Allan E. Calcitonin in the treatment of intractable pain from advanced malignancy. *Pharmatherapeutica* 1983;3:482–6.

590. Hano J, Bugajski J, Danek L, et al. The influence of serotonin on insulin-stimulated gastric secretion, blood glucose and serum electrolyte levels in the unanesthetized rat. *Arch Int Pharmacodyn Ther* 1975;216:28–39.

591. Hasking DJ, Denton LB, Codge B, Martin TJ. Functional significance of antibody formation after long-term salmon calcitonin therapy. *Clin Endocrinol [Oxf]* 1979;10:243–52.

592. Singer F, Fredericks RS, Minkin C. Salmon calcitonin therapy for Paget's disease of bone: the problem of acquired clinical resistance. *Arch Rheumatol* 1980;23:1148–54.

593. Heaney RP, Saville PD. Etidronate disodium in postmenopausal osteoporosis. *Clin Pharacol Ther* 1976;20:593–604.

594. Storm T, Thamsborg G, Steiniche T, Genant HK, Sorenson OH. The effects of etidronate therapy in postmenopausal osteoprotic women. *N Engl J Med* 1990;322:1265–71.

595. Hodsman AB. Effects of cyclical therapy for osteoporosis using an oral regimen of inorganic phosphate and sodium etidronate: a clinical and bone histomorphometric study. *Bone Miner* 1989;5:201–12.

596. Hesch RD, Heck J, Delling G, et al. Results of a stimulatory therapy of low bone metabolism in osteoporosis with (1-38)-hPTH and diphosphonate EHDP. *Klin Wochenschr* 1988; 66:976–84.

597. Mallette LE, LeBlanc AD, Pool JL, Mechanick JI. Cyclic therapy of osteoporosis with neutral phosphate and brief, high-dose pulses of etidronate. *J Bone Miner Res* 1989;4:143–8.

598. Anderson FC, Cope CD, Crilly RG, Hodsman AB, Wolfe BM. Preliminary observations of a form of coherence therapy for osteoporosis. *Calcif Tissue Int* 1984;36:341–3.

599. Smith ML, Fogelman I, Hart DM, Scott E, Bevan J, Leggate I. Effect of etidronate disodium on bone turnover following surgical menopause. *Calcif Tissue Int* 1989;44:74–9.

600. Watts NB, Herris ST, Genant HK, et al. Intermittent cyclical

etidronate therapy of postmenopausal osteoporosis. *N Engl J Med* 1990;323:73–9.

601. Valkema R, Papapoulas SE, Vismans FJ, et al. A four year continuous gain in bone mass in APD-treated osteoporosis. In: Christiansen C, Johansen JS, Riis BJ, eds, *Osteoporosis 1987.* Copenhagen: Osteopres, 1987;1172–6.

602. Bijvoet OLM, Valkema R, Lowik CWGM, Papapoulas SE. The use of bisphosphonates in osteoporosis. In: DeLuca HF, Mazess R, eds. *Osteoporosis: physiological basis, assessment and treatment.* New York: Elsevier, 1990;331–8.

603. Reid IR, King AR, Alexander CJ, Ibbertson HK. Prevention of steroid-induced osteoporosis with (3-amino-1-hydroxypropylidene)-1,1-bisphosphonate (APD). *Lancet* 1988;i:143–6.

604. Miller PD, Neal BJ, MacIntyre DO, Yanover MJ, Kowalski L. In: Christiansen C, Johansen JS, Riis BJ, eds. *Osteoporosis 1987,* Copenhagen: Osteopres, 1987.

605. Fleisch H. The possible use of bisphosphonates in osteoporosis. In: DeLuca HF, Mazess R, eds. *Osteoporosis: physiological basis, assessment and treatment.* New York: Elsevier, 1990;323–30.

606. Frijlink WB, TeVelde J, Bijvoet OLM, Heynen G. Treatment of Paget's disease of bone with (3-amino-1-hydroxypropylidene)-1,1-bisphosphonate (APD). *Lancet* 1979;i:799–803.

607. Singer FR, Ritch PS, Lad TE, et al. Treatment of hypercalcemia of malignancy with intravenous etidronate. *Arch Intern Med* 1991;151:471–476.

608. Jowsey J, Riggs BL, Kelly PJ, Hoffman DL, Bordier P. The treatment of osteoporosis with disodium ethane-1, 1-diphosphonate. *J Lab Clin Med* 1971;78:574–84.

609. Schneider VS, McDonald J. Skeletal calcium homeostasis and counter measures to prevent disuse osteoporosis *Calcif Tissue Int* 1984;36:151–4.

610. Flora L, Hassings GS, Cloyd GG, Bevan JA, Parfitt AM, Villaneuva AR. The long-term skeletal effects of EHDP in dogs. *Metab Bone Dis Rel Res* 1981;4:289–300.

611. Bijvoet OLM, Vellenga CJLR, Horinck HJ. Paget's disease of bones: assessment, therapy, and secondary prevention. In: Kleerekoper M, Krane SM, eds. *Clinical disorders of bone and mineral metabolism,* 1989;525–42.

612. Gallagher JC, Riggs BL, Recker RR, Goldgar D. The effect of calcitriol on patients with postmenopausal osteoporosis with special reference to fracture frequency. *Proc Soc Exp Biol Med* 1989;191:287–90.

613. Caniggia A, Nuti R, Love F, et al. The hormonal form of vitamin D in the pathophysiology and therapy of postmenopausal osteoporosis. *J Endocrinol Invest* 1984;7:373–8.

614. Gallagher JC, Jerpbak CM, Jee WSS, et al. 1,25-dihydroxyvitamin D$_3$ in patients with postmenopausal osteoporosis. *Proc Natl Acad Sci USA* 1982;79:3325–9.

615. Aloia JF, Vaswani A, Yeh JK, et al. Calcitriol in the treatment of postmenopausal osteoporosis. *Am J Med* 1988;84:401–8.

616. Ott S, Chesnut CH. Calcitriol treatment is not effective in postmenopausal osteoporosis. *Ann Intern Med* 1989;4:267–74.

617. Gallagher JC, Recker R. A comparison between high dose calcitriol and calcium supplements in osteoporosis. In: Norman AW, Schaefer K, Grigoleit HG, et al., eds. *Vitamin D, chemical, biochemical and clinical update.* Berlin: Walter de Gruyter, 1985.

618. Shwaki M, Orimo H, Ito H, et al. Long-term treatment of postmenopausal osteoporosis with active vitamin D$_3$, 1,alpha hydroxycholecalciferol and 1,25 dihydroxycholecalciferol. *Endocrinol Jpn* 1985;32:305–15.

619. Orimo H, Shwaki M, Hajeshi R, et al. Reduced occurrence of vertebral crush fractures in senile osteoporotics treated with 1,alpha(OH)-vitamin D$_3$. *Bone Miner* 1987;3:47–52.

620. Jensen GF, Christiansen C, Transbol I. Treatment of postmenopausal osteoporosis. A controlled therapeutic trial comparing oestrogen/gestagen, 1,25-dihydroxyvitamin D$_3$ and calcium. *Endocrinol (Oxf),* 1982;16:515–24.

621. Riggs BL, Nelson K. Effect of long-term treatment with calcitriol on calcium absorption and mineral metabolism in postmenopausal osteoporosis. *J Clin Endocrinol Metab* 1985;61:457–61.

622. Fujita T. Studies of osteoporosis in Japan. *Metabolism* 1990;39(4)(Suppl 1):39–42.

623. Fujita T, Inore T, Orimo H, et al. Clinical evaluation of the effect of calcitriol on osteoporosis. Multicenter double-blind study

using alfacalcitol as the control drug. *J Clin Exp Med* 1989;148:833–57.

624. Need AG, Horowitz M, Philcox JC, et al. 1,25-dihydroxycholecalciferol and calcium therapy in osteoporosis with calcium malabsorption. *Miner Electrolyte Metab* 1985;11:35–40.

625. Jensen GF, Meinecke B, Boesen J, et al. Does 1,25(OH)$_2$D$_3$ accelerate spinal bone loss? A controlled therapeutic trial in 70 year old women. *Clin Orthop* 1985;192:215–21.

626. Falch JA, Odegaard OR, Finnanger AM, et al. Postmenopausal osteoporosis: no effect of three years of treatment with 1,25-dihydroxycholecalciferol. *Acta Med Scand* 1987;221:199–204.

627. Christiansen C, Christiansen MS, Rodbro P. Effect of 1,25-dihydroxyvitamin D$_3$ in itself or combined with hormone treatment in preventing postmenopausal osteoporosis. *Eur J Clin Invest* 1984;11:305–9.

628. Tjellesen L, Christiansen C, Rodbro P. Effect of 1,25-dihydroxyvitamin D$_3$ on biochemical indices of bone turnover in postmenopausal women. *Acta Med Scand* 1984;215:411–5.

629. Canniggia A, Delling G, Nuti R, et al. Clinical, biochemical and histological results of a double-blind tiral with 1,25-dihydroxyvitamin D, estradiol and placebo in postmenopausal osteoporosis. *Acta Vitaminol Enzymol* 1984;6:117–30.

630. Tilyard M. Low dose calcitriol versus calcium in established osteoporosis. *Metabolism* 1990;39:50–2.

631. Raisz LG, Trumnel CL, Holick MF, et al. 1,25-dihydroxycholecalciferol: a potent stimulator of bone resorption in tissue culture. *Science* 1972;175:768–9.

632. Reynolds JJ, Holick MF, DeLuca HF. The role of vitamin D metabolites in bone resorption. *Calcif Tissue Res* 1973;12:295–301.

633. Price PA, Baukol SA. 1,25-dihydroxyvitamin D$_3$ increases synthesis of the vitamin D-dependent bone protein by osteosarcoma cells. *J Biol Chem* 1980;255:11660–6.

634. Prince CW, Butler WT. 1,25-dihydroxyvitamin D$_3$ regulates the biosynthesis of osteopontin on bone-derived cell attachment protein in clonal osteoblast-like osteosarcoma cells. *Collagen Rel Res* 1987;7:305–13.

635. Fujita T, Matsui T, Nakoa Y, et al. Lymphocyte subsets in osteoporosis. Effect of 1-alpha hydroxyvitamin D. *Miner Electrolyte Metab* 1984;10:375–8.

636. DeLuca HF. Osteoporosis and the metabolites of vitamin D. *Metabolism* 1990;39:3–9.

637. Marshall DH, Crilly RG, Nordin BEC. Plasma androstanedine and oestrone levels in normal and osteoporotic postmenopausal women. *Br Med J* 1977;2:1177–9.

638. Wild RA, Buchanan JR, Myers C, Lloyd T, Demers LM. Adrenal androgens, sex hormone binding globulin and bone density in osteoporotic menopausal women: is there a relationship? *Maturitas* 1987;9:55–61.

639. Davidson BJ, Ross RK, Paganini-Hill A, Hammond CD, Siiteri PK, Judd HL. Total and free androgens in postmenopausal women with hip fractures. *J Clin Endocrinol Metab* 1982; 54:115–20.

640. Taelman P, Kaufman JM, Janssen X, Vermuelan A. Persistence of increased bone resorption and possible role of dehydroepiandrosterone as a bone metabolism determinant in osteoporotic women in late post-menopause. *Maturitas* 1989;11:65–73.

641. Chesnut CH, Ivey JL, Gruber HE, et al. Stanozolol in postmenopausal osteoporosis: therapeutic efficacy and possible mechanisms of action. *Metabolism* 1983;32:571–580.

642. Dequeker J, Geusens P. Anabolic steroids and osteoporosis. *Acta Endocrinol (Copenh)* 1985;271(Suppl 110):45–52.

643. Need AG, Horowitz M, Morris HA, Walker CJ, Nordin BEC. Effects of nandroline therapy on forearm bone mineral content in osteoporosis. *Clin Orthop* 1987;225:273–8.

644. Chesnut CH, Nelp WB, Baylink DJ, Denney JD. Effect of methandrostanolene on postmenopausal bone wasting as assessed by changes in total bone mineral mass. *Metabolism* 1977;26:267–77.

645. Need AG, Challerton BE, Walker CJ, Stenner TA, Horowitz M, Nordin BEC. Comparison of calcium, calcitriol, ovarian hormones and nandrolone in the treatment of osteoporosis. *Maturitas* 1986;8:275–80.

646. Johannsen JS, Hassager C, Podephant J, et al. Treatment of post-

menopausal osteoporosis. Is the anabolic steroid nandrolone decanoate a candidate? *Bone Miner* 1989;6:77–86.

647. Aloia JF, Kapoer A, Vaswani A, Cohn SH. Changes in body composition following therapy of osteoporosis with methandrostaenelone. *Metabolism* 1981;30:1076–9.

648. Hassager C, Podenphant J, Riis BJ, Johansen JS, Jensen J, Christiansen C. Changes in soft tissue body composition and plasma lipid metabolism during nandrolone decanoate therapy in postmenopausal women. *Metabolism* 1989;38:238–42.

649. Vashnaiv R, Gallagher JA, Beresford JN, Poser JW, Russell RGG. Direct effect of stanozolol and estrogens on human bone cells in culture. In: Christiansen C, et al, eds, *Osteoporosis*, Denmark: Aalborg Stiftsbogtrykkeri, 1984;485–8.

650. Cuch M, Preston FE, Malia RG, Graham R, Russell G. Changes in plasma osteocalcin concentration following treatment with stanazolol. *Clin Chem Acta* 1986;158:43–57.

651. Taggart H, Appledorn-Bowden D, Haffner S, et al. Reduction in high-density lipoproteins by anabolic-steroid (stanozolol) therapy for postmenopausal osteoporosis. *Metabolism* 1982;31:1147–50.

652. Frost HM. Treatment of osteoporosis by manipulation of coherent bone cell populations. *Clin Orthop* 1979;143:227–44.

653. Largent EJ. Metabolism of inorganic fluorides. In: Vischer TL, ed. *Fluoridation as a Public Health Measure*, Bern, Switzerland: Hans Huber 1954;178–89.

654. Roholm K. *Fluorine intoxication: a clinical-hygienic study; with a review of the literature and some experimental investigations.* London: H.K. Lewis 1937.

655. Singh A, Jolly SS, Bansal BC, Mathur CC. Endemic fluorosis: epidemiological, clinical and biochemical study of chronic fluorine intoxication in Panjab (India). *Medicine (Baltimore)* 1963;42:229–46.

656. Leone NC, Stevenson CA, Hilbish TF, Sosman MC. A roentgenologic study of a human population exposed to high-fluoride domestic water: a ten year study. *Am J Roentgenol Rad Ther Nucl Med* 1955;74:874–85.

657. Bernstein DS, Sadowsky N, Hegsted DM, Guri CD, Stare FJ. Prevalence of osteoporosis in high and low fluoride areas in North Dakota. *JAMA* 1966;198:499–504.

658. Rich C, Ensinck J. Effect of sodium fluoride on calcium metabolism of human beings. *Nature* 1961;191:184–5.

659. Rich C, Ensinck J, Invanovich P. The effects of sodium fluoride on calcium metabolism of subjects with metabolic bone disease. *J Clin Invest* 1964;43:545–56.

660. Bernstein DS, Cohen P. Use of sodium fluoride in the treatment of osteoporosis. *J Clin Endocrinol Metab* 1967;27:197–210.

661. Baylink DJ, Bernstein DS. The effects of fluoride therapy on metabolic bone disease: a histologic study. *Clin Orthop Rel Res* 1967;55:51–85.

662. Cohen MB, Rubini ME. The treatment of osteoporosis with sodium fluoride. *Clin Orthop Rel Res* 1965;43:545–56.

663. Lukert BP, Bolinger RE, Meek JC. Acute effect of fluoride on [45]calcium dynamics in osteoporosis. *J Clin Endocrinol Metab* 1967;27:828–35.

664. Jowsey J, Schenk RK, Reutter FW. Some results of the effect of fluoride on bone tissue in osteoporosis. *J Clin Endocrinol Metab* 1968;28:869–74.

665. Jowsey J, Riggs BL, Kelly PJ, Hoffman DL. Effect of combined therapy with sodium fluoride, vitamin D and calcium in osteoporosis. *Am J Med* 1972;53:43–59.

666. Chlud K. Zur behandlung der osteoporose mit einem protrahiert wirksamen natrium-fluoride-praparat. *Z Rheumatol* 1977;36:126–39.

667. Baud CA, Lagier R, Bang S, Boivin G, Gossi M, Tochon-Danguy HJ. Treatment of osteoporosis with NaF, calcium or/and phosphorus, and vitamin D: histological morphometric and biophysical study of the bone tissue. In: Courvoisier B, Donath A, Baud CA, eds. *Fluoride and bone: Proceedings of the Second Symposium CEMO, Nyon, Switzerland.* Bern, Switzerland: Hans Huber 1978;238–41.

668. Hansson T, Roos B. Osteoporosis: effect of combined therapy with sodium fluoride, calcium, and vitamin D on the lumbar spine in osteoporosis. *Am J Roentgenol, Rad Thera Nucl Med* 1976;126:1294–7.

669. Briancon D, Meunier PJ. Treatment of osteoporosis with fluoride, calcium, and vitamin D. *Orthop Clin North Am* 1981;12:629–48.

670. Harrison JE, McNeill KG, Sturtridge WC, et al. Three-year changes in bone mineral mass of postmenopausal osteoporotic patients based on neutron activation analysis of the central third of the skeleton. *J Clin Endocrinol Metab* 1981;52:751–8.

671. Ryckwaert A, Kuntz D, Teyssedou JP, Tun Chot S, Bordier P, Hioco D. Etude histologique de l'os chez des sujet osteoporotiques en triatement prolonge par le fluorure de sodium. *Rev Rhum Mal Osteoartic* 1972;39:627–34.

672. Merz WA, Schenk RK, Reutter FW. Paradoxical effects of vitamin D in fluoride-treated senile osteoporosis. *Calcif Tissue Res* 1970;4:49–50.

673. Schenk RK, Merz WA, Reutter FW. Fluoride in osteoporosis: quantitative histological studies on bone structure and bone remodelling in serial biopsies of the iliac crest. In: Vischer TL, ed. *Fluoride in medicine.* Bern, Switzerland: Hans Huber, 1970;153–68.

674. Thiebaud M, Zender R, Courvoisier B, Baud CA, Jacot C. The action of fluoride on diffuse bone atrophies. In: Vischer TL, ed. *Fluoride in medicine.* Bern, Switzerland: Hans Huber, 1970;136–42.

675. Inkovaara J, Heikinheimo R, Jarvinen K, Kasurinen U, Hanhijarvi H, Iisalo E. Prophylactic fluoride treatment and aged bones. *Br Med J* 1975;3:73–4.

676. Parsons V, Mitchell CJ, Reeve J, Hesp R. The use of sodium fluoride, vitamin D and calcium supplements in the treatment of patients with axial osteoporosis. *Calcif Tissue Res* 1977;22:236–40.

677. Hauswaldt C, Fuchs C, Hesch RD, Kobberling J, Unger KO. Histomorphometrische Untersuchungen an beckenkammbiopsien bei fluorid-langzeittherapie der Osteoporose. *Deutsche Medizinische Wochenschrift* 1977;102:1177–80.

678. Dambacher MA, Lauffenburger T, Lammle B, Haas HG. Long term effects of sodium fluoride in osteoporosis. In: Courvoisier B, Donath A, Baud CA, eds. *Fluoride and bone: Proceedings of the Second Symposium CEMO, Nyon, Switzerland.* Bern, Switzerland: Hans Huber, 1978;290–2.

679. Hansson T, Roos B. Osteoporoses: effect of combined therapy with sodium fluoride, calcium, and vitamin D on the lumbar spine in osteoporosis. *Am J Roentgenol Rad Ther Nucl Med* 1976;126:1294–7.

680. Spencer H, Lewin I, Fowler J, Samachson J. Effect of sodium fluoride on calcium absorption and balances in man. *Am J Clin Nutr* 1969;22:381–90.

681. Schenk RK, Merz WA, Reutter FW. Fluoride in osteoporosis: quantitative histological studies on bone structure and bone remodelling in serial biopsies of the iliac crest. In: Vischer TL, ed. *Fluoride in medicine,* Bern, Switzerland: Hans Huber, 1970;153–68.

682. Haas HG, Lauffenburger T, Guncaga J, Lentner C, Ohal AJ, Dambacher MA. Bone turnover in osteoporosis, studied with sodium fluoride (abstract). *Eur J Clin Invest* 1973;3:235.

683. Olah AJ, Reutter FW, Dambacher MA. Effects of combined therapy with sodium fluoride and high doses of vitamin D in osteoporosis. A histomorphometric study of the iliac crest. In: Courvoisier B, Donath A, Baud CA, eds. *Fluoride and bone: Proceedings of the Second Symposium CEMO, Nyon, Switzerland.* Bern, Switzerland: Hans Huber, 1978;242–8.

684. Reutter FW, Olah AJ. Bone biopsy findings and clinical observations in long term treatment of osteoporosis with sodium fluoride and vitamin D3. In: Courvoisier B, Donath A, Baud CA, eds. *Fluoride and bone: Proceedings of the Second Symposium CEMO, Nyon, Switzerland.* Bern, Switzerland: Hans Huber, 1978;249–55.

685. Riggs BL, Hodgson SF, Hoffman DL, Kelly PJ, Johnson KA, Taves D. Treatment of primary osteoporosis with fluoride and calcium: clinical tolerance and fracture occurrence. *JAMA* 1980;243:446–9.

686. Riggs BL, Seeman E, Hodgson SF, Taves DR, O'Fallon WM. Effect of the fluoride/calcium regimen on vertebral fracture occurrence in postmenopausal osteoporosis: comparison with conventional therapy. *N Engl J Med* 1982;306:446–50.

687. Hodsman AB, Drost DJ. The response of vertebral bone mineral density during the treatment of osteoporosis with sodium fluoride. *J Clin Endocrinol Metab* 1989;69:932–8.

688. Ringe JD, Kruse HP, Kuhlencordt F. Long term treatment of primary osteoporosis by sodium fluoride. In: Courvoisier B, Donath A, Baud CA, eds. *Fluoride and bone: Proceedings of the Second Symposium CEMO, Nyon, Switzerland*. Bern, Switzerland: Hans Huber, 1978;228–32.

689. Aloia JF, Zanzi I, Vaswani A, Ellis K, Cohn SH. Combination therapy for osteoporosis with estrogen, fluoride, and calcium. *J Am Geriatr Soc* 1982;30:13–7.

690. Vose GP, Keele DK, Milner AM, Rawley R, Roach TL, Sprinkle EE III. Effect of sodium fluoride, inorganic phosphate, and oxymetholone therapies in osteoporosis: a six-year progress report. *J Gerontol* 1978;33:204–12.

691. Mamelle N, Meunier PJ, Dusen R, et al. Risk benefit ratio of sodium fluoride treatment in primary vertebral osteoporosis. *Lancet* 1988;ii:361–5.

692. Kleerekoper M. *Ann Intern Med* 1990; in press.

693. Riggs B. Treatment of osteoporosis with sodium fluoride: an appraisal. *Bone Miner Res* 1983;2:366–93.

694. Pak CYC, Sakhaee K, Gallagher C, et al. Allowment of therapeutic fluoride levels in serum without major side-effects, using a slow-release preparation of sodium preparation of sodium fluoride in osteoporosis. *J Bone Miner Res* 1986;1:563–71.

695. O'Duffy JD, Wahner HW, O'Fallon WM, et al. Mechanism of acute lower extremity pain syndrome in fluoride-treated osteoporotic patients. *Am J Med* 1986;80:561–6.

696. Budden FH, Bayley TA, Harrison JE, et al. The effect of fluoride on bone histology in postmenopausal osteoporosis depends on adequate fluoride absorption and retention. *J Bone Miner Res* 1988;3:127–32.

697. Vigorita VJ, Suda MK. The microscopic morphology of fluoride-induced bone. *Clin Orthop* 1983;177:274–282.

698. Gutteridge DH, Price RI, Nicholson GC, Kent GN, Retallack RW, Michell P. Fluoride in osteoporosis-vertebral but not femoral fracture protection. *Calcif Tissue Int* 1984;36:481.

699. Gutteridge DH, Price RI, Nicholson GC, et al. Fluoride in osteoporotic vertebral fractures trabecular increase, vertebral protection, femoral fractures. In: Christiansen C, ed. *Osteoporosis*. Denmark: Osteopres, Aalborg Stiftsbogtrykkeri, 1984;705–7.

700. Hedlund LR, Gallagher JC. Increased incidence of hip fracture in osteoporotic women treated with sodium fluoride. *J Bone Miner Res* 1989;4:223–5.

701. Riggs BL, Baylink DJ, Kleerekoper M, Lane JM, Melton LJ, Meunier PJ. Incidence of hip fractures in osteoporotic women treated with sodium fluoride. *J Bone Miner Res* 1987;2:123–6.

702. Farley JR, Tarbaux N, Hall S, Baylink DJ. Evidence that fluoride-stimulated 3[H]-thymidine incorporation in embryonic chick calvarial cell cultures is dependent on the presence of a bone cell mitogen, sensitive to changes in the phosphate concentration, and modulated by systemic skeletal effectors. *Metabolism* 1988;37:988–95.

703. Lundy MW, Lau KH, Blair HC, Baylink DJ. Chick osteoblasts contain fluoride-sensitive acid phosphatase activity. *J Histochem Cytochem* 1988;36:1175–80.

704. Wergedal JE, Lau KH, Baylink DJ. Fluoride and bovine bone extract influence cell proliferation and phosphatase activities in human bone cell cultures. *Clin Orthop* 1988;233:274–82.

705. Selye M. On stimulation of new bone formation with parathyroid extract and irradiated ergosterol. *Endocrinology* 1932;16:547–58.

706. Kalu DN, Pennock J, Doyle FH, Foster GV. Parathyroid hormone and experimental osteosclerosis. *Lancet* 1970;i:1363–6.

707. Tam CS, Heerscyhe JNM, Murray TM, Parsons JA. Parathyroid hormone stimulates the bone apposition rate independently of its resorptive action: differential effects of intermittent and continuous administration. *Endocrinology* 1982;110:506–12.

708. Hefti E, Trechsel U, Bonjour JP, Fleisch H, Schenk R. Increase of whole body calcium and skeletal mass in normal and osteoporotic adult rats treated with parathyroid hormone. *Clin Sci* 1982;62:389–96.

709. Gunness-Hey M, Hock JM. Increased trabecular bone mass in rats treated with human synthetic parathyroid hormone. *Metab Bone Dis Rel Res* 1984;5:177–81.

710. Podbesek R, Edouard C, Meunier PJ, et al. Effects of two treatment regimens with synthetic human parathyroid hormone fragment on bone formation and the tissue balance of trabecular bone in greyhounds. *Endocrinology* 1983;112:1000–6.

711. Kream BE, Rowe DW, Gworek SC, Raisz LG. Parathyroid hormone alters collagen synthesis and procollagen mRNA levels in fetal rat calvaria. *Proc Natl Acad Sci USA* 1983;77:5654.

712. Hummert J, Hock JM, Fonseca J, Raisz LG. Resorption is not essential for the stimulation of bone growth by hPTH 1–34 in rats in vivo (abstract). *J Bone Miner Res* 1986;1:83.

713. Hock JM, Gera I, Fonseca J, Raisz LG. Human parathyroid hormone (1–34) increases bone mass in ovariectomized or archidectomized rats. *Endocrinology* 1988;122:2899–904.

714. Parsons JA, Reit B. Chronic response of dogs to parathyroid infusion. *Nature* 1974;250:254–7.

715. Reeve J, Meunier PJ, Parsons JA, et al. Anabolic effect of human parathyroid hormone fragment on trabecular bone in involutional osteoporosis: a multicentre trial. *Br Med J* 1980;280:1340–1344.

716. Slovik DM, Neer RM, Potts JT Jr. Short-term effects of synthetic human parathyroid hormone (1–34) administration on bone mineral metabolism in osteoporotic patients. *J Clin Invest* 1981;68:1261–71.

717. Neer RM, Slovik DM, Tully G, Adams J, Holick M, Potts JT Jr. Interaction of synthetic human parathyroid hormone fragment 1–34 with other agents in osteoporotic patients. In: DeLuca H, et al, eds. *Osteoporosis*, Baltimore: University Park Press, 1981;467–70.

718. Slovik DM, Rosenthal DI, Doppelt SH, et al. Restoration of spinal bone in osteoporotic men by treatment with parathyroid hormone (1–34) and 1,25-dihydroxyvitamin D. *J Bone Miner Res* 1986;1:377.

719. Reeve J, Hesp R, Williams D, et al. Anabolic effect of low doses of a fragment of human parathyroid hormone on the skeleton in postmenopausal osteoporosis. *Lancet* 1976;i:1035–8.

720. Hesch RD, Busche U, Prokop M, Delling G, Rittinghause EF. Increase of vertebral density by combination therapy with pulsatile 1–38hPTH and sequential addition of calcitonin nasal spray in osteoporotic patients. *Calcif Tissue Int* 1989;44:176–80.

721. Reeve J, Bradbeer JN, Arlot M, et al. hPTH 1-34 Treatment of osteoporosis with added hormone replacement therapy: biochemical, kinetic and histological responses. *Osteoporosis Int* 1991;1:(in press).

722. Hesp R, Hulme P, Williams D, Reeve J. The relationship between changes in femoral bone density and calcium balance in patients with involutional osteoporosis treated with human parathyroid hormone fragment (hPTH 1-34). *Metab Bone Dis Rel Res* 1981;2:331–334.

723. Reeve J, Davies UM, Hesp R, McNally E, Katz D. Human parathyroid peptide treatment of osteoporosis substantially increases spinal trabecular bone. *Br Med J* 1990;301:314–318 and 477.

724. Frost HM. Coherence treatment of osteoporosis. *Orthop Clin North Am* 1981;12:649–69.

725. Anderson C, Cope RDT, Crilly RJ, Hodsman AB, Wolfe BMJ. Preliminary observations of a form of coherence therapy for osteoporosis. *Calcif Tissue Int* 1984;36:341–3.

726. Woodson GC. Coherence therapy with phosphate and etidronate for osteoporosis: preliminary results. In: Christiansen C, Johansen JS, Riis BJ, eds. *Osteoporosis 1987*, Aalborg, Denmark: Norhaven AS, 1987;1188–9.

727. Miller PD, Neal BJ, McIntyre DO, Yanover MJ, Kowalski L. The effect of coherence therapy with phosphate and etidronate on axial bone mineral density in postmenopausal osteoporosis. In: Christiansen C, Johansen JS, Riis BJ, eds. *Osteoporosis 1987*. Aalborg, Denmark: Norhaven AS, 1987;884–5.

728. Mallette LE, LeBlanc AD. Cyclic therapy of osteoporosis: use of a brief, high-dose pulse of etidronate as a terminator of osteoclast activity. In: Christiansen C, Johansen JS, Riis BJ, eds. *Osteoporosis 1987*. Aalborg, Denmark: Norhaven AS, 1987;994–46.

729. Hodsman AB. Effects of cyclical therapy of osteoporosis using an oral regimen of inorganic phosphate and sodium etidronate: a clinical and bone histomorphometric study. *Bone Miner* 1989;5:201–12.

730. Parfitt AM. ADFR and coherence therapy for osteoporosis. In:

DeLuca HF, Mazess R, eds. *Osteoporosis, physiological basis, assessment and treatment,* New York: Elsevier, 1990;315–20.

731. Marie PJ, Coulin F. Mechanisms underlying the effects of phosphate and calcitonin on bone histology in postmenopausal osteoporosis. *Bone* 1986;7:17–22.

732. Rasmussen H, Bordier P, Marie P, et al. Effect of combined therapy with phosphate and calcitonin on bone volume in osteoporosis. *Metab Bone Dis Rel Res* 1980;2:107–11.

733. Aloia JF, Vaswani A, Meunier PJ. Coherence treatment of postmenopausal osteoporosis with growth hormone and calcitonin. *Calcif Tiss Int* 1987;40:253–9.

734. Pedrazzoni M, Palummeri E, Pioli G, et al. Involutional osteoporosis and ADFR treatment: a controlled pilot study. *Curr Therap Res* 1989;45:188–197.

735. Halse J, Melsen F, Mosekilde L. Iliac crest bone mass and remodelling in acromegaly. *Acta Endocrinol* 1981;96:18–22.

736. Riggs BL, Randall RV, Wahner HW, Jowsey J, Kelly PJ, Singh M. The nature of the metabolic bone disorder in acromegaly. *J Clin Endocrinol Metab* 1972;34:911–8.

737. Aloia JF, Roginsky MS, Jowsey J, Dombrowski CS, Shukla KK, Cohn SH. Skeletal metabolism body composition in acromegaly. *J Clin Endocrinol Metab* 1972;35:543–51.

738. Halse J, Gordelaze JO. Total and non-dialyzable urinary hydroxyproline in acromegaly and control subjects. *Acta Endocrinol* 1981;96:451–7.

739. Brixen K, Nielson HK, Mosekilde L, Flyvbjerg A. A short course of recombinant human growth hormone treatment stimulates osteoblasts and activates bone remodeling in normal human volunteers. *J Bone Miner Res* 1990;5:609–18.

740. Aloia JF, Zanzi I, Ellis K, et al. Effects of growth hormone in osteoporosis. *J Clin Endocrinol Metab* 1976;43:992–9.

741. Aloia JF, Vaswani A, Kapoor A, Yeh JK, Cohn SV. Treatment of osteoporosis with calcitonin, with and without growth hormone. *Metabolism* 1985;34:124–9.

742. Rudman D, Felter AG, Nagraj HS, et al. Effects of human growth hormone in men over 60 years old. *N Engl J Med* 1990;323:1–6.

743. Turken S, Seldin D, Lindsay R. Effects of tamoxifen on spinal bone density. *J Natl Cancer Inst* 1989;81:1086–8.

744. Love RR, Mazess RB, Tormey DL, Barden HS, Newcomb PA, Jordan VC. Bone mineral density in women with breast cancer treated with adjuvant tamoxifen for at least two years. *Breast Cancer Res Treat* 1988;12:297–301.

745. Dupont WD, Page DL. Menopausal estrogen replacement therapy and breast cancer. *Arch Intern Med* 1991;151:67–72.

746. Mack TM, Henderson BE, Gerkins VR, et al. Reserpine and breast cancer in a retirement community. *N Engl J Med* 1975;292:1366–71.

747. Casagrande J, Gerkins V, Henderson BE, et al. Brief communication: exogenous estrogens and breast cancer in women with natural menopause. *J Natl Cancer Inst* 1976;56:839–41.

748. Byrd BF Jr, Burch JC, Vaughn WK. The impact of long term estrogen support after hysterectomy. *Ann Surg* 1977;185:574–9.

749. Wynder EL, MacCormack FA, Stellman SD. The epidemiology of breast cancer in 785 United States Caucasian women. *Cancer* 1978;41:2341–54.

750. Ravnihar B, Seigel DG, Lindtner J. An epidemiologic study of breast cancer and benign breast neoplasias in relation to the oral contraceptive and estrogen use. *Eur J Cancer Clin Oncol* 1979;15:395–405.

751. Vakil DV, Morgan RW, Halliday M. Exogenous estrogens and development of breast and endometrial cancer. *Cancer Detect Prev* 1983;6:415–24.

752. Horwitz RI, Stewart KR. Effect of clinical features on the association of estrogens and breast cancer. *Am J Med* 1984;76:192–8.

753. Buring JE, Hennekens CH, Lipnick RH, et al. A prospective cohort study of postmenopausal hormone use and risk of breast cancer in US women. *Am J Epidemiol* 1987;125:939–47.

754. Hunt K, Vessey M, McPherson K, Coleman M. Long-term surveillance of mortality and cancer incidence in women receiving hormone replacement therapy. *Br J Obstet Gynecol* 1987;94:620–35.

755. Rohan TE, McMichael AJ. Non-contraceptive exogenous oestrogen therapy and breast cancer. *Med J Aust* 1988;148:217–21.

756. Dupont WD, Page DL, Rogers LW, Parl FF. Influence of exogenous estrogens, proliferative breast disease, and other variables on breast cancer. *Cancer* 1989;63:948–57.

757. Mills PK, Beeson WL, Phillips RL, Fraser GE. Prospective study of exogenous hormone use and breast cancer in Seventh-Day Adventists. *Cancer* 1989;64:591–7.

758. Lindsay R, et al. *Osteoporosis 1987,* 508–12.

759. Overgaard K, Riis BJ, Christiansen C, Hansen MA. Effect of salcatonin given intranasally on early postmenopausal bone loss. *Br Med J* 1989;299:477–479.

760. Jacobsen SJ, Goldberg J, Miles TP, et. al. Regional variation in the incidence of hip fracture in U.S. white women aged 65 years and older. *J Am Med Assoc* 1990;264:500–502.

761. Proceedings of the International Workshop on Fluoride and Bone. *Journal of Bone and Mineral Research.* Murray TM, Singer FR, eds. New York: Mary Ann Liebert, Inc., pp. S1–S239.

762. Orcel PH, de Vernejoul MC, Prier A, et. al. Stress fractures of the lower limbs in osteoporotic patients treated with fluoride. *J Bone Min Res* 1990;5(Suppl):191–194.

763. Schnitzler CM, Sing JR, Mesquita JM, et. al. Risk factors for the development of stress fractures during fluoride therapy for osteoporosis. *J Bone Min Res* 1990;5(Suppl):195–199.

764. Schulz EE, Flowers C, Sauser DD, et. al. The causes of bone scintigram hot spots in fluoride-treated osteoporotic patients. *J Bone Min Res* 1990;5(Suppl):201–204.

765. Carter DR, Beaupre GS. Effects of flouride treatment on bone strength. *J Bone Min Res* 1990;5(Suppl):177–184.

766. Delmas PD, Dupuis J, Duboeuf F, Chapuy MC, Meunier PJ. Treatment of vertebral osteoporosis with disodium monofluorophosphate: comparison with sodium fluoride. *J Bone Min Res* 1990;5(Suppl):143–147.

767. Elmerson S, Zetterberg C, Anderson GBJ. Ten-year survival after fractures of the proximal end of the femur. *Gerontology* 1988;34:186–191.

768. Glajchen N, Ismail F, Epstein S, et. al. The effect of chronic caffeine administration on serum markers of bone mineral metabolism and bone histomorphometry in the rat. *Calcif Tiss Int* 1988;43:277–280.

769. Lindsay R, Cosman F, Herrington BS, Himmelstein S. Bone mass and body composition in normal women. *J Bone Min Res* 1991;(in press).

Disorders of Bone and Mineral Metabolism,
edited by Fredric L. Coe and Murray J. Favus,
© 1992 by Raven Press, Ltd. All rights reserved.

CHAPTER 38

Secondary Forms of Osteoporosis

Robert Marcus

On the surface it would appear a simple task to designate a disease as primary or secondary. However, the nomenclature of osteoporosis remains ambiguous. *Primary osteoporosis* is by tradition a condition of reduced bone mass and fractures found in menopausal women (postmenopausal osteoporosis) or in older men and women ("senile" osteoporosis). *Secondary osteoporosis* has referred to bone loss resulting from specific, well-defined clinical disorders, such as thyrotoxicosis and hyperadrenocorticism.

Albright and Reifenstein (1) concluded in 1948 that osteoporosis was composed of two separate entities, one related to menopausal estrogen loss and the other to aging. Recent support for this concept has been published by Riggs and associates (2), who proposed that primary osteoporosis represents two fundamentally different conditions: *type I osteoporosis,* a loss of trabecular bone after menopause, and *type II osteoporosis,* a loss of cortical and trabecular bone in men and women, related to long-term age-related bone loss. Whereas the type I disorder is considered to be directly related to lack of endogenous estrogen, type II osteoporosis would reflect long-term remodeling efficiency, adequacy of dietary calcium and vitamin D, intestinal mineral absorption, renal mineral handling, and parathyroid hormone (PTH) secretion.

Compelling proof that these two entities are truly distinct remains to be obtained, but separate consideration of osteoporosis due to estrogen deficiency allows a sensible and unified approach to understanding the pathophysiology of this condition. Consequently, several conditions legitimately considered to be secondary forms of osteoporosis are treated in this volume as categories of primary osteoporosis. These include the osteopenias re-

sulting from exercise-related amenorrhea and from prolactin-secreting tumors. In addition, the pathophysiology of several other secondary osteoporoses are sufficiently entwined with disorders of intestinal and renal function that they are also separately considered. Thus the specific clinical entities discussed in this chapter (Table 1) will not include all secondary forms of osteoporosis.

THE ROLE OF BONE REMODELING

To understand the mechanisms by which osteoporosis develops, it is essential to keep in mind the central importance of bone remodeling, a continuous process of destruction and renewal that takes place throughout life. The characteristics of the remodeling cycle and the dynamics of its two major phases, resorption and formation, are discussed in Chapter 15 and will not be reiterated here. However, a few general points should prove helpful.

First, like any biological process, remodeling appears to be intrinsically inefficient. That is, the amount of bone replaced by formation is not always equal to the amount previously removed. This imbalance is small for any normal bone remodeling event, and unless remodeling dynamics are perturbed, may be manifest only after many years. The best evidence for remodeling imbalance is the fact that the mean wall thickness of completed trabecular osteons decreases with age (3,4). It is not certain whether all remodeling events lead to loss of bone, or whether the inefficiency itself appears as an age-related phenomenon. Nonetheless, the implications of remodeling inefficiency are profound. Since bone remodels throughout life, age-related bone loss might properly be viewed as a normal, predictable phenomenon, beginning shortly after cessation of growth. Alterations in remodeling activity may be seen as the final common pathway through which diverse stimuli, such as dietary

R. Marcus: Stanford University School of Medicine, Stanford, California 94304; Aging Study Unit, Geriatrics Research Education, and Clinical Center, Veterans Administration Medical Center, Palo Alto, California 94304

TABLE 1. *Representative examples of secondary osteoporosis*

Cause	BRU birthrate[a]	Resorption	Formation[b]
Glucocorticoids	Probably increased	Normal to increased	Decreased
Hyperthyroidism	Increased	Increased	Increased[c]
Immobilization	Early increase	Increased then normal	Decreased
Heparin	Probably increased	Probably increased	Uncertain
Hypervitaminosis A	Probably increased	Increased	Uncertain
Anticonvulsants	Probably increased	Increased	Increased[c]

[a] Refers to activation, or birthrate, or bone remodeling units.
[b] Refers to total bone-forming activity.
[c] Despite an increase in overall formation, osteoblastic function for individual bone remodeling units may be impaired.

or hormonal deficiency, drugs, and disease states affect the rate of bone loss.

For many years, understanding of osteoporosis was predicated on two competing, and apparently irreconcilable models, one involving an increase in bone resorption, the other a decrease in formation. The naivete of this dichotomy is now evident. Total body remodeling balance encompasses the activation frequency, or birthrate, of new remodeling units, as well as the net activity of each of these units. The latter reflects the balance of individual resorption and formation phases. Thus an acceleration in total bone loss could result from several discrete perturbations of remodeling activity. These are shown schematically in Fig. 1.

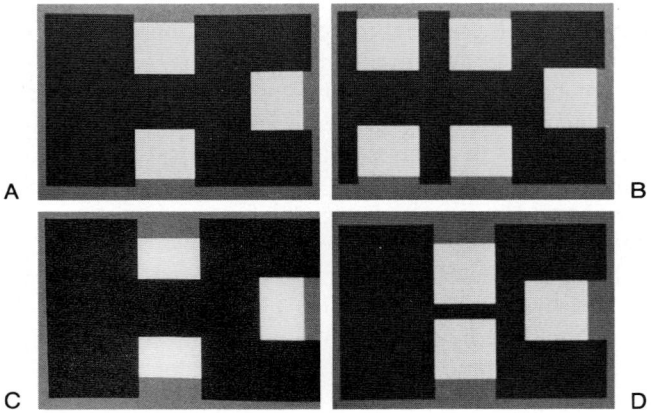

FIG. 1. Schematic model of perturbations in bone remodeling. **A:** Normal trabecular bone surface. Osteoclastic resorption has removed divots of bone from three sites; these have been replaced, but a small deficit persists at each site. **B:** An increased number of active remodeling units is shown. There will be an increase in the overall rate of bone loss, even though there has been no change in the depth to which osteoclasts resorb or in the efficiency of osteoblast response within any individual remodeling site. **C:** Effect of decreased osteoblast efficiency. Even if osteoclast function and the number of active remodeling units remain stable, bone loss increases. **D:** Effect of increased osteoclast resorption depth. If osteoblast response does not increase accordingly, accelerated bone loss occurs.

In this chapter we consider specific osteoporotic conditions and attempt to relate the clinical abnormalities within the context of remodeling dynamics wherever possible. Examples of increased birthrate of remodeling units (thyrotoxicosis) and decreased osteoblast efficiency (glucocorticoids and immobilization) can easily be found (Table 1). Estrogen-dependent bone loss characteristic of type I osteoporosis is typified by increased osteoclastic activity. In several cases, however, systematic analysis has not been possible, and the mechanisms of bone loss remain incompletely understood.

A final point on remodeling concerns the concept of *remodeling space.* This term was first applied by Jaworski (5) to bone that is temporarily missing because formation has not yet replaced that which was resorbed. This transient deficit includes the lacunar space and osteoid tissue awaiting mineralization and was calculated by Parfitt (6) to be about 7.5 g of calcium, or 12.5 cm^3 of bone when remodeling is normal. When bone turnover increases, commensurate expansion of the remodeling space achieves a new stable deficit. When turnover slows, remodeling space contracts. This principle must be remembered when considering the effects of disease on bone mass, since some measurable losses represent simple expansions of the remodeling space that predictably improve on successful treatment. Conversely, deficits arising from failure of osteoblasts to restore resorbed bone are likely to be permanent.

GLUCOCORTICOIDS

As early as 1932, Harvey Cushing described the occurrence of osteoporosis in patients with adrenal hyperfunction (7). Over succeeding decades, the devastating skeletal effects of excess glucocorticoids have been amply confirmed (8–12). Published experience with this condition reflects a bias toward patients with rheumatoid arthritis. Since local and generalized bone resorption are common manifestations of even untreated rheumatoid disease (13–15), it can sometimes be difficult to know whether bone loss is related to disease activity or to therapy. However, osteopenia is commonly observed in steroid-treated patients, even at low dose and regardless of the underlying disease, so the conclusion that it is a complication of chronic steroid therapy is beyond dispute. Indeed, glucocorticoid osteoporosis is probably the most common cause of "secondary" osteoporosis.

Bone loss due to glucocorticoid excess is diffuse, affecting both the cortical and axial skeleton, although it appears that axial loss is more substantial (16,17). Even within the appendicular skeleton, loss is greater in regions invested with higher amounts of trabecular bone, such as ribs and metaphyses, than in long-bone diaphyses. Mineral loss is highest during the first 3 months of treatment, despite maintenance of steroid dose level (18).

The histomorphometric features of glucocorticoid osteoporosis have been well characterized (19–24). Although an increased prevalence of resorption lacunae and osteoclasts is frequently observed (21,23), the most impressive findings point to a major impairment in bone formation. Static measures of bone-forming activity, such as osteoid surface prevalence and volume, are increased (21,23), indicating an overall increase in bone turnover. However, dynamic measures of bone formation, such as mineral apposition rate, are profoundly reduced (23), indicating that remodeling has been uncoupled. Dempster et al. (24) recently provided additional insight into the suppression of bone formation by demonstrating that the longevity (Sigma$_f$) of active osteoblasts and the mean wall thickness of completed trabecular osteons are decreased in steroid-treated patients. One may therefore consider steroid osteopenia to be the consequence of two discrete changes in bone remodeling: an increase in the birthrate of remodeling units and an exaggeration of remodeling imbalance.

In vitro activities of glucocorticoids are complex and vary among species. Glucocorticoid actions on bone cells have been reviewed by Feldman and Krishnan (25). The observation in several laboratories that corticosteroids do not directly stimulate bone resorption (26,27) has fostered the popular view that effects of glucocorticoids on bone resorption in vivo probably represent a response to increased circulating levels of PTH. By this formulation, glucocorticoids act initially to depress intestinal calcium absorption and increase urinary calcium excretion, leading to compensatory hypersecretion of PTH. PTH then increases bone turnover by activating the formation of new remodeling units. At the same time, the depressive effect of glucocorticoids on osteoblasts directly uncouples remodeling, so that bone loss accelerates (Fig. 2). This model is so well accepted and so often cited that it is reasonable to examine its elements in a critical fashion.

Clear and impressive support for the notion that glucocorticoids depress intestinal calcium absorption has been provided by several laboratories (21,28–31), al-

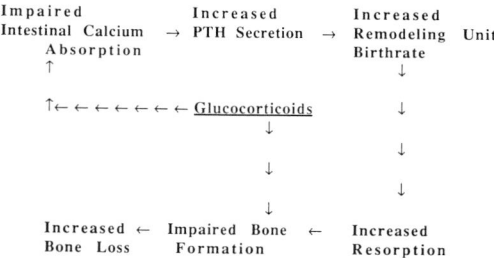

FIG. 2. Schematic representation of a PTH-based model for glucocorticoid osteoporosis.

though the mechanisms remain controversial. Considerable attention, with conflicting results, has been given to the suggestion (32) that steroids interfere with normal metabolism of vitamin D. Several groups have reported that steroid-treated patients show reduced serum levels of 25-hydroxyvitamin D [25(OH)D] (22,31,33), whereas normal values have been found by others (21,34–37). Similarly, glucocorticoids have been reported to enhance the peripheral metabolism and decrease the circulating level of 1,25-dihydroxyvitamin D [1,25(OH)$_2$D] (38,39). However, Seeman et al. (33) found normal 1,25(OH)$_2$D levels and no alterations in the production or clearance rates of this metabolite in patients with chronic glucocorticoid excess. In this careful study, 6 patients with endogenous Cushing's syndrome were studied before and several months following surgical cure, and 8 patients with exogenous glucocorticoid excess, average dose 50 mg of prednisone per day, were studied before and 1 month after institution of steroid therapy for rheumatic diseases. Although a slight reduction in 25(OH)D was found, average levels in the patients were still 23 ng/mL, a value that is unlikely to be of pathophysiological importance.

Animal studies do not support an important role for aberrant vitamin D metabolism in glucocorticoid action. Cortisone-treated rats exhibit normal conversion of radiolabeled vitamin D to 25(OH)D (29,39), and other evidence indicates that glucocorticoids directly inhibit intestinal calcium transport by mechanisms that are independent of the vitamin D system (29,30,39,40).

Less evidence is available concerning the effects of glucocorticoids on renal calcium handling. Laake (41) reported that renal tubular reabsorption of calcium is impaired in steroid-treated patients. More recently, Suzuki et al. (42) evaluated mineral metabolism in a group of 44 patients treated with steroids for periods ranging from 10 days to 4 years. Fasting calcium excretion was twice as high in the steroid group as in a simultaneous group of normal controls. This was accompanied by rises in serum immunoreactive PTH and in nephrogenous cyclicAMP (ncAMP) excretion, and there were significant positive correlations between ncAMP and steroid dose, and between ncAMP and calcium excretion. Patients showing obvious increases in urinary excretion parameters generally received more than 10 mg/day of prednisone equivalent for at least 2 months. The authors interpreted their data to indicate that glucocorticoid therapy decreased tubular calcium reabsorption despite the presence of increased levels of PTH, which should actually have led to increased mineral conservation. They also suggested that whereas enhanced urinary calcium and impaired intestinal absorption both contribute to negative calcium balance, changes in gut calcium absorption are not reliably seen at low doses of corticosteroid, so that at doses of prednisolone below 15 mg/day the renal effect may be of primary importance.

Central to the overall model is whether PTH secretion is increased in steroid-treated patients. Once again, the literature is mixed. Elevated immunoreactive PTH levels have been reported from several laboratories, in both humans (21,22,31,43,44) and animals (45). On the other hand, other investigators have reported normal values (31,33,37). Although differences in assay sensitivity, antiserum, and other technical factors could explain some of these discrepancies, it is not immediately clear that this is the case. In fact, Dykman et al. (46) described one series of steroid-treated patients in whom PTH levels were clearly normal, whereas the same laboratory had previously reported elevated values in a similar group of patients (21). Thus although a PTH-based model of steroid osteopenia is attractive, sufficient ambiguity remains that it would be premature to consider it validated at the present time. If these ambiguities are ever to be clarified, it will be important for future studies to deal effectively with such issues as steroid dose and treatment duration that confound interpretation of current literature.

It may prove useful to consider some alternative models. It is possible that glucocorticoids do not lead to PTH hypersecretion, but amplify the responsiveness of bone cells to normal levels of PTH. PTH-dependent cAMP formation in bone cells is enhanced by glucocorticoids (47–49) through a direct action on coupling of the guanyl nucleotide-regulatory protein to adenylate cyclase (49), and Yamamoto et al. (50) showed recently that glucocorticoids also increased the availability of PTH receptors in rat osteosarcoma cells. Although glucocorticoids appear not to stimulate bone resorption directly in certain cultured rodent models, direct action in humans and primates has not been excluded. Deficiency of other steroid hormones might also be involved in bone loss. For example, circulating estrogens and androgens may be decreased in patients with endogenous Cushing's syndrome, and Crilly et al. (51) found that fasting plasma estrone, estradiol, androstenedione, and testosterone were below normal postmenopausal levels in a group of steroid-treated elderly women. In addition, Smals et al. (52) and MacAdams et al. (53) showed that men with endogenous Cushing's disease and men taking chronic glucocorticoids show depressed circulating testosterone levels.

Treatment

Therapy of established steroid osteoporosis remains a frustrating and generally unrewarding experience. Attempts can be made to reduce the overall level of bone remodeling activity by increasing dietary calcium and providing supplemental vitamin D in hopes of suppressing parathyroid function. However, as long as glucocorticoids continue to be taken, it remains a formidable challenge to overcome the suppressive effects on osteoblast function. The cardinal principle, therefore, must be to reduce steroids to a minimum. Reid et al. (54) suggested that dose was the major determinant of bone loss. This is particularly true early in therapy, when mineral loss is highest. Some evidence suggests that the effects of glucocorticoids are most reversible in children (55), but Bressot et al. (22) clearly showed the capacity of adults with Cushing's syndrome to improve following surgical cure.

Attempts have been made to develop glucocorticoids that are less toxic to bone. Deflazacort, a derivative of prednisolone, has been reported to be less potent than prednisone in altering calcium metabolism (56,57). Whether doses of this agent that are reasonable from the perspective of mineral metabolism will provide adequate therapeutic anti-inflammatory or immunosuppressive action, however, remains to be settled. Deflazacort is not currently available for general use in the United States.

Hahn et al. (21) reported that treatment with 25(OH)D at an average daily dose of 40 µg and calcium, 500 mg/day, increased intestinal calcium absorption and decreased PTH levels after 6 months. In addition, after 1 year of therapy a 13% increase in metaphyseal forearm bone mass was achieved. No such changes occurred in a simultaneous control group.

In a double-blinded randomized clinical trial this same group (46) found that $1,25(OH)_2D$, 0.4 µg/day, also increased calcium absorption and decreased serum PTH levels. However, as opposed to their previous experience with 25(OH)D, no gain in forearm mineral was observed. The authors concluded that $1,25(OH)_2D$ should not be used for treatment of glucocorticoid osteopenia.

Braun et al. (37) evaluated 1α-hydroxyvitamin D_3, 2 µg/day, in a 6-month trial. Treatment with this agent increased intestinal calcium absorption and urinary calcium excretion, and suppressed immunoreactive PTH (iPTH) and urinary hydroxyproline excretion. Treatment was also associated with a decrease in resorption activity on biopsy.

Another pharmacological approach to steroid osteoporosis is the use of bisphosphonates. Although Jee et al.

(58) had demonstrated the ability of dichloromethane diphosphonate to give protection against glucocorticoid bone loss in rabbits, few human data have been available until recently. Reid et al. (59) have now reported a prospective randomized trial of a new bisphosphonate (3-amino-1-hydroxypropylidene)-1, 1-bisphosphonate (APD), 150 mg/day plus calcium, 1 g/day, versus calcium alone, in a group of 40 adults receiving glucocorticoids for a variety of conditions over a 5- to 6-year period. Vertebral trabecular mineral, determined by computed tomography, showed a 20% increase over a year's time in the APD group, but showed no significant change in the controls. Similarly, the mean radiographic metacarpal area increased by 1.2% in the treated group, compared to a progressive decrease in the controls. The APD subjects also showed a significant reduction in resorption surfaces and osteoclast numbers on iliac crest biopsy, and these changes were accompanied by reductions in fasting urine hydroxyproline, serum alkaline phosphatase activity, and serum osteocalcin levels. Of particular interest was the finding of no significant side effects of the medication, including no evidence for the osteomalacia that may confound treatment with other bisphosphonates.

Other pharmacologic approaches have been suggested, but sufficient data are not yet available to consider them established. Baylink (60) outlined a rational basis for counteracting the effects of steroids that involved administration of thiazide diuretics to reverse the increase in urinary calcium, and sodium fluoride to promote osteoblast activity. The presence of hypogonadism should also be kept in mind. Given the evidence cited above that steroid therapy may reduce endogenous reproductive steroids, and given the known influence of the latter on skeletal maintenance, it would appear to be appropriate to replace androgen or estrogen when deficiency is demonstrated.

Finally, resistance exercise can attenuate or prevent steroid-dependent muscle loss in animals and humans (61). One might also predict that an exercise program would provide skeletal benefits to patients. The difficulty with applying this information to humans, however, is that the types of exercise regimens necessary to attenuate bone loss are unlikely to be tolerated by chronically ill patients, particularly those with rheumatoid arthritis or obstructive airway disease.

HYPERTHYROIDISM

The skeletal consequences of thyrotoxicosis were first noted in 1891 by von Recklinghausen (62), who described a young woman with sustained hyperthyroidism and bone pain in whom postmortem examination revealed widespread skeletal softening and deformity. Subsequently, there has emerged a substantial literature that clearly documents an important role for thyroid hor-

mone in the regulation of skeletal turnover. Consequently, both thyroid insufficiency and excess lead to predictable changes in bone mass.

The mechanisms by which thyroid hormone alters bone turnover have received considerable attention. Early proposals included primary actions on renal calcium handling and modulation of bone cell responsiveness to PTH. However, the most parsimonious explanation for the observed changes in mineral metabolism in states of altered thyroid function is that thyroid hormone directly influences bone (63). From an extensive histomorphometry literature, it is possible to conclude that the primary effect of thyroid hormone is to increase the birthrate of new bone remodeling units, leading to an overall increase in remodeling activity, and therefore, to an increase in remodeling space (23,64,65). One can predict that any intervention that increases or decreases thyroid status will be accompanied by appropriate changes in remodeling space and measurable changes in bone mineral content.

Extensive clinical data confirm that patients with thyrotoxicosis have a decrease in bone mineral density. Although most reports have concentrated on the appendicular, cortical skeleton, hyperthyroidism is a recognized cause of vertebral compression fractures (66,67) and has been associated with a decrease in lumbar spine mineral density as well (16,68). Previous suggestions that hyperthyroid bone is uniquely sensitive to the effects of PTH are probably explained by suppression of PTH secretion by increased plasma-ionized calcium activity, with secondary up-regulation of PTH target tissue responsiveness. Increased bone resorption is accompanied by biochemical evidence for accelerated bone turnover, such as increased urinary excretion of calcium and hydroxyproline, and increased serum levels of alkaline phosphatase activity and osteocalcin (69–72). Modest hypercalcemia may occur, but parathyroid hormone secretion is suppressed (69,70), resulting in low serum levels of 1,25(OH)$_2$D (71).

Consensus has not been reached on the prevalence of low bone mass in hyperthyroidism. Smith et al. (74) and Ikkos et al. (75) both reported that bone mineral content was significantly reduced in groups of hyperthyroid patients older than 50 years. In a relatively small series, Linde and Friss (76) reported a significant decrease in bone mass in thyrotoxic women, but not in men, compared to a control group. Seeman et al. (16) found that the mineral densities of the lumbar spine and mid- and distal radius were below age-predicted values by −0.82, −0.70, and −0.67 standard deviation, respectively. Krølner et al. (68) reported median values for lumbar spine mineral in a group of 25 thyrotoxic adults that were 12.6% lower than those of a control group. However, only one patient had a lumbar mineral content that was lower than 2 standard deviations below the mean for age and sex.

On biopsy, trabecular bone volume may be low, but is often normal. Prevalence of resorption and osteoid surfaces is increased. However, an increase in the mineral apposition rate and in the fraction of surfaces taking up tetracycline excludes osteomalacia (23,64,71,73). Eriksen et al. (65) conducted a detailed analysis of resorption and formation rates in hyperthyroidism. Bone resorption was much faster than normal, 3.8 versus 1.1 mm/day. Initial formation rates were also rapid, but the total formation period, designated Sigma$_f$, 109 days, was significantly shortened from the control value of 151 days. Direct measurements of mean wall thickness were normal. However, this may have been confounded by a relatively short period between onset of symptoms and biopsy. Further analysis indicated that completed mean wall thickness of actively remodeling osteons was reduced, suggesting that part of the mineral deficit in hyperthyroidism is irreversible and not simply an expansion of the remodeling space.

The reversibility of the bone mass deficit remains uncertain. There have been some reports of increased bone density after correction of hyperthyroidism. Ikkos et al. (75) found that all treated patients had normal bone mass, and Linde and Friss (76) reported similar findings for women. Fraser et al. (67) observed a return of BMC (bone mineral content) to normal values following treatment, particularly in young patients. Conversely, Montz et al. (77) found no recovery of mineral deficit in their patients when studied as long as 9 years after treatment. Using neutron activation analysis to measure body calcium, Harrison and McNeill (78) reported no improvement in the calcium deficit after treatment. However, this same group (79) did subsequently show an increase in bone mass after restoration of the euthyroid state.

Toh and associates (80) conducted a longitudinal study of 23 men with Graves's disease. Bone mineral content of the mid-radius was measured each year following successful treatment of the thyrotoxicosis. Prior to treatment a 17% reduction of bone mineral content was observed compared to a group of normal controls matched for age and weight. One year later, an additional decrease in BMC from entry values was observed. By 2 years, however, BMC had increased to levels that did not differ significantly from baseline, but were still 17% less than control values. This trajectory did not differ in subjects below age 55 years, nor was it influenced by mode of treatment for the Graves's disease.

Recently, concern has been raised that chronic use of even mildly excessive doses of thyroid hormone also promotes bone loss. For example, Ettinger and Wingerd (81) showed a decrease in metacarpal cortical thickness in women taking 3 or more grains equivalent of thyroid hormone replacement per day. Fallon et al. (82) reported the occurrence of fractures in a small number of hypothyroid adults who had been treated with excess thyroid hormone. Ross et al. (83) demonstrated a decrease in cortical bone mineral density in a group of patients who were receiving suppressive doses of thyroxine.

Coindre et al. (84) conducted a cross-sectional analysis of iliac crest biopsies from hypothyroid adults stratified according to duration of therapy. Prior to treatment, trabecular bone volume did not differ from age-predicted norms. Resorption surfaces were significantly decreased, but osteoid surfaces were normal. The cortical elements of the specimen showed increased thickness but a normal degree of porosity. During the first month of therapy the prevalence of resorbing surfaces increased, in many cases to an abnormal extent. This was observed as early as 7 days after initiation of thyroid hormone and was accompanied by an increase in cortical porosity. After 6 months of treatment, trabecular bone volume (TBV) was significantly lower than predicted norms, with 6 of 14 patients showing values (<14%) that are associated with increased fracture risk. Five subjects were studied longitudinally with two biopsies. In these subjects, TBV decreased from 21% to 13.5%, a loss of one-third of their initial trabecular bone. It is important to note that uniform treatment was prescribed to all cases, a combination of 100 μg of 1-thyroxine and 20 μg of triiodothyronine daily. Serum thyroxine and triiodothyronine levels were within the normal range in all cases. Thus, startling changes in bone histomorphometry were produced in the absence of clinical or biochemical signs of hyperthyroidism. The authors propose three explanations for their results. First, they suggest that hypothyroid bone may be hyperresponsive to thyroid hormone. Second, the triiodothyronine component of the replacement regimen may have been excessive. Finally, a transient relative excess of thyroid hormone early in treatment may have initiated a burst of remodeling activity whose residual effects would persist for several months, even after termination of the temporary hyperthyroid state.

Paul et al. (85) compared the mineral density of the lumbar spine and proximal femur (dual photon absorptiometry) in 31 clinically euthyroid women who had received thyroxine therapy for more than 5 years to that of a group of control subjects matched for age, weight, and height. The thyroxine-treated women had received thyroid replacement therapy for 5 to 23 years, at doses of 0.1 to 0.3 mg/day (average dose = 0.175 mg/day). Serum thyroxine levels in the treated group were significantly higher than those of the controls, with frequent values above the normal range, and were associated with significant reductions in serum TSH (thyroid-stimulating hormone) concentrations. Lumbar spine densities were similar in thyroxine-treated and control women. However, mineral density at the proximal femur was significantly decreased. At the femoral neck, bone density was 12.8% lower in the treated group, and a 10% mineral deficit was observed at the trochanter. Women showing suppressed serum TSH levels had a trend toward lower femur mineral content. No relationship was observed between duration of therapy and bone density. It should be pointed out that 12 of the 31 women treated had been hypothyroid after treatment for Graves's disease or Hashimoto's thyroiditis. It is possible, therefore, that some of the observed bone mineral deficit could have occurred as a result of a previous hyperthyroid state rather than being necessarily a consequence of replacement therapy.

In summary, the published evidence indicates that even minimally excessive thyroid hormone replacement on a chronic basis can decrease cortical bone mass, thus raising important questions about appropriate lifelong replacement doses, particularly for young patients. These data should provoke caution in the use of traditional modes of suppressive therapy for thyroid nodules. Proper interpretation of studies such as these requires keeping in mind the concept of remodeling space. Predictable changes in bone density will be observed simply by increasing or restricting the remodeling space. However, after some months, a new equilibrium will be achieved. To know the clinical impact of such changes, it will be necessary to carry out studies over longer periods than have heretofore been reported, but for the present, the lowest possible dose of thyroid hormones to achieve a euthyroid state or to suppress thyroid gland activity is advisable.

IMMOBILIZATION

More than 100 years ago the German scientist Julius Wolff described the capacity of bone mass to change in amount and distribution to accommodate the mechanical stresses imposed on it. The nature and mechanisms of these adjustments have been a matter of intense study and have been distilled recently into general hypotheses of bone mass regulation by Frost (86) and by Carter (87). According to these models, mechanical loading is the primary regulator of bone mass, diet, and hormonal milieu providing modulating influences. Consequently, the loss of bone during periods of decreased mechanical loading, such as immobilization or weightlessness, is predictable, and were it not for such complications as kidney stones, hypercalcemia, and fracture, would be appropriate.

Rapid and diffuse bone loss is a well-known consequence of immobilization. Recognition of this phenomenon is traditionally credited to Fuller Albright et al. (88), who reported a young boy who developed hypercalcemia after immobilization for fracture, and who underwent two unsuccessful parathyroid explorations before resumption of weight-bearing activity resolved the hypercalcemia. Subsequent observations of children and adults paralyzed by poliomyelitis confirmed that bone loss from immobilization is rapid and substantial (89). Experimental studies in immobilized humans were undertaken during the 1940s, when Dietrick, Whedon, and

colleagues (90) imposed an immobilization protocol on volunteers and reported a prompt and sustained increase in urinary calcium excretion and a deterioration in calcium balance. These findings have been replicated in many studies of immobilized patients, volunteers, and experimental animals.

When healthy adults are placed at bed rest, hypercalciuria develops early and persists for months (91,92). Peak calcium excretion is achieved by 6–7 weeks, and begins thereafter to subside. Increased fecal calcium has also been observed, and calcium balance approximates −200 mg/day, representing a loss of whole body mineral of about 0.5% each month. Early studies showed maintenance of forearm mineral density but a 25–40% depletion of calcaneal mineral during bed rest (91,92). Radiokinetic studies demonstrated an increase in bone turnover rate, with a greater increase in resorption than in mineral accretion (93). Remineralization of the calcaneus began as soon as ambulation resumed.

The critical importance of gravitational stress to the maintenance of bone mass can be seen in data from the *Gemini* and *Skylab* space flights (94). Even though the astronauts engaged in frequent strenuous exercise during these missions, weightless orbit led to impressive hypercalciuria and negative calcium balance. Bone mineral density of the calcaneus showed losses as high as 7.9%, with the greatest change occurring in the crew members showing the greatest increase in urinary calcium. Losses of 5–8% were also reported following the 175-day Salut-6-Soyuz flight. In the American experience, duration of space flight has been relatively brief, and the astronauts recovered bone mass after resumption of their usual high levels of physical activity. There is concern, however, that more prolonged missions would lead to more severe and irreversible bone loss. For a review of the skeletal consequences of space flight, see Anderson and Cohn (94).

Although the effects of weightlessness represent a formidable challenge for the development of space flight strategy, the complications of bed rest and immobilization are of more immediate concern to physicians. Indeed, Krølner and Toft (95) reported that just a few weeks of simple "therapeutic" bed rest was sufficient to permit significant loss of axial bone mineral. Thirty-four patients hospitalized with back pain due to intervertebral disc disease were evaluated by dual-photon absorptiometry on admission to hospital, at the end of the bed-rest period (11–61 days), and several months after re-ambulation. During recumbency, lumbar spine mineral decreased by 0.9% per week, that is, 45% per year! Re-ambulation completely restored axial mineral content by 4 months. It should be noted that this particular group consisted of reasonably healthy patients, with no underlying restriction to mobility. Such optimistic results would probably not obtain in the setting of chronic disability. For example, a woman afflicted with severe rheumatoid arthritis would return, at best, to limited assisted ambulation, and would have a high probability of spending additional periods of time at bed rest over a span of years. It is likely that her bone density would follow a downward course punctuated by discrete episodes of immobilization-related accelerated loss.

The hormonal and metabolic consequences of immobilization have recently been characterized. Stewart et al. (96) evaluated a group of spinal cord trauma patients during the initial weeks after admission to a rehabilitation hospital, approximately 1 month after the initial traumatic event. Although mean serum calcium levels were normal, fasting and 24-h urinary calcium excretion were grossly elevated. Serum inorganic phosphorus levels were elevated, as was the renal phosphorus threshold (TmP/GFR). Plasma levels of immunoreactive parathyroid hormone and $1,25(OH)_2D$ and urinary nephrogenous cAMP excretion were suppressed. The authors reasonably concluded that a primary loss of mineral from bone had suppressed the parathyroid–vitamin D axis. Most of these patients remained normocalcemic during the period of study, but some patients, usually children and adults under 25 years, develop hypercalcemia, even to lethal degrees. The restriction of hypercalcemia to younger patients undoubtedly reflects the lower intrinsic level of bone turnover in adults. In fact, when older individuals with increased bone turnover are immobilized, such as patients with multiple myeloma or Paget's disease following a fracture, hypercalcemia commonly develops.

The fundamental alterations in remodeling dynamics that underlie immobilization osteopenia are not well defined. Histomorphometric data from immobilized subjects are sparse and restricted largely to patients with spinal cord trauma (97). Trabecular bone loss is at first extremely rapid, resulting in a substantial deficit by 6 months that subsequently stabilizes. Resorption activity appears to be increased during the initial few months, but later normalizes. Bone-forming activity is profoundly reduced, both with respect to static parameters and in tetracycline-related dynamic measurements.

A possible relationship of these changes to an increase in endogenous cortisol secretion deserves consideration, in view of the similarity of the histologic findings to those of glucocorticoid osteoporosis. Indeed, elevated urinary and plasma cortisol levels have been observed with space flight and would be anticipated in patients with spinal trauma. However, cortisol excess is not observed during experimental bed rest and therefore cannot entirely account for mineral loss.

Prevention and treatment of immobilization osteopenia remains an enormous challenge. In healthy subjects at bed rest, 4 h of daily ambulation corrected negative calcium balance (94). A variety of exercise regimens have been incorporated into space flight routines, including rowing, bungee cord exercises, bicycle ergom-

etry, and treadmill running, with marginal success. Experience shows that it is difficult and awkward to achieve the magnitude of skeletal loading that is produced so easily when gravity is present. For example, Issekutz et al. (98) tested the effects of bicycle ergometers and compression harnesses on bed-rested men. Ergometer exercise had no effect on mineral loss, and the results of compression for up to 21 days were inconclusive. Thus it appears that static compression will not inhibit bone loss. Donaldson et al. (91) used a harness system to generate cyclic compression equivalent to walking on subjects who remained at bed rest. Intermittent longitudinal compression by this device did not significantly reduce mineral loss, and it is likely that major portions of the load were reduced by friction between the body and bed and were not transmitted to the skeleton (R. Whalen, personal communication). On the other hand, standing, with simple periodic shifts in position, appears to limit mineral depletion. Issekutz et al. (98) permitted bed-rest volunteers to stand "passively" for up to 3 h each day in 30-min intervals, and urinary calcium decreased in most subjects.

Pharmacological approaches to preventing and treating bone loss in immobilized patients have been very discouraging. Hulley et al. (92) treated immobilized volunteers with supplemental phosphorus. Although reductions in urinary calcium were observed, increased fecal losses led to no change in balance, and loss of calcaneal mineral was not reduced. Anti-resorptive drugs, such as calcitonin and bisphosphonates, have also proved disappointing, and little attention has been given to agents, such as fluoride, that might promote osteoblast function. Immobilized patients are occasionally placed on thiazide diuretics to reduce hypercalciuria and the risk of renal stone. Particularly during the early period of increased bone resorption, this may lead to hypercalcemia and must therefore be done only with great caution.

HEPARIN

Long-term administration of subcutaneous heparin enjoyed a brief vogue more than 20 years ago as a treatment strategy for patients with ischemic heart disease. Although cardiac ischemia is not currently viewed as an indication for heparin therapy, occasional patients needing sustained anticoagulation cannot be managed with oral anticoagulants and receive chronic heparin. The majority of these are pregnant women with recurrent thromboembolism or cardiac prostheses, for whom concern over the rare fetal warfarin syndrome requires that heparin be used during the first trimester and after week 36.

A connection between heparin therapy and osteoporosis was first suggested by an anonymous physician speaking from the audience during a heparin symposium in

1963 (99). Griffith and Silverglade (99) reported the first series of patients documenting such a relationship, and concluded that dose was more important to the development of osteoporosis than treatment duration. Of 117 patients, osteoporosis was observed in 60% of those receiving greater than 15,000 units/day, whereas no cases occurred in individuals who received less than 10,000 units/day. Subsequent literature on this subject has been restricted largely to individual case reports, although a few small series have been reported. Rupp et al. (100) followed 25 patients with recurrent thromboembolic disease who were administered heparin by continuous infusion through an implantable pump. Doses were adjusted to reach plasma concentrations of about 0.2 units/mL. Over the duration of 105 weeks of treatment 6 patients developed demineralization and compression fractures of the spine. Over this same period, single-photon absorptiometry showed no reduction in forearm bone mineral.

In contrast, DeSwiet and colleagues (101) followed metacarpal and phalangeal cortical areas in 20 women taking heparin for 6 weeks prior to delivery, or from weeks 4–26 prior to delivery until 6 weeks postpartum. Women had therefore received a total of 6–32 weeks of treatment at 10,000 units twice daily by subcutaneous injection, followed by 8000 units twice daily after delivery. The authors found a clear decrease in cortical bone areas with prolonged therapy and concluded that 20 weeks of heparin therapy at doses greater than 20,000 units/day lead frequently to bone demineralization. Moreover, the authors found persistent cortical bone deficits 24 weeks after stopping the drug. It is not immediately clear why the patients of Rupp et al. showed effects only on the vertebral skeleton, whereas those of DeSwiet and colleagues experienced decreases in appendicular bone. It is possible that pregnancy-dependent adjustments in mineral metabolism placed the women in the latter study at greater risk for deleterious effects of heparin.

Little information is available concerning the effect of heparin on bone remodeling in humans. Zimran et al. (102) reported the histomorphometric findings of a single patient thought to have heparin-induced osteoporosis. This young pregnant woman received treatment for 7 months at a daily dose of 15,000 units, and iliac crest biopsy was taken 6 weeks postpartum. Although the patient had experienced two compression fractures, her trabecular bone volume, 18%, was fairly normal. The most striking abnormalities were an elevation in the prevalence of osteoid surfaces (42%) and a reduction in active resorption surfaces and osteoclast numbers. The authors interpreted this biopsy to show increased bone formation and decreased bone resorption, indicative of recovery from her osteoporotic state.

Unfortunately, several issues limit the interpretation of these data. First, the biopsy values were compared to normative data from another laboratory and may therefore be affected by a systematic reader bias. This is particularly likely to confound the assessment of resorption surfaces, which were said to be one of the major abnormalities in this case. Second, by comparing the patient to a normal control population, it is impossible to distinguish effects of heparin from those of pregnancy. Third, although the inference was drawn that hyperosteoidosis represented an increase in bone formation, one cannot reach conclusions about rates from static surface markers. In fact, dynamic measurements derived from tetracycline labeling were not increased in this case.

Several lines of experimental evidence support the conclusion that the skeletal effects of heparin are multiple and involve both an enhancement of resorption and a depression of formation.

Resorptive Effects

Goldhaber (103) was the first to demonstrate that heparin could enhance the PTH-dependent resorption. The suggestion that heparin directly stimulates bone resorption was first put forth by Asher and Nichols (104), who proposed that this effect was due to activation of bone collagenase activity. Although subsequent experience with bone collagenase suggested that this activity might be nothing more than an artifact of bacterial contamination (105), recent immunohistochemical evidence (106) confirms the presence of collagenase in osteoblasts and shows that this activity is stimulated by adding heparin to the culture medium.

On the basis of these experiments as well as data from other laboratories, it is possible to conclude that collagenase is present in osteoblasts and that its production and secretion are promoted by heparin. Stimulation of collagenase synthesis by heparin appears to be specific for bone cells and has not been found to occur in fibroblasts or other cell types (106). However, heparin does bind to and enhance the activity of several collagenases. Indeed, heparin binding is a distinctive property that underlies the use of heparin–Sepharose affinity chromatography in collagenase purification.

The possible links between collagenase production and bone resorption have been a matter of controversy and remain to be clarified. Shen et al. (107) have recently demonstrated that many bone resorbing factors stimulate bone cell collagenase production in vitro, whereas interferon-γ, a known inhibitor of resorption, inhibits this effect. Moreover, stimulation of collagenase production correlated well with known resorptive potency, indicating a close link between collagenase production and stimulation of resorption.

Sakamoto and Sakamoto (106) have advanced a comprehensive hypothesis that encompasses major recent advances in our knowledge of bone resorption, and, in particular, is consistent with compelling evidence that bone resorption in response to PTH and other bone-resorbing agents does not reflect primary actions on osteoclasts, but requires an initial interaction with osteoblasts. By this formulation, the earliest events in bone resorption include a morphologic change in osteoblasts that exposes a greater surface area for resorbing activity to take place, and, simultaneously, osteoblastic synthesis and secretion of collagenase, prostaglandins, and other agents that either contribute directly to resorption or assist in the recruitment of osteoclasts to the resorbing surface. The next event is digestion of matrix collagen by the secreted collagenase, followed by osteoclast accumulation and resorption of mineral and other matrix components. If validated, this model would provide a relatively straightforward explanation for the effects of heparin on bone. However, at the present time additional substantiation is required before it can be embraced. For comprehensive treatment of this hypothesis, the reader is referred to Sakamoto and Sakamoto (106).

Effects on Bone Formation

Thompson (108) studied the effects of heparin on rat bone in vivo. The animals were treated with vehicle or heparin, 400 units/day by subcutaneous injection. At the end of 8 weeks, conversion of [^{3}H]proline to hydroxyproline, an index of collagen formation, was decreased by 20% in the heparin-treated rats. This was associated with a decrease in cross-sectional bone area of 12.5% and in an 8% reduction in breaking strength.

Effects on Other Systems

Recent evidence also suggests that extraskeletal actions of heparin might be involved in heparin osteoporosis. The possibility of interference with the parathyroid–vitamin D axis was suggested by van der Vijgh et al. (109), who showed that heparin inhibits 25(OH)D 1α-hydroxylase activity in renal homogenates from Japanese quail. In this regard, Aarskog and colleagues (110) reported a single case of severe vertebral osteoporosis in a pregnant woman who had received high doses of heparin during her last trimester. Although serum levels of 25(OH)D were normal, she had an unexpectedly low level of circulating 1,25(OH)$_2$D. In a follow-up study, this group (111) evaluated 1,25(OH)$_2$D levels in 10 women treated with 5000 units of heparin three times daily between weeks 8 and 33 of gestation. Third-trimester blood samples were compared to those of a group of 22 healthy pregnant controls. All subjects received supplemental vitamin D at 400 IU/day. Control values of 1,25(OH)$_2$D were 92.8 ± 14 pg/mL, whereas values in the heparin-treated women were significantly reduced at 68 ± 9 pg/mL.

Natural heparin, a product of mast cells, is a heterogeneous collection of glycosaminoglycans that vary widely in molecular size (112). It contains alternating chains of hexuronic acid and hexosamine units. The latter vary greatly, some being N-sulfated and others N-acetylated, with some chains escaping sulfation entirely or in part. The biological activity of heparin as an anticoagulant depends on its interaction with antithrombin III, and there is great diversity in the capacity of different natural heparin fragments to carry out this activity. Only about one-third of the heparins in a commercial preparation accounts for most of the anticoagulant activity. Various semisynthetic and synthetic heparin analogs and sulfated polysaccharides have been manufactured, and these possess considerable diversity in anticoagulant activity. The relationship of heparin fragments and analogs to bone metabolism is not known.

In contemporary therapeutics, heparin is commonly prescribed for only a few days, prior to sustained oral warfarin therapy. Since production of the γ-carboxyglutamic acid-enriched osteoblast peptide, osteocalcin, is exquisitely sensitive to warfarin inhibition, it is relevant to consider whether a patient whose remodeling activity is stimulated first by heparin may later be subject to impaired bone formation while taking warfarin. There is currently no published evidence regarding this hypothetical interaction.

In 1968, Frame and Nixon (113) put forth the interesting observation that mast cell prevalence was higher in the bone marrow of osteoporotic patients than in control specimens. They speculated that heparin, a major secretory product of mast cells, may play a role in the pathogenesis of primary osteoporosis. In fact, mast cell accumulation can be observed following the application of several agents known to stimulate bone resorption, such as PTH and fracture (114). Although these data are provocative, several important factors confound their interpretation. First, other biologically active agents, such as histamine, are also secreted by mast cells, so mediator specificity would need to be established. Second, it is not clear whether mast cell accumulation in osteoporosis should be considered a primary abnormality, or whether it represents a response to injury, such as microfracture or inflammation. However, the fact that patients with systemic mastocytosis develop osteoporosis (115) does support the Frame and Nixon hypothesis and should foster additional work in this area.

VITAMIN A

Clinical vitamin A intoxication has been of interest to the medical community since it was first reported to follow the ingestion of polar bear liver in 1857 (116). Clinical features of hypervitaminosis A include weakness, fatigue, emotional lability, musculoskeletal aching, headache, and pseudotumor cerebri. Skeletal aspects of this syndrome were first enumerated by Josephs (117), and include osteopenia, epiphyseal mottling, accelerated skeletal maturation, and hypercalcemia. Toomey and Morissette (118) later described a characteristic feature of this syndrome, periosteal new bone formation, which, in close apposition to the cortex gives an appearance of hyperostosis. This finding is most commonly observed in the ulna, metacarpals and metatarsals, and skull.

Biochemical findings of hypervitaminosis A include elevated levels of serum alkaline phosphatase activity, representing a combination of hepatic and bone enzyme, and hypercalcemia, particularly in children. The reason for this age predilection must be related in part to the rapid growth of the young skeleton, where normal mineral deposition may be as much as several hundred milligrams of calcium each day. Interruption of such rapid deposition is more likely to overwhelm renal excretory capacity and result in hypercalcemia. On the other hand, adults are certainly not immune from hypercalcemia. Frame and associates (119) reported three cases of hypercalcemic hypervitaminosis A in males aged 7, 16, and 46 years. In each case, serum vitamin A levels exceeded 400 IU/dL (normal < 300 IU/dL). Two diagnostic points are raised by this study. Although vitamin A intoxication can be the sole etiologic factor, in some instances excessive consumption of vitamin D may be an additional basis for hypercalcemia. Further, although periosteal calcification is an uncommon finding in most types of hypercalcemia, it is frequently observed in hypervitaminosis A.

Few humans with hypervitaminosis A have been studied with contemporary methods, so specific information concerning remodeling dynamics remains incomplete. Jowsey and Riggs (120) reported a single patient from whom rib biopsies were taken before and months after discontinuing massive ingestion of vitamin A. On the initial biopsy, a severalfold increase in resorption area was observed, and this resolved on the follow-up specimen. Bone formation surfaces were normal while the patient took vitamin A and increased sevenfold on recovery. The authors concluded that the primary effect of vitamin A is to stimulate bone resorption. Although speculative, the possibility that vitamin A initiates an increase in birthrate of remodeling units appears to be highly likely.

Whereas vitamin A is critical for normal skeletal growth and differentiation, excessive quantities of either retinol or retinoic acid profoundly alter bone metabolism and morphology. Vitamin A directly resorbs bone in vitro, an effect that is additive to that of PTH, and is inhibited by hydrocortisone (121). In addition, several inhibitory activities of vitamin A on bone have been described. Pennypacker et al. (122) observed that vitamin A prevents accumulation of cartilage-specific proteoglycans in murine limb bud cultures. DeSimone and Reddi (123) used a demineralized matrix-implantation model of bone formation to examine the effects of exogenous retinoic acid during critical stages of endochondral bone differentiation in vivo. The temporal sequence of cellular events in bone growth is well characterized in this model, comprising four specific phases of differentiation: cell proliferation, chondrogenesis, bone formation, and mineralization. Animals received retinoic acid treatment (80 mg/kg body weight) 3 days after matrix implantation. No changes in body weight or serum calcium were observed, but vitamin A reduced mesenchymal cell proliferation by 50%. On day 7 sulfate incorporation into proteoglycans (a marker of chondrogenesis) was only 27% of control activity. On day 11 alkaline phosphatase activity was 60% of control, and incorporation of ^{45}Ca was 50% reduced. Thus retinoic acid inhibited bone differentiation at multiple sites.

Multiple skeletal lesions can be found in animals intoxicated with vitamin A. In young turkeys a lesion resembling rickets has been reported (124), although most other species show osteoporosis. Hough et al. (125) reported a careful study of experimental hypervitaminosis A. Young rats given 10,000 IU/day retinyl palmitate grew normally but developed impressive skeletal abnormalities, including osteoporosis, increased bone resorption, increased prevalence and size of osteoclasts, cartilage degeneration, and increased vascular penetration of the bony metaphyses. In addition, a previously undescribed lesion was reported: On low power, trabecular bone appeared to show widespread osteocytic osteolysis, but on closer examination, the lesions were actually composed of highly vascularized lacunae. The rats in this study did not become hypercalcemic, but dose-related increases in hydroxyproline excretion were observed. Total serum alkaline phosphatase activity was elevated, although no determinations of the bone isoenzyme were reported. Finally, circulating levels of immunoreactive PTH and vitamin D metabolites were indistinguishable from control values.

The cellular basis for vitamin A actions on the skeleton is unclear. In vitro, retinol, retinoic acid, and other retinoids can directly resorb bone at concentrations that are easily achieved by clinical dosage. Although specific high-affinity intracellular binding proteins for retinol (CRBP) and retinoic acid (CRABP) are thought likely to mediate the actions of these vitamers in a wide variety of tissues (126), such binding proteins have not yet been described for bone cells. A number of remarkable interactions between vitamin A and other bone-regulating agents has been described. For example, since retinol and calcitriol each stimulate bone resorption and inhibit bone collagen synthesis, it is of interest that both agents increase the production of IL-1, a potent bone resorber, by murine macrophages and human circulating monocytes (127). It has also been shown that retinol regulates the cell content of calcitriol receptors (128), although the direction in which regulation occurs is highly dependent on species (129).

Uncontrolled use of large doses of vitamin A is extremely common in the United States, and its sale in drug and health food stores is subject to little real scrutiny. Recent evidence suggesting a relationship between protection from cancer and the consumption of vitamin A and beta-carotene (130,131), as well as the medically sanctioned use of vitamin A and its retinoid congeners to treat such skin diseases as acne, psoriasis, and wrinkles make it likely that the frequency of hypervitaminosis A will continue to rise. Although osteoporosis has not been described with retinoid use, hyperostosis and premature epiphyseal closure have each been described in patients treated with 13-*cis*-retinoic acid for dermatologic conditions (132,133).

ANTICONVULSANT MEDICATION

An association of skeletal abnormalities with chronic anticonvulsant therapy was recognized fairly recently, having been described by Schmid (134) and Kruse (135) approximately 20 years ago. Confirmation of this relationship has appeared in many epileptic populations worldwide, and this subject has been reviewed extensively by Hahn and Avioli (136). In its most florid presentation, patients are found to have osteopenia, fractures, hypocalcemia, hypophosphatemia, and muscle weakness. In severely affected children, radiologic evidence of rickets is also found. More commonly, only minimal biochemical abnormalities can be demonstrated, including increased circulating levels of PTH (137–140) and a subtle deficit in cortical bone mass (139,141–143). In general, patients with more severe disease have taken more than one anticonvulsant drug, usually phenytoin in combination with a barbiturate. Severity of bone disease is related to medication dose as well as duration of therapy (136).

The alterations in bone remodeling due to anticonvulsant medications have been elucidated by Mosekilde and Melsen (144) and by Weinstein et al. (140). Although anticonvulsant bone disease has been considered to be a form of osteomalacia, it is clear from these two excellent studies that the characteristic lesion in most patients is *not* malacia, but a high-turnover osteoporosis.

Mosekilde and Melsen (144) evaluated iliac crest biopsies from 20 epileptic adults treated with anticonvulsants for at least 10 years. All had taken phenytoin, and an unspecified number had received other drugs as well. Compared to a control group, the patients had significant reductions in serum and urinary calcium, and elevated serum alkaline phosphatase activities. On biopsy, trabecular bone volume was similar to control values, but relative osteoid volume, prevalence of bone-forming surfaces, and the fraction of surfaces labeled with tetracycline were all significantly increased. Prevalence of resorbing surfaces was also increased. Despite the abundant osteoid, mineral apposition rate was normal, and although the thickness of osteoid seams was slightly higher in the patient group, it was not abnormal.

Weinstein et al. (140) described the biochemical features of 120 epileptic patients who had received anticonvulsant medication for an average of 18 years, and reported iliac crest histomorphometry on a subgroup of 20 patients whose cortical bone density, serum-ionized calcium, or immunoreactive PTH were abnormal. The patient group had a significantly decreased serum-ionized calcium activity and an increase in iPTH. On biopsy, trabecular bone volume was normal, and significant increases were observed for osteoid volume and osteoid surface prevalence. Osteoid seam width was normal, and mineralization rates were consistently normal or increased. Thus, in two major studies, anticonvulsant bone disease proved to be a high-remodeling state reminiscent of primary hyperparathyroidism and not compatible with osteomalacia.

The mechanisms by which anticonvulsant medications interfere with bone and mineral metabolism remain unclear. Hahn et al. (145) demonstrated that these agents induce an acceleration in hepatic metabolism of vitamin D to inactive polar metabolites, and subsequently demonstrated a decrease in circulating 25(OH)D in long-term epileptics (143). Similar decreases in 25(OH)D were also reported by Stamp et al. (146). This finding could explain the biochemical and histological changes described above. With a decrease in available 25(OH)D, production of 1,25(OH)$_2$D would be constrained, and intestinal calcium absorption would decrease. This would lead to compensatory hypersecretion of PTH, which would then support blood calcium levels at the expense of increased bone remodeling.

Although this is an attractive model, recent studies raise serious concerns about its validity for most patients. Wark et al. (147) monitored 25(OH)D concentrations in nonepileptic post-myocardial infarction patients placed on phenytoin, 400 mg/day. After 2 years, mean 25(OH)D levels were no different from control values, and 1 month after stopping the medication no changes in 25(OH)D were observed. The authors concluded that phenytoin alone does not produce a significant effect on circulating 25(OH)D. In the study of Weinstein et al. (140), the 20 subjects with bone disease had serum 25(OH)D levels that were not significantly different from normal. Although 7 patients had levels below 20 ng/mL that might be considered marginal, there was no correlation between 25(OH)D concentration and the abnormalities in mineral metabolism.

The basis for these discrepancies in 25(OH)D level is not immediately clear, although Weinstein et al. (140) pointed out that those studies in which decreases were observed had been conducted at relatively northern latitudes (e.g., Great Britain and St Louis, Missouri) compared to studies in which normal levels were found (Australia and Augusta, Georgia), so that anticonvulsant drugs might compound the effects of marginal sunlight exposure on vitamin D production. Thus vitamin D sufficiency may still play a role in anticonvulsant bone disease in areas of limited UV exposure, or for institutionalized patients who have restricted access to sunshine.

An alternative model for the effects of anticonvulsants is a primary inhibition of intestinal calcium absorption by the drugs, leading to compensatory hypersecretion of PTH. Koch et al. (148) showed that modest doses of phenytoin directly impaired intestinal calcium transport. In addition, Harrison and Harrison (149) showed that phenytoin and phenobarbital in combination inhibited the action of vitamin D on gut calcium transport. Finally, Hahn and Halstead (139) showed that increased levels of vitamin D metabolites are required to maintain normal intestinal calcium absorption in anticonvulsant-treated patients.

Several effects of phenytoin on cellular functions outside the intestine may also contribute to disordered mineral metabolism. Jenkins et al. (150) and Hahn et al. (151) showed that both phenytoin and phenobarbital inhibit bone responses to PTH. Phenytoin was the more potent agent and suppressed the PTH-sensitive adenylate cyclase complex in calvaria, whereas phenobarbital appeared to work by a different mechanism. Dietrich and Duffield (152) showed that phenytoin directly inhibits collagen synthesis in bone cultures. Moreover, lysosomal enzyme release was also inhibited, suggesting that the drug may produce a state of PTH resistance in bone.

Treatment of anticonvulsant bone disease is relatively straightforward and effective. Although vitamin D deficiency may not be the primary cause of disordered calcium homeostasis, therapy with modest doses of the vitamin is generally sufficient to normalize the abnormalities. Christiansen et al. (141) treated patients with 2000–4000 IU/day and demonstrated increased bone mineral content. Hahn and Halstead (139) administered 4000 IU/day for 4 months and reported significant improvement in calcium absorption, PTH levels, and urinary hydroxyproline. However, occasional patients do require higher doses of the vitamin to induce resolution of radiologic abnormalities.

Of greater controversy is the question of routine prophylaxis. Barden et al. (153) showed that institutionalized adults were relatively protected from bone loss if supplied with a daily vitamin supplement. Hahn and Avioli (136) point out that the economic impact of pathological bone fractures far exceeds the cost of a vitamin D supplement. Furthermore, at doses of up to 2000 IU/day, the risks of vitamin overdose is very small. Thus it seems reasonable to administer prophylaxis to all patients at high risk for bone disease, including institutional-

ized, frail, poorly mobile individuals, and patients at northern latitudes. Hahn and Avioli (136) proposed that 25(OH)D levels might be a useful index of prophylaxis need. In view of the data of Wark et al. (147) and Weinstein et al. (140), however, the relationship of 25(OH)D status to bone disease must be considered tenuous. Moreover, since elevations in alkaline phosphatase activity largely reflect a hepatic effect (136), and since accurate ionized calcium levels are not widely available, it is difficult to advocate any biochemical abnormality as a useful risk marker. Therefore, I consider it not an unreasonable strategy to recommend vitamin D prophylaxis for all patients.

REFERENCES

1. Albright F, Reifenstein EC Jr. The parathyroid glands and metabolic bone disease: selected studies. Baltimore: Williams & Wilkins 1948;162.
2. Riggs BL, Wahner HW, Seeman E, et al. Changes in bone mineral density of the proximal femur and spine with aging: differences between the postmenopausal and senile osteoporosis syndromes. J Clin Invest 1982;70:716–23.
3. Lips P, Courpron P, Meunier PJ. Mean wall thickness of trabecular bone packets in the human iliac crest: changes with age. Calcif Tissue Res 1978;26:13–17.
4. Kragstrup J, Melsen F, Mosekilde L. Thickness of bone formed at remodeling sites in normal human iliac trabecular bone: variations with age and sex. Metab Bone Dis Relat Res 1983;5:17–21.
5. Jaworski ZFG. Parameters and indices of bone resorption. In: Meunier PJ. Bone histomorphometry, 2nd international workshop, Armour Montague, 1976.
6. Parfitt AM. Morphologic basis of bone mineral measurements: transient and steady state effects of treatment in osteoporosis. Miner Electrolyte Metab 1980;4:273–87.
7. Cushing H. The basophil adenomas of the pituitary body and their clinical manifestations. Bull Johns Hopkins Hosp 1932;50:137–95.
8. Curtiss PH, Clark WS, Herndon CH. Vertebral fractures resulting from prolonged cortisone and corticotrophin therapy. JAMA 1954;156:467–9.
9. Soffer LJ, Iannaccone A, Gabrilove JL. Cushing's syndrome: a study of fifty patients. Am J Med 1961;30:129.
10. McConkey B, Fraser GM, Bligh AS. Osteoporosis and purpura in rheumatoid disease: prevalence and relation to treatment with corticosteroids. Q J Med 1962;31:419–27.
11. Saville PD, Kharmosh O. Osteoporosis of rheumatoid arthritis: influence of age, sex and corticosteroids. Arthritis Rheum 1967;423–30.
12. Adinoff AD, Hollister JR. Steroid-induced fractures and bone loss in patients with asthma. N Engl J Med 1983;309:265–8.
13. Skibsted O, Gotfredsen A, Christiansen C. The effect of glucocorticoids on bone mass in rheumatoid arthritis patients: influence of menopausal state. Arthritis Rheum 1985;28:369–75.
14. Reid DM, Kennedy NSJ, Smith MA, Tothill P, Nuki G. Total body calcium in rheumatoid arthritis: effects of disease activity and corticosteroid treatment. Br Med J 1982;285:330–2.
15. Kennedy AC, Smith DA, Buchanan WW, Anderson JB, Jasani MK. Bone loss in patients with rheumatoid arthritis. Scand J Rheumatol 1975;4:73–9.
16. Seeman E, Wahner HW, Offord KP, Kumar R, Johnson WJ, Riggs BL. Differential effects of endocrine dysfunction on the axial and the appendicular skeleton. J Clin Invest 1982;69:1302–9.
17. Dykman TR, Gluck OS, Murphy WA, Hahn TJ, Hahn BH. Evaluation of factors associated with glucocorticoid-induced osteo-

penia in patients with rheumatic diseases. *Arthritis Rheum* 1985;28:361–7.

18. Rickers H, Deding A, Christiansen C, Rodbro P, Naestoft J. Corticosteroid-induced osteopenia and vitamin D metabolism: effect of vitamin D₂, calcium, phosphate, and sodium fluoride administration. *Clin Endocrinol* 1982;16:409–15.

19. Frost HM, Villanueva AR. Human osteoblastic activity. III. The effect of cortisone on lamellar osteoblastic activity. *Henry Ford Hosp Bull* 1961;9:97–100.

20. Jowsey J, Riggs BL. Bone formation in hypercortisonism. *Acta Endocrinol (Copenh)* 1970;63:21–8.

21. Hahn TJ, Halstead LR, Teitelbaum SL, Hahn BH. Altered mineral metabolism in glucocorticoid-induced osteopenia: effect of 25-hydroxyvitamin D administration. *J Clin Invest* 1979;64:655–65.

22. Bressot C, Meunier PJ, Chapuy MC, Lejeune E, Edouard C, Darby AJ. Histomorphometric profile, pathophysiology and reversibility of corticosteroid-induced osteoporosis. *Metab Bone Dis Relat Res* 1979;1:303–11.

23. Meunier PJ, Bressot C. Endocrine influences on bone cells and bone remodeling evaluated by clinical histomorphometry. In: Parsons JA, ed. *Endocrinology of calcium metabolism.* New York: Raven Press, 1982;445–65.

24. Dempster DW, Arlot MA, Meunier PJ. Mean wall thickness and formation periods of trabecular bone packets in corticosteroid osteoporosis. *Calcif Tissue Int* 1983;35:410–7.

25. Feldman D, Krishnan AV. Glucocorticoid effects on calcium metabolism and bone in the development of osteopenia. In: Christiansen C, Johansen JS, Riis BJ, eds. *Osteoporosis 1987.* Viborg, Denmark: Osteopress, 1987;1006–13.

26. Raisz LG, Trummel CL, Wener JA, Simmons H. Effect of glucocorticoids on bone resorption in tissue culture. *Endocrinology* 1972;90:961–7.

27. Stern PH. Inhibition by steroids of parathyroid hormone-induced ⁴⁵Ca release from embryonic rat bone in vitro. *J Pharmacol Exp Ther* 1969;168:211–7.

28. Wajchenberg GL, Pereira VG, Kieffer J, Ursic S. Effect of dexamethasone on calcium metabolism and ⁴⁷Ca kinetics in normal subjects. *Acta Endocrinol* 1969;61:173–92.

29. Kimberg DV, Baerg RD, Gershon E, Gracidusius RT. Effect of cortisone treatment on the active transport of calcium by the small intestine. *J Clin Invest* 1971;50:1309–21.

30. Lukert BP, Stanbury SW, Mawer EB. Vitamin D and intestinal transport of calcium: effects of prednisolone. *Endocrinology* 1973;93:718–22.

31. Klein RG, Arnaud SB, Gallagher JC, DeLuca HF, Riggs BL. Intestinal calcium absorption in exogenous hypercortisolism: role of 25-hydroxyvitamin D and corticosteroid dose. *J Clin Invest* 1977;60:253–9.

32. Avioli LV, Birge SJ, Lee SW. Effects of prednisone on vitamin D metabolism in man. *J Clin Endocrinol Metab* 1968;28:1341–6.

33. Seeman E, Kumar R, Hunder GG, Scott M, Heath H III, Riggs BL. Production, degradation, and circulating levels of 1,25-dihydroxyvitamin D in health and in chronic glucocorticoid excess. *J Clin Invest* 1980;66:664–9.

34. Aloia JF, Roginsky FM, Ellis K, Shukla K, Cohn S. Skeletal metabolism and body composition in Cushing's syndrome. *J Clin Endocrinol Metab* 1974;39:981–5.

35. Hahn TJ, Halstead LR, Haddad JG Jr. Serum 25-hydroxy-vitamin D concentrations in patients receiving chronic corticosteroid therapy. *J Lab Clin Med* 1977;90:399–404.

36. Chesney RW, Hamstra AJ, Mazeso RB, DeLuca HF. Reduction of serum 1,25-dihydroxyvitamin D₃ in children receiving glucocorticoids. *Lancet* 1978;2:1123–5.

37. Braun JJ, Birkenhager-Frenkel DH, Rietveld AH, Juttmann JR, Visser TJ, Birkenhager JC. Influence of 1α-(OH)D₃ administration on bone and bone mineral metabolism in patients on chronic glucocorticoid treatment; a double blind controlled study. *Clin Endocrinol* 1983;18:265–73.

38. Carre M, Ayigbede O, Miravet L, Rasmussen H. The effect of prednisone upon the metabolism and action of 25-hydroxy- and 1,25-dihydroxyvitamin D₃. *Proc Natl Acad Sci USA* 1974;71:2996–3000.

39. Favus MJ, Kimberg DV, Millar GN, Gershon E. Effects of corti-

sone administration on the metabolism and localization of 25-hydroxy-cholecalciferol in the rat. *J Clin Invest* 1973;52:1328–35.

40. Kimberg DV. Effects of vitamin D and steroid hormones on the active transport of calcium by the intestine. *N Engl J Med* 1969;280:1396–1405.

41. Laake H. The actions of corticosteroids on the renal reabsorption of calcium. *Acta Endocrinol* 1960;34:60–4.

42. Suzuki Y, Ichikawa Y, Saito E, Homma M. Importance of increased urinary calcium excretion in the development of secondary hyperparathyroidism of patients under glucocorticoid therapy. *Metabolism* 1983;32:151–6.

43. Fucik RF, Kukreja SC, Hargis GK, Bowser EN, Henderson WJ, Williams GA. Effect of glucocorticoids on function of the parathyroid glands in man. *J Clin Endocrinol Metab* 1975;40:152–5.

44. Lukert BP, Adams JS. Calcium and phosphorus homeostasis in man: effect of corticosteroids. *Arch Intern Med* 1976;136:1249–53.

45. Williams GA, Peterson WC, Bowser EN, Henderson WJ, Hargis GK, Martinez NJ. Interrelationship of parathyroid and adrenocortical function in calcium homeostasis in the rat. *Endocrinology* 1974;95:707–12.

46. Dykman TR, Haralson KM, Gluck OS, et al. Effect of oral 1,25-dihydroxyvitamin D and calcium on glucocorticoid-induced osteopenia in patients with rheumatic diseases. *Arthritis Rheum* 1984;27:1336–43.

47. Chen TL, Feldman D. Glucocorticoid receptors and actions in subpopulations of cultured rat bone cells. *J Clin Invest* 1979;63:750–8.

48. Catherwood BD. 1,25-Dihydroxycholecalciferol and glucocorticosteroid regulation of adenylate cyclase in an osteoblast-like cell line. *J Biol Chem* 1985;260:736–43.

49. Rodan SB, Rodan GA. Dexamethasone effects on β-adrenergic receptors and adenylate cyclase regulatory proteins, Gₛ and Gᵢ in ROS 17/2.8 cells. *Endocrinology* 1986;118:2510–8.

50. Yamamoto I, Potts JT Jr, Segre GV. Glucocorticoids increase parathyroid hormone receptors in rat osteoblastic osteosarcoma cells (ROS 17/2). *J Bone Miner Res* 1988;3:707–12.

51. Crilly RG, Marshall DH, Nordin BEC. Metabolic effects of corticosteroid therapy in post-menopausal women. *J Steroid Biochem* 1979;11:429–33.

52. Smals AGH, Kloppenborg PWC, Benraad TJ. Plasma testosterone profiles in Cushing's syndrome. *J Clin Endocrinol Metab* 1977;45:240–5.

53. MacAdams MR, White RH, Chipps BE. Reduction of serum testosterone levels during chronic glucocorticoid therapy. *Ann Intern Med* 1986;104:648–51.

54. Reid DM, Kennedy NSJ, Smith MA, Tothill P, Nuki G. Total body calcium in rheumatoid arthritis: effects of disease activity and corticosteroid treatment. *Br Med J* 1982;285:330–2.

55. Pocock NA, Eisman JA, Dunstan CR, Evans RA, Thomas DH, Huq NL. Recovery from steroid-induced osteoporosis. *Ann Intern Med* 1987;107:319–23.

56. Caniggia A, Marchetti M, Gennari C, Varrimo A, Nicolis FB. Effects of a new glucocorticoid, oxazacort, on some variables connected with bone metabolism in man: a comparison with prednisone. *Int J Clin Pharmacol* 1977;15:126–34.

57. Hahn TJ, Halstead LR, Strates B, Imbimbo B, Baran DT. Comparison of subacute effects of oxazacort and prednisone on mineral metabolism in man. *Calcif Tissue Int* 1980;31:109–15.

58. Jee WSS, Black HE, Gotcher JE. Effect of dichloromethane diphosphonate on corticosteroid-induced bone loss in young adult rabbits. *Clin Orthop* 1981;156:39–51.

59. Reid IR, Alexander CJ, King AR, Ibbertson HK. Prevention of steroid-induced osteoporosis with (3-amino-1-hydroxypropylidene)-1, 1-bisphosphonate (APD). *Lancet* 1988;1:143–6.

60. Baylink DJ. Glucocorticoid-induced osteoporosis. *N Engl J Med* 1983;309:306–8.

61. Horber FF, Scheidegger JR, Grunig BE, Frey FJ. Evidence that prednisone-induced myopathy is reversed by physical training. *J Clin Endocrinol Metab* 1985;61:83–8.

62. Von Recklinghausen, FC. Die fibrose oder deformierende Ostitis, die Osteomalazie und die osteopastische Karzinose in inhren gegenseitigen Beziehungen. In: *Festschrift Rudolph Virchow zu seinem 71 Geburtstage.* Berlin: G Reimer, 1891;1–89.

63. Mundy GR, Shapiro JL, Bandelin JC, Canalis EM, Raisz LG. Direct stimulation of bone resorption by thyroid hormones. *J Clin Invest* 1976;58:529–34.

64. Melsen F, Mosekilde L. Morphometric and dynamic studies of bone changes in hyperthyroidism. *Acta Pathol Microbiol Scand Sec A*, 1977;85:141–50.

65. Eriksen EF, Mosekilde L, Melsen F. Trabecular bone remodeling and bone balance in hyperthyroidism. *Bone* 1985;6:421–8.

66. Koutras DA, Pandos PG, Koukoulommati AS, Constantes J. Radiological signs of bone loss in hyperthyroidism. *Br J Radiol* 1973;46:6950–698.

67. Fraser SA, Anderson JB, Smith DA, et al. Osteoporosis and fractures following thyrotoxicosis. *Lancet* 1971;1:981–4.

68. Krølner B, Jorgensen JV, Nielsen SP. Spine bone mineral content in myxoedema and thyrotoxicosis: effects of thyroid hormone(s) and antithyroid treatment. *Clin Endocrinol* 1983;18:439–46.

69. Bouillon R, DeMoor, P. Parathyroid function in patients with hyper- or hypothyroidism. *J Clin Endocrinol Metab* 1974; 38:999–1004.

70. Mosekilde L, Christensen MS. Decreased parathyroid function in hyperthyroidism: inter-relationships between serum parathyroid hormone, calcium–phosphorus metabolism and thyroid function. *Acta Endocrinol* 1977;84:566–75.

71. Jastrup B, Mosekilde L, Melsen F, Lund B, Lund BJ, Sorensen OH. Serum levels of vitamin D metabolites and bone remodeling in hyperthyroidism. *Metabolism* 1982;31:126–32.

72. Garrell DR, Delmas PD, Malaval L, Tourniaire J. Serum bone Gla protein: a marker of bone turnover in hyperthyroidism. *J Clin Endocrinol Metab* 1986;62:1052.

73. Meunier PJ, Bianchi GGS, Edouard CM, Bernard JC, Courpron P, Vignon GE. Bony manifestations of thyrotoxicosis. *Orthop Clin North Am* 1972;3:745–74.

74. Smith DA, Fraser SA, Wilson GM. Hyperthyroidism and calcium metabolism. *Metabolism* 1973;2:333–54.

75. Ikkos DG, Katsichtis P, Mtalles K, et al. Osteoporosis in thyrotoxicosis. *Lancet* 1971;2:1159.

76. Linde J, Friss T. Osteoporosis in hyperthyroidism estimated by photon absorptiometry. *Acta Endocrinol* 1979;91:437–48.

77. Montz R, Hehrmann C, Schneider V, et al. Calcium stoffwechsel bei hyperthreose. *Radiologie* 1974;14:166–72.

78. Harrison JE, McNeill KG. Partial body calcium measurements by in vitro neutron activation analysis. *AJR* 1976;126:1308.

79. Bayley TA, Harrison JE, McNeill KG, et al. Effect of thyrotoxicosis and its treatment on bone mineral and muscle mass. *J Clin Endocrinol Metab* 1980;50:916–22.

80. Toh SH, Claunch BC, Brown PH. Effect of hyperthyroidism and its treatment on bone mineral content. *Arch Intern Med* 1985;145:883–6.

81. Ettinger B, Wingerd J. Thyroid supplements: effect on bone mass. *West J Med* 1982;136:473–6.

82. Fallon MD, Perry HM, Bergfeld M, et al. Exogenous hyperthyroidism with osteoporosis. *Arch Intern Med* 1983;143:442–4.

83. Ross DS, Neer RM, Ridgway EC, et al. Subclinical hyperthyroidism and reduced bone density as a possible result of prolonged suppression of the pituitary-thyroid axis with L-thyroxine. *Am J Med* 1987;82:1167.

84. Coindre J-M, David J-P, Riviere L, et al. Bone loss in hypothyroidism with hormone replacement: a histomorphometric study. *Arch Intern Med* 1986;146:48–53.

85. Paul TL, Kerrigan J, Kelly AM, Braverman LE, Baran DT. Long-term L-thyroxine therapy is associated with decreased hip bone density in premenopausal women. *JAMA* 1988;259:3137–41.

86. Frost HM. The mechanostat: a proposed pathogenic mechanism of osteoporoses and the bone mass effects of mechanical and nonmechanical agents. *Bone Miner* 1987;2:73–85.

87. Carter DR. Mechanical loading history and skeletal biology. *J Biomech* 1987;20:1095–109.

88. Albright F, Burnett CH, Cope O, Parson W. Acute atrophy of bone (osteoporosis) simulating hyperparathyroidism. *J Clin Endocrinol Metab* 1941;1:711–6.

89. Whedon GD, Schorr E. Metabolic studies in paralytic acute anterior poliomyelitis. II. Alterations in calcium and phosphorus metabolism. *J Clin Invest* 1957;36:966–81.

90. Dietrick JE, Whedon GD, Short E. Effects of immobilization upon various metabolic and physiologic functions in normal men. *Am J Med* 1948;4:3–36.

91. Donaldson CL, Hulley SB, Vogel JM, Hattner RS, Eayers JH, McMillan DE. Effect of prolonged bed rest on bone mineral. *Metabolism* 1970;19:1071–84.

92. Hulley SB, Vogel JM, Donaldson CL, Bayers JH, Friedman RJ, Rosen SN. Effect of supplemental oral phosphate on the bone mineral changes during prolonged bed rest. *J Clin Invest* 1971;50:2506–18.

93. Lockwood DR, Vogel JM, Schneider VS, Hulley SB. Effect of the diphosphonate EHDP on bone mineral metabolism during prolonged bed rest. *J Clin Endocrinol Metab* 1975;41:533–41.

94. Anderson SA, Cohn SH. Bone demineralization during space flight. *Physiologist* 1985;28:212–7.

95. Krølner B, Toft B. Vertebral bone loss: an unheeded side effect of therapeutic bed rest. *Clin Sci* 1983;64:537–40.

96. Stewart AF, Adler M, Byers CM, Segre GV, Broadus AE. Calcium homeostasis in immobilization: an example of resorptive hypercalciuria. *N Engl J Med* 1982;306:1136–40.

97. Minaire P, et al. Quantitative histological data on disuse osteoporosis. *Calcif Tissue Res* 1974;17:57–73.

98. Issekutz B, Blizzard J, Birkhead N, Rodahl K. Effect of prolonged bed rest on urinary calcium output. *J Appl Physiol* 1966; 21:1013–20.

99. Griffith GC, Silverglade A. Symposium on heparin. *Am J Cardiol* 1964;14:1–2.

100. Rupp WM, McCarthy HB, Rohde TD, Blackshear PJ, Goldenberg FJ, Buchwald H. Risk of osteoporosis in patients treated with long-term intervenous heparin therapy. *Curr Surg* 1982;39:419–22.

101. DeSwiet M, Dorrington Ward P, Fidler J, et al. Prolonged heparin therapy in pregnancy causes bone demineralization. *Br J Obstet Gynecol* 1983;90:1129–34.

102. Zimran A, Shilo S, Fisher D, Bab I. Histomorphometric evaluation of reversible heparin-induced osteoporosis in pregnancy. *Arch Intern Med* 1986;146:386–8.

103. Goldhaber P. Heparin enhancement of factors stimulating bone resorption in tissue culture. *Science* 1965;147:407–8.

104. Asher JD, Nichols G Jr. Heparin stimulation of bone collagenase activity. *Fed Proc* 1965;24:211.

105. Sodek J, Heersche JNM. Uptake of collagenolytic enzymes by bone cells during isolation from embryonic rat calvaria. *Calcif Tissue Int* 1981;33:255–60.

106. Sakamoto S, Sakamoto M. Bone collagenase, osteoblasts and cell-mediated bone resorption. In: Peck WA, ed. *Bone Miner Res* 1986;4:49–102.

107. Shen V, Kohler G, Jeffrey JJ, Peck WA. Bone-resorbing agents promote and interferon-g inhibits bone cell collagenase production. *J Bone Miner Res* 1988;3:657–66.

108. Thompson RC. Heparin osteoporosis: an experimental model using rats. *J Bone Joint Surg* 1973;55-A:606–12.

109. van der Vijgh WJF, Kruik AJB, Jongen MJM, Lips P, Netelenbos JC. Inhibition of 25(OH)D 1α-hydroxylase in kidney homogenates of Japanese quail by heparin. *Calcif Tissue Int* 1983; 35(suppl):A50, *Abstract* 192.

110. Aarskog D, Aksnes L, Lehmann V. Low 1,25-dihydroxyvitamin D in heparin-induced osteopenia. *Lancet* 1980;2:650.

111. Aarskog D, Aksnes L, Markestad T, Ulstein M, Sagen N. Heparin-induced inhibition of 1,25-dihydroxyvitamin D formation. *Am J Obstet Gynecol* 1984;148:1141–2.

112. Vinazzer HA. Heparin fractions and analogues. In: Poller L, ed. *Recent Advances in Blood Coagulation*. Edinburgh: Churchill Livingstone 1985;169–89.

113. Frame B, Nixon RK. Bone marrow mast cells in osteoporosis of aging. *N Engl J Med* 1968;279:626–30.

114. Jowsey J. *Metabolic diseases of bone*. Saunders monographs in clinical orthopedics, vol 1. Philadelphia: WB Saunders, 1977;74–5.

115. Poppel MH, Gruber WF, Silber R, Holder AK, Christmanh RO. Roentgen manifestations of urticaria pigmentosa (mastocytosis). *AJR* 1959;82:239–49.

116. Kane EK. *Arctic explorations*, vol 1. Hartford, Conn: American Publishing, 1857;392–3. Reprinted by the Arno Press, New York, and The New York Times, 1971.

117. Josephs HW. Hypervitaminosis A and carotenemia. *Am J Dis Child* 1944;67:33–43.

118. Toomey JA, Morissette RA. Hypervitaminosis A. *Am J Dis Child* 1947;73:473–80.

119. Frame B, Jackson CE, Reynolds WA, Umphrey JE. Hypercalcemia and skeletal effects in chronic hypervitaminosis A. *Ann Intern Med* 1974;80:44–8.

120. Jowsey J, Riggs BL. Bone changes in a patient with hypervitaminosis A (letter). *J Clin Endocrinol Metab* 1968;28:1833–5.

121. Raisz LG. Bone resorption in tissue culture: factors influencing the response to parathyroid hormone. *J Clin Invest* 1965;44:103–16.

122. Pennypacker JP, Lewis CA, Hassell JR. Altered proteoglycan metabolism in mouse limb mesenchyme cell cultures treated with vitamin A. *Arch Biochem Biophys* 1978;186:351.

123. DeSimone DP, Reddi AH. Influence of vitamin A on matrix-induced endochondral bone formation. *Calcif Tissue Intl* 1983; 35:732–9.

124. Metz AL, Walser MM, Olson WG. The interaction of dietary vitamin A and vitamin D related to skeletal development in the turkey poult. *J Nutr* 1985;115:929–35.

125. Hough S, Avioli LV, Muir H, et al. Effects of hypervitaminosis A on the bone and mineral metabolism of the rat. *Endocrinology* 1988;122:2933–9.

126. Chytil F, Ong DE. Cellular retinol- and retinoic acid-binding proteins in vitamin A action. *Fed Proc* 1979;38:2510–4.

127. Trechsel U, Evequoz F, Hodler B, Fleisch H. Similarity of the effects of $1,25(OH)_2D$ and retinoic acid on interleukin (IL) 1, 2 and 3 production. *7th Annual meeting, American Society for Bone and Mineral Research,* Washington DC, 1985, abstract 279.

128. Petkovich PM, Heersche JNM, Tinker DO, Jones G. Retinoic acid stimulates 1,25-dihydroxyvitamin D_3 binding in rat osteosarcoma cells. *J Biol Chem* 1984;259:8274–80.

129. Chen TL, Feldman D. Retinoic acid modulation of $1,25(OH)_2D_3$ receptors and bioresponse in bone cells: species differences between rat and mouse. *Biochem Biophys Res Commun* 1985;132:74–80.

130. Wald N, Idle M, Boreham JB, Bailey A. Low serum-vitamin-A and subsequent risk of cancer. *Lancet* 1980;2:813–5.

131. Shekelle RB, Liu S, Raynor WJ Jr, Lepper M, Maliza C, Rossof AH. Dietary vitamin A and risk of cancer in the Western Electric study. *Lancet* 1981;2:1185–9.

132. Pittsley RA, Yoder FW. Retinoid hyperostosis: skeletal toxicity associated with long-term administration of 13-*cis* retinoic acid for refractory icthyosis. *N Engl J Med* 1983;308:1012–4.

133. Milstone LM, McGuire J, Ablow RC. Premature epiphyseal closure in a child receiving oral 13-*cis* retinoic acid. *J Am Acad Dermatol* 1982;7:663–6.

134. Schmid F. Osteopathien bei antiepileptischer Dauerbehandlung. *Fortschr Med* 1967;85:381.

135. Kruse R. Osteopathien bei antiepiliptischer längzeit-Therapie. *Monatsschr Kinderheilkd* 1968;116:378–80.

136. Hahn TJ, Avioli LV. Anticonvulsant-drug-induced mineral disorders. In: Roe DA, Campbell TC, eds. *Drugs and nutrients: the interactive effects. Drugs and the pharmaceutical sciences,* vol 21. New York: Marcel Dekker, 1984;409–27.

137. Bouillon R, Reynaert J, Claes JH, Lissens W, DeMoor P. The effect of anticonvulsant therapy on serum levels of 25-hydroxyvitamin D, calcium, and parathyroid hormone. *J Clin Endocrinol Metab* 1975;41:1130–5.

138. Mosekilde L, Christensen MS, Lund B, Sorenson OH, Melsen F. The interrelationships between serum 25-hydroxycholecalciferol, serum parathyroid hormone and bone changes in anticonvulsant osteomalacia. *Acta Endocrinol* 1977;84:559–65.

139. Hahn TJ, Halstead LR. Anticonvulsant drug-induced osteomalacia: alterations in mineral metabolism and response to vitamin D_3 administration. *Calcif Tissue Int* 1979;27:13–8.

140. Weinstein RS, Bryce GF, Sappington LJ, King DW, Gallagher BB. Decreased serum ionized calcium and normal vitamin D metabolite levels with anticonvulsant drug treatment. *J Clin Endocrinol Metab* 1984;58:1003–9.

141. Christiansen C, Rodbro P, Lund P. Incidence of anticonvulsant osteomalacia and effect of vitamin D: controlled therapeutic trial. *Br Med J* 1973;4:695–701.

142. Christiansen C, Rodbro P, Nielsen CT. Iatrogenic osteomalacia in epileptic children: a controlled therapeutic trial. *Acta Paediatr Scand* 1975;64:219–24.

143. Hahn TJ, Hendin BA, Scharp CR, Boisseau VC, Haddad JG Jr. Serum 25-hydroxycalciferol levels and bone mass in children on chronic anticonvulsant therapy. *N Engl J Med* 1975;292:550–4.

144. Mosekilde L, Melsen F. Dynamic differences in trabecular bone remodeling between patients after jejuno-ileal bypass for obesity and epileptic patients receiving anticonvulsant therapy. *Metab Bone Dis Relat Res* 1980;2:77–82.

145. Hahn TJ, Birge SJ, Scharp CR, Avioli LV. Phenobarbital induced alterations in vitamin D metabolism. *J Clin Invest* 1972; 51:741–8.

146. Stamp TCB, Round JM, Rowe DJF, Haddad JG Jr. Plasma levels and therapeutic effect of 25-hydroxycholecalciferol in epileptic patients taking anticonvulsant drugs. *Br Med J* 1972;4:9–12.

147. Wark JD, Larkins RG, Perry-Keene D, Peter CT, Ross DL, Sloman JG. Chronic diphenylhydantoin therapy does not reduce plasma 25-hydroxy-vitamin D. *Clin Endocrinol* 1979;11:267–74.

148. Koch HC, Kraft D, von Herrath D. Influence of diphenylhydantoin and phenobarbital on intestinal calcium transport in the rat. *Epilepsia* 1972;13:829–41.

149. Harrison HC, Harrison HE. Inhibition of vitamin D-stimulated active transport of calcium of rat intestine by diphenyhydantoin–phenobarbital treatment. *Proc Soc Exp Biol Med* 1976; 153:220–4.

150. Jenkins MV, Harris M, Wills MR. The effect of phenytoin on parathyroid extract and 25-hydroxycholecalciferol-induced bone resorption: adenosine 3′,5′-cyclic monophosphate production. *Calcif Tissue Res* 1974;16:163–7.

151. Hahn TJ, Scharp CR, Richardson CA, Halstead LR, Kahn AJ, Teitelbaum SL. Interaction of diphenylhydantoin (phenytoin) and phenobarbital with hormonal mediation of fetal rat bone resorption in vitro. *J Clin Invest* 1978;62:406–14.

152. Dietrich JW, Duffield R. Effects of diphenylhydantoin on synthesis of collagen and noncollagen protein in tissue culture. *Endocrinology* 1980;106:606–10.

153. Barden HS, Mazess RB, Rose PG, McAweeney W. Bone mineral status measured by direct photon absorptiometry in institutionalized adults receiving long-term anticonvulsant therapy and multivitamin supplementation. *Calcif Tissue Int* 1980;31:117–21.

Disorders of Bone and Mineral Metabolism,
edited by Fredric L. Coe and Murray J. Favus,
© 1992 by Raven Press, Ltd. All rights reserved.

CHAPTER 39

Bone Disease in Chronic Renal Failure and After Renal Transplantation

Eduardo Slatopolsky and James Delmez

The term *renal osteodystrophy* is used in a generic sense to include all skeletal disorders that occur in patients with renal failure, including osteitis fibrosa, osteomalacia, osteosclerosis, growth retardation, and osteoporosis.

The association of renal failure with hyperplasia of the parathyroid glands, abnormal vitamin D metabolism, and skeletal abnormalities has been known for many years (1–4). It is not surprising that metabolic bone diseases develop in patients with chronic renal disease because the kidney plays a major role in mineral homeostasis. It maintains external balance for phosphorus, calcium, and magnesium, synthesizes 1,25-dihydroxyvitamin D [1,25(OH)$_2$D] (calcitriol), degrades and removes parathyroid hormone (PTH) from the circulation, and is the main organ responsible for the excretion of aluminum. Under normal conditions small amounts of aluminum that may be ingested are rapidly eliminated in the urine. In renal failure, if the ingestion or exposure to aluminum is increased, the inability of the diseased kidney to excrete aluminum imposes a serious risk in dialysis patients. Now that the lives of patients with chronic renal failure can be prolonged through better conservative therapy, readily available dialysis, and successful renal transplantation, the morbidity associated with disordered divalent ion metabolism and bone disease has assumed greater clinical significance. Currently, the clinical features of renal osteodystrophy are better defined, several abnormal mechanisms have been clarified, and a rational approach to the prevention and treatment of renal osteodystrophy is possible.

SECONDARY HYPERPARATHYROIDISM AND OSTEITIS FIBROSA

Hyperplasia of the parathyroid glands and high levels of serum immunoreactive PTH (iPTH) are among the most consistent pathogenetic factors affecting divalent ion metabolism in patients with chronic renal failure. Increased levels of iPTH have been reported in patients with only mildly abnormal renal function (5,6), as shown in Fig. 1.

Although it is well accepted that the main factor leading to the development of secondary hyperparathyroidism is hypocalcemia, recent studies have demonstrated that hyperparathyroidism may develop in the absence of hypocalcemia (7). Osteitis fibrosa represents the skeletal abnormalities secondary to high levels of circulating parathyroid hormone. The factors that contribute to hypocalcemia and secondary hyperparathyroidism include (a) phosphate retention, (b) decreased synthesis of calcitriol, (c) skeletal resistance to the calcemic action of PTH, (d) an increased "set point" for calcium-regulated PTH secretion, and (e) impaired degradation of PTH secondary to reduced renal function (Fig. 2).

Phosphate Retention

Phosphate retention plays a key role in the pathogenesis of secondary hyperparathyroidism (8–10). Reiss et al. (11) reported that an oral load of phosphorus, providing 1.0 g of elemental phosphorus, led to an increase in serum phosphorus, a fall in ionized calcium levels, and an increase in serum iPTH in normal subjects. Several investigators have shown that long-term feeding of animals with a diet high in phosphate can produce parathy-

E. Slatopolsky and J. Delmez: The Renal Division, Department of Internal Medicine, and Chromalloy American Kidney Center, Washington University School of Medicine, St. Louis, Missouri 63110

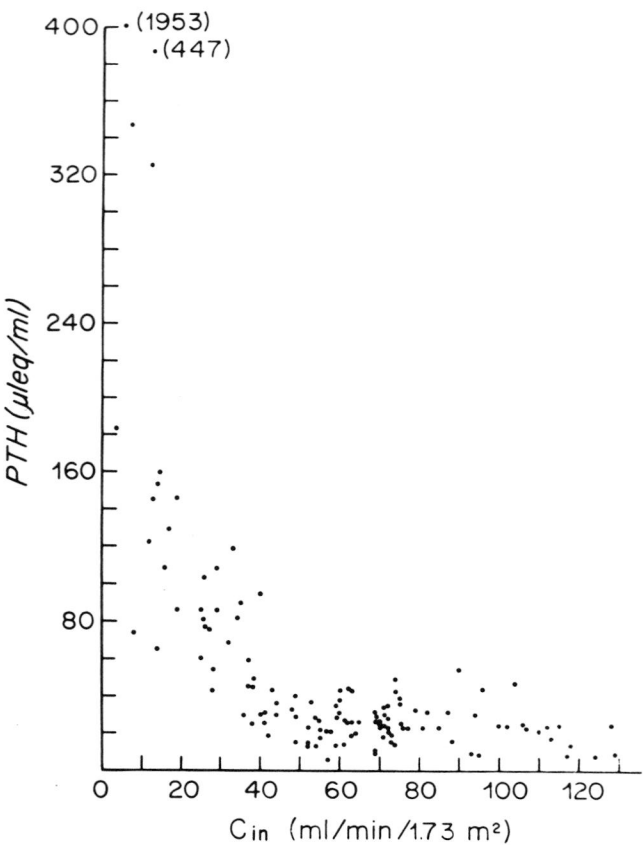

FIG. 1. Relationship between serum iPTH and the renal clearance of inulin in patients with varying levels of renal function. (From C. D. Arnaud, *Kidney Int,* 1973;4:89–95.)

roid hyperplasia, increased levels of iPTH, and a mild reduction in serum calcium levels (12,13). Studies in experimental renal failure have shown that the restriction of dietary phosphate in proportion to the decrease in glomerular filtration rate (GFR) can prevent the development of secondary hyperparathyroidism in azotemic dogs followed for 2 months (9). Subsequent studies (14) showed a substantial reduction of serum iPTH levels in animals with renal failure treated with a proportional phosphate restricted diet for 2 years. Llach et al. (15) indicated that a reduction in dietary phosphate intake in proportion to the decrease in GFR over a 2-month period in humans with creatinine clearances of 50–90 mL/min was associated with a decrease in serum iPTH to normal levels. When phosphate intake was reduced in patients with more advanced renal insufficiency, serum iPTH fell substantially but remained above normal levels (16). Other studies have shown that serum iPTH levels correlate positively with the degree of hyperphosphatemia in patients undergoing dialysis, (17) an observation providing support for a role of hyperphosphatemia in causing parathyroid hypersecretion, particularly in patients with advanced uremia. Thus phosphate

loading could cause a small fall in the level of ionized calcium, or it may decrease the renal production of 1,25(OH)$_2$D$_3$ (18), which may permit more secretion of PTH at any given levels of serum calcium (19). As renal disease advances and GFR falls below 25 mL/min, hyperphosphatemia is usual (20); under such circumstances, hypocalcemia is more directly related to a markedly increased level of serum phosphorus. Although high concentrations of serum phosphate (7–9 mg/dL) precipitate calcium in soft tissues, the mechanism by which mild hyperphosphatemia affects the concentration of ionized calcium in serum is not known. It may decrease the release of calcium from bone (21) or affect the activity of the renal enzyme 1-hydroxylase responsible for the conversion of 25(OH)D to 1,25(OH)$_2$D$_3$ (18). In healthy men, Portale et al. (22) found that when dietary phosphorus was restricted and then supplemented, an increase and then a decrease in plasma calcitriol was observed. This phenomenon was associated with an increase or a decrease in the production rate of calcitriol with no change in its metabolic clearance rate. The same investigators (23) have clearly demonstrated that in normal men, dietary phosphorus can finely regulate the serum concentration of calcitriol, and this regulation is mediated by the concentration of serum phosphorus. It is important to emphasize that correction of hyperphosphatemia alone will not totally reverse secondary hyperparathyroidism in patients with advanced renal failure (GFR less than 15 mL/min), because many other factors are responsible for the increased PTH levels in blood.

Altered Vitamin D Metabolism

The kidney is the major site for conversion of vitamin D to its active metabolite 1,25(OH)$_2$D$_3$ (24). Thus alterations in mineral homeostasis and skeletal disease can be expected in advanced renal failure. Because one of the main actions of vitamin D is to stimulate intestinal transport of calcium, it is easy to understand why the absorption of calcium from the intestine is decreased in patients with far-advanced renal insufficiency and low levels of 1,25(OH)$_2$D$_3$. The evidence that altered vitamin D metabolism contributes to abnormal calcium metabolism in advanced renal failure is considerable. Metabolic balance studies usually show the fecal losses of calcium are equal to or greater than dietary intake in patients with advanced renal insufficiency (25), and radioisotope techniques also show reduced intestinal absorption of calcium in most patients with advanced renal failure (26). Currently, there is controversy concerning the level of renal insufficiency at which vitamin D metabolism becomes abnormal. This information will be of considerable importance in elucidating the pathogenesis of secondary hyperparathyroidism in uremia. Slatopolsky et al. (27) compared the levels of 1,25(OH)$_2$D$_3$ and iPTH in a group of adults with normal renal function, patients with mild decreases in GFR (GFR between 40 and 60 mL/min), patients with advanced renal failure (GFR between 5 and 20 mL/min), and patients on dialysis. The plasma levels of $1,25(OH)_2D_3$ were normal or even slightly elevated in patients with creatinine clearances greater than 40 mL/min and low in patients with more advanced renal disease. Cheung et al. (28) found similar results. Other investigators, however, found low circulating levels of calcitriol in patients with moderate renal insufficiency (29–31). If one assumes that a patient with a GFR of 50 mL/min has lost roughly one-half of the renal mass, yet maintains normal levels of $1,25(OH)_2D_3$, one has to conclude that the production of $1,25(OH)_2D_3$ per unit of renal mass is greatly increased. This could be due to secondary hyperparathyroidism, which is usually present in patients with mild renal insufficiency. However, studies by Taylor et al. (32) in the dog showed that after unilateral nephrectomy, the remaining kidney increased the production of $1,25(OH)_2D_3$ even in the absence of PTH. Moreover, patients with a mild degree of renal insufficiency do not have calcium malabsorption. Coburn et al. (26) measured intestinal calcium absorption using ^{47}Ca isotope techniques in patients with different degrees of renal insufficiency. They found that patients with mild renal failure (serum creatinine less than 2.5 mg/dL) had calcium absorption values no different from those observed in normal volunteers. Malluche et al. (33) also studied calcium absorption in a large group of patients with renal disease. They found that as GFR decreased, there was a concomitant decline in the absorption of calcium. However, this abnormality became evident only at GFR values below 50 mL/min. The results obtained in patients with a GFR greater than 60 mL/min were not different from those obtained in patients with normal renal function. Thus there is no good evidence for calcium malabsorption or low serum levels of $1,25(OH)_2D_3$ in the majority of patients with early renal insufficiency.

Although the levels of $1,25(OH)_2D_3$ in most patients with advanced renal failure (GFR less than 20 mL/min) are low, many patients lack histologic features of vitamin D deficiency. Thus reduced synthesis of $1,25(OH)_2D_3$ may not be the only factor responsible for the development of osteomalacia in this group of patients (34,35). Perhaps normal or elevated serum phosphorus levels may protect some uremic patients from osteomalacia. The role of decreased generation of other vitamin D sterols, particularly $24,25(OH)_2D_3$, in the pathogenesis of renal osteodystrophy remains uncertain. The kidney is the organ primarily responsible for the formation of $24,25(OH)_2D_3$, but there is evidence that this metabolite may also be produced in the intestine and bone (36). Studies by Olgaard et al. (37) in uremic dogs indicated that the administration of $24,25(OH)_2D_3$ alone did not have any beneficial effect.

Skeletal Resistance to the Calcemic Action of Parathyroid Hormone

Skeletal resistance to the calcemic action of PTH may be an important cause of hypocalcemia in patients with renal insufficiency. The calcemic response to the infusion of parathyroid extract is significantly less in hypocalcemic patients with renal failure than in normal subjects or patients with hypoparathyroidism (38). The finding of a delayed recovery from EDTA-induced hypocalcemia in patients with mild renal insufficiency, despite a greater augmentation in serum iPTH levels, compared with results in normal subjects, indicates that the skeletal resistance to endogenous PTH appears early in the course of renal insufficiency (39). Such data suggest that higher circulating levels of PTH may be needed to maintain normal serum calcium levels in patients with renal failure.

The concept of skeletal resistance to PTH as an important factor in the development of secondary hyperparathyroidism has been challenged. Kaplan et al. (40) fed dogs with chronic renal failure a low-phosphate diet and prevented the development of secondary hyperparathyroidism. Nonetheless, these animals developed skeletal resistance to the calcemic action of PTH. Thus despite the presence of skeletal resistance to PTH, the dogs did not develop secondary hyperparathyroidism. However, Llach et al. (15) found that dietary phosphate restriction improved the calcemic response to a standardized infusion of PTH in patients with mild renal insufficiency. It is possible that alterations in vitamin D metabolism could be responsible for the resistance to the calcemic action of PTH seen in uremia. In dogs with acute renal failure (41), treatment with $1,25(OH)_2D_3$ results in partial correction of the blunted calcemic response to parathyroid extract. Other observations suggest that hyperphosphatemia accounts for the skeletal resistance to parathyroid extract in rats with acute renal failure (36). Results of studies in bone–organ culture systems indicate that the serum of uremic patients can inhibit PTH-stimulated release of calcium from the bone (21).

Galceran et al. (43) studied the calcemic effects of PTH in dogs before and after the induction of chronic renal failure. The administration of calcitriol did not improve the calcemic response to PTH (Fig. 3). However, when the uremic dogs underwent a parathyroidectomy 24 h before the infusion of PTH, the calcemic response returned to normal. Therefore, despite low levels of $1,25(OH)_2D_3$ and maintenance of a uremic environment, disappearance of PTH from the circulation restored the calcemic response to exogenous PTH to normal. These results clearly demonstrated that low levels of circulating calcitriol are not responsible for the skeletal resistance to PTH in uremia. These results suggest that desensitization to high levels of endogenous PTH pre-

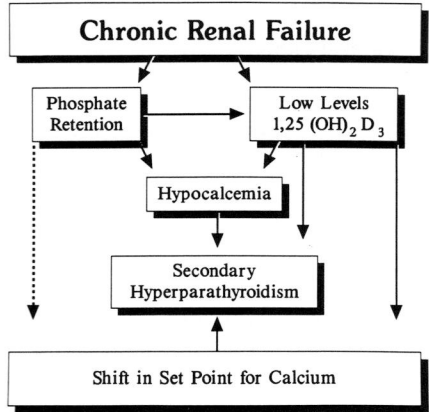

Chronic Renal Failure

Phosphate Retention

Low Levels 1,25 (OH)₂D₃

Hypocalcemia

Secondary Hyperparathyroidism

Shift in Set Point for Calcium

FIG. 2. Diagrammatic representation of the factors involved in the pathogenesis of secondary hyperparathyroidism.

vents a normal calcemic response to the administration of exogenous PTH in uremia.

Altered Calcium-Regulated PTH Secretion

Calcium is an inhibitor of the adenylate cyclase activity of isolated parathyroid membranes (44–48). Membranes prepared from hyperplastic glands are less susceptible to the inhibition of enzyme activity by calcium than are membranes prepared from normal human parathyroid tissue (47). This suggests that the set point for calcium to inhibit parathyroid adenylate cyclase may be elevated above normal in hyperfunctioning human parathyroid glands. In addition to the altered set point for the inhibition by calcium of parathyroid adenylate cyclase in membranes obtained from hyperfunctioning human glands, there is an altered set point for PTH secretion. This is defined as the calcium ion concentration causing

a 50% decrease in hormone secretion (49–53). The degree of suppression of hormone secretion with increasing calcium is apparently less for cells obtained from all types of hyperplastic glands than for cells from normal glands (53).

Several investigators (54–56) have provided evidence that vitamin D metabolites directly affect regulation of PTH secretion. In 1974, Oldham et al. (57) isolated a calcium-binding protein in porcine parathyroid glands with properties similar to those of the calcium-binding protein found in mammalian intestinal mucosa. The administration of $25(OH)D_3$ to rachitic puppies increased the calcium-binding protein in the parathyroid glands. Subsequently, Brumbaugh et al. (58) demonstrated specific binding of $1,25(OH)_2D_3$ to cytosolic and nuclear receptors of the chick parathyroid glands in vivo and in vitro in the rat. Chertow et al. (54) performed studies in vivo in the rat and in vitro with bovine parathyroid gland slices. These investigators clearly demonstrated an inhibitory effect of $1,25(OH)_2D_3$ on PTH release. After these initial publications, a series of papers appeared in the literature suggesting that $1,25(OH)_2D_3$ did not have a direct effect on the secretion of parathyroid hormone (59,60). Because of these controversial results, Golden et al. (61) studied in great detail the effect of $1,25(OH)_2D_3$ on parathyroid hormone secretion in vitro, using bovine parathyroid gland slices and isolated dispersed bovine parathyroid cells. The results failed to demonstrate an effect of $1,25(OH)_2D_3$ on PTH secretion by the isolated bovine parathyroid cells or by bovine parathyroid slices. It must be emphasized that the parathyroid glands used in these studies were obtained from normal cows that were not depleted of $1,25(OH)_2D_3$, and this may have had an effect on the outcome of the results. Moreover, the studies were performed in vitro and the incubations were conducted over a 4-h period. Studies by Oldham and collaborators (19) in vitamin D–deficient dogs

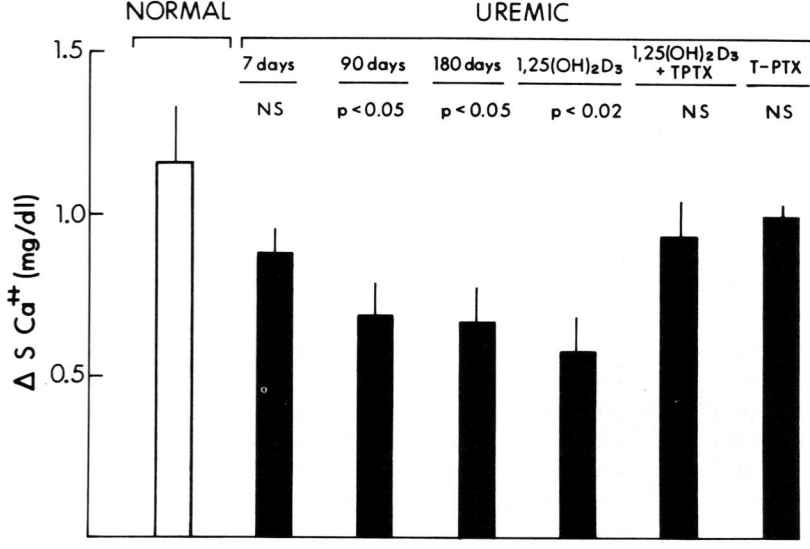

FIG. 3. Calcemic response to the administration of parathyroid hormone in a group of dogs before and after the induction of renal failure. After 90 days of renal insufficiency, the dogs had a blunted calcemic response to PTH. The administration of $1,25(OH)_2D_3$ did not improve the calcemic response. A T-PTX 24 hours before the administration of exogenous PTH returned the calcemic response to normal. (From Galceran et al. *Kidney Int*, 1987;32:801–7.)

clearly indicated that higher concentrations of calcium were necessary to suppress the release of parathyroid hormone in these animals. When similar studies were performed in the same animals after $1,25(OH)_2D_3$ was given to the dogs, the parathyroid glands appeared to be more sensitive to mild increments in serum calcium.

The low levels of $1,25(OH)_2D_3$ observed in patients with advanced renal insufficiency (27,28,62) could potentially play a role in the abnormal behavior of the parathyroid glands. Slatopolsky et al. (63) performed studies in dialysis patients using intravenous $1,25(OH)_2D_3$. Twenty patients with hypocalcemia maintained on chronic hemodialysis were selected for the study. Calcitriol was given intravenously at the end of each dialysis for a period of 8 weeks. The dose was 0.5 μg initially and gradually was increased to a maximum of 4.0 μg per treatment. All patients had a substantial decrease in the levels of PTH during $1,25(OH)_2D_3$ treatment. The mean decrement in PTH was 70.1%. After 3 weeks of treatment, there was a gradual rise in the levels of ionized calcium. Concomitantly, there was a significant decrease in the levels of i-PTH. After $1,25(OH)_2D_3$ was discontinued, PTH subsequently increased in all patients. They also observed that early during the administration of

$1,25(OH)_2D_3$, before a significant increase in ionized calcium levels occurred, there was a decrease in the levels of iPTH (Fig. 4). Thus these studies demonstrated that $1,25(OH)_2D_3$ has a potent suppressive effect on the release of PTH. It is likely that the effects were due mainly to an elevation of serum calcium levels to the upper limits of normal. However, it would seem that in addition to the calcemic effect, $1,25(OH)_2D_3$ directly modified the secretion of PTH. Further evidence has been provided from in vitro and in vivo studies. Primary cultures of bovine parathyroid cells have been used to demonstrate that $1,25(OH)_2D_3$ inhibits the release of PTH (64,65), decreases the levels of pre-pro PTH mRNA (66), and blocks transcription of the PTH gene (67). Silver et al. (68) confirmed inhibition of transcription in vivo by the administration of a dose of $1,25(OH)_2D_3$ that did not raise serum calcium levels. Thus there is now full agreement between investigators on the critical role of calcitriol on the regulation of PTH synthesis and secretion. Delmez et al. (69) have demonstrated that the administration of intravenous calcitriol in dialysis patients suppressed PTH independent of changes in ionized serum calcium levels and returned the abnormal "set point" for calcium toward normal (Fig. 5).

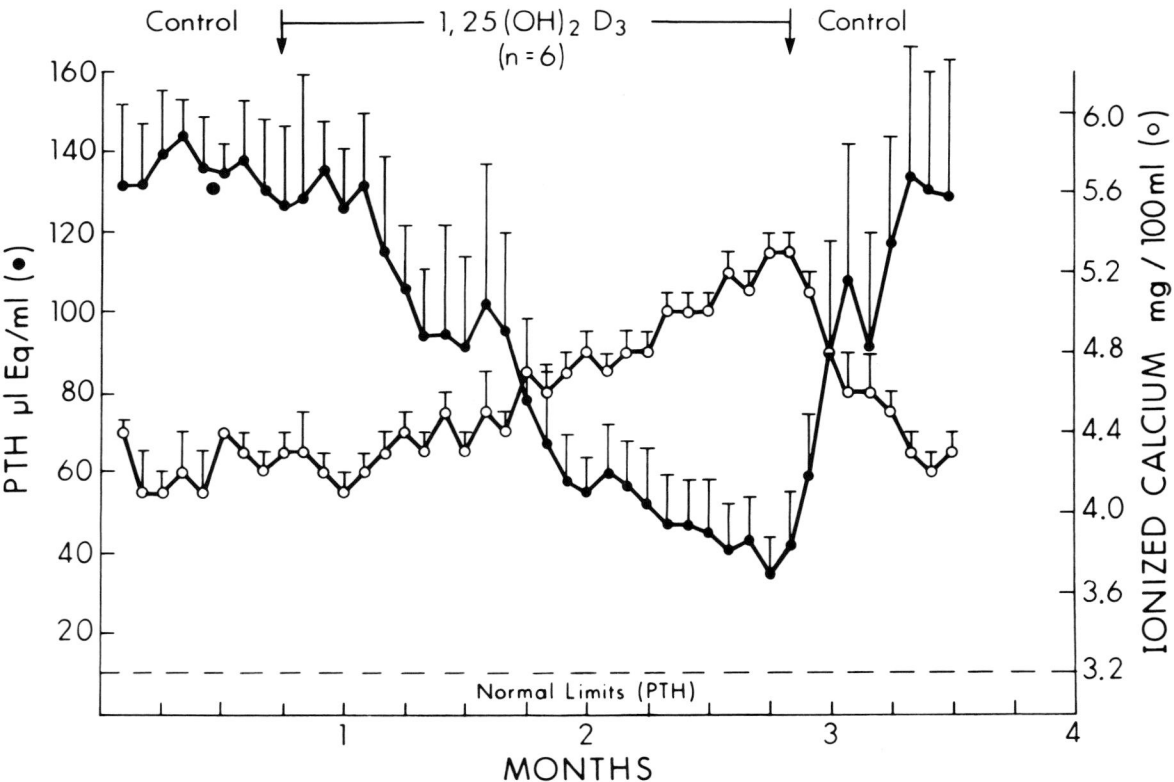

FIG. 4. Temporal relationship between ionized calcium and serum iPTH, before, during, and after intravenous $1,25(OH)_2D_3$ administration in patients with moderate secondary hyperparathyroidism. The maximum decrement in iPTH was 73.5%. In the first 3 weeks of treatment with $1,25(OH)_2D_3$ there was no change in ionized calcium; however, iPTH decreased from 132 ± 20 to 95 ± 20 μEq/mL. (From E. Slatopolsky et al., *J Clin Invest* 1984;74:2136–43.)

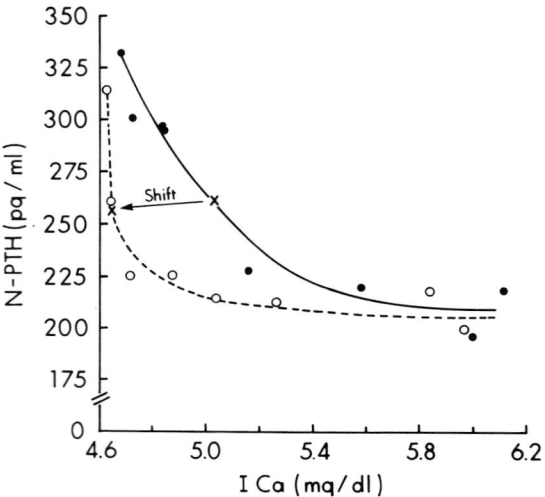

FIG. 5. Effects of intravenous 1,25(OH)$_2$D$_3$ on PTH secretion during a calcium infusion in a representative patient. During the control infusion (●) the set point (×) of ICa was 5.04 mg/dL. After 2 weeks of IV 1,25(OH)$_2$D$_3$ the PTH levels (○) fell despite a lower ICa value and the set point decreased to 4.64 mg/dL. (From J. Delmez et al., *J Clin Invest* 1989;83:1349–55.)

Role of Reduced Degradation of PTH

Increased secretion of PTH is the major factor responsible for high plasma levels of iPTH in patients with renal insufficiency. Since the kidney plays an important role in the degradation of PTH, this could be a factor contributing to the high levels of PTH in uremia (70). Because the kidney may be the only organ removing the carboxyl-terminal fragments of PTH from the circulation (71), the level of these fragments is greatly increased in renal failure. Measurements of iPTH specific for the carboxyl fractions reveal values that are much higher in uremic patients than in patients with primary hyperparathyroidism (72). However, the kidney also plays a role in the degradation of the intact 1-84 PTH molecule, and studies of the metabolic clearance of bovine PTH 1-84 suggest that it is decreased in patients with renal failure (73).

OSTEOMALACIA

Osteomalacia is another important feature of the skeletal disease in some patients with advanced renal failure. Bone biopsies show an increase in the osteoid seam width and impaired mineralization activity. The pathogenesis of decreased skeletal mineralization in patients with chronic renal failure is not clear. It is conceivable that altered vitamin D metabolism leads to impaired mineralization of bone. Whether 1,25(OH)$_2$D$_3$ directly stimulates bone mineralization or leads to mineral deposition by increasing the levels of calcium and phosphate

in the extracellular fluid surrounding bone is controversial. Although the plasma levels of 1,25(OH)$_2$D$_3$ are reduced in patients with advanced renal insufficiency, overt osteomalacia is found in only a small fraction of patients (34). Moreover, osteomalacia may be absent even in anephric patients (35). Thus other factors appear to participate in the pathogenesis of osteomalacia in uremic patients. One factor that may influence the development of osteomalacia is the level of plasma phosphorus. Hypophosphatemia per se can produce severe osteomalacia even in patients with normal renal function. Alterations in collagen synthesis and maturation may also contribute to the development of osteomalacia. Experimental studies in uremic rats have shown a preponderance of immature soluble collagen that fails to mineralize normally. Treatment of such uremic animals with 25(OH)D can normalize collagen maturation (74). Bone crystal formation also is affected in patients with renal insufficiency. Immature bone contains large quantities of amorphous calcium phosphate. Other abnormalities in the bone of uremic patients include an increase in magnesium and pyrophosphate content and decreased amounts of carbonate. A combination of these factors may play a role in bone maturation and contribute to the development of uremic osteomalacia. Acidosis may also contribute to the pathogenesis of renal osteodystrophy. Administration of bicarbonate and correction of the acidosis in azotemic patients can reduce fecal calcium, improve calcium balance, (75) and therefore may be of therapeutic benefit.

It is now clear that the retention of aluminum plays an important role in the development of osteomalacia. In patients with advanced renal failure treated with dialysis, the major source of aluminum may be from the dialysate. In geographical areas with a high aluminum content in the tap water used for dialysate, the incidence of osteomalacia appears to decrease with subsequent deionization treatment (76). However, recent evidence in the United States suggests that the main source of aluminum accumulation is the ingestion of phosphate binders containing aluminum. Finally, evidence suggests that a lack of PTH, as has been seen in uremic patients after total parathyroidectomy, can precipitate the development of osteomalacia (77,78).

BONE HISTOLOGY

Secondary Hyperparathyroidism (High-Turnover Bone Disease)

Examination of bone is often important for the diagnosis and management of patients with renal osteodystrophy (Figs. 6 and 7). The most common histological finding is osteitis fibrosa secondary to high circulating levels of PTH. In these patients the histological findings are osteoclastosis and increased bone resorption surfaces

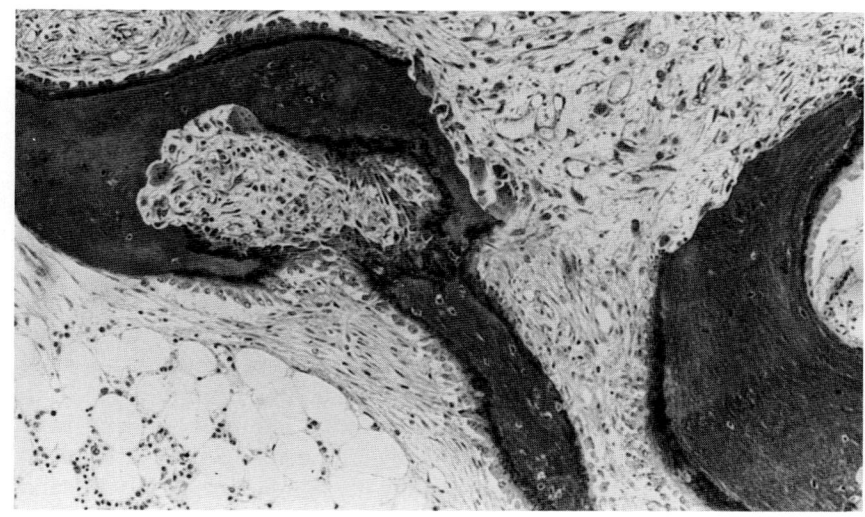

FIG. 6. Baseline bone biopsy from a patient on chronic maintenance dialysis exhibiting signs of marked secondary hyperparathyroid bone disease. Features include irregular trabecular structure, increased osteoid surface and volume, abundance of osteoblasts and osteoclasts, and marked bone marrow fibrosis. Mineralized bone histology. Undecalcified 3-μm-thick section. Modified Masson-Goldner trichrome. Original magnification ×12. (Courtesy of Dr. Malluche.)

(as reflected by many Howship lacunae). Osteoblastic activity is also substantially increased in patients with osteitis fibrosa. The total number of osteoblasts is usually increased, and a large percentage of the surface of bone is involved in bone formation. Bone biopsies characteristically show increased bone turnover, as indicated from double tetracycline labeling and increased quantities of woven osteoid. This differs from normal lamellar osteoid in that it exhibits a haphazard arrangement of collagen fibers. Woven osteoid can be mineralized, but the calcium may be deposited as amorphous calcium phosphate rather than as hydroxyapatite. The excess deposition of calcium phosphate in woven osteoid may explain the presence of osteosclerosis in some uremic patients.

Osteomalacia (Low-Turnover Bone Disease)

This form of bone disease is characterized by a reduction in the number of bone-forming and bone-resorbing cells in association with an accumulation of lamellar osteoid or unmineralized bone collagen detectable in a large proportion of the trabecular bone. Osteoidosis, however, does not indicate the presence of osteomalacia or defective mineralization. The amount of osteoid present in bone depends on the rate and extent of its formation by osteoblasts and the rate and extent of calcification. Thus, to make the histological diagnosis of osteomalacia, an abnormal mineralization front must be present. Osteoidosis, with a decreased calcification front has been taken to be evidence for osteomalacia. The use of double tetracycline labeling in conjunction with quantitative histomorphometric techniques provides the best method for identification of defective mineralization. The bone turnover rate (measured with double tetracycline labeling) is normal or increased in patients with osteitis fibrosa, whereas it is below normal in patients with osteomalacia. Dialysis patients with pure osteomalacia usually show little or no evidence of secondary hyperparathyroidism (79). Osteomalacia in patients

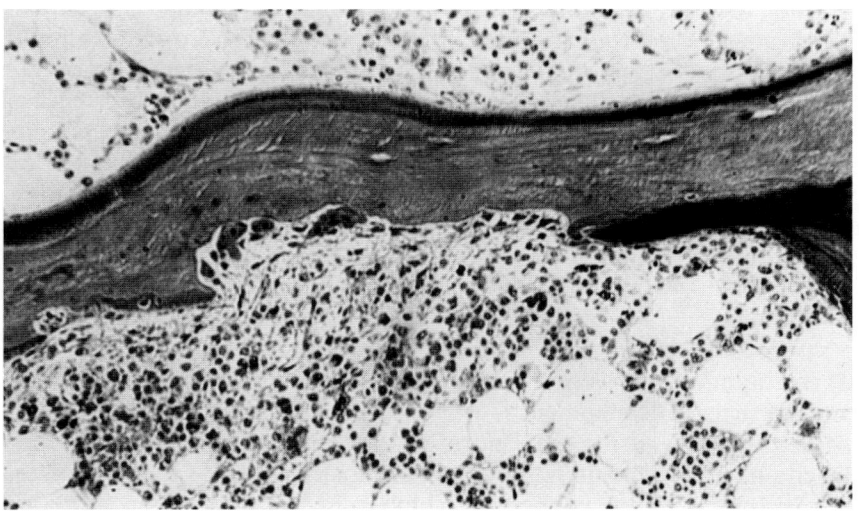

FIG. 7. Bone biopsy in the same patient as Fig. 6. 1 year after therapy with oral 1,25(OH)$_2$D$_3$ therapy. There was a decrease in the severity of hyperparathyroidism with decreased osteoid volume and surface, reduction in the number of osteoblasts and osteoclasts, and less marrow fibrosis. Mineralized bone histology. Undecalcified 3-μm-thick section. Modified Masson-Goldner trichome. Original magnification ×20. (Courtesy of Dr. Malluche.)

with chronic renal disease can result from vitamin D deficiency or from hypocalcemia and/or hypophosphatemia. However, in patients maintained on chronic hemodialysis, aluminum toxicity currently accounts for most of the osteomalacic lesions. In these patients, stainable aluminum deposits at the bone–osteoid surface are usually seen. A disorder termed *aplastic* or *adynamic* refers to bone histology exhibiting normal amounts of osteoid, no tissue fibrosis, diminished number of osteoblasts and osteoclasts, and low rates of bone formation. Patients with this lesion may have had a high exposure to aluminum.

Mixed Lesion

Some patients demonstrate histological evidence of both osteitis fibrosa and osteomalacia on bone biopsy. This pattern is termed a *mixed lesion* of renal osteodystrophy (80). Such patients frequently have biochemical findings characteristic of high PTH in addition to features that are associated with impaired bone formation and mineralization. Tetracycline studies reveals a decrease in the double-labeled lamellar osteoid seams. Usually, there is an increased number of osteoblasts, osteoclasts, and moderate peritrabecular fibrosis. Mixed renal osteodystrophy is seen in patients with previously established osteitis fibrosa who are developing aluminum-related bone disease. A large number of patients with mixed lesions have significant stainable aluminum at the mineralization front.

CLINICAL AND BIOCHEMICAL FEATURES OF ALTERED DIVALENT-ION METABOLISM

Alterations in mineral homeostasis may appear early in the course of renal insufficiency, and their identification should assist the physician in the introduction of prompt treatment to prevent renal osteodystrophy. On the other hand, symptoms from altered divalent-ion metabolism usually appear only in patients with advanced renal failure. Bone pain can develop and slowly progress to the point where the patient becomes bedridden. Moreover, this can occur whether the skeletal abnormality is osteitis fibrosa or osteomalacia. The bone pain is generally vague and commonly is located in the lower back, hips, knees, and legs. Low back pain may arise from collapse of a vertebral body, and sharp chest pain may result from spontaneous rib fractures. However, physical findings frequently are lacking. Muscular weakness, when present, usually is proximal; it appears slowly and progresses. Plasma levels of muscle enzymes, creatinine phosphokinase and transaminase, usually are normal, and the electromyographic changes are nonspecific. The pathogenesis of such muscle weakness is uncertain. In patients with such myopathy, electron micrographic

studies have revealed localized disorganization of the myofibrils and dispersion of Z bands. These changes revert to normal following treatment with 25(OH)D (81). The muscular weakness has also been attributed to secondary hyperparathyroidism on a neuropathic basis (82). Finally, we have seen the resolution of muscle weakness following treatment of aluminum excess with chelation therapy. Pruritus, an especially common symptom in uremic patients with severe secondary hyperparathyroidism, has been attributed to increased levels of calcium in the skin. Moreover, pruritus can develop in uremic patients receiving pharmacological doses of vitamin D and during the infusion of calcium. In patients with chronic renal failure, peripheral ischemic necrosis and vascular calcification have been reported. The lesions may involve the tips of the toes and fingers, where the skin becomes violaceous. Ulceration and scar formation may occur, with clear demarcation of the lesions from the surrounding skin. Most patients with such problems have concomitant severe secondary hyperparathyroidism, and some have benefited from subtotal parathyroidectomy (Fig. 8).

Acute pain and swelling around one or more joints may develop in uremic patients. This syndrome of calcified periarthritis, which may be caused by the deposition of hydroxyapatite crystals, is associated with marked hyperphosphatemia (83). Abnormal collagen metabolism, as is believed to exist in uremic bone, may also occur in tendon and may predispose to spontaneous tendon rupture.

Patients maintained on chronic dialysis for more than 5 years may develop amyloid deposition in bone and soft tissues. This type of amyloid is comprised of β_2-microglobulin (84). Since β_2-microglobulin, a polypeptide, is degraded by the kidney, the serum levels increase substantially in renal failure. Amyloid deposition in the musculoskeletal system may cause symptoms that could be confused with those of renal osteodystrophy. A common manifestation is the development of the carpal tunnel syndrome, with entrapment of the median nerve by fibrous and amyloid tissue. In addition, erosive arthritis of the shoulders and interphalangeal joints and knees are frequently seen. X-rays may demonstrate the presence of cysts in the humerus (Figs. 9 and 10), femoral head, acetabulum carpal and tarsal bones. Fractures can develop in bones affected and weakened by these cystic changes (85). Currently, it is not entirely known why all dialysis patients are not affected by amyloidosis or if certain methods of dialysis will influence the natural history of this disorder. Unfortunately, the clinical management of this pathological condition is unsatisfactory. It is likely, however, that early transplantation would prevent its development.

Skeletal deformities are common in growing azotemic children. Bowing of the tibiae and femor and deformities due to slipped epiphyses are not uncommon. Children

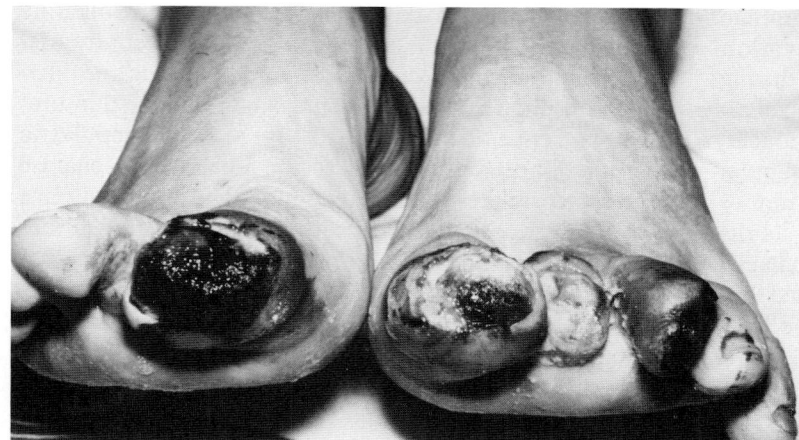

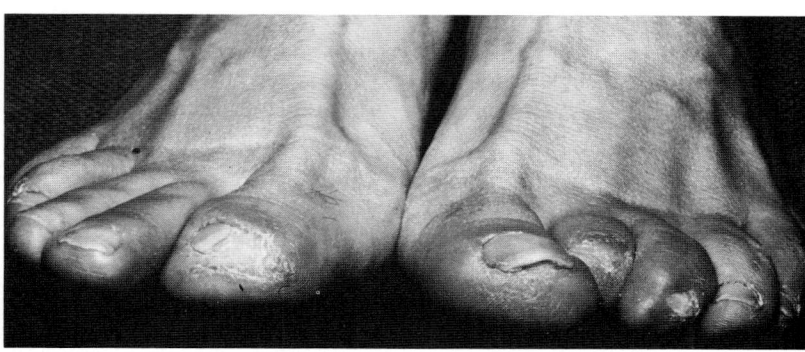

FIG. 8. A: Necrosis of the toes, 5 months after renal transplantation, in a patient with long history of chronic renal failure. **B:** Complete healing of lesions in same patient 3 months after subtotal parathyroidectomy. (From S. G. Massry et al., *Arch Intern Med.* 1969;124:431–9.)

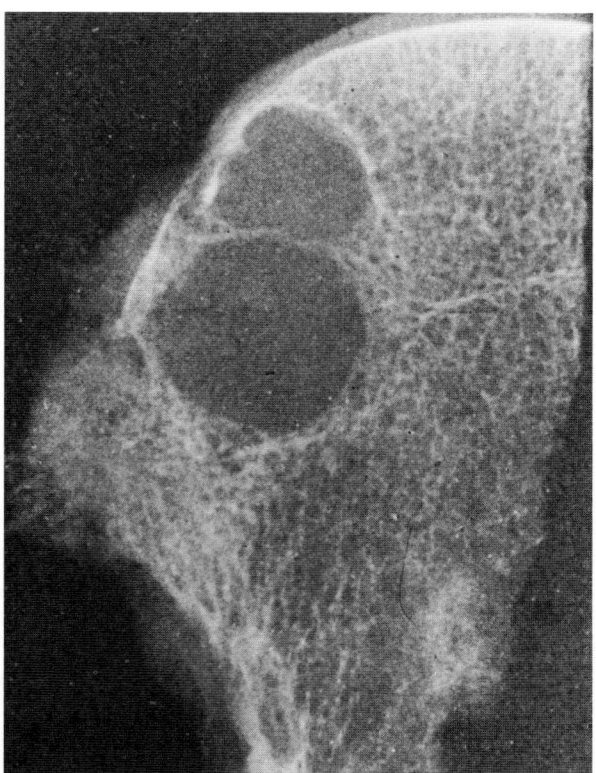

FIG. 9. Two large cysts in the head of the humerus [From A. Alfrey, AKF, *Nephrol Lett,* 1989;6:(4).]

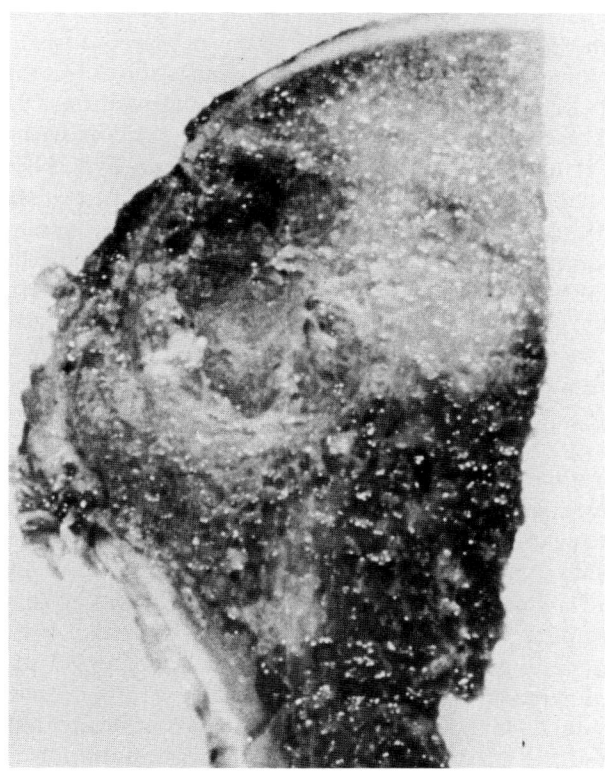

FIG. 10. Gross appearance of the bone shown in radiograph (Fig. 9). Cystic lesions are filled with β_2-microglobulin amyloid. [From A. Alfrey, AKF, *Nephrol Lett* 1989;6:(4).]

with renal rickets sometimes exhibit typical radiographic findings of vitamin D deficiency. Growth retardation usually is seen in young children both before and during maintenance hemodialysis. Several factors, such as malnutrition, chronic acidosis, and severe osteomalacia, may contribute to the retarded growth. Caloric supplementation, correction of acidosis, and addition of $1,25(OH)_2D_3$ may improve the growth rate. In adults with renal failure, particularly those with osteomalacia, marked skeletal deformities, with lumbar scoliosis, thoracic kyphosis, and deformities of the thoracic cage, may be observed.

From the biochemical point of view, one of the early changes in patients with renal insufficiency (GFR between 60 and 80 mL/min) is the presence of elevated levels of circulating iPTH. As the disease progresses (GFR less than 30 mL/min), hypocalcemia may be present. Alterations in circulating ionized calcium levels are seen earlier than in total calcium values. This is because of an increase in the complexed fraction of blood calcium. However, the serum calcium levels usually remain close to normal in patients with advanced renal insufficiency with values below 7.5 mg/dL noted infrequently. Usually, hypocalcemia is most marked in patients with severe osteomalacia or profound metabolic acidosis. Occasionally, hypercalcemia may be observed in uremic patients, particularly in those undergoing long-term dialysis. This can arise from severe secondary hyperparathyroidism, ingestion of large amounts of calcium or vitamin D, unrelated diseases such as sarcoidosis or malignancy, or from a "pure" mineralization defect that is believed to arise from aluminum accumulation (79).

Hyperphosphatemia is common in patients with a GFR less than 25 mL/min. The degree of hyperphosphatemia depends on the amount of phosphate ingested in the diet, the fraction absorbed by the intestine, and the quantity excreted into the urine. Obviously, if the patient ingests phosphate binders, the serum phosphorus may remain normal despite advanced renal insufficiency. PTH can also influence the concentration of serum phosphate ion. Although PTH decreases the reabsorption of phosphorus by the renal tubule, it mobilizes phosphorus from bone. Thus patients with severe hyperparathyroidism and advanced renal insufficiency usually have high serum concentrations of phosphate. Hypermagnesemia occurs in renal patients when the GFR falls below 15 mL/min. Intake of magnesium-containing antacids by patients with severe renal failure can lead to an abrupt and marked hypermagnesemia. Increased serum magnesium is usually associated with an increased content of magnesium in bone, which may, in turn, decrease crystal formation. In patients receiving chronic hemodialysis, with a dialysate magnesium concentration of 1.5 mEq/L, hypermagnesemia with blood levels of 2.5 to 3.0 mEq/L is common. Serum alkaline phosphatase activity is often increased in uremic patients with osteitis fibrosa,

osteomalacia, or mixed lesions. Although serum alkaline phosphatase activity is composed of isozyme activity arising from intestine, liver, kidney, and bone, routine alkaline phosphatase measurements, when increased in uremic patients, usually suggest increased osteoblastic activity. In dialysis patients, serum alkaline phosphatase activity correlates with the extent of bone osteoid surface covered with osteoblasts, resorbing surfaces, the number of osteoclasts, and the percentage of osteoid seams that take up tetracycline (86,87). Coexistent liver disease, however, should be excluded as a cause of elevated alkaline phosphatase in uremic patients. Bone Gla protein, also known as osteocalcin, synthesized by the osteoblast is a marker of bone formation. However plasma levels are increased when renal function is impaired. In dialysis patients there is a good correlation between the levels of osteocalcin, PTH, and alkaline phosphatase. Patients with high bone turnover and severe secondary hyperparathyroidism usually have high levels of circulating osteocalcin.

RADIOGRAPHIC FEATURES OF RENAL OSTEODYSTROPHY

Standard radiographic methods, as applied in clinical practice, often are inconsistent in identifying progression of renal osteodystrophy. Techniques to increase the sensitivity of x-ray studies (which are particularly applicable for views of the hands) include the use of fine-grained film (i.e., Kodak M industrial film or mammography film). The main radiographic feature of secondary hyperparathyroidism is increased bone resorption, most commonly seen on the subperiosteal surfaces of bone. Erosions that occur in conjunction with formation of new bone may appear as cysts or osteoclastomas (brown tumors). The presence of subperiosteal erosions correlates with serum iPTH and histomorphometric features of osteitis fibrosa on biopsy (86,87). Subperiosteal erosions of the phalanges (detected by fine-grained hand radiographs) may be the most sensitive radiographic sign of secondary hyperparathyroidism (Fig. 11). The tuft of the terminal phalanx of the second or third digit commonly shows resorption, and there may be collapse of the overlying soft tissue, so that the finger appears clubbed. Bone erosions also may occur at the proximal end of the tibia, the neck of the femur or humerus, and the inferior surface of the distal end of the clavicle. In the skull there is a mottled and granular appearance, with areas of resorption commonly associated with areas of osteosclerosis. The lamina dura of the teeth often shows erosions in primary hyperparathyroidism but is uncommonly affected by secondary hyperparathyroidism. Osteosclerosis, another feature of osteitis fibrosa, is due to an increase in the thickness and number of trabeculae in spongy bone and accounts for the typical "rugger jersey"

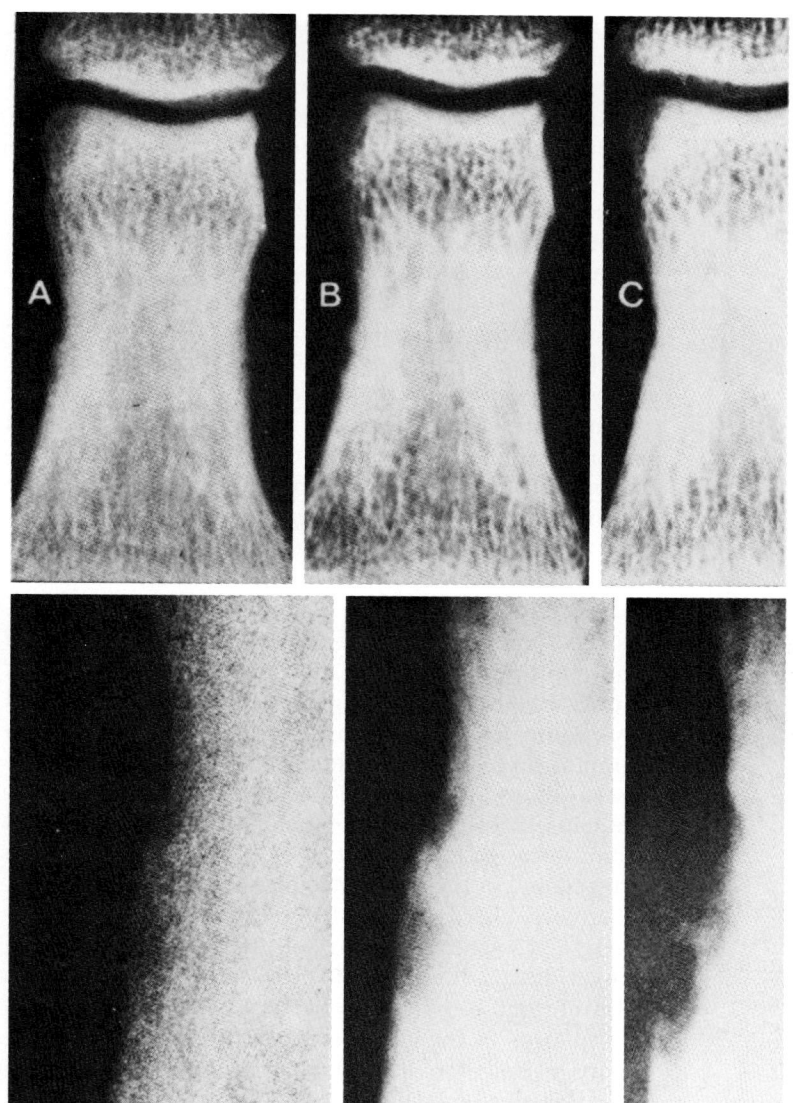

FIG. 11. Serial radiographs of the right index finger of a 43-year-old man with chronic renal failure under treatment with peritoneal dialysis. These views illustrate the value of fine-grain film and the use of simple magnification techniques to detect changes in periosteal resorption. The upper panels are magnified ×3, the lower ×12. **A:** The periosteal resorption at the midshaft is poorly identified, owing to the large-grain film (Kodak dental film). **B:** The radiolucent areas in the cortex are more clearly visualized, but only the higher magnification shows convincingly that there is an intact periosteal layer of bone covering these juxtaperiosteal resorption cavities. **C:** Six months later, juxtaperiosteal resorption had progressed to periosteal resorption. (B and C, Kodak M-film). (Reproduced from H. E. Meema and S. Meema, *Clin Orthop* 1978;130:297–310.)

appearance of the spine. Although the Looser zone or pseudofracture is considered pathognomonic of rickets in children or of osteomalacia in the adult, the x-ray features of osteomalacia often are less distinctive than those of secondary hyperparathyroidism. The typical x-ray feature of rickets (i.e., widening of the epiphyseal growth plate) cannot develop after epiphyseal closure, and hence this radiographic sign of defective bone mineralization is limited to children. With mechanical stress on the skeleton affected by rickets or osteomalacia, a Looser zone may extend across a bone and produce a true fracture (88). Features such as increased haziness or indistinctiveness of the trabeculae, biconcavity of the vertebral bodies (particularly in association with normal bone density), and deformities of long bones are said to be typical of osteomalacia, but these findings are uncommon and may not be easily recognized. Furthermore, uremic patients with osteomalacia commonly have sec-

ondary hyperparathyroidism with concomitant x-ray features of the latter. Thus the definitive diagnosis of osteomalacia requires a bone biopsy.

EXTRASKELETAL CALCIFICATIONS

The factors that predispose the appearance of soft-tissue calcification include an increase in the circulating calcium–phosphate product in plasma, the degree of secondary hyperparathyroidism, the magnitude of alkalosis, and local tissue injury (89). Three major varieties include (1) calcification of medium-sized arteries, (2) articular or tumoral calcification, and (3) visceral calcification affecting the heart, lung, and kidney. Arterial calcification often involves the media of the vessel. These calcifications are diffuse and continuous along the vessels, and their appearance contrasts to the regular dis-

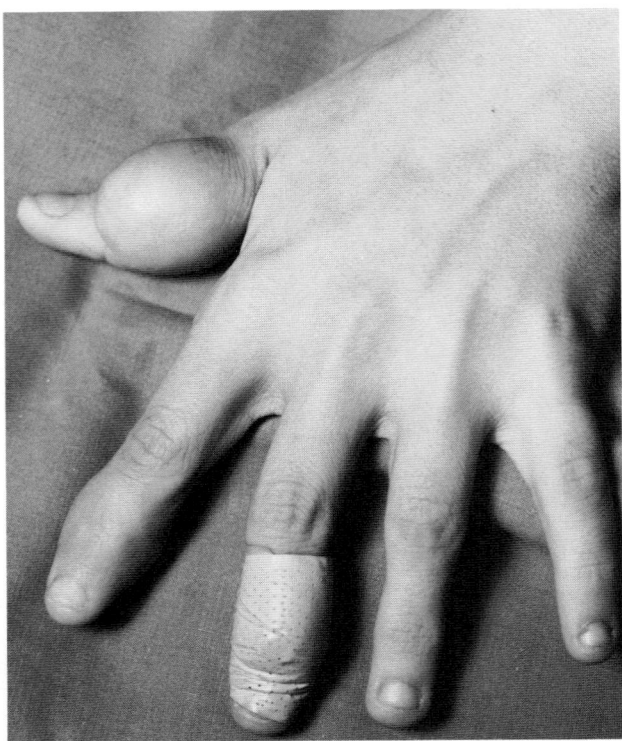

FIG. 12. Severe metastatic calcification of the left thumb in a patient maintained on chronic dialysis with a high Ca-P product.

crete appearance of calcified intimal plaques. Such medial calcification of the vessels may be seen first in the dorsalis pedis artery, where it appears as a ring or tube as it descends between the first and second metatarsals. Other sites commonly involved are the ankles, abdominal aorta, feet, pelvis, hands, and wrists (Fig. 12).

THERAPEUTIC APPROACH TO RENAL OSTEODYSTROPHY

Phosphate Retention

Hyperphosphatemia is a major factor accounting for the development and maintenance of secondary hyperparathyroidism in uremia. High serum phosphorus levels also contribute to the development of soft-tissue calcification in patients with advanced uremia. Thus restriction of dietary phosphorus and prevention of hyperphosphatemia are critical in the management of renal bone disease.

The intake of phosphorus depends primarily on meat and dairy products in the diet. The usual phosphorus intake by normal adults in the United States is 1.0–1.4 g/day. One can lower the dietary intake of phosphorus by restricting the intake of dairy products and by rigid adherence to a low-protein diet. However, there would be great difficulty in lowering phosphorus intake in pro-

portion to the reduced GFR in patients with advanced renal failure by use of dietary manipulation alone. Moreover, low-phosphate diets are generally unpalatable to the tastes of most people living in the United States, and aluminum-containing compounds that reduce the intestinal absorption of phosphorus are often prescribed (90). These compounds include aluminum hydroxide and aluminum carbonate gels, which are available in liquid, tablet, and capsule form. The capsules are less effective than liquid gels in binding phosphorus (91), but patient compliance is easier to achieve with capsules than with either the liquid or the tablets. The goal of such therapy in dialysis patients is to reduce serum phosphorus to near normal in patients treated conservatively; predialysis serum phosphorus levels are ideally maintained at 5.0–5.5 mg/dL. In patients with creatinine clearances below 10 mL/min and in those undergoing treatment with dialysis, dietary phosphorus should be restricted to 800–900 mg/day. One to three capsules of aluminum hydroxide or aluminum carbonate are often taken with each meal.

It was generally assumed that aluminum hydroxide and aluminum carbonate are nonabsorbable and safe. However, reported data suggest that orally administered aluminum may be absorbed in significant amounts in humans and in experimental animals, and such treatment can lead to increased plasma and tissue aluminum content (92,93). It is clear that dialysis dementia (93) and some forms of low bone turnover osteodystrophy (94) are related to the tissue accumulation of aluminum. Therefore, alternative binders of phosphorus in the gut have been sought. Clarkson et al. (95) demonstrated that a high dietary intake of calcium carbonate in patients with chronic renal failure decreased the absorption of phosphorus in the gastrointestinal tract. Subsequently, many investigators have shown that calcium carbonate is an effective phosphate binder (96–98) (Fig. 13). However, the administration of calcium carbonate is not completely free of side effects. Transient episodes of hypercalcemia have been observed frequently by several investigators (96–98). In the United States most patients undergo hemodialysis with dialysate containing 3.0–3.5 mEq/L of calcium. Since a positive calcium balance is induced during dialysis with dialysate calcium levels above 3.5 mEq/L, the administration of large amounts of calcium carbonate could increase the risk of hypercalcemia and extraskeletal calcifications. Several investigators (99–101) have attempted to decrease the incidence of hypercalcemic episodes by diminishing the amount of calcium in the dialysate. Slatopolsky et al. (101) evaluated the effect of long-term administration of calcium carbonate (mean dose, 10.5 g/day, range 2.5–28 g/day) in conjunction with use of a dialysate with the calcium lowered to 2.5 mEq/L in the management of hyperphosphatemia in patients undergoing maintenance hemodialysis. They confirmed the effectiveness of calcium carbonate as a phosphate binder.

TABLE 1. *Guidelines for management of renal osteodystrophy*

Control of Serum Phosphorus (target 4.5–5.5 mg/dL)
Restrict dietary phosphorus (P) intake to 0.7–0.9 g/day.
Individualize dosage of phosphate binders and ingest with meals: calcium carbonate, calcium acetate, aluminum hydroxide, or aluminum carbonate.
Minimize exposure to aluminum-containing compounds.
Avoid hypophosphatemia.

Adequate Calcium Intake
Give oral calcium supplements providing 1–2 g/day, when serum P is controlled.
Dialysate Ca should be 6.0–6.5 mg/dL (3.0–3.25 mEq/L).
In patients ingesting large doses of $CaCO_3$, dialysate Ca may be reduced to 5.0 mg/dL (2.5 mEq/L).

Use of Vitamin D Sterols
INDICATIONS FOR TREATMENT
Hypocalcemia in the presence of adequate P control
Overt second-degree hyperparathyroidism (high iPTH and high alkaline phosphatase with bone erosions) and serum Ca < 11.0 mg/dL
Osteomalacia not related to aluminum
Advanced renal failure in children
Concomitant anticonvulsant therapy
Proximal myopathy
Prophylaxis in dialysis patients (cost-benefit ratio not established)

TYPES AND APPROXIMATE DAILY DOSES
Vitamin D_2 or D_3: 10,000–200,000 IU/day (0.25–5.0 mg/day)
Dihydrotachysterol: 0.25–2.0 mg/day
Calcifediol, 25(OH)D_3: 25–100 μg/day
Calcitriol, 1,25(OH)$_2D_3$
 Oral: 0.25–1.0 μg/day
 IV: 1.0–3.0 μg thrice weekly

Parathyroidectomy
INDICATIONS: Evidence of second-degree hyperparathyroidism (x-ray erosions, biopsy: osteitis fibrosa, and markedly elevated iPTH) and exclusion of aluminum-related bone disease.
In this setting, the following may improve with parathyroidectomy:
Persistent hypercalcemia (serum Ca > 11.5–12.0 mg/dL)
Progressive or symptomatic extraskeletal calcification (particularly with serum Ca × P product > 75 mg/dL)
Pruritus not responsive to other treatment
Calciphylaxis (ischemic ulcers and necrosis)
Symptomatic and persistent hypercalcemia after renal transplantation

Management of Aluminum Overload
INDICATIONS FOR TREATMENT: Symptoms of osteomalacia, myopathy, or encephalopathy plus evidence of Al overload proven by bone biopsy.
Substitute $CaCO_3$ for Al-containing phosphorus binders.
Deferrioxamine infusions for Al chelation (1.0–3.0 g, once weekly).

Other Treatment Considerations
Purification of water for dialysate preparation: Aluminum conc. < 10 μg/L and removal of fluoride, calcium, and magnesium.
Normalized acid-base status.
Appropriate dialysate magnesium: 0.6–1.0 mg/dL (0.5–0.7 mEq/L).
Avoid unnecessary treatment with phenytoin, barbiturates, or glutethimide.

Source: Modified from J. W. Coburn et al., in M. H. Maxwell and C. R. Kleeman, eds., *Clinical disorders of fluid and electrolyte metabolism,* 3rd ed., McGraw-Hill, New York, 1980.

Moreover, the development of hypercalcemia was greatly minimized by the concomitant reduction of calcium concentration in the dialysate. It is important to emphasize that patients maintained on a dialysate concentration of 2.5 mEq/L may develop severe secondary hyperparathyroidism with the administration of small amounts of calcium carbonate. Therefore, the use of a dialysate formulated in this manner should be restricted to these patients who demonstrate compliance with the ingestion of the prescribed doses of calcium carbonate. When calcium carbonate is prescribed as a phosphate binder, it must be ingested with a meal, both to increase the efficiency of phosphate binding and to minimize the absorption of calcium and the consequent risk of hyper-

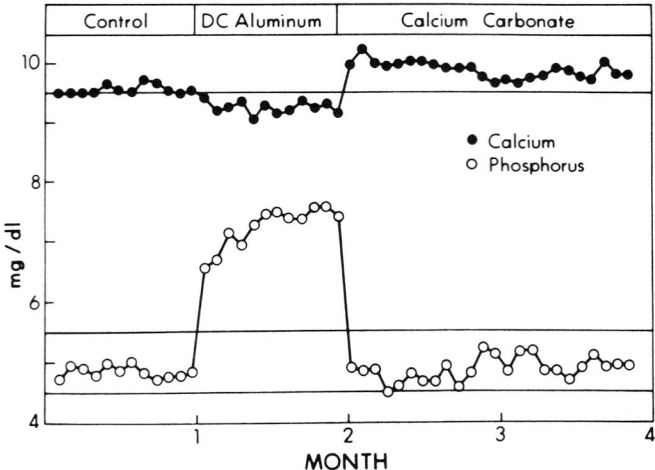

FIG. 13. Temporal relationship between serum calcium and phosphorus in a group of 20 patients maintained on chronic dialysis. During the control part of the studies, the patients ingested phosphate binders containing aluminum. In the second part the aluminum binders were discontinued. In the third part of the study, the patients received calcium carbonate as a phosphate binder. (From E. Slatopolsky et al., *N Engl J Med* 1986;315:157–61.)

calcemia (102). We recommend that dietitians determine the total amount of phosphorus ingested over 24 h and during each meal. There is both patient to patient variability and variability from meal to meal in the same patient. Thus, to prevent the development of hypercalcemia, it is important to prescribe calcium carbonate according to the amount of phosphorus ingested with each meal. The dose of calcium carbonate ingested with each meal should be adjusted to match the phosphorus intake at that time. In general, 1.0–2.0 g of calcium carbonate with each meal would be a reasonable initial dose. Sheikh et al. (103) demonstrated that calcium acetate may bind phosphorus more efficiently than calcium carbonate or calcium citrate. These investigators found that calcium acetate bound 1.0 ± 0.1 mg of phosphorus per milligram of calcium absorbed. This was better than both calcium carbonate (0.57 ± 0.5 mg of phosphorus per milligram of calcium absorbed) and calcium citrate (0.47 ± 0.5 mg of phosphorus per milligram of calcium absorbed). If these results are confirmed by others, calcium acetate may prove to be a clinically useful phosphate binder. Recently, it has been shown (104) that calcium citrate increases aluminum absorption. Thus this salt should not be given to patients with renal failure if there is any potential that they may also ingest aluminum-containing drugs.

If the serum calcium reaches a concentration of 11.0 mg/dL, the amount of calcium carbonate given should not be increased further. In the small number of patients who still have hyperphosphatemia, the patient should receive phosphate binders containing aluminum.

Calcium Supplements

Since impaired calcium absorption exists in patients with advanced renal failure, including those undergoing dialysis, and since their diets generally contain suboptimal quantities of calcium, oral calcium supplements are usually necessary. Studies of net intestinal calcium absorption suggest that a neutral or positive calcium balance can be achieved in uremic patients when supplemental calcium increases the total elemental calcium intake above 1.5 g/day (95,105).

Long-term treatment with large doses of oral calcium supplements has been reported to reduce the incidence of bone resorption lesions, fractures, and episodes of pseudogout or extraskeletal calcification (95). Another study showed lower plasma levels of alkaline phosphatase and iPTH in uremic patients receiving calcium supplements compared to controls (106).

Treatment with oral calcium supplements is not without risk. Calcium supplements should not be given to a patient with marked hyperphosphatemia because of the risk of increasing the Ca × P product and the consequent predisposition for the development of extraskeletal calcification. Hypercalcemia clearly can develop in uremic patients during oral therapy with calcium salts. Calcium carbonate is currently the first choice as a source of supplemental calcium, because it contains a high fraction of calcium and is inexpensive, tasteless, and relatively well tolerated. Calcium carbonate contains 40% elemental calcium. Calcium carbonate is available in several proprietary preparations, including Os-cal, Titralac, and Tums.

Concentration of Calcium in the Hemodialysis Dialysate

A number of studies have observed an effect on different dialysate calcium levels on the progress of renal bone disease. With the use of dialysate calcium levels lower than 6.0 mg/dL (3 mEq/L), evidence of progressive bone disease has been suggested by a progressive increase in plasma alkaline phosphatase (107) and bone deterioration on radiographs (108,109). This, in part, was due to the flux of diffusable calcium from the serum to the dialysate. From such information it was generally recommended that the dialysate calcium concentration be 3.0–3.5 mEq/L. However, such data were obtained in patients ingesting aluminum-containing phosphate binders. In uremic patients ingesting large doses of calcium carbonate as a phosphate binder, there is considerable risk of hypercalcemia with the use of such dialysate. Under these circumstances, lowering the dialysate calcium to 2.5 mEq/L may confer an additional level of safety (99–101).

Use of Vitamin D Sterols

Despite dietary phosphate restriction, the use of phosphate binders, the choice of an appropriate level of calcium in dialysate, and an intake of adequate amounts of dietary calcium, a significant number of uremic patients still develop skeletal disease. A growing understanding of the kidney's role in producing $1,25(OH)_2D_3$ has created interest in the use of active vitamin D sterols in such patients.

When uremic patients have evidence of overt secondary hyperparathyroidism (e.g., bone erosions, high iPTH levels, and increased alkaline phosphatase), treatment with a vitamin D sterol often leads to improvement. Thus treatment with vitamin D_2 (110) dihydrotachysterol (111,112), $25(OH)D_3$ (calcifidiol) (113,114), 1α-hydroxyvitamin D_3 (alfacalcidiol) (115), and $1,25(OH)_2D_3$ (calcitriol) (116,117) can improve symptoms, the radiographic appearance of bone, skeletal histology, and can lower the serum levels of alkaline phosphatase and iPTH.

Vitamin D administration is not without hazard. Hypercalcemia can develop even in anephric patients and may require several weeks for resolution (118). Such hypercalcemia develops as a consequence of high blood levels of $25(OH)D_3$ in the face of normal levels of $1,25(OH)_2D_3$ (119). Vitamin D sterols should not be used when hyperphosphatemia is present because the increase in $Ca \times P$ product can predispose to the development of extraskeletal calcification.

Although there is an apparent block in the 1-hydroxylation of $25(OH)D_3$, considerable data indicate that uremic patients can respond favorably to this sterol when it is given in doses of less than 100 μg/day. A reversal of symptoms of bone disease and improvement of histological evidence of severe secondary hyperparathyroidism in bone have been observed in adults (120) and children (113) given $25(OH)D_3$. Preliminary results from a six-center study indicate improvement in symptoms of bone pain, a fall in alkaline phosphatase, and a decrease in the degree of osteitis fibrosa during treatment of uremic patients with $25(OH)D_3$ (114). Hypercalcemia developed in some patients which was associated with the increase in the plasma level of $25(OH)D$ to supranormal levels of 200–300 ng/mL (114). However, another study showed improved bone mineralization during treatment with $25(OH)D_3$ in quantities that did not increase plasma levels of $25(OH)D_3$ to the normal range (121).

Results of several clinical trials indicate efficacy of $1,25(OH)_2D_3$ in treating patients with symptomatic renal osteodystrophy. These clinical evaluations have shown a decrease in bone pain, improvement in muscle strength, and decrease in plasma alkaline phosphatase (116,117,122). Studies of bone histology have revealed a prominent decrease in marrow fibrosis and other features of secondary hyperparathyroidism (123,124). In addition, bone mineralization improved in some patients with osteomalacic lesions (124,125), although these effects occurred more slowly. A decrease in serum phosphorus levels has been observed, particularly early in the course of treatment in patients who exhibited a favorable response. Increments in serum phosphorus levels have also been noted later in the course of treatment. Studies in uremic children indicate that treatment with $1,25(OH)_2D_3$ may increase the growth rate, particularly after plasma alkaline phosphatase and serum iPTH have substantially decreased toward normal (126).

The quantities of $1,25(OH)_2D_3$ utilized in these trials have varied from 0.14 to 1.5 μg/day, and the major side effect of such treatment has been the development of hypercalcemia. From results in a small number of patients with symptomatic bone disease, it has been suggested that a smaller dose of 0.5 μg/day may be efficacious and may result in a lower incidence of hypercalcemia (127). Hypercalcemia may occur after many weeks or months of treatment in patients who have a favorable response and may be heralded by a fall in plasma alkaline phosphatase to normal. Significant hypercalcemia may appear sooner in patients with aluminum-related bone disease or in those with severe secondary hyperparathyroidism who have serum calcium levels that are slightly above normal before treatment (118). The latter patients usually have massive parathyroid hyperplasia, and subtotal parathyroidectomy may be indicated.

Slatopolsky et al. (63) demonstrated that the intravenous administration of calcitriol markedly reduced the serum levels of PTH in hemodialysis patients. These results suggested that the suppression of PTH during intravenous administration of calcitriol was greater than that occurring after raising serum calcium levels with oral calcium carbonate (Fig. 14). It would seem that the greater suppressive effects of intravenous calcitriol versus oral calcitriol may relate to the high concentrations of calcitriol in serum following intravenous administration. Studies in vitro have clearly demonstrated that the suppression of PTH secretion by calcitriol is dose dependent (64).

The role of $1,25(OH)_2D_3$ treatment in the prophylaxis of skeletal disease for patients undergoing dialysis or those with mild renal failure remains controversial. It has been suggested that renal function may decrease in patients during treatment with $1,25(OH)_2D_3$ (128), although this may be related to hypercalcemia or phosphate retention. Recently, Baker et al. (129) demonstrated a beneficial effect of calcitriol in patients with moderate renal insufficiency. Further studies are needed to establish the prophylactic role of $1,25(OH)_2D_3$ in renal failure. Whether a deficiency of $24,25(OH)_2D_3$ plays a role in the pathogenesis of renal osteodystrophy

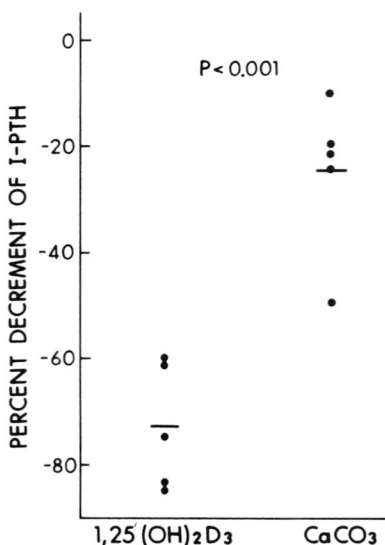

FIG. 14. Effects of intravenous 1,25(OH)$_2$D$_3$ or calcium carbonate on iPTH in 5 patients. A 73.5 ± 5.08% decrease in the levels of iPTH was observed during intravenous 1,25(OH)$_2$D$_3$ administration. The administration of calcium carbonate decreased the levels of iPTH by only 25 ± 6.65% ($p < 0.001$). The increment in serum calcium was the same (peak 10.9 ± 0.3) with both medications. (From E. Slatopolsky *J Clin Invest* 1984;2136–43.)

remains to be shown. Olgaard et al. (37) demonstrated that when given alone, 24,25(OH)$_2$D$_3$ does not have beneficial effects in uremic dogs.

Parathyroidectomy

The types of treatment discussed previously often lead to improvement of calcium and phosphorus homeostasis, reversal of symptoms of bone disease, and suppression of parathyroid secretion. However, such measures may be unsuccessful, and certain features of secondary hyperparathyroidism may necessitate parathyroid surgery. When this problem becomes a consideration, there should be ample evidence for the presence of severe secondary hyperparathyroidism, (e.g., very high levels of serum iPTH with bone erosions or the presence of osteitis fibrosa on bone biopsy). Also, it is important that aluminum-related bone disease be excluded. The features that may indicate the need for parathyroid surgery include (1) persistent hypercalcemia, particularly when symptomatic; (2) intractable pruritus that does not respond to dialysis or other medical treatment; (3) progressive extraskeletal calcifications that occur in conjunction with a Ca × P product that is consistently greater than 75–80, despite appropriate phosphate restriction; (4) severe and progressive skeletal pain or fractures; and (5) the appearance of calciphylaxis (ischemic lesions of soft tissue and skin and vascular calcification) (130–132).

Persistent and significant hypercalcemia (serum calcium level greater than 12.0 mg/dL) that occurs in association with symptoms of nausea or vomiting or evidence of ulcer disease may indicate a need for subtotal parathyroidectomy. Hypercalcemia can also develop in uremic patients who lack evidence of secondary hyperparathyroidism, and parathyroid surgery should not be undertaken unless bone erosions and elevated serum iPTH levels are documented.

The presence of marked hyperphosphatemia and overt secondary hyperparathyroidectomy in a noncompliant uremic patient presents a difficult therapeutic dilemma for the physician. Parathyroid surgery may lead to a transient lowering of blood phosphorus and even to the resolution of ectopic calcifications, but secondary hyperparathyroidism may recur, with all its manifestations, unless the patient follows the prescribed treatment with dietary phosphorus restriction and phosphate-binders compounds.

After parathyroid surgery, the treatment of hypocalcemia may pose a problem, although this may be less serious when some parathyroid tissue is left in place. The preoperative presence of skeletal erosions is frequently followed by severe hypocalcemia. The postoperative treatment of such patients with 1,25(OH)$_2$D$_3$, intravenous infusions of calcium gluconate and oral calcium supplements may be needed. Tetany and even seizures can occur during the postoperative period. Serum levels of phosphorus and magnesium may decrease after parathyroid surgery, and aluminum-containing phosphate binders should be withheld if the serum phosphorus falls below 2.5 mg/dL. However, serum phosphorus should not be allowed to increase above 4.5 mg/dL because of the risk of aggravating hypocalcemia. Rapid remineralization of the skeleton is usually occurring during this period, and blood calcium will usually begin to rise after the "hungry" bones have been repleted with calcium. A fall in the elevated plasma alkaline phosphatase toward normal may be a clue that rapid skeletal remineralization is nearly completed and indicates that calcium supplements and vitamin D dosage may be reduced or discontinued.

At time of parathyroidectomy four parathyroid glands should be identified, with the selection of one gland that is to be partially resected. A part of this gland is removed, leaving 60–80 mg of viable tissue in place. After the frozen sections are available from the first gland, each of the other three glands may be removed. The remnant parathyroid tissue left in situ may undergo hyperplasia leading to the reappearance of overt secondary hyperparathyroidism. The management of such a situation may be difficult. A second surgical procedure may be associated with greater technical difficulties and significant complications compared with the initial operation. Because of the difficulty and risk of a second surgical procedure, total parathyroidectomy with autotransplantation of some parathyroid tissue to the forearm has been recommended (133). Such tissue transplanted to the forearm may be more accessible for subsequent surgical removal. Another risk of parathyroid surgery is the development of hypoparathyroidism. To avoid this, parathyroid tissue should be frozen and stored to be implanted later if hypocalcemia persists. It would seem that a total parathyroidectomy has little place in the management of renal bone disease, since it may predispose uremic patients to the development of an isolated mineralizing defect.

The availability of highly active forms of vitamin D has made the need for parathyroid surgery less urgent (63). Whether one or more of the vitamin D analogs may be effective in leading to long-term suppression of the parathyroid glands must await further clinical evaluation.

Aluminum Accumulation

The presence of excessive quantities of trace metals, particularly aluminum, in the water used to prepare dialysate can cause bone disease in uremic patients (93). When a dialysis unit encounters an unusually high incidence of overt skeletal disease, the purity of the water supply should be tested and the methods of water treatment reevaluated. The amount of aluminum in the dialysate should not exceed 10 μg/L. However, it has become apparent in the United States that the main source of aluminum responsible for the development of bone disease is the ingestion of phosphate binders containing aluminum. Several reports have shown that deferrioxamine (DFO), a chelating agent, is useful as a diagnostic tool as well as therapeutic agent for patients with aluminum accumulation (134–136). When DFO is given intravenously in the dose of 20–30 mg/kg, an increase in the levels of serum aluminum is produced. If the increment in serum aluminum observed after the administration of DFO is greater than 250 μg/L, it is likely that the patient is at risk for the development of bone disease secondary to aluminum accumulation. Aluminum can be deposited in the mineralization front at the interface between bone and osteoid and may impair the normal mineralization of bone. Most of these patients also have low levels of circulating i-PTH. Although the "DFO test" may be a useful noninvasive tool in the diagnosis of aluminum accumulation, bone histomorphometry with special staining for aluminum is the definitive test in the diagnosis of aluminum-induced osteomalacia. If a patient requires DFO treatment for aluminum-induced osteomalacia, the usual dose of DFO is 2–3 g/week for 6–12 months. A second bone biopsy after 1 year can conclusively determine the effectiveness of the treatment. The use of dialyzers utilizing polysulfone membranes or cartridges containing activated colloidin-coated charcoal greatly increases the removal of aluminum during hemodialysis (137,138).

SPECIFIC CONSIDERATIONS IN CONTINUOUS AMBULATORY PERITONEAL DIALYSIS

The previous sections refer predominantly to patients treated conservatively or with chronic hemodialysis. In 1978, Popovich et al. (139) described a novel form of dialysis, termed *continuous ambulatory peritoneal dialysis* (CAPD) wherein 2 L of dialysate is instilled into the peritoneal cavity. Over the next 4–8 h solutes diffuse from the circulation to the dialysate at a rate inversely proportional to their molecular weight and proportional to the concentration gradient. The dialysate is then externally drained and a fresh solution is infused. Generally, four such exchanges are performed a day, 7 days a week. This results in a weekly clearance of small molecular weight solutes, such as urea (molecular weight 60 D), which is only 60% of that seen with chronic hemodialysis (140). However, the weekly clearance of larger molecules, such as vitamin B_{12} (molecular weight 1355 D), is threefold greater than that achieved with standard hemodialysis (140). For a variety of reasons, CAPD has grown in popularity in a number of countries. In the United States, approximately 10% of patients with end-stage renal failure are treated with CAPD. In the United Kingdom, almost 50% of such patients are undergoing CAPD.

The general principles of the pathogenesis and treatment of renal osteodystrophy are the same in chronic hemodialysis and in CAPD patients. Nonetheless, there are several unique features of CAPD that deserve attention. (For more extensive reviews, see Refs. 141 and 142.)

Mineral Metabolism

Unlike hemodialysis, CAPD is associated with a daily loss of 5–10 g of protein into the dialysate. Balance studies suggest that patients treated with CAPD should ingest 1.25 to 1.5 g/kg of protein per day to maintain nitrogen balance (143). This is considerably greater than the 0.9–1.0 gm/kg per day usually prescribed to hemodialysis patients. The higher protein intake generally necessitates a greater ingestion of phosphorus on the order of 900 mg/day or more. Assuming a 70% absorption of phosphorus by the intestine, dialysate removal of this anion is insufficient to maintain normal phosphorus levels. For example, we have previously shown that only 308 ± 2 mg of phosphorus is removed per day when the phosphorus levels of patients on CAPD were 5.2 ± 0.4 mg/dL (144). Blumenkrantz et al. (143), in short-term balance studies, found a net positive phosphorus balance of 708 ± 152 mg/day. Hence administration of phosphorus binders is essential in well-nourished patients on CAPD. Although it has been estimated that CAPD removes, on a weekly basis, approximately twice as much aluminum as does hemodialysis (141), it is likely that long-term administration of phosphorus binders containing aluminum will lead to aluminum toxicity (145,146). Calcium carbonate is an alternative phosphorus binder. However, when serum ionized calcium levels are maintained at the upper limits of normal with calcium supplements, there is a positive mass transfer of about 10 mg/day from a dialysate containing 3.5 mEq/L of calcium into the patient (144). This positive calcium balance may account for the relatively frequent episodes of hypercalcemia in patients treated with CAPD and oral calcium carbonate (147,148). Dialysate solutions containing 2.5 mEq/L calcium are now available. In the future it is conceivable that solutions with even lower concentrations of calcium may be warranted. A slow efflux of calcium into the dialysate would be countered by the absorption of phosphorus binders containing calcium. A very low concentration of calcium in the dialysate in hemodialysis would likely be hazardous because the inherent rapid fluxes could cause marked hypocalcemia.

The original concentration of magnesium in the dialysate was 1.5 mEq/L. This led to a daily removal of 30–50 mg into the dialysate (143,144). Because the removal of magnesium is less than that absorbed by the gastrointestinal tract, patients treated in this manner are in positive magnesium balance and hypermagnesemic. The long-term consequences of this are unknown. Dialysate solutions containing 0.5 mEq/L magnesium are now widely available and have been reported to reduce magnesium levels to normal (149). Magnesium salts, in conjunction with a low dialysate magnesium concentration, have been advocated by some as an alternative phosphorus binder in CAPD patients (149). Others (150), however, found that gastrointestinal side effects limited their usefulness.

Parathyroid Hormone

Unlike hemodialysis, a substantial amount of iPTH is removed during treatment with CAPD (144). Polyacrylamide gel electrophoresis of the dialysate shows a pattern similar to that seen in serum. Therefore, most of the iPTH removed during CAPD is comprised of biologically inactive carboxy-terminal fragments (144). Whether the clearance rate for iPTH of approximately 1.5 mL/min (144) contributes to the decline in iPTH levels reported by some (151) is unknown. However, others (152) noted a variable effect of CAPD on iPTH levels that correlated with the degree of fibrosis on bone histology (153).

Assuming that a portion of patients on CAPD develop progressive hyperparathyroidism despite good calcium and phosphorus control, issues arise concerning optimal management. Unlike hemodialysis, intravenous calcitriol is not feasible in CAPD. Delmez et al. (154) administered intraperitoneal calcitriol nightly to 11 CAPD patients for a period of 3 months. They found a profound fall in iPTH levels to approximately 50% of pretreatment values. The major, if not sole effect of intraperitoneal calcitriol in suppressing iPTH was felt to be due to increases in ionized calcium concentrations. Whether intraperitoneal calcitriol is superior to the oral form is unknown. However, because of cost and ease of administration, a course of oral calcitriol should be attempted before embarking on an intraperitoneal route of administration.

Vitamin D

Patients with nephrotic syndrome and normal renal function have low levels of 25(OH)D (155). Because patients on CAPD lose a comparable amount of protein into the dialysate per day, one would expect that levels of this metabolite would also be low. Unfortunately, the data are conflicting with both normal (144,152) and low (151,156–159) levels reported. A possible explanation for these discrepancies may be variability in the amount of sunlight exposure. Cassidy et al. (160) found a seasonal variation in the levels of 25(OH)D. Only one of 21 patients had low values during the summer, whereas 6 were low during the winter months. Although it is clear that 25(OH)D and vitamin D–binding protein are lost into the dialysate, it is likely that patients can maintain normal 25(OH)D levels if there is adequate substrate availability.

EFFECTS OF RENAL TRANSPLANTATION ON BONE AND MINERAL METABOLISM

The attainment of a normal metabolic environment with a successful renal transplant should result in the resolution of the multiple abnormalities of uremic osteodystrophy. That this is not always the case is a reflection of the extent of preexisting bone disease, the effects of immunosuppression, and alterations in renal function. Despite a wealth of information concerning the natural history of mineral metabolism post-transplant, the data are often conflicting. Undoubtedly, this is due to the diversity of regimens employed by dialysis and transplant teams from center to center and from decade to decade. In addition, there is considerable variability in the diagnostic tools and criteria employed in the evaluation of mineral metabolism in this growing population of patients. Nonetheless, an understanding of the pathophysiology and significance of these abnormalities may lead to improved methods of prevention and treatment.

Disorders of Calcium Metabolism

By far the most common abnormality of calcium metabolism is hypercalcemia, for which the reported incidence ranges from 10 to 50%. Parfitt (161) categorizes post-transplant hypercalcemia into early severe, transient, and persistent. Severe hypercalcemia, noted within the first few months after transplantation, is usually due to severe hyperparathyroidism. Schwartz et al. (162) reported calcium levels of 12–15 mg/dL in 7 of 34 patients. Radiographic evidence of osteitis fibrosa correlated with the severity of the hypercalcemia. The impaired renal function associated with the hypercalcemia improved in those 5 patients who subsequently underwent parathyroidectomy. David et al. (163) reported similar findings. The mechanism for severe hypercalcemia early in the course of transplantation is probably sustained secretion of parathyroid hormone by the hyperplastic glands. The animal model that mimics this clinical state was developed by Gittes and Radde (164). These investigators transplanted 20–80 isologous functional parathyroid glands into normal rats leading to sustained hypercalcemia. Presumably, despite suppression of parathyroid hormone secretion in individual cells by hypercalcemia, the basal nonsuppressible release of the hormone by the large number of cells led to parathyroid hormone excess. It is likely that as hyperparathyroidism is more aggressively treated in patients undergoing dialysis, early severe hypercalcemia is currently rather uncommon. This is supported by the more recent experience of Cundy et al. (165), who reported an infrequent occurrence of sustained hypercalcemia within the first 50 days of transplantation.

Multiple factors are probably involved in the generation of transient hypercalcemia following renal transplantation. Alfrey et al. (166) described mild hypercalcemia developing in 7 of 17 transplant patients. This occurred $1\frac{1}{2}$–6 months post-transplant in association with probable phosphorus depletion due to the use of antacids which bound phosphorus. Replacing the antacids with phosphorus supplements normalized the serum phosphorus and corrected the hypercalcemia. It was postulated that phosphorus depletion unmasked the hyperparathyroidism present at time of renal transplant. Christensen et al. (167) found mild transient hypercalcemia in approximately 10% of transplant patients. This spontaneously resolved 2–65 months (mean 19 months) after onset. The parathyroid hormone levels were elevated in half the patients in this group and lower than those with persistent hypercalcemia. Hence prolonged secretion of parathyroid hormone may play a role in the development of transient hypercalcemia in some patients. Another factor may be that of a rapid reduction of the dose of steroids. Ulmann et al. (168) noted transient hypercalcemia in 20 of 44 patients at a time when the

steroid dose was reduced. Geis et al. (169) correlated the rise in serum calcium levels with the tapering of the dose of steroids. David et al. (163) found that radiographic evidence of soft-tissue calcification was more common in those patients who subsequently developed hypercalcemia post-transplant than those remaining normocalcemic. Such a mechanism was thought to be operative in a patient described by Hornum (170). Presumably, hypercalcemia was a result of the mobilization of metastatic deposits to the extracellular space. It should be noted, however, that the hypercalcemic patients also demonstrate higher levels of parathyroid hormone compared to those with normocalcemia. Hence the presence of metastatic calcification may simply reflect prior poor control of mineral metabolism and may not be a significant pathogenetic factor in the development of hypercalcemia. A final cause for transient post-transplant hypercalcemia is the treatment of patients with metabolites of vitamin D that have a prolonged half-life. Cundy et al. (171) emphasized the need to utilize only metabolites with short duration of action in those dialysis patients awaiting transplantation.

Post-transplant persistent hypercalcemia is arbitrarily defined as hypercalcemia of greater than 1 year's duration. It is clear, however, that the duration of the hypercalcemia (which is usually mild) may be of the order of several years. Chatterjee et al. (172) reported mild, asymptomatic, and persistent hypercalcemia in 16 of 60 transplant patients. The majority developed hypercalcemia within the first 6 months. The duration of hypercalcemia ranged from 1 to 7 years with a mean of 3 years. In at least some, there did not seem to be a trend for the calcium levels to fall. Interestingly, parathyroid hormone levels were elevated in only half of these patients. Christensen et al. (167), however, found persistent hypercalcemia in 7 of 174 patients and hyperparathyroidism in the 5 in whom it was measured. None had radiographic evidence of osteitis fibrosa on standard radiograms. Parfitt et al. (173) reported an prevalence of persistent hypercalcemia in 11.7% of transplanted patients which he attributed to hyperparathyroidism. It is likely that the persistent hypercalcemia and hyperparathyroidism is due to hyperplasia of the parathyroid gland. McCarron et al. (174) evaluated 15 patients with persistent post-transplant hypercalcemia with infusions of disodium EDTA or calcium to acutely change calcium levels. They found a good correlation between the changes in parathyroid hormone induced with either infusion and gland volume measured at time of parathyroidectomy. A more recent study (175) in transplant patients undergoing parathyroidectomy has shown that the right-sided glands tend to enlarge to a greater size than those on the left. However, there is great variability from patient to patient.

Most patients with persistence hypercalcemia have excellent function of the renal allograft and therefore probably normal levels of calcitriol (176). Both in vivo (177) and in vitro (178) experiments have demonstrated that calcitriol inhibits parathyroid hyperplasia but does not induce dedifferentiation. Parfitt (161) suggests that the long lifespan of normal parathyroid cells (approximately 36 years) contributes to the very slow involution of the gland following transplantation.

With the induction of a more normal mineral and vitamin D metabolism following a successful transplant, it is likely that the sensitivity of the parathyroid gland to hypercalcemic suppression also improves. However, McCarron (174) found that patients with persistent hypercalcemia and hyperparathyroidism post-transplant demonstrated a reduced sensitivity to calcium. It is possible that the parathyroid gland continues to somewhat insensitive to the suppressant effects of calcium in post-transplant. Elevated levels of parathyroid hormone have been found in the states of glucocorticoid excess (179–182). More recently, studies in cultured parathyroid cells have shown that glucocorticoids blunt the suppressant effect of calcitriol on pre-proparathyroid hormone gene transcription (183) and parathyroid hormone secretion (184). The latter effects are depicted in Fig. 15. The mechanism does not appear to involve changes in calcitriol receptor content. Korkor (185) found an increased receptor number for calcitriol in transplant patients undergoing parathyroidectomy compared to dialysis patients. The former group, however, had fewer calcitriol receptors than determined in glands in patients with primary hyperparathyroidism and normal renal function.

In summary, the prevalence and severity of hypercalcemia in the post-transplant period is predominantly a function of the degree of hyperparathyroidism at the time of transplant and the level of renal function. The failure of hypercalcemia to resolve after many years of an apparent normalization of vitamin D metabolism suggests that the process of involution of the parathyroid gland is quite slow. It is also possible that steroids impair the suppress effect of calcitriol on parathyroid hormone secretion.

Treatment of Hypercalcemia following Renal Transplant

Patients who develop severe hypercalcemia (calcium levels greater than 12–13 mg/dL) in the early post-transplant period may develop impaired renal function (162,163,167) and require an emergent subtotal parathyroidectomy. For the majority of patients who demonstrate only mild hypercalcemia, the decision to perform a subtotal parathyroidectomy depends on the clinical situation. If evidence of persistence or worsening of osteitis fibrosa is noted on bone radiographs, surgery may be warranted. Although rare, renal calculi and nephrocalcinosis may develop in the renal allograft (186,187). When occurring in the setting of hypercalcemia and hyperparathyroidism, a subtotal parathyroidectomy may preserve renal function or avoid urological procedures. Parathyroid surgery may also be required when hypercalcemia is thought to be contributing to hypertension or when patients develop evidence of calciphylaxis (188). In the majority of hypercalcemic patients whose condition does not fulfill these criteria, careful monitoring of the clinical status may suffice.

Administration of oral phosphorus supplementation may lower calcium levels in those patients who develop phosphorus depletion by use of phosphorus binders. There is little evidence, however, that routine prescribing of phosphorus supplements would be beneficial in those patients with hypercalcemia and mild hypophosphatemia. The potential risks of renal stones, progression of renal insufficiency, and worsening of parathyroid hyperplasia argue against its use.

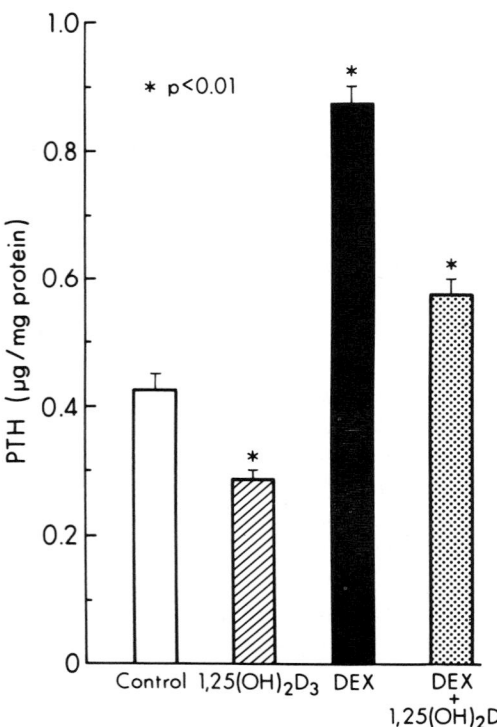

FIG. 15. Effects of 1,25(OH)$_2$D$_3$, dexamethasone (DEX), and the combination of the two steroids on PTH secretion in vitro. With 1,25(OH)$_2$D$_3$ alone, there was a decrease in PTH secretion. With DEX alone there was an increase in PTH secretion that remained greater than baseline even in the presence of 1,25(OH)$_2$D$_3$. (Modified from Ref. 184.)

Disorders of Phosphorus Metabolism

Persistent hypophosphatemia occurs in 20–35% of transplant recipients with good renal function. A major factor in the pathogenesis appears to be an inappropriate phosphaturia. Both PTH-dependent and PTH-independent mechanisms for this disorder have been described. Graf et al. (189) noted a low maximal tubular phosphorus reabsorption corrected for glomerular filtration rate (TmP/GFR) in 80% of patients with well-functioning renal allografts. There was a significant correlation between the TmP/GFR and serum levels of parathyroid hormone. Ward et al. (190) also found a correlation between tubular reabsorption of phosphorus and parathyroid hormone levels as well as urinary cyclic AMP excretion rates. Geis et al. (169) reported an increase in the tubular reabsorption of phosphorus in 7 transplant patients following parathyroidectomy. However, the tubular reabsorption of phosphorus normalized in only 2 patients. Although hyperparathyroidism may play a role in some patients with hypophosphatemia, more recent studies suggest an important role for a selective renal phosphate leak unrelated to parathyroid hormone excess. Rosenbaum et al. (191) found no differences in parathyroid hormone levels between normo- and hypophosphatemic transplant patients despite a marked decrease in TmP/GRF in the latter group. A continuous infusion of calcium suppressed parathyroid hormone levels in all hypophosphatemic patients but decreased urinary phosphorus excretion in only half of those studied.

The etiology of the parathyroid hormone-independent hypophosphatemia in renal transplant patients is unclear. Clearly, however, the presence of one kidney lowers the TmP/GFR. Pabico et al. (192) found a low TmP/GFR of 2.5 mg/dL in renal transplant donors 5–12 years following uninephrectomy. Comparable falls in TmP/GFR have been noted by others (168,191). It is unlikely, however, that the presence of one kidney fully explains post-transplant hypophosphatemia. Despite comparable renal function, hypophosphatemic transplant patients demonstrate a lower TmP/GRF than that of the donors (168,191). A possible etiology may be that of a relative deficiency of calcitriol. Graf et al. (189) administered 1α-vitamin D to 19 transplant patients with good renal function, normal parathyroid hormone levels, and a low TmP/GFR. Following 3 weeks of treatment, TmP/GFR rose in all patients in association with increased phosphorus levels. There was no correlation with TmP/GFR and parathyroid hormone levels either before or after treatment. Unfortunately, calcitriol levels were not measured. However, others (193,194) have shown that calcitriol values are normal in transplant patients with evidence of a renal phosphate leak. Since hypophosphatemia is a potent stimulus for calcitriol synthesis (23), it is possible that a relative deficiency of calcitriol plays a role in the inappropriate phosphaturia following successful renal transplant.

Although a renal phosphorus leak is of primary importance in the development of hypophosphatemia, there is also evidence of intestinal malabsorption of phosphorus in transplant patients. Farrington et al. (195) reported impaired intestinal absorption of phosphorus following transplantation despite normal absorption of calcium. The fractional absorption of phosphorus, however, was not different in those with low and normal levels of phosphorus.

Treatment of Hypophosphatemia in Renal Transplant Patients

The vast majority of patients with hypophosphatemia are asymptomatic and the major concern is that they will eventually develop osteomalacia. Moorhead et al. (196) in the United Kingdom found radiographic evidence of osteomalacia in 5 of 7 transplant patients with persistence hypophosphatemia. More recently, Felsenfeld et al. (197) in the United States performed bone biopsies in 10 patients with comparable phosphorus levels. No changes of osteomalacia were detected. Whether these divergent data reflect differences in methodology or vitamin D metabolism in the two countries is unknown. Nonetheless, due to concerns of stimulating PTH secretion, it would seem inadvisable to routinely prescribe oral supplementation of phosphorus in the asymptomatic patient with mild to moderate hypophosphatemia. In the normocalcemic patient with clinical evidence of sequelae from hypophosphatemia, judicious administration of vitamin D or one of its metabolites may be indicated. In this setting, careful monitoring of serum and urine calcium as well as renal function is mandatory.

Effects of Transplantation on Renal Osteodystrophy

The long-term effects of transplantation on renal osteodystrophy is predominantly a function of the type and severity of the bone disease prior to surgery, the level of renal function, and the dose of immunosuppression therapy (especially steroids). Pierides et al. (198) performed serial bone biopsies in 33 patients. In those 16 patients with osteomalacia, complete resolution of the bone disease occurred in 81% by 1 year and in virtually all by 2 years. Presumably, this improvement was due to a large excretion of aluminum by the transplanted kidney (199) with improvement in the aluminum-associated osteomalacia (200). In contrast, the changes of osteitis fibrosa resolve more slowly. Pierides et al. (198) noted persistence of this lesion in 55% of transplant patients 1 year after surgery. By 2 years, almost one-half of patients still had evidence of mild osteitis fibrosa. These results are consistent with the known slow rate of involution of the parathyroid glands. Carroll et al. (201) reported that the majority of bone biopsies in patients with good renal function do not show resolution of osteitis fibrosa until 4 or more years after transplantation. Predictably, those with impaired renal function showed slower and more incomplete correction. More recently, Alsina et al. (202) correlated the levels of intact parathyroid hormone with the uptake of [⁹⁹Tc]methylene diphosphonate in bone scans of patients with renal transplants.

The effect of renal transplantation on bone mass has been studied by several investigators. Eastell et al. (203) found an insignificant decline in total body calcium measured by neutron activation analysis in 10 patients. They attribute the earlier findings (204,205) of a 5–7% loss in bone mass in the first-year post-transplant to the higher doses of steroids.

Effects of Cyclosporine on Renal Osteodystrophy

Cyclosporine is increasingly utilized as a potent immunosuppressive agent in renal transplantation. However, little is known concerning its effects on mineral and bone metabolism. It is likely, however, that the associated lowered steroid dose, nephrotoxicity (206), distal renal tubular acidosis (207), and potential for magnesium wasting (208) may affect the metabolic milieu of the bone. In addition, cyclosporine affects cytokine production (209). Reports of in vivo inhibition of bone resorption and stimulation of formation (210), induction of severe osteopenia in normal rats (211), and accelerated bone resorption in the oophorectomized rat (212) suggests a major role of cyclosporine at the level of the bone. This contention is supported by in vitro data on cultured neonatal mouse calvaria (213), which showed an inhibition of bone resorption by the drug. Unfortunately, data concerning the effects of cyclosporine on mineral metabolism in renal transplant patients are quite limited. Two groups (214,215) have noted higher levels of alkaline phosphatase in patients receiving cyclosporine than in those given conventional therapy with azathioprine. These data suggested an activation of osteoblast activity by cyclosporine. Preliminary work by Aubia et al. (216), however, suggested that transplant patients treated with cyclosporine demonstrate an increased number of both osteoblasts and osteoclasts per millimeter of trabecular surface on bone biopsy compared to those receiving azathioprine. They suggest that cyclosporine may interfere in some way with bone healing.

Effects of Renal Transplantation on Serum Osteocalcin Levels

Following a successful renal transplant, there is a rapid fall in osteocalcin levels (217,218). There are probably several reasons for this initial decline. Restoration of renal function would increase the metabolic clearance rate of this vitamin K–dependent bone protein (219). In addition, a fall in parathyroid hormone secretion may lead to lower rates of osteocalcin synthesis and/or release. Finally, since glucocorticoids are known to lower osteocalcin levels (220), it is likely that high doses of steroids, usually administered early in the post-transplant period, contributes to the decline. After the first month, however, osteocalcin levels either do not change or may rise (217,218) for up to 1 year. During this period osteocalcin concentrations correlate predominantly with serum parathyroid hormone and alkaline phosphatase levels. This suggests that osteocalcin, like alkaline phosphatase, is a measure of parathyroid hormone mediated effects on bone turnover in renal transplant patients.

Growth of Children following Renal Transplantation

Normal or accelerated "catch-up" growth has been described in children transplanted at an early age (221,222). Factors that influence growth favorably include low steroid doses and normal renal function (221–223). Whether a regimen of alternate-day steroids is superior to daily low-dose steroids is controversial. However, it should be noted that growth remains stunted in the majority of children having undergone renal transplantation (224).

Osteonecrosis following Renal Transplantation

Osteonecrosis (also termed idiopathic ischemic necrosis, avascular necrosis, and aseptic necrosis) is a frequent cause of major disability in transplant patients. The incidence ranges from 3 to 41% in different centers with a mean of 15% (225). The femoral head is most commonly involved, but the process may also affect the femoral condyle, distal tibia, talus, humeral head, distal humerus, proximal radius, and proximal ulna (225). One-half to two-thirds of patients who develop osteonecrosis in one hip will develop it in the other. Although the highest incidence is found in the first 3 years after renal transplantation, patients may remain at risk for osteonecrosis up to 6 years post transplant (226).

Factors Involved in the Development of Osteonecrosis

Because osteonecrosis has been described in patients with a wide variety of disease processes treated with corticosteroids, it is reasonable to incriminate this drug in its development (227). However, the evidence to support this contention is conflicting. As reviewed by Meakin et al. (228), the studies showing a correlation with steroid dose are countered by an equal number of studies that could demonstrate no relationship. In one study, however, the incidence of osteonecrosis decreased from 24% to 1.5% when the total steroid dose was decreased three-fold during the first 3 weeks of transplantation (229). More recently, Landmann et al. (230) compared the effect of cyclosporine and low-dose corticosteroids with that of azathioprine and high-dose steroid therapy on the development of osteonecrosis. In the former group 1 of 96 developed osteonecrosis of the femoral head, whereas 15 of 174 encountered this problem in the latter group. Lausten et al. (231) described similar findings. They proposed that cyclosporine led to a decreased incidence of rejection, a reduction in corticosteroid dosage, and hence a reduced incidence of osteonecrosis. Sutherland et al. (232) found no difference in the occurrence of osteonecrosis in patients treated with cyclosporine (3%) or azathioprine (6%). The maintenance steroid dose was relatively low in both groups.

A variety of hypotheses have been offered to explain the role of steroids in the pathogenesis of osteonecrosis in renal transplant recipients. It is possible that steroids, by inhibiting osteoblast function (see Chapter 22), may lead to osteopenia, microfractures of the trabecular bone, and impairment of the local blood supply to bone. Presumably, a vicious cycle of microfractures leading to ischemia, which further affects bone integrity, would ensue. This concept is supported by studies of bone histology in transplant patients (233). A greater severity of osteopenia was noted in those with osteonecrosis compared to those without osteonecrosis. These pathological findings are shown in Fig. 16.

An alternative explanation of the role of steroids in the development of osteonecrosis implicates impaired blood flow to bone as an initiating event. Wilkes and Visscher (234) have shown that the bone circulation functions as a Starling resistor. This consists of a rigid canister through which passes a flexible thin-walled tube. Hence flow in the tube is determined not only by the driving pressure outside the canister, but also by the pressure inside the canister. Changes of pressure within the closed compartment would lead to a reciprocal change in flow within the tube. Although the clinical data concerning the effects of steroids on bone marrow pressure are limited, animal studies suggest a possible effect. Wang et al. (235) injected large doses of cortisone to rabbits, which subsequently developed osteonecrosis of the femoral head. An increase in the marrow fat-cell volume in the order of 25% was noted. Although marrow pressures were not measured, the authors suggested that compression of the sinusoidal vascular bed may lead to ischemia of bone cells. These data are consistent with the findings of Hungerford (236), who found elevated bone marrow pressures in patients with osteonecrosis due to a variety of causes. Core decompression of the femoral head and neck during the early ischemic phase led to a relief of symptoms and an arrest of the disease process.

Steroids could also impair blood flow to bones by causing fat embolization (237). It is postulated that subchondral arteriolar embolization would diminish blood flow and lead to ischemic necrosis of the bone. Fisher and Bickel (238) studied 77 patients with osteonecrosis and found abnormal lipid levels in the majority of patients and histological evidence of fat emboli in half of the femoral heads. Parfrey et al. (239), however, could not find evidence of either fatty infiltration of the liver or an increased amount of fat in the femoral heads in transplant patients with osteonecrosis.

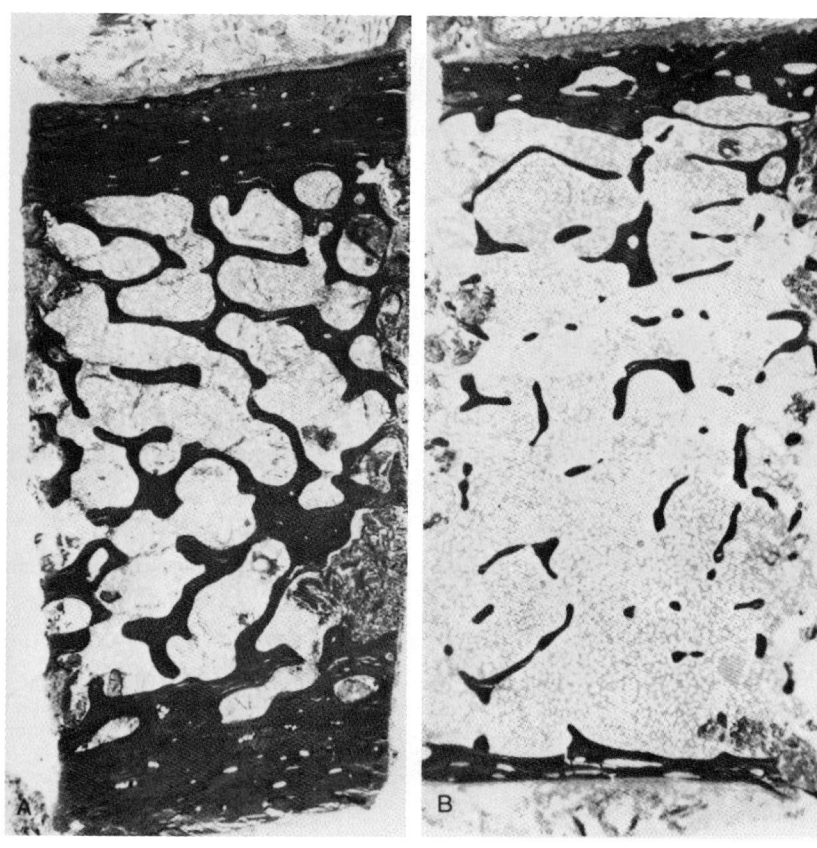

FIG. 16. Bone histology from a normal individual (**A**) and a renal transplant patient with osteonecrosis (**B**). Note the marked reduction in the amount of trabecular bone in B. (From Ref. 233.)

It is likely that the condition of the bone at time of transplantation and the persistence of hyperparathyroidism in the post-transplant period are contributing factors in the development of osteonecrosis. Although Gottlieb et al. (240) were unable to correlate abnormalities seen in standard radiographs or bone mineral content measured by photon absorptiometry with the subsequent development of post-transplant osteonecrosis, others have been more successful. Lindsay et al. (204) found an inverse correlation between peripheral bone mineral content and the development of osteonecrosis. Radiographic evidence of osteopenia and subperiosteal resorption before transplantation may also predispose patients to the evolution of osteonecrosis (241). Because transplant patients with osteonecrosis have more severe osteopenia but equally reduced rates of bone formation and calcification compared to those without osteonecrosis, Nielsen et al. (242) reasoned that those affected must have had a greater degree of osteopenia at the time of transplantation. Chatterjee et al. (172) determined that patients with persistent hypercalcemia and hyperparathyroidism post transplant had a high incidence of osteonecrosis, but others (239,243) have been unable to find a relationship between osteonecrosis and either hyperparathyroidism or hypercalcemia. Although it is theoretically attractive to postulate that the combination of heightened bone resorption due to hyperparathyroidism and steroid-induced impaired bone formation would predispose to osteonecrosis, definitive evidence of this link has not been shown.

Another potential risk factor for the development of osteonecrosis is the magnitude of weight gain after transplantation. Metselaar et al. (226) found that an increase in body weight of greater than 10% 180 days post transplant rendered patients at a relative risk of developing osteonecrosis 2.5 times that of patients with no weight gain. Because the cumulative steroid dose was not different in the two groups, the authors speculate that individual sensitivity to steroids rather than absolute cumulative dose is involved in the development of osteonecrosis. An alternative explanation is that excessive weight gain increases the trauma to weight-bearing bone and may increase the risk for microfractures. More recently, a role for iron overload as a risk factor in the genesis of osteonecrosis has been proposed. Parfrey et al. (239) found a 50% prevalence of parenchymal iron on liver biopsy 1 year after transplant in those with osteonecrosis compared to 15% in those without this problem. It is possible that multiple blood transfusions led to iron overload, which caused marrow fibrosis and osteopenia. This would make the femoral head more vulnerable to osteonecrosis in a manner similar to that seen with Bantu iron overload.

Prevention and Treatment of Osteonecrosis

Since there are undoubtedly multiple factors involved in the development of osteonecrosis, preventive measures are largely empirical. Common sense, however, dictates that aggressive efforts should be applied to control renal osteodystrophy while patients are treated with dialysis. In addition, the steroid doses should be minimized within the constraints of preservation of renal function post transplant. Scholz et al. (244) reported a 6.5% incidence of osteonecrosis in patients treated with vitamin D (ergocalciferol) compared to a 26.7% incidence in a matched control group. Although to our knowledge, this finding has not been confirmed by others, it may be reasonable to administer vitamin D cautiously to patients treated at transplant centers experiencing a continued high incidence of osteonecrosis.

Pain and restriction of joint movement, particularly in the hips, should alert the clinician to the possibility of osteonecrosis. Standard radiographs should be obtained, but a normal study does not preclude the diagnosis. It appears that bone scans diagnose an earlier stage of osteonecrosis than radiographs. Once diagnosed, the treatment largely depends on the extent of destruction. Early lesions may be treated with a reduction in weight bearing or core decompression. In advanced lesions, hip replacement is usually necessary. Several authors report markedly improved functional capacity and relief of pain and few complications in patients treated with this approach (229,245–247).

ACKNOWLEDGMENTS

This work was supported by U.S. Public Health Service NIADDK Grants AM-09976, AM-07126, and RR 00036. The authors wish to express their appreciation to Mrs. Patricia Shy and Mrs. Donna Morgan for their excellent assistance in the preparation of this manuscript.

REFERENCES

1. Albright F, Drake TG, Sulkowitch HW. Renal osteitis fibrosa cystica: report of case with discussion of metabolic aspects. *Johns Hopkins Med J* 1937;60:377–85.
2. Follis RH Jr, Jackson DA. Renal osteomalacia and osteitis fibrosa in adults. *Johns Hopkins Med J* 1943;72:232–41.
3. Stanbury SW, Lumb GA. Metabolic studies of renal osteodystrophy. In: Calcium, phosphorus and nitrogen metabolism in rickets, osteomalacia, and hyperparathyroidism complicating chronic uremia and in the osteomalacia of the adult Fanconi syndrome. *Medicine* 1962;42:1–31.
4. Dent CE, Harper CM, Philpot GR. Treatment of renal-glomerular osteodystrophy. *Q J Med* 1961;30:1–31.
5. Reiss E, Canterbury JM, Egdahl RH. Measurement of serum parathyroid hormone in renal insufficiency. *Trans Assoc Am Physicians* 1968;81:104–14.
6. Arnaud CD. Hyperparathyroidism and renal failure. *Kidney Int* 1973;4:89–95.
7. Lopez-Hilker S, Galceran T, Chan YL, Rapp N, Martin K, Slatopolsky E. Hypocalcemia may not be essential for the development of secondary hyperparathyroidism in chronic renal failure. *J Clin Invest* 1986;78:1097–102.
8. Slatopolsky E, Caglar S, Pennell JP, et al. On the pathogenesis of hyperparathyroidism in chronic experimental insufficiency in the dog. *J Clin Invest* 1971;50:492–9.
9. Slatopolsky E, Caglar S, Gradowska L, Canterbury J, Reiss E,

Bricker NS. On the prevention of secondary hyperparathyroidism in experimental chronic renal disease using "proportional reduction" of dietary phosphorus intake. *Kidney Int* 1972;2:147–51.

10. Slatopolsky E, Bricker NS. The role of phosphorus restriction in the prevention of secondary hyperparathyroidism in chronic renal disease. *Kidney Int* 1973;4:141–5.

11. Reiss E, Canterbury MJ, Bercovitz MA, Kaplan EL. The role of phosphate in the secretion of parathyroid hormone in man. *J Clin Invest* 1970;49:2146–9.

12. LaFlame GH, Jowsey J. Bone and soft tissue changes with oral phosphate supplements. *J Clin Invest* 1972;51:2834–9.

13. Jowsey J, Reiss E, Canterbury JM. Long-term effects of high phosphate intake on parathyroid hormone levels and bone metabolism. *Acta Orthop Scand* 1974;45:801–6.

14. Rutherford WE, Bordier P, Marie P, et al. Phosphate control and 25-hydroxycholecalciferol administration in preventing experimental renal osteodystrophy in the dog. *J Clin Invest* 1977;60:332–41.

15. Llach F, Massry SG, Koffler A, et al. Secondary hyperparathyroidism in early renal failure: role of phosphate retention. *Kidney Int* 1977;12:459–63.

16. Fotino S. Phosphate excretion in chronic renal failure: evidence for a mechanism other than circulating parathyroid hormone. *Clin Nephrol* 1977;8:499–503.

17. Fournier AE, Arnaud CD, Johnson WJ, Taylor WF, Goldsmith RS. Etiology of hyperparathyroidism and bone disease during chronic hemodialysis. II. Factors affecting serum immunoreactive parathyroid hormone. *J Clin Invest* 1971;50:599–605.

18. Tanaka Y, DeLuca HF. The control of 25-dihydroxyvitamin D metabolism by inorganic phosphorus. *Arch Biochem Biophys* 1973;159:566–70.

19. Oldham SB, Smith R, Hartenbower DL, et al. The acute effects of 1,25-dihydroxycholecalciferol on serum immunoreactive parathyroid hormone (i-PTH) in the dog. *Endocrinology* 1979;104:248–54.

20. Goldman R, Bassett SH. Phosphorus excretion in renal failure. *J Clin Invest* 1954;33:1623–8.

21. Raiz LG, Niemann I. Effect of phosphate calcium and magnesium on bone resorption and hormonal response in tissue culture. *Endocrinology* 1969;85:446–52.

22. Portale A, Halloran BP, Murphy MM, Morris RC. Oral intake of phosphorus can determine the serum concentration of 1,25 dihydroxyvitamin D by determining its production rate in humans. *J Clin Invest* 1986;77:7–12.

23. Portale A, Halloran BP, Morris RC. Physiologic regulation of the serum concentration of 1,25-dihydroxyvitamin D by phosphorus in normal men. *J Clin Invest* 1989;83:1494–9.

24. Fraser DR, Kodicek E. Unique biosynthesis by kidney of a biologically active vitamin D metabolite. *Nature* 1970;228:764–6.

25. Liu SH, Chu HI. Studies of calcium and phosphorus metabolism with special reference to the pathogenesis and effect of dihydrotachysterol and iron. *Medicine* 1943;22:103–61.

26. Coburn JW, Koppel MH, Brickman AS, et al. Study of intestinal absorption of calcium in patients with renal failure. *Kidney Int* 1973;3:264–72.

27. Slatopolsky E, Gray R, Adams ND, et al. The pathogenesis of secondary hyperparathyroidism in early renal failure. In: Norman A, ed. *4th International workshop in vitamin D.* Berlin: Walter de Gruyer, 1979;1209–13.

28. Cheung AK, Manolagas SC, Cathewood BD, et al. Determination of serum 1,25(OH)$_2$D$_3$ levels in renal disease. *Kidney Int* 1983;24:104–9.

29. Chesney RW, Hamstra AJ, Mazess RB, Rose P, DeLuca HF. Circulating vitamin D metabolite concentrations in childhood renal disease. *Kidney Int* 1982;21:65–72.

30. Juttmann JR, Burman JC, Dekam E, Wisser TJ, Birkenhager JC. Serum concentrations of metabolites of vitamin D in patients with renal failure. *Clin Endocrinol* 1981;14:225–32.

31. Wilson L, Felsenfeld A, Drezner MK, et al. Altered divalent ion metabolism in early renal failure: role of 1,25(OH)$_2$D$_3$. *Kidney Int* 1985;27:565–70.

32. Taylor CM, Caverzacio J, Jung A, Treschel U, Fleisch H, Bonfour JP. Unilateral nephrectomy and 1,25-dihydroxyvitamin D$_3$. *Kidney Int* 1984;24:37–42.

33. Malluche H, Werner E, Ritz E. Intestinal absorption of calcium and whole-body calcium retention in incipient and advanced renal failure. *Miner Electrolyte Metab* 1978;1:263–70.

34. Sherrard DJ, Baylink DJ, Wergedal JE, Maloney N. Quantitative histological studies on the pathogenesis of uremic bone disease. *J Clin Endocrinol* 1974;39:119–35.

35. Bordier PJ, Tun-chot S, Eastwood JB, Fournier A. Lack of histological evidence of vitamin D abnormality in the bones of anephric patients. *Clin Sci* 1973;44:33–41.

36. Garabedian M, Pavlovitch H, Fellot L, Balsan S. Metabolism of 25-hydroxyvitamin D$_3$ in anephric rats: a new active metabolite. *Proc Natl Acad Sci USA* 1974;71:554–7.

37. Olgaard K, Finco D, Schwartz J, et al. Effect of 24,25(OH)$_2$D$_3$ on PTH levels and bone histology in dogs with chronic uremia. *Kidney Int* 1984;26:791–7.

38. Evanson JM. The response to the infusion of parathyroid extract in hypocalcemic states. *Clin Sci* 1966;31:63–73.

39. Llach F, Massry SG, Singer FR, Kurokawa K, Kaye JH, Coburn JW. Skeletal resistance of endogenous parathyroid hormone in patients with early renal failure: a possible cause for secondary hyperparathyroidism. *J Clin Endocrinol Metab* 1975;41:339–45.

40. Kaplan MA, Canterbury JM, Gavellas GA, et al. The calcemic and phosphaturic effects of parathyroid hormone in the normal and uremic dog. *Metabolism* 1978;27:1785–92.

41. Massry SG, Stein R, Garty J, et al. Skeletal resistance to the calcemic action of parathyroid hormone in uremia: role of 1,25(OH)$_2$D$_3$. *Kidney Int* 1975;1:467–74.

42. Somerville P, Kaye M. Evidence that resistance to the calcemic action of parathyroid hormone in rats with acute uremia is caused by phosphate retention. *Kidney Int* 1979;16:552–60.

43. Galceran T, Martin KJ, Morrissey J, et al. Role of 1,25 dihydroxyvitamin D on the skeletal resistance to parathyroid hormone. *Kidney Int* 1987;32:801–7.

44. Dufresne LR, Gitelman HJ. A possible role of adenyl cyclase in the regulation of parathyroid activity by calcium. In: Talmadge RV, Munson PL, eds. *Calcium, parathyroid hormone and the calcitonins.* Amsterdam: Excerpta Medica, 1972;202.

45. Matsuzaki S, Dumont JE. Effect of calcium ion on horse parathyroid gland adenyl cyclase. *Biochim Biophys Acta* 1972;284:227–34.

46. Rodriguez JH, Morrison A, Slatopolsky E, Klahr S. Adenylate cyclase of human parathyroid gland. *J Clin Endocrinol Metab* 1978;47:319–25.

47. Bellorin-Font E, Martin KJ, Freitag JJ, et al. Altered adenylate cyclase kinetics in hyperfunctioning human parathyroid glands. *J Clin Endocrinol Metab* 1981;52:499–507.

48. Ontjes DA, Mahafdfee DD, Wells SA. Adenylate cyclase activity in human parathyroid tissues: reduced sensitivity to suppression by calcium in parathyroid adenomas as compared with normal glands from normocalcemic-subjects or noninvolved glands from hyperparathyroid subjects. *Metabolism* 1978;30:406–11.

49. Habener JF. Responsiveness of neoplastic and hyperplastic parathyroid tissue to calcium in vitro. *J Clin Invest* 1978;62:436–50.

50. Brown EM, Brennan MF, Hurwitz S, et al. Dispersed cells prepared from human parathyroid glands: distinct calcium sensitivity of adenomas vs. primary hyperplasia. *J Clin Endocrinol Metab* 1978;46:267–75.

51. Brown EM. Set-point for calcium: its role in normal and abnormal parathyroid secretion. In: Cohn DV, Talmadge RV, Matthews JL, eds. *Hormonal control of calcium metabolism.* Amsterdam: Excerpta Medica, 1981;35–41.

52. Brown EM, Wilson RE, Eastman RC, Pallota J, Marynick SP. Abnormal regulation of parathyroid hormone release by calcium in secondary hyperparathyroidism due to chronic renal failure. *J Clin Endocrinol Metab* 1982;54:172–9.

53. Brown EM. Four-parameter model of the sigmoidal relationship between parathyroid hormone release and extracellular calcium concentration in normal and abnormal parathyroid tissue. *J Clin Endocrinol Metab* 1983;56:572–81.

54. Chertow BS, Baylink DJ, Wergedal MH, Su MMH, Norman AW. Decrease in serum immunoreactive parathyroid hormone in rats and in parathyroid hormone secretion in vivo by 1,25-dihydroxycholecalciferol. *J Clin Invest* 1975;56:668–78.

55. Au WYW, Bukowsky A. Inhibition of PTH secretion by vitamin

D metabolites in organ cultures of rat parathyroids. *Fed Proc* 1976;35:530–1.

56. Dietel M, Dorn G, Montz R, et al. Influence of vitamin D₃, 1,25-dihydroxyvitamin D₃ and 24,25-dihydroxyvitamin D₃ on parathyroid hormone secretion, adenosine 3′, 5′-monophosphate release, and ultrastructure of parathyroid glands in organ culture. *Endocrinology* 1979;105:237–45.

57. Oldham SB, Fischer JA, Shen LH, et al. Isolation and properties of a calcium-binding protein from porcine parathyroid glands. *Biochemistry* 1974;13:4790–6.

58. Brumbaugh PF, Hughes MR, Haussler MR. Cytoplasmic and nuclear binding components for 1α,25-dihydroxyvitamin D₃ in chick parathyroid glands. *Proc Natl Acad Sci USA* 1975; 72:4871–5.

59. Llach F, Coburn JW, Brickman AD, et al. Acute actions of 1,25-dihydroxyvitamin D₃ in normal man, effect on calcium and parathyroid status. *J Clin Endocrinol Metab* 1977;4:1054–60.

60. Tanaka Y, DeLuca HF, Ghazarian JG, et al. Effects of vitamin D and its metabolites on serum parathyroid hormone levels in the rat. *Miner Electrolyte Metab* 1979;2:20–5.

61. Golden P, Greenwalt A, Martin K, et al. Lack of a direct effect of 1,25-dihydroxycholecalciferol on secretion of parathyroid hormone. *Endocrinology* 1980;107:602–7.

62. Christiansen C, Christiansen MS, Melsen F, et al. Mineral metabolism in chronic renal failure with special reference to serum concentrations of 1,25(OH)₂D₃ and 24,25(OH)₂D₃. *Clin Nephrol* 1981;15:18–22.

63. Slatopolsky E, Weerts C, Thielan J, Horst R, Harter H, Martin K. Marked suppression of secondary hyperparathyroidism by intravenous administration of 1,25-dihydroxycholecalciferol in uremic patients. *J Clin Invest* 1984;74:2136–43.

64. Cantley LK, Russell J, Lettieri D, Sherwood LM. 1,25-dihydroxyvitamin D₃ suppresses PTH secretion from bovine parathyroid cells in culture. *Endocrinology* 1985;117:2114–9.

65. Chan YL, McKay C, Dye E, Slatopolsky E. The effect of 1,25 dihydroxycholecalciferol on parathyroid hormone secretion by monolayer cultures of bovine parathyroid cells. *Calcif Tissue Int* 1986;38:27–32.

66. Silver J, Russell L, Lettieri D, Sherwood LM. Regulation by vitamin D metabolites of messenger RNA coding for pre-pro-parathyroid hormone in isolated parathyroid cells. *Proc Natl Acad Sci USA* 1984;82:4270–3.

67. Russell J, Lettieri D, Sherwood LM. Suppression by 1,25(OH)₂D₃ of transcription of the parathyroid hormone gene. *Endocrinology* 1986;119:2864–6.

68. Silver J, Naveh-Manly T, Mayer H, Schmeizer HJ, Popovtzer MM. Regulation by vitamin D metabolites of parathyroid hormone gene transcription in vivo in the rat. *J Clin Invest* 1986;78:1296–301.

69. Delmez J, Tindira C, Grooms P, Dusso A, Windus DW, Slatopolsky E. Parathyroid hormone suppression by intravenous 1,25 dihydroxyvitamin D: a role for increased sensitivity to calcium. *J Clin Invest* 1989;83:1349–55.

70. Hruska KA, Kopelman R, Rutherford WE, Klahr S, Slatopolsky E. Metabolism of immunoreactive parathyroid hormone in the dog: the role of the kidney and the effects of chronic renal disease. *J Clin Invest* 1975;56:39–46.

71. Martin KJ, Hruska KA, Lewis J, Anderson C, Slatopolsky E. The renal handling of parathyroid hormone: role of peritubular uptake and glomerular filtration. *J Clin Invest* 1977;60:808–14.

72. Freitag J, Martin KJ, Hruska KA, et al. Impaired parathyroid hormone metabolism in patients with chronic renal failure. *N Engl J Med* 1978;298:29–32.

73. Hruska K, Korkor A, Martin K, Slatopolsky E. The peripheral metabolism of parathyroid hormone: role of the liver and kidney and the effect of chronic renal failure. *J Clin Invest* 1981;67:885–92.

74. Russell JE, Avioli LV. 25-Hydroxycholecalciferol-enhanced bone maturation in the parathyroprivic state. *J Clin Invest* 1975;56:792–8.

75. Litzow JR, Lemann J Jr, Lennon EJ. The effect of treatment of acidosis on calcium balance in patients with chronic azotemic renal disease. *J Clin Invest* 1967;46:280–8.

76. Ward MK, Feest TG, Ellis HA, et al. Osteomalacic dialysis osteo-

dystrophy: evidence for a water borne etiological agent, probably aluminum. *Lancet* 1978;1:841–5.

77. Teitelbaum SL, Bergfeld MA, Freitag J, Hruska KA, Slatopolsky E. Do parathyroid hormone and 1,25-dihydroxyvitamin D modulate bone formation in uremia? *J Clin Endocrinol Metab* 1980;51:247–51.

78. Felsenfeld AJ, Harrelson JM, Gutman RA, et al. Osteomalacia after parathyroidectomy in patients with uremia. *Ann Intern Med* 1982;96:34–9.

79. Coburn JW, Brickman AS, Sherrard DJ, Wong EGC, Singer FR, Norman AW. Defective skeletal mineralization in uremia without relation to vitamin D, serum Ca or P. *Kidney Int* 1977;12:455–9.

80. Sherrard DJ, Baylink DJ, Wergedal JE, et al. Quantitative histological studies on the pathogenesis of uremic bone disease. *J Clin Endocrinol Metab* 1974;39:119–35.

81. Schoenfeld PJ, Martin JA, Barnes B, Teitelbaum SL. Amelioration of myopathy with 25-dihydroxyvitamin D₃ therapy (25(OH)D₃) in patients on chronic hemodialysis. Abstract book. *3rd Workshop on vitamin D,* Asilomar, 1977;160.

82. Mallette LE, Patten BM, Engel WK. Neuromuscular disease in secondary hyperparathyroidism. *Ann Intern Med* 1975;82:474–9.

83. Mirahmadi KS, Coburn JW, Bluestone R. Calcific periarthritis and hemodialysis. *JAMA* 1973;223:548–52.

84. Kleinman KS, Coburn JW. Amyloid syndromes associated with hemodialysis. *Kidney Int* 1989;34:567–75.

85. DiRaimondo CR, Cassey TT, DiRaimondo CV, et al. Pathologic fractures associated with idiopathic amyloidosis of bone in chronic hemodialysis patients. *Nephron* 1986;43:22–7.

86. Hruska KA, Teitelbaum SL, Kopelman R, et al. The predictability of the histologic features of uremic bone disease by non-invasive techniques. *Metab Bone Dis Relat Res* 1978;1:39–44.

87. Ritz E, Malluche HH, Bommer J, et al. Metabolic bone disease in patients on maintenance hemodialysis. *Nephron* 1974;12:393–7.

88. Parfitt AM. Clinical and radiographic manifestations of renal osteodystrophy. In: David DS, ed. *Calcium metabolism in renal failure and nephrolithiasis.* New York: John Wiley & Sons, 1977;150.

89. Parfitt AM. Soft tissue calcification in uremia. *Arch Intern Med* 1969;124:544–52.

90. Fournier AE, Johnson WJ, Taves DR, Beabout JW, Arnaud CD, Goldsmith RS. Etiology of hyperparathyroidism and bone disease during chronic hemodialysis. I. Association of bone disease with potentially etiologic factors. *J Clin Invest* 1971;50:592–8.

91. Rutherford E, Mercado A, Hruska K, et al. An evaluation of a new and effective phosphorus binding agent. *Trans Am Soc Artif Intern Organs* 1973;19:446–9.

92. Berlyne GM, Ben-Ari J, Pest D, et al. Hyperaluminaemia from aluminum resins in renal failure. *Lancet* 1970;2:494–9.

93. Alfrey AC, LeGendre GR, Kaehny WD. Dialysis encephalopathy syndrome: possible aluminum intoxication. *N Engl J Med* 1976;294:184–7.

94. Ward MK, Feest TG, Ellis HA, et al. Osteomalacic dialysis osteodystrophy: evidence for a water-borne aetiological agent, probably aluminum. *Lancet* 1978;1:841–5.

95. Clarkson EM, Eastwood JB, Koutsaimanis KG, DeWarner HE. Net intestinal absorption of calcium in patients with chronic renal failure. *Kidney Int* 1973;3:258–63.

96. Morniere PH, Roussel A, Tahiri Y, et al. Substitution of aluminum hydroxide by high doses of calcium carbonate in patients on chronic hemodialysis: disappearance of hyperaluminemia and equal control of hyperparathyroidism. *Proc Eur Dial Transplant Assoc* 1982;19:784–787.

97. Slatopolsky E, Weerts C, Lopez S, et al. Calcium carbonate is an effective phosphate binder in dialysis patients. *N Engl J Med* 1986;315:157–61.

98. Salusky IB, Coburn JW, Foley, et al. Effects of oral calcium carbonate on control of serum phosphorus and changes in plasma aluminum levels after discontinuation of aluminum-containing gels in children receiving dialysis. *J Pediatr* 1986;108:767–70.

99. Mactier RA, VanStone J, Cox A, VanStone M, Twardowski Z. Calcium carbonate is an effective phosphate-binder when dialysate calcium concentration is adjusted to control hypercalcemia. *Clin Nephrol* 1987;28:222–6.

100. Sawyer N, Noonan K, Altmann P, Marsh F, Cunningham J. High-dose calcium carbonate with stepwise reduction in dialysate calcium concentration: effective phosphate control and aluminum avoidance in haemodialysis patients. *Nephrol Dial Transplant* 1988;3:1–5.

101. Slatopolsky E, Weerts C, Norwood K, et al. Long-term effects of calcium carbonate and 2.5 mEq/liter calcium dialysate on mineral metabolism. *Kidney Int* 1989;36:897–903.

102. Schiller LR, Santa Ana CA, Sheikh MS, Emmett M, Fordtran JS. Effect of the time of administration of calcium acetate on phosphorus binding. *N Engl J Med* 1989;320:1110–1113.

103. Sheikh MS, Maguire JA, Emmett M, et al. Reduction of dietary phosphorus absorption by phosphorus binders: a theoretical, in vitro and in vivo study. *J Clin Invest* 1989;83:66–73.

104. Slanina P, Frech W, Ekstrom LG, Loof L, Slorach S, Cedergren A. Dietary citric acid enhances absorption of aluminum in antacids. *Clin Chem* 1986;32:534–41.

105. Kopple JD, Coburn JW. Metabolic studies of low protein diets in uremia. II. Calcium, phosphorus and magnesium. *Medicine* 1973;52:597–607.

106. Meyrier A, Marsac J, Richet G. The influence of a high calcium carbonate intake on bone disease in patients undergoing hemodialysis. *Kidney Int* 1973;4:146–53.

107. Curtis JR, DeWardener HE, Gower PE, Eastwood JB. The use of calcium carbonate and calcium phosphate without vitamin D in the management of renal osteodystrophy. *Proc Eur Dial Transplant Assoc* 1970;7:141–4.

108. Mirahmadi KS, Duffy BS, Shinaberger JH, et al. A controlled evaluation of clinical and metabolic effects of dialysate calcium levels during regular hemodialysis. *Trans Am Soc Artif Intern Organs* 1971;17:118–20.

109. Goldsmith RS, Johnson WJ. Role of phosphate depletion and high dialysate calcium in controlling dialytic renal osteodystrophy. *Kidney Int* 1973;4:154–60.

110. Stanbury SW, Lumb GA. Parathyroid function in chronic renal failure: a statistical survey of the plasma biochemistry in azotemic renal osteodystrophy. *Q J Med* 1966;35:1–26.

111. Kaye M, Chatterjee G, Cohen GF, Sagar S. Arrest of hyperparathyroid bone disease with dihydrotachysterol in patients undergoing chronic hemodialysis. *Ann Intern Med* 1970;73:225–31.

112. Kaye M, Sagar S. Effect of dihydrotachysterol on calcium absorption in uremia. *Metabolism* 1972;21:815–20.

113. Witmer G, Margolis A, Fontaine O, et al. Effects of 25-hydroxycholecalciferol on bone lesion of children with terminal renal failure. *Kidney Int* 1976;10:395–403.

114. Recker R, Schoenfeld P, Letteri J, Slatopolsky E, Goldsmith R, Brickman A. The efficacy of calcifediol in renal osteodystrophy. *Arch Intern Med* 1978;138:857–61.

115. Papapoulos SE, Brownjohn AM, Goodwin FJ, et al. The effect of 1α-hydroxycholecalciferol on secondary hyperparathyroidism of chronic renal failure. In: Norman AW, Schaefer K, Coburn JW, et al., eds. *Vitamin D biochemical, chemical and clinical aspects related to calcium metabolism.* Berlin: Walter de Gruyter, 1977;693–7.

116. Brickman AS, Sherrard DJ, Jowsey J, et al. 1,25-Dihydroxycholecalciferol: effect on skeletal lesions and plasma parathyroid hormone in uremic osteodystrophy. *Arch Intern Med* 1974;134:883–9.

117. Silverberg DS, Bettcher KB, Dossetor JB, et al. Effect of 1,25-dihydroxycholecalciferol in renal osteodystrophy. *Can Med Assoc J* 1975;112:190–4.

118. Counts SG, Baylink DJ, Shen FH, Sherrard DJ, Hickman RO. Vitamin D intoxication in an anephric child. *Ann Intern Med* 1975;82:196–203.

119. Hughes MR, Baylink DJ, Jones PG, et al. Radioligand receptor assay for 25-hydroxyvitamin D_2D_3. *J Clin Invest* 1976;58:61–70.

120. Teitelbaum SL, Bone JM, Stein PM, et al. Calcifediol in chronic renal insufficiency: skeletal response. *JAMA* 1976;235:164–9.

121. Eastwood JB, Stamp TCB, DeWardener HE, et al. The effect of 25-hydroxyvitamin D_3 in osteomalacia of chronic renal failure. *Clin Sci Mol Med* 1977;52:499–504.

122. Coburn JW, Brickman AS, Sherrard DJ, et al. Clinical efficacy of 1,25-dihydroxyvitamin D_3 in renal osteodystrophy, In: Norman AW, Schaefer K, Coburn JW, et al., eds. *Vitamin D: biochemical, chemical and clinical aspects related to calcium metabolism.* Berlin, Walter de Gruyter, 1977;657–61.

123. Sherrard DJ, Coburn JW, Brickman AS, et al. A histologic comparison of 1,25(OH)$_2$-vitamin D treatment with calcium supplementation in renal osteodystrophy. In: Norman AW, Schaefer K, Coburn JW, et al., eds. *Vitamin D: biochemical and clinical aspects related to calcium metabolism.* Berlin: Walter de Gruyter, 1977;719.

124. Sherrard DJ, Brickman AS, Coburn JW, Singer FR, Maloney N. Skeletal response to treatment with 1,25-dihydroxyvitamin D in renal failure. *Contrib Nephrol* 1980;18:92–8.

125. Eastwood JB, Phillips ME, DeWardener HE, et al. Biochemical and histological effects of 1,25-dihydroxycholecalciferol in the osteomalacia of chronic renal failure. In: Norman AW, Schaefer K, Grigoleit HG, et al., eds. *Vitamin D and problems related to uremic bone disease.* Berlin: Walter de Gruyter, 1975;595–9.

126. Chesney RW, Moorthy AW, Eisman JA, et al. Increased growth after long-term oral 1,25-vitamin D_3 in childhood renal osteodystrophy. *N Engl J Med* 1978;298:238–41.

127. Ahmed KY, Wills MR, Varghese Z, Meinhard EA, Moorhead JF. Long-term effects of small doses of 1,25-dihydroxycholecalciferol in renal osteodystrophy. *Lancet* 1978;1:629–32.

128. Christiansen C, Rodbro P, Christiansen MS, Hartnack B, Transbol I. Deterioration of renal function during treatment of chronic renal failure with 1,25-dihydroxycholecalciferol. *Lancet* 1978;2:700–8.

129. Baker LRI, Abrams SM, Roe CS, et al. 1,25(OH)$_2D_3$ administration in moderate renal failure: a prospective double-blind trial. *Kidney Int* 1989;35:661–9.

130. Wilson RE, Hampers CL, Bernstein DS, Johnson JW, Merrill JP. Subtotal parathyroidectomy in chronic renal failure. *Ann Surg* 1971;174:640–9.

131. Katz AD, Kaplan L. Parathyroidectomy for hyperplasia in renal disease. *Arch Surg* 1973;107:51–9.

132. David SD. Calcium metabolism in renal failure. *Am J Med* 1975;58:48–56.

133. Wells SA Jr, Gunnells JC, Shelburne JD, Schneider AB, Sherwood LM. Transplantation of the parathyroid glands in man: clinical indications and results. *Surgery* 1975;78:34–41.

134. Ackrill P, Day JP, Gargstang FM, et al. Treatment of fracturing renal osteodystrophy by desferrioxamine. *Proc Eur Dial Transplant Assoc* 1982;19:203–7.

135. Milliner DS, Nebeker HG, Ott SA, et al. Use of the desferrioxamine infusion test in the diagnosis of aluminum-related osteodystrophy. *Ann Intern Med* 1984;101:775–80.

136. Malluche HH, Smith AJ, Abreo K, et al. The use of desferrioxamine in the management of aluminum accumulation in bone in patients with renal failure. *N Engl J Med* 1984;311:140–4.

137. Molitoris BA, Alfrey AC, Alfrey PS, et al. Rapid removal of DFO-chelated aluminum during hemodialysis using polysulfone dialyzers. *Kidney Int* 1988;34:98–101.

138. Delmez J, Weerts C, Lewis-Finch J, Windus S, Slatopolsky E. Accelerated removal of deferoxamine mesylate-chelated aluminum by charcoal hemoperfusion in hemodialysis patients. *Am J Kidney Dis* 1989;13:308–11.

139. Popovich RP, Moncrief JW, Nolph KD, Ghods AJ, Twardowski ZJ, Pyle WK. Continuous ambulatory peritoneal dialysis. *Ann Intern Med* 1978;88:449–56.

140. Popovich RP, Pyle WK, Moncrief JW. Kinetics of peritoneal transport. In: Nolph KD, ed. *Peritoneal dialysis,* vol 2. Hingham, Mass: Martinus Nijhoff, 1981;79–123.

141. Delmez J. Control of mineral metabolism in CAPD patients. *Blood Purif* 1989;7:167–80.

142. Delmez J. Bone and mineral metabolism in continuous ambulatory peritoneal dialysis. In: Twardowski ZJ, Khanna R, Nolph KD, Stein J, Brenner B, eds. *Contemporary issues in nephrology,* vol 21. New York: Churchill Livingstone, 1990;191–209.

143. Blumenkrantz MJ, Kopple JD, Moran JD, Coburn JW. Metabolic balance studies and dietary protein requirements in patients undergoing continuous ambulatory peritoneal dialysis. *Kidney Int* 1982;21:849–61.

144. Delmez JA, Slatopolsky E, Martin KJ, Gearing BK, Harter HR. Minerals, vitamin D and parathyroid hormone in continuous ambulatory peritoneal dialysis. *Kidney Int* 1982;21:862–7.

145. Salusky IB, Coburn JW, Brill J. Bone disease in pediatric patients undergoing dialysis with CAPD or CCPD. *Kidney Int* 1988; 33:975–82.

146. Joffe P, Olsen F, Heaf JG, Gammelgaard B, Podenphant J. Aluminum concentrations in serum, dialysate, urine and bone among patients undergoing continuous ambulatory peritoneal dialysis (CAPD). *Clin Nephrol* 1989;32:133–8.

147. Salusky IB, Coburn JW, Foley J, Nelson P, Fine RN. Effect of oral calcium carbonate on control of serum phosphorus and changes in plasma aluminum levels after discontinuation of aluminum-containing gels in children receiving dialysis. *J Pediatr* 1984;105:767–70.

148. Delmez JA, Gearing BK. Renal osteodystrophy and aluminum bone disease in CAPD patients. In: Khanna R, Nolph KD, Prowant, Twardowski ZJ eds. *Advances in continuous ambulatory peritoneal dialysis.* Toronto: University of Toronto Press, 1987;38–45.

149. Shah GM, Winer RL, Catler RE, et al. Effects of magnesium-free dialysate on magnesium metabolism during continuous ambulatory peritoneal dialysis. *Am J Kidney Dis* 1987;10:268–75.

150. Jennings AE, Bodvarsson M, Galicka-Piskorska G, et al. Use of magnesium hydroxide and low magnesium dialysate does not permit reduction of aluminum hydroxide during continuous ambulatory peritoneal dialysis. *Am J Kidney Dis* 1986;8:192–5.

151. Gokal R, Ramos JM, Ellis HA, et al. Histological renal osteodystrophy, and 25 hydroxycholecalciferol and aluminum levels in patients on continuous ambulatory peritoneal dialysis. *Kidney Int* 1983;23:15–21.

152. Kurtz SB, McCarthy JT, Kumar R. Hypercalcemia in continuous ambulatory peritoneal dialysis patients: observations on parameters of calcium metabolism. In: Gahl GM, Kessel M, Nolph KD, eds. *Advances in peritoneal dialysis.* Amsterdam: Excerpta Medica, 1981;467–72.

153. Delmez JA, Fallon MD, Bergfeld MA, Gearing BK, Dougan CS, Teitelbaum SL. Continuous ambulatory peritoneal dialysis and bone. *Kidney Int* 1986;30:379–84.

154. Delmez JA, Dougan CS, Gearing BK, et al. The effects of intraperitoneal calcitriol on calcium and parathyroid hormone. *Kidney Int* 1987;31:795–9.

155. Goldstein DA, Haldimann B, Sherman D, Norman AW, Massry SG. Vitamin D metabolites and calcium metabolism in patients with nephrotic syndrome and normal renal function. *J Clin Endocrinol Metab* 1981;52:116–20.

156. Alon U, Shany S, Chaimovitz C. Losses of 25-hydroxyvitamin D in peritoneal fluid: possible mechanism for bone disease in uremic patients treated with chronic ambulatory peritoneal dialysis. *Miner Electrolyte Metab* 1983;9:82–6.

157. Buccianti G, Bianchi ML, Valenti G. Progress of renal osteodystrophy during continuous ambulatory peritoneal dialysis. *Clin Nephrol* 1984;6:279–83.

158. Tielemans C, Aubry C, Dratwa M. The effects of continuous ambulatory peritoneal dialysis on renal osteodystrophy. In: Gahl GM, Kessel M, Nolph KD, eds. *Advances in peritoneal dialysis.* Amsterdam: Excerpta Medica, 1981;454–60.

159. Zucchelli P, Catizone L, Casanova S, Fusavoli M, Fabbri L, Ferrari G. Renal osteodystrophy in CAPD patients. *Miner Electrolyte Metab* 1984;10:326–32.

160. Cassidy MJD, Own JP, Ellis HA, et al. Renal osteodystrophy and metastatic calcification in long-term continuous ambulatory peritoneal dialysis. *Q J Med* 1985;213:29–48.

161. Parfitt AM. Hypercalcemia hyperparathyroidism following renal transplantation: differential diagnosis, management, and implications for cell population control in the parathyroid gland. *Miner Electrolyte Metab* 1982;8:92–112.

162. Schwartz H, David DS, Riggio RR, et al. Hypercalcemia after renal transplantation. *Am J Med* 1970;49:42–51.

163. David DS, Sakai S, Brennan L, et al. Hypercalcemia after renal transplantation. *N Engl J Med* 1973;289:398–400.

164. Gittes RF, Radde IC. Experimental model for hyperparathyroidism: effect of excessive numbers of transplanted isologous parathyroid glands. *J Urol* 1966;95:595–603.

165. Cundy T, Kanis JA, Heynen G, et al. Calcium metabolism and hyperparathyroidism after renal transplantation. *Q J Med* 1985;205:67–78.

166. Alfrey AC, Jenkins D, Groth CG, Schorr WS, Gecelter L, Ogden DA. Resolution of hyperparathyroidism, renal osteodystrophy and metastatic calcification after renal homotransplantation. *N Engl J Med* 1968;279:1349–56.

167. Christensen MS, Nielsen HE, Torring S. Hypercalcemia and parathyroid function after renal transplantation. *Acta Med Scand* 1977;201:35–9.

168. Ulmann A, Chkoff N, Lacour B. Disorders of calcium and phosphorus metabolism after successful kidney transplantation. In: Hamburger J, Crosnier JP, Grunfeld J-P, Maxwell MH, eds. *Advances in nephrology.* Chicago: Year Book Medical Publishers, 1983;331–40.

169. Geis WP, Popovtzer MM, Corman JL, Halgrimson CG, Groth CG, Starzl TE. The diagnosis and treatment of hyperparathyroidism after renal homotransplantation. *Surg Gynecol Obstet* 1973;137:997–1010.

170. Hornum I. Post-transplant hypercalcemia due to mobilization of metastatic calcifications. *Acta Med Scand* 1971;189:199–205.

171. Cundy T, Kanis JA, Fhaher L, Clemens TL, O'Riordan JLH. The use of metabolites and analogues of vitamin D in prospective renal transplant recipients. *Clin Nephrol* 15:240–5.

172. Chatterjee SN, Friedler RM, Berne TV, Oldham SB, Singer FR, Massry SG. Persistent hypercalcemia after successful renal transplantation. *Nephron* 1976;17:1–7.

173. Parfitt AM, Kleerekoper M, Cruz C. Reduced phosphate reabsorption unrelated to parathyroid hormone after renal transplantation: implications for the pathogenesis of hyperparathyroidism in chronic renal failure. *Miner Electrolyte Metab* 1986;12:356–62.

174. McCarron DA, Muther RS, Lenfesty B, Bennett WM. Parathyroid function in persistent hyperparathyroidism: relationship to gland size. *Kidney Int* 1982;22:662–70.

175. McCarron DA, Lenfesty B, Narasimhan N, Barry JM, Vetto RM, Bennett WM. Anatomical heterogeneity of parathyroid glands in posttransplant hyperparathyroidism. *Am J Nephrol* 1988;8:388–91.

176. Lucas PA, Woodhead JS, Brown RC. Vitamin D_3 metabolites in chronic renal failure and after renal transplantation. *Nephrol Dial Transplant* 1988;3:70–6.

177. Szabo A, Merke J, Beier E, Mall G, Ritz E. 1,25(OH)$_2$ vitamin D_3 inhibits parathyroid cell proliferation in experimental uremia. *Kidney Int* 1989;35:1049–56.

178. Nygren P, Larsson R, Johansson H, Ljunghall S, Rastad J, Akerstrom G. 1,25(OH)$_2$D$_3$ inhibits hormone secretion and proliferation but not functional dedifferentiation of cultured bovine parathyroid cells. *Calcif Tissue Int* 1988;43:213–8.

179. Fucik RF, Kukreja SC, Hargis GK, Bowser EN, Henderson WJ, Williams GA. Effect of glucocorticoids on function of the parathyroid glands in man. *J Clin Endocrinol Metab* 1974;40:152–5.

180. Lukert BP, Adams JS. Calcium and phosphorus homeostasis in man: effect of glucocorticoids. *Arch Intern Med* 1976;136:1249–53.

181. Hahn TJ, Halstead LR, Teitelbaum SL, Hahn BH. Altered mineral metabolism in glucocorticoid-induced osteopenia: effect of 25-hydroxyvitamin D administration. *J Clin Invest* 1979;64:655–65.

182. Williams GA, Peterson WC, Bowser EN, Henderson WJ, Hargis GK, Martinez NJ. Interrelationship of parathyroid and adrenocortical function in calcium homeostasis in the rat. *Endocrinology* 1973;95:707–12.

183. Russell J, Lettieri D, Sherwood LM. Dexamethasone reverses the suppressive effects 1,25-(OH)$_2$D$_3$ on pre-pro PTH gene transcription. In: Cohn DV, Martin TJ, Meunier PJ, eds. *Calcium regulation and bone metabolism: basic and clinical aspects.* New York: Elsevier Science, 1987;475–8.

184. Sugimoto T, Brown AJ, Ritter C, Morrissey J, Slatopolsky E, Martin KJ. Combined effects of dexamethasone and 1,25-dihydroxyvitamin D_3 on parathyroid hormone secretion in cultured bovine parathyroid cells. *Endocrinology* 1989;125:638–41.

185. Korkor AB. Reduced binding of [^{3}H]1,25-dihydroxyvitamin D_3 in the parathyroid glands of patients with renal failure. *N Engl J Med* 1987;316:1573–7.

186. Leapman SB, Vidne BA, Butt KMH, Waterhouse K, Kountz SL. Nephrolithiasis and nephrocalcinosis after renal transplantation: a case report and review of the literature. *J Urol* 1976;115:129–32.

187. Hayes JM, Streem SB, Graneto D, Hodge EE, Steinmuller DR, Novick AC. Renal transplant calculi: a reevaluation of risks and management. *Transplantation* 1989;47:949–52.

188. Gipstein RM, Coburn JW, Adams DA, et al. Calciphylaxis in man. *Arch Intern Med* 1976;136:1272–80.

189. Graf H, Kovarik J, Stummvoll HK, Wolf A, Pinggerra WF. Handling of phosphate by the transplanted kidney. *Proc Eur Dial Transplant Assoc* 1979;16:624–8.

190. Ward HN, Pabico RC, McKenna BA, Freeman RB. The renal handling of phosphate by renal transplant patients: correlation with serum parathyroid hormone (S_{PTH}), cyclic 3' 5'-adenosine monophosphate (cAMP) urinary excretion, and allograft function. *Adv Exp Med Biol* 1977;81:173–81.

191. Rosenbaum RW, Hruska KA, Korkor A, Anderson C, Slatopolsky E. Decreased phosphate reabsorption after renal transplantation: evidence for a mechanism independent of calcium and parathyroid hormone. *Kidney Int* 1981;19:568–78.

192. Pabico RC, McKenna BA, Freeman RB. Renal function before and after unilateral nephrectomy in renal donors. *Kidney Int* 1975;8:166–75.

193. Madsen S, Olgaard K, Lund BI, Lund BJ, Sorensen OH. Pathogenesis of hypophosphataemia in kidney necrograft recipients: a controlled trial. *Proc Eur Dial Transplant Assoc* 1979;16:618–23.

194. Garabedian M, Silve C, Levy D, Ulmann A, Broyer M, Balsan S. Chronic hypophosphatemia in kidney transplanted children and young adults. *Miner Electrolyte Metab* 1979;2:225–6.

195. Farrington K, Varghese Z, Newman SP, Ahmed KY, Fernando ON, Moorhead JF. Dissociation of absorptions of calcium and phosphate after successful cadaveric renal transplantation. *Br Med J* 1979;1:712–4.

196. Moorhead JF, Ahmed KY, Varghese Z, Wills MR, Baillod RA, Tatler GLV. Hypophosphataemic osteomalacia after cadaveric renal transplantation. *Lancet* 1974;1:694–7.

197. Felsenfeld AJ, Gutman RA, Drezner M, Llach F. Hypophosphatemia in long-term renal transplant recipients: effects on bone histology and 1,25-dihydroxycholecalciferol. *Miner Electrolyte Metab* 1986;12:333–41.

198. Pierides AM, Ellis HA, Peart KM, Simpson W, Uldall PR, Kerr DNS. Assessment of renal osteodystrophy following renal transplantation. *Proc Eur Dial Transplant Assoc* 1974;11:481–7.

199. Boukari M, Jaudon MC, Rottembourg PFJ, Luciani J, Legrain M, Galli A. Kinetics of serum and urinary aluminum after renal transplantation. *Lancet* 1978;2:1044.

200. Ihle BU, Buchanan RC, Stevens B, Becker GJ, Kincaid-Smith P. The efficacy of various treatment modalities of aluminum associated bone disease. *Proc Eur Dial Transplant Assoc* 1982;19:195–202.

201. Carroll RN, Williams ED, Aung T, Yeboah E, Shackman R. The effects of renal transplantation on renal osteodystrophy. *Proc Eur Dial Transplant Assoc* 1973;10:446–52.

202. Alsina J, Gonzalez MT, Bonnin R, et al. Long-term evolution of renal osteodystrophy after renal transplantation. *Transplant Proc* 1989;21:2151–8.

203. Eastell R, Kennedy NSJ, Smith MA, Tothill P, Anderson JL. Changes in total body calcium after renal transplantation: effect of low-dose steroid regime. *Nephron* 1985;40:139–42.

204. Lindsay R, McPherson SG, Anderson JB, Smith DA. The value of bone density measurements in predicting the risk of developing avascular necrosis following renal transplantation. In: *Proceedings of the XIth European symposium on calcified tissues.* Copenhagen: FADL Publishing, 1975;242–6.

205. Aird EGA, Pierides AM. Photon absorptiometry of bone after successful renal transplantation. *Br J Radiol* 1977;50:350–6.

206. Myers BD, Ross J, Newton L, Leutscher J, Perlroth M. Cyclosporine-associated chronic nephropathy. *N Engl J Med* 1984;311:699–705.

207. Stahl RAK, Kanz L, Maier B, Schollmeyer P. Hyperchloremic metabolic acidosis with high serum potassium in renal transplant recipients: a cyclosporine A associated side effect. *Clin Nephrol* 1986;25:245–8.

208. June CH, Thompson CB, Kennedy MS, Nims J, Thomas ED. Profound hypomagnesemia and renal magnesium wasting associated with the use of cyclosporine for marrow transplantation. *Transplantation* 1985;39:620–4.

209. Espevik T, Figari IS, Shalaby MR, et al. Inhibition of cytokine production by cyclosporin A and transforming growth factor β. *J Exp Med* 1987;166:571–6.

210. Orcel P, Bielakoff J, Modrowski D, Miravet L, De Vernejoul MC. Cyclosporin A induces in vivo inhibition of resorption and stimulation of formation in rat bone. *J Bone Miner Res* 1989;4:387–91.

211. Movsowitz C, Epstein S, Fallon M, Ismail F, Thomas S. Cyclosporin-A in vivo produces severe osteopenia in the rat: effect of dose and duration of administration. *Endocrinology* 1988;123:2571–7.

212. Movsowitz C, Epstein S, Ismail F, Fallon M, Thomas S. Cyclosporin A in the oopohorectomized rat: unexpected severe bone resorption. *J Bone Miner Res* 1989;4:393–398.

213. Klaushofer K, Hoffman O, Stewart PJ, et al. Cyclosporine A inhibits bone resorption in cultured neonatal mouse calvaria. *J Pharmacol Exp Ther* 1987;243:584–90.

214. Calne RY. Cyclosporin in cadaveric renal transplantation: 5-year follow-up of a multicentre trial. *Lancet* 1987;2:506–7.

215. Rambuske M, Ritz E, Pomer S, Mohring K, Rohl L. Alkaline phosphate levels in renal transplant recipients receiving cyclosporin or azathioprine steroids. *Lancet* 1988;1:248.

216. Aubia J, Masramon J, Seranno S, Lloveras J, Marinoso LL. Bone histology in renal transplant patients receiving cyclosporin. *Lancet* 1988;1:1048–9.

217. Boiskin I, Epstein S, Ismail F, Thomas SB, Raja R. Serum osteocalcin and bone mineral metabolism following successful renal transplantation. *Clin Nephrol* 1989;31:316–22.

218. Schmidt H, Stracke H, Schatz H, Scheuermann EH, Fassbinder W, Schoeppe W. Osteocalcin serum levels in patients following renal transplantation. *Klin Wochenschr* 1989;67:297–303.

219. Delmas PD, Wilson DM, Mann KG, Riggs BL. Effect of renal function on plasma levels of bone gla-protein. *J Clin Endocrinol Metab* 1983;57:1028–30.

220. Lukert BP, Higgins JC, Stoskopf MM. Serum osteocalcin is increased in patients with hyperparathyroidism and decreased in patients receiving glucocorticoids. *J Clin Endocrinol Metab* 1986;62:1056–8.

221. Potter DP, Belzer FO, Rames L, Holliday MA, Kountz SL, Najarian JS. The treatment of chronic uremia in childhood. I. Transplantation. *Pediatrics* 1970;45:432–43.

222. McEnery PT, Gonzalez LL, Martin LW, West CD. Growth and development of children with renal transplants: use of alternate-day steroid therapy. *J Pediatr* 1973;183:806–14.

223. Ettenger RB, Blifeld C, Prince, et al. The pediatric nephrologist's dilemma: growth after renal transplantation and its interaction with age as a possible immunologic variable. *J Pediatr* 1987;111:1022–5.

224. Rizzoni G, Broyer M, Guest G, Fine R, Holliday MA. Growth retardation in children with chronic renal disease: scope of the problem. *Am J Kidney Dis* 1986;7:256–61.

225. Ibels LS, Alfrey AC, Huffer WE, Weil R III. Aseptic necrosis of bone following renal transplantation: experience in 194 transplant recipients and review of the literature. *Medicine* 1978;57:457–81.

226. Metselaar HJ, van Steenberge JP, Bijnen AB, Jeekel JJ, van Linge B, Weimar W. Incidence of osteonecrosis after renal transplantation. *Acta Orthop Scand* 1985;56:413–5.

227. Slatopolsky E, Martin K. Glucocorticoids and renal transplant osteonecrosis. In: Avioli L, Gennari C, Imbimbo B, eds. *Glucocorticoid effects and their biological consequences.* New York: Plenum Press, 1984;353–9.

228. Meakin CJ, Hopson CN, First MR. Avascular (aseptic) necrosis of bone following renal transplantation (editorial). *Int J Artif Organs* 1985;8:19–20.

229. Harrington KD, Murray WR, Kountz SL, Belzer FO. Avascular necrosis of bone after renal transplantation. *J Bone Joint Surg* 1971;53-A:203–15.

230. Landmann J, Renner N, Bachter A, Thiel G, Harder F. Cyclosporin A and osteonecrosis of the femoral head. *J Bone Joint Surg* 1987;62-A:795–800.

231. Lausten GS, Jensen JS, Olgaard K. Necrosis of the femoral head after renal transplantation. *Acta Orthop Scand* 1988;59:650–4.

232. Sutherland DER, Payne WD, Fryd DS, et al. Comparison of cyclosporine and azathioprine for immunosuppression in diabetic

and nondiabetic renal allograft recipients. *Transplant Proc* 1985;17:1204–11.

233. Melsen F, Nielsen H. Osteonecrosis following renal allotransplantation. *Acta Pathol Microbiol Scand* 1977;85:99–104.

234. Wilkes CH, Visscher MB. Some physiological aspects of bone marrow pressure. *J Bone Joint Surg* 1975;57-A:49–57.

235. Wang GJ, Sweet DE, Reger SI, Thompson RC. Fat cell changes as a mechanism of avascular necrosis of the femoral head in cortisone-treated rabbits. *J Bone Joint Surg* 1977;59-A:729–35.

236. Hungerford DS. Pathogenetic considerations in ischemic necrosis of the bone. *Can J Surg* 1981;24:583–588.

237. Jones JP Jr, Engleman EP, Najarian JS. Systemic fat embolism after renal homotransplantation and treatment with corticosteroids. *N Engl J Med* 1965;273:1453–8.

238. Fisher DEI, Bickel WH. Corticosteroid-induced avascular necrosis: a clinical study of 77 patients. *J Bone Joint Surg* 1971;53-A:859–64.

239. Parfrey PS, Farge D, Parfrey NA, Hanley JA, Guttman RD. The decreased incidence of aseptic necrosis in renal transplant recipients: a case control study. *Transplantation* 1986;41:182–7.

240. Gottlieb MN, Stephens MK, Lowrie EG, et al. A longtitudinal study of bone disease after successful renal transplantation. *Nephron* 1978;22:239–48.

241. Patton PR, Pfaff WW. Aseptic necrosis after renal transplant. *Surgery* 1988;103:63–8.

242. Nielsen HE, Melsen F, Christensen MS. Aseptic necrosis of bone following renal transplantation: clinical and biochemical aspects and bone morphometry. *Acta Med Scand* 1977;202:27–32.

243. Conceicao SC, Wilkinson R, Feest TG, Owen JP, Dewar J, Kerr DNS. Hypercalcemia following renal transplantation: causes and consequences. *Clin Nephrol* 1981;16:235–44.

244. Scholz D, Mebel J, Topelmann I, Grossmann I, Scholze J, Mrochen H. Prevention of osteonecrosis following renal transplantation by using vitamin D_2 (ergocalciferol). *Proc Eur Dial Transplant Assoc* 1983;20:331–7.

245. Harris RR, Niemann KMW, Diethelm AG. Skeletal complications after renal transplantation. *South Med J* 1974;67:1016–9.

246. Bradford DS, Morrow CE, Sutherland DER, Simmons RL, Najarian JS, Janes P. Osteonecrosis and total hip arthroplasty in renal transplant recipients. *Transplant Proc* 1983;15:1105–6.

247. Chmell SJ, Schwartz CM, Giacchino JL, Ing TS. Total hip replacement in patients with renal transplants. *Arch Surg* 1983;118:489–95.

Disorders of Bone and Mineral Metabolism,
edited by Fredric L. Coe and Murray J. Favus.
© 1992 by Raven Press, Ltd. All rights reserved.

CHAPTER **40**

Bone Disease Resulting From Inherited Disorders of Renal Tubule Transport and Vitamin D Metabolism

Michael J. Econs and Marc K. Drezner

Although vitamin D deficiency was by far the most common form of rickets and osteomalacia early in this century, supplementation of foods with ergocalciferol has virtually eliminated this disease in developed countries. With the disappearance of this disorder it became apparent that there were other forms of rickets/osteomalacia that did not respond to physiologic doses of vitamin D. In 1937 Albright et al. (1) reported that administration of vitamin D in pharmacologic doses healed the rickets in patients affected with such a disorder. Thus, they postulated that these diseases resulted from an end organ resistance to vitamin D and accordingly named them vitamin D resistant rickets. Further research over the past two decades indicates, however, that these diseases comprise a large group of disorders with diverse pathophysiologies (Table 1). Moreover, although end organ resistance to the active form of vitamin D, calcitriol, does occur (e.g., vitamin D dependent rickets, type II), the majority of these syndromes are not vitamin D resistant diseases per se.

In this chapter we present up-to-date information regarding the familial "vitamin D resistant" rachitic/osteomalacic disorders, a group of genetic diseases characterized by: (i) renal tubular defects that result in decreased reabsorption of phosphate and/or other solutes; (ii) decreased renal 25-hydroxyvitamin D-1α-hydroxylase; and/or (iii) end organ resistance to calcitriol. Recent studies of these disorders have provided extensive information regarding the genetic abnormalities and physiologic derangements which underlie their phenotypic expression. An enlightened insight into effective therapy of these diseases has resulted.

DISORDERS OF RENAL TUBULAR FUNCTION

X-Linked Hypophosphatemic Rickets

X-linked hypophosphatemic rickets/osteomalacia is the most common "vitamin D resistant" disease in man. The syndrome occurs as an X-linked dominant disorder with complete penetrance of a renal tubular abnormality resulting in phosphate wasting and consequent hypophosphatemia. Additional characteristic features of the disease include growth retardation, osteomalacia, and rickets in growing children. The clinical expression of the disease is widely variable, ranging from a simple biochemical defect to severe bone disease. The mildest abnormality is hypophosphatemia without clinically evident bone disease (2–4). Generally, this may be detected at birth. However, its presence and/or other features of the disease may not become apparent until age 6 to 12 months or older (5). The most common clinically evident manifestation of X-linked hypophosphatemia (XLH) is short stature. This height deficiency is a consequence of abnormal lower extremity growth, averaging 15% below normal. In contrast, upper segment growth is not affected.

The majority of affected children exhibit clinical evidence of rickets, varying from enlargement of the wrists and/or knees to a lateral collapse of both chest walls (Harrison's sulcus) and rachitic rosary. Bowing of the lower extremities is often an associated abnormality. Such defects may result in waddling gait and, in severely affected patients, genu varum or valgum (6). In addition,

M. J. Econs and M. K. Drezner: Departments of Medicine and Cell Biology, Duke University Medical Center, Durham, North Carolina 27710.

TABLE 1. *Rachitic/osteomalacic disorders secondary to inherited disorders of renal tubular transport and vitamin D metabolism*

Disorders of renal tubule function
X-linked hypophosphatemic rickets/osteomalacia (XLH)
Hereditary hypophosphatemic rickets with hypercalciuria (HHRH)
Adult hypophosphatemic rickets (AHR)
Fanconi's syndrome, type I (FS I)
    Familial idiopathic
    Cystinosis (Lignac-Fanconi disease)
    Hereditary fructose intolerance
    Tyrosinemia
    Galactosemia
    Glycogen storage disease
    Wilson's disease
    Lowe's syndrome
Fanconi's syndrome, type II (FS II)

Decreased renal 25-hydroxyvitamin D-1α-hydroxylase activity
Vitamin D dependent rickets, type I (VDDR I)
Pseudohypoparathyroidism

End-organ resistance to calcitriol
Vitamin D dependent rickets, type II (VDDR II)

---

x-ray examination reveals expanded areas of proliferating non-mineralized cartilage in epiphyseal regions and lateral curvature of the femora and/or tibia. Evidence of secondary hyperparathyroidism is notably absent. These changes often occur within the first year of life and are generally associated with an elevated serum concentration of alkaline phosphatase and osteocalcin (biochemical markers of the active rickets) and increased bone turnover.

Additional early signs of the disease may include late dentition, skull deformities, and "sitting" deformities of the legs. The skull deformities are manifest as a frontal bossing with flattening at the back and the leg abnormalities as anterior bowing at the lower ends of the tibiae (which result from sitting cross-legged). In severely affected children, abnormalities of the maxillofacial region, poor dental development, and spontaneous tooth abscesses often follow (7). Strikingly absent are common features of vitamin D deficiency and hypophosphatemia, most notably muscle weakness.

Adults with XLH may be asymptomatic or present with severe bone pain. On clinical examination they often display evidence of inactive post-rachitic deformities, such as bowed legs or short stature. However, radiographic or biochemical abnormalities typical of active bone disease are generally absent. In contrast, a relatively small group of adults present with post-rachitic deformities and "active" osteomalacia, characterized on x-ray examination by pseudofractures, coarsened trabeculation, rarified areas, and/or non-union fractures, and biochemically by an elevated serum alkaline phosphatase. Occasionally adults exhibit osteosclerosis. Symptoms at presentation often do not correlate with the apparent activity of the disease. Many adults also develop bone overgrowth at the site of muscle attachments and around joints which causes significant limitation of motion, particularly at the hips (8,9). Such overgrowth has resulted in complete fusion of the sacroiliac joints (10). In rare instances this overgrowth leads to spinal cord compression requiring surgical intervention. Indeed, these enthesopathic changes are the primary cause of morbidity in affected adults.

In general, females present less often than males with clinically evident bone disease. However, when present the disease in females may be equally severe (4,6) and males without apparent bone disease have also been reported (5). In spite of these differences, bone biopsy reveals osteomalacia in affected subjects, the severity of which bears no relationship to sex or clinical disability.

The bone disease in XLH is marked by a reduced rate of formation, diffuse patchy hypomineralization, a decrease in mineralizing surfaces, and a unique increase in perilacunar areas of absent mineralization (11). In teeth the formation and mineralization of interglobular dentine is abnormal (12). This leads to frequent tooth abscesses in many individuals.

Abnormal Growth

Several factors undoubtedly contribute to the short stature which commonly affects patients with XLH. Refractory hypophosphatemia, however, is most likely a primary cause of this abnormality. This is supported by the normal growth realized during the infancy of affected patients in whom the onset of hypophosphatemia is delayed until age 6–12 months, as well as the normal growth evidenced in affected subjects who maintain a normal serum phosphorus concentration secondary to coincident hypoparathyroidism or chronic renal failure. Moreover, a role for hypophosphatemia in the growth failure has been reinforced by the results of therapeutic intervention. In this regard, several investigators have reported that administration of phosphate in sufficient amounts (in conjunction with vitamin D or calcitriol) to restore the serum phosphorus concentration to normal (for a significant portion of the day) improves the linear growth rate to near normal or normal (13–17). However, a significant proportion of affected youths do not attain normal growth rate in spite of "adequate" treatment and fail to achieve an adult stature comparable to nonaffected members of their respective kindreds (18). Thus, complementary factors must influence the growth potential in patients with XLH.

Biochemical Characteristics

As previously noted, the primary biochemical abnormality of XLH is hypophosphatemia. In order to determine if a low serum phosphorus concentration is present, consideration must be given to the variable normal range which occurs as a function of age and sex. In addition, attention must be directed to the age when hypophosphatemia first appears. In this regard, some investigators have found low serum phosphorus levels in affected subjects from birth (19) while others have not observed consistently decreased values until after 6 months of age (5). Nevertheless, in every reported instance the hypophosphatemia in XLH is associated with increased urinary phosphate excretion. Moreover, gastrointestinal phosphate malabsorption is present, a factor that contributes to the evolution of the hypophosphatemia (20–23).

In contrast, the serum calcium concentration in affected subjects is normal despite mild gastrointestinal malabsorption of calcium. However, as a consequence of this defect, urinary calcium is low. Commensurate diminished bone mineralization preserves a slightly positive calcium balance (20,21). Such adequate maintenance of calcium homeostasis results in normal serum parathyroid hormone levels. Indeed, multiple laboratories, employing a variety of antisera with varying antigenic specificity, have reported normal circulating levels of immunoreactive parathyroid hormone (20,21,24–26). Accordingly, urinary cyclic AMP excretion is uniformly normal (27).

Recently several investigators have also reported a normal serum 25(OH)D concentration in patients with XLH (20,21,28). In addition, multiple laboratories have observed that untreated youths and adults have normal serum 1,25(OH)$_2$D levels (29–31). However, an elevation of this active vitamin D metabolite would be anticipated in the setting of hypophosphatemia and phosphate depletion, factors which increase calcitriol production in several animal species (32–34) and man (35,36). The paradoxical occurrence of hypophosphatemia and normal serum 1,25(OH)$_2$D levels in affected subjects is consistent with a defect in production of this active vitamin D metabolite, most likely due to diminished 25(OH)D-1α-hydroxylase activity. This supposition is supported by recent studies which show that the serum calcitriol in patients with XLH increases far less than that in normals in response to pharmacological stimulation with exogenous parathyroid hormone (37). However, the defect is not complete since administration of calcitonin results in a normal increment in the circulating concentration of 1,25(OH)$_2$D (unpublished observations).

In contrast, the serum calcitriol level in affected subjects treated with vitamin D alone or vitamin D [or 25(OH)D] and phosphates is low (31,38,39). The cause of this depression remains uncertain but the serum 1,25(OH)$_2$D levels are negatively correlated with the serum 25(OH)D concentrations in treated subjects (31).

Investigation of serum electrolytes, other than calcium and phosphorus, has revealed no abnormalities. Similarly, blood pH, bicarbonate, and blood urea nitrogen are normal. In contrast, although urinary amino acid excretion in most kindreds is normal, mild glycinuria and renal glycosuria have been reported in affected members of several families (4,40). Additionally, the serum alkaline phosphatase activity is often elevated and is associated in children (but less often in adults) with the presence of active bone disease. The biochemical characteristics of XLH, as well as those of the other disorders discussed in this chapter, are summarized in Table 2.

Genetics

With the recognition that hypophosphatemia is the definitive marker for XLH, whether occurring in appar-

TABLE 2. Comparison of abnormalities characteristic of the hereditary rachitic/osteomalacic disorders

	Phosphopenic					Calciopenic	
	XLH	HHRH	AHR	FS I	FS II	VDDR I	VDDR II
Biochemistries							
Calcium	N	N	N	N	N	↓	↓
Phosphorus	↓	↓	↓	↓	↓	↓	↓
Alkaline phosphatase	↑	↑	↑	↑	↑	↑	↑
Parathyroid hormone	N	↓	N	N	↓	↑	↑
25(OH)D	N	N	N	N	N	N	N
1,25(OH)$_2$	RD	↑	RD	RD	↑	↓	↑
Renal Function							
Urinary phosphorus	↑	↑	↑	↑	↑	↑	↑
Urinary calcium	↓	↑	↓	↓	↑	↓	↓
Gastrointestinal Function							
Calcium absorption	↓	↑	↓	↓	↑	↓	↓
Phosphorus absorption	↓	↑	↓	↓	↑	↓	↓

XLH, X-linked hypophosphatemic rickets; HHRH, hereditary hypophosphatemic rickets with hypercalciuria; AHR, adult hypophosphatemic rickets; FS I, Fanconi's syndrome type I; FS II, Fanconi's syndrome, type II; VDDR I, vitamin D dependent rickets, type I; VDDR II, vitamin D dependent rickets, type II.

N, normal; RD, decreased relative to the serum phosphorus concentration; ↑, increased; ↓, decreased.

ent isolation or in association with evident bone disease, Winters et al. (3) and Burnett et al. (4) suggested that this disease is transmitted as an X-linked dominant disorder. Evidence supporting their conclusion included: observations that: (i) the disorder is transmitted from generation to generation without interruption; and (ii) the segregation ratios in the progeny of affected parents are, with minor exceptions, those anticipated for such a gene. Indeed, in the few published reports where the paradoxic occurrence of male to male transmission has been reported, the existent disease differs appreciably from XLH. Recognition of an X-linked dominant mode of transmission, of course, provided explanation for the lesser severity of disease in affected females. In this regard, random inactivation of X chromosomes in heterozygous females has been proposed. However, such genetic transmission did not explain the rare sporadic occurrence of disease which is phenotypically identical to XLH. At least 10 such patients have been reported (41) and the disorder in these instances likely results from a new mutation. Accordingly, children of a propositus with sporadic new disease manifested evidence of XLH in a pattern consistent with a dominant gene on the X chromosome (42). On the assumption that each of the sporadic cases reported represents a new mutation, the rate of mutation per gene per generation is 6.4×10^{-6} and 5.3×10^{-6} for males and females, respectively (42), estimates similar to those for other hereditary diseases.

Localization of the gene responsible for XLH on the X chromosome led to many attempts at identification of the genetic defect. However, despite the use of a variety of biochemical techniques, the abnormal gene underlying X-linked hypophosphatemia has not been elucidated. Efforts in this regard have been hindered by uncertainty about the gene function and the tissue in which the abnormality is expressed. Nevertheless, since reverse (indirect) genetics, using restriction fragment length polymorphisms (RFLPs), has been used successfully to locate and ultimately clone disease genes under such circumstances, efforts to map the XLH gene locus have recently been initiated. In 1986 Read et al. (43) provided initial evidence that the Xp22.1 region of the X chromosome harbored the genetic abnormality underlying XLH. They studied 15 small families of which 11 proved informative for linkage of the XLH locus to the DNA probe DXS41 [$Z(\theta) = 4.82$; $\theta = 0.10$], which localized to this region. In addition, they reported data consistent with similar linkage to DXS43 [$Z(\theta) = 1.96$; $\theta = 0.15$], which is telomeric to DXS41 in the same region of the X chromosome. Subsequently, Thakker et al. (44,45) and Machler et al. (46) confirmed these observations and documented association of additional polymorphic DNA probes, DXS197 [$Z(\theta) = 1.29$; $\theta = 0.09$] and DXS207 [$Z(\theta) = 1.29$; $\theta = 0.09$], with the XLH gene. Further, using multipoint mapping techniques in their respective studies, they determined the most likely order of

the markers to be Xpter-*DXS85-(DXS43/DXS197)-XLH-DXS41*-Xcen and Xpter-*(DXS207/DXS43)-XLH-DXS41*-Xcen, respectively. While these data have provided important new information regarding the XLH gene locus, the relatively small number of informative matings within the pedigrees available for study prevented definitive determination of gene order along the Xp22-p21 section of the X chromosome. Further, the absence of tightly linked ($\theta < 0.01$) highly informative polymorphic probes for analysis has limited progress in identification and characterization of the XLH gene region. More recently, however, Econs et al. (47,48) have expanded these gene localization and mapping studies to include five large kindreds with over 100 affected individuals. Their efforts resulted in the creation of a detailed map around the XLH gene and the definition of more closely linked flanking markers. In this regard, they confirmed linkage between XLH and DXS41 [$Z(\theta) = 8.31$; $\theta = 0.06$] and DXS43 [$Z(\theta) = 5.94$; $\theta = 0.05$] and established tight linkage with DXS365 [$Z(\theta) = 13.98$; $\theta = 0.00$] and other closely linked markers, DXS257 [$Z(\theta) = 8.09$; $\theta = 0.06$], DXS451 [$Z(\theta) = 13.19$; $\theta = 0.03$], and the 5′ untranslated portion of the glycine receptor, GLR [$Z(\theta) = 7.91$; $\theta = 0.07$]. Moreover, using linkage data from the CEPH reference pedigrees and their XLH kindreds, as well as analysis of individual cross over pairs, they determined a locus order along Xp22.1 of Xcen-*DXS319-DXS451-DXS41-XLH-DXS257-DXS43/GLR-DXS43-GLR-DXS315*-Xtel. These efforts promise to define the tightly linked flanking markers essential to successful localization and cloning of the XLH gene. Such investigation may ultimately permit accurate identification of the pathophysiological defect underlying this disease.

Pathophysiology

The pathogenesis of XLH remains a subject of considerable controversy. However, investigators generally agree that the primary inborn error of this disorder results in an expressed abnormality in the renal proximal tubule (and perhaps the intestine) which impairs phosphate reabsorption (and absorption). This defect has been indirectly identified in affected patients (49–51) and directly demonstrated in the brush border membranes of the proximal nephron in the Hyp-mouse, the murine homologue of the human disease (52–55). Specifically this defect manifests as an abnormality of the sodium dependent, arsenate inhibitable component of phosphate transport.

However, this proposed defect, and the resultant hypophosphatemia that develops as a consequence, do not account for the full spectrum of biochemical and skeletal abnormalities which constitute the X-linked hypophosphatemic syndrome. Most notably, treatment of patients with XLH with phosphorus (and/or vitamin D), while correcting phosphate deficiency, does not restore bone mineralization to normal, indicating that renal phosphate wasting and hypophosphatemia alone do not underlie the abnormal bone calcification in XLH (20,56). Therefore, several investigators have proposed that additional abnormalities may contribute to the pathogenesis of this disease. In this regard, a variety of recent studies indicate that abnormal vitamin D metabolism is a part of the XLH syndrome. Data supporting this conclusion include the presence in affected subjects of: (i) a normal circulating level of the active vitamin D metabolite, $1,25(OH)_2D$ (29–31); (ii) a significantly reduced increment of the serum calcitriol level in response to parathyroid hormone stimulation compared to that in age-matched controls (37); and (iii) a subnormal increase of the serum $1,25(OH)_2D$ concentration after dietary phosphorus deprivation. While these data are in accord with the presence of an apparent defect in calcitriol production (and/or metabolism), they do not establish: (i) if the abnormality represents a defect in enzyme [25(OH)D-1α-hydroxylase] function (which may be a primary or acquired derangement secondary to the abnormal phosphate transport); or (ii) whether this defect or the abnormal phosphate transport is primary or secondary to the elaboration of an hormonal factor. However, recent studies in the Hyp- and Gy-mouse have provided data indicating that the abnormal renal phosphate transport and vitamin D metabolism may be interrelated and due to an hormonal abnormality.

Animal Models of X-Linked Hypophosphatemic Rickets

Eicher et al. (57) and Lyon et al. (58) have reported the discovery of two genetically distinct murine homologues of XLH, the Hyp- and Gy-mice. The mutant *Hyp* and *Gy* alleles have been transferred to the C57BL6J and B_6C_3H inbred strains of mice, respectively. The mutations in each of these models is X-linked dominant and detailed linkage studies indicate that they occur in alleles which are at closely linked, but physically separate, sites near the distal end of the murine X chromosome.

The biochemical abnormalities which have been documented in Hyp-mice are remarkably similar to those in humans with XLH. Indeed, these mutants manifest hypophosphatemia (57,59), an increased fractional urinary excretion of phosphate (57), normal immunoassayable parathyroid hormone (57,60) and a normal circulating level of calcitriol (59) (in spite of the decreased serum phosphorus concentration). In contrast, Gy-mice, while exhibiting similar characteristics of phosphate homeostasis and a normal parathyroid hormone concentration, maintain an appropriately elevated serum $1,25(OH)_2D$ level (61,62). These observations suggest that disease in the Hyp-mouse and in humans is due to a defect in an homologous gene which has withstood evolutionary alteration. The relationship between the genetic defect in Gy-mice and in man, however, is not equally certain. Thus, only the Hyp-mouse has provided a model in which to elucidate the basic defect(s) underlying the X-linked hypophosphatemic disorders in humans.

In this regard, investigations of the Hyp-mouse have confirmed that aberrant regulation of renal 25(OH)D-1α-hydroxylase activity underlies abnormal $1,25(OH)_2D$ production in the X-linked hypophosphatemic syndrome. Whereas renal homogenates from phosphate-depleted mice have profoundly increased enzyme activity compared to that of normals, enzyme function in the Hyp-mouse kidney is no different from normal and far below that in the kidneys of their phosphate-depleted counterparts (59). In further studies several investigators (63,64) established that this apparent abnormality did not represent altered enzyme responsiveness to hypophosphatemia alone but is indicative of a more generalized defect. Their investigations illustrated that in Hyp-mice calcium depletion and/or parathyroid hormone or cyclic AMP administration did not normally stimulate enzyme function. In contrast, Nesbitt et al. (65) recently reported that calcitonin stimulation in Hyp-mice elicits a normal increment of renal 25(OH)D-1α-hydroxylase activity. This paradoxical response indicates that the abnormal parathyroid hormone (cyclic AMP) and phosphate-regulated activity in Hyp-mice (and affected patients) may be localized in the proximal convoluted tubule, the PTH-dependent site of enzyme function (66,67). In contrast, the normal calcitonin-responsive 25(OH)D-1α-hydroxylase is likely located in the proximal straight tubule (68). Moreover, since defective phosphate transport in Hyp-mice occurs in the proximal convoluted tubules (60,69), aberrant enzyme function at this site may result from the abnormal phosphate transport and/or consequent changes in the intracellular milieu. Under these circumstances, the enzyme dysfunction in Hyp-mice (and patients with XLH) may not be a genetically determined abnormality of 25(OH)D-1α-hydroxylase structure/function, but rather an acquired aberration secondary to the primary genetic abnormality.

More recently, Seino et al. (70) found that the defective calcitriol production in Hyp-mice is more complex. They reported that mutant mice exhibit a more rapid turnover of $1,25(OH)_2D$ than normals. Tenenhouse and co-workers (71,72) confirmed these observations in their study of renal homogenates from Hyp-mice. These in vitro preparations have elevated 24-hydroxylase activity, an enzyme essential to turnover of the calcitriol.

Collectively, these observations indicate that the aberrant vitamin D metabolism in the hypophosphatemic syndrome may be secondary to multifactorial influences. More importantly, however, the various investigations have provided the basis for a unified hypothesis which can account for the multiple derangements characteristic of XLH. In this regard, the concept seems attractive that abnormal phosphate transport may result in aberrant regulation of 1,25(OH)$_2$D production and these interrelated abnormalities, in turn, may underlie the pathogenesis of XLH.

Nevertheless, these data provide no information which establishes if the primary defect in phosphate transport is the consequence of: (i) an intrinsic renal abnormality resulting in an alteration of the proximal tubule brush border membrane, or (ii) production of a humoral factor. Studies by Tenenhouse and co-workers (53,54) and Dobre et al. (55), however, suggest that the abnormality is a consequence of a membrane defect in the proximal convoluted tubule. In these investigations proximal tubule cells from Hyp-mice, grown in primary culture, exhibit abnormalities in phosphate transport most consistent with a defect in the high capacity/low affinity NaPi transport system. Additionally, Ecarot-Charrier et al. (73) have reported data which suggest that osteoblasts from Hyp-mice similarly exhibit an intrinsic abnormality. In contrast, Meyer et al. (74,75) demonstrated that parabiotic union of normal and Hyp-mice results in transfer of the defect in renal phosphate reclamation to the normal mouse, an observation which suggests the presence of an hormonal abnormality. Most recently, Nesbitt et al. (76) have employed cross-transplantation of kidneys in normal and Hyp-mice in an effort to resolve this apparent discrepancy. In these studies, they observed that normal mice with mutant kidney grafts display a serum phosphorus concentration and fractional excretion of phosphate no different from those of normal mice with normal kidney grafts or sham operated normals. In accord, transplantation of normal kidneys to Hyp-mice fails to normalize the serum phosphorus concentration or the renal phosphate handling of the mutants. These data illustrate that the Hyp phenotype is neither transferred nor corrected by renal transplantation. Such observations favor the hypothesis that the Pi transport defect in Hyp-mice, and most probably in XLH, does not result from an intrinsic renal defect but more likely a hormonal influence.

Treatment

In past years, physicians employed pharmacologic doses of vitamin D as the cornerstone for treatment of XLH (41,42,77). However, long-term observations indicate that this therapy fails to cure the disease and poses the serious problem of recurrent vitamin D intoxication and renal damage (78–80). Indeed, such treatment results only in incomplete healing of the rachitic abnormality, while hypophosphatemia and impaired growth remain without significant improvement. Similar unresponsiveness prevails upon the use of 25(OH)D.

More recently, choice of therapy for this disease has been markedly influenced by an understanding of the pathogenetic factors underlying the disease. With recognition that phosphate depletion is an important contrib-

uting element, physicians began to devise treatment strategies which employed oral phosphate supplementation to overcome the renal phosphate wasting and increase the serum phosphorus concentration into or near the normal range. By necessity such therapeutic regimens included pharmacologic amounts of vitamin D to prevent the secondary hyperparathyroidism attendant upon oral phosphorus administration (5,56,81). Since this combination therapy results in radiographic healing of the rachitic lesions and occasionally accelerated growth in affected subjects, many physicians claim that such treatment is of universal benefit and heals the bone disease of XLH. However, radiographic examination of bone offers only an incomplete evaluation of therapeutic effect. Thus, the efficacy of this therapy remains uncertain. In fact, in subsequent studies several investigators reported that the bone biopsy evidence of osteomalacia in affected subjects does not remit in response to long-term therapy with phosphorus and vitamin D (20,82). With this recognition, renewed efforts to define a more optimal therapeutic regimen for XLH became apparent.

In this regard, recent studies have offered new hope for successful therapy of XLH. Capitalizing on the observation that a relative deficiency of 1,25(OH)$_2$D may contribute to the pathogenesis of the disease, several investigators tested the efficacy of new combination drug regimens: 1,25(OH)$_2$D or 1α(OH)D$_3$ and phosphorus. This treatment strategy directly addresses the combined calcitriol and phosphorus deficiency characteristic of the disorder. In general, several reports indicate that patients respond well to this therapeutic regimen (15,41,56,82,83). However, healing of the associated rickets and osteomalacia, as well as acceleration of growth velocity, is not a universal outcome in affected subjects. Nevertheless, 1,25(OH)$_2$D$_3$ and phosphorus is the conventional current treatment for XLH.

In the majority of affected children the goal of therapy is to improve growth velocity, normalize the lower extremity defect, if present, and/or heal the attendant bone disease. Generally the treatment regimen includes a period of titration to achieve a maximum dose of calcitriol, 40–60 ng/kg/day in two divided doses, and phosphorus, 1–2 g/day in 4–5 divided doses. Occasionally patients will prove refractory to such therapeutic intervention and maximally tolerated amounts of calcitriol and phosphorus are required with daily dose limits of 3 μg and 3 g, respectively.

Use of calcitriol/phosphorus combination therapy involves a significant risk of toxicity that is generally expressed as abnormalities of calcium homeostasis and/or detrimental effects on renal function. The occurrence of hypercalcemia, nephrocalcinosis, and diminished creatinine clearance necessitates appropriate restriction of therapy and in some cases discontinuation of therapy. Throughout the treatment course careful attention to renal function, as well as serum and urine calcium is extremely important. Nevertheless, in spite of these varied complications of therapy, treatment of XLH often proceeds with limited interruptions. Moreover, the improved outcome of this therapeutic intervention, compared to that achieved by previous regimens, justifies the aggressive approach that constitutes the current "conventional therapy."

Indications for therapy in adults with XLH are less clear. The occurrence of intractable bone pain and refractory non-union fractures often respond to treatment with calcitriol and phosphorus. However, data remain unclear regarding the effects of treatment on fracture incidence (which may not be increased in untreated patients), enthesopathy, and dental abscesses. Therefore, the decision to treat affected adults must be individualized.

Hereditary Hypophosphatemic Rickets with Hypercalciuria (HHRH)

This recently described rare genetic disease is marked by hypophosphatemic rickets with hypercalciuria (84). The cardinal biochemical features of the disorder include hypophosphatemia due to increased renal phosphate clearance and normocalcemia. In contrast to other diseases in which renal phosphate transport is limited, patients with HHRH exhibit increased $1,25(OH)_2D$ production. The resultant elevated serum calcitriol levels enhance the gastrointestinal calcium absorption which in turn increases the filtered renal calcium load and inhibits parathyroid secretion (84). These events cause the characteristic hypercalciuria observed in affected patients.

The clinical expression of the disease is heterogeneous. In general children become symptomatic between the ages of six months and seven years. Initial symptoms consist of bone pain or deformities of the lower limbs (or both), which progressively interferes with gait and physical activity. The bone deformities vary from genu varum or genu valgum to anterior external bowing of the femur and coxa vara. Additional salient features at presentation include short stature with disproportionately short lower limbs, muscle weakness, and radiologic signs of rickets or osteopenia (or both). These various symptoms (and signs) may exist separately or in combination and may be present in a mild or severe form.

A large number of apparently unaffected relatives of patients with HHRH exhibit an additional mode of disease expression. These subjects, although without evidence of bone disease, manifest hypercalciuria, as well as a pattern of biochemical abnormalities similar to those of children with rickets and osteomalacia (85). Quantitatively, however, the abnormalities are milder, and the relevant biochemical values intermediate between those observed in family members with HHRH and those in normal relatives. The absence of bone disease in these patients may be explained by relatively mild hypophos-

phatemia compared to the severe phosphate depletion evidenced in patients with the full spectrum of the disorder. Although X-linked transmission of the disorder has been ruled out, the mode of genetic transmission for HHRH/hypercalciuria remains unknown.

Pathophysiology

Liberman and co-workers (84–86) have presented data which indicate that the primary inborn error underlying this disorder is an expressed abnormality in the renal proximal tubule which impairs phosphate reabsorption. They propose that this pivotal defect in turn stimulates renal $25(OH)D\text{-}1\alpha\text{-hydroxylase}$, thus promoting the production of $1,25(OH)_2D$ and increasing its serum and tissue levels. As a result intestinal calcium and phosphorus absorption are augmented and the renal filtered calcium load increased. The enhanced intestinal calcium absorption also suppresses parathyroid function. In addition, prolonged hypophosphatemia diminishes osteoid mineralization resulting in rickets and/or osteomalacia.

The proposal that abnormal phosphate transport results in increased calcitriol production remains untested. Indeed, the elevation of $1,25(OH)_2D$ in patients with HHRH is a unique phenotypic manifestation of the disease which distinguishes it from other disorders in which abnormal phosphate transport is likewise manifest. Recently, however, Davidai et al. (61,62) observed that a murine homologue of the hypophosphatemic disorders, the Gy-mouse, exhibits elevated serum $1,25(OH)_2D$ similar to patients with HHRH. In this animal model renal $25(OH)D\text{-}1\alpha\text{-hydroxylase}$ is normally responsive to hormonal/metabolic modulation. Moreover, in the baseline state the Gy-mice exhibit increased enzyme activity secondary to normally maintained phosphate-regulated function [an absent/mutated action in Hyp-mice (see above)]. These observations provide evidence that abnormal phosphate transport may be associated with biochemically diverse disease. Most likely, such heterogeneity results from disease at variable anatomical sites along the proximal convoluted tubule which uniformly impairs phosphate transport but not $25(OH)D\text{-}1\alpha\text{-hydroxylase}$ activity.

Treatment

In accord with the hypothesis that a singular defect in renal phosphate transport underlies HHRH, patients have been treated successfully with high doses of phosphorus (1–2.5 g/d in 5 divided doses) alone. Within several weeks after initiation of therapy, bone pain disappears and muscular strength improves substantially. Moreover, the majority of treated subjects exhibit accelerated linear growth and radiologic signs of rickets are completely absent within 4–9 months. Concordantly, serum phosphorus values increase toward normal, the

1,25(OH)$_2$D concentration decreases, and alkaline phosphatase activity declines to normal. Despite this favorable response, limited investigation indicates that the osteomalacic component of the bone disease does not exhibit normalization. Further studies will be necessary, therefore, to determine if phosphorus alone will be sufficient treatment for this rare disorder.

Adult Hypophosphatemic Rickets (AHR)

In some patients older than 15 years of age, an acquired form of hypophosphatemic osteomalacia occurs (87). The pathogenesis of this disorder is unclear but involves renal phosphate loss secondary to abnormal proximal tubule function. Serum levels of PTH and 25(OH)D are normal, whereas that of 1,25(OH)$_2$D is low or inappropriately normal. Presenting symptoms in affected patients include debilitating bone pain, a significant myopathy, and Looser's zones on bone x-rays. Usually the inheritance is sporadic, but a propositus occasionally passes the disease in an X-linked dominant mode, suggesting that spontaneous mutation may cause expression of the disease. Alternatively, the disorder may represent tumor-induced osteomalacia in a patient with an as yet undetected benign growth or malignancy. Treatment with oral phosphate supplements and vitamin D or 1,25(OH)$_2$D$_3$ is indicated.

Autosomal Dominant Hypophosphatemic Rickets

In addition to the more common X-linked hypophosphatemic rickets, an autosomal dominantly inherited form of the disease has been documented (88). Patients affected with this disorder display clinical, biochemical, and radiographic abnormalities indistinguishable from those of individuals with XLH. However, transmission of the disease is clearly autosomal dominant and in a few instances penetrance of the hypophosphatemic trait is delayed.

Nonrachitic Hypophosphatemic Osteomalacia

Several reports document a rare form of hypophosphatemic disease in which rickets is rarely a complication and the associated bone disease is invariably osteomalacia. In 1977 Frymoyer and Hodgkin (89) described such a syndrome in a 133 member kindred with renal phosphate wasting transmitted in an X-linked dominant fashion. All 13 affected children did not exhibit radiographic evidence of rickets despite hypophosphatemia. In contrast, adults with this disease displayed clear evidence of osteomalacia and were disabled by progressive bowing (an unusual finding in X-linked hypophosphatemia). Additional characteristics of the disease process

were indistinguishable from those in patients with XLH and included: (i) normocalcemia, (ii) renal phosphate wasting, (iii) a unique enthesopathy, and (iv) radiographic evidence of osteosclerosis and pseudofractures (89). At present it remains unclear if this X-linked disease is a forme fruste of XLH the expression of which is modified by unknown factors. Alternatively the disorder may be due to mutation of a different gene on the X chromosome (analogous to the *Hyp* and *Gy* mutations in the mouse) or mutation of a different site within the same gene. Additional biochemical and genetic investigations will be necessary to determine if two separate and unique forms of X-linked hypophosphatemic rickets do indeed exist.

More recently, Scriver et al. (90,91) reported a similar syndrome which they named hypophosphatemic nonrachitic bone disease. Affected subjects with this disease exhibited evidence of mild renal phosphate wasting and hypophosphatemia. Associated with these cardinal abnormalities were modest shortening of stature and bowing of the lower extremities, as well as dental abnormalities similar to, but less severe than, those in patients with XLH (92). Extensive studies revealed infrequent radiographic evidence of rickets in diseased children. Although the genetic transmission of this disorder could not be determined in all instances, apparent male to male inheritance of the disease ruled out X-linked dominant transmission and suggested autosomal dominant passage in some families.

Fanconi's Syndrome

Rickets and osteomalacia are frequently associated with Fanconi's syndrome, a disorder characterized by phosphaturia and consequent hypophosphatemia, aminoaciduria, renal glycosuria, albuminuria, and proximal renal tubular acidosis (93–97). Although a wide diversity of congenital diseases are associated with this syndrome (Table 1), damage to the proximal tubule represents the common underlying mechanism of disease. Resultant dysfunction results in renal wasting of those substances primarily reabsorbed at the proximal tubule. The associated bone disease in this disorder is likely secondary to hypophosphatemia and/or acidosis, abnormalities which occur in association with abnormally (Fanconi's syndrome, type I) or normally regulated (Fanconi's syndrome, type II) vitamin D metabolism.

Fanconi's Syndrome, Type I and Rachitic/Osteomalacic Disease

Renal phosphate wasting and hypophosphatemia are the hallmark abnormalities of this disease. Indeed, occurrence of abnormal bone mineralization appears dependent upon the phosphate loss. Thus, disease subtypes in which isolated wasting of amino acids, glucose, or potassium occur are not associated with rickets and/or osteomalacia. In many respects this disorder resembles the more common genetic disease, X-linked hypophosphatemic rickets. Thus, in the majority of patients studied, affected subjects similarly exhibit abnormal vitamin D metabolism. Consequently, serum $1,25(OH)_2D$ levels are overtly decreased or abnormally low relative to the prevailing serum phosphorus concentration (98–102). The cause of the aberrantly regulated calcitriol biosynthesis, however, remains unknown. Although it may be due to the abnormal renal phosphate transport, as suspected in patients with XLH, additional components of the syndrome, such as proximal tubule damage and acidosis, may play important roles. Indeed, the acidosis may contribute to the bone disease as well.

In this regard, several studies indicate that acidosis may exert multiple deleterious effects on bone. In some cases the negative sequelae may be related to the loss of bone calcium which occurs secondary to calcium release for use in buffering (96,102). Alternatively, several investigators (103,104) have reported that acidosis may impair bone mineralization secondary to a direct inhibition of renal $25(OH)D\text{-}1\text{-}\alpha\text{-hydroxylase}$ activity. Others dispute these findings (105,106) and acidosis does not cause rickets or osteomalacia alone but only in association with phosphate wasting. Thus, acidosis cannot be viewed as an independent variable underlying the bone disease in Fanconi's syndrome, type I. Indeed, Brenner et al. (107) reported that the rachitic/osteomalacic component of this disorder occurs only in patients with type II renal tubular acidosis and phosphate wasting. In contrast, those with type I and IV renal tubular acidosis displayed no evidence of abnormal bone mineralization. Thus, the interplay of acidosis and phosphate depletion on bone mineralization in this disorder remains poorly understood. Most likely, however, hypophosphatemia and abnormally regulated vitamin D metabolism are the primary factors underlying rickets and osteomalacia in this form of Fanconi's syndrome.

Fanconi's Syndrome, Type II and Rickets/ Osteomalacia Disease

Tieder et al. (108) have described two siblings (from a consanguineous mating) who presented with classic characteristics of Fanconi's syndrome, including renal phosphate wasting, renal glycosuria, generalized aminoaciduria, and increased urinary excretion of uric acid. However, in these patients the serum calcitriol levels were appropriately elevated (relative to the decreased serum phosphorus concentration) and urine calcium was increased despite normal serum parathyroid hormone levels and cyclic AMP excretion. Furthermore, treatment with phosphate alone reduced the serum $1,25(OH)_2D$ concentration in these patients into the normal range and eliminated the associated hypercal-

ciuria. In many regards, this syndrome resembles the genetic disease, HHRH and as such represents a variant of Fanconi's syndrome to which we have referred to as type II. The bone disease in affected subjects appears due to the exclusive effects of hypophosphatemia. In any case, the existence of this variant form of disease is likely the result of renal damage in a different segment of the proximal tubule or involvement of a different mechanism at the same site (108). Further studies will be necessary to distinguish these possibilities.

Treatment

Ideally treatment of the bone disease in Fanconi's syndrome should be directed towards correcting the cause of the pathophysiologic defect influencing proximal renal tubular function. Unfortunately, in many cases the primary abnormality has not been defined. Moreover, efforts to decrease the tissue levels of toxic metabolites by dietary (such as in fructose intolerance) or pharmacologic means (such as in cystinosis and Wilson's syndrome) have met with variable success. Indeed, it remains unknown if the proximal tubule damage is reversible upon relief of the acute toxicity. Regardless, in instances when specific therapies are not available or do not lead to normalization of the primary defect, therapy must be directed at raising the serum phosphorus concentration, replacing calcitriol (in type I disease) and reversing an associated acidosis. The use of phosphorus and calcitriol has been discussed extensively as a therapeutic intervention for XLH. Experience in the management of Fanconi's syndrome with phosphorus and calcitriol, however, is limited. In general such replacement therapy leads to substantial improvement or resolution of the bone disease (109). However, growth and development, abnormalities more likely associated with the underlying genetic disease, remain substantially impaired (109). Thus, more efficacious treatment would be directed at the specific pathophysiologic disruption causing the various diseases rather than the secondary manifestations. Therefore, only further research into the causes of these disorders will permit improvements in therapy.

DECREASED RENAL 25-HYDROXYVITAMIN D-1α-HYDROXYLASE

Vitamin D Dependent Rickets, Type I (Pseudovitamin D Deficiency)

Vitamin D dependent rickets, type I is a rare disorder that is characterized by presentation of patients with the symptoms and signs of vitamin D deficiency rickets. Most remarkably, affected patients present with these abnormalities despite an adequate intake of vitamin D and without a therapeutic response to an accepted vitamin D replacement therapy. Family studies reveal that the disorder is a genetic disease with inheritance consistent with an autosomal recessive trait. Fraser and Salter (110) and Prader et al. (111) initially identified this unique form of vitamin D resistant rickets and named the condition hereditare pseudomanglerachitis. Others subsequently referred to the disorder as hypocalcemic vitamin D resistant rickets (112), vitamin D dependency rickets (113,114), vitamin D dependency rickets (115), or *vitamin D dependent rickets, type I* (116–118).

At birth affected individuals are generally healthy. However, within the first year of life clinical symptoms appear and include hypocalcemic tetany, muscular hypotonia and weakness, motor retardation, and stunted growth (119). With progression patients develop thickening of the wrists and ankles, frontal bossing, and a widened anterior fontanel on physical examination. In addition, rachitic rosary and bowing of the femurs may manifest, as well as enamel hypoplasia of the teeth.

Radiographs reveal classic signs of vitamin D-deficiency rickets. These include irregular fraying at the provisional zone of calcification and metaphyseal widening at the distal ends of the radius and ulna. Further, untreated youths often develop coarse trabeculation of metaphyses.

The cardinal biochemical abnormalities of this disease include hypocalcemia, hypophosphatemia, and an elevated plasma alkaline phosphatase activity. As a result of the hypocalcemia, affected patients exhibit an elevated circulating level of immunoreactive parathyroid hormone (120) and consequently increased urinary cyclic AMP excretion, generalized aminoaciduria, and diminished renal tubular reabsorption of phosphate (121). Intestinal absorption of calcium is below normal levels and urinary calcium is accordingly quite low. No data regarding gastrointestinal phosphate absorption are available. Mild acidosis with hyperchloremia is occasionally observed.

Pathophysiology

Definition of the pathophysiological basis for vitamin D dependent rickets, type I was a consequence of the early observation that pharmacologic doses of vitamin D are necessary to effect biochemical and radiographic resolution of the disease. Study of the circulating levels of the vitamin D metabolites in affected subjects provided insight to the cause of this disparate therapeutic response and to the underlying defect. These investigations revealed that serum 25(OH)D levels are normal in untreated subjects (122) whereas circulating concentrations of 1,25(OH)$_2$D are profoundly decreased (123). Such observations suggest that a defect in renal 25(OH)D-1α-hydroxylase activity is manifest in subjects with this disease. This presumed abnormality, although not tested directly, has been substantiated by a variety of experiments which document that classic stimuli of enzyme activity do not influence the serum 1,25(OH)$_2$D levels in affected patients. Thus the serum calcitriol concentration remains low after successful treatment with vitamin D or 25(OH)D (124) in spite of a normal serum level of calcium and phosphorus and an elevated serum 25(OH)D. Moreover, administration of parathyroid hormone to diseased subjects fails to normally increase the already low serum 1,25(OH)$_2$D concentration (unpublished observations). Consistent with these data, physiologic doses of calcitriol promote complete healing of the bone disease whereas pharmacologic doses of vitamin D or 25(OH)D, 100–300 times the recommended amount, are required to achieve similar effects (125).

The recent discovery of a porcine homologue of the human disease permitted direct testing of the proposed pathophysiological defect. In this animal model the mode of inheritance and the clinical, radiological and biochemical abnormalities are similar to those in patients with vitamin D dependent rickets, type I. In this regard, affected piglets exhibit not only hypocalcemia and hypophosphatemia but elevated 25(OH)D and diminished or undetectable 1,25(OH)$_2$D levels as well. Moreover, these animals display a normal concentration of specific [^{3}H]1,25(OH)$_2$D$_3$ binding sites in vitamin D target tissues and have no detectable 25(OH)D-1α-hydroxylase activity in renal cortical homogenates (126,127). Thus, there is strong evidence that the disease in affected pigs (and likely in humans) results from a genetic defect in the renal 25(OH)D-1α-hydroxylase system which is responsible for the low circulating levels of 1,25(OH)$_2$D and the consequent rachitic disease.

Treatment

Vitamin D dependent rickets, type I responds to vitamin D in pharmacologic amounts. Such beneficial therapeutic effect results from elevation of circulating 25(OH)D which occurs without concomitant alteration of the depressed 1,25(OH)$_2$D levels. The 25(OH)D, at high concentrations, may activate the specific intracellular receptors for 1,25(OH)$_2$D (despite the lesser affinity for the precursor), drive the local production of the active metabolite in some tissues in a paracrine or autocrine manner or act through an unknown metabolite on target tissues. In any case, successful treatment generally requires 20,000–100,000 U/d of vitamin D$_2$, a dose 50–2500 fold greater than the physiologic requirement. In response to this regimen the biochemical and clinical abnormalities of the disorder remit. Alternatively, pharmacologic amounts of 25(OH)D (0.1–1 mg/d) may be employed to effect healing of the rachitic disease.

Treatment with 1,25(OH)$_2$D, however, is the optimal regimen in patients with vitamin D dependent rickets, type I. Fraser et al. (117) and Prader et al. (119) treated patients with physiologic doses of calcitriol (1 g/d) and observed both normalization of the hypocalcemia within a few days after initiation of treatment and healing of the bone disease after several weeks. Similar therapeutic benefit has been reported in response to administration of low dose $1\alpha(OH)D_3$ (1–3 g/d), an analogue of $1,25(OH)_2D_3$. Moreover, Delvin et al. (128) observed that long-term therapy (4–27 months) with physiologic doses of calcitriol (0.5–1.0 g/d) produced beneficial results in nine affected patients. Several, however, required higher doses (2–3 g/d) during the active phase of healing. As expected, treatment with $1,25(OH)_2D_3$ increases the serum level of this metabolite to normal. In addition, the serum 25(OH)D concentration decreases while the circulating level of $24,25(OH)_2D$ increases. After continuous treatment the serum $24,25(OH)_2D$ concentration gradually declines and in association with healing of the bone normalizes. These observations leave open the question whether the therapeutic response to $1,25(OH)_2D_3$ is merely the result of replacing the deficient vitamin D metabolite or involves a complementary effect of $24,25(OH)_2D$ on bone mineralization. Regardless, in the majority of affected patients therapy with vitamin D or its metabolites must be continued for life in order to prevent relapse of hypocalcemia and subsequent bone disease (122). However, in a minority of subjects with a syndrome clinically identical to vitamin D dependent rickets, type I, cessation of treatment evokes no reappearance of biochemical or radiographic signs of rickets (129,130).

END ORGAN RESISTANCE TO CALCITRIOL

Vitamin D Dependent Rickets, Type II

In 1978 Brooks et al. (131) described a patient with hypocalcemia, secondary hyperparathyroidism, osteomalacia, and elevated levels of $1,25(OH)_2D$. Treatment with vitamin D improved the hypocalcemia and resulted in a further increase of calcitriol. Thus, the term *vitamin D dependent rickets, type II* was adopted to describe this disorder in which an apparent peripheral resistance of target organs to $1,25(OH)_2D$ is manifest. Based on additional case reports in which approximately one-half of affected subjects do not respond to any form of vitamin D therapy, Liberman and Marx (125) suggested this disorder represents "hereditary resistance to $1,25(OH)_2D$." Since only 50 known patients with this phenotypically heterogeneous disease are on record, the mode of inheritance remains unknown. Indeed, in some instances the onset is sporadic (132). However, several reports document familial occurrence with a transmission pattern characteristic of an autosomal recessive trait (125). In this regard, parental consanguinity and multiple siblings with the same defect occur in about one-half of the reported kindreds. There is a striking clustering of patients close to the Mediterranean and most of the patients reported from Europe and North America are descendants of families originating around the Mediterranean. Notable exceptions are several kindreds reported from Japan (133,134).

The clinical, radiological, and biochemical characteristics common to all patients with this disease are rickets and/or osteomalacia of varying severity, hypocalcemia and secondary hyperparathyroidism, increased serum $1,25(OH)_2D$ levels (both prior to and during therapy with calciferol preparations) and unresponsiveness to physiologic doses of vitamin D or its active metabolites. Affected children appear normal at birth and in general exhibit evidence of the disease in infancy (125). However, presentation is occasionally delayed to later in childhood (125), adolescence (131), or even adult age (132). All patients with delayed disease expression have been normocalcemic and only mildly affected. Additional heterogeneity confounds the clinical presentation of this disorder. Approximately two-thirds of affected kindreds exhibit hair loss varying from alopecia areata to alopecia universalis. The alopecia may be present at birth or develop during the first months of life. Its presence usually signals the presence of a severe form of the disease characterized by early onset and total refractoriness to treatment with $1,25(OH)_2D$. A minority of subjects present with additional ectodermal anomalies including multiple milia, epidermal cysts, and oligodontia (135).

Pathogenesis

Although secondary hyperparathyroidism, hypocalcemia, and hypophosphatemia have been proposed as synergistic factors that contribute to the elevated levels of $1,25(OH)_2D$ characteristic of vitamin D dependent rickets, type II, the sustained increase of serum calcitriol, observed in patients in whom these biochemical abnormalities were corrected by treatment with vitamin D or 25(OH)D (136,137), indicates that other factors are of greater significance in the pathogenesis of this disease. In this regard, several investigators suggested that abnormal vitamin D receptor function and consequent defective $1,25(OH)_2D$ feedback inhibition of renal 25(OH)D-1α-hydroxylase activity may be the primary pathogenetic defect. Recognition of a decreased serum $24,25(OH)_2D$ concentration in affected subjects, in spite of increased $1,25(OH)_2D$ levels, is consistent with this possibility since abnormal vitamin D receptor function would preclude induction of 25(OH)D-24R-hydroxylase.

With the realization that cells (dermal fibroblasts, keratinocytes, and peripheral blood monocytes) which are easily procured contain receptors for $1,25(OH)_2D$, studies designed to characterize the proposed vitamin D receptor defect have been possible. Using a variety of methods to define hormone–receptor interaction, the existence of the abnormality has been confirmed and five specific intracellular defects identified (125).

Hormone Binding Negative

This is the most common abnormality observed thus far. In affected patients high concentrations of $1,25(OH)_2D$ do not evoke a biological response in spite of normal amounts of receptor. The in vitro studies performed in cells from these subjects reveal no evidence of $[^3H]1,25(OH)_2D$ binding to the available receptors (138). Thus, the apparent defect is a focal abnormality in the hormone binding domain and not receptor deletion. Not surprisingly patients with this disorder exhibit, in general, complete refractoriness to treatment with high doses of vitamin D or active metabolites. Recent studies indicate that in at least one large family the defect results from a nonsense mutation which causes a premature termination signal within the steroid binding domain of the $1,25(OH)_2D$ receptor (139,140). The consequent truncated molecule is unable to bind calcitriol and is thus nonfunctional.

Defect in Hormone Binding Capacity

This abnormality represents a less common defect of the hormone binding domain. Studies of cells from affected patients reveal a decrease in the number of available $1,25(OH)_2D$ binding sites. Indeed, binding capacity is reduced by approximately 90% in spite of apparent normal affinity. In patients with this abnormality therapeutic trials with high doses of calcitriol over prolonged periods produced no calcemic response (137).

Defect in Hormone Binding Affinity

A less severe form of the disease results as a consequence of abnormal receptor affinity for $1,25(OH)_2D$. In cells from these subjects $[^3H]1,25(OH)_2D$ binding affinity is reduced 20–30 fold while binding capacity is maintained at normal levels. High dose vitamin D or calcitriol therapy in patients with this defect results in complete remission of the disease (141).

Deficient Hormone–Receptor Nuclear Localization

In this unusual form of the disease $1,25(OH)_2D$ interaction with the receptor appears normal. Indeed, radiolabeled hormone binds with normal affinity to soluble receptors that have normal binding capacity. Moreover, the hormone–receptor complex is apparently structurally unaltered and binds to heterologous DNA. However, bound $[^3H]1,25(OH)_2D$ does not localize in the nuclei of intact cells (142,143). Thus, hormone driven events do not occur. For reasons that are poorly understood, the defect does not preclude successful treatment of affected subjects with high doses of vitamin D or its active metabolites (142–144).

Decreased Affinity of the Hormone–Receptor Complex

Most recently characterization of several kindreds with vitamin D dependent rickets, type II revealed that in some affected subjects there is apparent normal binding of $1,25(OH)_2D$ to the cell receptor and subsequent localization and binding of the hormone–receptor complex in cell nuclei. However, detailed study of binding to heterologous DNA provided evidence of diminished affinity for the complex (145,146). In concert, high doses of vitamin D or its metabolites elicits essentially no biological response in patients with this defect. Moreover, cells from these patients similarly are unresponsive to such stimuli in vitro. Recent studies indicate that this disorder is heterogeneous and results from multiple single nucleotide mutations in exons encoding the receptor (147). Each of these alterations changes the structure of the zinc binding fingers of the receptor and thereby negatively influences the DNA binding domain(s).

The epidermal abnormalities associated with vitamin D dependent rickets, type II, most notably alopecia, likely result from the $1,25(OH)_2D$ resistance that characterizes the syndrome. In support of this recent reports indicate that: (i) outer root sheath cells of the hair follicle in rats harbor calcitriol receptors; and (ii) the epidermis and hair follicles contain a vitamin D dependent calcium binding protein. However, the absence of similar defects in other states of $1,25(OH)_2D$ deficiency suggests that these epidermal abnormalities occur as a consequence of absent calcitriol dependent effects on hair follicle differentiation during fetal development.

Treatment

Although current data indicate that the response to treatment in patients with vitamin D dependent rickets, type II depends upon the nature of the underlying abnormality, observations are preliminary and the predictive therapeutic value of the in vitro $1,25(OH)_2D$ bioresponse unproven. Nevertheless, it does appear that patients with type C (deficient affinity) and type D (deficient nuclear localization) defects will respond to high dose vitamin D with complete clinical and biochemical remission. In contrast, most patients with types A (receptor negative), B (low capacity), and E (receptor positive) abnormalities remain refractory to therapeutic intervention. Until further information regarding the validity of these conclusions is available, however, every patient with vitamin D dependent rickets, type II should receive a trial of therapy. Such treatment should include: (i) vitamin D_2 (400,000–1,200,000 U/d) or 25(OH)D (0.05–1.5 mg/d) in the mildest cases or $1,25(OH)_2D$ (5–60 g/d) in more severe cases; and (ii) supplemental calcium (1–3 g/d). Therapeutic trials should be no less than 6 months in order to permit recovery from the hypocalcemia attendant upon bone hunger and should include close follow-up of bone x-rays and general indices of calcium and vitamin D homeostasis. Maintenance of the serum $1,25(OH)_2D$ at a concentration greater than 100 times the physiologic level throughout treatment is the goal of the treatment program. If the biochemical, clinical, and radiological abnormalities of the syndrome do not normalize under these conditions, failure of therapy may be considered. Under such circumstances, recent studies indicate a possible alternative therapeutic strategy. In this regard, remarkable clinical and biochemical remission occurred in severely affected patients treated with high dose oral calcium (148) or long-term intracaval infusion of calcium (149,150). Thus, clinical remission may be achieved by calcium administration in even the most vitamin D resistant patients with vitamin D dependent rickets, type II.

REFERENCES

1. Albright F, Butler AM, Bloom E. Rickets resistant to vitamin D therapy. *Am J Dis Child* 1937;54:529–44.
2. Graham JB, McFalls VW, Winters RW. Familial hypophosphatemia with vitamin D resistant rickets. II. Three additional kindreds of sex-linked dominant type with a genetic analysis of four such families. *Am J Hum Genet* 1959;11:311–32.
3. Winters RW, Graham JB, Williams TF, McFalls VW, Burnett CH. A genetic study of familial hypophosphatemia and vitamin D-resistant rickets with a review of the literature. *Medicine (Baltimore)* 1958;37:97–142.
4. Burnett CH, Dent CE, Harper C, Warland BJ. Vitamin D resistant rickets: analysis of 24 pedigrees and hereditary and sporadic cases. *Am J Med* 1964;36:222–32.
5. Harrison HE, Harrison HC, Lifshitz F, Johnson AD. Growth disturbance in hereditary hypophosphatemia. *Am J Dis Child* 1966;112:290–7.
6. Williams TF, Winters RW. Familial (hereditary) vitamin D-resistant rickets with hypophosphatemia. In: Stanbury JB, Wyngaarden JB, Fredrickson DS, eds. *The metabolic basis of inherited disease, 3rd ed.* New York: McGraw-Hill, 1465–85.
7. Tracey WE, Campbell RA. Dentofacial development in children with vitamin D resistant rickets. *J Am Dent Assoc* 1968;76:1026–31.
8. Polisson RP, Martinex S, Khoury M, et al. Calcification of entheses associated with X-linked hypophosphatemic osteomalacia. *N Engl J Med* 1985;313:1–6.
9. Hardy DC, Murphy WA, Siegel BA, Reid IR, Whyte MP. X-linked hypophosphatemia in adults: prevalence of skeletal radiographic and scintigraphic features. *Radiology* 1989;171:403–14.
10. Pierce DS, Wallace WM, Herndon CH. Long term treatment of vitamin D-resistant rickets. *J Bone Joint Surg* 1964;46A:979–86.
11. Marie PJ, Glorieux FH. Relation between hypomineralized periosteocytic lesions and bone mineralization in vitamin D-resistant rickets. *Calcif Tissue Int* 1983;35:443–8.
12. Tracy WE, Campbell RA. Dento-facial development in children with vitamin D-resistant rickets. *J Am Dent Assoc* 1968;76:1026–33.
13. Glorieux FH, Scriver CR, Reade TM, Goldman H, Roseborough A. The use of phosphate and vitamin D to prevent dwarfism and rickets in X-linked hypophosphatemia. *N Engl J Med* 1972;281:481–7.
14. Balsan S, Tieder M. Linear growth in patients with hypophosphatemic vitamin D-resistant rickets: influence of treatment regimen and parental height. *J Pediatr* 1990;116:365–71.
15. Rasmussen H, Pechet M, Anast C, Mazur A, Gertner J, Broadus AE. Long-term treatment of familial hypophosphatemic rickets with oral phosphate and 1-hydroxyvitamin D_3. *J Pediatr* 1981;99:16–25.
16. Chesney RW, Mazess R, Rose P, Hamstra AJ, DeLuca HF, Breed AL. Long-term influence of calcitriol (1,25-dihydroxyvitamin D_3) and supplemental phosphate in X-linked hypophosphatemic rickets. *Pediatrics* 1983;71:559–67.
17. Tsuru N, Chan JCM, Chinchilli VL. Renal hypophosphatemic rickets: growth and mineral metabolism after treatment with calcitriol (1,25-dihydroxyvitamin D_3) and phosphate supplementation. *Am J Dis Child* 1987;141:108–10.
18. Friedman NE, Drezner MK. Osteomalacia, genetic. In: Bardin CW, ed. *Current therapy in endocrinology and metabolism, 4th ed.* New York: B. C. Decker, 1991; 421–7.
19. Stickler GB. Familial hypophosphatemic vitamin D-resistant rickets. *Acta Paediatr Scand* 1969;58:213–9.
20. Lyles KW, Harrelson JM, Drezner MK. The efficacy of vitamin D_2 and oral phosphorus therapy in X-linked hypophosphatemic rickets and osteomalacia. *J Clin Endocrinol Metab* 1982;54:307–15.
21. Drezner MK, Lyles KW, Haussler MR, Harrelson JM. Evaluation of a role for 1,25-dihydroxyvitamin D_3 in the pathogenesis and treatment of X-linked hypophosphatemic rickets and osteomalacia. *J Clin Invest* 1980;66:1020–32.
22. Steindijk R. On the pathogenesis of vitamin D resistant rickets and primary vitamin D resistant rickets. *Helv Paediatr Acta* 1962;17:65–85.
23. Stickler GB. External calcium and phosphorus balances in vitamin D-resistant rickets. *J Pediatr* 1963;63:942–8.
24. Roof BS, Piel CF, Gordan GS. Nature of defect responsible for familial vitamin D-resistant rickets (VDRR) based on radioimmunoassay for parathyroid hormone (PTH). *Trans Assoc Am Physicians* 1972;85:172–80.
25. Fanconi A, Fischer JA, Prader A. Serum parathyroid concentrations in hypophosphatemic vitamin D-resistant rickets. *Helv Pediatr Acta* 1974;29:187–94.
26. Arnaud C, Glorieux FH, Scriver CR. Serum parathyroid hormone levels in acquired vitamin D deficiency of infancy. *Pediatrics* 1972;49:837–40.
27. Glorieux FH, Scriver CR. Loss of parathyroid hormone-sensitive component of phosphate transport in X-linked hypophosphatemia. *Science* 1972;173:997–1000.
28. Haddad JG, Chyu KJ, Hahn TJ, Stamp TCB. Serum concentrations of 25-hydroxyvitamin D in sex linked hypophosphatemic vitamin D-resistant rickets. *J Lab Clin Med* 1973;81:22–7.
29. Drezner MK, Haussler MR. Serum 1,25-dihydroxyvitamin D in bone disease. *N Engl J Med* 1979;300:435.
30. Delvin EE, Glorieux FH. Serum 1,25-dihydroxyvitamin D concentration in hypophosphatemic vitamin D resistant rickets. *Calcif Tissue Int* 1981;33:173–5.
31. Lyles KW, Clark AG, Drezner MK. Serum 1,25-dihydroxyvitamin D levels in subjects with X-linked hypophosphatemic rickets and osteomalacia. *Calcif Tissue Int* 1982;34:125–30.
32. Hughes MR, Brumbaugh PF, Haussler MR, Wergedal JE, Baylink DJ. Regulation of serum 1,25-dihydroxyvitamin D by calcium and phosphate in the rat. *Science* 1975;180:578–80.
33. Galante L, Colston KW, Evans IM, Byfield PGH, Matthews EW, MacIntyre I. The regulation of vitamin D metabolism. *Nature* 1973;244:438–40.
34. Haussler MR, Hughes M, Baylink D, Littledike ET, Cork D, Pitt M. Influence of phosphate depletion on the biosynthesis and circulating level of 1,25-dihydroxyvitamin D. *Adv Exp Med Biol* 1977;81:233–50.
35. Domininguez JH, Gray RW, Lemann J. Dietary phosphate deprivation in women and men: effects on mineral and acid balances, parathyroid hormone and the metabolism of 25(OH)D. *J Clin Endocrinol Metab* 1977;43:1056–68.
36. Gray RW, Wilz DR, Caldas AE, Lemann J. The importance of phosphate in regulating plasma $1,25(OH)_2D$ levels in humans. Studies in healthy subjects, in calcium stone formers and in patients with primary hyperparathyroidism. *J Clin Endocrinol Metab* 1977;45:299–306.
37. Lyles KW, Drezner MK. Parathyroid hormone effects on serum 1,25-dihydroxyvitamin D levels in patients with X-linked hypophosphatemic rickets: evidence for abnormal 25-hydroxyvitamin D-1-hydroxylase activity. *J Clin Endocrinol Metab* 1982;54:638–44.
38. Scriver CR, Reade TM, DeLuca HF, Hamstra AJ. Serum 1,25-di-

hydroxyvitamin D levels in normal subjects and in patients with hereditary rickets or bone disease. *N Engl J Med* 1978;299:976–9.

39. Chesney RW, Nazess RB, Rose P, Hamstra AJ, DeLuca HF. Supranormal 25-hydroxyvitamin D and subnormal 1,25-dihydroxyvitamin D: their role in X-linked hypophosphatemic rickets. *Am J Dis Child* 1980;134:140–3.

40. Fanconi G, Giradet P. Familairer persistierender phosphatdiabetes mit D-vitamin-resistenter rachitis. *Helv Paediatr Acta* 1952;7:14–41.

41. Rasmussen H, Anast C. Familial hypophosphatemic rickets and vitamin D-dependent rickets. In: *The metabolic basis of inherited disease, 5th ed.* Stanbury JB, Wyngaarden JB, Fredrickson DS, Goldstein JL, Brown MS, eds. New York: McGraw-Hill, 1983;1743–73.

42. Williams TF, Winters RW, Burnett CH. Familial (hereditary) vitamin D resistant rickets with hypophosphatemia. In: *The metabolic basis of inherited disease, 2nd ed.* Stanbury JB, Wyngaarden JB, Fredrickson DS, eds. New York: McGraw-Hill, 1979;1179–204.

43. Read AP, Thakker RV, Davies KE, et al. Mapping of human X-linked hypophosphatemic rickets by multilocus linkage analysis. *Hum Genet* 1986;73:267–70.

44. Thakker RV, Read AP, Davies KE, et al. Bridging markers defining the map position of X-linked hypophosphatemic rickets. *J Med Genet* 1987;24:756–60.

45. Thakker RV, Davies KE, Read AP, et al. Linkage analysis of two cloned DNA sequences, DXS197 and DXS207, in hypophosphatemic rickets families. *Genomics* 1990;8:189–93.

46. Machler M, Frey D, Gai A, Orth U, Wienker TF, Fanconi A, Schmid W. X-linked dominant hypophosphatemia is closely linked to DNA markers DXS41 and DXS 43 at Xp22. *Hum Genet* 1986;73:271–5.

47. Econs MJ, Pericak-Vance MA, Betz H, Bartlett RJ, Speer MC, Drezner MK. The human glycine receptor: a new probe that is linked to the X-linked hypophosphatemic rickets gene. *Genomics* 1990;7:439–41.

48. Econs MJ, Barker DF, Speer MC, Pericak-Vance MA, Fain P, Drezner MK. Multilocus mapping of the human X-linked hypophosphatemic rickets gene locus (Abstract). *J Bone Miner Res* 1990;5(Suppl 2):137.

49. Rupp W, Swoboda W. Untersuchungen des PO4-stoffwechsel bei vitamin D resistenter racitis ("phosphatdiabetes"). *Helv Paediatr Acta* 1955;10:135–47.

50. Winters RW, Graham JB, Williams TF, McFalls VW, Burnett CH. A genetic study of familial hypophosphatemia and vitamin D resistant rickets. *Trans Assoc Am Physicians* 1957;70:234–42.

51. Jackson WP, Dowdle E, Linder GC. Vitamin D-resistant osteomalacia. *Br Med J [Clin Res]* 1958;1:1269–74.

52. Tenenhouse HS, Scriver CR, McInnes RR, Glorieux FH. Renal handling of phosphate in vivo and in vitro by the X-linked hypophosphatemic male mouse: evidence for a defect in the brush border membrane. *Kidney Int* 1978;14:236–44.

53. Tenenhouse HS, Scriver CR. Renal brush border membrane adaptation to phosphorus deprivation in the Hyp/Gy mouse. *Nature* 1979;281:225–7.

54. Bell CL, Tenenhouse HS, Scriver CR. Primary cultures of renal epithelial cells from X-linked hypophosphatemic (Hyp) mice express defects in phosphate transport and vitamin D metabolism. *Am J Hum Genet* 1988;43:293–303.

55. Dobre C-V, Alvarez UM, Kruska KA. Primary culture of hypophosphatemic proximal tubule cells express defective adaptation to phosphate (Abstract). *J Bone Miner Res* 1990;5(Suppl 2):205.

56. Glorieux FH, Marie PJ, Pettifor JM, Delvin EE. Bone response to phosphate salts, ergocalciferol, and calcitriol in hypophosphatemic vitamin D resistant rickets. *N Engl J Med* 1980;303:1023–31.

57. Eicher EM, Southlard JL, Scriver CR, Glorieux FH. Hypophosphatemia: mouse model for human familial hypophosphatemic vitamin D-resistant rickets. *Proc Natl Acad Sci USA* 1976;73:4667–71.

58. Lyon MF, Scriver CR, Baker LRI, Tenenhouse HS, Kronick J, Mandla S. The *Gy* mutation: another cause of X-linked hypophosphatemia in the mouse. *Proc Natl Acad Sci USA* 1986;83:4899–903.

59. Lobaugh B, Drezner MK. Abnormal regulation of renal 25-hy-

60. Cogwell LD, Goldfarb S, Lau K, Slatopolsky E, Zalman SA. Evidence for an intrinsic renal tubular defect in mice with genetic hypophosphatemic rickets. *J Clin Invest* 1979;63:1203–10.

61. Davidai GA, Nesbitt T, Drezner MK. Normal regulation of calcitriol production in *Gy* mice: evidence for biochemical heterogeneity in the X-linked hypophosphatemic diseases. *J Clin Invest* 1990;85:334–9.

62. Davidai GA, Nesbitt T, Drezner MK. Variable phosphate-mediated regulation of vitamin D metabolism in the murine hypophosphatemic rachitic/osteomalacic disorders. *Endocrinology* 1991; in press.

63. Nesbitt T, Drezner MK, Lobaugh B. Abnormal parathyroid hormone stimulation of 25-hydroxyvitamin D-1α-hydroxylase activity in the hypophosphatemic mouse: evidence for a generalized defect of vitamin D metabolism. *J Clin Invest* 1986;77:181–7.

64. Tenenhouse H. Investigation of the mechanism for abnormal renal 25-hydroxyvitamin D₃-1α-hydroxylase activity in the X-linked Hyp mouse. *Endocrinology* 1984;115:634–9.

65. Nesbitt T, Lobaugh B, Drezner MK. Calcitonin stimulation of renal 25-hydroxyvitamin D-1α-hydroxylase activity in hypophosphatemic mice: evidence that the regulation of calcitriol production is not universally abnormal in X-linked hypophosphatemia. *J Clin Invest* 1987;79:15–9.

66. Kawashima H, Kurokawa K. Unique hormonal regulation of vitamin D metabolism in the mammalian kidney. *Miner Electrolyte Metab* 1983;9:227–35.

67. Kawashima H, Kurokawa K. Localization and hormone regulation of 25(OH)D₃-1α- and -24-hydroxylase in the mammalian kidney. In: Norman AW, Schaefer K, Herrath D, Grigoleit H-G, eds. *Vitamin D, chemical, biochemical, and clinical endocrinology of calcium metabolism.* Berlin: Walter de Gruyter; 1982;449–54.

68. Kawashima H, Torikae S, Kurokawa K. Calcitonin selective stimulates 25-hydroxyvitamin D₃-1α-hydroxylase in the proximal straight tubule of the rat kidney. *Nature (London)* 1981;291:327–9.

69. Giasson SD, Brunette MG, Danan G, Vigneault N, Carriere S. Micropuncture study of renal phosphorus transport in hypophosphatemic vitamin D-resistant rachitic mice. *Pflugers Arch* 1977;371:33–8.

70. Seino Y, Yamaaoka K, Ishida M, et al. Plasma clearance for high doses of exogenous 1,25-dihydroxy[22,23(n)-³H] cholecalciferol in X-linked hypophosphatemic mice. *Biomed Res* 1982;3:683–6.

71. Tenenhouse HS, Jones G. Effect of the X-linked *Hyp* mutation and vitamin D status on induction of renal 25-hydroxyvitamin D₃-24-hydroxylase. *Endocrinology* 1987;120:609–16.

72. Tenenhouse HS, Yip A, Jones G. Increased renal catabolism of 1,25-dihydroxyvitamin D₃ in murine X-linked hypophosphatemic rickets. *J Clin Invest* 1988;81:461–5.

73. Ecarot-Charrier B, Glorieux FH, Travers R, Desbarats M, Bouchard F, Hinek A. Defective bone formation by transplanted Hyp mouse bone cells into normal mice. *Endocrinology* 1988;123:768–73.

74. Meyer Jr RA, Meyer MH, Gray RW. Parabiosis suggests a humoral factor is involved in X-linked hypophosphatemia in mice. *J Bone Miner Res* 1989;4:493–500.

75. Meyer Jr RA, Tenenhouse HS, Meyer MH, Klugerman AH. The renal phosphate transport defect in normal mice parabiosed to X-linked hypophosphatemic mice persists after parathyroidectomy. *J Bone Miner Res* 1989;4:523–32.

76. Nesbitt T, Coffman TM, Drezner MK. Cross-transplantation of kidneys in normal and *Hyp*-mice: evidence that the *Hyp* phenotype is unrelated to an intrinsic renal defect (Abstract). *J Bone Miner Res* 1990;5(Suppl 2):205.

77. McNair SL, Stickler GB. Familial hypophosphatemic vitamin D-resistant rickets. *Acta Paediatr Scand* 1969;58:213–9.

78. Stickler GB, Jowsey J, Bianco AJ Jr. Possible detrimental effect of large doses of vitamin D in familial hypophosphatemic vitamin D resistant rickets. *J Pediatr* 1971;79:68–71.

79. Moncrief MW, Chance GW. Nephrotoxic effect of vitamin D therapy in vitamin D refractory rickets. *Arch Dis Child* 1969;44:571–9.

80. Paunier L, Kooh SW, Cohen PE, Gibson AAM, Fraser D. Renal function and histology after long term vitamin D therapy of vitamin D refractory rickets. *J Pediatr* 1968;73:833–44.

81. Wilson DR, York SE, Jaworski ZF, Yendt ER. Studies in hypophosphatemic vitamin D refractory osteomalacia in adults: oral phosphate supplements as an adjunct to therapy. *Medicine (Baltimore)* 1965;44:99–134.

82. Costa T, Marie PJ, Scriver CR, et al. X-linked hypophosphatemia: effect of calcitriol on renal handling of phosphate, serum phosphate and bone mineralization. *J Clin Endocrinol Metab* 1981;52:463–77.

83. Harrell RM, Lyles KW, Harrelson JM, Freedman NE, Drezner MK. Healing of bone disease in X-linked hypophosphatemic rickets/osteomalacia: induction and maintenance with phosphorus and calcitriol. *J Clin Invest* 1985;75:1858–64.

84. Tieder M, Modai D, Samuel R, et al. Hereditary hypophosphatemic rickets with hypercalciuria. *N Engl J Med* 1985;312:611–7.

85. Tieder M, Modai D, Shaked U, et al. "Idiopathic" hypercalciuria and hereditary hypophosphatemic rickets: two phenotypical expressions of a common genetic defect. *N Engl J Med* 1987;316:125–9.

86. Liberman UA. Inborn errors in vitamin D metabolism—Their contribution to the understanding of vitamin D metabolism. In: Norman AW, Schaefer K, Grigoleit H-G, Herrath DV, eds. *Vitamin D molecular, cellular and clinical endocrinology.* Berlin: Walter de Gruyter, 1988;935–47.

87. Dent CE, Stamp TCB. Hypophosphatemic osteomalacia presenting in adults. *Q J Med* 1971;40:303–29.

88. Harrison HE, Harrison HC. Rickets and osteomalacia. In: *Disorders of calcium and phosphate metabolism in childhood and adolescence.* Philadelphia: WB Saunders, 1979;141–256.

89. Frymoyer JW, Hodgkin W. Adult-onset vitamin D-resistant hypophosphatemic osteomalacia. *J Bone Joint Surg* 1977;59:101–6.

90. Scriver CR, MacDonald W, Reade T, Glorieux FH, Nogrady B. Hypophosphatemic nonrachitic bone disease: an entity distinct from X-linked hypophosphatemia in the renal defect, bone involvement, and inheritance. *Am J Med Genet* 1977;1:101–17.

91. Scriver CR, Reade T, Halal F, Costa T, Cole DEC. Autosomal hypophosphatemic bone disease responds to 1,25-$(OH)_2D_3$. *Arch Dis Child* 1981;56:203–7.

92. Schwartz S, Scriver CR, Reade TM, Shields ED. Oral findings in patients with autosomal dominant hypophosphatemic bone disease and X-linked hypophosphatemia: further evidence that they are different diseases. *Oral Surg Oral Med Oral Pathol* 1988;66:310–4.

93. De Toni G. Remarks on the relations between renal rickets (renal dwarfism) and renal diabetes. *Acta Paediatr Scand* 1933;16:479–84.

94. McCune DJ, Mason HH, Clarke HT. Intractable hypophosphatemic rickets with renal glycosuria and acidosis (the Fanconi syndrome). *Am J Dis Child* 1943;65:81–146.

95. Brewer ED. The Fanconi syndrome: clinical disorders. In: Gonick HC, Buckalew VM Jr, eds. *Renal tubular disorders.* New York: Marcel Dekker, 1985;475–544.

96. Chan JCM, Alon U. Tubular disorders of acid-base and phosphate metabolism. *Nephron* 1985;40:257–79.

97. Chesney RW. Fanconi syndrome and renal tubular acidosis. In: Favus MJ, ed. *Primer on metabolic bone diseases and disorders of mineral metabolism.* Kelseyville, CA: American Society for Bone and Mineral Research, 1990;190–4.

98. Chesney RW, Rosen JF, Hamstra AJ, DeLuca HF. Serum 1,25-dihydroxyvitamin D levels in normal children and in vitamin D disorders. *Am J Dis Child* 1980;134:135–9.

99. Steinherz R, Chesney RW, Schulman JD, DeLuca HF, Phelps M. Circulating vitamin D metabolites in nephropathic cystinosis. *J Pediatr* 1983;102:592–4.

100. Baran DT, Marcy TW. Evidence for a defect in vitamin D metabolism in a patient with incomplete Fanconi syndrome. *J Clin Endocrinol Metab* 1984;59:998–1001.

101. Chesney RW, Kaplan BS, Phelps M, DeLuca HF. Renal tubular acidosis does not alter circulating values of calcitriol. *J Pediatr* 1984;104:51–5.

102. Chevalier RL. Hypercalciuria in a child with primary Fanconi syndrome and hearing loss. *Int J Pediatr Nephrol* 1983;4:53–7.

103. Lee SW, Russell J, Avioli LV. 25-hydroxycholecalciferol to 1,25-dihydroxycholecalciferol: conversion impaired by systemic metabolic acidosis. *Science* 1977;195:994–6.

104. Brewer ED, Tsai HC, Szeto KS, Morris RC. Maleic acid induced impaired conversion of 25(OH)D3 to 1,25(OH)2D3: implications for Fanconi's syndrome. *Kidney Int* 1977;12:244–52.

105. Cunningham J, Avioli LV. Systemic acidosis and the bioactivation of vitamin D. In: Norman AW, et al., eds. *Vitamin D, chemical, biochemical and clinical endocrinology of calcium metabolism.* Berlin: Walter de Gruyter, 1982;443–7.

106. Kraut JA, Gordon EM, Ransom JC, Horst R, Slatopolsky E, Coburn JW, Kurokawa K. Effect of chronic metabolic acidosis on vitamin D metabolism in humans. *Kidney Int* 1983;24:644–8.

107. Brenner RJ, Spring DB, Sebastian A, McSherry EM, Genant HK, Palubinskas AJ, Morris RC. Incidence of radiographically evident bone disease, nephrocalcinosis, and nephrolithiasis in various types of renal tubular acidosis. *N Engl J Med* 1982;307:217–21.

108. Tieder M, Arie R, Modai D, Samuel R, Weissgarten J, Liberman UA. Elevated serum 1,25-dihydroxyvitamin D concentrations in siblings with primary Fanconi's syndrome. *N Engl J Med* 1988;319:845–9.

109. Schneider JA, Schulman JD. Cystinosis. In: Stanbury JB, Wyngaarden JB, Fredrickson DS, Goldstein JL, Brown MS, eds. *The metabolic basis of inherited disease, 5th ed.* New York: McGraw-Hill, 1983;1844–66.

110. Fraser D, Salter RB. The diagnosis and management of the various types of rickets. *Pediatr Clin North Am* 1958;5:417–35.

111. Prader AV, Illig R, Heierli E. Eine besondere form der primaren vitamin-D reistenten rachitis mit hypocalcamie und autosomaldominatem erbgang: die hereditare pseudo-mangelrachitis. *Helv Pediatr Scand* 1961;16:452–64.

112. Bergstrom WH, Gardner LI. Metabolic disorders with bone lesions. In: Baughan VC, McKay R, Nelson WE, eds. *Textbook of pediatrics.* Philadelphia: WB Saunders, 1975;1503–11.

113. Stoop JW, Schraagen JC, Tiddens HAMW. Pseudovitamin D deficiency rickets, report of four new cases. *Acta Pediatr Scand* 1967;56:607–16.

114. Matsuda I, Sugai M, Ohsawa T. Laboratory findings in child with pseudovitamin D deficiency rickets. *Helv Paediatr Acta* 1969;24:329–36.

115. Scriver CR. Vitamin D dependency. *Pediatrics* 1970;45:361–3.

116. Hamilton R, Harrison J, Fraser D, Raddle I, Morecki R, Paunier L. The small intestine in vitamin D dependent rickets. *Pediatrics* 1970;45:364–73.

117. Fraser D, Kooh SW, Kind HO, Holick MF, Tanaka Y, DeLuca HF. Pathogenesis of hereditary vitamin D dependent rickets: an inborn error of vitamin D metabolism involving defective conversion of 25-hydroxyvitamin D to 1,25-dihydroxyvitamin D. *N Engl J Med* 1973;289:817–22.

118. Rosen JF, Finberg L. Vitamin D-dependent rickets: action of parathyroid hormone and 25-hydroxycholecalciferol. *Pediatr Res* 1972;6:552–62.

119. Prader A, Kind GP, DeLuca HF. Pseudo-vitamin D deficiency (vitamin D dependency). In: Brickets H, Stern J, eds. *Inborn errors of calcium and bone metabolism.* Baltimore: University Park Press, 1976;115–23.

120. Arnaud C, Maijer R, Reade T, Scriver CR, Whelan DT. Vitamin D dependency: an inherited postnatal syndrome with secondary hyperparathyroidism. *Pediatrics* 1970;46:871–80.

121. Sovik O, Aksnes L, Apold J. Urinary cyclic AMP: high concentration in vitamin D-deficient and dependent rickets. *J Pediatr* 1976;89:946–9.

122. Fanconi A, Prader A. Die hereditare pseudomangelrachitis. *Helv Paediatr Acta* 1969;24:423–47.

123. Balsan S, Garabedian M, Leiberherr M, Gueris J, Ulmann A. Serum 1,25-dihydroxyvitamin D concentrations in two different types of pseudodeficiency rickets. In: Norman AW, et al., eds. *Vitamin D: basic research and its clinical application.* Berlin: Walter de Gruyter, 1979;1143–9.

124. Reade TM, Scriver CR, Glorieux FH, et al. Response to crystalline 1α-hydroxyvitamin D_3 in vitamin D dependency. *Pediatr Res* 1975;9:593–9.

125. Liberman UA, Marx SJ. Vitamin D dependent rickets. In: Favus

MJ, ed. *Primer on the metabolic bone diseases and disorders of mineral metabolism, 1st ed.* Kelseyville, CA: American Society for Bone and Mineral Research, 1990;178–82.

126. Fox J, Maunder EMW, Ranall VA, Care AD. Vitamin D dependent rickets type I in pigs. *Clin Sci* 1985;69:541–8.

127. Harmeyer JV, Grabe C, Winkley I. Pseudovitamin D deficiency rickets in pigs. An animal model for the study of familial vitamin D dependency. *Exp Biol Med* 1982;7:117–25.

128. Delvin EE, Glorieux FH, Marie PJ, Pettifor JM. Vitamin D-dependency: replacement therapy with calcitriol. *J Pediatr* 1981;99:26–34.

129. Vecchio F, Carnevale F, Paganetti G, DiBitonto G, Marinelli G. A case of pseudovitamin D deficiency-like rickets in an infant treated with 1,25-dihydroxycholecalciferol: preliminary note. *J Inherited Metab Dis* 1978;1:183–5.

130. Robinow M. Spontaneous recovery from severe rickets resembling pseudo-vitamin D deficiency rickets. *Birth Defects* 1978;10:179–86.

131. Brooks MH, Bell NH, Love L, et al. Vitamin D dependent rickets, type II, resistance of target organs to 1,25-dihydroxyvitamin D. *N Engl J Med* 1978;293:996–9.

132. Fujita T, Nomura M, Okajima S, Suzuya H. Adult-onset vitamin D-resistant osteomalacia with unresponsiveness to parathyroid hormone. *J Clin Endocrinol Metab* 1980;50:927–31.

133. Tsuchiya Y, Matsuo N, Cho H, et al. An unusual form of vitamin D-dependent rickets in a child: alopecia and marked end-organ hyposensitivity to biological active vitamin D. *J Clin Endocrinol Metab* 1980;51:685–90.

134. Tajkeda E, Kuroda Y, Saijo T, Naito E, Kobashi H, Yokota I, Miyao M. 1α-Hydroxyvitamin D₃ treatment of three patients with 1,25-dihydroxyvitamin D-receptor-defect rickets and alopecia. *Pediatrics* 1987;80:97–101.

135. Liberman UA, Samuel R, Halabe A, et al. End organ resistance to 1,25-dihydroxycholecalciferol. *Lancet* 1980;1:504–6.

136. Marx SJ, Liberman UA, Eil C, Gamblin GT, DeGrange DA, Balsan S. Hereditary resistance to 1,25-dihydroxyvitamin D. *Recent Prog Horm Res* 1984;40:589–620.

137. Balsan S, Garabedian M, Liberman UA, et al. Rickets and alopecia with resistance to 1,25-dihydroxyvitamin D: two different clinical courses with two different cellular defects. *J Clin Endocrinol Metab* 1983;57:803–11.

138. Liberman UA, Eil C, Marx SJ. Resistance to 1,25-dihydroxyvitamin D₃: association with heterogeneous defects in cultured skin fibroblasts. *J Clin Invest* 1983;71:192–200.

139. Ritchie HH, Hughes MR, Thompson ET, et al. An ochre muta-tion in the vitamin D receptor gene causes hereditary 1,25 dihydroxyvitamin D₃ resistant rickets in three families. *Proc Natl Acad Sci USA* 1989;86:9783–7.

140. Malloy PJ, Hochberg Z, Tiosano D, Pike JW, Hughes MR, Feldman D. The molecular basis of hereditary 1,25-dihydroxyvitamin D₃ resistant rickets in seven related families. *J Clin Invest* 1990;86:2071–9.

141. Castells S, Greig F, Fusi MA, et al. Severely deficient binding of 1,25-dihydroxyvitamin D to its receptor in a patient responsive to high doses of this hormone. *J Clin Endocrinol Metab* 1986;63:252–6.

142. Eil C, Liberman UA, Rosen JF, Marx SJ. A cellular defect in hereditary vitamin D-dependent rickets type II: defective nuclear uptake of 1,25-dihydroxyvitamin D in cultured skin fibroblasts. *N Engl J Med* 1981;304:1588–91.

143. Tajkeda E, Kuroda Y, Saijo T, Naito E, Kobashi H, Yokota I, Miyao M. 1α-Hydroxyvitamin D₃ treatment of three patients with 1,25-dihydroxyvitamin D-receptor-defect rickets and alopecia. *Pediatrics* 1987;80:97–101.

144. Marx SJ, Spiegel AM, Brown EM, et al. A familial syndrome of decrease in sensitivity of 1,25-dihydroxyvitamin D. *J Clin Endocrinol Metab* 1978;47:1303–10.

145. Hirst MA, Hochman HI, Feldman D. A kindred with normal 1,25-dihydroxyvitamin D₃ binding, but decreased receptor affinity for deoxyribonucleic acid. *J Clin Endocrinol Metab* 1985;60:490–5.

146. Liberman UA, Eil C, Marx SJ. Receptor positive hereditary resistance to 1,25-dihydroxyvitamin D: chromatography of hormone-receptor complexes on DNA-cellulose shows two classes of mutation. *J Clin Endocrinol Metab* 1986;62:122–6.

147. Hughes MR, Malloy PJ, Kieback DG, Kesterson RA, Pike JW, Feldman D, O'Malley BW. Point mutations in the human vitamin D receptor gene associated with hypocalcemic rickets. *Science* 1988;242:1702–5.

148. Sakati N, Woodhouse NTY, Niles N, Harji H, DeGrange DA, Marx SJ. Hereditary resistance to 1,25-dihydroxyvitamin D: clinical and radiological improvement during high-dose oral calcium therapy. *Hormone Res* 1986;24:280–7.

149. Weisman Y, Bab I, Gazit D, Spirer Z, Jaffe M, Hochberg Z. Long-term intracaval calcium infusion therapy in end-organ resistance to 1,25-dihydroxyvitamin D. *Am J Med* 1987;83:984–90.

150. Bliziotes M, Yergey AL, Nanes MS, et al. Absent intestinal response to calciferols in hereditary resistance to 1,25-dihydroxyvitamin D: documentation and effective therapy with high dose intravenous calcium infusion. *J Clin Endocrinol Metab* 1988;66:294–300.

Disorders of Bone and Mineral Metabolism,
edited by Fredric L. Coe and Murray J. Favus,
© 1992 by Raven Press, Ltd. All rights reserved.

CHAPTER 41

Bone Disease Due to Nutritional, Gastrointestinal, and Hepatic Disorders

Daniel D. Bikle

The mineral constituents of bone come from the diet and must be absorbed from the ingested food in the intestine. Vitamin D, through its active metabolite, 1,25-dihydroxyvitamin D [$1,25(OH)_2D$], regulates the intestinal absorption of the two major mineral constituents of bone, calcium and phosphate (see Chapter 3). Vitamin D, although synthesized in the skin under the influence of ultraviolet light, is also an important dietary constituent, especially under circumstances of reduced exposure to ultraviolet light (see Chapter 7). Vitamin D requires bile acids for its proper intestinal absorption, and its absorption is reduced under conditions leading to steatorrhea. Therefore, the bone is dependent on the adequate supply of calcium, phosphate, and vitamin D from the diet as well as their adequate absorption from the intestine.

In this chapter we emphasize the bone disease resulting from vitamin D deficiency secondary to nutritional inadequacy or disorders in the hepatogastrointestinal tract. Such conditions are associated with or lead to calcium and phosphate deficiencies as well. Six potential etiologies for vitamin D deficiency will be discussed (Fig. 1). First, vitamin D deficiency may result from inadequate intake of vitamin D in a person who otherwise fails to make sufficient quantities in the skin. This disorder of nutrition continues to haunt the very young and the very old even in First World countries. Second, vitamin D deficiency may result from failure to absorb adequate amounts of vitamin D from an otherwise appropriate diet. Absorption takes place in the jejunum and ileum, requires bile acids, and is affected by fat and pH. Partial gastrectomy, chronic pancreatic insufficiency, intrinsic

small bowel disease, disorders of the biliary tract, and surgical bypass procedures of the jejunum and ileum are the principal cause of this disturbance. Third, vitamin D that enters the body must be further metabolized to active metabolites. Diseases of the liver where the first step in this bioactivation takes place or drugs such as phenytoin that alter this first metabolic step lead to deficiency of the active metabolites. Fourth, the vitamin D metabolites undergo an enterohepatic circulation, being secreted in bile in conjugated form with subsequent reabsorption in the small intestine. Disruption of this pathway may contribute to the vitamin D deficiency in certain diseases of the liver and small intestine. Fifth, vitamin D and its metabolites are poorly soluble in water and must be transported in blood bound to proteins made in the liver. Decreased synthesis of these proteins may impair the delivery of the vitamin D metabolites to the target tissues. Finally, the diseased or surgically altered intestine may fail to respond normally to the active vitamin D metabolites with respect to calcium and phosphate absorption.

Clearly, one disease may affect bone adversely by several mechanisms involving aberrations in vitamin D absorption, metabolism, or function. In this chapter, specific disease entities are discussed individually even though different diseases may affect bone by similar or identical mechanisms. Since nutritional vitamin D deficiency provides the paradigm for the bone disease associated with most of the other disorders discussed in this chapter, it is discussed first and in greatest detail.

NUTRITIONAL VITAMIN D DEFICIENCY

Prevalence and Incidence

Vitamin D deficiency is uncommon in developed countries but continues to be a problem in the Third

D. D. Bikle: Department of Medicine, University of California, San Francisco and Veterans Administration Medical Center, San Francisco, 94121.

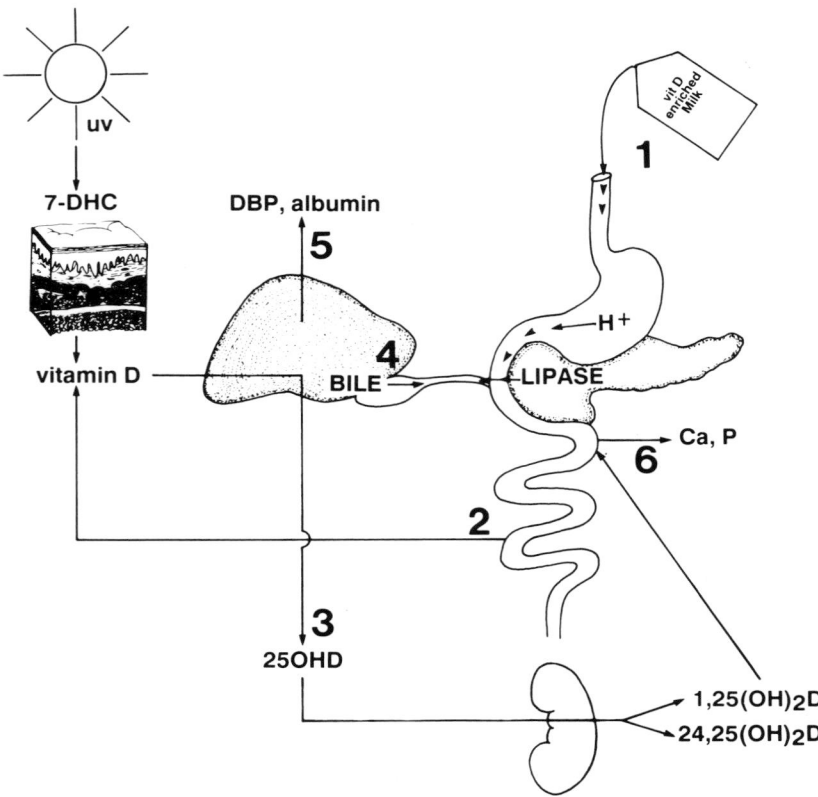

FIG. 1. Six steps in vitamin D absorption and handling that may be altered by hepatogastrointestinal disorders and so lead to bone disease: (1) decreased intake of vitamin D; (2) decreased absorption of vitamin D secondary to disorders in biliary secretion, pancreatic enzymes, enterocyte function, or intestinal anatomy; (3) abnormal production of 25(OH)D by the liver secondary to hepatic parenchymal disease or anticonvulsants; (4) disruption in the enterohepatic circulation of vitamin D metabolites and conjugates secondary to disorders in biliary secretion; (5) reduced delivery of vitamin D metabolites to target tissues secondary to decreased DBP and albumin synthesis; and (6) decreased response of the diseased intestine to 1,25(OH)$_2$D with respect to Ca and P absorption.

World. For example, Rab and Baseer (1) observed that 12.6% of mothers bringing their children to a pediatric outpatient clinic and 33% of pregnant females attending a prenatal clinic in Pakistan had biochemical evidence (low serum calcium, phosphate, or high serum alkaline phosphatase) for vitamin D deficiency that was corrected by vitamin D administration. Clinically significant bone disease was not observed. The likelihood of developing more severe vitamin D deficiency and clinically evident osteomalacia increases when Asians migrate to countries in northern latitudes, such as Great Britain (2,3).

Even in First World countries, two populations remain at risk: the very young and the very old. The American Academy of Pediatrics reported an incidence of 1 case of nutritional rickets per 2791 children (i.e., 0.036%) seen between 1956 to 1960 in 294 hospitals with approved residency programs in pediatrics in the United States (4). The children most at risk are born to mothers eating vegetarian diets who practice prolonged breast feeding without supplementation (5–7). The amount of vitamin D and vitamin D metabolites in human milk is low and varies according to the vitamin D status of the mother (8). The mothers of these children tend to be African-American and/or restrict their sun exposure and have received limited pre- and postnatal medical care (6). Infants born prematurely may be at greater risk than full-term infants for the development of rickets (9,10).

The elderly also are prone to develop vitamin D deficiency and bone disease. Aaron et al. (11) reported that 34% of 102 elderly females treated for fractures of the femoral neck (hip fractures) in Leeds had evidence of osteomalacia (increased osteoid, decreased calcification front) on iliac crest bone biopsy. In many of these patients, osteoporosis was also noted. This report was soon followed by others noting low 25-hydroxyvitamin D [25(OH)D] levels in such patients (12–14), but a correlation between the bone histology and the serum level of 25(OH)D has not been clearly established (15,16). Comparably low levels of 25(OH)D have been found in elderly patients who did not have hip fractures (17,18).

Clinical Presentation (Table 1)

The clinical presentation of vitamin D deficiency depends on the severity of the deficiency and the age of onset. In children whose epiphyses have not yet closed, both the cartilage and bone are involved. The result is rickets, and the clinical diagnosis is usually obvious if the disease is of sufficient severity to produce the characteristic skeletal features to be discussed below. On the other hand, adults who become vitamin D deficient develop osteomalacia. This has a more subtle presentation, often requiring a bone biopsy for diagnosis.

TABLE 1. *Clinical features of vitamin D deficiency*

	Rickets	Osteomalacia
A. *Presentation*		
Age	Infants, young children	Older adults
Asthenia	Common	Uncommon
Muscle weakness	Common	Uncommon
Bone pain	Common	Uncommon
Tetanus	Uncommon	Rare
Convulsions	Uncommon	Rare
Skeletal deformity	Common	Uncommon
Abnormal teeth	Common	Rare
B. *Biochemical changes*		
1. Serum		
Calcium	→ ↓	→ ↓
Phosphorus	↓	→ ↓
Alkaline phosphatase	↑ ↑	→ ↑
PTH	↑	↑
25(OH)D	↕	↕
24,25(OH)$_2$D	↓	↓
1,25(OH)$_2$D	→ ↓	→ ↓
2. Urine		
Calcium	↓	↓
Phosphorus	→	→
TmP/GFR	↓	↓
C. *Radiologic changes*		
Decreased bone density	Common	Common
Long-bone bowing	Common	Uncommon
Epiphyseal hypertrophy	Present	Absent
Metaphyseal flaring	Present	Absent
Pseudofractures	Uncommon	Uncommon
D. *Histologic changes*		
Osteoid	↑	↑
Trabecular bone volume	↓ →	↓ →
Active forming surface	↓	↓
Mineral apposition rate	↓	↓
Mineralization lag time	↑	↑
Epiphyseal plate	Hyperplasia / Disorganized / Abnormal matrix calcification	Closed

→, normal; ↑, increased; ↓, decreased.

Clinical Features of Vitamin D Deficiency *(Fig. 2)*

Infants and young children with rickets are usually listless, irritable, weak, and prone to recurrent respiratory infections (19). In severe cases, tetany, laryngeal stridor, and convulsions may occur. The skull may show widened sutures, asymmetric contours, and frontal bossing. The eruption of the teeth may be delayed, and when teeth do appear they are often poorly mineralized and prone to caries. The cartilaginous portion of the costochondral junctions, like that of the epiphyseal cartilage of the long bones, hypertrophies, producing the bilateral rows of nodular masses down the thorax known as the rachitic rosary. This may be accompanied by protrusion of the sternum. At the insertion of the diaphragm into the lower ribs, an indentation known as Harrison's groove may form. The laxity of the abdominal muscles results in a pot belly accompanied by a prominent lumbar lordosis. If the child can walk, it is often with a waddling gait because of the proximal muscle weakness. The long bones become bowed and their ends flared. In the digits, this produces the string-of-pearls deformity. Adults who develop vitamin D deficiency after childhood may present with proximal muscle weakness and bone pain, but the skeletal abnormalities so characteristic of childhood rickets are not observed.

Biochemical Features of Vitamin D Deficiency

Except when vitamin D deficiency is severe, the serum calcium level is normal or only slightly depressed. Urinary calcium levels can be quite low, however, reflecting the negative calcium balance of the patient. This is a useful and sensitive indicator of vitamin D deficiency in

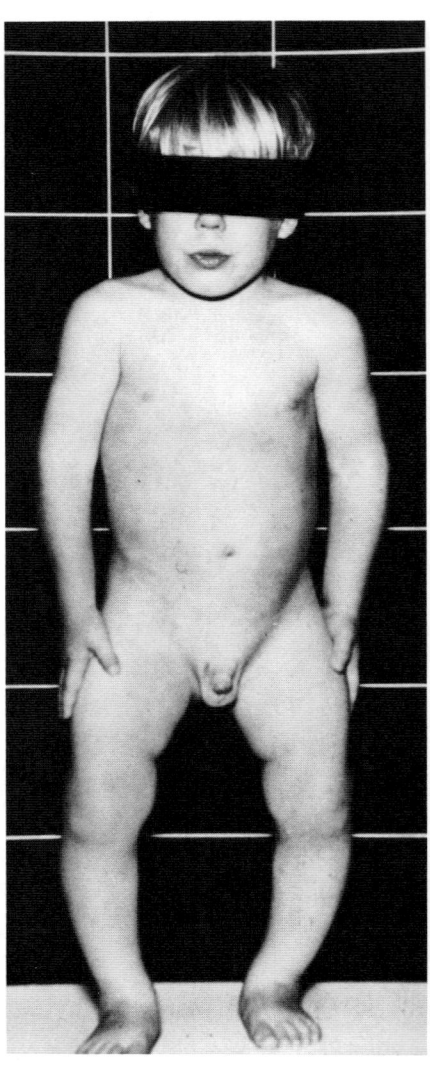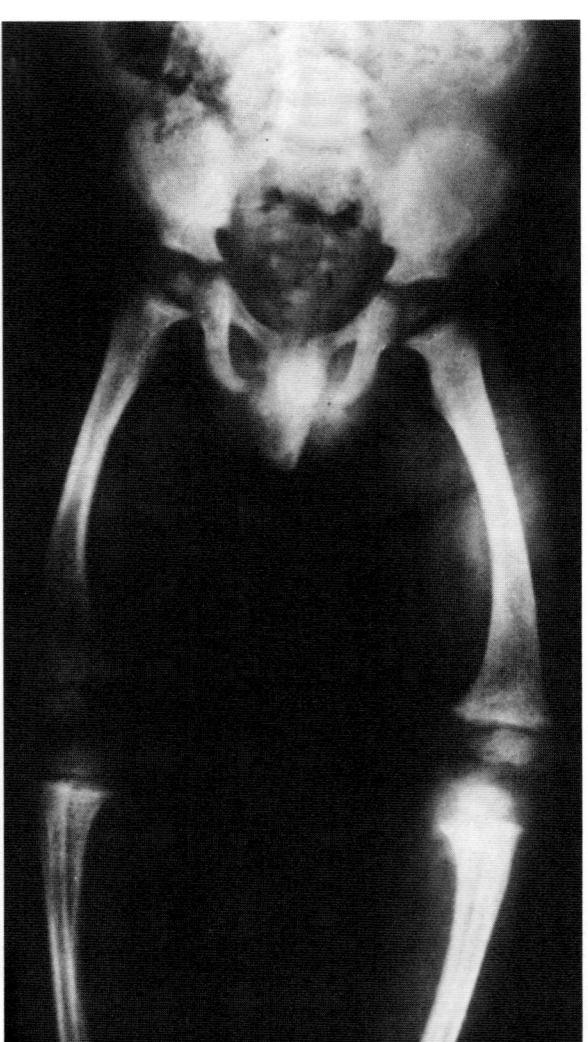

A

B

FIG. 2. Clinical (**A**) and radiologic (**B**) appearance of a young child with rickets. Note the bowing of the legs with flaring of the distal ends of the femora and proximal ends of the tibiae. (Reproduced, with permission, from D. D. Bikle, Osteomalacia and rickets, in *Cecil textbook of medicine,* J. B. Wyngaarden and L. H. Smith, eds., W.B. Saunders, Philadelphia, 1988, p. 1483.)

adults, especially since nutritional vitamin D deficiency is often accompanied by nutritional calcium deficiency (20). In contrast to serum calcium, the serum phosphorus level is almost invariably low and seems to correlate well with the extent of the bone disease (21). At least part of the reason the serum phosphorus level is low is the increased clearance of phosphorus by the kidney as a result of the secondary hyperparathyroidism. This may be accompanied by renal wasting of amino acids and bicarbonate as well (22). Adults with normal renal function also develop hypophosphatemia and renal phosphate wasting when they become vitamin D deficient. However, in the elderly, renal function is often impaired, obscuring these laboratory findings. Elevated serum alkaline phosphatase activity is a good indicator of vitamin D deficiency and rickets in children. In adults, how-

ever, the levels attained are less dramatic, and interpretation of an elevated level may be confounded by coexistent liver disease.

Parathyroid hormone (PTH) levels are increased in vitamin D deficiency. With the advent of assays that measure only the intact form of the hormone, not the circulating fragments that accumulate in renal failure, this measurement may become increasingly important in the assessment of the elderly, who often have reduced renal function. Many of the biochemical abnormalities that characterize vitamin D deficiency result at least in part from the associated hyperparathyroidism. The well-maintained serum calcium reflects the increased release of calcium from bone and the increased reabsorption of calcium in the kidneys in response to increased PTH. Similarly, increased clearance of phosphate by the kidneys during vitamin D deficiency is due in part to the action of PTH on that organ. PTH stimulates alkaline phosphatase in bone, which may account for the elevated serum alkaline phosphatase levels.

The most definitive biochemical marker for vitamin D deficiency is a low serum 25(OH)D level. 25(OH)D provides a good marker for the body stores of vitamin D for two reasons: It has a high affinity for the vitamin D binding protein (DBP), which circulates at a high molar excess to all the vitamin D metabolites (23), and it is produced from vitamin D in the liver at a rate that is substrate dependent and only loosely regulated (24,25). Thus much of the vitamin D that enters the body under normal conditions is converted to 25(OH)D, and most of the 25(OH)D circulates in the blood until metabolized further (26).

Circulating levels of the most potent metabolite of vitamin D, 1,25-dihydroxyvitamin D [1,25(OH)$_2$D], have not proven to be as good a marker for vitamin D deficiency as levels of 25(OH)D and may be normal even in the presence of frank osteomalacia (27). Unlike the hepatic production of 25(OH)D, the renal production of 1,25(OH)$_2$D is tightly regulated. In vitamin D deficiency, the low calcium and phosphorus levels and the high PTH levels all increase the efficiency of 1,25(OH)$_2$D production, maintaining the serum 1,25(OH)$_2$D level until the substrate 25(OH)D is de-

pleted. In contrast, the production of the other major renal metabolite of 25(OH)D, 24,25-dihydroxyvitamin D [24,25(OH)$_2$D], is inhibited when 1,25(OH)$_2$D production is stimulated so that 24,25(OH)$_2$D levels, like 25(OH)D levels, are low in vitamin D deficiency (14,16). All of these vitamin D metabolites are bound to DBP, so that if the DBP levels were decreased as in liver disease, the total vitamin D metabolite levels would also be decreased. However, in uncomplicated vitamin D deficiency the DBP levels are normal (28).

Radiologic Features of Vitamin D Deficiency

In growing children, the radiologic features of vitamin D deficiency are striking and distinctive, whereas in adults the appearance is more subtle and frequently indistinguishable from osteoporosis. The skeleton shows a generalized decrease in density both in cortical and cancellous bone. Vertebral osteopenia is more characteristic of osteomalacia in adults than it is of rickets in children (29). The cortices have a less distinct border in osteomalacia and rickets than in osteoporosis and seem to blend into the medullary bone. The trabeculae also are fuzzy in appearance, in contrast to their pencil-sharp appearance in osteoporosis. Such differences in appearance reflect the large amount of poorly mineralized osteoid lining the trabeculae of patients with rickets or osteomalacia,

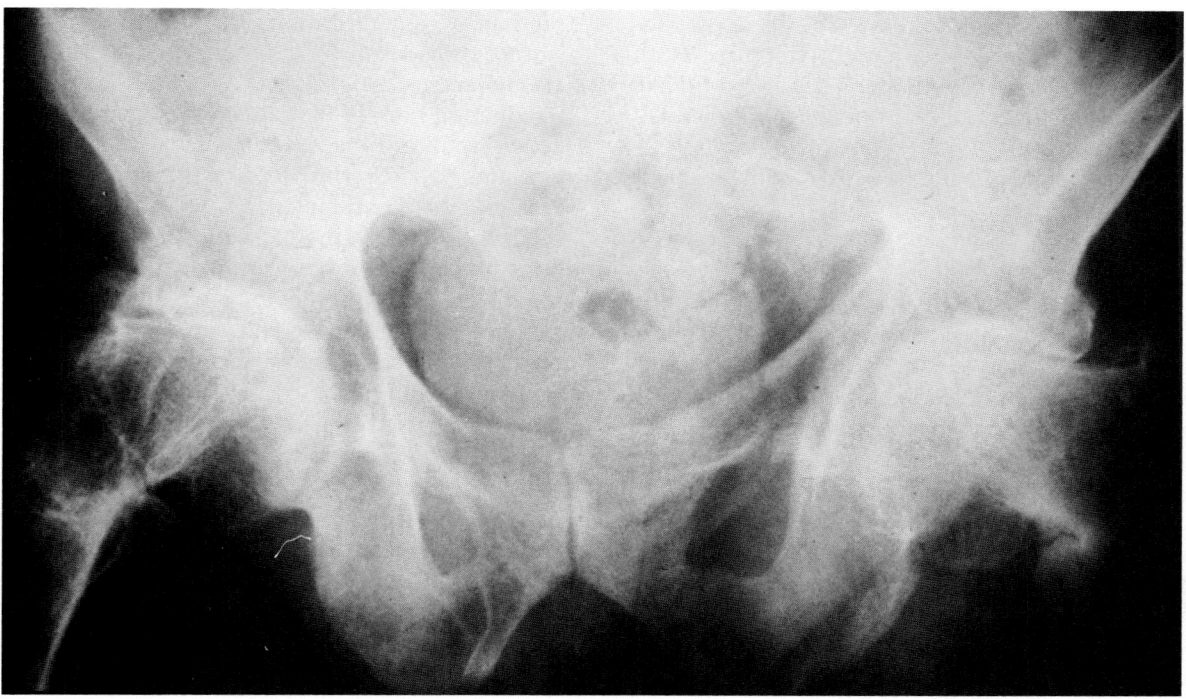

FIG. 3. Radiograph of the pelvis of an elderly female with severe osteomalacia. Note the deformity of the femoral neck bilaterally due to multiple pseudofractures. Note also the pseudofracture in the superior aspect of the left pubic ramus. (Reproduced with permission from D.D. Bikle, Osteomalacia and rickets, in *Cecil textbook of medicine*, J. B. Wyngaarden and L. H. Smith, eds., W.B. Saunders, Philadelphia, 1988, p. 1483.)

which is less radiopaque than normally mineralized bone. At least part of the osteopenia reflects the secondary hyperparathyroidism, which may also lead to erosion of the tufts, subperiosteal resorption, and loss of the distal ends of the clavicles (30,31). In children, the long bones are often bowed. Adults may also show deformities of the long bones because of multiple, often silent fractures, but this is uncommon.

The most distinctive radiologic features of rickets occur in the epiphyseal region. The axial height of the epiphyseal line is markedly increased, the radiolucent zone of the growth plate is greatly enlarged, and the zone of provisional calcification is expanded and irregular in outline with decreased density and fuzzy appearance. The epiphyseal plate is increased in width and cupped with flaring of the adjacent metaphyseal bone. These changes are most marked in the distal femur, proximal tibia, and distal radius (19). The severity of the observed lesions depends on the age at which the patient became vitamin D deficient—the younger the age, the more severe the changes in the epiphyseal region.

Perhaps the most pathognomonic feature of osteomalacia is the presence of Milkman's pseudofractures or Looser's zones (Fig. 3) (32). These are thin radiolucent bands perpendicular to the cortex found near the ends of the long bones, the neck of the femur, the pubic rami, the ribs, the clavicles, and the axillary side of the scapulae. Their exact etiology is not known, but they may represent microfractures that have failed to heal properly leaving a band of unmineralized osteoid. These pseudofractures may progress to complete fracture. Both pseudo- and complete fractures show enhanced uptake by bone-seeking isotopes, making bone scanning a sensitive means of detecting these lesions (33). Pseudofractures seldom are found in patients with osteomalacia unless the disease is severe, however (34).

Histologic Features of Bone in Vitamin D Deficiency

Although seldom necessary to diagnose childhood rickets, bone biopsy is often required to definitively determine the existence of osteomalacia in a patient who otherwise might be considered to have only osteoporosis. McKenna et al. (35) have compiled a diagnostic index (Table 2) based on clinical, biochemical, and radiologic features to help discriminate between osteomalacia and osteoporosis. Using their index a high score (>35%) points toward osteomalacia, whereas a low score (<15%) suggests osteoporosis. Intermediate scores indicate the need for a bone biopsy for definitive diagnosis.

The diagnostic histologic features of osteomalacia include a reduction in mineralization out of proportion to matrix formation (Fig. 4). This results in an accumulation of unmineralized osteoid. Diseases that result in high rates of bone remodeling, such as hyperparathyroidism and hyperthyroidism, may also resemble osteomala-

TABLE 2. *Osteomalacia/osteoporosis discriminant index*

Parameter	Score[a]
CLINICAL FEATURES	
Limb pain	1
Proximal myopathy	1
CHEMISTRY	
Calcium–phosphate product	
1.62–2.41 (mmol/L)	1
1.21–1.61	2
<1.21	3
Alkaline phosphatase	
(score only if LFTs normal)	
75–100 IU/L	1
101–200	2
201–300	3
>300	4
25(OH)D	
5–12.5 nmol/L	1
<5	2
RADIOLOGY	
Looser zone	1
Total score (maximum = 12)	

Source: From M. J. McKenna et al. (35); used with permission.
[a] 100 × *patient score* ÷ 12 = % index score. Interpretation of index score: >35% = osteomalacia, 15–35% = bone biopsy indicated for diagnosis, and <15% = no osteomalacia.

cia in that osteoid volume is increased. However, through the use of double-label tetracycline incorporation, the rate of bone mineralization and the extent of the active bone-forming surface can be determined. The product of mineralization rate and active bone-forming surface provides the rate of bone formation. Osteomalacia is characterized by low rates of bone formation due to a reduction both in the rate of bone mineralization and active bone-forming surface, whereas hyperparathyroidism and hyperthyroidism are characterized by an increase in these parameters.

Thus, to maximize the diagnostic information from a bone biopsy, one should administer tetracycline on two separate occasions (preferably two different tetracyclines such as oxytetracycline and demeclocycline) separated by a fixed period of time such as 2 weeks before the bone biopsy is obtained (36). The iliac crest is the most commonly used site for the biopsy, and transcortical biopsies can be obtained readily and safely under local anesthesia. Tetracycline is incorporated into bone at the calcification front, the zone separating the osteoid and mineralized bone that is currently undergoing active mineralization. Tetracycline fluoresces and can readily be detected in bone sections using fluorescence microscopy. Thus tetracycline marks the region of newly forming bone at the time the label was given. The mineral apposition rate is calculated from the distance between the two tetracycline labels divided by the time interval between the administration of the two labels. The fraction of bone surface undergoing active formation is de-

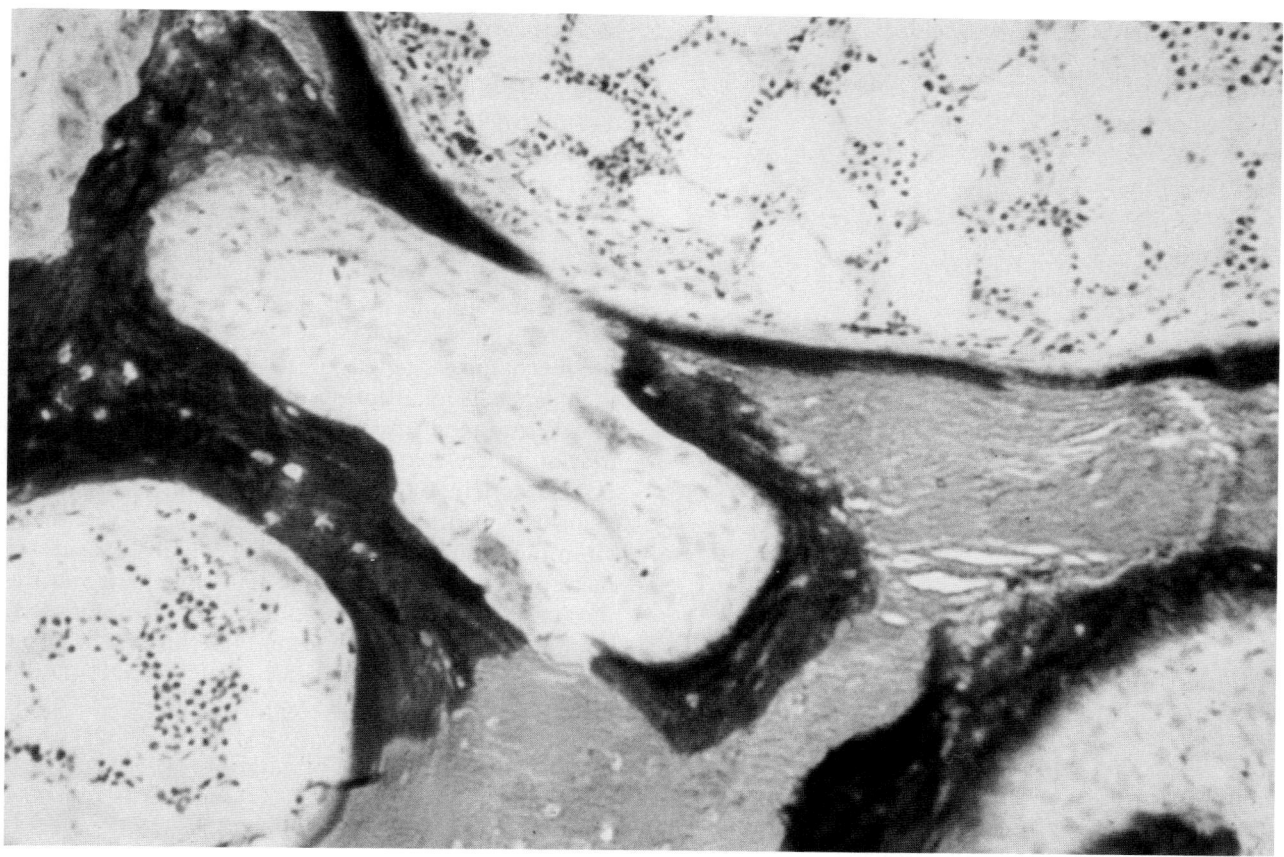

FIG. 4. Undecalcified bone biopsy section stained with Goldner's stain to reveal the extensive amount of osteoid lining the trabecular bone in this patient with severe osteomalacia.

termined by the fraction of total surface that incorporates the tetracycline labels. Mineralization lag time, the time required for newly formed matrix to undergo mineralization, is calculated as the quotient of the osteoid seam width divided by the mineral apposition rate corrected for the fraction of bone surface undergoing active mineralization. The prolongation of mineralization lag time in osteomalacia represents not only a mineralization defect but also a maturation defect of the matrix (32,37) (see Chapters 15 and 22).

Just as the progression of biochemical abnormalities of vitamin D deficiency has been divided into three stages in part related to the severity of the secondary hyperparathyroidism (38), the histologic appearance of the bone in vitamin D deficiency has been divided into three stages (Table 3) (39). In the first stage, osteoid surface and volume (but not osteoid seam width) are increased. Bone formation and bone resorption are also increased, presenting a picture much like hyperparathyroidism except that the mineralization lag time is prolonged. As the severity of the disease increases, osteoid surface, volume, and seam width increase further, while bone formation falls to zero (stage 3).

Although the histologic assessment of the epiphyseal plate region is not performed for the diagnosis of rickets, changes in this region of bone are highly characteristic. The normal epiphyseal plate has five zones (19): the resting zone adjacent to the epiphyseal nucleus, comprised of cartilage and sparse small cells; the proliferative zone, in which the cells line up in columns and tend to flatten out; the maturation zone, in which the cells enlarge and round up; the zone of provisional calcification, where the cartilage is invaded by vascular buds from the metaphysis and the bars of cartilage matrix begin to calcify; and the zone of primary spongiosa, which contains osteoblasts producing a seam of calcified osteoid around the bars of calcified cartilage (see Chapter 14). In rickets, the cells in the zone of maturation increase in number, resulting in elongation and disorganization of the columns, a disorganization that also affects the zone of provisional calcification and primary spongiosa. The increased number of cells not only increases the height of the epiphyseal region but increases its width. The failure to develop an organized calcified matrix contributes to the cupping and flaring of long bones presumably because of the lack of structural support in this region (19).

TABLE 3. *Three stages in the histologic diagnosis of osteomalacia in the adult*

Stage 1 (HVOi)
  Increased osteoid
  Increased or normal bone formation rate

Stage 2 (HVOii)
  Increased osteoid
  Osteoid seam width > 15 μm
  Mineralization lag time > 100 days
  Decreased bone formation rate

Stage 3 (HVOiii)
  Increased osteoid
  Osteoid seam width > 15 μm
  No incorporation of tetracycline labels
  Therefore, mineralization lag time is infinite and bone
    formation rate is zero.

Source: Adapted from Sudhaker Rao et al. (39); used with permission.

Pathogenesis

Vitamin D deficiency leads to a reduction in the availability of the ions required for bone mineralization as well as changes in the hormones regulating this mineralization. Of the ions, most attention has been paid to calcium and phosphate. Of the hormones, most attention has been paid to PTH and the vitamin D metabolites 25(OH)D, 1,25(OH)$_2$D, and 24,25(OH)$_2$D. Despite intense research interest for many years, the relative importance of these vitamin D regulated ions and hormones with respect to normal bone mineralization has not been completely clarified.

The requirement for calcium in bone mineralization independent of vitamin D has been emphasized by reports that calcium infusion can correct the mineralization defect in vitamin D deficiency (or resistance) in both humans (40,41) and rats (42,43) without the need to administer vitamin D. Furthermore, calcium deficiency without vitamin D deficiency has been shown to cause rickets in children (44,45), the rickets being cured with supplemental calcium (45). However, dietary calcium deficiency generally is considered to result in osteoporosis rather than in osteomalacia or rickets (46,47) (see Chapters 37 and 38).

Phosphate deficiency in the absence of vitamin D deficiency has also been reported to lead to osteomalacia and rickets (48–50), although concomitant vitamin D deficiency makes the bone disease much more severe (51). Phosphate deficiency in humans occasionally results from decreased dietary intake or overzealous use of phosphate binding antacids (50), but most cases of hypophosphatemia and osteomalacia or rickets result from renal phosphate wasting. Many of these patients have a disorder in renal phosphate transport, which also appears to involve vitamin D metabolism (see Chapter 37). This makes the interpretation that the hypophosphate-

mia is the sole reason for the mineralization defect somewhat problematic.

Despite reports of osteomalacia or rickets in isolated cases of calcium or phosphate deficiency, the effects seen on bone in states of vitamin D deficiency appear to extend beyond that of a failure to provide adequate amounts of calcium and phosphate for bone mineralization. Lester et al. (52) were able to raise rats on a vitamin D–deficient diet, which maintained normal serum levels of calcium and phosphate despite undetectable levels of 25(OH)D and 1,25(OH)$_2$D. They observed a decrease in the mechanical strength of the shaft along with enlargement and disorganization of the epiphyses of the long bones from these animals. Similarly, changes in the maturation of the matrix have been demonstrated in vitamin D deficiency which are not readily explained by changes in serum calcium and phosphate (53,54). Thus vitamin D and its metabolites are generally considered to have direct actions on bone. However, the nature of these actions and the metabolites responsible for mediating the effects of vitamin D on bone remain in dispute.

The major controversy is whether 1,25(OH)$_2$D mediates all actions of vitamin D on bone, or whether another metabolite, such as 24,25(OH)$_2$D or 25(OH)D, also plays a role. A number of carefully performed experiments using an analog of 25(OH)D that is resistant to 24-hydroxylation [24,24-difluoro 25(OH)D] suggest that 1,25(OH)$_2$D alone is sufficient to cure the bone disease of vitamin D deficiency (55,56). Other studies indicate that 24,25(OH)$_2$D alone, or in combination with 1,25(OH)$_2$D, is superior to 1,25(OH)$_2$D alone in curing rickets or osteomalacia (57–60). Definitive studies in humans have not been performed, and interpretation of studies in rats is complicated by the fact that these animals maintain adequate (for a human) serum phosphate levels even when vitamin D deficient. It seems likely that since 1,25(OH)$_2$D levels are often normal in patients with vitamin D deficiency and bone disease, whereas 25(OH)D and 24,25(OH)$_2$D levels are uniformly low, the bone disease of vitamin D deficiency in humans involves more than 1,25(OH)$_2$D deficiency.

Treatment and Prophylaxis

Treatment of nutritional vitamin D deficiency is straightforward in concept and involves ensuring adequate amounts of vitamin D. The amount of sunlight necessary to produce adequate amounts of vitamin D in the skin varies according to latitude, season, time of day, age, and skin pigment (61). Latitude, season, and time of day determine the intensity of the ambient ultraviolet radiation (290–315 nm), which converts the 7-dehydrocholesterol in the epidermis to previtamin D, which then isomerizes to vitamin D. The levels of 7-dehydrocholesterol in the epidermis fall with age (62). Increased melanin in the skin blocks the photosynthesis of previtamin D (63). Holick et al. (63) estimated that elderly people living in Boston in the summer would produce adequate amounts of vitamin D by exposing their hands, arms, and face to sunlight for 10–15 min two or three times per week. Sunscreens, of course, would block this (64).

Individuals who because of their disability or location cannot achieve this amount of sunlight may be treated with artifical ultraviolet radiation (65,66), although in a chronic care facility this is likely to prove impractical. Therefore, oral vitamin D is often used. The recommended daily allowance is 400 units (10 μg), although Parfitt et al. (67) suggest that older people may require somewhat higher amounts. The amount of vitamin D used to treat nutritional vitamin D deficiency is on the order of 1000–4000 units (25–100 μg) per day. Vitamin D_2 (ergocalciferol) is more readily available than the natural form, vitamin D_3 (cholecalciferol), but both are effective and readily absorbed from the intestine regardless of age (68). Use of the vitamin D metabolites 25(OH)D (calcifediol) and 1,25(OH)$_2$D (calcitriol) or the vitamin D analog dihydrotachysterol (DHT) is not warranted for nutritional vitamin D deficiency in patients with normal intestinal absorption and renal function. Larger doses of vitamin D will not help and can result in toxicity, manifesting as hypercalcemia, hypercalciuria, nephrocalcinosis, and nephrolithiasis. Some studies have even suggested that excessive amounts of vitamin D [or 1,25(OH)$_2$D] may actually inhibit bone mineralization, the very problem lower amounts of vitamin D is intended to treat (69,70). Since nutritional vitamin D deficiency is often accompanied by inadequate calcium intake, calcium supplementation of approximately 1 g/day may be required, adjusting the dose based on the urine calcium excretion. Successful treatment will restore serum and urine calcium and phosphorus levels to normal, normalize serum alkaline phosphatase, PTH, and 25(OH)D concentrations, and cure the bone disease.

GASTROINTESTINAL DISEASES

Gastrointestinal diseases lead to bone disease primarily through the malabsorption of vitamin D and calcium, although the presence of the disease may lead to reduced intake of vitamin D and calcium or limited exposure to sunlight. Each disease discussed below has its own subtle variations on this prevailing theme (Table 4).

Postgastrectomy Bone Disease

Incidence and Prevalence

In a study of 342 postgastrectomy patients and 180 unoperated patients with peptic ulcer disease of similar age, Eddy (71) observed osteopenia of the spine in 24%

of the post-gastrectomy patients compared to 4% of the unoperated controls. Pseudofractures and fractures were seen in 2.4 and 5.2% of gastrectomized patients, whereas none were seen in the controls. Bone pain or tenderness was observed in 26% of the gastrectomized patients compared to 4% of controls. Bone biopsies of 84 gastrectomized patients showed widened osteoid seams in 32%, compared to none of the 9 controls biopsied. A higher prevalence of spinal osteopenia (50%) was observed by Deller et al. (72) in a study of 100 unselected patients following partial gastrectomy; 22% of age-matched controls had spinal osteopenia. Twelve of 20 patients selected for bone biopsy because of the severity of their bone disease had increased osteoid seam width, and 17 of 20 had decreased trabecular bone volume. In contrast to the apparently high prevalence of bone disease among gastrectomized patients in these studies, two British studies showed a lower prevalence. In a survey of 1228 patients following partial gastrectomy, Paterson et al. (73) identified only 6 who had symptoms, biochemical features, and bone biopsy evidence of osteomalacia. Eighty-four of the patients were biopsied, but the criteria for diagnosing osteomalacia were not defined, and the prevalence of reduced trabecular bone volume or osteopenia was not reported. Tovey et al. (74) found osteomalacia in only 10 of 227 post-gastrectomy patients followed over a 25-year period; however, only 15 patients underwent bone biopsy. Thus osteopenia may develop in up to 50% of patients following partial gastrectomy, although the prevalence of frank osteomalacia appears to be less. The studies by Eddy (71) and Deller et al. (72) suggest that at least subtle forms of osteomalacia are found in 25% of patients when this is sought carefully.

Approximately 1 out of 5 postgastrectomy patients is female (73), yet females account for most cases of osteomalacia (29,75). The Billroth II procedure appears to cause more bone disease than the Billroth I procedure or vagotomy and pyloroplasty (71,72,76), although the differences are modest.

Clinical Features

Peptic ulcer disease leading to gastrectomy is a problem primarily of the middle-aged adult, and bone disease is not likely to develop for several years after the procedure. Therefore, the clinical presentation is often that of osteoporosis and osteomalacia in the elderly. Distinguishing between the bone disease accompanying the aging process and that due to gastrectomy is not always obvious, even with a bone biopsy, unless the biopsy shows frank osteomalacia. Bone pain or tenderness is generally found in patients in whom osteomalacia is eventually diagnosed. Symptomatic patients often provide a history of at least modest fat malabsorption (72,73,75,77) and milk intolerance (78).

Routine laboratory assessment reveals a reduction in

TABLE 4. *Bone disease associated with gastrointestinal disorders*

Prevalence	Clinical features	Pathogenesis	Treatment
1. Postgastrectomy			
Up to 50%	Older adults, females > males, bone pain common; ↓ Ca, P, 25(OH)D, ↑ alk. phosphatase, normal PTH, ↓ urine Ca; osteopenia by x-ray; ↑ osteoid, ↓ TBV	↓ Ca, vit. D absorption, ? 2° to ↓ acid and duodenal bypass	Vitamin D or calcifediol
2. Crohn's Disease			
~30%	Younger adults, steatorrhea, frequent ileal resection, frequent glucocorticoid use; ↓ 25(OH)D, Ca, P, alk. phosphatase often normal; osteopenia by x-ray; ↑ osteoid, ↓ TBV	↓ Ca, vit. D absorption 2° disruption of enterohepatic circulation and abnormal jejunal-ileal function; glucocorticoid use	Vitamin D or calcifediol
3. Celiac Disease			
? < 25%	Older children, younger adults, steatorrhea, response to gluten-free diet; ↓ 25(OH)D, ↑ alk. phosphatase	↓ Ca, vit. D absorption 2° abnormal enterocyte function from gliadin toxicity	Gluten-free diet
4. Pancreatic insufficiency			
Uncommon	Associated cholestasis or alcohol abuse, steatorrhea	May be due to associated conditions more than to fat malabsorption per se	Vitamin D, enzyme replacement
5. Jejuno-ileal Bypass			
Up to 60%	↓ Ca, Mg, albumin, ↓ 25(OH)D, ↑ alk. phosphatase, PTH; osteopenia uncommon; ↑ osteoid, ↓ bone formation	↓ Ca, vit. D absorption 2° bypass of distal small intestine	Vitamin D or calcifediol, restore normal anatomy

serum calcium and phosphate and an increase in alkaline phosphatase in 10–25% of patients following partial gastrectomy (73,79). Urinary calcium excretion tends to be low and phosphate clearance increased (79). PTH values are normal in most patients (80–82), although urinary cAMP levels may be increased (83,84), suggesting a functional hyperparathyroidism. 25(OH)D levels tend to be reduced in most studies (81–86). The significance of this observation is obscured by the fact that the transport proteins of the vitamin D metabolites, vitamin D binding protein, and albumin (87) are also reduced (84,86), and no correlation between 25(OH)D level and bone disease has been established (74). 1,25(OH)$_2$D levels are well maintained (80,81). Radiologic assessment demonstrates the frequent association of osteopenia with gastrectomy (82,83). Fractures and pseudofractures, including fractures of the hip (88), are less common but occur more frequently in these patients than in aged-matched controls (82,83).

As discussed above, the prevalence of bone disease on bone biopsy varies widely from study to study, reflecting the often subtle nature of the findings. Osteopenia as indicated by reduced trabecular bone volume, and osteomalacia, as indicated by increased osteoid volume and a reduced calcification front, frequently coexist (71,77,79). A recent report (80) using double-labeled tetracycline found normal mineral apposition rates, normal mineralization lag time, and slightly increased bone formation rates along with increased osteoid volume in 16 asymptomatic patients with partial gastrectomies. This suggests that most "osteomalacia" diagnosed in other studies not using tetracycline labeling may represent stage 1 vitamin D deficiency and/or secondary hyperparathyroidism. Some patients have increased marrow fibrosis and osteoclast numbers clearly indicating that secondary hyperparathyroidism occurs at least occasionally (75).

Pathogenesis

Both vitamin D [or 25(OH)D] absorption (89–91) and calcium absorption (81,92–94) are reduced in postgastrectomy patients, especially those who have evidence of bone disease. Such patients also tend to have mild degrees of fat malabsorption (71,72,89) in the absense of small bowel disease (71). Milk intolerance contributes to the reduced oral intake of vitamin D and calcium in at least some patients (78).

Normal calcium absorption has been thought to require the acid environment of the stomach for solubilization of calcium salts prior to their absorption in the small intestine. Thus procedures that reduce acid output would reduce calcium absorption. However, this concept has recently been tested (95,96), and it appears that gastric acid is not required for normal calcium absorption. The duodenum plays an important role in the vitamin D–regulated absorption of calcium (97), so that with duodenal bypass as in the Billroth II procedure, calcium absorption is likely to be reduced. Fat malabsorption would be expected to reduce calcium absorption both directly by the formation of calcium complexes and indirectly by the accompanying malabsorption of vitamin D.

Treatment

The osteomalacic component of the bone disease responds to vitamin D and calcium supplements (98), but the osteoporotic component may not (99,100). Distinguishing between these two components without a bone biopsy is difficult, and unless a biopsy is obtained that shows no osteomalacia, a clinical trial with vitamin D and calcium is indicated, especially if the serum 25(OH)D level is low. Since malabsorption of these substances is likely to accompany gastrectomy to a variable degree, the amount of either agent required to correct the deficiency will vary and needs to be established for each patient. Serum 25(OH)D levels are a good means to monitor the adequate absorption of vitamin D. If steatorrhea is a major problem, calcifediol [25(OH)D] rather than vitamin D should be used because it is better absorbed under these conditions (101).

Inflammatory Bowel Syndromes

Incidence and Prevalence

Of the two major forms of inflammatory bowel disease, Crohn's disease and ulcerative colitis, bone disease is most frequently associated with Crohn's disease (102). 30% of an unselected series of patient's with Crohn's disease had osteopenia (bone mineral density 2 SD below normal) demonstrated by single-photon absorptiometry of the radius or quantitative computed tomography of the spine (102). In an earlier study, 5% of such patients had the clinical features of osteomalacia (103). This may be an underestimate since 6 of 9 patients studied by

Driscoll et al. (104) and 9 of 25 patients studied by Compston et al. (105) had increased osteoid on their bone biopsies despite the fact that most of these patients had few clinical features of osteomalacia.

Clinical Features

The clinical features of bone disease in patient's with Crohn's disease are usually subtle. Most of these patients are young adults and have a variety of gastrointestinal and extragastrointestinal concerns that obscure symptoms of bone disease. Ileal resection, malabsorption, and glucocorticoid treatment are common and relevant to the bone disease that ensues. Routine serum biochemical measurements, including calcium, phosphorus, and magnesium, may be low and the alkaline phosphatase may be high, but these values generally are normal (104,106). However, serum 25(OH)D levels are reduced in up to 65% of patients (84,102,104), especially in those who have undergone ileal resection (102). Osteopenia is commonly observed both of cortical (102,106) and cancellous (102) bone, but less than 10% will have fractures or pseudofractures (102,103). Bone biopsy may be the only means of diagnosing osteomalacia in most of these patients. Bone biopsy frequently shows reduced trabecular bone volume and increased osteoid (104,105,107). However, one study using double tetracycline labeling failed to show a reduction in bone formation, mineral apposition, or mineralization lag time in 30 unselected patients (108), suggesting that stage 2 or 3 osteomalacia is uncommon. These patients also had normal vitamin D metabolites, inactive disease, and were not on glucocorticoid therapy, so that these results may not be applicable to sicker patients.

Pathogenesis

Patients with Crohn's disease have multiple reasons for developing bone disease. Vitamin D (101) and calcium (109) absorption are reduced. Vitamin D is absorbed primarily in the jejunum and ileum via a process expedited by bile salts and inhibited by fat (110). Therefore, disease or resection of this portion of the intestine will result in less vitamin D absorption. Concurrent use of cholestyramine or the development of hepatobiliary complications will reduce the available bile salts required for vitamin D absorption. Vitamin D metabolites undergoing enterohepatic circulation (111) cannot be reabsorbed properly by a diseased or resected ileum. Calcium malabsorption reflects both the state of vitamin D insufficiency and the steatorrhea. Dietary intake of nutrients, including milk products, is often low, compounding the problem of absorption. Glucocorticoid therapy is frequently used during active disease and can contribute to the calcium malabsorption (see Chapter 2) and bone loss (see Chapter 34).

Treatment

Vitamin D in doses of 4000–12,000 units (100–300 μg) per day is generally adequate therapy for patients with low serum 25(OH)D levels, although the appropriate dose must be determined for each patient (106). Calcifediol [25(OH)D] at doses starting with 50 μg three times per week may be used instead of vitamin D if vitamin D therapy is not effective. Dietary counseling to ensure that adequate calcium is also being ingested should be performed. Serum 25(OH)D and urine calcium levels provide good monitors of treatment. Vitamin D treatment will reduce the osteomalacic component of the bone disease (104), but available data are not sufficient to determine whether the osteoporotic component will improve.

Celiac Disease

Incidence and Prevalence

The prevalence of bone disease among patients with celiac disease appears to be less than that among patients with Crohn's disease or postgastrectomy. Presumably, this reflects early recognition of celiac disease and its effective treatment. Osteomalacia can be the presenting complaint (112), however. Of 9 untreated patients with celiac disease, Dibble et al. (84) found 2 with low (<5 ng/mL) 25(OH)D levels; 12 patients successfully treated with a gluten-free diet had normal 25(OH)D levels. A higher (3/7) prevalence of low 25(OH)D levels was found by Arnaud et al. (113) using a higher value of 25(OH)D as the lower limit of normal. Five of nine untreated patients studied by Melvin et al. (114) had osteomalacia on bone biopsy; two of these patients had fractures (ribs, spine).

Clinical Features

The finding of bone disease in patients with celiac disease is usually in association with malabsorption, although the steatorrhea may be occult (115). The upper small intestine is usually more affected than the ileum. Patients with osteomalacia have a greater likelihood of having reduced serum and urine calcium levels and elevated serum alkaline phosphatase (114).

Pathogenesis

Vitamin D and calcium absorption are abnormal in patients with celiac disease (114,116) as part of the general disorder in enterocyte function. Gluten-free diets will correct this disorder in most cases, although osteomalacia has been reported in one case otherwise successfully treated on a gluten-free diet (117).

Treatment

The treatment of choice is a gluten-free diet. This will correct the disorder in calcium metabolism in most cases. Vitamin D and calcium supplementation should be reserved for the person who fails to normalize serum calcium, phosphorus, alkaline phosphatase, and 25(OH)D levels or urine calcium excretion on a gluten-free diet.

Pancreatic Insufficiency

Incidence and Prevalence

Osteomalacia or rickets in patients with pancreatic insufficiency from a number of causes, including cystic fibrosis and total pancreatectomy, is unusual (118–121). Reduced 25(OH)D levels and osteopenia may be seen in nearly half of the patients, however, especially if the disease also involves other organs, such as the liver, biliary tract, or small bowel (84,122,123).

Clinical Features

The presence of bone disease in a patient presenting with malabsorption thought to be secondary to pancreatic insufficiency should lead to a search for complicating features such as alcohol abuse, cholestasis, cirrhosis, or intrinsic small bowel involvement. Current data are insufficient to determine the extent to which the osteopenia observed radiologically represents osteoporosis versus osteomalacia.

Pathogenesis

The infrequency of serious bone disease in patients with pancreatic insufficiency and steatorrhea who do not also have hepatic involvement, cholestasis, or small bowel disease indicates that steatorrhea per se is not sufficient to cause major impairment in vitamin D and calcium absorption. However, the steatorrhea resulting from the lack of pancreatic enzymes may be synergistic with malabsorption resulting from insufficient bile salts or intrinsic small bowel disease.

Treatment

Patients who have low 25(OH)D levels should be treated with sufficient amounts of vitamin D to restore their 25(OH)D levels to normal. The dose will vary from patient to patient. In patients with substantial amounts of steatorrhea, calcifediol [25(OH)D] may be required. The diet should be supplemented with enough calcium to raise urinary calcium to levels above 150 mg/day (adults). These patients may also require pancreatic enzyme replacement and supplementation with other fat-soluble vitamins.

Jejuno-ileal Bypass

Incidence and Prevalence

Fortunately, the popularity of the jejuno-ileal bypass as a treatment for massive obesity has waned because of the large number of undesirable side effects, of which bone disease is one. Bone disease is subtle and not usually appreciated by routine radiologic procedures (124,125). However, osteomalacia on bone biopsy has been found in up to 60% of unselected people evaluated several years after the procedure (124–130).

Clinical Features

Few patients present with bone pain or fractures, and radiologic evidence of osteopenia is generally not found (124,125). However, reductions in serum calcium and magnesium with an increase in serum alkaline phosphatase are found in approximately half the patients following this operation (124–128). Serum phosphorus is generally normal. At least part of the fall in serum calcium can be attributed to the fall in albumin. Serum 25(OH)D levels, which tend to be reduced in the obese patient prior to operation, fall even further in most individuals (124–128,131). On the other hand, serum 1,25(OH)$_2$D levels are generally well maintained (124,131; but see 128). PTH levels tend to be increased (124,128,129,131). Osteomalacia is found on bone biopsy in 12–60% (124–127), even when the more restrictive criteria incorporating the results from double tetracycline labeling are used (128–130).

Pathogenesis

The ileum and much of the jejunum are effectively cut off from the flow of nutrients by this procedure. This region of the intestine is most responsible for the absorption of vitamin D and the metabolites of vitamin D secreted in the bile. Malabsorption of vitamin D (124), calcium (132), and magnesium (133) have all been demonstrated. Fatty infiltration of liver is often found, but the degree to which liver disease contributes to the bone disease is not clear.

Treatment

Vitamin D and the analog of 1,25(OH)$_2$D, 1α-vitamin D, have been used successfully to treat the bone disease following jejuno-ileal bypass (134–136). However, since 1,25(OH)$_2$D levels are usually normal in these patients, vitamin D or calcifediol [25(OH)D] should be tried first using doses that normalize serum 25(OH)D levels. Calcium supplementation to normalize urine calcium levels is also indicated. Treatment failures may respond following antibiotic treatment of bacterial overgrowth in the bypassed segment (136). If these measures fail, reanastomosis of the bypassed segment may be required (137).

LIVER DISEASES

For this discussion on the relationship of liver disease to bone disease, three categories of liver disease are considered: chronic cholestatic diseases, of which the most common are primary biliary cirrhosis, chronic active hepatitis, and alcoholic cirrhosis (Table 5).

Chronic Cholestatic Diseases

Incidence and Prevalence

Primary biliary cirrhosis (PBC) is a disease primarily of the middle-aged female, an age at which postmenopausal osteoporosis is common and not readily distinguished from the osteoporosis of the liver disease. Both osteomalacia and osteoporosis occur in primary biliary cirrhosis, but estimates of the prevalence of these forms of bone disease vary widely. Some studies indicate that patients with PBC have primary osteomalacia (138,139), others find mostly osteoporosis (140–143), others find a high prevalence of both osteomalacia and osteoporosis (144,145), and still others find little of either (146–149). Although studies differ somewhat with respect to the severity of the disease in patients studied or in the criteria used to diagnose the bone disease, these differences do not fully account for the differences in results obtained. Since the more recent studies show the least amount of bone disease, it may be that with the heightened awareness of the potential for bone disease in patients with PBC more attention is being paid to nutritional factors that can prevent or forestall this complication.

In contrast to PBC, biliary atresia is a disease of infants and children. Children with this condition, even if surgically corrected, have a high likelihood of developing rickets (150), which is readily treated with vitamin D.

Clinical Features

Patients with PBC are often asymptomatic, although bone pain is common in patients subsequently shown to have osteomalacia on bone biopsy (138). Laboratory assessment tends to show normal or slightly reduced serum and urine calcium, normal serum phosphorus, and normal serum magnesium levels. PTH levels may be increased despite normal serum calcium and vitamin D metabolite levels (140,143,148,151). Alkaline phosphatase levels in serum are increased, but the source is the liver, not the bone. Serum 25(OH)D levels are normal in asymptomatic patients but may fall as the disease progresses (139,141,152). The 25(OH)D levels are not a good predictor of bone disease (138,141). Radiologic assessment is unlikely to demonstrate pseudofractures or osteoporosis beyond what is expected for age and sex, unless the patient has been treated in the past with glucocorticoid hormones (153). Bone biopsy is required to make a definitive diagnosis of osteomalacia. However, recent studies indicate that this diagnosis is being made less and less often in patients with PBC.

Pathogenesis

Bone disease in PBC has many potential etiologies. Intestinal malabsorption of calcium (154), phosphate

TABLE 5. *Bone disease associated with liver disorders*

Prevalence	Clinical features	Pathogenesis	Treatment
1. Primary Biliary Cirrhosis			
Common	1° females, bone pain, jaundice; ↓ Ca, 25(OH)D, ↑↑ alk. phosphatase (liver); osteopenia by x-ray; ↓ TBV more common than ↑ osteoid	↓ Ca, P, vit. D absorption ? 2° ↓ bile, ↑ urinary losses of vit. D conjugates, 25 hydroxylation of vit. D intact	OM responds to vit. D, OP does not
2. Chronic Active Hepatitis			
~50%	Patients often on glucocorticoids; bone disease usually asymptomatic; osteopenia by x-ray; ↓ TBV	Bone disease 2° to glucocorticoid use more than to liver disease	Ensure adequate nutrition limit glucocorticoid dose
3. Alcohol Abuse			
Most alcoholics with >10 yr ETOH abuse	Back pain, rib fractures; ↓ Ca, Mg, P, albumin, ↓ 25(OH)D, ↑ PTH; osteopenia, fractures by x-ray; ↓ TBV, ↓ bone formation	Poor diet, ETOH induced ↑ urinary losses of Ca, Mg, possible direct toxic affects of ETOH on bone	Stop ETOH ↑ Ca, Mg, P in diet, vit. D if ↓ 25(OH)D and OM on biopsy

(155), and vitamin D (139,156,157) have all been demonstrated to occur in these patients. Vitamin D absorption will be further impaired in patients treated with cholestyramine (158). Although some reports (159,160) indicate that the heptic hydroxylation of vitamin D to 25(OH)D is impaired, this does not appear to be a problem in most patients. 25(OH)D levels are readily increased with vitamin D therapy in most studies (139,160–162). Disruption of the enterohepatic circulation of the vitamin D metabolites with increased losses in the urine has been postulated to lead to vitamin D deficiency in PBC (111,163,164), but the significance of the enterohepatic circulation for the conservation of the vitamin D metabolites is not established (165). Finally, an abnormality in the bone forming cell itself, the osteoblast, has been postulated to account for the failure of adequate vitamin D and mineral levels to correct the reduction in bone formation seen in patients with PBC (140–142,146).

Treatment

When present, osteomalacia responds readily to vitamin D, calcifediol [25(OH)D], calcitriol [1,25(OH)$_2$D], or 1α(OH)D (145,166). However, osteoporosis has not been treated successfully with vitamin D or its metabolites (141,142,166). If the serum 25(OH)D level is reduced, vitamin D should be given to restore the level to normal. If vitamin D is ineffective, calcifediol should be tried. The rationale for using calcitriol or 1α(OH)D vitamin D in the absence of renal failure is weak. Such therapy ignores the potential benefit of 24,25(OH)$_2$D, which is low in patients with low 25(OH)D levels and which is increased by vitamin D or calcifediol therapy. Supple-

menting this regimen with calcium has been shown to increase the effectiveness of vitamin D therapy (167).

Chronic Active Hepatitis

Incidence and Prevalence

Patients with cryptogenic cirrhosis or chronic active hepatitis tend to have 25(OH)D levels below the normal range and comparable to levels seen in patients with alcoholic cirrhosis or PBC (84,152). Osteopenia demonstrated by bone densitometry of the radius or reduced trabecular bone volume on bone biopsy was found in 47% of patients with chronic active hepatitis treated with glucocorticoid hormones (168).

Clinical Features

The bone disease associated with chronic active hepatitis is usually asymptomatic. Many patients are treated with glucocorticoid hormones, which may account for much of the bone disease that manifests as osteopenia or osteoporosis. The reduction in 25(OH)D levels is accompanied by a reduction in DBP levels (84), suggesting that the free 25(OH)D level is normal in most patients. No osteomalacia was observed by Stellon et al. (168) in bone biopsies from 36 patients with chronic active hepatitis, although reduced trabecular bone volume was frequently seen.

Pathogenesis

The scarcity of data makes problematic the compilation of a pathogenetic mechanism for the bone disease in chronic active hepatitis. However, vitamin D deficiency secondary to malabsorption or impaired hepatic conversion to 25(OH)D does not appear to play a major role. Osteoporosis secondary to glucocorticoid therapy seems likely (see Chapter 38). Conceivably, patients with parenchymal liver disease are at increased risk for the development of bone disease when glucocorticoid therapy is used if the disease is accompanied by malabsorption, poor nutrition, or reduced sunlight exposure. This hypothesis is supported by the high incidence of osteoporosis in patients following liver transplantation, who routinely are placed on high doses of glucocorticoid hormones (169).

Treatment

Limiting the use of glucocorticoid therapy, ensuring adequate nutrition, and encouraging sunlight exposure are the recommended first steps. The role of vitamin D and calcium supplementation in patients requiring glucocorticoid therapy is not clear and cannot be recommended unless malabsorption of these substances is strongly suspected.

Alcohol-Induced Bone Disease

Incidence and Prevalence

Although listed with liver diseases, alcohol-induced bone disease is not restricted to those who develop cirrhosis. Saville (170) was the first to call attention to the high prevalence of osteopenia in alcoholics in his study of bone biopsies from cadavers in the New York City morgue. Spinal osteopenia may be observed in 50% of ambulatory male alcoholics by routine x-ray procedures (171), and fractures of ribs or vertebrae occur in nearly 30% of this population (172,173). Partial gastrectomy increases the likelihood of developing osteopenia and fractures (174,175). Bone densitometry and bone biopsy have demonstrated osteopenia in most patients with a prolonged history of heavy alcohol abuse (176–178). Osteoporosis is the disease usually found histologically (176–180), although osteomalacia does occur (181,182) and may be more likely in patients who have had a partial gastrectomy (183).

Clinical Features

Alcoholism is a subtle disease in most patients and may be missed unless the person is specifically questioned. The presentation is often that of idiopathic osteoporosis, discovered by chance on radiologic assessment for low back pain or pulmonary complaints. Aseptic necrosis of the hip is associated with alcoholism, but the incidence of this disease in alcoholics is low (182,184,185). Serum calcium, phosphorus, and magnesium tend to be low normal in the ambulatory alcoholic (176,177,180), although following a binge or with other alcohol-related medical problems serious enough to require hospitalization, serum levels of these minerals can be low enough to cause neuromuscular disturbances and rhabdomyolysis (186). Part of the reduction in serum calcium is accounted for by a reduction in albumin concentration. Serum PTH and urinary cyclic AMP levels may be elevated or high normal in part because of the lowered calcium and magnesium levels (176,180,187). 25(OH)D levels are usually low (138,151,176,180,181, 187), and correlate with the low albumin and DBP concentrations (188,189). 1,25(OH)₂D concentrations have variably been reported as low (181,190), normal (126), or high (187). Low levels of 1,25(OH)₂D are found in the alcoholics with the most liver disease, and like 25(OH)D levels, correlated with serum albumin and DBP (190). The free or unbound concentrations of the vitamin D metabolites are normal (189,190). It is now appreciated that much of the reduction in the total concentrations of the vitamin D metabolites is a direct result of the reduction in the circulating levels of the carrier proteins (191,192) (Fig. 5). The radiologic assessment of bone reveals osteopenia or osteoporosis. The cancellous bone of the spine is more affected than the cortical bone of the long bones (Fig. 6). Fractures are common, often following trauma, but pseudofractures are rare in this population. The bone biopsy usually reveals reduced trabecular bone volume with normal or decreased amounts of osteoid (176–180), although a few patients will have increased osteoid volume (181,182). Marrow fibrosis is uncommon. Bone formation and active bone resorption are generally reduced (176–182), although in younger patients high rates of bone turnover may be observed (187 and personal observation) (Fig. 7).

Pathogenesis

The original reports of low 25(OH)D levels in alcoholics led to suggestions that poor nutrition (193), decreased sunlight (194), vitamin D malabsorption (195), or defective hydroxylation of vitamin D to 25(OH)D (188,196) might be involved in alcoholic bone disease. Vitamin D deficiency could therefore account for the osteomalacia seen in some alcoholic patients. Hypophosphatemia due to poor intake, malabsorption, concomitant use of aluminum-containing antacids, or increased renal excretion (197) could enhance the mineralization defect. However, the infrequency of osteomalacia, the finding of normal free levels of the vitamin D metabolites, and the realization that low total concentrations of the vitamin D metabolites reflect decreased hepatic production of DBP and albumin, not decreased hepatic production of 25(OH)D, all indicate that for most people the bone disease is not one of vitamin D deficiency. Calcium deficiency from poor intake, malabsorption (198,199), or increased urinary excretion (200) could lead to osteoporosis, especially if associated with secondary hyperparathyroidism (176,180,187).

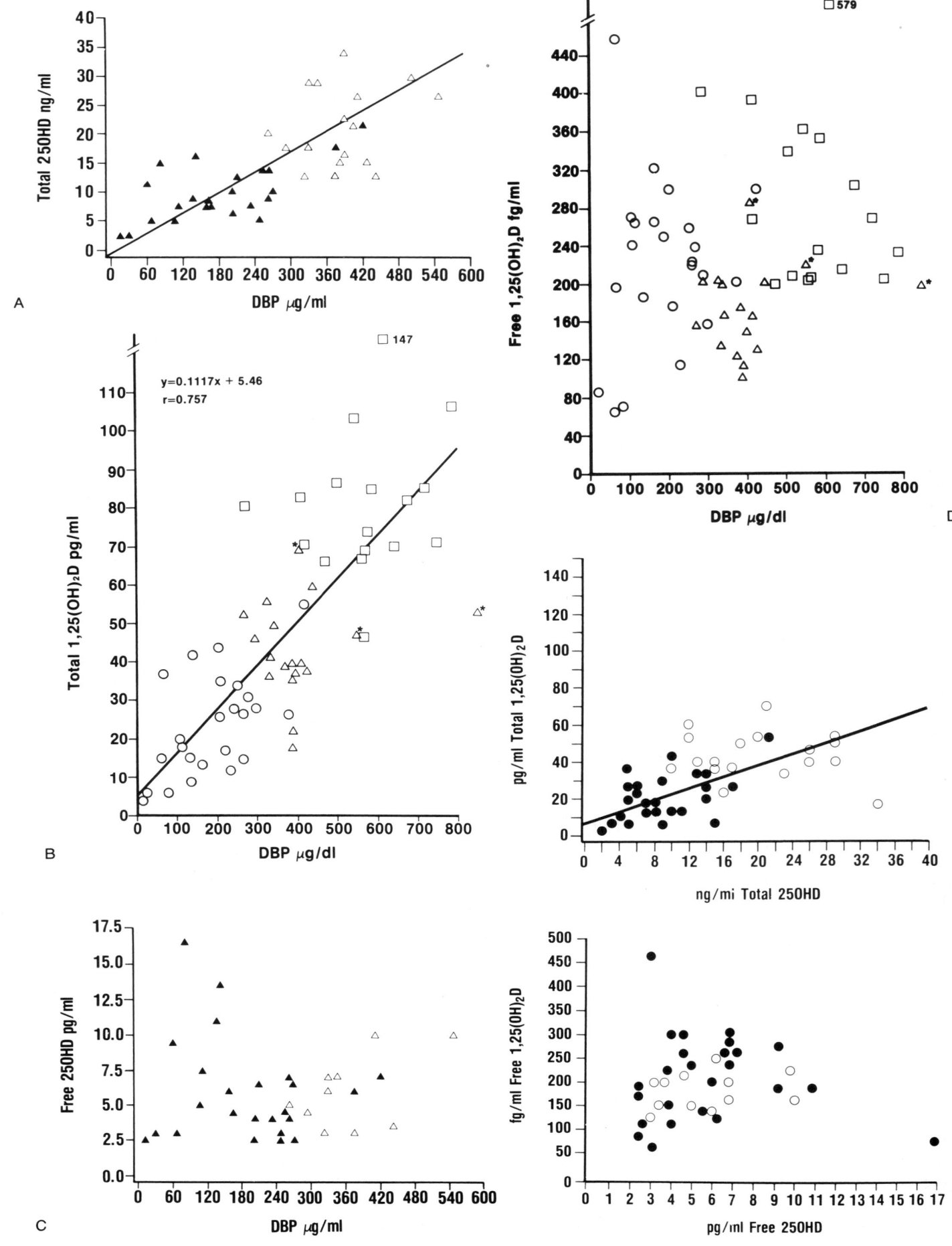

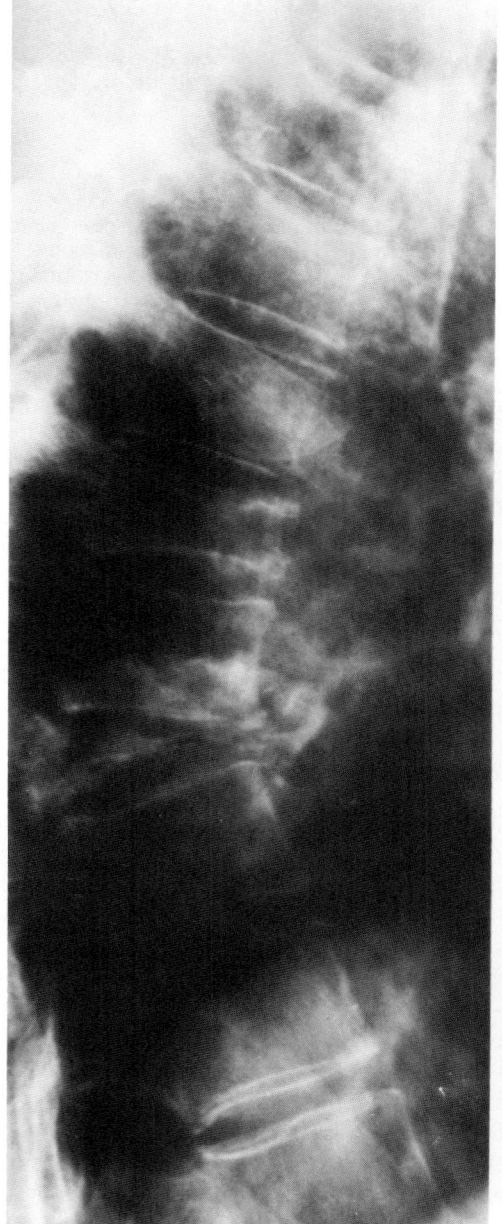
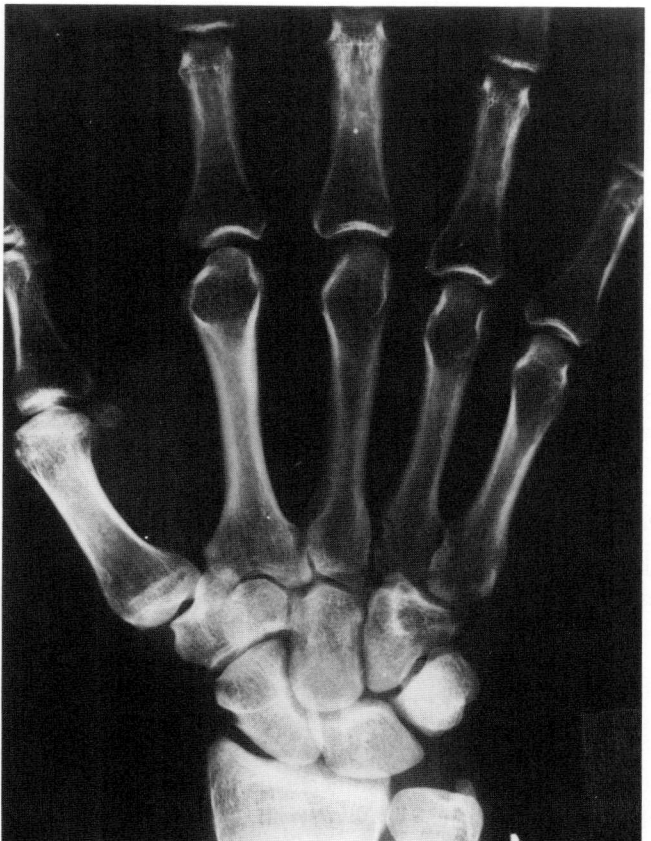

A   B

FIG. 6. Radiographs of the spine (**A**) and hand (**B**) of an alcoholic, showing severe demineralization and compression fractures of the spine with relatively little loss of cortical bone of the hands. (Reproduced with permission from D. D. Bikle et al., *Ann Intern Med* 1985;103:42–8.)

FIG. 5. Correlation of (**A**) total 25(OH)D and (**B**) 1,25(OH)$_2$D levels to DBP; lack of correlation of (**C**) free 25(OH)D and (**D**) 1,25(OH)$_2$D levels to DBP; (**E**), correlation of total 25(OH)D to total 1,25(OH)$_2$D levels, but (**F**) lack of a correlation between free 25(OH)D and 1,25(OH)$_2$D levels in normal individuals (○) and patients with liver disease (●). In **B** and **D**, data from pregnant women (△) are also included. These data demonstrate the dependence of total 25(OH)D and 1,25(OH)$_2$D concentrations on DBP levels that are reduced by liver disease. However, free concentrations of 25(OH)D and 1,25(OH)$_2$D are normal in most patients with liver disease. (Reproduced from the *Journal of Clinical Investigation,* 1984, vol. 74, pp. 1166–76, and 1986, vol. 78, pp. 748–52 by copyright permission of the American Society for Clinical Investigation.)

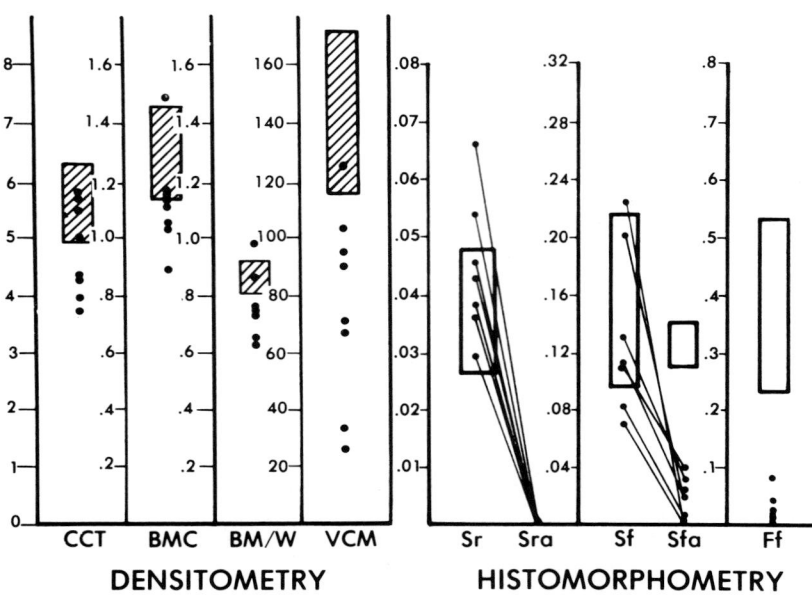

FIG. 7. Bone densitometry and histomorphometry of bone biopsies from alcoholics showing a greater decrease in vertebral bone density (VCM) than peripheral bone density (CCT, BMC, BM/W), reduced active bone resorption (Sra) and bone formation (Sfa) surfaces, and reduced bone formation rates (Ff). Total resorption (Sr) and formation (Sf) surfaces are normal. The rectangles contain the normal range. (Reproduced with permission from D. D. Bikle et al., *Ann Intern Med* 1985; 103:43–8.)

Mild degrees of hypomagnesemia could aggravate this picture (very low magnesium levels cause hypoparathyroidism). However, evidence for hyperparathyroidism is seldom seen on bone biopsies; rather, the picture is usually one of inactive bone. Failure to explain the bone disease of alcoholics on the basis of changes in the calciotropic hormones has led to the hypothesis that the prime offender is alcohol itself, causing a direct inhibition of bone cell activity (176,180,201).

Treatment

Alcoholics should discontinue their drinking habits, but thus far there is no convincing evidence that this will lead to a restoration of lost bone. Vitamin D therapy should be considered if the 25(OH)D levels are lower than what would be expected for the reduction in albumin and DBP. Such therapy will reverse osteomalacia if present and may help to restore bone mass (180). Vitamin D itself is effective in most subjects since malabsorption is usually not severe (196) and 25(OH)D production is usually intact (202). If oral vitamin D therapy does not raise 25(OH)D levels, calcifediol [25(OH)D] can be used. Ensuring adequate nutrition, including calcium, magnesium, and phosphate, is also appropriate. The degree to which osteoporosis can be reversed with current therapeutic measures remains unclear, however.

BONE DISEASE COMPLICATING THERAPY

In this chapter two iatrogenic bone diseases are considered: that attending long-term anticonvulsant therapy and that accompanying total parenteral nutrition (Table 6). Other forms of treatment that may aggravate or precipitate bone disease, such as glucocorticoid hormones, heparin, vitamin A, or hemodialysis, are covered in Chapters 38 and 39.

Anticonvulsant-Induced Bone Disease

Incidence and Prevalence

Following its original description in the German literature 20 years ago (203,204), the relationship between long-term anticonvulsant therapy and bone disease has been the subject of a voluminous literature. Initial reports indicated that 20–65% of epileptics receiving anticonvulsants developed signs of rickets or osteomalacia (205–208). The highest prevalence of bone disease occurred among institutionalized children (208,209). It soon became apparent that institutionalized patients have a high prevalence of bone disease regardless of whether they are taking anticonvulsants (210–212). Nevertheless, institutionalized patients are at substantial additional risk for the development of bone disease when treated with anticonvulsants (210). Outpatient studies have indicated a much lower prevalence of clinically significant bone disease (213–220), although biochemical abnormalities (reduced serum and urine calcium, reduced serum 25(OH)D, elevated serum PTH and alkaline phosphatase), reduced bone density, and increased osteoid on bone biopsy are observed in 10–44% of patients on long-term anticonvulsant therapy (210,212, 215–223).

Clinical Features

Bone disease is seldom symptomatic in outpatients treated with anticonvulsants. Institutionalized children have a high incidence of fractures regardless of whether

TABLE 6. *Bone disease associated with anticonvulsant therapy and TPN*

Prevalence	Clinical features	Pathogenesis	Treatment
1. Anticonvulsants			
Common in institutionalized children, uncommon in outpatients	Postseizure fractures, ↓ Ca, 25(OH)D, ↑ alk. phosphatase (liver); modest osteopenia on x-ray	↓ Efficiency of 25(OH)D production, ↑ vit. D clearance, ? direct effects on bone and gut	Vit. D, Ca supplementation
2. TPN			
Decreasing with newer TPN solutions osteopenia by	Bone pain; ↑ Ca, P, alk. phosphatase, normal 25(OH)D, ↓ 1,25(OH)$_2$D; and other x-ray; ↓ TBV, ↑ osteoid, ↓ bone formation	Aluminum contamination in casein hydrolysate as for components of TPN solution	Discontinue TPN, substitute purified casein hydrolysate

they are being treated with anticonvulsants (211), and the fracture may be the presenting complaint by which the metabolic bone disease is discovered. Serum and urine calcium are generally low or low normal. Since seizure can be caused by a low serum calcium concentration, it is important to check the serum calcium before assuming that new seizures represent failure of current anticonvulsant therapy (224). Serum phosphorus is generally normal but may be low. Elevated serum alkaline phosphatase is frequently observed, but much of the increase is derived from the liver, not the bone (221,222). PTH can be elevated and may be associated with increased urinary cAMP and hydroxyproline excretion (216,220,225–227). 25(OH)D and 24,25(OH)$_2$D levels are often low (210,215,216,218,221–223,228–233), but 1,25(OH)$_2$D levels are normal or even elevated (216,231–238). A modest reduction (10–15%) in bone density of the forearm is seen (212,215,219,222,223, 234), but radiologic evidence of rickets or osteomalacia (pseudofractures) is uncommon in the outpatient population. Bone biopsy specimens may show increased osteoid (217,218,220,226,235,236), but frank osteomalacia (decreased bone formation coupled with increased osteoid) is unusual (220,221,235,237). Rather, the increased osteoid probably reflects mild secondary hyperparathyroidism in most cases (236), although marrow fibrosis and increased osteoclast activity is rare. Trabecular bone volume is usually normal (235,236).

Pathogenesis

The high rate of bone disease in institutionalized patients, regardless of anticonvulsant therapy, emphasizes the importance of nutrition and sunlight, which can be lacking in those settings. However, anticonvulsant therapy clearly compounds this problem. Two of the most frequently used anticonvulsants, phenobarbital and phenytoin, induce liver drug metabolizing enzymes and in-

crease the metabolism and clearance of vitamin D (224,238,239). 25(OH)D clearance is not affected by these drugs, and its production from vitamin D may even be increased (224,238,239). Therefore, the low 25(OH)D levels frequently observed appear to be due primarily to reduced substrate (i.e., vitamin D) availability and can readily be corrected by increasing dietary intake of vitamin D (221,222) (Fig. 8). Anticonvulsants such as sodium valproate and carbamazepine that do not induce the hepatic drug metabolizing enzymes have less impact on serum calcium and 25(OH)D levels (229,240). In vitro studies suggest that phenobarbital and phenytoin have direct inhibitory effects on PTH-stimulated bone resorption (241) and intestinal calcium absorption (242), but the relevance of these studies to the in vivo situation in humans is unclear.

Treatment

Numerous studies point out that the well-nourished patient exposed to adequate amounts of sunlight will seldom develop clinically significant bone disease as a result of anticonvulsant therapy. This observation has caused one group to recommend that patients on anticonvulsants should not receive prophylaxis with vitamin D (243). If vitamin D is to be used, vitamin D$_2$ appears to be more effective in increasing bone density than equal amounts of vitamin D$_3$ (223), despite having less effect on elevating the serum vitamin D metabolite levels (244). Normal replacement doses (400 units/day) are usually not adequate (223,229); higher doses (4000 units or 100 μg per day) are generally required (224,245) and should be accompanied by adequate amounts of dietary calcium. Evaluating therapy by monitoring serum 25(OH)D, PTH, and serum and urine calcium is important because of individual variation in response to treatment. Monitoring alkaline phosphatase levels may be misleading because of the large hepatic component.

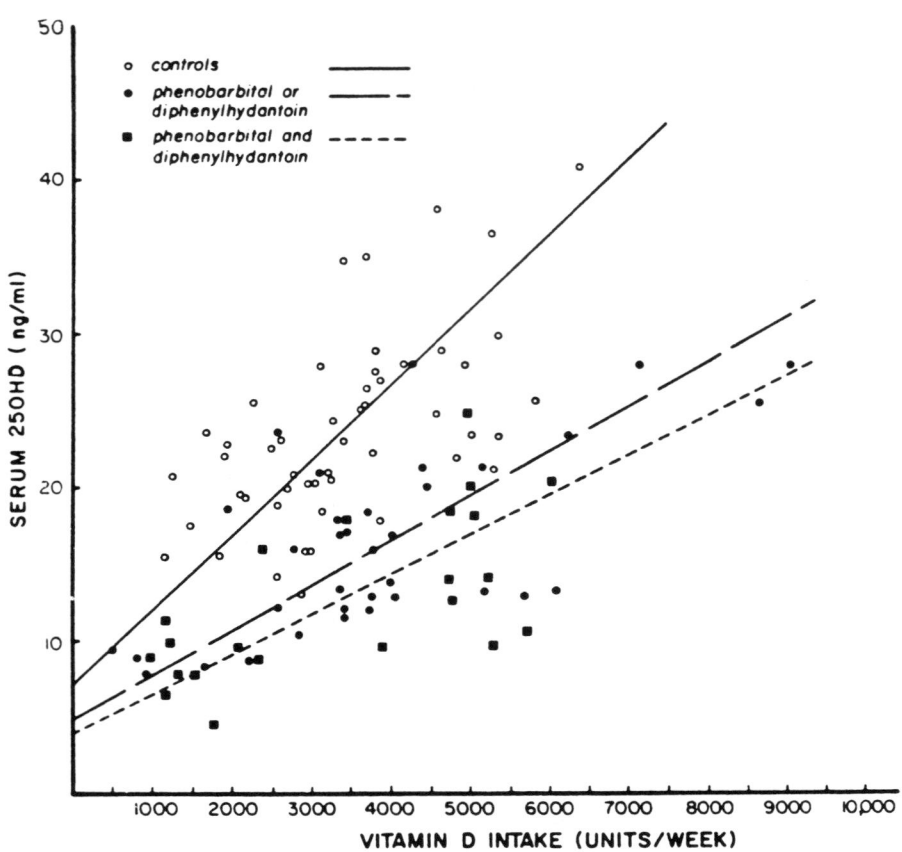

FIG. 8. Correlation of serum 25(OH)D levels to vitamin D intake in normals and patients taking anticonvulsants. The patients taking anticonvulsants had a lower 25(OH)D level for any given amount of vitamin D intake. (Reproduced with permission from Hahn et al., *N Engl J Med* 1975;292:550–4.)

Total Parenteral Nutrition and Bone Disease

Incidence and Prevalence

At the time (1980), the relationship between total parenteral nutrition (TPN) and bone disease was first described (246,247), 20–30% of patients on long-term TPN complained of bone pain often within a year of beginning treatment. Most of the patients who were biopsied showed evidence of osteomalacia (246,247) regardless of the presence of bone pain. In these early studies, casein hydrolysate was used as the source of amino acids. Casein hydrolysate was shown to contain high concentrations of aluminum (248), a contaminant strongly implicated in the osteomalacia associated with hemodialysis (see Chapter 39). Substituting purified amino acids for casein hydrolysate has markedly reduced the incidence of bone pain and prevalence of osteomalacia on bone biopsy, although osteopenia still occurs (249–251).

Clinical Features

When described initially, TPN-induced bone disease resulted in often severe bone pain primarily affecting the lower extremities, lower back, and ribs. Some patients could not walk as a result of the pain. This clinical picture is seldom seen with newer formulations of TPN solutions. In the initial studies (246,247,252,253), serum calcium, alkaline phosphatase, and phosphorus levels were high normal or frankly high. At least part of the increased alkaline phosphatase was hepatic in origin, as other liver function tests were abnormal (254). Hypercalciuria exceeding the infused amount of calcium was observed. PTH and $1,25(OH)_2D$ levels were low despite normal levels of 25(OH)D and adequate amounts of vitamin D in the TPN solution. Substituting purified amino acids for casein hydrolysate (249,250) results in lower serum calcium levels (which may even be abnormally low) and normal serum phosphorus, PTH, 25(OH)D, and $1,25(OH)_2D$ concentrations. Alkaline phosphatase continues to be elevated in these patients. Osteopenia may still be found radiologically. Bone biopsies in the original reports showed reduced trabecular bone volume, increased osteoid, and decreased mineralization characteristic of osteomalacia (247,255). More recent reports of patients on TPN supplemented with purified amino acids rather than casein hydrolysate show less of a mineralization defect, although reduced trabecular bone volume is still seen (250,251).

Pathogenesis

In the original studies by Shike et al. (247,253), vitamin D itself was implicated in the genesis of the bone disease, although the mechanism for this was obscure.

This explanation has given way to the hypothesis that aluminum is the likely culprit for many of the abnormalities. Aluminum contaminates not only casein hydrolysate, but also albumin, phosphate, and calcium solutions (256). However, casein hydrolysate appears to be the major source of aluminum contamination, and replacing this with purified amino acids has resulted in a marked reduction in aluminum concentrations in the blood, urine, and bone of patients receiving TPN (248). Changing from casein hydrolysate to purified amino acids has markedly reduced the amount of clinically evident bone disease and altered the morphologic picture from osteomalacia to mild osteopenia. However, TPN is still associated with bone disease. At least some of the patients presumably have subclinical bone disease before they begin TPN because of the underlying gastrointestinal disorder, which leads them to require TPN. Furthermore, the amino acids in the TPN solution may lead to excessive hypercalciuria and subtle hyperparathyroidism if the infused amounts are high (257).

Treatment

Discontinuing TPN, where feasible, may correct the bone disease (246). Adjusting the vitamin D, amino acid, and calcium concentration to achieve a positive calcium balance needs to be done in those patients who cannot discontinue TPN. Reducing the aluminum contamination of the solutions to the lowest possible level has proven to be of great importance. Other trace contaminants or deficiencies that affect on the skeleton may be found in the future.

REFERENCES

1. Rab SM, Baseer A. Occult osteomalacia amongst healthy and pregnant women in Pakistan. *Lancet* 1976;2:1211–3.
2. Stephens WP, Klimiuk PS, Warrington S, Taylor JL, Berry JL, Mawer EB. Observations on the natural history of vitamin D deficiency amongst Asian immigrants. *Q J Med* 1982;51:171–88.
3. Rashid A, Mohammed T, Stephens WP, Warrington S, Berry JL, Mawer EB. Vitamin D state of Asians living in Pakistan. *Br Med J* 1983;286:182–4.
4. American Academy of Pediatrics, Committee on Nutrition. Infantile scurvy and nutritional rickets in the United States. *Pediatrics* 1962;29:646.
5. Edidin DV, Levitsky LL, Schey W, Dumbovic N, Campos A. Resurgence of nutritional rickets associated with breast-feeding and special dietary practices. *Pediatrics* 1980;65:232–5.
6. Bachrach S, Fisher J, Parks JS. An outbreak of vitamin D deficiency rickets in a susceptible population. *Pediatrics* 1979; 64:871–7.
7. Curtis JA, Kooh SW, Fraser D, Greenberg ML. Nutritional rickets in vegetarian children. *Can Med Assoc J* 1983;128:150–2.
8. Hollis BW, Pittard WB III, Reinhardt TA. Relationships among vitamin D, 25-hydroxyvitamin D, and vitamin D-binding protein concentrations in the plasma and milk of human subjects. *J Clin Endocrinol Metab* 1986;62:41–4.
9. Seino Y, Shimotsuji T, Ishida M, Ishii T, Yabuuchi H. Rickets in infancy and childhood. *Endocrinol Jpn* 1979;1:95–100.
10. Hoff N, Haddad J, Teitelbaum S, McAlister W, Hillman LS. Serum concentrations of 25-hydroxyvitamin D in rickets of extremely premature infants. *J Pediatr* 1979;94:460–6.
11. Aaron JE, Gallagher JC, Anderson J, et al. Frequency of osteomalacia and osteoporosis in fractures of the proximal femur. *Lancet* 1974;1:229–33.
12. Brown IRF, Bakowska A, Millard PH. Vitamin D status of patients with femoral neck fractures. *Age Ageing* 1976;5:127–31.
13. von Knorring J, Slätis P, Weber TH, Helenius T. Serum levels of 25-hydroxyvitamin D, 24,25-dihydroxyvitamin D and parathyroid hormone in patients with femoral neck fracture in southern Finland. *Clin Endocrinol* 1982;17:189–94.
14. Hoikka V, Alhava EM, Savolainen K, Parviainen M. Osteomalacia in fractures of the proximal femur. *Acta Orthop Scand* 1982;53:255–60.
15. Lund B, Sørensen OH, Lund B, et al. Vitamin D metabolism and osteomalacia in patients with fractures of the proximal femur. *Acta Orthop Scand* 1982;53:251–4.
16. Lips P, Netelenbos JC, Jongen MJM, et al. Histomorphometric profile and vitamin D status in patients with femoral neck fracture. *Metab Bone Dis Relat Res* 1982;4:85–93.
17. Lund B, Sørensen OH, Christensen AB. 25-hydroxycholecalciferol and fractures of the proximal femur. *Lancet* 1975;2:300–2.
18. Bouillon RA, Auwerx JH, Lissens WD, Pelemans WK. Vitamin D status in the elderly: seasonal substrate deficiency causes 1,25-dihydroxycholecalciferol deficiency. *Am J Clin Nutr* 1987; 45:755–63.
19. Mankin HJ. Rickets, osteomalacia, and renal osteodystrophy: part 1. *J Bone Joint Surg* 1974;56:101–28.
20. Chapuy M-C, Chapuy P, Meunier PJ. Calcium and vitamin D supplements: effects on calcium metabolism in elderly people. *Am J Clin Nutr* 1987;46:324–8.
21. Lapatsanis P, Makaronis G, Vretos C, Doxiadis S. Two types of nutritional rickets in infants. *Am J Clin Nutr* 1976;29:1222–6.
22. Fraser D, Kooh SW, Scriver CR. Hyperparathyroidism as the cause of hyperaminoaciduria and phosphaturia in human vitamin D deficiency. *Pediatr Res* 1967;1:425–35.
23. Haddad JG. Transport of vitamin D metabolites. *Clin Orthop Relat Res* 1979;142:249–61.
24. Bolt MJG, Meredith SC, Rosenberg IH. Suppression of rat hepatic vitamin D-25-hydroxylase by cholecalciferol, but not by 25-hydroxy- or 1,25-dihydroxymetabolites. *Calcif Tissue Int* 1988;42:273–8.
25. Baran DT, Milne ML. 1,25 dihydroxyvitamin D increases hepatocyte cytosolic calcium levels: a potential regulator of vitamin D-25-hydroxylase. *J Clin Invest* 1986;77:1622–6.
26. Mawer EB, Backhouse J, Holman CA, Lumb GA, Stanbury SW. The distribution and storage of vitamin D and its metabolites in human tissues. *Clin Sci* 1972;43:413–31.
27. Eastwood JB, de Wardener HE, Gray RW, Lemann JL Jr. Normal plasma-1,25-(OH)$_2$-vitamin-D concentrations in nutritional osteomalacia. *Lancet* 1979;1:1377–8.
28. Bouillon R, van Baelen H, de Moor P. The measurement of the vitamin D-binding protein in human serum. *J Clin Endocrinol Metab* 1977;45:225–31.
29. Chalmers J, Conacher WDH, Gardner DL, Scott PJ. Osteomalacia: a common disease in elderly women. *J Bone Joint Surg* 1967;49B:403–23.
30. Fonseca V, Agnew JE, Nag D, Dandona P. Bone density and cortical thickness in nutritional vitamin D deficiency: effect of secondary hyperparathyroidism. *Ann Clin Biochem* 1988; 25:271–4.
31. Thalassinos NC, Wicht S, Joplin GF. Secondary hyperparathyroidism in osteomalacia. *Br Med J* 1970;1:76–9.
32. Frame B, Parfitt AM. Osteomalacia: current concepts. *Ann Intern Med* 1978;89:966–82.
33. McFarlane JD, Lutkin JE, Burwood MA. The demonstration by scintigraphy of fractures in osteomalacia. *Br J Radiol* 1977; 50:369–71.
34. Marel GM, McKenna MJ, Frame B. Osteomalacia. In: Peck WA, ed. *Bone and mineral research,* vol 4. Amsterdam: Elsevier, 1986;335–412.
35. McKenna MJ, Freaney R, Casey OM, Towers RP, Muldowney FP. Osteomalacia and osteoporosis: evaluation of a diagnostic index. *J Clin Pathol* 1983;36:245–52.
36. Recker RR, ed. *Bone histomorphometry: techniques and interpretation.* Boca Raton, Fla: CRC Press, 1983.

37. Baylink DJ, Morey ER, Ivey JL, Stauffer ME. Vitamin D and bone. In: Norman AW, ed. *Vitamin D: molecular biology and clinical nutrition.* New York: Marcel Dekker, 1980;387–453.

38. Arnaud C, Glorieux F, Scriver CR. Serum parathyroid hormone levels in acquired vitamin D deficiency in infancy. *Pediatrics* 1972;49:832–40.

39. Sudhaker Rao D, Villanueva A, Mathews M, et al. Histologic evolution of vitamin-D depletion in patients with intestinal malabsorption or dietary deficiency. In: Frame B, Potts JT Jr, eds. *Clinical disorders of bone and mineral metabolism.* Amsterdam: Excerpta Medica, 1983;224–6.

40. Popovtzer MM, Malthay R, Alfrey AC, et al. Vitamin D deficiency osteomalacia: healing of the bone disease in the absence of vitamin D with intravenous calcium and phosphorus infusion. In: Frame B, Parfitt AM, Duncan H, eds. *Clinical aspects of metabolic bone disease.* Amsterdam: Excerpta Medica, 1973;382–7.

41. Balsan S, Garabédian M, Larchet M, et al. Long-term nocturnal calcium infusions can cure rickets and promote normal mineralization in hereditary resistance to 1,25-dihydroxyvitamin D. *J Clin Invest* 1986;77:1661–7.

42. Miller SC, Miller MA, Omura TH. Dietary lactose improves endochondral growth and bone development and mineralization in rats fed a vitamin D-deficient diet. *J Nutr* 1988;118:72–7.

43. Holtrop ME, Cox KA, Carnes DL, Holick MF. Effects of serum calcium and phosphorus on skeletal mineralization in vitamin D-deficient rats. *Am J Physiol* 1986;251:E234–40.

44. Kooh SW, Fraser D, Reilly BJ, Hamilton JR, Gall DG, Bell L. Rickets due to calcium deficiency. *N Engl J Med* 1977; 297:1264–6.

45. Marie PJ, Pettifor JM, Ross FP, Glorieux FH. Histological osteomalacia due to dietary calcium deficiency in children. *N Engl J Med* 1982;307:584–8.

46. Heaney RP, Gallagher JC, Johnston CC, Neer R, Parfitt AM, Whedon GD. Calcium nutrition and bone health in the elderly. *Am J Clin Nutr* 1982;36:986–1013.

47. Nordin BEC. Osteomalacia, osteoporosis and calcium deficiency. *Clin Orthop* 1960;17:235–58.

48. Rowe JC, Wood DH, Rowe DW, Raisz LG. Nutritional hypophosphatemic rickets in a premature infant fed breast milk. *N Engl J Med* 1979;300:293–6.

49. Baylink D, Stauffer M, Wergedal J, Rich C. Formation, mineralization and resorption of bone in vitamin D deficient rats. *J Clin Invest* 1970;49:1122–34.

50. Lotz M, Zisman E, Bartter FC. Evidence for a phosphorus depletion syndrome in man. *N Engl J Med* 1968;278:409–14.

51. Harrison JE, Hitchman AJW, Hitchman A, Hasany SA, McNeill KG, Tam CS. Differences between the effects of phosphate deficiency and vitamin D deficiency on bone metabolism. *Metabolism* 1980;9:1225–33.

52. Lester GE, VanderWiel CJ, Gray TK, Talmage RV. Vitamin D deficiency in rats with normal serum calcium concentrations. *Proc Natl Acad Sci USA* 1982;79:4791–4.

53. Mechanic GL, Toverud SU, Ramp WK, Gonnerman WA. The effect of vitamin D on the structural crosslinks and maturation of chick bone collagen. *Biochim Biophys Acta* 1975;393:419–25.

54. Baylink D, Wergedal J, Thompson E. Loss of protein polysaccharides at sites where bone mineralization is initiated. *J Histochem Cytochem* 1972;20:279–92.

55. Parfitt AM, Mathews CHE, Brommage R, Jarnagin K, DeLuca HF. Calcitriol but no other metabolite of vitamin D is essential for normal bone growth and development in the rat. *J Clin Invest* 1984;73:576–86.

56. Brommage R, Jarnagin K, DeLuca HF, Yamada S, Takayama H. 1- but not 24-hydroxylation of vitamin D is required for skeletal mineralization in rats. *Am J Physiol* 1983;244 (*Endocrinol Metab* 7):E298–304.

57. Rasmussen H, Baron R, Broadus A, DeFronzo R, Lang R, Horst R. 1,25(OH)$_2$D$_3$ is not the only D metabolite involved in the pathogenesis of osteomalacia. *Am J Med* 1980;69:360–7.

58. Atkin I, Pita JC, Ornoy A, Agundez A, Castiglione G, Howell DS. Effects of vitamin D metabolites on healing of low phosphate, vitamin D-deficient induced rickets in rats. *Bone* 1985;6:113–23.

59. Ornoy A, Goodwin D, Noff D, Edelstein S. 24-25-dihydroxyvita-

60. Kraft K, Offerman G, Steldinger R, Gawlik D. Effect of 1,25(OH)$_2$D$_3$ and 24,25(OH)$_2$D$_3$ on experimental rickets. *Res Commun Chem Path Pharm* 1979;26:571–80.

61. Holick MF. Photosynthesis of vitamin D in the skin: effect of environmental and life-style variables. *Fed Proc* 1987;46:1876–82.

62. MacLaughlin J, Holick MF. Aging decreases the capacity of human skin to produce vitamin D$_3$. *J Clin Invest* 1985;76:1536–8.

63. Holick MF, MacLaughlin JA, Doppelt SH. Factors that influence the cutaneous photosynthesis of previtamin D$_3$. *Science* 1981;211:590–3.

64. Matsuoka LY, Ide L, Wortsman J, MacLaughlin JA, Holick MF. Sunscreens suppress cutaneous vitamin D$_3$ synthesis. *J Clin Endocrinol Metab* 1987;64:1165–8.

65. Corless D, Gupta SP, Switala S, et al. Response of plasma-25-hydroxyvitamin D to ultraviolet irradiation in long-stay geriatric patients. *Lancet* 1978;2:649–51.

66. Adams JS, Clemens TL, Parrish JA, Holick MF. Vitamin-D synthesis and metabolism after ultraviolet irradiation of normal and vitamin-D-deficient subjects. *N Engl J Med* 1982;306:722–5.

67. Parfitt AM, Gallagher JC, Heaney RP, Johnston CC, Neer R, Whedon GD. Vitamin D and bone health in the elderly. *Am J Clin Nutr* 1982;36:1014–31.

68. Clemens TL, Zhou X-Y, Myles M, Endres D, Lindsay R. Serum vitamin D$_2$ and vitamin D$_3$ metabolite concentrations and absorption of vitamin D$_2$ in elderly subjects. *J Clin Endocrinol Metab* 1986;63:656–60.

69. Wronski TJ, Halloran BP, Bikle DD, Globus RK, Morey-Holton ER. Chronic administration of 1,25-dihydroxyvitamin D$_3$: increased bone but impaired mineralization. *Endocrinology* 1986;119:2580–5.

70. Stickler GB, Jowsey J, Bianco AJ Jr. Possible detrimental effect of large doses of vitamin D in familial hypophosphatemic vitamin D-resistant rickets. *J Pediatr* 1971;79:68–71.

71. Eddy RL. Metabolic bone disease after gastrectomy. *Am J Med* 1971;50:442–9.

72. Deller DJ, Begley MD, Edwards RG, Addison M. Metabolic effects of partial gastrectomy with special reference to calcium and folic acid. *Gut* 1964;5:218–25.

73. Paterson CR, Woods CG, Pulvertaft CN, Fourman P. Search for osteomalacia in 1228 patients after gastrectomy and other operations on the stomach. *Lancet* 1965;2:1085–8.

74. Tovey FI, Karamanolis DG, Godfrey J, Clark CG. Post-gastrectomy nutrition: methods of outpatient screening for early osteomalacia. *Hum Nutr: Clin Nutr* 1985;39C:439–46.

75. Morgan DB, Hunt G, Paterson CR. The osteomalacia syndrome after stomach operations. *Q J Med* 1970;39:395–410.

76. Hoikka V, Alhava EM, Savolainen K, Karjalainen P, Parviainen M. The effect of partial gastrectomy on bone mineral metabolism. *Scand J Gastroenterol* 1982;17:257–61.

77. Garrick R, Ireland AW, Posen S. Bone abnormalities after gastric surgery: a prospective histological study. *Ann Intern Med* 1971;75:221–5.

78. Ekbom HR. Calcium studies in partially gastrectomized patients, with special reference to the oral intake of calcium. *Acta Med Scand* 1965;178:193–201.

79. Deller DJ, Edwards RG, Addison M. Calcium metabolism and the bone after partial gastrectomy. II. The nature and cause of the bone disorder. *Aust Ann Med* 1963;12:295–309.

80. Klein KB, Orwoll ES, Lieberman DA, Meier DE, McClung MR, Parfitt AM. Metabolic bone disease in asymptomatic men after partial gastrectomy with Billroth II anastomosis. *Gastroenterology* 1987;92:608–16.

81. Nilas L, Christiansen C. Influence of PTH and 1,25(OH)$_2$D on calcium homeostasis and bone mineral content after gastric surgery. *Calcif Tissue Int* 1985;37:461–6.

82. Kozawa K, Imawari M, Shimazu M, Kobori O, Osuga T, Morioka Y. Vitamin D status after total gastrectomy. *Dig Dis Sci* 1984;29:411–6.

83. von Lilienfeld-Toal H, Mackes KG, Kodrat G, Ochs H, Sonnenberg A. Plasma 25-hydroxyvitamin D and urinary cyclic AMP in

German patients with subtotal gastrectomy (Billroth II). *Dig Dis* 1977;22:633–6.

84. Dibble JB, Sheridan P, Losowsky MS. A survey of vitamin D deficiency in gastrointestinal and liver disorders. *Q J Med* 1984;209:119–34.

85. Schoen MS, Lindenbaum J, Roginsky MS, Holt PR. Significance of serum level of 25-hydroxycholecalciferol in gastrointestinal disease. *Dig Dis* 1978;23:137–42.

86. Imawari M, Kozawa K, Akanuma Y, Koizumi S, Itakura H, Kosaka K. Serum 25-hydroxyvitamin D and vitamin D-binding protein levels and mineral metabolism after partial and total gastrectomy. *Gastroenterology* 1980;79:255–8.

87. Bikle DD, Gee E, Halloran, Kowalski MA, Ryzen E, Haddad JG. Assessment of the free fraction of 25-hydroxyvitamin D in serum and its regulation by albumin and the vitamin D-binding protein. *J Clin Endocrinol Metab* 1986;63:954–9.

88. Nilsson BE. Conditions contributing to fracture of the femoral neck. *Acta Chir Scand* 1970;136:383–4.

89. Gertner JM, Lilburn M, Domenech M. 25-hydroxycholecalciferol absorption in steatorrhoea and postgastrectomy osteomalacia. *Br Med J* 1977;1:1310–2.

90. Thompson GR, Lewis B, Both CC. Vitamin-D absorption after partial gastrectomy. *Lancet* 1966;1:457–8.

91. Stamp TCB. Intestinal absorption of 25-hydroxycholecalciferol. *Lancet* 1974;2:121–3.

92. Gregory DH, van Uelft R. Calcium absorption following gastric resection. *Am J Gastroenterol* 1972;57:34–40.

93. Caniggia A, Gennari C, Cesari L. Intestinal absorption of ^{45}Ca and dynamics of ^{45}Ca in gastrectomy osteoporosis. *Acta Med Scand* 1964;176:599–605.

94. Harvald B, Krogsgaard AR, Lous P. Calcium deficiency following partial gastrectomy. *Acta Med Scand* 1962;172:497–503.

95. Bo-Linn GW, Davis GR, Buddrus DJ, Morawaki SG, Santa Ana C, Fordtran JS. An evaluation of the importance of gastric acid secretion in the absorption of dietary calcium. *J Clin Invest* 1984;73:640–7.

96. Recker RR. Calcium absorption and achlorhydria. *N Engl J Med* 1985;313:70–3.

97. Bikle DD, Morrissey RL, Zolock DT, Rasmussen H. The intestinal response to vitamin D. *Rev Physiol Biochem Pharmacol* 1981;89:63–143.

98. Morgan DB, Paterson CR, Woods CG, Pulvertaft CN, Fourman P. Osteomalacia after gastrectomy: a response to very small doses of vitamin D. *Lancet* 1965;2:1089–91.

99. Tougaard L, Rickers H, Rødbro P, et al. Bone composition and vitamin D after Pólya gastrectomy. *Acta Med Scand* 1977;202:47–50.

100. Alhava EM, Aukee S, Juuti M, Karjalainen P, Kettunen K. The effect of vitamin D$_2$ treatment on bone mineral after partial gastrectomy. *Scand J Gastroenterol* 1977;12:497–9.

101. Davies M, Mawer EB, Krawitt EL. Comparative absorption of vitamin D$_3$ and 25-hydroxyvitamin D$_3$ in intestinal disease. *Gut* 1980;21:287–92.

102. Compston JE, Judd D, Crawley EO, et al. Osteoporosis in patients with inflammatory bowel disease. *Gut* 1987;28:410–5.

103. Cooke WT. Survey of results of treatment of Crohn's disease. *Clinics Gastroenterol* 1972;1:521–31.

104. Driscoll RH Jr, Meredith SC, Sitrin M, Rosenberg IH. Vitamin D deficiency and bone disease in patients with Crohn's disease. *Gastroenterology* 1982;83:1252–8.

105. Compston JE, Ayers AB, Horton LW, Tighe JR, Creamer B. Osteomalacia after small-intestinal resection. *Lancet* 1978;1:9–12.

106. Sitrin M, Meredith S, Rosenberg IH. Vitamin D deficiency and bone disease in gastrointestinal disorders. *Arch Intern Med* 1978;138:886–8.

107. Genant HK, Mall JC, Wagonfeld JB, Horst JV, Lange LH. Skeletal demineralization and growth retardation in inflammatory bowel disease. *Invest Radiol* 1976;11:541–9.

108. Hessov I, Mosekilde L, Melsen F, et al. Osteopenia with normal vitamin D metabolites after small-bowel resection for Crohn's disease. *Scand J Gastroenterol* 1984;19:691–6.

109. Krawitt EL, Beeken WL, Janney CD. Calcium absorption in Crohn's disease. *Gastroenterology* 1976;71:251–4.

110. Avioli LV. Absorption and metabolism of vitamin D$_3$ in man. *Am J Clin Nutr* 1969;22:437–46.

111. Arnaud SR, Goldsmith RS, Lambert PW, Go VLW. 25 Hydroxyvitamin D: evidence of an enterohepatic circulation in man. *Proc Soc Exp Biol Med* 1975;149:570–2.

112. Hajjar ET, Vincenti F, Salti IS. Gluten-induced enteropathy. *Arch Intern Med* 1974;134:565–6.

113. Arnaud SB, Newcomer AD, Dickson ER, Arnaud CD, Go VLW. Altered mineral metabolism in patients with gastrointestinal (GI) diseases. *Gastroenterology* 1976;70:860.

114. Melvin KEW, Hepner GW, Bordier P, Neale G, Joplin GF. Calcium metabolism and bone pathology in adult coeliac disease. *Q J Med* 1970;39:83–113.

115. Jürgens JL, Scholz DA, Wolläger EE. Severe osteomalacia associated with occult steatorrhea due to nontropical sprue: report of five cases. *Arch Intern Med* 1956;98:774–82.

116. Thompson GR, Lewis B, Booth CC. Absorption of vitamin D$_3$-^{3}H in control subjects and patients with intestinal malabsorption. *J Clin Invest* 1966;45:94–102.

117. Hepner GW, Jowsey J, Arnaud C, et al. Osteomalacia and celiac disease: response to 25-hydroxyvitamin D. *Am J Med* 1978;65:1015–20.

118. Hubbard VS, Farrell PM, de Sant'Agnese PA. 25-hydroxycholecalciferol levels in patients with cystic fibrosis. *J Pediatr* 1979;94:84–6.

119. Scott J, Elias E, Moult PJA, Barnes S, Wills MR. Rickets in adult cystic fibrosis with myopathy, pancreatic insufficiency and proximal renal tubular dysfunction. *Am J Med* 1977;63:488–92.

120. Friedman HZ, Langman CB, Favus MJ. Vitamin D metabolism and osteomalacia in cystic fibrosis. *Gastroenterology* 1985;88:808–13.

121. Assan R, Alexandre JH, Tiengo A, Marre M, Costamailleres L, Lhomme C. Survival and rehabilitation after total pancreatectomy. *Diabetes Metab* 1985;11:303–9.

122. Hahn TJ, Squires AE, Halstead LR, Strominger DB. Reduced serum 25-hydroxyvitamin D concentration and disordered mineral metabolism in patients with cystic fibrosis. *J Pediatr* 1979;94:38–42.

123. Stead RJ, Houlder S, Agnew J, et al. Vitamin D and parathyroid hormone and bone mineralisation in adults with cystic fibrosis. *Thorax* 1988;43:190–4.

124. Teitelbaum SL, Halverson JD, Bates M, Wise L, Haddad JG. Abnormalities of circulating 25-OH vitamin D after jejunal-ileal bypass for obesity. *Ann Intern Med* 1977;86:289–93.

125. Rickers H, Christiansen C, Balslev I, Foltved H, Rødbro P, Christensen MS. Vitamin D and bone mineral after intestinal bypass operation for obesity. *Gut* 1983;24:67–72.

126. Sellin JH, Meredith SC, Kelly S, Schneir H, Rosenberg IH. Prospective evaluation of metabolic bone disease after jejunoileal bypass. *Gastroenterology* 1984;87:123–9.

127. Compston JE, Horton LWL, Laker MF, et al. Bone disease after jejuno-ileal bypass for obesity. *Lancet* 1978;2:127.

128. Mosekilde L, Melsen F, Hessov I, et al. Low serum levels of 1,25-dihydroxyvitamin D and histomorphometric evidence of osteomalacia after jejunoileal bypass for obesity. *Gut* 1980;21:624–31.

129. Parfitt AM, Pødenphant J, Villanueva AR, Frame B. Metabolic bone disease with and without osteomalacia after intestinal bypass surgery: a bone histomorphometric study. *Bone* 1985;6:211–20.

130. Melsen F, Mosekilde L. Trabecular bone mineralization lag time determined by tetracycline double-labeling in normal and certain pathological conditions. *Acta Pathol Microbiol Scand* [A] 1980;88:83–8.

131. Hey H, Stokholm KH, Lund Bj, Lund Bi, Sørensen OH. Vitamin D deficiency in obese patients and changes in circulating vitamin D metabolites following jejunoileal bypass. *Int J Obes* 1982;6:473–9.

132. Dano P, Christiansen C. Calcium absorption and bone mineral contents following intestinal shunt operation in obesity. *Scand J Gastroenterol* 1974;9:775–9.

133. Swenson SA Jr, Oberst B. Pre- and post-operative care of the patient with intestinal bypass for obesity. *Am J Surg* 1975;129:225–8.

134. Charles P, Mosekilde L, Søndergård K, Jensen FT. Treatment with high-dose oral vitamin D₂ in patients with jejunoileal bypass for morbid obesity: effects on calcium and magnesium metabolism, vitamin D metabolites, and faecal lag time. *Scand J Gastroenterol* 1984;19:1031–8.

135. Franck WA, Hoffman GS, Davis JS, Alpern HD, Olson JE. Osteomalacia and weakness complicating jejunoileal bypass. *J Rheumatol* 1979;6:51–6.

136. Compston JE, Chadha S, Horton LWL, Merrett AL. Post-gastrectomy osteomalacia. *Gut* 1980;21:A904.

137. Hey H, Lund Bi, Sørensen OH, Lund Bj. Delayed fracture healing following jejunoileal bypass surgery for obesity. *Calcif Tissue Int* 1982;34:13–15.

138. Long RG, Meinhard E, Skinner RK, Varghese Z, Wills MR, Sherlock S. Clinical, biochemical, and histological studies of osteomalacia, osteoporosis, and parathyroid function in chronic liver disease. *Gut* 1978;19:85–90.

139. Davies M, Mawer EB, Klass HJ, Lumb GA, Berry JL, Warnes TW. Vitamin D deficiency, osteomalacia, and primary biliary cirrhosis: response to orally administered vitamin D₃. *Dig Dis Sci* 1983;28:145–52.

140. Stellon AJ, Webb A, Compston J, Williams R. Low bone turnover state in primary biliary cirrhosis. *Hepatology* 1987;7:137–42.

141. Matloff DS, Kaplan MM, Neer RM, Goldberg MJ, Bitman W, Wolfe HJ. Osteoporosis in primary biliary cirrhosis: effects of 25-hydroxyvitamin D₃ treatment. *Gastroenterology* 1982;83:97–102.

142. Herlong HF, Recker RR, Maddrey WC. Bone disease in primary biliary cirrhosis: histologic features and response to 25-hydroxyvitamin D. *Gastroenterology* 1982;83:103–8.

143. Atkinson MJ, Vido I, Keck E, Hesch RD. Hepatic osteodystrophy in primary biliary cirrhosis: a possible defect in Kupffer cell mediated cleavage of parathyroid hormone. *Clin Endocrinol (Oxford)* 1983;19:21–8.

144. Bengoa JM, Sitrin MD, Meredith S, et al. Intestinal calcium absorption and vitamin D status in chronic cholestatic liver disease. *Hepatology* 1984;4:261–5.

145. Reed JS, Meredith SC, Nemchausky BA, Rosenberg IH, Boyer JL. Bone disease in primary biliary cirrhosis: reversal of osteomalacia with oral 25-hydroxyvitamin D. *Gastroenterology* 1980;78:512–7.

146. Hodgson SF, Dickson ER, Wahner HW, Johnson KA, Mann KG, Riggs BL. Bone loss and reduced osteoblast function in primary biliary cirrhosis. *Ann Intern Med* 1985;103:855–60.

147. Mitchison HC, Malcolm AJ, Bassendine MF, James OFW. Metabolic bone disease in primary biliary cirrhosis at presentation. *Gastroenterology* 1988;94:463–70.

148. Cuthbert JA, Pak CYC, Zerwekh JE, Glass KD, Combes B. Bone disease in primary biliary cirrhosis: increased bone resorption and turnover in the absence of osteoporosis or osteomalacia. *Hepatology* 1984;4:1–8.

149. Shih M-S, Anderson C. Does "hepatic osteodystrophy" differ from peri- and postmenopausal osteoporosis? A histomorphometric study. *Calcif Tissue Int* 1987;41:187–91.

150. Griffin JB, Smith CD, Bright GM. Bone disease in biliary atresia: a not uncommon complication. *Curr Surg* 1985;42:475–7.

151. Fonseca V, Epstein O, Gill DS, et al. Hyperparathyroidism and low serum osteocalcin despite vitamin D replacement in primary biliary cirrhosis. *J Clin Endocrinol Metabol* 1987;64:873–7.

152. Long RG, Skinner RK, Wills MR, Sherlock S. Serum-25-hydroxy-vitamin-D in untreated parenchymal and cholestatic liver disease. *Lancet* 1976;2:650–2.

153. Stellon AJ, Davies A, Compston J, Williams R. Osteoporosis in chronic cholestatic liver disease. *Q J Med* 1985;57:783–90.

154. Kehayoglou AK, Holdsworth CD, Agnew JE, Whelton MJ, Sherlock S. Bone disease and calcium absorption in primary biliary cirrhosis. *Lancet* 1968;1:715–9.

155. Long RG, Varghese Z, Wills MR, Sherlock S. Plasma calcium and magnesium fractions in liver disease. *Clin Chim Acta* 1978;84:239–45.

156. Sitrin MD, Bengoa JM. Intestinal absorption of cholecalciferol and 25-hydroxycholecalciferol in chronic cholestatic liver disease. *Am J Clin Nutr* 1987;46:1011–5.

157. Danielsson A, Lorentzon R, Larsson S-E. Intestinal absorption and 25-hydroxylation of vitamin D in patients with primary biliary cirrhosis. *Scand J Gastroenterol* 1982;17:349–55.

158. Thompson WG, Thompson GR. Effect of cholestyramine on absorption of vitamin D₃ and calcium. *Gut* 1969;10:717.

159. Wagonfeld JB, Nemchausky BA, Bolt M, Vander Horst J, Boyer JL, Rosenberg IH. Comparison of vitamin D and 25-hydroxy-vitamin-D in the therapy of primary biliary cirrhosis. *Lancet* 1976;2:391–4.

160. Skinner RK, Long RG, Sherlock S, Wills MR. 25-hydroxylation of vitamin D in primary biliary cirrhosis. *Lancet* 1977;1:720–1.

161. Hepner GW, Roginsky M, Moo H-F. Abnormal vitamin D metabolism in patients with cirrhosis. *Dig Dis* 1976;21:527–33.

162. Mawer EB, Klass HJ, Warnes TW, Berry JL. Metabolism of vitamin D in patients with primary biliary cirrhosis and alcoholic liver disease. *Clin Sci* 1985;69:561–70.

163. Wiesner RH, Kumar R, Seeman E, Go VLW. Enterohepatic physiology of 1,25-dihydroxyvitamin D₃ metabolites in normal man. *J Lab Clin Med* 1980;96:1094–100.

164. Jung RT, Davie M, Siklos P, Chalmers TM, Hunter JO, Lawson DEM. Vitamin D metabolism in acute and chronic cholestasis. *Gut* 1970;20:840–7.

165. Fraser DR, Kodicek E. Unique biosynthesis by kidney of a biologically active vitamin D metabolite. *Nature* 1970;228:764–6.

166. Long RG. Hepatic osteodystrophy: outlook good but some problems unsolved. *Gastroenterology* 1980;78:644–7.

167. Epstein O, Kato Y, Dick R, Sherlock S. Vitamin D, hydroxyapatite, and calcium gluconate in treatment of cortical bone thinning in postmenopausal women with primary biliary cirrhosis. *Am J Clin Nutr* 1982;36:426–30.

168. Stellon AJ, Davies A, Compston J, Williams R. Bone loss in autoimmune chronic active hepatitis on maintenance corticosteroid therapy. *Gastroenterology* 1985;89:1078–83.

169. Haagsma EB, Thijn CJP, Post JG, Slooff MJH, Gips CH. Bone disease after orthotopic liver transplantation. *J Hepatol* 1988;6:94–100.

170. Saville PD. Changes in bone mass with age and alcoholism. *J Bone Joint Surg* 1965;47A:492–9.

171. Spencer H, Rubio N, Rubio E, Indreika M, Seitam A. Chronic alcoholism: frequently overlooked cause of osteoporosis in men. *Am J Med* 1986;80:393–7.

172. Lindsell DRM, Wilson AG, Maxwell JD. Fractures on the chest radiograph in detection of alcoholic liver disease. *Br Med J* 1982;285:597–9.

173. Israel Y, Orrego H, Holt S, MacDonald DW, Meema HE. Identification of alcohol abuse: thoracic fractures on routine chest X-rays as indicators of alcoholism. *Alcoholism (NY)* 1980;4:420–2.

174. Nilsson BE, Westlin NE. Femur density in alcoholism and after gastrectomy. *Calcif Tissue Res* 1972;10:167–70.

175. Nilsson BE, Westlin NE. Changes in bone mass in alcoholics. *Clin Orthop* 1973;90:229–32.

176. Bikle DD, Genant HK, Cann C, Recker RR, Halloran BP, Strewler GJ. Bone disease in alcohol abuse. *Ann Intern Med* 1985;103:42–8.

177. de Vernejoul MC, Bielakoff J, Herve M, et al. Evidence for defective osteoblastic function: a role for alcohol and tobacco consumption in osteoporosis in middle-aged men. *Clin Orthop Relat Res* 1983;179:107–15.

178. Jorge-Hernandez JA, Gonzalez-Reimers CE, Torres-Ramirez A, et al. Bone changes in alcoholic liver cirrhosis: a histomorphometrical analysis of 52 cases. *Dig Dis Sci* 1988;33:1089–95.

179. Schnitzler CM, Solomon L. Bone changes after alcohol abuse. *S Afr Med J* 1984;66:730–4.

180. Mobarhan SA, Russell RM, Recker RR, Posner DB, Iber FL, Miller P. Metabolic bone disease in alcoholic cirrhosis: a comparison of the effect of vitamin D₂, 25-hydroxyvitamin D, or supportive treatment. *Hepatology* 1984;4:266–73.

181. Lalor BC, France MW, Powell D, Adams PH, Counihan TB. Bone and mineral metabolism and chronic alcohol abuse. *Q J Med* 1986;59:497–511.

182. Arlot ME, Bonjean M, Chavassieux PM, Meunier PJ. Bone histology in adults with aseptic necrosis. *J Bone Joint Surg* 1983;65A:1319–20.

183. Johnell O, Nilsson BE, Wiklund PE. Bone morphometry in alcoholics. *Clin Orthop Relat Res* 1982;165:253–8.

184. Solomon L. Idiopathic necrosis of the femoral head: pathogenesis and treatment. *Can J Surg* 1981;24:573–8.

185. Gold EW, Cangemi PJ. Incidence and pathogenesis of alcohol-induced osteonecrosis of the femoral head. *Clin Orthop* 1979; 143:222–6.

186. Pitts TO, Van Thiel DH. Disorders of divalent ions and vitamin D metabolism in chronic alcoholism. *Recent Dev Alcohol* 1986;4:357–77.

187. Feitelberg S, Epstein S, Ismail F, D'Amanda C. Deranged bone mineral metabolism in chronic alcoholism. *Metabolism* 1987; 36:322–6.

188. Roginsky MS, Zanzi I, Cohn SH. Skeletal and lean body mass in alcoholics with and without cirrhosis. *Calcif Tissue Res* 1976;21(suppl):386–91.

189. Bikle DD, Halloran BP, Gee E, Ryzen E, Haddad JG. Free 25-hydroxyvitamin D levels are normal in subjects with liver disease and reduced total 25-hydroxyvitamin D levels. *J Clin Invest* 1986;78:748–52.

190. Bikle DD, Gee E, Halloran B, Haddad JG. Free 1,25-dihydroxyvitamin D levels in serum from normal subjects, pregnant subject, and subjects with liver disease. *J Clin Invest* 1984;74:1966–71.

191. Bikle DD, Siiteri PK, Ryzen E, Haddad JG. Serum protein binding of 1,25-dihydroxyvitamin D: a reevaluation by direct measurement of free metabolite levels. *J Clin Endocrinol Metab* 1985;61:969–75.

192. Bikle DD, Gee E, Halloran B, Kowalski MA, Ryzen E, Haddad JG. Assessment of the free fraction of 25-hydroxyvitamin D in serum and its regulation by albumin and the vitamin D-binding protein. *J Clin Endocrinol Metab* 1986;63:954–9.

193. Leevy CM, Thompson A, Baker H. Vitamins and liver injury. *Am J Clin Nutr* 1970;23:493–9.

194. Jung RT, Davie M, Hunter JO, Chalmers TM, Lawson DE. Abnormal vitamin D metabolism in cirrhosis. *Gut* 1978;19:290–3.

195. Meyer M, Wechsler S, Shibolet S, Jedwab M, Edelstein S. Malabsorption of vitamin D in patients and rat with liver cirrhosis. In: Norman AW, Schaeffer K, Coburn JW, et al., eds. *Vitamin D: biochemical, chemical and clinical aspects related to calcium metabolism.* Berlin: Walter de Gruyter, 1977;831–3.

196. Lund B, Sørensen OH, Hilden M, Lund B. The hepatic conversion of vitamin D in alcoholics with varying degrees of liver affection. *Acta Med Scand* 1977;202:221–4.

197. Adler AJ, Gudis S, Berlyne GM. Reduced renal phosphate threshold concentration in alcoholic cirrhosis. *Miner Electrolyte Metab* 1984;10:63–6.

198. Krawitt EL. Ethanol inhibits intestinal calcium transport in rats. *Nature* 1973;243:88–9.

199. Garcia-Pascual B, Donath A, Courvoisier B. Plasma 25OHD, bone mass densitometry and ^{47}Ca intestinal absorption deficiency in chronic alcoholism. In: Norman AW, Schaefer K, Coburn JW, et al., eds. *Vitamin D: biochemical, chemical and clinical aspects related to calcium metabolism.* Berlin: Walter de Gruyter, 1977;819–21.

200. Linkola J, Fyhrquist F, Ylikahri R. Adenosine 3',5' cyclic monophosphate, calcium and magnesium excretion in ethanol intoxication and hangover. *Acta Physiol Scand* 1979;107:333–7.

201. Bikle DD. Effects of alcohol abuse on bone. *Compr Ther* 1988;14:16–20.

202. Posner DB, Russell RM, Absood S, et al. Effective 25-hydroxylation of vitamin D_2 in alcoholic cirrhosis. *Gastroenterology* 1978;74:866–70.

203. Schmid F. Osteopathien bei antiepileptischer Dauerbehandlung. *Fortschr Med* 1967;85:381–2.

204. Kruse R. Osteopathien bei antiepileptischer Langzeittherapie (vorläufige Mitteilung). *Monatsschr Kinderheilkd* 1968;116:378–83.

205. Dent CE, Richens A, Rowe DJ, Stamp T. Osteomalacia with long-term anticonvulsant therapy in epilepsy. *Br Med J* 1970;4:69–72.

206. Richens A, Rowe DJF. Disturbance of calcium metabolism by anticonvulsant drugs. *Br Med J* 1970;4:73–6.

207. Hunter J, Maxwell JD, Stewart DA, Parsons V, Williams R. Altered calcium metabolism in epileptic children on anticonvulsants. *Br Med J* 1971;4:202–4.

208. Tolman KG, Jubiz W, Sannella JJ, et al. Osteomalacia associated with anticonvulsant drug therapy in mentally retarded children. *Pediatrics* 1975;56:45–50.

209. Hunt PA, Wu-Chen ML, Handal NJ, et al. Bone disease induced by anticonvulsant therapy and treatment with calcitriol (1,25-dihydroxyvitamin D_3). *Am J Dis Child* 1986;140:715–8.

210. Offermann G, Pinto V, Kruse R. Antiepileptic drugs and vitamin D supplementation. *Epilepsia* 1979;20:3–15.

211. Sherk HH, Cruz M, Stambaugh J. Vitamin D prophylaxis and the lowered incidence of fractures in anticonvulsant rickets and osteomalacia. *Clin Orthop Relat Res* 1977;129:251–7.

212. Barden HS, Mazess RB, Chesney RW, Rose PG, Chun R. Bone status of children receiving anticonvulsant therapy. *Metab Bone Dis Relat Res* 1982;4:43–7.

213. Livingston S, Berman W, Pauli LL. Anticonvulsant drugs and vitamin D metabolism. *JAMA* 1973;224:1634–5.

214. Fogelman I, Gray JM, Gardner MD, et al. Do anticonvulsant drugs commonly induce osteomalacia? *Scott Med J* 1982; 27:136–42.

215. Pylypchuk G, Oreopoulos DG, Wilson DR, et al. Calcium metabolism in adult outpatients with epilepsy receiving long-term anticonvulsant therapy. *Can Med Assoc J* 1978;118:635–8.

216. Keck E, Gollnick B, Reinhardt D, Karch D, et al. Calcium metabolism and vitamin D metabolite levels in children receiving anticonvulsant drugs. *Eur J Pediatr* 1982;139:52–5.

217. Ashworth B, Horn DB. Evidence of osteomalacia in an outpatient group of adult epileptics. *Epilepsia* 1977;18:37–43.

218. Hoikka V, Savolainen K, Alhava EM, Sivenius J, Karjalainen P, Parviainen M. Anticonvulsant osteomalacia in epileptic outpatients. *Ann Clin Res* 1982;14:129–32.

219. Bogliun G, Beghi E, Crespi V, Delodovici L, d'Amico P. Anticonvulsant drugs and bone metabolism. *Acta Neurol Scand* 1986;74:284–8.

220. Weinstein RS, Bryce GF, Sappington LJ, King DW, Gallagher BB. Decreased serum ionized calcium and normal vitamin D metabolite levels with anticonvulsant drug treatment. *J Clin Endocrinol Metab* 1984;58:1003–9.

221. Hahn TJ, Hendin BA, Scharp CR, Haddad JG Jr. Effect of chronic anticonvulsant therapy on serum 25-hydroxycalciferol levels in adults. *N Engl J Med* 1972;287:900–4.

222. Hahn TJ, Hendin BA, Scharp CR, Boisseau VC, Haddad JG Jr. Serum 25-hydroxycalciferol levels and bone mass in children on chronic anticonvulsant therapy. *N Engl J Med* 1975;292:550–4.

223. Christiansen C, Rødbro P. Treatment of anticonvulsant osteomalacia with vitamin D. *Calcif Tissue Res* 1976;21(suppl):252–9.

224. Stamp TCB. Calcium and vitamin D metabolism during anticonvulsant therapy. In: Bickel H, Stern J, eds. *Inborn errors of calcium and bone metabolism.* Baltimore: University Park Press, 1976;256–66.

225. Tjellesen L, Gotfredsen A, Christiansen C. Different actions of vitamin D_2 and D_3 on bone metabolism in patients treated with phenobarbitone/phenytoin. *Calcif Tissue Int* 1985;37:217–22.

226. Nilsson OS, Lindholm TS, Elmstedt E, Lindbäck A, Lindholm TC. Fracture incidence and bone disease in epileptics receiving long-term anticonvulsant drug treatment. *Arch Orthop Trauma Surg* 1986;105:146–9.

227. Kruse K, Bartels H, Ziegler R, Dreller E, Kracht U. Parathyroid function and serum calcitonin in children receiving anticonvulsant drugs. *Eur J Pediatr* 1980;133:151–6.

228. Hahn TJ, Shires R, Halstead LR. Serum dihydroxyvitamin D metabolite concentrations in patients on chronic anticonvulsant drug therapy: response to pharmacologic doses of vitamin D_2. *Metab Bone Dis Relat Res* 1983;5:1–6.

229. Gough H, Goggin T, Bissessar A, Baker M, Crowley M, Callaghan N. A comparative study of the relative influence of different anticonvulsant drugs, UV exposure and diet on vitamin D and calcium metabolism in out-patients with epilepsy. *Q J Med* 1986;59:569–77.

230. Weisman Y, Fattal A, Eisenberg Z, Harel S, Spirer Z, Harell A. Decreased serum 24,25-dihydroxy vitamin D concentrations in children receiving chronic anticonvulsant therapy. *Br Med J* 1979;2:521–3.

231. Tjellesen L, Christiansen C. Serum vitamin D metabolites in epileptic patients treated with 2 different anti-convulsants: preliminary report. *Acta Neurol Scand* 1982;66:335–41.

232. Jubiz W, Haussler MR, McCain TA, Tolman KG. Plasma 1,25-dihydroxyvitamin D levels in patients receiving anticonvulsant drugs. *J Clin Endocrinol Metab* 1977;44:617–21.

233. Zerwekh JE, Homan R, Tindall R, Pak CY. Decreased serum 24,25-dihydroxyvitamin D concentration during long-term anticonvulsant therapy in adult epileptics. *Ann Neurol* 1982;12:184–6.

234. Wolschendorf K, Vanselow K, Moler WD, Schulz H. A quantitative determination of anticonvulsant-induced bone demineralization by an improved X-ray densitometry technique. *Neuroradiology* 1983;25:315–8.

235. Mosekilde L, Christensen MS, Lund B, Sørensen OH, Melsen F. The interrelationships between serum 25-hydroxycholecalciferol, serum parathyroid hormone and bone changes in anticonvulsant osteomalacia. *Acta Endocrinol* 1977;84:559–65.

236. Hoikka V, Savolainen K, Alhava EM, Sivenius J, Karjalainen P, Repo A. Osteomalacia in institutionalized epileptic patients on long-term anticonvulsant therapy. *Acta Neurol Scand* 1981;64:122–31.

237. Jowsey J, Arnaud SB, Hodgson SF, Johnson KA, Beabout JW, Wahner HW. The frequency of bone abnormality in patients on anticonvulsant therapy. *Electroencephalogr Clin Neurophysiol* 1978;45:341–7.

238. Matheson RT, Herbst JJ, Jubiz W, Freston JW, Tolman KG. Absorption and biotransformation of cholecalciferol in drug-induced osteomalacia. *J Clin Pharmacol* 1976;16:426–32.

239. Hahn TJ, Birge SJ, Scharp CR, Avioli LV. Phenobarbital-induced alterations in vitamin D metabolism. *J Clin Invest* 1972;51:741–8.

240. Davie MW, Emberson CE, Lawson DE, et al. Low plasma 25-hydroxyvitamin D and serum calcium levels in institutionalized epileptic subjects: associated risk factors, consequences and response to treatment with vitamin D. *Q J Med* 1983;52:79–91.

241. Hahn TJ, Scharp CR, Richardson CA, Halstead LR, Kahn AJ, Teitelbaum SL. Interaction of diphenylhydantoin (phenytoin) and phenobarbital with hormonal mediation of fetal rat bone resorption in vitro. *J Clin Invest* 1978;62:406–14.

242. Corradino RA. Diphenylhydantoin: direct inhibition of the vitamin D3-mediated calcium absorptive mechanism in organ-cultured duodenum. *Biochem Pharmacol* 1976;25:863–4.

243. Christiansen C, Rødbro P, Tjellesen L. Pathophysiology behind anticonvulsant osteomalacia. *Acta Neurol Scand* 1983;94(suppl):21–8.

244. Tjellesen L, Hummer L, Christiansen C, Rødbro P. Different metabolism of vitamin D_2/D_3 in epileptic patients treated with phenobarbitone/phenytoin. *Bone* 1986;7:337–42.

245. Hahn TJ, Halstead LR. Anticonvulsant drug-induced osteomalacia: alterations in mineral metabolism and response to vitamin D_3 administration. *Calcif Tissue Int* 1979;27:13–8.

246. Klein GL, Targoff CM, Ament ME, et al. Bone disease associated with total parenteral nutrition. *Lancet* 1980;2:1041–4.

247. Shike M, Harrison JE, Sturtridge WC, et al. Metabolic bone disease in patients receiving long-term total parenteral nutrition. *Ann Intern Med* 1980;92:343–50.

248. Klein GL, Alfrey AC, Miller NL, et al. Aluminum loading during total parenteral nutrition. *Am J Clin Nutr* 1982;35:1425–9.

249. Vargas JH, Klein GL, Ament ME, et al. Metabolic bone disease of total parenteral nutrition: course after changing from casein to amino acids in parenteral solutions with reduced aluminum content. *Am J Clin Nutr* 1988;48:1070–8.

250. Lipkin EW, Ott SM, Klein GL. Heterogeneity of bone histology in parenteral nutrition patients. *Am J Clin Nutr* 1987;46:673–80.

251. Shike M, Shils ME, Heller A, et al. Bone disease in prolonged parenteral nutrition: osteopenia without mineralization defect. *Am J Clin Nutr* 1986;44:89–98.

252. Klein GL, Horst RL, Norman AW, Ament ME, Slatopolsky E, Coburn JW. Reduced serum levels of 1α,25-dihydroxyvitamin D during long-term total parenteral nutrition. *Ann Intern Med* 1981;94:638–43.

253. Shike M, Sturtridge WC, Tam CS, et al. A possible role of vitamin D in the genesis of parenteral-nutrition-induced metabolic bone disease. *Ann Intern Med* 1981;95:560–8.

254. Klein GL, Coburn JW. Metabolic bone disease associated with total parenteral nutrition. *Adv Nutr Res* 1984;6:67–92.

255. Ott SM, Maloney NA, Klein GL, et al. Aluminum is associated with low bone formation in patients receiving chronic parenteral nutrition. *Ann Intern Med* 1983;93:910–4.

256. Sedman AB, Klein GL, Merritt RJ, et al. Evidence of aluminum loading in infants receiving intravenous therapy. *N Engl J Med* 1985;312:1337–43.

257. Bengoa JM, Sitrin MD, Wood RJ, Rosenberg IH. Amino acid-induced hypercalciuria in patients on total parenteral nutrition. *Am J Clin Nutr* 1983;38:264–9.

Disorders of Bone and Mineral Metabolism,
edited by Fredric L. Coe and Murray J. Favus,
© 1992 by Raven Press, Ltd. All rights reserved.

CHAPTER 42

Hereditary Metabolic and Dysplastic Skeletal Disorders

Michael P. Whyte

Physicians who care for patients with skeletal disorders frequently encounter individuals who represent the great diversity of hereditary metabolic and dysplastic bone diseases (1). Some of these conditions are merely radiologic curiosities; others are significant clinical problems (2). Some are associated with overt derangements in mineral homeostasis; others are diagnosed radiologically from characteristic disturbances of bone growth and modeling that may result in osteosclerosis or osteopenia (3,4). Several are important because they provide clues concerning normal mechanisms of mineral metabolism and skeletal homeostasis. For a few of these entities, the precise molecular defects are becoming understood (5). Cumulatively, the number of affected subjects is great.

This chapter reviews several of the more common or more revealing of the hereditary metabolic and dysplastic bone disorders. It begins with a discussion of three unusual forms of rickets/osteomalacia where defective skeletal mineralization occurs without decrements in either serum calcium or inorganic phosphate levels—hypophosphatasia, axial osteomalacia, and fibrogenesis imperfecta ossium. It then considers some of the derangements that are traditionally grouped together among the sclerosing bone dysplasias (Table 1)—osteopetrosis, carbonic anhydrase II deficiency, progressive diaphyseal dysplasia, pycnodysostosis, endosteal hyperostosis, and others (6). Then there is a discussion of an important (albeit sporadic) disorder—fibrous dysplasia (including McCune-Albright syndrome). Two afflictions that are

transmitted as autosomal dominant traits—fibrodysplasia ossificans progressiva, which is also called myositis ossificans progressiva, and pachydermoperiostosis—are reviewed. The chapter then concludes with a description of two conditions that are heritable and have well-characterized metabolic disturbances—osteogenesis imperfecta and tumoral calcinosis.

HYPOPHOSPHATASIA

This metabolic bone disease was characterized in 1948 by J. C. Rathbun, a Canadian pediatrician (7). He coined the term *hypophosphatasia* to describe an infant with developmental lethal rickets who had paradoxically low levels of alkaline phosphatase (ALP) activity in serum and in tissues obtained at autopsy. Hypophosphatasia is now recognized to be a heritable disorder in which the principal biochemical defect is a global deficiency of activity of the "tissue nonspecific" (liver/bone/kidney) isoenzyme of ALP (TNSALP) (8). The other major ALP isoenzymes found in man, placental ALP and intestinal ALP, have normal levels of activity in their proper tissue-specific distribution. In hypophosphatasia, defective mineralization of the skeleton occurs although, in contrast to most other forms of rickets or osteomalacia, neither serum levels of calcium or inorganic phosphate are reduced (8). Thus, hypophosphatasia is an instructive inborn error of metabolism that supports the long-held notion that ALP has a critical role in bone mineralization (9). As reviewed below, the physiologic role of TNSALP and the pathogenesis of hypophosphatasia are becoming understood and recent accumulating evidence incriminates point mutations in the "candidate" TNSALP gene as the most common molecular explanation for this condition (10–12).

M. P. Whyte: Division of Bone and Mineral Diseases, Departments of Medicine and Pediatrics, The Jewish Hospital of St. Louis, Washington University School of Medicine, St. Louis, Missouri 63110; Metabolic Research Unit, Shriners Hospital for Crippled Children, St. Louis, Missouri 63131.

TABLE 1. *Disorders that cause osteosclerosis*

Dysplasias	Metabolic
1. Craniodiaphyseal dysplasia	1. Carbonic anhydrase II deficiency
2. Craniometaphyseal dysplasia	2. Fluorosis
3. Dysosteosclerosis	3. Heavy metal poisoning
4. Endosteal hyperostosis (van Buchem's disease and sclerosteosis)	4. Hypervitaminosis A, D
5. Frontometaphyseal dysplasia	5. Hyper-, hypo-, and pseudo-hypoparathyroidism
6. Infantile cortical hyperostosis (Caffey's disease)	6. Hypophosphatemic osteomalacia
7. Melorheostosis	7. Milk-alkali syndrome
8. Metaphyseal dysplasia (Pyle's disease)	8. Renal osteodystrophy
9. Mixed sclerosing bone dystrophy	*Other*
10. Oculodento-osseous dysplasia	1. Axial osteomalacia
11. Osteodysplasia of Melnick and Needles	2. Fibrogenesis imperfecta ossium
12. Osteoectasia with hyperphosphatasia (hyperostosis corticalis)	3. Ionizing radiation
13. Osteopathia striata	4. Lymphomas
14. Osteopetrosis	5. Mastocytosis
15. Osteopoikilosis	6. Multiple myeloma
16. Progressive diaphyseal dysplasia (Engelmann's disease)	7. Myelofibrosis
17. Pycnodysostosis	8. Osteomyelitis
	9. Osteonecrosis
	10. Paget's disease
	11. Sarcoidosis
	12. Skeletal metastases
	13. Tuberous sclerosis

Source: From Whyte and Murphy (248), with permission.

Clinical Features

The clinical features of hypophosphatasia have been described thoroughly in the approximately 300 cases reported in the medical literature (8). Of interest, TNSALP is ubiquitous in human tissues and is especially rich in liver, bone, and kidney (13), yet hypophosphatasia seems to affect only the skeleton and dentition directly and does not cause significant hepatic or renal dysfunction. Any pathology at extraskeletal sites seems to be secondary to defects in the hard tissues themselves (8,14). Nevertheless, the severity of clinical expression is remarkably variable and spans intrauterine death from profound skeletal hypomineralization at one extreme and life-long absence of symptoms at the other (8,14). Six clinical types are distinguished. The age at which skeletal disease is first noted delineates perinatal (lethal), infantile, childhood, and adult hypophosphatasia (see below) (15). However, it is not unusual to encounter affected children and adults who have dental abnormalities only. They may have premature tooth loss yet their skeletal radiographs or biopsy specimens of bone are normal. Such subjects are classified as having "odonto-hypophosphatasia" (8). Lastly, there is a very rare variant "pseudohypophosphatasia" characterized by patients who have the clinical/radiologic/biochemical features of classic hypophosphatasia, yet their serum ALP activity is normal in routine clinical assays (8,16). As discussed below, these individuals have defects in TNSALP cellular localization and substrate specificity.

Because the severity of expression of hypophosphatasia is a continuum, the above clinical classification is imprecise and artificial, but it is important in that it provides some idea of the patient's prognosis (8,14). It should also prove helpful to understand the structure/function relationship of the TNSALP mutations to clinical/biochemical phenotype as the molecular basis for the various forms unfolds (12). Furthermore, although the inheritance pattern for the severe forms of hypophosphatasia is clearly autosomal recessive, the mode(s) of transmission of the more mild classifications is poorly understood and will require molecular insight (8,14).

Perinatal Hypophosphatasia

Perinatal hypophosphatasia is a lethal condition. As reviewed later, it can be detected in utero by ultrasound study which reveals profound skeletal hypomineralization and deformity (17). Accordingly, the intrauterine environment may not be protective for severe deficiency of TNSALP activity. Polyhydramnios can complicate the pregnancy and stillbirth is frequent. Severe skeletal hypomineralization accounts for *caput membranaceum* and fractures. The limbs are obviously short and deformed (8,14). Rarely, peculiar bony spurs jut out from the ends of the major long bones and may traverse the skin. Although clinically severe osteogenesis imperfecta (see section on "Osteogenesis Imperfecta," this chapter) or one of the lethal forms of dwarfism may be suspected from the physical features, these disorders should be readily distinguished from perinatal hypophosphatasia since serum ALP activity is not reduced. Furthermore, the radiologic features of perinatal hypophosphatasia are distinctive (see below).

Some affected newborns survive delivery but fail to gain weight, are irritable with a high-pitched cry, and have unexplained fever, seizures, anemia, and periods of apnea with cyanosis and bradycardia. They may also suffer intracranial hemorrhage. Respiratory compromise from severe rachitic deformity of the chest is typically fatal soon after birth (8,14).

Infantile Hypophosphatasia

Infantile hypophosphatasia, by definition, becomes clinically apparent sometime after birth but before 6 months of age. In many affected infants, including the subject reported by Rathbun (7), the disorder manifests as though it is a developmental problem (8). Psychomotor skills advance normally and the baby appears well at first, but at a few months of age there begins a "downhill" course characterized by poor feeding and failure to thrive. At this time, widened "fontanels" and hypotonia are discovered and rickets becomes clinically obvious. In many such infants, skeletal deformities then progress. Hypercalcemia and hypercalciuria evolve and may account for bouts of vomiting as well as the development of nephrocalcinosis and occasionally significant renal impairment. There may be seizures and spells of apnea. Despite the clinical impression based upon palpation of the skull or radiologic evidence that the fontanels are widely patent, a functional craniosynostosis is generally present. What might appear to be a widened "suture" is not the fibrous tissue that normally allows the skull to grow, but is actually a hypomineralized area of the calvarium. Skull growth may cease and lead to raised intracranial pressure. Proptosis, bulging of the anterior fontanel, and papilledema can occur from this complication. Mild hypertelorism and brachycephaly may also develop (8,14). Deformity of the chest appears to account for the recurrent pneumonias or respiratory failure that cause death in about 50% of affected infants (15).

Childhood Hypophosphatasia

Childhood hypophosphatasia has a very variable severity of expression, but the clinical manifestations are less marked than in the perinatal and infantile forms (8,14). Premature exfoliation of decidous teeth (i.e., before age 5 years) may be the only clinically apparent abnormality. Usually the incisors are lost first, but nearly the whole of the dentition can be shed prematurely. This complication occurs because of hypoplasia or aplasia of dental cementum which normally anchors the tooth root to the periodontal ligament (see below). Teeth are lost before the physiologic mechanism of root resorption by osteoclasts can take place. If skeletal radiographs also show signs of bone disease, then childhood hypophosphatasia is diagnosed. When rickets is present there is delayed walking and then a characteristic waddling gait. Rachitic

deformity will occasionally cause bowed legs or knock-knees. Short stature, beading of the costochondral junctions, dolichocephaly with frontal bossing, and enlargement of the wrists, knees, or ankles is present in the subjects who are more severely affected (8,14).

Adult Hypophosphatasia

Adult hypophosphatasia typically manifests first during middle age with recurrent, slowly-healing, metatarsal stress fractures (8,14,18). In severe cases, pseudofractures (Looser's zones) develop in the proximal femora (19). Chondrocalcinosis is a common radiologic finding, but calcium pyrophosphate deposition disease that results in attacks of overt arthritis (pseudogout) occurs only rarely. Loss or fracture of adult teeth may be an early expression of this form of the disease and can predate the onset of skeletal manifestations by decades. About 50% of patients give histories of early exfoliation of deciduous teeth and/or rickets. Thus, a significant number of cases of adult hypophosphatasia appear to reflect re-expression of the childhood form of the disease (18).

Odontohypophosphatasia

Odontohypophosphatasia signifies (as discussed) the patient with dental manifestations of hypophosphatasia in whom there is no evidence of skeletal disease (8).

Pseudohypophosphatasia

Pseudohypophosphatasia has been described convincingly in two subjects (16,20). Both presented with the typical clinical and radiologic manifestations of infantile hypophosphatasia, yet had serum ALP activity that was not reduced in routine clinical laboratory assays. In one case, serum ALP values were normal or actually elevated (20); in the other, they were low-normal and therefore clearly higher than the very low levels seen in classic infantile disease (16).

Radiologic Findings

Radiologic investigation of the skeleton of infants and children with hypophosphatasia does more than merely reveal that some type of rickets is present (3,4).

Perinatal hypophosphatasia has characteristic radiographic features. The bones can be so profoundly hypomineralized that their appearance is diagnostic (Fig. 1). In a few cases, only the skull base was seen. With somewhat less dramatic presentation, one observes marked osteopenia, but there is sufficient skeletal mineralization so that pronounced rachitic changes become apparent. A characteristic feature, radiolucent "tongues" extending from physes into the metaphyses, may be noted in major long bones. Fractures are not uncommon. In these sub-

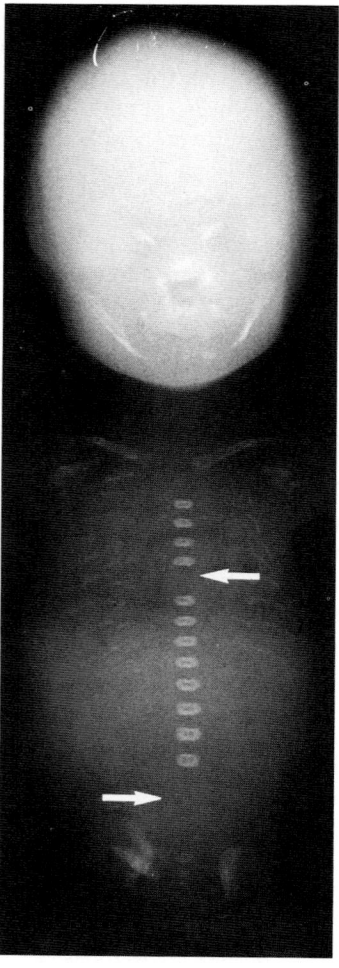

FIG. 1. Hypophosphatasia (perinatal form). This aborted fetus of 31 weeks gestation is profoundly hypomineralized with only a few areas of ossification apparent in the axial skeleton. Note the absence of several vertebrae (*arrows*).

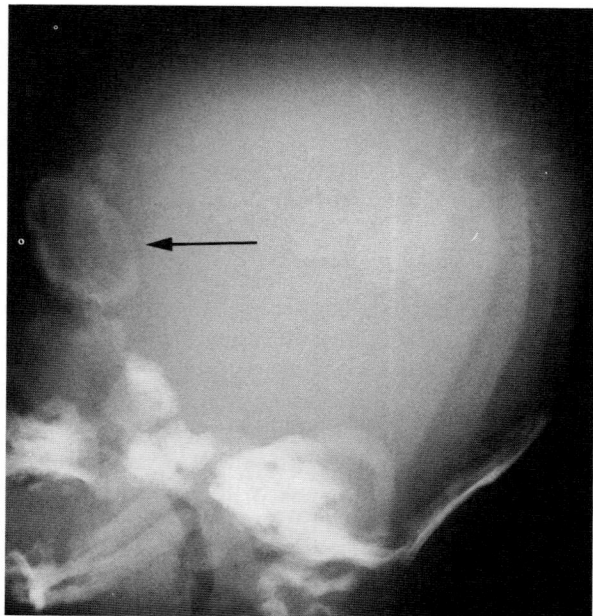

FIG. 2. Hypophosphatasia (perinatal form). The skull of this newborn shows characteristic marked hypomineralization. Ossification is apparent in only a few areas in the frontal bone (*arrow*), at the base, and in the occiput. From Whyte (250), with permission.

jects, calvarial bones can be mineralized only centrally and thereby produce the illusion that the skull sutures are widened (Fig. 2). Occasionally, highly unusual and unexplained radiologic signs are present like bony spurs at the ends of major long bones and individual vertebra that seem to be absent (Fig. 1) (3,4,8).

Infantile hypophosphatasia also has characteristic radiologic signs that are somewhat less severe but otherwise resemble those of the perinatal form (3,4,8). Of interest, one may see rather abrupt transition from relatively well-mineralized diaphyses to markedly hypomineralized metaphyses. This radiologic finding suggests that fairly sudden metabolic deterioration can occur in infantile hypophosphatasia and is consistent with the suggestion of Rathbun that this condition can be a developmental disorder (7). In infants who have an especially poor prognosis, in addition to the persistence of active rachitic disease, there may also be progressive skeletal demineralization with increasing deformity (21). Radio-

nuclide scanning of the skeleton can be helpful in searching for craniosynostosis since, if it is present, tracer uptake in the cranial "sutures" will be decreased though they are widely separated on conventional radiographs (22).

Childhood hypophosphatasia also features characteristic "tongues" of radiolucency that project from the physes into the metaphyses of long bones (Fig. 3). However, these areas of osteopenia are somewhat less pronounced than in the infantile form. There is no satisfactory explanation for this sign which appears to reflect a localized increased disturbance of endochondral bone formation. In subjects with relatively severe childhood hypophosphatasia, as well as those who survive the first year of life with the infantile form, true premature fusion of cranial sutures can occur. Radiographs of the skull may then demonstrate the typical "beaten-copper" appearance that results from this complication (3,4). Diminished mechanical stimulation of alveolar bone by properly anchored dentition can cause periodontal osteopenia. Dental radiographs may also reveal "shell teeth" characterized by enlarged pulp chambers and root canals. This finding can occur in other forms of rickets and is a reflection of defective dentinogenesis.

Adult hypophosphatasia often causes recurrent, poorly-healing stress fractures of the metatarsals (18). Osteopenia, chondrocalcinosis, and changes of pyrophosphate arthropathy may also evolve (Fig. 4) (8,18,23). Femoral pseudofractures develop in subjects

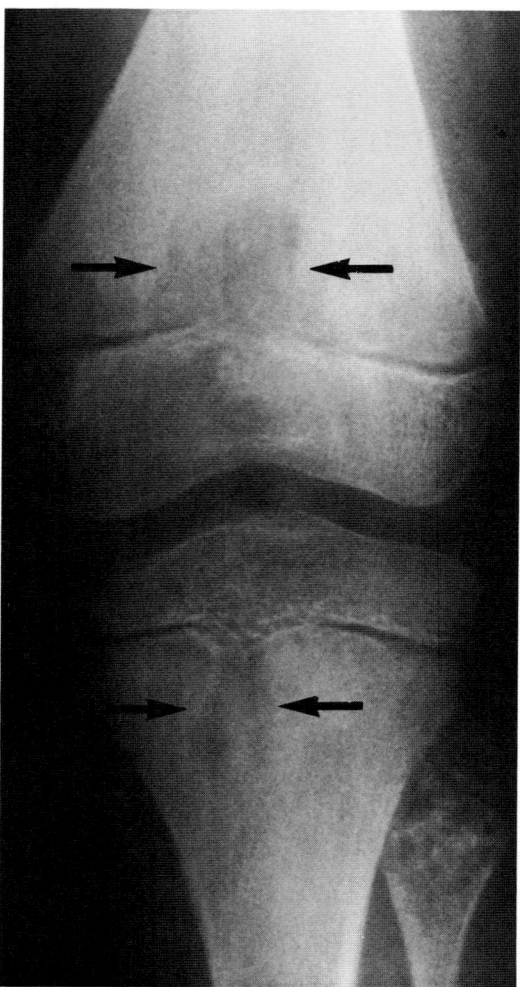

FIG. 3. Hypophosphatasia (childhood form). Although the growth plates are not widened as they are in most other forms of rickets, subtle but characteristic tongues of radiolucency (*arrows*) project into the femoral and tibial metaphyses in this boy aged 11 yr 4 mo. The head of the fibula is especially irregular.

who are relatively severely affected, and are located proximally and laterally rather than on the medial side as typically occurs in other forms of osteomalacia (Fig. 5) (19).

Laboratory Findings

Hypophosphat*asemia* (subnormal serum ALP activity for the patient's age and sex) is the biochemical hallmark of all clinical forms of hypophosphatasia except the very rare variant, pseudohypophosphatasia (8). The level of serum ALP activity in hypophosphatasia (referable to age-matched controls) generally reflects the clinical severity of the disorder. Subjects with perinatal or infantile disease have 2% to 12% of controls levels, whereas those with odontohypophosphatasia have just

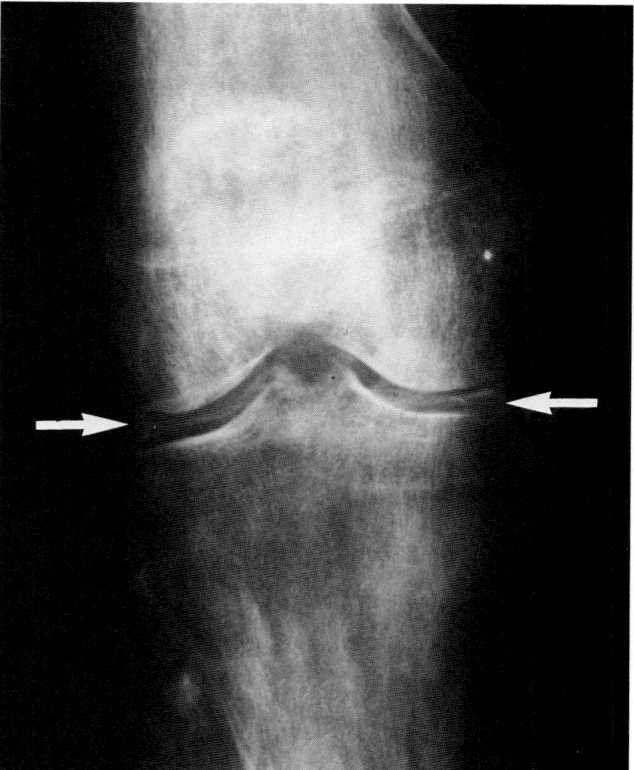

FIG. 4. Hypophosphatasia (adult form). The bones at the knee of this 65-year-old woman are considerably osteopenic. There is marked chondrocalcinosis of the articular cartilage (*arrows*).

mildly reduced levels (unpublished observations). However, the presence of hypophosphatasemia in hypophosphatasia becomes especially impressive when one recognizes that other forms of rickets or osteomalacia typically elevate serum ALP activity from increased amounts of "bone" ALP isoenzyme (13). Conditions other than hypophosphatasia may lower serum ALP activity, but they are usually clinically significant and readily diagnosed (8). Theoretically, a diagnosis of hypophosphatasia could be missed if a concomitant disorder substantially increased the serum level of one of the other ALP isoenzymes (e.g., placental ALP in pregnancy, or "placental-like" ALP with certain malignancies). Furthermore, increases to some degree in the serum level of the bone or liver form of TNSALP, as occurs with fracture or hepatitis, respectively, could obscure the diagnosis (13).

Hypercalcemia and hypercalciuria are common in infantile hypophosphatasia (8,14) and seem to stem from "dyssynergy" between gastrointestinal absorption of dietary calcium and defective bone mineralization. It may also be, however, that progressive skeletal demineralization, perhaps in part from immobilization, contributes to this biochemical complication in severely affected subjects (21).

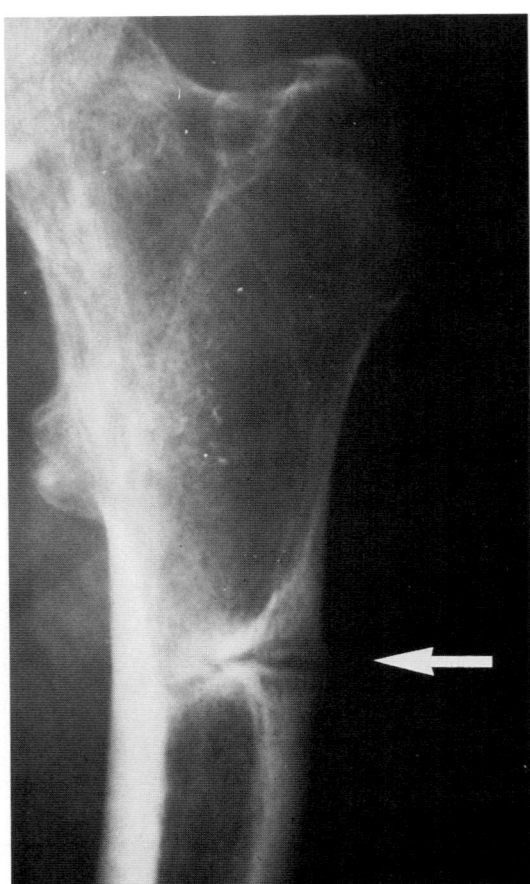

FIG. 5. Hypophosphatasia (adult form). A characteristic pseudofracture is present in the lateral cortex of the proximal femur (*arrow*).

$$O=P-O-P=O \quad \text{PPi}$$

$$NH_2CH_2CH_2-O-P=O \quad \text{PEA}$$

$$PLP$$

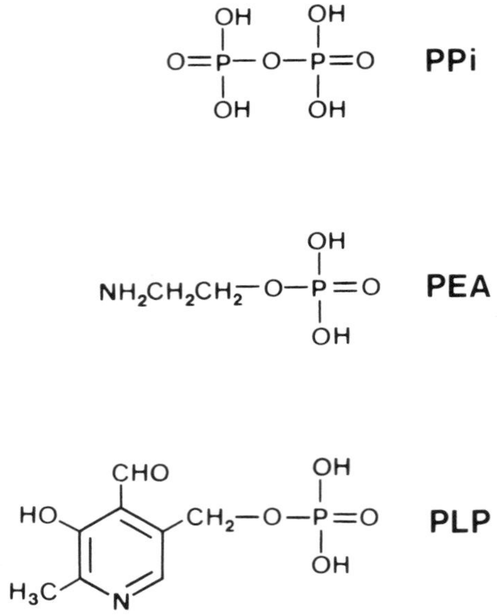

FIG. 6. Natural substrates for tissue nonspecific alkaline phosphatase. Inorganic pyrophosphate (PPi), phosphoethanolamine (PEA), and pyridoxal 5'-phosphate (PLP) accumulate endogenously in hypophosphatasia and therefore appear to be natural substrates for TNSALP.

Serum concentrations of 25(OH)D, 1,25(OH)$_2$D, and PTH are typically unremarkable unless there is hypercalcemia or renal compromise, in which case the levels change in the way that would normally occur with these disturbances (8).

Mild hyperphosphatemia is present in approximately half of all patients with either the childhood or the adult form of hypophosphatasia (9); almost invariably fasting serum inorganic phosphate concentrations are above the normal mean level. The hyperphosphatemia results from enhanced renal reclamation of inorganic phosphate from the glomerular filtrate, but further understanding of this phenomenon is necessary (9). The situation for perinatal and infantile hypophosphatasia requires investigation.

Three phosphocompounds [phosphoethanolamine (PEA), inorganic pyrophosphate (PPi), and pyridoxal 5'-phosphate (PLP)] that each appear to be natural substrates for TNSALP accumulate endogenously in hypophosphatasia (Fig. 6) (8,9,14). Assays are commercially available for urinary PEA and plasma PLP; quantitation of PPi remains a research technique. Although documen-

tation of phosphoethanolaminuria or inorganic pyrophosphaturia supports a diagnosis of hypophosphatasia, it is not pathognomonic (8). Other conditions, including several metabolic bone diseases, increase urinary PEA and PPi excretion. Furthermore, levels of PEA and PPi in urine are influenced by age and diet and can be normal in some hypophosphatasia cases (8,14). Of note, however, it is the endogenous accumulation of PPi that seems to be a key pathogenetic factor for the skeletal disease (see below). An increased plasma concentration of PLP is a specific and sensitive marker for hypophosphatasia (8,24). For accurate testing, multivitamins or vitamin B$_6$ (pyridoxine) supplementation must be avoided for several days. Even patients with odontohypophosphatasia have elevated plasma PLP levels (Fig. 7) (8). The greater the clinical severity, the greater the PLP increment. However, there is overlap of the plasma PLP levels among the various clinical forms.

Histopathologic Findings

Histopathologic abnormalities are noted principally in the skeleton and the teeth (8,14). Osteoidosis and abnormal patterns of tetracycline "labeling" on fluorescence microscopy (following oral administration of this antibiotic) occur in nondecalcified sections of bone in all clinical forms of the disease except odontohypophosphatasia (18). The degree of defective skeletal mineralization generally reflects the severity of clinical expression (8). Nevertheless, without histochemical evaluation of ALP

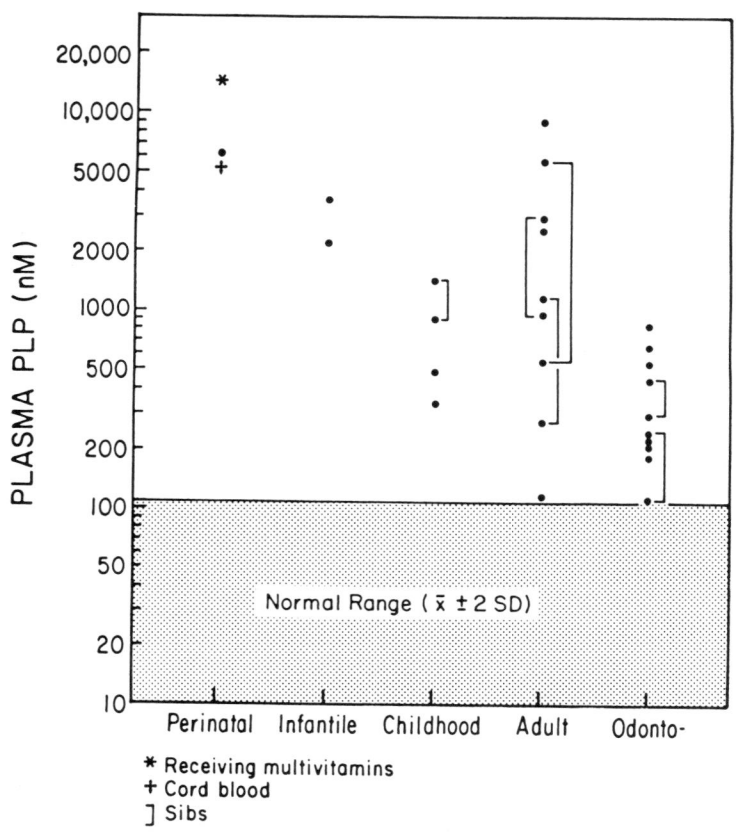

* Receiving multivitamins
+ Cord blood
] Sibs

FIG. 7. Plasma pyridoxal 5'-phosphate levels in hypophosphatasia. In all clinical forms of hypophosphatasia, plasma PLP levels are elevated. The degree of increment generally reflects the clinical severity (note: log scale). From Coburn and Whyte (251), with permission.

activity in bone, the findings are merely those of many other types of rickets or osteomalacia (14).

Electron microscopy of the skeleton of cases of lethal hypophosphatasia has disclosed collagen fibers and proteoglycan granules that are distributed normally in the matrix. Osteoblasts, chondrocytes, and matrix vesicles are present. However, the matrix vesicles have no ALP activity and are devoid of hydroxyapatite crystals. Only a few isolated crystals are observed outside of these extracellular structures (8,14).

The cranial "sutures" that appear to be widened are not composed of fibrous tissue, but are instead merely areas of hypomineralized membranous bone (15).

The histopathologic abnormalities of the dentition in hypophosphatasia involve primarily the cementum (8,14). Despite the presence of cells that appear to be cementoblasts, there is aplasia or hypoplasia and impaired calcification of this structure (Fig. 8). Excessively widened areas of predentin, increased amounts of interglobular dentin, and dental tubules that are large but few are additional findings. These changes appear to be analogous to the osteoidosis that is found in skeletal tissue (8). Pulp chambers may be enlarged as a result of retarded dentinogenesis and explain the radiologic sign of "shell teeth." Of interest, the dental aberrations impact the incisors most, but vary from tooth to tooth. Enamel does not seem to be affected directly.

Prevalence and Inheritance

Hypophosphatasia affects all races, but seems to be especially common among the Mennonites and Hutterites in Canada. In Canada, the incidence of the severe forms has been estimated to be about 1/100,000 live births (15).

It is well established that the perinatal and infantile forms of hypophosphatasia are inherited as autosomal recessive traits (1,8,14). Parents of such cases generally have low or low-normal levels of serum ALP activity and may have modest increments in urine PEA levels. Recent detailed studies of inbred Mennonite kindreds in Canada show that carriers of severe hypophosphatasia in that population also have somewhat greater serum levels of inorganic phosphate and excessive pre- and post-pyridoxine challenge plasma levels of PLP compared to unaffected family members (25).

The mode(s) of inheritance for odonto-, adult, and childhood hypophosphatasia is still unclear (14,18). Autosomal dominant transmission has been described in some kindreds with mild disease (18,23). Generation-to-generation occurrence of hypophosphatasemia, sometimes with clinical evidence of skeletal or dental disease in successive generations, is evidence for this type of inheritance pattern (8,14). Accordingly, these cases may reflect clinical expression in subjects who are heterozy-

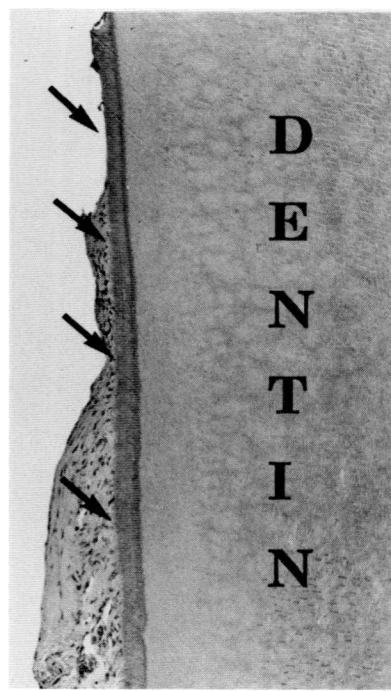 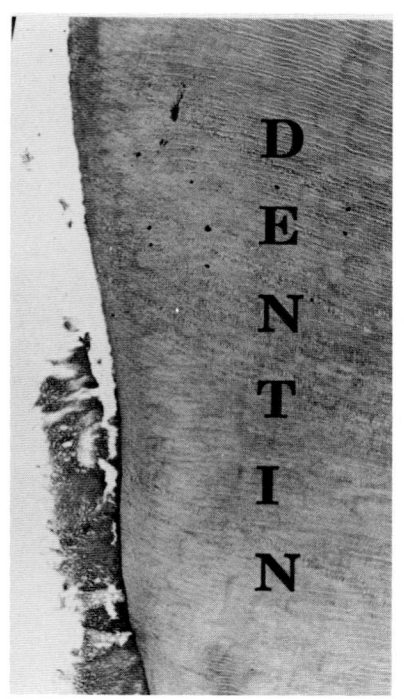

FIG. 8. Hypophosphatasia (dental pathology). **A:** Decalcified maxillary incisor from a child with X-linked hypophosphate*mia* is essentially normal and shows primary cementum (*arrows*) between the root surface and periodontal ligament. **B:** In this tooth from a subject with hypophosphatasia, cementum is absent (×150).

gotes for a molecular defect that conditions TNSALP biosynthesis. Homozygosity for such defects would presumably cause severe disease (8). It is notable however that vertical transmission of clinically apparent hypophosphatasia is somewhat unusual. Indeed, expression of the disease often runs "true-to-form," even when mild, within just one affected sibship (18,23). Thus, in some cases, mild disease may reflect mutations in two alleles that condition TNSALP biosynthesis (26). Skeletal mineralization is a complex process (9) and it may be that epigenetic factors also help to account for the extreme range of clinical expression of hypophosphatasia.

Biochemical/Genetic Defect

ALP [orthophosphoric monoester phosphohydrolase (alkaline optimum), EC 3.1.3.1] is found in nearly all living organisms (9,13). Early on, autopsy studies of subjects with lethal hypophosphatasia revealed a profound deficiency of ALP activity in liver, bone, and kidney, yet normal levels of ALP activity in intestine and placenta (fetal trophoblast) (8). The meaning of this observation became apparent during the 1960s and 1970s when protein analysis of ALPs purified from normal human tissues suggested that ALP in human liver, bone, and kidney is the product of one gene whereas intestinal and placental ALP are derived from two separate genes (13). Hypophosphatasia appeared to be an inborn error of metabolism that selectively involved the TNSALP isoenzyme. Recently, each of the ALP genes in man has been

cloned and sequenced (27). The TNSALP gene has been localized to the tip of the short arm of chromosome 1 (1p36.1–1p34) and exists as a single copy in the haploid genome. A fourth ALP locus encodes a placental-like (germ cell) ALP isoenzyme which is an oncofetal protein that serves as a useful tumor marker (27). The three tissue-specific ALPs are a multigene family that maps to the long arm of chromosome 2 (2q34–2q37) (27).

In 1987, linkage analysis of infantile hypophosphatasia with the Rh blood group locus on the short arm of chromosome 1 indicated that the genetic defect for severe hypophosphatasia in Canadian Mennonites was at the TNSALP locus (28). In 1988, homozygosity for a point mutation in the TNSALP gene that lead to a missense base change was identified in a severely affected infant from an inbred kindred in Nova Scotia (10). The base change predicted an alanine/threonine substitution in the mature protein near a metal binding site and functionally important arginine residue. Transfection studies following site-directed mutagenesis confirmed that this mutation inactivated the TNSALP enzyme (10). However, since consanguinity has been reported in just a minority of families where perinatal or infantile hypophosphatasia has occurred, different rather than identical allelic defects will likely explain most severe cases (8,14). Indeed, a preliminary report now indicates that such "compound heterozygosity" with a variety of such point mutations commonly causes severe disease (11,12). Furthermore, it appears that these mutations are also involved in some cases of mild disease (12). The genetic basis for hypophosphatasia may, however, be more complex. Regulatory defects of TNSALP gene expression may account for some cases. One child with infantile hypophosphatasia had dramatic clinical, radiologic, and histopathologic improvement following a period in which ALP was transiently synthesized in his skeleton and his serum ALP activity level corrected (29).

Other recent preliminary evidence shows that hypophosphatasia is associated with deficiency of bone ALP protein in serum and that the magnitude of the decrement reflects the clinical severity of the disorder (30). In pseudohypophosphatasia, essentially normal levels of bone ALP protein were found in the serum (see below).

As an "experiment of nature," hypophosphatasia shows clearly that TNSALP acts importantly in the formation of the skeleton and the dentition (9). Conversely, it also suggests that TNSALP is less critical in other tissues. Functioning of even TNSALP-rich organs like the liver and kidney does not appear to be disturbed.

The discoveries of endogenous accumulation of three phosphocompounds in hypophosphatasia has helped to elucidate the physiologic function of TNSALP (9). Although PEA was the first of the putative natural substrates identified (8), its metabolic origin is unclear. The liver has been suggested to be the source for plasma PEA. However, PEA is now recognized to be a component of the phosphatidylinositol anchor that links certain proteins, including the ALPs, to the cell surface (31). This suggests that there may be extracellular production of PEA. The discovery in 1985 that plasma levels of PLP (the principal cofactor form of vitamin B_6) are increased in hypophosphatasia indicated that TNSALP acts primarily as an *ecto*enzyme (8,9) (Fig. 9). The observation that individuals with hypophosphatasia typically do not manifest signs or symptoms of vitamin B_6 deficiency or toxicity was predictable if TNSALP functioned at cell surfaces (24). This clinical observation has been followed by a number of cell culture studies, including those utilizing TNSALP-deficient hypophosphatasia fibroblasts, which confirm that TNSALP acts physiologically as an PEA- and PLP-ectophosphatase (31). However, it was the discovery in 1965 that urinary PPi levels are elevated in hypophosphatasia that provided a possible explanation for not only the chondrocalcinosis, pseudogout, and pyrophosphate arthropathy, but more importantly for the bone disease as well. PPi is a potent inhibitor of biomineralization since it disrupts hydroxyapatite crystal formation (14). Understandably, endogenous accumulation of PPi would cause rickets or osteomalacia (9).

Pseudohypophosphatasia is a hypophosphatasia variant in which the cellular localization and substrate specificity of TNSALP is altered (32). Artificial substrates (e.g., para-nitrophenylphosphate) that are used in routine clinical assays performed at markedly alkaline pH produce normal serum levels of ALP activity. However, TNSALP activity against PEA and PLP at physiologic pH is localized intracellularly and is diminished in pa-

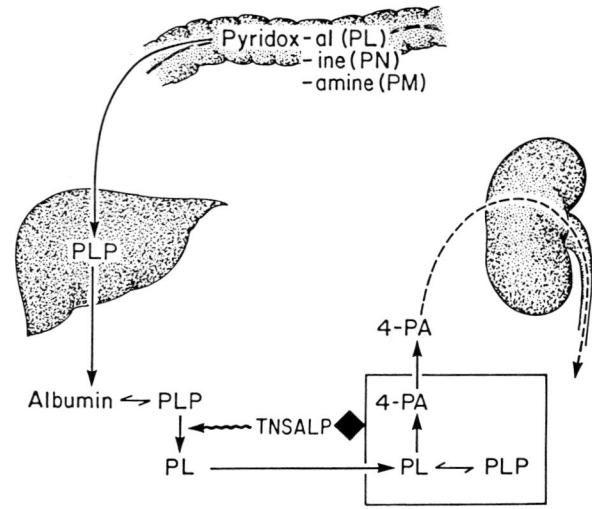

FIG. 9. Vitamin B_6 metabolism. Dietary forms of vitamin B_6—pyridoxal (PL), pyridoxine (PN), and pyridoxamine (PM)—are each converted to PLP in the liver. PLP then enters the circulation where it is largely bound to albumin. The small amount of unbound PLP must first be dephosphorylated to PL before it can enter tissues. Within cells PL is then rephosphorylated to the cofactor PLP form. PLP is ultimately degraded to 4-pyridoxic acid (4-PA) primarily in the liver. From Whyte (8), with permission.

tient fibroblasts (32). The molecular basis for this hypophosphatasia variant is not known.

Elucidation of the pathogenesis of hypophosphatasia has shown that the term "alkaline phosphatase" is a misnomer (9). This inborn error of metabolism demonstrates that TNSALP normally dephosphorylates physiologic concentrations of a variety of phosphocompounds at physiologic pH (Fig. 10). The term "alkaline phosphatase" was never used by its discoverer, Robert Robison (9,13). It was coined later when the enzyme's peculiar pH optimum was exploited during the development of clinical and research assays of its activity (9,13).

Treatment

Conventional medical therapy for the more common forms or rickets or osteomalacia (e.g., vitamin D sterols and mineral supplementation) should not be used for hypophosphatasia unless specific deficits are documented. Serum levels of calcium and inorganic phosphate and the principal vitamin D metabolites typically are not reduced (8). Because severely affected patients are predisposed to hypercalcemia and hypercalciuria, such treatment could potentially lead to nephrocalcinosis and renal compromise. Conversely, willingful restriction of sunshine exposure and vitamin D intake for one hypercalciuric child led to vitamin D deficiency rickets (8). In infantile hypophosphatasia, hypercalcemia will generally respond to reduced dietary calcium levels but

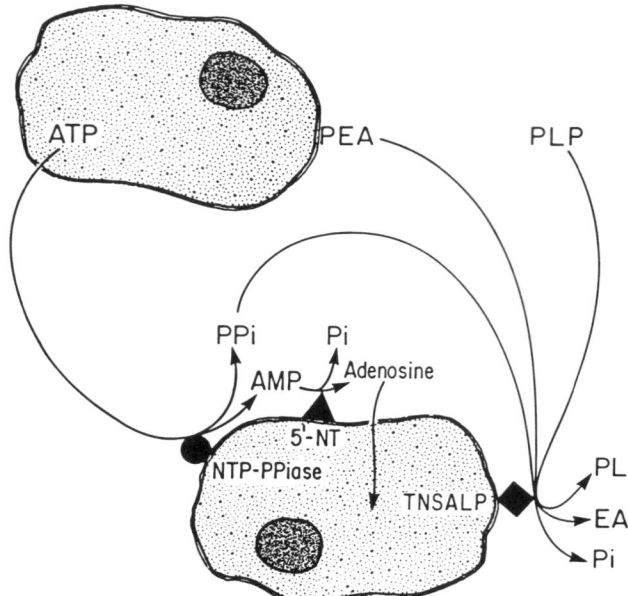

FIG. 10. Ectoenzyme role of tissue nonspecific alkaline phosphatase. Endogenous accumulation of PPi, PEA, and PLP in hypophosphatasia is due to deficient TNSALP ectophosphatase activity. Extracellular accumulation of PPi, an inhibitor of hydroxyapatite crystal formation, appears to cause the defective skeletal mineralization that is expressed as rickets in children or osteomalacia in adults. From Whyte (8), with permission.

glucocorticoid therapy may also be helpful. In the early literature, cortisone treatment reportedly corrected serum ALP activity levels and led to radiologic improvement in a few such patients. Unfortunately, this has not been a consistent finding (8,29).

Enzyme replacement therapy, using various sources of ALP, has also generally produced disappointing results. Intravenous infusions of plasma from patients with Paget's bone disease (8) or with purified human liver ALP (33) have transiently normalized serum ALP activity, but have not substantially altered skeletal mineralization. In one unusual case, however, serial intravenous infusions of pooled normal plasma was followed by normalization for several months of serum bone ALP activity and remarkable transient clinical and radiographic improvement (29). This therapeutic approach, however, was unsuccessful in a second infant (24).

Injections of the biologically active 1–34 fragment of bovine PTH, in hopes of stimulating skeletal ALP activity, was also without effect (29). Sodium fluoride, which can be mitogenic for osteoblasts and increase serum ALP activity, has not been rigorously tested (8). Interpretation of the results of any therapeutic trial for hypophosphatasia in infants or children can be difficult because there can be some natural fluctuation in the clinical/radiologic course of the disease (8,14).

Supportive therapy is important. Fractures usually mend, but slowly (18,19). In affected adults, insertion of load-sharing intramedullary rods, rather than load-sparing devices like plates, appears to be preferable for the acute or prophylactic treatment of pseudofractures and fractures (19). Expert dental care is especially important for young children, since their nutrition can be impaired by premature tooth loss. Soft diets and use of dentures may be necessary. Craniotomy can be life-saving for craniosynostosis.

Prognosis

Perinatal hypophosphatasia is a lethal disorder (8,14). Infantile hypophosphatasia often shows progressive clinical and radiologic deterioration and about 50% of patients succumb to the disease during the first year of life (15). The prognosis for the infantile form seems to improve after infancy (15). Childhood hypophosphatasia causes chronic symptoms that may improve somewhat when growth plates fuse after puberty. However, recurrence of skeletal complications during adult life is possible (18). In adults, once metatarsal stress fractures develop, they will be a recurrent problem. Femoral pseudofractures will persist unless there is complete fracture or orthopedic intervention (18,19,23).

Prenatal Diagnosis

Severely affected fetuses can be detected reliably in utero (17). The accuracy of prenatal diagnosis is optimum, however, with combined use of ultrasonography (with attention to the limbs as well as the skull), assay by an experienced laboratory of ALP activity in amniotic fluid cells, and radiologic study (17). Of note, a recent preliminary report cautions that bowed limbs may be detected by ultrasound in utero in subjects who later have only clinically mild hypophosphatasia (34).

AXIAL OSTEOMALACIA

Axial osteomalacia is another unusual disorder in which defective skeletal mineralization occurs although serum calcium and inorganic phosphate levels are typically normal. It is characterized radiologically by a coarsened pattern of the trabecular bone in the axial skeleton but unremarkable appearance of bones in the limbs (35–40). Fewer than 20 patients have been reported. Most cases have occurred sporadically, but an affected mother and son have been described (36).

Clinical Presentation

Affected individuals usually have been middle-aged or elderly men. A few middle-aged women have had the condition. It is likely, however, that radiologic manifestations are detectable considerably earlier in life (36).

The majority of patients have presented with vague, dull, chronic axial skeletal discomfort that typically affects the cervical region most severely. Long-term follow-up of one subject showed, however, that symptoms and radiologic findings did not change (38).

Radiologic Features

Abnormal findings are limited to the pelvis and spine where the coarsened trabecular pattern resembles other types of osteomalacia (Fig. 11) (2,3,40). The cervical spine and ribs seem to be most involved. Pseudofractures (Looser's zones), a radiologic hallmark of osteomalacia that can occur in the axial or appendicular skeleton, have not been noted. Two affected subjects reportedly had features of ankylosing spondylitis (37).

Laboratory Studies

Serum levels of inorganic phosphate tended to be low in four patients (28). In other affected subjects, osteomalacia occurred although levels of calcium, inorganic phosphate, 25(OH)D, and 1,25(OH)D were normal in the serum (27). Alkaline phosphatase activity (bone isoenzyme) in serum may be increased.

Histopathologic Findings

Findings from a limited number of patients show that, unlike in some other types of osteomalacia, corticomedullary junctions of iliac crest specimens are typically distinct though the cortices can be porous and wide. Trabeculae are of variable thickness and the total bone volume may be increased. Osteoidosis (increased width and extent of osteoid seams) is present. Polarized-light microscopy shows collagen with a normal lamellar pattern. Fluorescence microscopy following in vivo tetracycline labeling before bone biopsy confirms that defective skeletal mineralization is present. Fluorescent "labels" can be irregular, single, and wide (36). Osteoblasts have had the flat inactive-appearance of "lining" cells. They can have reduced Golgi zones and rough endoplasmic reticulum and increased amounts of glycogen in their cytoplasm. Osteoblasts do, however, stain intensely for alkaline phosphatase activity. Features of secondary hyperparathyroidism are absent (36).

Etiology and Pathogenesis

The histopathologic features suggest that axial osteomalacia may be due to an osteoblast defect (35). Electron microscopic studies of bone from one affected subject revealed that these cells were capable of forming matrix vesicles within abundant osteoid (36).

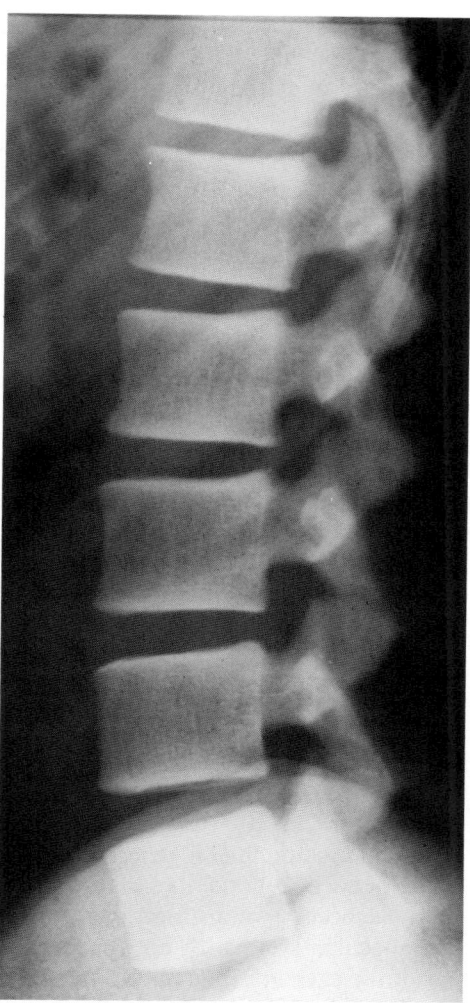

FIG. 11. Axial Osteomalacia. Lateral view of the lumbar spine of this 35-year-old black man shows generalized osteosclerosis due to thickening of the trabeculae. From Whyte et al. (36), with permission.

Treatment

Specific medical therapy is not available. The clinical course of axial osteomalacia, however, seems to be relatively benign. Methyltestosterone and stilbesterol have been used without apparent success (38). As much as 20,000 units/day of vitamin D_2 for three years was similarly without beneficial effect (38). Slight improvement in histological abnormalities in bone, but not in symptoms, was described for calcium and vitamin D_2 treatment during a study of four cases (37).

FIBROGENESIS IMPERFECTA OSSIUM

Fibrogenesis imperfecta ossium was delineated in 1950 (41). Fewer than 20 cases appear in the medical literature (40–51). The clinical, biochemical, radiologic, and histopathologic features of this sporadic condition have been carefully contrasted with those of axial osteomalacia (40). Although radiologic studies indicate that there is diffuse osteopenia, the coarse and dense appearance of trabecular bone in many areas explains why this entity is often grouped among the sclerosing bone disorders (Table 1).

Clinical Presentation

Fibrogenesis imperfecta ossium usually manifests first during middle age or later in life. Both sexes are affected. Gradual onset of intractable skeletal pain that rapidly progresses is the principal symptom. There is increasing immobility and a generally debilitating course. Patients typically become bedridden. Pathologic fractures are also a prominent clinical feature. Physical examination is remarkable for marked bony tenderness. Acute agranulocytosis (45) and macroglobulinemia (51) have been reported.

Radiologic Features

Radiologic abnormalities occur diffusely in the skeleton but spare the skull. Early on, there may merely be osteopenia and a slightly coarsened appearance to the trabecular bone (50). Subsequently, however, the features become more consistent with osteomalacia. Advanced changes include heterogeneous bone density with thinning of cortical bone. Eventually, corticomedullary junctions become indistinct as cortices are replaced by trabecular bone with an abnormal pattern. Some areas of the skeleton may have a mixed lytic and sclerotic appearance (50). Although bony contours are typically normal, deformities secondary to fractures can be present and periosteal reaction may involve the shafts of long bones. Pseudofractures also may develop. Some patients have a "rugger jersey" spine like that that occurs in renal osteodystrophy. In fibrogenesis imperfecta ossium and in axial osteomalacia, the distribution of the radiographic abnormalities (generalized versus axial) help to distinguish the two conditions (2,3,40).

Laboratory Findings

Calcium and inorganic phosphate levels are normal in serum, but alkaline phosphatase activity is increased. Hydroxyproline levels in urine are either normal or elevated (50). Typically, there is no evidence of renal tubular dysfunction or aminoaciduria.

Histopathologic Findings

Tetracycline labeling shows that the bony lesion is generalized and is a form of osteomalacia (50). The amount of affected bone varies considerably from site to site in the skeleton. Cortical bone in the diaphyses of the femora and tibiae can have the least abnormality. Unless bone tissue is examined with polarized-light or electron microscopy, fibrogenesis imperfecta ossium can be mistaken for osteoporosis or other forms of osteomalacia (50). Polarized-light microscopy, however, shows an absence of normal bone collagen birefringence. Electron microscopy reveals a "tangled" pattern of collagen fibrils that appear thin and randomly organized. In some regions, peculiar circular structures that are 300–500 nm in diameter have been noted in the matrix (47). Osteoblasts and osteoclasts may be abundant. Collagen synthesis in nonosseous tissues as well as in the subperiosteum appears to be normal.

Etiology and Pathogenesis

The etiology of fibrogenesis imperfecta ossium is not known. Since this condition has been reported only as sporadic cases, genetic factors have not been implicated for this acquired disorder. In one patient who also had a monoclonal gammopathy, it was postulated that a bone marrow toxin was being produced (see below) (48).

Treatment

There is no specific medical treatment. Temporary spontaneous improvement in symptoms may occur (50). Calcium supplementation together with vitamin D_2 or one of its active metabolites has been used, but no significant benefit was noted. In one affected subject, synthetic salmon calcitonin, $24,25(OH)_2D$, and sodium fluoride were also tested but without apparent success (50). However, a relatively recent case report indicated that melphalan and prednisone was an effective therapy (48).

OSTEOPETROSIS

Osteopetrosis is a generic term for a group of disorders that share a common pathogenesis characterized by failure of osteoclast-mediated resorption of bone. Description of the first case is credited to Albers-Schönberg who reported an affected adult in 1904 (52). More than 500 cases of "marble bone disease" are mentioned in the medical literature. Eight types have been identified in man based upon a clinical/genetic classification (Table 2). The two principal forms include a "benign" autosomal dominant type that is often asymptomatic (53) and a "malignant" autosomal recessive type that typically kills during infancy or childhood unless successfully treated (54). Benign osteopetrosis occurs with a prevalence estimated recently to be about 1:20,000; the malignant type is considerably rarer (55). Among the more unusual variants is the entity of "osteopetrosis with renal tubular acidosis" that was first reported as a syndrome

TABLE 2. *Forms of human osteopetrosis*

Type	Inheritance
Benign (Adult)	
Type I	AD
Type II	AD
Malignant	AR
Carbonic anhydrase II deficiency	AR
Intermediate	AR
Lethal	AR
Osteopetrosis with neuronal storage disease	AR
Transient infantile osteopetrosis	?

AD, autosomal dominant; AR, autosomal recessive.

simultaneously in 1972 in both the United States and Europe (56). In 1980, cerebral calcification was recognized to be its third distinguishing feature (57). Three years later, carbonic anhydrase II isoenzyme deficiency was discovered in three affected sisters from St. Louis (58). Accordingly, a detailed description of this new inborn error of metabolism is provided in the section on Carbonic Anhydrase II Deficiency in this chapter. Cases of "intermediate" osteopetrosis were delineated beginning in 1979 (59). This type first manifests during childhood with generally more mild symptoms and signs than occur in the malignant type. Survival beyond childhood appears to be possible, but its effect on longevity is uncertain (60,61). Intermediate osteopetrosis seems to be inherited as an autosomal recessive trait. In 1986, "lethal" osteopetrosis that presented with stillbirth was reported in two children of first cousins in Morocco (62). In 1987, the benign (adult) type of osteopetrosis was found in Denmark to occur in two distinct forms (55), and there has since been considerable investigation to distinguish their presentation and pathogenesis (63,64). Severe osteopetrosis that is accompanied by neuronal storage disease was reported in 1988 and seems to be inherited as an autosomal recessive trait (65). Lastly, in 1991 a form of "transient infantile" osteopetrosis was identified (66).

In many medical publications the term "osteopetrosis" is used to describe disorders where there is diffuse osteosclerosis on radiologic study. Such usage should now cease because the pathogenesis of the osteopetroses in man is now generally understood. Osteo*sclerosis* can be the outcome of combinations of disturbances in bone growth, modeling, and remodeling. For example, exuberant uncompensated bone formation, or mild yet chronically mismatched bone remodeling so that there is net formation of bone.

Osteopetrosis in man is caused by profound reduction or failure of osteoclast-mediated resorption of bone (67). Nevertheless, the mechanisms by which osteoclasts malfunction are poorly understood. The clinical/genetic nosology for the osteopetroses in man will certainly require revision in the near future. The molecular/biochemical basis for the various heritable types seems ripe for discov-

ery. However, it now appears increasingly likely that not all types of osteopetrosis have a genetic basis. Sporadic cases of marble bone disease are not uncommon and recent evidence suggests that for some of these patients there may be an infectious etiology (see below).

Clinical Presentation

Malignant (Infantile) Osteopetrosis

Malignant osteopetrosis is usually diagnosed during infancy (54). One of the earliest symptoms is nasal "stuffiness" due to underdevelopment of the paranasal and mastoid sinuses. Because cranial foramina also do not widen appropriately, there may be palsies of the optic, oculomotor, and facial nerves. Failure of the skeleton to model properly leads to inadequate space for marrow which is also often crowded by increased numbers of abnormal osteoclasts as well as fibrous tissue (see below). As a result, myelophthisic disturbances occur engendering extramedullary hematopoiesis and secondary hypersplenism. As leukopenia develops there are recurrent infections, and thrombocytopenia predisposes to bruising and bleeding. Understandably, affected children fail to thrive. Since the basal foramina do not widen properly, there eventually can be symptoms of ischemia due to arterial stenosis (68). Hydrocephalus and sleep apnea occur in some patients (69). Other neurological manifestations of malignant osteopetrosis are cerebral atrophy, irritability, developmental delay, dysarthria, and mental retardation (69). Vision can be impaired by retinal degeneration, chronic papilledema, and defective myelinization of the optic nerves (70). Individual teeth may be ankylosed within a sclerotic jaw and fail to erupt, or the failure of osteoclasts to resorb their roots can delay their shedding. Accordingly, osteomyelitis of the mandible is a frequent troublesome complication (71). The increased density of individual bones belies their mechanical properties—they are usually fragile and fracture is not uncommon. Because of the inability of osteoclasts to liberate mineral from the skeleton, some affected infants develop symptomatic hypocalcemia and associated rickets. On physical examination there is short stature, hepatosplenomegaly, knock-knee deformity, frontal bossing of a large head, strabismus, nystagmus, proptosis, optic atrophy, and perhaps papilledema. Children who do not respond to treatment (see below) often die during the first decade of life. Lethal complications include severe anemia, bleeding, pneumonia, and sepsis (54).

Intermediate Osteopetrosis

Intermediate osteopetrosis is characterized by short stature, macrocephaly with cranial nerve palsies, ankylosed teeth with osteomyelitis of the jaw, and recurrent fractures (60,61). Some affected subjects have mild or moderately severe anemia. Since few cases have been described and long-term follow-up is wanting, the prognosis is not well understood (Fig. 12 A and B).

Benign (Adult) Osteopetrosis

Benign osteopetrosis may be a developmental condition in which radiologic features unfold during childhood (53). Recent detailed kindred studies in Denmark indicate that two types of adult osteopetrosis in that country are distinguishable by their radiologic and biochemical features (55,63,64). Though most subjects with either of the two benign forms are asymptomatic (53), fractures do occur with increased frequency. Index cases are typically men, since they are more prone to suffer trauma (55). However, there may also be loss of vision, deafness, psychomotor delay, mandibular osteomyelitis, spondylolysis/spondylolisthesis, osteoarthritis, carpal tunnel syndrome, and hypogonadotropic hypogonadism (53,72). In some kindreds, nonpenetrance occurs; i.e.,

there are adults without skeletal radiologic abnormalities yet osteopetrosis is apparent in their offspring and predecessors (55). Accordingly, "skip generations" can occur. Conversely a severely affected child has been reported in two kindreds wherein osteopetrosis was otherwise benign (73).

Neuronal Storage Disease

Neuronal storage disease with osteopetrosis is an especially rare lethal syndrome in which the skeletal features of malignant osteopetrosis occur together with pronounced central nervous system changes including cerebral atrophy with ventricular dilatation, hypertonia, and seizures (65).

Lethal Osteopetrosis

Lethal osteopetrosis was described once and appears to be inherited as an autosomal recessive condition since

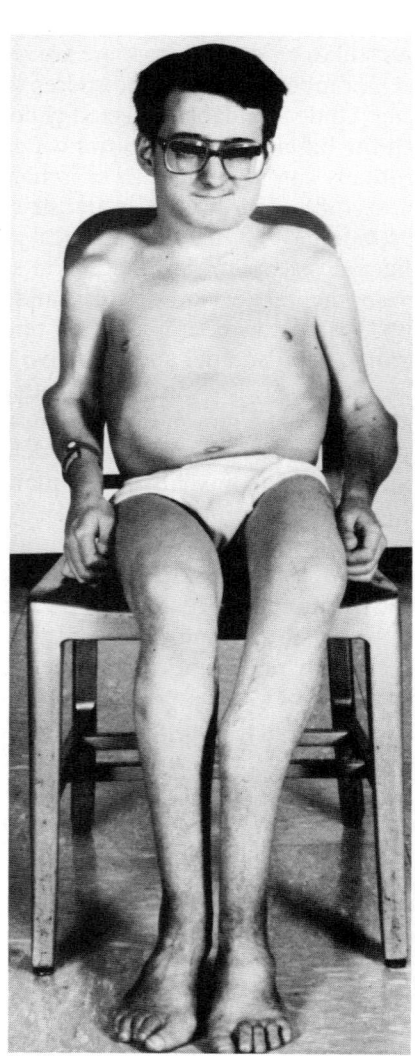
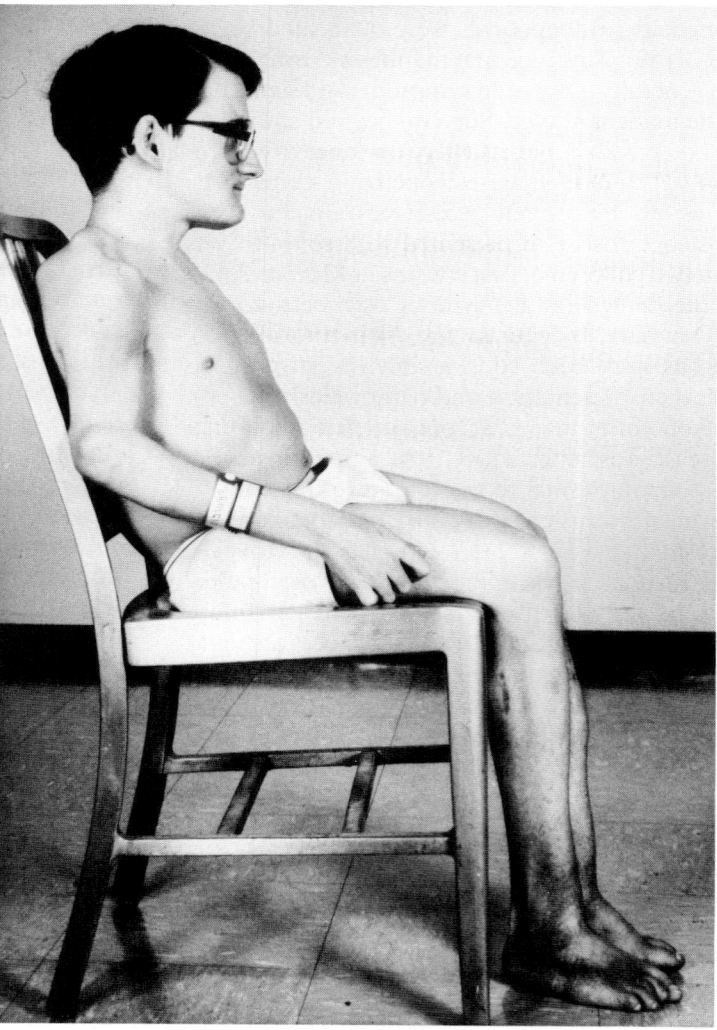

A   B

FIG. 12 A and B. Osteopetrosis (intermediate form). This 21-year-old man suffered from recurrent fracture, dental abscesses, and transfusion-dependent anemia.

the parents of the affected siblings were first cousins. It caused stillbirth but was detected in utero because of osteosclerosis and hydrocephaly (62).

Carbonic Anhydrase II Deficiency

Carbonic Anhydrase II Deficiency is reviewed in Section VI.

Transient Infantile Osteopetrosis

Transient infantile osteopetrosis has been described in one newborn who was suspected of having a dislocated hip but was well. Characteristic radiologic and histopathologic changes of osteopetrosis were documented (66). The condition resolved by 24 months of age.

Radiologic Features

Because all types of osteopetrosis in man cause universally defective bone resorption, the processes of skeletal modeling and remodeling are both disrupted (2,3). Together these aberrations engender the radiologic hallmark of generalized osteosclerosis (Fig. 13). The abnor-

mal modeling contributes to the symmetrically increased bone mass in part because tubulation of long bones does not occur properly, and also because characteristic abnormal widened contours of the long bones are produced (2,3). However, the severity of the resultant bony changes differs considerably according to the type of osteopetrosis. In the relatively severe cases, modeling defects produce broadened metadiaphyseal regions of the major long bones known as "Erlenmeyer flask deformity" (Fig. 14). An unexplained radiologic feature is the alternating dense/lucent bands that appear in the pelvis and at the ends of the major long bones in some patients. Rarely, the distal phalanges are resorbed. In the axial skeleton, the skull is thickened and dense especially at its base. The paranasal and mastoid sinuses are generally underdeveloped and underpneumatized. On lateral

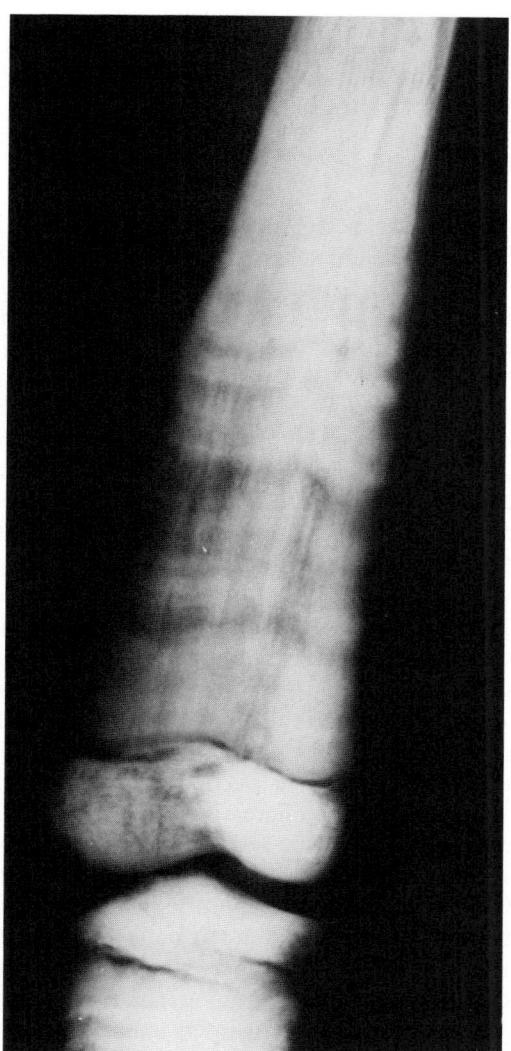

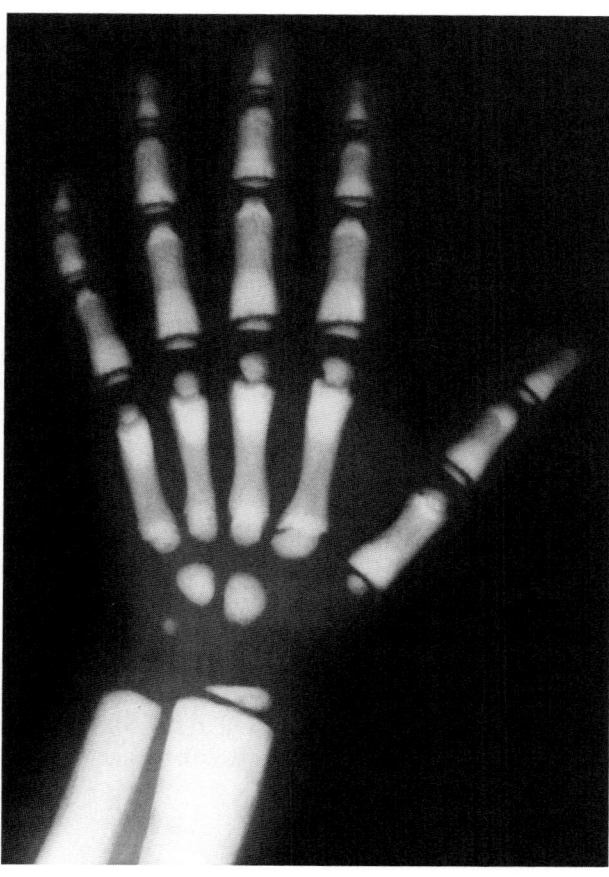

FIG. 13. Osteopetrosis (intermediate form). All of the bones of the forearm and hand of this boy aged 4 yr 9 mo show characteristic modeling defects and generalized osteosclerosis.

FIG. 14. Osteopetrosis (intermediate form). The distal femur of this 10-year-old boy shows a widened metadiaphyseal region (Erlenmeyer flask deformity) with characteristic alternating dense and lucent bands. From Whyte and Murphy (248), with permission.

view, one may see vertebrae with a "bone-in-bone" (endobone) or "sandwich" appearance. Rickets occurs in some children with severe osteopetrosis (see below) (74) and can cause confusion during attempted treatment. Within the past few years, reports of two types of benign osteopetrosis in Denmark indicate that the adult form is distinguished radiologically by either marked thickening and sclerosis of the cranial vault with diffuse sclerosis of vertebrae (type I), or selective thickening of the skull base with characteristic endobone formation in the spine (type II). Both types cause progressive osteosclerosis during childhood, yet skeletal modeling is not defective (75). Fractures are more common in type II disease (55).

Skeletal scintigraphy of patients with osteopetrosis has its customary utility to disclose fractures, osteomyelitis, etc. (76). Computed tomography has been reported to be the best technique for assessing optic nerve impingement by narrow foramena (77). Magnetic resonance imaging appears to be useful for determining the effects of bone marrow transplantation (see below), since engraftment will enlarge marrow spaces (78).

Laboratory Findings

Malignant osteopetrosis can be associated with hypocalcemia of sufficient severity to cause rickets (79). Diminished skeletal resorption together with ongoing bone formation seems to account for this disturbance in mineral homeostasis. Thus, serum calcium levels are conditioned principally by dietary calcium intake and absorption (80). Hypocalcemia causes secondary hyperparathyroidism with appropriately elevated serum $1,25(OH)_2D$ levels in such cases (81). Benign osteopetrosis is usually reported with normal levels of biochemical parameters that reflect mineral homeostasis. However, recent studies concerning the two forms of benign osteopetrosis describe increases in serum immunoreactive PTH levels in type II disease (55). Acid phosphatase activity that is tartrate-resistant and apparently originates from defective osteoclasts is often increased in the serum of patients with the various severe forms of osteopetrosis and those with type II benign disease (55). Recently, the intriguing observation has been made that the level of the "brain" isoenzyme of creatine kinase (EC 2.7.3.2) is frequently elevated in the serum of subjects with osteopetrosis (82), but not in other sclerosing bone disorders (83). It has been postulated that the relatively anaerobic environment within osteopetrotic bone alters the energy metabolism of cells within the marrow spaces to increase their dependence on creatine phosphate as a source of "high-energy phosphate" for intermediary metabolism.

Histopathologic Findings

In severe cases of osteopetrosis, the radiologic findings are characteristic (2,3). However, in the mild forms, the changes may not be diagnostic. Thus, it is especially noteworthy that the inability of osteoclasts to resorb bone engenders a pathognomonic histologic sign. This feature also provides unequivocal evidence of the pathogenesis of osteopetrosis (84,85). Osseous tissue that would normally be removed during skeletal modeling or remodeling instead persists life-long or is only very slowly resorbed. Accordingly, one sees primary spongiosa; i.e., the calcified cartilage deposited during endochondral bone formation, in appropriate specimens of bone. This primary spongiosa is detected as characteristic "islands" or "bars" of material encased within trabeculae. It becomes "trapped" in bone with distinctly different staining properties compared to lamellar bone throughout most parts of the adult skeleton during either epiphyseal (e.g., long bone) or apophyseal (e.g., iliac crest) skeletal formation (Color Plate A) (85). In other types of sclerosing bone dysplasia, some osteoclast activity occurs and this primary spongiosa is resorbed. Of note, however, recent reports concerning the two types of benign osteopetrosis indicate that cartilage bars may not persist lifelong when the disease is relatively mild. Primary spongiosa is seen in children but not always observed in affected adults in whom it is probably resorbed very gradually (55).

In the more common forms of osteopetrosis, osteoclasts are often increased in number (84). Malignant osteopetrosis typically shows numerous osteoclasts that are positioned correctly on the bony surfaces of trabecular bone or within Haversian canals (84). Nevertheless, ultrastructural abnormalities are present within these typically multinucleated cells. Electron microscopy often, but not invariably, discloses absence of a "ruffled border" of the plasma membrane where the cell is juxtaposed to the bone surface. This structure is characteristic of osteoclasts that are activity resorbing bone (84–86). Similarly, the osteoclasts found in malignant osteopetrosis generally lack a "clear zone" which is an organelle-free cytoplasmic area that is normally found adjacent to the ruffled border (86). Lastly, the numbers of nuclei can be unusually great. Benign osteopetrosis may also show osteoclasts that lack ruffled borders. Woven (disorganized) bone present throughout the skeleton and areas of osteoidosis are also common (55). The extremely unusual entity of lethal osteopetrosis is of particular interest because osteoclasts are rarely observed (62).

Though its pathogenesis is unclear, fibrous tissue often proliferates in the marrow spaces in severe osteopetrosis. This finding may, in part, be related to concomitant secondary hyperparathyroidism and can exacerbate the crowding of marrow cells (84,86).

Pathogenesis and Etiology

The cellular origin of the osteoclast is controversial, but is generally regarded to be a hematopoietic stem cell that is expressed in the monocyte/macrophage lineage (87). Hypothetically, fusion of tissue macrophages

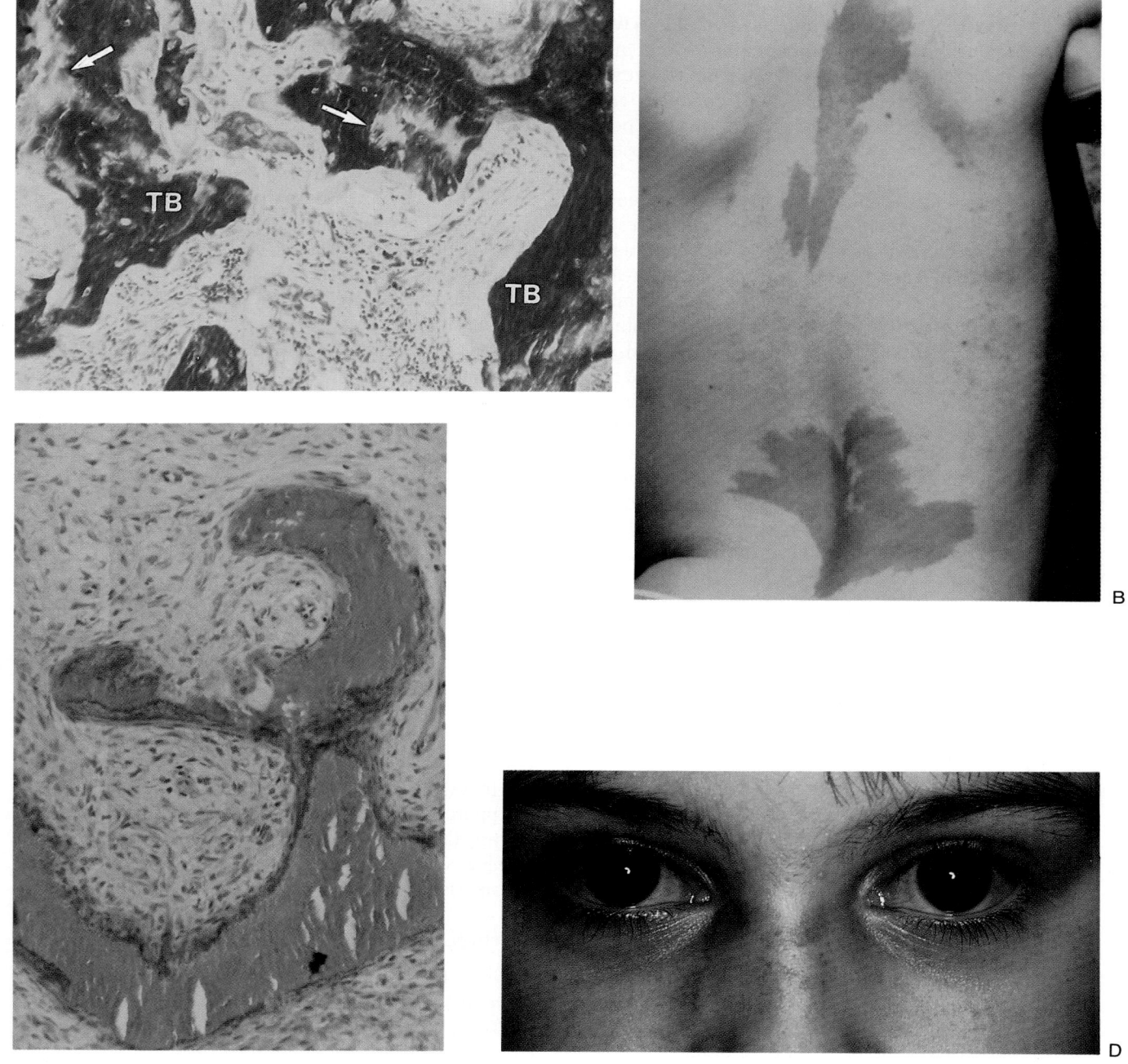

Color Plate A. Osteopetrosis (malignant form). Throughout darkly-blue-stained trabecular bone (TB) are characteristic light-staining "bars" of calcified primary spongiosa (*arrows*). Masson trichrome stain, ×250.

Color Plate B. McCune-Albright syndrome. Typical rough-border ("coast-of-Maine") pigmented café-au-lait spots are present on the back of this teenage boy.

Color Plate C. Fibrous dysplasia. Blue-staining trabecular bone is lined by darkly red-staining osteoid that is characteristically devoid of columnar-shaped osteoblasts. The marrow space is filled with swirls of fibrous tissue. Masson trichrome stain, ×250.

Color Plate D. Osteogenesis imperfecta. The sclerae of this $11\frac{1}{2}$-year-old-girl are markedly blue.

would then form the multinucleated osteoclast. This theory is supported by observations in two children with severe osteopetrosis who had dramatic improvement in their condition following successful bone marrow transplantation (see below). In each child, engrafted cells were demonstrated to be the precursors of their post-transplant functioning osteoclasts but not their osteoblasts (88,89).

Identification of two inheritance patterns for osteopetrosis (autosomal dominant and autosomal recessive) as well as characterization of a variety of clinical phenotypes show that several genetic abnormalities can greatly disrupt osteoclast-mediated bone resorption in man. However, the ultimate (molecular) basis for the heritable human types of osteopetrosis is yet to be understood. All forms that are genetically transmitted appear to be due to autosomal defects, but only for carbonic anhydrase II deficiency (see section on Carbonic Anhydrase II Deficiency, this chapter) has a specific biochemical disturbance been identified (58). Indeed, the heterogeneity of pathogenetic mechanisms among the many animal models for osteopetrosis also indicates that multiple biochemical/genetic defects will be found in humans (67). The pathogenesis of human osteopetrosis may include aberrations of osteoclast precursor cells themselves, or their microenvironment so that marrow elements fail to produce cytokines that foster stem cell maturation. Alternatively, mature osteoclasts could have defects within lysosomes so that degradation of osseous tissue is impaired, or they may not respond to hormonal stimulation or properly "recognize" osseous tissue. It could also be that in some patients the skeletal matrix itself is abnormal and refractory to resorption (67).

Subjects with malignant osteopetrosis have reportedly had aberrations of monocyte and granulocyte function detected in vitro (90). Nevertheless, disturbances indicative of clinically apparent immune deficiency are not common even in the severe forms (67). The hypothesis that defects in lysosome function may explain osteopetrosis with neuronal storage disease has come from several recent autopsy studies that describe degenerative neuronal changes characterized by diffuse axonal dystrophy and the presence of spheroidal bodies (65). Indeed, lysosomal abnormalities have been postulated for other clinical forms of osteopetrosis as well. Benign osteopetrosis may involve resistance to thyroid hormone and $1,25(OH)_2D$ in types I and II, respectively (55). Other investigations, including animal model studies, indicate that some patients may have disturbances in the generation of interleukin-2 (91), biosynthesize an abnormal PTH (92), or fail to elaborate factors essential for bone resorption such as superoxide (93). Evidence to support these pathogenetic mechanisms includes recent animal model studies in which bone resorption was successfully stimulated with macrophage colony-stimulating factor (94,95), with interleukin-2 (96), and by induction of superoxide with γ-interferon (97).

Finally, there is increasing evidence that some cases of osteopetrosis may have an infectious rather than genetic basis (98). Sporadic occurrences of osteopetrosis are not uncommon. Electron microscopy of several such cases has revealed viral inclusions in osteoclasts like those of the nucleocapsids of *Paramyxoviridae* (99). Respiratory syncytial virus or measles virus antigens have also been reported in osteoclasts (99). In 1990, a reverse transcriptase, like that made by retroviruses, was isolated from the supernatant of mononuclear blood cells in culture taken from a subject with benign osteopetrosis (98). Indeed, findings from animal model studies are also consistent with a retroviral etiology for some cases of benign or severe osteopetrosis. However, it is notable that viral inclusions in osteoclasts have been found in other bone disorders as well (e.g., Paget's bone disease, pycnodysostosis). Whether the viral inclusions reflect the etiology of the osteopetrosis or are an epiphenomenon remains unclear (99).

Treatment

As reviewed, the prognoses vary greatly for the different types of osteopetrosis and the pathogenetic defects seem to be diverse. Accordingly, a correct diagnosis from among the various clinical types is critical before treatment is undertaken. This is so because several therapeutic approaches (see below) have been used to increase skeletal resorption in this disorder. Some treatments, such as bone marrow transplantation, are hazardous and complex and would therefore be appropriate only for life-threatening or severely debilitating disease. It should be apparent that radiologic screening of the patient's family, together with careful assessment of how the patient's disease is progressing may be necessary to distinguish among the various clinical forms.

Marrow Transplantation

Since 1977, transplantation of HLA-identical bone marrow has been used to treat malignant osteopetrosis (100). Engraftment of allogeneic marrow has been shown in several affected subjects to result in significant clinical, laboratory, radiologic, and histopathologic improvement (85,88,89,100–103). Nevertheless, neurological abnormalities may persist despite successful transplantation. Subjects whose marrow space is overwhelmed by numerous osteoclasts and fibrous tissue seem more refractory to successful engraftment (84). Thus, histopathologic assessment of an iliac crest specimen may help to prognosticate the efficacy of marrow exchange. Accumulating experience indicates that successful transplantation and clinical improvement are more likely in young patients (<4 years of age) (103). As one would expect, however, not all subjects with malignant osteopetrosis respond to allogeneic marrow transplantation. Since there is likely heterogeneity for the pathogenesis of osteopetrosis, successful engraftment of normal osteoclasts could not be expected to benefit all patients (67,103). Marrow transplantation from HLA-nonidentical donors has been attempted for osteopetrosis, but requires further evaluation (102).

Dietary/Hormonal Treatment

Some success in treating osteopetrosis was reported in 1965 with a diet that was deficient in calcium (104). Paradoxically, recent findings caution that dietary calcium supplementation may occasionally be necessary for children with severe osteopetrosis to correct concomitant hypocalcemia that has caused rickets (79). Administration of a calcium-restricted diet has resulted in rickets in severe osteopetrosis that falsely suggested a beneficial response to marrow transplantation; the osteopenia in the region of the growth plates was from the mineralization defect, not from restoration of bone resorption (105).

$1,25(OH)_2D$ has been demonstrated to be important for the formation and activation of osteoclasts in several experimental systems (80). Recent observations indicate that some cases of osteopetrosis may involve resistance to $1,25(OH)_2D$ or defective $25(OH)D,1\alpha$-hydroxylase activity. Administration of high doses of $1,25(OH)_2D_3$ to a few severely affected patients seemed to have some therapeutic success (85). A preliminary report of an adult who had what appeared to be an intermediate form of osteopetrosis described decreased skeletal mass and improved hematopoiesis with long-term $1,25(OH)_2D_3$ treatment (106). The observation that intravenous infusions of PTH benefited a severely affected infant could be explained indirectly by enhanced renal $1,25(OH)_2D$ biosynthesis (92).

Supportive Therapy

Myelophthesis appears to explain much of the hematologic dysfunction in malignant osteopetrosis. Other factors, however, also exacerbate the anemia. Hemolysis can occur because myelophthisis engenders extramedullary hematopoiesis which in turn causes hypersplenism. Hemolysis also seems to result from other more poorly understood causes. It is important to recognize that high-dose glucocorticoid therapy helps to stabilize the hematologic status when there is pancytopenia and hepatosplenomegaly in malignant osteopetrosis (107). Furthermore, prednisone administration together with a low-calcium/high-phosphate diet has been reported to be effective overall treatment for severely affected subjects (108).

Hyperbaric oxygenation can be a significant adjunctive therapy for osteomyelitis. When dental sepsis is refractory to antibiotic and hyperbaric oxygen treatment, extraction of teeth may be necessary.

Surgical decompression of cranial nerves I and VII has benefited some subjects with associated palsies (69,77). Decompressive surgery for the optic nerve may help if the retina is spared as shown by electroretinography and slit-lamp examination (70).

Prenatal Diagnosis

Information concerning the prenatal diagnosis of osteopetrosis is generally wanting. The few relevant reports indicate that early in utero detection is often not possible by routine radiologic techniques. In 1943, a conventional x-ray examination reportedly detected unexpected osteopetrosis at 6 months gestation (109). Subsequently, however, malignant osteopetrosis was inapparent at 20 weeks gestation on routine radiographs (110). In 1986, ultrasonography was successful for prenatal diagnosis at 18 weeks gestation for the very rare "lethal" form (62).

CARBONIC ANHYDRASE II DEFICIENCY

Carbonic anhydrase II (CA II) isoenzyme deficiency was identified as an inborn error of metabolism in 1983 (58). In 1972, three independent publications from the United States and Europe delineated a new syndrome of osteopetrosis with renal tubular acidosis that was transmitted as an autosomal recessive trait (56). Cerebral calcification was found to be the third principal clinical feature in 1980 (57). However, the discovery three years later that an affected sibship from St. Louis had a marked deficiency of CA II in their red cells constituted the first elucidation of a fundamental biochemical defect for human osteopetrosis (58). In 1990, a preliminary report (see below) described a point mutation in a coding exon of the "candidate" CA II gene of one patient (111).

Clinical Presentation

More than 30 affected subjects have been reported in the medical literature (112,113). Most cases have occurred in the Mediterranean region or in the Middle East (112). Labor and delivery are usually uneventful and the disorder is typically not recognized until late in infancy or during early childhood. At that time, patients present with developmental delay, failure to thrive, short stature, or fracture (112). In some subjects, apathy, hypotonia, and muscle weakness may be due to the underlying renal tubular acidosis. Hypokalemic weakness or paralysis can rarely occur episodically and appears to be another manifestation of the kidney defect. Dental malocclusion is a frequent finding. Blindness can develop from compression of the optic nerves. Mental subnormality, to various degrees, is common but not invariable. In keeping with other forms of osteopetrosis, long bones are brittle and although most patients do not fracture, recurrent breaks may cause significant morbidity (112,113). The long-term consequences of CA II deficiency are not understood. Life span is not well studied, but may be normal. Case III among the St. Louis siblings (Fig. 15; extreme left) (57) is micrognathic and remains obese at 34 years of age and has developed severe sleep apnea. This complication has also been reported in malignant osteopetrosis (114).

Radiologic Features

Bony abnormalities have been noted at the time of diagnosis in all cases, though one newborn had only subtle radiographic signs (115). CA II deficiency resembles other forms of osteopetrosis except that cerebral calcification is present and the osteosclerosis, as well as the defects in skeletal modeling, can diminish gradually (57,115). This latter feature contrasts to the other types of osteopetrosis in which osteosclerosis may increase with aging (2,3). The cerebral calcification begins at about 5 years of age and becomes more pronounced during childhood. Computed tomography reveals that it affects cortical gray matter as well as the basal ganglia. This calcification is similar if not identical to that which is found in idiopathic hypoparathyroidism or in pseudohypoparathyroidism (116).

Laboratory Findings

Metabolic acidosis has been documented in affected neonates (115). Either proximal or distal renal tubular acidosis, or both types together, have been reported (117). There is, however, no further evidence of Fanconi's syndrome (112). When anemia is present, it is usually mild and has a nutritional basis.

Histopathologic Findings

The bone marrow is typically unremarkable. The cartilage "bars" that are characteristic of all human forms of osteopetrosis and reflect unresorbed primary spongiosa (see section on Osteopetrosis, this chapter) have been documented in iliac crest specimens from four affected subjects in two families with CA II deficiency (57).

Pathogenesis and Etiology

In 1983, deficiency of CA II was discovered in the erythrocyte lysates of each of three sisters (Fig. 15) with

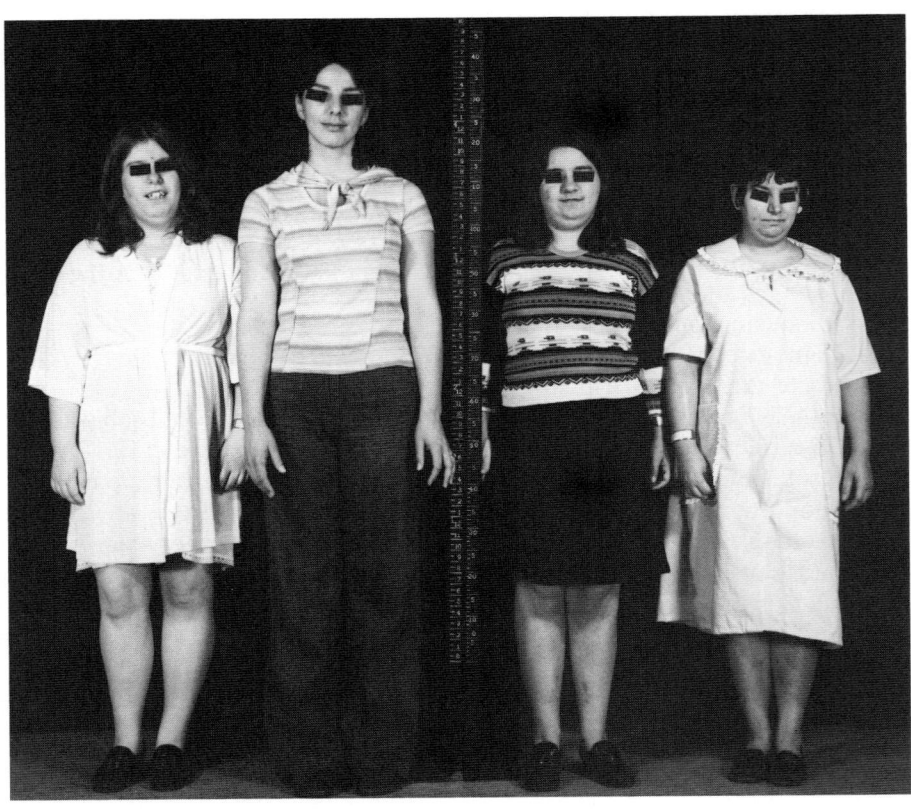

FIG. 15. Carbonic anhydrase II deficiency. Three of 4 sisters are affected and have short stature. From Whyte et al. (57), with permission.

the syndrome of osteopetrosis, renal tubular acidosis, and cerebral calcification (58). CA I levels were normal. CA II activity, protein, and immunoreactivity were profoundly deficient. In keeping with an inborn error of metabolism that was transmitted as an autosomal recessive trait, approximately half-normal CA II levels were found in their parents' erythrocytes (58). These findings were documented soon after in all of 21 patients available for study who represented 12 unrelated kindreds of diverse geographic and ethnic origins (56).

Autopsy findings in CA II deficiency have not been reported. Lack of CA II remains to be demonstrated directly in tissues other than blood. However, absence of CA II in patient urine supports the hypothesis that the enzyme is diminished in the kidney and that the deficiency is generalized (118). Furthermore, the pleotropic clinical manifestations of the syndrome (58), recent evidence of mutation in the CA II gene of one typical subject (see below), and the observations from a mouse model developed by mutagenesis (119) all indicate that a global deficiency of CA II activity will be found in affected subjects.

The discovery of CA II deficiency as a new inborn error of metabolism provides compelling evidence that CA II has an important function in bone and kidney and perhaps in the brain (56,58). CA II has the widest tissue distribution of the CAs and includes the kidney, brain, erythrocytes, and elsewhere (120). CA accelerates the association of CO_2 and H_2O to form H_2CO_3 which then rapidly dissociates to H^+ and HCO_3^-. CA II is a cytosolic isoenzyme and the most active CA. Thus, CA II acts critically in acid/base homeostasis.

Significantly, CA II is the CA isoenzyme found in osteoclasts (121). A variety of evidence indicates that the osteoclast must acidify its pericellular milieu if it is to be able to resorb bone (122). During skeletal resorption, the ruffled membrane of this cell forms an enclosure over the adjacent osseous tissue. This enclosure in effect becomes an extracellular lysosome in which the pH may decrease to as low as 5.5. Such potent acidification appears to be made possible by the H^+ pump that is responsible for acid secretion by the kidney tubule (123). At this high H^+ concentration, bone mineral is solubilized and concomitantly collagenases and other proteases become active in order to degrade the demineralized skeletal matrix (123). In CA II deficiency, absence of cytosolic CA II impairs the intracellular interaction of CO_2 and H_2O to form H_2CO_3 and thus disrupts production of H^+ for transport and acidification of the extracellular milieu. Ironically, osteoclast-mediated bone resorption is blocked despite a systemic metabolic acidosis stemming from the renal tubular defect that might otherwise be buffered by HCO_3^- release from the skeleton. Indeed, inhibition of CA activity by a variety of pharmacologic agents blunts skeletal resorption in vitro (124). The in vivo experience is controversial (125).

Erythrocytes from CA II deficiency patients appear to have sufficient CA activity from CA I to fulfill the minimum requirements at rest for respiratory gas exchange in the circulation (126). The observation that subjects with CA II deficiency enhance their bicarboniduria upon receiving an intravenous dose of the CA inhibitor, acetazolamide, indicates that a CA isoenzyme in addition to CA II functions in the kidney (117). Indeed, recently, CA IV was detected in the urine of CA II deficiency patients (118). Further studies will, however, be necessary to refine our understanding of the pathogenesis of the disturbed acid/base homeostasis (117,118). Why cerebral calcification occurs in this disorder is not understood. Recent development of a mouse model for CA II deficiency should enable these questions to be explored (119).

In the Middle East, consanguinity is a common etiologic factor for CA II deficiency. This fact also helps to explain the prevalence of the disorder in that region (115). The variable clinical severity of this condition noted among affected families and the somewhat widespread geographic distribution suggest, however, that there is some genetic heterogeneity (58). Be this as it may, variable clinical expression has been noted even within sibships and epigenetic factors appear to influence the severity of this disorder (113).

The locus of the CA II gene is on the long arm of chromosome 8 in man (58,120), and the cDNA and gene have been cloned and sequenced (120). The molecular defects that cause CA II deficiency now seem to be on the verge of discovery (111). Indeed, a preliminary report describes a missense mutation in a coding region of the CA II gene in the Belgian patient who was among the subjects initially reported with this disorder (111). Different allelic defects in the "candidate" CA II gene, however, will probably be found and help to explain some of the clinical heterogeneity (58).

Treatment

There is no established therapy for this disorder. Therapeutic trials have been attempted in only a few subjects. Whether the systemic acidosis should be treated is not at all clear. The outcome of long-term administration of alkali is unknown. Correction of the systemic metabolic acidosis could, in theory, negate its beneficial effect to stimulate mineral release from the skeleton in order to simultaneously provide bicarbonate buffer. Indeed, subjects may benefit from untreated acidosis since skeletal density may decrease over time (57).

Transfusion of CA II-replete red cells to case III of the affected sisters from St. Louis did not affect her systemic acidosis (127). This finding suggests that the acidification defect is intrinsic to the kidney since it is not remedial by correcting CA II deficiency in circulating erythrocytes. Although the seemingly satisfactory prognosis for

CA II deficiency together with the current risks of bone marrow transplantation preclude this procedure as a therapy, the above finding indicates that marrow engraftment that might favorably affect the skeleton would leave the renal tubular acidosis uncorrected (127).

Prenatal Diagnosis

Attempts to diagnose CA II deficiency in utero have not been reported.

PROGRESSIVE DIAPHYSEAL DYSPLASIA

Progressive diaphyseal dysplasia was first characterized in 1920 by Cockayne (128). It is also known, however, by the eponym Camurati-Engelmann disease. Englemann described the typical severe form in 1929 (129); Camurati found that it is transmitted as an autosomal dominant trait (130). More than 100 case reports appear in the medical literature. They reveal that progressive diaphyseal dysplasia is a developmental disorder where the clinical and radiologic penetrance is rather variable (131). Indeed, "skip generations" in which obligate carriers show no radiologic abnormalities have been described. The characteristic feature is new bone formation that gradually spreads along both the endosteal and periosteal surfaces of the diaphyses of major long bones (132). In severe cases, the osteosclerosis can be more generalized and involve the skull and axial skeleton.

Clinical Presentation

During childhood, patients develop limping or a waddling and broad-based gait. Leg pain is common and muscle wasting with decreased subcutaneous fat is noted in the limbs. The disorder is not infrequently mistaken for a form of muscular dystrophy until skeletal radiographs are examined (133). Severely affected subjects share a very similar body habitus that includes thin limbs with little muscle mass yet palpably thickened bones (Fig. 16). When the skull is involved, the head may be large with a prominent forehead and proptosis. Cranial nerve palsies and raised intracranial pressure can also occur. Delayed puberty may result from hypothalamic hypogonadotropic hypogonadism (personal observation). Physical findings also include palpable skeletal tenderness in affected areas. Occasionally, there is hepatosplenomegaly. Some patients have Raynaud's phenomenon and other findings suggestive of vasculitis (134,135). Although progressive osteosclerosis can occur, the clinical course is variable and affected subjects may have remission of symptoms during adulthood (135).

Radiologic Features

The principal radiologic feature is progressive endosteal and periosteal new bone formation of the major long bones (2,3,136). The tibiae and femora are involved most commonly. Less frequently, the humeri, radii, ulnae, and occasionally the short tubular bones are affected as well (Fig. 17). Gradually, hyperostosis that begins in diaphyses spreads to affect metaphyses as well. However, the epiphyses are spared. As subperiosteal bone formation continues, the diaphyseal shafts widen and develop irregular surfaces. The pelvis, clavicles, and scapulae can also become sclerosed. Expressivity is, however, very variable. The age-of-onset, affected skeletal sites, rate of progression, and severity of the osteosclerosis differ considerably from patient to patient. Radiologic findings may be limited to the long bones of the lower extremities when the disorder is relatively mild. Osteopenia is found in some regions of the skeleton in children with severe disease. Hyperostosis of the calvarium and the base of the skull can mimic craniodiaphyseal dysplasia (Table 1).

Bone scintigraphy typically shows increased accumulation of radionuclide in diseased areas. In general the clinical, radiologic, and scintigraphic findings are concordant (137). However, in some subjects, considerable radiologic abnormality can be present although bone scans are unimpressive. This situation appears to reflect advanced but quiescent disease. Conversely, a marked increase in radioisotope uptake in the skeleton despite few radiologic abnormalities seems to reflect early and active disease (137).

Laboratory Findings

Most routine biochemical parameters of bone and mineral homeostasis are unremarkable in progressive diaphyseal dysplasia. However, the urinary hydroxyproline levels are elevated in some subjects. Modest hypocalcemia and pronounced hypocalciuria does occur when the disease is severe. These latter findings probably reflect a markedly positive calcium balance (138). An elevated erythrocyte sedimentation rate together with mild anemia and leukopenia lend credence to the hypothesis that this is a systemic disease (see below) (134,135).

Histopathologic Findings

At the most peripheral regions of periosteal new bone formation there is disorganized "woven" osseous tissue. Centrally, this woven bone appears to undergo a process of remodeling and maturation until it is incorporated into the diaphyseal cortex by "cancellous compaction" (132).

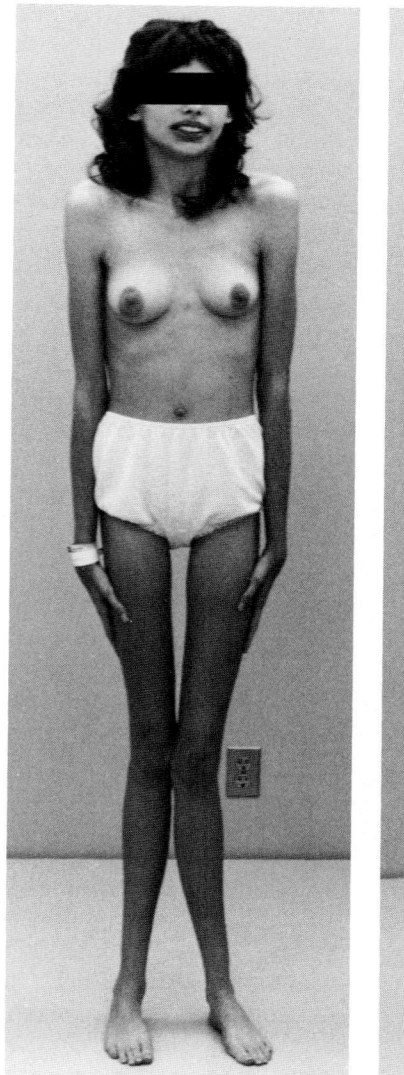 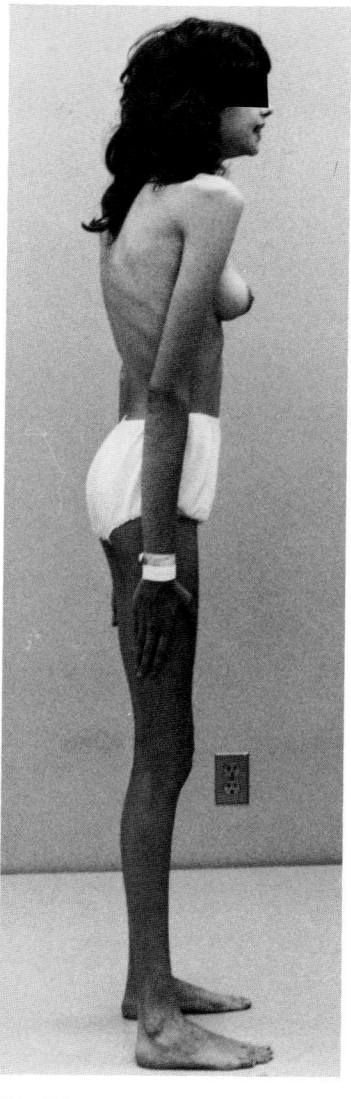

A   B

FIG. 16 A and B. Progressive diaphyseal dysplasia. This 17-year-old woman has the characteristic body habitus including thin extremities with lack of soft tissue mass and palpable thickening of the long bones.

Electron microscopy of muscle has revealed isolated muscle fiber atrophy together with accumulation of endomysial collagen fibrils. These histopathologic abnormalities are similar in both sporadic and familial cases (133). In one patient, type II muscle fiber atrophy was found on light microscopy, but degenerative changes were not present on electron microscopic study (139).

Etiology and Pathogenesis

Progressive diaphyseal dysplasia, like many of the other sclerosing bone disorders (Table 1), is caused by a gene defect at an autosomal locus that remains to be mapped and characterized. Especially mild cases have been reported to reflect a different (autosomal recessive) disorder called Ribbing's disease (140). However, mild

and severe cases can occur in the same kindred and reflect an autosomal dominant trait (M. P. Whyte and W. A. Murphy, unpublished observation). Accordingly, Ribbing's disease may reflect sporadic occurrence of mild progressive diaphyseal dysplasia. Some of the clinical and laboratory manifestations of progressive diaphyseal dysplasia, together with its ready responsiveness to glucocorticoid treatment, indicate that it is a heritable inflammatory connective tissue disease (134,135).

Treatment

Progressive diaphyseal dysplasia is a chronic and somewhat unpredictable condition. Symptoms may remit spontaneously during adolescence or early adult years. Since 1967, substantial evidence has accumulated that

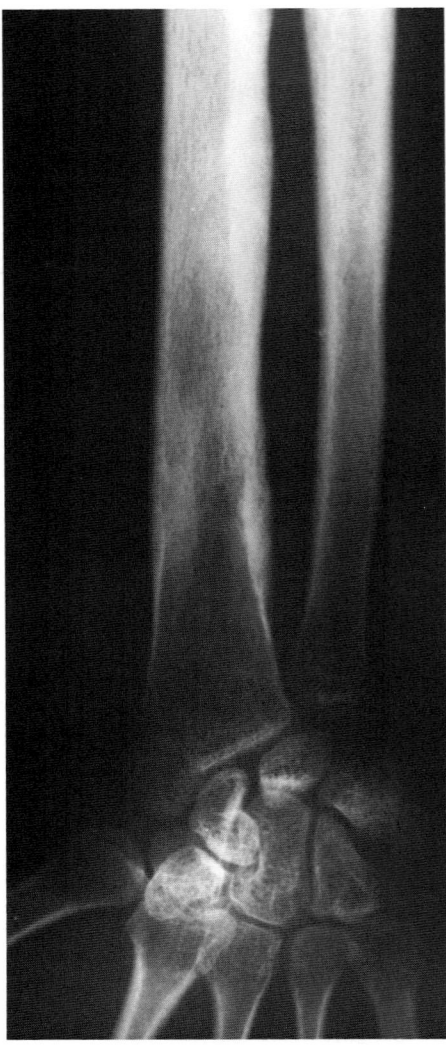

FIG. 17. Progressive diaphyseal dysplasia. The diaphyseal shafts of the radius and ulna of the patient depicted in Fig. 16 show characteristic endosteal and periosteal sclerosis.

shows that glucocorticoid therapy is quite helpful. Alternate-day, low-dose treatment with prednisone has been reported to relieve bone pain in most cases (141). Furthermore, there are a few descriptions of normalization of the histopathologic changes in affected bone (141). A preliminary report of intermittent use of the diphosphonate compound, disodium etidronate (Didronel), describes improved symptoms in one subject (142). Two adolescents with mild disease had complete relief of localized tibial pain after surgical removal of an affected area of diaphyseal bone and creation of a "cortical window" (personal observation) (132).

PYCNODYSOSTOSIS

This skeletal dysplasia was first characterized in 1962 (143). More than 100 cases representing 50 kindreds

have been reported. It is inherited as an autosomal recessive trait and parental consanguinity has been noted in about 30% of patients. Most case reports have come from the United States or Europe, but the disorder is found in Indonesia, Asian Indians, Israel, African blacks, and appears to be particularly prevalent in the Japanese (144). Pycnodysostosis is believed to have affected the French impressionist painter Henri de Toulouse-Lautrec (1864–1901) (145).

Clinical Presentation

Pycnodysostosis is typically diagnosed during infancy or early childhood. Affected subjects have a variety of dysmorphic features that include a small facies and chin, fronto-occipital prominence, beaked and pointed nose, relatively large cranium, and obtuse mandibular angle (146). Acro-osteolysis or aplasia of the terminal phalanges causes shortening of the fingers. The hands are small and square and the fingernails are hypoplastic. The thorax is narrow and there may be kyphoscoliosis, *pectus excavatum,* and a pronounced lumbar lordosis. There is disproportionate short stature. Adult height ranges between 4 ft 3 in and 4 ft 11 in. Physical examination also reveals a high-arch palate, dental malocclusion, ankylosed retained deciduous teeth, and bluish sclerae. The anterior fontanel and other cranial sutures remain patent (146). Recurrent fractures often involve the lower limbs and may result in *genu valgum* deformity. Generally, however, affected subjects are able to walk independently. There are descriptions of atypical individuals who have visceral manifestations and rickets. Mental retardation is present in about 10% of cases (146). Right heart failure may develop due to chronic upper airway obstruction from micrognathia in some patients. Recurrent respiratory infections may also be a troublesome complication.

Radiologic Features

Many of the radiologic features of pycnodysostosis are also found in osteopetrosis; e.g., both disorders cause generalized uniform osteosclerosis that appears during childhood and increases with age (2,3,147). Both conditions are associated with recurrent fracture. Nevertheless, the marked modeling defects of severe osteopetrosis do not occur in pycnodysostosis. The long bones are properly shaped but are radiodense because of thick cortices that narrow the medullary canals. Additional radiologic findings that help to distinguish pycnodysostosis from osteopetrosis include delayed closure of cranial sutures (especially the anterior fontanel) (Fig. 18), obtuse mandibular angle, wormian bones, gracile clavicles that are hypoplastic laterally, hypoplasia or aplasia of the distal phalanges (Fig. 19) and ribs, and partial absence of

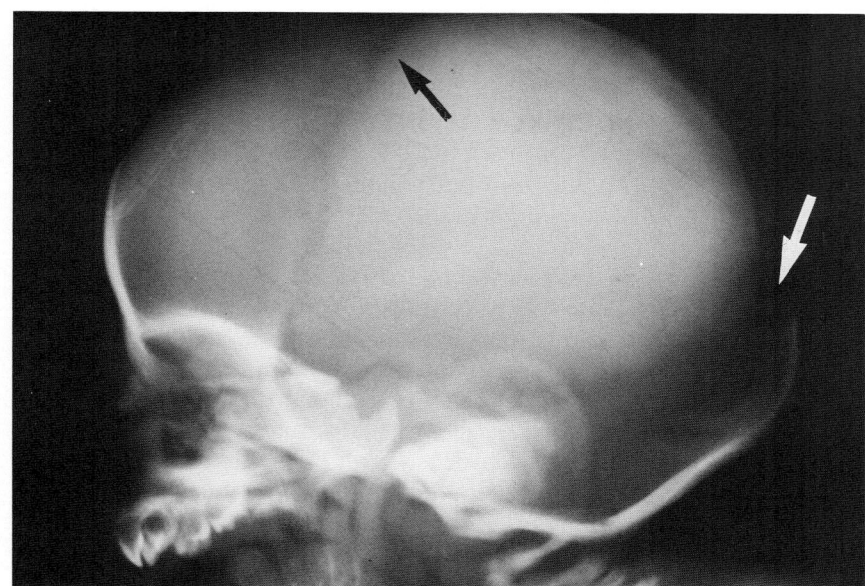

FIG. 18. Pycnodysostosis. This infant skull shows cranial sutures that are markedly widened (*arrows*); the base is sclerotic. Courtesy of Dr. William H. McAlister, St. Louis, MO. From Whyte and Murphy (248), with permission.

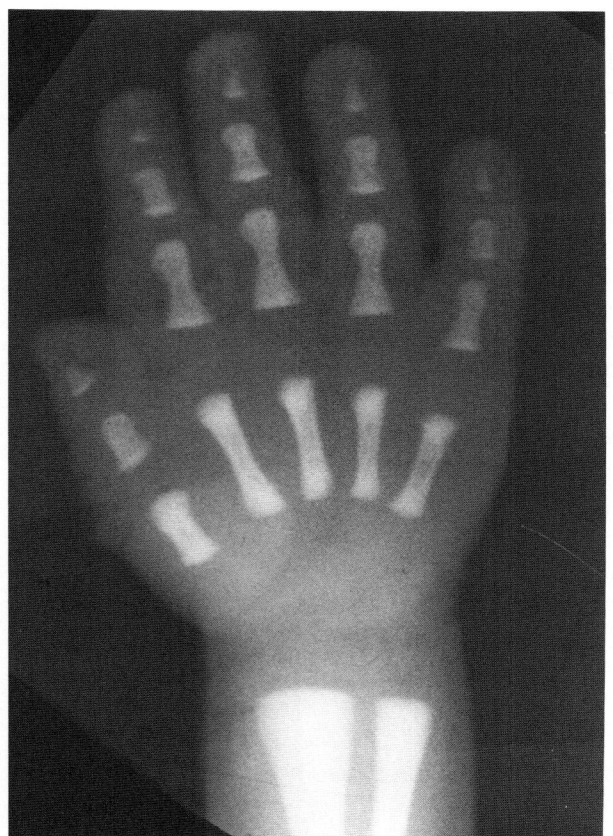

FIG. 19. Pycnodysostosis. The bones are sclerotic and the distal phalanges are hypoplastic. Courtesy of Dr. William H. McAlister, St. Louis, MO. From Whyte and Murphy (248), with permission.

the hyoid bone (147). In pycnodysostosis, the calvarium and the base of the skull are sclerotic and the orbital ridges are radiodense. Hypoplasia of sinuses, facial bones, and terminal phalanges is characteristic. Vertebrae are sclerotic with anterior and posterior concavities, yet the transverse processes are uninvolved. Lack of segmentation of the atlas and axis and lumbosacral spondylolisthesis are not uncommon. Madelung's deformity may affect the forearms. The endobones and radiodense striations that are characteristic of osteopetrosis are absent (2,3,147).

Laboratory Findings

Serum calcium and inorganic phosphate levels as well as alkaline phosphatase activity are typically normal. Anemia is not a feature of pycnodysostosis.

Histopathologic Findings

Cortical bone structure seems to be normal although there is the appearance of decreased osteoclastic and osteoblastic activity (148). Thus skeletal turnover may be decreased. Electron microscopy of osseous tissue from two affected subjects revealed changes that suggested that the degradation of collagen could be defective. It is uncertain if this observation reflects an abnormality in the bone matrix or in the osteoclast (149). In chondrocytes, abnormal inclusions have been described.

Etiology and Pathogenesis

The molecular basis for pycnodysostosis is unknown. Virus-like inclusions were found in the osteoclasts of two affected brothers (150). Absorption of dietary calcium has been noted to be markedly increased. Since both the size of the exchangeable calcium pool and the rate of bone accretion may be reduced (151), diminished rates of bone resorption may be a fundamental pathogenetic mechanism. This hypothesis would seem to be consistent with the histologic findings above.

Treatment

There is no effective medical therapy for pycnodysostosis. Fractures of the long bones are typically transverse, but heal at a satisfactory rate. However, delayed union and massive callus formation has been reported. Internal fixation of long bones is difficult because of their hardness. Extraction of teeth is similarly risky, since fracture of the jaw has occurred in some subjects (146). Osteomyelitis of the mandible may require treatment by a combined antibiotic/surgical approach. Perhaps, hyperbaric oxygenation would be helpful as it is in osteopetrosis.

ENDOSTEAL HYPEROSTOSIS

In 1955, van Buchem and colleagues described a new disease entity that they called hyperostosis corticalis generalisata (152). Subsequently, it appeared that this condition was one among several that could best be classified as endosteal hyperostosis. Van Buchem's disease is an autosomal recessive and clinically severe disorder (152). A less deforming autosomal dominant form of endosteal hyperostosis was designated the "Worth type" (152,153). Endosteal hyperostosis with syndactyly is also known as sclerosteosis. Van Buchem's disease is considerably rarer than the number of literature reports might suggest (154). Furthermore, it may reflect the same gene defect as sclerosteosis (see below).

Van Buchem's Disease

Clinical Presentation

Van Buchem's disease has been reported in children and adults. The incidence in males and females seems to be equal. During puberty, progressive asymmetrical enlargement of the jaw occurs. The adult mandible is markedly thickened with a wide angle; yet there is no prognathism and dental malocclusion is uncommon. Although some affected subjects are symptom-free, in the others recurrent facial nerve palsy, deafness, and/or optic atrophy from narrowing of cranial foramina occur as early as infancy. Long bones may be painful to applied pressure, but they are not fragile and joint range-of-motion is typically normal.

Radiologic Features

Endosteal cortical thickening produces a dense homogeneous diaphyseal cortex (2,3). Hyperostosis is selectively endosteal and the long bones are properly modeled. The medullary canal is narrowed. Generalized osteosclerosis may also affect the facial bones, base of the skull, vertebrae, ribs, and pelvis. The mandible becomes enlarged (Fig. 20).

Laboratory Findings

Alkaline phosphatase activity in serum may be increased. In such cases, it is primarily of skeletal origin. Calcium and inorganic phosphate levels in serum are unremarkable.

Histopathologic Findings

Van Buchem and colleagues indicated that the appearance of the excessive bone was essentially normal.

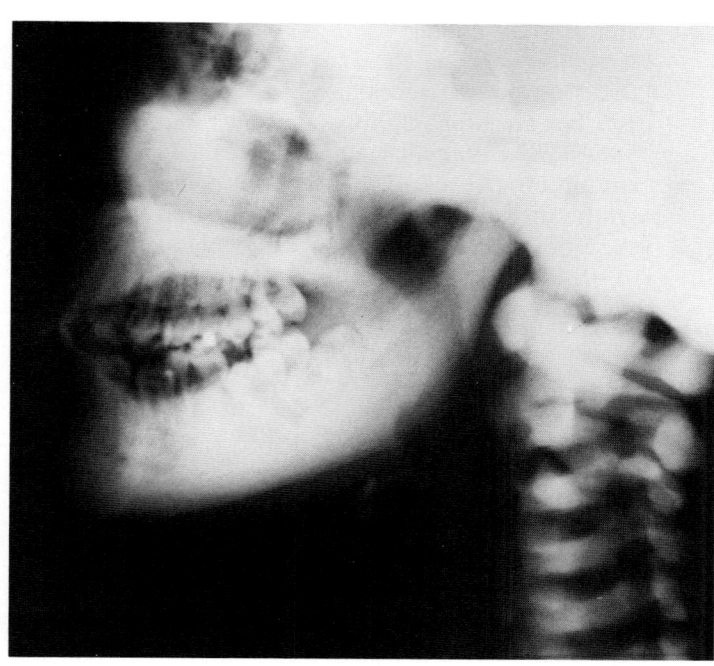

FIG. 20. Endosteal hyperostosis. The mandible and facial bones show dense sclerosis of all osseous structures. From Whyte and Murphy (248), with permission.

Etiology and Pathogenesis

Recently, evidence has been published which indicates that van Buchem's disease and sclerosteosis share the same genetic defect. Their clinical/radiologic differences may be explained by the effects of modifying genes (155).

Treatment

Surgical decompression of narrowed foramina may be helpful for cranial nerve palsies.

Sclerosteosis

Sclerosteosis (cortical hyperostosis with syndactyly) is transmitted as an autosomal recessive trait. It occurs with greatest prevalence in the Afrikaners of South Africa. Affected subjects from other regions are also often of Dutch ancestry (155).

Clinical Presentation

At birth, only syndactyly may be noted (156). It is the result of either bony or cutaneous fusion of the middle and index fingers and is of variable severity. However, during early childhood, overgrowth of the skeleton involves especially the skull and causes facial disfigurement. Soon after, affected subjects are noted to be distinctly tall and heavy. The term *gigantism* has been used to describe their appearance. The mandible has a square configuration. Facial palsy and deafness from cranial nerve entrapment can also be presenting problems. Raised intracranial pressure and headache may be complications of a small cranial cavity. The brain stem can

be compressed. Affected subjects are not fracture-prone, and their intelligence is normal. Life expectancy may be shortened (157).

Radiologic Features

In early childhood, unless syndactyly is present, the skeleton appears normal. The major radiologic aberration is developmental progressive bony thickening that widens the skull and causes prognathism of the mandible (2,3,158). Modeling defects occur in the long bones and their cortices are thickened. Syndactyly, typically involves the index and middle fingers. The vertebral pedicles, ribs, pelvis, and other tubular bones can become radiodense. Computed tomography has revealed that ossicle fusion and narrowing of the internal auditory canal and the cochlear aqueduct seem to explain the hearing loss.

Histopathologic Findings

In one affected subject from an American kindred, histomorphometric analysis of the calvarium following in vivo tetracycline labeling suggested that the rate of bone formation was increased. Osteoclastic bone resorption seemed to be quiescent (159).

Etiology and Pathogenesis

Uncoupling of bone remodeling with enhanced osteoblast activity and failure of osteoclasts to compensate for it appears to explain the osteosclerosis (159). No abnormality of pituitary function or of calcium homeostasis has been documented (160). The pathogenesis of the neurological defects has been discussed in some detail (159).

Sclerosteosis has, until recently (155), been differentiated from van Buchem's disease because affected subjects are excessively tall and have syndactyly. A recent comparison of the two conditions, however, suggests that both disorders may be caused by abnormalities in the same gene. The phenotypic variation perhaps results from epistatic effects of modifying genes (155).

Treatment

There is no specific medical treatment. Surgical correction of syndactyly is difficult if it is due to bony fusion. Correction of prognathism is complicated by the dense bone (161). Management of the neurological complications has been reviewed (159).

OSTEOPOIKILOSIS

Osteopoikilosis literally translated means "spotted bones." It is a radiologic curiosity that is transmitted as a highly penetrant autosomal dominant trait (162). In some kindreds, affected subjects also have connective tissue nevi known as *dermatofibrosis lenticularis disseminata*. These combined abnormalities constitute the Buschke-Ollendorff syndrome (163). Typically, the bony lesions of osteopoikilosis are asymptomatic but, when incorrectly diagnosed, rigorous and expensive studies for other disorders such as metastatic disease often precede the correct diagnosis (164).

Clinical Presentation

Musculoskeletal aches have been described in many cases but are probably unrelated. *Dermatofibrosis lenticularis disseminata* usually involves the lower trunk or extremities. This dermatosis appears typically as small asymptomatic papules. However, they are sometimes yellow or white discs or deep nodules, plaques, or streaks (163). Skin changes present before puberty; occasionally they are congenital.

Radiologic Features

Numerous small, variably-shaped (usually round or oval) foci of bony sclerosis within cancellous bone is the characteristic radiologic finding (2,3,165). The ends of the short tubular bones, the metaepiphyseal regions of the long bones, and the tarsal, carpal, and pelvic bones are commonly affected (Fig. 21). The foci may mimic metastatic lesions, but actually remain unchanged in shape and size for decades. Furthermore, radionuclide accumulation is not increased on bone scanning (164).

Histopathologic Studies

Dermatofibrosis lenticularis disseminata consists of excessive amounts of unusual markedly-branched, interlacing, broad elastin fibers in the dermis (164).

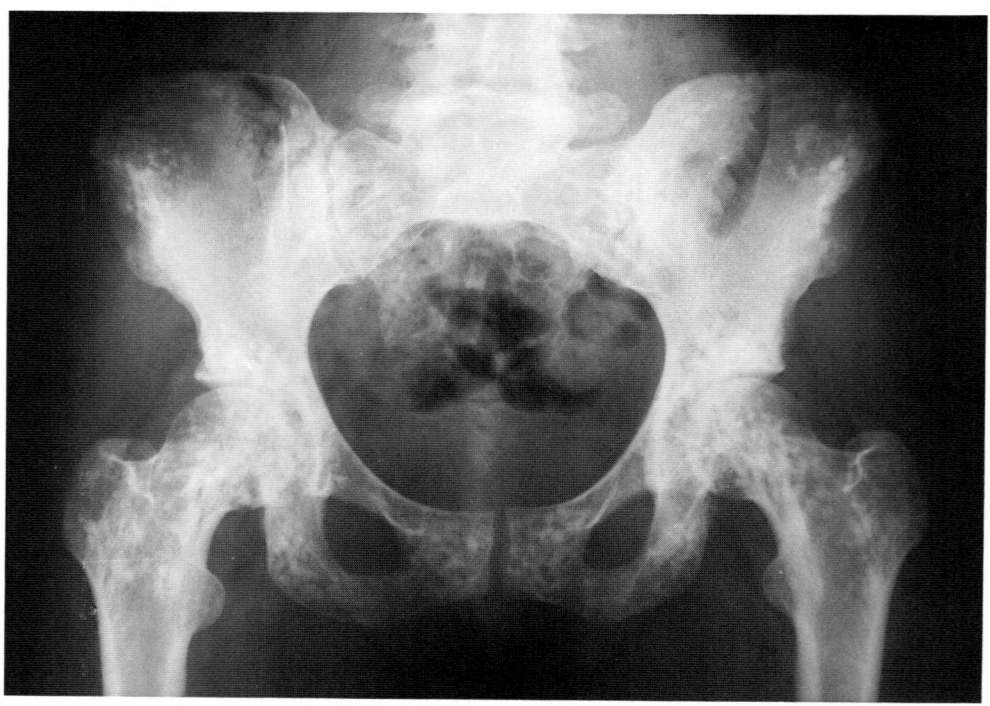

FIG. 21. Osteopoikilosis. The proximal femora and pelvis of this middle-aged woman show numerous characteristic round and oval punctate radiodensities.

The bony lesions are thickened trabeculae that merge with surrounding normal bone or are islands of cortical bone that include Haversian systems. Mature lesions appear as though they are remodeling slowly (166).

Treatment

Osteopoikilosis does not require treatment. However, family members at risk should be screened with a radiograph of the forearm and knee after childhood. If affected, they should be educated concerning the condition.

OSTEOPATHIA STRIATA

Osteopathia striata is characterized by linear striations in the ilium and the ends of long bones (2,3). When the striations occur as an isolated finding, like in osteopoikilosis, the condition is a radiographic curiosity. However, as discussed below, osteopathia striata is a feature of a variety of clinically important syndromes that include: osteopathia striata with focal dermal hypoplasia (Goltz's syndrome) and osteopathia striata with cranial sclerosis (167).

Clinical Presentation

When osteopathia striata occurs alone, it is transmitted as an autosomal dominant trait. Musculoskeletal symptoms that may have led to its discovery are proba-
bly unrelated. However, when there is cranial sclerosis, cranial nerve palsies are not uncommon (167). This disorder is also transmitted as an autosomal dominant trait. Goltz's syndrome is a serious X-linked recessive condition. The affected boys have widespread linear areas of dermal hypoplasia through which adipose tissue can herniate. In Goltz's syndrome, there can also be a variety of bony defects in the limbs (168).

Radiologic Features

Gracile linear striations of trabecular bone, particularly in the metaepiphyseal portions of the long bones and in the periphery of the iliac wings, is the characteristic radiologic feature (Fig. 22) (2,3). The tubular bones of the hands and feet and carpal and tarsal bones are less commonly and more subtly affected. The striations are unchanged in appearance for years. The skull may be diffusely sclerotic in some affected kindreds (Fig. 23). Radionuclide accumulation is not increased in the striations during bone scanning (164).

Histopathologic Findings

Histopathologic features have not been described.

Treatment

Although the characteristic skeletal features are unlikely to be misdiagnosed, radiologic screening of individuals at risk would seem prudent after childhood.

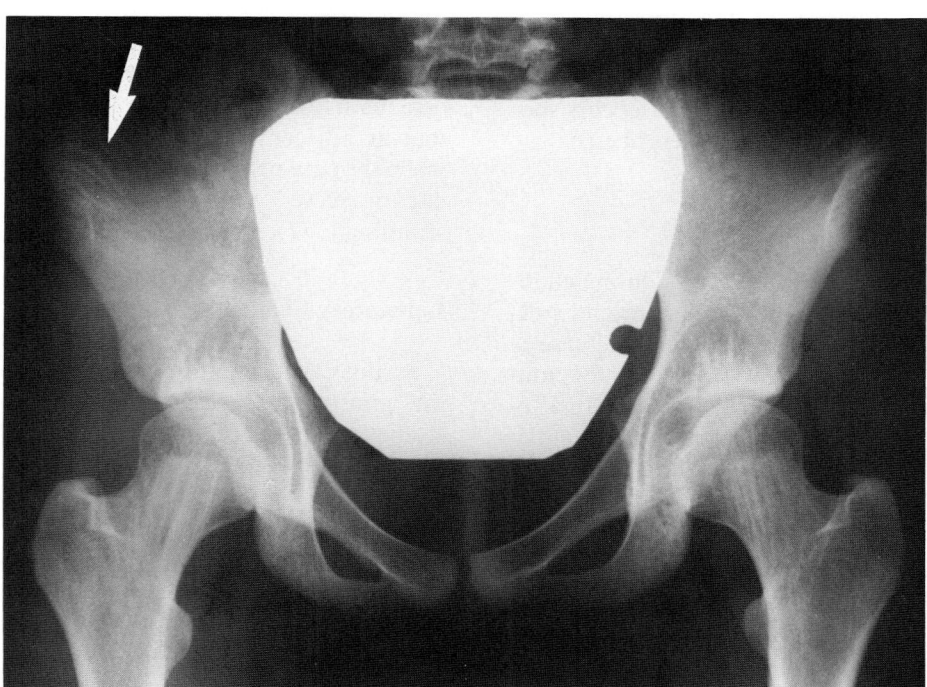

FIG. 22. Osteopathia striata. Characteristic fine linear striations are apparent in both femoral necks and especially in the right iliac wing (*arrow*) of this girl aged 15 yr 2 mo.

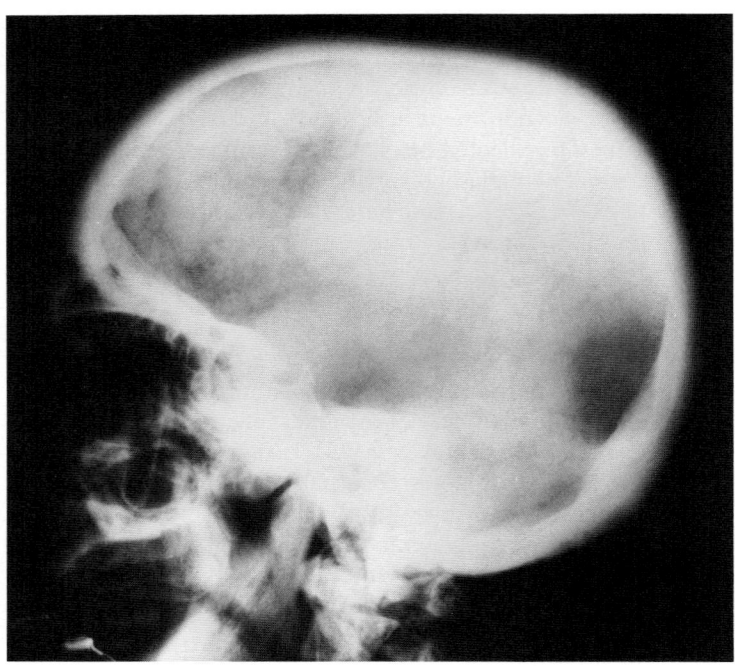

FIG. 23. Osteopathia striata with cranial sclerosis. The skull of this elderly man is diffusely dense, but there was no cranial nerve compression.

In one family with osteopathia striata and cranial sclerosis, prenatal diagnosis was reported by ultrasound examination (169).

MELORHEOSTOSIS

Melorheostosis, translated from Greek, depicts "flowing hyperostosis." The skeletal radiologic findings have understandably been likened to the appearance of melted wax that has dripped down the side of a candle. Since its first description in 1922 (170), about 200 cases have been reported (171,172). The disorder occurs sporadically; no Mendelian basis has been described.

Clinical Presentation

Melorheostosis characteristically presents during childhood. The major skeletal symptoms are pain and stiffness. Usually one limb is involved; bilateral disease is generally asymmetric. Of interest, it is common for cutaneous changes to overlie affected areas of bone. In a report of 131 patients, 17% had linear scleroderma-like areas and hypertrichosis (173). However, fibromas, capillary hemangiomas, fibrolipomas, lymphangiectasis, and arterial aneurysms also occur (174). Not infrequently, soft tissue abnormalities are noted before the hyperostosis is discovered. The skeletal abnormalities seem to progress most rapidly during childhood. In adulthood, melorheostosis may gradually extend or cease to progress (175). Nevertheless, pain seems to be more frequent in adults compared to children. Eventually, affected joints may become contracted and deformed.

Leg-length inequality results from the soft tissue contractures and from premature fusion of growth plates.

Radiologic Features

Dense, irregular, eccentric hyperostosis that affects both the cortex and medullary canal of an individual bone, or several adjacent bones, is the typical radiologic finding (Fig. 24) (2,3,172,176). The lower extremity is most commonly involved, but any anatomic region or bone can manifest the abnormalities. Furthermore, osseous tissue can also develop in areas of soft tissues that lie adjacent to involved skeletal sites, particularly when they are near joints. Melorheostotic bone accumulates increased amounts of radionuclide during bone scanning (177).

Laboratory Findings

Serum calcium and inorganic phosphate levels, alkaline phosphatase activity, and other routine laboratory studies are normal in melorheostosis.

Histopathologic Findings

Typically there is endosteal thickening of bone during infancy; periosteal new bone formation then follows during adulthood (172). Bony lesions consist of osteosclerosis with irregular thickened lamellae that can occlude Haversian systems. Marrow fibrosis may also be present (172). Of interest, unlike true scleroderma, the collagen of the scleroderma-like lesions is normal-

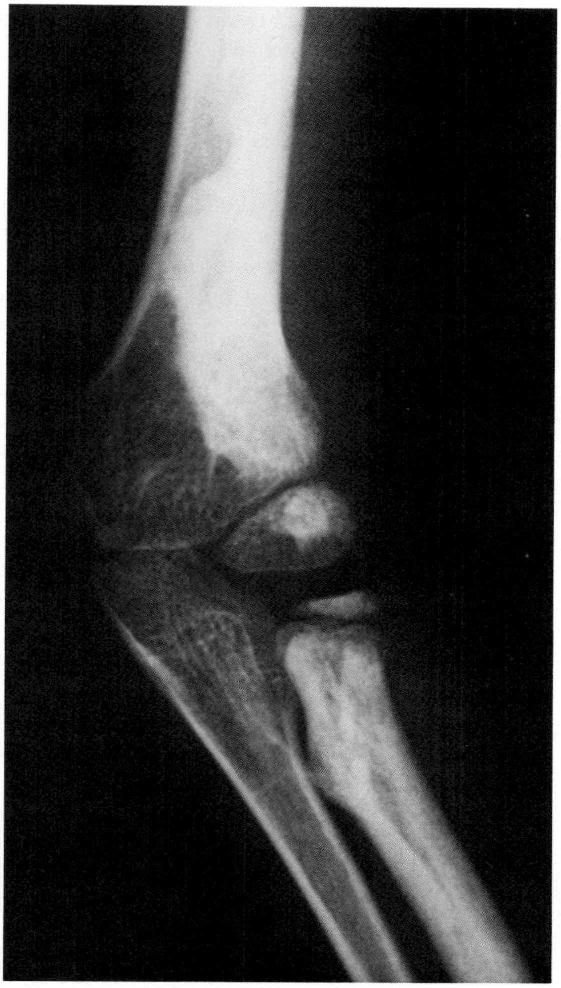

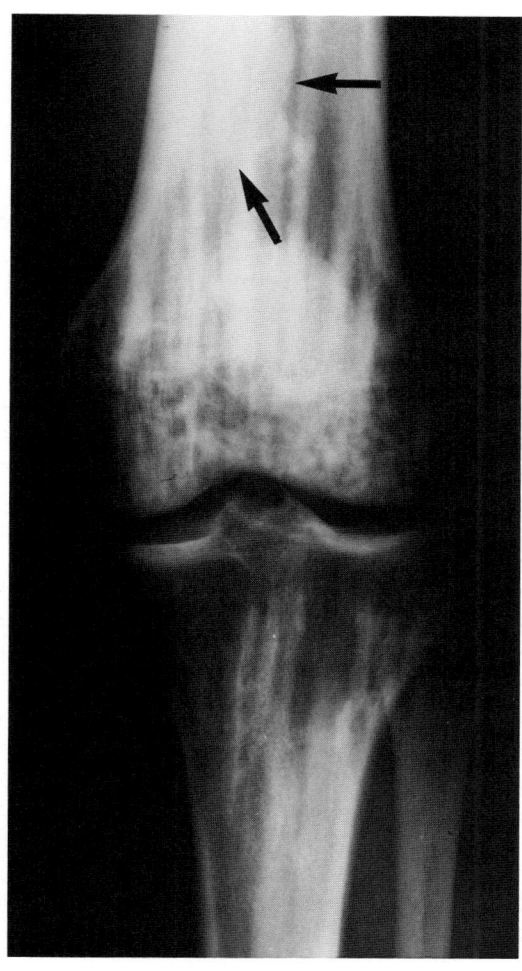

FIG. 24. Melorheostosis. Characteristic dense osteosclerosis involves areas of the distal humerus and radius, including their epiphyses, in this girl aged 7 yr 3 mo. The appearance of the osteosclerosis in the humerus is that of "dripping candle wax."

appearing. Thus, this dermatosis has been called "linear melorheostotic scleroderma" (173,178).

Etiology and Pathogenesis

Linear scleroderma may reflect a primary abnormality which then extends deep to involve the skeleton. The distribution of melorheostosis and its associated soft-tissue lesions within myotomes, sclerotomes, and dermatomes suggests that a mosaic defect may explain this sporadic condition (173,178).

Treatment

Surgical correction of contractures in children is difficult; recurrent deformity is not uncommon.

MIXED SCLEROSING BONE DYSTROPHY

Mixed sclerosing bone dystrophy is a rare skeletal dysplasia in which radiologic features of osteopoikilosis, osteopathia striata, melorheostosis, cranial sclerosis, and other skeletal abnormalities occur together in various combinations in one individual (Fig. 25) (179). Affected subjects may experience the symptoms and complications typically associated with the individual patterns of osteosclerosis. For example, melorheostosis may cause contractures, bone pain, etc., and cranial sclerosis can result in cranial nerve palsy. Bone scanning shows increased radionuclide uptake in the areas where osteosclerosis is greatest (179,180). Although the term "osteopetrosis" has been used to describe the generalized osteosclerosis of some affected subjects, histopathologic study has failed to show remnants of calcified primary

FIG. 25. Mixed sclerosing bone dystrophy. The bones of the left knee of this middle-aged man show osteopoikilosis of the distal femoral epiphysis, osteopathia striata of the distal femoral and proximal tibial metaepiphyses, and melorheostosis (*arrows*) of the distal femoral diaphysis. From Whyte and Murphy (248), with permission.

spongiosa (see section on Osteopetrosis, this chapter) (179,180). Delineation of this condition suggests a common pathogenesis for the component types of osteosclerosis. However, osteopoikilosis and most forms of osteopathia striata are heritable conditions, whereas mixed sclerosing bone dystrophy has been a sporadic disorder (179,180). There is no specific medical treatment. Surgical intervention may be necessary for contractures or neurovascular compression.

FIBROUS DYSPLASIA (McCUNE-ALBRIGHT SYNDROME)

Fibrous dysplasia is typically a sporadic, idiopathic, developmental bone disorder that may be monoostotic or polyostotic in skeletal distribution. It is characterized by an expanding fibrous lesion of bone-forming mesenchyme. The condition affects either sex and often results in deformity and fracture (181).

Clinical Presentation

Monoostotic fibrous dysplasia is more prevalent than the polyostotic variety. Disease that affects just one bone characteristically presents during the second or third decade of life, whereas polyostotic involvement typically manifests before 10 years of age and progresses until adulthood (181). For either type, an expansile bony lesion commonly causes deformity and there may be fracture. Occasionally, expanding bone will entrap a nerve. The skull and long bones are affected most often. Sarcomatous degeneration can occur (incidence < 1%) especially when the facial bones or femora are involved (182). The likelihood of malignant transformation appears to be increased by radiation exposure (183).

McCune-Albright syndrome refers to the rare subject who has polyostotic fibrous dysplasia, café-au-lait spots, and hyperfunction of one or more endocrine glands. Café-au-lait spots are characteristic, flat, hyperpigmented macules that have a rough border (Color Plate B) in McCune-Albright syndrome ("coast-of-Maine") compared to a smooth border ("coast-of-California") lesions of neurofibromatosis. The most common endocrinopathy is pseudo-precocious puberty in girls. However, thyrotoxicosis, Cushing's syndrome, acromegaly, hyperparathyroidism, hyperprolactinemia, or pseudo-precocious puberty in boys, and other endocrine problems have been reported (184–186). In especially rare individuals who have nearly panostotic skeletal involvement, renal phosphate wasting causes hypophosphatemic rickets or osteomalacia. A recent study revealed that affected girls commonly have thyroid dysfunction that may be occult but not rapidly progressive (185). Ultrasonography frequently revealed cystic thyroid abnormalities, as often occurs in the ovaries (185).

Radiologic Features

Any skeletal site can be affected (2,3). The femora, tibiae, ribs, and facial bones are involved most frequently. Small bones contain radiographic features of the disease in about 50% of individuals who have polyostotic involvement. In the long bones, the lesions are found either in the metaphysis or in the diaphysis. They are characterized by well-defined, thin cortices and have a "ground glass" appearance (Fig. 26). Occasionally, the involved area is lobulated and contains trabeculated foci of radiolucency. Skull involvement may produce features that resemble Paget's bone disease (Fig. 27). Fibrous dysplasia does not have a characteristic appearance on magnetic resonance imaging (187).

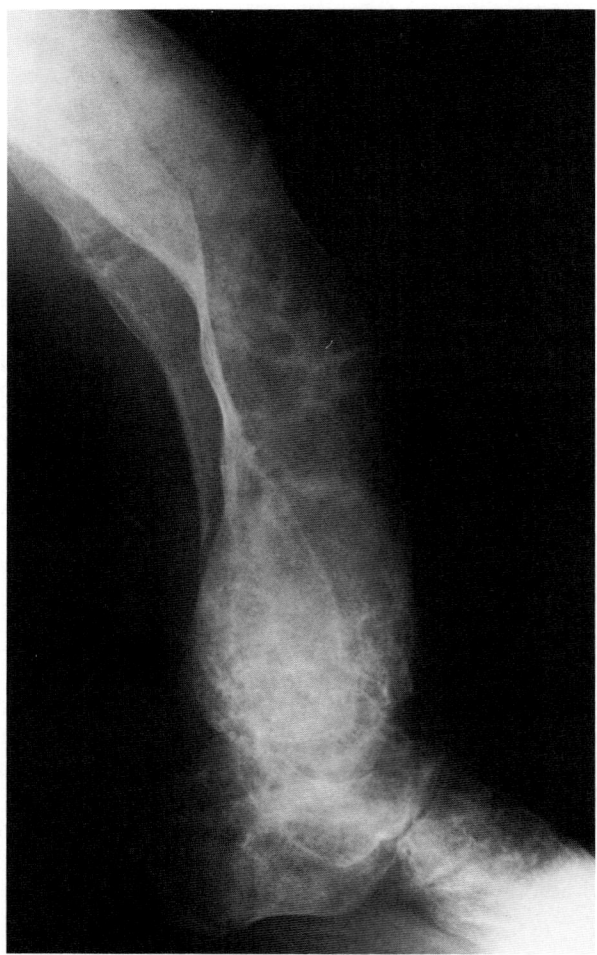

FIG. 26. McCune-Albright syndrome with renal phosphate wasting. The osteopenic and deformed bones of the left leg of this girl aged 11 yr 11 mo show the typical "ground-glass" appearance and thinned cortices.

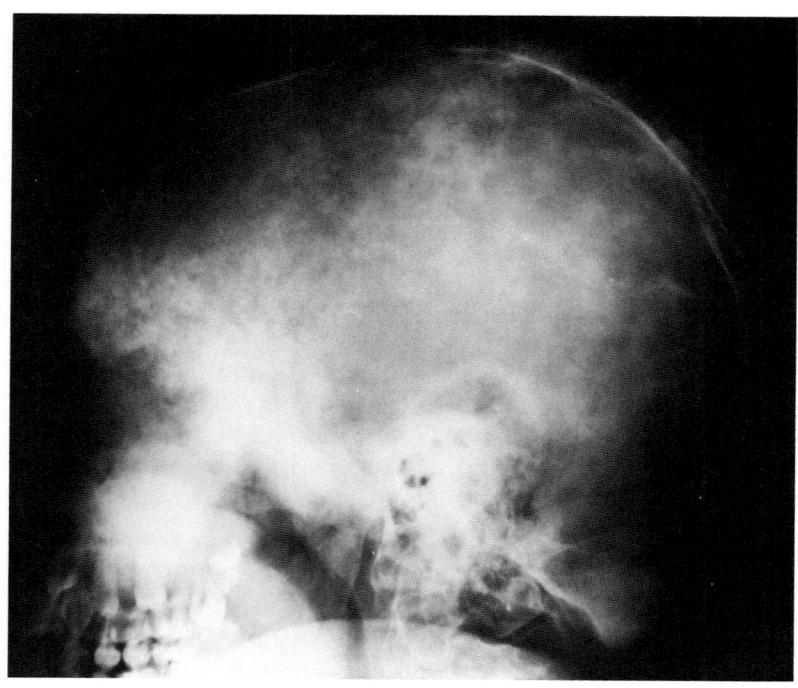

FIG. 27. McCune-Albright syndrome with renal phosphate wasting. The skull of this girl aged 11 yr 11 mo has a "cotton wool" appearance with areas of fluffy increased and decreased radiodensity reminiscent of advanced Paget's disease.

Laboratory Findings

Serum alkaline phosphatase activity not uncommonly is elevated, yet calcium and inorganic phosphate levels are typically normal.

Histopathologic Findings

Monoostotic and polyostotic lesions are well-defined anatomically, but do not have capsules. They share similar histological appearances. Spindle-shaped fibroblasts form "swirls" within the marrow space (Color Plate C). Trabeculae are haphazardly arranged and are composed of woven bone. When lesions are polyostotic, cartilage tissue is especially likely to be present. Cystic regions lined by multinucleated giant cells are also typical. The findings of fibrous dysplasia somewhat resemble the histopathologic changes of hyperparathyroidism (*osteitis fibrosa cystica*), but differ importantly in that osteoblasts are absent in fibrous dysplasia rather than plentiful in hyperparathyroidism.

Pathogenesis

The etiology of fibrous dysplasia, including the McCune-Albright syndrome, is not known. There is no evidence for an influence by Mendelian factors in fibrous dysplasia—the disorder occurs sporadically. McCune-Albright syndrome may, however, reflect an autosomal dominant mutation that is lethal except when it occurs by somatic mutation to cause mosaicism (188).

Further studies, however, are needed (1). The pathogenesis of the skeletal lesion seems to involve the formation of imperfect bone because mesenchymal cells do not differentiate properly to osteoblasts. The endocrine hyperfunction in the McCune-Albright syndrome appears to involve end-organ hyperactivity, but is also baffling (184,185,189). Recently, estrogen receptors have been identified in affected bone cells and may explain why skeletal lesions may progress during pregnancy (190). Recent investigation of growth hormone and prolactin hypersecretion indicates that some patients have disordered hypothalamic endocrine regulation, or perhaps an embryologic abnormality in pituitary cell differentiation and function (189). The complication of renal phosphate wasting in McCune-Albright syndrome seems in many ways analogous to tumor-induced ("oncogenic") rickets or osteomalacia (191). A phosphaturic factor may be elaborated from the fibrous tissue.

Treatment

Once formed, the skeletal lesions of fibrous dysplasia do not heal. There is no established drug therapy for the skeletal disease. In most patients with limited bony involvement, the radiologic appearance of osseous defects remains stable. However, in severely affected subjects, the lesions may progress and new ones can appear (2,3). Stress or fissure fractures can be difficult to detect and treat, but complete fractures generally mend well. When the skull is involved, neurological assessment and careful follow-up is necessary since nerve compression and deformity may respond to surgical intervention (192,193).

In the McCune-Albright syndrome, control of precocious puberty in affected girls has been achieved with the aromatase inhibitor, testolactone (194). Calcitriol and inorganic phosphate supplementation has not been thoroughly evaluated for the especially rare patient with hypophosphatemic bone disease.

FIBRODYSPLASIA OSSIFICANS PROGRESSIVA

Fibrodysplasia ossificans progressiva (myositis ossificans progressiva) is a rare heritable disorder characterized by congenital skeletal abnormalities of the hands and feet together with episodic soft tissue swellings that proceed to ossify. Ectopic bone formation occurs in aponeuroses, fascia, tendons, ligaments, and connective tissue within voluntary muscles. The condition was first described in 1692; more than 500 cases are reported in the medical literature (195,196). Descriptions of affected subjects most commonly concern caucasians, but the disorder has involved blacks (197). Sporadic occurrence is the usual observation, however, autosomal dominant transmission with very variable expressivity is established (1).

Clinical Presentation

Fibrodysplasia ossificans progressiva characteristically presents during the first decade of life with an episode of soft tissue swelling (196). In some cases, this event does not occur until early adulthood. Conversely, there are rare reports of in utero involvement. Tender, rubbery, induration within a muscle that is sometimes precipitated by trauma evolves during a few days and may persist for several weeks. Fever can occur during periods of swelling and the condition may be mistaken for an infectious process. The paraspinal and limb girdle muscles and the muscles of mastication are involved most frequently. Gradually, calcification develops within the inflamed region and it eventually becomes heterotopic bone. The episodes of soft tissue induration recur unpredictably, but most frequently prior to puberty (195,196).

Although the diagnosis of fibrodysplasia ossificans progressiva is established when characteristic swellings appear, the condition can be suspected strongly at birth if the typical congenital skeletal anomalies are present (196). The usual finding is *hallux valgus* with microdactyly (Fig. 28). Synostosis and hypoplasia of the phalanges with microdactyly of the thumb also occur.

Complications of the recurrent soft tissue swellings and ectopic bone formation include torticollis when there is involvement of a sternocleidomastoid muscle. The shoulder girdle and/or dorsum of the trunk are also frequently affected and decreased range-of-motion occurs particularly in the neck and shoulders. The frequency of scoliosis seems to be increased (198). Involve-

ment of the muscles of mastication can impair movement of the jaw and may ultimately compromise nutrition. As the thorax becomes deformed it engenders a form of restrictive "lung" disease that will eventually cause hypercapnia and predispose the patient to pneumonia. Deafness and alopecia also occur with increased prevalence. Secondary amenorrhea is not uncommon, but reproduction has been successful.

Laboratory Findings

Routine biochemical parameters of mineral metabolism are generally normal in fibrodysplasia ossificans progressiva except that serum alkaline phosphatase activity may be increased. The electrocardiogram may be abnormal perhaps from fibrodysplasia of the myocardium.

Radiologic Features

Skeletal anomalies, primarily in the fingers and especially in the toes, together with soft tissue ossification comprise the principal radiologic features of fibrodysplasia ossificans progressiva (3,4,199).

A variety of bony defects may occur in the extremities. Microdactyly most commonly of the big toe, but frequently involving the thumb, is a radiologic hallmark, but is not pathognomonic of the disorder (3). Four types of abnormalities of the big toe have been distinguished (200).

When progressive heterotopic ossification of fascia, tendons, aponeuroses, and other tissues occurs it begins early on in the neck and shoulders (Fig. 29). The lower extremities (Figs. 30 to 32) become affected relatively late. The paraspinal muscles are especially prone to calcification. Cervical vertebrae often become fused (Fig. 33). Portions of the skeleton may become osteopenic at sites of severe inflammatory swelling. Otherwise, the bones are well mineralized. Computed tomography to search for soft tissue calcification is the best technique for detecting an early lesion (201). However, increased uptake of tracer diphosphonate also occurs during bone scanning before calcification is demonstrable in the swellings by conventional radiographs (202).

Histopathologic Findings

The characteristic soft tissue mass of fibrodysplasia ossificans progressiva is initially composed of an edematous area within fascial planes of one or more voluntary muscles. Interestingly, smooth muscle is not affected. Soon after, interconnecting nodules of fibroblasts form. Later, in the center of this matrix of fibrous connective tissue, one may observe osteoid, bone, and sometimes cartilage (203). Eventually, the osseous lesions "mature"

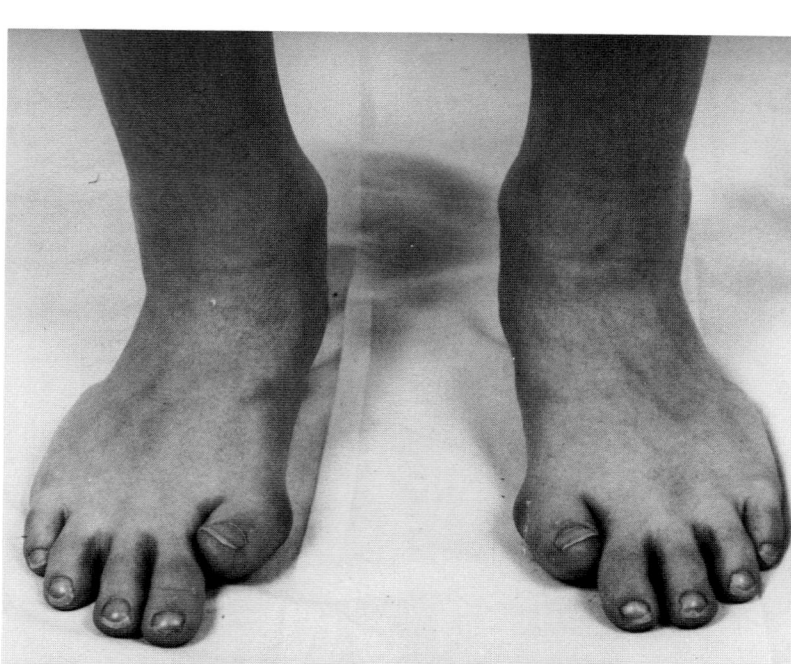

FIG. 28. Fibrodysplasia ossificans progressiva. Characteristic *hallux valgus* deformity in this 9-year-old mildly affected boy has been present life-long.

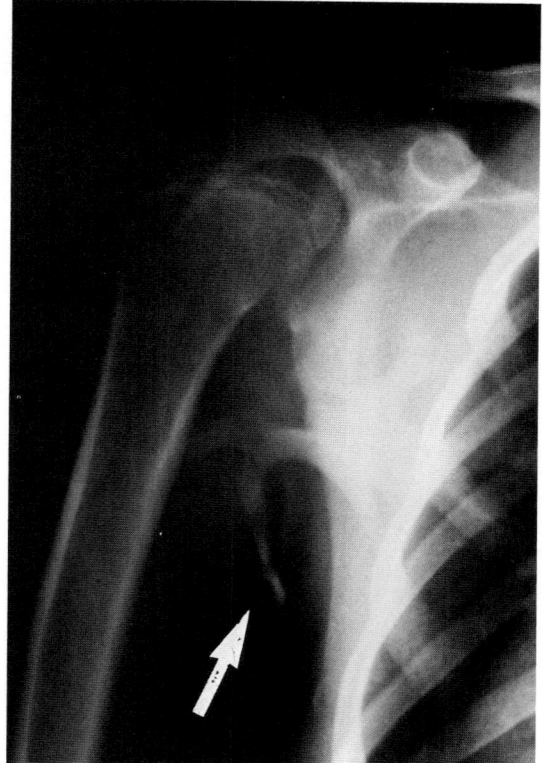

FIG. 29. Fibrodysplasia ossificans progressiva. A typical spur (*arrow*) of ectopic bone appears to originate from the right scapula of this $14\frac{1}{2}$-year-old boy.

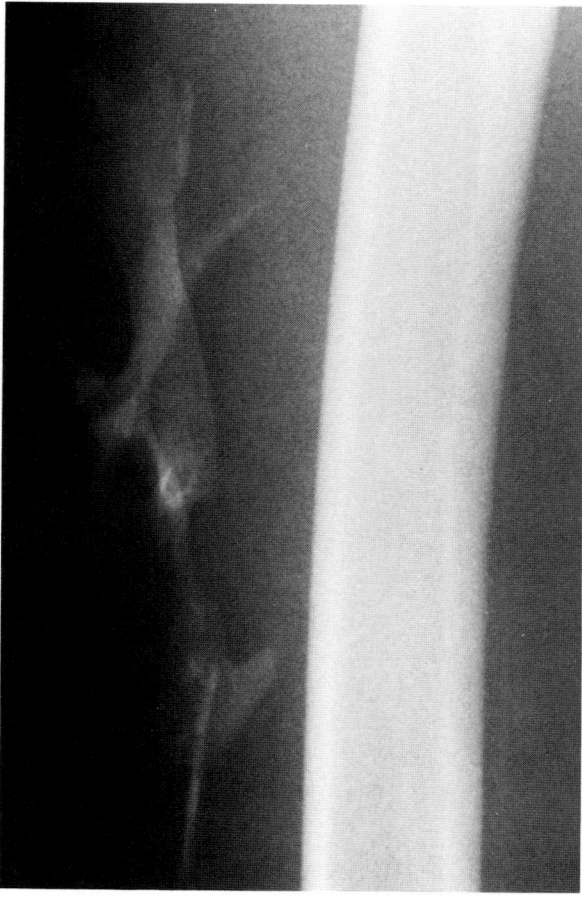

FIG. 30. Fibrodysplasia ossificans progressiva. Characteristic large plates and spicules of ectopic bone are present in the quadriceps muscle of this 11-year-old boy.

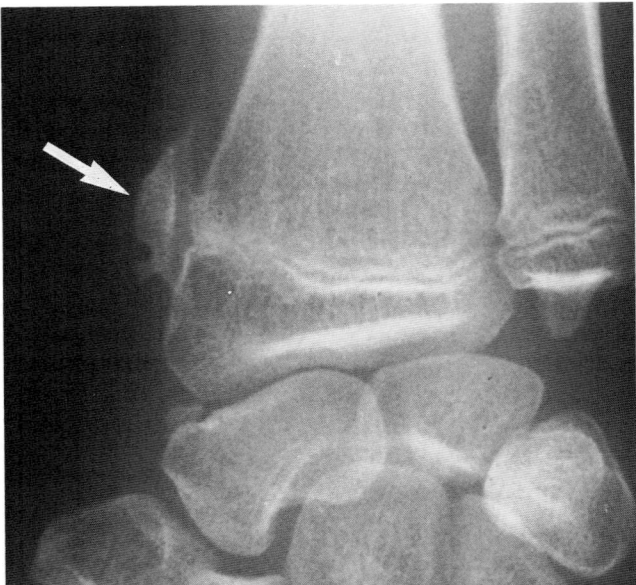

FIG. 31. Fibrodysplasia ossificans progressiva. This area of ectopic bone formation (*arrow*) developed within several weeks of radial artery puncture for blood gas determinations in this 16-year-old boy.

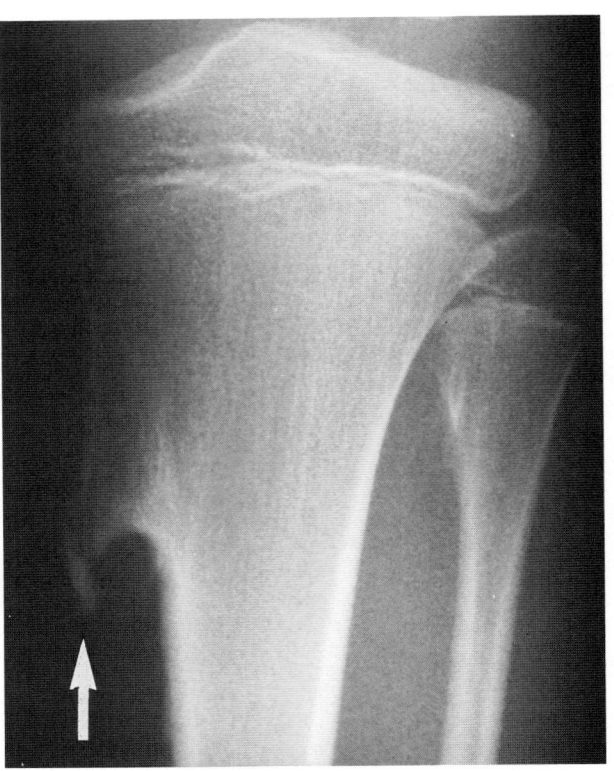

FIG. 32. Fibrodysplasia ossificans progressiva. A typical tibial spur (*arrow*) of ectopic bone has formed in this $7\frac{1}{2}$-year-old boy at the site of a tendon insertion.

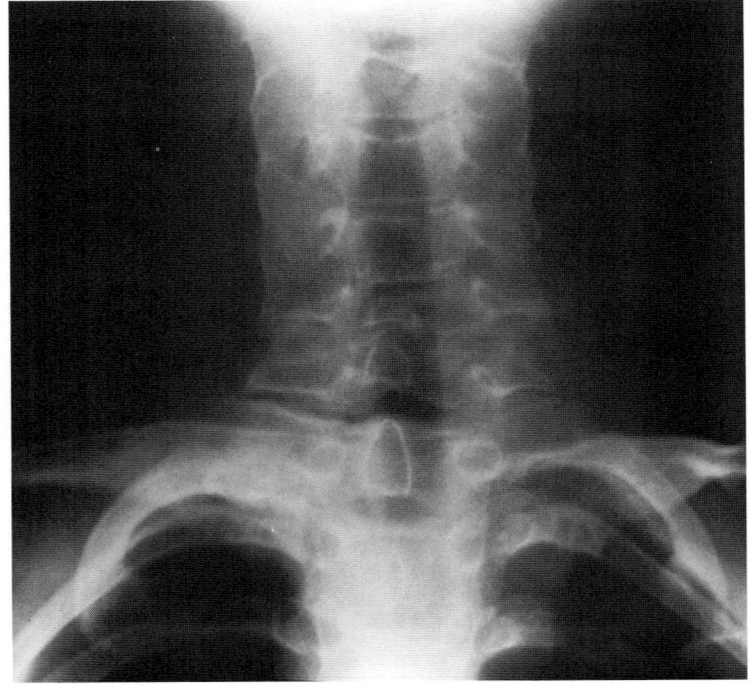

FIG. 33. Fibrodysplasia ossificans progressiva. Characteristic complete fusion of the cervical vertebrae is present in this $14\frac{1}{2}$-year-old boy.

and hematopoietic tissue appears within trabecular bone. The heterotopic ossification appears macroscopically as dense, flat, irregular areas within the connective tissue of facial planes. It may partly or completely surround a muscle (3,4).

Etiology and Pathogenesis

The autosomal locus for fibrodysplasia ossificans progressiva has not been identified within the human genome (1). Most cases appear to be sporadic. Increased paternal age seems to contribute importantly to the development of new dominant mutations (204), but banding studies have not revealed microscopic chromosomal defects.

The pathogenesis of this condition is also poorly understood (200). Debate persists as to whether the disorder primarily affects connective tissue and secondarily muscle, or if the fundamental defect is in muscle itself. The term *fibrodysplasia ossificans progressiva* is favored by those who believe that connective tissue is primarily involved; the term *myositis ossificans progressiva* suggests an underlying muscle disorder. The former definition is gaining increased acceptance (1). In its defense, computed tomography has revealed that the first pathologic swellings are within the fascial planes of muscle. However, investigators who favor a "myositis" emphasize that histologic and electromyographic aberrations occur in muscle before there is connective tissue proliferation.

Treatment

There is no established pharmacologic treatment for fibrodysplasia ossificans progressiva. The very variable clinical course of this disorder not only among patients, but for individuals as well, makes it very difficult to assess any attempted therapy. Corticosteroids, adrenocorticotrophic hormone, dietary calcium binders, and intravenous infusion of ethylenediaminetetraacetic acid (EDTA) have been tested with equivocal results (205). Oral administration of the diphosphonate, disodium etidronate (Didronel), has been evaluated as having a variable therapeutic outcome (206). Warfarin was given in one study in an attempt to inhibit vitamin K-dependent γ-carboxylation of osteocalcin and thereby reduce ectopic bone formation, but this drug also did not have clinical efficacy (207). Thus, medical intervention for fibrodysplasia ossificans progressiva remains supportive. Surgical release of joint contractures is typically unsuccessful. Indeed, such trauma puts the patient at risk of new swellings (Fig. 31). For this reason, intramuscular injections should not be administered if possible or given in the gluteus or quadriceps rather than into the deltoid

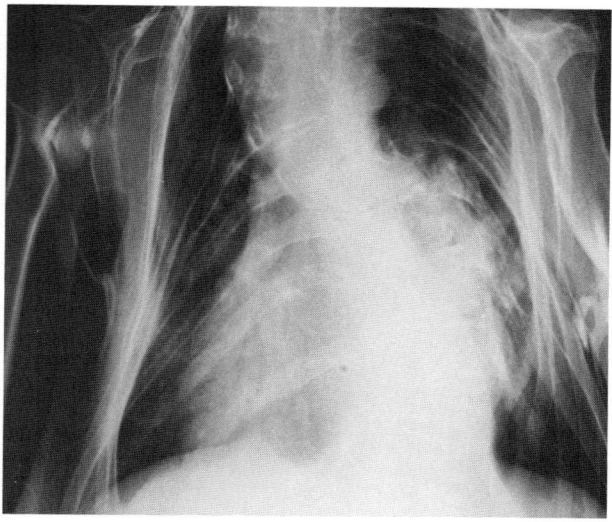

FIG. 34. Fibrodysplasia ossificans progressiva. The thorax of this 16-year-old boy is markedly narrowed by ectopic bone formation within the chest wall and together with scoliosis contributed to restrictive lung disease.

muscle. Dental problems should be addressed as early as possible since range-of-motion of the mandible may decrease. In some patients with severely compromised nutrition, surgical release of a frozen jaw has been successful. If such a procedure is contemplated, computed tomography should be performed since it will help to show soft tissue abnormalities and/or ossification that is not apparent by conventional radiography (201). Unfortunately, removal of the offending lesions may be followed by their recurrence. A brief course of high-dose disodium etidronate before and after surgery that will traumatize voluntary muscle may help to mitigate the ossification of trauma-induced swellings (206).

Prognosis

Despite widespread ectopic bone formation, some subjects live into the sixth decade. Most, however, develop restrictive ventilation from chest wall involvement and succumb to pulmonary complications with hypercapnia and pneumonia (Fig. 34) (196).

PACHYDERMOPERIOSTOSIS

Pachydermoperiostosis (hypertrophic osteoarthropathy: primary or idiopathic) is characterized by periosteal new bone formation that occurs prominently in the distal limbs; clubbing of the digits (Fig. 35); hyperhydrosis; and thickening of the skin, especially of the face and forehead. Autosomal dominant inheritance with variable expression is established, but autosomal recessive transmission may also occur (1).

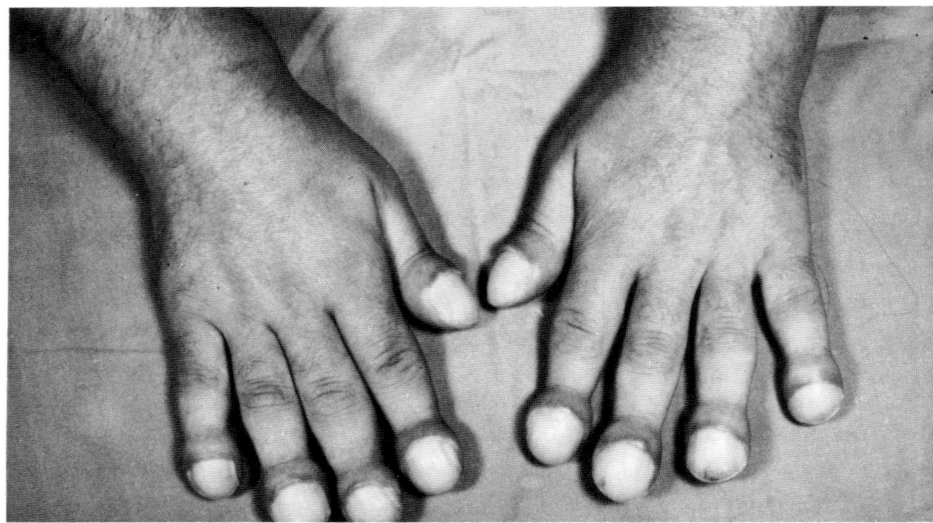

FIG. 35. Pachydermoperiostosis. Characteristic marked finger clubbing is present in this 33-year-old man. From Whyte and Murphy (248), with permission.

Clinical Presentation

The disorder is more prevalent in blacks than in whites. Men are generally more severely affected than women. In some patients, all three principal features (pachydermia, *cutis verticis gyrata,* periostitis) are present; other affected individuals have just one or two of these findings. The age at presentation is variable, but adolescence is when symptoms typically first manifest (208). Usually, the clinical picture unfolds over a decade, and the disorder then becomes quiescent (209). During its active phase, progressive gradual enlargement of the hands and feet causes a "paw-like" appearance and patients may be described as acromegalic. Arthralgias of the knees, ankles, elbows, and wrists are common. Occasionally, the small joints are also painful. Acro-osteolysis has also been reported. Chondrocalcinosis with calcium pyrophosphate crystals in synovial fluid has been documented in one affected subject. Symptoms of pseudogout can occur. Stiffness together with limited mobility of the axial and appendicular skeleton troubles some patients. Cranial nerves and major spinal nerves may become compressed. Cutaneous changes include coarsening, thickening, pitting, furrowing, and oiliness of especially the face and scalp. Fatigue is not unusual and myelophthisic anemia with extramedullary hematopoiesis has been described. Life expectancy is normal (209).

Radiologic Features

The principal radiologic abnormality of pachydermoperiostosis is severe periostitis that thickens and scleroses the distal aspects of the major tubular bones—typically the tibia, fibula, radius, and ulna (3,4) (Fig. 36). Occasionally, the phalanges, metacarpals, tarsals/metatarsals, clavicles, pelvis, and base of the skull are also affected. Clubbing is obvious and acro-osteolysis can occur. In older affected individuals, ankylosis of joints (especially in the hands and feet) may occur (3,4).

The principal differential diagnostic consideration for pachydermoperiostosis is a form of *secondary* hypertrophic osteoarthropathy (3,4). The latter condition can stem from pulmonary pathology or from disease elsewhere. Fortunately, the radiologic features of the primary and secondary conditions are, however, somewhat different. In pachydermoperiostosis, periosteal new bone proliferation is exuberant and has an irregular appearance (Fig. 36). Furthermore, it may be so extensive as to involve epiphyses. In hypertrophic pulmonary osteoarthropathy, the periosteal reaction usually has a smooth undulating appearance (210). Bone scanning in either condition reveals symmetrical, diffuse, regular uptake along the cortical margins of long bones, especially in the legs. This feature causes a "double stripe" sign.

Laboratory Findings

Synovial fluid typically shows no evidence of inflammation.

Histopathologic Findings

Periosteal new bone formation produces a rough surface over affected cortical bone (211). Since the newly formed osseous tissue then undergoes cancellous compaction, on routine light microscopy it may be difficult

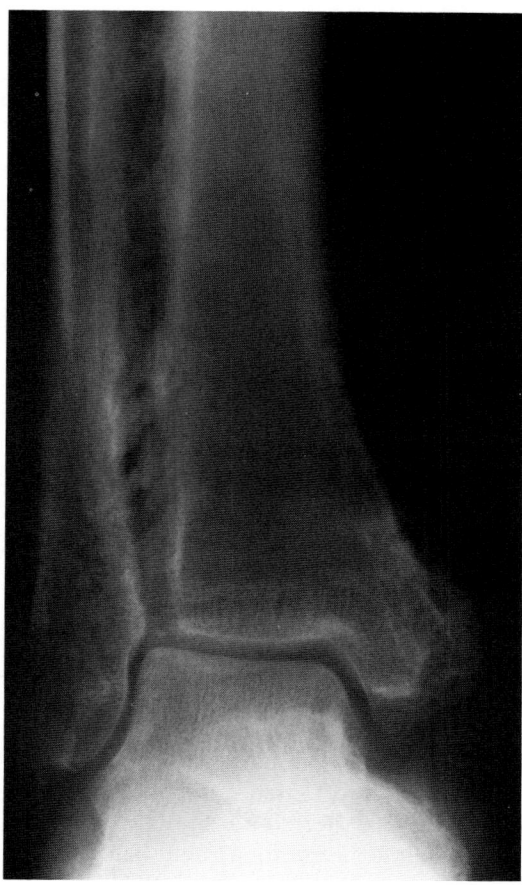

FIG. 36. Pachydermoperiostosis. Extensive shaggy periosteal reaction is present along the interosseous membrane between the tibia and fibula: note also the extensive proliferative bone formation along the medial malleolus. From Whyte and Murphy (248), with permission.

to distinguish maturing periosteal new bone from the original cortex (211). Mild cellular hyperplasia and thickening of blood vessels is found near synovial membranes (212). Electron microscopy reveals layered basement membranes.

Treatment

Colchicine was recently reported to be helpful for the arthralgias, clubbing, folliculitis, and pachyderma of one affected subject (213).

OSTEOGENESIS IMPERFECTA

Osteogenesis imperfecta ("brittle bone disease") is a heritable disorder of connective tissue characterized by disturbances in the quality or quantity of type I collagen throughout the body (214,215). Type I collagen is the most abundant protein in bone, but is also found in skin, sclerae, teeth, ligaments, and elsewhere (214). Thus, al-

though the major clinical manifestations are skeletal, tissues other than bone are defective as well. The cardinal clinical feature is recurrent fracture and skeletal deformity (216). However, many affected subjects also have dental disease (dentinogenesis imperfecta) caused by aberration in the formation of dentin. An important characteristic of osteogenesis imperfecta is the extremely variable severity of clinical expression. There may be stillbirth or life-long absence of symptoms (214–216).

Some forms of osteogenesis imperfecta are clearly inherited as autosomal dominant traits. Others have, until recently, been thought to reflect autosomal recessive transmission. The well-known classification system that was devised by Sillence for this disorder according to clinical features and apparent mode of genetic transmission has been useful for providing a framework for prognostication and has served as a foundation for biochemical/molecular studies (Table 3) (217). However, this long-standing nosology has significant exceptions and limitations. The clinical heterogeneity of osteogenesis imperfecta is now being clarified through identification of an ever increasing number and variety of molecular defects within the genes that encode the pro-α1 and pro-α2 chains of type I collagen (214,215). Furthermore, recent molecular findings provide important new insight into the genetic origins of the specific biochemical defects and the inheritance patterns for several Sillence types have been importantly modified (see below) (214,218).

Clinical Presentation

Generalized osteopenia can occur during childhood due to a variety of disorders including idiopathic juvenile osteoporosis, homocystinuria, Cushing's disease, etc. (3,4). Multiple fractures in infants and children may result from child abuse (219,220) and congenital indifference to pain (3,4). Nevertheless, osteogenesis imperfecta is usually readily diagnosed from its clinical/radiologic findings. The cardinal clinical feature that results from the generalized osteopenia is recurrent fracture and deformities of the long bones and vertebrae. Patients often, however, may also manifest ligamentous laxity with joint hypermobility, diaphoresis, easy bruisability, and dentinogenesis imperfecta. Hearing loss troubles about 50% of patients younger than age 30 years and is present in nearly all affected subjects who are older (221). Deafness typically reflects conductive or mixed hearing defects; less commonly it is the result of sensorineural disease (222). Other signs of osteogenesis imperfecta include sclerae with a blue or gray tint in most patients (Color Plate D), a head that appears to be disproportionately large compared to a small body size, a high-pitched voice, triangular-shaped face, short stature, scoliosis, and herniae. Mitral valve clicks are not uncommon, but car-

TABLE 3. *Clinical heterogeneity and biochemical defects in osteogenesis imperfecta (OI)*

OI type	Clinical features	Inheritance	Biochemical defects
I	Normal stature, little or no deformity, blue scleras, hearing loss in about 50% of individuals; dentinogenesis imperfecta is rare and may distinguish a subset.	AD	Decreased production of type I procollagen. Substitution for residue other than glycine in triple helix of $\alpha 1(I)$.
II	Lethal in the perinatal period, minimal calvarial mineralization, beaded ribs, compressed femurs, marked long bone deformity, platyspondyly.	AD (new mutation)	Rearrangements in the COL1A1 and COL1A2 genes. Substitutions for glycyl residues in the triple-helical domain of the $\alpha 1(I)$ $\alpha 2(I)$ chain.
		AR (rare)	Small deletion in $\alpha 2(I)$ on the background of a null allele.
III	Progressively deforming bones, usually with moderate deformity at birth. Scleras variable in hue, often lighten with age. Dentinogenesis common, hearing loss common. Stature very short.	AR	Frameshift mutation that prevents incorporation of pro$\alpha 2(I)$ into molecules. (noncollagenous defects).
		AD	Point mutations in the $\alpha 1(I)$ or $\alpha 2(I)$ chain.
IV	Normal scleras, mild to moderate bone deformity and variable short stature, dentinogenesis is common, and hearing loss occurs in some.	AD	Point mutations in the $\alpha 2(I)$ chain. Rarely, point mutations in the $\alpha 1(I)$ chain. Small deletions in the 2(1) chain.

Source: From Byers (214), with permission.

AD, autosomal dominant; AR, autosomal recessive; COL1A1, gene that encodes the $\alpha 1$ chain of type 1 collagen; COL1A2, gene that encodes the $\alpha 2$ chain of type 1 collagen.

diac disease is unusual. Patients with even the most severe skeletal deformities typically have normal intelligence. Thoracic deformity including *pectus excavatum* or *carinatum* may predispose affected subjects to pulmonary infection. The severity of clinical expression is, however, extremely variable (214–216). Indeed, some variability is often apparent among affected individuals in a single family or kindred.

The Sillence classification is based upon the clinical findings and the apparent mode of inheritance (Table 3) (217). Type I patients typically have readily apparent bluish discoloration of their sclerae that is especially prominent during childhood, (e.g.; Color Plate D), osteopenia with recurrent fracture but only mild skeletal deformity, and deafness that first manifests during early adulthood. Affected subjects are typically of normal height. Elderly women with this mild form of osteogenesis imperfecta are often diagnosed mistakenly as having postmenopausal or "involutional" osteoporosis. Indeed, the radiologic findings in these disorders could be indistinguishable. Once the correct diagnosis is suspected, the family history and scleral discoloration usually clarify the nature of their condition. In such cases, however, examination of a specimen of bone may also be helpful, since numerous cortical osteocytes occur in type I disease (see below) (223,224). Some clinicians subdivide this form of the disease into types I-A or I-B depending respectively upon the absence or more rarely the presence of dentinogenesis imperfecta. Type I osteogenesis imperfecta is transmitted as an autosomal dominant disorder, but approximately one-third of cases represent new mutations.

Type II osteogenesis imperfecta has come to be regarded as almost always lethal within the first few days or weeks of life (214). Affected newborns are often premature and small for gestational age. They have short bowed limbs, numerous fractures, a markedly soft skull, and a small thoracic cavity. Respiratory insufficiency is the usual cause of death.

Type III disease is characterized by skeletal disease that seems to become severe during childhood. There is progressive bony deformity from recurrent fractures that leads to short stature (217). These patients are often troubled by dental problems as well.

Type IV disease, until recently, was considered to be a relatively rare form of osteogenesis imperfecta. However, it is now believed to frequently account for instances of multigeneration involvement where genetic transmission occurs as an autosomal dominant trait (214). The sclerae are of normal color, but skeletal deformity, dental abnormalities, and deafness are characteristic.

Radiologic Features

Characteristic findings are observed in severely affected individuals (3,4). All three processes of skeletal development—growth, modeling, and remodeling—are adversely affected in such patients. Cardinal radiologic features, however, are the modeling defects of the long bones that help engender osteopenia which in turn accounts for skeletal deformity from fractures. Defective periosteal bone formation retards the circumferential growth of individual bones. This produces a gracile appearance with thin cortices. In some very severely affected newborns, there is micromelia from shortened long bones that appear as though they are "thick" in external diameter. Wormian bones in the skull of significant number and size is a common but not pathognomonic finding (Fig. 37) (225). Recurrent collapses also deform vertebrae. The pelvis can have a triradiate-shaped appearance. Bone "softening" also occurs from defects in skeletal remodeling and can cause *protrusio acetabuli* (Fig. 38). Platybasia and excessive pneumatization of the frontal and mastoid sinuses are observed when the disease is severe (3,4). Radiologic findings may evolve considerably during growth. This feature helps to define the "progressively-deforming" type III form of osteogenesis imperfecta. In these patients, "popcorn calcifications" reflect developmental defects stemming from the disruption of the epiphyses and metaphyses of major long bones, especially at the ankles and knees (226). Traumatic fragmentation of growth plate cartilage that is followed by disordered physeal maturation severely limits long bone growth and helps to account for the short stature. Such findings partially "resolve" at puberty once growth plates fuse and physeal cartilage fully mineralizes. Fractures in osteogenesis imperfecta are often transverse but heal at normal rates. Understandably, not all breaks are casted and with motion about the fracture site there may be exuberant bony callus formation. This finding has been mistaken for skeletal malignancy. Osteoarthritis is a common problem for ambulatory adults who have skeletal deformity. Platybasia may occasionally progress to basilar impression (227).

Laboratory Findings

Routine studies of mineral metabolism are typically unremarkable in osteogenesis imperfecta, except that elevations in serum alkaline phosphatase activity and urinary levels of hydroxyproline occur in some affected individuals. Recently, it has been found that subjects with severe disease are often hypercalciuric (228).

Histopathologic Findings

Specimens of bone may contain features that suggest an abnormal skeletal matrix, particularly in severely affected subjects. Disorganized ("woven") bone or abnormally thin collagen bundles within lamellar bone may be found on polarized-light microscopy. Numerous osteocytes are observed in the cortical osseous tissue in some patients. This finding appears to reflect reduced rates of bone formation by individual osteoblasts that subsequently become embedded relatively close to one another. Nevertheless, many osteoblasts are active at one time and the overall rate of skeletal remodeling in osteogenesis imperfecta is often rapid as shown by in vivo tetracycline labeling followed by fluorescence histomorphometry (229).

Pathogenesis/Etiology

Animal models and more recently a transgenic mouse model has been developed (230). The various clinical types of human osteogenesis imperfecta are described in Table 3 (214). Table 3 also summarizes what is now becoming understood of the numerous and varied mutations in the type I procollagen genes that cause this disorder (214,215). Included among the defects that lead to brittle bone disease are patients in whom rates of type I collagen synthesis are reduced. In most subjects there are molecular defects within the pro-α 1 or pro-α 2 genes that together encode type I collagen. Rarely, defects are found within both polypeptides in a given patient. The interested reader is referred elsewhere for detailed discussion of the numerous types of molecular/biochemical defects identified in osteogenesis imperfecta (214,215).

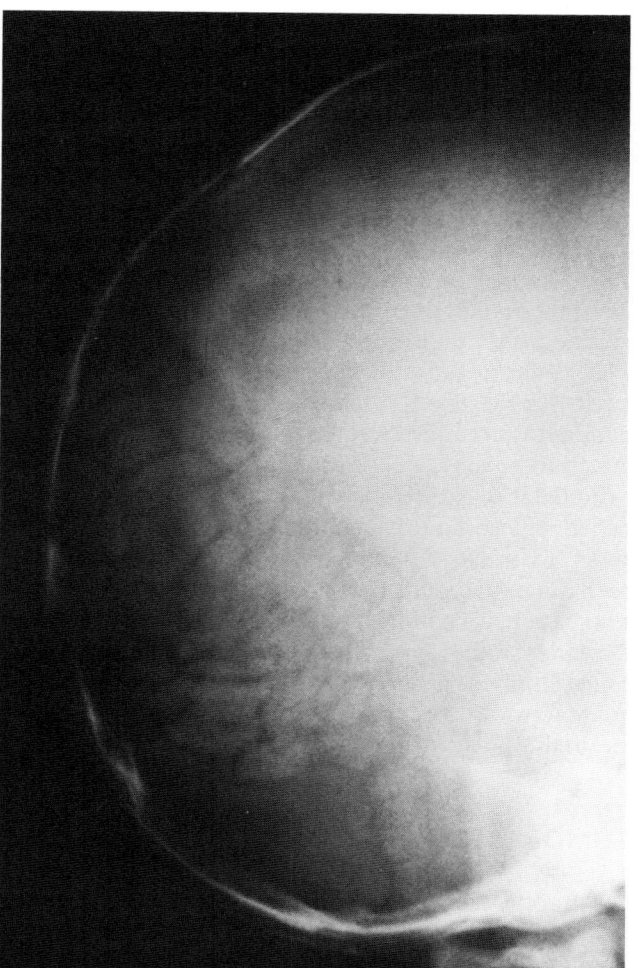

FIG. 37. Osteogenesis imperfecta. Numerous wormian bones are present in the posterior skull.

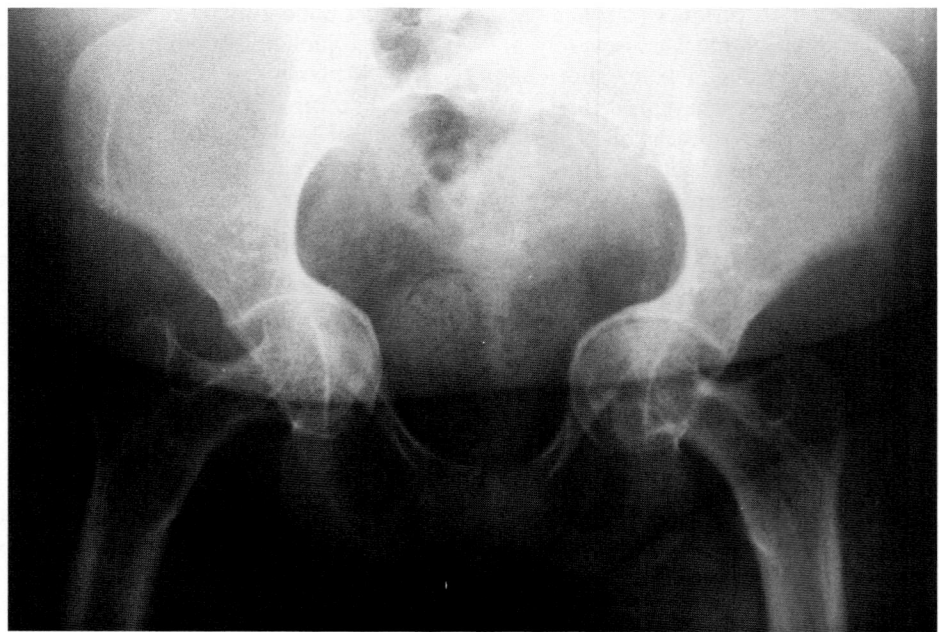

FIG. 38. Osteogenesis imperfecta. There is marked protrusio acetabuli from bone softening in this 19-year-old woman.

Treatment

Despite considerable progress in the elucidation of the biochemical/genetic defects that cause osteogenesis imperfecta, treatment remains supportive. There is no established medical therapy to improve the quantity or quality of skeletal tissue. Use of bisphosphonate compounds seems promising for increasing bone mass, but requires further study (231). Instead, expert orthopedic, dental, and rehabilitative care for recurrent fractures, limb deformities, kyphoscoliosis, dental sequelae, etc. is often needed. To prevent long bone deformities and fracture, correct deformities, and enhance the patient's ability to walk, intramedullary nailing with elongating and nonelongating rods has had success (232). Operative management of the unusual feature of basilar invagination has been clarified recently (227). Use of a "vacuum pants" orthosis can facilitate weight-bearing (233). A program for ambulation was described recently (234) and many of the rehabilitation considerations have been comprehensively reviewed (235,236). The clinical presentation and pathogenesis of deafness in osteogenesis imperfecta appears to be that of osteosclerosis (221,222). Stapedectomy may be helpful. Nevertheless, hearing loss can then progress because of sensorineural disease (222). Support groups, such as the Osteogenesis Imperfecta Foundation, Inc., in the United States and the Brittle Bone Society in the United Kingdom publish newsletters, hold educational and social gatherings, etc., that are important sources of information and comfort for patients and their families.

Genetic counseling is often helpful for families where osteogenesis imperfecta has occurred. When appropriate it should be periodically updated since progress in understanding the inheritance patterns for this variable disease is now quite rapid. Indeed, recent studies reveal that many cases of type II osteogenesis imperfecta result from new dominant mutations rather than autosomal recessive inheritance as previously thought (214,237). Furthermore, germline mosaicism may explain instances where there are affected siblings. Thus, the overall recurrence risk for type II disease is not the Mendelian 1:4 of pure autosomal recessive transmission, but is now estimated to be only 5% to 10% (214).

Prenatal diagnosis of severe disease is possible by a variety of techniques, including ultrasound examination at 14–18 weeks gestation. This routine technique has been quite successful and should be offered to all women who have had a child with osteogenesis imperfecta (214). Research studies have also shown that linkage analysis using family and fetal DNA samples can improve the prediction of recurrence risks in some informative kindreds.

TUMORAL CALCINOSIS

Tumoral calcinosis was first reported in 1899. More than 2,000 cases have been described. This disorder is a heritable condition characterized by masses of "metastatic calcification" in periarticular soft tissue around the major joints (1). Deposition of mineral does not typically occur in the vasculature or viscera. Usually, areas about the shoulders and hips are affected although additional joints may be involved (238). Hyperphosphatemia is an apparent pathogenetic factor in many cases (see below) (239,240), but it is important to recognize that periarticular metastatic calcification also occurs in disorders (Table 4) where hypercalcemia is the principal aberration in mineral homeostasis (e.g.; milk-alkali syndrome, sarcoidosis, and vitamin D intoxication).

Clinical Presentation

Most of the patients reported from North America have been black. There is no sex predominance. About one-third of cases reflect familial disease where autosomal recessive inheritance has usually been surmised, but autosomal dominant transmission has also been documented (1,238). The disorder characteristically presents in childhood, but periarticular masses have been recognized first in infancy or even in old age. Tumoral calcinosis is a life-long problem.

The masses are typically painless and grow at variable rates. One or two years after presentation, swellings can be the size of an orange or grapefruit. Deposits sometimes weigh as much as 1 kg. Often they are hard, lobulated, and adhere firmly to deep fascia. Occasionally, the ectopic calcification infiltrates into tendons and muscles (240). Joint range-of-motion is not restricted, because the deposits are extracapsular, unless the tumors are especially large. However, compression of neural structures may occur. The tumors can also ulcerate the skin and drain chalky fluid, and a sinus tract can form that becomes a conduit for infection. Additional complications of tumoral calcinosis are low-grade fever, regional lymphadenopathy, anemia, and splenomegaly. There is also a characteristic dental abnormality (i.e., short bulbous tooth roots and calcific deposits in often obliterated pulp chambers) (238). Some patients have features of *pseudoxanthoma elasticum* (i.e., cutaneous and vascular calcifications as well as angioid streaks in their retinas).

Radiologic Features

The deposits of metastatic calcification are usually large aggregations of densely-calcified, irregular lobules confined to soft tissues (Fig. 39) (3,4). The joints near the tumors, however, are normal. Radiolucent fibrous septae within the masses explain their lobulated appearance. Occasionally, fluid layers are seen within these structures. Periarticular masses that are indistinguishable from those that occur in tumoral calcinosis are also found in chronic renal failure when calcium and phosphate homeostasis is poorly controlled. Bone scanning is the best method to detect and localize the tumors.

Recently, a "diaphysitis" has been described in some patients with tumoral calcinosis. It can be confused with neoplasm or osteomyelitis (241). New bone formation occurs along the medullary canal perhaps from calcific myelitis. Computed tomography and magnetic resonance imaging are effective techniques for detecting this feature (241).

Laboratory Findings

Affected subjects are in positive calcium/phosphate balance. The chalky fluid within lesions is predominantly hydroxyapatite (242,243). Hyperphosphatemia and increased serum calcitriol levels are found in some patients (240,244). Hyperphosphatemic subjects usually are black, have a positive family history, manifest the disease before age 20 years, and are troubled by multiple lesions (240). Levels of calcium and alkaline phosphatase activity are usually normal in serum. Renal studies reflect both the calcium and the phosphate retention, and some affected individuals are frankly hypocalciuric. The TmP/GFR may be supranormal, but renal function is otherwise unremarkable.

Histopathologic Findings

The masses of tumoral calcinosis are essentially foreign body granuloma reactions that consist of multilocu-

TABLE 4. *Disorders associated with extraskeletal calcification and ossification*[a]

Metastatic calcification	Dystrophic calcification
Hypercalcemia	Calcinosis (universalis or circumscripta)
Milk-alkali syndrome	Childhood dermatomyositis
Hypervitaminosis D	Scleroderma
Sarcoidosis	Systemic lupus erythematosis
Hyperparathyroidism	Post-traumatic
Renal failure	Ectopic ossification
Hyperphosphatemia	Myositis ossificans (post-traumatic)
Tumoral calcinosis	Burns
Hypoparathyroidism	Surgery
Pseudohypoparathyroidism	Neurologic injury
Cell lysis following chemotherapy for leukemia	Fibrodysplasia (myositis) ossificans progressiva
Renal failure	

Source: From Whyte (249), with permission.

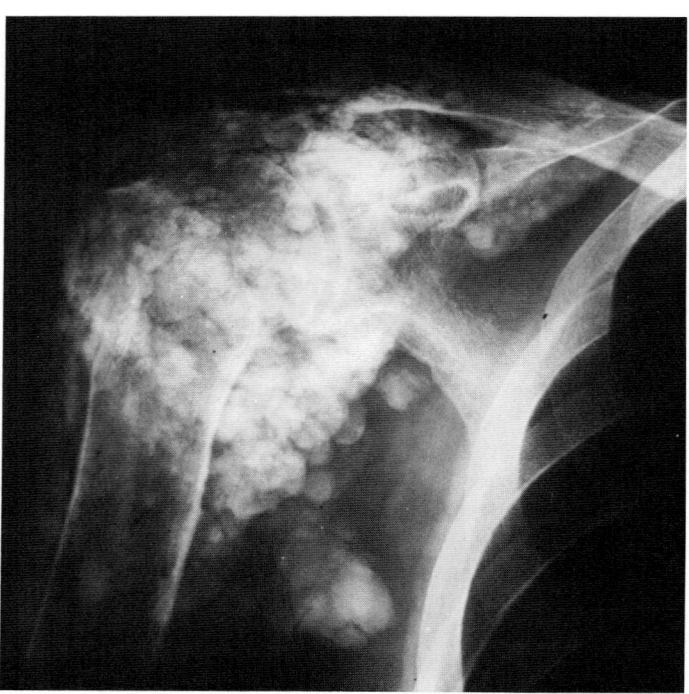

FIG. 39. Tumoral calcinosis. Typical lobular periarticular calcifications are present in the region of the right shoulder of this middle-aged man. From Whyte (249), with permission.

lar cystic structures. The cysts have tough connective tissue capsules and their fibrous walls contain numerous foreign body giant cells. They are filled with calcareous material in a viscous milky fluid. Occasionally, spicules of spongy bone and cartilage are noted.

Etiology/Pathogenesis

In normal individuals, calcium and inorganic phosphate levels in serum and extracellular fluid are sufficiently great that together they form a "metastable" solution, i.e., concentrations are too low for spontaneous precipitation of mineral, but sufficiently great to cause hydroxyapatite $[Ca_{10}(PO)_6(OH)_2]$ formation once crystal nucleation has begun (244,245). In healthy tissues, the presence of several inhibitors of mineralization such as inorganic pyrophosphate prevent precipitation from occurring inappropriately (244).

A significant number and variety of disorders cause extraskeletal deposition of calcium and phosphate where the mineral is precipitated as amorphous calcium phosphate or as hydroxyapatite crystals (Table 4). These conditions are different from disorders in which true bone tissue is formed (see section on Fibrodysplasia Ossificans Progressiva, this chapter). The pathogenesis involves a supranormal "calcium-phosphate solubility product" in extracellular fluid resulting in "metastatic" calcification, or "dystrophic" calcification in metabolically impaired or dead tissue despite normal serum levels of minerals (Table 4).

Metastatic calcification can result from hypercalcemia or hyperphosphatemia (especially both) of any etiology. Direct precipitation of mineral occurs when the calcium-phosphate solubility product in extracellular fluid is exceeded. A value of 75 for this parameter (mg/dL × mg/dL) is commonly taken as the level above which mineral deposition is likely to occur. The mineral precipitated in metastatic calcification is amorphous calcium phosphate initially, but hydroxyapatite crystals are formed soon after (242,243). There is a predilection for precipitation of mineral into certain tissues. The pattern varies somewhat for hypercalcemia versus hyperphosphatemia, but occurs irrespective of the specific underlying condition or mechanism for the disturbed ion level. Hypercalcemia typically results in mineral deposits within "acid-secreting" organs (i.e., kidneys, lungs, and stomach fundus). Additionally, however, the media of large arteries, elastic tissue of the endocardium (especially the left atrium), conjunctiva, and periarticular soft tissues are often affected. Why these sites are also predisposed is not well understood (244,245).

Hyperphosphatemia that is severe enough to cause metastatic calcification occurs in subjects with idiopathic hypoparathyroidism, pseudohypoparathyroidism, and following massive cell lysis with chemotherapy for leukemia. Renal failure commonly causes metastatic calcification; the pathogenesis may involve hyperphosphatemia, hypercalcemia, or both. Interestingly, ectopic calcification is more typical of pseudohypoparathyroidism (type I) than of idiopathic hypoparathyroidism despite comparable elevations in serum phosphate levels. Furthermore, the location of ectopic calcification in pseudohypoparathyroidism and hypoparathyroidism (e.g., basal ganglion region of the brain) is different from that which occurs from hypercalcemia. With hyperphosphatemia, calcification of periarticular subcutaneous tissues may be related to tissue trauma from the movement of joints.

The precise pathogenesis of tumoral calcinosis is not known, but it may lie within the renal tubule cell. Enhanced renal reclamation of filtered phosphate appears to be a fundamental pathogenetic factor. In hyperphosphatemic patients, enhanced renal tubular reabsorption of phosphate occurs independently of suppressed serum PTH levels (240,244). Furthermore, vitamin D metabolism is aberrant with apparently defective regulation of the renal 25-hydroxyvitamin D 1α-hydroxylase so that increased amounts of calcitriol are synthesized. In turn, there is enhanced absorption of dietary calcium and suppression of serum PTH levels (240,244). Since masses similar to those of tumoral calcinosis occur in disorders like sarcoidosis, hypervitaminosis D, or milk-alkali syndrome, the ectopic calcification of tumoral calcinosis is a nonspecific phenomenon. The masses may begin as calcific bursitis that extend into adjacent fascial planes as they grow. Tissue damage with fat necrosis may be a fundamental pathogenetic abnormality (243).

Treatment

Surgical removal of subcutaneous calcified masses may be helpful if they cause discomfort, interfere with function, or are cosmetically unacceptable. When surgical excision of a tumor is complete, it is believed to rarely occur at the same site.

Radiation therapy and cortisone treatment have not been effective. Use of phosphate-binding antacids together with dietary phosphate and calcium deprivation has been helpful (239). Although it might appear that if large apatite crystals were already in place phosphate-binding antacid therapy alone might not be very effective, a recent report describes dissolution of calcific tumors after aluminum hydroxide therapy (246). Nevertheless, use of such antacids to decrease extracellular fluid phosphate levels could help to prevent reformation of mineral deposits (239). Preliminary studies indicate that calcitonin therapy may also be efficacious, since it helps to minimize the hyperphosphatemia by enhancing renal clearance of phosphate (247).

REFERENCES

1. McKusick VA. *Mendelian inheritance in man: catalogs of autosomal dominant, autosomal recessive, and X-linked phenotypes,* 9th ed. Baltimore: Johns Hopkins University Press, 1990.
2. Beighton P. *Inherited disorders of the skeleton,* 2nd ed. Edinburgh: Churchill Livingstone, 1988.
3. Edeiken J, Dalinka M, Karasick D. *Edeiken's roentgen diagnosis of diseases of bone,* 4th ed. Baltimore: Williams & Wilkins, 1990.
4. Resnick D, Niwayama G. *Diagnosis of bone and joint disorders,* 2nd ed. Philadelphia: WB Saunders, 1988.
5. Scriver CR, Beaudet A, Sly WS, Valle D, eds. *The metabolic basis of inherited disease,* 6th ed. New York: McGraw-Hill, 1989.
6. Frame B, Honasoge M, Kottamasu SR. *Osteosclerosis, hyperostosis, and related disorders.* New York: Elsevier, 1987.
7. Rathbun JC. Hypophosphatasia, a new developmental anomaly. *Am J Dis Child* 1948;71:822–31.
8. Whyte MP. Hypophosphatasia. In: Scriver CR, Beaudet AL, Sly WS, Valle D, eds., *The metabolic basis of inherited disease,* 6th ed. New York: McGraw-Hill, 1989;2843–56.
9. Whyte MP. Alkaline phosphatase: physiologic role explored in hypophosphatasia. In: Peck WA, ed. *Bone and mineral research,* vol 6. Amsterdam: Elsevier Science, 1989;175–218.
10. Weiss MJ, Cole DEC, Ray K, et al. A missense mutation in the human liver/bone/kidney alkaline phosphatase gene causing a form of lethal hypophosphatasia. *Proc Natl Acad Sci USA* 1988;85:7666–9.
11. Weiss MJ, Ray K, Fallon MD, et al. Analysis of liver/bone/kidney alkaline phosphatase mRNA, DNA, and enzymatic activity in cultured skin fibroblasts from 14 unrelated patients with severe hypophosphatasia. *Am J Hum Genet* 1989;44:686–94.
12. Henthorn PS, Raducha MR, Lafferty MA, et al. Hypophosphatasia: point mutations at the human tissue nonspecific alkaline phosphatase gene locus in severely affected subjects (abstract). *Am J Hum Genet* (in press).
13. McComb RB, Bowers GN Jr, Posen S. *Alkaline phosphatase.* New York: Plenum, 1979.
14. Caswell AM, Whyte MP, Russell RGG. Hypophosphatasia and the extracellular metabolism of inorganic pyrophosphate: clinical and laboratory aspects. *Crit Rev Clin Lab Sci* 1991;28:175–232.
15. Fraser D. Hypophosphatasia. *Am J Med* 1957;22:730–46.
16. Moore CM, Wappner RS, Mulivor RA, Fedde KN, Coburn SP, Whyte MP. Pseudohypophosphatasia: clinical, radiographic, and biochemical characteristics of a second case (abstract). *Am J Hum Genet* 1990;47:A68.
17. Kousseff BG, Mulivor RA. Prenatal diagnosis of hypophosphatasia. *Obstet Gynecol* 1981;57:6(Suppl):9S–12S.
18. Whyte MP, Teitelbaum SL, Murphy WA, Bergfeld M, Avioli LV. Adult hypophosphatasia: clinical, laboratory and genetic investigation of a large kindred with review of the literature. *Medicine (Baltimore)* 1979;58:329–47.
19. Coe JD, Murphy WA, Whyte MP. Management of femoral fractures and pseudofractures in adult hypophosphatasia. *J Bone Joint Surg* 1986;68A:981–90.
20. Cole DEC, Stinson RA, Coburn SP, Ryan LM, Whyte MP. Increased serum pyridoxal-5′-phosphate in pseudohypophosphatasia (letter). *N Engl J Med* 1991;314:992–3.
21. Whyte MP, Valdes R Jr, McAlister WH, Ryan LM. Infantile hypophosphatasia: enzyme replacement therapy by intravenous infusion of alkaline phosphatase-rich plasma from patients with Paget's bone disease. *J Pediatr* 1982;101:379–86.
22. Sty JR, Boedecker RA, Babbitt DP. Skull scintigraphy in infantile hypophosphatasia. *J Nucl Med* 1979;20:305–6.
23. Whyte MP, Murphy WA, Fallon MD. Adult hypophosphatasia with chondrocalcinosis and arthropathy: variable penetrance of hypophosphatasemia in a large Oklahoma kindred. *Am J Med* 1982;72:631–41.
24. Whyte MP, Mahuren JD, Fedde KN, Cole FS, McCabe ERB, Coburn SP. Perinatal hypophosphatasia: tissue levels of vitamin B₆ are unremarkable despite markedly increased circulating concentrations of pyridoxal-5′-phosphate (evidence for an ectoenzyme role for tissue nonspecific alkaline phosphatase). *J Clin Invest* 1988;81:1234–9.
25. Chodirker BN, Coburn SP, Seargeant LE, Whyte MP, Greenberg CR. Increased plasma pyridoxal-5′-phosphate levels in carriers of infantile hypophosphatasia before and after pyridoxine loading. *J Inherited Metab Dis* 1990;13:891–6.
26. MacFarlane JD, Kroon HM, van der Harten JJ. Phenotypically dissimilar hypophosphatasia within two sibships. *Am J Med Genet* 1991 (in press).
27. Harris H. The human alkaline phosphatases: what we know and what we don't know. *Clin Chim Acta* 1990;186:125–320.

28. Chodirker BN, Evans JA, Lewis M, et al. Infantile hypophosphatasia—linkage with the RH locus. *Genomics* 1987;1:280-2.

29. Whyte MP, Magill LH, Fallon MD, Herrod HG. Infantile hypophosphatasia: normalization of circulating bone alkaline phosphatase activity followed by skeletal remineralization (evidence for an intact structural gene for tissue nonspecific alkaline phosphatase). *J Pediatr* 1986;108:82-8.

30. Whyte MP, Walkenhorst DA, Hill C, Fedde KN. Hypophosphatasemia in hypophosphatasia reflects proportionately decreased serum bone alkaline phosphatase antigen (abstract). *J Bone Miner Res* 1990;5:S171.

31. Fedde KN, Lane CC, Whyte MP. Alkaline phosphatase (tissue nonspecific isoenzyme) is a phosphoethanolamine and pyridoxal 5'-phosphatate ectophosphatase: normal and hypophosphatasia fibroblast study. *Am J Hum Genet* 1990;47:767-75.

32. Fedde KN, Cole DEC, Whyte MP. Pseudohypophosphatasia: aberrant localization and substrate specificity of alkaline phosphatase in cultured skin fibroblasts. *Am J Hum Genet* 1990;47:776-83.

33. Weninger M, Stinson RA, Plenk H Jr, Bock P, Pollak A. Biochemical and morphological effects of human hepatic alkaline phosphatase in a neonate with hypophosphatasia. *Acta Paediatr Scand Suppl* 1989;360:154-60.

34. Curry CJR, Smith JC, O'Lague P, Workman LA, Golbus MS. The prenatal diagnosis of autosomal dominant hypophosphatasia (abstract). *Am J Hum Genet* 1988;43:A230.

35. Frame B, Frost HM, Ormond RS, et al. Atypical axial osteomalacia involving the axial skeleton. *Ann Intern Med* 1961;55:632-9.

36. Whyte MP, Fallon MD, Murphy WA, et al. Axial osteomalacia: clinical, laboratory and genetic investigation of an affected mother and son. *Am J Med* 1981;71:1041-9.

37. Nelson AM, Riggs BL, Jowsey JO. Atypical axial osteomalacia: report of four cases with two having features of ankylosing spondylitis. *Arthritis Rheum* 1978;21:715-22.

38. Condon JR, Nassim JR. Axial osteomalacia. *Postgrad Med J* 1971;47:817-20.

39. Arnstein AR, Frame B, Frost HM. Recent progress in rickets and osteomalacia. *Ann Intern Med* 1967;67:1296-330.

40. Christman D, Wenger JJ, Dosch JC, et al. L'osteomalacie axiale anaylse comparee avec la fibrogenese imparfaite. *J Radiol* 1981;62:37-41.

41. Baker SL, Turnbull HM. Two cases of hitherto undescribed disease characterized by a gross defect in the collagen of the bone matrix. *J Pathol Bacteriol* 1950;62:132-4.

42. Baker SL, Dent CE, Friedman M, et al. Fibrogenesis imperfecta ossium. *J Bone Joint Surg* 1966;48B:804-25.

43. Thomas WC Jr, Moore T. Fibrogenesis imperfecta ossium. *Trans Am Clin Climatol Assoc* 1968;80:54-62.

44. Golding FC. Fibrogenesis imperfecta. *J Bone Joint Surg* 1968;50B:619-22.

45. Golde D, Greipp P, Sanzenbacher L, et al. Hematologic abnormalities in fibrogenesis imperfecta ossium. *J Bone Joint Surg* 1971;53A:365.

46. Frame B, Frost HM, Pak CYC, et al. Fibrogenesis imperfecta ossium, a collagen defect causing osteomalacia. *N Engl J Med* 1971;285:769-72.

47. Swan CHJ, Shah K, Brewer DB, et al. Fibrogenesis imperfecta ossium. *Q J Med* 1976;45:233-53.

48. Stamp TCB, Byers PD, Ali SY, Jenkins MV, Willoughby JMT. Fibrogenesis imperfecta ossium: remission with melphalan. *Lancet* 1985;1:582-3.

49. Byers PD, Stamp TCB, Stoker DJ. Fibrogenesis imperfecta (case report 296). *Skeletal Radiol* 1985;13:72-6.

50. Lang R, Vignery AM, Jensen PS. Fibrogenesis imperfecta ossium with early onset: observations after 20 years of illness. *Bone* 1986;7:237-46.

51. Stanley P, Baker SL, Byers PD. Unusual bone trabeculation in a patient with macroglobulinaemia simulating fibrogenesis imperfecta ossium. *Br J Radiol* 1971;44:305-13.

52. Albers-Schönberg H. Rontgenbilder einerseltenen, Knochenerkrankung. *Muench Med Wochenschr* 1904;51:365.

53. Johnston CC Jr, Lavy N, Lord T, Vellios F, Merritt AD, Deiss WP Jr. Osteopetrosis: a clinical, genetic, metabolic, and morphologic study of the dominantly inherited, benign form. *Medicine (Baltimore)* 1968;47:149-67.

54. Loria-Cortes R, Quesada-Calvo E, Cordero-Chaverri E. Osteopetrosis in children: a report of 26 cases. *J Pediatr* 1977;91:43-7.

55. Bollerslev J. Autosomal dominant osteopetrosis: bone metabolism and epidemiological, clinical and hormonal aspects. *Endocr Rev* 1989;10:45-67.

56. Sly WS. The carbonic anhydrase II deficiency syndrome: osteopetrosis with renal tubular acidosis and cerebral calcification. In: Scriver CR, et al., eds. *The metabolic basis of inherited disease,* 6th ed. New York: McGraw-Hill, 1989;2857-68.

57. Whyte MP, Murphy WA, Fallon MD, et al. Osteopetrosis, renal tubular acidosis and basal ganglia calcification in three sisters. *Am J Med* 1980;69:64-74.

58. Sly WS, Hewett-Emmett D, Whyte MP, Yu YSL, Tashian RE. Carbonic anhydrase II deficiency identified as the primary defect in the autosomal recessive syndrome of osteopetrosis with renal tubular acidosis and cerebral calcification. *Proc Natl Acad Sci USA* 1983;80:2752-6.

59. Beighton P, Hamersma H, Cremin BJ. Osteopetrosis in South Africa. The benign, lethal, and intermediate forms. *S Afr Med J* 1979;55:659-65.

60. Kahler SG, Burns JA, Aylsworth AS. A mild autosomal recessive form of osteopetrosis. *Am J Med Genet* 1984;17:451-64.

61. Horton WA, Schimek RN, Iyama T. Osteopetrosis: further heterogeneity. *J Pediatr* 1980;97:580-5.

62. El Khazan N, Faverly D, Vamos E, et al. Lethal osteopetrosis with multiple fractures in utero. *Am J Med Genet* 1986;23:811-9.

63. Bollerslev J, Kvetny J. Thyroid hormone resistance in blood monocyte cells and elevated serum T_3 in patients with autosomal dominant osteopetrosis. *Scand J Clin Lab Invest* 1988;48:795-9.

64. Bollerslev J, Steiniche T, Melsen F, Mosekilde L. Structural and histomorphometric studies of iliac crest trabecular and cortical bone in autosomal dominant osteopetrosis: a study of two radiological types. *Bone* 1989;10:19-24.

65. Jagadha V, Halliday WC, Becker LE, Hinton D. The association of infantile osteopetrosis and neuronal storage disease in two brothers. *Acta Neuropathol* 1988;75:233-40.

66. Monaghan BA, Kaplan FS, August CS, Fallon MD, Flannery DB. Transient infantile osteopetrosis. *J Pediatr* 1991;118:252-6.

67. Marks SC Jr. Osteopetrosis—multiple pathways for the interception of osteoclast function. *Appl Pathol* 1987;5:172-83.

68. Wilms G, Casaer P, Alliet P, Demaerel P, Smet M, Baert AL. Cerebrovascular occlusive complications in osteopetrosis major. *Neuroradiol* 1990;32:511-3.

69. Lehman RAW, Reeves JD, Wilson WB, Wesenberg RL. Neurological complications of infantile osteopetrosis. *Ann Neurol* 1977;2:378-84.

70. Ruben JB, Morris RJ, Judisch GF. Chorioretinal degeneration in infantile malignant osteopetrosis. *Am J Ophthalmol* 1990;110:1-5.

71. Osborn R, Boland T, DeLuchi S, Beirne OR. Osteomyelitis of the mandible in a patient with malignant osteopetrosis. *J Oral Pathol Med* 1985;40:76-80.

72. Mazur J, Wortsman J. Hypogonadotropic hypogonadism from osteopetrosis. *Clin Orthop* 1982;162:202-6.

73. Walpole IR, Nicoll A, Goldblatt J. Autosomal dominant osteopetrosis type II "malignant" presentation: further support for heterogeneity? *Clin Genet* 1990;38:257-63.

74. Oliveira G, Boechat MI, Amaral SM, Young LW. Osteopetrosis and rickets: an intriguing association. *Am J Dis Child* 1986;140:377-8.

75. Andersen PE Jr, Bollerslev J. Heterogeneity of autosomal dominant osteopetrosis. *Radiology* 1987;164:223-5.

76. Park H-M, Lambertus J. Skeletal and reticuloendothelial imaging in osteopetrosis: case report. *J Nucl Med* 1977;18:1091-5.

77. Al-Mefty O, Fox JL, Al-Rodhan N, Dew JH. Optic nerve decompression in osteopetrosis. *J Neurosurg* 1988;68:80-4.

78. Rao VM, Dalinka MK, Mitchell DG, et al. Osteopetrosis: MR characteristics at 1.5T'. *Radiology* 1986;161:217-20.

79. Kaplan F. Osteopetrorickets. *Clin Orthop* (in press).

80. Key LL, Carnes D, Cole S, et al. Treatment of congenital osteopetrosis with high dose calcitriol. *N Engl J Med* 1984;310:409-15.

81. Reeves JD, Arnaud S, Gordon S, et al. The pathogenesis of infantile malignant osteopetrosis: bone mineral metabolism and complications in five infants. *Metab Bone Dis Rel Res* 1981;3:135-42.

82. Yoneyama T, Fowler HL, Pendleton JW, et al. Elevated levels of creatine kinase BB isoenzyme in three patients with adult osteopetrosis (letter). *N Engl J Med* 1989;320:1294.

83. Whyte MP, Silva DP, Ladenson JH. Creatine kinase ("brain" isoenzyme) activity is elevated in the serum of select cases of osteopetrosis, but not in other sclerosing bone disorders (abstract). *J Bone Miner Res* 1990;5(Suppl 2):S239.

84. Teitelbaum SL, Coccia PF, Brown DM, Kahn AJ. Malignant osteopetrosis: a disease of abnormal osteoclast proliferation. *Metab Bone Dis Rel Res* 1981;3:99–105.

85. Key LL Jr. Osteopetrosis: a genetic window into osteoclast function. In: *Cases in metabolic bone disease.* 2(3), New York: Triclinica Communications, 1987.

86. Shapiro F, Glimcher MJ, Holtrop ME, Tashjian AH Jr, Brickley-Parsons D, Kewzora JE. Human osteopetrosis: a histological, ultrastructural, and biochemical study. *J Bone Joint Surg* 1980;62A:384–99.

87. Coccia PF. Cells that resorb bone (editorial). *N Engl J Med* 1984;310:456–8.

88. Coccia PF, Krivit W, Cervenka J, et al. Successful bone-marrow transplantation for infantile malignant osteopetrosis. *N Engl J Med* 1980;302:701–8.

89. Sorell M, Kapoor N, Kirkpatrick D, et al. Marrow transplantation for juvenile osteopetrosis. *Am J Med* 1981;70:1280–7.

90. Beard CJ, Key L, Newburger PE, et al. Neutrophil defect associated with malignant infantile osteopetrosis. *J Lab Clin Med* 1986;108:498–505.

91. Key LL, Ries WL, Schiff R. Osteopetrosis associated with interleukin-2 deficiency. *J Bone Miner Res* 1987;2(Suppl 1):85.

92. Glorieux FH, Pettifor JM, Marie PJ, et al. Induction of bone resorption by parathyroid hormone in congenital malignant osteopetrosis. *Metab Bone Dis Rel Res* 1981;3:143–50.

93. Reeves JD, August CS, Humbert JR, Weston WL. Host defense in infantile osteopetrosis. *Pediatr* 1979;64:202–6.

94. Yoshida H, Hayashi S, Kunisada T, et al. The murine mutation osteopetrosis is in the coding region of the macrophage colony stimulating factor gene. *Nature* 1990;345:442–4.

95. Felix R, Fleisch H, Cecchini M. Restoration of osteoclast formation and bone resorption in osteopetrotic OP/OP mice in vivo by recombinant human macrophage colony-stimulating factor (abstract). *J Bone Miner Res* 1990;5:S207.

96. Schneider GB, Kelly JD, Relfson M. Effects of interleukin-2 on bone resorption in osteopetrotic rats (abstract). *J Bone Miner Res* 1990;5(Suppl 2):207.

97. Key LL, Ries WL, Van Camp TM, Pitzer BL, Shepard A. Administration of interferon gamma to osteopetrotic mice stimulates bone resorption (abstract). *J Bone Miner Res* 1990;5(Suppl 2):S102.

98. Labat ML, Bringuier AF, Chandra A, Einhorn TA, Chandra P. Retroviral expression in mononuclear blood cells isolated from a patient with osteopetrosis (Albers-Schönberg disease). *J Bone Miner Res* 1990;5:425–35.

99. Mills BG, Yabe H, Singer FR. Osteoclasts in human osteopetrosis contain viral-nucleocapsid-like nuclear inclusions. *J Bone Miner Res* 1988;3:101–6.

100. Ballet J-J, Griscelli C, Coutris G, Milhaud G, Maroteaux P. Bone marrow transplantation in osteopetrosis (letter). *Lancet* 1977;2:137.

101. Kaplan FS, August CS, Fallon MD, Dalinka M, Axel L, Haddad JG. Successful treatment of infantile malignant osteopetrosis by bone-marrow transplantation: a case report. *J Bone Joint Surg* 1988;70A:617–23.

102. Orchard PJ, Dickerman JD, Mathews CHE, et al. Haploidentical bone marrow transplantation for osteopetrosis. *Am J Pediatr Hematol Oncol* 1987;9:335–40.

103. Cournot G, Thil Cl, Fischer A, Garabédian M. Osteopetrosis: the role of transplantation in marble bone disease. *Bone: Clinical and Biochemical News and Reviews* 1989;6:15–8.

104. Dent CE, Smellie JM, Watson L. Studies in osteopetrosis. *Arch Dis Child* 1965;40:7–15.

105. O'Meara A, Breatnach F, Kelleher J. Misleading radiology following bone marrow transplantation for infantile osteopetrosis. *Eur J Pediatr* 1990;149:447–50.

106. Delmas PD, Chapuy MC, Viala JJ, Meunier PJ. Improvement of adult congenital osteopetrosis with high doses of calcitriol (abstract 93). *J Bone Miner Res* 1987;2(Suppl 1).

107. Ozsoyla S. High dose intravenous methylprednisolone in treatment of recessive osteopetrosis (letter). *Arch Dis Child* 1987;62:214.

108. Dorantes LM, Mejia AM, Dorantes S. Juvenile osteopetrosis: effects on blood and bone of prednisone and low calcium, high phosphate diet. *Arch Dis Child* 1986;61:666–70.

109. Jenkinson EL, Pfisterer WH, Latteier KK, Martin M. A prenatal diagnosis of osteopetrosis. *Am J Radiol* 1943;49:455–62.

110. Golbus MS, Loerper MA, Hall BD. Failure to diagnose osteopetrosis *in utero* (letter). *Lancet* 1976;2:1246.

111. Venta PJ, Welty RJ, Johnson TH, Tashian RE. Human carbonic anhydrase II deficiency syndrome in a Belgian family appears to be caused by a destabilizing amino acid substitution (107 His → Tyr) (abstract). *Am J Hum Genet* 1990;47:A168.

112. Sly WS, Whyte MP, Sundaram V, et al. Carbonic anhydrase II deficiency in 12 families with the autosomal recessive syndrome of osteopetrosis with renal tubular acidosis and cerebral calcification. *N Engl J Med* 1985;313:139–45.

113. Strisciuglio P, Sartorio R, Pecoraro C, Lotito F, Sly WS. Variable clinical presentation of carbonic anhydrase deficiency: evidence for heterogeneity? *Eur J Pediatr* 1990;149:337–40.

114. Carter M, Stokes D, Wang W. Severe obstructive sleep apnea in a child with osteopetrosis. *Clin Pediatr* 1988;27:108–10.

115. Ohlsson A, Cumming WA, Paul A, Sly WS. Carbonic anhydrase II deficiency syndrome: recessive osteopetrosis with renal tubular acidosis and cerebral calcification. *Pediatrics* 1986;77:371–81.

116. Cumming WA, Ohlsson A. Intracranial calcification in children with osteopetrosis caused by carbonic anhydrase II deficiency. *Radiology* 1985;157:325–7.

117. Sly WS, Whyte MP, Krupin T, Sundarum V. Positive renal response to acetazolamide in carbonic anhydrase II-deficient patients. *Pediatr Res* 1985;19:1033–6.

118. Sato S, Zhu XL, Sly WS. Carbonic anhydrase isozymes IV and II in urinary membranes from carbonic anhydrase II-deficient patients. *Proc Natl Acad Sci USA* 1990;87:6073–6.

119. Lewis SE, Erickson RP, Barnett LB, et al. N-ethyl-N-nitrosurea-induced null mutation at the mouse car-2 locus: an animal model for human carbonic anhydrase II deficiency syndrome. *Proc Natl Acad Sci USA* 1988;85:1962–6.

120. Tashian RE, Hewett-Emmett D, Goodman M. On the evolution and genetics of carbonic anhydrase I, II, and III. In: Rattazzi ME, Scandalios JG, Whitt GS, eds. *Isoenzymes: current topics in biological and medical research,* vol 7. New York: Alan R Liss, 1983;79–100.

121. Sundquist KT, Leppilampi M, Järvelin K et al. Carbonic anhydrase isoenzyme in isolated rat peripheral monocytes, tissue macrophages, and osteoclasts. *Bone* 1987;8:33–8.

122. Baron R, Neff L, Louvard D, Courtoy PJ. Cell-mediated extracellular acidification and bone resorption: evidence for a low pH in resorbing lacunae and localization of a 100-kD lysosomal membrane protein on the osteoclast ruffled border. *J Cell Biol* 1985;101:2210–22.

123. Blair H, Teitelbaum SL, Ghiselli R, Gluck S. Osteoclastic bone resorption by a polarized vacuolar proton pump. *Science* 1989;245:855–7.

124. Raisz LG, Simmons HA, Thompson WJ, et al. Effects of a potent carbonic anhydrase inhibitor on bone resorption in organ culture. *Endocrinology* 1988;122:1083–6.

125. Gram J, Bollerslev J, Nielsen HK, Larsen HF, Mosekilde L. The effect of carbonic anhydrase inhibition on calcium and bone homeostasis in healthy postmenopausal women. *J Intern Med* 1990;228:367–71.

126. Dodgson SJ, Forster RE II, Sly WS, Tashian RE. Carbonic anhydrase activity of intact carbonic anhydrase II-deficient human erythrocytes. *J Appl Physiol* 1988;65:1472–80.

127. Whyte MP, Hamm LL, Sly WS. Transfusion of carbonic anhydrase-replete erythrocytes fails to correct the acidification defect in the syndrome of osteopetrosis, renal tubular acidosis, and cerebral calcification (carbonic anhydrase II deficiency). *J Bone Miner Res* 1988;3:385–8.

128. Cockayne EA. A case for diagnosis. *Proc R Soc Med* 1920;13:132–6.

129. Engelmann G. Ein fall von osteopathia hyperostotica (sclerotisans) multiplex infantilis. *Fortschr Geb Roentgenstr Nuklearmed Erganzungsband* 1929;39:1101–6.

130. Camurati M. Di un rar caso di osteite simmetrica ereditaria delgi arti inferiori. *Chir Organi Mov* 1922;6:662.

131. Hundley JD, Wilson FC. Progressive diaphyseal dysplasia. Review of the literature and report of seven cases in one family. *J Bone Joint Surg* 1973;55A:461–74.

132. Fallon MD, Whyte MP, Murphy WA. Progressive diaphyseal dysplasia (Engelmann's disease): report of a sporadic case of the mild form. *J Bone Joint Surg* 1980;62A:465–72.

133. Naveh Y, Ludatsheer R, Alon U, et al. Muscle involvement in progressive diaphyseal dysplasia. *Pediatrics* 1985;76:944–9.

134. Crisp AJ, Brenton DP. Engelmann's disease of bone—a systemic disorder? *Ann Rheum Dis* 1982;41:183–8.

135. Aggarwal P, Wali JP, Sharma SK. Progressive diaphyseal dysplasia: case report and literature review. *Orthopedics* 1990;13:901–4.

136. Kaftori JK, Kleinhaus U, Neveh Y. Progressive diaphyseal dysplasia (Camurati-Engelmann): radiographic follow-up and CT findings. *Radiology* 1987;164:777–82.

137. Kumar B, Murphy WA, Whyte MP. Progressive diaphyseal dysplasia (Englemann's disease): Scintigraphic-radiologic-clinical correlations. *Radiology* 1981;140:87–92.

138. Smith R, Walton RJ, Corner BD, et al. Clinical and biochemical studies in Engelmann's disease (progressive diaphyseal dysplasia). *Q J Med* 1977;46:273–94.

139. Yoshioka H, Mino M, Kiyosawa N, et al. Muscular involvement in progressive diaphyseal dysplasia. *Arch Dis Child* 1980;55:716–9.

140. Shier CK, Krasicky GA, Ellis BI, Kottamasu SR. Ribbing's disease: radiographic-scintigraphic correlation and comparative analysis with Engelmann's disease. *J Nucl Med* 1987;28:244–8.

141. Naveh Y, Alon U, Kaftori JK, et al. Progressive diaphyseal dysplasia: evaluation of corticosteroid therapy. *Pediatrics* 1985;75:321–3.

142. Guan DW, Mionuddin M, Pitcock J, et al. Intermittent diphosphonate in Engelmann's disease: a 5 year followup (abstract). *J Bone Miner Res* 1986;1:117.

143. Maroteaux P, Lamay M. La pycnodysostose. *Presse Med* 1962;70:999.

144. Sugiura Y, Yamada Y, Koh J. Pycnodysostosis in Japan: report of six cases and a review of Japanese literature. *Birth Defects* 1974;10(12):78–98.

145. Maroteaux P, Lamy M. The malady of Toulouse-Lautrec. *JAMA* 1965;191:715–7.

146. Elmore SM. Pycnodysostosis: a review. *J Bone Joint Surg* 1967;49A:153–62.

147. Wolpowitz A, Matisson A. A comparative study of pycnodysostosis, cleidocranial dysostosis, osteopetrosis and acro-osteolysis. *S Afr Med J* 1974;48:1011.

148. Soto TJ, Mautalen CA, Hojman D, et al. Pycnodysostosis, metabolic and histologic studies. In: *Birth Defects* 1969;5(4):109–15.

149. Everts V, Aronson DC, Beertsen W. Phagocytosis of bone collagen by osteoclasts in two cases of pycnodysostosis. *Calcif Tissue Int* 1985;37:25–31.

150. Beneton MNC, Harris S, Kanis JA. Paramyxovirus-like inclusions in two cases of pycnodysostosis. *Bone* 1987;8:211–7.

151. Cabrejas ML, Fromm GA, Roca JF. Pycnodysostosis. Some aspects concerning kinetics of calcium metabolism and bone pathology. *Am J Med Sci* 1976;271:215.

152. Van Buchem FSP, Prick JJG, Jaspar HHJ. *Hyperostosis corticalis generalisata familiaris (van Buchem's disease)*. Amsterdam: Excerpta, 1976.

153. Perez-Vicente JA, Rodriquez de Castro E, Lafuente J, et al. Autosomal dominant endosteal hyperostosis. Report of a Spanish family with neurological involvement. *Clin Genet* 1987;31:161–9.

154. Eastman JR, Bixler D. Generalized cortical hyperostosis (van Buchem disease): nosologic considerations. *Radiology* 1977;125:297–304.

155. Beighton P, Barnard A, Hamersma H, et al. The syndromic status of sclerosteosis and van Buchem disease. *Clin Genet* 1984;25:175–81.

156. Beighton P, Durr L, Hamersma H. The clinical features of scler-

157. Barnard AH, Hamersma H, Kretzmar JH, et al. Sclerosteosis in old age. *S Afr Med J* 1980;58:401–3.

158. Beighton P, Cremin BJ, Hamersma H. The radiology of sclerosteosis. *Br J Radiol* 1976;49:934–9.

159. Stein SA, Witkop C, Hill S, et al. Sclerosteosis, neurogenetic and pathophysiologic analysis of an American kinship. *Neurology* 1983;33:267–77.

160. Epstein S, Hamersma H, Beighton P. Endocrine function in sclerosteosis. *S Afr Med J* 1979;55:1105–10.

161. Ruckert EW, Caudill RJ, McCready PJ. Surgical treatment of van Buchem disease. *J Oral Maxillofac Surg* 1985;43:801–5.

162. Berlin R, Hedensio B, Lilja B, et al. Osteopoikilosis—a clinical and genetic study. *Acta Med Scand* 1967;18:305–14.

163. Uitto J, Starcher BC, Santa-Cruz DJ, et al. Biochemical and ultrastructural demonstration of elastin accumulation in the skin of the Buschke-Ollendorff syndrome. *J Invest Dermatol* 1981;76:284–7.

164. Whyte MP, Murphy WA, Seigel BA. 99m Tc-pyrophosphate bone imaging in osteopoikilosis, osteopathia striata, and melorheostosis. *Radiology* 1978;127:439–43.

165. Resnick D, Niwayama G. *Diagnosis of bone and joint disorders*, 2nd ed. Philadelphia: WB Saunders, 1988.

166. Lagier R, Mbakop A, Bigler A. Osteopoikilosis: a radiological and pathological study. *Skeletal Radiol* 1984;11:161–8.

167. Rabinow M, Unger F. Syndrome of osteopathia striata, macrocephaly, and cranial sclerosis. *Am J Dis Child* 1984;138:821–3.

168. Happle R, Lenz W. Striation of bones in focal dermal hypoplasia: manifestation of functional mosaicism? *Br J Dermatol* 1977;96:133–8.

169. Kornreich L, Grunebaum M, Ziv N, Shuper A, Mimouni M. Osteopathia striata, cranial sclerosis with cleft palate and facial nerve palsy. *Eur J Pediatr* 1988;147:101–3.

170. Léri A, Joanny J. Une affection non decrite des os. Hyperostose "en coulée" sur toute la longueur d'un membre ou "melorheostose." *Bull Mem Soc Hop Paris* 1922;46:1141–5.

171. Murray RO, McCredie J. Melorheostosis and sclerotomes: a radiological correlation. *Skeletal Radiol* 1979;4:57–71.

172. Campbell CJ, Papademetriou T, Bonfiglio M. Melorheostosis: a report of the clinical, roentgenographic, and pathological findings in fourteen cases. *J Bone Joint Surg* 1968;50A:1281–1304.

173. Miyachi Y, Horio T, Yamada A, et al. Linear melorheostotic scleroderma with hypertrichosis. *Arch Dermatol* 1979;115:1233–4.

174. Applebaum RE, Caniano DA, Sun C-C, et al. Synchronous left subclavian and axillary artery aneurysms associated with melorheostosis. *Surgery* 1986;99:249–53.

175. Colavita N, Nicolais S, Orazi C, Falappa PG. Melorheostosis: presentation of a case followed up for 24 years. *Arch Orthop Trauma Surg* 1987;106:123–5.

176. Resnick D, Niwayama G. *Diagnosis of bone and joint disorders*, 2nd ed. Philadelphia: WB Saunders, 1988.

177. Whyte MP, Murphy WA, Seigel BA. 99m Tc-pyrophosphate bone imaging in osteopoikilosis, osteopathia striata, and melorheostosis. *Radiology* 1978;127:439–43.

178. Wagers LT, Young AW Jr, Ryan SF. Linear melorheostotic scleroderma. *Br J Dermatol* 1972;86:297–301.

179. Whyte MP, Murphy WA, Fallon MD, et al. Mixed-sclerosing-bone dystrophy: report of a case and review of the literature. *Skeletal Radiol* 1981;6:95–102.

180. Pacifici R, Murphy WA, Teitelbaum SL, et al. Mixed-sclerosing-bone dystrophy: 42-year follow-up of a case reported as osteopetrosis. *Calcif Tissue Int* 1986;38:175–85.

181. Harris WH, Dudley HR Jr, Barry RJ. The natural history of fibrous dysplasia: an orthopedic, pathological, and roentgenographic study. *J Bone Joint Surg* 1962;44A:207–33.

182. Johnson CB, Gilbert EF, Gottlieb LI. Malignant transformation of polyostotic fibrous dysplasia. *South Med J* 1979;72:353–6.

183. Chetty R, Kalan MR, Kranold DH. Malignant transformation in fibrous dysplasia. *S Afr J Surg* 1990;28:80–2.

184. Harris RI. Polyostotic fibrous dysplasia with acromegaly. *Am J Med* 1985;78:538–42.

185. Feuillan PP, Shanker T, Rose SR, Jones J, Jeevanram RK, Nisula

BC. Thyroid abnormalities in the McCune-Albright syndrome: ultrasonography and hormonal studies. *J Clin Endocrinol Metab* 1990;71:1596–601.

186. Swislocki ALM, Camargo CA, Hoffman AR. McCune-Albright syndrome: a case of primary hypogonadism obscured by hyper-prolactinemic hypogonadotropic hypogonadism. *West J Med* 1990;153:653–6.

187. Norris MA, Kaplan PA, Pathria M, Greenway G. Fibrous dysplasia: magnetic resonance imaging appearance at 1.5 Telsa. *Clin Imaging* 1990;14:211–5.

188. Happle R. The McCune-Albright syndrome: a lethal gene surviving by mosaicism. *Clin Genet* 1986;29:321–4.

189. Cuttler L, Jackson JA, Saeed us-Zafar M, Levitsky LL, Mellinger RC, Frohman LA. Hypersecretion of growth hormone and prolactin in McCune-Albright Syndrome. *J Clin Endocrinol Metab* 1989;68:1148–54.

190. Kaplan FS, Fallon MD, Boden SD, Schmidt R, Senior M, Haddad JG. Estrogen receptors in bone in a patient with polyostotic fibrous dysplasia (McCune-Albright syndrome). *N Engl J Med* 1988;319:241–5.

191. Lever EG, Pettingale KW. Albright's syndrome associated with a soft-tissue myxoma and hypophosphatemic osteomalacia. Report of a case and review of the literature. *J Bone Joint Surg* 1983;65B:621–6.

192. Smith MD, Bohlman HH, Gideonse N. Fibrous dysplasia of the cervical spine: a fatal complication of treatment. *J Bone Joint Surg* 1990;72A:1254–8.

193. Chen Y-R, Noordhoff MS. Treatment of craniomaxillofacial fibrous dysplasia: how early and how extensive? *Plast Reconstr Surg* 1990;86:835–42.

194. Feuillan PP, Foster CM, Pescovits OH, et al. Treatment of precocious puberty in the McCune-Albright syndrome with the aromatase inhibitor testolactone. *N Engl J Med* 1986;315:1115–9.

195. Rogers JG, Geho WB. Fibrodysplasia ossificans progressiva: a survey of forty-two cases. *J Bone Joint Surg* 1979;61A:909–14.

196. Connor JM, Evans DAP. Fibrodysplasia ossificans progressiva: the clinical features and natural history of 34 patients. *J Bone Joint Surg* 1982;64B:76–83.

197. Connor JM, Beighton P. Fibrodysplasia progressiva in South Africa: case reports. *S Afr Med J* 1982;61:404–6.

198. Hsu LCS, Hsu KY, Leong JCY. Severe scoliosis associated with fibrodysplasia ossificans progressiva. *Spine* 1986;11:643–4.

199. Cremin B, Connor JM, Beighton P. The radiological spectrum of fibrodysplasia ossificans progressiva. *Clin Radiol* 1982;33:499–508.

200. Cole DEC, Cohen MM Jr. Mutations involving bone-forming cells. In: Hall BK, ed. *Bone: The osteoblast and osteocyte*, vol 1. Caldwell, NJ: Telford Press, 1990.

201. Reinig JW, Hill Sc, Fang M, et al. Fibrodysplasia ossificans progressiva: CT appearance. *Radiology* 1986;159:153–7.

202. Fang MA, Reinig JW, Hill SC, et al. Technetium-99m MDP demonstration of heterotopic ossification in fibrodysplasia ossificans progressiva. *Clin Nucl Med* 1986;11:8–9.

203. Sumiyoshi K, Tsuneyoshi M, Enjoji M. Myositis ossificans: a clinicopathologic study of 21 cases. *Acta Pathol Jpn* 1985;35:1109–22.

204. Rogers JG, Chase GA. Paternal age effect in fibrodysplasia ossificans progressiva. *J Med Genet* 1979;16:147–8.

205. Lutwak L. Myositis ossificans progressiva. Mineral, metabolic, and radioactive calcium studies of the effects of hormones. *Am J Med* 1964;37:269–93.

206. Smith R, Russell RGG, Wood CG. Myositis ossificans progressiva. Clinical features of eight patients and their response to treatment. *J Bone Joint Surg* 1976;58B:48–57.

207. Moore SE, Jump AA, Smiley JD. Effect of warfarin sodium therapy on excretion of 4-carboxy-L-glutamic acid in myositis ossificans progressiva. *Arthritis Rheum* 1986;29:344–51.

208. Rimoin DL. Pachydermoperiostosis (idiopathic clubbing and periostosis). Genetic and physiologic consideration. *N Engl J Med* 1965;272:923–31.

209. Herman MA, Massaro D, Katz S. Pachydermoperiostosis—clinical spectrum. *Arch Intern Med* 1965;116:919–23.

210. Ali A, Tetalman M, Fordham EW. Distribution of hypertrophic pulmonary osteoarthropathy. *AJR* 1980;134:771–80.

211. Vogl A, Goldfischer S. Pachydermoperiostosis: primary or idiopathic hypertrophic osteoarthropathy. *Am J Med* 1962;33:166–87.

212. Lauter SA, Vasey FB, Hüttner I, et al. Pachydermoperiostosis: studies on the synovium. *J Rheumatol* 1978;5:85–95.

213. Matucci-Cerinic M, Fattorini L, Gerini G, et al. Colchicine treatment in a case of pachydermoperiostosis with acroosteolysis. *Rheumatol Int* 1988;8:185–8.

214. Byers PH. Disorders of collagen biosynthesis and structure. In: Scriver CR, et al., eds. *The metabolic basis of inherited disease*, 6th ed. New York: McGraw-Hill, 1989;2805–42.

215. Prockop DJ, Baldwin CT, Constantinou CD. Mutations in type I procollagen genes that cause osteogenesis imperfecta. *Adv Hum Genet* 1990;19:105–32.

216. Albright JA, Millar EA. Osteogenesis Imperfecta (symposium). *Clin Orthop* 1981;159:1–156.

217. Sillence D. Osteogenesis imperfecta: an expanding panorama of varients. *Clin Orthop* 1981;159:11–25.

218. Byers PH, Tsipouras P, Bonadio JF, Starman BJ, Schwartz RC. Perinatal lethal osteogenesis imperfecta (OI type II): a biochemically heterogeneous disorder usually due to new mutations in the genes for type I collagen. *Am J Hum Genet* 1988;42:237–48.

219. Dent JA, Paterson CR. Fractures in early childhood: osteogenesis imperfecta or child abuse. *J Pediatr Orthop* 1991;11:184–6.

220. Ablin DS, Greenspan A, Reinhart M, Grix A. Differentiation of child abuse from osteogenesis imperfecta. *AJR* 1990;154:1035–46.

221. Pedersen U. Hearing loss in patients with osteogenesis imperfecta. *Scand Audiol* 1984;13:67–74.

222. Garretsen TJTM, Cremers CWRJ. Stapes surgery in osteogenesis imperfecta: analysis of postoperative hearing loss. *Ann Otol Rhinol Laryngol* 1991;100:120–30.

223. Revell PA. *Pathology of bone*. Berlin: Springer-Verlag, 1986.

224. Falvo KA, Bullough PG. Osteogenesis imperfecta: a histometric analysis. *J Bone Joint Surg [Am]* 1973;55:275–86.

225. Cremin B, Goodman H, Prax M, Spranger J, Beighton P. Wormian bones in osteogenesis imperfecta and other disorders. *Skeletal Radiol* 1982;8:35–8.

226. Goldman AB, Davidson D, Pavlor H, Bullough PG. "Popcorn" calcifications: a prognostic sign in osteogenesis imperfecta. *Radiology* 1980;136:351–8.

227. Harkey HL, Crockard HA, Stevens JM, Smith R, Ransford AO. The operative management of basilar impression in osteogenesis imperfecta. *Neurosurgery* 1990;27:782–6.

228. Chines A, Petersen DJ, Schranck F, Whyte MP. Hypercalciuria in children severely affected with osteogenesis imperfecta. *J Pediatr* (in press).

229. Baron R, Gertner JM, Lang R, Vighery A. Increased bone turnover with decreased bone formation by osteoblasts in children with osteogenesis imperfecta tarda. *Pediatr Res* 1983;17:204–7.

230. Bonadio J, Saunders TL, Tsai E, et al. Transgenic mouse model of the mild dominant form of osteogenesis imperfecta. *Proc Natl Acad Sci USA* 1990;87:7145–9.

231. Devogelaer JP, Malghem J, Maldague B, Nagant de Deuxchaisnes C. Radiological manifestations of bisphosphonate treatment with APD in a child suffering from osteogenesis imperfecta. *Skeletal Radiol* 1987;16:360–3.

232. Porat S, Heller E, Seidman DS, Meyer S. Functional results of operation in osteogenesis imperfecta: elongating and nonelongating rods. *J Pediatr Orthop* 1991;11:200–3.

233. Letts M, Monson R, Weber K. The prevention of recurrent fractures of the lower extremities in severe osteogenesis imperfecta using vacuum pants: a preliminary report in four patients. *J Pediatr Orthop* 1988;8:454–6.

234. Gerber LH, Binder H, Weintrob J, et al. Rehabilitation of children and infants with osteogenesis imperfecta. A program for ambulation. *Clin Orthop* 1990;251:254–62.

235. Marini JC. Osteogenesis imperfecta: comprehensive management. *Adv Pediatr* 1988;35:391–426.

236. Gerber LH, Binder H, Weintrob J, et al. Rehabilitation of children and infants with osteogenesis imperfecta. *Clin Orthop* 1990;251:254–62.

237. Wenstrup RJ, Willing MC, Starman BJ, Byers PH. Distinct biochemical phenotypes predict clinical severity in nonlethal vari-

ants of osteogenesis imperfecta. *Am J Hum Genet* 1990;46:975–82.

238. Lyles KW, Burkes EJ, Ellis GJ, et al. Genetic transmission of tumoral calcinosis: autosomal dominant with variable clinical expressivity. *J Clin Endocrinol Metab* 1985;60:1093–6.

239. Mozaffarian G, Lafferty FW, Pearson OH. Treatment of tumoral calcinosis with phosphorus deprivation. *Ann Intern Med* 1972;77:741–5.

240. Prince MJ, Schaefer PC, Goldsmith RS, Chausmer AB. Hyperphosphatemic tumoral calcinosis: association with elevation of serum 1,25-dihydroxycholecalciferol concentrations. *Ann Intern Med* 1982;96:586–91.

241. Martinez S, Vogler JB 3rd, Harrelson JM, Lyles KW. Imaging of tumoral calcinosis: new observations. *Radiology* 1990;174:215–22.

242. Boskey AL, Vigorita VJ, Sencer O, Stuchin SA, Lane JM. Chemical, microscopic and ultrastructural characterization of mineral deposits in tumoral calcinosis. *Clin Orthop* 1983;178:258–70.

243. Kindblom L-G, Gunterberg B. Tumoral calcinosis: an ultrastructural analysis and consideration of pathogenesis. *APMIS* 1988;96:368–76.

244. Lyles KW, Halsey DL, Friedman NE, Lobaugh G. Association of 1,25-dihydroxyvitamin D, phosphorus and parathyroid hormone in tumoral calcinosis: potential pathogenetic mechanisms for the disease. *J Clin Endocrinol Metab* 1988;68:88–92.

245. Anderson HC. Calcific diseases: a concept. *Arch Pathol Lab Med.* 1983;107:341–8.

246. Davies M, Clements MR, Mawer EB, Freemong AJ. Tumoral calcinosis: clinical and metabolic response to phosphorus deprivation. *Q J Med* 1987;242:493–503.

247. Salvi A, Cerudelli B, Cimino A, Zuccato F, Giustina G. Phosphaturic action of calcitonin in pseudotumoral calcinosis (letter). *Horm Metab Res* 1983;15:260.

248. Whyte MP, Murphy WA. Osteopetrosis and other sclerosing bone disorders. In: Alvioli LV, Krane SM, eds. *Metabolic bone disease,* 2nd ed. Philadelphia: WB Saunders, 1990;616–58.

249. Whyte MP. Extraskeletal (ectopic) calcification and ossification. In: Favus M, et al., eds. *Primer in the metabolic bone diseases and disorders of mineral metabolism.* Richmond: Byrd Press, 1990;261–9.

250. Whyte MP. Heritable metabolic and dysplastic bone diseases. *Endocrinol Metab Clin North Am* 1990;19:133–73.

251. Coburn SP, Whyte MP. Role of phosphatases in the regulation of vitamin B_6 metabolism in hypophosphatasia and other disorders. In: Leklem JE, Reynolds RD, eds. *Clinical and physiological applications of vitamin B_6.* New York: Alan R. Liss, 1988;65–93.

CHAPTER **43**

Paget's Disease of Bone

Roy D. Altman

Paget's disease of bone is a remodeling disease of isolated areas of the skeleton. The initial event involves active resorption. This is followed by deposition of bone that is disorganized, often enlarged, interspersed with areas of fibrosis, and structurally weak. Paget's disease is a localized bone disease that may have widespread distribution in contrast to a generalized disease such as hyperparathyroidism. Prior names include *osteitis deformans, osseous dystrophy, rarefying osteitis with distortion and thickening of bone,* and *hereditary heterogenous osteopathy* (1).

BACKGROUND

Sir James Paget (1814–1899) was one of several children of an affluent business family from Yarmouth, England. He was a celebrated surgeon with accompanying fame in surgical pathology. He skillfully combined his clinical skills with descriptive pathology (2). At age 30 he was elected a Fellow of the Royal College of Surgeons in London, was appointed professor of anatomy and pathology at the Royal College of Surgeons three years later, received fellowship at the Royal Society when he was 37 years old; was knighted at age 43, and became surgeon to Queen Victoria and the Prince of Wales when he was 53.

During a postmortem examination in his freshman year of medical school, he identified little white specks in the muscles of a 45-year-old man, performed light microscopy, and sketched an encysted spiral worm that was later named *Trichina spiralis.*

He later joined the faculty at St. Bartholomew's Hospital in London and was given the task of cataloguing 3520 surgical specimens. While working on that project, he collected and collated an additional 2298 specimens.

Seven years later he completed his assignment, a catalog not previously accomplished, and became the acknowledged master of surgical pathology. In 1851 he entered private practice, and in 1878 ceased to operate as an active surgeon, participating as a consultant on difficult cases.

His notes define metastatic tumors to ovaries and dermatofibrosarcoma protuberans long before description by Krukenberg (3). Other diseases associated with Paget's original descriptions include carpal tunnel syndrome, Paget's disease of the breast, Paget's disease of the anus, Paget van Schrotter syndrome, Paget's abscess, Paget's quiet necrosis, and Paget's disease of bone. Additionally, Paget seemed to have described postsurgical toxic shock syndrome (4).

Paget's disease of bone is not a disease of recent origin. There is paleopathologic evidence from Anglo-Saxon skulls (5), American-Indian skeletons found in the Illinois River Valley region (6), and a parietal bone from an Egyptian tomb (7).

Although isolated case reports in the midnineteenth century describe what is now called Paget's disease (8–10), the classic clinical description by Sir James Paget and the excellent pathologic description by (Sir) Henry Butlin clarified this entity in 1876 in a presentation to the Royal Medical Chirurgical Society of London (11).

Paget followed the evolution of the disease in his original patient for 22 years until the patient's death related to an osteoid cancer (presumably pagetic sarcoma). Paget felt that the basic pathologic process was one of chronic inflammation of infectious origin, naming the condition *osteitis deformans.* Paget's name was later associated with the disease because similar terminology had been used previously for other conditions of bone.

Beethoven's deafness may have been due to Paget's disease (12). His autopsy, performed by Wagner and Rokitansky, was inconclusive (13): There was no otosclerosis, and thickening of the calvarum was not described. Unfortunately, the specimen bottle containing his tem-

R. D. Altman: Department of Medicine, University of Miami School of Medicine, Miami, Florida 33101; Arthritis Section, Miami Veterans Administration Medical Center, Miami, Florida 33101

poral bones are missing from the National Museum in Vienna and reexamination is not feasible.

EPIDEMIOLOGY

There is a slight male predominance (3 men:2 women). The youngest convincing case of Paget's disease reported was an 18-year-old man (13). Variations in the prevalence of Paget's disease in different areas of the world are striking. The disease appears to have its greatest frequency in Eastern and Western Europe, in addition to regions inhabited by emigrants from these areas to Australia, New Zealand, South Africa, and areas of South America. The disease is distinctly uncommon in African blacks, Orientals (14), Asian-Indians, and Scandinavians.

Most prevalence studies are based on radiographs, commonly of the pelvis. In 1932, Schmorl found Paget's disease in 3% of an autopsy series (15). More recent studies place the prevalence ranges between 3.5 and 4.5% of the population in high-prevalence regions of the world, with a high of 8.3% in a part of Lancashire, England (16), to 0.4% in Sweden (17). In a survey of Paget's disease on pelvic roentgenograms in the United States, the prevalence was 3.9% in Caucasians of Brooklyn and 0.9% in Caucasians of Atlanta (18). Similarly, 1000 pelvic roentgenograms revealed no Paget's disease in Lexington, Kentucky and 1.1% pelvic Paget's disease in Providence, Rhode Island (19). A Philadelphia survey of 333 diphosphonate bone scans found Paget's disease in 2.1% (20).

In an epidemiologic survey, 13.8% of patients with Paget's disease had relatives with Paget's disease (21). Approximately half of those relatives were from successive generations and half were siblings. The disease has been reported in monozygotic twins (22,23). Familial cases had an earlier onset than isolated cases.

An autosomal dominant pattern has been suggested (21,24). Some family studies suggest an HLA association with linkage disequilibrium (24,25). Others are unable to document an HLA association (26,27). We have seen two families with Paget's disease in the spouses. There is no seasonal predominance for discovery of the disease.

It has been proposed that Paget's disease is acquired through ingestion of contaminated tissues from bovine meat (28), but adequate documentation is lacking. Evidence for the relation of Paget's disease to maintaining pets, such as dogs, has also been inconclusive (29,30). Evidence that Paget's disease may exist in animals other than humans are not convincing. A childhood osseosis condition called juvenile Paget's disease appears to be a separate entity.

Survival in Paget's disease is normal. Most deaths relate indirectly to malignancy (31). No population studies have examined disability, impact of disease on daily living activity, health assessment, or other social parameters.

ETIOLOGY

It is interesting to follow the myriad listing of the etiology of Paget's disease. Only a condition of unknown etiology could generate so many possible causes. Original confusion with von Recklinghausen's hyperparathyroidism was dissipated by Mandle (32). Possible etiologies have included trauma, endocrine, nonspecific chronic inflammation, heredity, vascular compromise from arteriosclerosis with resultant arteriovenous fistulas, and mechanical factors of stress and strain. An endocrine etiology, such as increased parathyroid hormone and reduced calcitonin, is unsupported on clinical and experimental grounds.

Sir James Paget named this disease osteitis deformans in the belief that the basic process was inflammatory and had an infectious origin (11). Infection with inflammation was also suspected by Looser (33) and Erdheim (34).

The most convincing data relate to a possible viral etiology. Ultrastructural studies of involved bone in pagetic patients have revealed nuclear and cytoplasmic inclusions (35) (Fig. 1). Osteoclastic nuclei contain microfilaments that are tubular in appearance and are arranged in semiorganized bundles. In the cytoplasm, the tubules are scattered randomly. They have not been found in bone cells of patients with other skeletal disorders, with the exception of giant-cell tumors of bone. The cytoplasmic tubules are similar to those seen in inclusion body myositis. Their morphologic appearance resembles nuclei of cells infected with paramyxoviruses such as parainfluenza, mumps, and measles; they are similar in appearance to cultured cells infected with respiratory syncytial virus (RSV) (36). This tubular morphologic finding has raised the question as to whether Paget's disease is a slow virus infection of bone. Other slow virus infections of humans have similarly demonstrated a long clinical latent period, absence of an acute inflammatory response, a slowly progressive course, restriction of disease to a single organ system, patchy distribution in the body, and genetic predisposition. Support for a viral infection comes from a study demonstrating increased serum binding of poly I:C from 25% of patients with Paget's disease (37). Increased measles antibodies were not found by complement fixation by some (38,39) but were found by others (40,41). Titers of RSV antibodies were similar to controls (41). Immunohistologic studies of bone biopsy specimens grown in culture from 30 patients have demonstrated evidence for both measles and RSV antigens in pagetic bone (42). After receiving disodium etidronate (EHDP) therapy, immunocytologic analysis showed persistence of nuclear and cytoplasmic staining in markedly altered osteoclasts (43); this suggests virus rather than distortion of cellular components.

As stated above, morphology and some immunology suggest a viral infection; however, the suggestion of dif-

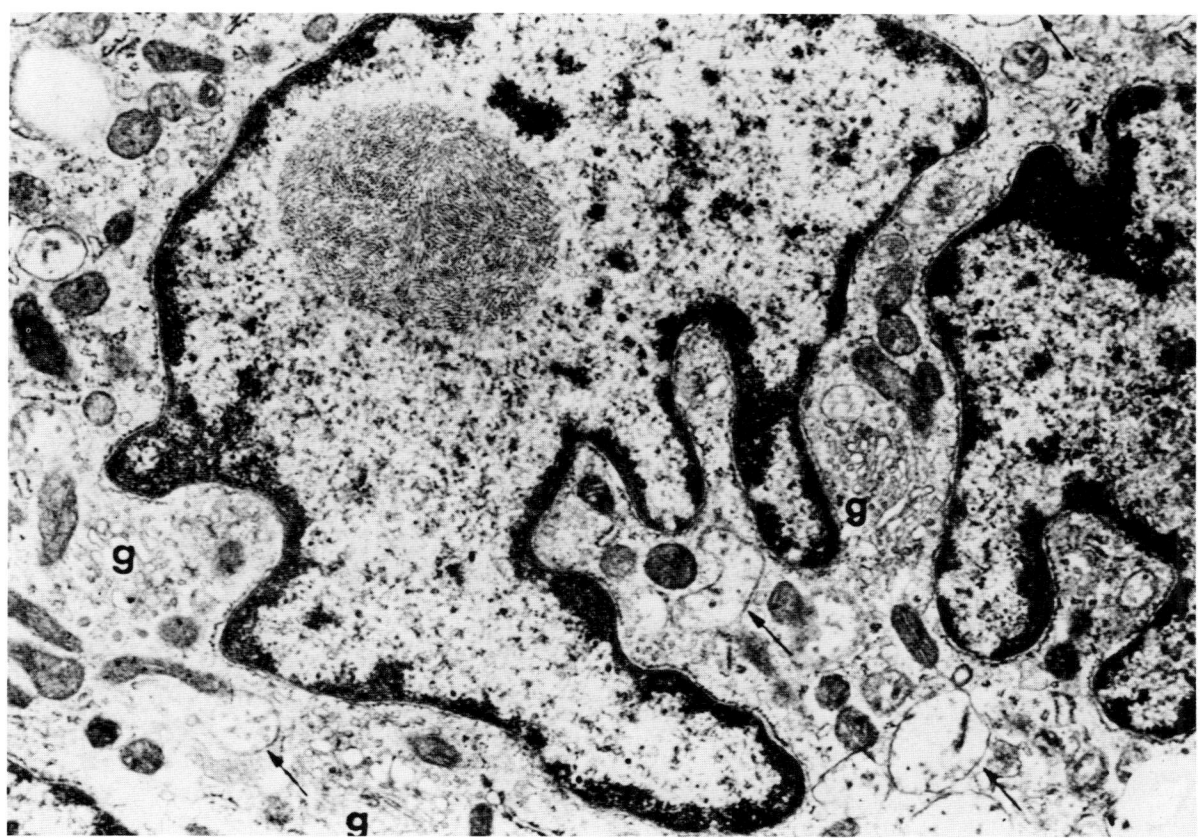

FIG. 1. Electron microscopic view of an osteoclast nucleus from pagetic bone. The nucleus contains an inclusion composed of numerous microfilaments in a paracrystalline arrangement that have a diameter of about 150 Å. Numerous swollen mitochondria (*arrows*) and well-developed Golgi zones (g) are noted (×7000). (Courtesy of A. Rebel.)

ferent RNA viruses (measles is a morbillivirus and RSV is a pneumovirus) seems incompatible. It is proposed that the real villain is a previously uncharacterized virus, perhaps of the pneumovirus family (42).

The hypothesis of a viral infection in Paget's disease involves infestation by a slow virus at an early age, probably under the age of 30. The slow virus would isolate to particular areas of the skeleton by growth pattern and/or blood supply. As the metabolic activity of the skeleton decreases with age, the infested osteoclasts increase their metabolic activity. This increased activity may be due to oncogenes; or perhaps to signals from osteoblasts. Eventually, the disease is evidenced some 20–40 years following the initial infestation.

ANATOMY AND PATHOPHYSIOLOGY

Gross Pathology

Flat Bones

The pelvis may be broadened and thickened. The vertebral bodies may be enlarged and/or broadened or flat-tened, concaved, or wedged. Scapulae may be broadened and thickened similar to the pelvis. The skull is widened, enlarged, knobby, and distorted. The cortex is thickened, the base of the skull is flat. Both the inner and outer tables of the skull are broadened and thickened and may be irregular.

Long Bones

Long bones bow in planes related to the pull of muscles and in response to gravity (e.g., anterior and lateral bow to femur). The cortex is thick, with an elevated periosteum and possible marrow compromise. The bones are heavy and of variable strength: friable to "rock hard." This variation of both softer or harder than normal may involve different areas of the same bone. Both the overly rigid and the softened bone are at risk for fracture.

Microscopic Pathology

The disease is characterized by an active histologic picture (Figs. 2 to 4). The bone histology is characterized by three phases. Initially, bone resorption is prominent

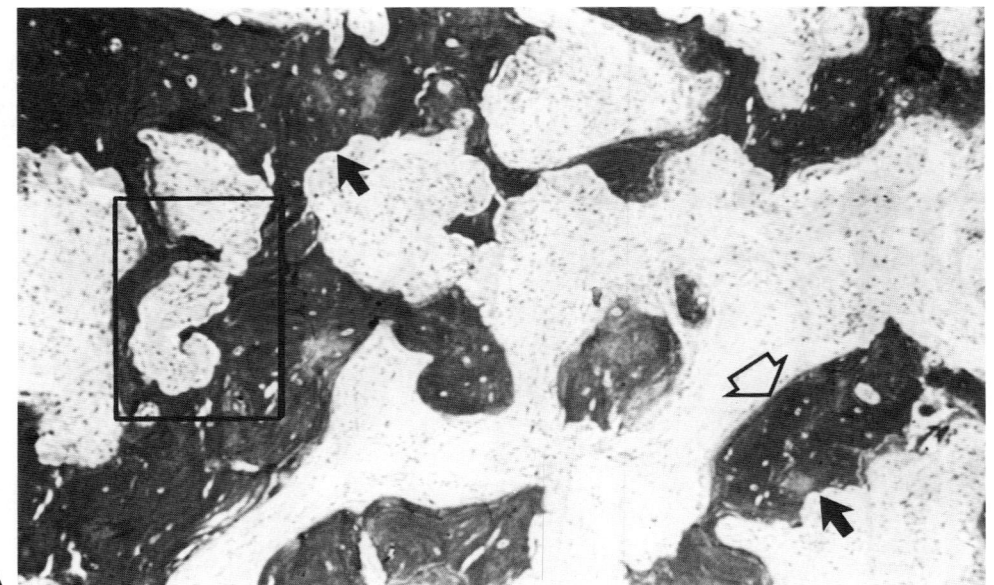

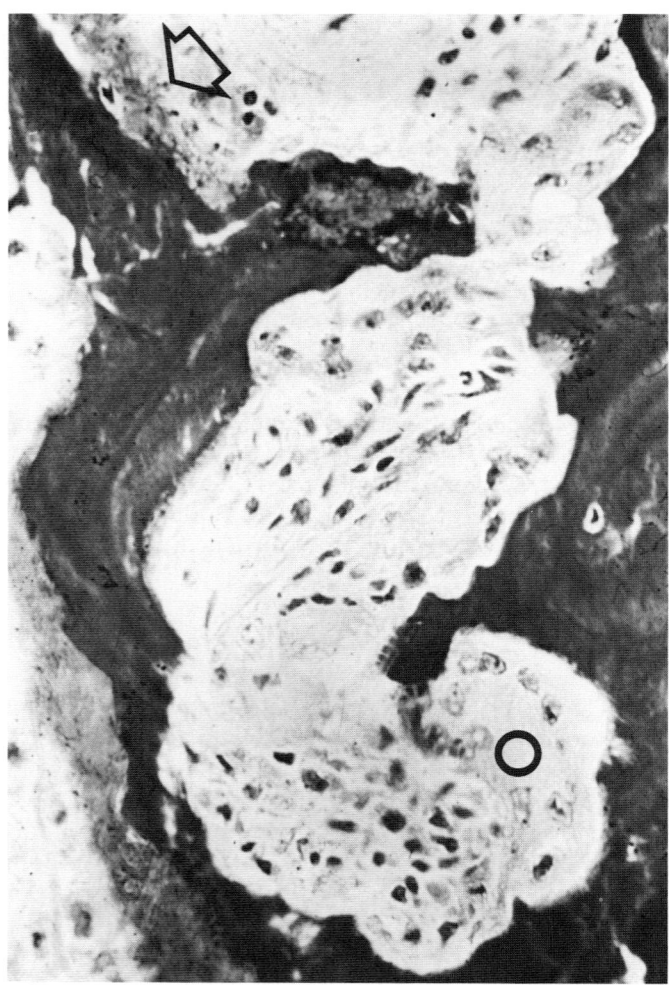

FIG. 2. Light microscopic examination of Paget's bone from an iliac crest biopsy. **A:** Scalloped edges indicating active osteoclastic activity (*arrows*). There are irregular osteoid seams with widened osteocyte lacunae and poorly mineralized osteoid (*wide arrow*) interspersed with fibrosis (×200). **B:** Magnified section shows scalloping is in contrast with a larger osteoclast (○) containing 14 nuclei (×400).

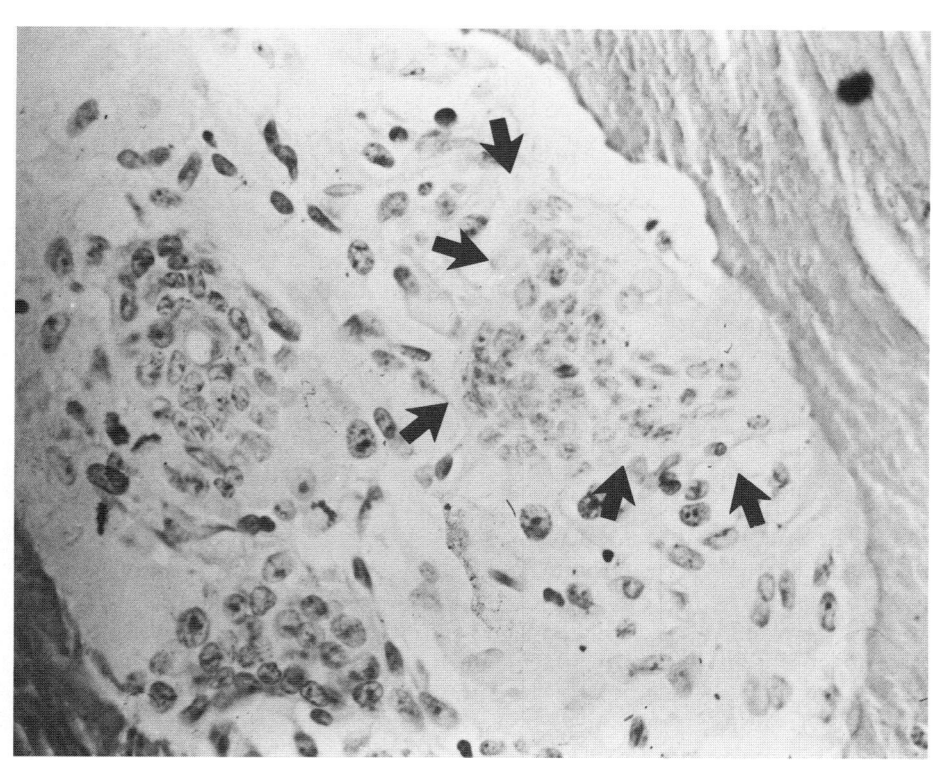

FIG. 3. Light microscopic section shows scalloped bone from an osteoclast containing about 75 nuclei (*arrows*) (×700).

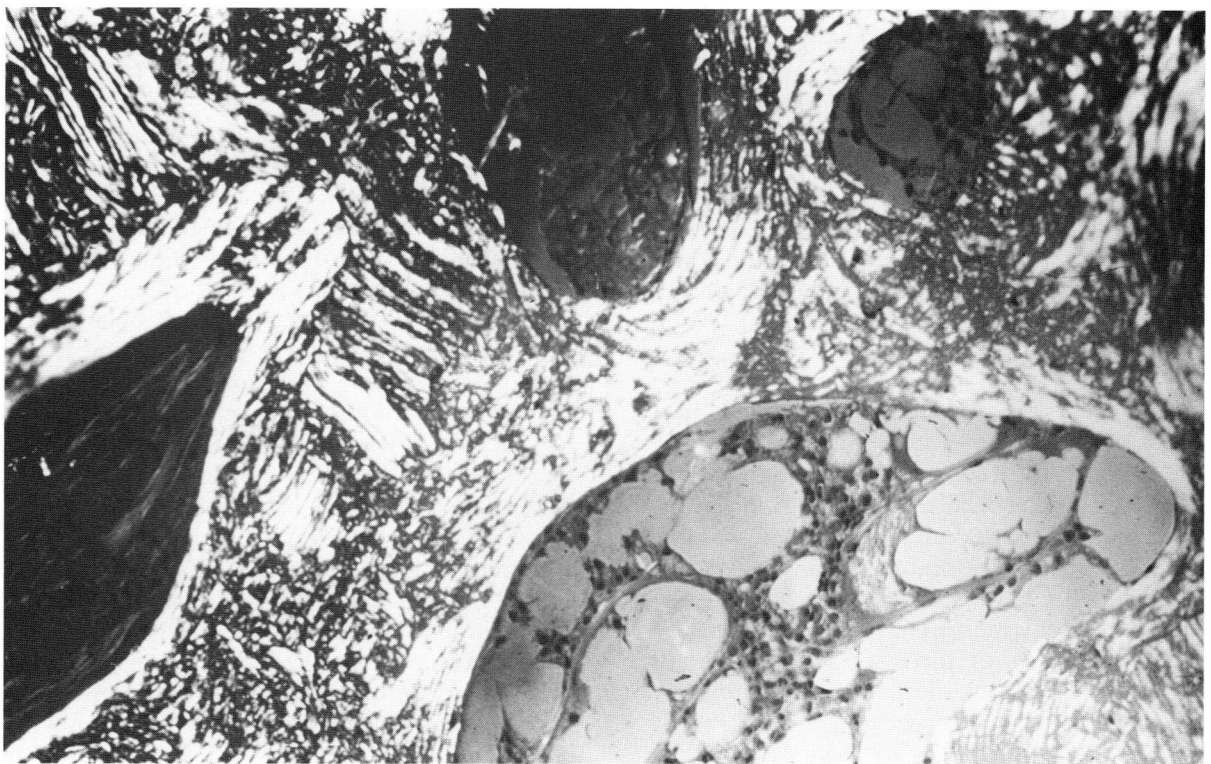

FIG. 4. Polarizing light microscopic view of pagetic bone. Note the wide osteoid seams and heavy calcification (birefringent areas). The collagen is aligned in short, irregular bundles in a "mosaic" pattern that is characteristic of Paget's disease (×100).

and there is marked hypervascularization (*osteolytic phase*). This stage is followed by a period of very active bone formation and resorption (*mixed phase*). There is both endosteal and periosteal new bone. After considerable remodeling, the haversian system is often disorganized or haphazard. It leaves a characteristic mosaic of cement lines typical of this disease. Woven bone may be prominent. Osteoid seams are widened. The lamellar pattern reflects shortened collagen fibrils. Fibrous connective tissue may replace normal marrow. The final, *sclerotic phase* is marked by a more normal marrow with decreased vascularity and fibrosis. Resorption decreases and bone becomes inactive and less vascular.

Schmorl (15) was the first to recognize that Paget's disease began with localized osteolysis characterized by an increase in the number of osteoclasts in Howship's lacunae. He then noted an increase in blood vessels and the development of connective tissue within the marrow. He felt that repair was evidenced by proliferation of osteoblasts on the surface of previously resorbed bone and on the trabeculae of newly formed bone in the fibrous marrow.

Pagetic bone demonstrates marked hyperplasia of arterial capillaries, their number increasing with the duration of disease (44). The marrow sinuses and venous system of bone marrow increase as an apparent consequence of stasis, resulting from the increasing arterial blood flow. Much of the active phase is present in the haversian system. The haversian canals become enlarged with ready communication to the medullary canal.

There is an increased birthrate of the basic multicellular bone units (45). Resorption by the basic multicellular units are greater than normal, which creates a "large tunnel." Although osteoblasts perform normal function in tunnel repair, the quantities of osteoid synthesized is often not adequate to fill the cavities. This may be due to uneven structures left by the osteoclasts. Biopsy may show Paget's disease before the bone scan or radiograph.

Osteoclasts and Resorption of Bone

Osteoclasts are probably developed from bone marrow-derived monocyte/macrophage precursors. Turnover of bone begins with activation of osteoclasts, perhaps in response to activated osteoblasts. Pagetic osteoclasts are often large, attaining sizes of over 200 μm in diameter. As many as 150 nuclei—many picnotic—have been counted in a single osteoclast.

Accelerated osteoclastic activity is demonstrated by resorptive surfaces that are increased seven times normal, the number of osteoclasts per square millimeter is increased 10 times normal (pagetic 3.18 ± 2.30 mm^{-2} versus nonpagetic 0.33 ± 0.23 mm^{-2}), and the erosion rate of bone is often over 9 μm/day (normal 1 μm/day) (45). Osteoclasts are also present in large numbers that range from 1.6 to 6.7 mm^{-2} of biopsied involved iliac crest (46). However, great variation in size and number of nuclei exist. Nearly half the osteoclasts are not attached to bone, which indicates their mobility. Resorption surface was three times that found in hyperparathyroidism (45).

Scanning electron microscopy has revealed that resorption surfaces extend irregularly in multiple directions and are unusually deep (47). Osteoclastic lacunae were irregular. Mineralizing fronts extended over bone surfaces and are abnormally thick.

In general, under electron microscopy, osteoclasts have mostly normal characteristics. They have well-developed ruffled borders with an adjacent clear zone on attached osteoclasts. The cytoplasm contains abundant mitochondria, vacuoles, free ribosomes, a small Golgi apparatus associated with a nucleus, and very little rough endoplasmic reticulum. As above, nuclei are abnormal, containing nuclear inclusions in various size and arrangements (35,48). The individual microfilaments in the nucleus average 15 mm in diameter and are in a hexagonal arrangement when tightly packed in a paracrystalline array. In the cytoplasm, they are often found in random strands or loose bundles. Giant osteoclasts isolated from pagetic bone tested by enzyme histochemistry (49) revealed acid phosphatase, succinic dehydrogenase, and several esterases in both osteoclasts and monocytes.

Osteoblasts and Deposition of Bone

The coupling of resorption and formation of bone matrix is maintained in Paget's disease (50). Quantitative bone histomorphometry shows increased trabecular bone area, forming surfaces, and osteoid area. The linear rate of matrix formation is elevated. There is increased subperiosteal density of bone tissue and hypertrophy of bone matrix. Trabeculae are thick and numerous (45). There is poor definition of the boundary between cortical and medullary bone, and trabecular bone volume is more than twice normal. Active osteoblastic activity is demonstrated by trabecular osteoid volume that is more than twice normal. Trabecular osteoid surface is increased two to four times normal. The thickness index of the osteoid borders are decreased almost 20% indicating that the osteoid borders are extended but thin. Both endosteal and epiphyseal bone units are involved, which causes the bone to become thick as well as long.

It appears the pagetic osteoblasts produce an excess of collagen matrix that is quickly synthesized in an anarchic fashion to produce a woven bone in a typical "mosaic" that can be visualized best under polarizing light. This is rapidly mineralized and at the expense of lamellar bone. Alkaline phosphatase is identified only in osteoblasts. The calcification rate is nearly twice normal and is faster than the increase in osteoblastic appositional rate, producing an excess of heavily calcified collagen matrix. In addition, there are isolated areas of poorly mineralized osteoid. Coupled with the high formation rate, the bone may show histologic findings suggestive of osteomalacia (51). Dissimilar to osteomalacia, the calcification rate is faster than the osteoblastic appositional rate.

Paradoxically, there are interspersed areas of increased medullary fibrosis. Fibrosis may be diffuse or may only affect the periphery of the alveolar cavities with adipose tissue in their center. Degree of marrow fibrosis is directly related to hyperosteoclastosis.

Extensive new bone formation is reflected by tetracycline label that occupies 80% of the total trabecular osteoid surface, and there is an increase in distance between fluorochrome stains on double tetracycline labeling. The osteone system loses its regular appearance. Patches of bone have scalloped contours and interlock by polycyclic cement lines. Collagen fibers form woven bone alternating with short lamellar bands. The periosteocytic lacunae are enlarged.

The histologic mosaic collagen in Paget's disease is heavily calcified, and total body calcium is often increased. The alternating heavily calcified and fibrotic areas of long bone produce the radiographic appearance of coarse trabeculation, characteristic of this disease. Examination of resting bone by scanning electron microscopy shows complex scaffolding of vascular channels. Resting fronts were small and irregular.

By transmission electron microscopy, osteocytic lacunae of lamellar bone appear normal with occasional enlargement adjacent to Howship's lacunae. Osteocytic lacunae of woven bone vary in size. Osteocytes adjacent to bone accretion surfaces are large and fill their lacunae. They contain a well-developed endoplasmic reticulum and round nucleus. Those distant from accretion surfaces are in smaller lacunae and contain less cytoplasm and organelles. Areas of inactive bone contain empty lacunae or degenerating osteocytes with picnotic nuclei.

Uninvolved Bone, Bone Matrix, and Teeth

In 40% of iliac crest bone biopsied from uninvolved bone of pagetic patients, trabecular bone volume is normal, resorption surfaces and periosteocytic lacunar size are increased, osteoid surfaces are increased, thickness of osteoid seams are reduced, and calcification rate is normal—characteristics of increased remodeling and suggestive of secondary increased parathyroid activity (45).

The teeth may be involved. New cementum shows curvilinear markings (52) and a mosaic pattern similar to the adjacent bone. The lamina dura is often thinned. Mandibular and maxillary histologic appearance is sometimes confused with fibrous dysplasia or sometimes a localized fibroosteoma. In contrast to Paget's disease, fibrous dysplasia is often unilateral and uncommonly expands after age 30.

CLINICAL SYNDROME

Paget's disease is most often asymptomatic and without clinical findings. In the estimated 20% (53) of patients that are symptomatic, clinical manifestations often reflect complications of the disease (Table 1). By necessity, this discussion will include pathophysiology. A patient with severe disease is pictured in Fig. 5.

The clinical features have changed little from Sir James Paget's early observations, a credit to his astuteness. Paget's description of the clinical findings has been summarized as follows (54):

TABLE 1. Complications of Paget's disease of bone

Symptoms or findings	Pathologic anatomy
Bone pain	Unknown, periostitis, "bone angina," osteomalacia
Deformity	Softened bone, gravity, muscular pull
Fracture	Advancing osteolytic wedge, structurally weak bone, stress fracture of bowed extremity, compression fracture vertebra
Secondary osteoarthritis	Juxta-articular Paget's disease, change in joint congruity, altered gait dynamics
High-output cardiac state	Extensive skeletal involvement (i.e., over one-third of the skeleton, serum alkaline phosphatase > 4 × upper normal value)
Malignancy	Sarcomatous degeneration of involved bone; metastatic malignant disease to pagetic bone
Dizziness/headache	Unknown, massive skull involvement platybasia (with occipital headache)
Hearing loss	Eighth nerve compression, otosclerosis, invasion of cochlea by pagetic bone
Change in mental status	Platybasia with high-pressure hydrocephalus
Paraparesis/paraplegia	Cord compression, spinal artery "steal" syndrome
Back pain	Altered gait dynamics, secondary osteoarthritis, active spinal Paget's disease, spinal stenosis, lateral recess syndrome
Hypercalcemia	Hyperparathyroidism, immobilization, fracture immobilization
Visual loss	Rupture of angioid streak of fundus, optic nerve entrapment

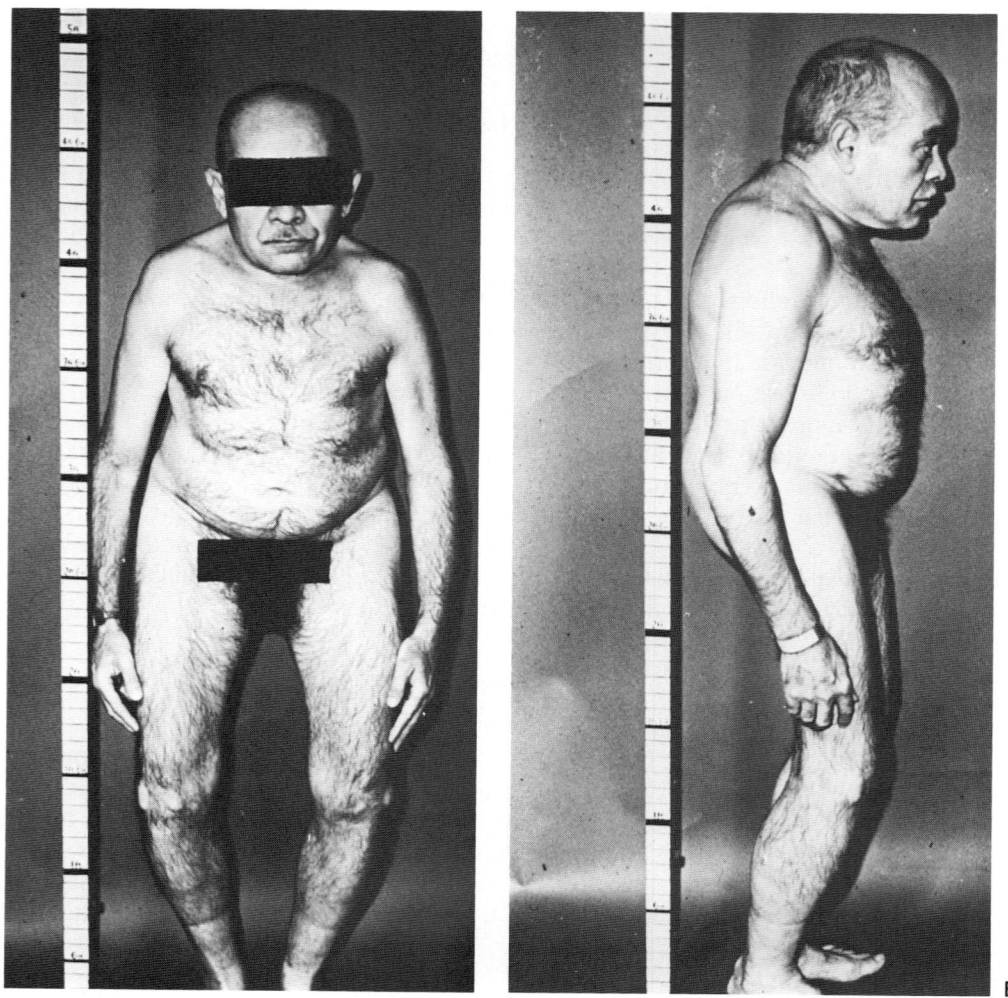

FIG. 5A and **B:** These photographs of a patient with severe Paget's disease demonstrate many clinical characteristics. At age 40 the patient was 5 ft 8 in. tall. At the time of the photograph, age 61, he was 4 ft 9 in. tall. There is an anthropoid appearance with simian posturing. Skull: Enlarged, frontal bossing with short neck, suggesting platybasia. Trunk: Short dorsal and lumbar region with accentuated dorsal kyphosis and flared pelvis. Extremities: Anterior and lateral bow to thighs, legs, and arms. Functional flexion contracture at hips, knees, and elbows.

It begins in middle age or later, is very slow in progress, may continue for many years without influence on the general health, and may give no other trouble than those which are due to the changes of shape, size, and direction of the diseased bones. Even when the skull is hugely thickened and all its bones exceedingly altered in structure, the mind remains unaffected. The disease affects most frequently the long bones of the lower extremities and the skull, and is usually symmetrical. The bones enlarge and soften, and those bearing weight yield and become unnaturally curved and misshapen. The spine, whether by yielding to the weight of the overgrown skull, or by change in its own structures, may sink and seem to shorten with greatly increased dorsal and lumbar curves; the pelvis may become wide, the necks and femora may become nearly horizontal, but the limbs, however misshapen, remain strong and fit to support the trunk. In its earlier periods, and sometimes through all its course, the disease is attended with pains in the affected bones, pains widely various in severity and variously described as rheumatic, gouty, or neuralgic, not especially nocturnal or periodical. It is not attended by fever. No characteristic conditions of urine or feces have been found in it. It is not associated with syphilis or any other known constitutional disease, unless it be cancer. In three out of the five well-marked cases that I have seen or read of, cancer appeared late in life; a remarkable proportion, possibly not more than might have occurred in accidental coincidences, yet suggesting careful inquiry.

Paget felt that those portions of the skeleton most subject to stress and strain show the greatest evidence of involvement (55). There is a tendency to involve the right side of the body more than the left. Paget's disease may involve a single bone. One of our patients had solitary involvement of the third middle phalanx of the right hand.

TABLE 2. *Paget's disease: reason for consultation*

Reason	Number of patients	Percent	Time present prior to consultation (mean years)
Back pain	98	(34)	7.8
Hip pain	65	(22)	9.0
Bone pain	33	(11)	4.0
Headache	29	(10)	7.8
Knee pain	18	(6)	5.4
Hearing loss	7	(2)	9.1
Neck pain	5	(2)	4.0
No symptoms[a]	8	(3)	<1.0
Other	27	(9)	6.5
	290		6.2

[a] Incidental diagnosis of Paget's disease prompted consultation.

In addition to the above, general symptoms may include dizziness, stiffness, weakness, and fatigability. There may be a tendency to somnambulance, limitation of joint motion, flattening of the chest with kyphosis, shortened torso, and prominence of pelvis (Fig. 5). The shortened stature from dorsal and lumbar compression may lead to restrictive lung disease.

Despite vague symptoms, patients consult the physician for a variety of specific problems, often related to pain. Reasons for consultation in 290 patients are listed in Table 2.

Pain

Pain is not usually due to the Paget's disease per se. It is most commonly related to osteoarthritis that may or may not have been precipitated by the Paget's disease. When pain is directly due to Paget's disease, it is aching, poorly described, and occasionally continuous at night. It is suggested that some of the bone pain in Paget's disease is analogous to the pain of osteomalacia. The nighttime tendency may separate Paget's disease pain from that of osteoarthritis but may confuse it with pain associated with malignancy. A pagetic femur or tibia may be more painful with weight bearing. Similarly, pressure on the periosteum may aggravate Paget's disease pain. Rapidly increasing focal bone pain should alert one to the possibility of malignancy or may herald an impending fracture. Unfortunately, physical examination most often does not clarify the cause of pain and additional studies are often needed.

Deformity

The spectrum of deformity may involve asymptomatic localized change to symptomatic gross deformity. When diffusely involved, the patient has an enlarged skull, short stature, Simian posturing, stands bent forward (Fig. 5), and walks with a distinct limp (antalgia) that simulates the gait of a patient with ankylosing spondylitis of Marie Strümpell.

Skull

Localized changes of the skull may reveal knobby deformity, frontal bossing, or diffuse enlargement. This is often associated with dilated scalp veins (56). Enlargement of the zygoma, mandible, or maxilla may give the face a grotesque appearance. Maxillary disease exceeds mandibular involvement 2:1, and both may disrupt the lamina dura, causing teeth to loosen. Gums become swollen and infected. The skull may become thickened, softened, and enlarged and may have the gross appearance of an inverted triangle. (See also "Skull Symptoms" below.)

Axial Skeleton

An accentuated dorsal kyphosis may result from both spinal enlargement and compression fractures. There may be straightening or reversal of the normal lumbar lordosis. Both dorsal and lumbar spine often undergo shortening and rotoscoliosis. These spinal changes may give the patient an anthropoid appearance.

Simian posturing is accentuated by weight-bearing-induced axial (or medial) migration of the femoral heads into the softened pagetic pelvis. This migration (protusio acetabuli) results in functional flexion contractures of the hips and accentuates the short stature.

Peripheral Skeleton

Long bones involved with Paget's disease often soften and become deformed or bow from the stress of weight bearing and/or the force of the attached muscles. Deformity of an arm or forearm may cause a functional extension contracture at the elbow, restricting activities of daily living such as the ability to comb one's hair, shave, or eat. The lower extremities develop an anterior and lateral bow. The Simian posturing is accentuated by the "bowed leg" appearance. Although the involved femur and/or tibia is enlarged or elongated, the bowing results in functional flexion contracture at the knees. This is despite the fact that the knee is often hyperextended 5–10 degrees. If only one lower extremity is bowed, the heel will be raised off the ground, resulting in an abnormal gait. If the lateral bow is severe, the ankle is sharply everted when the foot touches the ground.

Gait analysis in patients with Paget's disease and lower extremity deformity revealed a decrease in velocity and cadence and an increase in stride time and double-limb support time (57). The leg was flexed during stance and flexed less than would be expected during swing. When varus was present there was increased adduction moment. Patterns of ground-reaction force was similar when compared to normal, but the magnitudes of forces were reduced.

Fractures

The true fracture rate in Paget's disease is unknown. One or more completed fractures were present in 18% of 1339 patients in a review of the literature (58). Eight percent of 300 patients (59) were diagnosed as having Paget's disease when seen for a pathologic fracture through pagetic bone.

Fractures may not be complete (Fig. 6). In Paget's disease, fracture can occur with compression of a vertebrae. Many patients with Paget's disease have significant coexistent osteoporosis of the spine and osteoporotic compression fractures. Similarly, pagetic or osteoporotic ribs may fracture with little or undetected trauma. Incomplete or stress fracture of long bones are often asymptomatic but may be a reason for sudden onset of pain, particularly in the lateral upper femur or upper anterior tibia. Fortunately, these incomplete fractures rarely advance to completion.

Any pagetic bone may fracture. The most common sites of fracture involve femur, tibia, lumbar spine, humerus, and dorsal spine in decreasing frequency (60). Pathologic fractures may occur from minimal trauma. Completed fractures of long bones are usually transverse (i.e., perpendicular to the external cortex) (Fig. 7). There is frequently wide separation of the fragments without comminution. Femoral fractures tend to occur through the shaft just distal to the lesser trochanter. Tibial fractures tend to occur in the upper one-third of the shaft. We have seen two avulsion fractures of the tibial tubercle.

In a British study, nonunion fractures were reported as high as 40%, particularly subtrochanteric fractures and those of the upper femoral shaft (61). Callus, however, is usually abundant. Interestingly, callus may be involved with the pagetic process (Fig. 7) (61,62). Early fixation of the fracture is encouraged as a means of reducing the risk

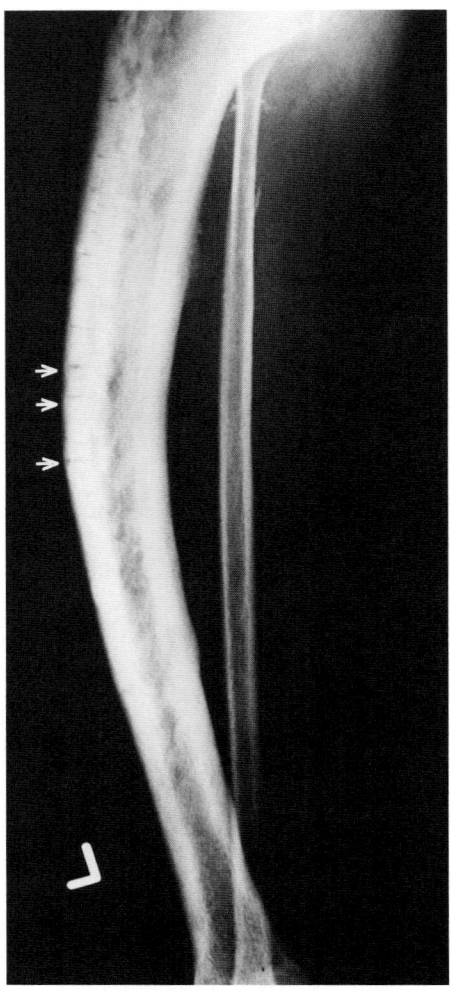

FIG. 6. Lateral radiograph of leg. There is a marked anterior bow to the tibia. The cortex is thickened throughout the tibia, expanding centrally toward the medullary canal and outward toward the periosteum. There are multiple stress or microfractures of the anterior cortex (*arrows*). Nonthickened cortex has a coarse trabecular pattern. There is arterial calcification and sparing of the fibula.

of nonunion. Fractures may be the herald of sarcoma and careful review of the radiography is needed.

Osteoarthritis

As stated above, osteoarthritis is probably the most common cause of pain in Paget's disease. Paget's disease may cause osteoarthritis by the following mechanisms:

1. *Uniform bony enlargement.* Pagetic bone may become enlarged, altering the congruity of "fit" between joint surfaces. For example, femoral head enlargement (Fig. 8) may exceed the acetabular space. Conversely, acetabular enlargement may also narrow the space allotted to the femoral head (Fig. 9), usually from an axial impingement.

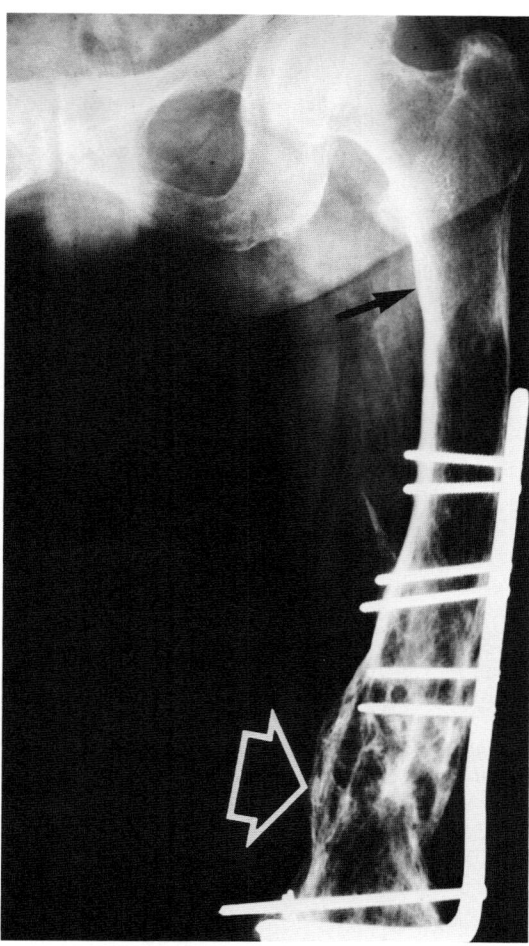

FIG. 7. Radiograph demonstrates a transverse fracture of the lower femur through severely osteopenic bone (*large arrow*). Plate and screws were used for stabilization. The fracture has healed with callus that is pagetic in appearance. The area above the fracture demonstrates the coarse trabecular pattern of Paget's disease. The upper midshaft demonstrates an "advancing" osteolytic wedge (*small arrow*). The more normal appearing proximal femur, osteolytic wedge of the midshaft, and more distal coarse trabeculation suggests an inverted "flame sign."

2. *Uneven bony enlargement.* Joint surfaces are subjected to uneven pressures, perhaps on an uneven base of pagetic subchondral bone.
3. *Altered joint biodynamics.* Alteration arises from bowed, softened long bones.
4. *Softened pelvis.* As above, migration of bones produces protrusion that alters joint dynamics and joint congruity.

Low back pain is common in patients with Paget's disease. Back pain accounts for the clinical presentation in 30% of patients (63,64). The origin of back pain is often difficult to determine in many patients (65,66). In only 3 of 25 patients (12%) with lumbrosacral Paget's disease did low back pain evaluation comfortably sug-

gest Paget's disease as the major cause of pain, in contrast to other causes such as osteoarthritis (67). Pain in the remaining patients (88%) were indistinguishable from osteoarthritis. Osteoarthritis coexisted, or was contiguous but at different levels of the spine, which made clinical separation difficult. In 6 patients (24%), it appeared the osteoarthritis was caused by Paget's disease. Some back pain was felt to be from altered biodynamics of gait due to Paget's disease of the pelvis and/or lower extremities (i.e., bowing, pelvic softening, or unequal leg length). Lumbar canal stenosis can be correlated with the degree of symptoms and findings (67,68).

High Cardiac Output

Metabolically active pagetic bone is highly vascular. Blood flow increases to the entire area of involvement, including skin and soft tissues. Although it has been suggested that Paget's disease of 35% of the skeleton was needed for a high cardiac output (69), our own studies and those of Wootton et al. (70) suggest a relation to the degree of disease activity as expressed by chemistries rather than percent of skeletal involvement. However, patients with more than 15% of the skeleton involved showed cardiac enlargement and depressed myocardial contractility by echocardiogram (71,72).

Skeletal blood flow doubles from 300 mL/min or 6% of the blood volume per minute, to about 12% of the blood volume per minute when the serum alkaline phosphatase is elevated four times the upper normal limits (70). Uncommonly, the demand for blood stresses the heart greatly enough to exceed the cardiac capability and precipitates congestive heart failure.

Resting blood flow of Paget's disease involving one extremity was tested by water plethysmography (73). The pagetic limb flow was 14.2 ± 2.95 SE mL/min × 100 mL of extremity in contrast to 2.5 ± 0.7 mL/min in the uninvolved limb. Cutaneous vessels were considered dilated because epinephrine iontophoresis that normally suppresses flow to the skin only decreased the pagetic limb flow to 3.6 ± 1.5 mL/min. Local heating of the pagetic extremity did not increase flow appreciably; this suggested that increased skin blood tissue flow may account for much of the increased cardiac output in Paget's disease. Hyperperfusion of pagetic bone rather than anatomic arteriovenous shunts was suggested by a flow study using microparticles (74).

Increased demand of blood by pagetic bone is accentuated by increased blood flow to the involved area. The involved extremity is commonly palpably warm to the touch and may be as much as 8 degrees warmer than the contralateral uninvolved side. The increased warmth can be demonstrated by thermography. This sometimes results in breakdown of the skin over an involved tibia that is refractory to local skin care, topical steroids, or

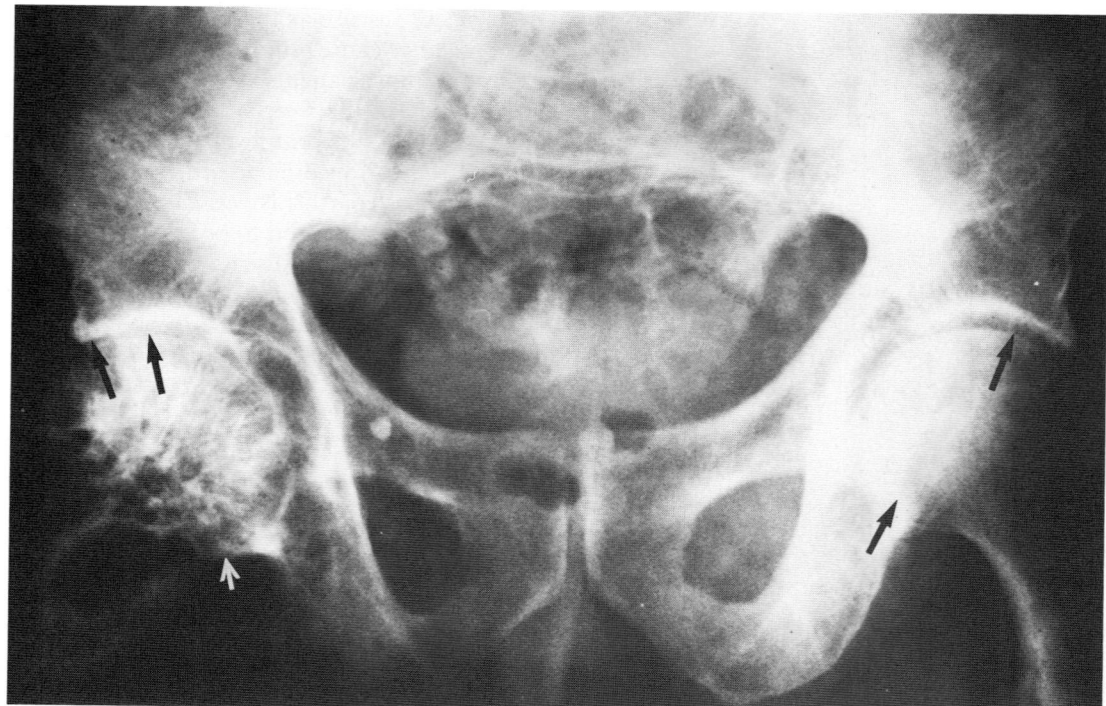

FIG. 8. Radiograph of the pelvis shows diffuse sacral and pelvic Paget's disease with sclerotic changes of the left pelvic brim and mixed sclerotic and fibrotic changes of the right pelvic brim. Paget's disease involves the proximal right femur. The diameter of the right proximal femoral head is 0.8 cm wider than the left (*black arrows*). The radiographic joint space is narrowed in the superior plane (*white arrow*).

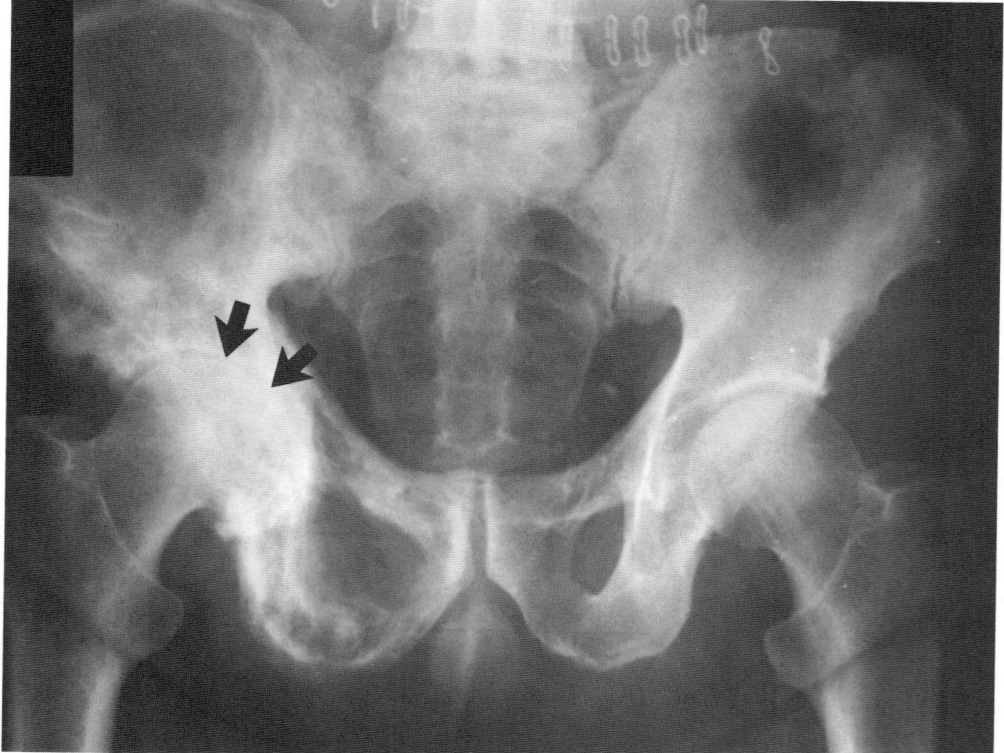

FIG. 9. Radiograph of the pelvis shows right hemispheric Paget's disease. The ilium has "whorls" of coarse trabeculation. The iliopectineal line is thickened and has migrated axially (protrusio acetabuli). The radiographic joint space of the right hip is narrowed, particularly in the axial plane (*arrows*).

antibiotics. Increased flow to the scalp will cause dilated scalp veins (56).

Paget's disease has been associated with calcific aortic stenosis. Advanced grades of calcific aortic valve disease relate to more extensive Paget's disease. Combined mitral valve calcification and heart block has been reported (75). Diffuse calcification of blood vessels has also been associated with Paget's disease.

Sarcoma and Other Tumors

Sir James Paget's original patient developed bone sarcoma. Bone sarcoma is estimated to occur in approximately 1% of patients with Paget's disease. This represents a 40-fold increase in bone sarcomas when compared to a nonpagetic adult population. It is most often heralded by increasing pain, sometimes associated with swelling or fracture. Pagetic sarcomas comprise about 5% of registered osteogenic sarcomas and causes approximately 100 deaths in the United States each year. There is a male predominance for all sites except the skull, and involvement above the waist occurs more commonly in younger persons. Most patients with sarcoma have oligo-ostotic disease. Sarcomas have been noted most often in the spine, skull (Fig. 10), pelvis, femur, tibia, and humerus. Average survival is 9 months, shorter than the nonpagetic bone sarcoma survival time. However, we have had one patient who had an excisional biopsy of the skull and subsequent radiation that survived at least 24 years, without known recurrence of the tumor.

Pagetic sarcomas are often multifocal in origin (76). Three families were found in which two members had pagetic sarcomas (77). Also, one family had three members suffering from pagetic sarcomas.

Ultrastructural examination has demonstrated five cell types exist in these sarcomas: osteoblast, chondro-

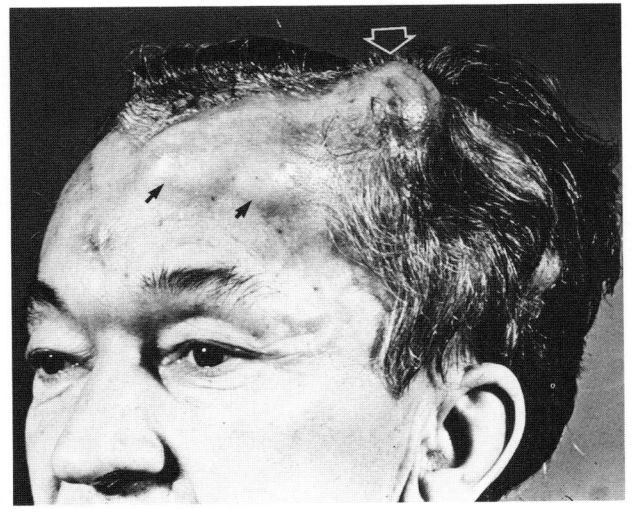

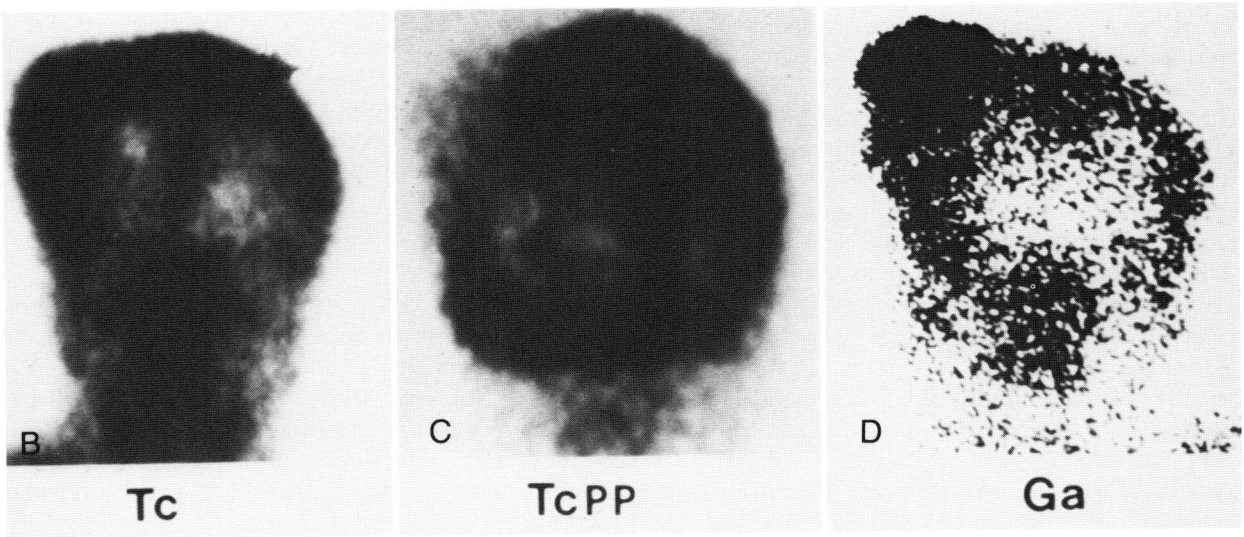

FIG. 10. A: Photograph of patient with sarcoma of the skull showing large, knobby deformity of the skull (*arrows*). The skin over the upper lesion is ulcerating. B: [99mTc] pertechnetate early phase posterior scintigram of the skull localizes the nuclide suggesting increased blood flow to the deforming lesion C: Bone scanning with [99mTc] diphosphonate shows a posterior scintigram of the skull at 4 h. The deforming lesion fails to localize the nuclide suggesting the sarcoma contains few bone forming cells. D: 67Ga posterior scintigram of the skull localizes to the deforming area suggesting intense cellular activity. The lack of localization of the bone scanning nuclide to an area of clinically active Paget's disease is compatible with pagetic sarcoma.

blast, osteocyte, undifferentiated cells (stem-cell type), and myofibroblasts (78). Hence Barry has suggested the title *Paget's sarcoma.* Pagetic sarcomas often emphasize the nonosteoblast cell lines that may account for their resistance to therapy. It may also account for the frequent lack of localization of the nuclide on bone scan (Fig. 10C). Sarcoma may be suspected by a marked increase in urinary cetyl pyridium chloride–precipitable uronic acid (79).

Some of these tumors may actually be giant-cell reparative granulomas (80). Giant-cell tumors can occur in pagetic lesions and are sometimes familial and associated with geographic clustering (81).

Numerous tumors may metastasize to pagetic bone, presumably because of high perfusion and abnormal structure of the pagetic lesion (82–84). Prostatic carcinoma is most common, but breast, renal cell, and bronchogenic carcinoma have been seen. The differential between a blastic metastatic lesion and Paget's disease is often difficult and may require biopsy. There are several reports of multiple myeloma within the pagetic lesion.

Skull Symptoms

Skull symptoms may include headaches, tinnitus, vertigo, rushing sensations, and "noise" in the head. Invasion of the cochlea by Paget's disease may cause vertigo and unsteady gait and balance. By auscultation over the involved skull, one may hear breath sounds from the nasopharynx and/or the flow of blood through the calvarium.

Skull enlargement can be elicited historically by change in hat size. The clinician may wish to measure skull circumference on initial examination and remeasure at periods of 6–12 months thereafter. Women's hats are based on circumference. Interpretation of change in men's hat size is more difficult because men's hats are based on the AP distance plus the right–left side of skull distance (measured by a caliper—the sum divided by 2).

Diffuse headaches may result in "rushing sensations," because of increased blood flow. The heavy, softened skull appears to "settle" on the top of the neck (Fig. 5) around the foramen magnum, causing platybasia. This may result in refractory occipital headaches.

Occasionally, a rather abrupt change in mental states may be due to obstruction of spinal fluid flow through the area of the foramen magnum. The hydrocephalis dementia complex of communication hydrocephalus from platybasia has been described. This has responded to ventriculoatrial shunt (85,86).

Maxillary exceeds mandibular involvement 2:1 in Paget's disease (87), and both may disrupt the lamina dura, loosen teeth, as well as cause unsightly deformity. Patients with Paget's disease suffer greater difficulty at dental extraction and more post-extraction complica-

TABLE 3. *Oral changes of Paget's disease*

Overview
  Maxilla 6: mandible 1: both 1
  Alveolar ridge evidenced
  Palate flattened
  Teeth loose or migrate

Radiograph
  Loss of lamina dura
  Hypercementosis (ankylosis)
  Roots replaced/resorbed
  Pulpal calcification

Pathology
  Cemental resorption
  Pagetic changes of tooth

Complications
  Firm teeth (may crumble)
  Migration/loosening teeth
  Pulpal calcification
  Ankylosis—extraction
  Neurologic pain
  Salivary calculi (18%)
  Sarcoma

Differential diagnosis
  Chronic sclerosing osteomyelitis
  Fibrosis dysplasia
  Ossifying fibroma

Source: After Smith and Eveson (87).

tions than is normally expected (88). Mouth pain from gingivitis with infection may be superimposed on loosened teeth. Oral changes in Paget's disease are reflected in Table 3.

Hearing Loss

Hearing loss may be severe but is most often moderate. Hearing loss may be caused by pagetic involvement of the middle ear with resultant otosclerosis. More commonly, sensorineural deafness results from pagetic involvement of the petrous ridge, which may cause VIII cranial nerve compression and/or invasion of the semicircular canals and cochlea. The bones of the middle ear may be involved with Paget's disease giving functional otosclerosis. Sensorineural hearing loss may not be due to the Paget's disease per se (89). Tinnitis and/or vertigo were seen in about 20% of patients with hearing loss.

Visual Loss

Visual loss may be due to angioid streaks or pagetic bony impingement of the optic nerve. Angioid streaks are fibrovascular changes of the superficial (Bruch's) membrane of the eye. They occur in about 15% of pagetic patients and are usually associated with skull involvement and active disease (90). Partial or complete blindness can occur from rupture of this highly vascular structure.

Pagetic enlargement of the orbit may interfere with muscular function to the eye or may actually compress the optic nerve. Facial nerve paralysis has been related to "crocodile tears" in Paget's disease (91).

Neural Compression

In addition to compression of the optic (II) and auditory (VIII) cranial nerves noted above, other forms of neural compression can occur. Paraparesis/paraplegia in Paget's disease is most often related to Paget's disease of dorsal or cervical vertebrae. It has been theorized to be secondary to a "spinal artery steal" syndrome rather than direct neural compression (92). Improvement with therapy might be related to decreased perfusion of the pagetic vertebrae with resultant return of blood flow to the small vessels of the spinal cord. This is perhaps a more tenable hypothesis than retraction of bone around the cord or decreased edema of the periosteal tissues.

Potential neurologic manifestations have been listed (93) in Table 4. Neural compression of the lumbar spine may cause spinal stenosis or a spinal lateral recess impingement. These may result in a cauda equina syndrome with pseudoclaudication or prominent unilateral radiculopathy. Pseudoclaudication is most often associated with good pedal pulses.

Hypercalcemia

The not uncommon coexistence of Paget's disease and hyperparathyroidism (94–96) leads to speculation about secondary hyperparathyroidism. Patients with severe Paget's disease may develop immobilization hypercalcemia, perhaps related to continued osteoclastic activity with reduced new bone formation. Fracture and immobilization hypercalcemia are often accentuated by high calcium intake (97).

TABLE 4. *Neurologic manifestations of Paget's disease*

I. Cranial manifestations
  1. Changes in head size, shape, and thickness, nodular enlargement, enlargement of zygoma
  2. Abnormal brain scan
  3. Radiographic abnormalities (e.g., osteoporosis circumscripta)
  4. Giant-cell tumor of bone
  5. Sarcomas—with or without intracranial extension
II. Intracranial
  1. Brain—intracranial extension of malignant skull tumors with increased intracranial pressure, seizures, hemiplegia, etc.
        Hypertensive hemorrhage
        Pituitary insufficiency
        Aneurysms—middle meningeal artery
  2. Cranial nerves
        I. Anosmia
       II. Exophthalmus
          Optic atrophy (bony impingement)
          Angioid streaks (blindness)
          Corneal opacities
    III, IV, VI. Extraocular muscle palsies
       V. Trigeminal neuralgia
     VII. Hemifacial spasm
    VIII. Deafness, vertigo
  IX, X, XI, XII. Deficits
III. Craniospinal junction
  Basilar impression associated with:
    Occipital neuralgia
    Lower cranial nerve signs
    Medullary compression
    Cerebellar compression
    Syringomyelia with ventricular obstruction
    Hydrocephalus—dementia complex
    Vertebrobasilar insufficiency
IV. Spinal compression by pagetic bone, fracture/dislocation, epidural fat calcification, vascular occlusion, spinal artery "steal"
  1. Cervical region; involvement of axis or atlas, atlanto-axial fractures and dislocations
  2. Thoracic: myeloradicular syndromes
  3. Lumbar
      Pseudo-intermittent claudication of cauda equina entrapment
      Radicular compression
      Neurologic deficit without myelographic compression
V. Pain: Associated with local disease, malignant degeneration, fractures, and dislocation.

Source: After Schmidek (93).

Miscellaneous Arthropathies

We have seen one patient with rupture of the ulna extensor tendons over the wrist similar to that seen in rheumatoid arthritis. It was associated with a markedly bowed pagetic ulna. Rheumatoid arthritis has occurred in no greater frequency in Paget's disease.

In our own population, gout was present in 11 of 290 patients (59). Gout was felt to be increased in Paget's disease (20), based on positive bone scans in 6 of 26 patients (23%) with gout compared to a base of 2.1% Paget's disease in the population scanned. There has been no reported increased of pseudogout in Paget's disease.

The association of renal lithiasis to Paget's disease seems due to the serendipity of detecting asymptomatic Paget's disease by obtaining pelvic radiographs for renal lithiasis. The association to arteriosclerosis may simply be a factor of the population at risk for both conditions.

LABORATORY ANALYSIS

Metabolic turnover of bone is active in Paget's disease and may be reflected in several methods.

Alkaline Phosphatase

Anabolic bone activity may be detected by measuring the serum alkaline phosphatase. The value of the serum alkaline phosphatase as a diagnostic tool was first proposed by Kay in 1929 (98). There are higher values in Paget's disease than in any other condition (99). The elevation of the serum alkaline phosphatase is a function of the extent and activity of the Paget's disease. There is no diurnal variation in alkaline phosphatase (60). Early in disease there may be an upward trend and cyclic fluctuations. Alkaline phosphatase may vary over long periods of time in individuals (100). However, the serum alkaline phosphatase most often remains stable over long periods of time. The serum alkaline phosphatase may eventually decrease, probably as the disease moves into a healed, sclerotic, inactive phase. Rapid rises in serum alkaline phosphatase may be indicative of malignant degeneration of Paget's disease, but more often pagetic sarcomas are associated with low levels of alkaline phosphatase.

Serum alkaline phosphatase includes a set of enzymes acting on phosphorus–oxygen bonds in an alkaline medium and includes at least some pyrophosphatase activity. Separation of an elevated serum alkaline phosphatase of bone or liver origin is sometimes problematic. Heat fractionation and isoenzyme determination have failed to consistently differentiate serum alkaline phosphatase from bone or liver sources. Serum alkaline phosphatase from liver, kidney, bone, and pagetic bone ap-

pear to be products of the same structural gene (101). Hepatic alkaline phosphatase is normally secreted in the bile, and elevation in alkaline phosphatase reflects biliary or canalicular obstruction. A search for elevation of other liver function tests such as SGOT or AST, SGPT, or ALT may suggest liver origin of the alkaline phosphatase. Elevation of other enzymes that are normally secreted in the bile (i.e., serum 5′-nucleotidase or leucine aminopeptidase) may also suggest an increased alkaline phosphatase of hepatic origin. An increase in enzymes that represents increased bone metabolism—such as isocitric dehydrogenase, acid phosphatase, imidopeptidase, and proline imidopeptidase—may be associated with increased alkaline phosphatase of bony origin. The origin of increased alkaline phosphatase may ultimately need to be correlated with the bone scan since the bone scan also reflects anabolic activity of bone.

Hydroxyproline and Other Collagen Markers

In humans, the amino acid hydroxyproline is found almost exclusively in collagen. Measurement of the total urine hydroxyproline is a useful index of bone collagen turnover and correlates well with the alkaline phosphatase. Collagen fragments containing hydroxyproline are produced in bone by collagenolytic activity of osteoclasts through enzymatic degradation. These fragments are not reutilized for synthesis, are then transported to the vascular system, and are excreted in the urine in large amounts by patients with Paget's disease.

Elevations of hydroxyproline excretion are determined from urine that is traditionally collected over a 24-h period on the third day of a gelatin-free diet. Patients are instructed to avoid foods such as red meats, animal skins, Jell-o, canned foods, and ice cream. The urine collection should be iced and probably should contain an acid preservative such as sodium azide.

Peak total hydroxyproline urine excretion may be from midnight to 8:00 A.M. and lowest from noon to 8:00 P.M., which suggests greater bone turnover at night (102). However, in an unpublished study, we have shown that a carefully collected 2-h urine specimen predicts the 24-h collection even though hydroxyproline/creatinine ratios were altered by the diurnal variation in creatinine excretion.

Both catabolic and anabolic collagen turnover may be determined by urine hydroxyproline. In vivo incorporation of [14C]L-proline into urine hydroxyproline suggests that the urine fragments of collagen were recently synthesized and degraded or rapidly synthesized but not incorporated into tropocollagen molecule (103). Recent synthesis is also supported by isolation of a urinary polypeptide containing equal amounts of glycine, proline, and 4-hydroxyproline—suggesting that the origin is from the N-terminal propeptide of type I collagen (104).

Although normal collagen is produced (105), pagetic bone synthesizes three to four times more protein and collagen per milligram than normals (106).

Other markers of collagen metabolism in Paget's disease are an increased urinary excretion of hydroxylysine and its collagen-derived glycosides (50), serum and urine procollagen fragments, serum osteocalcin (107), proline iminopeptidase (108,109), serum type I procollagen carboxyterminal peptide (110), and type III procollagen amino-terminal peptide (111). A portion of the urinary 4-hydroxyproline and hydroxylysine is in 5000-D peptides related to collagen synthesis. Suppressive therapy of Paget's disease lowers these values. Moreover, collagen cross-linking compounds that are specific for destruction of bone collagen in Paget's disease may be detected in urine by 3-hydroxypyridinium and dihydroxylysinonorleucine (112).

Suppression of Paget's disease by therapy decreases resorption and then formation is suggested by the initial decrease in hydroxyproline excretion prior to decrease in serum alkaline phosphatase (50,108).

Other Measurements

The marked acceleration of bone metabolism in Paget's disease is not usually reflected in changes of serum (bound or unbound), calcium, or inorganic phosphate. Calcium accumulates in the bone, as evidenced by calcium balance studies. Hypercalcemia has occurred in Paget's disease, usually with immobilization of patients with severe and active Paget's disease, acutely following fractures, malignancy in bone, and coincident hyperparathyroidism. The association of Paget's disease to hyperparathyroidism was first recognized by Albright et al. in 1934 (113).

Osteocalcin (γ-carboxyglutamic acid, bone Gla protein BCP) is increased in Paget's disease and is a nonspecific reflection of increased bone metabolism (114). Serum osteocalcin levels were elevated in 25 of 49 patients (53%) with Paget's disease: values were as high as 4.2 times normal (115). In another study, osteocalcin levels were modestly elevated at 22.7 ± 6.1 mg/mL (116). These levels were low when compared to secondary hyperparathyroidism and untreated metastatic bone disease. The levels were similar to those requiring open reduction for fracture or with primary hyperparathyroidism. These measurements were not felt to have more diagnostic value than the serum alkaline phosphatase, elevated in 48 of 49 patients (115).

Elevated levels of serum acid phosphatase may occur in severe Paget's disease (117) and probably is related to osteoclastic bone resorption (118). Calcitonin levels are not different in Paget's disease compared to age- and sex-matched controls (119). There was no correlation between calcitonin levels and alkaline phosphatase. In a study from Sheffield, England, patients with Paget's disease had lower circulating concentrations of 24,25-dihydroxycholecalciferol compared to age-matched controls (120).

During therapy with disodium etidronate there may be a rise in plasma phosphate. This is due to an increase in renal tubular reabsorption of phosphate (121). Intracellular phosphate and intracellular ATP did not change significantly. Serum prostaglandin E levels are normal in Paget's disease (122).

Urinary glycosaminoglycans (uronic acid and hexosamine) were not increased in Paget's disease unless sarcomatous change had occurred (79). There was no advantage of this analysis over the hydroxyproline/creatinine ratio that was similarly reduced in neoplastic disease (i.e., increased urine creatinine). The hydroxyproline/creatinine ratio is felt to be of diagnostic value in suspected tumor and Paget's disease.

Higher levels of plasma fibronectin were found in the arm with humeral, ulnar, and radial Paget's disease compared to venous blood from the contralateral uninvolved arm (123). Hyperuricemia was found in 11% of 290 patients.

Nonspecific antibodies to type II and IX collagen were found in approximately one-half of the patients with Paget's disease (124). Elevated serum monoclonal IGM proteins were found in 5 of 26 patients with active Paget's disease, suggesting disordered immune regulation, possibly of viral origin (125).

IMAGING

Radiography and Magnetic Resonance Imaging

Radiographic and clinical studies have outlined the distribution of Paget's disease: the pelvis is involved in approximately 80% of patients with Paget's disease, and the skull, spine, and femur follow in frequency (with variations of order depending on the study) (Table 5).

There are four radiographic appearances to bone involvement, including *osteolytic, osteoblastic, fibrotic,* and *sclerotic* phases. These roughly correspond to the morbid anatomy (126–130). The radiographic appearance of the lesion and the site involved does not correlate with symptoms (128).

1. *Osteolytic.* The normal osseous pattern disappears with cyst formation in the early, or osteolytic, phase (Fig. 7). In the tubular bone, a V-shaped lytic area demarcates abnormal bone and may advance along the shaft of a long bone being replaced by a disorganized, fluffy, course trabecular pattern—the so-called *flame sign.* The lytic areas of long bones correspond to maplike changes of the skull called *osteoporosis circumscripta.*

TABLE 5. *Radiographic and symptomatic distribution of Paget's disease*

Site	Radiographic[a] Guyer et al. (1864 patients) (%)	Radiographic[b] Buchoff and Altman (50 patients) (%)	Buchoff[b] Primary site of pain
Pelvis[c]	76	58	24
Lumbar spine[c]	33	30	8
Sacrum[c]	28	30	—
Femora[c]	25	60	17
Skull	28	37	5
Scapula	26	7	—
Dorsal spine	20	18	—
Humerus	—	18	3
Cervical spine	14	—	—
Ribs	3	—	—
Tibia	—	70	8
Clavicle	—	4	—
Fibula	—	1	—

[a] After Guyer et al. (272).
[b] After Buchoff and Altman (128).
[c] All patients had at least one of these sites.

2. *Osteoblastic.* The normal bone is eventually replaced by alternating radiodense and radiolucent areas, giving the bone a coarse trabecular pattern (Figs. 11 and 12). This is particularly common in the pelvis, proximal femur, and spine.
3. *Fibrotic.* Radiolucent areas may predominate with sparse radiodense changes (Fig. 13).
4. *Sclerotic.* The bone may be extremely radiodense without lucency, particularly the thickened cortex of

long bones and occasionally of vertebrae, giving an "ivory bone" appearance (Fig. 14).

Skull

Skull involvement may be reflected by diffuse cortical thickening, spotty osteoblastic "cotton-wool" lesions, osteoporosis circumscripta (Fig. 15), and platybasia. The earliest changes on skull roentgenogram include dimin-

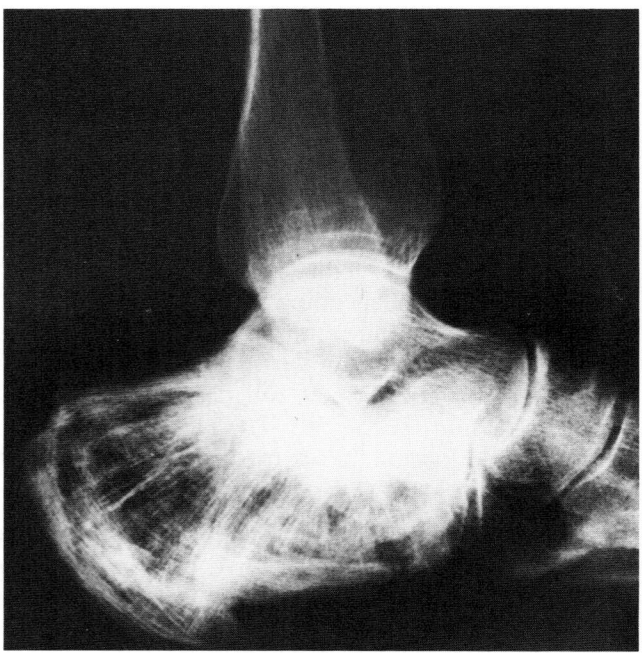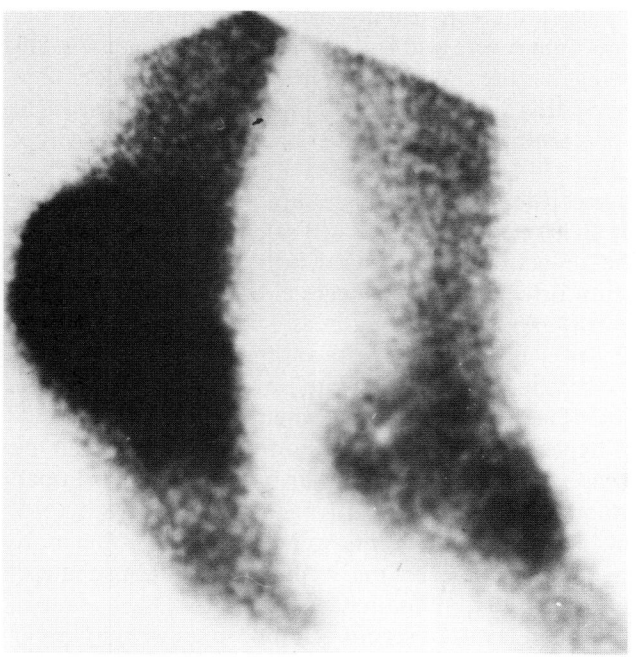

FIG. 11. A: Radiograph of foot shows diffuse coarse trabeculation of the calcaneous. This radiographic pattern should not be confused with other diseases. Subperiosteal new bone has the appearance of Paget's disease. **B:** ⁹⁹ᵐTc-labeled diphosphonate bone scan localizes to the area of Paget's disease of the foot in a diffuse pattern. The intensity of uptake appears to overlap with uninvolved tibia, talus, and navicular bones.

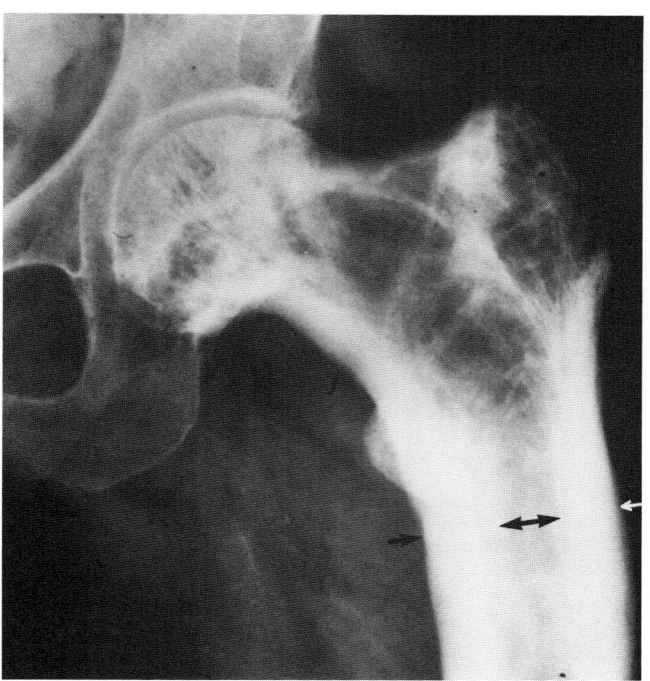

FIG. 12. Radiograph of the proximal femur shows markedly thickened cortex (*arrows*), narrowed medullary canal, fibrotic changes in the trochanteric region, and coarse trabeculation of the femoral head.

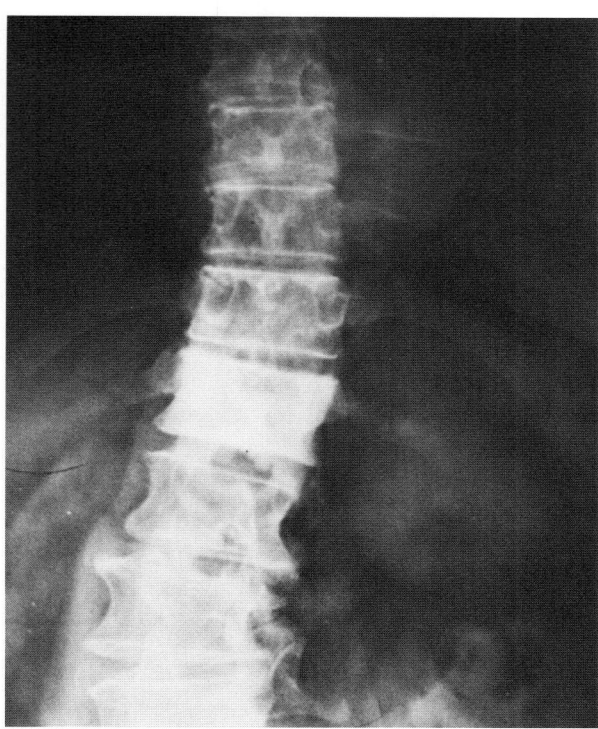

FIG. 14. Anterior–posterior radiograph of the lower dorsal and upper lumbar spine shows intense radiodensity of the twelfth thoracic vertebra, an "ivory vertebra" of blastic Paget's disease.

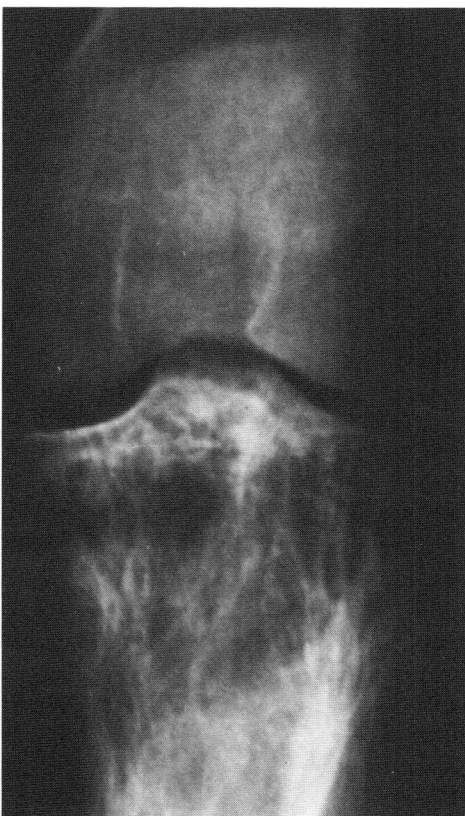

FIG. 13. Radiograph of the proximal tibia shows widening of the tibial plateaus with radiolucent areas interspersed with sparse trabeculae.

ished density of the diploe and thinning of the outer table of bone from within (131). The lytic phase begins in the frontal or occipital area and may progress to involve the entire calvarium. Suture lines and vessels do not restrain progression and are eventually obliterated as the disease progresses from lytic to mixed and sclerotic phases. With progression, the calvarium thickens. The outer tables extend externally and internally because of new bone on the periosteal surface and widening of the diploe (Fig. 16). Sclerotic areas of new bone condense into a cotton-wool appearance. Continued coalescence leads to mottling. Thickened trabeculae impinge on the marrow space. Gravity and muscular pull on the softened skull provide mechanical stress that invaginates the base of the skull and produces platybasia. The inward expansion may impinge on the vault size, reducing the area available for the brain. Cortical atrophy is commonly demonstrated by computed tomography (CT) or magnetic resonance imaging (MRI) but is not usually excessive for age. One must carefully examine the inner and outer table of the cortex for disruption suggestive of malignancy.

Special views of the skull may be needed to demonstrate Paget's disease invasion of the petrous ridge or cochlea. This may require the Towne's view, radiographic tomograms, computed tomography, or high-resolution computed tomography (132). Similar studies may be

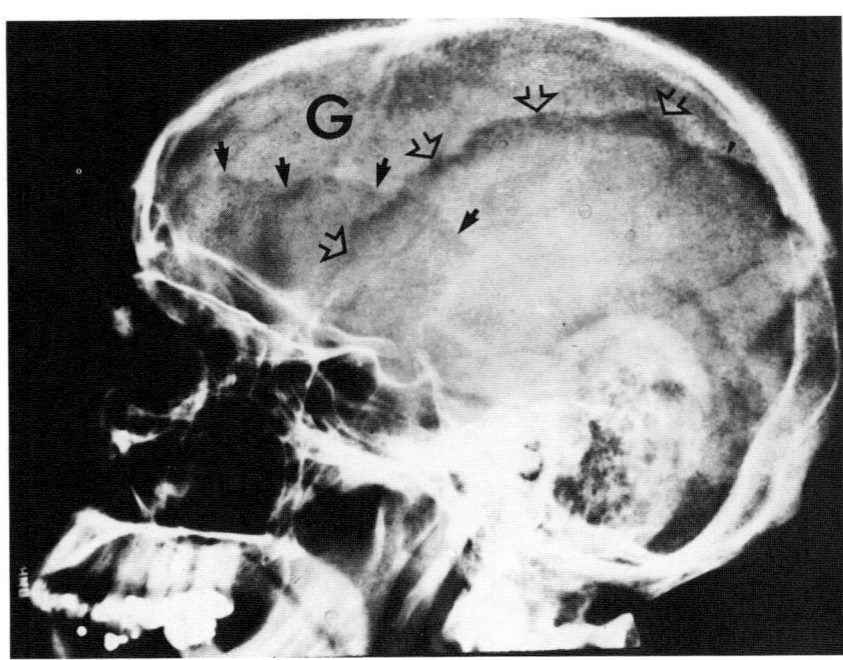

FIG. 15. Lateral radiograph of the skull shows a ground-glass appearance with overlapping osteoporosis circumscripta of both tables of bone (*narrow arrows*, right temporal bone; *wide arrows*, left temporal bone).

needed to demonstrate optic nerve compression by Paget's disease of the orbit. Other cranial nerve impingement is rare.

Platybasia with change in mental status may raise the issue of hydrocephalus. Computer tomography or MRI may be needed to evaluate outflow obstruction of spinal fluid. In these cases, cortical atrophy is associated with dilatation of all ventricles of the brain. MRI of pagetic skull allows evaluation of the bony calvarium as well as excellent definition of the soft tissues (133). Cerebrospinal flow can be assessed by MRI.

Radiographically, Paget's disease of the maxilla or

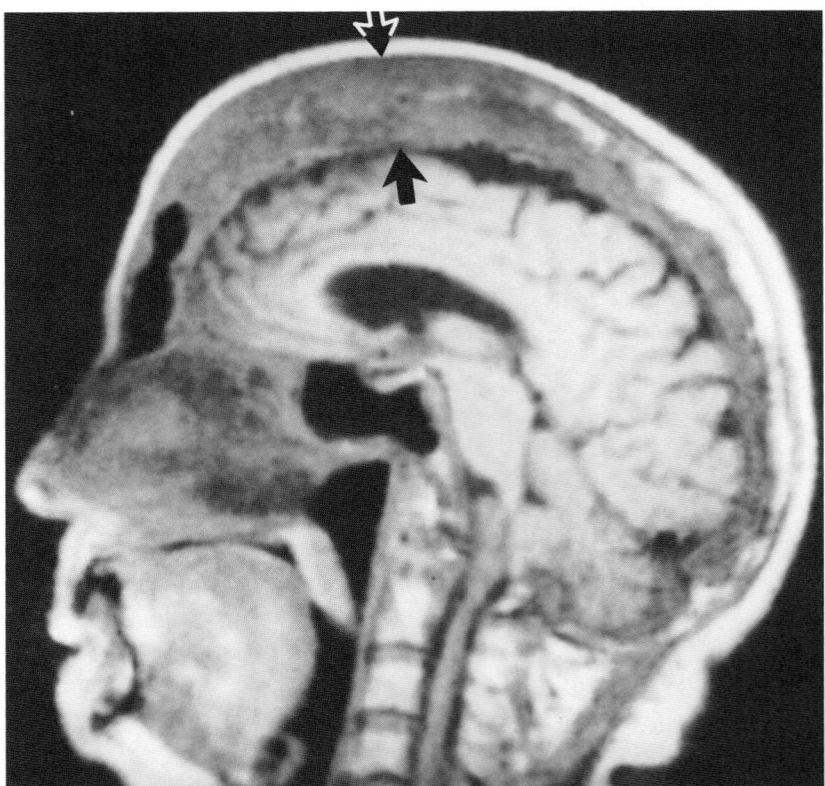

FIG. 16. Sagittal section of skull as produced by magnetic resonance imaging shows an enlarged lateral ventricle, cortical atrophy, and wide, thick skull mostly composed of wide diploic areas (*arrows*). Platybasia without cord impingement is present.

mandible may be confused with fibrous dysplasia of bone. Interestingly, Paget's disease rarely involves both the mandible and maxilla. Resorption of the lamina dura may be present about the teeth.

If small, spotty osteoblastic lesions may give the skull a ground-glass appearance. Larger blastic lesions may be reminiscent of those seen in metastatic blastic carcinoma (e.g., prostate or breast). Radiographically, Paget's disease should not be confused with hyperostosis frontalis interna.

Spine

Lumbar vertebrae are involved more often than cervical or dorsal vertebrae (Table 6). One or more vertebrae may be involved. The involved vertebra is often enlarged in all planes. Widening of the vertebra without similar enlargement of the posterior neural arch leads to loss of lordosis or kyphosis. It may be radiodense (ivory vertebra) (Fig. 14) or porotic. There is often cortical thickening of the upper and lower vertebral plates with coarse, vertically arranged trabeculae—the so-called "picture frame" vertebra (Fig. 17). Porotic vertebrae may collapse into the typical "codfish vertebra" pattern associated with osteoporosis.

Anteroposterior and lateral radiographs of the vertebral column often strikingly contrasts the abnormal vertebrae (Figs. 14 and 17). Oblique views of the spine may demonstrate Paget's disease of the facet from facet osteoarthritis (Fig. 18). Cord impingement syndromes may require computed tomography, MRI (Fig. 19), or contrast myelography.

The enthesopathy, ankylosing hyperostosis [diffuse idiopathic skeletal hyperostosis (DISH)], may develop radiographic characteristics of Paget's disease (59,134).

The mottled change visible on radiography may require MRI to separate signals of tumor from those of Paget's disease; the T1 and T2 mixed appearance of Paget's disease contrasts with the high signal on T2 and low signal on T1 of tumor.

Pelvis

Pelvic changes are characteristic. Most often involvement is bilateral with adjacent disease of the sacrum (Fig.

TABLE 6. Radiographic spinal distribution of Paget's disease

Vertebrae	Percent[a]
Cervical 1–7	5
Dorsal 1–12	12
Lumbar 1	9
Lumbar 2	17
Lumbar 3	22
Lumbar 4	24
Lumbar 5	12

Source: After Guyer et al. (272).
[a] Percent of 1163 involved vertebrae.

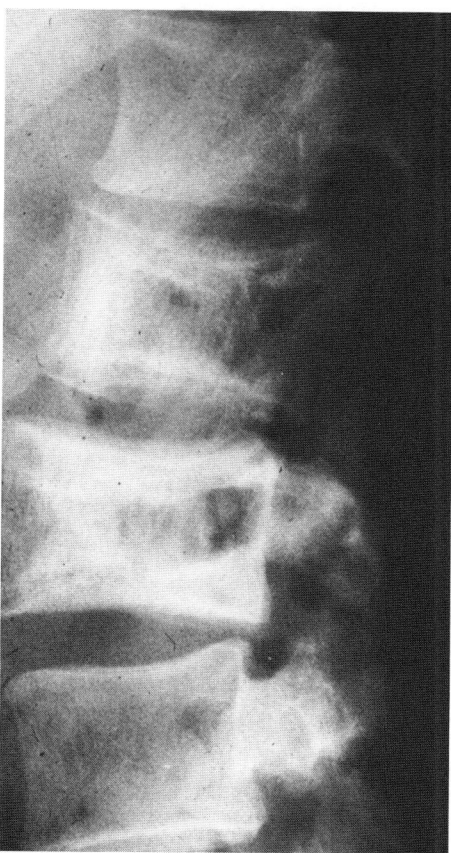

FIG. 17. Lateral radiograph of the lumbar spine shows Paget's disease of the second and third lumbar vertebrae. The third lumbar vertebra is enlarged in the anteroposterior and superior–inferior planes. The thick cortices of the involved vertebrae surround mixed changes of the body of the vertebrae, giving them a "picture-frame" appearance.

8). The sacroiliac joints are often disrupted or fused by CT but rarely symptomatic. The ilei may be porotic, diffusely radiodense, or have "whorls" of coarse trabeculation (Fig. 9). The ileopectineal line is often thickened and sclerotic in appearance (*Brim sign*) (Fig. 20) (135). Similarly, the pubis may be involved. The softened pelvis migrates axially, giving the pelvic brim a triangular appearance or *triradiate* deformity (136). Patchy sclerotic areas may cause difficulty in separating blastic tumors from coexistent Paget's disease.

Extremities

Four radiographic appearances of tubular bones include homogeneous sclerosis, trabecular coarsening, cortical thickening, and lysis (137). Tubular bones demonstrate thickened cortex with both new subperiosteal bone and narrowing of the medullary canal (Fig. 6). The shaft of the long bone can demonstrate the flame sign discussed above (Fig. 7). Proximal or distal areas of long bones demonstrate coarse trabeculation (Fig. 8).

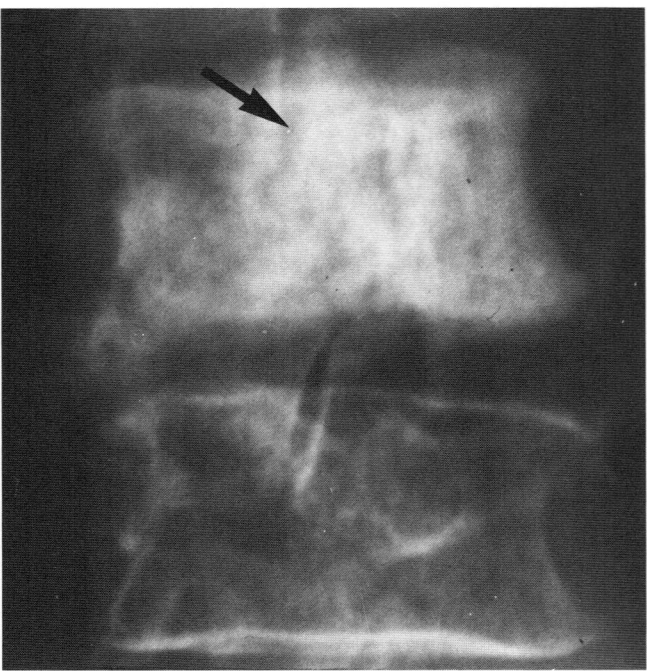

FIG. 18. Oblique radiograph of the lumbar spine shows sclerotic changes of the third lumbar vertebra with enlargement and sclerosis of the superior facet. The radiographic facet joint (*arrow*) is preserved.

Juxta-articular subchondral bone is often enlarged. If on only one side of the articulation, the normal congruity between surfaces is altered (i.e., the pagetic side of the articulation is larger than the nonpagetic side). Evidence of joint space narrowing is common. Some osteophytic growth is also common.

Long bones are often bowed because of muscle pull or gravity. Microfracture can be noted on the convex side of the bow, surrounded by reactive bone. Articular chondrocalcinosis does not occur more frequently in Paget's disease than the general population (59,138). As many as 20% of cases involve the foot (139).

Sarcoma

Radiographically, pagetic sarcomas can be suspected if there is disruption of the cortex and fluffy calcifications with a soft-tissue mass effect surrounding the involved bone (Fig. 21). Bone destruction and new bone formation may be present. Early signs are subcortical medullary bone destruction, followed by cortical bone loss and evidence of a soft-tissue mass. Osteolysis rather than osteosclerosis is the major radiographic characteristic of sarcoma (140). Additionally, a soft-tissue mass, bony spiculation, and a nonunion fracture may be seen (141).

When sarcoma is discovered, there is often radiographic evidence of metastases, particularly to the lungs. Giant-cell tumors most often occur in the skull or facial bones and in elderly patients with polyostotic Paget's disease. These are most often benign in appearance. Radiographically, giant-cell tumors are lytic expansile lesions with a soft tissue mass. Pagetic fat-filled marrow spaces can simulate tumor (142).

Fractures

Various forms of fractures can be visualized on the roentgenogram. Vertebral compression fractures can be seen. Cortical stress or incompleted fractures are most

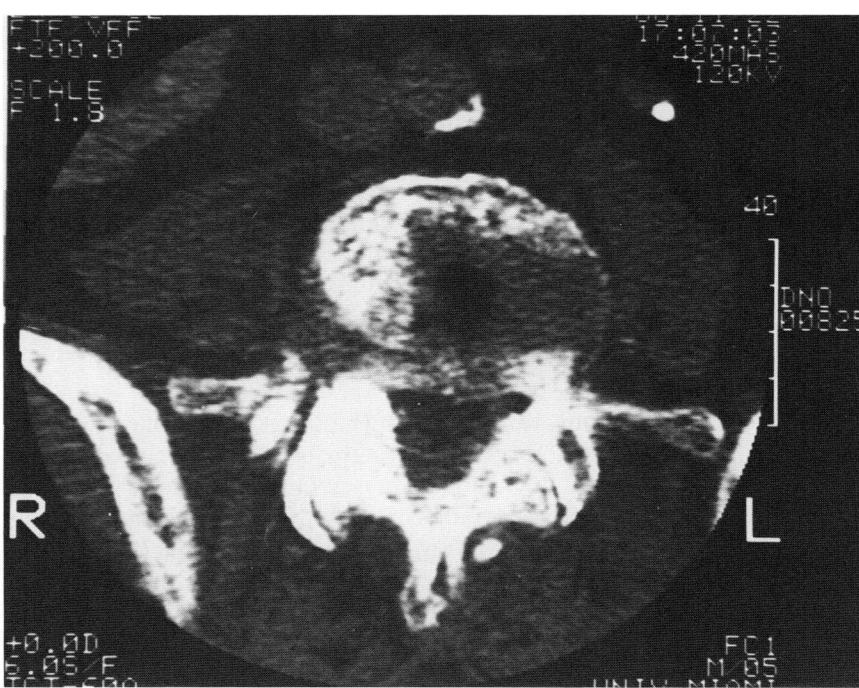

FIG. 19. Axial view of the fifth lumbar vertebra by computed tomography shows pagetic coarse trabeculation of the spine laminae and facets with pagetic changes of the superior facets and spine from the first sacral vertebra. The iliac crests similarly demonstrate coarse trabeculation of Paget's disease. The disc space is partially deteriorated, demonstrating a vacuum phenomenon. The facets are hypertrophied, showing osteoarthritis by joint space narrowing, osteophyte formation, and subchondral sclerosis.

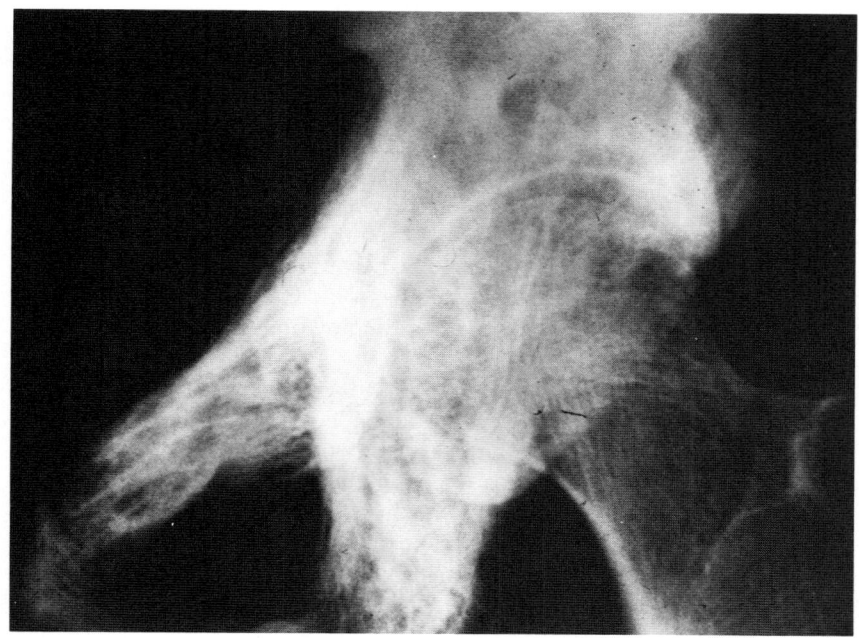

FIG. 20. Radiograph of the innominate bone showing thickening of the iliopectineal line, the Brim sign.

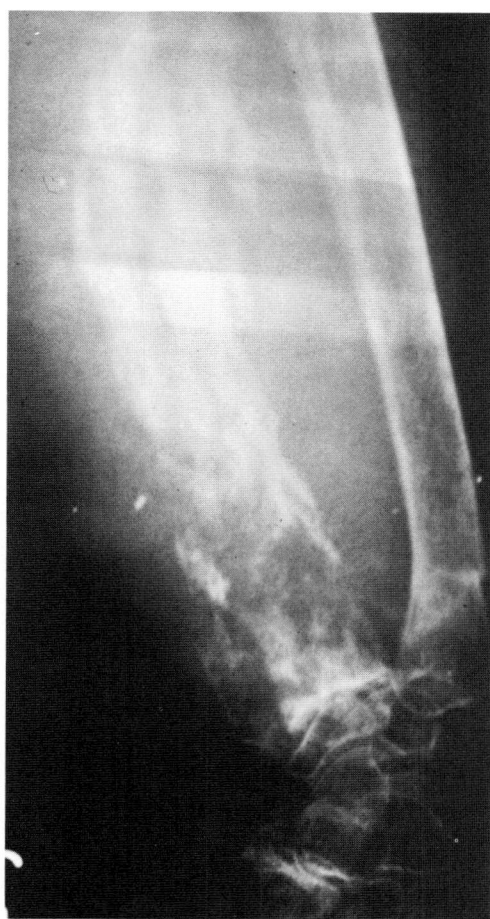

FIG. 21. Radiograph from a woman who presented with a sudden onset of left forearm pain. The cortex of the radius is disrupted and fragmented. There is a mass effect beyond the confines of the radius containing bone spicules. This gross disruption of bone is common in sarcomatous changes of Paget's disease.

notable in the lateral femur or anterior tibia, appearing as multiple or single horizontal, radiolucent lines (Fig. 6). Their placement on the convex surface of the bone separates these from the concave surface location of Looser zones, seen in osteomalacia.

Completed fractures of the femur are commonly subtrochanteric in location (Fig. 7) (143). Fracture callus occasionally takes on the radiographic appearance of Paget's disease (Fig. 7).

Bone Scanning

Bone scanning is presently based on a pertechnetate-labeled diphosphonate with a strong tendency to localize at sites of blastic activity of bone, or inflammatory/damaged soft tissue. It is also influenced by blood flow. In Paget's disease, early phase pertechnetate scanning demonstrates highly vascular bone and surrounding tissues. Early phase radionuclide studies show increased flow (144) while later phase studies localize the nuclide to new bone formation. The unique diffuse cortical uptake separates the bone scan of Paget's disease from other diseases (Figs. 11B, 22, and 23). Nonpagetic metastatic diseases isolate the nuclide to localized areas on bones, usually not as intense or as extensive as Paget's disease. Osteomalacia, renal osteodystrophy, hyperthyroidism, hypertrophic osteoarthropathy, or osteomyelitis rarely extend in the diffuse manner of Paget's disease.

All pagetic sites do not accumulate the radionuclide equally. There are differences in scintigraphic activity at each anatomic site. Disease recurrence has been detected by nuclear scan as early as 6 months prior to increase in alkaline phosphatase (145).

Khairi reported that 20% of Paget's disease sites could only be detected by scan. Others also report the bone

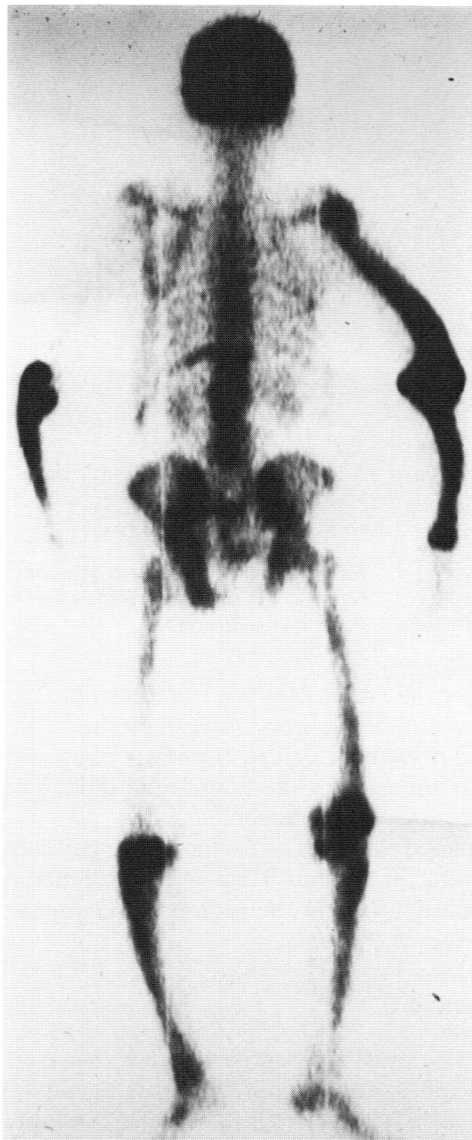

FIG. 22. 99mTc-labeled diphosphonate bone scans localize to the areas of active bone deposition and are well suited for detection of active areas of Paget's disease. This posterior scintigram shows intense uptake of Paget's disease in the skull, left scapula, right humerus, right radius, left ulna, several dorsal and lumbar vertebrae, left twelfth rib, right and left hemipelvis, sacrum, proximal left femur, diffuse right femur, right patella, and both tibias. Although if an isolated finding, the uptake of the left twelfth rib could be confused with metastatic carcinoma, the diffuse uptake of the other areas is typical of Paget's disease. The pattern of nuclear uptake reflects the bony deformity.

studies (128). In 5% the scan was positive when the radiograph had been read as uninvolved, most often involving scapulae or clavicles. In less than 1% did the radiograph reveal Paget's disease that the nuclide did not localize.

Diphosphonate bone scanning continues to be of value for patients receiving diphosphonates as suppressive therapy, even by quantitative techniques (148,149). However, it is expected that the nuclide will less consistently localize to radiographic Paget's disease in patients receiving suppressive therapy due to suppressed activity of disease.

Our studies have found a poor correlation of pain to the intensity of radionuclide uptake. Those lesions present on the bone scan but not apparent on radiograph tend to be less symptomatic (150). The most intense lesions by radionuclide uptake may be the most symptomatic. Increased uptake of technetium-labeled diphosphonate in bone is inversely related to the intensity of the renal image (151).

Quantitative radionuclide bone scanning has been applied to total body scans and is proposed as a method of following patients under therapy for their Paget's disease (149,152). Several quantitative techniques for isolated areas of involvement have been proposed, which are generally based on a timed acquisition of the nuclide at the

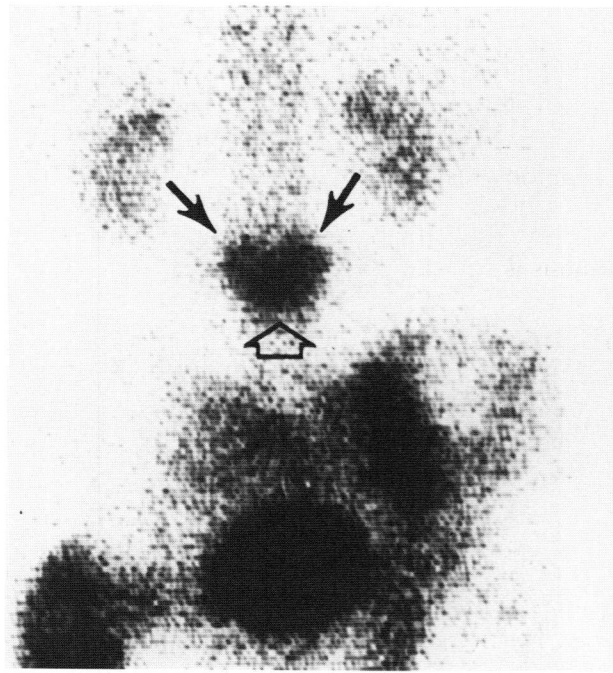

FIG. 23. 99mTc-labeled diphosphonate localizes to the body of the involved vertebra (*wide arrow*) as well as the superior facets of the posterior neural arch (*narrow arrows*) provides a "Y-like" configuration. Paget's disease is also present in the right hemipelvis, sacrum, proximal left femur, and left and right humeri.

scan more sensitive than roentgenogram (146). Increased sensitivity of the bone scan over the radiograph was stressed in a study in which 94.5 sites were recognized by bone scan, but only 74% were recognized by radiograph (147). In a review of 290 pagetic sites in 50 patients, bone scan and radiograph correlated in 95% of

site being studied and a blank or control site. Not all sites change or change equally under therapy.

Diminished [^{99m}Tc]sulfur colloid activity of the bone marrow was noted in Paget's disease (153). Similarly, decreased uptake of [^{131}I]indium WBC scintiscan can be seen in Paget's disease of bone (154). Sulfur colloid gastrointestinal bleeding studies may be falsely positive in the presence of symmetric bone marrow activity of Paget's disease (155). Delayed images may be of value. Lesions seen by radiograph and not by Na^{18}F bone scan were asymptomatic (156). However, lesions seen by Na^{18}F bone scan and radiograph were symptomatic.

Gallium readily localizes to active Paget's disease. Reduction of activity of bone was better demonstrated by radiolabeled gallium than by radiolabeled diphosphonates, perhaps because gallium uptake more specifically reflects cellular activity (157). Recurrence could not be predicted by reactivation of radionuclide uptake of symptomatic Paget's disease at an individual site (158).

If an area of expected active Paget's disease fails to accumulate the nuclide, sarcomatous change may be suspected (Fig. 10B). Nevertheless, photon deficiency in Paget's disease may be present early in the disease even without sarcoma (159). Paget's disease of the skull can cause falsely positive brain scans. Intense extracerebral perfusion can mask an underlying intracerebral perfusion deficiency, such as occlusion of the middle cerebral artery (160).

DIAGNOSIS

Clinical Features

Symptoms may be present for a period of years before the diagnosis is made (Table 7). However, the majority of patients have no apparent clinical abnormalities. The diagnosis is occasionally apparent from classic features on clinical examination, such as a large skull with frontal bossing and dilated scalp veins, short stature with Simian posturing, and lateral/anterior bow to an extremity.

In trying to separate the findings of osteoarthritis from Paget's disease, one may wish to place lidocaine into the suspected joint, such as a hip or a knee. If there is prompt relief of pain, the symptoms are most likely osteoar-thritic in origin. Joint analgesia is not expected to relieve Paget's disease pain of bony origin.

Serum Alkaline Phosphatase Measurement

Most of the time, the diagnosis of Paget's disease is suggested during pursuit of a serum alkaline phosphatase elevation. (See the laboratory section above.)

Radiograph

The roentgenographic features of Paget's disease are most often diagnostic. Only rarely will the initial lytic phase present some difficulty.

Pelvic Paget's disease can mimic osteoblastic metastases. However, the accentuated trabecular pattern, enlargement of the involved bone, thickening of the iliopectineal line, triangular appearance of the pelvic brim, and diffuse distribution of Paget's disease in the pelvis are characteristic.

The picture frame vertebra with condensation of the vertebral cortex, ivory vertebra, and the coarse trabecular pattern separate Paget's disease from vertebral hemangioma, the "rugger-jersey" spine of renal osteodystrophy, and osteoporosis. The ivory vertebra may mimic blastic skeletal metastases and lymphoma. Long-bone epiphyseal involvement, widespread sclerosis, bony enlargement, thickened cortex, bowing, sharply demarcated bone lysis, and an advancing osteolytic wedge are characteristic of Paget's disease.

However, increased skeletal density may be seen in blastic bone metastases (e.g., prostatic carcinoma), myelofibrosis, fluorosis, malignant mastocytosis, renal osteodystrophy, fibrous dysplasia of bone, and tuberous sclerosis. Examination and laboratory testing may be needed to separate these diseases. Axial osteomalacia, osteogenesis imperfecta ossium, familial idiopathic hyperphosphatasia, and hyperostosis frontalis may on occasion be difficult to separate from Paget's disease.

Bone Scan

The bone scan is helpful in outlining the extent of bony involvement in Paget's disease. Because Paget's

TABLE 7. *Reason for diagnosis in 290 patients*

	Number of patients	Time symptoms present (mean ± SD)
Symptoms suggestive of Paget's disease	119	6.8 ± 7.6
Elevated serum alkaline phosphatase	47	7.2 ± 10.2
Radiograph showing Paget's disease	84	13.1 ± 11.3
Pathologic fracture	6	15.5 ± 11.3
Other	21	15.0 ± 11.0

disease rarely adds new bones with time, repeat bone scan is uncommonly needed. Spread within the involved bone does occur; this can be evaluated by radiograph and occasionally by bone scan.

Bone Biopsy

In Paget's disease, the radiograph is characteristic and most often confirms diagnosis. However, bone biopsy may be needed if malignant transformation or another tumor metastatic to bone is suspected. Biopsy of the osteolytic wedge is unnecessary and should be avoided because of increased risk of fracture (161).

TREATMENT

General Measures

The patient should be advised that Paget's disease is rarely a serious illness. Most often symptoms are mild and readily suppressed by a therapeutic program. In the patients with symptomatic disease, an array of physical, medicinal, and surgical measures are often effective in disease control. Death from Paget's disease is almost limited to the less than 1% of patients that develop sarcomatous changes of the pagetic lesion.

Orthopedic Measures

Mechanical devices such as orthotics often correct symptoms related to bowed lower extremities or pelvic deformity. Often a heel lift, or occasionally a medial wedge to the heel and sole, will suffice. Orthopedic procedures indicated for Paget's disease may include osteotomy for tibial or femoral deformity, open or closed reduction for fracture, joint arthroplasty for secondary osteoarthritis, and spinal decompression for symptoms and signs of cord compression.

Tibial osteotomy can reduce bone pain and improve ambulatory ability (162). Osteotomies as well as nonsurgical fractures may require plates or intramedullary rods for stabilization. Because pagetic fractured bone by osteotomy or trauma is often soft and tends to bow, the plate or intramedullary rod is often left in place indefinitely for continued stabilization. Fractures most often heal without event; however, occasional nonunion occurs. The fracture callus is often pagetic.

During orthopedic surgery, pagetic bone may be hard and difficult to cut, or may be soft and bleed excessively. Medicinal therapy prior to orthopedic surgery may reduce the excessive bleeding. In general, total joint replacement has been successful. However, loosening is more common than the nonpagetic population, perhaps due to the softened bone and bowed extremities (163).

Arthrodesis is occasionally indicated. There is a single report of Paget's disease extending from the femur to the previously uninvolved tibia following knee arthrodesis (164).

Anti-inflammatory Drugs

High-dose salicylates have been used for their analgesic and anti-inflammatory properties. In addition, they retard collagen production and reduce hydroxyproline excretion in pagetic patients (165). Suppression of prostaglandin levels by indomethacin and other anti-inflammatory agents is felt to decrease skeletal vascularity and bone resorption (122).

In many patients with Paget's disease, pain is related to secondary osteoarthritis. Symptoms related to osteoarthritis may respond to anti-inflammatory agents.

Guidelines for Suppressive Medicinal Therapy

Patients should have symptoms or progressive complications of Paget's disease, demonstration of active disease by an elevated serum alkaline phosphatase, and radiographic evidence of Paget's disease at the symptomatic site to receive suppressive medicinal therapy. Because there are no uniformly accepted guidelines for the therapy of Paget's disease, the author's indications for therapy are outlined in Table 8. Most would agree that pain related to Paget's disease and not due to another phenomenon, such as secondary osteoarthritis, indicates the need for suppressive therapy.

One should be cautious in the therapy of lumbar spine involvement with Paget's disease. Although back pain is a common complaint in patients with Paget's disease, it is an uncommon cause of symptoms. Back pain is often due to an arthritic process. The arthritic process may have resulted from the Paget's disease.

Paraparesis or paraplegia may relate to Paget's disease of the dorsal or cervical spine. These patients are often poor surgical candidates for decompression because of coexistent multiple medical problems. These syndromes have often been reversed, at least in part, by medicinal therapy. The improvement is probably due to reversal of a "spinal artery steal" syndrome rather than alteration of bone from the spinal canal.

Pagetic bone has sometimes been described by orthopedic surgeons as structurally soft and highly vascular. Pretreatment with one of the suppressive agents appears to decrease the vascularity of the pagetic bone and may limit blood loss during orthopedic surgery. The treated bone is more likely to heal normally.

The long-bone osteolytic phase of Paget's disease may require high-quality radiographs for diagnosis. This complication is not common, occurring in about 10% of

TABLE 8. *Indications for medicinal therapy of Paget's disease*[a]

	Calcitonins	Diphosphonates
Bone pain due to Paget's disease	+	+
Spinal Paget's disease with paraparesis/paraplegia	+	+
Preoperative orthopedic surgery	+	+
Immobilization hypercalcemia	+	−
Nonunion pagetic fracture	−	+
Osteolytic wedge of long bone on x-ray	+	?
Skull symptoms: headache, dizziness (not platybasia)	+	+
High-output cardiac failure	+	+
Prevent progression of disease (i.e., not correction of existing defect)		
Hearing loss (Paget's disease of the skull)	+	+
Osteoarthritis (juxta-articular Paget's disease)	+	+
Deformity (Paget's disease of long bones)	+	+
Asymptomatic increase in serum alkaline phosphatase without complication listed above	−	−

[a] +, useful; −, not indicated.

radiographs in our series. Calcitonin consistently induces radiographic "healing" during therapy (161). However, withdrawal of calcitonin is often followed by rapid progression of osteolysis, implying that therapy should not be discontinued. Disodium etidronate inconsistently induces radiographic healing and is sometimes associated with progression.

A possible set of indications of suppressive therapy for Paget's disease are dependent on the hypothesis that suppressive therapy will prevent additional complications of the pagetic process. It can be argued that suppressive therapy inhibits disease activity and that progressive abnormalities may at least in part be retarded or prevented. However, none of these therapies are expected to correct existing hearing loss, deformity, or osteoarthritis.

Activity of disease should be followed by periodic testing of Paget's disease of bone, namely the serum alkaline phosphatase and, if possible, urine total peptide hydroxyproline excretion. Follow-up radiographs are occasionally necessary, while follow-up bone scans are uncommonly needed.

The question has been raised as to whether suppression of Paget's disease by medications could prevent sarcoma. This does not appear to be the case, as we have observed three sarcomas in patients on calcitonin, two in patients on etidronate disodium, and one in a patient on plicamycin.

Calcitonin

Calcitonin, a recently discovered hormone, demonstrates dramatic effectiveness in the therapy of Paget's disease. Calcitonin is a 32-amino acid hormone of the thyroid C cells. It has been demonstrated to lower plasma inorganic calcium concentration by action on the bone and kidney. It inhibits osteoclastic bone resorption (166) with loss of the ruffled resorption surface of osteoclasts within 1 h, having some effect within 15 min

(167,168). In Paget's disease, calcitonin induces a more normal bony histologic picture, with more lamellar than woven bone. Calcitonin caused a reduction in osteoclast size and number, a decrease in bone density and resorption, and an increase in lamellar bone (169). There may be an increase in surface covered with osteoid. This effect is proposed to be mediated by cyclic AMP accumulation (170) and results in reduction in the number of osteoclasts (171). Even though there is no deficiency of calcitonin in Paget's disease (119), calcitonin has been demonstrated to suppress clinical and chemical disease. In rats, calcitonin did not interfere with net collagen, calcifying callus, or mechanical strength of healing fractures (172).

Response to Calcitonin

Reduction of symptoms during synthetic salmon or synthetic human calcitonin therapy may occur by the end of the first month of therapy, sometimes occurring dramatically in the first few weeks. Calcitonin analgesia may be independent of its effects on bone turnover and may precede the change in hydroxyproline (173).

In a retrospective review of 45 patients with hearing loss due to Paget's disease (174), the hearing loss was less than 1 dB in the calcitonin-treated group. Not all studies documented reduced hearing loss with calcitonin, but in a negative study, the group was small (175). Spastic paraparesis resolves or improves with SCT therapy, even after failure of decompression laminectomy (176,177). Cauda equina syndrome was reversed in additional patients with Paget's disease, treated with SCT (178).

Calcitonin reduced the increased skeletal blood flow of Paget's disease (179). Cardiac index fell toward normal during treatment with calcitonin, but exacerbated in three of nine patients when therapy was discontinued (180). Increased cardiac output of Paget's disease is not always responsive to calcitonin (181). Radiologic improvement has been noted with calcitonin therapy

(182–185), particularly in healing the lytic phase in long bones (161).

Chemical and clinical relapse do not necessarily coincide; indeed, most patients have a considerable delay in exacerbation of symptoms after withdrawal of calcitonin. Following discontinuation of SCT, symptomatic improvement persisted in 10 of 13 patients, for up to 1 year (186). Hydroxyproline remained depressed for up to 1 year, but alkaline phosphatase returned to pretreatment values within 6 months.

Calcitonin is probably not anti-inflammatory, as suggested by a patient with Paget's disease who developed rheumatoid arthritis while on calcitonin therapy (187). Based on serum calcitonin levels, it was felt that parenteral calcitonin two to four times daily would be more effective than once daily in Paget's disease (188). In the uncomplicated patient with Paget's disease, the drug could be discontinued after 2 years of therapy. Because the cessation of calcitonin leads to a recurrence of the osteolytic phase (189), in the presence of a lytic bony lesion, calcitonin probably should be continued indefinitely.

Antibodies and Resistance

Antibodies have been demonstrated in patients receiving porcine calcitonin (190,191), salmon calcitonin (192), and synthetic human calcitonin (193). Others feel that there has not been a detectable antibody to human calcitonin (194). In many cases, resistance to calcitonin appears related to high titers of neutralizing antibodies (192,195). Binding antibodies developed in 60% of those treated with SCT (196).

However, antibodies also occur without clinical resistance (190,191,193) and are not present in all patients with resistance to calcitonin (197). Primary and secondary resistance to calcitonin occurs with all calcitonins, but antibody-based clinical resistance was felt to be uncommon (198). Resistance to calcitonin may be an induced phenomenon; this is supported by a study demonstrating in vitro escape of calcitonin-induced bone resorption (199), perhaps suggesting down-regulation of surface receptors.

If resistance to salmon calcitonin is suspected, one can test for a calcitonin effect on serum calcium. Serum calcium is determined after an overnight fast. Synthetic salmon calcitonin (100 IU) is injected intramuscularly and serum calcium is determined 3–6 h after the injection. Breakfast is allowed. If the calcitonin is effective, a decrease of 0.5 mg/dL or more in serum calcium is seen. A decrease of 0.3 mg/dL or less of serum calcium is seen in calcitonin resistance. Treatment response has been reported to be better if disodium etidronate is used before calcitonin (200).

It has been suggested that the lack of response to calcitonin is due to low plasma vitamin A (201). It was also felt that combining ascorbic acid with calcitonin provided a greater degree of pain relief, but the percent of responders did not change and the urine hydroxyproline was unchanged in the early period of therapy (202).

Porcine Calcitonin

Lyophilized porcine calcitonin is a partially purified extract. Doses of 8 Medical Research Council (MRC) units were effective and reduced bone turnover in short-term trials (203,204). Although considerable variation occurs, porcine calcitonin suppresses alkaline phosphatase to about 50% of pretreatment values. Porcine calcitonin gave pain relief, more often in the lower extremities (205). Circulating antibodies were not related to response or lack of same. Chemical exacerbation often occurs between 6 and 12 months. It has been suggested that very small doses of porcine calcitonin are effective in Paget's disease (certainly of economic importance) (206), but confirmation of these results are needed.

Salmon Calcitonin

Similarly, parenteral synthetic salmon calcitonin (Calcimar, Miacalcin) suppresses the chemical expressions of Paget's disease to about 50% of pretreatment levels, with a slight loss of effect after 3–6 months. After 18–24 months, chemical exacerbation often occurs (194). Most patients will have chemical exacerbation within 6 months of calcitonin discontinuation. Antibodies may be present without clinical resistance. They are not present in all patients with resistance to salmon calcitonin.

The author proposes the initial dose of synthetic salmon calcitonin as 100 (MRC) units or 0.5 mL of Calcimar subcutaneously or intramuscularly daily for the first month. The dose can be decreased or the interval between doses increased depending on the severity of disease and response to therapy.

Even though there is no histologic confirmation, clinical benefit and chemistries can be controlled in many patients on as little as 50 units, two or three times weekly. Salmon calcitonin (Calcimar) should be refrigerated. It is supplied as 400 units per 2-mL vial.

Synthetic salmon calcitonin nasal spray was effective in 17 patients with Paget's disease who were untreated previously: alkaline phosphatase decreased 31 ± 5% (SEM), and hydroxyproline decreased 37 ± 7% in 1 year. Adverse effects were minimal (207).

Synthetic salmon calcitonin 200 units by nasal spray decreased hydroxyproline excretion within 8–16 h but was not as effective as synthetic salmon calcitonin 100 IU intramuscularly (208). It was ineffective in others. In this study, nasal synthetic salmon calcitonin was mildly effective and more convenient than parenteral synthetic salmon calcitonin, but dose response and efficacy relative to parenteral synthetic salmon calcitonin have not been established, raising questions of cost-effectiveness (209).

Human Calcitonin

Synthetic human calcitonin (Cibacalcin) does not lose its suppressive chemical effect in most patients while the drug is administered; however, the net chemical suppression of chemistries, for unexplained reasons, is often somewhat less than might be expected with synthetic salmon calcitonin. Synthetic human calcitonin has been of value in patients resistant to synthetic salmon calcitonin (210,211). Synthetic human calcitonin was not radiographically effective at less than 0.5 mg daily (212).

Synthetic human calcitonin is supplied as five doses of 0.5 mg per container dispensed. Each dose is supplied with dessicated calcitonin in a vial connected to a syringe containing diluent. Similar to synthetic salmon calcitonin, the initial dose of synthetic human calcitonin is a single dose daily of 0.5 mg for the first month, with increase in the interval between doses depending on the clinical and chemical response.

Miscellaneous Programs

A proposed therapy combines drugs to decrease endogenous parathyroid hormone excretion and increase endogenous calcitonin (213). A 30% decrease in chemistries was demonstrated in 75 patients. The program included calcium supplement plus a thiazide diuretic with or without a low-phosphorus diet and aluminum hydroxide (phosphorus binder).

Better bone was felt to be produced by a synthetic analog of eel calcitonin even though alkaline phosphatase and hydroxyproline did not change (214). Combined plicamycin and calcitonin have been proposed for severely afflicted patients.

Adverse Reactions to Calcitonin

The most important adverse reactions to the calcitonins are gastrointestinal (nausea, vomiting, diarrhea, abdominal pain, cramps); vascular symptoms (flushing of face, tingling of hands and feet); local reactions at the injection sites (pain, erythema, pruritis); and other reactions, such as urinary frequency, rash, unpleasant metallic taste, rhinorrhea, and occasional angioedema (Table 9). Most symptoms occur within several minutes of injection and last about 1 hour.

Adverse reactions are most common during the initial period of therapy and tend to decrease or disappear with continued administration. These reactions are more common with synthetic human calcitonin than synthetic salmon calcitonin (215). Flushing occurs in 20 to 30% of patients. It involves a feeling of warmth, predominantly in the face and hands and occurs within minutes of injection, usually lasting about an hour (171). Occa-

TABLE 9. *Adverse reactions of Pagetic suppressive agents*

Calcitonin
GASTROINTESTINAL
Nausea and vomiting
Abdominal cramps
Diarrhea

VASCULAR
Facial flush
Hand/feet dysesthesias (tingling)
Pain at injection site with/without erythema
Urinary frequency
Rhinorrhea

DERMATOLOGIC
Exanthem
Angiodema

OTHER
Hyperparathyroidism
Sterile abscess at injection site

Disodium etidronate
Cramps
Diarrhea
Hyperphosphatemia
Bone pain
Fractures(?)

Plicamycin
Nausea and vomiting
Hypercalcemia
Anemia, leukopenia, thrombocytopenia, hemorrhagic, disorder, coagulation defect
Increased creatinine clearance
Increased liver function tests
Skin reactions

sionally, patients paradoxically complain of feeling cold. We have seen one patient with sterile abscesses at the injection site. Hyperparathyroidism, thought to be secondary to calcitonin therapy, has been reported. Nasal calcitonins produce fewer systemic adverse reactions but may cause nasal irritation and occasional nasal ulceration.

Synthetic salmon calcitonin therapy in Paget's disease reduced plasma urate and increased uric acid excretion independent of other effects of calcitonin. Hypouricemia may be observed (216).

Diphosphonates

Newer suppressive agents for Paget's disease are diphosphonates. The diphosphonates or bisphosphonates are pyrophosphate analogs that replace the central oxygen of pyrophosphate with a carbon. Therefore, they are resistant to pyrophosphatase activity such as contained in the serum alkaline phosphatase. Diphosphonates inhibit the precipitation of calcium phosphate, block the transformation of amorphous calcium phosphate to hydroxyapatite, and inhibit aggregation of calcium apatite crystals into clusters (217). In addition, they retard dissolution of calcium crystals, disaggregate apatite crystal clusters, peptidize crystals (transform crystals into a colloidal state), and form polynuclear complexes in the presence of calcium. Diphosphonates can inhibit both soft and hard tissue calcification and bone resorption.

Another effect of diphosphonates may be present. Implants of bone matrix from rats treated with disodium etidronate 20 times the level used in humans produced 40% less ash than controls, implying a direct effect of diphosphonates on protein metabolism of all bone cells (218). Diphosphonates have a direct effect on macrophage function.

Diphosphonate treatment in Paget's disease shows reduced osteoclastic resorption accompanied by gradual replacement of irregular woven bone by lamellar tissue (43). In pagetic bone there is a reduced appositional rate, regular lamellar texture, and reduced marrow fibrosis. After treatment, the bone was more normal in quantity, quality, and metabolism.

Iliac crest bone biopsies were performed on patients with Paget's disease treated with disodium etidronate 5 mg/kg per day for 6 months (43,219,220). There was a marked antiosteoclastic effect that persisted after cessation of treatment. Nonpagetic osteoclasts were less affected but there was a transient decrease in calcification rate. Osteoclasts degenerated after diphosphonates, but the nucleocapsid-like inclusions of remaining osteoclastic nuclei do not. All diphosphonates appear to work by similar mechanisms (221), and pagetic osteoclasts appear particularly sensitive to the diphosphonates (219). Mineralization at low-dose disodium etidronate is most often normal, but in a study from Glasgow, Scotland, 9 of 13 patients on disodium etidronate 5 to 8 mg/kg per day developed focal mineralization defects of pagetic as well as nonpagetic iliac crest bone biopsies (222). High-dose oral disodium etidronate (20 mg/kg per day), even for 2–4 weeks, has demonstrated appreciable mineralization defects in bone biopsy of 11 patients (223).

Disodium Etidronate

Short- and long-term clinical and chemical suppression of Paget's disease was demonstrated in several studies utilizing disodium etidronate (Didronel) at doses of 5 mg/kg per day for periods of 6 months (224,225). Pain from long bones responded more completely than pain from central bones (224). Larger doses of disodium etidronate caused greater suppression of alkaline phosphatase and hydroxyproline (226). Continuation of therapy beyond 6 months did not provide increased clinical or chemical effectiveness. Higher doses can be used for shorter periods of time but are not usually necessary in the initial course of therapy. Clinical improvement may occur after the first month of therapy, yet is often not apparent until 3–6 months or until after therapy has

been discontinued. Prolonged clinical and chemical remission from disodium etidronate can occur (219,220, 226–230). The duration of response may be related to the initial dose of medication but probably correlates to the pretreatment level of hydroxyproline excretion and serum alkaline phosphatase.

Repeat therapy with disodium etidronate can be variable but most often is with 5 mg/kg per day for a 6-month period of each year or 20 mg/kg per day for 1 month of every 4 months (231). Lytic Paget's disease may be healed by disodium etidronate (232), and disodium etidronate may also retard hearing loss (233).

At very high doses in animals, disodium etidronate was shown to inhibit vitamin D absorption from the gastrointestinal tract—a phenomenon not yet demonstrated in humans. During fracture healing there is prompt bone healing with calcified callus during disodium etidronate therapy (234).

Disodium etidronate decreased nuclide accumulation in pagetic lesions by qualitative and quantitative techniques (149,235). Cardiac index falls during therapy with disodium etidronate and persists for 24 weeks (180). In our own studies, cardiac index dropped most impressively with doses of disodium etidronate 20 mg/kg per day for 3 months. Response persisted for 6 months in this group but only for 3 months with lesser doses.

Rapid improvement in paraparesis due to Paget's disease at the sixth thoracic vertebra was reported in a patient who initially responded to calcitonin and subsequently to a single dose of intravenous disodium etidronate 4.3 mg/kg over 3 hours. Investigationally, intravenous disodium etidronate has been administered in high doses with dramatic benefit to severely afflicted patients with Paget's disease (236).

Therapy with disodium etidronate seems to produce three types of responses (62):

1. Prolonged clinical and chemical improvement after a single course of disodium etidronate. This varies from 15 to 40% of patients. Seventy-six percent of these patients tend to have pretreatment alkaline phosphatase and hydroxyproline of between two and four times the upper normal.
2. Those requiring and responding to retreatment. About 45% of the disodium etidronate–treated patients are involved: these patients have modest disease and require retreatment less than once yearly.
3. Those eventually becoming resistant to disodium etidronate. This involves about 15% of patients. They have the most severe disease clinically and chemically. Their initial response to therapy is excellent but transient. At first, response to retreatment is good, but this is quickly followed by resistance to retreatment with 5 mg/kg per day. Retreatment is clinically indicated more often than once a year because of ac-

tive disease with transient clinical and chemical responses. Resistance to doses above 5 mg/kg per day is often accompanied by increasing bone pain.

The usual dose of disodium etidronate for Paget's disease is 5 mg/kg per day or 400 mg daily for a 40 kg (88 lb) to 80-kg (176-lb) patient. The drug is supplied in 200- and 400-mg tablets. The entire disodium etidronate dose should be administered at one time, midway between breakfast and lunch (or at bedtime), with either water, or black coffee. The empty stomach is needed since disodium etidronate adheres to food, milk, or dairy products, all of which prevent absorption.

Adverse Drug Reactions to Disodium Etidronate

Adverse reactions to disodium etidronate include abdominal cramps, diarrhea, hyperphosphatemia, increasing bone pain, and a possible increase in fractures (Table 9). Abdominal symptoms often subside by altering dose or time of drug administration. Hyperphosphatemia appears to be due to a direct renal effect of disodium etidronate in humans and does not occur in animals (121). Hyperphosphatemia in humans is not related to changes in parathyroid hormone, vitamin D, calcitonin, or calcium homeostasis. These adverse reactions have been reported with low-dose disodium etidronate (5 mg/kg per day) (222).

In the United States, there appears to be regional differences in the frequency of adverse reactions, such as bone pain. It is tempting to attribute these differences to climate (sun exposure—vitamin D) or hereditary factors. It is still uncertain if vitamin D supplements will alter the mineralization defect induced by disodium etidronate (237,238).

The risk of fracture related to disodium etidronate was reviewed in a retrospective survey of 737 patients (239). Fracture rate was equal to that of the normal aging population. Elevation of pretreatment hydroxyproline was a strong predictor of fracture rate. Fracture rates were higher in those receiving high-dose disodium etidronate for prolonged periods of time, but fracture rate decreased in all disodium etidronate–treated groups with time and was in the range of fracture frequency of the aging population.

Dichloromethylene Diphosphonate (MDCl₂)

Other diphosphonates have been investigated in therapy of Paget's disease. MDCl₂ has been of particular interest of because it does not impair mineralization, as evidenced by double tetracycline labeling (240). Reduced hydroxyproline, alkaline phosphatase, urine calcium, number of pagetic bone osteoclasts, bone scans, and pain is common by 9 months. MDCl₂ provided more complete biochemical suppression of Paget's disease than disodium etidronate and was associated with

more prolonged responses irrespective of dose regimen (241). Also, MDCl₂ was effective in patients resistant to disodium etidronate. Short-term high doses (1600 mg for 1 month) were felt to produce effects for at least 1 year (242). Short-term MDCl₂ intravenously (300 mg daily for 5 days) was as effective as oral MDCl₂ (1.6 g daily for 6 months), suggesting an alternative mode of therapy (243).

Hyperparathyroidism has been found in patients treated with MDCl₂. Treatment-induced increase in serum parathyroid hormone was noted in 13 of 19 patients and was associated with high 1,25 dihydrocholecalciferol. In a 6-month study using 400–2400 mg MDCl₂ daily, the authors felt that dietary vitamin D prevented secondary hyperparathyroidism (244). Others reported similar results (245).

MDCl₂ was added to human calcitonin therapy, effecting a decrease in chemistries from 40 to 60% of pretreatment values (246). However, it is uncertain if there was an additive effect or just strong response to the MDCl₂. MDCl₂ seemed to exaggerate the early hypercalcemic effect that precedes the hypocalcemic effect of calcitonin (247).

Concern for an unusual toxicity to this drug has not been supported, and research continues outside the United States. No chromosomal abnormalities were noted in 10 patients treated with MDCl₂ after 2–6 months therapy (248).

Aminohydroxypropylidene Diphosphonate (APD)

3 - Amino - 1,hydroxypropylidene - 1 - bisphosphonate (APD, AHPnBP) (AREDIA) is without appreciable effect on bone mineralization at doses in which it is a potent inhibitor of bone resorption. It appears to be 100 times more potent than disodium etidronate in its effect on osteoclasts.

APD produced rapid and dramatic biochemical responses in Paget's disease (249,250). Oral APD 500 mg daily for 4–12 months was clinically effective in 34 of 39 (87%) patients (251). Alkaline phosphatase decreased to 50% and hydroxyproline decreased to 40% of pretreatment values.

Because it remains in bone for a long period of time, it was also found effective orally at 1200 mg/day for 5 consecutive days (252). Benefits persisted for 6 months.

Oral APD 400 mg daily for 3 months was effective for up to 18 months in 16 of 24 patients with disodium etidronate–resistant, very active Paget's disease (alkaline phosphatase 20 times normal) (253).

A single infusion of 60 mg of APD was effective in 10 of 11 patients at 1 year, the exception having remarkably active disease (254). APD was infused at 25 mg/day for 7 days in 9 patients with benefit (255). At these doses, however, chemical relapse was noted in 75% within 3 months. Oral and parenteral APD were compared in 42 patients (256). Both 400 mg orally for 1 month and 25–

50 mg intravenously for 5 days suppressed Paget's disease for 6 months. APD therapy and clinical response correlated with a decrease quantitative uptake of [^{99m}Tc]disodium etidronate (257). Retreatment was effective, but prior therapy for Paget's disease predicted a lesser response.

Adverse reactions have been reported (249,258). Fever was present in 30–40%, usually less than 39.2°C for only the first 2 days of therapy (259). Parathyroid hormone levels increase transiently during therapy. Total body calcium increases. Peripheral blood lymphocytes decrease 30% for the first 1–3 days. There is mild and transient nausea. Plasma calcium decreases, serum zinc transiently decreases, and C-reactive protein rises. Decrease in lymphocytes could represent their local recruitment.

Other Diphosphonate Programs

Diphosphonates have been combined with calcitonin (260); this program seemed of particular value in severely afflicted patients. The effects of disodium etidronate and SCT were additive in a trial comparing the two drugs separately and in combination, achieving a decrease of 71% in alkaline phosphatase and 69% in hydroxyproline (261).

There is clinical and laboratory evidence that when used sequentially, disodium etidronate should precede, rather than follow, calcitonin (200). New and promising diphosphonates are under development (262,263). A new diphosphonate, SR41 319B, or (4-chlorophenyl) thiomethylene disodium bisphosphonate, has shown promise in preliminary studies (264).

Plicamycin

The first agent that seemed to attack the progression of Paget's disease effectively was plicamycin (Mithramycin). This drug is not presently approved by the U.S. Food and Drug Administration for use in Paget's disease. Plicamycin is a yellow crystalline antibiotic derived from the microorganism *Streptomyces tanashiensis*. It is an inhibitor of deoxyribonucleic acid (DNA)–directed ribonucleic acid (RNA) synthesis, probably by binding to, but not altering DNA (265). Plicamycin probably works by affecting the osteoclast directly, the more rapidly metabolizing the bone cells. However, a suppressive effect on the osteoblast may also occur.

Interest in plicamycin followed a report of intravenous administration of 25 μg/kg per day for 10 days, resulting in clinical and chemical benefit in two patients (266). Clinical response to plicamycin is often dramatic. Another trial utilizing smaller doses (10–15 μg/kg per day for 10 days) showed similar results (226). Additional studies utilized plicamycin (25 mg/kg) intravenously by slow drip once every 2–3 weeks (267); cessation of therapy resulted in recurrence of symptoms and elevated chemistries. By all of these methods, pain seems dramatically associated with a drop in temperature over involved skin, decrease in cardiac output, reduced quantitative radionuclide bone scans, reduced hydroxyproline, and eventually reduced alkaline phosphatase. No roentgenographic improvement was noted. Prolonged remission of disease has been reported (268). Plicamycin decreased accumulation of radionuclide bone scanning agent using quantitative techniques (146). In resistant patients, combination with disodium etidronate was effective (269).

During administration of plicamycin, serum calcium invariably decreases, often dramatically. Patients on plicamycin may have hypocalcemic-associated tetany. Many patients develop nausea. In addition, intravenous plicamycin has been hematotoxic, dermatotoxic, hepatotoxic, and nephrotoxic (Table 9). This is despite the reduced dose of plicamycin used for Paget's disease compared to therapy of malignancy or hypercalcemia associated with malignancy. Patients must be monitored carefully and provided with calcium supplementation and antiemetics.

Widespread use of plicamycin has been limited because of concern about serious side effects. Many physicians reserve plicamycin for the most seriously affected patients, especially patients that do not respond to alternative therapies.

Other Medications

Many other therapeutic modalities have been proposed for Paget's disease, including actinomycin, radiotherapy, and colchicine. Large infusions of glucagon have produced relief of bone pain and reduction in alkaline phosphatase and urine hydroxyproline (270). Relapse occurred upon discontinuation and nausea occurred at high doses.

Sodium fluoride at 120 mg/day for 1 year reduced bone pain and normalized alkaline phosphatase and hydroxyproline levels in five patients (271). It was felt that fluoride stabilized bone crystal by converting hydroxyapatite to fluoroapatite, thus preventing crystal dissolution. Preliminary results suggest parenteral oral gallium nitrate may be of value.

CONCLUDING REMARKS

Paget's disease of bone is characterized by change in the morphology of local areas of the skeleton. It was clinically and histologically defined just over 100 years ago by Sir James Paget, a famous physician of his time and a major contributor to medical science.

Characterization of the disease includes rapid bone turnover from activated, large, distorted osteoclasts and overworked osteoblasts. This results in disorganized, heavily calcified fibrotic, enlarged, and softened bone.

The disease may originate from bone infected with a slow virus. Prevalence in the United States is somewhere between 1 and 3% and involves men more often than women, both over the age of 40.

Most patients with the disease are asymptomatic. When symptomatic, though, patients may have bone pain, osteoarthritis, hearing loss, skull symptoms, hypercalcemia, or sarcoma in the pagetic lesion. These patients are generally not very ill. The laboratory reflects increased serum alkaline phosphatase, urine hydroxyproline, and many other measures of bone turnover. Radiographs are characteristic and findings are rarely confused with other diseases. The bone scan mirrors the sites of involvement and is often positive before the radiograph. Bone biopsy is only needed if tumor is suspected.

Dramatic advances in therapy have provided physical measures (e.g., heel lift), orthopedic measures (e.g., hip prosthesis), and medications that appear to effectively alter the course of the disease. Both calcitonins and diphosphonates seem safe and effective in the majority of patients.

Despite the fact that Paget's disease is uncommon, interest into its pathogenesis and therapy continue. Much understanding about bone metabolism and disease in general has been generated by research into Paget's disease. At present the majority of research into therapy is directed at suppression of disease. Perhaps in the future, the etiology or pathogenesis can be altered. Even with the present state of knowledge, in most of these patients, it is rewarding to care for Paget's disease of bone for both the physician and patient.

REFERENCES

1. Sugarbaker ED. Osteitis deformans (Paget's disease of bones). *Am J Surg* 1940;48:417.
2. Shenoy BV, Scheithauer BW. Paget's perspectives in pathology. *Mayo Clin Proc* 1988;63:184–92.
3. Krukenberg F. Ueber das fibrosarcoma ovarii mucocellulare (carcinomatodes). *Arch Gynakol* 1896;50:287–321.
4. Severino LJ. Scarlatina after operations (letter to the editor). *JAMA* 1983;249:589.
5. Wells C, Woodhouse N. Paget's disease in an Anglo-Saxon. *Med Hist* 1975;19:396–400.
6. Denninger HS. Paleopathological evidence of Paget's disease. *Ann Med Hist* 1933;5:73–81.
7. Hutchinson J. On osteitis deformans. *Illus Med News* 1889;2:169.
8. Wrany. Spongrose Hyperostose des Schadels, des Beckins und des linken oberschenkels. *Vjsch Prakt Heilk* 93:79–95, quoted by Paget, 1877.
9. Wilks S. Case of osteoporosis, or spongy hypertrophy of the bones (calvaria, clavicle, or femoris and rib, exhibited at the Society). *Trans Pathol Soc Lond* 1869;20:273.
10. Czerny V. Eine Lakale Maladie des Unterschenkels. *Wien Med Wochenschr* 1873;23:895–925.
11. Paget J. On a form of chronic inflammation of bones (osteitis deformans). *Med Chir Trans* 1877;60:37–63.
12. Sellars SL. Beethoven's deafness. *SA Med J* 1974;48:1585–8.
13. Wagner M. Report of a case of Paget's disease in an eighteen-year-old male with a review of the literature. *Wis Med J* 1947;46:1098.
14. Snapper I. *Medical clinics on bone diseases*. New York: Interscience, 1949;174.
15. Schmorl G. Uber osteitis deformans Paget. *Virchow Arch Pathol Anat* 1932;283:694–737.
16. Barker DJP, Chamberlain AT, Guyer PB, Gardner MJ. Paget's disease of bone: the Lancashire focus. *Br Med J* 1980;4:1105–7.
17. Detheridge FM, Guyer PB, Barker DJP. European distribution of Paget's disease of bone. *Br Med J* 1982;285:1005–8.
18. Guyer PB, Chamberlain AT. Paget's disease of bone in two American cities. *Br Med J* 1980;281:985.
19. Rosenbaum HD, Hanson DJ. Geographic variation in the prevalence of Paget's disease of bone. *Radiology* 1969;92:959–63.
20. Lluberas-Acosta G, Hansell JR, Schumacher HR Jr. Paget's disease of bone in patients with gout. *Arch Intern Med* 1986;146:2389–92.
21. Sofaer JA, Holloway SM, Emery AEH. A family study of Paget's disease of bone. *J Epidemiol Community Health* 1983;37:226–31.
22. Aschner BM, Hurst LA, Roizin L. Genetic study of Paget's disease in monozygotic twin brothers. *Acta Genet Med Gemell* 1952;1:67.
23. Melick RA, Martin TJ. Paget's disease in identical twins. *Aust NZ J Med* 1975;5:564–5.
24. Fotino M, Haymovits A, Falk CT. Evidence for linkage between HLA and Paget's disease. *Transplant Proc* 1977;IX:1867–8.
25. Tilyard MW, Gardner RJM, Milligan L, Cleary TA, Stewart RDH. A probable linkage between familial Paget's disease and the HLA loci. *Aust NZ J Med* 1982;12:498–500.
26. Cullen P, Russell RGG, Walton RJ, Whiteley J. Frequencies of HLA-A and HLA-B: histocompatibility antigens in Paget's disease of bone. *Tissue Antigens* 1976;7:55–6.
27. Altman RD, Winchester R. HLA-A,B,C,D,Dr loci in Paget's disease. [Unpublished data.]
28. Piga AM, Lopez-Abente G, Ibanez AE, Vadillo AG, Lanza MG, Jodra VM. Risk factors for Paget's disease: a new hypothesis. *Int J Epidemiol* 1988;17:198–201.
29. O'Driscoll JB, Anderson DC. Past pets and Paget's disease. *Lancet*, Oct 26, 1985.
30. Barker DJP, Detheridge FM. Dogs and Paget's disease. *Lancet*, Nov 30, 1985.
31. Barker DJP. The epidemiology of Paget's disease of bone. *Br Med Bull* 1984;40(4):396–400.
32. Mandle F. Therapeutucher Versuch bei einem Falle von Osteitis Fibrosa generalizste mittels extinpation eines Epithelkorperchentumors. *Zentralbl Chir* 1926;53:260.
33. Looser E. Schweigerishe Mediyensacje. *Wochenschrift* 1926;7:598.
34. Erdheim J. Beitrage zur Pathologeischen. *Anatomie* 1935;96:1.
35. Rebel A, Malkani K, Basle M, Bregeon CH. Particularites ultrastructuales des osteoclastes de la maladie de Paget. *Rev Rheum* 1974;41:767–71.
36. Howatson AF, Fornasier VL. Microfilaments associated with Paget's disease of bone: comparison with nucleocapsids of measles virus and respiratory syncytial virus. *Intervirology* 1982;18:150–9.
37. Kalmakoff J, Maskill WJ, Thongkraja P, Palmer DG. Antibodies against double-stranded RNA in patients with rheumatoid arthritis, osteoarthrosis and Paget's disease of bone. *Aust NZ J Med* 1981;11:173–8.
38. Singer FR. Paget's disease of bone: a slow virus infection? *Calcif Tissue Int* 1980;31:185–7.
39. Basle M, Kouyoumdjian S, Pouplard A, Rebel A, Filmon R. Maladie osseuse de Paget. *Pathol Biol* 1983;31:41–4.
40. Morgan-Capner P, Robinson P, Clewley G, Darby A, Pettingale K. Measles antibody in Paget's disease. *Lancet* 1981;8222:733.
41. Stroop WG, Baringer JR. Persistent, slow and latent viral infections. *Prog Med Virol* 1982;28:1.
42. Mills BG, Singer FR, Weiner LP, Suffin SC, Stabile E, Holst P. Evidence for both respiratory syncytial virus and measles virus antigens in the osteoclasts of patients with Paget's disease of bone. *Clin Orthop* 1984;183:303–11.
43. Basle MF, Rebel A, Renier JC, Audram M, Filmon R, Malkani K. Bone tissue in Paget's disease treated with ethane-1, hydroxy-1,1 diphosphonate (EHDP) (structure, ultrastructure and immunocytology). *Clin Orthop Relat Res* 1984;184:281–8.

44. Demmler K. Die vaskularisation des Paget-knochens. *Dtsch Med Wochenschr* 1974;99:91–5.

45. Meunier PJ, Coindre JM, Edouard CM, Arlot ME. Bone histomorphometry in Paget's disease. *Arthritis Rheum* 1980;23:1095–103.

46. Bordier P, Woodhouse NJY, Joplin GF, Tun Chot S. Quantitative bone histology in Paget's disease of bone. *J Bone Joint Surg* 1972;54B:553–4.

47. Chappard D, Alexandre C, Laborier JC, Robert JM, Riffat G. Paget's disease of bone: a scanning electron microscopic study. *J Submicrosc Cytol* 1984;16(2):341–8.

48. Mills BG, Singer FR. Nuclear inclusions in Paget's disease of bone. *Science* 1976;194:201–2.

49. Basle MF, Mazaud P, Malkani K, Chretien MF, Moreau MF, Rebel A. Isolation of osteoclasts from pagetic bone tissue morphometry and cytochemistry on isolated cells. *Bone* 1988;9:1–6.

50. Krane SM. Skeletal metabolism in Paget's disease of bone. *Arthritis Rheum* 1980;23:1087–94.

51. Williams ED, Barr WT, Rajan KT. Relative vitamin D deficiency in Paget's disease. *Lancet* 1981;1:384–5.

52. Rushton MA. The dental tissue in osteitis deformans. *Guy's Hosp Rep* 1938;88:163.

53. Barry HC. *Paget's disease of bone.* London: E&S Livingstone, 1969;82.

54. Woodhouse NJY. Paget's disease of bone. *Clin Endocrinol Metab* 1972;1:125–41.

55. Bhardwaj OP. Monostotic Paget's disease of bone. *J Indian Med Assoc* 1964;43:341.

56. Altman RD, Gray RG. Scalp vein sign in Paget's disease of bone. *J Rheumatol* 1982;9:624–6.

57. Gainey JC, Kadaba MP, Wootten ME, et al. Gait analysis of patients who have Paget disease. *J Bone Joint Surg* 1989;71A(4):568–79.

58. Altman RD, Ciliberti E. Orthopedic events in Paget's disease of bone. [Unpublished report].

59. Altman RD, Collins B. Musculoskeletal manifestations of Paget's disease of bone. *Arthritis Rheum* 1980;23:1121–7.

60. Altman RD, Howell DS. A 6 month double blind trial of EHDP and placebo in osteoarthritis. [Unpublished trial].

61. Dove J. Complete fractures of the femur in Paget's disease of bone. *J Bone Joint Surg* 1980;62B:12–7.

62. Altman RD. Long-term follow-up of therapy with intermittent etidronate disodium in Paget's disease of bone. *Am J Med* 1985;79:583–9.

63. Altman RD, Collins B. Arthritic manifestations of Paget's disease of bone. *Arthritis Rheum* 1980;23:648.

64. Dickson DD, Camp JD, Ghormley RK. Osteitis deformans: Paget's disease of bone. *Radiology* 1945;44:449–70.

65. Brown MD. The source of low back pain and sciatica. *Semin Arth Rheum* 1989;18(4, suppl 2):67–72.

66. Jayson MIV. Vascular damage, fibrosis, and chronic inflammation in mechanical back problems. *Semin Arth Rheum* 1989;18(4, suppl 2):73–6.

67. Altman RD, Brown M, Gargano F. Low back pain in Paget's disease of bone. *Clin Orthop* 1987;217:152–61.

68. Weisz GM. Lumbar spinal canal stenosis in Paget's disease. *Spine* 1983;8:192–8.

69. Howarth S. Cardiac output in osteitis deformans. *Clin Sci* 1953;12:271–5.

70. Wootton R, Reeve J, Veall N. The clinical measurement of skeletal blood flow. *Clin Sci Mol Med* 1976;50:261–8.

71. Plaza I, Arnalich F, Sobrino JA, Oliver J, Vazquez JJ, Puig JG. Hallazgos ecocardiográficos en la osteitis deformante. *Rev Esp Cardiol* 1982;35:23–9.

72. Arnalich F, Plaza I, Sobrino JA, et al. Cardiac size and function in Paget's disease of bone. *Int J Cardiol* 1984;5:491–505.

73. Heistad DD, Abboud FM, Schmid PG, Mark AL, Wilson WR. Regulation of blood flow in Paget's disease of bone. *J Clin Invest* 1975;55:69–74.

74. Rhodes BA, Greyson ND, Hamilton CR, White RI, Giargiana FA, Wagner HN. Absence of anatomic arteriovenous shunts in Paget's disease of bone. *N Engl J Med* 1975;287:686–9.

75. King M, Huang JM, Glassman E. Paget's disease with cardiac calcification and complete heart block. *Am J Med* 1969;46:302–4.

76. Choquette D, Haraoui B, Altman RD, Pelletier JP. Simultaneous multifocal sarcomatous degeneration in Paget's disease of bone. *Clin Orthop* 1983;179:308–11.

77. Barry HC. *Paget's disease of bone.* London: E&S Livingstone, 1969;144.

78. Reddick RL, Michelitch HJ, Levine AM, Triche TJ. Osteogenic sarcoma. *Cancer* 1980;45:64–71.

79. Bower L, Manley G. Urinary excretion of glycosaminoglycans and hydroxyproline in Paget's disease of bone, compared with neoplastic invasion of bone. *J Clin Pathol* 1981;34:1097–101.

80. Upchurch KS, Simon LS, Schiller AL, Rosenthal DL, Campion EW, Krane SM. Giant cell reparative granuloma of Paget's disease of bone: a unique clinical entity. *Ann Intern Med* 1983;98:35–40.

81. Jacobs TP, Michelsen T, Polay JS, Dadamo C, Canfield E. Giant cell tumor in Paget's disease: familial and geographic clustering. *Cancer* 1979;44:742.

82. Burgerer FA, Perry PE. Solitary renal cell carcinoma metastases in Paget's disease simulating sarcomatous degeneration. *AJR* 1977;128:853.

83. Agha FP, Norman A, Hirsehl S, Klein R. Paget's disease: coexistence with metastatic carcinoma. *NY State J Med* 1976;76:734.

84. Jacobsen HG, Siegleman SS. Some miscellaneous solitary bone lesions. *Semin Roentgenol* 1966;1:314.

85. Hens L, van den Bergh R. Hydrocephalus-dementia-complex in Paget's disease. *Clin Neurol Neurosurg* 1979;81:255–63.

86. Goldhammer Y, Braham J, Kosary IZ. Hydrocephalic dementia in Paget's disease of the skull: treatment by ventriculoatrial shunt. *Neurology* 1979;29:513–6.

87. Smith BJ, Eveson JW. Paget's disease of bone with particular reference to dentistry. *J Oral Pathol* 1981;10:233–47.

88. Sofaer JA. Dental extractions in Paget's disease of bone. *Int J Oral Surg* 1984;13:79–84.

89. Harner SG, Rose DE, Facer GW. Paget's disease and hearing loss. *Otolaryngology* 1978;86:869–74.

90. Clarkson JG, Altman RD. Angioid streaks. *Surv Ophthalmol* 1982;25:235–46.

91. Downey R, Siris ES, Antunes JL. "Crocodile tears" and Paget's disease: case report. *Neurosurgery* 1980;7(6):621–2.

92. Herzberg L, Bayliss E. Spinal-cord syndrome due to noncompressive Paget's disease of bone: a spinal-artery steal phenomenon reversible with calcitonin. *Lancet* 1980;2:13–5.

93. Schmidek HH. Neurologic and neurosurgical sequelae of Paget's disease of bone. *Clin Orthop Relat Res* 1977;127:70–7.

94. Avramides A, Leonidas J-R, Chen C-K, Nicastri A. Coexistence of Paget's disease and hyperparathyroidism. *NY State J Med* 1981;81:660–2.

95. Martin MM, Barr AB, Howe JS. Coexisting hyperparathyroidism and Paget's disease. *Arch Intern Med* 1964;114:482–6.

96. Gay JDL, Poznanski WJ. Hyperparathyroidism in Paget's disease of bone. *Clin Invest Med* 1983;6:97–101.

97. Auld WHR, Simpson RH, Smyth M. Hypercalcemia in Paget's disease of bone. *Lancet,* March 10, 1979.

98. Kay HD. Plasma phosphatase in osteitis deformans and in other diseases of bone. *Br J Exp Pathol* 1929;10:253.

99. Albright F, Reifenstein EC Jr. *The parathyroide glands and metabolic bone disease.* Baltimore: Williams & Wilkins, 1948.

100. Woodard HQ. Long term studies of the blood chemistry in Paget's disease of bone. *Cancer* 1959;12:1226.

101. Seargeant LE, Stinson RA. Evidence that three structural genes code for human alkaline phosphatases. *Nature* 1979;281:152–4.

102. Mautalen CA. Circadian rhythm of urinary total and free hydroxyproline excretion and its relation to creatinine excretion. *J Lab Clin Med* Jan 1970;11–8.

103. Krane S, Munoz AJ, Harris ED Jr. Collagen-like fragments: excretion in urine of patients with Paget's disease of bone. *Science* 1967;157(67):713–5.

104. Szymanowicz A. Polymorphism of urinary 4-hydroxyproline-containing polypeptides. *J Chromatogr* 1981;225:55–63.

105. Quelch KJ, Murphy WH, Melick RA. Analysis of collagen from normal and abnormal human bone. *Aust J Exp Biol Med Sci* 1984;62(part 3):309–15.

106. Cheung HS, Singer FR, Mills B, Nimni ME. In vitro synthesis of normal bone (type I) collagen by bones of Paget's disease patients. *Proc Soc Exp Biol Med* 1980;163:547–52.

107. Gundberg CM, Lian JB, Gallop PM, Steinberg JJ. Urinary Y-carboxyglutamic acid and serum osteocalcin as bone markers: studies in osteoporosis and Paget's disease. *J Clin Endocrinol Metab* 1983;57:1221–5.

108. Russell RGG, Beard DJ, Cameron EC, et al. Biochemical markers of bone turnover in Paget's disease. *Metab Bone Dis Relat Res* 1981;4/5:255–262.

109. Whiteley J, Francis MJO, Walton RJ, Smith R. Serum proline imino-peptidase activity in normal adult subjects and in patients with Paget's disease of bone. *Clin Chim Acta* 1976;71:157–63.

110. Simon LS, Krane SM, Wortman PD, Krane IM, Kovitz KL. Serum levels of type I and III procollagen fragments in Paget's disease of bone. *J Clin Endocrinol Metab* 1984;58:110–20.

111. Taubman MB, Kammerman S, Goldberg B. Radioimmunoassay of procollagen in serum of patients with Paget's disease of bone. *Proc Soc Exp Biol Med* 1976;152:284–7.

112. Gunja-Smith Z, Boucek RJ. Collagen cross-linking compounds in human urine. *Biochem J* 1981;197:759–62.

113. Albright F, Aub JC, Bauer. Hyperparathyroidism: a common and polymorphic condition as illustrated by seventeen proved cases from one clinic. *J Am Med Assoc* 1934;102:1276.

114. Coulton LA, Preston CJ, Couch M, Kanis JA. An evaluation of serum osteocalcin in Paget's disease of bone and its response to diphosphonate treatment. *Arthritis Rheum* 1988;31(9):1142–7.

115. Wilkinson MR, Wagstaffe C, Delbridge L, Wiseman J, Posen S. Serum osteocalcin concentrations in Paget's disease of bone. *Arch Intern Med* 1986;146:268–71.

116. Slovik DM, Gundberg CM, Neer RM, Lian JB. Clinical evaluation of bone turnover by serum osteocalcin measurements in a hospital setting. *J Clin Endocrinol Metab* 1984;59:228–30.

117. Sullivan TJ, Gutman EB, Gutman AB. Theory and appreciation of the serum acid phosphatase determination in metastatic prostatic carcinoma; early effects of castration. *J Urol* 1942;48:426.

118. Vaes G. The role of lysosomes and their enzymes in the development of bone resorption induced by parathyroid hormone. In: Talmage RV, Relanger LF, eds. *Parathyroid hormone and thyrocalcitonin (calcitonin).* International Congress Series 159. Montreal: Excerpta Medica, 1968.

119. Kanis JA, Heynen G, Walton RJ. Plasma calcitonin in Paget's disease of bone. *Clin Sci Mol Med* 1977;52:329–32.

120. Guillard-Cumming DF, Bear DJ, Douglas DL, et al. Abnormal vitamin D metabolism in Paget's disease of bone. *Clin Endocrinol* 1985;22:559–66.

121. Walton RJ, Russell RGG, Smith R. Changes in renal and extrarenal handling of phosphate induced by disodium etidronate (EHDP) in man. *Clin Sci Mol Med* 1975;49:45–56.

122. Baran DT, Jaffe BM, Avioli LV. Plasma prostaglandin E levels in Paget's disease: effect of indomethacin. *Calcif Tissue Int* 1979;29:5–6.

123. Cutolo M, Accardo S, Zardi L. Different fibronectin concentrations in plasma samples drawn from the affected and unaffected arms of a pagetic patient. *J Rheumatol* 1985;12(1):176–8.

124. Charriere G, Hartmann DJ, Vignon E, Ronziere MC, Herbage D, Ville G. Antibodies to types I, II, IX, and XI collagen in the serum of patients with rheumatic diseases. *Arthritis Rheum* 1988;31:325–32.

125. Buxbaum JN, Kammerman S. Immunoglobulin abnormalities in Paget's disease of bone. *Clin Exp Immunol* 1984;55:200–4.

126. Seaman WB. The roentgen appearance of early Paget's disease. *AJR* 1951;66:587–94.

127. Pugh DG. The roentgenologic diagnosis of diseases of bone. In: Robbins LL, ed. *Golden's diagnostic roentgenology,* vol 2. Baltimore: Williams & Wilkins, 1952;415.

128. Buchoff HS, Altman RD. Paget's disease: correlation of pain, x-rays and bone scans. *Arthritis Rheum* 1981;24(suppl):572.

129. Barry HC. Sarcoma in Paget's disease of bone in Australia. *J Bone Joint Surg* 1961;43-A:1122.

130. Bauer GCH, Wendeberg B. External counting of ^{47}Ca and ^{85}Sr in studies of localised skeletal lesions in man. *J Bone Joint Surg* 1959;41B:558.

131. Olmstead WW. Some skeletogenic lesions with common calvarial manifestations. *Radiol Clin North Am* 1981;19:703–13.

132. Lloyd GAS, Phelps PD, Du Boulay GH. High-resolution computerized tomography of the petrous bone. *Br J Radiol* 1980;53:631–41.

133. Tjon-a-Tham RTO, Bloem JL, Falke THM, et al. Magnetic resonance imaging in Paget disease of the skull. *AJNR* 1985;6:879–81.

134. Lagier R and Baud CA. Diffuse enthesopathic hyperostosis: anatomical and radiological study on a macerated skeleton. *Fortschr Rontgenstr* 1978;129:588–97.

135. Marshall TR, Ling JT. The brim sign: a new sign found in Paget's disease (osteitis deformans) of the pelvis. *Am J Roentgenol Rad Ther Nucl Med* 1963;90:1267–70.

136. Chakravorty NK. Triradiate deformity of the pelvis in Paget's disease of bone. *Postgrad Med J* 1980;56:213–5.

137. Friedman AC, Orcutt J, Madewell JE. Paget's disease of the hand: radiographic spectrum. *AJR* 1982;138:691–3.

138. Boussina I, Gerster JC, Epiney JU, Fallet GH. A study of the incidence of articular chondrocalcinosis in Paget's disease of bone. *Scand J Rheumatol* 1976;5:33–5.

139. Rubin RP, Adler JJ, Adler D. Paget's disease of the calcaneus. *J Am Podiatry Assoc* 1983;73:263–7.

140. Price CHG, Goldie W. Paget's sarcoma of bone. *J Bone Joint Surg* 1967;51B:205.

141. McKenna RJ, Schwinn CP, Soong KY, Higinbothosa NL. Osteogenic sarcoma arising in Paget's disease. *Cancer* 1964;17:42.

142. Jaffe HL. Paget's disease of bone. *Arch Pathol* 1933;15:83.

143. Grundy M. Fractures of the femur in Paget's disease of bone, their etiology, and treatment. *J Bone Joint Surg* 1970;52B:252.

144. Boudreau RJ, Lisbona R, Hadjipavlou A. Observations on serial radionuclide blood-flow studies in Paget's disease: concise communication. *J Nucl Med* 1983;24:880–5.

145. Vellenga CJLR, Pauwels EKJ, Bijvoet OLM, Hosking DJ, Frijlink WB. Bone scintigraphy in Paget's disease treated with combined calcitonin and diphosphonate (EHDP). *Metab Bone Dis Relat Res* 1982;4:103–11.

146. Lentle BC, Russell AS, Heslip PG, Percy JS. The scintigraphic findings in Paget's disease of bone. *Clin Radiol* 1976;27:129–35.

147. Fogelman I, Carr D. A comparison of bone scanning and radiology in the assessment of patients with symptomatic Paget's disease. *Eur J Nucl Med* 1980;5:417–21.

148. Smith ML, Fogelman I, Ralston S, Boyce BF, Boyle IT. Correlation of skeletal uptake of ^{99m}Tc-diphosphonate and alkaline phosphatase before and after oral diphosphonate therapy in Paget's disease. *Metab Bone Dis Relat Res* 1984;5:167–70.

149. Sankey R, Serafini A, Altman RD, Miale A. Computer analysis of radiostrontium deposition in Paget's disease. *Am Assoc Nucl Med* (abstr), 1972.

150. Vellenga CJLR, Pauwels EKJ, Bijvoet OLM, Frijlink WB, Mulder JD, Hermans J. Untreated Paget disease of bone studied by scintigraphy. *Radiology* 1984;153:799–805.

151. Winter PF, Johnson PM. Significance of renal visualization during bone scanning in Paget's disease. *Nuklearmedizin* 1976;15:131–4.

152. Waxman AD, Ducker S, McKee D, Siemsen JK, Singer FR. Evaluation of ^{99m}Tc diphosphonate kinetics and bone scans in patients with Paget's disease before and after calcitonin treatment. *Radiology* 1977;125:761–4.

153. Fletcher JW, Butler RL, Henry RE, Solaric-George E, Donati RM. Bone marrow scanning in Paget's disease. *J Nucl Med* 1973;14:928–30.

154. Dunn EK, Vaquer RA, Strashun AM. Paget's disease: a cause of photopenic skeletal defect in indium-111 WBC scintigraphy. *J Nucl Med* 1988;29:561–3.

155. Veluvolu P, Ilsithman AT, Collier BD, Whalen JP, Bell RM. False-positive technetium-99m sulfur colloid gastrointestinal bleeding study due to Paget's disease. *Clin Nucl Med* 1988;13:465–6.

156. Khairi MRA, Wellman HN, Robb JA. Paget's disease of bone (osteitis deformans): symptomatic lesions and bone scan. *Ann Intern Med* 1973;79:348–51.

157. Waxman AD, McKee D, Siemsen JK, Singer FR. Gallium scanning in Paget's disease of bone: effect of calcitonin. *Am J Roentgenol* 1980;134:303–6.

158. Vellenga CJLR, Pauwels EKJ, Bijvoet OLM, Frijlink WB. Scintigraphic aspects of the recurrence of treated Paget's disease of bone. *J Nucl Med* 1981;22:510–7.

159. Jaspers MMJR, Pauwels EKJ, Harinck HIJ, Blom J. Photon-defi-

cient bone scan lesion as a precursor of active Paget's disease. *Diagn Imaging Clin Med* 1984;54:144–8.

160. Hofstetter KR, Patton DD, Henry RE. Cerebral perfusion deficit masked by Paget's diseases of skull. *J Nucl Med* 1978;19:197–9.

161. Eisman JA, Martin TJ. Osteolytic Paget's disease. *J Bone Joint Surg* 1986;68A(1):112–7.

162. Meyers MH, Downey, Singer FR. Osteotomy for tibia vara in Paget's disease under cover of calcitonin. *J Bone Joint Surg* 1978;60A(6):810–4.

163. McDonald DJ, Sim FH. Total hip arthroplasty in Paget's disease. *J Bone Joint Surg* 1987;69A(5):766–72.

164. O'Driscoll SW, Hastings DE. Extension of monostotic Paget disease from the femur to the tibia after arthrodesis of the knee. *J Bone Joint Surg* 1989;71A(1):129–32.

165. Nagant de Deuxchaisnes C, Krane SM. Paget's disease of bone: clinical and metabolic observations. *Medicine* 1964;43:233–66.

166. Holtrop ME, Raisz LG, Simmons HA. The effects of parathyroid hormone, colchicine, and calcitonin on the ultrastructure and the activity of osteoclasts in organ culture. *J Cell Biol* 1974;60:341–55.

167. Kallio DM, Garant PR, Minkin C. Ultrastructural effects of calcitonin on osteoclasts in tissue culture. *J Ultrastruct Res* 1972;39:205–16.

168. Chambers TJ, Dunn CJ. Osteoclast activity is determined by intracellular cAMP levels. In: Silbermann M, Slavkin HC, eds. *Current advances in skeletogenesis.* Amsterdam: Excerpta Medica, New York: Elsevier, 1982;154–9.

169. Fornasier VL, Stapleton K, Williams CC. Histologic changes in Paget's disease treated with calcitonin. *Hum Pathol* 1978;9:455–61.

170. Peck WA, Burks JK, Wilkins J, Rodan SB, Rodan GA. Evidence for preferential effects of parathyroid hormones calcitonin and adenosine on bone and periosteum. *Endocrinology* 1977;100:1357–66.

171. MacIntyre I, Evans IMA, Hobitz HHG. Chemistry, physiology, and therapeutic applications of calcitonin. *Arthritis Rheum* 1980;23:1139–47.

172. Paavolainen P, Taivainen T, Michelsson JE, Lalla M, Penttinen R. Calcitonin and fracture healing, an experimental study on rats. *J Orthop Res* 1989;7:100–6.

173. Gennari C, Bocchi L, Orso CA, Francini G, Civitelli R, Maioli E. The analgesic effect of calcitonin in active Paget's disease of bone and in metastatic bone disease. *Orthopedics* 1984;7(9):1449–52.

174. El Sammaa M, Linthicum F Jr, House HP, House JW. Calcitonin as treatment for hearing loss in Paget's disease. *Am J Otol* 1986;7(4):241–3.

175. Walker GS, Evanson JM, Canty DP, Gill NW. Effect of calcitonin on deafness due to Paget's disease of skull. *Br Med J* 1979;2(6186):364–5.

176. Melick RA, Eberling P, Hjhorth RJ. Improvement in paraplegia in vertebral Paget's disease treated with calcitonin. *Br Med J* 1976;1(6010):627–8.

177. Ravichandran G. Neurologic recovery of paraplegia following use of salmon calcitonin in a patient with Paget's disease of spine. *Spine* 1979;4(1):37–40.

178. Walpin LA, Singer FR. Paget's disease: reversal of severe paraparesis using calcitonin. *Spine* 1979;4(3):213–9.

179. Wootton R, Reeve J, Spellacy E, Tellez-Yudilevich M. Skeletal blood flow in Paget's disease of bone and its response to calcitonin therapy. *Clin Sci Mol Med* 1978;54:69–74.

180. Henley JW, Croxson RS, Ibbertson HK. The cardiovascular system in Paget's disease of bone and the response to therapy with calcitonin and diphosphonate. *Aust NZ J Med* 1979;9:390–7.

181. Crosbie WA, Mohamedally SM, Woodhouse NJY. Effect of salmon calcitonin on cardiac output, oxygen transport and bone turnover in patients with Paget's disease. *Clin Sci Mol Med* 1975;48:537–40.

182. Woodhouse NJY, MacIntyre I, Joplin GF, Doyle FH. Radiological regression in Paget's disease treated by human calcitonin. *Lancet* 1972;2:992–4.

183. Murphy WA, Whyte MP, Haddad JG Jr. Paget bone disease: radiologic documentation of healing with human calcitonin therapy. *Radiology* 1980;136:1–4.

184. Whyte MP, Daniels EH, Murphy WA. Osteolytic Paget's bone disease in a young man. *Am J Med* 1985;78:326–32.

185. Nagant de Deuxchaisnes C, Rombouts-Lindemans C, Haux JP, Malghem J, Maldague B. Roentgenologic evaluation of the efficacy of calcitonin in Paget's disease of bone. In: MacIntyre I, Szelke M, eds. *Molecular endocrinology.* Amsterdam: Elsevier/North-Holland, 1977;213–33.

186. Avramides A. Paget's disease of bone: treating Paget's disease with calcitonin. *Curr Concepts Bone Dis* 1976;1:2–5.

187. Woodhouse NJY. Historical and epidemiological aspects of Paget's disease. In: MacIntyre I, ed. *Human calcitonin and Paget's disease.* Bern: Hans Huber, 1976;50–65.

188. Chapuy MC, Meunier PJ, Alexandre C. Comparison of the acute effects of human and salmon calcitonins in Pagetic patients: relation with plasma calcitonin levels. *Metab Bone Dis Relat Res* 1980;2:93–7.

189. Doyle FH, Banks LM, Pennock JM. Radiologic observations on bone resorption in Paget's disease. *Arthritis Rheum* 1980;23:1205–14.

190. Hosking DJ, Denton LB, Cadge B, Martin TJ. Functional significance of antibody formation after long-term salmon calcitonin therapy. *Clin Endocrinol* 1979;10:243–52.

191. Martin TJ, Jerums G, Melick RA, Xipell JM, Arnott R. Clinical, biochemical and histological observations on the effect of porcine calcitonin in Paget's disease of bone. *Aust NZ J Med* 1977;7:36–43.

192. Singer RF, Aldred JP, Neer RM, Krane SM, Potts JT Jr, Bloch KJ. An evaluation of antibodies and clinical resistance to salmon calcitonin. *J Clin Invest* 1972;51:2331–8.

193. Dietrich FM, Fischler JA, Bijvoet OLM. Formation of antibodies to synthetic human calcitonin during treatment of Paget's disease. *Acta Endocrinol* 1979;92:468–76.

194. Singer FR. Human calcitonin treatment of Paget's disease of bone. *Clin Orthop* 1977;127:86–91.

195. Haddad JG Jr, Caldwell JG. Calcitonin resistance: clinical and immunologic studies in subjects with Paget's disease of bone treated with porcine and salmon calcitonin. *J Clin Invest* 1972;51:3133–41.

196. DeRose J, Singer F, Avramides A, et al. Response of Paget's disease to porcine and salmon calcitonins. *Am J Med* 1974;56:858–66.

197. Singer FR, Fredericks RS, Minkin C. Salmon calcitonin therapy for Paget's disease of bone. *Arthritis Rheum* 1980;23:1148–54.

198. Martin TJ. Treatment of Paget's disease with the calcitonins. *Aust NZ J Med* 1979;9:36–43.

199. Raisz LG, Wener JA, Trummel CL, Feinblatt JD, Av WYW. Induction of inhibition and escape as phenomena of bone resorption. In: *Calcium, parathyroid hormone and the calcitonins. Proceedings 4th parathyroid conference,* 1972;446–53.

200. Perry HM III, Droke DM, Avioli LV. Alternate calcitonin and etidronate disodium therapy for Paget's bone disease. *Arch Intern Med* 1984;144:929–33.

201. Hamdy RC, Brown IRF, Howells DW, Nisbet JA. Vitamin A and Paget's disease. *Lancet* 1982;2:1103–4.

202. Smethurst M, Basu TK, Gillett MB, et al. Combined therapy with ascorbic acid and calcitonin for the relief of bone pain in Paget's disease. *Acta Vitaminol Enzymol* 1981;3:8–11.

203. Shai F, Baker RK, Wallach S. The clinical and metabolic effects of porcine calcitonin on Paget's disease of bone. *J Clin Invest* 1971;50:1927–40.

204. Haddad JG Jr, Birg SJ, Avioli LV. Effects of prolonged thyrocalcitonin administration on Paget's disease of bone. *N Engl J Med* 1970;283(11):549–55.

205. Plehwe WE, Hudson J, Clifton-Bligh P, Posen S. Porcine calcitonin in the treatment of Paget's disease of bone. *Med J Aust* 1977;1:577–81.

206. Milhaud G. Low-dose calcitonin in Paget's disease. *Lancet* 1978;1:1153.

207. Reginster JY, Jeugmans-Huynen AM, Albert A, Denis D, Franchimont P. One year's treatment of Paget's disease of bone by synthetic salmon calcitonin as a nasal spray. *J Bone Miner Res* 1988;3(3):249–52.

208. Gonzalez D, Vega E, Ghiringhelli G, Mautalen C. Comparison of the acute effect of the intranasal and intramuscular administration of salmon calcitonin in Paget's disease. *Calcif Tissue Int* 1987;41:313–5.

209. D'Agostino HR, Barnett CA, Zielinski XJ, Gordan GS. Intrana-

sal salmon calcitonin treatment of Paget's disease of bone. *Clin Orthop Relat Res* 1988;230:223–8.

210. Rojanasathit S, Rosenberg E, Haddad JG Jr. Paget's bone disease: response to human calcitonin in patients resistant to salmon calcitonin. *Lancet* 1974;2:1412–5.

211. Altman RD, Collins-Yudiskas B. Synthetic human calcitonin in refractory Paget's disease of bone. *Arch Intern Med* 1987;147:1305–8.

212. Doyle FH, Pennock J, Greenberg PB, Joplin GF, MacIntyre I. Radiological evidence of a dose-related response to long-term treatment of Paget's disease with human calcitonin. *Br J Radiol* 1974;47:1.

213. Evans RA, Dunstan CR, Wong SYP, Hills E. Long-term experience with a calcium-thiazide treatment for Paget's disease of bone. *Miner Electrolyte Metab* 1982;8:325–33.

214. Vattimo A, Martini G. Dynamic radionuclide study in Paget's disease before and after (Asu) E-calcitonin treatment. *J Nucl Med Allied Sci* 1984;28(3):217–20.

215. Gennari C, Passeri M, Chierichetti SM, Piolini M. Side-effects of synthetic salmon and human calcitonin. *Lancet,* Mar 12, 1983.

216. Gattereau A, Vinay P, Bielmann P, Davignon J, Lemieux G, Gougoux A. Effect of acute administration of salmon and human calcitonin on blood urate and renal excretion of uric acid in patients with Paget's disease of bone. *J Clin Endocrinol Metab* 1979;49(4):635–7.

217. Fleisch H. Experimental basis for the clinical use of diphosphonates in Paget's disease of bone. *Arthritis Rheum* 1980;23:1162–71.

218. Bauer FCH, Nilsson OS, Tornkvist H, Lindholm TC, Lindholm TS. Effect of a diphosphonate on the osteoinductive activity of rat bone matrix. *Clin Orthop* 1984;185:266–9.

219. Alexandre C, Meunier PJ, Edouard C, Khairi RA, Johnston CC. Effects of ethane-1 hydroxy-1, 1-diphosphonate (5 mg/kg/day dose) on quantitative bone histology in Paget's disease of bone. *Metab Bone Dis Relat Res* 1981;4/5:309–16.

220. Johnston CC Jr, Khairi MRA, Meunier PJ. Use of etidronate (EHDP) in Paget's disease of bone. *Arthritis Rheum* 1980;23:1172–6.

221. Raisz LG. New diphosphonates to block bone resorption. *N Engl J Med* 1980;302:347–8.

222. Boyce BF, Fogelman I, Ralston S, Smith L, Johnston E, Boyle IT. Focal osteomalacia due to low-dose diphosphonate therapy in Paget's disease. *Lancet* 1984;1(8321):821–4.

223. Gibbs CJ, Aaron JE, Peacock M. Osteomalacia in Paget's disease treated with short term, high dose sodium etidronate. *Br Med J* 1986;292:1227–9.

224. Altman RD, Johnston CC, Khairi MRA, Wellman H, Serafini AN, Sankey RR. Influence of disodium etidronate on clinical and laboratory manifestations of Paget's disease of bone (osteitis deformans). *N Engl J Med* 1973;289:1379–84.

225. Alexandre CM, Chapuy MC, Vignon E, Edouard C, Johnston CC, Meunier PJ. Treatment of Paget's disease of bone with ethane-1, hydroxy-1, 1 diphosphonate (EHDP) at a low dosage (5 mg/kg/day). *Clin Orthop* 1983;174:193–205.

226. Russell AS, Lentle BC. Mithramycin therapy in Paget's disease. *Can Med Assoc J* 1974;110:397–400.

227. Siris ES, Canfield RE, Jacobs TP, Stoddart E, Spector PJ. Clinical and biochemical effects of EHDP in Paget's disease of bone: patterns of response to initial treatment and to long-term therapy. *Metab Bone Dis Relat Res* 1981;4/5:301–8.

228. Altman RD, Collins B. Disodium etidronate (EHDP) in Paget's disease (Pag D): 11 year study of 93 patients. *Arthritis Rheum* 1983;25S:9.

229. Krane SM. Etidronate disodium in the treatment of Paget's disease of bone. *Ann Intern Med* 1982;96:619–25.

230. Canfield R, Rosner W, Skinner J, et al. Diphosphonate therapy of Paget's disease of bone. *J Clin Endocrinol Metab* 1977;44:96–106.

231. Siris ES, Canfield RE, Jacobs TP, Baquiran DC. Long-term therapy of Paget's disease of bone with EHDP. *Arthritis Rheum* 1980;23:1177–84.

232. Murphy WA, Whyte MP, Haddad JG Jr. Healing of lytic Paget bone disease with diphosphonate therapy. *Radiology* 1980;134:635–7.

233. Lando M, Hoover LA, Finerman G. Stabilization of hearing loss in Paget's disease with calcitonin and etidronate. *Arch Otolaryngol Head Neck Surg* 1988;114:891–4.

234. Finerman GAM, Gonick HC, Smith RK, Mayfield JM. Diphosphonate treatment of Paget's disease. *Clin Orthop* 1976;120:115–24.

235. Vellenga CJLR, Pauwels EKJ, Buvoet OLM, Hosking DJ. Evaluation of scintigraphic and roentgenologic studies in Paget's disease under treatment. *Radiol Clin* 1976;45:292–301.

236. Charhon S, Chapuy MC, Valentin-Opran A, Meunier PJ. Intravenous etidronate for spinal cord dysfunction due to Paget's disease. *Lancet* 1982;1:391–2.

237. Ralston SH, Boyce BF, Cowan RA, et al. The effect of 1-hydroxyvitamin D_3 on the mineralization defect in disodium etidronate-treated Paget's disease—a double-blind randomized clinical study. *J Bone Miner Res* 1987;2(1):5–12.

238. Menczel J, Singer L, Ophaug RH. An investigation of calcium intake, 1-alpha(OH)D_3, and etidronate of bone. *Bone* 1987;8:91–4.

239. Johnston CC Jr, Altman RD, Canfield RE, Finerman GA, Taulbee JD, Ebert ML. Review of fracture experience during treatment of Paget's disease of bone with etidronate disodium (EHDP). *Clin Orthop* 1983;172:186–94.

240. Meunier PJ, Alexandre C, Edouard C, et al. Effects of disodium dichloromethylene diphosphonate on Paget's disease of bone. *Lancet* 1979;2:489–92.

241. Gray RES, Yates AJP, Preston CJ, Smith R, Russell RGG, Kanis KA. Duration of effect of oral diphosphonate therapy in Paget's disease of bone. *Q J Med (NS)* 1987;64(245):755–67.

242. Chapuy MC, Charhon SA, Meunier PJ. Sustained biochemical effects of short treatment of Paget's disease of bone with dichloromethylene diphosphonate. *Metab Bone Dis Relat Res* 1983;4:325–8.

243. Yates AJP, Gray RES, Urwin GH, et al. Intravenous clodronate in the treatment and retreatment of Paget's disease of bone. *Lancet* June 29, 1985;1474–7.

244. Delmas PD, Chapuy MC, Vignon E, et al. Long term effects of dichloromethylene diphosphonates in Paget's disease of bone. *J Clin Endocrinol Metab* 1982;54:837–44.

245. Douglas DL, Duckworth T, Kanis JA, et al. Biochemical and clinical responses to dichloromethylene diphosphonate (Cl_2MDP) in Paget's disease of bone. *Arthritis Rheum* 1980;23:1185–92.

246. Adami S, Guarrera G, Salvagno G, et al. Sequential treatment of Paget's disease with human calcitonin and dichloromethylene diphosphonate (Cl_2MDP). *Metab Bone Dis Relat Res* 1984;5:265–7.

247. Delmas PD, Chapuy MC, Meunier PJ. Paradoxical acute hypercalcemic effect of salmon calcitonin in patients having Paget's disease of bone after treatment with dichloromethylene diphosphonate. *Horm Metab Res* 1984;16:258–61.

248. Borgstrom GH, Elomaa I, Blomqvist C, Porkka L. Cytogenetic investigations of patients on clodronate therapy for Paget's disease of bone. *Bone* 1987;8(suppl 1):S85–6.

249. Bijvoet OLM, Frijlink WB, Jie K, et al. APD in Paget's disease of bone. *Arthritis Rheum* 1980;23:1193–204.

250. Heynen G, Delwaide P, Bijvoet OLM, Franchimont P. Clinical and biological effects of low doses of (3 amino-1 hydroxypropylidene)-1, 1-bisphosphonate (APD) in Paget's disease of bone. *Eur J Clin Invest* 1982;11:29–35.

251. Mautalen CA, Gonzalez D, Ghiringhelli G. Efficacy of the bisphosphonate APD in the control of Paget's bone disease. *Bone* 1985;6:429–32.

252. Thiebaud D, Jaeger P, Burckhardt P. Paget's disease of bone treated in five days with AHPrBP (APD) per Os. *J Bone Miner Res* 1987;2(1):45–52.

253. Delmas PD, Chapuy MC, Edouard C, Meunier PJ. Beneficial effects of aminohexane diphosphonate in patients with Paget's disease of bone resistant to sodium etidronate. *Am J Med* 1987;83:276–82.

254. Thiebaud D, Jaeger P, Gobelet C, Jacquet AF, Burckhardt P. A single infusion of the biphosphonate AHPrBP (APD) as treatment of Paget's disease of bone. *Am J Med* 1988;85:207–12.

255. Vega AE, Gonzalez D, Ghiringhelli G, Mautalen C. Intravenous aminopropylidene bisphosphonate (APD) in the treatment of Paget's bone disease. *J Bone Miner Res* 1987;2(4):267–71.

256. Atkins RM, Yates AJP, Gray RES, et al. Aminohexane diphosphonate in the treatment of Paget's disease of bone. *J Bone Miner Res* 1987;2(4):273–9.

257. Vellenga CJLR, Pauwels EKJ, Bijvoet OLM, Harinck HIJ, Frijlink WB. Quantitative bone scintigraphy in Paget's disease treated with APD. *Br J Radiol* 1985;58:1165–72.

258. Adami S, Bhalla AK, Dorizzi R, et al. The acute-phase response after bisphosphonate administration. *Calcif Tissue Int* 1987;41:326–31.

259. Frijlink WB, Te Velde J, Bijvoet OLM, Heynen G. Treatment of Paget's disease with (3-amino-1-hydroxypropylidene)-1, 1-bisphosphonate (A.P.D.). *Lancet,* Apr 14, 1979.

260. Hosking DJ. Calcitonin and diphosphonate in the treatment of Paget's disease of bone. *Metab Bone Dis Relat Res* 1981;4/5:317–26.

261. O'Donoghue DJ, Hosking DJ. Biochemical response to combination of disodium etidronate with calcitonin in Paget's disease. *Bone* 1987;8:219–25.

262. Reginster JY, Jeugmans-Huynen AM, Denis AAD, et al. Biological and clinical assessment of a new bisphosphonate, (chloro-4 phenyl) thiomethylene bisphosphonate, in the treatment of Paget's disease of bone. *Bone* 1988;9:349–54.

263. Francis MD, Ferguson DL, Tofe AJ, Bevan JA, Michaels SE. Comparative evaluation of three diphosphonates: in vitro adsorption (C-14 Labeled) and in vivo osteogenic uptake (Tc-99m complexed). *J Nucl Med* 1980;21:1185–9.

264. Nagant de Deuxchaisnes C, Devogelaer JP, Malgehm J, Maldague B, Cornet F. The effect of the (4-chlorophenyl) thiomethylene disodium bisphosphonate or SR 41319B in Paget's disease of bone: a radiological study. *Satellite workshop on molecular and cell biology,* Sirmione, Italy, Oct 4, 1987.

265. Kennedy BJ. Metabolic and toxic effects of mithramycin during tumor therapy. *Am J Med* 1970;49:494–503.

266. Ryan WG, Schwartz TB, Perlia CP. Effects of mithramycin on Paget's disease of bone. *Ann Intern Med* 1969;70:549–57.

267. Elias EG, Evans JT. Mithramycin in the treatment of Paget's disease of bone. *J Bone Joint Surg* 1972;54A:1730–5.

268. Ryan WG, Fordham EW. Mithramycin and Paget's disease revisited. *Ann Intern Med* 1984;100:771.

269. Ryan WG, Schwartz TB. Mithramycin treatment of Paget's disease of bone. *Arthritis Rheum* 1980;23:1155–61.

270. Condon JR. Glucagon in the treatment of Paget's disease of bone. *Br Med J* 1971;4:719.

271. Avioli LV, Berman MI. Role of magnesium metabolism and the effects of fluoride therapy in Paget's disease of bone. *J Clin Endocrinol* 1968;28:700.

272. Guyer PB, Chamberlain AT, Ackery DM, Chir B, Rolfe EB. The anatomic distribution of osteitis deformans. *Clin Orthop Relat Res* 1981;156:141–4.

Disorders of Bone and Mineral Metabolism,
edited by Fredric L. Coe and Murray J. Favus,
© 1992 by Raven Press, Ltd. All rights reserved.

CHAPTER 44

Primary Cystic and Neoplastic Diseases of Bone

Robert E. Turcotte, Lester E. Wold, and Franklin H. Sim

The diagnosis and management of bone tumors, either benign or malignant, is a major challenge for the physician. Primary bone tumors are rare, and benign bone tumors outnumber malignant tumors (1,2). Currently, it is estimated that 2100 new cases of malignant bone tumors will be diagnosed in the United States, and approximately 1300 patients will die of them (3). Compounding the diagnostic problem that bone tumors pose because of the infrequency with which they are encountered in practice is the large number of tumor types and subtypes.

Although plain radiographs remain the most effective tool for the diagnosis of a bone tumor, the findings are rarely characteristic enough to exclude the need for other diagnostic studies (4,5). Modern imaging techniques, including computed tomography (CT) and magnetic resonance imaging (MRI), are very useful in determining the extent of the tumor and its relationship to adjacent anatomic structures, but these techniques offer little aid in the differential diagnosis of primary osseous neoplasms. The diagnostic dilemma may remain unresolved after biopsy because pathologists may disagree about the classification of the process (2,6,7).

Experience gained by exposure to many osseous lesions permits the oncologist, orthopedic surgeon, radiologist, and pathologist to recognize and deal adequately with these tumors. A multidisciplinary approach is the cornerstone of modern treatment of bone tumors. All members of the team—physicians, nurses, and social workers—bring their own expertise to help solve the problem posed by patients with osseous tumors, as no one person can address all facets of the care of patients with these lesions.

This chapter provides an overview of the most frequent primary bone tumors. For more detailed information, the reader is referred to the many references listed at the end of the chapter.

STAGING AND BIOPSY

The clinician must answer many questions about the diagnosis and treatment of an osseous lesion. Is the lesion a tumor or not? If it is a tumor, is it benign or malignant? Usually, the clinical history and the physical findings are nonspecific and of little help in answering these questions. The patient's age and the location of the lesion provide helpful information. The best diagnostic aid is the plain roentgenogram. The presence of a large, radiographically lytic lesion that is poorly defined and involves the cortex is suggestive of a malignancy. A small lesion with a well-defined sclerotic margin and an intact cortex is suggestive of a benign process. Although not absolutely diagnostic, certain radiologic patterns can be recognized that are characteristic of certain tumors.

After an osseous lesion has been identified radiographically, the local extent of the tumor and the presence or absence of spread should be determined. This determination is particularly helpful if the tumor is suspected to be malignant. CT, MRI, bone scan using technetium or gallium, and angiography are all useful for this purpose (8–11). A CT scan of the chest remains the best tool to detect lung metastasis that is not visible on the chest roentgenogram (12). Regional lymph nodes are rarely the site of metastasis in primary malignant bone tumors.

Staging studies (CT, MRI, and bone scan) are best performed before biopsy because any surgical procedure may affect the quality of the study and thus its interpretation. In addition, these studies are very helpful in the determination of the region of the tumor to be biopsied.

R. E. Turcotte: Department of Orthopedics, Mayo Clinic and Mayo Foundation, Rochester, Minnesota 55905.

L. E. Wold: Section of Surgical Pathology, Mayo Clinic and Mayo Foundation, Rochester, Minnesota 55905.

F. H. Sim: Department of Orthopedics, Mayo Clinic and Mayo Foundation, Rochester, Minnesota 55905.

Stage	Grade	Site
IA	Low (G_1)	Intracompartmental (T_1)
IB	Low (G_1)	Extracompartmental (T_2)
IIA	High (G_2)	Intracompartmental (T_1)
IIB	High (G_2)	Extracompartmental (T_2)
III	Any (G) Regional or distant metastasis	Any (T)

FIG. 1. Surgical staging system for bone tumors (adopted by the Musculoskeletal Tumor Society). (From Ref. 14.)

Biopsy specimens should be taken only by experienced surgeons who are ready to provide the definitive treatment, even if the tumor is malignant. A poorly planned biopsy may affect subsequent surgical therapy and patient outcome (13). The surgeon should plan the initial biopsy in a manner that will not preclude subsequent surgical approaches to all lesions considered in the radiographic differential diagnosis. The biopsy specimen should be taken from a representative area of the tumor and in a quantity and quality sufficient to satisfy the pathologist. To avoid the risk of a pathologic fracture, the surgeon should avoid breaking the integrity of the bone if a soft-tissue mass is present. The biopsy specimen should be interpreted without delay by a pathologist who is experienced in bone pathology.

Biopsy and identification of the bone tumor complete the staging process. The staging system proposed by Enneking et al. in 1980 (14,15) and accepted by the Musculoskeletal Tumor Society is now widely used (Fig. 1). This system correlates with the prognosis and the local recurrence rate according to the treatment (Fig. 2). Once the diagnosis and stage of the tumor are known, the plan of treatment, often including multiple therapeutic modalities (16–18), can be undertaken.

BENIGN BONE TUMORS

Osteochondroma

Osteochondroma is the most frequent benign tumor of bone, accounting for 36% of the benign lesions in the Mayo Clinic series. Its incidence is underestimated because many of the patients are asymptomatic. More males than females are affected (60% versus 40%), and half of the patients are less than 20 years old.

The osteochondroma has two parts: (1) a bony stalk that may be long and narrow (pedunculated) or broad and flat (sessile) and (2) a cartilaginous cap that covers the tumor. The lesion generally develops at the end of a long bone and grows away from the adjacent joint (Fig. 3). The lesion enlarges by enchondral ossification from the cartilaginous cap, and growth usually ceases with skeletal maturity.

Osteochondroma is most frequently solitary; however, multiple osteochondromas may be encountered. Multiple osteochondromas have a strong familial tendency (19,20). Although the potential for malignant degenera-

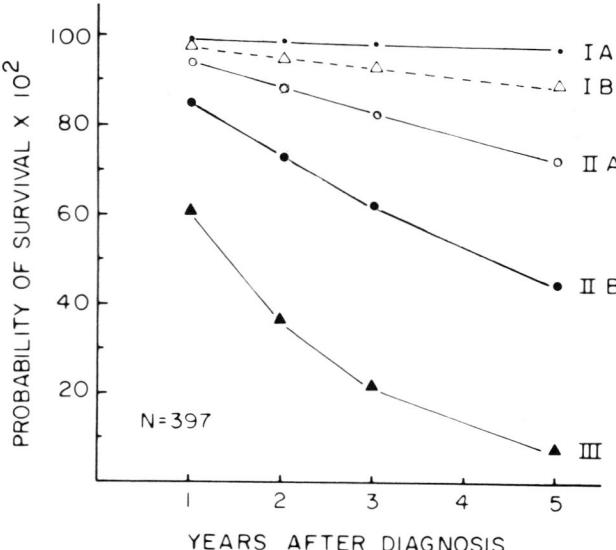

FIG. 2. Probability of survival in 397 cases of bone tumors according to surgical staging system.

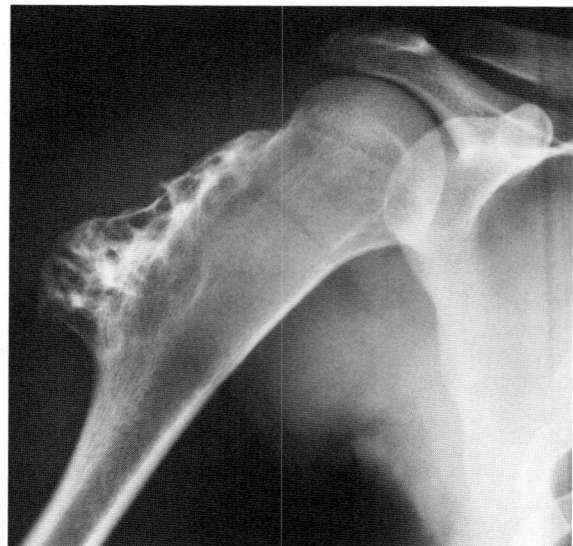

FIG. 3. Sessile osteochondroma of proximal humerus. Large stalk communicates with medullary cavity of bone. Tumor has well-outlined margin along its soft-tissue border. Cartilaginous cap is thin and has no evidence of calcification.

tion of a single osteochondroma into chondrosarcoma is less than 1% (21), the risk for patients with multiple osteochondromatosis is more likely about 10%, and thus these patients need to be followed up more closely.

On plain roentgenograms, the cortex and the spongiosa of the stalk are seen in continuity with those from the host bone. The cartilaginous cap is thicker in adolescents but is usually 2–3 mm thick in adults. The finding of a cartilaginous cap more than 2 cm in diameter is highly suggestive of malignant transformation. Calcific deposits may be present in the cartilaginous cap, but if these deposits are extensive and irregular or if there are associated myxoid cystic changes in the cap, malignant degeneration should be excluded.

At low magnification, the cartilaginous cap consists of chondrocytes arranged in parallel clusters, similar to that seen in a growth plate. There are underlying regions of endochondral ossification.

Most osteochondromas can be confidently diagnosed on the basis of the radiographic appearance and do not need to be removed. However, if the tumor causes pain, produces cosmetic defects, or is growing rapidly, excision is performed at the junction of its stalk and the host bone. Osteochondroma that is suspected of malignant transformation should be excised with a wider margin, after biopsy confirmation of the malignant change (22).

Chondroma

Chondromas are benign tumors consisting of mature cartilage. They may be centrally located in bone (enchondroma) or arise on the surface of the bone (periosteal chondroma). They represent 12% of the benign bone tumors in the Mayo Clinic files. Men and women are affected in equal numbers, and chondromas can occur in a person of any age. Half of the tumors affect tubular bones of the hands and feet, although they can be seen in any bone. They are the most frequent bone tumors found in the hand (23).

Most chondromas are asymptomatic and found incidentally on roentgenograms. At presentation, if the patient has pain, a malignancy must be ruled out. Pathologic fractures may occur at the site of the chondroma.

On plain roentgenograms, enchondroma is a lytic lesion that most frequently involves the diaphysis (Fig. 4). Frequently, the lesion contains areas of stippled or matted calcific deposits and may even be heavily calcified. Calcific deposits are less conspicuous in chondromas of small bones of the hands and feet. In long bones, the cortex may be expanded, but endosteal scalloping and breakthrough of the cortex are signs of malignancy. Periosteal chondromas are well-demarcated, saucer-shaped erosions of the outer cortex with extension into the soft tissues seen on plain roentgenograms (24,25). The inner aspect of the bone is uninvolved. Periosteal chondromas are frequently seen in the proximal humerus.

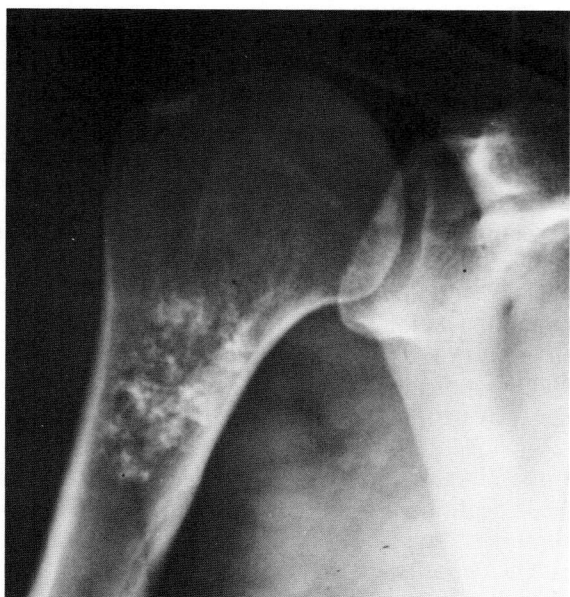

FIG. 4. Chondroma of proximal humerus. Lesion is well calcified. There is no scalloping of cortex by tumor.

Chondromas are hypocellular lesions composed of mature hyaline cartilage arranged in lobules. Enchondroma of the hands and feet, multiple enchondromatosis, and periosteal chondromas have greater cellularity and greater nuclear atypia than do chondromas of long bones (26,27). Small areas of calcific deposits are seen throughout the lesion. Evidence of ossification is seen less often than calcific deposits.

Chondroma most frequently occurs as a solitary lesion, but occasionally multiple chondromas are found and they often involve one extremity. This syndrome is called *Ollier's disease* or *dyschondroplasia.* When multiple enchondromas are associated with soft-tissue hemangiomas, it is known as *Maffucci's syndrome* (28). Patients with Ollier's disease or Maffucci's syndrome need to be followed up closely because the risk of malignant degeneration into chondrosarcoma is approximately 33%. The risk of solitary enchondroma degeneration is very low (less than 1%).

The treatment of patients with asymptomatic, nonaggressive-appearing lesions is conservative. Radiographic follow-up of the patient every few months to ensure that the lesion is stable is recommended initially. Patients with multiple chondromas must be followed up more closely. If any lesion becomes painful or enlarged, a biopsy is mandatory to exclude malignant transformation. For a symptomatic chondroma, thorough curettage and bone grafting are advised. If a pathologic fracture occurs at the site of a chondroma, the fracture should be allowed to heal before curettage and bone grafting are performed.

Chondromyxoid Fibroma

Chondromyxoid fibroma is a rare benign tumor of bone that is seen more often in males than females. At presentation, patients most frequently are in the second and third decades of life. The most frequent site of involvement is the metaphysis of the long bones. The lower extremities are more often affected than the upper extremities. The tibia is the most frequent site, accounting for 33% of all sites. The symptoms are nonspecific. Pain is often of long duration and is the most frequent complaint. Local swelling is occasionally reported.

Radiographically, chondromyxoid fibroma typically presents as a small (usually less than 5 cm) eccentric, round-or-oval lesion that is sharply circumscribed by a sclerotic margin. There is generally no evidence of matrix calcification on plain roentgenograms. The involved bone may show some fusiform enlargement, and pseudocalcific deposits are frequently seen and explained on the basis of the scalloping of the inner surface of the bone. The overlying cortex may rarely be broken, allowing a soft-tissue extension. Although commonly round, the tumor may be elongated along the long axis of the bone. The growth plate is usually spared (Fig. 5).

At low magnification, a lobular pattern of growth is seen in the tumor. There is a sharp demarcation from the adjacent bone. Chondromyxoid fibroma is composed of three components in variable amounts: cartilage, fibrous tissue, and myxoid stroma. Characteristically, there is a "condensation" of nuclei at the periphery of the lobules. Because of the presence of chondroid and myxoid re-

gions, chondrosarcoma should be considered in the pathologic differential diagnosis (26).

The recommended treatment of this benign condition includes curettage and bone grafting. A recurrence rate of 25% has been reported with this treatment. En bloc excision is preferred for a lesion in an expendable bone; radiation therapy is not suggested. Malignant transformation is exceedingly rare.

Osteoid Osteoma

Osteoid osteoma is a small, nonprogressive benign lesion. It represents 12% of benign bone tumors in the Mayo Clinic series (2). Although the tumor can occur in a person of any age, 80% of the patients are between 5 and 20 years old. Males outnumber females by 3 to 1. Osteoid osteomas can affect any bone, but the ends of long bones seem to be involved more frequently (29,30).

The symptoms associated with this lesion are somewhat characteristic. Pain is the main feature and is often worse at night. It is relieved by salicylates or other prostaglandin inhibitors. Referred pain and muscular atrophy may result in misdiagnosis of a neurologic disorder. In a young patient with a painful, atraumatic scoliosis, the clinician must rule out osteoid osteoma as the cause. The lesion will usually be found in the apical arch of the vertebra at the concave side of the curve (31,32).

Radiographically, the lesion is seen as a small radiolucent nidus (usually less than 1 cm) surrounded by a large halo of sclerotic bone (Fig. 6). If the nidus is larger than 1.5 cm, the lesion is designated as an osteoblastoma (33–35). The nidus can be difficult to see on plain roentgenograms, and often, bone scans, tomograms, or CT scans will help localize it. The sclerotic reaction around the nidus is not always present, particularly when the tumor is located in cancellous bone or near the articular surface. Technetium bone scans will always show an increase in uptake and are reliable means of localizing the lesion.

Grossly, the nidus is more red than the surrounding bone and is often described as a "small cherry." The nidus is composed of tightly woven osteoid trabeculae lined by osteoblasts. Some loose fibrovascular connective tissue is seen among the trabeculae.

Treatment includes surgical excision of the nidus. Because the sclerotic bone that surrounds the nidus does not need to be removed completely, a well-planned surgical approach is essential. Identification of the nidus is confirmed by roentgenograms before and after en bloc removal, together with confirmation by the pathologist. Preoperative bone scanning or the use of tetracycline has been useful in identifying the nidus during operation. Bone grafting may be necessary, depending on the size of the bony defect left by the resection. Recurrence of symptoms is most often due to incomplete excision of the nidus.

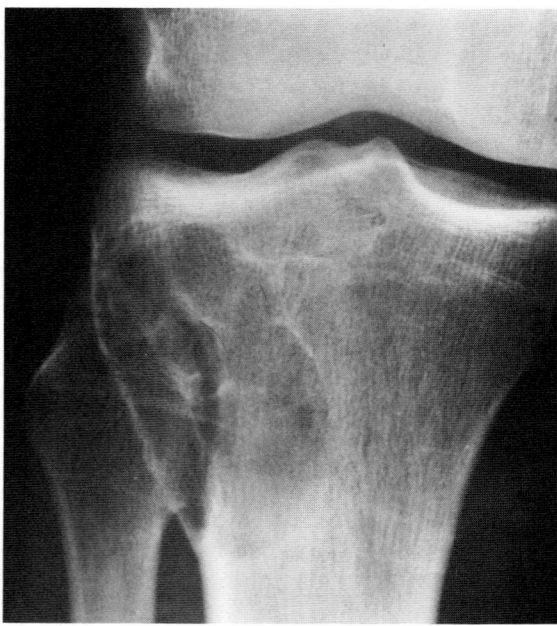

FIG. 5. Chondromyxoid fibroma seen as expansile lytic lesion of proximal tibia. Margins are sclerotic, and periosteum is intact.

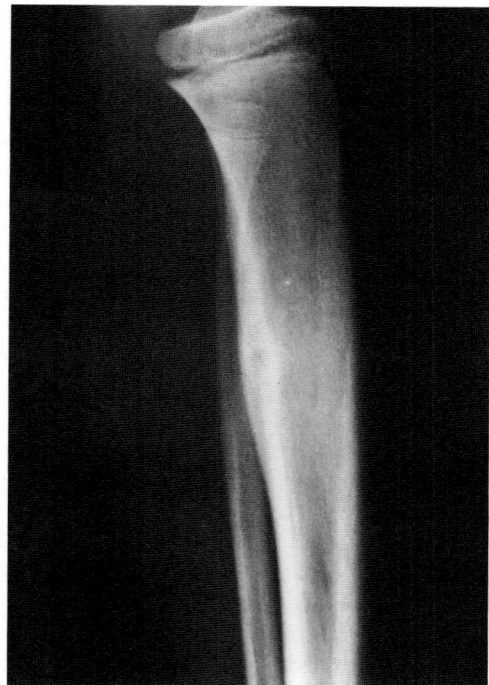

FIG. 6. Osteoid osteoma of posterior tibial cortex. Nidus is surrounded by thick cortical bone reaction.

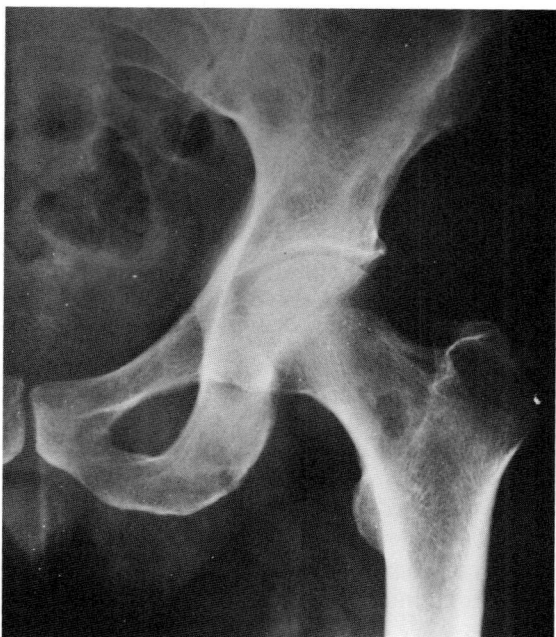

FIG. 7. Osteoblastoma of left femoral neck seen as lytic lesion with well-defined margins.

Osteoblastoma

Osteoblastoma is a rare tumor, accounting for approximately 4% of all benign bone tumors. There is a strong preponderance of males (78%). Eighty-four percent of the people affected are less than 30 years of age. Almost any bone may be involved, but there is a high predilection for the spinal column and sacrum. Multifocal osteoblastomas have also been reported (2).

Although the histologic appearance of osteoblastoma is similar to that of osteoid osteoma, the classic symptoms and radiographic evidence of peripheral sclerotic bone reaction, as well as the limited growth potential of osteoid osteoma, are not features of osteoblastoma (33,34,36). Pain is generally described as dull aching and is of long duration. Scoliosis and neurologic deficits due to impingement of the cord or nerve by the tumor may be seen with vertebral lesions (37).

The radiologic features are not characteristic. They may show a well-circumscribed region of bony destruction up to many centimeters in diameter that may or may not be surrounded by a dense sclerotic bone (Fig. 7). Occasionally, the bone will be expanded and the tumor delineated by a thin rim of periosteal bone formation. Approximately 25% of tumors show radiographic features of malignancy. Seventy-six percent of osteoblastomas involving the long bone are located in the diaphysis.

Radiographically, osteoid osteomas have been classified as lesions smaller than 1.5 cm and osteoblastomas as lesions greater than 1.5 cm (38). Histologically, osteoblastomas show abundant osteoid production arranged in a haphazard fashion. The bony trabeculae are surrounded by plump osteoblasts. Among the bony trabeculae is a loose fibrovascular connective tissue that often contains many benign giant cells.

The usual treatment includes curettage with bone grafting. En bloc resection may be performed when the lesion is in expendable bone. The chance for malignant transformation is very low (39). Radiation therapy is not recommended.

Benign Fibrous Lesions of Bone

There is a wide range of fibrous lesions of bone. Numerous terms have been used to describe these lesions, some of which represent different stages of evolution of the same process. Fibroma of bone generally includes nonossifying or nonosteogenic fibroma, metaphyseal fibrous defects, cortical fibrous defects, and xanthogranuloma (40). Periosteal desmoid is a less cellular variant, occurring more superficially on the bone (41,42).

These lesions of bone probably represent a defect in ossification rather than a true neoplastic process because they are generally self-limited (43–46). Fibromas are common, having been found in 30–40% of children more than 2 years old. The rarity of these lesions in the mature skeleton attests to their spontaneous resolution. Only a few of these fibrous lesions will require operation. In some patients, these fibrous lesions may involve many bones and be associated with a familial onset or some extraskeletal abnormalities. Males predominated in most series.

Most of these fibromas are located in the metaphysis of the long bone. When seen initially, they are closely related to the epiphyseal plate, although they may "migrate" toward the diaphysis with maturation. The great majority of patients with these lesions are asymptomatic, but pain or pathologic fractures may occur (47).

The roentgenographic appearance is characteristic. The lesion is seen as an eccentric, multiloculated lesion surrounded by a sclerotic rim of bone. The cortex is intact but may show some thinning and some bulging. The long axis of the fibroma is parallel to the axis of the bone.

Microscopically, these lesions are composed of fibrous connective tissue arranged in whole bundles. Benign giant cells and lipid-ladened histiocytes are seen in variable numbers. Hemosiderin-ladened macrophages are scattered among spindle-shaped stromal cells. Mitotic figures may be found, but the nuclei do not show atypical features.

If the lesion does not cause symptoms and the roentgenographic appearance is characteristic, operation is not needed, but roentgenograms should be taken periodically. If the diagnosis is uncertain or if the lesion is painful, biopsy followed by curettage and bone grafting will be curative. As suggested by Arata et al. (48), if the fibroma is large and involves more than 50% of the diameter of the bone, an operation may be indicated to prevent pathologic fracture. If such fracture occurs, conservative measures usually will allow bony union, but most frequently, the defect will persist and operation is indicated if the defect remains large. Radiation therapy is contraindicated.

Giant-Cell Tumor

Giant-cell tumor is a benign, locally aggressive tumor that accounts for 20% of all benign bone tumors. More females than males are affected. Eighty-five percent of patients are older than 20 years, and the tumor most frequently occurs in persons who are in the third and fourth decades of life. Age is helpful in differentiating a giant-cell tumor from an aneurysmal bone cyst; the latter occurs most commonly in persons who are less than 20 years old. Giant-cell tumor involves the epiphysis and the metaphysis of the long bone and usually extends close to the articular surface. The most frequent locations are the distal femur and the proximal tibia, which account for 50% of all sites. The distal radius and sacrum are the next most frequent sites (2). The vertebrae are not frequently involved, but when they are, the body of the vertebra is the usual location. This may also help in differentiating the tumor from an aneurysmal bone cyst, which usually involves the posterior elements of the vertebra.

Pain and swelling are the usual presenting complaints (49–52). Neurologic deficits are frequently present when the vertebral column is involved (sacrum 86%, spinal column 40%) (R. E. Turcotte et al., unpublished data).

Giant-cell tumor may have a very aggressive radiographic appearance. It presents as a purely lytic, eccentric lesion involving the epiphysis and extending to the subarticular region. Usually, there is no sclerotic rim of bone demarcating the tumor, and the outline of the tumor is ill-defined. As the lesion enlarges, it loses its eccentricity and involves the entire end of the bone. It frequently breaks through the cortex and extends into the soft tissues. There is no periosteal reaction (Fig. 8). In the spinal column and sacrum, the tumor has the appearance of a large eccentric lytic lesion involving the vertebral body. There is usually a large soft-tissue mass that can impinge on the nerve root or the cord.

Microscopically, the tumor is composed of round-to-oval mononuclear cells containing an oval-shaped nucleus. Mitotic figures are common. Numerous giant cells are uniformly scattered among the stromal cells. The nuclei of giant cells are similar to those of the stromal cells.

Histologic grading of giant-cell tumor has not uniformly been useful in predicting the biologic behavior of the tumor (53,54). Although most giant-cell tumors are benign, malignant variants have been described. They are believed to be a separate clinical entity consisting of a sarcoma that either is juxtaposed to zones of typical benign giant-cell tumor or occurs at a site of previously documented benign giant-cell tumor (2). Most fre-

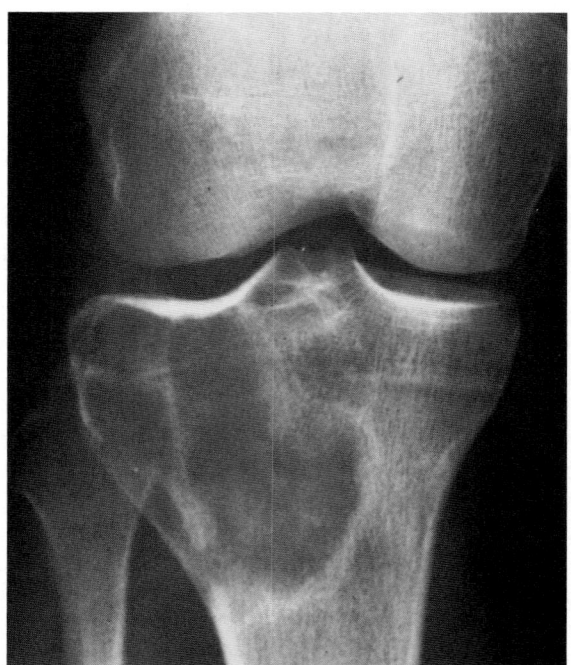

FIG. 8. Giant-cell tumor of proximal tibia of 23-year-old man. Tumor expands into metaphysis and extends to subchondral bone.

quently, malignant variants occur after radiation of a benign giant-cell tumor (53), and their incidence ranges from 1 to 15% (55–58).

Rarely, benign giant-cell tumors metastasize to the lungs. Rock et al. (59) reported 8 cases in a series of 411 cases of benign giant-cell tumors from the Mayo Clinic. The histologic appearance of these metastatic lesions is indistinguishable from that of the primary tumor. Giant-cell tumor may infrequently be multicentric (60–62).

The treatment of patients with giant-cell tumor remains very controversial (63–65). Complete removal of the tumor with a margin of normal tissue has always achieved the best tumor control (55,66). Because these tumors involve the articular ends of major bones, resection usually requires a major reconstructive procedure and produces a functional deficit in the young adult. Curettage associated with either bone grafting or methyl methacrylate provides a way to remove the tumor and retain the joint (67–79). Local recurrence rates are between 25 and 35% with these techniques (66). The risks of malignant transformation or metastasis by a recurrent tumor are negligible. Radiation therapy should not be used routinely.

MALIGNANT BONE TUMORS

Osteosarcoma

Osteosarcoma is characterized by malignant sarcomatous stromal cells producing osteoid. It accounts for 20% of all malignant primary bone tumors and is second in frequency only to multiple myeloma. Slightly more males than females are affected, and the peak age at onset is the second decade of life. Usually, the tumor involves the metaphysis of long bones, although any bone may be involved. The knee region is the most frequent location, accounting for 50% of all sites (80,81).

The vast majority of osteosarcomas arise in bone free of preexisting lesions (82). Although "secondary" osteosarcomas arising from benign conditions, such as fibrous dysplasia (83) or bone infarct, have been reported, the most frequently noted benign preexisting condition is Paget's disease. Osteosarcoma arising in Paget's disease has an extremely poor prognosis.

Patients with osteosarcoma most commonly present with pain of short duration and swelling in the region of the tumor. When the diagnosis is delayed, the skin over the lesion is distended and the superficial venous network is prominent. Pathologic fractures may occur, most commonly after open biopsy. With the exception of elevated erythrocyte sedimentation rate and high serum alkaline phosphatase concentration, all laboratory data are generally normal.

Many variants of osteosarcoma have been recognized on the basis of clinical, radiographic, and pathologic features (84). The radiographic and pathologic features of these types and the prognosis associated with them vary widely.

Conventional osteosarcoma is a high-grade intramedullary sarcoma accounting for 85% of all osteosarcomas. The radiographic appearance is usually that of a mixed lytic and sclerotic lesion involving the metaphysis. The margins are not well defined, and the cortex is commonly breached. A periosteal reaction is usually manifested as nonneoplastic bone deposited by the elevated periosteum. This reaction gives rise to the well-known Codman's triangle and sunburst appearance. A soft-tissue extension of the tumor is often present as a mixed ossified mass (Fig. 9). Occasionally, the tumor may cross the epiphyseal plate or invade the joint. The histologic appearance is highly variable from tumor to tumor as well as from region to region within a given tumor, but the hallmark is the production of osteoid by sarcomatous stromal cells (85). This osteoid may be calcified or uncalcified. Histologically, conventional osteosarcomas can be divided into three categories (osteoblastic, chondroblastic, and fibroblastic), depending on the predominant histologic pattern evident.

Telangiectatic osteosarcoma is a variant of conventional intramedullary osteosarcoma and comprises less than 3% of all osteosarcomas (86). Radiographically, the tumor presents as a large lytic lesion with indistinct borders. Grossly, the tumor is a large cystic blood-filled cavity with multiple septa. Osteoid production is minimal, and the septa contain malignant stromal cells. Benign giant cells are commonly present. The main radio-

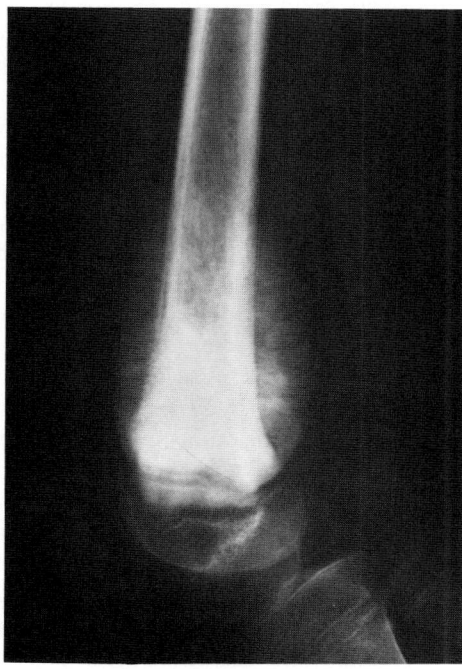

FIG. 9. Osteosarcoma of distal femur. Large osteoblastic lesion with sunburst periosteal reaction.

graphic and pathologic differential diagnosis is that of an aneurysmal bone cyst. Prognosis is similar to that in conventional osteosarcoma, and the primary reason for differentiating this entity is the potential for confusing it with an aneurysmal bone cyst.

Low-grade central osteosarcoma generally involves the metaphysis of long bones. Patients on the average are older than those with conventional osteosarcoma, having a peak incidence in the third decade of life. Radiographically, the lesion may easily be confused with fibrous dysplasia, but usually the margins are less well demarcated. The cortex may be permeated by the tumor or even transgressed. This lesion also frequently extends into the subchondral region. Microscopically, the tumor is composed of a fibroblastic stroma that consists of spindled cells with slight nuclear atypia and produces osteoid. These lesions are slow growing and have a much better prognosis than does conventional osteosarcoma.

Parosteal osteosarcoma is a low-grade subtype of osteosarcoma, accounting for approximately 4% of all osteosarcomas. Most (70%) patients are females, and the peak incidence is in the third and fourth decades of life. The tumor arises at the surface of the long bones, most often at the posteromedial aspect of the distal femur. Localized swelling, slowly enlarging, is the most frequent complaint and is usually present for a long time before the patient seeks medical attention.

Radiographically, the lesion is seen as a dense mass applied to the surface of the affected bone and *not* involving the medullary canal. The tumor may encircle the bone, but a space of 2–3 mm may be found between the tumor and the underlying bone. The tumor is heavily ossified, although peripheral lobules are less mineralized. There is no Codman's triangle. The differential diagnosis includes osteochondroma and myositis ossificans (87).

Histologically, the spindled stromal cells show slight cytologic atypia. Parallel bone trabeculae course through the spindled stroma. The low-power pattern may mimic that of fibrous dysplasia; however, osteosarcoma may show more cytologic atypia at the periphery of the lesion. Cartilaginous regions are often found at the periphery of the tumor, and the chondrocytes usually show minimal nuclear atypia. Prognosis is very good, with more than 80% of the patients surviving when treatment is adequate. Occasionally, local recurrent lesions may have more pronounced histologic and cytologic atypia than the original lesion.

Periosteal osteosarcoma is a subtype of osteosarcoma arising on the surface of the cortex, most commonly involving the shaft of the femur and the tibia (88). The roentgenographic appearance typically is that of a radiolucent defect on a saucer-shaped depression at the surface of the bone. The endosteum is uninvolved. A sunburst pattern of periosteal reaction may be present and extend into the soft tissues. Histologically, the tumor is lobulated, and cartilaginous differentiation is prominent. The cells are usually moderately atypical. With appropriate surgical treatment, the prognosis is better than that for conventional osteosarcoma.

High-grade surface osteosarcoma is a rare surface osteosarcoma with a prognosis similar to that for conventional intramedullary sarcoma. Classically, the medulla is uninvolved. Separation of periosteal and high-grade surface osteosarcoma may be difficult radiographically, but the latter is usually less well ossified and demarcated. The histologic appearance is similar to that of conventional osteosarcoma. Metastasis from all osteosarcomas occurs via the hematogenous route, with the lungs being the most frequent site of metastatic spread; bone is second in frequency.

In the past decade, improvements in chemotherapeutic regimens (89–91), better understanding of orthopedic oncologic principles (92), and improved orthopedic reconstructive techniques (93) have resulted in increased enthusiasm for limb-sparing surgical approaches in the treatment of osteosarcoma (94–101). Proper patient selection techniques are mandatory. Despite the difficulty, satisfactory margins need to be obtained with the limb-salvage procedure because local recurrences are associated with a poorer prognosis. The local recurrence rate after a limb-salvage procedure is reported to be between 4 and 6%, which is comparable to the rates achieved with wide amputation. Furthermore, Simon et al. (102) have recently shown that osteosarcomas of the distal femur treated either by amputation or by limb salvage have comparable late results. Although limb-preserving surgery is most easily accomplished when the tumor is entirely confined to the bone (stage IIA), small soft-tissue extension of the tumor does not preclude using this technique. A large soft-tissue mass closely related to major vascular or nerve structures is the most frequent reason precluding the conservation of the limb. Patient age is also an important consideration inasmuch as many of the limb-salvaging techniques are more easily accomplished in patients who have achieved skeletal maturity.

The type of reconstruction depends on many factors (100), including patient's age, tumor location, prognosis, patient's expectations, and patient's activities. The usual options are endoprosthesis, allograft replacement (103–106), resection arthrodesis, or leaving the limb flail.

For young patients with tumors in the knee region, rotation-plasty has given reliable results (107). This technique involves an "en bloc" resection of the tumor coupled to a fusion of the residual femur and tibia. The leg is rotated 180 degrees on the femur, so that the foot is facing backward. The ankle joint then functions as the knee. The patient is fitted with a special prosthesis, and gait analysis has demonstrated a walking pattern similar to that in below-knee amputation. Emotional acceptance by the patient is surprisingly good. Expandable endoprostheses are currently under investigation and may be another option in the future (108).

Current results with modern approaches are encouraging, the 5-year survival rates being more than 60%. Prevention and treatment of the metastasis are the most difficult problems to resolve. The surgical excision of pulmonary metastatic lesions, even if multiple, has proven to be a useful adjunctive therapy (109–111). Most of the metastatic lesions are located at the periphery of the lung, and young patients tolerate surgical excision well. Early detection is possible utilizing CT scans so that early treatment can be initiated. In a recent study, Glasser et al. (109) showed that patients with lung metastasis (stage III) have a 5-year disease-free survival of 22% with this aggressive treatment approach.

Patients with osteosarcoma are best treated by a multidisciplinary approach. Initially, the malignant character of the lesion must be recognized on the plain radiographs. Then the tumor must be staged with the aid of CT and MRI. The last step is biopsy, which should give the pathologist a sample representative of the tumor. Careful planning of the biopsy site is critical in order to respect the oncologic principle that may allow the patient to be a candidate for a limb-salvage procedure.

Amputation remains the "standard" surgical treatment for osteosarcoma (112). In the past, some authors (113) have advocated that amputation should be performed one joint above the affected bony segment, but currently, with reliable staging, amputation can be safely performed 8–10 cm above the most proximal extent of the lesion. Historically, amputation alone gave an overall 5-year survival rate of 20% (98,114). Most patients experienced lung metastasis despite adequate local tumor control, thus reflecting the failure to control the early systemic spreading of the disease.

In the early 1970s, studies reported increased survival of patients treated with multidrug chemotherapy (115,116). Currently, chemotherapy is one of the cornerstones in the treatment of patients with osteosarcoma. Neoadjuvant chemotherapy or chemotherapy given before the definitive surgical treatment remains somewhat controversial (91,117). Chemotherapy has been more accepted during the last few years and is usually given for 2–3 months before operation. The chemotherapy serves many purposes. It allows immediate treatment of the tumor, which is considered a systemic disease. If operation is to be performed first, a delay would be necessary to permit wound healing, which may be delayed by complications. It also allows evaluation of the response of the tumor to chemotherapy. Tumors showing less than 90% necrosis after the preoperative courses of chemotherapy are associated with a poorer prognosis than tumors showing greater than 90% necrosis. For patients who are "nonresponders" to the regimen used before operation,

other chemotherapeutic agents may be used postoperatively in an attempt to increase the effectiveness of the treatment. When a limb-salvaging procedure is contemplated, the neoadjuvant chemotherapy will often reduce the volume of the soft-tissue mass associated with the tumor, and the tumor will undergo extensive ossification that renders the operation more feasible. Unfortunately, the effects of delaying the operation for patients who will be poor responders to the neoadjuvant treatment are not known.

Radiation therapy has been used to control local disease. Experience has shown that osteosarcoma is relatively radioresistant, and the frequent severe side effects associated with its use have also brought this modality into disrepute.

Patients with local recurrence are usually treated by high amputation. Patients with nonresectable metastatic bone lesions are given radiation therapy in addition to chemotherapy.

Ewing's Sarcoma

Ewing's sarcoma is a malignant bone tumor composed of small, round cells of uncertain origin. Recently, a neuroectodermal origin has been proposed after Ewing's sarcoma cells have been found to possess a reciprocal translocation between the long arms of chromosomes 11 and 22 [t(11;22)(q23;q11)], as does the lesion termed *primitive neuroepithelioma* (118–122).

Ewing's sarcoma accounts for 5% of primary bone sarcomas. Patients in the first and second decades of life are most frequently affected, and in more than 90% of the patients, the onset is before the age of 30 years. Slightly more males than females are affected by this tumor. The most frequent locations are the pelvic girdle and long bones of the lower extremity, accounting for more than 60% of all sites (123). The shoulder girdle is another common location.

At presentation, signs and symptoms are slightly more characteristic of Ewing's sarcoma than for other bone sarcomas. Pain and swelling are almost always present, often for many months before the diagnosis is made. Low-grade fever may be present. Anemia, leukocytosis, an elevated erythrocyte sedimentation rate, and an increased lactic dehydrogenase level may be found. Rarely, a patient will have a pathologic fracture at presentation.

Factors associated with a poorer prognosis include pelvic location of the tumor, young age in males, and local recurrence (124). Metastatic lesions are hematogenous, with more than 50% affecting the lungs. The skeleton is also frequently involved, particularly the spinal column and the skull.

At presentation, Ewing's sarcoma rarely shows diagnostic radiographic features. The tumor is best described as a lytic lesion with a moth-eaten pattern involving the bone. Some blastic areas may be present. In long bones, the diaphysis is usually affected near its metaphyseal end. The lesion is poorly defined at its periphery, and the entire medullary canal is occasionally involved. The cortex is usually eroded and permeated by the process. Periosteal reaction is common and can be of the classic onionskin appearance produced by a layered deposition of subperiosteal bone. Although commonly described in Ewing's sarcoma, this feature is not pathognomonic of it. A sunburst pattern also may be found, as in osteosarcoma (Fig. 10). A large soft-tissue mass is frequently identified with the aid of CT or MRI.

Osteomyelitis must always be considered in the differential diagnosis because the clinical findings, the roentgenographic pattern, and the gross appearance may be identical to those in osteomyelitis.

A rare subtype of Ewing's sarcoma is the so-called subperiosteal Ewing sarcoma. This subtype occurs at the surface of the bone and may show little involvement of the medullary cavity. On plain radiographs, the tumor is usually seen as a saucer-shaped lytic lesion at the surface of the bone.

Grossly, Ewing's sarcoma is a gray or white tumor. It is usually very soft and has a semiliquid consistency, suggestive of pus. Histologically, the tumor is cellular, being composed of sheets of small cells with round-to-oval dark nuclei. Cytoplasmic borders are indistinct. These small cells are monotonous in their cytologic characteristics, and they do not produce matrix. Ewing's sarcoma must be differentiated from other small-cell tumors, including lymphoma (125,126), small-cell osteosarcoma, and metastatic neuroblastoma. The cytologic monotony of Ewing's sarcoma and the absence of reticulin fibers help to make the diagnosis. In addition, glycogen frequently can be identified in the cells utilizing periodic acid–Schiff stain (127); however, glycogen is not a constant feature of Ewing's sarcoma of bone with this histochemical technique.

Ewing's sarcoma is a radio-sensitive tumor, and until recently, the standard treatment has been radiation therapy to the entire bone to achieve local tumor control. The dosage used has varied (4000–6000 cGy) according to different protocols (128). Radiation therapy has been associated with local complications, including limb-length inequality, pathologic fracture, joint ankylosis, and post-radiation sarcoma. Dosages of more than 4500 cGy do not provide better local control of the tumor but significantly increase the local complication rate. Chemotherapy has been used to achieve systemic control of the disease. Recently, new chemotherapeutic modalities have dramatically improved survival rates and lowered the incidence of complications in the treatment of this disease (129–133).

Despite all these improvements, the 5-year survival rate is between 60 and 70% and the local recurrence rate associated with the standard regimen is between 10 and 20% (134). In more than 90% of the patients, local recurrences were associated with a fatal outcome (135,136).

Although the role of operation in Ewing's sarcoma has been limited, recent data suggest that surgical resection of the affected region of bone improves survival. Currently, it is widely accepted that surgical resection should be performed for tumors located in expendable bones such as the rib and fibula. Primary amputation, although rarely performed, may be indicated for tumors of the distal tibia and foot in a young patient.

The surgical approach to patients with Ewing's sarcoma has evolved during the last 10 years on the basis of a better understanding of oncologic surgical principles and major innovations in surgical techniques, which have permitted wide resection of the tumor with preservation of the limb. Reconstruction of the surgical defect created by the resection is now standardized, and functional results are more predictable. Furthermore, achieving adequate margins with the resection has made it possible to avoid radiation therapy and some of its complications.

Operation should probably be contemplated when the resection (a) will not produce important functional deficits and (b) is easy to perform and will not necessitate major reconstructive techniques. Sites that usually fulfill these criteria include ribs, clavicle, fibula, hand, foot, and lower part of the scapula. The role of operation is

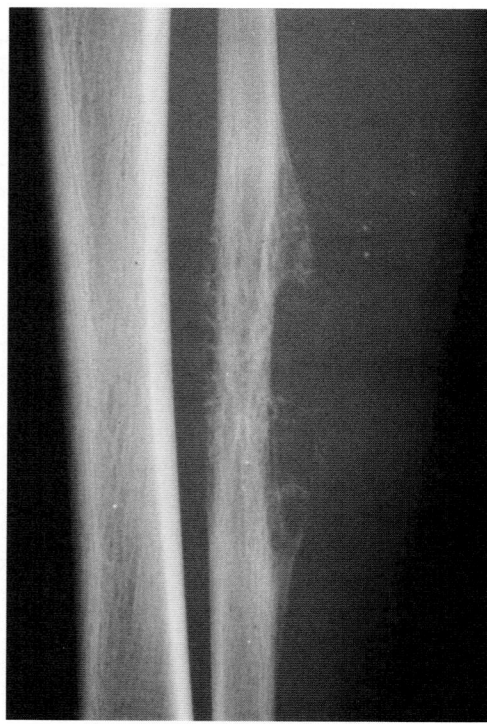

FIG. 10. Ewing's sarcoma of fibula showing lytic lesion of diaphysis with periosteal reaction (sunburst and Codman's triangle).

still debatable for tumors of the femur, tibia, and humerus. Ewing's sarcoma of the pelvis poses a specific challenge because results of conventional treatment are not as good as they are for Ewing's sarcoma at other sites, primarily because of the large tumor volume of pelvic tumors (137). Frequently, the large soft-tissue mass associated with these lesions responds to chemotherapy or to radiation by shrinking sufficiently to allow limb-salvage surgery to be performed. Tumors limited to the ilium probably should be resected, but for tumors in the acetabulum or the sacroiliac joint, the primary role of operation is still to be defined. Further studies are needed to clarify the exact role of operation as the primary treatment for Ewing's sarcoma.

Fibrosarcoma

Fibrosarcoma of bone is a rare lesion, representing 3% of all malignant bone tumors in the Mayo Clinic files. The tumor is characterized by the proliferation of malignant fibroblastic cells without the production of cartilage or osteoid. Males and females are affected in equal numbers, and there is an even distribution of patients among the age decades from the end of the second decade to the seventh decade. The long tubular bones are affected in 50% of the patients. Although fibrosarcomas usually arise de novo, approximately 23% occur in bones previously affected by radiation therapy, Paget's disease, or bone infarct (138). Symptoms, including pain and swelling, are nonspecific and of short duration.

On plain radiographic studies, fibrosarcoma is seen as a lytic lesion usually involving the metaphysis. The tumor frequently destroys the cortex and may show soft-tissue extension. High-grade lesions will show a permeative pattern at their periphery (Fig. 11). None of these findings is specific for fibrosarcoma, as osteolytic osteosarcoma can have the same radiographic features. Both tumors may present with periosteal reaction. CT or MRI is useful to determine the extent of the tumor inside the bone and in the surrounding soft tissues.

Histologically, the tumor is characterized by spindle-shaped malignant cells, arranged in a herringbone pattern. Collagen production by the malignant cells may be abundant but varies widely from tumor to tumor. In general, the most poorly differentiated tumors produce the least collagen. Although low-grade fibrosarcoma of bone may be identified, nearly two-thirds of the tumors are high-grade (poorly differentiated). A well-differentiated fibrosarcoma may be difficult to distinguish from a benign fibrous lesion (40).

Fibrosarcoma metastasizes by hematogenous dissemination. Lungs are the most frequently involved organs. Adequate treatment for fibrosarcoma requires a resection with at least a wide margin. Amputation is considered when a large soft-tissue mass is present.

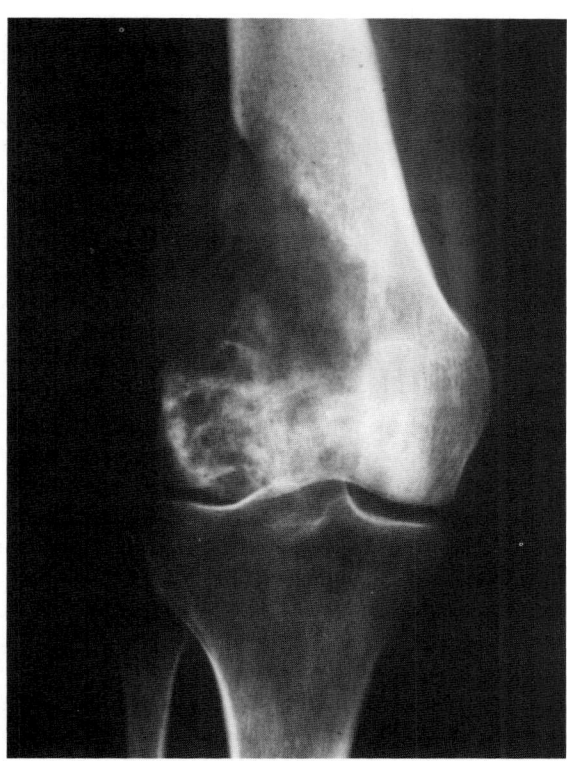

FIG. 11. Fibrosarcoma of distal femur showing large lytic lesion with permeative margins. No periosteal reaction is seen.

Radiation therapy has not been effective for this tumor, and it is reserved for patients with inoperable lesions. Chemotherapy needs to be evaluated further to establish its role in these high-grade tumors. The overall survival for patients with fibrosarcoma is approximately 30%, but survival is much better for patients with low-grade lesions than for patients with high-grade tumors.

Chondrosarcoma

Chondrosarcoma, a tumor composed of malignant chondrocytes producing a chondroid matrix (26), accounts for 11% of malignant bone tumors. Most tumors occur in adults, with a peak incidence during the fifth and sixth decades. More men than women are affected.

Chondrosarcoma may arise either de novo (primary chondrosarcoma) or in a prior benign condition (secondary chondrosarcoma). Primary chondrosarcomas are more frequent and comprised 76% of the Mayo Clinic series. Secondary chondrosarcoma most commonly complicates osteochondroma and enchondroma (139). The probability of such a "malignant degeneration" is small, probably less than 1%. However, in familial multiple osteochondromatosis and in Ollier's disease or multiple enchondromatosis, the risk is much higher, and these patients need to be followed up more closely. Chondrosarcomas can arise from within the bone (central chondrosarcoma) or from the surface of the bone (periosteal chondrosarcoma or peripheral chondrosarcoma).

Although chondrosarcomas may involve any bone, the most frequent locations are the pelvis, the ribs, and the proximal femur and humerus (140–142). The tumor usually grows slowly, and pain may have been present for months or years before the patient seeks medical attention. Occasionally, patients will present with a huge tumor that causes few symptoms.

On plain roentgenograms, the central chondrosarcoma is seen as a large lytic lesion containing multiple areas of matted calcific deposits that can be discrete or confluent. In general, endosteal erosion or scalloping is present and occasionally frank cortical breakthrough may be associated with soft-tissue extension of the tumor (Fig. 12A). CT and MRI are very useful to evaluate the cortical integrity and the medullary or soft-tissue extent of the tumor, particularly for pelvic tumors. They are the most useful tools for detecting local recurrence.

Peripheral chondrosarcoma usually appears as a soft-tissue mass arising from the surface of the bone and containing numerous calcific deposits. When the mass is large, it may be difficult to establish if the chondrosarcoma arose centrally and expanded into soft tissues or arose peripherally and subsequently invaded the bone.

Grossly, the tumor is lobulated, semitranslucent, gray-white hyaline cartilage. Frequently, the center of the tumor undergoes degenerative myxoid changes and has a semiliquid consistency. Calcific deposits are found in the chondroid matrix. Whether central or peripheral, the tumors show similar histologic features. The tumors may be divided into three grades of malignancy, which histologically are separated, depending on the cellularity of the lesion and the cytologic atypia evident. Most (90%) of the lesions are low grade (grade 1 or 2). Because osteosarcoma may show abundant cartilage matrix production, the finding of even a minimal amount of osteoid precludes the diagnosis of chondrosarcoma.

Three subtypes of chondrosarcoma have been identified (143). The early dedifferentiated chondrosarcoma accounts for approximately 10% of all chondrosarcomas (144). It is a high-grade lesion associated with a poor prognosis (Fig. 12B). Elderly patients who, at presentation, have a calcified osseous tumor with a soft-tissue mass containing a large unmineralized component should be carefully evaluated to exclude this diagnosis. Microscopically, the lesion is composed of lobules of ordinary low-grade (grade 1 or 2) chondrosarcoma immediately adjacent to zones of highly anaplastic spindle cells (grade 3 or 4).

Mesenchymal chondrosarcoma, a rare subtype of chondrosarcoma (Fig. 12C), is composed of areas of low-grade chondrosarcoma mixed with areas of highly cellular tumor composed of round-to-ovoid small cells (145,146). It tends to affect younger people, 80% being less than 40 years old. There is also a female preponder-

ance. Approximately one-third of mesenchymal chondrosarcomas arise in soft tissues (147). The overall prognosis is poor, but patients may live for long periods after diagnosis before the tumor recurs or metastasizes.

Clear-cell chondrosarcoma, a third variant of chondrosarcoma, is generally of a lower grade and associated with a better prognosis than the two chondrosarcoma variants previously described (148). Typically, it affects the end of the long bones and extends to the articular cartilage. Radiographically, the appearance may be similar to that of chondroblastoma, producing a lytic expansion at the epiphysis. The tumor is often well demarcated by a sclerotic rim of reactive bone (Fig. 12D). Microscopically, the tumor is composed of cells with abundant clear cytoplasm. Benign, multilobulated giant cells are usually found, and sometimes areas of low-grade conventional chondrosarcomas or reactive bone formation are present.

Surgical resection remains the sole effective treatment for all types of chondrosarcoma. Chemotherapy and radiation therapy, either by external-beam irradiation or by radioactive isotopes (sulfur-35), have not been very effective, although they may be utilized when the lesion is high grade or in a surgically inaccessible location.

Staging of the tumor is the first step in determining the appropriate treatment options for patients with chondrosarcoma. Local extension within the bone and surrounding soft tissues must be assessed by either CT or MRI in order to plan the operation. Large soft-tissue masses or extension to neurovascular structures may preclude limb salvage and thus mandate an amputation. Although soft-tissue masses are common with chondrosarcoma, the tumor usually does not invade the surrounding structures but rather pushes them away as it expands. Because chondrosarcoma has a high rate of local recurrence, a wide margin is mandatory at operation. The local recurrence rate is directly proportional to the size of the soft-tissue extent of the tumor (141). Frequently, for pelvic and spinal tumors, marginal resection is the best that can be achieved.

As with all potentially malignant primary bone tumors, the diagnostic biopsy in patients with suspected chondrosarcoma should be well planned. There is a pronounced tendency for chondrosarcoma to seed the biopsy track. The biopsy specimen must be representative of the tumor and should include any portion that radiographically suggests the possibility of being high grade (usually in a peripheral zone where the tumor is less calcified).

The same reconstructive techniques as used for osteosarcomas are valid for chondrosarcomas (149,150). Because many lesions involve the proximal femur or humerus, custom prosthetic replacements are frequently done (100,151–154). For pelvic lesions, internal hemipelvectomy with or without hip fusion has yielded satisfactory results (155).

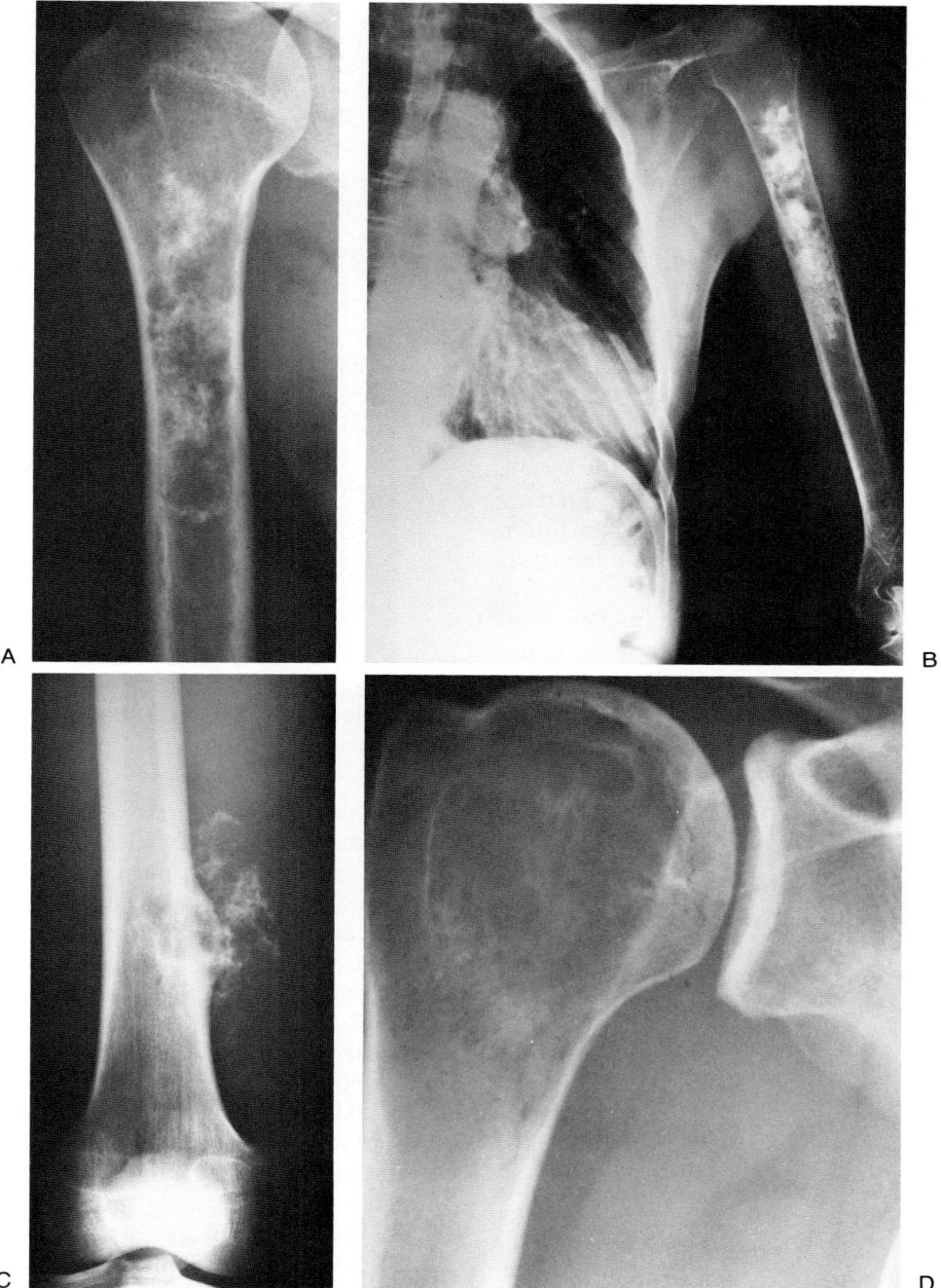

FIG. 12. A: Low-grade chondrosarcoma of humeral shaft. Cartilaginous lesion is large. There is scalloping of cortex, but cortex is not broken through by tumor. **B:** Dedifferentiated chondrosarcoma presenting as partially calcified lesion extending down humeral shaft. Cortex is permeated, but soft-tissue mass is not well seen on plain roentgenogram. **C:** Mesenchymal chondrosarcoma of distal femur extending into soft tissues. **D:** Clear-cell chondrosarcoma of proximal humerus. Tumor extends to subchondral bone and is poorly marginated. There is no evidence of matrix calcification.

Patients with chondrosarcoma should be followed up for at least 10 years, as this tumor is generally a slowly progressing one. Prognosis is directly related to the histologic grade of the lesion. Patients with grade 1 tumors have a 10-year survival of approximately 85%; grade 2, 50%; and grade 3, 30%. Metastasis occurs by hematogenous dissemination, with the lungs being the primary site for metastatic involvement. An aggressive approach for pulmonary metastasis (as is used for osteosarcoma) is recommended. Low-grade chondrosarcoma has a low rate of metastasis, and failure to control the disease locally is the usual cause of death from the disease. Grade 3 chondrosarcoma has a metastatic rate of more than 50%, and it is usually the cause of death. In patients surviving more than 10 years with or without evidence of disease, as many as 20% are expected to die because of the chondrosarcoma (R. E. Turcotte et al., unpublished data). Peripheral chondrosarcoma has a better prognosis than the central type.

LESIONS SIMULATING BONE TUMORS

Unicameral Bone Cysts

Simple bone cysts are common, benign fluid-filled cystic lesions of bone. They are most frequently seen in persons who are in the first two decades of life, and more males than females are affected. The origin of the tumor is still debated (156,157); possibilities include disturbance of the growth plate, retrophyseal and venous flow obstruction, and synovial cysts. The most frequent location is the proximal part of long tubular bones (45,95,158–161). The proximal humerus and femur account for 50–90% of the sites.

Although asymptomatic lesions may be identified radiographically, pain is usually the reason for the patient seeking medical attention, with pathologic fracture frequently being the cause of the pain.

Radiographically, the simple bone cyst is seen as a large frequently multiloculated radiolucency, which often is near the growth plate and extends to the medullary canal of the shaft (162). The bone may be slightly expanded, and the cortices are intact but thin (Fig. 13).

Histologically, the lining of the tumor is composed of fibroconnective tissue containing giant cells, pigments of hemosiderin, and some inflammatory cells. The cavity is filled with protein-rich fluid (163).

The treatment of simple bone cysts remains controversial (164–168). Curettage with bone grafting has been the standard treatment of choice for large or symptomatic cysts, but Scaglietti et al. (169,170) have obtained good results and fewer complications from an injection of methylprednisolone into the cyst. If a pathologic fracture occurs, union will usually be achieved by conservative measures. Only 15% of the cysts are expected to regress after a fracture. If the cyst becomes larger, treatment is often indicated.

Aneurysmal Bone Cyst

Aneurysmal bone cyst represents a reactive nonneoplastic process (158). Frequently, areas of aneurysmal bone cyst may be found in association with benign bone tumors such as giant-cell tumor, chondroblastoma, and chondromyxoid fibroma, as well as with fibrous dyspla

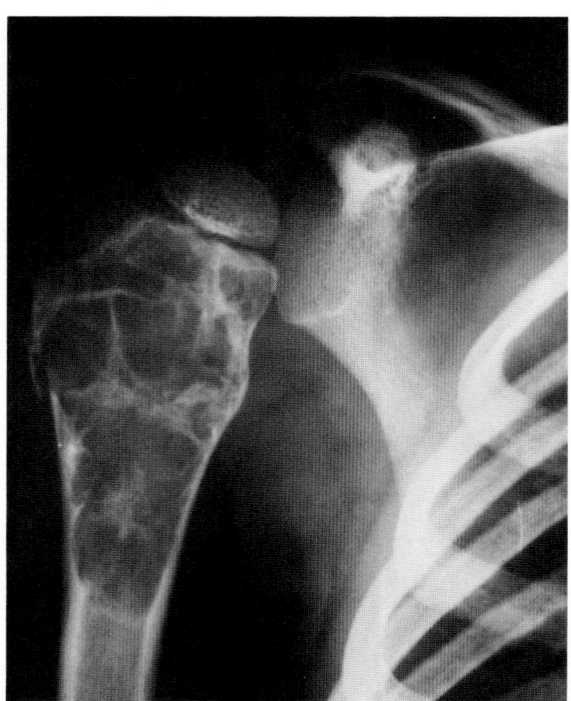

FIG. 13. Large multiloculated simple bone cyst of proximal humerus showing pathologic fracture.

sia. Because of its aggressive radiographic appearance and potentially rapid clinical evolution, aneurysmal bone cyst may be mistaken for a malignant neoplasm clinically and radiographically.

The exact cause of aneurysmal bone cyst remains unknown. Some authors have suggested that increased vascular pressure inside the bone from altered vascular dynamics may be the underlying cause. Others have suggested that the cystlike lesion results from the local production of fibrinolytic substances that destroy the bone. Although frequently identified as accompanying benign tumors, these lesions may arise de novo (2).

The peak incidence is in persons who are in the second decade of life, with more than 75% of the affected patients being less than 20 years old (171). In contrast, 80% of the patients with giant-cell tumor, which may mimic an aneurysmal bone cyst histologically, are more than 20 years of age. Pain and swelling are the common manifestations. With spinal lesions, nerve root or spinal cord impingement may be encountered.

On plain roentgenograms, an aneurysmal bone cyst is usually seen located in the metaphysis of long bones, but when the growth plate is closed, the cyst may extend into the epiphysis. Twenty percent of the cysts occur in the spinal column, and these usually involve the posterior elements. An aneurysmal bone cyst may involve more than one adjacent spinal segment. The tumor is seen as a rapidly expansile eccentric lytic lesion which is usually delimited by a thin rim of sclerosis or periosteal new

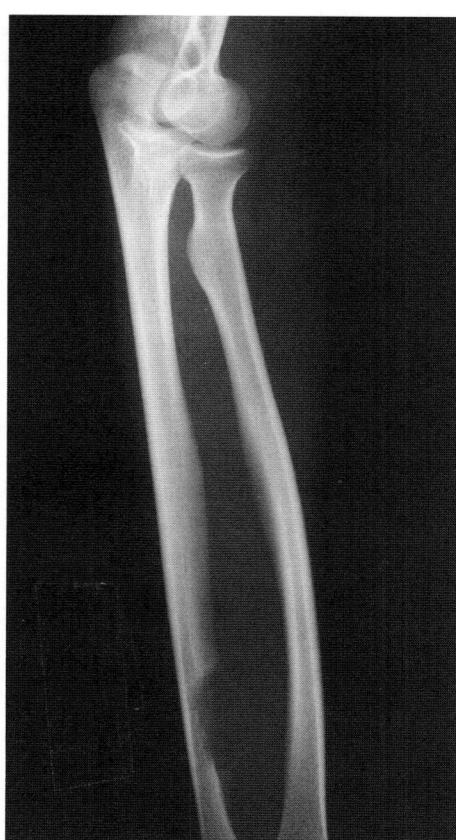

FIG. 14. Lytic bone cyst of distal ulna showing well-defined margins, bone loculations, and thin layer of periosteal new bone formation. This is characteristic of aneurysmal bone cyst.

bone formation (Fig. 14). The characteristic ballooning expansion of the lesion is not always present. The aneurysmal bone cyst may also have a very aggressive appearance, with cortical destruction, soft-tissue mass, and Codman's triangle, suggestive of a malignant tumor (172).

Grossly, the tumor appears as a bag filled with unclotted blood and internally divided by numerous septa. Microscopically, these septa are thin, lack any endothelial lining, and are covered by a stroma of spindle cells that lack atypia or pleomorphism. Mitotic figures may be present. Bony trabeculae are frequently found in the septa and are referred to as "fiberosteoid." Histologically, benign multinucleated giant cells are seen to be nearly uniformly present. Because areas of aneurysmal bone cyst may be found with other bone tumors, the specimen must be examined thoroughly to exclude an underlying lesion when an aneurysmal bone cyst is identified histologically.

Treatment of an aneurysmal bone cyst depends on its location (63). "En bloc" resection is preferred for lesions involving an expendable bone such as the rib or fibula (173). When such a resection cannot be performed be-

cause the aneurysmal bone cyst is located in a large bone or near a joint and treatment would result in a significant loss of function, then curettage with bone grafting is selected. When curettage and grafting are employed, a recurrence rate of 29% (generally within 2 years of operation) can be anticipated. Treatment of local recurrences is usually similar to that of the primary cyst, although more extensive wide resection with reconstruction may be necessary. After curettage and bone grafting, the persistence of a nonprogressive cystic area in an asymptomatic patient can be treated by close observation only.

Although good results have been reported with radiation therapy (174), its use is not recommended for a patient with an aneurysmal bone cyst because of the potential malignant transformation of irradiated bone.

Fibrous Dysplasia

Fibrous dysplasia is a developmental abnormality of bone characterized by fibrous replacement of a portion of the medullary cavity. The dysplasia may affect one (monostotic) bone or several (polyostotic) bones. The polyostotic disease is usually more severe and manifests itself at a younger age than the monostotic form. It is also less frequent, accounting for 11% of all tumors in the Mayo Clinic files. Brown or yellow skin patches with an irregular "coast-of-Maine" outline may occasionally be found in association with polyostotic fibrous dysplasia. Albright's syndrome is a severe form of polyostotic disease associated with patches of cutaneous pigmentation and endocrine abnormalities, especially precocious puberty in girls.

Both sexes are affected in equal numbers, and the disease has its onset during infancy. Symptoms frequently begin before the age of 30 years. Many of the patients remain asymptomatic. Pain and a limp are the usual complaints and are often secondary to an undisplaced pathologic fracture. Leg-length inequality may be present and is the consequence of the bony deformations that can be associated with fibrous dysplasia, most often a "shepherd-crook" deformity of the proximal femur.

In the long bone, there is a predilection for the metaphysis. Any bone can be involved by fibrous dysplasia. In the monostotic form, the upper end of the femur is the site of more than a third of the lesions. Other frequent sites are the ribs, base of the skull, and jawbone.

On plain roentgenograms, the lesion is seen as a radiolucent defect that may be transparent or have a ground-glass appearance. The lesion is usually well circumscribed by a rim of sclerotic bone (175). The cortex may be thinned and expanded, but it is not broken through, and there is no soft-tissue mass. A periosteal reaction is unusual when there is no fracture (Fig. 15). The radiographic differential diagnosis includes unicameral bone cyst and nonossifying fibroma.

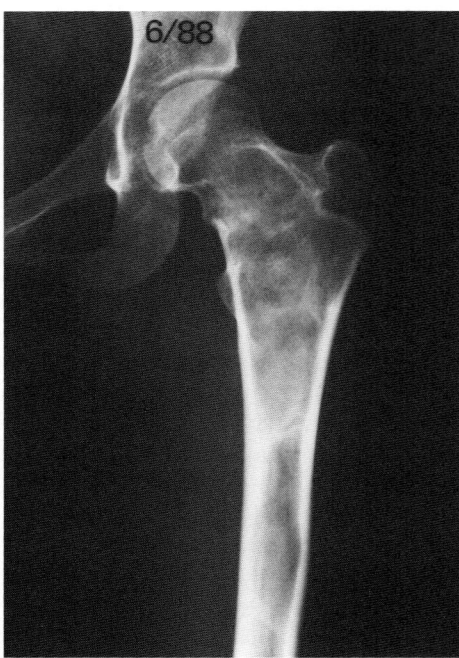

FIG. 15. Classic ground-glass appearance of fibrous dysplasia of femur. Pathologic fracture through femoral neck can be seen.

Grossly, the lesion is composed of dense fibrous tissue and often contains small osteoid trabeculae, giving the lesion a gritty consistency. Microscopically, lesional tissue consists of benign-appearing fibroblasts producing a dense collagenous matrix. Trabeculae of bone or osteoid are interspaced in the stroma and are randomly arranged. They are not bordered by osteoblasts. Mitotic figures are sometimes present, as are regions of xanthic degeneration.

Treatment is usually conservative. The goal is to prevent a worsening of the deformity. Most lesions will stabilize after puberty, although symptoms may start in adulthood.

Operation should be considered when the deformity of bone increases, when the pain does not respond to conservative management, or when pathologic fracture is impending. Curettage with bone grafting is the preferred method of treatment. Preventive internal fixation and corrective osteotomies may also be needed. Recurrence of the lesion is infrequent but is more common in younger patients.

Radiation therapy should not be used. Cases of spontaneous malignant transformation have been described (83,176,177).

Osteofibrous Dysplasia

Osteofibrous dysplasia, or Campanacci's disease (178), has recently been recognized as an entity distinct from fibrous dysplasia. Classically, it involves the cortex of the tibia or the fibula in patients younger than 10 years of age. The disease is ordinarily monostotic and often produces a severe bowing deformity.

On plain roentgenograms, the lesion of the tibia is seen located in the diaphysis, involving the anterior cortex and producing multiple lucent areas surrounded by dense sclerotic bone. Anterior bowing is common. The radiographic differential diagnosis primarily involves adamantinoma. Patient age is a helpful distinguishing criterion because osteofibrous dysplasia occurs nearly exclusively in persons who are in the first two decades of life, with adamantinoma most commonly occurring after 20 years of age.

Histologically, osteofibrous dysplasia resembles fibrous dysplasia, showing a benign, fibrous stroma containing few bony trabeculae; the main differentiating feature is the presence of numerous osteoblasts rimming the trabeculae in osteofibrous dysplasia.

Treatment is usually conservative and directed toward the prevention of increased deformity and pathologic fracture. Surgical treatment, if necessary, should be delayed until the patient is more than 10 years old because the disease or deformity may recur.

Osteomyelitis

Osteomyelitis can mimic any bone tumor clinically and radiographically (179,180). The most valid example is Ewing's sarcoma, which may present with fever, leukocytosis, lytic defects, and periosteal new bone formation. It is more difficult to differentiate subacute or chronic osteomyelitis from a bone tumor than it is to differentiate the acute form from a bone tumor.

On roentgenograms, osteomyelitis usually involves the metaphysis. The roentgenogram may show areas of permeated bone, including the cortex. In more chronic osteomyelitis, mixed areas of blastic and lytic qualities may be found. Periosteal reaction can produce Codman's triangle and onionskin patterns of periosteal new bone formation (Fig. 16). The presence of a sequestrum and lucent serpiginous track allows the distinction from a primary neoplasm of bone.

The final diagnosis of osteomyelitis rests on the growth of a microorganism from either blood or bone cultures. When all culture results are negative, the diagnosis rests on the finding of inflammatory cells, granulation tissue, and pus at microscopy.

Rarely, a squamous cell carcinoma develops in a chronic draining sinus of long-standing duration. This squamous cell carcinoma commonly involves the underlying bone.

Hyperparathyroidism

Between 30% and 40% of patients with hyperparathyroidism may have bony lesions. Because of early diagno-

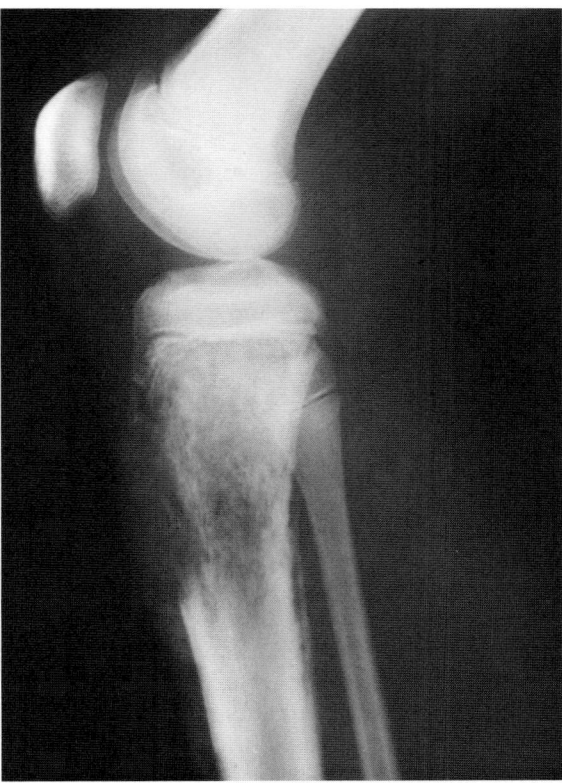

FIG. 16. Osteomyelitis of tibia that can easily be interpreted as malignant tumor such as Ewing's sarcoma or osteosarcoma.

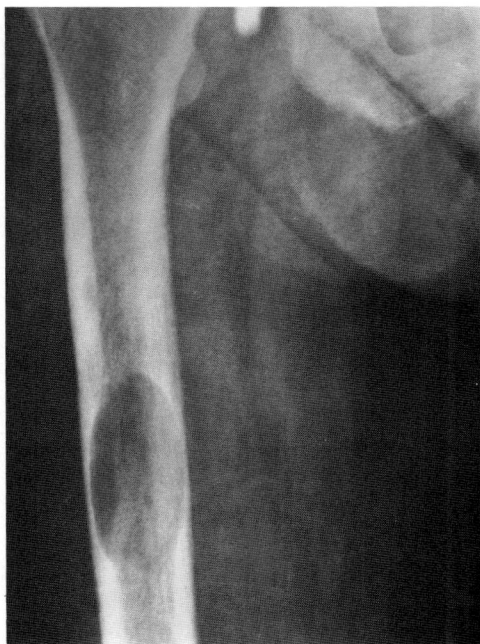

FIG. 17. Lytic lesion of midshaft of femur. Lesion is somewhat well defined but does not elicit a bone reaction. Diagnosis was brown tumor of hyperthyroidism.

sis of the condition and improved treatment, severe bony involvement is rarely encountered.

The main radiographic finding is a diffuse demineralization of the entire skeleton. Osteomalacia, osteoporosis, and multiple myeloma may produce a similar appearance on roentgenograms. The presence of nephrocalcinosis, soft-tissue calcific deposits, and salt-and-pepper calvarium is suggestive of the diagnosis. Early signs of increased bone resorption can be seen classically at the radial aspect of the second phalanx of the second and third fingers, the distal phalangeal tufts, and the distal ends of both clavicles.

Occasionally, pronounced local resorption produces a cystlike defect that may expand the contours of the bone and simulate a neoplasm, the so-called brown tumor. On plain radiographs, the brown tumor may have the appearance of a giant-cell tumor or even an aneurysmal bone cyst. When the location is not typical for giant-cell tumor (Fig. 17), the clinician should consider the possibility that the patient suffers from a metabolic abnormality. Histologically, the lesion consists of a proliferative fibroblastic tissue containing many osteoclast-like giant cells. The presence of numerous multinucleated giant cells may result in a mistaken diagnosis of giant-cell tumor. The presence of bony trabeculations, osteoclast tunneling, and fibrous stroma helps differentiate giant-cell tumor from hyperparathyroidism. The histology of hy-

perparathyroidism is not specific, and the most reliable way to confirm the diagnosis is by the determination of serum calcium and phosphorus levels as well as determination of parathyroid hormone.

The treatment of patients with bone lesions of hyperparathyroidism is usually surgical resection of the abnormal parathyroid glands (see Chapters 24 and 31). The correction of the biochemical abnormalities will allow the brown tumors to heal.

Bone Infarcts

Bone infarcts occur in deep-sea divers and in patients with sickle-cell anemia. Atherosclerosis, trauma, and immobilization also have been cited as possible causes. Bone infarcts can also be found in middle-aged persons without any known predisposition (181). Although bone infarcts are often an incidental finding on roentgenograms taken for another purpose, half of the patients with bone infarcts have a history of dull-aching pain (181).

The most frequent locations are the proximal tibia, distal femur, ilium, and calcaneus. Bone infarcts may involve multiple bones in the same patient. The lesion is usually metaphyseal and may be symmetrical. Early, there are no radiographic findings. Later, an area of bone rarefaction becomes apparent, the result of ischemic necrosis. Slowly, the lesion appears irregularly denser as new bone is deposited over the necrotic trabeculae. Spotty calcific deposits can also be seen and are produced by the deposition of calcium salt in the necrotic fatty marrow. This radiographic appearance may simu-

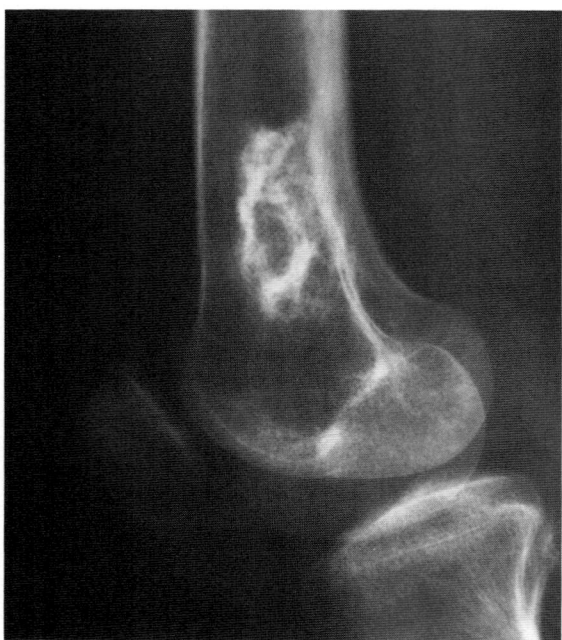

FIG. 18. Characteristic aspect of bone infarct showing fuzzy sclerotic halo with radiotransparent center.

late that of an enchondroma. However, the margins are more easily defined with a bone infarct than with an enchondroma, and the calcific deposits are less regularly dispersed than with an enchondroma. When well organized, the lesion has the typical appearance of a moderately thick serpentine border frequently outlining a central elongated area of lucency (Fig. 18). The radiographic differential diagnosis includes enchondroma, chondrosarcoma, osteoid osteoma, and osteoblastoma.

Histologically, bone infarcts are characterized by necrotic osseous trabeculae with amorphous mineralization in the degenerative marrow. New bone deposition also can be seen at the periphery of the lesion.

Treatment is conservative. Malignant bone tumors are rare but have been reported to arise in old bone infarct.

Bone Island

Bone islands represent small areas of benign osteosclerosis. They are more frequent in adults than in children. They are asymptomatic and discovered incidentally. They may appear or disappear on serial roentgenograms. The pelvis, femur, humerus, and ribs are the most frequent locations.

Usually, the islands are round or oval and seldom exceed 1 cm in diameter. They are uniformly dense, and they do not deform the contours of the bone (182). They must be differentiated from osteoid osteoma or osteoblastic metastasis. The technetium bone scan may show an increased uptake (183).

The histologic appearance of a bone island is one of a medullary lesion composed of mature compressed lamellar bone. Haversian systems may be present, as in cortical bone.

Massive Osteolysis

Massive osteolysis (Gorham's disease or disappearing bone disease) is a rare and poorly understood disease characterized by progressive and extensive resorption of bone. The process can be limited to a single bone or may cross a joint to affect the nearby bones. The most frequent locations affected are the shoulder and hip girdles (184,185).

Pain, deformity, weakness, and pathologic fractures are the usual complaints. Massive osteolysis most commonly affects children and young adults. There is no sex predilection. Despite the relentless progression of the disease, suggestive of a malignancy, the process usually, but unpredictably, ceases.

Early, the only roentgenographic findings may be some radiolucent areas in the bone involving both spongiosa and cortex. When massive osteolysis involves a long bone, a characteristic concentric shrinkage of the shaft is seen, and this has been compared to the end of a sucked candy (Fig. 19). There is no periosteal reaction or sclerotic margins that delimit the disease.

The course of the disease is unpredictable. Whole bone may disappear, and joints or intervertebral disks seem unable to limit the process.

Histologically, the disease is indistinguishable from hemangioma of bone. It is composed of cavernous vascular spaces. The endothelial cell lacks atypia or pleomorphism.

Appropriate treatment is unknown; however, radiation therapy has been employed with some success. Although benign, massive osteolysis has been responsible for a few deaths, usually due to extensive involvement of the thorax with resulting problems of pulmonary function.

Histiocytosis X

Under the name histiocytosis X, suggested by Lichtenstein (186,187), are grouped three related entities. The first is eosinophilic granuloma of bone, which is usually solitary, self-limited, and curable. The second is the Hand-Schüller-Christian syndrome, which is the disseminated form of the disease. The third subtype is the fulminating Letterer-Siwe disease, which is highly fatal.

Many hypotheses have been proposed to explain the causes of these diseases. Although often considered a malignant disease, histiocytosis X lacks certain histologic criteria, and the rate of spontaneous remission remains high for some forms of the disease.

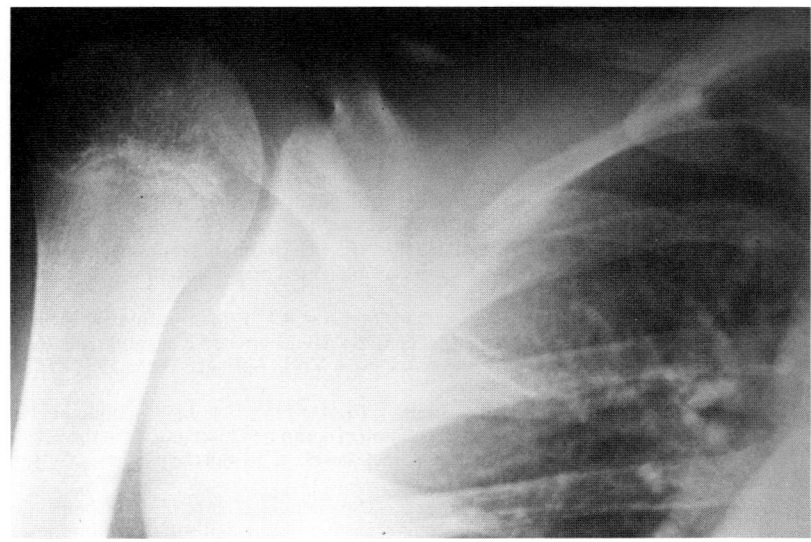

FIG. 19. Disappearing bone disease involving midportion of right clavicle of 15-year-old boy. Within months, the whole clavicle disappeared. Note the "sucked-candy" appearance of the bone ends.

Latest studies suggest that the disease has an immunologic basis. Deficiency in circulating suppressor T lymphocytes has been found as well as an increase in the ratio of helper T lymphocytes to suppressor T lymphocytes in the peripheral blood. It is still not clear if these findings are the cause or the result of the disease.

Eosinophilic granuloma is a form of histiocytosis X limited to bone (188). One or more bones may be affected. Patients are usually less than 30 years of age, and the highest incidence is in patients between the age of 5 and 10 years. The prognosis is very good and there is a high rate of cure.

In the Hand-Schüller-Christian syndrome, the disease affects the bone and the visceral organs. The onset is usually in children between the ages of 5 and 10 years, but middle-aged adults also may be affected occasionally. The manifestations are varied, and the prognosis depends on the degree of involvement and the age of the patient; young patients have a worse prognosis. The disease may be chronic.

Letterer-Siwe disease is characterized by a fulminating onset in children younger than 2 years. Severe multisystem involvement is frequent. Despite modern treatments, mortality rates as high as 20% are reported, and in some series, 50% of the survivors remain disabled.

Localized pain is the usual complaint when there are bone lesions. When there is spinal involvement, a neurologic deficit may be encountered. Pathologic fracture may occur. The locations most frequently affected are the skull and the femur for patients younger than 20 years. For older persons, the ribs and jaws are frequent sites of involvement.

The roentgenographic appearance of the bone lesions is similar in all the subtypes of histiocytosis X. The lesion is seen as a radiolucent defect with a geographic pattern. In adult patients, a thin, sclerotic rim of bone may encir-

cle the defect occasionally. Endosteal scalloping and cortical expansion may also be found. Uneven destruction of cortical surfaces may produce the classic "hole in a hole" radiographic appearance. This is most frequently seen for skull lesions. A periosteal reaction is common (Fig. 20). Occasionally, the vertebral involvement will result in total collapse of the vertebral body, the so-called vertebra plana. Bone scans, using either technetium or gallium, are unreliable in detecting the lesions because of the high rate of false negative results (189,190). The radiographic bone survey is the method of choice to exclude involvement of multiple bones.

When the lesions have a typical appearance, as do those in the skull, in vertebra plana, or in polyostotic disease, a biopsy is usually not necessary. Differential diagnosis of solitary lesions may be difficult. Ewing's sar-

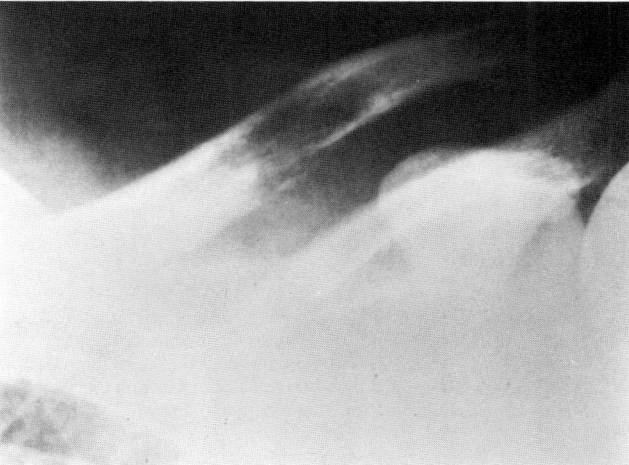

FIG. 20. Eosinophilic granuloma of clavicle presenting as poorly marginated aggressive lytic lesion. Differential diagnosis includes osteomyelitis and Ewing's sarcoma.

coma and osteomyelitis are to be ruled out, so a biopsy is often necessary.

Histologically, the pathognomonic features of eosinophilic granuloma are foci of proliferating histiocytes. These foci lack atypia, but mitotic figures are common. Multinucleated giant cells can be encountered as well as areas of necrosis. Inflammatory cells are nearly always present. Characteristically, the histiocytes contain "bean-shaped" nuclei, which have a central groove when viewed en face. Ultrastructurally, the histiocytes contain cytoplasmic inclusions called *Bierbeck granules*. These granules are also characteristic of Langerhans' cells of skin.

Treatment of eosinophilic granuloma remains controversial (191–193). The natural history of the lesion is poorly understood. When an eosinophilic granuloma is diagnosed, a bone survey should be done to exclude multiple osseous sites of involvement, and a general workup should be done to eliminate the possibility of systemic disease.

Patients with asymptomatic lesions probably should be observed at regular intervals. Patients with symptomatic lesions that need to be biopsied or that compromise the structural integrity of the bone can be treated by curettage and bone grafting. The local recurrence rate is low with this treatment. Radiation therapy using low doses (300–600 cGy) is also a successful method. It has its best use when the lesions are multiple or difficult to reach, as in the spinal column. Recently, local injections of methylprednisolone, as done for simple bone cysts, have been very successful (194,195). Treatment of the disseminated forms of histiocytosis X is more difficult and includes corticosteroids and chemotherapy and is beyond the scope of this chapter.

SUMMARY

The management of patients with primary cystic and neoplastic diseases of bone remains a challenge. The first hurdle is recognition of the existence of the lesion. Once the lesion is discovered, a systematic approach to evaluation is important. The problem is magnified by the great diversity of benign and malignant bone tumors, as well as by nonneoplastic lesions that simulate them.

REFERENCES

1. Dahlin DC. *Bone tumors: general aspects and data on 6,221 cases*, 3rd ed. Springfield, Ill: Charles C Thomas, 1978.
2. Dahlin DC, Unni KK. *Bone tumors: general aspects and data on 8,542 cases*, 4th ed. Springfield, Ill: Charles C Thomas, 1986.
3. Silverberg ES, Lubera JA. Cancer statistics, 1989. *CA* 1989;39:3–20.
4. Edeiken J. *Roentgen diagnosis of diseases of bone (Golden's diagnostic radiology series, section 6)*, vol 1, 3rd ed. Baltimore: Williams & Wilkins, 1981.
5. Greenfield GB. *Radiology of bone diseases*, 3rd ed. Philadelphia: JB Lippincott, 1980.
6. Hajdu SI. *Pathology of soft tissue tumors*. Philadelphia: Lea & Febiger, 1979.
7. Lichtenstein L. *Bone tumors*, 4th ed. St. Louis, Mo: Kimpton, 1972.
8. Hudson TM, Hamlin DJ, Enneking WF, Pettersson H. Magnetic resonance imaging of bone and soft tissue tumors: early experience in 31 patients compared with computed tomography. *Skeletal Radiol* 1985;13:134–46.
9. Levine E. Computed tomography of musculoskeletal tumors. *CRC Crit Rev Diagn Imaging* 1981;16:279–309.
10. Lukens JA, McLeod RA, Sim FH. Computed tomographic evaluation of primary osseous malignant neoplasms. *Am J Roentgenol* 1982;139:45–8.
11. Sim FH, Berquist TH, McLeod RA. Primary tumours of bone and soft tissue. In: Galasko CSB, Isherwood I, eds. *Imaging techniques in orthopaedics*. New York: Springer-Verlag, 1989;283–91.
12. Chang AE, Schaner EG, Conkle DM, Flye MW, Doppman JL, Rosenberg SA. Evaluation of computed tomography in the detection of pulmonary metastases: a prospective study. *Cancer* 1979;43:913–16.
13. Mankin HJ, Lange TA, Spanier SS. The hazards of biopsy in patients with malignant primary bone and soft-tissue tumors. *J Bone Joint Surg [Am]* 1982;64:1121–7.
14. Enneking WF, Spanier SS, Goodman MA. Current concepts reviews: the surgical staging of musculoskeletal sarcoma. *J Bone Joint Surg [Am]* 1980;62:1027–30.
15. Enneking WF, Spanier SS, Goodman MA. A system for the surgical staging of musculoskeletal sarcoma. *Clin Orthop* 1980; 153:106–20.
16. Sim FH. Principles of surgical treatment. In: Sim FH, ed. *Diagnosis and treatment of bone tumors: a team approach (a Mayo Clinic monograph)*. Rochester, Minn: Mayo Foundation, 1983;23–35.
17. Sim FH, Irwin RB, Dahlin DC. Management of benign bone tumors in children. *Progr Pediatr Hematol Oncol* 1979;2:233–56.
18. Sim FH, Unni KK, Wold LE, McLeod RA. Benign tumors. In: Sim FH, ed. *Diagnosis and treatment of bone tumors: a team approach (a Mayo Clinic monograph)*. Rochester, Minn: Mayo Foundation, 1983;107–51.
19. Jaffe HL. Hereditary multiple exostosis. *Arch Pathol* 1943; 36:335–57.
20. Solomon L. Hereditary multiple exostosis. *Am J Hum Genet* 1964;16:351–63.
21. Harsha WN. The natural history of osteocartilaginous exostoses (osteochondroma). *Am Surg* 1954;20:65–72.
22. Morton KS. On the question of recurrence of osteochondroma. *J Bone Joint Surg [Br]* 1964;46:723–5.
23. Takigawa K. Chondroma of the bones of the hand: a review of 110 cases. *J Bone Joint Surg [Am]* 1971;53:1591–600.
24. deSantos LA, Spjut HJ. Periosteal chondroma: a radiographic spectrum. *Skeletal Radiol* 1981;6:15–20.
25. Rockwell MA, Saiter ET, Enneking WF. Periosteal chondroma. *J Bone Joint Surg [Am]* 1972;54:102–8.
26. Lichtenstein L, Bernstein D. Unusual benign and malignant chondroid tumors of bone: a survey of some mesenchymal cartilage tumors and malignant chondroblastic tumors, including a few multicentric ones, as well as many atypical benign chondroblastomas and chondromyxoid fibromas. *Cancer* 1959;12:1142–57.
27. Lichtenstein L, Hall JE. Periosteal chondroma: a distinctive benign cartilage tumor. *J Bone Joint Surg [Am]* 1952;34:691–7.
28. Lewis RJ, Ketcham AS. Maffucci's syndrome: functional and neoplastic significance: case report and review of the literature. *J Bone Joint Surg [Am]* 1973;55:1465–79.
29. Jaffe HL, Lichtenstein L. Osteoid-osteoma: further experience with this benign tumor of bone. With special reference to cases showing the lesion in relation to shaft cortices and commonly misclassified as instances of sclerosing non-suppurative osteomyelitis or cortical-bone abscess. *J Bone Joint Surg* 1940; (ns)22:645–82.
30. Swee RG, McLeod RA, Beabout JW. Osteoid osteoma: detection, diagnosis, and localization. *Radiology* 1979;130:117–23.
31. Keim HA, Reina EG. Osteoid-osteoma as a cause of scoliosis. *J Bone Joint Surg [Am]* 1975;57:159–63.

32. Sim FH, Dahlin DC, Stauffer RN, Laws ER Jr. Primary bone tumors simulating lumbar disc syndrome. *Spine* 1977;2:65–74.
33. Byers PD. Solitary benign osteoblastic lesions of bone: osteoid osteoma and benign osteoblastoma. *Cancer* 1968;22:43–57.
34. Dahlin DC, Johnson EW Jr. Giant osteoid osteoma. *J Bone Joint Surg [Am]* 1954;36:559–72.
35. Sim FH, Dahlin DC, Beabout JW. Osteoid-osteoma: diagnostic problems. *J Bone Joint Surg [Am]* 1975;57:154–9.
36. Lichtenstein L, Sawyer WR. Benign osteoblastoma: further observations and report of twenty additional cases. *J Bone Joint Surg [Am]* 1964;46:755–65.
37. Marsh BW, Bonfiglio M, Brady LP, Enneking WF. Benign osteoblastoma: range of manifestations. *J Bone Joint Surg [Am]* 1975;57:1–9.
38. McLeod RA, Dahlin DC, Beabout JW. The spectrum of osteoblastoma. *Am J Roentgenol* 1976;126:321–35.
39. Schajowicz F, Lemos C. Malignant osteoblastoma. *J Bone Joint Surg [Br]* 1976;58:202–11.
40. Sim FH, Wold LE, Swee RG. Fibrous tumors of bone. *Instr Course Lect* 1984;33:40–59.
41. Bufkin WJ. The avulsive cortical irregularity. *Am J Roentgenol Radium Ther Nucl Med* 1971;112:487–92.
42. Kimmelstiel P, Rapp I. Cortical defect due to periosteal desmoids. *Bull Hosp Joint Dis* 1951;12:286–97.
43. Caffey J. On fibrous defects in cortical walls of growing tubular bones: their radiologic appearance, structure, prevalence, natural course, and diagnostic significance. *Adv Pediatr* 1955;7:13–51.
44. Simon H. Medial distal metaphyseal femoral irregularity in children. *Radiology* 1968;90:258–60.
45. Sontag LW, Pyle SI. The appearance and nature of cyst-like areas in the distal femoral metaphyses of children. *Am J Roentgenol Radium Ther* 1941;46:185–8.
46. Young DW, Nogrady MB, Dunbar JS, Wiglesworth FW. Benign cortical irregularities in the distal femur of children. *J Can Assoc Radiol* 1972;23:107–15.
47. Barnes GR Jr, Gwinn JL. Distal irregularities of the femur simulating malignancy. *Am J Roentgenol Radium Ther Nucl Med* 1974;122:180–5.
48. Arata MA, Peterson HA, Dahlin DC. Pathological fractures through non-ossifying fibromas: review of the Mayo Clinic experience. *J Bone Joint Surg [Am]* 1981;63:980–8.
49. Dahlin DC, Cupps RE, Johnson EW Jr. Giant-cell tumor: a study of 195 cases. *Cancer* 1970;25:1061–70.
50. Goldenberg RR, Campbell CJ, Bonfiglio M. Giant-cell tumor of bone: an analysis of two hundred and eighteen cases. *J Bone Joint Surg [Am]* 1970;52:619–63.
51. Larsson S-E, Lorentzon R, Boquist L. Giant-cell tumor of bone: a demographic, clinical, and histopathological study of all cases recorded in the Swedish Cancer Registry for the years 1958 through 1968. *J Bone Joint Surg [Am]* 1975;57:167–73.
52. Sung HW, Kuo DP, Shu WP, Chai YB, Liu CC, Li SM. Giant-cell tumor of bone: analysis of two hundred and eight cases in Chinese patients. *J Bone Joint Surg [Am]* 1982;64:755–61.
53. Dahlin DC. Giant cell tumor of bone: highlights of 407 cases. *Am J Roentgenol* 1985;144:955–60.
54. Jaffe HL, Lichtenstein L, Portis RB. Giant cell tumor of bone: its pathologic appearance, grading, supposed variants and treatment. *Arch Pathol* 1940;30:993–1031.
55. Campanacci M, Giunti A, Olmi R. Giant-cell tumours of bone: a study of 209 cases with long-term follow-up in 130. *Ital J Orthop Traumatol* 1975;1:249–77.
56. Duncan CP, Morton KS, Arthur JF. Giant cell tumour of bone: its aggressiveness and potential for malignant change. *Can J Surg* 1983;26:475–7.
57. McGrath PJ. Giant-cell tumour of bone: an analysis of fifty-two cases. *J Bone Joint Surg [Br]* 1972;54:216–29.
58. Sanerkin NG. Malignancy, aggressiveness, and recurrence in giant cell tumor of bone. *Cancer* 1980;46:1641–9.
59. Rock MG, Pritchard DJ, Unni KK. Metastases from histologically benign giant-cell tumor of bone. *J Bone Joint Surg [Am]* 1984;66:269–74.
60. Averill RM, Smith RJ, Campbell CJ. Giant-cell tumors of the bones of the hand. *J Hand Surg* 1980;5:39–50.
61. Peimer CA, Schiller AL, Mankin HJ, Smith RJ. Multicentric giant-cell tumor of bone. *J Bone Joint Surg [Am]* 1980;62:652–6.
62. Sim FH, Dahlin DC, Beabout JW. Multicentric giant-cell tumor of bone. *J Bone Joint Surg [Am]* 1977;59:1052–60.
63. Jacobs PA, Clemency RE Jr. Closed cryosurgical treatment of giant cell tumor, aneurysmal bone cyst and other lesions of bone (abstract). *Orthop Trans* 1983;7:195–6.
64. Malawer MM, Zielinski CJ. Giant cell tumor of bone: cryosurgery and 'en-bloc' resection, current concepts and recommendations for treatment (abstr). *Orthop Trans* 1983;7:492.
65. Marcove RC, Weis LD, Vaghaiwalla MR, Pearson R. Cryosurgery in the treatment of giant cell tumors of bone: a report of 52 consecutive cases. *Clin Orthop* 1978;134:275–89.
66. McDonald DJ, Sim FH, McLeod RA, Dahlin DC. Giant-cell tumor of bone. *J Bone Joint Surg [Am]* 1986;68:235–42.
67. Baddeley S, Cullen JC. The use of methylmethacrylate in the treatment of giant cell tumours of the proximal tibia. *Aust NZ J Surg* 1979;49:120–2.
68. Camargo FP, Camargo OP. Surgical treatment of benign cavitary bone lesions employing methyl methacrylate cement and polyethylene prosthesis: an experience with 135 cases. In: Enneking WF, chairman. *Abstracts of the international symposium on limb salvage in musculoskeletal oncology* (Bristol-Myers/Zimmer orthopaedic symposium in cooperation with the Orthopaedic Research and Education Foundation). Park Ridge, Ill: American Orthopaedic Association, 1985;vi–15.
69. Conrad EU, Enneking WF, Springfield DS. Giant cell tumor treatment with curettage and cementation. In: Enneking WF, chairman. *Abstracts of the international symposium on limb salvage in musculoskeletal oncology* (Bristol-Myers/Zimmer orthopaedic symposium in cooperation with the Orthopaedic Research and Education Foundation). Park Ridge, Ill: American Orthopaedic Association, 1985.
70. Johnston J. Treatment of giant cell tumor of bone by aggressive curettement and packing with bone cement. In: Enneking WF, chairman. *Abstracts of the international symposium on limb salvage in musculoskeletal oncology* (Bristol-Myers/Zimmer orthopaedic symposium in cooperation with the Orthopaedic Research and Education Foundation). Park Ridge, Ill: American Orthopaedic Association, 1985;vi–13.
71. Manley PA, McKeown DB, Schatzker J, Palmer NC, Carman S. Replacement of epiphyseal bone with methylmethacrylate: its effect on articular cartilage. *Arch Orthop Trauma Surg* 1982;100:3–10.
72. Persson BM, Wouters HW. Curettage and acrylic cementation in surgery of giant cell tumors of bone. *Clin Orthop* 1976;120:125–33.
73. Persson BM, Ekelund L, Lövdahl R, Gunterberg B. Favourable results of acrylic cementation for giant cell tumors. *Acta Orthop Scand* 1984;55:209–14.
74. Taminiau AHM, Wouters HW. Treatment of giant cell tumors by curettage and acrylic cementation. In: Enneking WF, chairman. *Abstracts of the international symposium on limb salvage in musculoskeletal oncology.* (Bristol-Myers/Zimmer orthopaedic symposium in cooperation with the Orthopaedic Research and Education Foundation). Park Ridge, Ill: American Orthopaedic Association, 1985;vi–6.
75. Vidal MMJ, Mimran R, Allieu Y, Jamme M, Goalard G. Plastie de comblement par métacrylate de méthyle traitement de certaines tumeurs osseuses bénignes. *Montpellier Chir* 1969;15:389–96.
76. Wilkins RM, Okada Y, Gorski JP, Sim FH, Chao EY. Methyl methacrylate replacement of subchondral bone: a biomechanical, biochemical, and morphologic analysis. In: Enneking WF, chairman. *Abstracts of the international symposium on limb salvage in musculoskeletal oncology* (Bristol-Myers/Zimmer orthopaedic symposium in cooperation with the Orthopaedic Research and Education Foundation). Park Ridge, Ill: American Orthopaedic Association, 1985;vi-7–vi-8.
77. Willert HG. Clinical results of the temporary acrylic bone cement plug in the treatment of bone tumors: a multicentric study. In: Enneking WF, chairman. *Abstracts of the international symposium on limb salvage in musculoskeletal oncology* (Bristol-Myers/Zimmer orthopaedic symposium in cooperation with the Ortho-

paedic Research and Education Foundation). Park Ridge, Ill: American Orthopaedic Association, 1985.

78. Willert GH, Enderle A. Temporary bone cement plug: an alternative treatment of large cystic tumorous bone lesions near the joint. In: Kotz R, ed. *Proceedings of the 2nd international workshop on the design and application of tumor prostheses for bone and joint reconstruction.* Wien: Egerman, 1983;69–72.

79. Wouters HW. Tumeur à cellules géantes de l'extrémité distale du fémur avec fracture intra-articulaire de genou: traitée par excochléation et remplissage avec du ciment osseux. *Rev Chir Orthop* 1974;60(suppl 2):316.

80. Campanacci M, Cervellati G. Osteosarcoma: a review of 345 cases. *Ital J Orthop Traumatol* 1975;1:5–22.

81. Dahlin DC, Coventry MB. Osteogenic sarcoma: a study of six hundred cases. *J Bone Joint Surg [Am]* 1967;49:101–10.

82. Pritchard DJ, Finkel MP, Reilly CA Jr. The etiology of osteosarcoma: a review of current considerations. *Clin Orthop* 1975;111:14–22.

83. Perkinson NG, Higinbotham NL. Osteogenic sarcoma arising in polyostotic fibrous dysplasia: report of a case. *Cancer* 1955; 8:396–402.

84. Dahlin DC, Unni KK. Osteosarcoma of bone and its important recognizable varieties. *Am J Surg Pathol* 1977;1:61–72.

85. Dahlin DC. Pathology of osteosarcoma. *Clin Orthop* 1975; 111:23–32.

86. Matsuno T, Unni KK, McLeod RA, Dahlin DC. Telangiectatic osteogenic sarcoma. *Cancer* 1976;38:2538–47.

87. Ackerman LV. Extra-osseous localized non-neoplastic bone and cartilage formation (so-called myositis ossificans): clinical and pathological confusion with malignant neoplasms. *J Bone Joint Surg [Am]* 1958;40:279–98.

88. Unni KK, Dahlin DC, Beabout JW. Periosteal osteogenic sarcoma. *Cancer* 1976;37:2476–85.

89. Bleyer WA, Haas JE, Feigl P, et al. Improved three-year disease-free survival in osteogenic sarcoma: efficacy of adjunctive chemotherapy. *J Bone Joint Surg [Br]* 1982;64:233–8.

90. Link MP. The role of adjuvant chemotherapy in the treatment of osteosarcoma of the extremity: preliminary results of the Multi-Institutional Osteosarcoma Study. In: *Proceedings of the National Institutes of Health consensus development conference on limb-sparing treatment: adult soft tissue and osteogenic sarcomas,* Dec 1984;74.

91. Rosen G, Caparros B, Huvos AG, et al. Preoperative chemotherapy for osteogenic sarcoma: selection of postoperative adjuvant chemotherapy based on the response of the primary tumor to preoperative chemotherapy. *Cancer* 1982;49:1221–30.

92. Eckhardt JJ, Eilber FR, Grant TT, Mirra JM, Weisenberger TH, Dorey FJ. The UCLA experience in the management of stage IIB osteogenic sarcoma. In: *Proceedings of the National Institutes of Health consensus development conference on limb-sparing treatment: adult soft tissue and osteogenic sarcomas,* Dec 1984;61.

93. Packard AG Jr. Prosthetic replacement of the proximal half of the humerus. *Clin Orthop* 1973;93:250–2.

94. Marcove RC, Rosen G. En bloc resections for osteogenic sarcoma. *Cancer* 1980;45:3040–4.

95. Marcove RC, Miké V, Hajek JV, Levin AG, Hutter RVP. Osteogenic sarcoma under the age of twenty-one: a review of one hundred and forty-five operative cases. *J Bone Joint Surg [Am]* 1970;52:411–23.

96. Miké V, Marcove RC. Osteogenic sarcoma under the age of 21: experience at Memorial Sloan-Kettering Cancer Center. *Progr Cancer Res Ther* 1978;6:283–92.

97. Sim FH, Bowman WE Jr, Wilkins RM, Chao EYS. Limb salvage in primary malignant bone tumors. *Orthopedics* 1985;8:574–81.

98. Sim FH, Ivins JC, Pritchard DJ. Surgical treatment of osteogenic sarcoma at the Mayo Clinic. *Cancer Treat Rep* 1978;62:205–11.

99. Sim FH, Ivins JC, Taylor WF, Chao EYS: Limb-sparing surgery for osteosarcoma: Mayo Clinic experience. *Cancer Treat Symp* 1985;3:139–54.

100. Sim FH, Beauchamp CP, Chao EYS. Reconstruction of musculoskeletal defects about the knee for tumor. *Clin Orthop* 1987;221:188–201.

101. Taylor WF, Ivins JC, Dahlin DC, Edmonson JH, Pritchard DJ. Trends and variability in survival from osteosarcoma. *Mayo Clin Proc* 1978;53:695–700.

102. Simon MA, Aschliman MA, Thomas N. Limb-salvage treatment versus amputation for osteosarcoma of the distal end of the femur. *J Bone Joint Surg [Am]* 1986;68:1331–7.

103. Czitrom AA, Langer F, McKee N, Gross AE. Bone and cartilage allotransplantation: a review of 14 years of research and clinical studies. *Clin Orthop* 1986;208:141–5.

104. Mankin HJ, Fogelson FS, Thrasher AZ, Jaffer F. Massive resection and allograft transplantation in the treatment of malignant bone tumors. *N Engl J Med* 1976;294:1247–55.

105. Parrish FF. Allograft replacement of all or part of the end of a long bone following excision of a tumor: report of twenty-one cases. *J Bone Joint Surg [Am]* 1973;55:1–22.

106. Wilson PD. Follow-up study of the use of refrigerated homogenous bone transplants in orthopaedic operations. *J Bone Joint Surg [Am]* 1951;33:307–22.

107. Kotz R, Salzer M. Rotation-plasty for childhood osteosarcoma of the distal part of the femur. *J Bone Joint Surg [Am]* 1982;64:959–69.

108. Lewis MM. The use of an expandable internal prosthesis in the management of malignant bone tumors in childhood. *Proceedings of Musculoskeletal Tumor Society,* Kansas City, Mo, May 1983.

109. Glasser DB, Lane JM, Bain M, et al. Long term survival in metastatic osteosarcoma: 85 consecutive patients. *Orthop Trans* 1987;11:495–6.

110. Spanos PK, Payne WS, Ivins JC, Pritchard DJ. Pulmonary resection for metastatic osteogenic sarcoma. *J Bone Joint Surg [Am]* 1976;58:624–8.

111. Telander RL, Pairolero PC, Pritchard DJ, Sim FH, Gilchrist GS. Resection of pulmonary metastatic osteogenic sarcoma in children. *Surgery* 1978;84:335–40.

112. Cortes EP, Holland JF, Wang JJ, et al. Amputation and Adriamycin in primary osteosarcoma. *N Engl J Med* 1974;291:998–1000.

113. Enneking WF, Kagan A. "Skip" metastases in osteosarcoma. *Cancer* 1975;36:2192–205.

114. Gehan EA, Sutow WW, Uribe-Botero G, Romsdahl M, Smith TL. Osteosarcoma: the M.D. Anderson experience, 1950–1974. *Progr Cancer Res Ther* 1978;6:271–82.

115. Friedman MA, Carter SK. The therapy of osteogenic sarcoma: current status and thoughts for the future. *J Surg Oncol* 1972;4:482–510.

116. Jaffe N, Frei E III, Traggis D, Bishop Y. Adjuvant methotrexate and citrovorum-factor treatment of osteogenic sarcoma. *N Engl J Med* 1974;291:994–7.

117. Rosen G, Marcove RC, Caparros B, Nirenberg A, Kosloff C, Huvos AG. Primary osteogenic sarcoma: the rationale for preoperative chemotherapy and delayed surgery. *Cancer* 1979;43:2163–77.

118. Aurias A, Rimbaut C, Buffe D, Zucker JM, Mazabraud A. Translocation involving chromosome 22 in Ewing's sarcoma: a cytogenetic study of four fresh tumors. *Cancer Genet Cytogenet* 1984;12:21–5.

119. Douglass EC, Valentine M, Green AA, Hayes FA, Thompson EI. t(11;22) and other chromosomal rearrangements in Ewing's sarcoma. *J Natl Cancer Inst* 1986;77:1211–3.

120. Israel MA, Thiele C, Whang-Peng J, Kao-Shan C-S, Triche TJ, Miser J. Peripheral neuroepithelioma: genetic analysis of tumor derived cell lines. *Progr Clin Biol Res* 1985;175:161–70.

121. Prieto F, Badía L, Montalar J, Massuti B. Translocation (11;22) in Ewing's sarcoma. *Cancer Genet Cytogenet* 1985;17:87–9.

122. Turc-Carel C, Philip I, Berger MP, Philip T, Lenoir GM. Chromosome study of Ewing's sarcoma (ES) cell lines: consistency of a reciprocal translocation t(11;22) (q24;q12). *Cancer Genet Cytogenet* 1984;12:1–19.

123. Dahlin DC, Coventry MB, Scanlon PW. Ewing's sarcoma: a critical analysis of 165 cases. *J Bone Joint Surg [Am]* 1961;43:185–92.

124. Pritchard DJ, Dahlin DC, Dauphine RT, Taylor WF, Beabout JW. Ewing's sarcoma: a clinicopathological and statistical analysis of patients surviving five years or longer. *J Bone Joint Surg [Am]* 1975;57:10–6.

125. Dahlin DC. Bone and soft-tissue sarcomas: is it worthwhile to differentiate Ewing's sarcoma and primary lymphoma of bone? *Proc Natl Cancer Conf* 1972;7:941–5.

126. Reimer RR, Chabner BA, Young RC, Reddick R, Johnson RE.

Lymphoma presenting in bone. Results of histopathology, staging, and therapy. *Ann Intern Med* 1977;87:50–5.

127. Schajowicz F. Ewing's sarcoma and reticulum-cell sarcoma of bone: with special reference to the histochemical demonstration of glycogen as an aid to differential diagnosis. *J Bone Joint Surg [Am]* 1959;41:349–56.

128. Razek A, Perez CA, Tefft M, et al. Intergroup Ewing's sarcoma study: local control related to radiation dose, volume, and site of primary lesion in Ewing's sarcoma. *Cancer* 1980;46:516–21.

129. Bacci G, Picci P, Gitelis S, Borghi A, Campanacci M. The treatment of localized Ewing's sarcoma: the experience at the Instituto Ortopedico Rizzoli in 163 cases treated with and without adjuvant chemotherapy. *Cancer* 1982;49:1561–70.

130. Chan RC, Sutow WW, Lindberg RD, Samuels ML, Murray JA, Johnston DA. Management and results of localized Ewing's sarcoma. *Cancer* 1979;43:1001–6.

131. Rosen G, Caparros B, Mosende C, McCormick B, Huvos AG, Marcove RC. Curability of Ewing's sarcoma and considerations for future therapeutic trials. *Cancer* 1978;41:888–99.

132. Rosen G, Caparros B, Nirenberg A, et al. Ewing's sarcoma: ten-year experience with adjuvant chemotherapy. *Cancer* 1981; 47:2204–13.

133. Zucker JM, Henry-Amar M. Therapeutic controlled trial in Ewing's sarcoma: report on the results of a trial by the clinical cooperative group on radio- and chemotherapy of the E.O.R.T.C. *Eur J Cancer* 1977;13:1019–23.

134. Telles NC, Rabson AS, Pomeroy TC. Ewing's sarcoma: an autopsy study. *Cancer* 1978;41:2321–9.

135. Johnson RE, Pomeroy TC: Evaluation of therapeutic results in Ewing's sarcoma. *Am J Roentgenol* 1975;123:583–7.

136. Macintosh DJ, Price CHG, Jeffree GM. Ewing's tumour: a study of behaviour and treatment in forty-seven cases. *J Bone Joint Surg [Br]* 1975;57:331–40.

137. Li WK, Lane JM, Rosen G, et al. Pelvic Ewing's sarcoma: advances in treatment. *J Bone Joint Surg [Am]* 1983;65:738–47.

138. Furey JG, Ferrer-Torells M, Reagan JW. Fibrosarcoma arising at the site of bone infarcts: a report of two cases. *J Bone Joint Surg [Am]* 1960;42:802–10.

139. Dahlin DC, Salvador AH. Chondrosarcomas of bones of the hands and feet: a study of 30 cases. *Cancer* 1974;34:755–60.

140. Barnes R, Catto M. Chondrosarcoma of bone. *J Bone Joint Surg [Br]* 1966;48:729–64.

141. Campanacci M, Guernelli N, Leonessa C, Boni A. Chondrosarcoma: a study of 133 cases, 80 with long term follow-up. *Ital J Orthop Traumatol* 1975;1:387–414.

142. Gilmer WS Jr, Kilgore W, Smith H. Central cartilage tumors of bone. *Clin Orthop* 1963;26:81–102.

143. Dahlin DC. Chondrosarcoma and its "variants." *Monogr Pathol* 1976;17:300–7.

144. Dahlin DC, Beabout JW. Dedifferentiation of low-grade chondrosarcomas. *Cancer* 1971;28:461–6.

145. Dahlin DC, Henderson ED. Mesenchymal chondrosarcoma: further observations on a new entity. *Cancer* 1962;15:410–7.

146. Salvador AH, Beabout JW, Dahlin DC. Mesenchymal chondrosarcoma: observations on 30 new cases. *Cancer* 1971;28:605–15.

147. Guccion JG, Font RL, Enzinger FM, Zimmerman LE. Extraskeletal mesenchymal chondrosarcoma. *Arch Pathol* 1973; 95:336–40.

148. Unni KK, Dahlin DC, Beabout JW, Sim FH. Chondrosarcoma: clear-cell variant. A report of sixteen cases. *J Bone Joint Surg [Am]* 1976;58:676–83.

149. Lettin AWF. Fibular replacement of the upper humerus after segmental resection for chondrosarcoma. *Proc R Soc Med* 1964;57:90–2.

150. Sim FH. Chondrosarcoma. In: Uhthoff HK, Stahl E, eds. *Current concepts of diagnosis and treatment of bone and soft tissue tumors.* New York: Springer-Verlag, 1984;405–10.

151. Salzer M, Knahr K, Locke H, et al. A bioceramic endoprosthesis for the replacement of the proximal humerus. *Arch Orthop Trauma Surg* 1979;93:169–84.

152. Sim FH, Chao EYS. Hip salvage by proximal femoral replacement. *J Bone Joint Surg [Am]* 1981;63:1228–38.

153. Sim FH, Chao EYS, Pritchard DJ, Salzer M. Replacement of the proximal humerus with a ceramic prosthesis: a preliminary report. *Clin Orthop* 1980;146:161–74.

154. Sim FH, Beauchamp CP, Chao EYS. Joint arthrodesis: with particular reference to knee arthrodesis using a porous-coated intercalary prosthesis. In: Combs R, ed. *Bone tumour management.* Greenborough, Kent: Butterworth, 1987.

155. Enneking WF, Dunham WK. Resection and reconstruction for primary neoplasms involving the innominate bone. *J Bone Joint Surg [Am]* 1978;60:731–46.

156. Cohen J. Etiology of simple bone cyst. *J Bone Joint Surg [Am]* 1970;52:1493–7.

157. Morton KS. The pathogenesis of unicameral bone cyst. *Can J Surg* 1964;7:140–50.

158. Campanacci M, Capanna R, Picci P. Unicameral and aneurysmal bone cysts. *Clin Orthop* 1986;204:25–36.

159. Cohen J. Unicameral bone cysts: a current synthesis of reported cases. *Orthop Clin North Am* 1977;8(4):715–36.

160. Garceau GJ, Gregory CF. Solitary unicameral bone cyst. *J Bone Joint Surg [Am]* 1954;36:267–80.

161. Smith RW, Smith CF. Solitary unicameral bone cyst of the calcaneus: a review of twenty cases. *J Bone Joint Surg [Am]* 1974;56:49–56.

162. Jaffe HL, Lichtenstein L. Solitary unicameral bone cyst: with emphasis on the roentgen picture, the pathologic appearance and the pathogenesis. *Arch Surg* 1942;44:1004–25.

163. Cohen J. Simple bone cysts: studies of cyst fluid in six cases with a theory of pathogenesis. *J Bone Joint Surg [Am]* 1960;42:609–16.

164. Neer CS II, Francis KC, Marcove RC, Terz J, Carbonara PN. Treatment of unicameral bone cyst: a follow-up study of one hundred seventy-five cases. *J Bone Joint Surg [Am]* 1966;48:731–45.

165. Neer CS II, Francis KC, Johnston AD, Kiernan HA Jr. Current concepts on the treatment of solitary unicameral bone cyst. *Clin Orthop* 1973;97:40–51.

166. Oppenheim WL, Galleno H. Operative treatment versus steroid injection in the management of unicameral bone cysts. *J Pediatr Orthop* 1984;4:1–7.

167. Spence KF, Sell KW, Brown RH. Solitary bone cyst: treatment with freeze-dried cancellous bone allograft. A study of one hundred seventy-seven cases. *J Bone Joint Surg [Am]* 1969; 51:87–96.

168. Spence KF Jr, Bright RW, Fitzgerald SP, Sell KW. Solitary unicameral bone cyst: treatment with freeze-dried crushed cortical-bone allograft. A review of one hundred and forty-four cases. *J Bone Joint Surg [Am]* 1976;58:636–41.

169. Scaglietti O, Marchetti PG, Bartolozzi P. The effects of methylprednisolone acetate in the treatment of bone cysts: results of three years follow-up. *J Bone Joint Surg [Br]* 1979;61:200–4.

170. Scaglietti O, Marchetti PG, Bartolozzi P. Final results obtained in the treatment of bone cysts with methylprednisolone acetate (Depo-Medrol) and a discussion of results achieved in other bone lesions. *Clin Orthop* 1982;165:33–42.

171. Tillman BP, Dahlin DC, Lipscomb PR, Stewart JR. Aneurysmal bone cyst: an analysis of ninety-five cases. *Mayo Clin Proc* 1968;43:478–95.

172. Zimmer WD, Berquist TH, Sim FH, et al. Magnetic resonance imaging of aneurysmal bone cyst. *Mayo Clin Proc* 1984;59:633–6.

173. Sim FH. Aneurysmal bone cyst. In: Uhthoff HK, Stahl E, eds. *Current concepts of diagnosis and treatment of bone and soft tissue tumors.* New York: Springer-Verlag, 1984;255–60.

174. Nobler MP, Higinbotham NL, Phillips RF. The cure of aneurysmal bone cyst: irradiation superior to surgery in an analysis of 33 cases. *Radiology* 1968;90:1185–92.

175. Harris WH, Dudley HR Jr, Barry RJ. The natural history of fibrous dysplasia: an orthopaedic, pathological, and roentgenographic study. *J Bone Joint Surg [Am]* 1962;44:207–33.

176. Coley BL, Stewart FW. Bone sarcoma in polyostotic fibrous dysplasia. *Ann Surg* 1945;121:872–81.

177. Schwartz DT, Alpert M. The malignant transformation of fibrous dysplasia. *Am J Med Sci* 1964;247:1–20.

178. Campanacci M. Osteofibrous dysplasia of long bones: a new clinical entity. *Ital J Orthop Traumatol* 1976;2:221–37.

179. Cabanela ME, Sim FH, Beabout JW, Dahlin DC. Osteomyelitis appearing as neoplasms: a diagnostic problem. *Arch Surg* 1974;109:68–72.

180. Elliott GR. Chronic osteomyelitis presenting distinct tumor for-

mation simulating clinically true osteogenic sarcoma. *J Bone Joint Surg* 1934;16:137–44.

181. Bullough PG, Kambolis CP, Marcove RC, Jaffe HL. Bone infarctions not associated with Caisson disease. *J Bone Joint Surg [Am]* 1965;47:477–91.

182. Onitsuka H. Roentgenologic aspects of bone islands. *Radiology* 1977;123:607–12.

183. Davies JAK, Hall FM, Goldberg RP, Kasdon EJ. Positive bone scan in a bone island: case report. *J Bone Joint Surg [Am]* 1979;61:943–5.

184. Bullough PG. Massive osteolysis. *NY State J Med* 1971;71:2267–78.

185. Johnson PM, McClure JG. Observations on massive osteolysis: a review of the literature and report of a case. *Radiology* 1958;71:28–41.

186. Lichtenstein L. Histiocytosis X: integration of eosinophilic granuloma of bone, "Letterer-Siwe disease," and "Schüller-Christian disease" as related manifestations of a single nosologic entity. *Arch Pathol* 1953;56:84–102.

187. Lichtenstein L. Histiocytosis X (eosinophilic granuloma of bone, Letterer-Siwe disease, and Schüller-Christian disease): further observations of pathological and clinical importance. *J Bone Joint Surg [Am]* 1964;46:76–90.

188. Schajowicz F, Slullitel J. Eosinophilic granuloma of bone and its relationship to Hand-Schüller-Christian and Letterer-Siwe syndromes. *J Bone Joint Surg [Br]* 1973;55:545–65.

189. Gerrard MP, Hendry MH, Eden OB. Comparison of radiographic and sciyntigraphic assessment of skeletal lesions in histiocytosis X. *Workshop on the childhood histiocytoses: concepts and controversies,* May 16–17, 1985, The Children's Hospital of Philadelphia Children's Cancer Research Center, Philadelphia, Pa.

190. Siddiqui AR, Tashjian JH, Lazarus K, Wellman HN, Baehner RL. Nuclear medicine studies in evaluation of skeletal lesions in children with histiocytosis X. *Radiology* 1981;140:787–9.

191. Broadbent V, Pritchard J. Histiocytosis X: current controversies. *Arch Dis Child* 1985;60:605–7.

192. Mickelson MR, Bonfiglio M. Eosinophilic granuloma and its variations. *Orthop Clin North Am* 1977;8(4):933–45.

193. Winkelmann RK, Burgert EO. Therapy of histiocytosis X. *Br J Dermatol* 1970;82:169–75.

194. Capanna R, Springfield DS, Ruggieri P, et al. Direct cortisone injection in eosinophilic granuloma of bone: a preliminary report on 11 patients. *J Pediatr Orthop* 1985;5:339–42.

195. Cohen M, Zornoza J, Cangir A, Murray JA, Wallace S. Direct injection of methylprednisolone sodium succinate in the treatment of solitary eosinophilic granuloma of bone: a report of 9 cases. *Radiology* 1980;136:289–93.

Subject Index

A

Absorptive hypercalciuria, 687
Acetazolamide
    calcium, 15–16
    phosphate excretion, 30
Acid-base balance
    calcium, 14–15
    kidney, 734–735
        ammonia excretion, 735
        fixed acid metabolism, 734–735
        hydrogen ion excretion, 735
        liver, 734
        lung, 734
        phosphate reabsorption, systemic, 26
        renal phosphate excretion, 25–26
Acid mucopolysaccharide, calcium oxalate
    crystallization inhibitor, 784
Acidic fibroblast growth factor, 255
    bone matrix, 255
Acromegaly
    bone biopsy, 463–464
    histomorphometry, 463–464
Actin, serum calcium, mRNA levels, 86
Actin binding, vitamin D-binding protein,
    202
Activation, remodeling, 356–359
Acute renal failure, 440
Adaptive remodeling, 355
Addison's disease, 440
Adenylate cyclase
    bioamine hormone receptor, periodically
        recurring regions of hydrophobicity,
        137–138
    G protein, 140
    guanine nucleotide guanosine
        triphosphate, 138
    parathyroid hormone
        effect specificity, 134–135
        stimulation, 127–130
    polypeptide hormone receptor,
        periodically recurring regions of
        hydrophobicity, 137–138
Adenylate-cyclase-linked receptor
    gene structure, 138
    purification, 137–138
ADFR
    bone mass, 871–872
    osteoporosis, 871–872
ADP-ribosylation, 140
    G protein, 140
    pertussis toxin, 140
Adult, calcium metabolism, integration,
    417–428

Adult hypophosphatemic rickets, 942
    alkaline phosphatase, 937
    calcium, 937
    calcium absorption, 937
    1,25-dihydroxyvitamin D, 937
    25-hydroxyvitamin D, 937
    parathyroid hormone, 937
    phosphorus, 937
    phosphorus absorption, 937
    urinary calcium, 937
    urinary phosphorus, 937
Age
    bone, 374
    cancellous bone
        packet wall thickness, 371
        volume, 371
    remodeling, 370–373
Akaline phosphatase, subperiosteal bone, 257
Albumin, plasma carrier features, 202
Alcohol, osteoporosis, 850
Alcohol-induced bone disease, 440, 964,
        965–968
    clinical features, 965, 966, 967, 968
    incidence, 965
    pathogenesis, 965–968
    prevalence, 965
    treatment, 968
Alcohol withdrawal, hypophosphatemia, 590
Alcoholism, 440
    bone biopsy, 470
    histomorphometry, 470
    hypophosphatemia, 590
Alkaline phosphatase
    adult hypophosphatemic rickets, 937
    bone matrix, 251
    calbindin, 167
    child, normal values, 408
    1,25-dihydroxyvitamin D_3, 167
    Fanconi's syndrome, 937
    hereditary hypophosphatemic rickets with
        hypercalciuria, 937
    hypophosphatasia, 977
    kidney, 259
    liver, 259
    matrix vesicle, inorganic phosphate
        generation, 333
    Paget's disease, 1042
    pseudovitamin D deficiency, 937
    vitamin D dependent rickets
        type I, 937
        type II, 937
    X-linked hypophosphatemic rickets, 937

Allopurinol
    calcium oxalate stone, 785–787
    uric acid calculus, 804–805
Altered divalent-ion metabolism
    biochemical features, 912–914
    clinical features, 912–914
Aluminum, dialysis
    accumulation, 921
    deferrioxamine, 921
Aluminum carbonate
    dialysis dementia, 916
    renal osteodystrophy, 916
Aluminum hydroxide
    dialysis dementia, 916
    renal osteodystrophy, 916
Amiloride
    calcium, 16
    idiopathic hypercalciuria, 702
Amino acid, 733
Aminoglycoside nephropathy, 440
Aminohydroxypropylidene diphosphonate,
        Paget's disease, 1057–1058
Ammonia, hyperchloremic acidosis, 741–742
Ammonia excretion, renal tubular acidosis
        type I, 738
Amorphous calcium phosphate theory, bone
        mineral phase, 267
    alternative theories, 267–269
    limitations, 267–269
Amphotericin nephropathy, 440
Amyloid, dialysis, 912
Anabolic agent, osteoporosis, 869–870
Anatrophic nephrolithotomy, staghorn
        calculus, 660, 661
Androgen
    bone resorption, 298–299
    osteoporosis, 869
Androstanedione, osteoporosis, 869
Aneurysmal bone cyst, 1078–1079
Angiogenesis, growth plate, 343–344
Angiogenic (growth) factor, growth plate,
        capillary invasion, 343–344
Angiotension, calcium, 14
Anorexia, hypercalcemia, 510
Anti-inflammatory drug, Paget's disease,
        1052
Anti-receptor monoclonal antibody,
        1,25-dihydroxyvitamin D_3 receptor,
        174
Anticonvulsant medication
    bone disease, 968–969
    bone biopsy, 464
    clinical features, 968–969

Anticonvulsant medication, bone disease
  (contd.)
    histomorphometry, 464
    incidence, 968
    pathogenesis, 969
    prevalence, 968
    treatment, 969
    osteoporosis, 900–901
Antidiuresis, nephron
    calcium reabsorption, 42
    chloride reabsorption, 42
    magnesium reabsorption, 42
    sodium reabsorption, 42
    water reabsorption, 42
Antiestrogen
    hypercalcemia, 508
    hypercalcemic flare, 540
Antimicrobial agent, struvite calculus,
    817–818
AP-1-binding protein complex,
    1,25-dihydroxyvitamin D₃
    responsive element, 183
Apatite, 269
    calcium oxalate crystallization promoter,
      794–796
    cell interactions, 795–796
    in vitro experiments, 794–795
Apical ectodermal ridge, 221
Appendicular skeleton
    adult, 224
    development, 221
Apposition rate, osteoid thickness, 487
Arteriovenous fistula, percutaneous
    nephrostolithotomy, 634, 635
Arthropathy, Paget's disease, 1042
Articular cartilage, 315
Ascorbic acid, 708
    oxalate analysis, 712–713
Ascorbic acid metabolism, pathway, 708
Asymptomatic osteosclerosis, 870
Atrial natriuretic factor, phosphate excretion,
    29
Atypical insufficiency fracture, transileal
    bone biopsy, 471
Autoimmune polyglandular syndrome type I,
    hypocalcemia, 573–574
Autosomal dominant hypophosphatemic
    rickets, 942
Avian egg-laying, 1,25-dihydroxyvitamin D₃
    biosynthesis, 166
Axial osteomalacia, 439, 986–987
    clinical presentation, 986–987
    etiology, 987
    histopathologic findings, 987
    laboratory studies, 987
    pathogenesis, 987
    radiologic features, 987
    treatment, 987
Axial skeleton
    adult, 224–225
    development, 220–221
    Paget's disease, 1035
Axial weakness, 438

B
Back pain, 437
Band keratopathy, 438

Bartter's syndrome, hypocalciuria, 16
Basic fibroblast growth factor, 255
    bone matrix, 255
    growth plate, 343
Basic multicellular unit, 356
Basolateral membrane
    calcium
        Ca-Na exchange system, 6
        calcium exit, 6–8
        calcium ATPase, 7
    phosphate transport, 24
Benign osteopetrosis, 990
Berylliosis, 567
Bicarbonate
    biochemical sites of excess, 731
    reactions generating excess, 730
Bicarbonate generation, renal tubular
    acidosis, decreased, 736
Bicarbonate reabsorption
    renal acid excretion, 729–730
    renal tubular acidosis, decreased, 735–736
Biglycan, 244–245, 246, 246–250
    immunohistochemical localization, 246
    schematic representation, 245
Biliary atresia, 439
Bioamine hormone receptor, adenylate
    cyclase, periodically recurring regions
    of hydrophobicity, 137–138
Bioassay
    parathyroid hormone, 113
        adenylate cyclase activity, 113
        cyclic AMP production, 113
        glucose-6–phosphate dehydrogenase
          activity, 113
        parathyroid hormone related polypeptide,
          113
Biochemical abnormality, renal
    osteodystrophy, 115–117
Biochemical marker, bone matrix protein,
    258–259
Biologically induced mineralization, bone
    calcification, 274
Biomechanical competence, remodeling,
    364–367
Bisphosphonate
    bone loss, 866–867
    bone resorption inhibition, 515, 516
    osteoporosis, 866–867
Blood-bone barrier, plasma mineral level, 369
Blood calcium ion level, 757
Blue sclera, 438
Bone. See also Specific type
    age, 374
        histomorphometry, 483–485
    anatomy, 219–239
    benign fibrous lesions, 1069–1070
    calcium, distribution determinants, 419
    embryology, 219–239
    eroded surface, 230, 231
    fiber-mineral composite, functional
      adaptation, 226–227
    forming surface, 229–230, 231
    Howship's lacuna, 230, 231
    lining cell, 232
    macroscopic organization, 222–225
    matrix-mineral composite, 225–226
    mechanical properties, 226, 227

    mechanical strength, 226, 227
    mechanostat, 238
        setpoint change, 238–239
    microcrack, 364, 366
    microdamage, 364, 365
    microstructure, 219–239
    mineral content separation, 268
    osteoid surface, 229–230, 231
    parathyroid hormone
        anabolic actions, 124–125
        catabolic actions, 123–124
        coupling, 124
    parathyroid hormone binding site, 136
    primary hyperparathyroidism, 495–496
    resorbing surface, 230, 231
    resting surface, 229, 230
    RGD-containing protein, RGD region
        predicted conformation, 250
    strain, 237–238
    stress, 237–238
    structural adaptation to mechanical usage,
      237–239
        safety margin, 238
    structural organ, 222–225
    as tissue, 225–227
    transitional zone, 229
Bone balance, histomorphometry, 483–485
Bone biopsy, 455–471. See also Specific type
    acromegaly, 463–464
    alcoholism, 470
    anticonvulsant drug-induced bone disease,
      464
    arrangements, 456–457
    gastrointestinal disease, 468
    glucocorticoid, 464
    hemodialysis, 466–467
    hepatic osteodystrophy, 471
    hypophosphatasia, 470
    immobilization, 464
    indications, 455
    limitations, 455–456
    mastocytosis, 465
    osteogenesis imperfecta, 470
    osteomalacia, 468, 469
    osteoporosis, 465–466
    Paget's disease, 469–470
    postmenopausal osteoporosis, 465–466
    primary hyperparathyroidism, 463, 496,
      497
    renal osteodystrophy, 466–468
    requirements, 455
    specimen evaluation, 458–460
        examination list, 458
    thyrotoxicosis, 468–469
Bone calcification, 269–273
    biologically induced mineralization, 274
    chondrocyte, 319
    collagen
        calcium, 278
        chondroblast, 278
        osteoblast, 278
        phosphate, 278
    collagen fibril, 271, 279–284
        phosphoprotein, 280–283
    crystal formation, 276
        alignment, 276
        collagen, 276–279

nucleation site, 277
orientation, 276
postulated role, 276–279
solid mineral phase, 276
diagrammatic representation, 277
embryo, 274
extracellular compartments, 277
growth plate, vasculature, 318
heterogeneous nucleation, 274
homogeneous nucleation, 274
independent nucleation sites, 271
intracellular compartments, 277
matrix-mediated mineralization, 274
mechanism, 273–279
membrane phospholipid, 334
calcium phosphate-phospholipid
complex, 334
metastable equilibrium, 274
metastable solution, 274
metastable state, 274
phase transformation, 273
phosphoprotein, recent data, 284
state of aggregation, 273
Bone cell, 230–234
Bone collagen, soft tissue collagen,
comparison, 244
Bone crystal
heterogeneous sample, 267
size, 266
Bone cyst, 440
aneurysmal, 1078–1079
unicameral, 1078
Bone densitometry, 446–451
bone mass assessment, 446–447
primary hyperparathyroidism, 496
principles, 446
Bone deposition, Paget's disease, 1032–1033
Bone disease
anticonvulsant medication, 968–969
clinical features, 968–969
incidence, 968
pathogenesis, 969
prevalence, 968
treatment, 969
clinical approach, 435–441
clinical findings, 436–440
gastrointestinal disease, 959–963
laboratory approach, 435–441
liver disease, 963–968
physical findings, 437
recognition, 436–440
symptoms, 436–440
total parenteral nutrition, 970–971
clinical features, 970
incidence, 970
pathogenesis, 970–971
prevalence, 970
treatment, 971
Bone envelope, 227–229. See also Specific
type
Bone formation
alternative models, 477
cell cycle, cellular activity, 257–258
cellular biology, 241–259
enchondral calcification, postnatal, 314
histomorphometry, indices, 481–483
model, 479

molecular biochemistry, 241–259
off-time, 230
patterns, 241, 243
prenatal, 313–314
rate, in canine skeleton, 375
Bone-forming cell, mineralized matrix
non-structural components, 241, 242
organic composition, 241, 242
Bone gene, structural features, 253
Bone gene transcribed product, structural
features, 253
Bone growth
fracture healing, 314
growth plate, role, 313
Bone histogenesis, 221–222
Bone histology
malignancy-associated hypercalcemia, 541
osteomalacia, 911–912
secondary hyperparathyroidism, 910–911
Bone histomorphometry, normal values,
460–463
race, 461–462
Bone infarct, 1081–1082
Bone island, 1082
Bone loss
bisphosphonate, 866–867
calcium, 847–848
1,25-dihydroxyvitamin D, 847
estrogen, 845–846
menopause, 845–846
metabolic defect, 847
osteoporosis, 844–850
Bone marrow, osteoclast, 290
Bone mass
ADFR, 871–872
estradiol, 842, 843
menopause, 841–844, 845–847
osteoporosis
consolidation, 840–841
control of peak, 839–841
genetic factors, 839–840
sexual maturation, 402–403
Bone mass assessment
bone densitometry, 446–447
indications, 450–451
noninvasive techniques, 448
Bone mass quantitation, fracture, 450
normal vs. osteoporotic groups, 450
predictive value, 450
risk factor value, 450
Bone matrix
acidic fibroblast growth factor, 255
alkaline phosphatase, 251
basic fibroblast growth factor, 255
cartilage, 256
circulation, proteins adsorbed, 251–252
degradation, 293
1,25-dihydroxyvitamin D₃, 256
enzyme, 251
enzyme inhibitor, 251
estrogen, 256
functions, 259
growth factor, 242, 250–251
synthesis, 255
turnover, 255
insulin-like growth factor, 255
mineralization, 252–253

parathyroid hormone, 256
platelet-derived growth factor, 256
somatomedin, 255
transforming growth factor-beta, 255–256
Bone matrix formation, regulation, 255–257
local factors, 255–256
systemic factors, 256–257
Bone matrix gene expression, subperiosteal
bone, pattern, 254
Bone matrix protein
biochemical marker, 258–259
molecular biology, 253–255
Bone metabolism, kidney transplantation,
922–928
Bone mineral age, 266
Bone mineral phase
amorphous calcium phosphate theory, 267
alternative theories, 267–269
limitations, 267–269
biological functions, 265–266
changes over time, 266–267
collagen, location, 273
location, 269–273
nature, 266–267
theories, 267–269
Bone mineralization, race, 405
Bone pain, 436
Bone remodeling, 355–376
activation, 356–359
age, 370–373
animal models, 374–376
biomechanical competence, 364–367
calcium, 847–848
epidemiological data, 847–848
calcium stress, 369
cancellous bone, 374
cell cycle, analogy between, 475–476
cellular mechanism, 356–364
concepts, 475–478
cycle
cancellous bone, 357, 358
cortical bone, 357
cycle in detail, 477–478
cycle-period relationship, 476
definition, 355–356
formation, 364
bone structural unit, 364
cancellous osteon, 364
closing cone, 364
Haversian system, 364
mineralization lag time, 364
packet, 364
secondary osteon, 364
trabecular osteon, 364
functional significance, 364–370
historical perspective, 355–356
menopause, 370–372, 845–847
microcrack, 364–367
mineral homeostasis, 367–370
calcium, 368–369
vitamin D, 368
normal, 844
osteoclast, 287–288, 844
osteoporosis, 844–850
phosphate homeostasis, 368–369
quantal remodeling theory, 476
race, 370–373

Bone remodeling (contd.)
  resorption, 358, 359, 360, 361
    coupling, 363
      1,25-dihydroxyvitamin D, 363
      Haversian system, 359, 361
      interleukin-1, 363
      parathyroid hormone, 363
    reversal, 359-363
    sex, 370-373
    skeletal envelope
      tissue balance, 373
      variation, 373-374
    skeleton, 236-237
    vs. modeling, 235
    three levels of organization, 476-477
Bone remodeling unit, 356
Bone resorption
  androgen, 298-299
  cell interactions, 289
  cytokine, 297
  enzyme inhibitor, 300
  estrogen, 298-299
  glucocorticoid, 298
  growth factor, 297-298
  hormone analog, 299-300
  interleukin-1, 297
  ion transport inhibitor, 300-301
  lining cell, 288
  local inhibitors, 299
  local stimulators, 295-298
  monocyte-macrophage, 289
  nonsteroidal anti-inflammatory drug, 296
  osteoblast, 288
  osteoclast
    factors halting, 298-299
    mechanisms, 287-301
    regulation, 287-301, 293-295
    significance, 287-288
  osteocyte, 288
  Paget's disease, 1032
  parathyroid hormone, 295-296
  pathologic agents, 299-301
  pathologic regulators, 295
  pharmacologic agents, 299-301
  phosphate compound, 300
  physiologic regulators, 295
  prostaglandin, 296-297
  prostaglandin E2, 296-297
  prostaglandin F2alpha, 296
  retinol, 297
  systemic stimulators, 295-298
  thyroid hormone, 297
  vitamin A, 297
  vitamin D, 296
Bone resorption inhibition
  bisphosphonate, 515, 516
  etidronate, 515, 517
  gallium nitrate, 515, 517
  mithramycin, 515, 516
  phosphate, 516
  plicamycin, 515, 516
  prostaglandin inhibitor, 516
  WR2721, 515, 517
Bone sample
  compositional studies, 266-267
  structural studies, 266-267
Bone scan, 451-453

Bone sialoprotein, 246-250
  biochemical features, 246
Bone surface, 229-230. See also Specific type
Bone tissue, material properties, 226
Bone tumor, 1065-1078
  benign, 440, 1066-1071
  biopsy, 1065-1066
  lesions simulating, 1078-1084
  malignant, 440, 1071-1078
  staging, 1065-1066
Bony island, 314
Brachydactyly, pseudohypoparathyroidism,
  575, 576, 577, 579
Brush-border membrane, phosphate
  transport, 20-23
  ADP-ribosylation, 22-23
  allosteric regulation by H^+, 21-22
  allosteric regulation by Na^+, 21-22
  covalent modification, 22-23
  endocytosis, 23
  exocytosis, 23
  lipid microenvironment, 23
  membrane lipid orientation, 23
  membrane recycling, 23
  Na^+-phosphate cotransporter regulation,
    21-23
  phosphorylation, 22-23
  sodium-phosphate cotransporter, 20-21
  thiol redox, 22-23
Brush-border membrane vesicle, phosphate
  uptake, time course, 70
Burkitt's lymphoma
  serum calcium, 551
  serum creatinine, 551
  serum phosphorus, 551
Burn, hypophosphatemia, 591

C

Cafe-au-lait spot, 440
Calbindin
  alkaline phosphatase, 167
  collagen, 167
  fibronectin, 167
  matrix gla protein, 167
  osteocalcin, 167
  osteopontin, 167
Calcification, pathological, 436
Calcified bone, collagen fibril, 269-272
Calcitonin
  bone resorption inhibition, 515-516
  calcium, 13-14, 83
  calcium homeostasis, 87
  child, normal values, 408
  extracellular fluid calcium concentration,
    89
  mineral metabolism during growth,
    399-400
  osteoporosis, 864-866
  Paget's disease, 1053-1055
    adverse reactions, 1055
    antibodies, 1054
    human calcitonin, 1055
    porcine calcitonin, 1054
    resistance, 1054
    response, 1053-1054
    salmon calcitonin, 1054-1055

  parathyroid hormone secretion, 99
  phosphate excretion, 29
  pregnancy, 386-387
  serum calcium, mRNA levels, 86
  urine Mg^{2+} excretion, 51-52
Calcitonin gene transcription,
  1,25-dihydroxyvitamin D_3, 89
Calcitriol
  dialysis, 919
  end organ resistance, 945-947
  osteoporosis, 867-869
Calcium
  acetazolamide, 15-16
  acid-base, 14-15
  adult hypophosphatemic rickets, 937
  amiloride, 16
  angiotension, 14
  basolateral membrane
    Ca-Na exchange system, 6
    calcium exit, 6-8
  bone, distribution determinants, 419
  bone loss, 847-848
  calcitonin, 13-14, 83
  catecholamine, 14
  chlorothiazide, 16
  daily intake, 3
  1,25-dihydroxyvitamin D_3, 83
  epithelial transport, characteristics, 3-9
  extracellular fluid, 419-428
    1,25-dihydroxyvitamin D/d3/D excess,
      424
    distribution determinants, 419
    metabolic acidosis, 424-425
    normal, 421-422
    parathyroid hormone excess, 423-424
    renal failure, 426-428
    respiratory acidosis, 425-426
    very low calcium diet, 422-423
  Fanconi's syndrome, 937
  ferrocyanide, 15
  gastrointestinal tract, distribution
    determinants, 419
  glomerular filtration, 9
  glucagon, 14
  glucocorticoid, 14
  gluconate, 15
  growth hormone, 14
  hereditary hypophosphatemic rickets with
    hypercalciuria, 937
  hypercalcemia, 15
    excessive gastrointestinal absorption
      therapy, 517-518
  inorganic phosphate, 12
  insulin, 14
  intestinal absorption, 57-67
    androgen, 66
    basolateral membrane exit, 60-61
    brush-border influx, 58-60
    calcitonin, 65
    calcium and magnesium cotransport, 69
    calcium secretion, 63
    cellular events, 61-62
    cellular transport, 57-62
    cellular transport mechanisms, 58-62
    chlorthalidone, 66
    dietary intake and aging, 67
    diuretic, 66

estrogen, 66
factors affecting, 63–67
furosemide, 66
glucocorticoid, 65
growth hormone, 65–66
hormones, 65–66
lactose, 66–67
luminal factors, 66–67
nonsaturable components, 57, 58
nonsaturable transport, 63–64
oxalate, 66
paracellular transport, 63–64
parathyroid hormone, 65
pathways, 57–64
phytate, 66
saturable components, 57, 58
saturable transport, 57–62
thiazide, 66
thyroid hormone, 65
transcytotic calcium transport, 62
vitamin D, 62–63, 69
ion, 15
kidney, 3–16
distribution determinants, 419
loop diuretic, 15
magnesium, 15
mineralocorticoid, 14
osmotic diuretic, 15
osteoporosis, 847–848, 849, 856–858
dietary, 856–858
supplementation, 856–858
parathyroid hormone, 13, 14, 86–93
parathyroid hormone secretion, sigmoidal
relationship, 96
phosphate excretion, 30
phosphate ultrafilterability, 17
potassium-sparing diuretic, 16
protein intake, 12–13
proximal convoluted tubule, 9–10
pseudovitamin D deficiency, 937
recommended daily intake, 403
remodeling, 847–848
epidemiological data, 847–848
renal excretion, 3
renal handling, 3–16
dietary factors, 11–13
diuretics, 15–16
enteral factors, 11–13
factors, 11–16
hormonal factors, 13–14
metabolic perturbation, 14–15
parenteral factors, 11–13
sodium, 11–12
spironolactone, 16
sulfate, 15
thiazide, 16
thyroid hormone, 14
trabecular bone volume, 870
triamterene, 16
vitamin D, 13, 14
vitamin D dependent rickets
type I, 937
type II, 937
X-linked hypophosphatemic rickets, 937
Calcium absorption
adult hypophosphatemic rickets, 937
endocytotic, vesicular pathway, 8–9

Fanconi's syndrome, 937
hereditary hypophosphatemic rickets with
hypercalciuria, 937
intestinal epithelium
cellular pathways, 60
paracellular pathways, 60
pseudovitamin D deficiency, 937
transcellular pathway, 5–8
calbindin-D, 5–6
luminal entry, 5
schematics, 5
transcytoplasmic calcium buffering, 5–6
transcytoplasmic calcium ferrying, 5–6
vitamin D, 62–63
vitamin D dependent rickets
type I, 937
type II, 937
X-linked hypophosphatemic rickets, 937
Calcium ATPase, 6
basolateral plasma membrane, 7
proximal tubule, 7
Calcium balance, magnesium deficiency,
598–600
Calcium channel, voltage-sensitive, 96–97
Calcium flux
between body compartments, 420
pool integration, 419–428
Calcium homeostasis
calcitonin, 87
parathyroid hormone, 87, 571–573
principles, 493–494
Calcium hyperabsorption, idiopathic calcium
oxalate urolithiasis, 718
Calcium ion, matrix vesicle, 332–333
Calcium kinetics
hypocalcemia, 571, 572
idiopathic hypercalciuria, 700
normal, 571, 572
Calcium metabolism
abnormal, pathogenesis, 565–566
adult, integration, 417–428
hormonal control, 842, 843
kidney transplantation, 923–924
menopause
mineral homeostasis, 842, 843
skeletal homeostasis, 842, 843
race, 405–406
sarcoidosis, 565–566
Calcium nephrolithiasis
parathyroidectomy, 678–680
hypercalciuria after, 680
recurrent, 679
primary hyperparathyroidism, 671–684
biochemical parameters, 678
brushite, 675–676
calcitriol, 681
calcium intake, 680
calcium oxalate, 675–676
clinical features, 672
diagnosis, 676–677
drug therapy, 681
estrogen, 681
ethacrynic acid, 681
fluid intake, 681
furosemide, 681
historical aspects, 671

hypercalciuria, 674–675
hypercalciuria after surgery, 680
hyperuricosuria, 675
incidence, 671–672
medical treatment, 680–681
natural history, 679
parathyroidectomy, 677–680
phosphate, 681
protein intake, 680
recurrence, 679
renal tubular acidosis, 675
sodium intake, 680–681
stone pathogenesis, 674–676
surgery, 677–680
surgery complications, 677–678
urine pH, 675
Calcium oxalate
calcium oxalate crystallization inhibitor,
758–761
relative supersaturation, 685, 686
Calcium oxalate crystal formation,
hyperoxaluric state, 710–711
Calcium oxalate crystallization inhibitor,
757–784
acid mucopolysaccharide, 784
calcium oxalate, 758–761
calcium phosphate, 758
citrate, 779–783
thiazide, 782–783
treatment, 781–783
urine citrate levels, 780–781
urine crystallization, 780
defined, 761–784
fish antifreeze protein, 779
gallstone, 779
glycosaminoglycan, 784
macromolecule, 761–762
magnesium, 783
nephrocalcin, 762–776
air-water interface, 765, 768
amino acid composition, 765
carbohydrate composition, 765
cell culture, 762–765
crystal adsorption, 771–772
electrophoretic mobility, 764, 766
high-performance liquid
chromatography, 765, 767
human urinary inhibitor, 765, 767, 768
human urine, 765–768
kidney tissue culture inhibitor, 764, 766
Langmuir adsorption coefficients, 769
Langmuir-type adsorption plot, 765, 768
Langmuir-type adsorption therm plot,
764, 766
multiple DEAE elution peaks, 772–774
proximal tubule origin, 774–775
rat kidney, 768–769
rat urine, 768–769
renal production sites, 770
SDS-polyacrylamide gel
electrophoretogram, 765, 767
sedimentation equilibrium
centrifugation, 765, 767
stone-former urine, 769–770
surface pressure curve, 765, 768
Toyo-Soda column, 765, 767

Calcium oxalate crystallization inhibitor, nephrocalcin (contd.)
  urine protein crystal growth inhibitor, 769
  UV absorption spectrum, 764, 765
  pancreatic stone, 779
  pyrophosphate, 783–784
  RNA, 784
  saliva, 779
  Tamm-Horsfall glycoprotein, 776–779
    aggregation effects, 774
    clinical studies, 777–779
    crystal formation promotion, 776
    crystal growth inhibition, 776
    growth effects, 774
    nucleation inhibition, 776
    zero growth conditions, 777, 778
  thiazide-potassium-citrate treatment, 782–783
  undefined, 758–761
  urine, 758–761
Calcium oxalate crystallization promoter, 784–796
  apatite, 794–796
    cell interactions, 795–796
    in vitro experiments, 794–795
  uric acid, 785–794
    allopurinol, 785–787
    citrate, 787–788
    clinical evidence, 785–788
    heterogeneous nucleation, 790–792
    hyperuricosuria, 788
    mechanism studies, 788–794
    urate reduction, 792–794
    uric acid reduction, 792–794
Calcium oxalate dihydrate, 710
Calcium oxalate monohydrate, 710
Calcium oxalate salt, 707
Calcium oxalate stone
  allopurinol, 785–787
  uric acid, 785
Calcium oxalate urolithiasis, enteric hyperoxaluria, small bowel resection, 713
Calcium phosphate
  amorphous, 267
  calcium oxalate crystallization inhibitor, 758
Calcium reabsorption
  intercellular pathway, 3–5
    active, 4
    diffusion, 4–5
    equilibrium concentration, 4
    passive, 4
    schematics, 4
    solvent drag/convection, 3–4
    transepithelial electrochemical gradient, 4
  nephron, 9
Calcium receptor
  diacylglycerol concentration, 97
  divalent cation, 97
  evidence, 96–97
  inositol triphosphate concentration, 97
  intracellular calcium, 97

Calcium secretion
  mannitol, 63–64
  polyethylene glycol 900, 63–64
Calcium stress, remodeling, 369
Calcium supplement
  dialysis, 918
  renal failure, 918
  renal osteodystrophy, 918
Calcium transport
  1,25-dihydroxyvitamin D$_3$, 166
  nephron, 9–11
    collecting duct, 11
    descending limb of Henle's loop, 10
    distal convoluted tubule, 10–11
    glomerular filtration, 9
    proximal convoluted tubule, 9–10
    proximal straight tubule, 10
    thin ascending limb of Henle's loop, 10
    thick ascending limb of Henle's loop, cellular mechanisms, 43–44
Calcium uptake, intestinal epithelial basolateral membrane vesicle
  A23187, 60, 61
  ATP, 60, 61
Calculus. See Kidney stone
Cambrian layer, 228
Cancellous bone, 223
  age
    packet wall thickness, 371
    volume, 371
  basic structural units, 357
  loss mechanisms, 372
  normal, 846
  osteoporotic, 846
  remodeling, 374
  remodeling cycle, 357, 358
  sex
    packet wall thickness, 371
    volume, 371
Cancer, serum mineral disorder, 539–558
Carbonic acid
  hydrogen ion, 293
  proton pump, 293
Carbonic anhydrase II deficiency, 440, 995–998
  clinical presentation, 995–996
  etiology, 996–997
  histopathologic findings, 996
  laboratory findings, 996
  pathogenesis, 996–997
  radiologic features, 996
  treatment, 997–998
delta-Carboxy glutamic acid (gla)-containing protein, 249–250
Carboxyl (53–84) radioimmunoassay, intact parathyroid hormone immunometric assay, 117–118
Cardiac output, Paget's disease, 1037–1039
Cartilage
  bone matrix, 256
  noncollagenous protein, 330
  parathyroid hormone, 126
Cartilage canal, 314–315
Cartilage septal calcification
  features, 337

mechanisms, 337
  theories, 337
CAT reporter gene
  cyclic AMP response element, 99
  forskolin, 99
Catecholamine
  calcium, 14
  phosphate excretion, 29
Celiac disease, 439, 960, 962
  clinical features, 961
  incidence, 961
  pathogenesis, 961
  prevalence, 961
  treatment, 961
Cell cycle
  bone formation, cellular activity, 257–258
  remodeling, analogy between, 475–476
Cellular calcium, parathyroid hormone, 133
Child
  1,25-dihydroxyvitamin D, normal values, 408
  hypophosphatasia, 979, 981
  mineral metabolism, 395–410
    acid phosphatase normal values, 409
    alkaline phosphatase normal values, 408, 409
    bone density normal values, 409
    calcitonin normal values, 408, 409
    calcium-regulating hormones, 407
    magnesium normal values, 407–408
    mineral absorption, 406
    mineral renal handling, 406–407
    normal values, 407–410
    osteocalcin normal values, 409
    parathyroid hormone normal values, 409
    phosphorus normal values, 407–408
    serum calcium normal values, 407–408
    stable isotope studies, 406
    study methodology, 406–407
    urinary hydroxyproline normal values, 409
    vitamin D metabolite normal values, 408, 409
  osteocalcin, normal values, 408
  phosphorus, normal values, 408
Chlorothiazide, calcium, 16
Chlorthalidone, idiopathic hypercalciuria, 702
Cholecalciferol, osteoporosis, 867
Cholestatic disease, chronic, 963–964
  clinical features, 963
  incidence, 963
  pathogenesis, 963–964
  prevalence, 963
  treatment, 964
Cholesterol, sterol structures, 150
Chondrocalcin, growth plate, 335, 336
Chondrocalcin hypothesis, growth plate, 334–338
  large proteoglycans, 334
  original observations, 334–335
Chondrocyte
  bone calcification, 319
  growth plate, 316
  hypertrophy, 319
  proliferation, 319

Chondroma, 1067
Chondromyxoid fibroma, 1068
Chondrosarcoma, 1075–1078
  radiography, 445
Chromatin-associated receptor fraction,
    vitamin D, 168
Chromosomal gene, 1,25-dihydroxyvitamin
    D_3 receptor, 180–181
Chronic active hepatitis, 964–965
  clinical features, 964
  incidence, 964
  pathogenesis, 964–965
  prevalence, 964
  treatment, 965
Chronic lymphocytic leukemia
  hypophosphatemia, 557
  osteomalacia, 557
Chronic renal failure, 440
Chvostek's sign, 438
  hypocalcemia, 576, 577
Chylomicron, 200
  transport, 200
  vitamin D, oral route, 200
Circulation, bone matrix, proteins adsorbed,
    251–252
Cisplatin nephropathy, 440
  hypocalciuria, 16
Citrate, calcium oxalate crystallization
    inhibitor, 779–783
  thiazide, 782–783
  treatment, 781–783
  urine citrate levels, 780–781
  urine crystallization, 780
Citric acid cycle, 731–732
Collagen, 227
  assessment, 258
  bone calcification
    calcium, 278
    chondroblast, 278
    osteoblast, 278
    phosphate, 278
  bone mineral phase, location, 273
  calbindin, 167
  1,25-dihydroxyvitamin D_3, 167
  endogenous protein, 241–244
  growth plate, 322–326
    collagen type II, 324
    collagen type IX, 324–325
    collagen type X, 325, 326
    collagen type XI, 325–326
    functional role, 322–323
    genetically distinct types, 323–324
  types, 243
Collagen fibril, 225, 226, 325
  bone calcification, 279–284
    phosphoprotein, 280–283
  calcified bone, 269–272
  osteoid bone, 269–272
Collagen marker, Paget's disease, 1042–1043
Collecting duct system, magnesium, 45–46
Colles' fracture, osteoporosis, 838–839
  epidemiology, 838–839
Compact bone, 223, 228
Computerized tomography, 449–450
Connecting tubule, magnesium, 45–46

Continuous ambulatory peritoneal dialysis,
    921–922
  mineral metabolism, 921–922
  parathyroid hormone, 922
  vitamin D, 922
Cortical bone, 223
  basic structural units, 357
  osteoclast, 359
  remodeling cycle, 357
Cortico-endosteal envelope, 229
Cortisol, parathyroid hormone secretion, 99
Creatinine, primary hyperparathyroidism,
    525
Creatinine clearance
  lactation, 385, 387
  pregnancy, 385, 387
Crohn's disease, 960
  incidence, 961
  prevalence, 961
Crystal formation, bone calcification, 276
  alignment, 276
  collagen, 276–279
  nucleation site, 277
  orientation, 276
  postulated role, 276–279
  solid mineral phase, 276
Crystal proliferation, enzymatic regulator,
    333
Crystallization
  kidney stone formation, 613–616
    liquid-phase behavior, 614–616
    surface events, 616
  urolithiasis, 613–616
    liquid-phase behavior, 614–616
    surface events, 616
Cutis verticis gyrata, 1014
Cyclic AMP
  hypocalcemia, 126
  parathyroid hormone secretion, 97–98
Cyclic AMP response element, CAT reporter
    gene, 99
Cyclic GMP, 138–139
Cyclosporine, renal osteodystrophy, 926
Cyclosporine nephropathy, 440
Cystic fibrosis, 439
Cystic parathyroid adenomatosis, primary
    hyperparathyroidism, 499
Cystine
  cystine calculus
    conversion, 808
    solubility alteration, 807, 808
  urinary pH, solubility, 807, 808
Cystine calculus, 806–810
  cystine
    conversion, 808
    solubility alteration, 807, 808
  diagnosis, 807
  dietary therapy, 807–808
  extracorporeal shock wave lithotripsy,
    809–810
  history, 806
  irrigant dissolution, 808–809
  kidney transplantation, 810
  lithotomy, 809–810
  pathophysiology, 806
  percutaneous nephrolithotomy, 809–810

presentation, 806–807
  treatment, 807–810
Cytochrome P450, vitamin D_3-25-
    hydroxylase, 153
Cytokine, bone resorption, 297
Cytosol alanine:glyoxylate aminotransferase
    deficiency, 721

D
Decorin, 244–245, 246–250
  immunohistochemical localization, 246
  schematic representation, 245
7-Dehydrocholesterol, sterol structures, 150
Dermal fibroblast, parathyroid hormone
    binding site, 136
Dermatofibrosis lenticularis disseminata,
    1004
Dexamethasone, parathyroid hormone
    secretion, 99
Diabetes
  25-hydroxyvitamin D_3 metabolism, 156
  vitamin D, free sterol concentration, 210
Diabetic ketoacidosis, hypophosphatemia,
    590–591
Diacylglycerol
  calcium receptor, 97
  phosphatidylinositol metabolism, 131
Dialysis. See also Continuous ambulatory
    peritoneal dialysis aluminum
    accumulation, 921
    deferrioxamine, 921
  amyloid, 912
  calcitriol, 919
  calcium supplement, 918
  chronic, 912
  parathyroidectomy, 920–921
  phosphorus, 916–918
  radiographic features, 914–915
  secondary hyperthyroid bone disease, 911
  serum calcium, 916–918
  vitamin D sterol, 919–920
Dialysis dementia
  aluminum carbonate, 916
  aluminum hydroxide, 916
Diaphysis, 228
Dichloromethylene diphosphonate, Paget's
    disease, 1057
Diet
  idiopathic calcium oxalate urolithiasis,
    717–718
  oxalate, 711–712
Dietary calcium intake, urine calcium
    excretion, 687, 688
Dietary protein intake, urinary calcium
    excretion idiopathic hypercalciuria,
    697
  normal, 697
Dietary purine, uric acid calculus, 804
Dietary supplementation, struvite calculus,
    817
2,8-Dihydroxyadenine calculus, 821
1,25-Dihydroxyvitamin D
  adult hypophosphatemic rickets, 937
  bone loss, 847
  child, normal values, 408

1,25-Dihydroxyvitamin D (contd.)
  Fanconi's syndrome, 937
  free sterol concentration
    age, 205–206
    hormones, 206
    ions, 206
    race, 205–206
    sex, 205–206
    vitamin D deficiency, 206–207
    vitamin D intoxication, 207–208
  hereditary hypophosphatemic rickets with
      hypercalciuria, 937
  lymphoma, malignancy-associated
      hypercalcemia, 548, 549
  plasma, 196, 197–198
    kinetics, 198
    plasma concentrations, 197–198
    sources, 197
  pseudovitamin D deficiency, 937
  renal disease, 210
  vitamin D dependent rickets
    type I, 937
    type II, 937
  X-linked hypophosphatemic rickets, 937
24,25-Dihydroxyvitamin D, plasma, 198
25,26-Dihydroxyvitamin D, plasma
    concentrations, 198
1,25-Dihydroxyvitamin D₃
  alkaline phosphatase, 167
  bone matrix, 256
  calcitonin gene transcription, 89
  calcium, 83
  calcium transport, 166
  collagen, 167
  1,25-dihydroxyvitamin D₃ receptor,
      175–176
  1,25-dihydroxyvitamin D₃ receptor
      regulation, 176–177
  discovery, 164–165
  extracellular fluid calcium concentration,
      89
  fibronectin, 167
  genomic mechanism of action, current
      view, 181–184
  as hormonal signal, 165–166
  25-hydroxyvitamin D₃ metabolism, 155
  hypocalcemia, 126
  matrix gla protein, 167
  mineral homeostasis, 149
  monoclonal antibody, 170–171
  mRNA level
    actin, 89
    calcitonin, 89
    parathyroid hormone, 89
    somatostatin, 89
    thyroglobulin, 89
  osteocalcin, 167
  osteocalcin gene promoter, induction,
      181–183
  osteopontin, 167
  paracrine system, activated macrophages,
      156–158
  parathyroid cell, 94, 95
  parathyroid hormone gene, 1,25-
      dihydroxyvitamin D₃ receptor, 89
  parathyroid hormone mRNA, parathyroid
      cells, 88–89

  parathyroid hormone secretion,
      parathyroid cells, 88–89
  protein induction, 166–167
  renal failure, 907
  serum calcium, 165
  serum phosphorus, 165
  tissue distribution
    autoradiographic analysis, 170
    biochemical analysis, 170
    immunohistochemical analysis, 170
  transcription, 166
1,25-Dihydroxyvitamin D₃ biosynthesis
  avian egg-laying, 166
  estrogen, 166
  growth, 166
  lactation, 166
  pregnancy, 166
  prolactin, 166
1,25-Dihydroxyvitamin D₃ catabolism, 158
  pathway, 158
1,25-Dihydroxyvitamin D₃ formation, kidney
  hormones, 165, 166
  mineral ions, 165, 166
1,25-Dihydroxyvitamin D₃ receptor, 89–93
  anti-receptor monoclonal antibody, 174
  biochemical properties, 172–177
  cellular distribution, 167–171
  chromosomal gene, 180–181
  1,25-dihydroxyvitamin D₃, 175–176
  discovery, 167–169
  expression regulation, 171–172
  hereditary 1,25-dihydroxyvitamin D₃-
      resistance
    mutant transcriptional activity, 186–187
    phenotypic defects, 185
  human chromosomal gene, 180–181
  intracellular biology, 174–175
  intracellular properties, 172–177
  molecular biology, 177–181
  molecular cloning, 177–178
    orphan receptor gene, 178–179
    retinoid receptor gene, 178–179
    steroid receptor gene, 178–179
    thyroid receptor gene, 178–179
  mouse 3T6 fibroblast, 177
  osteocalcin gene activation, 184
  physical features, 172–174
  structural organization, 174
1,25-Dihydroxyvitamin D₃ receptor
    chromosomal gene, genetic lesions,
    185–186
1,25-Dihydroxyvitamin D₃ receptor mRNA,
    parathyroid hormone mRNA, 89–93
1,25-Dihydroxyvitamin D₃ receptor
    regulation, 1,25-dihydroxyvitamin D₃,
    176–177
1,25-Dihydroxyvitamin D₃-responsive
    element
  AP-1–binding protein complex, 183
  nucleotide sequence, 183
  properties, 183–184
  structure, 183–184
1,25-Dihydroxyvitamin D₃ synthesis,
    153–158
  extrarenal, 156–158
Diphosphonate
  Paget's disease, 1055–1058
  primary hyperparathyroidism, 533–534

Diphosphonate retention, radionuclide bone
    imaging, 452
Disappearing bone disease, 1082
Disodium etidronate, Paget's disease,
    1056–1057
  adverse reactions, 1055, 1057
Disseminated candidiasis, 567
Disseminated coccidiomycosis, 567
Distal convoluted tubule
  magnesium, 45–46
  Mg²⁺ fractional reabsorption
    arginine vasopressin, 51
    calcitonin, 51
    glucagon, 51
    parathyroid hormone, 51
  phosphate reabsorption, 19
Distal hydrogen-ion secretion, 738
Distal tubule
  phosphate reabsorption, 19
  renal tubular acidosis, 737
Diuretic. See also Specific type
  phosphate excretion, 30
  renal calcium, 15–16
Divalent cation, calcium receptor, 97
Drug-induced osteomalacia, 439
Dual energy X-ray absorptiometry, 446,
    447–449
Dual photon absorptiometry, 446, 447–449
Dyschondroplasia, 1067

E
Ecto-phosphatase, matrix vesicle, 333
Ectopic calcification, radiography, 445
Ectopic hyperparathyroidism, 542
Electrohydraulic lithotripsy, percutaneous
    nephrostolithotomy, 632–633
Embryo
  17 days, 220
  28 days, 221
  bone calcification, 274
  fourth week, 221
Enchondral calcification, bone formation,
    postnatal, 314
Endochondral ossification, 222
  schematic diagrams, 223
Endocrine disorder
  magnesium deficiency, 601–602
  vitamin D, free sterol concentration, 210
Endocytosis, vesicular pathway, calcium
    absorption, 8–9
Endogenous protein, 241–251
  collagen, 241–244
Endoplasmic reticulum, phosphatidylinositol
    metabolism, 131
Endosteal envelope, 229
Endosteal hyperostosis, 1002–1004
  van Buchem's disease, 1002, 1003
Endothelial cell stimulating angiogenic
    factor, growth plate, 344
Energetics, growth plate, 320–322
Enteric hyperoxaluria, 440, 713–717
  calcium oxalate urolithiasis, small bowel
      resection, 713
  fatty acid malabsorption, 714
  gastrointestinal disorder, 713

small bowel bypass
  steatorrhea, 717
    treatment, 717
  steatorrhea, 714
    treatment, 716–717
  uric acid excretion, 714–715
Enzymatic regulator, crystal proliferation, 333
Enzyme, bone matrix, 251
Enzyme inhibitor
  bone matrix, 251
  bone resorption, 300
Epidermal nevus syndrome
  hypophosphatemia, 557
  osteomalacia, 557
Epinephrine, phosphate excretion, 29
Epiphyseal bone, 314, 315
Epiphyseal plate, 225
Epiphysis, 224, 225, 314
Epithelial transport, calcium, characteristics, 3–9
Ergocalciferol, 150
Eroded surface, bone, 230, 231
Estradiol
  bone mass, 842, 843
  skeletal mass, 842
Estrogen
  bone loss, 845–846
  bone matrix, 256
  bone resorption, 298–299
  1,25-dihydroxyvitamin D_3 biosynthesis, 166
  hypercalcemia, 508
  hypercalcemic flare, 540
  mineral metabolism during growth, 401–402
  osteoporosis, 859–864, 865
    bone mass, 860
    breast cancer, 862, 864
    endometrial carcinoma, 861–862, 863
    hip fracture, 860–861, 862
    ischemic heart disease, 861
    long-term prevention, 856–857
    prescription, 862–864
    progestin, 862
    radiographic changes, 861
    skeleton, 860
  parathyroid hormone
    secretion, 99
    skeleton, 846
  primary hyperparathyroidism, 532–533
Ethacrynic acid, 440
  phosphate excretion, 30
Etidronate
  bone resorption inhibition, 515, 517
  osteoporosis, 866–867, 868, 869
Ewing's sarcoma, 1073–1075
Exercise, osteoporosis, prevention, 858–859
Exon, 254
External remodeling, 355
Extracellular calcium
  inositol 1,4,5-triphosphate, 97
  inositol tetrakisphosphate, 97
  parathyroid hormone gene transcription, 96
  parathyroid hormone secretion, 96
    cellular events, 98

Extracellular fluid, calcium, 419–428
  calcitonin, 89
  1,25-dihydroxyvitamin D_3, 89
  1,25-dihydroxyvitamin D_3 excess, 424
  distribution determinants, 419
  metabolic acidosis, 424–425
  normal, 421–422
  parathyroid hormone, 89
  parathyroid hormone excess, 423–424
  renal failure, 426–428
  respiratory acidosis, 425–426
  very low calcium diet, 422–423
Extracellular fluid volume, phosphate excretion, 29
Extracellular magnesium
  inositol 1,4,5-triphosphate, 97
  inositol tetrakisphosphate, 97
Extracorporeal shock wave lithotripsy, 642–667, 643–648
  bilateral simultaneous, 647
  complications, 647–648
  cystine calculus, 809–810
  gravel passage, 646
  hydrodynamic shock wave, 642–643
  impacted stones, 646
  indications, 648–667
  kidney stone, 625–626
    adjunctive procedures, 650
    compared by stone number, 653
    cystoscopy, 651, 653
    development, 625–626
    further procedure frequency, 654
    historical aspects, 625–626
    multiple treatments, 652
    nonstaghorn renal calculus, 649–654
    nonsurgical complications, 651
    outcome, 652
    postoperative stay length, 651
    stone basketing, 651, 653
    stone location, 649
    stone size, 649
    treatment morbidity, 650
    ureteral stent, 651, 653
    ureteroscopy, 651, 653
  low-density calculus, 646–647
  multiple stones, 646
  patient positioning, 643–645, 646
  principles, 643–647
  proximal ureteral calculus, 662–666
  radiolucent calculus, 646–647
  shock wave dosage, 647
  solitary stones, 645–646
  staghorn calculus, 654–662, 815
  steinstrasse, 647
  stones larger than 2 cm, 646
  struvite calculus
    combination treatment, 815–816
    monotherapy, 815
  theoretical aspects, 642–643
  ureteral calculus, distal, 666
Extraskeletal calcification, 915–916
  associated disorders, 1019

F
Fall
  annual risk, 837
  extrinsic factors altering risk, 837

  intrinsic factors altering risk, 837
  osteoporosis, 859
  osteoporotic hip fracture, 835–836, 837, 838
Familial hypocalciuric hypercalcemia, 440, 508–509, 535–536
  hypocalciuria, 16
  vitamin D, free sterol concentration, 211
Familial primary hyperparathyroidism, primary hyperparathyroidism, 499
Fanconi's syndrome, 439, 942–943
  alkaline phosphatase, 937
  calcium, 937
  calcium absorption, 937
  1,25-dihydroxyvitamin D, 937
  25-hydroxyvitamin D, 937
  hypophosphatemia, 557
  osteomalacia, 557
  parathyroid hormone, 937
  phosphorus, 937
  phosphorus absorption, 937
  rachitic/osteomalacic disease, 942–943
  treatment, 943
  type I, 942–943
  type II, 943
  urinary calcium, 937
  urinary phosphorus, 937
  vitamin D, free sterol concentration, 211
Fatty acid, 733–734
Fatty acid malabsorption, enteric hyperoxaluria, 714
Femur, 224
  properties, 226
Ferredoxin reductase, 154
Ferrocyanide, calcium, 15
Fetus, mineral metabolism, 388–389
Fibril, collagen, 225, 226
Fibroblast, parathyroid hormone, 127
Fibroblast model, vitamin-D_3-resistant, 185
Fibrodysplasia ossificans progressiva, 1010–1013
  clinical presentation, 1010, 1011
  etiology, 1013
  histopathologic findings, 1010
  laboratory findings, 1010
  pathogenesis, 1013
  prognosis, 1013
  radiologic features, 1010, 1011, 1012
  treatment, 1013
Fibrogenesis imperfecta ossium, 439, 987–988
  clinical presentation, 988
  etiology, 988
  histopathologic findings, 988
  laboratory findings, 988
  pathogenesis, 988
  radiologic features, 988
  treatment, 988
Fibronectin, 246–250
  biochemical features, 246
  calbindin, 167
  1,25-dihydroxyvitamin D_3, 167
Fibrosarcoma, 1075
Fibrous dysplasia, 993, 1008–1010, 1079–1080
  clinical presentation, 1008
  histopathologic findings, 1009
  laboratory findings, 1009

Fibrous dysplasia (contd.)
  pathogenesis, 1009
  radiologic features, 1008
  treatment, 1009–1010
Fibrous dysplasia syndrome, 440
Filamentous zone, osteoclast, 233, 234
Fish antifreeze protein, calcium oxalate
      crystallization inhibitor, 779
Fixed acid production, renal acid excretion,
      730–734
  acid ash, 730
  amino acid, 733
  biochemical reactions, 730–732
  citric acid cycle, 731–732
  fatty acid, 733–734
  fatty acid oxidation, 732
  fixed ash, 730
  foodstuff metabolism, 733–734
  gluconeogenesis, 732
  glucose, 733
  glycolysis, 731
  organic anions, 734
  urea cycle, 732
Flank tenderness, 440
Flat bone, adult, 224–225
Flavoprotein cytochrome P450 reductase,
      154
Flexible nephroscopy, percutaneous
      nephrostolithotomy, 633–634
Fluoride, osteoporosis, 870–871
Fluorosis, 870
Foodstuff metabolism, 733–734
Formation, remodeling, 364
  bone structural unit, 364
  cancellous osteon, 364
  closing cone, 364
  Haversian system, 364
  mineralization lag time, 364
  packet, 364
  secondary osteon, 364
  trabecular osteon, 364
Forming surface, bone, 229–230, 231
Forskolin, CAT reporter gene, 99
Fracture
  annual U.S. cost, 833
  bone mass quantitation, 450
    normal vs. osteoporotic groups, 450
    predictive value, 450
    risk factor value, 450
  epidemiology, 832–839
  Paget's disease, 1036, 1037
  pathological, 436
  postmenopausal osteoporosis, 832
  sodium fluoride, 870–871
Fracture healing
  bone growth, 314
  skeleton, 237
Free sterol concentration
  1,25-dihydroxyvitamin D
    age, 205–206
    hormones, 206
    ions, 206
    race, 205–206
    sex, 205–206
    vitamin D deficiency, 206–207
    vitamin D intoxication, 207–208
  25-hydroxyvitamin D
    age, 205–206

    ions, 206
    race, 205–206
    sex, 205–206
    vitamin D deficiency, 206–207
    vitamin D intoxication, 207–208
  vitamin D metabolite, 203–211
    estimated, 203–204
    measured, 204
    vitamin D deficiency, 206–207
    vitamin D intoxication, 207–208
Furosemide
  NaCl transport, 44
  phosphate excretion, 30

G
G protein
  adenylate cyclase, 140
  ADP-ribosylation, 140
  alpha subunits, 141
    primary structure, 141
  beta unit, 141
  functional classification, 140
  gamma unit, 141
  parathyroid hormone, 141–142
    guanine nucleotides, 141
  phospholipase C, 140
  transmembrane signaling, 138–139
    features, 139
G-protein action, schema, 139
G-protein-linked receptor, model, 137, 138
Gallium nitrate, bone resorption inhibition,
      515, 517
Gallstone, calcium oxalate crystallization
      inhibitor, 779
Gastrectomy, 439
  vitamin D, free sterol concentration, 209
Gastrointestinal disorder
  bone biopsy, 468
  bone disease, 959–963
  enteric hyperoxaluria, 713
  histomorphometry, 468
  magnesium deficiency, 601
  vitamin D, free sterol concentration, 209
Gastrointestinal tract
  calcium, distribution determinants, 419
  parathyroid hormone, 127
Gastrointestinal transport, oxalate transport,
      710
Gene
  exon, 254
  intron, 254
  promoter, 254
  structural organization, 254
Genetic disorder, vitamin D, free sterol
      concentration, 211
Gestation, mineral metabolism, 383–389
Giant-cell tumor, 1070–1071
  parathyroid hormone binding site, 136
Gigantism, sclerosteosis, 1003
Glomerular filtration
  calcium, 9
  magnesium, 41, 42
  urinary calcium excretion
    idiopathic hypercalciuria, 695
    normal, 695

Glomerular filtration rate
  hyperphosphatemia, 914
  secondary hyperparathyroidism, 906–907
Glucagon, calcium, 14
Glucocorticoid
  bone biopsy, 464
  bone resorption, 298
  calcium, 14
  histomorphometry, 464
  osteoporosis, 890–893
    intestinal calcium absorption, 891
    parathyroid hormone, 892–893
    vitamin D metabolism, 891–892
  phosphate excretion, 29
  progressive diaphyseal dysplasia, 999–1000
Glucocorticoid osteoporosis, 890–893
  treatment, 892–893
Gluconate, calcium, 15
Glucose, 733
Glucose-6-phosphatase deficiency, 803
Glycogen storage disease, type I, 803
Glycolysis, 731
Glycoprotein, 245–250, 246–250
  biochemical features, 246
Glycosaminoglycan
  calcium oxalate crystallization inhibitor,
      784
  growth plate, 335–338
  struvite calculogenesis, 812, 813
Glyoxylate, 708
Glyoxylate metabolism, 721
Gorham's disease, 1082
Gout, 802–803
Granulomatous disease, 439, 567
  hypercalcemia, 506–507
Groove of Ranvier, 315
Growth
  1,25-dihydroxyvitamin D₃ biosynthesis,
      166
  mineral metabolism, 395–396
    calcitonin, 399–400
    calcium, 403–404
    challenges, 396
    control, 396–402
    growth hormone, 400–401
    hormonal control, 398–402
    integration, 396–402
    intestine, 396–398
    kidney, 396–397
    magnesium, 404–405
    nutrition, 403–405
    parathyroid hormone, 398–399
    phosphorus, 403, 404
    sex steroid, 401–402
    vitamin D, 399, 403, 404
  skeletal changes, 395–396
    endochondral ossification, 395
    intramembranous ossification, 395
  skeleton, 234–235
Growth center, ectopic, 314
Growth factor
  bone matrix, 242, 250–251
    synthesis, 255
    turnover, 255
  bone resorption, 297–298
Growth hormone
  calcium, 14
  growth plate, skeletal growth, 339–340

mineral metabolism during growth, 400–401
osteoporosis, 872
phosphate reabsorption, 28–29
Growth plate
anatomy, 314–318
angiogenesis, 343–344
angiogenic (growth) factor, capillary invasion, 343–344
basic fibroblast growth factor, 343
biochemistry, 313–344
of structural macromolecules, 322–330
biology, 313–344
bone calcification, vasculature, 318
bone growth, role, 313
chemistry, 313–344
chondrocalcin, 335, 336
chondrocalcin hypothesis, 334–338
large proteoglycans, 334
original observations, 334–335
chondrocyte, 316
classification, 313–314
closure, 315
collagen, 322–326
collagen type II, 324
collagen type IX, 324–325
collagen type X, 325, 326
collagen type XI, 325–326
functional role, 322–323
genetically distinct types, 323–324
endothelial cell stimulating angiogenic factor, 344
energetics, 320–322
function, 313–314
glycosaminoglycan, 335–338
growth hormone, skeletal growth, 339–340
heparin-binding growth factor, 343–344
histology, 314–318
insulin-like growth factor, 340
insulin-like growth factor-I, 340
growth regulation, 341
insulin-like growth factor-I binding protein, 340–341
low-molecular-weight angiogenic factor, 344
lower cell zones, 316–317
matrix vesicle, rachitic rat, 332
matrix vesicle hypothesis, 331–334
mineral formation in vitro, 331
mineral formation in vivo, 331
mineral phase elemental analysis, 330–331
mineralization mechanisms, 330–338
mineralized tissue study difficulties, 318–319
morphology, 315–316
multiplication stimulating activity, 340
noncollagenous protein
anchorin CII, 329
function, 329–330
structure, 329–330
normal physiology, 318–322
oxygenation, 320–322
parathyroid hormone, 341–342
physiologic functions, 318
Poole-Hunter ion-exchange hypothesis, 335–338
postnatal mammalian, 315
proteoglycan, 326–329, 335–338

core protein domain structure, 327
function, 326–327
interactions, 329
organization, 327–329
structure, 327–329
somatomedin, 340
transforming growth factor, 342–343, 343
upper cell zones, 316
vitamin D, 341–342
Growth retardation, renal tubular acidosis type I, 740
Gs unit, structural features, 141
Guanine nucleotide, phospholipase C, 141
Guanine-nucleotide-binding protein, 138–142
Guanine nucleotide guanosine triphosphate, adenylate cyclase, 138
Guanosine diphosphate, 138

H
Haversian bone, 223
ulna, 367
Haversian envelope, 228–229
Haversian system, ulna, 367
Hearing loss, Paget's disease, 1040
Heart myocyte, Na^+/Ca^{2+} exchanger, 7–8
Height loss, 440
Hematopoietic stem cell, osteoclast, derivation, 289–290
Hemodialysis
bone biopsy, 466–467
histomorphometry, 466–467
Henle's loop
magnesium reabsorption
arginine vasopressin, 50
calcitonin, 50
glucagon, 50
luminal magnesium, 47–48
parathyroid hormone, 50
peritubular magnesium, 47–48
magnesium transport
characteristics, 43
micropuncture experiments, 43
thick ascending limb, 43–45
transepithelial transport, 43–45
Heparin, 439
osteoporosis
bone formation, 898
bone remodeling, 897
mast cell, 898
parathyroid hormone, 898
pregnancy, 896
resorptive effects, 897–898
vitamin D, 898
Heparin-binding growth factor, growth plate, 343–344
Hepatic osteodystrophy
bone biopsy, 471
histomorphometry, 471
Hepatitis, 964–965
clinical features, 964
incidence, 964
pathogenesis, 964–965
prevalence, 964
treatment, 965
Hepatobiliary disorder, vitamin D, free sterol concentration, 209

Hereditary 1,25-dihydroxyvitamin D_3 resistance, 184–187
1,25-dihydroxyvitamin D_3 receptor mutant transcriptional activity, 186–187
phenotypic defects, 185
Hereditary hypercalciuria, renal tubular acidosis type I, pathophysiology, 748
Hereditary hypophosphatemic rickets with hypercalciuria, 439, 941–942
alkaline phosphatase, 937
calcium, 937
calcium absorption, 937
1,25-dihydroxyvitamin D, 937
25-hydroxyvitamin D, 937
parathyroid hormone, 937
pathophysiology, 941
phosphorus, 937, 941–942
phosphorus absorption, 937
treatment, 941–942
urinary calcium, 937
urinary phosphorus, 937
Heterogeneous nucleation, bone calcification, 274
Heterogeneous nucleation theory, 790–792
Hip fracture, osteoporosis
epidemiology, 833–837
falls, 834–836, 837, 838
incidence, 833, 834, 835
survival, 837
Histiocytosis X, 1082–1084
Histomorphometry
acromegaly, 463–464
alcoholism, 470
anticonvulsant drug-induced bone disease, 464
birthrate, 478
bone age, 483–485
bone balance, 483–485
bone formation, indices, 481–483
gastrointestinal disease, 468
geometric aspects of bone structure, 480–481
glucocorticoid, 464
hemodialysis, 466–467
hepatic osteodystrophy, 471
hypophosphatasia, 470
immobilization, 464
individual values, 479–480
interpretation principles, 478–480
lifespan, 478
mastocytosis, 465
mean values, 479–480
osteogenesis imperfecta, 470
osteoid accumulation kinetics, 485–487
osteomalacia, 468, 469
osteoporosis, 465–466
Paget's disease, 469–470
pathogenetic significance, 475–487
physiologic significance, 475–487
postmenopausal osteoporosis, 465–466
primary hyperparathyroidism, 463, 526–527
renal osteodystrophy, 466–468
resorption depth, 483–485
significance of particular measurements, 480–487
space-time relationship, 478
steady states, 478–479

Histomorphometry (contd.)
    tetracycline labeling, 481–483
    thyrotoxicosis, 468–469
    topological aspects of bone structure,
        480–481
    transient states, 478–479
    wall thickness, 483–485
Histoplasmosis, 567
Homogeneous nucleation, bone calcification,
    274
Hormonal control, magnesium transport,
    48–53
    distal convoluted tubule, 51
    Henle's loop, 48–51
    overall kidney function, 51–53
    proximal convoluted tubule, 48
    thick ascending limb, 48–51
Hormone action, phosphatidylinositol
    pathway, 130–133
Hormone analog, bone resorption, 299–300
Howship's lacuna, bone, 230, 231
HTLV-I leukemia, malignancy-associated
    hypercalcemia, 548
HTLV-I lymphoma, malignancy-associated
    hypercalcemia, 548
Human gene
    1,25-dihydroxyvitamin D_3 receptor,
        180–181
    osteocalcin, structural organization, 182
Humoral factor, malignancy-associated
    hypercalcemia, 549
Humoral hypercalcemia of malignancy, 439,
    503–504
    biochemical findings, 542
    causes, 504–505
    malignancy-associated hypercalcemia,
        542–548
    parathyroid hormone related peptide of
        malignancy, 503
Hungry bone syndrome, hypocalcemia, 579
Hyaluronan, 244–245, 246
    biochemical features, 246
    schematic representation, 245
Hydrogen ion
    biochemical sites of excess, 731
    carbonic acid, 293
    proton pump, 293
    reactions generating excess, 730
Hydroxamic acid
    I_{50} urease values, 818
    struvite calculus, 819
Hydroxyapatite, 227
Hydroxyproline, Paget's disease, 1042–1043
25-Hydroxyvitamin D
    adult hypophosphatemic rickets, 937
    Fanconi's syndrome, 937
    free sterol concentration
        age, 205–206
        ions, 206
        race, 205–206
        sex, 205–206
        vitamin D deficiency, 206–207
        vitamin D intoxication, 207–208
    hereditary hypophosphatemic rickets with
        hypercalciuria, 937
    plasma, 196–197
        kinetics, 197

        plasma concentrations, 197
        quantitation, 198
        sources, 196–197
    pseudovitamin D deficiency, 937
    renal disease, 209–210
    vitamin D dependent rickets
        type I, 937
        type II, 937
    X-linked hypophosphatemic rickets, 937
25-Hydroxyvitamin D-1 alpha-hydroxylase,
    decreased renal, 943–945
25-Hydroxyvitamin D_3-1 alpha-hydroxylase,
    properties, 155
25-Hydroxyvitamin D_3-24-hydroxylase,
    properties, 155
25-Hydroxyvitamin D_3-26,23-lactone
    biological activity, 158
    physiological functions, 158
25-Hydroxyvitamin D_3 catabolism, 158
    pathway, 158
25-Hydroxyvitamin D_3 formation, 153–155
25-Hydroxyvitamin D_3 metabolism
    diabetes, 156
    1,25-dihydroxyvitamin D_3, 155
    kidney, 155–156
    parathyroid hormone, 155–156
    regulation, 155–156
    serum calcium, 156
    serum phosphate, 156
Hyperalimentation, hypophosphatemia, 589
Hypercalcemia
    anorexia, 510
    antiestrogen, 508
    calcium, 15
        excessive gastrointestinal absorption
            therapy, 517–518
    causes, 494
    clinical features, 510–511
    differential diagnosis, 494–510
    estrogen, 508
    granulomatous disease, 506–507
    immobilization, 509
    immunoreactive parathyroid hormone
        differential diagnosis, 114–115, 117
        renal failure, 117
    infant, 568
    kidney transplantation, 923–924
        hypercalcemia after, 924
        post-transplant persistent, 923–924
    lithium, 507–508
    lymphoma, 567–568
    malignancy, 502–505
        humoral, 503–504
        pathophysiological mechanisms,
            502–503
        renal calcium excretion, 15
    management, 511–518
    medication-induced, 507–508
    milk-alkali syndrome, 508
    multiple causes in the same person, 510
    nonmalignant causes, 549
    nonparathyroid endocrine disorder, 505
    nonparathyroid tumor, 114–115
    Paget's disease, 1041
    parenteral nutrition, 509
    pathogenesis, 564–565

    polyuria, 510
    primary hyperparathyroidism, 494–502
    renal disease
        acute, 509
        chronic, 509
        solid tumor, 567–568
        thiazide diuretic, 507
        thyrotoxicosis, 505
        tuberculosis, 566
        tumors associated, 539, 540
        vitamin A, 508
        vitamin D, 505–507
            malignancy-associated, 507
        vitamin D metabolism, 564
        vitamin D toxicity, 506, 508
        William's syndrome, 568
Hypercalcemia of malignancy
    humoral, 503–504
    pathophysiological mechanisms, 502–503
    renal calcium excretion, 15
Hypercalciuria
    absorptive, 687
    mechanisms, 687–700, 701
    prevalence, 686–687
    primary hyperparathyroidism, 674–675
        renal stones, 674–675
    quantitative definition, 685–686
    renal, 687
    tuberculosis, 566
    Wilson's disease, 752
Hyperchloremic acidosis
    ammonia, 741–742
    urine anion gap, 743
    urine pH, 741–742
Hyperchloremic metabolic acidosis, 737–739
    pathophysiology, 737–739
Hypermagnesemia
    causes, 605–606
    renal failure, 606
    symptoms and signs, 606
Hyperostosis syndrome, 440
Hyperoxaluria, 707–722
    clinical disorders complicated by, 713–717
    primary. See Primary hyperoxaluria
Hyperoxaluric state, 707–722
    calcium oxalate crystal formation, 710–711
Hyperparathyroidism, 1080–1081
    primary. See Primary hyperparathyroidism
    secondary. See Secondary
        hyperparathyroidism
    vitamin D, free sterol concentration, 210
Hyperphosphatasia, 439
Hyperphosphatemia, 594–597
    acute, 576
    causes, 594–595
    clinical consequences, 596
    definition, 594
    gastrointestinal causes, 595
    glomerular filtration rate, 914
    hypocalcemia, 551
    increased release of intracellular
        phosphorus, 595–596
    pharmacologic causes, 595
    renal causes, 595
    resulting from redistribution, 595
    treatment, 596–597

complications, 597
side effects, 597
Hypertension
parathyroid hormone, 126–127
primary hyperparathyroidism, 126–127
Hyperthyroidism, 440
osteoporosis, 893–895
bone mass, 893–894
bone mineral density, 893
Hypertonic chondrocyte, osteogenic cell, 317
Hypertrophic osteoarthropathy, 1013
Hyperuricosuria, 440
causes, 804
low urinary volumes, 802
Hypervitaminosis A, osteoporosis, 898–900
biochemical findings, 899
retinoic acid, 899
retinol, 899
Hypocalcemia
acute, 576–577
autoimmune polyglandular syndrome type
I, 573–574
calcium homeostatic response, 574
calcium kinetics, 571, 572
cardiovascular effects, 577, 578
causes, 573–577
Chvostek's sign, 576, 577
classification, 572
cyclic AMP, 126
diagnostic algorithm, 579
1,25-dihydroxyvitamin D₃, 126
due to cancer, 549–551
hungry bone syndrome, 579
hyperphosphatemia, 551
hypoparathyroidism, surgery, 579
idiopathic hypoparathyroidism, 573–574
immunoreactive parathyroid hormone,
differential diagnosis, 113–114
laboratory studies, 579–582
leukemia, 550
management, 577
mechanisms, 571–573
from osteoblastic metastasis, 550–551
pancreatitis, 576
parathyroid hormone, 126
paresthesias, 577
pseudohypoparathyroidism, 574–576
recalcification tetany, 579
treatment
immediate, 582
long-term, 582–583
Trousseau's sign, 577–578
tumor-lysis syndrome, 551
vitamin D analog, 582
Hypocalciuria
Bartter's syndrome, 16
cisplatin nephropathy, 16
familial hypocalciuric hypercalcemia, 16
Hypokalemia, renal tubular acidosis type I,
739–740
Hypomagnesemia, 440
Hypoparathyroidism, 439
forms, 573–574
hypocalcemia, surgery, 579
radiography, 444
vitamin D, free sterol concentration,
208–209

Hypophosphatasia, 439, 977–986
adult, 979, 981, 982
alkaline phosphatase, 977
biochemical/genetic defect, 984–985
bone biopsy, 470
child, 979, 981
clinical features, 978–979
dental pathology, 979, 984
histomorphometry, 470
histopathologic findings, 982–983
hypophosphatemia, 981
infantile, 979
inheritance, 983–984
laboratory findings, 981–982
osteoidosis, 982
perinatal, 978–979, 980
plasma pyridoxal 5'-phosphate, 982, 983
prenatal diagnosis, 986
prevalence, 983–984
prognosis, 986
radiologic findings, 979–981
treatment, 985–986
Hypophosphatemia, 587–594
alcohol withdrawal, 590
alcoholism, 590
burn, 591
causes, 588
alcoholic patient, 590
decreased gastrointestinal absorption,
588
decreased renal tubular reabsorption,
588
redistribution, 588
severe, 588, 589
chronic lymphocytic leukemia, 557
clinical consequences, 591–592
definition, 587
diabetic ketoacidosis, 590–591
epidermal nevus syndrome, 557
Fanconi's syndrome, 557
hyperalimentation, 589
hypophosphatasia, 981
incidence, 587
kidney transplantation, 591, 924–925
treatment, 925
leukemia, 591
linear sebaceous nevus syndrome, 557
mesenchymal tumor, 551–555
clinical features, 551–553
pathogenesis, 553–555
treatment, 555
myeloma, 557
nutritional recovery syndrome, 590–591
oat-cell carcinoma, 557
phosphate-binding antacid, 589–590
phosphate replacement therapy, 593–594
phosphorus-containing preparation, 593
prostate cancer, 555–556
respiratory alkalosis, 588–589
treatment, 592–594
complications, 594
side effects, 594
Hypophosphatemic rickets with
hypercalciuria, vitamin D, free sterol
concentration, 211
Hypotension, parathyroid hormone, 126
cardiovascular effects, 126–127

Hypoxanthine guanine
phosphoribosyltransferase deficiency,
803

I

Iatrogenic magnesium excess, 440
Idiopathic calcium oxalate urolithiasis,
717–720
calcium hyperabsorption, 718
causes of hyperoxaluria, 717
diet, 717–718
magnesium, 720
orthophosphate, 719
oxalate excretion, 718
oxalate transport, 718
potassium citrate, 719–720
pyridoxine, 720
treatment, 719
diet, 719
medication, 719
Idiopathic hypercalciuria, 439
amiloride, 702
chlorthalidone, 702
indapamide, 702
intestinal calcium absorption, 689–693
nephrogenous cyclic AMP excretion, 692
pathogenesis, 685–703
serum 1,25-dihydroxyvitamin D, 690–691
serum parathyroid hormone
concentration, 692
serum phosphate, 692
skeleton, 698–700
sodium cellulose phosphate, 703
thiazide diuretic, 702
treatment, 701–703
medications, 702
nutritional, 701–702
urinary calcium excretion, 693–698
urinary cyclic AMP excretion, 692
vitamin D, free sterol concentration, 211
Idiopathic hypocitraturic calcium-oxalate
nephrolithiasis, renal tubular acidosis
type I, hypocitraturic, 748
Idiopathic hypoparathyroidism,
hypocalcemia, 573–574
Imaging
percutaneous nephrostolithotomy, 628
ureteroscopy, 636–637
Immobilization, 439
bone biopsy, 464
histomorphometry, 464
osteoporosis, 895–896
bed rest, 895–896
bone loss, 895
hormonal consequences, 896
metabolic consequences, 896
pharmacological approaches, 896
remodeling, 896
weightlessness, 895
Immobilization hypercalcemia, 509
Immobilization osteopenia, 895–896
Immunoassay
parathyroid hormone, 111–113
clinical applications, 113–118
clinical utility, 116

Immunoassay, parathyroid hormone (contd.)
  mid-region tyrosyl analogue, 112
  NH$_2$ region, 112
  vitamin D-binding protein, 202
Immunoreactive parathyroid hormone,
    107–110, 112–119
  circulating form, 109
  clearance, 109
  elution patterns, 110
  hypercalcemia
    differential diagnosis, 114–115, 117
    renal failure, 117
  hypocalcemia, differential diagnosis,
      113–114
  malignancy associated hypercalcemia,
      114–115
  primary hyperparathyroidism, 114–115
  renal osteodystrophy, staging, 115–117
  serum calcium
    hypocalcemic states, 114–115
    primary hyperparathyroidism, 114–115
Immunoreactive parathyroid hormone
    metabolism, 109
Immunoreactive parathyroid hormone
    secretion, 109
Indapamide, idiopathic hypercalciuria, 702
Infant, hypercalcemia, 568
Infantile hypophosphatasia, 979
Inflammatory bowel syndrome, 439, 960,
      961–962
  clinical features, 961
  incidence, 961
  pathogenesis, 961
  prevalence, 961
  treatment, 962
Inorganic phosphate, calcium, 12
Inorganic phosphorus absorption, intestinal
    epithelium, 70
Inorganic phosphorus secretion, intestinal
    epithelium, 70
Inositol 1,4,5–triphosphate
  extracellular calcium, 97
  extracellular magnesium, 97
Inositol phosphate, active, cellular
    consequences, 132
Inositol tetrakisphosphate
  extracellular calcium, 97
  extracellular magnesium, 97
Inositol triphosphate concentration, calcium
    receptor, 97
Insulin
  calcium, 14
  phosphate excretion, 29
Insulin-like growth factor
  bone matrix, 255
  growth plate, 340
Insulin-like growth factor-I, growth plate, 340
  growth regulation, 341
Insulin-like growth factor-I binding protein,
    growth plate, 340–341
Insulin-like growth factor-II, 363
Intact parathyroid hormone immunometric
    assay
  carboxyl (53–84) radioimmunoassay,
      117–118

mid (44–68) parathyroid hormone
    radioimmunoassay, 117–118
Intercellular pathway, calcium reabsorption,
      3–5
  active, 4
  diffusion, 4–5
  equilibrium concentration, 4
  passive, 4
  schematics, 4
  solvent drag/convection, 3–4
  transepithelial electrochemical gradient, 4
Interleukin-1, bone resorption, 297
Internal remodeling, 355
Internephron heterogeneity, phosphate
    reabsorption, 18
Intestinal absorption
  calcium, 57–67
    androgen, 66
    basolateral membrane exit, 60–61
    brush-border influx, 58–60
    calcitonin, 65
    calcium and magnesium cotransport, 69
    calcium secretion, 63
    cellular events, 61–62
    cellular transport, 57–62
    cellular transport mechanisms, 58–62
    chlorthalidone, 66
    dietary intake and aging, 67
    diuretic, 66
    estrogen, 66
    factors affecting, 63–67
    furosemide, 66
    glucocorticoid, 65
    growth hormone, 65–66
    hormones, 65–66
    idiopathic hypercalciuria, 689–693
    isotopic calcium, 690
    lactose, 66–67
    luminal factors, 66–67
    menopause, 842
    nonsaturable components, 57, 58
    nonsaturable transport, 63–64
    normal, 689–693
    oxalate, 66
    paracellular transport, 63–64
    parathyroid hormone, 65
    pathways, 57–64
    phytate, 66
    saturable components, 57, 58
    saturable transport, 57–62
    thiazide, 66
    thyroid hormone, 65
    transcytotic calcium transport, 62
    urinary calcium excretion, 687, 688
    vitamin D, 62–63, 69
  magnesium
    driving forces, 68
    in humans, 68–69
    transport pathways, 68
    vitamin D, 68
  oxalate, 712
  phosphorus, 69–79
    brush-border phosphorus influx, 71
    calcium and phosphorus cotransport, 72
    cellular transport events, 70–71
    colon, 74

diffusional phosphorus movement, 72
    ileum, 74
    inorganic phosphorus transport
        pathways, 69–74
    jejunum, 74
    Na-P cotransporter, 71
    pH, 71
    phosphate depletion, 72
    proximal small intestine, 73–74
    segmental calcium transport, 73–74
    segmental phosphorus transport, 73–74
    vitamin D, 71–72
Intestinal epithelial basolateral membrane
    vesicle, calcium uptake
  A23187, 60, 61
  ATP, 60, 61
Intestinal epithelium
  calcium absorption
    cellular pathways, 60
    paracellular pathways, 60
  inorganic phosphorus absorption, 70
  inorganic phosphorus secretion, 70
Intestine, mineral metabolism during growth,
      397–398
Intracellular calcium
  calcium receptor, 97
  parathyroid hormone, changes, 133–135
Intracellular pH
  phosphate excretion, 26
  phosphate reabsorption, 26
Intramembranous ossification, 222
  photomicrograph, 222
Intranephron heterogeneity, phosphate
    reabsorption, 18
Intron, 254
Invading capillary complex, 318
Ion, calcium, 15
Ion reservoir, 265
Ion transport inhibitor, bone resorption,
      300–301
Isoproterenol, phosphate excretion, 29
Isotopic calcium, intestinal calcium
    absorption, 690
Isozyme
  kidney, 259
  liver, 259

J
Jejuno-ileal bypass, 960, 962–963
  clinical features, 963
  incidence, 962–963
  pathogenesis, 963
  prevalence, 962–963
  treatment, 963
Juvenile osteoporosis, 439

K
Kidney
  acid-base balance, 734–735
    ammonia excretion, 735
    fixed acid metabolism, 734–735
    hydrogen ion excretion, 735
  alkaline phosphatase, 259

calcium, 3–16
  distribution determinants, 419
  1,25-dihydroxyvitamin D_3 formation
    hormones, 165, 166
    mineral ions, 165, 166
  growth mineral metabolism, 396–397
  25-hydroxyvitamin D_3 metabolism,
    155–156
  isozyme, 259
  parathyroid hormone, 125–126
    acid-base handling, 125–126
    calcium-conserving, 125
    cyclic AMP excretion, 125
    1,25-dihydroxyvitamin D_3 formation,
      125
    negative calcium balance, 125
    phosphaturic agent, 125
  parathyroid hormone binding site, 136
  primary hyperparathyroidism, 496–498
Kidney stone. See also Specific type
  asymptomatic, treatment indications, 667
  cystine
    clinical features, 627
    radiographic features, 627
  extracorporeal shock wave lithotripsy,
    625–626
    adjunctive procedures, 650
    compared by stone number, 653
    cystoscopy, 651, 653
    development, 625–626
    further procedure frequency, 654
    historical aspects, 625–626
    multiple treatments, 652
    nonstaghorn renal calculus, 649–654
    nonsurgical complications, 651
    outcome, 652
    postoperative stay length, 651
    stone basketing, 651, 653
    stone location, 649
    stone size, 649
    treatment morbidity, 650
    ureteral stent, 651, 653
    ureteroscopy, 651, 653
  historical background, 625–626
  new removal techniques, 626–677
  percutaneous nephrostolithotomy
    adjunctive procedures, 650
    compared by stone number, 653
    cystoscopy, 651, 653
    further procedure frequency, 654
    multiple treatments, 652
    nonstaghorn renal calculus, 649–654
    nonsurgical complications, 651
    outcome, 652
    postoperative stay length, 651
    stone basketing, 651, 653
    stone location, 649
    stone size, 649
    treatment morbidity, 650
    ureteral stent, 651, 653
    ureteroscopy, 651, 653
  percutaneous techniques, 625–626
  surgical techniques, 625–626
    perioperative antibiotic indications, 627
    preoperative evaluation, 627

Kidney stone disruption, 625–667. See also
  Specific type
Kidney stone dissolution, 625–667
Kidney stone formation
  crystallization, 613–616
    liquid-phase behavior, 614–616
    surface events, 616
  nucleation, 620–622
  physical-chemical processes, 613–624
  solution chemistry, 616–620
    adsorption, 619–620
    citrate ion concentration, 619
    crystal growth, 622–623
    EQUIL, 616–620
    ions, 617–618
    magnesium ion concentration, 619
    oxalate concentration, 618–619
    particle growth, 622–623
    pool diagram, 617
    relative supersaturation, 618–619
    speciation, 616–168
  surface chemistry, 616–620
    adsorption, 619–620
    citrate ion concentration, 619
    EQUIL, 616–620
    ions, 617–618
    magnesium ion concentration, 619
    oxalate concentration, 618–619
    pool diagram, 617
    relative supersaturation, 618–619
    speciation, 616–168
Kidney transplantation
  bone metabolism, 922–928
  calcium metabolism disorder, 923–924
  cystine calculus, 810
  hypercalcemia, 923–924
    hypercalcemia after, 924
    post-transplant persistent, 923–924
  hypophosphatemia, 591, 924–925
    treatment, 925
  mineral metabolism, 922–928
  osteonecrosis, 926–928
    factors, 926–928
    prevention, 928
    treatment, 928
  phosphorus metabolism disorder, 924–925
    treatment, 925
  post transplantation, 440
  renal osteodystrophy, 925–926
    growth of children following, 926
    serum osteocalcin, 926
Kyphosis, 438
  differential diagnosis, 852

L

Lactation
  creatinine clearance, 385, 387
  1,25-dihydroxyvitamin D_3 biosynthesis,
    166
  mineral metabolism, 389–391
    bone calcium, 390–391
    calcium absorption, 390
    hormonal changes, 389–390
    urinary calcium excretion, 390
Lamella, 227, 228

Lanthanum, 96
Lasix, 440
Lavage chemolysis, struvite calculus, 816–817
Leprosy, 567
Lesch-Nyhan syndrome, 803
Leukemia
  hypocalcemia, 550
  hypophosphatemia, 591
Limb bud, 221
Linear sebaceous nevus syndrome
  hypophosphatemia, 557
  osteomalacia, 557
Lining cell
  bone, 232
  bone resorption, 288
Lipoprotein, 200
  transport, 200
  vitamin D, oral route, 200
Lithium, hypercalcemia, 507–508
Lithium carbonate, 440
Lithotomy, cystine calculus, 809–810
Lithotripter, 644
  extracorporeal shock wave lithotripsy
    complications, 647–648
Liver
  acid-base balance, 734
  alkaline phosphatase, 259
  isozyme, 259
  parathyroid hormone binding site, 136
  vitamin D_3-25-hydroxylase, 153
Liver disease, bone disease, 963–968
Local osteolytic hypercalcemia
  biochemical findings, 542
  malignancy-associated hypercalcemia,
    540–542
  osteoclast activating factor, 540
Long bone
  adult, 224
  development, 223
  tissue organization at ends, 314–315
Loop diuretic, calcium, 15
Low back pain, 437
Low-molecular-weight angiogenic factor,
  growth plate, 344
Luminal pH, phosphate reabsorption, 25–26
Lung, acid-base balance, 734
Lymphoma
  1,25-dihydroxyvitamin D, malignancy-
    associated hypercalcemia, 548, 549
  hypercalcemia, 567–568
Lysosomal enzyme
  osteoclast, polarized secretion, 293
  parathyroid hormone
    cathepsin B, 108
    cathepsin D, 108
Lysozyme, proteoglycan disaggregation, 339

M

Macromolecule, calcium oxalate
  crystallization inhibitor, 761–762
Maffucci's syndrome, 1067
Magnesium
  calcium, 15
  calcium oxalate crystallization inhibitor,
    783

Magnesium (*contd.*)
  collecting duct system, 45–46
  connecting tubule, 45–46
  distal convoluted tubule, 45–46
  glomerular filtration, 41, 42
  idiopathic calcium oxalate urolithiasis, 720
  intestinal absorption
    driving forces, 68
    in humans, 68–69
    transport pathways, 68
    vitamin D, 68
  parathyroid hormone secretion, 99
  primary hyperoxaluria, 722
  proximal convoluted tubule, 42
  proximal tubule, 42–43
    water removal, 42
  recommended daily intake, 403
  renal handling, 41–46
  requirements, 404–405
  terminal nephron segment, 45–46
    renal handling, 45–46
  tubular handling, 42
Magnesium deficiency, 598–605
  calcium balance, 598–600
  causes, 600–603
  clinical consequences, 604–605
  endocrine disorder, 601–602
  gastrointestinal disorder, 601
  parathyroid hormone, 599–600
  potassium balance, 598–600
  renal disorder, 601, 602–603
  symptoms, 603–604
  treatment, 605
Magnesium disorder, 597–606. *See also*
    Specific type
Magnesium excess, 605–606
  causes, 605
  renal failure, 606
  symptoms and signs, 606
Magnesium excretion, regulation, 41–53
Magnesium reabsorption, Henle's loop
  arginine vasopressin, 50
  calcitonin, 50
  glucagon, 50
  luminal magnesium, 47–48
  parathyroid hormone, 50
  peritubular magnesium, 47–48
Magnesium transport
  hormonal control, 48–53
    distal convoluted tubule, 51
    Henle's loop, 48–51
    overall kidney function, 51–53
    proximal convoluted tubule, 48
    thick ascending limb, 48–51
  loop of Henle
    characteristics, 43
    micropuncture experiments, 43
    thick ascending limb of Henle's loop,
      43–45
    transepithelial transport, 43–45
  nephron
    acute phosphate loading, 47–48
    calcium loading, 46
    factors, 46–48
    factors increasing magnesium excretion,
      46–48

furosemide, 48
NaCl reabsorption, 47
peritubular magnesium, 46
Malabsorption state, 439
Male hypogonadism, 439
Malignancy-associated hypercalcemia,
    114–115, 502–505, 539–549
  bone histology, 541
  causes, 540–549
  HTLV-I leukemia, 548
  HTLV-I lymphoma, 548
  humoral, 503–504
  humoral factor, 549
  humoral hypercalcemia of malignancy,
    542–548
  immunoreactive parathyroid hormone,
    114–115
  local osteolytic hypercalcemia, 540–542
    osteoclast activating factor, 540
  pathophysiological mechanisms, 502–503
  prostaglandin, 549
  signs and symptoms, 539–540
  skeletal metastasis, 543–544
Malignant osteopetrosis, 989
Malignant tumor, 440
Mammalian growth plate
  biochemistry, 313–344
  biology, 313–344
  chemistry, 313–344
Mannitol
  calcium secretion, 63–64
  phosphate excretion, 30
Marrow, 223
Marrow transplantation, osteopetrosis,
    994–995
Mastocytosis, 439
  bone biopsy, 465
  histomorphometry, 465
Matrix apposition, mineral apposition, 486
Matrix gla protein, 249–250
  calbindin, 167
  1,25-dihydroxyvitamin D$_3$, 167
  osteocalcin, comparison, 249
Matrix-mediated mineralization, bone
    calcification, 274
Matrix vesicle
  alkaline phosphatase, inorganic phosphate
    generation, 333
  calcium ion, 332–333
  ecto-phosphatase, 333
  growth plate, rachitic rat, 332
  nucleotide triphosphate
    pyrophosphohydrolase, inorganic
    phosphate generation, 333
  peptidase, inorganic phosphate generation,
    333
  phosphate ion, 332–333
  protease, inorganic phosphate generation,
    333
  structure, 331–332
Matrix vesicle hypothesis, growth plate,
    331–334
McCune-Albright syndrome, 993, 1008–1010
  clinical presentation, 1008
  histopathologic findings, 1009

  laboratory findings, 1009
  pathogenesis, 1009
  radiologic features, 1008
  treatment, 1009–1010
Mechanistic urolithiasis, 623–624
  EQUIL, 623
Mechanostat, bone, 238
  setpoint change, 238–239
Medullary canal, 224
Medullary cavity, 224
Melorheostosis, 1006–1007
  clinical presentation, 1006
  etiology, 1007
  histopathologic findings, 1006–1007
  laboratory findings, 1006
  pathogenesis, 1007
  radiologic features, 1006, 1007
  treatment, 1007
Membrane phospholipid, bone calcification,
    334
  calcium phosphate-phospholipid complex,
    334
Membranous bone, 222
Menopause
  bone loss, 845–846
  bone mass, 841–844, 845–847
  calcium metabolism
    mineral homeostasis, 842, 843
    skeletal homeostasis, 842, 843
  cellular changes, 845
  intestinal calcium absorption, 842
  osteoporosis, 841–844
  primary hyperparathyroidism, 528
  remodeling, 370–372, 845–847
  urinary calcium, 842
Menstrual cycle, vitamin D, free sterol
    concentration, 211
Mesenchymal tumor
  hypophosphatemia, 551–555
    clinical features, 551–553
    pathogenesis, 553–555
    treatment, 555
  osteomalacia, 551–555
    clinical features, 551–553
    pathogenesis, 553–555
    treatment, 555
Metabolic bone disease, radionuclide bone
    imaging, 452
Metacarpal bone,
    pseudohypoparathyroidism, 575, 576,
    577, 579
Metaphyseal bone, 315
Metaphyseal junction, 316, 317
Metaphysis, 224, 314
Metastable equilibrium, bone calcification,
    274
Metastable solution, bone calcification, 274
Metastable state, bone calcification, 274
Methylene blue, struvite calculus, 818
Mg^{2+} fractional reabsorption, distal
    convoluted tubule
  arginine vasopressin, 51
  calcitonin, 51
  glucagon, 51
  parathyroid hormone, 51

Microcrack
  osteon, 367
  remodeling, 364–367
beta-Microglobulin, 363
Mid (44–68) parathyroid hormone
      radioimmunoassay, intact parathyroid
      hormone immunometric assay,
      117–118
Milk alkali syndrome, 439
  hypercalcemia, 508
Mineral apposition
  matrix apposition, 486
  mineralization lag time, 486
Mineral formation, proteoglycan, 338–339
Mineral growth inhibition, 338–339
Mineral homeostasis
  1,25-dihydroxyvitamin D_3, 149
  remodeling, 367–370
    calcium, 368–369
    vitamin D, 368
Mineral metabolism
  child, 395–410, 406–410
    acid phosphatase normal values, 409
    alkaline phosphatase normal values, 409
    bone density normal values, 409
    calcitonin normal values, 409
    calcium-regulating hormones, 407
    magnesium normal values, 407–408
    mineral absorption, 406
    mineral renal handling, 406–407
    normal values, 407–410
    osteocalcin normal values, 409
    parathyroid hormone normal values, 409
    phosphorus normal values, 407–408
    serum calcium normal values, 407–408
    stable isotope studies, 406
    study methodology, 406–407
    urinary hydroxyproline normal values,
      409
    vitamin D metabolite normal values, 409
  continuous ambulatory peritoneal dialysis,
      921–922
  fetus, 388–389
  gestation, 383–389
  growth, 395–396
    calcitonin, 399–400
    calcium, 403–404
    challenges, 396
    control, 396–402
    growth hormone, 400–401
    hormonal control, 398–402
    integration, 396–402
    intestine, 396–398
    kidney, 396–397
    magnesium, 404–405
    nutrition, 403–405
    parathyroid hormone, 398–399
    phosphorus, 403, 404
    sex steroid, 401–402
    vitamin D, 399, 403, 404
  kidney transplantation, 922–928
  lactation, 389–391
    bone calcium, 390–391
    calcium absorption, 390
    hormonal changes, 389–390
    urinary calcium excretion, 390

parturition, 389
placenta, 387–388
    active calcium transport, 387
    ATPases, 388
    calcium bidirectional fluxes, 387–388
    calcium-binding protein, 388
    hormonal regulation, 388
    maternal serum calcium concentration,
      388
    placental calcium transport regulation,
      388
    uteroplacental blood flow, 388
  pregnancy, 383–389
    calcitonin, 386–387
    changes, 384
    hormones regulating mineral
      homeostasis, 385–387
    integration, 384
    intestine, 384
    kidney, 384
    parathyroid hormone, 385
    vitamin D, 385–386, 387
  race, 405–406
Mineral metabolism disorder
  clinical approach, 435–441
  clinical findings, 436–440
  laboratory approach, 435–441
  physical findings, 437
  recognition, 436–440
  symptoms, 436–440
Mineralization lag time, mineral apposition,
      486
Mineralocorticoid, calcium, 14
Mithramycin, bone resorption inhibition,
      515, 516
Mixed function oxidase, characteristics,
      153–154
Mixed sclerosing bone dystrophy, 1007–1008
Modeling
  osteoclast, 287–288
  skeleton, 235–236
    diagram, 235
    vs. remodeling, 235
Molecular cloning, 1,25-dihydroxyvitamin
      D_3 receptor, 177–178
  orphan receptor gene, 178–179
  retinoid receptor gene, 178–179
  steroid receptor gene, 178–179
  thyroid receptor gene, 178–179
Monoclonal antibody
  1,25-dihydroxyvitamin D_3, 170–171
  parathyroid hormone receptor, 137
Monocyte, parathyroid hormone binding
      site, 136
Monocyte-macrophage, bone resorption, 289
Monovalent cation hyperexcretion, renal
      tubular acidosis type I, 739–740
Mouse 3T6 fibroblast, 1,25-
      dihydroxyvitamin D_3 receptor, 177
mRNA, subperiosteal bone,
      immunohistochemical localization,
      247
mRNA level, 1,25-dihydroxyvitamin D_3
  actin, 89
  calcitonin, 89
  parathyroid hormone, 89

somatostatin, 89
thyroglobulin, 89
Multiple endocrine neoplasia
  primary hyperparathyroidism, 499
  type I, 534–535
  type II, 535
Multiple myeloma, 439, 803–804
Multiplication stimulating activity, growth
      plate, 340
Muscle weakness, 437
Myeloid metaplasia, 803–804
Myeloma
  hypophosphatemia, 557
  osteomalacia, 557
Myeloproliferative disorder, 803–804
Myositis ossificans, 439
Myositis ossificans progressiva, 1013

N
Na^+/Ca^{2+} exchanger
  functional expression, 7
  heart myocyte, 7–8
  hydropathy map, 7
  model, 7
  molecular cloning, 7
  renal basolateral membrane, 8
Neonatal hypocalcemia, 440
Neonate, primary hyperparathyroidism, 499
Nephrocalcin
  calcium oxalate crystallization inhibitor,
      762–776
    air-water interface, 765, 768
    amino acid composition, 765
    carbohydrate composition, 765
    cell culture, 762–765
    crystal adsorption, 771–772
    electrophoretic mobility, 764, 766
    high-performance liquid
      chromatography, 765, 767
    human urinary inhibitor, 765, 767, 768
    human urine, 765–768
    kidney tissue culture inhibitor, 764, 766
    Langmuir adsorption coefficients, 769
    Langmuir-type adsorption plot, 765, 768
    Langmuir-type adsorption therm plot,
      764, 766
    multiple DEAE elution peaks, 772–774
    proximal tubule origin, 774–775
    rat kidney, 768–769
    rat urine, 768–769
    renal production sites, 770
    SDS-polyacrylamide gel
      electrophoretogram, 765, 767
    sedimentation equilibrium
      centrifugation, 765, 767
    stone-former urine, 769–770
    surface pressure curve, 765, 768
    Toyo-Soda column, 765, 767
    urine protein crystal growth inhibitor,
      769
    UV absorption spectrum, 764, 765
  defined, 762
Nephrogenous cyclic AMP excretion
  idiopathic hypercalciuria, 692
  normal, 692

Nephrolithiasis, 435
    management, 626
    noncalcium, 801–822
    pathogenesis, 685–703
    renal tubular acidosis type I
        alkaki, 749
        clinical features, 744
        genetic considerations, 750
        hypercalciuria, 746–747
        hyperuricosuria, 747
        hypocitraturia, 744–746
        incidence, 744
        lithogenesis, 747–748
        nephrocalcinosis, 744
        pathophysiology, 744–748
        potassium, 749
        prevalence, 744
        stone number, 744
        stone type, 744
        treatment, 748–750
    urinary calcium excretion, 685, 686
    Wilson's disease, 752–753
Nephron
    antidiuresis
        calcium reabsorption, 42
        chloride reabsorption, 42
        magnesium reabsorption, 42
        sodium reabsorption, 42
        water reabsorption, 42
    calcium reabsorption, 9
    calcium transport, 9–11
        collecting duct, 11
        descending loop of Henle, 10
        distal convoluted tubule, 10–11
        glomerular filtration, 9
        proximal convoluted tubule, 9–10
        proximal straight tubule, 10
        thick ascending limb of loop of Henle, 10
        thin ascending limb of loop of Henle, 10
    magnesium transport
        acute phosphate loading, 47–48
        calcium loading, 46
        factors, 46–48
        factors increasing magnesium excretion, 46–48
        furosemide, 48
        NaCl reabsorption, 47
        peritubular magnesium, 46
Nephroscopy
    flexible, features, 633
    percutaneous nephrostolithotomy, 631, 632
        closed irrigating system, 631
        open irrigating system, 631
    rigid, characteristics, 631, 633
Nephrostomy tube, percutaneous nephrostolithotomy, 634
Neurofibromatosis, 439
Neuromuscular irritability, 438
Neuronal storage disease, osteopetrosis, 990
Neuronal tissue, parathyroid hormone, 127
Noncalcium nephrolithiasis, 801–822
Noncalcium stone, 440
Noncollagenous protein, 244–251
    cartilage, 330
    growth plate
        anchorin CII, 329

    function, 329–330
    structure, 329–330
Nonparathyroid endocrine disorder, hypercalcemia, 505
Nonparathyroid tumor, hypercalcemia, 114–115
Nonrachitic hypophosphatemic osteomalacia, 942
Nonsteroidal anti-inflammatory drug, bone resorption, 296
Norepinephrine, phosphate excretion, 29
Normocalcemic hyperparathyroidism, surgery, 679–680
Nuclear receptor, steroid-response gene
    carboxy-terminal steroid-binding region, 180
    DNA-binding domain, 179–180
Nucleation
    kidney stone formation, 620–622
    urolithiasis, 620–622
Nucleotide triphosphate
    pyrophosphohydrolase, matrix vesicle, inorganic phosphate generation, 333
Nutritional recovery syndrome, hypophosphatemia, 590–591

O

Oat-cell carcinoma
    hypophosphatemia, 557
    osteomalacia, 557
Odontohypophosphatasia, 979, 984
Ollier's disease, 1067
Organic anions, 734
Orthophosphate, 16
    idiopathic calcium oxalate urolithiasis, 719
    primary hyperoxaluria, 721–722
Osmotic diuretic, calcium, 15
Osseous abnormality, renal osteodystrophy, 115–117
Ossification
    associated disorders, 1019
    endochondral, 222
    intramembranous, 222
Osteitis fibrosa, 466
    osteomalacia, bone biopsy, 912
    renal failure, 905–910
Osteitis fibrosa cystica. See Primary hyperparathyroidism
Osteoarthritis, Paget's disease, 1036–1037, 1038
Osteoblast, 230–232, 232
    bone resorption, 288
    Paget's disease, 1032–1033
    parathyroid hormone, 124
    ultrastructure, 241, 242
Osteoblast-like cell, parathyroid hormone, cytosolic calcium, 133
Osteoblastic tumor metastasis, 440
Osteoblastoma, 1069
Osteocalcin, 249–250, 258–259
    calbindin, 167
    child, normal values, 408
    1,25-dihydroxyvitamin D_3, 167
    human gene, structural organization, 182
    matrix gla protein, comparison, 249

Osteocalcin gene activation, 1,25-dihydroxyvitamin D_3 receptor, 184
Osteocalcin gene promoter, 1,25-dihydroxyvitamin D_3, induction, 181–183
Osteochondroma, 1066–1067
Osteoclast
    basolateral surfaces, 292
    bone marrow, 290
    bone resorption
        factors halting, 298–299
        mechanisms, 287–301
        regulation, 287–301, 293–295
        significance, 287–288
    cortical bone, 359
    filamentous zone, 233, 234
    functional morphology, 290, 291
    hematopoietic stem cell, derivation, 289–290
    lysosomal enzyme, polarized secretion, 293
    mechanism of action, 290–293
    modeling, 287–288
    oxygen-derived free radical, 293
    Paget's disease, 1032
    parathyroid hormone, 123
        function increases, 123–124
        number increases, 123–124
    podosome, 233, 234
    remodeling, 287–288, 844
    ruffled border, 233, 234, 290, 292–293
    spleen cell, 290
    time-lapse sequence, 362
    transport, 293
    vitronectin receptor, 291
Osteoclast nucleus, pagetic bone, 1028, 1029
Osteoclastic resorption, 372
Osteocyte, 232–234
    bone resorption, 288
    function, 233–234
Osteocyte cell body, 232
Osteocyte lacunocanalicular network, plasma mineral level, 369
Osteofibrous dysplasia, 1080
Osteogenesis imperfecta, 439, 993, 1015–1018
    biochemical defects, 1015, 1016
    bone biopsy, 470
    clinical heterogeneity, 1015, 1016
    clinical presentation, 1015–1016
    etiology, 1016, 1017
    histomorphometry, 470
    histopathologic findings, 1017
    laboratory findings, 1017
    pathogenesis, 1016, 1017
    radiologic features, 1016–1017, 1018
    treatment, 1018
Osteogenic cell
    hypertonic chondrocyte, 317
    progenitor cell, 317
Osteogenic sarcoma, radiography, 445
Osteoid accumulation kinetics, histomorphometry, 485–487
Osteoid bone, collagen fibril, 269–272
Osteoid osteoma, 1068, 1069
Osteoid surface
    bone, 229–230, 231
    osteoid thickness, 487

Osteoid thickness
  apposition rate, 487
  osteoid surface, 487
Osteoidosis, hypophosphatasia, 982
Osteolysis, massive, 1082
Osteomalacia
  bone biopsy, 468, 469
  bone histology, 911–912
  chronic lymphocytic leukemia, 557
  epidermal nevus syndrome, 557
  Fanconi's syndrome, 557
  histomorphometry, 468, 469
  linear sebaceous nevus syndrome, 557
  mesenchymal tumor, 551–555
    clinical features, 551–553
    pathogenesis, 553–555
    treatment, 555
  myeloma, 557
  oat-cell carcinoma, 557
  osteitis fibrosa, bone biopsy, 912
  prostate cancer, 555–556
  radiography, 444
  renal failure, 910
    aluminum, 910
Osteomalacia/osteoporosis discriminant
    index, vitamin D deficiency, 956
Osteomyelitis, 1080
Osteon, microcrack, 367
Osteonecrosis, kidney transplantation,
    926–928
  factors, 926–928
  prevention, 928
  treatment, 928
Osteonectin, 245–246, 246–250, 259
  biochemical features, 246
  subperiosteal bone, immunohistochemical
    localization, 247
Osteonectin molecule, schematic
    representations, 248–249
Osteopathia striata, 1005–1006
  clinical presentation, 1005
  radiologic features, 1005
  treatment, 1005–1006
Osteopenia, 831
  radiography, 444
Osteopetrosis, 440, 988–995
  adult, 990
  benign, 990
  clinical presentation, 989–991
  dietary treatment, 995
  etiology, 992–994
  forms, 988–989
  histopathologic findings, 992
  hormonal treatment, 995
  infantile, 989, 993
  intermediate, 989–990, 991
  laboratory findings, 992
  lethal, 990–991
  malignant, 989, 993
  marrow transplantation, 994–995
  neuronal storage disease, 990
  pathogenesis, 992–994
  prenatal diagnosis, 995
  radiologic features, 991–992
  supportive therapy, 995
  transient infantile, 991
  treatment, 994–995

Osteopoikilosis, 1004–1005
  clinical presentation, 1004
  histopathologic studies, 1004–1005
  radiologic features, 1004
  treatment, 1005
Osteopontin, 246–250
  biochemical features, 246
  calbindin, 167
  1,25-dihydroxyvitamin D_3, 167
  subperiosteal bone, immunolocalization,
    251
Osteoporosis, 435. See also Primary
    osteoporosis; Secondary osteoporosis
  alcohol, 850
  anabolic agent, 869–870
  androgen, 869
  androstanedione, 869
  anticonvulsant medication, 900–901
  asymptomatic woman assessment,
    853–856
    bone mass, 853–856
  bisphosphonate, 866–867
  bone biopsy, 465–466
  bone loss, 844–850
  bone mass
    consolidation, 840–841
    control of peak, 839–841
    genetic factors, 839–840
  calcitonin, 864–866
  calcitriol, 867–869
  calcium, 847–848, 849, 856–858
    dietary, 856–858
    supplementation, 856–858
  cholecalciferol, 867
  clinical characteristics, 851–852
  Colles' fracture, 838–839
    epidemiology, 838–839
  dietary factors, 847–850
  differential diagnosis, 852
  epidemiology, 832–839
  estrogen, 859–864, 865
    bone mass, 860
    breast cancer, 862, 864
    endometrial carcinoma, 861–862, 863
    hip fracture, 860–861, 862
    ischemic heart disease, 861
    long-term prevention, 856–857
    prescription, 862–864
    progestin, 862
    radiographic changes, 861
    skeleton, 860
  etidronate, 866–867, 868, 869
  exercise, prevention, 858–859
  factors, 833
  fall, 859
  fluoride, 870–871
  glucocorticoid, 890–893
    intestinal calcium absorption, 891
    parathyroid hormone, 892–893
    vitamin D metabolism, 891–892
  growth hormone, 872
  heparin, 896–898
    bone formation, 898
    bone remodeling, 897
    mast cell, 898
    parathyroid hormone, 898
    pregnancy, 896

    resorptive effects, 897–898
    vitamin D, 898
  hip fracture
    epidemiology, 833–837
    falls, 834–836, 837, 838
    incidence, 833, 834, 835
    survival, 837
  histomorphometry, 465–466
  historical aspects, 831
  hyperthyroidism, 893–895
    bone mass, 893–894
    bone mineral density, 893
  hypervitaminosis A, 898–900
    biochemical findings, 899
    retinoic acid, 899
    retinoil, 899
  immobilization, 895–896
    bed rest, 895–896
    bone loss, 895
    hormonal consequences, 896
    metabolic consequences, 896
    pharmacological approaches, 896
    remodeling, 896
    weightlessness, 895
  laboratory investigation, 852–853
  menopause, 841–844. See also
    Postmenopausal osteoporosis
  parathyroid hormone, amino-terminal
    fragment, 871
  pathophysiology, 839–844
  phenytoin, 900–901
  phosphate, 850
  physical activity, 850–851
    prevention, 858–859
  physical examination, 851
  prevention, 856–872
  primary, 831–873
    definition, 831
  radiography, 444, 445, 445–446
    spinal fracture, 445–446
  radiologic evaluation, 853
  regional, 439
  remodeling, 844–850, 889–890
    perturbations, 890
  risk factors, 832, 854
  senile, 847
  sodium, 850
  sodium fluoride, 870–871
  treatment, 856–872
  type I, 889
  type II, 847, 889
  vertebral fracture, 837–838
    epidemiology, 837–838
    incidence, 838
    prevalence, 839
  vitamin A, 898–900
  vitamin D_3, 867
  vs. other metabolic bone disorders,
    831–832
Osteosarcoma, 1071–1073
Osteosarcoma cell, parathyroid hormone
    binding site, 136
Osteosclerosis
  causes, 978
  radiography, 445
Oxalate, 707
  diet, 711–712

Oxalate (*contd.*)
  functions, 709
  intestinal absorption, 712
  measurement, 712–713
Oxalate absorption, factors influencing, 714
Oxalate excretion, idiopathic calcium oxalate
    urolithiasis, 718
Oxalate metabolism, 707–709
Oxalate production, 707–709
  metabolic pathways, 707–708, 709
Oxalate transport, 709–710
  gastrointestinal transport, 710
  idiopathic calcium oxalate urolithiasis, 718
  renal clearance, 709–710
  renal transport, 710
Oxygen-derived free radical, osteoclast, 293
Oxygenation, growth plate, 320–322

P
Pachydermia, 1014
Pachydermoiperiostosis, 1013–1015
  clinical presentation, 1014
  histopathologic findings, 1014–1015
  laboratory findings, 1014
  radiologic features, 1014
  treatment, 1015
Pagetic bone, 1029–1033
  osteoclast nucleus, 1028, 1029
Paget's disease, 440, 1027–1059
  alkaline phosphatase, 1042
  aminohydroxypropylidene diphosphonate,
      1057–1058
  anatomy, 1029–1033
  anti-inflammatory drug, 1052
  arthropathy, 1042
  axial skeleton, 1035
  bone biopsy, 469–470, 1052
  bone deposition, 1032–1033
  bone matrix, 1033
  bone resorption, 1032
  bone scanning, 1049–1051, 1051–1052
  calcitonin, 1053–1055
    adverse reactions, 1055
    antibodies, 1054
    human calcitonin, 1055
    porcine calcitonin, 1054
    resistance, 1054
    response, 1053–1054
    salmon calcitonin, 1054–1055
  cardiac output, 1037–1039
  clinical features, 1051
  clinical syndrome, 1033–1042
  collagen marker, 1042–1043
  complications, 1033
  deformity, 1034, 1035
  diagnosis, 1051–1052
  dichloromethylene diphosphonate, 1057
  diphosphonate, 1055–1058
  disodium etidronate, 1056–1057
    adverse reactions, 1055, 1057
  epidemiology, 1028
  etiology, 1028–1029
  flat bones, 1029
  fracture, 1036, 1037
  gross pathology, 1029

  hearing loss, 1040
  histomorphometry, 469–470
  historical aspects, 1027–1028
  hydroxyproline, 1042–1043
  hypercalcemia, 1041
  laboratory analysis, 1042–1043
  long bones, 1029
  magnetic resonance imaging, 1043–1049
  medicinal therapy indications, 1052–1053
  microscopic pathology, 1029–1032
  neurologic manifestations, 1041
  orthopedic measures, 1052
  osteoarthritis, 1036–1037, 1038
  osteoblast, 1032–1033
  osteoclast, 1032
  pain, 1035
  pathophysiology, 1029–1033
  peripheral skeleton, 1035–1036
  plicamycin, 1058
    adverse reactions, 1055, 1058
  radiography, 1043–1049, 1051
  sarcoma, 1039–1040
  serum alkaline phosphatase, 1051
  skull, 1035
    oral changes, 1040
    symptoms, 1040
  suppressive medicinal therapy guidelines,
      1052–1053
  teeth, 1033
  treatment, 1052–1058
  tumor, 1039–1040
  uninvolved bone, 1033
  visual loss, 1040–1041
Paget's disease of bone, radiography, 445
Pancreatic insufficiency, 439, 960, 962
  clinical features, 962
  incidence, 962
  pathogenesis, 962
  prevalence, 962
  treatment, 962
Pancreatic stone, calcium oxalate
    crystallization inhibitor, 779
Pancreatitis, hypocalcemia, 576
Paracrine system, 1,25-dihydroxyvitamin D$_3$,
    activated macrophages, 156–158
Parathyroid adenoma, 107
  parathyroid cell, 99
  parathyroid localization test, 531–532
  primary hyperparathyroidism,
      preoperative localization, 512–513
Parathyroid carcinoma, primary
    hyperparathyroidism, 498–499
Parathyroid cell, 87
  1,25-dihydroxyvitamin D$_3$, 94, 95
  parathyroid adenoma, 99
  primary parathyroid hyperplasia, 99
  proliferation regulation, 99–100
  protein kinase C, 97
  secondary parathyroid hyperplasia, 99
Parathyroid crisis, 498
Parathyroid disorder, radiography, 443–444
Parathyroid gene promoter, 86–87
Parathyroid gland, 83
  parathyroid hormone degradation,
      parathyroid gland dysfunction,
      109–110

  parathyroid hormone secretion
    exocytosis, 96
    extracellular fluid, 96
    hypocalcemia, 96
  radionuclide bone imaging, 452–453
Parathyroid hormone
  adenylate cyclase
    effect specificity, 134–135
    stimulation, 127–130
  adenylate cyclase assay, 129–130
  adult hypophosphatemic rickets, 937
  amino acid sequence, 128, 544
  assay, 111–118
  bioassay, 113
    adenylate cyclase activity, 113
    cyclic AMP production, 113
    glucose-6–phosphate dehydrogenase
        activity, 113
  bone
    anabolic actions, 124–125
    catabolic actions, 123–124
    coupling, 124
  bone matrix, 256
  bone resorption, 295–296
  calcium, 13, 14, 86–93
  calcium homeostasis, 87, 571–573
  carboxyl fragment, 107
  cartilage, 126
  cellular calcium, 133
  circulating forms, 107
  continuous ambulatory peritoneal dialysis,
      922
  estrogen, skeleton, 846
  extracellular fluid calcium concentration,
      89
  Fanconi's syndrome, 937
  fibroblast, 127
  G protein, 141–142
    guanine nucleotides, 141
  gastrointestinal tract, 127
  growth plate, 341–342
  hereditary hypophosphatemic rickets with
      hypercalciuria, 937
  hydrolysis of phosphoinositides, 131
  25-hydroxyvitamin D$_3$ metabolism,
      155–156
  hypertension, 126–127
  hypocalcemia, 126
  hypotension, 126
    cardiovascular effects, 126–127
  immunoassay, 111–113
    clinical applications, 113–118
    clinical utility, 116
    mid-region tyrosyl analogue, 112
    NH2 region, 112
  immunoheterogeneity sources, 107–111
  immunoheterogeneous, 111–112
  immunoreactive. *See* Immunoreactive
      parathyroid hormone
  initial hypocalcemic actions, 130
  intracellular calcium, changes, 133–135
  intracellular processing, 93–94, 95
  intraglandular degradation, 108–109
  kidney, 125–126
    acid-base handling, 125–126
    calcium-conserving, 125

cyclic AMP excretion, 125
1,25-dihydroxyvitamin D₃ formation,
125
negative calcium balance, 125
phosphaturic agent, 125
lysosomal enzyme
cathepsin B, 108
cathepsin D, 108
magnesium deficiency, 599–600
mechanisms of action, 127–142
middle fragment, 107
mineral metabolism during growth,
398–399
neuronal tissue, 127
non-cyclic AMP-mediated actions, 131
osteoblast, 124
osteoblast-like cell, cytosolic calcium, 133
osteoclast, 123
function increases, 123–124
number increases, 123–124
osteoporosis, amino-terminal fragment,
871
parathyroid gland, 107–110
phosphate reabsorption, 27–28
adenylate cyclase, 27–28
bicarbonate reabsorption, 27
cyclic AMP-dependent protein
phosphorylation, 27
fluid reabsorption, 27
Na⁺ reabsorption, 27
phosphate transport rate, 28
proximal tubule, 27
phosphatidylinositol hydrolysis, 131–132,
132–133
phosphatidylinositol pathway, 130–133
phospholipase C, effect specificity, 134–135
physiological actions, 123–127
pregnancy, 385
primary hyperparathyroidism, 126–127,
500–501
prostaglandin E2, 124
protein structure, 128
pseudovitamin D deficiency, 937
radioimmunoassay, 579–581
second messengers other than cyclic AMP,
130
serum calcium
malignancy-associated hypercalcemia,
542–543
mRNA levels, 86
primary hyperparathyroidism, 542–543
size, 544
skeletal resistance to calcemia action,
907–908
structure-activity relationships, 129
target tissue actions, 123–142
two-site, noncompetitive, 112, 113
urinary cyclic AMP, 128
urine Mg²⁺ excretion, 51–52
vitamin D dependent rickets
type I, 937
type II, 937
X-linked hypophosphatemic rickets, 937
Parathyroid hormone analogue, 135–136
Parathyroid hormone antagonist, 129,
135–136

Parathyroid hormone binding site
autoradiographic studies, 136
bone, 136
dermal fibroblast, 136
giant cell tumor, 136
kidney, 136
liver, 136
monocyte, 136
osteosarcoma cell, 136
renal membrane, 136
Parathyroid hormone biosynthesis, 93–94, 95
Parathyroid hormone degradation
parathyroid gland, parathyroid gland
dysfunction, 109–110
secondary hyperparathyroidism, 910
Parathyroid hormone gene, 83–86
chromosomal location, 83–84
1,25-dihydroxyvitamin D₃ receptor, 89
promoter sequences, 85–86
structure, 85
transcription, extracellular calcium, 96
transcription regulation, 86–93
extracellular calcium concentration, 86
vitamin D response element, 85
Parathyroid hormone-like protein, 545–549
amino acid sequence, 544
size, 544
structures, 545
Parathyroid hormone metabolism
hepatic, 111
peripheral, 110–111, 111
extracellular calcium, 111
hormone cleavage sites, 111
liver, 111
Parathyroid hormone mRNA
1,25-dihydroxyvitamin D₃, parathyroid
cells, 88–89
1,25-dihydroxyvitamin D₃ receptor
mRNA, 89–93
Parathyroid hormone production, regulation,
100–101
levels, 100
time sequences, 100
Parathyroid hormone receptor, 135–138
asymmetric, 137
criteria, 135
hydrodynamic properties, 137
ligand, 135
monoclonal antibody, 137
purification, 136–137
subtypes, 136
Parathyroid hormone-related peptide of
malignancy
assay, 503
humoral hypercalcemia of malignancy, 503
Parathyroid hormone-related polypeptide,
bioassay, 113
Parathyroid hormone-related protein,
545–549
amino acid sequence, 544
size, 544
structures, 545
Parathyroid hormone secretion, 95–99
calcitonin, 99
calcium, sigmoidal relationship, 96
cellular events, 101

cortisol, 99
cyclic AMP, 97–98
dexamethasone, 99
1,25-dihydroxyvitamin D₃, parathyroid
cells, 88–89
estrogen, 99
extracellular calcium, 96
cellular events, 98
magnesium, 99
parathyroid gland
exocytosis, 96
extracellular fluid, 96
hypocalcemia, 96
secondary hyperparathyroidism, altered
calcium regulators, 908–909
serum calcium, 95
Parathyroid hormone synthesis, cellular
events, 101
Parathyroid hormone(1–25), 129
Parathyroid hormone(1–34), 128
stepwise deletion from carboxyterminal
end, 129
Parathyroid hormone(3–34), 129
Parathyroid hormone(7–34)amide, 129
Parathyroid localization test, 531–532
parathyroid adenoma, 531–532
sensitivity, 531–532
specificity, 531–532
Parathyroid poisoning, 498
Parathyroidectomy
calcium nephrolithiasis, 678–680
hypercalciuria after, 680
recurrent, 679
dialysis, 920–921
efficacy, 531
primary hyperparathyroidism, 531
renal failure, 920–921
safety, 531
secondary hyperparathyroidism, 920–921
Parenteral nutrition, hypercalcemia, 509
Parturition, mineral metabolism, 389
Pathological calcification, 436
Pathological fracture, 436
Peptic ulcer disease, 959
Peptidase, matrix vesicle, inorganic
phosphate generation, 333
Percutaneous nephrolithotomy
cystine calculus, 809–810
staghorn calculus, 814
struvite calculus
combination treatment, 815–816
monotherapy, 814–815
Percutaneous nephrostolithotomy, 627–635
angle of entry, 629, 630
arteriovenous fistula, 634, 635
complications, 634–635
electrohydraulic lithotripsy, 632–633
flexible nephroscopy, 633–634
imaging, 628
indications, 648–667
kidney stone
adjunctive procedures, 650
compared by stone number, 653
cystoscopy, 651, 653
further procedure frequency, 654
multiple treatments, 652

Percutaneous nephrostolithotomy, kidney
stone (contd.)
  nonstaghorn renal calculus, 649–654
  nonsurgical complications, 651
  outcome, 652
  postoperative stay length, 651
  stone basketing, 651, 653
  stone location, 649
  stone size, 649
  treatment morbidity, 650
  ureteral stent, 651, 653
  ureteroscopy, 651, 653
  nephroscope, 631, 632
  nephroscopy
    closed irrigating system, 631
    open irrigating system, 631
  nephrostomy tube, 634
  patient positioning, 628
  portable C-arm and image table, 628, 629
  renal access, 628–630
  renal puncture techniques, 629–630
  staghorn calculus, access, 630
  ultrasonic lithotripsy, 631–632
  ureteral catheter, 627–628
Perichondrium, 315
Perinatal hypophosphatasia, 978–979, 980
Periosteal envelope, 227–228
Periosteum, 227–228
Periostitis, 1014
Peripheral skeleton, Paget's disease,
    1035–1036
Pertussis toxin, 98
  ADP-ribosylation, 140
pH, phosphate ultrafilterability, 17
Phenytoin, osteoporosis, 900–901
Pheochromocytoma, 440
Phosphate
  bone resorption inhibition, 516
  osteoporosis, 850
  primary hyperparathyroidism, 533
  renal handling, 16–31
  renal osteodystrophy, retention, 916–918
  renal threshold concentration, 19
Phosphate-binding antacid,
    hypophosphatemia, 589–590
Phosphate composition, plasma, 16–17
Phosphate compound, bone resorption, 300
Phosphate deficiency, 439
Phosphate disorder, 587–597. See also
    Specific type
Phosphate excretion
  acetazolamide, 30
  atrial natriuretic factor, 29
  calcitonin, 29
  calcium, 30
  catecholamine, 29
  diuretic, 30
  epinephrine, 29
  ethacrynic acid, 30
  extracellular fluid volume, 29
  furosemide, 30
  glucocorticoid, 29
  insulin, 29
  intracellular pH, 26
  isoproterenol, 29
  mannitol, 30

  norepinephrine, 29
  thiazide, 30
  thyroid hormone, 29
  vitamin D metabolite, 28
Phosphate homeostasis, remodeling, 368–369
Phosphate ion, matrix vesicle, 332–333
Phosphate molecule, 17
Phosphate production, nonenzymatic routes,
    333–334
Phosphate reabsorption
  acid-base balance, systemic, 26
  distal convoluted tubule, 19
  distal tubule, 19
  growth hormone, 28–29
  internephron heterogeneity, 18
  intracellular pH, 26
  intranephron heterogeneity, 18
  luminal pH, 25–26
  parathyroid hormone, 27–28
    adenylate cyclase, 27–28
    bicarbonate reabsorption, 27
    cyclic AMP-dependent protein
        phosphorylation, 27
    fluid reabsorption, 27
    Na$^+$ reabsorption, 27
    phosphate transport rate, 28
    proximal tubule, 27
  proximal tubule, 19, 20
  saturability, 17–18
Phosphate replacement therapy,
    hypophosphatemia, 593–594
  phosphorus-containing preparation, 593
Phosphate retention, secondary
    hyperparathyroidism, 905–906
Phosphate transport
  basolateral membrane, 24
  brush border membrane, 20–23
    ADP-ribosylation, 22–23
    allosteric regulation by H$^+$, 21–22
    allosteric regulation by Na$^+$, 21–22
    covalent modification, 22–23
    endocytosis, 23
    exocytosis, 23
    lipid microenvironment, 23
    membrane lipid orientation, 23
    membrane recycling, 23
    Na$^+$-phosphate cotransporter regulation,
        21–23
    phosphorylation, 22–23
    sodium-phosphate cotransporter, 20–21
    thiol redox, 22–23
  cellular mechanisms, 19–20
  nephron sites, 18–19
  proximal convoluted tubule, 18–19
  transcellular, 24
Phosphate ultrafilterability
  calcium, 17
  pH, 17
  protein binding, 17
Phosphate uptake, brush-border membrane
    vesicle, time course, 70
Phosphatidylinositol, 131–135
Phosphatidylinositol hydrolysis, parathyroid
    hormone, 131–133
Phosphatidylinositol metabolism
  diacylglycerol, 131

  endoplasmic reticulum, 131
  pathways, 131
  protein kinase C, 131
Phosphatidylinositol pathway
  hormone action, 130–133
  parathyroid hormone, 130–133
Phosphoibosyl pyrophosphate synthetase,
    803
Phospholipase C, 138–139
  G protein, 140
  guanine nucleotide, 141
  parathyroid hormone, effect specificity,
      134–135
Phosphoprotein, 280–283
  bone calcification, recent data, 284
Phosphorus, 17
  adult hypophosphatemic rickets, 937
  child, normal values, 408
  dialysis, 916–918
  Fanconi's syndrome, 937
  hereditary hypophosphatemic rickets with
      hypercalciuria, 937, 941–942
  intestinal absorption, 69–79
    brush-border phosphorus influx, 71
    calcium and phosphorus cotransport, 72
    cellular transport events, 70–71
    colon, 74
    diffusional phosphorus movement, 72
    ileum, 74
    inorganic phosphorus transport
        pathways, 69–74
    jejunum, 74
    Na-P cotransporter, 71
    pH, 71
    phosphate depletion, 72
    proximal small intestine, 73–74
    segmental calcium transport, 73–74
    segmental phosphorus transport, 73–74
    vitamin D, 71–72
  pseudovitamin D deficiency, 937
  recommended daily intake, 403
  requirements, 403, 404
  vitamin D dependent rickets
    type I, 937
    type II, 937
  X-linked hypophosphatemic rickets, 937
Phosphorus absorption
  adult hypophosphatemic rickets, 937
  Fanconi's syndrome, 937
  hereditary hypophosphatemic rickets with
      hypercalciuria, 937
  pseudovitamin D deficiency, 937
  vitamin D dependent rickets
    type I, 937
    type II, 937
  X-linked hypophosphatemic rickets, 937
Phosphorus metabolism disorder, kidney
    transplantation, 924–925
  treatment, 925
Phosphotriamide, I_{50} urease values, 818
Placenta, mineral metabolism, 387–388
  active calcium transport, 387
  ATPases, 388
  calcium bidirectional fluxes, 387–388
  calcium-binding protein, 388
  hormonal regulation, 388

maternal serum calcium concentration, 388
placental calcium transport regulation, 388
uteroplacental blood flow, 388
Plasma
1,25-dihydroxyvitamin D, 196, 197–198
kinetics, 198
plasma concentrations, 197–198
sources, 197
24,25-dihydroxyvitamin D, 198
25-hydroxyvitamin D, 196–197
kinetics, 197
plasma concentrations, 197
quantitation, 198
sources, 196–197
phosphate composition, 16–17
vitamin D, 195–196
cholecalciferol, 195
ergocalciferol, 195
kinetics, 196
metabolites, 196
plasma concentrations, 196
sources, 195–196
vitamin D-binding protein, concentration by disorder, 207
vitamin D metabolite, concentration by disorder, 207
vitamin D sterol, 195–198
assays, 198–200
chromatographic techniques, 198–199
extraction techniques, 198
physicochemical assays, 199
quantitation, 199–200
radioimmunoassays, 200
receptors, 200
saturation analysis, 199–200
vitamin D, 199
Plasma binding protein
chylomicron, 200
lipoprotein, 200
saturation analysis, 199–200
vitamin D sterol, 200–202
Plasma calcium concentration, determinants, 417–419
Plasma concentrations, 25,26–dihydroxyvitamin D, 198
Plasma (inorganic) phosphate, 16–17
Plasma membrane Ca^{2+} ATPase-pump, teratoma, 6
structure, 6
Plasma mineral level
blood-bone barrier, 369
osteocyte lacunocanalicular network, 369
Plasma phosphate concentration, 17
urinary phosphate excretion rate, 17–18
Plasma phosphorus concentration, 17
Plasma pyridoxal 5'-phosphate, hypophosphatasia, 982, 983
Platelet-derived growth factor, bone matrix, 256
Plicamycin
bone resorption inhibition, 515, 516
Paget's disease, 1058
adverse reactions, 1055, 1058
Podosome, osteoclast, 233, 234
Polycythemia rubra vera, 803–804

Polyethylene glycol 900, calcium secretion, 63–64
Polypeptide hormone receptor, adenylate cyclase,
periodically recurring regions of hydrophobicity, 137–138
Polyuria, 437–438
hypercalcemia, 510
Poole-Hunter ion-exchange hypothesis, growth plate, 335–338
Post-renal transplantation, 440
Postgastrectomy bone disease, 959–961
clinical features, 959–960
incidence, 959
pathogenesis, 960–961
prevalence, 959
treatment, 961
Postmenopausal osteoporosis, 439
bone biopsy, 465–466
fracture, 832
histomorphometry, 465–466
Potassium, renal tubular acidosis type I, 739–740
Potassium balance, magnesium deficiency, 598–600
Potassium citrate, idiopathic calcium oxalate urolithiasis, 719–720
Potassium-sparing diuretic, calcium, 16
Potassium transport, thick ascending limb of Henle's loop, cellular mechanisms, 43–44
Pregnancy
creatinine clearance, 385, 387
1,25-dihydroxyvitamin D_3 biosynthesis, 166
mineral metabolism, 383–389
calcitonin, 386–387
changes, 384
hormones regulating mineral homeostasis, 385–387
integration, 384
intestine, 384
kidney, 384
parathyroid hormone, 385
vitamin D, 385–386, 387
primary hyperparathyroidism, 499, 536
skeleton
calcium, 383
dietary calcium, 383–384
mother, 383–387
phosphorus, 383
Preproparathyroid hormone, amino acid sequence, 83, 84
Previtamin D_3, sterol structures, 150
Primary aldosteronism, 440
Primary biliary cirrhosis, 439
Primary hyperoxaluria, 440, 720–722
enzymatic defects, 720
magnesium, 722
medical treatment, 721–722
natural progression, 720
orthophosphate, 721–722
pyridoxine, 721–722
renal failure, 722
type 2 L-glyceric aciduria, 720–721
type I glycolic aciduria, 720, 721

Primary hyperparathyroidism, 439
acute, 498–499
asymptomatic, 498–499, 523–536
biochemical findings, 542
biochemical indices, 500
biochemical measurements, 529
bone, 495–496
bone biopsy, 463, 496, 497
bone densitometry, 496
calcium nephrolithiasis, 671–684
biochemical parameters, 678
brushite, 675–676
calcitriol, 681
calcium intake, 680
calcium oxalate, 675–676
clinical features, 672
diagnosis, 676–677
drug therapy, 681
estrogen, 681
ethacrynic acid, 681
fluid intake, 681
furosemide, 681
historical aspects, 671
hypercalciuria, 674–675
hypercalciuria after surgery, 680
hyperuricosuria, 675
incidence, 671–672
medical treatment, 680–681
natural history, 679
parathyroidectomy, 677–680
phosphate, 681
protein intake, 680
recurrence, 679
renal tubular acidosis, 675
sodium intake, 680–681
stone pathogenesis, 674–676
surgery, 677–680
surgery complications, 677–678
urine pH, 675
classification, 524–525
clinical forms, 498–500
clinical presentation, 672–674
clinical spectrum, 500
creatinine, 525
cystic parathyroid adenomatosis, 499
diagnosis, 500–502
diphosphonate, 533–534
estrogen, 532–533
evaluation, 500–502
familial forms, 499, 534–536
familial primary hyperparathyroidism, 499
features, 524
histomorphometry, 463, 526–527
hypercalcemia, 494–502
hypercalciuria, 674–675
renal stones, 674–675
hypertension, 126–127
immunoreactive parathyroid hormone, 114–115
kidney, 496–498
medical management, 513–514, 532–534
indications, 523–529
menopause, 528
multiple endocrine neoplasia, 499
natural history, 524–526, 529
neonate, 499

Primary hyperparathyroidism (*contd.*)
  parathyroid adenoma, preoperative
      localization, 512–513
  parathyroid carcinoma, 498–499
  parathyroid hormone, 126–127, 500–501
  parathyroidectomy, 531
  phosphate, 533
  pregnancy, 499, 536
  radiography, 443, 444, 495
  serum, 525
  signs and symptoms, 495–498
  single-photon absorpiometry, forearm
      bone densitometry, 529
  surgical treatment, 511–512
    complication rate, 530
    criteria, 524
    indications, 529–532
    insidious nature, 530
    parathyroid localization test, 531–532
    physiologic derangements, 530
    prolonged observation problems, 532
  treatment, 511–514
  vs. acute primary hyperparathyroidism,
      498–499
  vs. parathyroid carcinoma, 498–499
  without physiologic derangements,
      523–524
Primary osteoporosis, 831–873
  defined, 831, 889
Primary parathyroid hyperplasia,
    parathyroid cell, 99
Primary radiographic bone abnormality, 436
Primitive bone, 222
Primitive neuroepithelioma, 1073
Progressive diaphyseal dysplasia, 998–1000
  clinical presentation, 998, 999
  etiology, 999
  glucocorticoid, 999–1000
  histopathologic findings, 998–999
  laboratory findings, 998
  pathogenesis, 999
  radiologic features, 998
  treatment, 999–1000
Prolactin, 1,25-dihydroxyvitamin D_3
    biosynthesis, 166
Promoter, 254
Propionohydroxamic acid, struvite calculus,
    819
Prostaglandin
  bone resorption, 296–297
  malignancy-associated hypercalcemia, 549
Prostaglandin E_2
  bone resorption, 296–297
  parathyroid hormone, 124
Prostaglandin F_{2alpha}, bone resorption, 296
Prostaglandin inhibitor, bone resorption
    inhibition, 516
Prostate cancer
  hypophosphatemia, 555–556
  osteomalacia, 555–556
Protease
  matrix vesicle, inorganic phosphate
      generation, 333
  proteoglycan degradation, 339

Protein. *See also* Endogenous protein
  subperiosteal bone, immunohistochemical
      localization, 247
Protein binding, phosphate ultrafilterability,
    17
Protein induction, 1,25-dihydroxyvitamin
    D_3, 166–167
Protein intake, calcium, 12–13
Protein kinase C
  parathyroid cell, 97
  phosphatidylinositol metabolism, 131
Proteoglycan, 244–245, 246
  biochemical features, 246
  growth plate, 326–329, 335–338
    core protein domain structure, 327
    function, 326–327
    interactions, 329
    organization, 327–329
    structure, 327–329
  mineral formation, 338–339
  schematic representation, 245
Proteoglycan condensation site, 337
Proteoglycan degradation, protease, 339
Proteoglycan disaggregation, lysozyme, 339
Proton pump
  carbonic acid, 293
  hydrogen ion, 293
Proximal convoluted tubule
  calcium, 9–10
  magnesium, 42
  phosphate transport, 18–19
Proximal tubule
  calcium ATPase, 7
  magnesium, 42–43
    water removal, 42
  phosphate reabsorption, 19, 20
  renal tubular acidosis, 737
Pseudo-pseudohypoparathyroidism,
    radiography, 444
Pseudohyperparathyroidism, 542
Pseudohypoparathyroidism
  brachydactyly, 575, 576, 577, 579
  hypocalcemia, 574–576
  metacarpal, 575, 576, 577, 579
  radiography, 444
  vitamin D, free sterol concentration,
      208–209
Pseudohypophosphatasia, 440, 979, 984
Pseudovitamin D deficiency, 943–945
  alkaline phosphatase, 937
  calcium, 937
  calcium absorption, 937
  1,25-dihydroxyvitamin D, 937
  25-hydroxyvitamin D, 937
  parathyroid hormone, 937
  pathophysiology, 944
  phosphorus, 937
  phosphorus absorption, 937
  treatment, 944–945
  urinary calcium, 937
  urinary phosphorus, 937
Puberty, vitamin D, free sterol concentration,
    211
Purine degradation, pathway, 821
Purine metabolism, 801, 802

Pycnodysostosis, 1000–1002
  clinical presentation, 1000
  etiology, 1002
  histopathologic findings, 1002
  laboratory findings, 1002
  pathogenesis, 1002
  radiologic features, 1000–1002
  treatment, 1002
Pyridoxal metabolism, 985
Pyridoxamine metabolism, 985
Pyridoxine
  idiopathic calcium oxalate urolithiasis, 720
  primary hyperoxaluria, 721–722
Pyridoxine metabolism, 985
Pyrophosphate, calcium oxalate
    crystallization inhibitor, 783–784

Q
Quantal remodeling theory, remodeling, 476

R
Race
  bone histomorphometry, normal values,
      461–462
  bone mineralization, 405
  calcium metabolism, 405–406
  mineral metabolism, 405–406
  remodeling, 370–373
Rachitic/osteomalacic disease, Fanconi's
    syndrome, 942–943
Radial immunodiffusion, vitamin D-binding
    protein, 202
Radiography, 443–446
  chondrosarcoma, 445
  ectopic calcification, 445
  hypoparathyroidism, 444
  osteogenic sarcoma, 445
  osteomalacia, 444
  osteopenia, 444
  osteoporosis, 444, 445, 445–446
    spinal fracture, 445–446
  osteosclerosis, 445
  Paget's disease of bone, 445
  parathyroid disorder, 443–444
  primary hyperparathyroidism, 443, 444,
      495
  pseudo-pseudohypoparathyroidism, 444
  pseudohypoparathyroidism, 444
  renal osteodystrophy, 444
  rickets, 444
  secondary hyperparathyroidism, 444
Radioimmunoassay
  parathyroid hormone, 579–581
  vitamin D-binding protein, 203
Radionuclide bone imaging, 451–453
  diphosphonate retention, 452
  metabolic bone disease, 452
  parathyroid, 452–453
  principles, 451–452
  vs. X-ray, 452
Recalcification tetany, hypocalcemia, 579
Receptor-effector coupling, 138–142
Relative supersaturation, calcium oxalate,
    685, 686

Remodeling, osteoporosis, 889–890
  perturbations, 890
Remodeling space, 890
Renal acid excretion, 729–736
  bicarbonate reabsorption, 729–730
  fixed acid production, 730–734
    acid ash, 730
    amino acid, 733
    biochemical reactions, 730–732
    citric acid cycle, 731–732
    fatty acid, 733–734
    fatty acid oxidation, 732
    fixed ash, 730
    foodstuff metabolism, 733–734
    gluconeogenesis, 732
    glucose, 733
    glycolysis, 731
    organic anions, 734
    urea cycle, 732
Renal basolateral membrane, Na$^+$/Ca^{2+}
    exchanger, 8
Renal calcium excretion, hypercalcemia of
    malignancy, 15
Renal clearance, oxalate transport, 709–710
Renal colic, 436
  operative intervention, 806
Renal disease
  1,25-dihydroxyvitamin D, 210
  25-hydroxyvitamin D, 209–210
  hypercalcemia
    acute, 509
    chronic, 509
  vitamin D, free sterol concentration,
    209–210
Renal disorder, magnesium deficiency, 601,
    602–603
Renal excretion, calcium, 3
Renal failure, 905–922
  acute, 440
  calcium supplement, 918
  chronic, 440
  1,25-dihydroxyvitamin D$_3$, 907
  hypermagnesemia, 606
  magnesium excess, 606
  osteitis fibrosa, 905–910
  osteomalacia, 910
    aluminum, 910
  parathyroidectomy, 920–921
  primary hyperoxaluria, 722
  secondary hyperparathyroidism, 905–910
  skeletal resistance to parathyroid hormone
    calcemic action, 907–908
  vitamin D metabolism, 906–907
  vitamin D sterol, 919–920
Renal hypercalciuria, 687
Renal insufficiency, renal tubular acidosis
    type I, 740
Renal membrane, parathyroid hormone
    binding site, 136
Renal osteodystrophy
  aluminum carbonate, 916
  aluminum hydroxide, 916
  biochemical abnormality, 115–117
  bone biopsy, 466–468
  calcium supplement, 918
  cyclosporine, 926

defined, 905
histomorphometry, 466–468
immunoreactive parathyroid hormone,
    staging, 115–117
kidney transplantation, 925–926
  growth of children following, 926
  serum osteocalcin, 926
mixed lesion, 912
osseous abnormality, 115–117
phosphate, retention, 916–918
radiographic features, 914–915
radiography, 444
secondary hyperparathyroidism, 920–921
treatment, 916–922
  guidelines, 917
vitamin D sterol, 919–920
Renal phosphate excretion
  acid-base, 25–26
  characteristics, 17–24
  clearance characteristics, 17–18
  dietary effects, 24–25
  growth hormone, 28–29
  hormones, 27–28
  regulation, 24–31
Renal transport, oxalate transport, 710
Renal tubular acidosis
  bicarbonate generation, decreased, 736
  bicarbonate reabsorption, decreased,
    735–736
  classification, 735–736, 737
  distal, classifications, 742
  distal tubule, 737
  incomplete, urinary pH, 738–739
  pathophysiology, 729–736
  proximal tubule, 737
  variant pathophysiology, 735
  Wilson's disease, 752
Renal tubular acidosis type I, 440, 736–750
  ammonia excretion, 738
  clinical manifestations, 736
  diagnosis, 740–743
  etiology, 736–737
  growth retardation, 740
  hereditary hypercalciuria,
    pathophysiology, 748
  hypokalemia, 739–740
  idiopathic hypocitraturic calcium-oxalate
    nephrolithiasis, hypocitraturic, 748
  monovalent cation hyperexcretion,
    739–740
  nephrolithiasis
    aklaki, 749
    clinical features, 744
    genetic considerations, 750
    hypercalciuria, 746–747
    hyperuricosuria, 747
    hypocitraturia, 744–746
    incidence, 744
    lithogenesis, 747–748
    nephrocalcinosis, 744
    pathophysiology, 744–748
    potassium, 749
    prevalence, 744
    stone number, 744
    stone type, 744
    treatment, 748–750

nosology, 736–737
potassium, 739–740
presentation, 740–741
renal insufficiency, 740
sodium, 740
transport defect, 737–738
urine acidification, 738, 741–743
  tests, 742–743
urine anion gap, 743
Renal tubular acidosis type II, 439, 750–752
  etiology, 750
  hypercalciuria, 750–751
  metabolic acidosis pathophysiology, 750
  nephrocalcinosis, 750–751
  nephrolithiasis, 750–751
  nosology, 750
Renal tubular function disorder, 935–943
Resorbing surface, bone, 230, 231
Resorption, remodeling, 358, 359, 360, 361
  coupling, 363
  1,25-dihydroxyvitamin D, 363
  Haversian system, 359, 361
  interleukin-1, 363
  parathyroid hormone, 363
Resorption depth, histomorphometry,
    483–485
Respiratory alkalosis, hypophosphatemia,
    588–589
Resting surface, bone, 229, 230
Reticulum, 224
Retinoic-acid-receptor gene
  amino acid sequences, 178
  structural organization, 178
Retinol, bone resorption, 297
Reversal, remodeling, 359–363
RGD-containing protein, 246–250
  biochemical features, 246
  bone, RGD region predicted
    conformation, 250
Ribbing's disease, 999
Rickets, 149, 435, 438
  radiography, 444
RNA, calcium oxalate crystallization
    inhibitor, 784
Rocket immunoelectrophoresis, vitamin
    D-binding protein, 203
Ruffled border, osteoclast, 233, 234, 290,
    292–293

S
Saliva, calcium oxalate crystallization
    inhibitor, 779
Sarcoidosis, 439, 563–566
  calcium metabolism, 565–566
  clinical findings, 566
  pathophysiology, 563–564
  treatment, 566
  vitamin D metabolism, 564–565
Sarcoma, Paget's disease, 1039–1040
Saturation analysis
  plasma binding protein, 199–200
  vitamin D-binding protein, 202
    ligand, 202
Sclera, blue, 438

Sclerosteosis, 1003–1004
  clinical presentation, 1003
  etiology, 1003–1004
  gigantism, 1003
  histopathologic findings, 1003
  pathogenesis, 1003–1004
  radiologic features, 1003
  treatment, 1004
Seco-steroid, vitamin D, 150
Secondary hyperparathyroidism
  bone histology, 910–911
  factors, 905, 908
  glomerular filtration rate, 906–907
  parathyroid hormone degradation, 910
  parathyroid hormone secretion, altered
    calcium-regulated, 908–909
  parathyroidectomy, 920–921
  pathogenesis, 905, 908
  phosphate retention, 905–906
  radiography, 444
  renal failure, 905–910
  renal osteodystrophy, 920–921
  vitamin D metabolism, 906–907
  vitamin D sterol, 919–920
Secondary osteoporosis, 889–901
  defined, 889
  examples, 890
Secondary parathyroid hyperplasia,
    parathyroid cell, 99
Secondary polycythemia, 803–804
Serum, primary hyperparathyroidism, 525
Serum alkaline phosphatase, Paget's disease,
    1051
Serum calcium
  actin, mRNA levels, 86
  Burkitt's lymphoma, 551
  calcitonin, mRNA levels, 86
  dialysis, 916–918
  1,25-dihydroxyvitamin D$_3$, 165
  25-hydroxyvitamin D$_3$ metabolism, 156
  immunoreactive parathyroid hormone
    hypocalcemic states, 114–115
    primary hyperparathyroidism, 114–115
  parathyroid hormone
    malignancy-associated hypercalcemia,
      542–543
    mRNA levels, 86
    primary hyperparathyroidism, 542–543
  parathyroid hormone secretion, 95
  tumor-lysis syndrome, 551
Serum creatinine
  Burkitt's lymphoma, 551
  tumor-lysis syndrome, 551
Serum 1,25-dihydroxyvitamin D
  idiopathic hypercalciuria, 690–691
  normal, 690–691
Serum mineral disorder, cancer, 539–558
Serum mineral level, abnormal, 435–436
Serum osteocalcin, 926
Serum parathyroid hormone concentration
  idiopathic hypercalciuria, 692
  normal, 692
Serum phosphate
  25-hydroxyvitamin D$_3$ metabolism, 156
  idiopathic hypercalciuria, 692
  normal, 692

Serum phosphorus
  Burkitt's lymphoma, 551
  1,25-dihydroxyvitamin D$_3$, 165
  tumor-lysis syndrome, 551
Sessile osteochondroma, 1066
Sex
  cancellous bone
    packet wall thickness, 371
    volume, 371
    remodeling, 370–373
Sex steroid, mineral metabolism during
    growth, 401–402
Sexual maturation, bone mass, 402–403
Sialoprotein, 259
  subperiosteal bone, immunolocalization,
    251
Silica stone, 820–821
Silicone-induced granuloma, 567
Single photon absorpiometry, primary
    hyperparathyroidism, forearm bone
    densitometry, 529
Single photon absorptiometry, 446, 447
Skeletal envelope
  location, 373
  remodeling
    tissue balance, 373
    variation, 373–374
Skeletal growth factor, 361–363
Skeletal mass, estradiol, 842
Skeletal metastasis, malignancy-associated
    hypercalcemia, 543–544
Skeletal tissue, origins, 220
Skeleton
  bone formation rate, canine, 375
  developmental biology. See also Specific
    type
  fracture healing, 237
  growth, 234–235, 395–396
    endochondral ossification, 395
    intramembranous ossification, 395
  idiopathic hypercalciuria, 698–700
  intermediary organization, 234–237
  modeling, 235–236
    diagram, 235
    vs. remodeling, 235
  pregnancy
    calcium, 383
    dietary calcium, 383–384
    mother, 383–387
    phosphorus, 383
  remodeling, 236–237
    vs. modeling, 235
  vitamin A, cellular basis, 899–900
Skin, vitamin D$_3$, 153
Skull, Paget's disease, 1035
  oral changes, 1040
  symptoms, 1040
Small bowel bypass, enteric hyperoxaluria
  steatorrhea, 717
  treatment, 717
Sodium
  calcium, 11–12
  osteoporosis, 850
  renal tubular acidosis type I, 740
Sodium cellulose phosphate, idiopathic
    hypercalciuria, 703
Sodium chloride transport, furosemide, 44

Sodium fluoride
  fracture, 870–871
  osteoporosis, 870–871
  trabecular bone volume, 870
Sodium transport, thick ascending limb of
    Henle's loop, cellular mechanisms,
    43–44
Soft tissue collagen, bone collagen,
    comparison, 244
Solid tumor, hypercalcemia, 567–568
Solution chemistry
  kidney stone formation, 616–620
    adsorption, 619–620
    citrate ion concentration, 619
    crystal growth, 622–623
    EQUIL, 616–620
    ions, 617–618
    magnesium ion concentration, 619
    oxalate concentration, 618–619
    particle growth, 622–623
    pool diagram, 617
    relative supersaturation, 618–619
    speciation, 616–168
  urolithiasis, 616–620
    adsorption, 619–620
    citrate ion concentration, 619
    crystal growth, 622–623
    EQUIL, 616–620
    ions, 617–618
    magnesium ion concentration, 619
    oxalate concentration, 618–619
    particle growth, 622–623
    pool diagram, 617
    relative supersaturation, 618–619
    speciation, 616–168
Somatomedin
  bone matrix, 255
  growth plate, 340
Somite, 221
  differentiation, 220
  formation, 220
Spironolactone, calcium, 16
Spleen cell, osteoclast, 290
Spongiosa
  primary, 316
  secondary, 316
Spongious bone, 223
Sprue, 439
Staghorn calculus, 654–662
  anatrophic nephrolithotomy, 660, 661
  classification, 656
  complete, stone-free rates, 658, 660
  distribution, 656
  extracorporeal shock wave lithotripsy,
    654–662, 815
  length of postoperative stay
    renal anatomy, 656, 659
    stone volume, 656, 659
  partial, stone-free rates, 658, 660
  percutaneous nephrolithotomy, 814
  percutaneous nephrostolithotomy, access,
    630
  pretreatment consideration, 655–656
  procedure number
    renal anatomy, 656, 658
    stone volume, 656, 658
  stone composition, 659, 661

Steatorrhea, enteric hyperoxaluria, 714
Steinstrasse, extracorporeal shock wave
    lithotripsy, 647
Steroid-induced osteoporosis, 439
    treatment, 890–893
Steroid-receptor gene
    amino acid sequences, 178
    structural organization, 178
Steroid-response gene
    nuclear receptor
        carboxy-terminal steroid-binding region,
            180
        DNA-binding domain, 179–180
        structural organization, 179–180
Sterol transport, vitamin D-binding protein,
    201–202
Stoichiometry, struvite calculus, 810–811
Strain, bone, 237–238
Stress, bone, 237–238
Struvite calculus, 654–655, 810–820
    antimicrobial agent, 817–818
    bacteriology, 811–812
    clinical manifestations, 812–813
    dietary supplementation, 817
    extracorporeal shock wave lithotripsy
        combination treatment, 815–816
        monotherapy, 815
    glycosaminoglycan, 812, 813
    hydroxamic acid, 819
    lavage chemolysis, 816–817
    methylene blue, 818
    open surgical procedures, 814
    percutaneous nephrolithotomy
        combination treatment, 815–816
        monotherapy, 814–815
    propionohydroxamic acid, 819
    recurrence rate, 655
    stoichiometry, 810–811
    substrate depletion, 817
    treatment, 813–820
    urease inhibitor, 818–820
    urinary acidification, 816
Subarticular growth center, 315
Subperiosteal bone
    akaline phosphatase, 257
    bone matrix gene expression, pattern, 254
    mRNA, immunohistochemical
        localization, 247
    osteonectin, immunohistochemical
        localization, 247
    osteopontin, immunolocalization, 251
    protein, immunohistochemical
        localization, 247
    sialoprotein, immunolocalization, 251
Substrate depletion, struvite calculus, 817
Sulfate, calcium, 15
Surface chemistry
    kidney stone formation, 616–620
        adsorption, 619–620
        citrate ion concentration, 619
        EQUIL, 616–620
        ions, 617–618
        magnesium ion concentration, 619
        oxalate concentration, 618–619
        pool diagram, 617
        relative supersaturation, 618–619
        speciation, 616–168

urolithiasis, 616–620
    adsorption, 619–620
    citrate ion concentration, 619
    EQUIL, 616–620
    ions, 617–618
    magnesium ion concentration, 619
    oxalate concentration, 618–619
    pool diagram, 617
    relative supersaturation, 618–619
    speciation, 616–168
Syndactyly, 1003, 1004
Syndrome of calcified periarthritis, 912

T
Tamm-Horsfall glycoprotein, calcium
    oxalate crystallization inhibitor,
    776–779
    aggregation effects, 774
    clinical studies, 777–779
    crystal formation promotion, 776
    crystal growth inhibition, 776
    growth effects, 774
    nucleation inhibition, 776
    zero growth conditions, 777, 778
Teratoma, plasma membrane Ca^{2+}
    ATPase-pump, 6
    structure, 6
Terminal nephron segment, magnesium,
    45–46
    renal handling, 45–46
Testosterone, mineral metabolism during
    growth, 401–402
Tetany, 438
Tetracycline labeling, histomorphometry,
    481–483
Thiazide, 440
    calcium, 16
    phosphate excretion, 30
Thiazide diuretic, 440
    hypercalcemia, 507
    idiopathic hypercalciuria, 702
Thiazide-potassium-citrate treatment,
    calcium oxalate crystallization
    inhibitor, 782–783
Thick ascending limb of Henle's loop
    calcium transport, cellular mechanisms,
        43–44
    potassium transport, cellular mechanisms,
        43–44
    sodium transport, cellular mechanisms,
        43–44
Thrombospondin, 246–250
    biochemical features, 246
Thyroid disease, vitamin D, free sterol
    concentration, 210
Thyroid hormone
    bone resorption, 297
    calcium, 14
    phosphate excretion, 29
Thyroid-hormone-receptor gene
    amino acid sequences, 178
    structural organization, 178
Thyrotoxicosis, 893
    bone biopsy, 468–469
    histomorphometry, 468–469
    hypercalcemia, 505

Tibia, 225
Tirameterene, 820
Tissue distribution, 1,25-dihydroxyvitamin
    D_3
    autoradiographic analysis, 170
    biochemical analysis, 170
    immunohistochemical analysis, 170
Tissue nonspecific alkaline phosphatase
    ectoenzyme role, 986
    natural substrates, 977, 984–985
Total parenteral nutrition, 439
    bone disease, 970–971
        clinical features, 970
        incidence, 970
        pathogenesis, 970–971
        prevalence, 970
        treatment, 971
Trabecular bone, 223, 224
Trabecular bone volume
    calcium, 870
    sodium fluoride, 870
    vitamin D, 870
Trace mineral, requirements, 404–405
Transcellular pathway, calcium absorption,
    5–8
    calbindin-D, 5–6
    luminal entry, 5
    schematics, 5
    transcytoplasmic calcium buffering, 5–6
    transcytoplasmic calcium ferrying, 5–6
Transcription, 1,25-dihydroxyvitamin D_3,
    166
Transcription regulation, parathyroid
    hormone gene, 86–93
    extracellular calcium concentration, 86
Transepithelial voltage, 9
Transforming growth factor, growth plate,
    342–343, 343
Transforming growth factor-beta, bone
    matrix, 255–256
Transient infantile osteopetrosis, 991
Transileal biopsy specimen, 230, 231, 232,
    233
Transileal bone biopsy, atypical insufficiency
    fracture, 471
Transileal closed needle bone biopsy,
    457–458
Transitional envelope, 229
Transmembrane signaling, G protein,
    138–139
Transport, osteoclast, 293
Transport defect, renal tubular acidosis type
    I, 737–738
Triamterene, calcium, 16
Trousseau's sign, 438
    hypocalcemia, 577–578
Tuberculosis, 566–567
    hypercalcemia, 566
    hypercalciuria, 566
    pathogenesis, 567
    treatment, 567
Tumor, Paget's disease, 1039–1040
Tumor-associated osteomalacia, 439
Tumor-lysis syndrome
    hypocalcemia, 551
    serum calcium, 551

Tumor-lysis syndrome (contd.)
  serum creatinine, 551
  serum phosphorus, 551
Tumoral calcinosis, 439
  clinical presentation, 1019
  etiology, 1020–1021
  histopathologic findings, 1019–1020
  laboratory findings, 1019
  pathogenesis, 1020–1021
  radiologic features, 1019, 1020
  treatment, 1021

U
Ulcerative colitis, 960
  incidence, 961
  prevalence, 961
Ulna
  Haversian bone, 367
  Haversian system, 367
Ultrasonic lithotripsy, percutaneous
    nephrostolithotomy, 631–632
Ultrasonic lithotrite, characteristics, 631, 633
Ultrasound, 453
Unicameral bone cyst, 1078
Urate renal calculus, 801–806
  pathophysiology, 801–804
Urea, molecular structure, 818
Urease
  organisms producing, 812
  urine, biochemical changes, 811
Urease inhibitor, 818
  struvite calculus, 818–820
Uremic osteodystrophy, 435
Ureteral calculus, 662–667
  distal, 666
  extracorporeal shock wave lithotripsy,
      distal, 666
  intervention indications, 662
  proximal, 662–666
  treatment options, 662
  ureteroscopy, distal, 666
Ureteral catheter, percutaneous
    nephrostolithotomy, 627–628
Ureteral perforation, ureteroscopy, 642
Ureteral stent, ureteroscopy, 641–642
  indications for internal, 641
Ureteroscopy, 635–642
  complications, 642
  guide wires, 637
  imaging, 636–637
  indications, 636, 648–667
  instrumentation, 637–638
  irrigant choice, 640
  passing ureteroscope, 638–640
  patient positioning, 637
  stone removal techniques, 640–641
    basket, 640–641
    electrohydraulic probe, 641
    pulsed-dye laser, 641
    ultrasonic lithotripsy, 641
  ureteral calculus, distal, 666
  ureteral dilation, 637
  ureteral perforation, 642
  ureteral stent, 641–642
    indications for internal, 641
  ureteroscope, 637–638

Uric acid
  calcium oxalate crystallization promoter,
      785–794
    allopurinol, 785–787
    citrate, 787–788
    clinical evidence, 785–788
    heterogeneous nucleation, 790–792
    hyperuricosuria, 788
    mechanism studies, 788–794
    urate reduction, 792–794
    uric acid reduction, 792–794
  calcium oxalate stone, 785
    daily balance, 801–802
    daily input and output, 801–802
    low urinary volumes, 802
    renal handling, 801, 803
    urinary pH, saturation curve, 802, 803
Uric acid calculus, 785
  allopurinol, 804–805
  decreased, 804
  dietary purine, 804
  increasing urinary volume, 804
  operative intervention, 806
  presentation, 804
  treatment, 804
  urinary alkalinization, 805–806
Uric acid excretion, enteric hyperoxaluria,
    714–715
Urinary acidity
  low urinary volumes, 802
  struvite calculus, 816
Urinary alkalinization, uric acid calculus,
    805–806
Urinary calcium, 571
  adult hypophosphatemic rickets, 937
  Fanconi's syndrome, 937
  hereditary hypophosphatemic rickets with
      hypercalciuria, 937
  menopause, 842
  pseudovitamin D deficiency, 937
  vitamin D dependent rickets
    type I, 937
    type II, 937
  X-linked hypophosphatemic rickets, 937
Urinary calcium excretion
  dietary calcium intake, 687, 688
  dietary protein intake
    idiopathic hypercalciuria, 697
    normal, 697
  factors decreasing, 695
  factors increasing, 695
  glomerular filtration
    idiopathic hypercalciuria, 695
    normal, 695
  idiopathic hypercalciuria, 693–698
  intestinal calcium absorption
    hypercalciuria, 687, 688
    normal, 687, 688
  nephrolithiasis, 685, 686
  normal, 685, 686, 693–698
  urinary PO4 excretion
    idiopathic hypercalciuria, 700
    normal, 700
  urinary potassium excretion, 698
    idiopathic hypercalciuria, 699
    normal, 699
  urinary SO4 excretion

    idiopathic hypercalciuria, 697
    normal, 697
  urinary sodium excretion
    idiopathic hypercalciuria, 696
    normal, 696
Urinary cyclic AMP, parathyroid hormone,
    128
Urinary cyclic AMP excretion
  idiopathic hypercalciuria, 692
  normal, 692
Urinary oxalate excretion, dietary factors, 712
Urinary pH
  cystine, solubility, 807, 808
  hyperchloremic acidosis, 741–742
  normal diurnal variation, 804
  uric acid, saturation curve, 802, 803
Urinary phosphate excretion rate, plasma
    phosphate concentration, 17–18
Urinary phosphorus
  adult hypophosphatemic rickets, 937
  Fanconi's syndrome, 937
  hereditary hypophosphatemic rickets with
      hypercalciuria, 937
  pseudovitamin D deficiency, 937
  vitamin D dependent rickets
    type I, 937
    type II, 937
  X-linked hypophosphatemic rickets, 937
Urinary potassium excretion, urinary
    calcium excretion, 698
  idiopathic hypercalciuria, 699
  normal, 699
Urinary sodium excretion, urinary calcium
    excretion
  idiopathic hypercalciuria, 696
  normal, 696
Urinary uric acid, saturation measurements,
    789
Urine
  calcium oxalate crystallization inhibitor,
      758–761
  urease, biochemical changes, 811
Urine acidity, renal tubular acidosis type I,
    738, 741–743
  tests, 742–743
Urine anion gap
  hyperchloremic acidosis, 743
  renal tubular acidosis type I, 743
Urine citrate, low, 440
Urine citrate excretion, 780–781
Urine inorganic pyrophosphate excretion,
    783
Urine Mg^{2+} excretion
  calcitonin, 51–52
  parathyroid hormone, 51–52
  vasopressin, 51–52
Urolithiasis
  crystallization, 613–616
    liquid-phase behavior, 614–616
    surface events, 616
  cystine
    clinical features, 627
    radiographic features, 627
  mechanistic, 623–624
  nonspecific abnormalities favoring, 714
  nucleation, 620–622
  physical-chemical processes, 613–624

secondary to drug crystalluria, 820–821
solution chemistry, 616–620
   adsorption, 619–620
   citrate ion concentration, 619
   crystal growth, 622–623
   EQUIL, 616–620
   ions, 617–618
   magnesium ion concentration, 619
   oxalate concentration, 618–619
   particle growth, 622–623
   pool diagram, 617
   relative supersaturation, 618–619
   speciation, 616–168
surface chemistry, 616–620
   adsorption, 619–620
   citrate ion concentration, 619
   EQUIL, 616–620
   ions, 617–618
   magnesium ion concentration, 619
   oxalate concentration, 618–619
   pool diagram, 617
   relative supersaturation, 618–619
   speciation, 616–168

V

Van Buchem's disease, 1002–1004
   clinical presentation, 1002
   endosteal hyperostosis, 1002, 1003
   etiology, 1003
   histopathologic findings, 1002–1003
   laboratory findings, 1002
   pathogenesis, 1003
   radiologic features, 1002, 1003
   treatment, 1003
Vasopressin, urine Mg^{2+} excretion, 51–52
Versican, 244–245, 246
   schematic representation, 245
Vertebra, anatomy, 224–225
Vertebral crush fracture
   clinical characteristics, 851–852
   differential diagnosis, 852
   rib angulation, 852
Vertebral fracture, osteoporosis, 837–838
   epidemiology, 837–838
   incidence, 838
   prevalence, 839
Visual loss, Paget's disease, 1040–1041
Vitamin A
   bone resorption, 297
   hypercalcemia, 508
   osteoporosis, 898–900
   skeleton, cellular basis, 899–900
Vitamin A toxicity, 440
Vitamin B_6 metabolism, 985
Vitamin D
   bone resorption, 296
   calcium, 13, 14
   calcium absorption, 62–63
   chemistry, 150
   chromatin-associated receptor fraction, 168
   chylomicron, oral route, 200
   continuous ambulatory peritoneal dialysis, 922
   diabetes mellitus, free sterol concentration, 210

endocrine disorder, free sterol concentration, 210
familial hypocalciuric hypercalcemia, free sterol concentration, 211
Fanconi's syndrome, free sterol concentration, 211
gastrectomy, free sterol concentration, 209
gastrointestinal disorder, free sterol concentration, 209
genetic disorder, free sterol concentration, 211
growth plate, 341–342
hepatobiliary disorder, free sterol concentration, 209
history of discovery, 149–150
hypercalcemia, 505–507
   malignancy-associated, 507
hyperparathyroidism, free sterol concentration, 210
hypoparathyroidism, free sterol concentration, 208–209
hypophosphatemic rickets with hypercalciuria, free sterol concentration, 211
idiopathic hypercalciuria, free sterol concentration, 211
lipoprotein, oral route, 200
menstrual cycle, free sterol concentration, 211
metabolism, 149–160
mineral metabolism during growth, 399
photoproduction, 152
plasma, 195–196
   cholecalciferol, 195
   ergocalciferol, 195
   kinetics, 196
   metabolites, 196
   plasma concentrations, 196
   sources, 195–196
pregnancy, 385–386
pseudohypoparathyroidism, free sterol concentration, 208–209
puberty, free sterol concentration, 211
recommended daily intake, 403
renal disease, free sterol concentration, 209–210
requirements, 403, 404
seco-steroid, 150
thyroid disease, free sterol concentration, 210
trabecular bone volume, 870
vitamin D dependent rickets type I, free sterol concentration, 211
vitamin D dependent rickets type II, free sterol concentration, 211
X-linked hypophosphatemia, free sterol concentration, 211
Vitamin D absorption, steps, 952
Vitamin D analog, hypocalcemia, 582
Vitamin D-binding protein
   actin binding, 202
   assays, 202–203
   immunoassay, 202
   ligand-binding characteristics, 201
   physicochemical features, 201
   plasma, concentration by disorder, 207
   plasma carrier features, 202

   plasma kinetics, 201
   radial immunodiffusion, 202
   radioimmunoassay, 203
   rocket immunoelectrophoresis, 203
   saturation analysis, 202
   ligand, 202
   sterol transport, 201–202
   tissue distribution, 201
Vitamin D catabolism, 158
Vitamin D deficiency, 439
   biochemical features, 953–955
   clinical presentations, 952–953, 954
   histologic features, 956–958
   incidence, 951–952
   nutritional, 951–959
   osteomalacia/osteoporosis discriminant index, 956
   pathogenesis, 958
   prevalence, 951–952
   prophylaxis, 958–959
   radiologic features, 955–956
   treatment, 958–959
Vitamin D dependent rickets
   type I, 439, 943–945
      alkaline phosphatase, 937
      calcium, 937
      calcium absorption, 937
      1,25-dihydroxyvitamin D, 937
      25-hydroxyvitamin D, 937
      parathyroid hormone, 937
      pathophysiology, 944
      phosphorus, 937
      phosphorus absorption, 937
      treatment, 944–945
      urinary calcium, 937
      urinary phosphorus, 937
      vitamin D free sterol concentration, 211
   type II, 439, 945–947
      alkaline phosphatase, 937
      calcium, 937
      calcium absorption, 937
      deficient hormone-receptor nuclear localization, 946
      1,25-dihydroxyvitamin D, 937
      hormone binding affinity defect, 946
      hormone binding capacity defect, 946
      hormone binding negative, 946
      25-hydroxyvitamin D, 937
      parathyroid hormone, 937
      pathogenesis, 945–946
      phosphorus, 937
      phosphorus absorption, 937
      treatment, 946–947
      urinary calcium, 937
      urinary phosphorus, 937
      vitamin D free sterol concentration, 211
Vitamin D metabolism
   abnormal, pathogenesis, 564–565
   hypercalcemia, 564
   regulation, 154
   renal failure, 906–907
   sarcoidosis, 564–565
   secondary hyperparathyroidism, 906–907
Vitamin D metabolite. *See also* Specific type
   free sterol concentration, 203–211
      estimated, 203–204
      measured, 204

Vitamin D metabolite, free sterol
    concentration (*contd.*)
  vitamin D deficiency, 206–207
  vitamin D intoxication, 207–208
  phosphate excretion, 28
  plasma, concentration by disorder, 207
  plasma carrier features, 202
Vitamin D preparation, characteristics, 582
Vitamin D response element, parathyroid
    hormone gene, 85
Vitamin D sterol
  dialysis, 919–920
  plasma, 195–198
    assays, 198–200
    chromatographic techniques, 198–199
    extraction techniques, 198
    physicochemical assays, 199
    quantitation, 199–200
    radioimmunoassays, 200
    receptors, 200
    saturation analysis, 199–200
    vitamin D, 199
  plasma binding protein, 200–202
  renal failure, 919–920
  renal osteodystrophy, 919–920
  secondary hyperparathyroidism, 919–920
Vitamin D synthesis, 151–153
Vitamin D therapy, associated disorders,
    208–210
Vitamin D toxicity, 439, 568
  hypercalcemia, 506, 508
Vitamin D$_2$, 150
  metabolic transformations, 151
Vitamin D$_3$
  genomic mechanism of action, 163–169

contemporary research, 169–177
  historical considerations, 163–169
  metabolic transformations, 150
  osteoporosis, 867
  skin, 153
  sterol structures, 150
Vitamin D$_3$-25-hydroxylase
  characteristics, 153–155
  cytochrome P450, 153
  liver, 153
  regulation, 154–155
  subcellular distribution, 153
  tissue distribution, 153
Vitamin-D$_3$-dependent rickets type II,
    184–187
Vitamin D$_3$ endocrine system, 159
Vitamin D$_3$ hormone, cellular response,
    molecular mechanisms, 163–188
Vitamin D$_3$ metabolism, 164
Vitamin D$_3$ metabolite, sterol structures, 150
Vitamin-D$_3$-resistant fibroblast model, 185
Vitamin D$_3$-responsive element, localized,
    182
Vitronectin receptor, osteoclast, 291

W

Wall thickness, histomorphometry, 483–485
Weddellite, 710
Whewellite, 710
William's syndrome, 440
  hypercalcemia, 568
Wilson's disease, 752–753
  hypercalciuria, 752

nephrolithiasis, 752–753
renal abnormalities, 752
renal tubular acidosis, 752
Woven bone, 222
WR2721, bone resorption inhibition, 515,
    517

X

X-linked hypophosphatemia, vitamin D, free
    sterol concentration, 211
X-linked hypophosphatemic rickets, 439,
    935–941
  abnormal growth, 936
  alkaline phosphatase, 937
  animal models, 939–940
  biochemistry, 936–937
  calcium, 937
  calcium absorption, 937
  clinical evidence, 935–936
  1,25-dihydroxyvitamin D, 937
  genetics, 937–938
  25-hydroxyvitamin D, 937
  parathyroid hormone, 937
  pathophysiology, 938–939
  phosphorus, 937
  phosphorus absorption, 937
  short stature, 935
  treatment, 940–941
  urinary calcium, 937
  urinary phosphorus, 937
Xanthine lithiasis, 821–822
Xylitol, 708–709